Saunders Manual of

SMALL ANIMAL PRACTICE

Saunders Manual of

SMALL ANIMAL PRACTICE

Stephen J. Birchard, D.V.M., M.S., Diplomate, A.C.V.S.
Associate Professor and Head
Small Animal Surgery Section
Department of Veterinary Clinical Sciences
The Ohio State University
Columbus, Ohio

Robert G. Sherding, D.V.M., Diplomate, A.C.V.I.M.
Professor of Small Animal Internal Medicine
Chair, Department of Veterinary Clinical Sciences
The Ohio State University
Columbus, Ohio

■ *Original Artwork by Felecia J. Paras*

W.B. SAUNDERS COMPANY
A Division of Harcourt Brace & Company
Philadelphia   London   Toronto   Montreal   Sydney   Tokyo

W.B. SAUNDERS COMPANY
A Division of Harcourt Brace & Company

The Curtis Center
Independence Square West
Philadelphia, Pennsylvania 19106

Library of Congress Cataloging-in-Publication Data

Saunders manual of small animal practice / [edited by]
Stephen J. Birchard, Robert G. Sherding.—1st ed.

p.   cm.

ISBN 0–7216–3219–X

1. Pet medicine—Handbooks, manuals, etc.   2. Dogs—Diseases—
  Handbooks, manuals, etc.   3. Cats—Diseases—Handbooks,
  manuals, etc.   I. Birchard, Stephen J.
  II. Sherding, Robert G.   III. Title: Manual of small animal
  practice.

SF981.S34 1994

636.089—dc20   92–4856

Saunders Manual of Small Animal Practice   ISBN 0–7216–3219–X

Printed in the United States of America.

Last digit is the print number: 9   8   7   6   5   4   3   2   1

We dedicate this book to our families

To my wife, Susan Crisp;
my children, Justin and Mary Elizabeth;
my parents, Robert and San Chica;
and my brother, Thomas

SJB

To my parents, Robert and Janet

RGS

Contributors

Nancy L. Anderson, D.V.M.
College of Veterinary Medicine, The Ohio State University, Columbus, Ohio. *Basic Husbandry and Medicine of Pocket Pets*

Richard K. Anderson, D.V.M.
Staff Dermatologist, Angell Memorial Animal Hospital, Boston, Massachusetts. *Scabies, Notoedric Mange, and Cheyletiellosis*

Dennis N. Aron, D.V.M.
Departments of Small Animal Medicine and Anatomy and Radiology, College of Veterinary Medicine, University of Georgia, Athens, Georgia. *Luxation, Subluxation, and Shearing Injuries of the Tarsal Joint*

Michael S. Bauer, D.V.M., Diplomate, A.C.V.S.
Associate Professor of Small Animal Surgery, Veterinary Teaching Hospital, Colorado State University, Ft. Collins, Colorado. *Open Wound Management*

Karin Muth Beale, D.V.M., Diplomate, A.C.V.D.
Formerly Assistant Professor of Dermatology, University of Florida, Gainesville, Florida; Dermatologist, Gulf Coast Veterinary Specialists, Houston, Texas. *Dermatophytosis*

Jamie R. Bellah, B.S.V.Sc., D.V.M., Diplomate, A.C.V.S.
Associate Professor of Surgery and Chief, Small Animal Surgery, College of Veterinary Medicine, University of Florida, Gainesville, Florida. *Surgery of Intertriginous Dermatoses*

Larry Berkwitt, D.V.M., Diplomate, A.C.V.I.M.
Staff Internist, Darien Animal Hospital, Darien, Connecticut. *Diagnostic Methods for Respiratory Disorders*

David S. Biller, D.V.M., Diplomate, A.C.V.R.
Assistant Professor, College of Veterinary Medicine;

Radiologist, Veterinary Teaching Hospital, The Ohio State University, Columbus, Ohio. *Radiographic and Ultrasonographic Techniques*

Stephen J. Birchard, D.V.M., M.S., Diplomate, A.C.V.S.
Associate Professor and Head, Small Animal Surgery Section, Department of Veterinary Clinical Sciences, The Ohio State University, Columbus, Ohio. *Thyroid Gland, Selected Skin Graft and Reconstructive Techniques, Principles of Thoracic Surgery, Liver and Biliary Surgery, Diseases and Surgery of the Exocrine Pancreas, Peritonitis*

Cynthia L. Bishop, D.V.M.
Seattle, Washington. *Avian Infectious Diseases*

Dale E. Bjorling, D.V.M., M.S.
Associate Professor and Chair, Department of Surgical Sciences, School of Veterinary Medicine, The University of Wisconsin-Madison, Madison, Wisconsin. *Management of Thoracic Trauma, Surgery of the Kidney and Ureter, Surgery of the Urethra*

John D. Bonagura, D.V.M., Diplomate, A.C.V.I.M.
Professor, Veterinary Clinical Sciences, College of Veterinary Medicine, The Ohio State University; Cardiologist, Veterinary Teaching Hospital, Columbus, Ohio. *Radiographic Evaluation, Drugs for Treatment of Cardiovascular Diseases, Heart Failure, Valvular Heart Disease, Cardiomyopathy, Vascular Diseases, Congenital Heart Disease, Bronchopulmonary Disorders, Respiratory Infection*

Harry W. Boothe, D.V.M., M.S.
Professor of Surgery, Department of Small Animal Medicine and Surgery; Professor of Surgery, Texas Veterinary Medical Center, College of Veterinary

Medicine, Texas A&M University, College Station, Texas. *Surgery of Otitis Media and Otitis Interna, Surgery of the Prostate Gland, Surgery of the Testis and Scrotum, Surgery of the Penis and Prepuce*

Randy J. Boudrieau, D.V.M., Diplomate, A.C.V.S.
Tufts University School of Veterinary Medicine, North Grafton, Massachusetts. *Delayed Union, Nonunion, and Malunion*

Bernard M. Bouvy, D.V.M.
Department of Surgical Sciences, School of Veterinary Medicine, The University of Wisconsin-Madison, Madison, Wisconsin. *Neoplasia of Thoracic and Pelvic Limbs*

Ronald M. Bright, D.V.M., M.S., Diplomate, A.C.V.S.
Professor and Director of Surgical Services, Department of Urban Practice, College of Veterinary Medicine, University of Tennessee; General Surgeon, Veterinary Teaching Hospital, College of Veterinary Medicine, Knoxville, Tennessee. *Surgery of the Esophagus, Diseases of the Stomach, Surgery of the Stomach, Surgery of the Intestines, Anorectal Surgery*

Marjory Brooks, D.V.M., Diplomate, A.C.V.I.M.
Research Scientist, Comparative Hematology Laboratory, Wadsworth Center for Laboratories and Research, New York State Department of Health, Albany, New York. *Coagulation Disorders*

Susan A. Brown, D.V.M.
Midwest Avian and Exotic Animal Hospital, Westchester, Illinois. *Ferrets*

Steven C. Budsberg, D.V.M., M.S.
College of Veterinary Medicine and Veterinary Teaching Hospital, University of Georgia, Athens, Georgia. *Orthopedic Disorders of the Distal Extremities*

C. A. Tony Buffington, D.V.M., Ph.D., D.A.C.V.N.
Associate Professor of Veterinary Clinical Sciences, College of Veterinary Medicine, The Ohio State University; Head of Nutrition Support Service, Veterinary Teaching Hospital, Columbus, Ohio. *Critical Care Techniques*

Clay A. Calvert, D.V.M., Diplomate, A.C.V.I.M.
Associate Professor, College of Veterinary Medicine, Internist, Department of Small Animal Medicine, University of Georgia, Athens, Georgia. *Heartworm Disease*

Marcia Carothers, D.V.M.
Veterinary Referral Clinic, Cleveland, Ohio. *Disorders of the Parathyroid Gland and Calcium Metabolism, Respiratory Neoplasia*

Dennis J. Chew, D.V.M.
Professor, Department of Clinical Science, College of Veterinary Medicine, The Ohio State University, Columbus, Ohio. *Fluid Therapy for Dogs and Cats, Disorders of the Parathyroid Gland and Calcium Metabolism*

David M. Clark, D.V.M., Diplomate, A.C.V.S.
Formerly, Associate Professor, College of Veterinary Medicine; Chief, Small Animal Surgery, Boren Veterinary Medical Teaching Hospital, Oklahoma State University, Stillwater, Oklahoma. *Degenerative Joint Disease, Immune-Mediated Joint Disease*

Susan Phillips Cohen, M.S.W.
Director of Counseling and Chairperson, Carola Warburg Rothschild Society for the Human-Animal Bond, The Animal Medical Center, New York, New York. *Care of the Grieving Client*

C. Guillermo Couto, D.V.M., Diplomate, A.C.V.I.M. (Oncology and Internal Medicine)
Associate Professor, Department of Veterinary Clinical Sciences, College of Veterinary Medicine; Chief, Oncology and Hematology Service, Veterinary Teaching Hospital, The Ohio State University, Columbus, Ohio. *Rickettsial Diseases, Tumors of the Skin and Subcutaneous Tissues*

Laine A. Cowan, D.V.M., M.S.
Assistant Professor, Small Animal Internal Medicine, Veterinary Medical Teaching Hospital, Kansas State University, Manhattan, Kansas. *Diseases of the Urinary Bladder, Urethral Diseases*

M. Susan Crisp, D.V.M., Diplomate, A.C.V.I.M. (Internal Medicine)
Assistant Professor, Department of Veterinary Clinical Sciences, College of Veterinary Medicine; Director, Intensive Care Unit, Veterinary Teaching Hospital, The Ohio State University, Columbus, Ohio. *Critical Care Techniques*

Steven E. Crow, D.V.M., Diplomate, A.C.V.I.M. (Internal Medicine and Oncology)
Staff Oncologist and Internist, Sacramento Animal Medical Group, Carmichael, California. *Pericardial Disease and Cardiac Neoplasia*

Charles E. DeCamp, D.V.M., M.S.
Associate Professor, Department of Small Animal Clinical Sciences, College of Veterinary Medicine; Section Chief of Surgery and Anesthesia, Veterinary Medical Center, Michigan State University, East Lansing, Michigan. *Open Fractures*

R. Tass Dueland, D.V.M., M.S., Diplomate, A.C.V.S.
Department of Surgical Sciences, School of Veterinary Medicine, The University of Wisconsin-Madison, Madison, Wisconsin. *Orthopedic Disorders of the Stifle*

Karen R. Dyer, D.V.M.
Department of Small Animal Clinical Sciences, Virginia-Maryland Regional College of Veterinary Medicine, Virginia Polytechnic Institute and State University, Blacksburg, Virginia. *Peripheral Nerve Disorders*

Joan Dziezyc, D.V.M., Diplomate, A.C.V.O.
Associate Professor, Department of Small Animal Medicine and Surgery, College of Veterinary Medicine; Ophthalmologist, Veterinary Teaching Hospital, Texas A&M University, College Station, Texas. *Diseases of the Retina, Choroid, and Optic Nerve*

Erick L. Egger, D.V.M.
Associate Professor, Department of Clinical Sciences, College of Veterinary Medicine; Veterinary Teaching Hospital, Colorado State University, Ft. Collins, Colorado. *Fractures of the Tibia and Fibula*

William R. Fenner, D.V.M., Diplomate, A.C.V.I.M. (Neurology)
College of Veterinary Medicine, The Ohio State University, Columbus, Ohio. *Diagnostic Approach to Neurologic Disease; Diseases of the Brain; Seizures, Narcolepsy, and Cataplexy*

Roger B. Fingland, D.V.M., M.S.
Associate Professor of Surgery and Head, Small Animal Surgery, Department of Clinical Sciences, College of Veterinary Medicine, Kansas State University, Manhattan, Kansas. *Diagnosis and Surgical Management of Obstructive Airway Diseases, Surgery of the Urinary Bladder, Surgery of the Ovaries and Uterus, Surgery of the Vagina and Vulva*

S. Dru Forrester, D.V.M., M.S., Diplomate, A.C.V.I.M. (Internal Medicine)
Assistant Professor, Department of Small Animal Clinical Sciences; Small Animal Internist, Veterinary Teaching Hospital, Virginia-Maryland Regional College of Veterinary Medicine, Virginia Polytechnic Institute and State University, Blacksburg, Virginia. *Diseases of the Kidney and Ureter*

Theresa W. Fossum, D.V.M., M.S., Diplomate, A.C.V.S.
Assistant Professor, Department of Small Animal Medicine and Surgery, College of Veterinary Medicine, Texas A&M University, College Station, Texas. *Pleural Effusion*

Donald Gillespie, D.V.M.
Veterinarian, Montgomery Zoo, Montgomery, Alabama. *Reptiles*

Margi Gilmour, D.V.M., Diplomate, A.C.V.O.
Staff Ophthalmologist, Coral Springs Animal Hospital, Coral Springs, Florida. *Diseases of the Lens*

Stephen D. Gilson, D.V.M.
Moon Valley Animal Hospital, Veterinary Surgical Referral Service, Phoenix, Arizona. *Principles of Oncology*

Mary B. Glaze, D.V.M., M.S.
Associate Professor of Veterinary Ophthalmology, Veterinary Clinical Sciences; Veterinary Ophthalmologist, Veterinary Teaching Hospital and Clinics, Louisiana State University, Baton Rouge, Louisiana. *Diseases of the Orbit*

Joanne C. Graham, D.V.M.
Formerly, Oncology Resident, College of Veterinary Medicine, University of Illinois; Currently, Veterinary Poison Information Specialist, National Animal Poison Control Center, University of Illinois, Urbana, Illinois. *Soft Tissue Sarcomas and Mast Cell Tumors*

Thomas K. Graves, D.V.M.
Department of Small Animal Clinical Sciences, College of Veterinary Medicine, Michigan State University, East Lansing, Michigan. *Thyroid Gland*

Craig E. Griffin, D.V.M., Diplomate, A.C.V.D.
Director, Animal Dermatology Clinic, San Diego, California. *Flea Allergy Dermatitis*

Amy M. Grooters, D.V.M.
Clinical Instructor, Internal Medicine, Department of Veterinary Clinical Sciences, College of Veterinary Medicine, The Ohio State University, Columbus, Ohio. *Diseases of the Ovaries and Uterus, Diseases of the Vagina and Vulva*

Paul R. Haider, A.H.T., A.A., A.S.
Woodland, California. *Radiographic and Ultrasonographic Techniques*

Robert L. Hamlin, D.V.M., Ph.D., Diplomate, A.C.V.I.M. (Cardiology and Internal Medicine)
Professor, Veterinary Physiology and Pharmacology, College of Veterinary Medicine, The Ohio State University, Columbus, Ohio. *Physical Examination*

Cheryl S. Hedlund, D.V.M., M.S., Diplomate, A.C.V.S.
Professor and Chief, Companion Animal Surgery and Anesthesia, Department of Veterinary Clinical Sciences, School of Veterinary Medicine, Louisiana State University, Baton Rouge, Louisiana. *Surgical Management of Chronic Nasal Cavity and Paranasal Sinus Disease*

Karen Helton-Rhodes, D.V.M., Diplomate, A.C.V.D.
Dermatology, Service Head, The Animal Medical Center, New York; Clinical Instructor, Comparative Dermatology, New York University Hospital, New York, New York. *Immune-Mediated Dermatoses*

Elizabeth V. Hillyer, D.V.M.
Animal Medical Center, New York, New York. *Avian Dermatology, Ferrets*

Paul E. Howard, D.V.M., M.S., Diplomate, A.C.V.S.
Vermont Veterinary Surgical Center, Burlington, Vermont. *Fractures and Dislocations of the Mandible, Fractures of the Maxilla, Neoplasms of the Maxilla and Mandible*

John A. E. Hubbell, D.V.M., M.S., A.C.V.A.
Associate Professor of Veterinary Clinical Sciences, Assistant Dean for Academic Affairs, College of Veterinary Medicine; Member, Section of Anesthesia, Veterinary Teaching Hospital, The Ohio State University, Columbus, Ohio. *Practical Methods of Anesthesia*

Kenneth A. Johnson, M.V.Sc., Ph.D., F.A.C.V.Sc., Diplomate, A.C.V.S.
Associate Professor of Surgery, Department of Surgical Sciences; School of Veterinary Medicine, University of Wisconsin-Madison; Associate Professor of Orthopaedics, Veterinary Medical Teaching Hospital, University of Wisconsin-Madison, Madison, Wisconsin. *Pelvic Fractures, Osteomyelitis*

Susan E. Johnson, D.V.M., M.S., Diplomate, A.C.V.I.M.
Associate Professor, Department of Veterinary Clinical Sciences, College of Veterinary Medicine; Internist, Veterinary Teaching Hospital, The Ohio State University, Columbus, Ohio. *Diseases and Surgery of the Exocrine Pancreas, Diseases of the Esophagus and Disorders of Swallowing, Diseases of the Stomach, Diseases of the Intestines, Disease of the Liver and Biliary Tract*

Denise Jones, D.V.M.
Clinical Instructor, Outpatient Clinic, Veterinary Teaching Hospital, The Ohio State University, Columbus, Ohio. *History and Physical Examination*

Renee L. Kaswan, D.V.M.
Professor of Ophthalmology, College of Veterinary Medicine, University of Georgia, Athens, Georgia. *Diseases of the Lacrimal Apparatus*

Nancy D. Kay, D.V.M., Diplomate, A.C.V.I.M.
Private Practice, Oakland, California. *Diseases of the Prostate Gland*

Thomas J. Kern, D.V.M.
Associate Professor of Ophthalmology, Department of Clinical Sciences, College of Veterinary Medicine, Veterinary Medical Teaching Hospital, Cornell University, Ithaca, New York. *Diseases of the Cornea and Sclera*

Susan Kirschner, D.V.M., Diplomate, A.C.V.O.
Staff Ophthalmologist, The Animal Medical Center, New York, New York. *Diseases of the Eyelid*

Gail A. Kunkle, D.V.M.
Professor, Department of Small Animal Clinical Sciences, College of Veterinary Medicine; Service Chief, Dermatology, Veterinary Medical Teaching Hospital, University of Florida, Gainesville, Florida. *Necrotizing Skin Diseases*

Kenneth W. Kwochka, D.V.M., Diplomate, A.C.V.D.
Associate Professor of Dermatology, Department of Veterinary Clinical Sciences, College of Veterinary Medicine; Chief of Dermatology Service, Veterinary Teaching Hospital, College of Veterinary Medicine, The Ohio State University, Columbus, Ohio. *Keratinization Defects*

Mary Anna Labato, D.V.M., Diplomate, A.C.V.I.M.
Clinical Assistant Professor, Department of Medicine, School of Veterinary Medicine, Tufts University; Staff Clinician, Foster Hospital for Small Animals, School of Veterinary Medicine, Tufts University, North Grafton, Massachusetts. *Micturition Disorders*

George E. Lees, D.V.M., M.S., Diplomate, A.C.V.I.M. (Internal Medicine)
Professor of Medicine, Department of Small Animal Medicine and Surgery; Small Animal Internist, Texas Veterinary Medical Center, College of Veterinary Medicine, Texas A&M University, College Station, Texas. *Diseases of the Kidney and Ureter*

Linda B. Lehmkuhl, D.V.M.
Clinical Instructor and Cardiology Resident, Department of Veterinary Clinical Science, College of Veterinary Medicine, The Ohio State University, Columbus, Ohio. *Cardiomyopathy*

Timothy M. Lenehan, D.V.M., Diplomate, A.C.V.S.
Veterinary Surgical Specialists, San Diego, California. *Osteochondrosis*

Patricia J. Luttgen, D.V.M., M.S.
Associate Professor of Neurology and Neurosurgery, College of Veterinary Medicine, Colorado State University, Ft. Collins, Colorado. *Spinal Cord Disorders*

Paul A. Manley, D.V.M., M.Sc., Diplomate, A.C.V.S.
Associate Professor, Department of Surgical Sciences, School of Veterinary Medicine, University of Wisconsin-Madison, Madison, Wisconsin. *Pelvic Fractures, Amputation of the Digit, Pediatric Fractures, Lyme Disease*

Sandra Manfra Marretta, D.V.M., Diplomate, A.C.V.S., A.V.D.C.
Assistant Professor, Small Animal Surgery and Dentistry, College of Veterinary Medicine, University of Illinois, Urbana, Illinois. *Oropharynx*

Kurt J. Matushek, D.V.M., M.S., Diplomate, A.C.V.S.
Assistant Editor, American Veterinary Medical Association, Schaumburg, Illinois. *Fractures and Dislocations of the Carpus*

Scott McDonald, D.V.M.
Midwest Avian and Exotic Animal Hospital, Westchester, Illinois. *Avian Digestive System Disorders*

Margaret C. McEntee, D.V.M.
Clinical Instructor, Oncology, Veterinary Teaching Hospital, North Carolina State University, Raleigh, North Carolina. *Diseases of the Spleen*

Matthew W. Miller, D.V.M.
Assistant Professor, College of Veterinary Medicine; Staff Cardiologist, Texas Veterinary Medical Center, Texas A&M University, College Station, Texas. *Congenital Heart Disease*

Michael S. Miller, M.S., V.M.D., Diplomate, A.B.V.P.
Vice President, Staff Consultant, Department of Cardiology, Cardiopet, Inc., Floral Park; Staff Clinician, A & A Veterinary Hospital, Franklin Square, New York. *Electrocardiography, Disorders of Cardiac Rhythm*

Nicholas J. Millichamp, B. Vet. Med., Ph.D., M.R.C.V.S., Diplomate, A.C.V.O.
Ophthalmologist, Veterinary Teaching Hospital; Associate Professor, Department of Small Animal Medicine and Surgery, College of Veterinary Medicine, Texas A&M University, College Station, Texas. *Diseases of the Retina, Choroid, and Optic Nerve*

Cecil P. Moore, D.V.M., M.S., Diplomate, A.C.V.O.
Associate Professor, Department of Veterinary Medicine and Surgery, College of Veterinary Medicine; Section Head of Ophthalmology Service, Veterinary Teaching Hospital, College of Veterinary Medicine, University of Missouri, Columbia, Missouri. *Conjunctiva*

Peter Muir, B.V.Sc., M.A.C.V.Sc., M.R.C.V.S.
Department of Surgical Sciences, School of Veterinary Medicine, University of Wisconsin-Madison, Madison, Wisconsin. *Pelvic Fractures*

William W. Muir, III, D.V.M., Ph.D.
Chairman, Department of Veterinary Clinical Sciences, College of Veterinary Medicine, The Ohio State University, Columbus, Ohio. *Drugs for Treatment of Cardiovascular Diseases, Cardiopulmonary Cerebral Resuscitation*

Holly S. Mullen, D.V.M.
Senior Staff Surgeon, The Animal Medical Center, New York, New York. *Adrenal Gland*

Alan C. Mundell, D.V.M., Diplomate, A.C.V.D.
Private Dermatology Referral Practice, Animal Dermatology Service, Seattle, Washington. *Mycobacteriosis, Demodicosis*

Wendy Myer, D.V.M., M.S.
Associate Professor, Department of Veterinary Clinical Sciences, The Ohio State University, Columbus, Ohio. *Radiographic Evaluation, Diagnostic Imaging of the Respiratory System*

Richard W. Nelson, D.V.M.
Associate Professor, Department of Medicine, School of Veterinary Medicine, University of California, Davis, Davis, California. *Diabetes Mellitus, Pancreatic Beta Cell Neoplasia*

Rhett Nichols, D.V.M.
College of Veterinary Medicine, Mississippi State University, Mississippi State, Mississippi. *Adrenal Gland*

James O. Noxon, D.V.M., Diplomate, A.C.V.I.M. (Internal Medicine)
Department of Clinical Sciences, College of Veterinary Medicine, Colorado State University, Ft. Collins, Colorado. *Otitis Externa*

Richard R. Nye, D.V.M.
Midwest Avian and Exotic Animal Hospital, Westchester, Illinois. *Avian Respiratory System*

Gregory K. Ogilvie, D.V.M., Diplomate, A.C.V.I.M. (Internal Medicine and Oncology)
Head, Medical Oncology, Veterinary Teaching Hospital; Associate Professor of Oncology, Comparative Oncology Unit, Department of Clinical Sciences, College of Veterinary Medicine and Biomedical Sciences, Colorado State University; Ft. Collins, Colorado. *Lymphoid Neoplasia*

Barbara L. Oglesbee, D.V.M.
College of Veterinary Medicine and Veterinary Teaching Hospital, The Ohio State University, Columbus, Ohio. *Avian Techniques, Avian Infectious Diseases, Avian Digestive System Disorders*

Deborah A. O'Keefe, D.V.M., M.S.
Assistant Professor, College of Veterinary Medicine, University of Illinois, Urbana, Illinois. *Soft Tissue Sarcomas and Mast Cell Tumors*

Marvin L. Olmstead, D.V.M., Diplomate, A.C.V.S.
Department of Veterinary Clinical Sciences, College of Veterinary Medicine, The Ohio State University, Columbus, Ohio. *Coxofemoral Joint*

Rodney L. Page, D.V.M., M.S.
Associate Professor, School of Veterinary Medicine, North Carolina State University, Raleigh, North Carolina. *Diseases of the Spleen, Principles of Oncology*

Robert B. Parker, D.V.M., Diplomate, A.C.V.S.
Associate Professor and Chief, Small Animal Surgery, College of Veterinary Medicine; Staff Orthopedic Surgeon, Veterinary Medical Teaching Hospital, University of Florida, Gainesville, Florida. *Fractures of the Humerus*

Nigel R. Perkins, B.V.Sc.(Hons.), M.S., Diplomate, A.C.T.
Clinical Instructor, Theriogenology, College of Veterinary Medicine, The Ohio State University, Columbus, Ohio. *Infertility, Intersex Abnormalities*

Steven W. Petersen, D.V.M.
Formerly, Chief Resident, Small Animal Surgery, School of Veterinary Medicine, University of Wisconsin-Madison, Madison, Wisconsin; Staff Surgeon, Alameda East Veterinary Hospital, Denver, Colorado. *Surgery of Skeletal Muscle and Tendons*

Janet L. Peterson, D.V.M.
Clinical Instructor and Resident, Small Animal Medicine, The Ohio State University, Columbus, Ohio. *Tumors of the Skin and Subcutaneous Tissues, Adrenal Gland*

Mark E. Peterson, D.V.M.
The Animal Medical Center, New York, New York. *Thyroid Gland, Hypothalamus and Pituitary Gland, Adrenal Gland*

James Prueter, D.V.M., Diplomate, A.C.V.I.M.
Hospital Director of Operation, Veterinary Referral Clinic, Cleveland, Ohio. *Diagnostic Methods for Respiratory Disorders*

Katherine E. Quesenberry, D.V.M.
Animal Medical Center, New York, New York. *Avian Neurologic Disorders, Rabbits*

John F. Randolph, D.V.M., Diplomate, A.C.V.I.M.
Associate Professor, Department of Clinical Sciences, College of Veterinary Medicine, Cornell University; Small Animal Internist, Veterinary Teaching Hospital, Cornell University, Ithaca, New York. *Hypothalamus and Pituitary Gland*

Rose E. Raskin, D.V.M., Ph.D., Diplomate, A.C.V.P.
Assistant Professor, Department of Physiological Sciences, College of Veterinary Medicine, University of Florida, Gainesville, Florida. *Erythrocytes, Leukocytes, and Platelets*

John R. Reed, M.S., D.V.M., Diplomate, A.C.V.I.M. (Cardiology)
Staff Cardiologist, Sacramento Animal Medical Group, North Highlands, California. *Pericardial Disease and Cardiac Neoplasia.*

Wayne S. Rosenkrantz, D.V.M., Diplomate, A.C.V.D
Assistant Clinical Instructor, Summer Preceptor Program, University of California, Davis; Partner-Owner of Animal Dermatology Clinics of Garden Grove and San Diego, California. *Miliary Dermatitis and Eosinophilic Granuloma Complex*

Edmund J. Rosser, Jr., D.V.M., Diplomate, A.C.V.D.
Associate Professor of Dermatology, College of Veterinary Medicine, Department of Small Animal Clinical Sciences, Veterinary Medical Center, Michigan State University, East Lansing, Michigan. *Pyoderma*

Walter J. Rosskopf, D.V.M.
Avian and Exotic Animal Hospital, Hawthorne, California. *Avian Obstetrical Medicine*

James K. Roush, D.V.M., M.S., Diplomate, A.C.V.S.
Assistant Professor, Small Animal Surgery, College of Veterinary Medicine, Kansas State University, Manhattan, Kansas. *Diseases Affecting Developing Bone*

John Rush, D.V.M., M.S., Diplomate, A.C.V.I.M. (Cardiology)
Assistant Professor, Tufts University, School of Veterinary Medicine; Head Cardiologist and Co-Director of the Intensive Care Unit/Emergency Services, Foster Hospital for Small Animals, Tufts University, School of Veterinary Medicine, North Grafton, Massachusetts. *Heart Failure*

S. Kathleen Salisbury, D.V.M., M.S.
Associate Professor, Small Animal Surgery, School of Veterinary Medicine, Purdue University; Purdue University Veterinary Teaching Hospital, West Lafayette, Indiana. *Pancreatic Beta Cell Neoplasia*

Randall H. Scagliotti, D.V.M.
Sacramento Animal Medical Group, Carmichael, California. *Neuro-Ophthalmology*

Vicki J. Scheidt, D.V.M.
Dermatologist, Referral Practice, Hanover, New Hampshire. *Feline Symmetric Alopecia*

Eric R. Schertel, D.V.M., Ph.D.
Division of Thoracic and Cardiovascular Surgery, Department of Surgery, College of Medicine; Department of Veterinary Clinical Sciences, College of Veterinary Medicine, The Ohio State University, Columbus, Ohio. *Surgical Correction of Patent Ductus Arteriosus, Shock, Principles of Thoracic Surgery*

Mary P. Schick, D.V.M.
Veterinary Dermatology Referral Practitioner, Atlanta Animal Allergy and Dermatology, Roswell, Georgia. *Skin Biopsy, Pinnal Diseases*

Robert O. Schick, D.V.M.
Veterinary Dermatology Referral Practitioner, Atlanta Animal Allergy and Dermatology, Roswell, Georgia. *Skin Biopsy, Pinnal Diseases*

Lynn P. Schmeitzel, D.V.M.
Associate Professor, Department of Urban Practice, College of Veterinary Medicine, University of Tennessee, Knoxville, Tennessee. *Growth Hormone–Responsive Alopecia and Sex Hormone–Associated Dermatoses*

Linda G. Shell, D.V.M., Diplomate, A.C.V.I.M. (Neurology)
Associate Professor, Section Chief, Small Animal Medicine, Virginia-Maryland Regional College of Veterinary Medicine, Virginia Polytechnic Institute and State University, Blacksburg, Virginia. *Otitis Media and Otitis Interna, Peripheral Nerve Disorders*

G. Diane Shelton, D.V.M., Ph.D.
Associate Clinical Professor, Department of Pathology; Director, Comparative Neuromuscular Laboratory, University of California, San Diego, School of Medicine, San Diego, California. *Neuromuscular Disorders*

Robert G. Sherding, D.V.M., Diplomate, C.V.I.M.
Professor of Small Animal Internal Medicine, and Chair, Department of Veterinary Clinical Sciences, The Ohio State University, Columbus, Ohio. *Section 2, Infectious Diseases; Respiratory Infection, Diseases of the Esophagus and Disorders of Swallowing, Diseases of the Stomach, Diseases of the Intestines, Disease of the Liver and Biliary Tract, Diseases and Surgery of the Exocrine Pancreas, Anorectal Diseases*

Peter Shires, B.V.Sc., M.S., Diplomate, A.C.V.S.
Professor, Small Animal Surgery, and Orthopedic Surgeon, Veterinary Medical Teaching Hospital, Virginia-Maryland Regional College of Veterinary Medicine, Virginia Polytechnic Institute and State University, Blacksburg, Virginia. *Fractures of the Femur and Patella*

David Sisson, D.V.M., Diplomate, A.C.V.I.M. (Cardiology)
Associate Professor, College of Veterinary Medicine, University of Illinois; Director, Cardiology Service, Veterinary Medical Teaching Hospital, University of Illinois; Urbana, Illinois. *Valvular Heart Disease*

Daniel D. Smeak, D.V.M.
Associate Professor of Surgery, College of Veterinary Medicine, The Ohio State University, Columbus, Ohio. *Selected Skin Graft and Reconstructive Techniques, Surgery of the External Ear Canal and Pinna*

Francis W. K. Smith, Jr., D.V.M., Diplomate, A.C.V.I.M.
Chief of Medicine, Cardiopet, Inc., Floral Park, New York. *Electrocardiography, Disorders of Cardiac Rhythm*

Mark M. Smith, V.M.D., Diplomate, A.C.V.S.
Associate Professor, Department of Small Animal Clinical Sciences, Virginia-Maryland Regional College of Veterinary Medicine, Virginia Polytechnic Institute, Blacksburg, Virginia. *Fractures of the Skull, Neoplasia of the Axial Skeleton*

Susan F. Soderberg, D.V.M., Diplomate, A.C.V.I.M.
Northeast Veterinary Hospital, Detroit; East Detroit Animal Hospital, Eastpointe, Michigan. *Diseases of the Scrotum and Testes, Diseases of the Penis and Prepuce*

Rebecca L. Stepien, D.V.M., M.S., Diplomate, A.C.V.I.M.
Cardiologist, Department of Small Animal Medicine and Surgery, The Royal Veterinary College, University of London, England. *Vascular Diseases*

Elizabeth Arnold Stone, D.V.M., M.S., Diplomate, A.C.S.
Professor, College of Veterinary Medicine; Staff Surgeon, Veterinary Teaching Hospital, College of Veterinary Medicine, North Carolina State University, Raleigh, North Carolina. *Mammary Gland Neoplasia*

Steven F. Swaim, D.V.M., M.S.
Professor of Surgery, College of Veterinary Medicine, Auburn University; Scott-Ritchey Research Center and Department of Small Animal Surgery and Medicine, Auburn, Alabama. *Closure of Traumatic Wounds Using Adjacent Skin*

Robert A. Taylor, D.V.M., M.S., Diplomate, A.C.V.S.
Alameda East Veterinary Hospital, Denver, Colorado. *Scapulohumeral Luxation*

James P. Thompson, D.V.M., Ph.D.
Associate Professor, Department of Small Animal Clinical Sciences; Director, Immunology Laboratory, Veterinary Medical Teaching Hospital, University of Florida, Gainesville, Florida. *Systemic Immune-Mediated Diseases*

Walter R. Threlfall, D.V.M., M.S., Ph.D.
Professor, Department of Veterinary Clinical Sciences, The Ohio State University, Columbus, Ohio. *Infertility, Intersex Abnormalities*

Larry Patrick Tilley, D.V.M., Diplomate, A.C.V.I.M. (Internal Medicine)
President, Chief Medical Officer, Department of Cardiology, Cardiopet, Inc., Floral Park, New York. *Electrocardiography, Disorders of Cardiac Rhythm*

James Tomlinson, D.V.M., M.V.Sci., Diplomate, A.C.V.S.
Associate Professor of Surgery, College of Veterinary Medicine, University of Missouri, Columbia, Missouri. *Fractures and Growth Deformities of the Radius and Ulna*

Thomas M. Turner, D.V.M.
Assistant Professor, Department of Orthopaedic Surgery, Rush Presbyterian St. Luke's Medical Center, Chicago; Staff Surgeon, Berwyn Veterinary Associates, Berwyn, Illinois. *Fractures of the Shoulder*

David M. Vail, D.V.M., M.S., Diplomate, A.C.V.I.M. (Oncology)
Assistant Professor of Oncology, Department of Medical Sciences, School of Veterinary Medicine; Associate Member, Wisconsin Comprehensive Cancer Center, Department of Human Oncology, School of Medicine, University of Wisconsin-Madison, Madison, Wisconsin. *Lymphoid Neoplasia*

Tom Van Gundy, D.V.M., M.S.
Staff Surgeon, Akron Veterinary Surgical Associates,
Metropolitan Veterinary Hospital, Akron, Ohio. *Disorders
of the Parathyroid Gland and Calcium Metabolism*

S.D. Wagner, D.V.M., M.S.
Small Animal Hospital, College of Veterinary Medicine,
Iowa State University, Ames, Iowa. *Fractures and
Dislocation of the Spine*

**Larry J. Wallace, D.V.M., M.S., Diplomate,
A.C.V.S.**
Department of Small Animal Clinical Sciences, College of
Veterinary Medicine, University of Minnesota, St. Paul,
Minnesota. *Traumatic Luxation of the Elbow Joint*

Ken Warthen, D.V.M.
Featherquest Farms, Pembroke, Virginia. *Avian Digestive
System Disorders*

Richard W. Woerpel, D.V.M., M.S.
Avian and Exotic Animal Hospital, Hawthorne, California.
Avian Obstetrical Medicine

Patricia D. White, D.V.M., M.S.
Formerly, Research Fellow, College of Veterinary
Medicine, The Ohio State University, Columbus, Ohio;
Currently, Atlanta Veterinary Skin and Allergy Clinic,
Avondale Estates, Georgia. *Atopy*

Stephen D. White, D.V.M.
Associate Professor, Department of Clinical Sciences,
College of Veterinary Medicine and Biomedical Sciences;
Dermatologist, Veterinary Teaching Hospital, Colorado
State University, Ft. Collins, Colorado. *Food
Hypersensitivity*

**David A. Wilkie, D.V.M., M.S. Diplomate,
A.C.V.O.**
Assistant Professor and Head, Ophthalmology, Department
of Veterinary Clinical Sciences, The Ohio State
University, Columbus, Ohio. *Introduction to
Ophthalmology, Diseases of the Lens, Uvea, Glaucoma*

Preface

Producing a book that concisely covers nearly all common diseases treated in small animal practice seemed an almost insurmountable task. When considering the number of new veterinary textbooks that have been written, how could we possibly hope to create a book that condenses all pertinent information into one volume? It certainly provided us with a significant challenge, but one that we felt was possible to meet. Although many good quality veterinary texts are available, we saw a need for an accessible, concise, and usable book that provided a broad scope of practical information. We spent many hours quizzing practitioners to determine the kind of reference book that would best meet their needs, especially considering their busy schedules and shortage of time. We hope we have succeeded in designing a book that can rapidly provide practical information to the busy practitioner. We do not see this as a book that sits on a shelf collecting dust; we see it as one that is open on a counter in a treatment room with veterinarians and technicians flipping its pages frequently during the day.

Saunders Manual of Small Animal Practice is organized, with some exceptions, in a systems approach. We believe that one of the most exciting aspects of this book is that information on medical and surgical treatment of diseases is combined into one volume. Medical chapters discuss etiology, clinical signs, diagnosis, and treatment; surgical chapters discuss anatomy, preoperative considerations, procedures, and postoperative care. The emphasis is on diseases of the dog and cat, but an entire section is also devoted to exotic species, recognizing their increasing importance as pets. Some chapters are focused on general methods of patient management in small animal practice, such as anesthetic and radiologic techniques and critical care. A chapter has also been included to help the veterinarian deal with grieving clients.

We have employed several methods to make this a usable book. Color has been added to highlight major titles and key points in the chapters, making important information easy to find. Contributors have attempted to adhere to a standardized outline format to give the chapters consistency. Bulleted charts are used to list items such as the differential diagnoses and treatment options. Surgical procedures are numbered sequentially. Extensive cross referencing of information helps make the book more user friendly. Illustrations, all drawn by a single artist, give consistency to the chapters and allow a better understanding of anatomy and of surgical technique.

We recognize the need to keep this book concise and in one volume. Some information had to be left out. There is very little discussion of the pathophysiology of diseases. Readers will have to refer to other texts for this information. Uncommon diseases, rarely performed surgical techniques, and surgical procedures that require specialty training and facilities are not discussed extensively.

Many excellent texts are available for those seeking more in-depth discussions of certain diseases or treatments.

We are grateful to many people for their help with this book. The section editors and chapter authors provided the backbone of this book with their excellent contributions. We particularly appreciate their willingness to conform to a standardized outline format that was somewhat nontraditional. We also would like to thank the staff at W.B. Saunders, especially Mary Anne Folcher, Linda R. Garber, and Ray Kersey. A special note of thanks and gratitude goes to Linda Mills, former editor at Saunders. We sincerely appreciate her devotion to this project, including countless hours organizing material, working with authors, and generally taking care of the unbelievable number of ''loose ends.'' Special thanks also to our departmental secretary and assistant Kim Hammer, and to the very talented artist, Felecia J. Paras, for her beautiful illustrations.

We welcome comments and critiques from the readers to help us identify the strengths and weaknesses of the book. We need input to ''fine tune'' the manual for future editions and thus allow it to become the best possible book for small animal practitioners.

Contents

S E C T I O N 8

Patient Management

Stephen J. Birchard

1

History and Physical Examination

Denise Jones

Veterinarians are faced with many diagnostic challenges daily in the clinical setting. By far the most important diagnostic tool that veterinarians possess is their ability to obtain a complete history and thorough physical examination. This information, when accurately interpreted, lays the foundation for a logical diagnostic and therapeutic plan. However, if the history or physical examination is performed haphazardly, the clinician may be led astray from the patient's pertinent problem and the appropriate diagnosis. In the modern clinical setting, the veterinarian can perform an array of diagnostic tests, spend much of the client's money, and still overlook the definitive diagnosis, if shortcuts are taken with the initial data collection. The ability to collect information is an art and must be approached systematically and thoroughly.

GENERAL HISTORY

- Approach the history so that both objective and subjective information are obtained. Objective data consist of the signalment, environment, diet, and medical history. For a patient's first visit, the length of ownership and the place of origin are included.
- Subjective data include a description of the primary complaint and a historical overview of the patient's general health. The client often may not realize how a seemingly unimportant observation may be related to the primary problem.

Signalment

- The signalment consists of the patient's age, species, breed, and gender. Note whether the patient is intact or neutered.
- Verify that previously recorded data are correct and up to date. As examples, the patient may have been neutered since its last visit and the physical examination may indicate that the recorded age is questionable.

Environment

- Gather environmental information as a routine part of the patient's history. In many circumstances, the knowledge of where the pet is kept becomes a vital clue in diagnosis.
- Determine whether the pet is free roaming or confined to a yard or house. If the patient is confined to a yard, question the client specifically as to whether the yard is fenced, whether the pet is chained, and whether an escape has been possible in the recent past. The free-roaming or recently escaped pet may have had access to toxins or have been subject to trauma, which is unlikely for an indoor pet. For a dyspneic patient, diaphragmatic hernia ranks higher on the differential diagnosis list for a free-roaming pet than for a strictly indoor pet.
- Determine the geographic origin of the pet and any record of recent travels. This information becomes paramount, if the patient has been exposed to diseases endemic to certain regions but not prevalent

1

in the current environment, such as systemic mycoses and rickettsial diseases.

■ Determine the pet's water source and the access to any toxins or ingestible foreign bodies. Source of water may be important if the pet has access to toilet-bowl water treated with cleansers or deodorants or if the pet has limited access to water. This information is unimportant if the presenting complaint does not suggest toxicity or foreign body ingestion.

Dietary History

■ Always include dietary information in the routine data base. Question the owner about the patient's appetite and evidence of any weight gain or loss. Also note whether the owner watches the pet eat.
■ Determine the following pertinent facts in the dietary history:
  • Type of diet (e.g., dry, moist, semimoist, and table food)
  • Brand name of food
  • Type of snacks
  • Method of feeding (i.e., free-choice or individual meals)
  • Amount.

Preventative Health Care Status

■ Evaluate the preventative health care status of the patient. Review the patient's medical record prior to taking the history because this information may have been previously obtained.
■ Record the previous vaccinations received and the dates of each. Avoid simply asking if the patient is current on vaccinations because many clients are unfamiliar with vaccination recommendations. Inform the client of what vaccinations are available as well as the indications and booster intervals for each (see sec. 2, chs. 1 to 11).
■ For the feline patient, discuss the subject of feline leukemia virus (FLV), including the dates and results of previous testing as well as vaccination dates. Exposure to FLV-positive patients may also be relevant.
■ For the canine patient, record heartworm test dates and results. If the patient is receiving heartworm preventative note the type, frequency, and dose (see sec. 6, ch. 10).

Prior Medical History: Previous Illnesses and Surgeries

■ Often the patient's prior or ongoing health problems play a role in its presenting ailment; therefore, review the information previously recorded in the medical chart and discuss previous problems managed by another veterinarian.
■ Record the dates of the previous illness or surgery, followed by a brief description of the problem, how it was managed, and what level of response was seen.
■ Discern the relevance of these problems prior to acquiring a detailed account of each event; other-

wise, the history may become unnecessarily lengthy and confusing.

Primary Complaint

■ Use the history to identify and localize the primary problem. Much of this information is subjective, based mostly on the client's interpretation of their pet's clinical symptoms and behavior. One must be aware that some clients are extremely observant of their pet and others are not. The astute clinician collects all data and subjectively analyzes this information in respect to the client's perceptivity.
■ Encourage the client to describe the patient's problem from its onset so that a chronologic picture is obtained.
■ Avoid leading questions so that a deceptive history is not obtained. For example, ask if there has been any change in frequency of defecation. Do not ask if the patient is defecating more frequently than normal.
■ Certain data are essential to the clinician's diagnostic and therapeutic approach. This information aids in ranking the differential diagnoses in order of preference.
  • Determine the last period of normalcy. This information influences how rapidly or aggressively the problem is to be approached.
  • Determine the onset (acute vs. chronic) of the problem. For example, intestinal intussusception is a likely differential for a puppy presenting with an acute episode of frequent vomiting. A gastric foreign body is more likely in a similar patient with chronic intermittent vomiting.
  • Determine treatments and response to those treatments. For example, a dog presenting with pruritus unresponsive to previous treatment with corticosteroids is a more likely candidate for food allergy dermatitis than for atopy. Determine what medication was given, the dosage, the duration of treatment, and the level of response observed.
  • Determine the duration and progression of the clinical signs. The data are also mandatory in therapeutically approaching some problems. For example, a patient presenting with a history of seizures is managed more aggressively when the seizures are increasing in frequency and length than when they have been the same for months or years.
  • Determine the intervening signs that may also provide a clue to the most likely differential diagnosis. For example, a cat with chronic diarrhea and intermittent episodes of fever is considered a more likely candidate for infectious disease than for dietary intolerance.
■ Further define and localize the problem, if possible, depending on the nature of the problem. With a case of diarrhea, for example, it is preferable to characterize the diarrhea as initiating in the small or large bowel before proceeding to a diagnostic or therapeutic plan. Questions regarding frequency, appearance (color and consistency), and presence or absence of straining are helpful to localize this problem. Specific

questions are further detailed under the body systems section that follows.

HISTORY ORIENTED BY BODY SYSTEMS

For a complete history, include a system-by-system review of the patient's general health. This can be approached by the experienced clinician as the physical examination is performed. The novice may prefer to obtain the entire history before proceeding with the physical examination. Develop a consistent and systematic method. One method is to begin with questions concerning the patient's head and proceed caudally, as demonstrated in the following text. It is left to the clinician's discretion as to how in-depth the client is questioned on systems that do not appear to affect the primary complaint. Apply the general principles described in the previous section in the approach to all body systems (e.g., onset and duration).

Eyes

- Ask if any ocular discharge has been noted. If so, describe the discharge (serous, mucoid, mucopurulent) and determine if it has been unilateral or bilateral.
- Determine the presence of ocular pain or discomfort as indicated by blepharospasm, face rubbing or pawing, or photophobia.
- Ask about ocular redness, swelling, and asymmetry.
- Ask if the owner has noticed a color change in the pet's eye. This change can occur with anterior uveitis and iriditis, in which hyphema may be present or the iridial color may be altered. A localized color change in the iris may occur with an iris cyst or melanoma.
- Ask if visual disturbances have been noted, as with an acute onset of blindness.

See also sec. 11.

Head, Neck, Ears, Nose, and Oral Cavity

- Record any history of swelling and asymmetry of the head and neck region.
- Inquire about head shaking, ear scratching, and otic discharge or odor that may indicate the possibility of otitis or a foreign body in the ear. Determine if hearing loss has been noted.
- Ask if any nasal discharge has been present. Note the character of any such discharge (serous, mucoid, mucopurulent, hemorrhagic) as well as whether it has been unilateral or bilateral. Record any history of sneezing, nose rubbing, nasal asymmetry, and stridor.
- Request information relating to the oral cavity, such as odor, difficulty eating or swallowing, presence of abnormal swellings involving the gingiva or tongue, and changes in gingival pigmentation. Ask if there has been any change in the patient's bark or meow.

Cardiopulmonary System

- Ask if exercise intolerance, weakness, or fainting has been observed. These may indicate cardiopulmonary disease.

KEY POINT ► Differentiate syncope from seizures based on the client's description of the event.

- Characterize coughing as productive or nonproductive, moist or dry, harsh or honking. Some clients may confuse a productive cough with vomiting; therefore, ask if abdominal heaving occurs prior to the production of fluid or foam or if coughing and gagging are more typical. A description of the fluid may help if bile is present. The circumstances under which the cough occurs are often relevant. For example, cough associated with tracheal collapse is often elicited with excitement or pulling on the patient's collar. Coughing secondary to congestive heart failure may be exacerbated with the pet in a sternal position.
- Determine if dyspnea has been observed. If the owner describes difficult breathing, discern whether it is panting or true dyspnea.

See sec. 6.

Skin

An accurate and a detailed history is vital in a successful approach to a dermatologic problem. Some clinicians prefer to use a standardized dermatologic history form prior to questioning the owner. The following questions are included on such a form or answered directly by the client.

- Any observation of hair loss? Was the hair involved undercoat or maincoat?
- Is there evidence of pruritus (scratching, biting, licking)?
  - If so, how severe? Mild, moderate, or severe?
  - Continuous or seasonal? If seasonal, when?
  - Has the owner noticed fleas? What is the treatment for fleas?
  - What type of bedding does the pet use?
  - Any exposure to feathers?
  - What type of carpet in the house (wool, synthetic, cotton)?
  - Of what does the diet consist? Treats? Toys?
  - Any indoor plants?
  - Is the pruritus worse indoors or outdoors?
  - Is there any exposure to tobacco smoke?
  - Has the pet ever had any drug reactions? (describe)
- Any odor noticed? (description of odor)
- Any pigment changes of the skin or hair? (describe)
- Any textural changes of the skin or haircoat? (describe)
- Any presence of dandruff? If so, what areas are involved?
- How often is the patient groomed (clipped, brushed, combed)?
- How often is the patient bathed? Last bath? Product used?
- Other pets in household? Are they affected?
- Do any members of the household have skin problems?
- Do any of the pet's close relatives have skin problems?

■ Any previous treatment? When was the pet last treated? What was the name of the drug, the dose, the route of administration, and the frequency of treatment? What level of response was noted?

See sec. 5.

Digestive System

Most problems related to the digestive system are clinically manifested as regurgitation vomiting, diarrhea, constipation, weight loss, or their combination. Frequently, the clinician is required to determine which symptom is actually being exhibited because the client may incorrectly interpret what is observed. For example, a client often assumes that the patient is constipated if it is observed straining to defecate, when diarrhea may be the actual cause. The following specific information is included in approaching a digestive system problem:

■ Dietary history is reviewed as previously described. Specifically ask about treats or access to garbage.
■ Environmental history is recorded as previously described.
  • Specifically, any exposure to toxins or plants?
  • Specifically, any toys or other objects that the pet may have ingested?
■ Vaccination status is noted.
■ Has any vomiting been observed (onset, progression)?
  • Has the owner actually observed the pet vomiting?
  • How frequently is the pet vomiting?
  • What is the relationship of vomiting to eating, if any?
  • What is produced when the pet vomits? Describe the vomitus—digested or undigested food, fluid, foam, and color.
  • Is any retching or abdominal component observed?
■ Is any diarrhea observed (onset, progression)?
  • Has the owner witnessed the patient defecating?
  • How frequently does the animal defecate?
  • Is the stool persistently loose?
  • What is the owner's description of the stool in regard to color and consistency (formed but soft, cow patty–like, watery)?
  • Is there any blood or mucus present?
  • What volume of stool is produced?
  • Does the animal strain while defecating?
  • Does the animal consume its own stool?
■ Does the owner believe that the patient is constipated?
  • How long since the last observed bowel movement?
  • Consistency of last stool?
  • Does the owner witness all eliminations (leash walks, access to yard, or free roaming)?

See also sec. 7.

Urinary System

Often, the client complaint may be that the pet is urinating quite excessively. The following questions help to distinguish whether excessive urination is due to polyuria or to pollakiuria.

■ Has there been any change in the quantity of water that the pet consumes?
■ Are there other pets in the household that have access to the same water source?
■ Has there been any change in frequency of urination?
■ Is the pet urinating inside the house?
  • Are these urinations observed?
  • Do they occur while the animal is awake or asleep?
  • Does the patient seem to be consciously aware of the act?
  • Does the animal dribble urine without seeming to be aware?
■ What quantity of urine is produced?
■ Does the animal appear to strain while urinating?
■ Has the owner noticed any blood in the urine? Before, after, or during urination?

See also sec. 8.

Genital System

The reproductive status of the patient was previously noted. If the patient is intact, consider the following questions.

■ If female, when was the patient's last heat cycle?
■ Was she bred or is there any possibility of an incidental breeding?
■ Was the heat cycle normal in respect to the expected interval since previous estrus and the duration?
■ Has the animal been previously bred? Was the breeding successful? Difficulty whelping?
■ Has any vulvar discharge been noted (describe amount, consistency, color, odor)?
■ If male, has the patient been used for breeding? When?
■ Any litters sired?
■ Any preputial or penile discharge (describe amount, consistency, color, odor)?
■ For both the male and female dog, has the patient been tested for brucellosis? When? Was the mate previously tested?

See also sec. 8.

Musculoskeletal System

■ History relating to the musculoskeletal system focuses on lameness. When lameness has been observed, discern if the patient has been bearing weight versus not bearing weight. Determine whether any lameness has been previously observed in the other limbs; determine whether there are any other signs of illness in addition to the lameness.
■ Ascertain any possibility of trauma preceding the lameness. In some cases, the client may have witnessed the traumatic incident. In others, the patient may have been unsupervised during the time in question. If the animal was free roaming and unobserved, determine for how long and the probability of exposure to automobiles or other sources of trauma.
■ Determine if the client has observed loss of muscle mass, asymmetry of the limbs, or swollen joints.
■ Ask if the patient has demonstrated any difficulty on

rising, climbing stairs, or descending stairs. Determine if these signs improve or worsen with exercise.

■ In regions endemic for Lyme disease, ask if any ticks have been observed on the pet.

See also sec. 9.

Nervous System

Many questions related to the nervous systems may have been previously asked while approaching the other body systems. Because all the body systems rely on the central nervous system (CNS) for their ability to function normally, diseases of the CNS may be reflected by abnormalities in the individual systems (e.g., blindness and hearing loss). In the case of a presenting complaint of rear limb "weakness," the clinician does not know if the primary problem is related to the musculoskeletal system or to the nervous system until the history and physical examination are completed. Consider the following points in regard to the nervous system:

■ Ask if any behavioral changes, such as aggression and dementia, have been observed.

■ Record any history of seizures, including their duration and the time interval between them. A description of the seizure is obtained.

■ Determine if any abnormalities in posture or ambulation have been observed, such as the pet's tendency to fall to one side, to circle to one side, to knuckle over, or to drag its toes.

See also sec. 10.

Swelling or Masses

Ask if any abnormal swellings have been observed that have not been previously mentioned. Note the location, how long the mass or swelling has been present, and any change in appearance or size.

PHYSICAL EXAMINATION: GENERAL OBSERVATION OF PATIENT

■ To begin the physical examination, watch the patient as it comes into the room.

■ Continue the visual evaluation of the patient while the history is collected. Observe the general body condition and abnormalities in behavior, attitude, posture, ambulation, and respiratory pattern. During this time, the patient may be placed on the examination table or allowed to roam the examination room.

Vital Signs

Record the vital signs and current body weight initially on every patient.

■ Body temperature
  • Obtain the rectal temperature early in the course of the examination to help avoid an elevation of temperature that may result from anxiety or ex-

citement. In emergency situations, early attention is given to hypothermia and/or hyperthermia.
  • Note any blood or melena that may be present on the thermometer.

■ Pulse or heart rate
  • Record the pulse rate and evaluate the pulse quality.
  • Determine the presence of arrhythmias and pulse deficits.

■ Respiratory rate
  • Evaluate the respiratory pattern as the rate is taken.
  • When moderate or severe dyspnea is present, caution is taken before continuing with the remainder of the examination. The additional stress of restraint and examination may result in life-threatening respiratory compromise. Oxygen therapy is often warranted followed by a rapid oral examination and thoracic auscultation to help determine the source of the dyspnea and appropriate emergency therapy. After the respirations are stable, continue with the remainder of the physical examination.

■ Hydration
  • Note if the eyes appear sunken or if the third eyelids are protruding bilaterally.
  • Note if the mucous membranes are dry or tacky.
  • Evaluate skin turgor by gently lifting the skin over the dorsal thorax. Geriatric or cachectic patients may appear to be dehydrated, based on their skin turgor alone because of the loss of the skin's natural elasticity.

PHYSICAL EXAMINATION: BODY SYSTEMS APPROACH

The physical examination should follow the same logical pattern as the history. A consistent approach is taken so that no part of the examination is overlooked. For example, analyze one body system at a time, starting with the patient's head, and proceed caudally. Many parts of the examination may involve verification of what the client has observed; therefore, some of the data collected may seem repetitive.

Head

■ Examine the head carefully for any evidence of asymmetry or localized swellings. Visual examination and palpation of these areas may be necessary to discover subtle swellings or masses. Palpation is necessary to assess the nature of any swelling or mass (firm or fluctuant, mobile or attached).

■ Evaluate the posture of the head and neck. Ventroflexion may be observed in cats with hypokalemia, chronic organophosphate toxicity, thiamine deficiency, and polymyopathies. A reluctance to lift the head may be noticed in a dog with cervical intervertebral disc protrusion. In that case, it may be beneficial to gently manipulate the head dorsally and ventrally and to either side, to look for evidence of pain or resistance.

Eyes

- Initially determine if abnormalities are present unilaterally or bilaterally. If only one eye is affected, examine the normal eye first.
- Observe size and symmetry of the eyes. Congenital microphthalmia or acquired phthisis bulbi results in a smaller than normal eye, whereas, chronic glaucoma results in a larger than normal eye.
- Examine the position of the eyes for evidence of enophthalmos, exophthalmos, or strabismus. Enophthalmos may be secondary to microphthalmia, loss of the orbital fat pad (e.g., cachexia), Horner's syndrome, dehydration, or acute ocular pain (e.g., anterior uveitis). Exophthalmos may due to space-occupying lesions of the orbit (neoplasia, abscess, cellulitis), buphthalmos (glaucoma), myositis, or breed predisposition.
- Look for evidence of ocular discharge and characterize any discharge as serous, mucoid, or mucopurulent.
- Note any swelling or masses involving the eyelids as well as distichiasis, entropion, or ectropion.
- Evaluate the conjunctiva for hyperemia, chemosis, pallor, or jaundice of the underlying sclera. The superior conjunctiva is more reliable for evaluating hyperemia than the inferior conjunctiva, which may normally appear reddened. Note any abnormal pigmentation or masses involving the sclera or conjunctiva.
- Protrusion of the third eyelid may be a reflection of enophthalmos or Haw's syndrome in cats. Note any masses associated with the nictitans or prolapse of the gland of the nictitans. Apply gentle pressure to the superior globe to aid in exposing the nictitans. Apply topical anesthesia and grasp the third eyelid gently with forceps, so that the posterior surface of the third eyelid can be examined for foreign bodies or follicular hyperplasia.
- Examine the cornea for cloudiness, pigmentation, vascularization, or obvious defects.
- Evaluate the anterior chamber for the presence of aqueous flare, hypopyon, hyphema, or abnormal masses. If a slit lamp is not available, use a magnifying lens and a penlight to produce a narrow beam of light so that subtle aqueous flair can be detected when the anterior chamber is viewed from a lateral aspect.
- Evaluate the pupil size and symmetry and the direct and consensual pupillary light reflexes. A darkened room aids in this examination. Persistent pupillary membranes may also be identified.
- Evaluate the iris for pigmentary changes, hyperemia, roughening, swelling, or synechia. Any of these changes can be seen with anterior uveitis. Iridial tumors or cysts may occasionally be found.
- Evaluate the lens via direct or indirect ophthalmoscopy for lenticular sclerosis, cataract, or displacement.
- For a complete fundic examination, dilate the pupil with a short-acting mydriatic. Evaluate the fundus for vascularity, areas of hemorrhage, pigmentary changes, chorioretinal dysplasia or hypoplasia, or retinal detachment. Evaluate the optic disc as to color, size, vascularity, fissures or colobomas, or abnormal masses. Practice and experience are the keys to informative retinal examinations.
- Evaluate vision by dropping a cotton ball in front of the patient or by rolling a cotton ball across the table or floor. Evaluate the menace response. Remember that young puppies and kittens normally do not respond appropriately to menace.

See also sec. 11.

Oral Cavity

- Perform a thorough oral examination if the patient's demeanor allows (Fig. 1). If this examination is specifically indicated but cannot be performed, owing to the patient's aggression, sedation is indicated.
- Always carefully evaluate the mucous membranes for color, moisture, and capillary refill time in order to assess the hydration status. The presence of hyperemia, congestion, cyanosis, jaundice, pallor, or petechia can provide vital clues as to the patient's problem. Note gingival masses, ulcerations, or pigmentary changes.
- Examine the teeth for the presence of calculus or exudate at the gingival margin. Digital pressure applied to the gingiva may aid in expressing exudate when a tooth root abscess is suspected.
- Examine the tongue for evidence of trauma or masses when unexplained oral hemorrhage has been observed. In the feline patient that presents for vomiting, examine the sublingual area for evidence of a linear foreign body, using one of the following two methods.
  - Open the patient's mouth and, with the middle finger of the hand depressing the mandible, apply

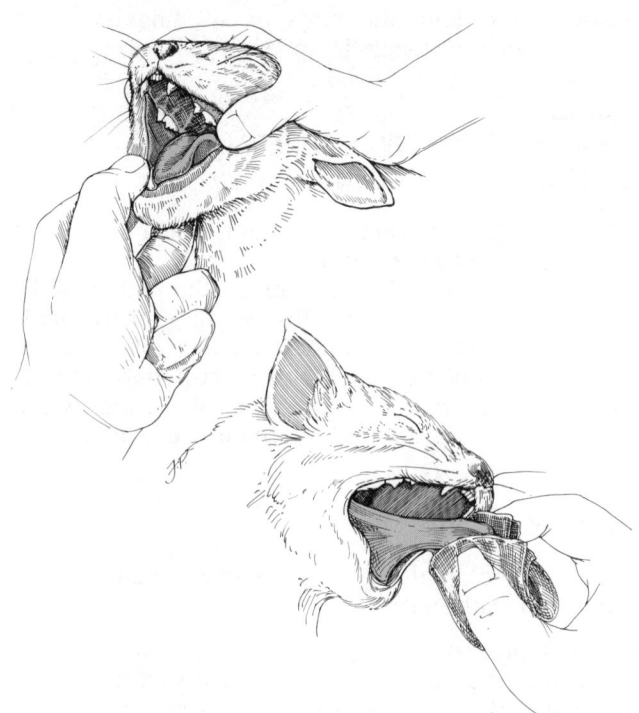

Figure 1. Oral examination of the feline mouth and tongue.

pressure between the mandibular rami from the ventral aspect. In this manner, the tongue is elevated so that the sublingual surface can be seen (Fig. 1, top).
- Occasionally, string can be overlooked with this first method. The sublingual tissue can overlap a thin string that has been drawn taut so that it is not visualized. In this case, the second method is to grasp the tongue, with a 4 × 4-inch sponge, for example, and pull the tongue out and over, so that it can be seen more completely (Fig. 1, bottom).
■ The hard palate is examined in the neonate for clefts. The soft palate is evaluated for elongation or masses.
■ Examine the pharyngeal region for asymmetry, masses, or foreign bodies or for evidence of inflammation or trauma. Examine the tonsils for enlargement. Depress the caudal aspect of the tongue to see the caudal pharynx.

See sec. 7, ch. 1.

Nose

■ Examine the nose for asymmetry or swelling. If a mass or swelling is present, it is carefully palpated to determine whether it is firm or fluctuant.
■ Note any evidence of nasal discharge. Examine the nares closely to determine if the discharge is unilateral or bilateral and to characterize it as serous, mucoid, mucopurulent, or hemorrhagic. It may be beneficial to gently swab the external nares to detect a subtle discharge.
■ If either nasal swelling or discharge is present, evaluate the patency of each nostril by wiping the examination table with an alcohol swab and positioning the patient's nose close to the table to observe condensation of the patient's breath on the surface. Alternately, place a wisp of cotton in front of each nostril to observe movement from airflow, and note any stridor.

See sec. 6, ch. 18.

Ears

■ Inspect both the external and inner surfaces of the pinna for skin lesions, hair loss, erythema, or swelling.
■ Examine the external ear canals for erythema, discharge, and odor prior to an otoscopic examination. Palpate the ear canal cartilages for masses, pain, or other abnormalities.
■ An otoscopic exam is invaluable is assessing an ear-related problem.
- Otoscopic technique requires practice to be successful. Sedation of the pet may be required.
- Lift the pinna and gently place the otoscopic cone in the vertical canal from a dorsal approach and direct it ventrally (Fig. 2). As the otoscope is guided deeper into the vertical canal, pull the pinna and otoscope horizontally to bring the horizontal ear canal and tympanic membrane into view.
- Examine both the horizontal and vertical canals for masses, foreign bodies, discharges, and para-

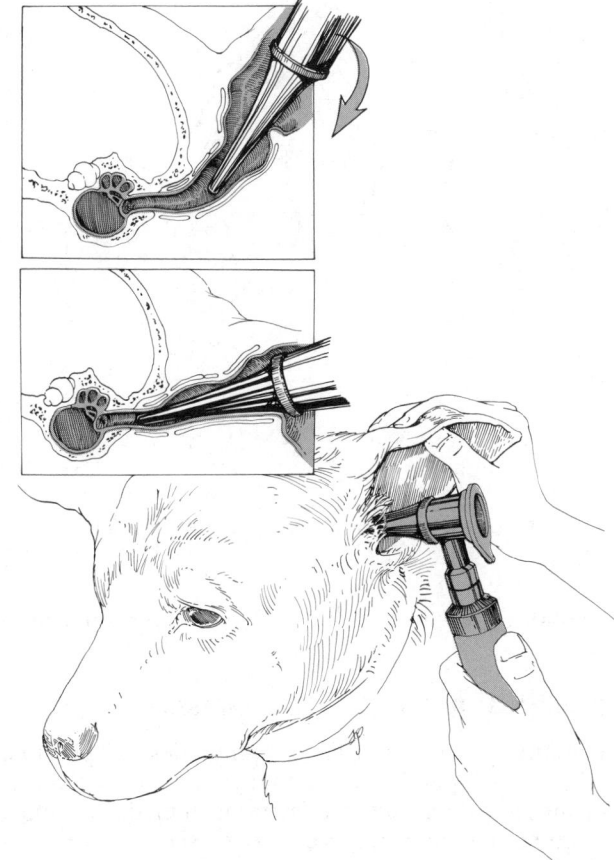

Figure 2. Otoscopic examination.

sites (ear mites and ticks). Assess the tympanic membrane for rupture or evidence of otitis media (erythema or protrusion).

See sec. 5, chs. 21 and 22.

Neck

■ Palpate the paratracheal area from the larynx to the thoracic inlet.
- In middle-aged to older cats, this palpation is especially important because of the increased incidence of hyperthyroidism. Place the thumb and forefinger on either side of the trachea and slide them down the length of the trachea to detect a thyroid nodule (Fig. 3). The normal thyroid is not palpable.
- In dogs, palpation may detect thyroid carcinoma.
■ Palpate the trachea for collapse, soft cartilage, or flattening.
■ Attempt to elicit a cough by gently encircling the trachea with one hand and applying pressure on the tracheal muscle dorsally. If a cough is produced by this method, it suggests tracheal collapse or tracheobronchitis. Conduct this part of the examination after the thorax has been auscultated because it may induce paroxysms of coughing.
■ Evaluate the jugular veins for distension or a jugular pulse extending more than one third the way up the neck. It may be necessary to moisten this area with

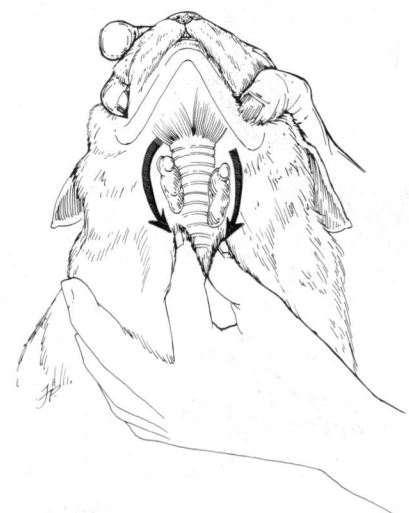

Figure 3. Paratracheal palpation of the thyroid.

alcohol or to clip the hair to detect these abnormalities.

Lymph Nodes and Subcutaneous Masses

■ Palpate all the external lymph nodes, if possible (Fig. 4). Generalized lymphadenopathy usually indicates a systemic disease (systemic fungal infections, immune-mediated diseases, neoplasia), whereas local lymph node enlargement usually indicates a regional infection (abscess).
- The mandibular lymph nodes are located at the angle of the mandible. These are slightly cranial and ventral to the parotid and submaxillary salivary glands. The nodes are generally smooth and ovoid in contrast to the irregular texture of the salivary glands. Practice may be necessary to distinguish these lymph nodes from salivary glands.
- The superficial cervical or prescapular lymph nodes can usually be palpated just in front of the cranial

border of the scapula. These lymph nodes may be grasped by palpating beneath the scapular border. They may be more difficult to palpate in the obese or heavily muscled patient.
- The axillary lymph nodes are not always palpable because of their disc-like shape and surrounding musculature.
- The superficial inguinal lymph nodes are located at the junction of the abdominal wall and the medial thigh and may be difficult to palpate in the obese patient.
- The popliteal lymph nodes are usually palpable caudal to the stifle joint. The surrounding subcutaneous fat may make these nodes seem larger than their actual size, especially those in cats.

■ Palpate the trunk and extremities for abnormal masses or swelling. When a mass is found, note the location, size, and consistency. Determine which tissues are involved (dermal-epidermal, subcutaneous, underlying tissue). Note whether the mass is freely movable or attached to the underlying muscle, fascia, or bone.

Skin

■ Inspect the general appearance of the haircoat for luster and fullness and areas of hair loss. Note a symmetric alopecic pattern as seen with endocrinopathy. Inspect areas of alopecia for the remains of broken hairs as seen with pruritic or psychogenic conditions. Note the presence of erythema.

■ When approaching a pet with a dermatologic problem, examine all areas of the body. Location of skin lesions often aid in the diagnosis. For example, localized demodicosis is typified by alopecic patches involving the head and forelegs. Sarcoptic mange is typically represented by scaling and partial alopecia of the pinnae, elbows, and hocks. Do not overlook the interdigital areas and the foot pads. Examine mucocutaneous junctions (lips, anus, vulva, prepuce,

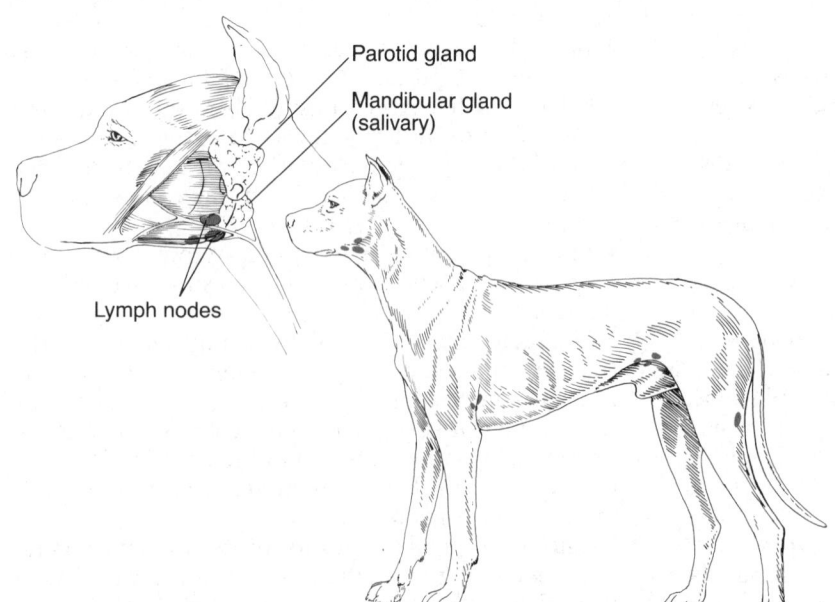

Parotid gland

Mandibular gland (salivary)

Lymph nodes

Figure 4. Commonly palpated lymph nodes.

and so forth) for evidence of immune-mediated diseases.

■ Identify all skin lesions and categorize them as primary or secondary. Primary lesions include papules, pustules, nodules, wheals, macules, and vesicles. Common secondary lesions are scales, crusts, ulcers, excoriations, lichenifications, hyperpigmentations, and hyperkeratoses.

■ Note any evidence of external parasites. If fleas are not seen, search the patient for flea dirt, especially in the tail head region. A flea comb is often helpful in discovering small amounts of flea dirt.

See sec. 5.

Thorax

■ As previously described, evaluate the respiratory rate, rhythm, and effort.

■ Palpate the thorax for evidence of fractured ribs, congenital malformations (pectus excavatum), subcutaneous emphysema, and masses. Palpate the areas between the fourth and sixth intercostal spaces on either side of the thorax for the point of maximum intensity (PMI) of the heart beat and for cardiac thrills.

■ Auscultation is performed in a quiet room with a calm patient. The patient is standing independently during the examination, so that the heart is in its normal position. Evaluate the heart independently from the lungs.

• Artifactual sounds must be recognized and disregarded. These include rumbles due to shivering and crackles from the stethoscope rubbing against the hair. Close the patient's mouth for short periods of time to reduce the upper respiratory noises.

• Auscultate the heart initially over the PMI and identify the first and second heart sounds. Characterize the cardiac rhythm. Sinus arrhythmias are typified by increases in cardiac rate during inspiration and decreases during expiration. Evaluate

the femoral pulses for quality and deficits while auscultating heart. Note split heart sounds, murmurs, and clicks. Auscultate all cardiac valve areas, because some murmurs are localized, such as the mitral, aortic, and pulmonic on the left hemithorax and the tricuspid on the right (Fig. 5).

• Note muffled heart sounds that may be due to obesity, pleural effusion, pericardial effusion, thoracic mass, or diaphragmatic hernia.

• Pulmonary auscultation requires practice and persistence. Normal bronchovesicular sounds may be intensified in the nervous or tachypneic patient. These sounds are heard equally on both sides of the chest. Abnormally quiet or dull areas are suggestive of pleural effusion, pneumothorax, thoracic mass, and pulmonary consolidation. Crackles or rales are produced by air passage through partially obstructed bronchi because of the accumulation of fluid or mucus or the thickening of the bronchial wall.

■ Percussion is a technique for evaluating the resonance (pitch and tone) of sound produced by a series of quick taps of uniform force at various points on the chest wall using a finger or a percussion hammer. Increased resonance (tympany) is indicative of pneumothorax, and decreased resonance (dull sounding) suggests pleural effusion, diaphragmatic hernia, large pulmonary mass, or area of consolidation.

See sec. 6.

Abdomen

■ Examine the external appearance of the abdomen for distension or asymmetry. If distension appears, perform percussion to determine if it is a result of peritoneal effusion, air (gastric dilatation or volvulus), obesity, or a mass.

■ Palpate the abdomen systematically proceeding in a cranial-to-caudal direction so that nothing is overlooked (Fig. 6). For small animals, use a one-handed

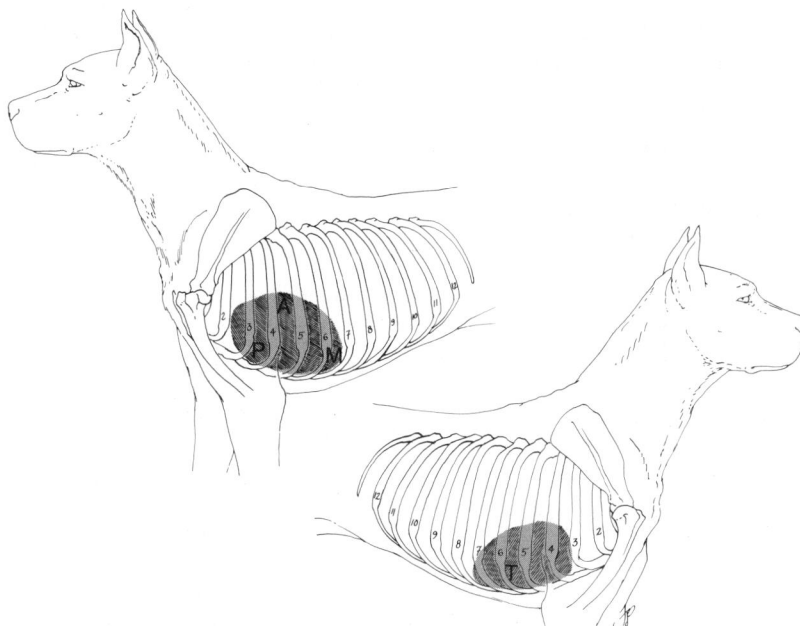

Figure 5. Location of pulmonary (P), aortic (A), mitral (M), and tricuspid (T) valves of the canine heart.

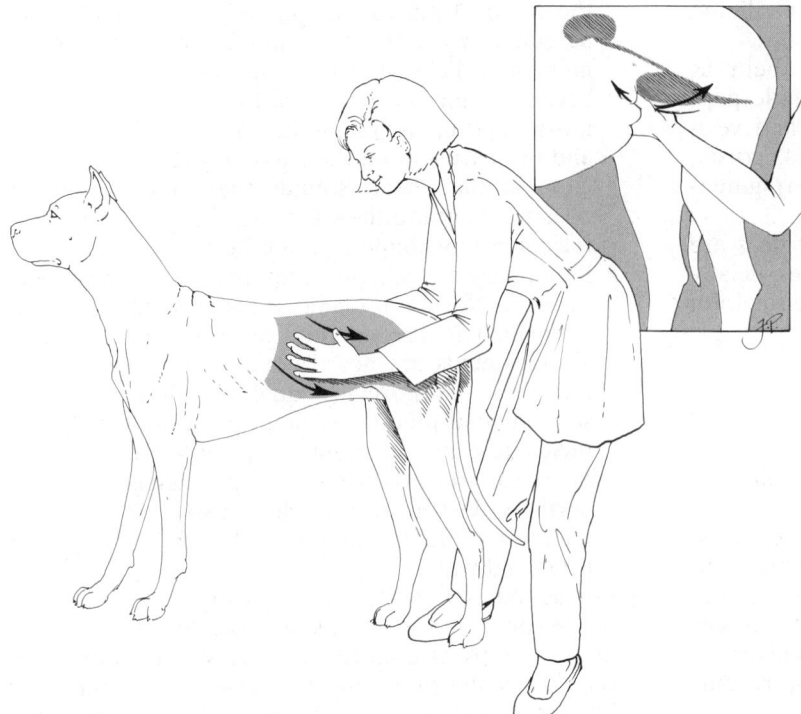

Figure 6. Abdominal palpation can be performed with two hands or with one hand (inset).

technique. With larger patients, two hands are needed, one on either side of the abdomen. In either case, the patient is standing. Gentle, but steady, pressure yields the best results.

■ Palpate the cranial abdomen for evidence of gastric distension (see also sec. 7, ch. 5). The normal stomach is rarely palpable. Tympany indicates the presence of gastric dilatation or volvulus and is pursued aggressively. Overeating may result in a doughy or fluid-filled stomach in the left middle region of the cranial abdomen.

■ The liver may be difficult to palpate in the normal patient (see also sec. 7, ch. 8). The caudal edges are barely palpable, smooth, and well-defined. Hepatomegaly results in a liver that extends past the costal arch. The edges may be rounded, rather than sharp. Palpation with the animal in lateral recumbency or standing on the hind legs may be helpful.

■ The spleen is located in the midabdomen and may not always be palpable (see also sec. 3, ch. 4). If splenomegaly is present, it is usually palpable. Determine if the spleen is irregular or if a palpable mass is present.

■ Other organs in the midabdomen include the mesenteric lymph nodes and intestines. The mesenteric lymph nodes are not usually palpable unless markedly enlarged, as with lymphosarcoma.

■ Palpate the thickness of the bowel wall and the presence of gas, fluid, foreign bodies, or masses (see also sec. 7, ch. 6). Plication and clumping of the intestines may be appreciated in the presence of a string foreign body.

■ The kidneys can be palpated in the feline patient in the dorsal region of the abdomen. The right kidney tends to be farther cranial in position than the left and may actually be obscured by the last ribs. Elevate

the cat's thorax with one hand, while palpating with the other. This maneuver allows the kidneys to fall into a palpable position (Fig. 7). Palpate both kidneys and compare them for size, shape, firmness, and surface irregularities. The left kidney is especially movable. Care must be taken not to mistake it for a midabdominal mass. The kidneys are not as readily palpable in the dog. Sometimes, the caudal poles or lateral aspect can be identified. Kidney palpation is also discussed in sec. 8, ch. 1.

■ Palpate the colon in the dorsal-caudal abdomen, and note the presence of feces. If indecision exists as to whether the palpable structure is feces or a mass, apply gentle pressure to test for deformability of the stool. Evaluate quantity and consistency of the feces to aid in the diagnosis of constipation.

Figure 7. Renal palpation in the cat.

- The urinary bladder can usually be palpated in the central caudal abdomen (see also sec. 8, ch. 3). The patient does not usually resist palpation of the normal bladder. Assess size, turgidity, and thickness of the bladder wall. The normal urinary bladder is thin walled. Careful palpation may reveal cystic calculi.
- The normal uterus usually cannot be palpated (see also sec. 8, ch. 14). If it is markedly enlarged, because of pyometra or late pregnancy, the uterus is found in the mid-to-ventral abdomen, often extending from the pelvic inlet to the diaphragm. The uterus often is tubular in shape in the case of pyometra or late pregnancy. In midgestation, the individual fetuses may be palpated.
- The prostate can occasionally be palpated in the caudal abdomen central to the colon and caudal to the urinary bladder (see also sec. 8, ch. 8). If found in this location, evaluate the prostate for size, shape, and surface irregularities.

External Genitalia

- In the female patient, palpate the mammary glands carefully for masses. If the history indicates a possibility of pseudopregnancy, gently express the nipples for signs of discharge or milk. In the nursing bitch or queen, examine the mammary glands for abnormal swelling, firmness, or heat, as seen with abscessed glands.
- In the female patient, examine the vulva for conformational abnormalities, swelling, or discharge. Determine the color, consistency, and odor of the discharge. Examine the vulvar mucous membranes for evidence of jaundice, cyanosis, petechia, or ulceration. In dystocia, a vaginal examination is indicated.
- In the male canine, examine the prepuce and penis. Retract the preputial sheath caudal to the bulb so that the entire penis can be examined for any signs of trauma or masses. Inspect the penis for jaundice, cyanosis, petechia, or ulceration. Examine the tip of the feline penis for evidence of obstruction (discoloration or the presence of "sand"), if so indicated by the history.
- In the male intact patient, palpate both testicles for symmetry, firmness, and irregularity. If both testicles are not present in the scrotum, examine the inguinal region for the presence of a retained testicle and palpate the abdomen for masses.

See sec. 8.

Rectal Examination

- A rectal examination is indicated in all mature intact male dogs to evaluate the prostate. The normal prostate is palpable via a rectal examination, bilobed (characterized by the presence of the median raphe), smooth, and nonpainful. If the prostate is enlarged, it may extend slightly over the brim of the pelvis or fall into the abdomen, as previously described.
- In female dogs, abnormal masses associated with the uterus or urethra may sometimes be detected on rectal palpation.

- During a rectal examination, palpate the sublumbar lymph nodes in the dorsal aspect of the pelvic canal. Enlargement is usually suggestive of metastatic neoplasia.
- Note the symmetry of the pelvis for palpable fractures during the rectal examination. This is always indicated in a trauma victim. Evaluate abnormal masses in the pelvic canal for size, position, and consistency.
- During the rectal examination, observe the perineal region for herniations or abnormal masses.
- Evaluate the anal sacs for evidence of distension or masses.
- Note the consistency of any fecal material and anal tone.

Musculoskeletal System

- Initially evaluate the musculoskeletal system by observing for lameness with the patient in motion. Observe the patient's posture with special attention to the head carriage, arching of the back, or stilted gait.
- A complete musculoskeletal examination in not necessary unless evidence of lameness is noted in the history or the initial observation of the patient.
- If lameness is present, examine the affected limb systematically to attempt to localize the area involved. First, examine the foot for evidence of traumatized or abnormal toenails or nail beds and evaluate each interdigital area for evidence of erythema, swelling, or draining tracts, which may be indicative of a foreign body. Palpate each toe individually and note swelling or pain.
- Palpation proceeds proximally. Evaluate each long bone for pain, swelling, abnormal masses, or palpable fractures.
- Evaluate each joint for evidence of effusion, soft tissue swelling, crepitation, or pain with flexion and extension.
- In examining the stifle, note the position of the patella in extension and flexion. If the patella is in its normal location, attempt to luxate it medially and laterally. Extension of the stifle usually aids in mobilizing the patella. Palpate the stifle for evidence of a cranial drawer sign.
- Evaluate each coxofemoral joint for a positive Ortolani sign, if the patient's breed is at risk for hip dysplasia (see sec. 9, ch. 14 for more details).
- Palpate the vertebral column for signs of a pain response. Pressure applied to either side of the dorsal spinal process of each vertebra may be necessary to elicit pain.

See sec. 9, ch. 5.

Nervous System

- As with the musculoskeletal system, a complete neurologic examination is not necessary unless specifically indicated by the history or the general physical examination. The details of the neurologic examination are discussed in section 10, chapter 1. A brief overview of the basic principles necessary to localize the lesion is addressed here.

- Observe mental status and behavior as previously described.
- Evaluate the gait and posture while the patient is walking and standing. Particular attention is given to strength, symmetry, and coordination.
- Always perform a complete cranial nerve examination when evaluating any neurologic problem (see sec. 10, chs. 1 and 2).
- Evaluate and compare postural reactions in all limbs, including proprioception, "wheelbarrowing," hopping, extensor postural thrust, and placing reaction.
- Evaluate and compare spinal reflexes with the calm patient in lateral recumbency. Important segmental reflexes include the triceps, biceps, patellar, and cranial tibial reflexes, as well as the flexor (withdrawal) reflexes of the thoracic and pelvic limbs. Evaluate the panniculus reflex by pricking the thoracic or lumbar skin.

See sec. 10, ch. 4.

Supplemental Readings

Bistner SI, Shaw D: Examination of the eye. Vet Clin North Am [Small Anim Pract] 11:595–622, 1981.

Crow SE, Walshaw SO: Restraint of dogs and cats. *In* Crow SE, Walshaw SO, eds.: *Manual of Clinical Procedures in the Dog and Cat.* Philadelphia: J.B. Lippincott, 1987, p 3–14.

McCurnin DM, Poffenbarger EM: *Small Animal Physical Diagnosis and Clinical Procedures.* Philadelphia: W.B. Saunders, 1991.

Schaer M: The medical history, physical examination, and physical restraint. *In* Sherding RG, ed.: *The Cat: Diseases and Clinical Management.* New York: Churchill Livingstone, 1989, p 7–22.

2 Practical Methods of Anesthesia

John A. E. Hubbell

Anesthesia is an integral part of the practice of companion animal medicine. In addition to surgical applications, some form of anesthesia may be required for a wide variety of procedures, such as radiography, endoscopy, cerebrospinal fluid collection, and bone marrow aspiration. The keys to successful anesthesia are as follows:

1. An understanding of what is "normal" in the various species.

2. A working knowledge of the pharmacology of anesthetic drugs.

3. A systematic evaluation and re-evaluation of the patient's status (monitoring) during the period of anesthesia.

The understanding of what is "normal" comes with experience. Several excellent texts describe the pharmacology of anesthetic drugs (see Supplemental Readings at the end of this chapter). Monitoring is a matter of establishing a routine and maintaining the discipline to adhere to the routine. This chapter suggests some basic anesthetic techniques and protocols that can be used in small animal practice.

GENERAL PRINCIPLES

Preoperative Assessment (Table 1)

- A history of vomiting or a recent meal is an indication for postponing surgery or using techniques that produce rapid induction to allow rapid endotracheal intubation to minimize the potential for aspiration of gastric contents.
  - On an elective basis, withhold food 6 to 8 hours prior to the administration of anesthetic drugs.
  - Do not withhold water.
  - Potential problems that are discovered from the history include exercise intolerance or cough, as an indicator of cardiorespiratory dysfunction; polyuria or polydipsia, as an indicator of endocrine or renal dysfunction; or any other recent change in the animal's physical status.
- Perform a physical examination with emphasis on the cardiovascular and respiratory systems (Table 2 provides normal values).
  - Evaluate traumatized patients more extensively because of the potential for blood loss, cardiac arrhythmias (ventricular tachycardia), and thoracic trauma (pneumothorax).
  - Evaluate abnormalities discovered after auscultation, percussion, palpation, and examination of mucous membranes with ancillary tests, such as thoracic radiography and electrocardiography.

- The pertinent abnormalities associated with each metabolic disease are discussed with the disease syndrome.
- Weigh the animal. Estimate the lean body weight if the animal is obese in order to more accurately calculate correct anesthetic drug doses.
- Determine a packed cell volume and total plasma protein level to establish a baseline for reference if hemorrhage occurs. Check the renal function with blood urea nitrogen (BUN) or creatinine concentrations in older (>7 years) animals. Increases in BUN or creatinine values may indicate the need for a more careful perianesthetic fluid management to prevent further renal dysfunction (see Table 2).

Intravenous Catheterization

Place an intravenous catheter prior to induction of anesthesia to provide a convenient pathway for the

TABLE 1. Preanesthetic Checklist

History and Physical Examination
Age
Body weight
Temperature
Auscultation
Respiratory rate
Pulse rate, rhythm, and strength
Hydration, mucous membrane color, and capillary refill time
Mentation
Current medication history
Cardiopulmonary, renal, and nervous system disease history

Laboratory Data
Packed cell volume
Total plasma protein
Blood urea nitrogen, creatinine, or Azostick if > 7 years
Other tests optional dependent on primary disease

Drugs
Appropriate anesthetic drugs
Sufficient oxygen supply
Emergency drugs
   Atropine or glycopyrrolate
   Lidocaine
   Epinephrine
   Sodium bicarbonate
   Intravenous fluids
   Dopamine
   Doxapram

Equipment
Syringes, needles, and catheters
Leak-tested anesthetic machine
Cuffed endotracheal tubes
Optional monitoring equipment
   Electrocardiogram
   Blood pressure monitor (pulse detector)
   Stethoscope

TABLE 2. Normal Values

	Dogs		Cats	
	Awake	**Anesthetized (if different)**	**Awake**	**Anesthetized (if different)**
Temperature (degrees F)	99.5–102.5		100–102.5	
Heart rate (beats/min)	70–180	60–180	145–200	100–200
Respiratory rate (breaths/minute)	20–40	8–20	20–40	10–30
Capillary refill time (seconds)	<1.5		<1.5	
Packed cell volume (%)	35–54		27–46	
Total plasma protein (gm/100 ml)	5.7–7.3		6.3–8.3	
Total leukocytes (6,000–17,000/μl)	6–18		6–20	
Albumin (gm/100 ml)	2.1–3.6		2.3–3.6	
Sodium (mEq/L)	140–155		149–162	
Potassium (mEq/L)	3.8–5.3		3.6–5.4	
Chloride (mEq/L)	105–121		105–135	
Calcium (mg/100 ml)	8.8–11.3		8.3–11.3	
Creatinine (mg/100 ml)	0.3–1.3		0.8–1.8	
Blood urea nitrogen (mg/100 ml)	8–25		15–35	
Arterial pH	7.30–7.43		7.27–7.40	
Arterial pCO_2 (mm Hg)	30–49		35–49	
Arterial pO_2 (mm Hg)	91–97	90–500 (> 50% inspired O_2)	91–97	100–500 (> 50% inspired O_2)
Arterial HCO_3 (mEq/L)	18–22		18–25	
Arterial base excess (mEq/L)	−3–+3		−6–+1.5	
CO_2 combining power (mEq/L)	15–25		16–30	

administration of the drugs, to allow for fluid or blood administration if required, and to ensure access to the vascular space if an emergency occurs.

Endotracheal Intubation

A patent airway is essential to any anesthetic protocol.

■ Place a cuffed endotracheal tube in the trachea soon after induction of anesthesia for optimal protection.
■ Alternatively, use drugs that maintain the swallowing reflex (ketamine, tiletamine-zolazepam).
■ Clean, thoroughly rinse, and dry endotracheal tubes between uses. Sterilization of endotracheal tubes between uses is not necessary on a routine basis. Use chemical sterilization if a known pathogen is present. Glutaraldehyde is a safe disinfectant if the tubes are thoroughly rinsed following sterilization.
■ See Table 3 for the range of sizes of endotracheal tubes for dogs and cats.

PRODUCING A TRACTABLE ANIMAL

Many procedures, such as radiography and cystocentesis, do not require complete anesthesia. In these instances, the combination of appropriate sedation and

TABLE 3. Approximate Endotracheal Tube Sizes

	Weight (kg)	Cuffed Tube Diameter (mm)
Dogs	3–7	3.0–5.0
	7–15	5.0–7.5
	15–30	7.5–9.5
	> 30	9.5–12.0
Cats		2.5–4.0

physical restraint can facilitate the completion of the procedure with minimal stress to the patient and minimal drug-induced cardiopulmonary depression. The choice of drugs is based on species, the patient's temperament, physical status, the veterinarian's familiarity with the drug, and the intended purpose. The agents that follow are employed as components of many anesthetic protocols.

The doses of drugs alone and in combination are listed in Table 4 (dogs) and Table 5 (cats).

Tranquilizers

■ Acepromazine
  • A potent phenothiazine tranquilizer that produces sedation in the dog. It also has antiemetic and antiarrhythmic properties.
  • Not an analgesic itself, but it may potentiate other drugs that are analgesics.
  • Produces hypotension through alpha-adrenergic blockade, particularly in large doses.
  • Potentiates hypothermia.
  • Epinephrine reversal (i.e., hypotension after epinephrine administration) can occur.
  • Calms excitable dogs. Aggressive dogs or cats may not become tractable. Combine with opioids or cyclohexamines to produce the desired effect (see Tables 4 and 5).
  • Avoid in animals with epilepsy, shock, bleeding disorders (inhibition of platelet function), or liver disease.
  • Reduce the dose or choose another agent in stressed or older animals because effects may be exaggerated. Cats are calmed but usually still resist restraint.
■ Xylazine
  • An alpha$_2$-adrenergic agonist that produces sedation with muscle relaxation and analgesia.

TABLE 4. Anesthetic Drugs and Doses in Dogs

Drug	Intravenous Dose (mg/kg)	Intramuscular or Subcutaneous Dose (mg/kg)
Anticholinergics		
Atropine	0.02–0.04	0.02–0.04
Glycopyrrolate	0.005–0.01	0.005–0.01
Tranquilizer/Sedatives		
Acepromazine	0.05–0.2	0.1–0.3
Xylazine	0.4–1.0	1.0–2.0
Diazepam	0.1–0.25	0.1–0.25
Midazolam	0.05–0.2	0.1–0.2
Analgesics		
Morphine	NR*	0.2–0.5
Oxymorphone	0.01–0.04	0.1–0.3
Fentanyl	0.002–0.005	0.004–0.008
Meperidine	0.4–2.0	1.0–4.0
Fentanyl/droperidol (Innovar-Vet)	1 ml/20–30 kg	1 ml/10 kg
Butorphanol	0.1–0.2	0.1–0.4
Nalbuphine	0.5–2.0	0.5–2.0
Buprenorphine	0.005	0.005
Anesthetics		
Tiletamine/zolazepam (Telazol)	0.5–4.0	4–10
Thiamylal	6–10	NR
Thiopental	6–10	NR
Etomidate	1.0–4.0	NR
Propofol	4–8	NR
Combinations		
Acepromazine/oxymorphone	0.05–0.1/0.01–0.02	0.1–0.2/0.1–0.2
Acepromazine/butorphanol	0.05–0.1/0.1–0.2	0.1–0.2/0.1–0.2
Acepromazine/ketamine	0.05–0.1/2.0–5.0	0.1–0.2/5–10
Xylazine/ketamine	0.1–0.8/1.0–5.0	0.3–1.5/5–10
Diazepam/ketamine (50:50)	1 ml/10 kg	NR

*NR, not recommended.

TABLE 5. Anesthetic Drugs and Doses in Cats

Drug	Intravenous Dose (mg/kg)	Intramuscular or Subcutaneous Dose (mg/kg)
Anticholinergics		
Atropine	0.02–0.04	0.02–0.04
Glycopyrrolate	0.005–0.01	0.005–0.01
Tranquilizer/Sedatives		
Acepromazine	0.05–0.2	0.1–0.3
Xylazine	0.4–1.0	0.8–1.8
Diazepam	0.1–0.25	0.1–0.25
Midazolam	0.05–0.2	0.1–0.2
Analgesics*		
Oxymorphone	0.01–0.04	0.05–0.1
Butorphanol	0.05–0.2	0.1–0.3
Nalbuphine	0.5–1.5	0.5–1.5
Buprenorphine	0.005	0.005
Anesthetics		
Ketamine	4–10	10–20
Tiletamine/zolazepam (Telazol)	0.5–4.0	4–12
Thiamylal	6–10	NR†
Thiopental	6–10	NR
Etomidate	1.0–4.0	NR
Propofol	4–8	
Combinations		
Acepromazine/oxymorphone	0.05–0.07/0.05–0.08	0.1–0.2/0.05–0.8
Acepromazine/butorphanol	0.05–0.07/0.07–0.15	0.1–0.2/0.1–0.2
Acepromazine/ketamine	0.05–0.1/4.0–8.0	0.1–0.2/7–15
Xylazine/ketamine	0.1–0.8/4.0–8.0	0.3–1.5/7–15
Diazepam/ketamine (50:50)	1 ml/10 kg	NR

*Higher doses can be associated with nervousness and excitement.
†NR, not recommended.

- Produces an obtunded state from which the patient is difficult to arouse.
- Produces analgesia for minor procedures. Is not usually sufficient for surgery.
- Produces profound cardiopulmonary depression, including bradycardia, first- and second-degree atrioventricular blockade, catecholamine sensitization, and decreased respiratory rate.
- Combine with an anticholinergic (atropine or glycopyrrolate).
- Do not use in patients with pre-existing cardiac, liver, or kidney disease, or with shock.
- Reverse effects with yohimbine or tolazoline.
- Vomiting occurs in approximately 25% of dogs and 50% of cats.
- See Tables 4 and 5 for doses.
- ■ Diazepam and midazolam
  - Benzodiazepine derivatives that produce mild sedation in dogs and cats. Neither is effective in calming an excited patient when used alone. Both are anticonvulsants.
  - Use to enhance tractability in depressed patients or in combination with other agents (primarily opioids).
  - Administer diazepam intramuscularly or slowly, intravenously with caution. The drug is solubilized in a propylene glycol base that can produce bradycardia and hypotension.
  - Administer water-soluble midazolam via IV, SC, or IM route.
  - Use in patients with cardiorespiratory compromise or other metabolic disease. Both agents produce minimal cardiopulmonary side effects and provide muscle relaxation.
  - Use both drugs as premedicants to parenteral or inhalation anesthesia.
  - Occasionally, paradoxical responses, including disorientation and aggression, occur.
  - Diazepam can be given as an appetite stimulant in cats.
  - See Tables 4 and 5 for doses and suggested combinations.

Analgesic Drugs

- ■ Opioids
  - Use in dogs and cats to augment the effects of sedatives and tranquilizers and to provide analgesia.
  - Minimal or no sedation produced when administered alone, except for morphine and meperidine. Use in combination with tranquilizers or sedatives.
  - Use lower doses in cats compared with dogs (Tables 4 and 5), because higher doses have the potential to cause excitement and disorientation.
  - Morphine, oxymorphone, fentanyl, and meperidine are opioid agonist drugs frequently used in small animal practice. Fentanyl in combination with droperidol (Innovar-Vet, Pitman-Moore) is a proprietary combination that is widely used in the dog, particularly in aggressive animals. Regulations require rigorous record keeping and security.
  - Butorphanol, nalbuphine, and buprenorphine are opioid agonist/antagonist or partial agonist drugs.

This classification means that these compounds produce analgesia but have less addictive potential.
- Vagal tone is increased (bradycardia), and respiration is depressed.
- Sensations of touch or vision are not diminished. Sensitivity to sound may be increased.
- May cause vomiting and defecation.
- Reverse agonists and agonist/antagonists with naloxone. Partial reversal of the respiratory and central nervous system depressant effects of agonists can be accomplished with agonist/antagonists. Reported to reverse the deleterious effects of the agonists, while providing the animal with some analgesia.

Dissociative Anesthetics

- ■ Ketamine and tiletamine/zolazepam
  - Ketamine and tiletamine/zolazepam (Telazol, A.H. Robbins) produce a unique form of sedation/anesthesia that has been called dissociative anesthesia.
  - Both maintain swallowing and ocular reflexes, increase muscle tone, and produce amnesia, superficial analgesia, and catatonia.
  - Both stimulate the cardiovascular system resulting in increases in heart rate and arterial blood pressure.
  - Both produce an apneustic (breath-holding) respiratory pattern. The intensity is dose related.
  - Use low doses of ketamine (up to 6 mg/kg, IM) in the cat to produce an obtunded state with malleable rigidity of the limbs, dilated pupils, and hypersalivation. Use higher doses (14 to 20 mg/kg, IM) to intensify the effect so that surgery can be performed.
  - Use Telazol to produce a state similar to that of ketamine with the addition of muscle relaxation. Approved for IM use in both the dog and the cat. Provides helpful restraint in both the dog and cat at low doses (2 to 4 mg/kg, IM). Higher doses can produce a state resembling general anesthesia but are associated with prolonged recoveries that can be stormy, particularly in the dog.
  - Use ketamine in combination with other agents (acepromazine, diazepam, xylazine) in both the dog and the cat. Do not give ketamine alone in the dog, because of the drug's ability to produce muscle rigidity and seizure activity. See Tables 4 and 5 for doses.

INJECTABLE DRUGS FOR SHORT-TERM ANESTHESIA

A variety of injectable drugs and drug combinations can be utilized for short-term anesthesia or restraint (Tables 6 and 7). Many of these combinations employ the drugs previously described, because the prior or coadministration of sedatives or tranquilizers with drugs that produce anesthesia allows a reduction in the dose of the anesthetic drug. Anesthetic drugs tend to produce more depression of cardiopulmonary function than do sedatives or tranquilizers, thus the patient

TABLE 6. Suggested Anesthetic Protocols for Dogs

Patient Agent	Dose	Comments
Healthy (Elective Procedure)		
Acepromazine	0.02 mg/kg, SQ or IM	Total dose not to exceed 4 mg
Thiamylal	6–10 mg/kg, IV	Give 6 mg/kg initially, increase in 2 mg/kg increments
Halothane* (or)	0.5–3.5%, inhaled	Adjust to anesthetic depth
Methoxyflurane*	0.3–3%, inhaled	Adjust to anesthetic depth
Aged Patient		
Intravenous fluids		
Diazepam/ketamine	1 ml/10 kg (50:50 v/v mixture, IV)	Short duration of action
Halothane* (or)	0.5–3.5%, inhaled	
Methoxyflurane* (or)	0.3–3%, inhaled	
Isoflurane*	0.5–3.5%, inhaled	
Patient in Pain		
Acepromazine	0.01–0.02 mg/kg, IM	Can be mixed with oxymorphone
Oxymorphone	0.05–0.02 mg/kg, IM	Watch for bradycardia
Intravenous fluids		
Thiamylal	4–8 mg/kg, IV	Dose is reduced after premedicant Start with 4 mg/kg
Halothane* (or)	0.5–3.5%, inhaled	
Methoxyflurane* (or)	0.3–3%, inhaled	
Isoflurane*	0.5–3.5%, inhaled	
Critical Patient		
Diazepam and	0.02 mg/kg, IV	Give slowly
Thiamylal (or)	2.0–6.0 mg/kg, IV	Give to effect
Diazepam/ketamine	1 ml/10 kg (50:50 v/v mix)	
Halothane* (or)	0.5–3.5%, inhaled	
Isoflurane*	0.5–3.5%, inhaled	

*Concentration required is dependent on fresh gas flow rate. The lower the flow rate, the higher the concentration required.

TABLE 7. Suggested Anesthetic Protocols for Cats

Patient Agent	Dose	Comments
Healthy (Elective Procedure)		
Acepromazine (with)	0.01–0.02 mg/kg, SQ or SC, IM	Mix acepromazine with ketamine
Ketamine (and)	4–8 mg/kg, IM	
Thiamylal (or)	5–10 mg/kg, IV	Give to effect
Tiletamine/zolazepam (with)	3–5 mg/kg, IM	Tiletamine/zolazepam may be sufficient for intubation
Thiamylal	3–7 mg/kg, IV	
Halothane* (or)	0.5–3.5%, inhaled	
Methoxyflurane*	0.3–3.5%, inhaled	
Aged or Renally Compromised Patient		
Midazolam (with)	0.1–0.2 mg/kg, IM	Drugs can be mixed
Oxymorphone		
Intravenous fluids	0.05 mg/kg, IM	
Ketamine (or)	1–2 mg/kg, IV	
Thiamylal	3–7 mg/kg, IV	
Halothane* (or)	0.5–3.5%, inhaled	
Isoflurane*	0.5–3.5%, inhaled	
Critical Patient		
Intravenous fluids		
Diazepam/ketamine	0.5 ml/5 kg of a 50:50 mixture, IV	Administer slowly
Halothane* (or)	0.5–3.0%, inhaled	
Isoflurane*	0.5–3.5%, inhaled	

*Use a nonrebreathing anesthetic system (Bain or Ayres T-piece)

benefits from the decreased dose. Thiobarbiturates are the primary addition to the list of drugs already discussed. Newer drugs, such as etomidate and propofol, offer potential advantages, such as less cardiopulmonary effects and lack of cumulative effects, but are expensive. Although endotracheal intubation is not required for the delivery of injectable anesthetic drugs, patients can benefit from intubation for protection of the airway and for oxygen supplementation.

Thiobarbiturates (Thiamylal and Thiopental)

- Sedative/hypnotic agents that produce short-term intravenous anesthesia.
- Barbiturates produce central nervous system depression that ranges from drowsiness to coma.
- Not good analgesics at subhypnotic doses. When doses are increased to produce unconsciousness, anesthesia is produced.
- Cause respiratory depression and some arterial blood pressure depression.
- Sensitize the heart to catecholamine-induced arrhythmias. Ventricular bigeminy is noted but resolves without treatment.
- Duration of effect primarily determined by redistribution away from the brain into muscle and lean body tissues. Level and duration of anesthesia produced by a given dose is dependent upon what other drugs have been administered, the rate administered, and the level of awareness of the animal at the time administered.
- Use with caution in patients with pre-existing cardiovascular disease, hypotension, or shock.
- Administer to effect, beginning with doses in the range of 4 to 6 mg/kg, increasing in 2 mg/kg increments. Onset of action is within 30 seconds.
- Do not mix with other drugs because of extreme alkalinity. Can cause sloughing of tissues if administered perivascularly.
- Use for induction to inhalation anesthesia. Compatible with all of the agents previously described. Reduce the dose by approximately half if sedatives/tranquilizers are given prior to administration.
- Duration of action is prolonged by hypoproteinemia and acidosis. Shorten duration by promoting diuresis—administer IV fluids—and by alkalinizing the urine—administer sodium bicarbonate, 2 mEq/kg.

Ketamine

- Use in combination with sedatives and tranquilizers to provide short-term injectable anesthesia.
- Administer ketamine with diazepam in a 50:50 volume/volume mixture intravenously, at a dose of 1 ml/10 kg. Given for brief periods (5 to 10 minutes) of restraint. Provides enough analgesia for minor surgical procedures. Readminister as needed to effect. Works well in depressed or geriatric patients. May not be effective in young, excited, or aggressive animals. Produces moderate muscle relaxation, cardiopulmonary support, and increased salivation. Ocular and swallowing reflexes are maintained, but orotracheal intubation can be accomplished.
- Use ketamine with acepromazine to produce a quie-

ter recovery than that with ketamine with diazepam but with less muscle relaxation. Usually produces enough anesthesia for minor surgery but visceral analgesia is not prominent.
- Use ketamine with xylazine to produce muscle relaxation, sedation, and analgesia that are improved over other combinations. Bradycardia and depression of cardiac contractility and respiration occur. Coadminister an anticholinergic. Use in young animals with good cardiopulmonary reserve. Avoid in animals with pre-existing cardiovascular disease, particularly those with cardiac conduction abnormalities.

Tiletamine/Zolazepam

- Use intravenously or intramuscularly to produce anesthesia.
- Produces muscle relaxation and support of hemodynamics but also produces respiratory depression.
- Maintains oropharyngeal reflexes. Recovery is prolonged with increasing doses. Recovery is usually uneventful in the cat but may be stormy in the dog.
- Administer low doses of acepromazine to quiet the difficult recovery.

Etomidate

- A nonbarbiturate hypnotic that can be utilized for short-term IV anesthesia.
- Produces a hypnotic state with little cardiovascular effect.
- Etomidate is expensive. Limit to patients with significant cardiovascular and respiratory disease.
- Recovery can be stormy, with vomiting and muscle tremors. Premedicate the animal with sedatives or tranquilizers to minimize these effects.

Propofol

- A phenolic compound that produces hypnosis. Currently, this drug is undergoing clinical trials.
- Depresses hemodynamics comparable to thiobarbiturates.
- Depresses respiration and commonly causes a short period of apnea.
- Noncumulative, so that recovery following multiple doses occurs within the same time frame as that following a single dose.
- Relatively insoluble. Formulated in a mixture of soybean oil, egg phosphatide, and glycerol.

Anticholinergics

- Used to reduce salivation, block vagal inhibition of the heart, and quiet the digestive tract if indicated.
- Not innocuous. Respiratory dead space is increased (bronchodilation). Ventricular arrhythmias are more likely to occur.
- Use if bradycardia occurs or is likely to occur.
- Not routinely indicated in anesthesia. Myocardial oxygen consumption is increased owing to tachycardia. Secretions become more viscous.
- Glycopyrrolate is more potent and has a longer duration of action than atropine. Does not cross the placental or blood-brain barrier.

■ Give intramuscularly, subcutaneously, or intravenously when expediency is important. Atropine dose is 0.02 to 0.04 mg/kg. Glycopyrrolate dose is 0.01 mg/kg.

ANESTHESIA FOR MAJOR PROCEDURES

Anesthesia for major procedures, requiring optimal hypnosis, analgesia, and muscle relaxation for relatively long periods, usually incorporates the inhalant anesthetics. Although inhalant drugs can be given as the sole source of anesthesia, injectable drugs are usually given to facilitate induction and endotracheal intubation. The injectable drugs and drug combinations previously described, with the possible exception of xylazine-ketamine combinations, can be utilized to induce anesthesia. Xylazine-ketamine combinations produce significant cardiopulmonary depression that can be extreme when inhalant anesthetic drugs are added.

Inhalant Anesthetics

■ Inhalant anesthetics have several advantages including the coadministration of oxygen, the ease with which anesthesia depth is changed, and the fact that recovery is not dependent upon metabolism. The agents are primarily eliminated by exhalation. Administer via breathing circuits, with circle anesthetic systems being the most common.
■ Circle anesthetic systems
  • A carbon dioxide absorber removes carbon dioxide from the exhaled gas.
  • Exhaled gas is rebreathed, making the system an economic one.
  • Use 3 to 6 ml/kg/minute as the minimum fresh gas flow rate for oxygen. This rate matches the animal's metabolic need for oxygen. Increase the fresh gas flow rate for oxygen to 10 to 20 ml/kg/minute, if nitrous oxide is given. Add the nitrous oxide flow to this. The pop-off valve in the circle system needs to be open to vent the excess gas at this flow rate.
■ Nonrebreathing anesthetic systems (Bain and Ayres T-piece)
  • Use for patients less than 5 to 7 kg, because less resistance to respiration is produced.
  • Use a fresh gas flow of 1.5 times the minute ventilation (approximately 150 ml/kg/minute). Fresh gas flow rates are higher because the fresh gas removes carbon dioxide from the system.
■ Scavenging equipment
  • Use of inhalation anesthetics mandates the removal of expired and waste gases from the operating room environment.
  • Exhaust waste gases via suction systems or vent them to the outside via a hole in an exterior wall.
  • Directing gases to the floor is insufficient.
  • Use activated charcoal canisters as alternatives to absorb halogenated compounds. Not effective for nitrous oxide.

■ Methoxyflurane
  • Once the most commonly used agent in small animal practice.
  • Most potent of the inhalation agents and least volatile.
  • Induction and recovery can be prolonged owing to high blood solubility.
  • Best muscle relaxant of the commonly used inhalation agents.
  • Produces dose-dependent respiratory and cardiovascular depression.
  • Administered using vaporizer in-the-circle or vaporizer out-of-the-circle apparatuses.
  • Maximum attainable concentration at room temperature is approximately 3%.
  • Relatively inexpensive.
  • Use for long procedures in which muscle relaxation is important (orthopedics).
  • Highly metabolized but the clinical relevance of this quality is questionable.
  • Administer at concentrations of 3% for induction followed by maintenance at 0.3 to 1.5%.
  • No longer used in human beings because it is associated with postanesthetic renal failure. This has not been a problem in normal animals, however. Avoid, if possible, in animals with renal disease or those receiving nephrotoxic drugs.
■ Halothane
  • A halogenated hydrocarbon that produces anesthesia when administered at concentrations of 0.5 to 3%, depending on the fresh gas flow rate.
  • Induction and recovery are more rapid than those with methoxyflurane. Can be used for mask or chamber induction of anesthesia.
  • Use precision vaporizers in out-of-the-circle configuration. Can be administered using wickless in-the-circle vaporizers.
  • Maximum attainable concentration at room temperature is approximately 30%.
  • Produces dose-dependent cardiopulmonary depression with moderate degrees of muscle relaxation. Adequate ventilation is usually maintained. Potentiates ventricular arrhythmias in susceptible patients. Cardiac contractility and cardiac output are depressed.
  • Termination of clinical effects is primarily due to redistribution and exhalation of the gas, which is metabolized by the liver.
  • Incriminated in a syndrome characterized by hepatic failure in human beings. Not shown to occur in animals.
■ Isoflurane
  • Halogenated ether that produces anesthesia when inhaled in concentrations of 1.0 to 3.0%.
  • Produces very rapid induction and recovery; relatively insoluble in blood.
  • Vapor pressure similar to that of halothane.
  • Use in precision out-of-the-circle vaporizers. Can be employed in wickless in-the-circle vaporizers.
  • Better maintenance of cardiac output but produces respiratory depression similar to that for halothane. Arterial blood pressure is usually more

depressed than that with halothane. Ventricular arrhythmias are not enhanced.
- Use in patients with metabolic disease, in geriatric patients, and in patients prone to cardiac arrhythmias. Expensive but provides significant advantages.
- Is minimally metabolized (<1%).
■ Nitrous oxide
- A nonirritant gas that produces some analgesia when inhaled in concentrations of 50 to 70%.
- Cannot produce anesthesia when administered alone. Can reduce the required concentration of the other, more potent, gases (halothane, isoflurane) by approximately a third when coadministered.
- Coadministration speeds the uptake of the second gas and thus speeds the induction to anesthesia.
- Recovery can be complicated by diffusion hypoxia. Oxygen should be supplemented for 3 to 5 minutes after cessation of nitrous oxide administration.
- Total fresh gas flow rate must be increased if nitrous oxide is given.
- Not employed widely in veterinary practice because of its limited potency and potential problems with hypoxia.

KEY POINT ▶ Do not use in patients with pneumothorax, gastric torsion, or intestinal obstruction because it will diffuse into closed gas spaces and enlarge them.

MONITORING THE ANESTHETIZED PATIENT

Monitoring is the cornerstone of safe anesthetic practice. Because irreversible central nervous system changes can occur within 4 to 5 minutes of cardiac arrest, a convenient monitoring interval of 5 minutes seems appropriate. The skills needed in basic monitoring of anesthetized patients parallel those needed in performing a physical examination.

Anesthetic Record

■ Prompts the anesthetist to evaluate the patient at regular intervals. Serves as a legal document.
■ Contains the following information, at minimum:
- Summary of preoperative physical examination
- Purpose of anesthesia
- Drugs administered including dose, route, and time
- Regular recording of heart or pulse rate and respiratory rate.

Heart Rate

■ Measured by auscultation using an esophageal (Mallinckrodt) or precordial stethoscope.
■ Palpate a peripheral pulse to determine heart rate and provide additional subjective information concerning the strength of cardiac contraction. Feel the pulse on the ventral side of the tongue (lingual pulse). Alternatively, use the femoral pulse if the animal's head is covered.

■ Administer anticholinergics (atropine or glycopyrrolate) if the heart rate falls to less than 60 beats per minute in dogs and 90 beats per minute in cats.
■ Evaluate the patient for hypotension or anesthetic plane that is too light, if the heart rate is greater than 150 in dogs or 180 in cats.
■ Evaluate patients with irregular heart beats or heart beats of variable intensity with an electrocardiogram for abnormal cardiac rhythms.

Respiratory Rate

■ Measure respiratory rate by watching the movements of the chest wall or the rebreathing bag of the anesthetic machine.
- Most anesthetics are respiratory depressants.
- Increases in rate or depth of panting usually indicate a plane of anesthesia that is too light.
- Check the anesthetic depth in patients with irregular respirations. Can be a sign of excessive medullary depression. An apneustic pattern is expected after ketamine or tiletamine administration.

Capillary Refill Time and Mucous Membrane Color

■ Gives further information on homeostasis.
■ Capillary refill time should be less than 1.5 to 2 seconds.
■ May be altered by the anesthetic agent chosen.

Other Monitors

■ Assess jaw tone to determine the degree of muscle relaxation present. This is an index of anesthetic depth.
- Gently push the jaws apart, and note the resistance to movement.
- Halothane produces less muscle relaxation in an equivalent degree of anesthesia compared with other agents.
- Dissociative agents do not produce muscle relaxation.
■ Pinch a toe and look for a withdrawal response to check the depth of anesthesia prior to incision.

Monitoring Equipment

A wide variety of instruments are available to aid in monitoring patients.

■ Stethoscopes
- Use esophageal stethoscopes (Mallinckrodt) to hear heart and respiratory sounds. Amplified stethoscopes are also available.
■ Electrocardiograms (ECGs)
- Use ECG to measure heart rate and to determine if cardiac arrhythmias are present.
- ECGs do not always ensure that the heart is beating.
■ Blood pressure monitoring
- Use Doppler flow probes (Parks Electronics) to detect peripheral pulses. Place the probe over a peripheral artery. An audible signal is created, as pulses of blood pass under the probe and the

sound waves emitted by the Doppler are altered. Place an occlusive cuff proximal to the Doppler probe to obtain an estimate of systolic arterial blood pressure. This monitor is reliable as a pulse detector but unreliable as an estimator of blood pressure.

- Oscillometric units (Dinamap; Criticon) can record heart rate and estimate systolic, mean, and diastolic blood pressures. The units inflate an occlusive cuff and slowly release pressure. Characteristic pressure fluctuations during deflation are utilized to estimate blood pressures. These monitors are expensive and tend to lose accuracy as blood pressure falls.
- Dorsal pedal artery can be catheterized with an over-the-needle catheter to directly measure arterial blood pressures. Connect an aneroid manometer to the catheter as a simple way to determine the mean arterial blood pressure. Use a pressure transducer to make more definitive measurements.

■ Blood gas analysis
  - More definitive monitoring of respiratory and metabolic integrity is accomplished by measuring arterial pH and blood gas values.

See section 1, chapter 5 for the treatment of acid-base disorders.

RECOVERY AND POSTOPERATIVE COMPLICATIONS

Watch the patient after anesthesia until it can remain in sternal recumbency without being assisted.

■ If reversible drugs have been given, the administration of antagonists speeds recovery. Antagonists are not administered indiscriminantly.
■ Doxapram (1.0 to 5.0 mg/kg) is a nonspecific stimulant of respiration and the central nervous system. Doxapram can be given to effect arousal in an emergency, but it can also produce excitement.
■ Animals recovering from isoflurane anesthesia may go through a period of emergence delirium. This period apparently results from a rapid return to consciousness with disorientation. The animal may or may not be in pain. Many animals respond to a reassuring voice and petting. Provide analgesia and/or sedation for animals that do not respond to these actions.
■ Check the animal's temperature. Most animals lose body heat during anesthesia.
  - Some animals do not return to consciousness until body temperature is restored to 95 to 97°F.
  - Warm animals by placing them on recirculating, warm-water heating pads or by providing radiant heat from a lamp.
  - Take care to not burn the patient, particularly when heating lamps are placed.
  - Oxygen utilization increases dramatically with shivering. Monitor the patient, and provide oxygen if necessary.
■ Leave the endotracheal tube in place until the animal regains the oropharyngeal reflexes (i.e., begins to swallow). Give oxygen if necessary.
■ Remove intravenous catheters, if no longer necessary, after the patient is rewarmed and conscious. Postoperative hypotension can occur, particularly if the patient does not rapidly return to consciousness.
■ Monitor the patient periodically until it can stand unassisted.

Supplemental Readings

Lumb WV, Jones EW: *Veterinary Anesthesia, 2nd edition.* Philadelphia: Lea & Febiger, 1984.

Muir WW, Hubbell JAE, Skarda R: *Handbook of Veterinary Anesthesia.* St. Louis: C.V. Mosby, 1989.

Sawyer, DC: *The Practice of Small Animal Anesthesia.* Philadelphia: W.B. Saunders, 1982.

Short CE: *Principles and Practice of Veterinary Anesthesia.* Baltimore: Williams & Wilkins, 1987.

3 Critical Care Techniques

M. Susan Crisp

This chapter describes commonly used techniques in emergency and critical care medicine. See appropriate chapters for information on the diseases that require critical care.

INTRAVENOUS CATHETERIZATION BY CUTDOWN

Indication

For intravenous administration of drugs and/or fluids in animals that cannot be catheterized percutaneously.

KEY POINT ▶ In an animal with cardiopulmonary arrest, rapidly proceed with cutdown procedure after one to two unsuccessful attempts at percutaneous placement.

Objective

To establish a vascular access for the administration of fluids and drugs.

Equipment

- Minor surgical pack
  - Scalpel blade (#10) and handle
  - Mosquito forceps
  - Mayo scissors
- Intravenous catheter
  - Jelco (Pittman-Moore) or Angiocath (Becton, Dickinson & Co.) over-the-needle catheter (18 to 22 gauge).
- Silk or chromic catgut 3–0 or 4–0 suture

Technique

In an emergency situation, when time is critical (e.g., cardiac arrest; see sec. 6, ch. 15), modify the sterile procedure described next by doing the following: use the jugular or cephalic vein; dispense with aseptic preparation—simply clip the area and swab with alcohol; secure the catheter with tape and leave the incision open; place a sterile intravenous catheter in another vein; and remove the catheter after successful cardiopulmonary resuscitation (CPR).

1. Use the jugular, cephalic, or lateral saphenous vein for catheterization.
2. Prepare the catheterization site for an aseptic procedure, including field drapes, cap, mask, and gloves.
3. Make a 2- to 4-cm skin incision parallel and slightly lateral to the vein to be catheterized.
4. Locate the vein and dissect it from surrounding tissues with mosquito forceps (Fig. 1A).
5. Place two stay sutures around the vein. Pass a double strand of suture underneath the vein and cut the looped end to result in two equal strands around the vein (Fig. 1B).
6. Insert the over-the-needle catheter into the vein while stabilizing the vessel with the stay sutures.
7. Tie the stay sutures around the catheterized vein (Fig. 1C). Tie one suture just below the catheter hub; tie the other suture more proximally. Connect the catheter to a syringe or fluid-administration set.
8. Close the skin incision in a routine fashion.

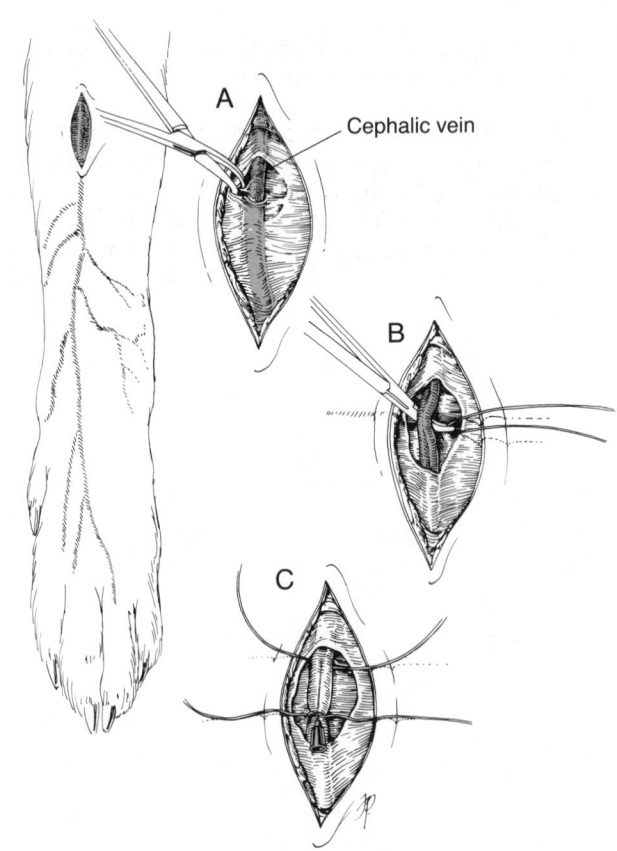

Figure 1. Intravenous catheterization by cutdown. *A,* Dissection of cephalic vein; *B,* threading for two stay sutures; *C,* catheter placement relative to stay sutures.

9. Place an antiseptic ointment and a sterile bandage over the catheterization site.
10. Change the catheter after 3 days to help prevent thrombophlebitis and infection.

CENTRAL VENOUS PRESSURE MEASUREMENT

Indications

- For determination of increased venous pressure associated with right-sided heart dysfunction or pericardial disease.
- For monitoring of fluid therapy in animals in hypovolemic shock (see sec. 6, ch. 14).
- For monitoring of poor-risk surgical patients during anesthesia and surgery.

Objectives

- Central venous pressure (CVP) in dogs and cats is normally 0 to 5 cm H_2O. The rate of fluid administration can be adjusted to maintain the normal CVP.
- The trend of the CVP changes is more valuable than the absolute measurements. Adjust the treatment (IV fluid administration) based on the changes in the CVP values.

Equipment

- Jugular catheters (I-Cath, Delmed, Inc.; 18.5-gauge, 22-gauge; 8-inch or 12-inch length)
- Water manometer (Central Venous Pressure Monitor, American Pharmaseal Co.)
- Three-way stopcock
- Intravenous extension set
- Sterile isotonic fluid

Technique

1. Aseptically prepare the right or left jugular vein area for catheterization.
2. Place the intravenous catheter. The tip of the catheter is advanced to about the second intercostal space—just proximal to the right atrium. Secure the catheter to the neck and cover with a sterile, padded bandage.
3. Place an extension set on the catheter and connect to a stopcock. Connect the manometer to the stopcock and connect the fluid bag to the stopcock via a fluid administration set (Fig. 2). Do not allow air bubbles into the system.
4. Place the manometer so that the 0 level is approximately at the level of the right atrium (sternal recumbency—level of thoracic inlet; lateral recumbency—level of sternum).
5. Flush the intravenous line to remove any obstructions. Turn the stopcock so that it is closed to the patient and open from the IV fluid bag to the manometer. Fill the manometer to above 15 cm H_2O (Fig. 3A).
6. Turn the stopcock so that it is closed to the IV fluid administration set and open from the manometer to the patient (Fig. 3B).
7. Allow the fluid level in the manometer to equilibrate

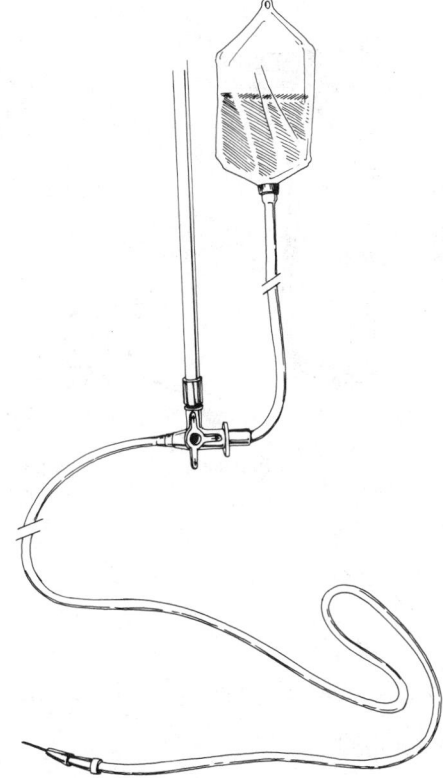

Figure 2. Manometer, stopcock, and catheter for central venous pressure measurement.

with the right atrium; read the resultant value from the meniscus of the column of fluid.
8. Adjust the stopcock to open the fluid line between the fluid bag and the IV catheter (closed to the manometer) (Fig. 3C).

TEMPORARY TRACHEOSTOMY

Indications

- For upper airway obstruction (e.g., acute laryngeal edema, brachycephalic syndrome, laryngeal paralysis, and pharyngeal or laryngeal foreign body or neoplasia).
- For facilitation of artificial respiration in animals exhibiting hypoventilation.
- For insurance of a patent airway either before or after major surgery of the upper airways.

Objectives

- To establish a patent airway.
- To maintain patency of the airway by frequent cleaning or replacement of the tracheostomy tube.

Equipment

- Minor surgical pack (see IV cutdown procedure)
- Shiley (Shiley, Inc.) or Portex (Portex, Inc.) tracheostomy tubes (Fig. 4)
- Suture
  - 3–0 or 4–0 polypropylene or nylon (Prolene or Ethilon; Ethicon)

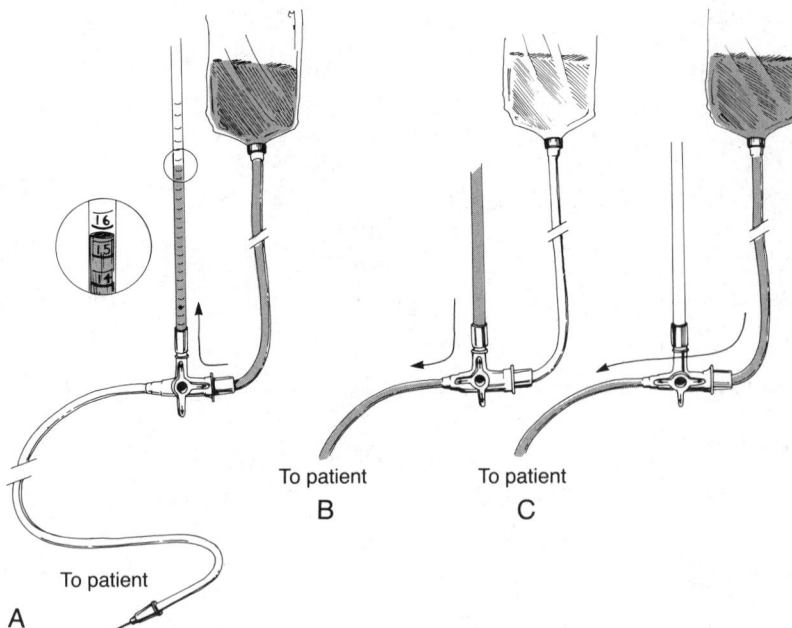

Figure 3. Central venous pressure measurement. See text for details.

- 3–0 absorbable (Vicryl; polydioxanone suture, PDS)
■ Umbilical tape

Technique

1. Place the animal in ventral recumbency with the head extended and a rolled towel or sandbag under the neck.
2. Prepare the ventral cervical area for aseptic surgery. If this is an emergency situation, simply clip the hair and swab with alcohol.
3. Make a 6- to 8-cm skin incision in the ventral cervical midline from the caudal aspect of the larynx caudally.
4. Expose the sternohyoideus and sternothyroideus muscles.

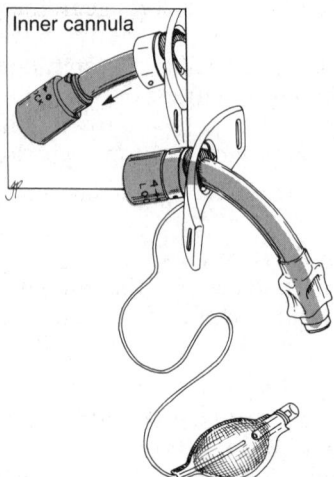

Inner cannula

Figure 4. Shiley tracheostomy tube showing replaceable inner cannula.

KEY POINT ▶ Divide the muscles precisely on the midline to prevent excessive hemorrhage and poor exposure.

5. Make a transverse incision in the annular ligament between the third and fourth tracheal rings or caudal to the obstruction. Incise one half to two thirds of the circumference of the trachea. Avoid trauma to the recurrent laryngeal nerves. Place nonabsorbable stay sutures on the third and fourth tracheal rings to allow separation of the rings. Leave long tags on the stay sutures (Fig. 5A).
6. Place the tracheostomy tube through the incision and pass caudally. Do not use too large a tube because improper fit can produce pressure necrosis of the dorsal and/or ventral tracheal mucosa (Fig. 5B).
7. Secure the tracheostomy tube passing umbilical tape around the animal's neck. Close the muscle layer with 3–0 Vicryl or PDS in a simple continuous pattern. Close the subcutaneous layer in the same fashion as for the muscle; close the skin up to the level of the tube in a routine fashion.
8. Do not bandage the tracheostomy tube because this interferes with the replacement of the tube when it becomes obstructed with mucus.

Postoperative Care and Complications

■ Check the tube for patency every 1 to 2 hours or more frequently, if necessary.
■ Clean the tube every 2 hours or more frequently, if necessary. When a double-lumen tube (Shiley) is used, remove inner cannula, clean off mucus with hydrogen peroxide, and rinse with distilled water or sterile saline. Disinfect cannula by soaking in chlorhexidine (Nolvasan) solution for 5 minutes. Rinse again with sterile saline and replace inside the outer cannula.

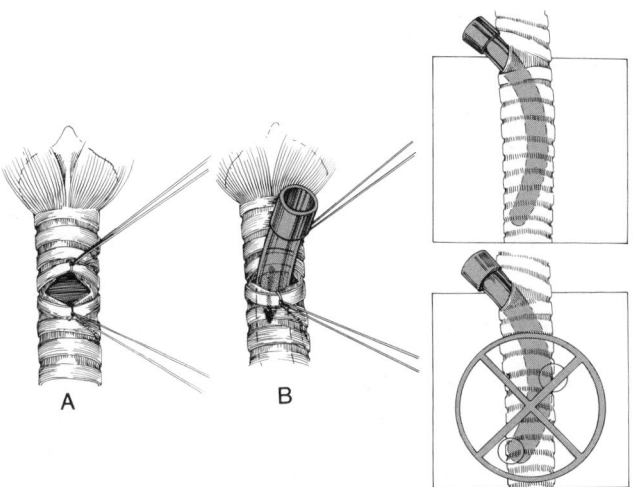

Figure 5. Placement of tracheostomy tube. *A*, Stay sutures retract tracheal rings; *B*, tube should slip easily through the incision. Note that a tube that is too large can cause pressure necrosis of the tracheal mucosa.

- If a single-lumen tracheostomy tube is in place, change the tube every 2 hours. One tube is kept in cold sterilization (Nolvasan); the other tube is kept in the patient. At the time of tube change, prepare the replacement tube by rinsing with sterile saline to *completely* remove all disinfectant. Remove the soiled tracheostomy tube from the patient. By utilizing the tracheal ring stay sutures, open the tracheal stoma and insert the clean tube. Clean the soiled tube with hydrogen peroxide, rinse with distilled water, and place in cold sterilization until next tube change.
- Do not apply active suction to the tracheostomy tube unless necessary. Suctioning shortly after eating can induce vomiting.
- Acetylcysteine (a mucolytic agent) is contraindicated because it is irritating to the tracheal mucosa.
- Keep the animal well hydrated to decrease the viscosity of secretions. Humidify inspired air, if possible.
- Monitor the animal for subcutaneous emphysema by palpating the head, neck, and body. Monitor the ventral neck area for evidence of irritation due to serum discharge. Apply petrolatum (Vaseline) to the area, if necessary.
- After removal, temporarily cover the tracheal stoma to be sure the animal will be able to ventilate adequately without the tube. Allow the incision to heal as an open wound. Lightly bandage the wound, if necessary, to prevent self-trauma.

OXYGEN THERAPY VIA NASAL CATHETER
Indications

- For severe, acute respiratory or cardiovascular failure (dysfunction) causing hypoxia and hypoxemia
- For ventilation-perfusion mismatches (e.g., pneumonia, pneumothorax, and airway obstruction)
- For supportive care for animals in shock
- For any disease causing hypoxia ($PaO_2 < 70$ mm Hg with normal packed cell volume (PCV); $PaO_2 < 80$ mm Hg with PCV <20%)
- Hypoventilation is *not* an indication for nasal oxygen. Animals with poor ventilation require tracheal intubation and positive pressure ventilation.

Objectives

- To elevate arterial oxygen by increasing the inspired concentration of oxygen.
- To provide a nasal catheter that is effective yet comfortable for the patient.

Equipment

- Nasal catheter: 5- to 8-Fr. infant feeding tube (Davol) or 5- to 8-Fr. red rubber feeding tube and urethral catheter (Sovereign)
- Monofilament 2–0 or 3–0 nylon suture
- Adhesive tape
- Lidocaine (2%) or proparacaine (Ophthaine) 0.5%
- Sterile lubricant (K-Y jelly)
- Elizabethan collar (optional)

Technique

1. With the animal's nose pointing upward, instill 1 ml of lidocaine (dogs) or 5 drops of proparacaine (cats) into one nostril. Repeat after 1 minute.
2. Measure the tube from the external nares to carnassial tooth.
3. Lubricate catheter tip with sterile lubricant (K-Y jelly).
4. Insert the catheter into the ventral nasal meatus to the level of the carnassial tooth. Direct the tube caudomedially ventral to the alar fold. As the nasal planum is pressed upward (Fig. 6A), direct the tube ventrally and caudally to allow entry into the ventral nasal meatus (Abood, 1991).
5. Apply tape to the catheter, in butterfly fashion, and suture to the skin immediately adjacent to the alar fold (Fig. 6B).
6. Position the tube between the animal's eyes and secure it to the top of the head in a similar fashion (see Fig. 6B).
7. Connect extension tubing to the nasal catheter. Humidify the oxygen through a bubble humidifier (Chemetron Medical Products) attached to an oxygen wall outlet or, if oxygen is not available through a wall outlet, construct a humidifier. Attach an IV administration set to the extension set (on the nasal catheter). Place the opposite end in a fluid administration bottle that is half filled with sterile saline or water. Attach an oxygen line to the vent hole in the lid of the bottle, and bubble oxygen through the liquid.
8. Administer oxygen at a flow rate of 50 to 100 ml/min/kg to maintain tracheal concentrations of greater than, or equal to, 40%.

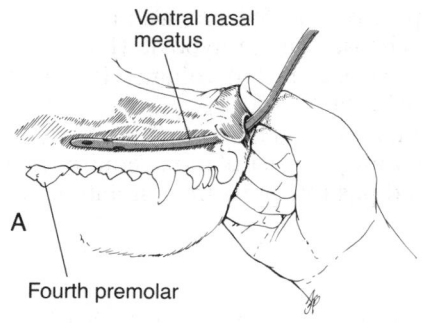

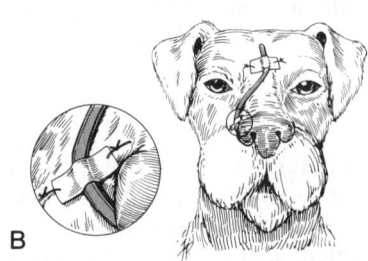

Figure 6. *A*, Placement of nasal catheter; *B*, method of securing the nasal catheter.

Postoperative Care and Complications

- Prevent dislodgement of the tube by placing an Elizabethan collar, if necessary.
- Nasal hemorrhage may occur if the catheter is improperly placed.
- Gagging may occur if the catheter is placed too far caudally.
- Gastric distension can occur if the flow rate is too high or the catheter is placed too far caudally.

THORACOCENTESIS

Indications

- For pneumothorax, if causing a clinical problem
- For hydrothorax

Objectives

- To evacuate fluid or air from the pleural space
- To avoid iatrogenic pneumothorax or trauma to the lungs, heart, and intercostal blood vessels

Equipment

- Sterile butterfly needle (19 to 22 gauge) for small or thin animals; over-the-needle catheter (20 to 22 gauge) for large or obese animals
- Intravenous extension set
- Three-way stopcock
- Syringe

Technique

1. The animal is either standing or in sternal recumbency.
2. Clip and aseptically prepare the appropriate site on the thoracic wall.
3. Generally, perform the thoracocentesis between the seventh and ninth intercostal spaces. Based upon radiographic evaluation, it may sometimes be necessary to enter the thorax at a different space.
4. To avoid the intercostal vessels and nerve, which lie along the caudal border of each rib, place the needle just cranial to the rib.
5. To evacuate pleural air, perform the thoracocentesis in the dorsal half of the thorax; to evacuate pleural fluid, perform the thoracocentesis in the ventral half of the thorax.
6. Connect the tubing of the butterfly needle to the stopcock or connect the catheter to the extension set and place the stopcock at the end of the extension set. Turn off the stopcock toward the patient.
7. Carefully place the needle into the pleural space. A slight "pop" can usually be felt when the pleura is entered. When the needle is into the thorax, angle the needle so that the point is facing slightly cranially or caudally and not aiming directly at the lung. A friction rub will be felt with each inspiration, if the needle is touching the lung.
8. Connect a syringe to the stopcock. Open the stopcock from the patient to the syringe. Apply gentle negative pressure (3 to 5 units) to evacuate the thorax.
9. If no air or fluid is obtained, redirect the needle or tap one or two alternative areas.

CHEST TUBE PLACEMENT

Indications

- For persistent pneumothorax or hydrothorax requiring repeated thoracocentesis
- For more complete evacuation of the thorax than that possible with thoracocentesis
- For tension pneumothorax
- For postoperative thoracotomy (see sec. 6, ch. 25)
- For administration of intrathoracic medications

Objectives

- To aseptically place an indwelling thoracic drain tube without causing iatrogenic trauma to thoracic viscera
- To minimize iatrogenic pneumothorax
- To place the tube such that it effectively drains the pleural fluid or air

Equipment

- Chest tubes
  - Argyle trocar catheter (Sherwood)
  - Red rubber feeding tube and urethral catheter (Sovereign)
- Minor surgical pack plus Kelly or Carmalt hemostatic forceps
- Three-way stopcock and Pharmaseal plastic tubing connector (Baxter)
- Monofilament nylon 2–0 or 3–0 suture
- Bandage material
- Antiseptic ointment

Technique

1. Provide local or general anesthesia depending upon the patient's status and compliance. If local

anesthesia (2% lidocaine) is used, infiltrate the area of the skin incision and the chest wall at the point of tube entry including the parietal pleura.

2. Place the animal in lateral or sternal recumbency.

3. Clip and aseptically prepare the lateral thoracic wall from the fifth to the twelfth ribs.

4. Select an appropriately sized chest tube, i.e., approximately the diameter of a main stem bronchus.

5. Measure and mark the chest tube from the skin incision (tenth intercostal space) to the point of the ipsilateral elbow.

6. Cut additional holes in the chest tube and be certain that the last hole will be within the thoracic cavity.

7. Make a stab incision in the skin over the tenth intercostal space in the dorsal third of the thorax and insert the tube through the incision into the subcutis (Fig. 7A).

8. Advance the tube subcutaneously in a cranioventral direction and enter the thoracic cavity at the seventh or eighth intercostal space, at the level of the junction between the dorsal third and middle third of the thorax (Fig. 7B).

9. Avoid the caudal border of the rib to prevent the possibility of trauma to the intercostal vessels and nerve.

10. To enter the thoracic cavity, grasp the trocar chest tube firmly in one hand so that the hand acts as a guard to prevent the trocar from penetrating too deeply into the chest cavity. Hold the chest tube perpendicular to the thoracic wall and firmly "smack" the tube through the thoracic wall with the other hand (Fig. 7C).

11. Once the tube is through the thoracic wall, place the tube parallel to the chest wall. While holding on to the trocar, advance the chest tube into the thoracic cavity to the premeasured point. Direct the tube ventrally to evacuate fluid and dorsally to evacuate air (Fig. 7D).

12. Quickly remove the trocar and clamp the tube to limit the development of pneumothorax.

13. Place one or two cerclage sutures around the tube in the subcutaneous tunnel.

14. Place a pursestring suture around the tube at the skin incision site.

15. Secure the tube with a Chinese finger trap suture. Place an anchoring suture through the skin adjacent to the tube's exit. Tie a square knot and leave long suture tags. Place a surgeon's throw over the top of the tube and pull snugly enough to slightly indent the tube. Cross the suture material underneath the tube, and place another surgeon's throw over the top of the tube as before. Continue this pattern 5 to 10 times and end with a square knot on top of the tube (Fig. 8).

16. Place a Pharmaseal plastic tubing connector into the flared end of the chest tube. Cut the flared end from a red rubber feeding tube, and place it over the other end of the tubing connector. Attach a stopcock to the narrow end of the cut red rubber feeding tube. Place ligatures around all connections from the chest tube to the stopcock (Fig. 9).

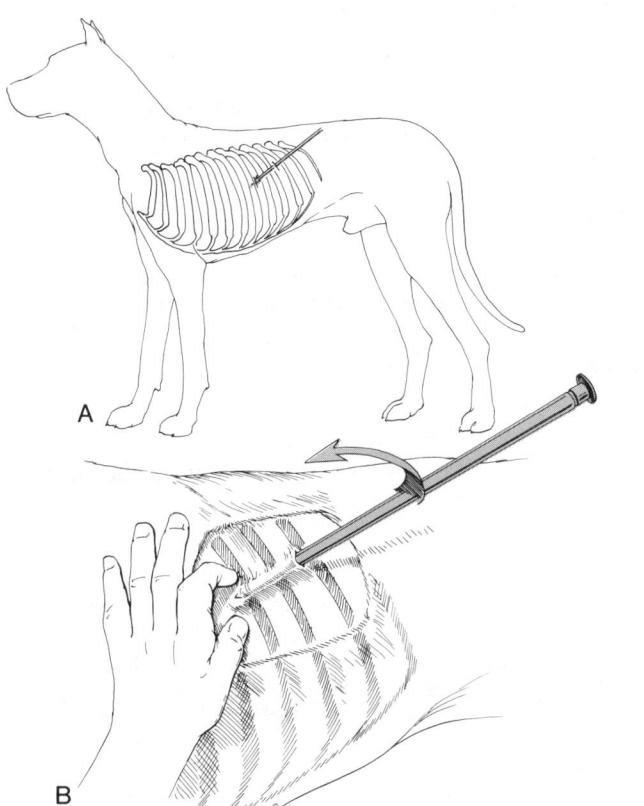

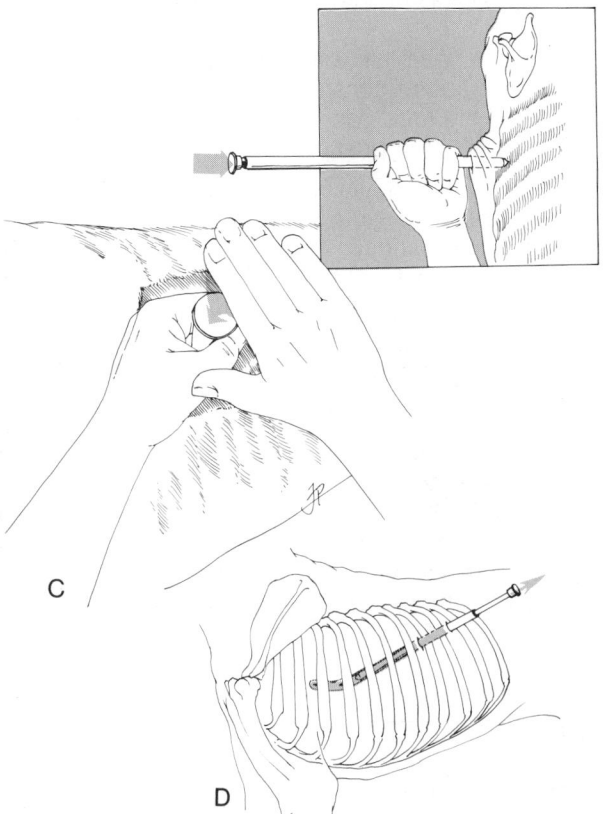

Figure 7. Chest tube placement. *A,* General view of direction and angle of chest tube placement; *B,* subcutaneous advancement of the tube to the entrance into thoracic wall; *C,* entering thoracic cavity; *D,* removing trochar once tube is in place.

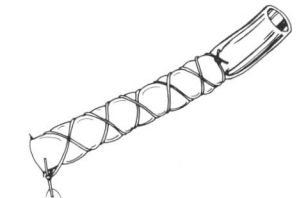

Figure 8. Chinese finger trap suture.

17. Place antiseptic ointment and a 4 × 4-gauze over the tube exit site.
18. Wrap the thoracic wall with Kling and Vet-Wrap and place the bandage material around one or both front legs to prevent bandage slippage. Apply a small amount of Elasticon at the cranial edge of the bandage for adherence to the haircoat.
19. Apply gentle suction (3 to 5 cc pressure) or attach the chest tube apparatus to a continuous suction unit (Pleur-Evac, Deknatel, Pfizer Inc.).
20. If a trocar catheter is unavailable, a red rubber feeding tube can be utilized for thoracic drainage. The tip of the catheter is grasped in the tip of Kelly or Carmalt forceps and advanced through the subcutaneous tissue as previously described. The technique for placement into the thoracic cavity is the same as that for the trocar catheter. Once the thoracic wall is penetrated, spread the tips of the forceps to allow passage of the tube into the thoracic cavity. The remainder of the technique is the same as that for the trocar catheter.

Postoperative Care and Complications

KEY POINT ▶ Animals with indwelling chest tubes require constant supervision. Damage to the tube can cause life-threatening tension pneumothorax.

■ Use an Elizabethan collar on the animal if necessary to prevent damage to the tube.
■ Change the bandage every other day or more often if necessary. Check the position of the tube during bandage changes. Radiograph the thorax if necessary to check tube position in the pleural space.
■ The chest tube itself can create pleural effusion. Pleural effusion ≤ 1 to 2 ml/kg/24 hours can be attributed to the presence of the chest tube. When the effusion has decreased to this volume, remove the chest tube.
  • Remove the sutures and pull the chest tube from the thorax smoothly and quickly. The tip of the tube can be cultured, if necessary.
  • Apply antiseptic ointment and a light bandage to the skin incision.

ABDOMINOCENTESIS

Indications

■ For determination of organ damage associated with abdominal trauma

■ For evaluation of any disease causing the development of peritoneal fluid

Objectives

■ To aseptically obtain fluid from the abdominal cavity for analysis and/or culture
■ To avoid causing trauma to any of the abdominal viscera

Equipment

■ Butterfly needle (19 to 22 gauge) or needle and intravenous extension set
■ 12-cc syringe

Technique

1. The animal can be standing or in lateral recumbency.
2. Aseptically prepare a small area (approximately 6 cm^2) in each of the four abdominal quadrants.
3. Slowly insert the needle into the abdominal cavity, until it is felt to enter the peritoneal cavity.
4. Let the fluid drain by gravity flow or connect the syringe to the butterfly needle and gently aspirate. Do not drain all of the fluid out of the abdomen, if it is ascitic.
5. Place fluid in ethylenediaminetetra-acetic acid (EDTA) and clot tubes for analysis. Save some fluid for Gram staining and bacterial culture.

DIAGNOSTIC PERITONEAL LAVAGE

Indications

■ For early detection of organ damage in an animal with an acute abdomen, when abdominocentesis results are negative.

Objectives

■ To obtain fluid or debris from the abdomen
■ To avoid causing trauma to the abdominal viscera

Equipment

■ Local anesthetic (2% lidocaine)
■ Scalpel blade (# 15) and handle
■ Peritoneal dialysis catheter (Travenol Laboratories, Inc.)

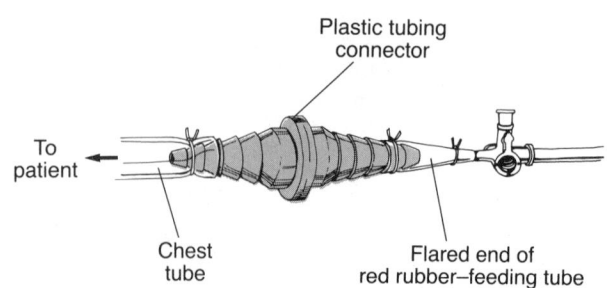

Figure 9. Pharmaseal plastic tubing connector and attachment to chest tube.

■ Intravenous extension set
■ 500 ml of sterile saline
■ 12-cc syringe

Technique

1. Place the animal in dorsal recumbency.
2. Empty the urinary bladder.
3. Aseptically prepare the abdomen (a 6-cm² area caudal to the umbilicus).
4. Infiltrate the subcutaneous tissue, rectus fascia, and peritoneum with 2% lidocaine.
5. Make a stab incision with the scalpel 1 to 2 cm caudal to the umbilicus—through the skin, subcutaneous tissue, and fascia down to the level of the linea alba.
6. Aim the catheter in a dorsocaudal direction. With one hand, grasp the catheter and stylet to guard against penetrating too deeply into the abdomen (see Fig. 7C on chest tube placement). Use a controlled push to advance the catheter and stylet through the linea alba. Once the peritoneal cavity has been entered, hold the stylet and advance the catheter off the stylet to the dorsal lumbar region. Be sure all fenestrations are within the abdominal cavity. If a celiotomy scar is present, enter the abdomen off the midline. The abdominal organs may have adhesions with the scar.
7. Infuse 20 ml/kg of sterile saline into the peritoneal cavity through the catheter.
8. Plug the catheter and gently roll the dog or cat from side to side.
9. Aspirate the fluid from the abdomen through the catheter and save a sample for analysis.
10. Fluid analysis (Crane, 1986).

    • PCV >2% or RBC count ≥ 200,000 mm³ indicates significant hemorrhage—PCV > 1% but <2% is equivocal, and PCV < 1% is insignificant.
    • The normal neutrophil count is <500/mm³. The neutrophil count after uncomplicated abdominal surgery can be 750 to 1500/mm³ but may be higher if peripheral leukocytosis exists. Leukocyte response requires 2 to 4 hours for intraperitoneal accumulation following irritation or sepsis.
    • Biochemical tests can be performed to check for the presence of urea, creatinine, bilirubin, amylase, or lipase. The Azostick (for urea) or Ictotest (for bilirubin) (Ames Laboratories) can be employed as a rapid test.
    • Examine the fluid microscopically for the presence of bacteria or vegetable material.
    • Submit an aliquot of the lavage fluid for bacterial culture and sensitivity testing.

11. If the results are equivocal, the catheter can be sutured in place. Lavage and aspiration can be repeated several hours later.
12. After the catheter is removed, close the incision routinely.

KEY POINT ▶ This procedure is contraindicated in patients with ileus or gravid uterus.

NUTRITIONAL MANAGEMENT OF THE CRITICAL CARE PATIENT

Animals require energy, proteins, minerals, and vitamins for normal body metabolism. If these are not ingested by the animal, they are provided by the animal's own body tissue. Nutritional support via enteral or parenteral feeding can prevent this "autodigestion" and subsequent complications, including impaired immunity, muscular weakness, decreased wound strength, decreased resistance to infection, and death.

Indications for Nutritional Support: Patient Selection

History

■ Recent weight loss
■ Decreased food intake
■ Increased nutrient needs—recent trauma or surgery, burns, fever
■ Increased losses—vomiting, diarrhea, burns
■ Homemade diet that may be nutritionally incomplete or imbalanced.

Physical Examination

■ Underweight
  • Loss of subcutaneous fat
  • Muscle wasting
  • Hair that is easily plucked.
■ Overweight
  • Edema
  • "Overcoat syndrome" or a disproportionate loss of lean body tissue that leaves an overcoat of fat, giving the impression of a better body condition than what actually exists.
■ Inability to eat

Absence of Indication for Starvation

■ There are no indications for starvation.

Route Selection

See Figure 10.

What to Feed: Categories of Enteral Diets

Polymeric or intact macronutrients (protein, fat, carbohydrate, caloric density ~ 1 kcal/ml) for patients with normal or near-normal gastrointestinal function.

■ High fat (>50% of kcal; caloric density ~ 1.5 kcal/ml) for high-energy needs, volume restriction, diarrhea caused by high-carbohydrate (>50% kcal) products.
■ Fiber-containing diets for improved feces consistency compared with those resulting from high-carbohydrate diets.

Defined-formula diets or diets specifically modified for patients with impaired organ function.

■ *Impaired gastrointestinal function, including >2 weeks' anorexia.* Diet contains peptides, medium-

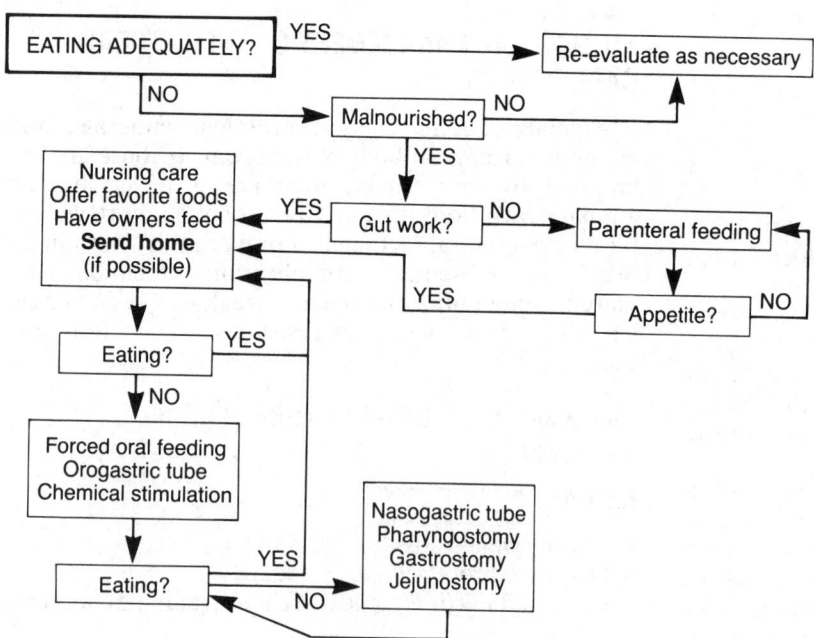

Figure 10. Route selection for nutritional support.

chain triglycerides, and glucose polymers' versus intact macronutrient sources. Usually causes diarrhea if given longer than 2 to 3 days.

- *Impaired liver function.* Diet with reduced protein (<18% of kcal). High branched–chain and aromatic amino acid content formulas are available, but their efficacy is questionable.
- *Impaired kidney function.* A diet of reduced protein (<18% of kcal). Formulas supplemented with alpha-ketoacids of some essential amino acids are available, but their efficacy is disputed.
- Stress diets are of high branched–chain amino acid content and high (>1 kcal/ml) caloric density. Efficacy is disputed.

Nutrient Modifications for Specific Disease Problems

Energy

- Total calories (<1 kcal/ml)
  - Restricted—obesity, uncontrollable hyperglycemia (rare)
  - Increased (>1 kcal/ml)—disease-induced increases in requirements from severe trauma, burns, sepsis, hyperthyroidism
- Carbohydrate
  - Increased (>50% of kcal)—prolonged anorexia (>2 weeks), fat maldigestion, malabsorption
  - Decreased (<30% of kcal)—diarrhea, glucose intolerance
- Fat
  - Increased (>50% of kcal)—diarrhea due to high-carbohydrate feedings, increased energy needs
  - Decreased (<30% of kcal)—same as increased carbohydrate
  - Triglycerides. Long chain—adequate pancreatic and intestinal function. Medium chain—severely impaired pancreatic or intestinal function, chylothorax, or lymphangiectasia

Protein

- Total intake
  - Restricted (<18% of kcal)—impaired liver or kidney function
- Increased (>22% of kcal)—losses via intestinal tract, draining wounds, trauma
- Form
  - Intact—adequate pancreatic and intestinal function
  - Hydrolyzed—intact protein not tolerated
- Specific amino acids for cats
  - Arginine—recommend 2.5 mg/kcal/day. Current formulas are supplemented with 1 mg/kcal/day.
  - Taurine—not necessary for short-term feeding. Add 0.1 mg/kcal/day for long-term feeding.

Electrolytes

Electrolytes (sodium, potassium, chlorine) ~40 mEq/L have been adequate. Adjust amounts based on laboratory determinations.

Minerals and Vitamins

Minerals and vitamins—National Research Council (NRC) recommendations in the absence of specific information to the contrary

Osmolality

- Normal serum albumin of <650 mOsm/kg
- Hypoalbuminemia of 250 to 650 mOsm/kg, depending on severity. The lower the serum albumin level, the lower the diet osmolality.

Feeding Rates for Enteral Diets

The calculations for feeding liquid diets follow. If the tube size is ≥14 Fr., blenderized commercial canned pet food may be fed.

KEY POINT ▶ Proceed with feeding only as patient tolerance allows.

Bolus Feeding

Day 1
First feeding	Water
Subsequent feedings	$(0.5 \times BEE^*)/A^\dagger$
Last feeding	BEE/A

Day 2
First feeding	BEE/A
Subsequent feedings	$\left[BEE + \dfrac{(GEE\ddagger - BEE)}{2}\right]/A$
Last feeding	GEE/A

Day 3
First feeding	GEE/A
Subsequent feedings	GEE/A

Continuous (Hourly Rate)

Day 1
First 12 hours	Water at $0.5 \times BEE/24$ hours
Second 12 hours	$0.5 \times BEE/24$

Day 2
First 12 hours	BEE/24
Second 12 hours	$\left(BEE + \dfrac{GEE - BEE}{2}\right)/24$

---

*BEE (basal energy estimate), found in Figure 11.
†A = Number of feedings per day.
‡GEE (goal energy estimate) = BEE × stress estimate (see Fig. 11).

Day 3
GEE rate/24

For formulas containing 1.5 kcal/ml, divide energy needs by 1.5 to get volume to feed. Use this value to replace energy needs in the previously listed calculations.

Sample Calculation. A moderately stressed 30-lb dog's energy needs are estimated at 500 (basal) × 1.5 = 750 kcal/day. (Round off calculations to the nearest 5.) For four-times daily feeding, the schedule is as follows:

Day 1
Feeding	1	Water	$(0.5 \times 500) \div 4 =$	65 ml
	2	Diet	same as feeding 1	65 ml
	3	Diet	same as feeding 1	65 ml
	4	Diet	$500 \div 4$	125 ml
		Total		320 ml (255 kcal)

Day 2
Feeding	1	$500 \div 4$	125 ml
	2	$\dfrac{500 + \dfrac{750 - 500}{2}}{4}$	160 ml
	3	Same as feeding 2	160 ml
	4	$750 \div 4$	190 ml
	Total		635 ml (635 kcal)

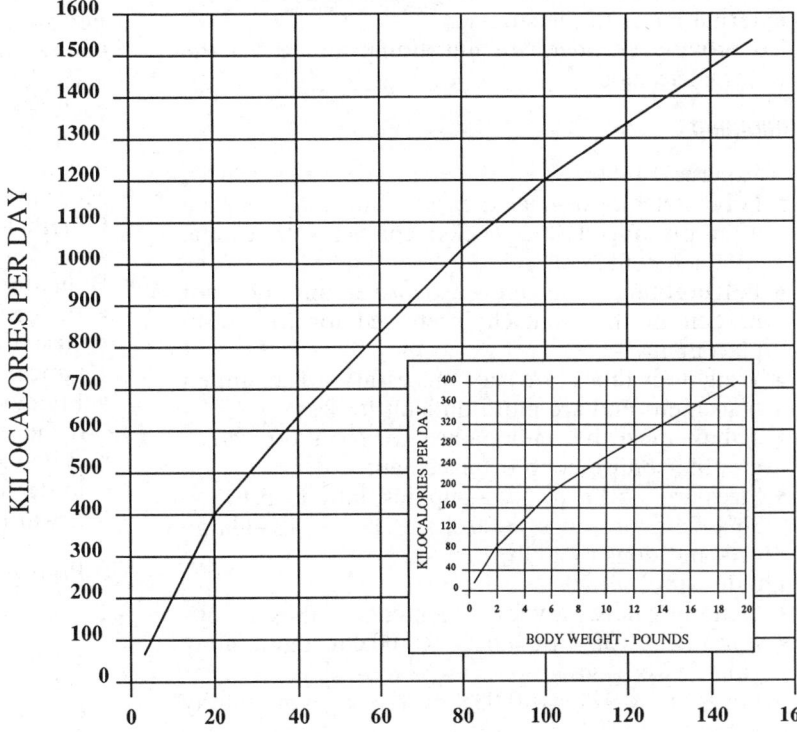

Figure 11. Graph for calculating caloric requirements to fill basal energy needs and to meet increased needs of stress. (BEE, basal energy estimate.)

How much to feed (kcal/day)
A. To meet basal needs-see graph:

KILOCALORIES PER DAY

BODY WEIGHT - POUNDS

B. **To meet increased needs of stress**
  1. Mild stress-25% increase above BEE
  2. Moderate stress-50% increase above BEE
  3. Severe stress-100% increase above BEE

Day 3

| All feedings | 750 ÷ 4 | 190 ml |
| | *Total* | 760 ml (760 kcal) |

For continuous feeding, the schedule is as follows:

Day 1

12 hours	Water	(0.5 × 500) ÷ 24 =	10 ml/hr = 120 ml
12 hours	Diet	As above	10 ml/hr = 120 ml
		Total	240 ml (120 kcal)

Day 2

12 hours	Diet	500 ÷ 24	20 ml/hr = 240 ml
12 hours	Diet	$500 + \dfrac{\frac{750 - 500}{2}}{24}$	25 ml/hr = 300 ml
		Total	540 ml (540 kcal)

Day 3

| | Diet | 750 ÷ 24 | 30 ml/hr = 720 ml |
| | | | (720 kcal) |

FEEDING DEVICES

Nasogastric Tube

Indications

See general indications for nutritional support. See Figure 10.

Objectives

- To successfully pass a nasogastric tube from the external nares to the stomach
- To provide an adequate nutritional intake via the nasogastric tube

Equipment

- Nasogastric tubes
  - Polyvinylchloride—inexpensive but may harden after prolonged (>2 weeks) contact with canine stomach contents.
  - Polyurethane, silicone—expensive but do not harden in the stomach; preferred for long-term placement.
  - Weighted tubes are not necessary to maintain placement and are more difficult to pass.
  - Tubes must be radiopaque to facilitate radiographic confirmation of placement.
  - Sizes are 3.5 Fr. × 15"—puppies, kittens; 5 Fr. × 36"—cats and dogs (≤20 lb); 8 Fr. × 42"—large cats and dogs (>20 lb).
- Guide wire
  - Generally necessary for placement of tubes in dogs
  - For 5 Fr. × 36", use 0.025" × 100 cm angiography guide wire
  - For 8 Fr. × 42", use 0.035" × 120 cm angiography guide wire
- 2% lidocaine or 0.5% proparacaine
- Lubricant (K-Y jelly)
- Monofilament nylon 2-0 or 3-0 suture
- Adhesive tape
- Elizabethan collar

Technique

1. Lubricate angiography guide wire with mineral oil to use as stylet.
2. Before passing the tube, measure the distance from the external nares to the last rib (level of the stomach) and mark the tube.
3. Ensure patency of the nostrils.
4. Apply lubricant to the catheter tip.
5. With the animal's nose pointed upward, instill 1 ml of lidocaine (dogs) or 5 drops of proparacaine (cats) into one nostril.
6. Hold the animal's head in a normal, neutral position to avoid tracheal intubation.
7. Insert the catheter into the ventral nasal meatus. Direct the tube caudomedially, ventral to the alar fold. As the nasal planum is pushed upward, direct the tube ventrally and caudally to allow entry into the ventral nasal meatus (see Fig. 6).
8. Once the tube is believed to be in the stomach, a small bolus of water (3-6 ml) is injected into the tube. The animal is observed for coughing. Tube position can be confirmed by radiography.
9. Apply tape to the catheter in butterfly fashion and suture to the skin immediately adjacent to the alar fold (see Fig. 6*B*). Bring the tubing between the animal's eyes, and suture with butterfly tape to the top of the animal's head (see Fig. 6). An Elizabethan collar or bucket may be needed to protect the tube from removal.

Postoperative Care and Complications

Feeding Instructions

- Check the position of continuous feeding tubes at least daily; check the position of bolus tubes before each feeding.
- Urine glucose initially is checked 2 to 4 times daily because of the high-carbohydrate content of the diet.
- Measure body weight daily.
- Other laboratory determinations ordered as necessary.
- Bolus feeding instructions for *each feeding*
  - Inject a small bolus of air through the tube and auscultate over the cranial abdomen for sounds indicating the tube is properly placed.
  - Inject water through the tube to produce coughing if the tube is improperly placed.
  - When satisfied that the animal can be fed, place it in sternal or right lateral recumbency. The solution is warmed and fed slowly.

KEY POINT ▶ If the animal vomits, stop feeding.

  - After feeding, flush the tube with 1 to 2 ml of warm water. Cap the tube so that a column of water is left to prevent food from drying and occluding the tube.
  - Observe the animal for discomfort, colic, or diarrhea for a few minutes.
  - Record all feedings (Fig. 12).

Complications of enteral feeding are listed in Table 1.

FOOD INTAKE RECORD

INSTRUCTIONS:
1. Weigh the food and container using the gram scale that is located on the counter in the ICU. Record this weight in the "offered" column.
2. When uneaten food is removed from cage, weigh as above (the food and container!). Record this weight in the "removed" column.
3. Subtract amount that was removed from amount that was offered. Record this weight in the "eaten" column.
4. Write down what was fed (and if it was canned, dry, liquid, etc.) in the last column.

		AMOUNT OF FOOD (grams)			
DATE/TIME	INITIALS	offered	removed	eaten	What was fed?
	example:	100	25	75	Chicken baby food

Figure 12. Example of a food intake record chart as used by the Nutritional Support Service of The Ohio State University Veterinary Hospital.

Pharyngostomy Tube

Indications

- See general indications for nutritional support.
- See Figure 10.
- When the nasal passages or oral cavity must be by-passed because of trauma, tumors, and other oronasal disorders.
- For tracheal intubation and anesthesia during oral surgery

Objectives

■ To pass a tube from the piriform recess to the midthoracic esophagus
■ To provide adequate nutritional intake via the pharyngostomy tube

TABLE 1. Complications of Enteral Feeding and Their Management

Clogged tube	Flush with water; replace tube if necessary.
Aspiration of stomach contents	Stop feeding.
Vomiting and bloating	Reduce flow rate; stop feeding.
Diarrhea	Reduce flow rate; add fat or fiber, dilute solution, add antidiarrheal drug.
Hyperglycemia and glucosuria	Reduce flow rate; administer insulin.

Equipment

- Minor surgial pack
- Red rubber feeding tube and urethral catheter (Sovereign)
- Monofilament 2-0 or 3-0 nylon suture
- Adhesive tape

Technique

1. Anesthetize the patient and place in lateral recumbency.
2. Measure the tube from the piriform recess to the seventh or eighth rib, and mark the tube.
3. Aseptically prepare the left or right lateral cervical area.
4. Place an oral speculum.
5. Palpate the piriform recess with a finger in the mouth, just cranial to the hyoid apparatus (Fig. 13A).
6. Place a hemostat or right-angle forceps in the mouth with the tip in the piriform recess (Fig. 13B).
7. Make a stab incision in the skin over the tip of the forceps. Advance the forceps through the skin incision.
8. Grasp the end of the feeding tube with the forceps and pull out through the mouth (Fig. 13C).
9. Turn the tube around and direct it down the

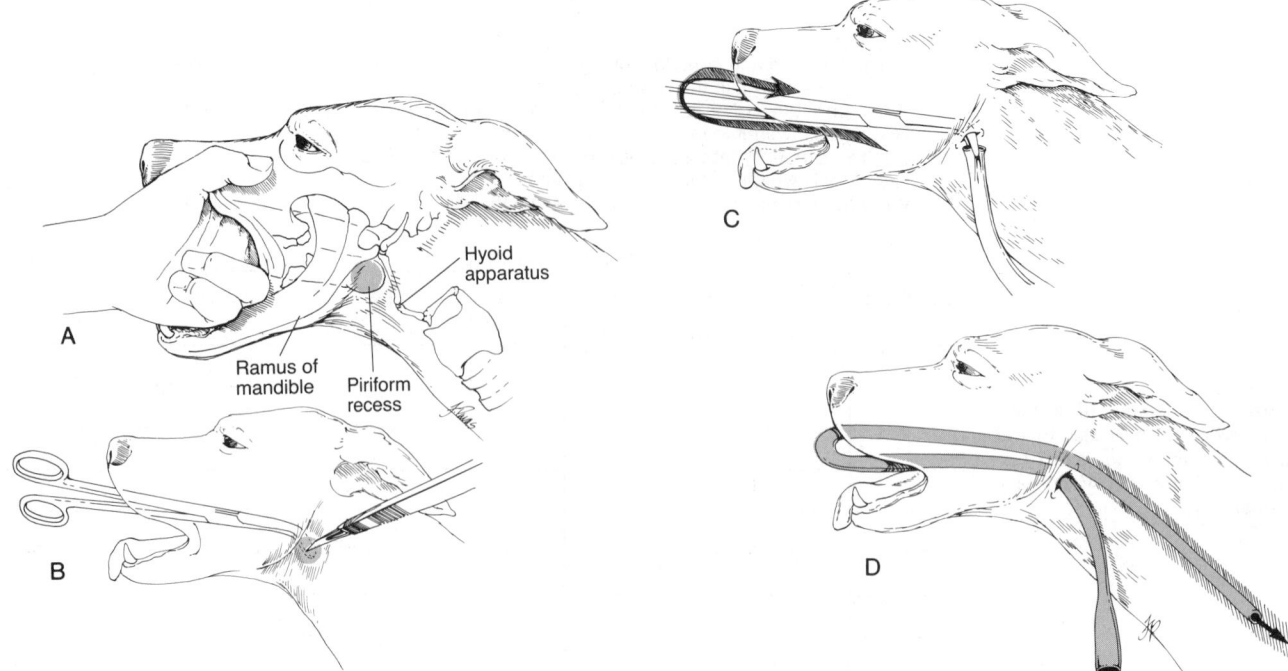

Figure 13. Placement of pharyngostomy tube. *A,* Palpation of piriform recess; *B,* make stab incision over tip of the hemostat; *C,* pull the feeding tube through the stab incision, and direct the tube down the esophagus (*D*).

esophagus. Examine the larynx to ensure proper placement of the tube (Fig. 13*D*).

10. Advance the tube to the level of the mid-to-caudal thoracic esophagus.

11. Secure the external portion of tube to the neck using the Chinese finger trap suture (see Chest Tube Placement, in this chapter).

12. Place a light bandage around the neck to help protect the tube, and place a cap in the end of the tube. A hypodermic needle cap may also be used.

Postoperative Care and Complications

- See Nasogastric Tube in this chapter for feeding instructions and complications of enteral feeding.
- Complications of pharyngostomy tube include hemorrhage due to trauma to the internal carotid artery, dislodgement of the tube due to the animal's intolerance, laryngeal irritation, gagging and coughing, and inadvertent placement into the trachea.

Percutaneous Endoscopic Gastrostomy (PEG) Tube

Indications

- See Indications for Nutritional Support for route.
- See Figure 10.
- To provide nutrition in patients in which the nasal passages, oral cavity, or esophagus is by-passed.
- To provide advantages over pharyngostomy tube including better animal tolerance of the device and fewer complications.

Objectives

- To allow access to the stomach for nutritional support
- To provide a leakage-free chronic indwelling gastric catheter

Equipment

- Endoscope
- Grasping forceps
- Bard urologic catheter (14 Fr. Pezzer mushroom-tip model)
- Indwelling catheter (14 gauge), needle (16 gauge) (Sovereign)
- Three-way stopcock
- Suture (Vetafil) 2-0 (2 ft.)
- #11 blades (2)
- 20 gauge × 1-inch needle
- 1¼-inch rubber tubing (2)
- 1-inch tape
- Cast padding (3-inch)
- Kling (3-inch)
- Vet Wrap (4-inch)
- Stockinette (cut to fit for "sweater")
- Scissors
- Hemostats
- Nolvasan

Technique

1. To prepare materials

   • Soak two 1¼-inch pieces of tubing in Nolvasan solution for at least 10 minutes prior to procedure.

TABLE 2. Manufacturers of Nutritional Devices and Dietary Products

Argyle Quest (A)*
1831 Olive
St. Louis, MO 63103
314/241-5700

Clintech Nutrition (A,B)*
Three Parkway North
Ste. 500
Deerfield, IL 60015
708/940-5000
800/323-5493

Corpak Company (A,B)*
160 West Hintz Road
Wheeling, IL 60090
312/537-4601
800/323-6305

ENtech, Inc. (A)*
8 Route 22 East
Lebanon, NJ 08833
201/236-6500

Kendall-McGaw Laboratories (A)*
2525 McGaw Avenue
Irvine, CA 92714
714/600-2147
800/854-6851

Mead Johnson
Nutritionals (B,D,E,F)*
2404 Pennsylvania St.
Evansville, IN 47721
812/426-6000

Navaco Laboratories (B,D,E,F)*
P.O. Box 23162
Phoenix, AZ 86063
602/269-1430
800/528-3358

O'Brien/KMI (B)*
320 Charles Street
Cambridge, MA 02141
617/868-6400
800/237-3535

Ross Laboratories (A,B,C,D,F)*
625 Cleveland Avenue
Columbus, OH 43216
614/227-4000

Sherwood Medical (A,B,D,E,F)*
1831 Olive Street
St. Louis, MO 63103
314/621-7788

Upjohn Pharmaceuticals (B)
P.O. Box 2034
2605 E. Kilgore
Kalamazoo, MI 49002
800/253-8600

Biosearch Medical Products (A,B)*
35 Industrial Parkway
Somerville, NJ 08876
201/772-5000
800/526-5976

Cook Critical Care (A)*
925 South Curry Pike
Bloomington, IN 47402
812/339-2235
800/457-4500

Davol Inc. (A)*
100 Sockanossett Crossroad
Cranston, RI 02920
401/463-7000

Ethox Corporation (A)*
251 Seneca Street
Buffalo, NY 14204-2088
716/842-4000
800/521-1022

Lederle Laboratories (B)*
North Middletown Road
Pearl River, NY 10965-1299
914/732-5000
800/533-3753

Medovations Inc. (A)*
102 East Keefe Avenue
Milwaukee, WI 53212
414/265-7620

Norwich Eaton
Pharmaceuticals, Inc. (B)*
P.O. Box 191
Norwich, NY 13815-0231
607/335-2111

Pet-Ag, Inc. (B)*
30W432 Rt. 20,
Elgin, IL 60120
708/741-3131

Sandoz Nutrition (B,D,E,F)*
5320 W. 23rd Street
Minneapolis, MN 55440
612/925-2100

Superior Healthcare Group (A)*
Nutrition Systems Division
Cumberland Industrial Park
Cumberland, RI 02864
401/333-6061

*A, tubes; B, feeding products; C, guidewires; D, carbohydrate modules; E, fat modules; F, protein modules.

- Using a #11 blade, cut an approximate 1 cm slice (stab) through the center of these tubing pieces
- Remove the distal tip (nipple) from the mushroom end to make an open-ended tube.

- Remove the flared end (opposite the mushroom end), and cut this end at a 60° angle.
- Place one of the 1¼-inch pieces of tubing over the gastrostomy tube and fit snugly up against the mushroom end (optional).

2. Place animal in right lateral recumbency, and insert endoscope.
3. Distend stomach with air using endoscope.
4. Locate skin incision site over the gastric fundus on the left side caudal to the last rib by pressing the finger and using the endoscope for visual guidance. Be sure the penetration site is far enough away from pylorus.
5. Insert an over-the-needle IV catheter through body wall into the distended stomach while viewing through the endoscope. Withdraw the needle, leaving the cannula in place in the stomach (Fig. 14 A).
6. Thread Vetafil suture material through the cannula into the stomach.
7. Using grasping forceps via the channel of the endoscope, grasp the Vetafil suture and withdraw the entire endoscope, along with the luminal end of the suture, out through the mouth (Fig. 14B). Continue holding the percutaneous end of the suture so that it remains in place through the body wall.
8. Withdraw the cannula from the animal's body wall while leaving the suture in place (Fig. 14C). Slide the cannula, narrow end first, over the suture coming out of the mouth (Fig. 14D).
9. Tie the end of the suture coming out of the mouth to the proximal end of the gastrostomy tube and pull the tube up into the end of the cannula to fit together snugly (Fig. 14E).
10. Lubricate the cannula and gastrostomy tube.
11. Pull the percutaneous end of the suture until the gastrostomy tube is pulled all the way out through the body wall and the mushroom end is up against the inside wall (mucosal surface) of the stomach (Fig. 14F).
12. Check the position with the endoscope.
13. Slide the other piece of 1¼-inch rubber tubing over the outside of the tube for a snug fit (not too tight) against the body wall (Fig. 14G).
14. Butterfly a 1-inch piece of tape around the PEG tube above small piece of rubber tubing to secure in place.
15. Put three-way stopcock on the end of the PEG tube, and put a light bandage around part of the tube to secure in place, leaving the end out for accessibility.
16. Put the stockinette sweater on the animal.

Postoperative Care and Complications

- See Nasogastric Tube in this chapter for feeding instructions and complications of enteral feeding.
- Allow 24 hours before beginning feeding.
- To remove the tube place moderate traction on the tube and cut the tube as close to the skin as possible.

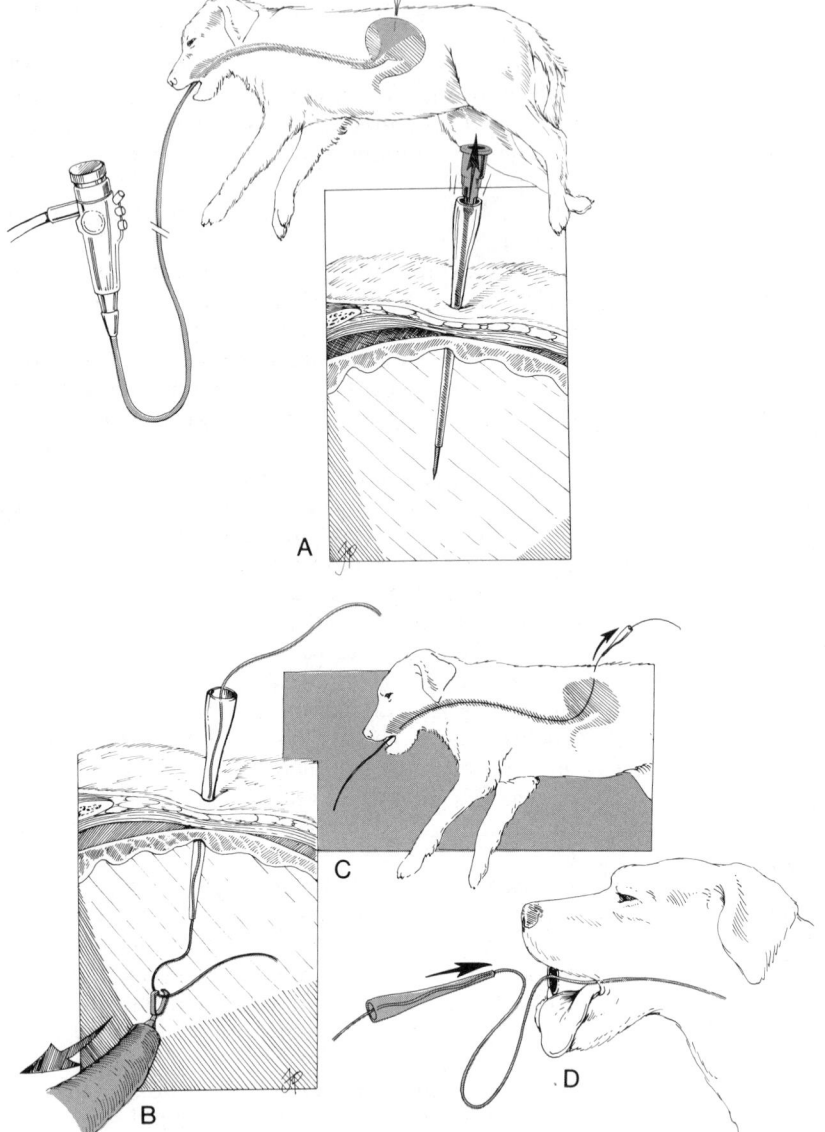

Figure 14. Placement of percutaneous endoscopic gastrostomy (PEG) tube. *A,* Over-the-needle catheter is placed through the skin and into the air-distended stomach; *B,* suture threaded through the catheter is grasped by endoscopic forceps and pulled out through the mouth (*C*); *D,* over-the-needle catheter is threaded onto the suture, which is tied to the gastrostomy tube

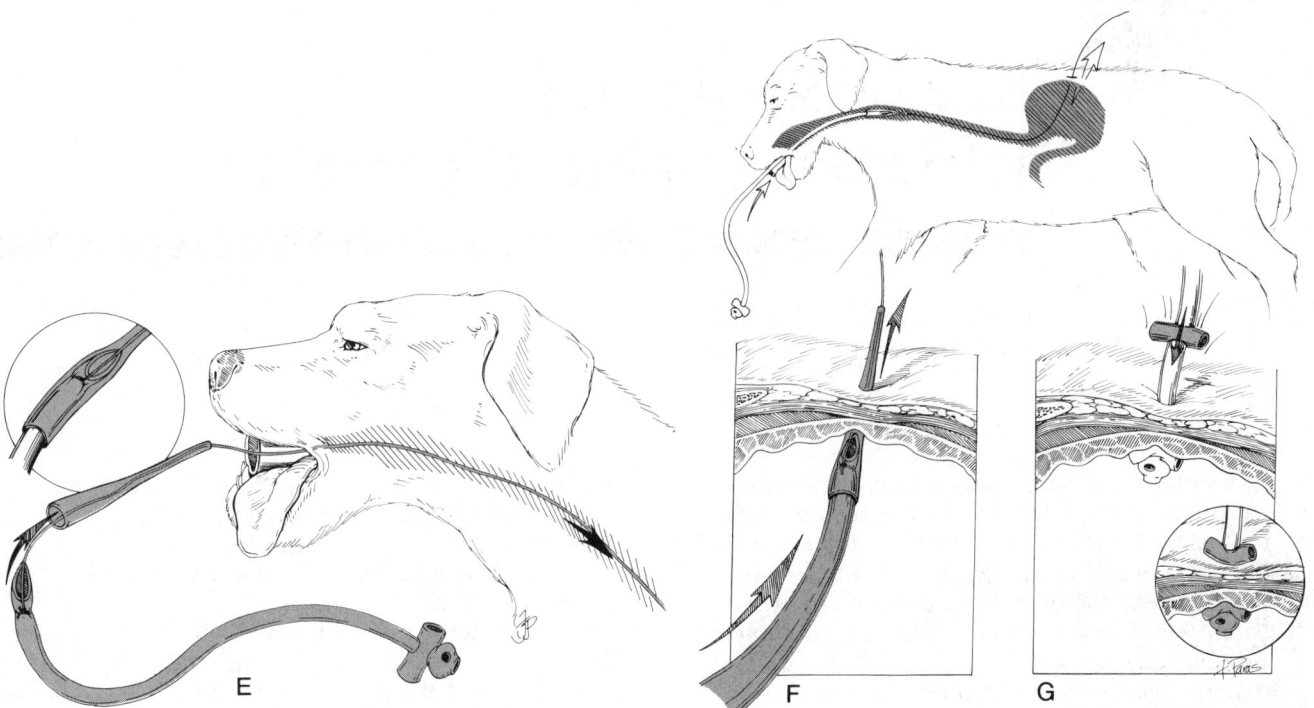

Figure 14 *Continued (E)* and subsequently pulled into the stomach and out the gastric and body wall. The flange at the end of the gastrostomy tube should press snugly against the gastric mucosa. See text for *F* and *G*.

Force the tip of the tube completely into the stomach using a cotton-tipped applicator. The tip eventually migrates down the intestinal tract and passes in the feces. In cats and small dogs, consider the endoscopic removal of the tip to prevent intestinal obstruction.

■ Complications of PEG tubes include mutilation of the tube by the animal; leakage of liquid diet intraperitoneally or subcutaneously (very rare using described technique); and obstruction of the pylorus, subsequent to the migration of the tip of the tube (also very rare).

Supplemental Readings

Abood SK, Buffington CA: Improved nasogastric intubation technique for administration of nutritional support in dogs. J Am Vet Med Assoc 199:577, 1991.

Crane SW: Diagnostic peritoneal lavage. *In* Kirk RW, ed.: *Current Veterinary Therapy IX*. Philadelphia: W.B. Saunders, 1986, p 3.

Grandage J: The oral cavity and pharynx. *In* Slatter DH, ed.: *Textbook of Small Animal Surgery*. Philadelphia: W.B. Saunders, 1985, p 639.

Nelson AW: Lower respiratory system. *In* Slatter DH, ed.: *Textbook of Small Animal Surgery*. Philadelphia: W.B. Saunders, 1985, p 1007.

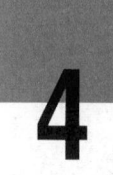

4 Radiographic and Ultrasonographic Techniques

David S. Biller
Paul R. Haider

The purpose of the radiograph is to provide a lasting record of maximum information. The sequence of the major operations involved in transforming the altered morphology and tissue density within a diseased animal into a two-dimensional, black-and-white radiograph and then reaching a diagnosis is complex and includes the following steps: (1) making a properly exposed and positioned radiograph; (2) recording the x-ray picture with the assistance of accessory equipment; (3) reviewing radiographs in proper conditions and in a systematic and detailed manner; (4) recognizing lesions—therefore (requiring) a knowledge of normal radiographic anatomy and its variation by age, species, and breed and the ability to recognize and understand artifacts; and (5) evaluating radiographic abnormalities with respect to clinical and laboratory findings.

Dr. Peter Suter

X-RAY MACHINE

mAs and kVp

- The *mA (milliamperage)* × *seconds (time)* = *mAs* affects the degree of blackness (density) of the radiograph with no effect on contrast. A direct relationship exists between mA and radiographic density. Time and mA both influence the number of x-rays produced but have no effect on the penetrating ability of the beam. To quickly check the adequacy of the mAs on a film, hold the film up to room light and place a white sheet of paper about 1 inch behind the film. Place a finger between film and paper. If the finger can be readily seen through the film in the black area (most exposed), the mAs needs to be increased.
- The *kVp (kilovolt peak)* is the only machine factor that influences radiographic contrast and has some control over the amount of radiographic density (blackness). The contrast can be expressed as being low, which means that there are many gray scales (long scale) between the extremes of black and white. The term high contrast means that there are few gray scales (short scale). Lowering the kVp increases the contrast, and raising the kVp reduces the contrast.
- mAs/kVp relationship

  - The mAs and kVp have to be in balance.
  - As mAs increases, kVp must decrease.
  - As kVp increases, mAs must decrease.
  - This adjustment keeps the density on the film at a constant level.
- To change density while in the 40- to 100-kVp range, the kVp may be increased or decreased by 10% to double or half the original film density. This change may also be accomplished by doubling or halving the mAs. To change density in the ≥100 kVp range, the kVp may be increased or decreased by 15% to double or half the original film density.

Recommendations

- The *300 mA machine* has adjustable mA stations of 25, 50, 100, 200, and 300 and two (1 and 2 mm or smaller) focal spots.
- An ideal kVp range of 40 to 120 that is adjustable in 1 or 2 kVp per step.
- A *timing device* is necessary to control the duration of an x-ray exposure. Modern x-ray machines have electronic timers with ranges that can control motion in the patient and prevent blurring. With a timed exposure of 1/120 second, all significant motion is stopped.
- The *line voltage compensator* is automatic or manual.
- The *tube stand* moves along the full length of the table and has an adjustable height from 0 to 60 inches (152 cm). The tube is able to rotate 90° around the vertical axis and 180° around the horizontal axis.
- The *table* is 5 to 6 feet in length with a top that has floating motion in four directions.
- The *collimator* at the region of interest decreases scatter radiation and increases film quality. A helpful guideline is to always leave a clear margin of collimation on every film. The collimator is lighted and has a centering mark. A high-quality, dial-adjustable, multileaf lead shutter collimator is highly recommended.
- The *filters* have the primary function of reducing patient radiation dose by removing scatter radiation and increasing (mean beam energy) quality. Most x-ray equipment has inherent filtration equal to 1.5- to 2.0-mm aluminum. Increased film quality can be obtained by adding an additional 2.0-mm aluminum filtration. Total filtration must be at least 2.5-mm aluminum.

■ The *grids* consist of a flat plate with a series of lead foil strips separated by transparent spacers. They are made in various sizes and improve the diagnostic quality of radiographs by absorbing the greater part of the scatter radiation. Grids are positioned between the patient and cassette, usually under the table, and generally are used only for body parts thicker than 10 cm. Reciprocating grid (Potter-Buckey diaphragm) includes a mechanism utilized to move the grid during exposure, in order to eliminate grid lines from the radiograph. This grid is optional equipment but recommended for the best quality radiographs.

Grids can be classified in two ways: the number of lines per inch and the ratio of lead strip height to the space between the lead strips. Generally, high-ratio grids absorb scatter better but are more expensive. More lines per inch gives better quality, because the lead strips are narrower and therefore lines become less prominent; however, they cost more. The most common grid is an 8:1 with 103 lines per inch.

A grid is not used with machines of less than 100 mA because the exposure is too prolonged and motion is a problem. Machines with mA of 100 to 300 use a grid with a ratio of 8:1 and a 40-inch focal film distance. Machines with 400 mA can use a grid of 10:1; 500 mA, a 12:1 grid; 800 mA, 15:1 grid. All have a focal film distance of 40 inches. More exposure mAs (not kVp) is needed when using a grid. The higher the grid ratio the more critical is the x-ray tube alignment. Always stay within the focal zone of the grid. This is usually written on the grid and is 36 to 42 inches in most instances.

■ The *exposure switches* include the two-position exposure switch on the console and two-position exposure foot switch, with a cord of sufficient length.
■ The *high-frequency x-ray machines* have a few advantages over single-phase x-ray machines. A 150-mA high-frequency generator can produce a quantity of x-rays equal to that of a 300-mA, single-phase x-ray machine. Many of the units can employ 110 voltage. They are reliable, with less down time than single-phase machines. Their cost, at present, is greater than that of single-phase machines but most likely will decrease in the future.
■ For a listing of X-ray machine manufacturers see Table 1.

ACCESSORY RADIOGRAPHIC EQUIPMENT

Screen

The screen is a suspension of phosphor crystals in a binder. The phosphor in the screen converts x-ray photons into visible light, to which the film is more sensitive. A latent image is created by exposure of the film to this light. This technique reduces x-ray exposure to the patient by at least 10 times and the time of x-ray exposure, thus decreasing the chance of blurring.

■ Screen speed is dependent upon the thickness of phosphor layer, size of phosphor crystals, and efficiency of phosphor crystals at absorbing x-rays and converting them to light.
■ Screen classification varies as each company has a slightly different system for labeling screen speed. Resolution ability of the screen is inversely related to speed. Increased speed gives decreased resolution. A technique chart must be available for each screen speed. Par speed is the starting point for comparison of screens. High speed has a speed two times that of par speed. Ultra (super) speed is four times par speed. High detail speed is half that of par speed.
■ Types of screens
  • Calcium tungstate screens reduce the amount of radiation necessary to expose film by 10 times. They are also less expensive than rare earth screens. Calcium tungstate emits a broad spectrum of light in the ultraviolet and blue range.
  • Rare earth screens are more expensive than calcium tungstate screens. The light emitted is a narrow spectrum in the green or blue range. The major advantage of rare earth over calcium tungstate screens is that rare earth screens are fast, because of a more efficient production of light. Therefore, they decrease the production of scatter, the exposure time, the radiation dosage, the chance of motion and subsequent blurring, and the wear and tear on the x-ray tube.
■ System speed is the speed of film and screen in combination. It is not an additive system. A very low system speed results when screens and films with different color spectrum sensitivities are put together. Ask the film dealer what speed system you have with your particular screens and film. The higher the system speed number, the more sensitive it is and the less radiation necessary to make an exposure. System speeds can vary from 50 to 3200 and higher. The higher the system speed number, the less radiation to the patient and to anyone within the room; however, the lower the system speed number, the better the resolution qualities. When

TABLE 1. X-Ray Machine Manufacturers

Summit Industries Inc. 2901 W. Lawrence Ave. Chicago, IL 60625 800/729-9729	X-ray Marketing Associates 1205 Lakeview Ct. Romeoville, IL 60441 800/325-8880
Dxeaco 1367 Sadlier Circle South Dr. Indianapolis, IN 46239 800/223-4173	Kramex Corp. 481 Sylvan St Saddle Brook, NJ 07662 201/845-5156
Universal/Allied Imaging Inc. 4014 W. Grand Ave. Chicago, IL 60651 312/276-4400	Control-X Inc. West Pointe Business Park 2289 W. Brooke Dr. Columbus, OH 43228 614/777-0476
Bennett X-ray Corp. 54 Railroad Ave. Copiague, NY 11726 516/691-6100	Trans-Continental X-Ray Corp. 2000 S. 25th Ave. Broadview, IL 60153 708/345-3050
Amrad 2020 North Janice Ave. Melrose Park, IL 60160 800/323-2213	Fischer Imaging 12300 North Grant St. Denver, CO 80241 303/452-6800

you know the system speed, changing the technique chart is simpler. If the system speed doubles, change the mAs on the technique chart by half. If the system speed decreases by 50%, double the mAs on the technique chart.

- Exposure time
  - Always use the shortest exposure times possible to eliminate blurring. For thoracic radiographs, exposure times of $\frac{1}{60}$ of a second or shorter stop the effects of respiratory and heart motion. For abdominal radiograph, employ exposure times of $\frac{1}{40}$ second or shorter in order to eliminate gastrointestinal motion. For an extremity radiograph, exposure times of $\frac{1}{20}$ second or shorter eliminate the effects of patient motion.
- Rare earth screens have a system speed that allows the shortest exposure times possible to eliminate motion problems and to lower radiation exposure to patient and personnel. Generally, when using a 300-mA machine, a 400 to 800 speed system with an 8:1, 103 lines per inch grid gives good quality radiographs of large breed dogs. With the table top, this system also is useful for small dogs and cats. In a feline practice, a slower system, such as 100 to 250 speed system, provides excellent quality. As the crystal size gets larger, the system gets faster but resolution is reduced.
- Clean screens with the product recommended by the manufacturer on a regular schedule (monthly) and whenever debris is noted on the radiographs.

Film

Radiographic film provides a permanent record containing the maximum amount of diagnostic information. Film is made of a light-sensitive emulsion, composed of gelatin and silver halide with other ingredients attached to a plastic (polyester) base. The silver halides are sensitive to light and change when exposed to light to produce a latent image. The process of developing changes silver ions into black silver, thus producing the radiographic image. Fixer removes all the unexposed silver from the film. The emulsion may be attached to one or both sides of the base. X-ray film may be divided into blue- or green-sensitive (orthochromatic) film, into different speeds, and into screen vs. nonscreen. Films vary in their contrast—some films appear more black and white after exposure and development. Use the film that is recommended by your screen manufacturer to match the spectrum of light produced by your screens. Choose a film that results in the contrast range that is most pleasing to you. Use a film that gives you a system speed that results in quality radiographs. Make sure to match films, screens, and processing chemicals.

Film must be sensitive to the type of light emitted by the screens in use. Film speed determines the amount of light required to produce an image on the radiograph. Fast film has large crystals (silver halide), requires less exposure, and produces a grainy image. Slow film has small crystals, requires greater exposure, and produces a less grainy or sharper-defined image.

Screen film is manufactured with crystals that are sensitive to fluorescent light. Nonscreen film is a direct exposure type film and is manufactured to be sensitive to x-rays. Nonscreen film requires ten to 25 times more radiation than screen film.

Film is available in both metric and nonmetric measurements. The most common sizes used in small animal practice are $8'' \times 10''$, $10'' \times 12''$, and $14'' \times 17''$.

X-ray film is sensitive not only to light and x-ray photons but also to humidity, chemicals, and physical stress. Film is stored on end to reduce pressure on the face of the film. High humidity causes film fogging, and low humidity causes film static; therefore, between 30 and 40% humidity is appropriate for film storage. Storage temperature should not exceed 50 to 70° F. Store the film away from developing chemicals and ionizing radiation. No undue pressure can be exerted on the film when loading or unloading film. Film and screen companies are provided in Table 2.

Cassettes and Miscellaneous Accessories

Cassettes are used primarily to contain and protect film. Two basic types are available: rigid cassettes that contain both the film and screen and cardboard cassettes that hold nonscreen film.

- Rigid cassettes protect both screens and film from physical damage and film from exposure to light. The cassette provides snug contact between the film and screens. The front of the cassette is usually a rigid plastic, aluminum, or other substance that absorbs relatively few x-ray photons. Usually, a small rectangle in the corner of the cassette acts to shield the film from x-rays to allow an unexposed area for film identification. The back of the cassette is lined with lead to absorb backscatter radiation. The back of the cassette is also equipped with latches to provide a lightproof seal.
- Cassette for a nonscreen film only protects the film from light exposure. It is usually made from cardboard.
- Cassettes are numbered. When defects are noted on a radiograph, they can be traced to the correct

TABLE 2. Film and Screen Companies

Eastman Kodak Company Health Sciences Division Rochester, NY 14650 800/926-1519	3 M Medical Imaging System 3 M Center Building 223-2S St. Paul, MN 55144-1000 612/733-1110
E. I. Du Pont De Nemours and Co., Inc. Medical Products Department Barley Mill Plaza Wilmington, DE 800/535-7605	Konica Medical Corporation 411 Newark Pompton Turnpike Wayne, NJ 07470 201/633-1500
Agfa Gavert Corp. 2803 Butterfield Rd. Suite 200 Oak Brook, IL 60521 708/593-8787	Picker International Inc. 595 Miner Rd. Highland Heights, OH 44143 216/473-3000
Fuji Medical Systems 90 Viaduct Rd. Stanford, CT 06907 800/431-1850	

TABLE 3. Radiographic Accessory Companies

Cone Instruments 5201 Naimen Parkway Solon, OH 44139 800/321-6964	Burkhart Roentgen, Inc. 3 River Rd. South Cornwall Bridge, CT 06754 800/872-9729
Wolf X-ray Corp. 420 Hempstead Turnpike West Hempstead, NY 11552 516/485-7000	Shielding International Inc. 182 Earl St. P. O. Box 578 Madras, OR 97741-0069 800/292-2247
Atomic Products Corp. P. O. Box 702 Shirley, NY 11967-0917 516/924-9000	Tab 1545 Waukegan Rd. Glenview, IL 60025 312/998-6150
Infab Corp. 3651 Via Pescador Camarillo, CA 93012 805/987-5255	Victoreen Inc. 100 Voice Rd. Carle Place, NY 11514-1593 516/741-6360
Bar-ray Products, Inc. 237 Twenty-fifth St. Brooklyn, NY 11232 718/965-7000	Medical I.D. Systems Inc. 3954 44th St. Grand Rapids, MI 49512 616/698-0535
Fischer Industries, Inc. P. O. Box 570 2630 Kaneville Ct. Geneva, IL 60134 800/356-5911	S. & S. X-ray Products Inc. 1101 Linwood St. Brooklyn, NY 11208 800/221-6634
Hale X-ray Company Inc. 222-224 E. 14th St. Cincinnati, OH 45210 513/241-4357	Picker International Inc. 595 Miner Rd. Highland Heights, OH 44143 216/473-3000

cassette. Dropping a cassette causes warping and results in poor film screen contact and a distorted radiographic image.

- Use the screen cleaner that is recommended by your screen manufacturer.
- Safety devices (lead aprons, lead gloves, glasses, and lead thyroid shield) are needed.
- Film markers consist of right and left lead film markers; Mitchell markers (for horizontal radiographs); and time markers (for upper gastrointestinal and intravenous urography radiographs).
- A device capable of measuring body part thickness and determining kVp for exposure is needed.
- Positioning devices include sponge wedges; sandbags; Plexiglas trough; rope; and tape.
- Film filing envelopes are needed.
- Contrast media including positive—barium suspension and iodinated agents—and negative—CO_2 (subject to availability).
- Monitoring devices (film badges) for employees and room monitoring and film viewer (at least one double bank) and hot light (high-intensity light) are needed.
- Radiographic accessory companies are listed in Table 3.

CHECKING X-RAY MACHINE ACCURACY

mA Station Check

An aluminum step wedge can be utilized to check mA station (setting) accuracy. Use the step wedge to determine if your mA stations are linear—it cannot determine if all your mA stations are off by the same amount. A step wedge gives a general idea about the mA stations. A step wedge is inexpensive ($100) and easy to use. Place the step wedge on a loaded cassette; make many separate exposures of the step wedge, changing mA but always having the same mAs and kVp. If you cannot keep the same mAs throughout all the mA stations, do as many as possible at one mAs setting then go back and check the rest at another mAs.

Example

25 mA	$\frac{1}{10}$ sec	2.5 mAs	70 kVp
50 mA	$\frac{1}{20}$ sec	2.5 mAs	70 kVp
100 mA	$\frac{1}{40}$ sec	2.5 mAs	70 kVp
300 mA	$\frac{1}{120}$ sec	2.5 mAs	70 kVp
100 mA	$\frac{1}{60}$ sec	1.7 mAs	70 kVp
200 mA	$\frac{1}{120}$ sec	1.7 mAs	70 kVp

Compare the densities of all exposures. They should be the same for all mA stations taken at the same mAs. An exposure that varies from the average shows that there is a problem with that mA station. This test does not tell you if all the mA stations are accurate, but it does tell you if a particular station has a problem. A digital electronic mA checking device is the most accurate way to compare your mA stations.

kVp Check

The only accurate way to check kVp is the Wisconsin test cassette ($1300). The Wisconsin test cassette has many kVp settings listed on the front of the cassette. Under each of these settings is a certain amount of material to attenuate the beam. After exposure and processing, this film provides information to determine if the kVp settings are accurate. Another less accurate way to obtain a general check of kVp accuracy is to vary mAs and kVp. Go through all the kVp settings employing density changing factors to keep the densities the same throughout all these exposures.

Example

100 mAs at 50 kVp
50 mAs at 55 kVp
25 mAs at 61 kVp
12.5 mAs at 67 kVp
6.2 mAs at 74 kVp
3.1 mAs at 81 kVp
1.5 mAs at 90 kVp
0.8 mAs at 99 kVp
0.4 mAs at 108 kVp
0.2 mAs at 124 kVp

If your mA stations and kVp settings are working correctly, these exposures have the same density but the contrast range of each is different. Remember to employ density changing factors when necessary.

Exposure Timer Check (Single-Phase Machine)

A spinning top test tool is needed. It can be purchased from the same company as the machine or from an accessory company. This tool is inexpensive ($50) and easy to use. It is a flat metal spinning top with a hole in one side. The top is set on a loaded cassette and spun. Take an exposure at $\frac{1}{120}$ second. Move the top over to another corner of the film, and spin again at $\frac{1}{60}$ second. This maneuver is repeated at $\frac{1}{40}$ and $\frac{1}{30}$ second. At $\frac{1}{120}$ second, only one dot should be seen; at $\frac{1}{60}$, two dots; at $\frac{1}{40}$, three dots; and at $\frac{1}{30}$, four dots. If more or less dots are on the film than expected, the timer is not accurate.

Line Voltage

Line voltage is the amount of current coming into the machine. This amount of current may vary, depending upon electrical wiring, consistency of voltage in the area, and usage of current on the same circuit in the particular practice. Almost all machines for small animal have a line voltage check device. Some have a meter and a dial to adjust line voltage and do not permit exposure until the voltage is manually adjusted. Other machines have an automatic line voltage adjustment. Almost all equipment in small animal practice utilizes 120 volts (i.e., right out of the socket).

FILM PROCESSING
Manual Processing

Film developing is a chemical process and is therefore dependent upon both time and temperature.

- Advantages
  - Less expensive set-up costs than those of automatic processor. Average set-up cost is $300 to $1000.
  - No special electrical or structural changes are necessary for the darkroom.
- Disadvantages
  - Valuable technician time is needed to develop films (i.e., increased labor costs).
  - Quality is not consistent, due to human error, compared with automatic processors.
  - Longer time needed to prepare diagnostic films compared with automatic processors..
- Accessories
  - Developing tanks
  - Two stirring paddles
  - Two thermometers
  - Film developing hangers of different sizes
  - Chemicals
  - Adjustable mixing valve for measuring water temperature
  - Timer
  - Dust-free drying cabinet or area
- Darkroom safelight must produce enough illumination in the darkroom so that a person can see to process radiographic film (load and unload cassettes) without unwanted density (fog) to the film. Safelights utilize a wavelength of light different from that to which the film is sensitive. A Wratten 6B filter is adequate for blue-sensitive film. A GBX-2 filter is employed with green-sensitive or both green- and blue-sensitive films. Usually, 15-watt bulbs are used with safelights. The safelight is about 4 feet away from the film-handling area. No system is 100% safe; therefore, expose the film no longer than necessary.

- A radiograph is a legal document and must therefore have permanent labeling. This labeling must include the hospital or veterinarian's name, the date the radiograph was taken, and the owner's name or animal's file number. The radiograph is also labeled with right or left, dorsovental/ventrodorsal (DV/VD), time marker on contrast studies, and Mitchell marker, when a horizontal beam is utilized. Basic types of permanent marking systems are available:
  - Lead letters and numbers in a holder with the hospital or veterinarian's name. Placed on the cassette during exposure.
  - Radiopaque marking tape (lead-impregnated tape). Information may be written on the tape and the tape is placed on the cassette prior to exposure.
  - A darkroom printer transfers data from a card to the corner of the x-ray film that was shielded from radiation during exposure. This system requires cassettes with special windows. The film is removed from the cassette, and the corner of the film where it was blocked from light exposure is imprinted by exposing the patient information on a 5″ × 7″ card onto the film.
- Silver recovery from fixer solutions by either manual or automatic systems is done. Fixer solutions may be sold to companies for silver recovery. Alternatively, you may purchase a system (metallic replacement process, electrolytic recovery, or chemical precipitation) for silver recovery in your practice. Exposed developed and undeveloped film may also be sold for silver recovery. Usually, the supplier of the x-ray films or processing solutions can be consulted, to determine if silver recovery is feasible and who to contact.
- Procedure for manual film processing
  - Check temperatures, turn off room lights, use safelights, and agitate (mix) solutions well.
  - Place the film on development hangers, making sure all four corners are attached.
  - Set and start time, depending upon the temperature in the developing tank.
  - Place the hanger with the film into the developing tank. Rap hard against the tank wall to dislodge air bubbles. Agitate by pulling film out of the developer, and let the developer drain to one lower corner. Return film to the developer. Repeat agitation every minute. Manufacturers recommend a specific temperature for the developed solution that they produce, usually 68°F (20°C). Adjust for change in temperature (increased temperature, decreased time and vice versa). The place of purchase for chemicals can provide a time temperature development chart.

Example

60°F	8.5 minutes
65°F	6.0 minutes
68°F	5.0 minutes
70°F	4.5 minutes
75°F	3.5 minutes

- At the end of the developing time, remove the hanger from the developer and drain over rinse tank. Agitate film in rinse water for 30 seconds.

- Place the hanger with film in fixer at the end of developing time.
- Set the timer—fixer time equals twice the development time.
- Agitate film every 2 to 3 minutes while in the fixer.
- At the end of fixation time, remove film from fixer and drain.
- Place the hanger in wash water at the end of fixer time.
- Agitate after 2 to 3 minutes.
- Wash for 15 to 30 minutes, depending upon water flow and temperature in wash tank.
- No less than four water changes per hour in the wash tank are recommended.
- At the end of the wash, remove from water and drain.
- Place film in drier cabinet or hang up to dry.

Automatic Processing

- Processors are a good investment for most veterinary practices. New, small, table top models are priced from $3500. Most of these processors develop an excellent quality film in 90 to 210 seconds. They can use cold water for processing; therefore, no special needs exist for plumbing. They are also easy to maintain. If your small animal practice is processing seven to ten films a day, consider an automatic processor.
- Advantages
  - Highly repeatable results
  - Short waiting time for diagnostic films
  - Ability to process large quantity of films quickly and accurately
  - Good quality control
  - Smaller dark room necessary
- Disadvantages
  - Machine is expensive.
  - Darkroom structural changes are expensive.
  - Needs daily and weekly maintenance.
  - Repairs can be expensive.
- Equipment includes processor, safe light, water for processing, chemicals, sponges to clean rollers of processor, and processor cleaning solution.
- Table top film processors are easy to install. Need no special plumbing or wiring. Different models process films as fast as 90 seconds or as long as 3½ minutes. Most are made for easy care and cleaning. They are relatively inexpensive (from $3000 to $7000).
- Large, hard-wired, 90-second film processors need special plumbing and electrical wiring, but they are able to process large quantity of films. They need special cleaning and repairs and are expensive ($15,000 to $25,000).
- The more a processor is used, the less problems it will have. It is made to be used on a 24-hour basis. Chemical buildup on rollers can cause film artifacts. Rollers age and crack, if oxidized chemicals are left on them.
- Clean processors often.
  - Any processor needs cleaning daily when not in use. Take out the rollers and wash down with a sponge and water. Dry and replace rollers. Clean chemical tanks. Once a month, clean with proces-

TABLE 4. Automatic Processors Companies

AFP Imaging Corp. 250 Clearbrook Rd. Elmsford, NY 10523 800/592-6666	JNO. V. Doehren Co. 1450 N. McLean Blvd. Elgin IL 60123 708/931-0075
Agfa Gavert Corp. 2803 Butterfield Rd. Oak Brook, IL 60521 414/274-9116	Konica Medical Corp. 411 Newark Pompton Turnpike Wayne, NJ 07470 201/633-1500
All Pro Imaging Corp. 70 Cantiague Rock Rd. P. O. Box 870 Hicksville, NY 11802 516/433-7676	Kramex Corp. 481 Sylvan St. Saddlebrook, NJ 07662 201/845-5156
Eastman Kodak Co. Health Sciences Division Rochester, NY 14650 800/926-1519	Picker International 595 Miner Rd. Highland Heights, OH 44143 216/473-3000
Fischer Industries Inc. 2630 Kaneville Ct. Geneva, IL 60134 708/232-2803	

sor cleaning solution. Cleaning a processor takes about 15 minutes a day but saves in wasted film and time.
- Check to see if standby set up is available on the processor you wish to purchase. This function helps to conserve water, energy, and chemicals.
- Automatic processor companies are given in Table 4.

Darkroom

Recommendations

- Darkroom location. Close to water and drains for plumbing purposes: close to radiographic area to reduce unnecessary walking and to increase efficiency.
- Basic darkroom layout (Figs. 1 and 2). Darkrooms do not have to take up much room but are at least 6 by 8 feet. Many darkrooms are located where a bathroom might have been located. This eliminates the process of bringing in new plumbing and electrical outlets. Try to include a sink for cleaning up and processor maintenance. Keep wet and dry areas separate to eliminate contamination of screens and unexposed film by chemicals. Always have good ventilation to keep heat, humidity, and chemical fumes from destroying film and to reduce exposure of personnel to chemical fumes. Paint all walls white to reflect light from the safelights and for a brighter working environment. Use an adequate number and type of safelights. Make sure all the safelights are 40 inches from the working area to prevent film fogging.

TECHNIQUE CHARTS

One needs to have a working knowledge of equipment (tube rating charts and anode cooling curves). Always select the shortest possible exposure times.

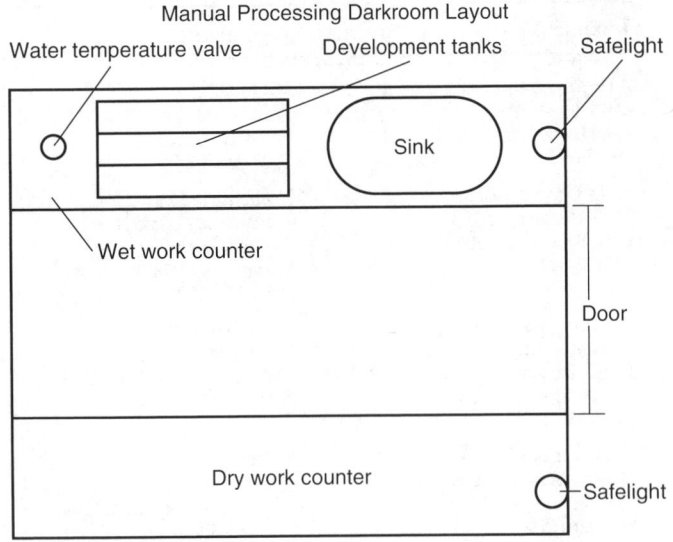

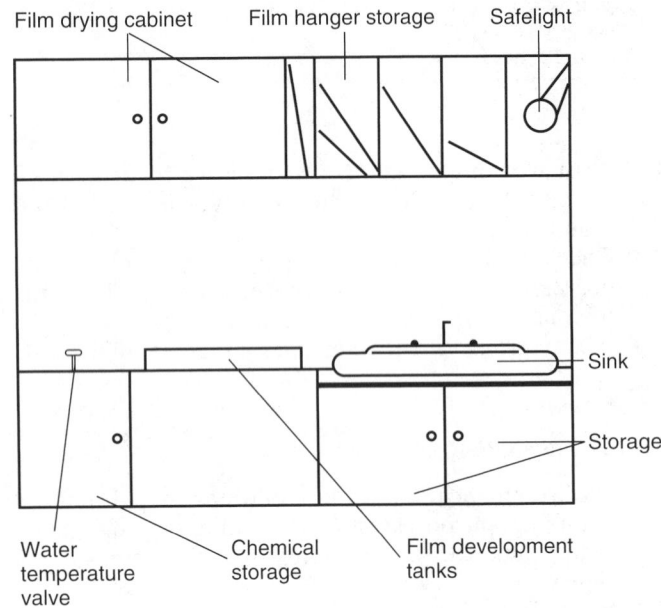

Figure 1. Floor plan for a darkroom using manual (wet tank) processing.

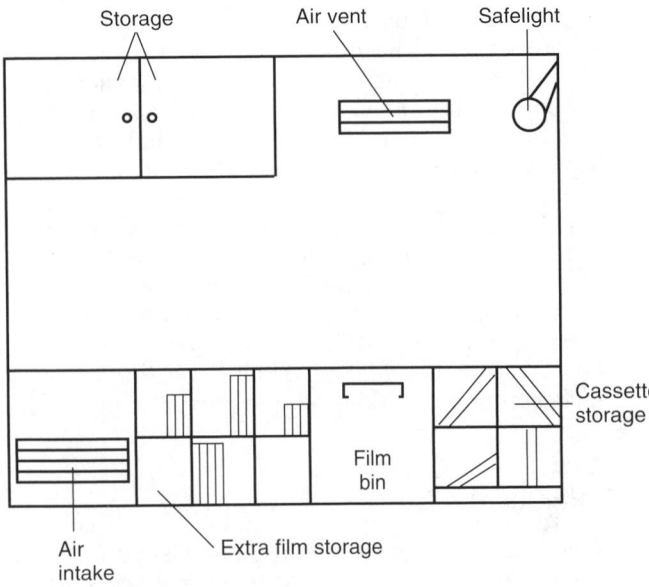

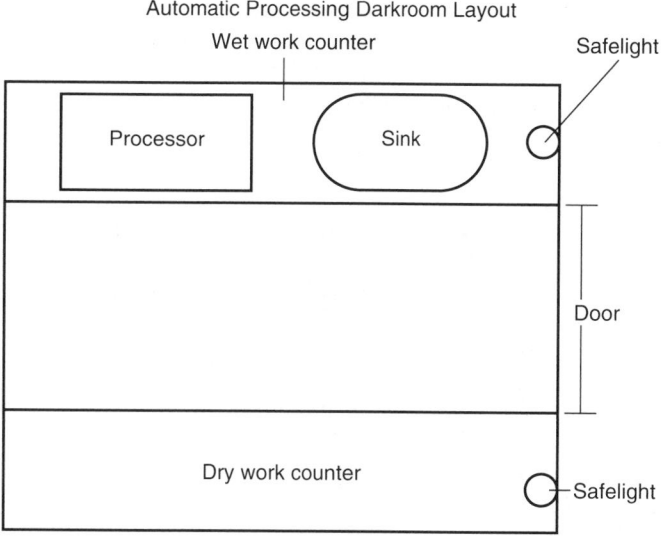

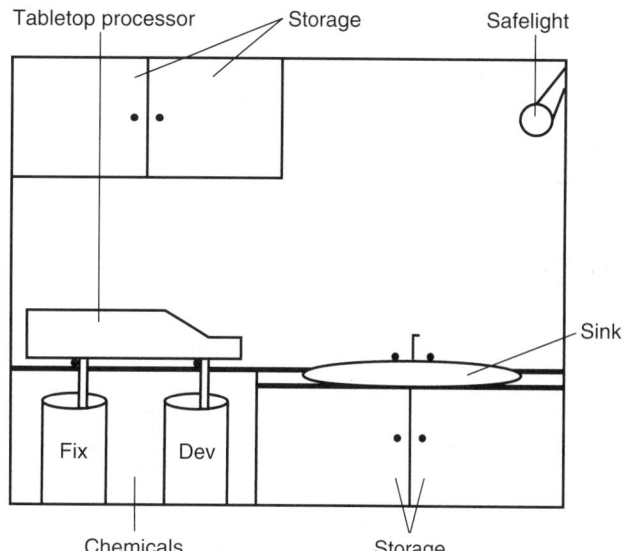

Figure 2. Floor plan for a darkroom using automatic processing.

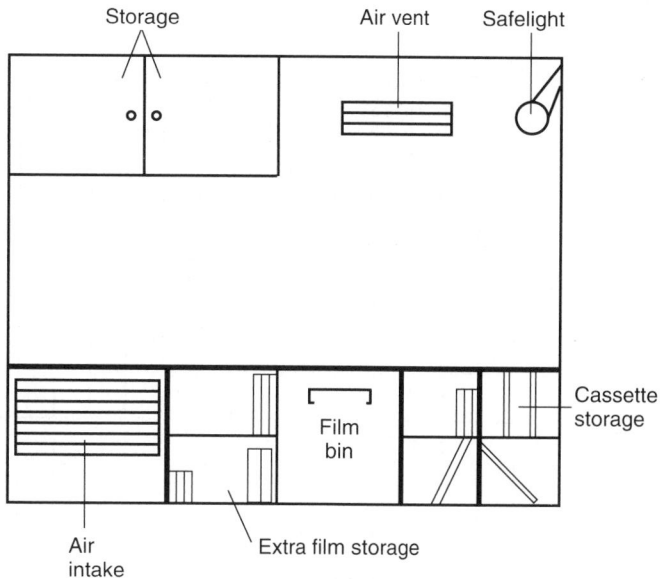

This entails the highest mA value to achieve the shortest exposure times. A constant focal film distance is recommended. The same film, screens, and darkroom technique are utilized.

Technique Chart (Figure 3)

- Thorax-grid
  - Use a dog of average size and body condition for all measurements.
  - Take a lateral measurement across the chest at the widest point.
  - Find that measurement on your technique chart.
  - Underneath this lateral measurement, set your kVp at 95—a value in the middle of the ideal kVp parameters for a thorax.
  - Fill out your chart according to the kVp per cm increments.
  - Once the kVp values have been assigned, take three chest films at different mAs values. You may begin with 0.8, 1.6, and 3.2 for a rare earth system, and 5, 10, and 20 mAs for calcium tungstate, for example. Select the mAs value at 95 kVp that provides you with the best technique.

- Abdomen-grid
  - Follow the first four steps under Thorax Grid.
  - Set your kVp at 85.
  - Fill out the chart according to the kVp per cm increments.
  - Double the mAs value for the thorax technique.
- Spine-grid
  - Follow the first four steps under Thorax Grid.

- Set your kVp at 65.
- Fill out the chart according to the kVp per cm increments.
- Set the mAs value at a number four times that value for the abdomen. This section also works for femur, humerus, shoulder, and pelvis.
- Thorax, abdomen, and spine-table top (Figure 4)
  - On the grid chart for thorax, abdomen, and spine, find the last kVp setting for 11 cm.
  - Decrease the kVp as the thickness decreases. For example, if 74 kVp is at 11 cm, use 72 kVp at 10 cm, 70 kVp at 9 cm, and so forth.
  - Adjust the mAs by reducing to half (possibly more dependent upon type of grid) the mAs value for the base techniques for the thorax, abdomen, and spine. If films are still overexposed, reduce the mAs in half again.
- Extremity chart-table top see Figure 4
  - Measure a normal dog carpus. The average is 4 to 5 cm.
  - Underneath that measurement, set your kVp at 60 (a value in the middle of your ideal kVp parameters for extremities).
  - Fill out the chart, according to the kVp per cm increments.
  - Take films at three different mAs values (0.8, 1.6, and 3.2 with rare earth, and 5, 10 and 20 with calcium tungstate). Continue selecting mAs values until an appropriate exposure has been made. Your table top extremity chart is now complete. Employ this chart for all extremities distal to and including the elbow and stifle.

Making of a Technique Chart (Grid)

Ideal Parameters	kVp per cm Increments		Appreciable Difference
Thorax — 90 to 100 kVP Abdomen — 80 to 90 kVp Spine Skull — 60 to 80 kVp Pelvis Extremities — 50 to 70 kVp	40 to 80 range = 2 kVp per cm 80 to 100 kVp range = 3 kVp per cm ≥100 kVp = 4 kVp per cm		Amount of kVp change necessary to see a change in technique per kVp range 40 - 60 kVp = 2 - 4 kVp 60 - 80 kVp = 4 - 6 kVp 80 - 100 kVp = 6 - 8 kVp ≥100 kVp = 10 - 12 kVp
	Chart Factors		
	Thorax ___ mAs ___ kVp base technique Abdomen - 2 X thoracic mAs, minus 10 kVp Spine - 4X abdomen mAs, minus 20 kVp		

Thorax	11	12	13	14	15	16	17	18	19	20	21	22	23	24	25	26	27	28	29	30	cm
																					kVp
																					mAs

Abdomen	11	12	13	14	15	16	17	18	19	20	21	22	23	24	25	26	27	28	29	30	cm
																					kVp
																					mAs

Spine Skull Pelvis	11	12	13	14	15	16	17	18	19	20	21	22	23	24	25	26	27	28	29	30	cm
																					kVp
																					mAs

Figure 3. Technique chart to use with a grid.

Table Top Technique Chart
(Without Grid)

Thorax _____ mAs

1	2	3	4	5	6	7	8	9	10	cm
										kVp

Abdomen _____ mAs

1	2	3	4	5	6	7	8	9	10	cm
										kVp

Spine ⎫
Skull ⎬ _____ mAs
Pelvis ⎭

1	2	3	4	5	6	7	8	9	10	cm
										kVp

Extremities _____ mAs

1	2	3	4	5	6	7	8	9	10	cm
										kVp

Figure 4. Technique chart. For table top exposures, take the Buckey grid technique and reduce mAs by 50 to 75%. Continue kVp down from Buckey chart.

- For the nonscreen film technique chart, the mAs in your technique chart may vary up or down from the example (Fig. 5).
- The technique chart is set up to take radiographs of normal animals. Different animals may have the same lateral thoracic measurement but different body types (obese, emaciated). The emaciated animal may be overexposed with the technique from the chart, therefore, you need to decrease the exposure (kVp). The obese animal may be underexposed following the chart technique, therefore, you have to increase the exposure (kVp).
  - The technique may need to be increased (2 to 30%) for numerous reasons, e.g., obesity, pregnancy, ascites, pleural effusion, disease processes that increase lung opacity (e.g., pneumonia and atelectasis), and positive contrast studies.
  - The technique may need to be decreased (2–30%) for numerous reasons, including emaciation, pneumothorax, emphysema, gastric dilatation, and volvulus.

POSITIONING AND TECHNIQUE

Measuring for Radiographic Studies

- Measure all animals standing
- Measurements for thorax, abdomen, and thoracolumbar spine are all taken at the same place on the animal. Observe the back of the animal from above, looking for the widest point across the ribs and take a lateral measurement. The DV/VD measurement is made at the same point. The widest point is usually over the thoracolumbar junction.
- Measurements for the pelvis are taken across the wings of the ilium. This is a very accessible area to measure, giving highly repeatable results.
- Extremities are measured at the widest point.
- Make sure all personnel measure all areas at the same point, or the technique will vary from one study to the next.

Thorax

Thorax is taken at full inspiration. Film includes diaphragm to thoracic inlet. In a large dog, this may take two radiographs for both lateral and DV/VD. Short exposure times of 1/60 second or less compensate for cardiac and respiratory motion. High kVp, low mAs technique increases latitude (increased shades of gray).

- For the lateral (right or left) measurement, elevate the sternum to the same plane as the spine. Pull the animal's legs cranially to reduce soft tissue over the cranial thorax. Include the sternum, and take the radiograph during peak inspiration (Fig. 6).
- For the DV/VD, the sternum is superimposed over the spine. Center the beam at the caudal border of the scapula; center the beam on the spine. Take the radiograph during peak inspiration. VD radiographs are preferable to DV for evaluation of the accessory lung lobe and the caudal mediastinum. DV radiographs are preferred if evaluation of the caudal pulmonary vessels is important. The dog's disposi-

Figure 5. Technique chart to use with nonscreen film. Use a lateral measurement across the skull to set technique. Always use 50 kVp for the best contrast.

Kodak X-omat TL Nonscreen Technique Chart Using a 30-inch Focal Film Distance

Nasal, Dental, and High Detail Studies

1	2	3	4	5	6	7	8	9	10	11	cm
50	100	125	150	200	250	300	350	400	450	500	mAs

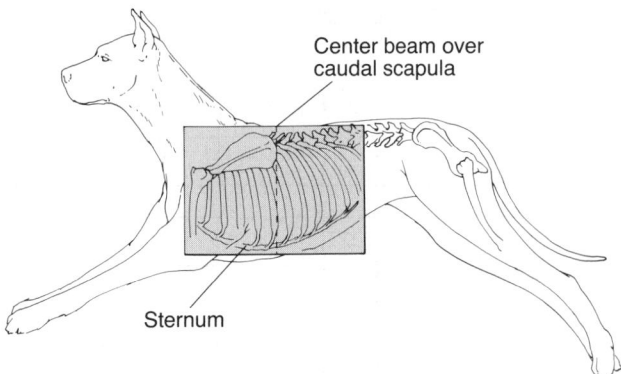

Figure 6. Positioning for lateral thoracic radiograph.

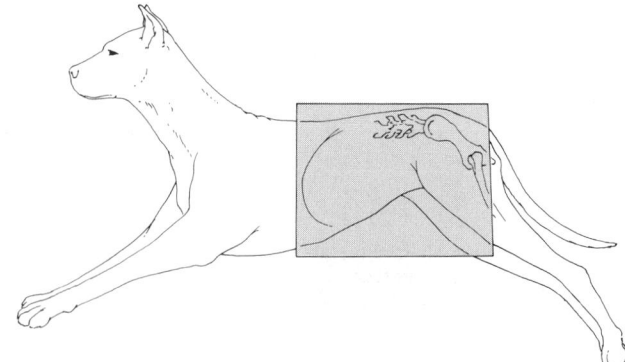

Figure 8. Positioning for lateral abdominal radiograph.

tion, clinical status (heart failure, pulmonary edema, pleural effusion), or position of previous radiographs help choose between VD and DV thoracic radiographs (Fig. 7).

Abdomen

For the abdomen, ideally, food is withheld from the animal for at least 12 hours. The animal is encouraged to defecate and urinate prior to being radiographed. Radiographs include the diaphragm to the pelvic canal. Measure over the widest portion of the abdomen (costal arch). Use ¼₀ second or less to reduce motion; use a kVp in the 70 to 90 range for maximum latitude.

- For a lateral (right or left), the legs are pulled caudally but not enough to stretch the abdominal musculature taut. Place the edge of the cassette 1 to 2 inches cranial to the xiphoid and the cranial edge of the acetabulum. Palpate the greater trochanter. Take the radiograph at peak expiration (Fig. 8).
- The VD/DV is the same as that for lateral abdomen (Fig. 9).
- Horizontal beam is used to check for free abdominal air. Animal is placed in left lateral recumbency for

10 minutes prior to radiography. Air is demonstrated around the right liver lobes. The technique is similar to the vertical beam technique in that distance remains at 40 inches. Remember to reduce the mAs if a grid is not used.

- A wooden spoon can be used to compress the abdomen for separation of structures. The spoon can separate the colon from the urinary bladder to demonstrate the uterus, for example. Remember to reduce the kVp, because you are decreasing the thickness of the tissue being radiographed.

Extremities

For radiography of the extremities, the animal needs a clean, dry, hair coat. Splints and bandages are removed if possible. The limb to be radiographed is placed closest to the film. Employ a high mAs and low kVp (50 to 70) technique to produce high-contrast radiographs. Collimate closely. Table top (nongrid) techniques are utilized on parts less than 10 cm-thick. Anesthesia or tranquilizers are provided whenever possible. Use positioning devices. The part to be radiographed is measured over the thickest area. If the part thickness varies greatly, two exposures (e.g.,

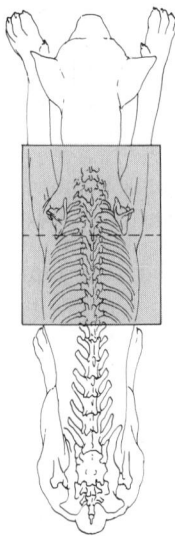

Figure 7. Positioning for dorsoventral (DV) or ventrodorsal (VD) thoracic radiograph.

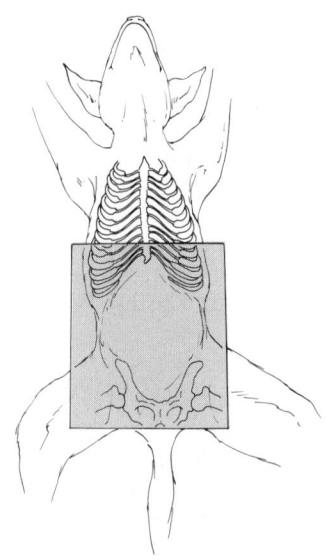

Figure 9. Positioning for ventrodorsal (VD) abdominal radiograph.

lateral pelvis and femur) may be necessary. In the case of moderate variation, choose the greater measurement to set the exposure and "hot light" the slightly over-exposed areas on the film. When long bones are being radiographed, the joints proximal and distal are included. Never hesitate to make a film of the opposite limb for comparison.

Scapula and Shoulder Joint

- Caudocranial. The animal is in dorsal recumbency, with the sternum rotated away from the side being radiographed. The leg is fully extended. Center the x-ray beam mid scapula. For the shoulder joint, center the beam at the point of flexion for the joint.
- Mediolateral (ML). The animal is in lateral recumbency, with the down side to be radiographed. The leg is extended about 45° from the vertebral column. The opposite leg is flexed and placed over the thorax. Pull the head and neck back so that the cervical spine and trachea are not overlapping the joint space.

Humerus

- Caudocranial. The animal is in dorsal recumbency, with the legs extended. The sternum is rotated away from the side being radiographed. Center the x-ray beam at the mid humerus. Radiograph includes both the shoulder and elbow joints.
- Mediolateral. The animal is positioned similar to that of the ML view of the scapula and the shoulder joint. The x-ray beam is centered mid humerus. The radiograph includes both shoulder and elbow joints.

Elbow Joint

- Craniocaudal. The animal is in sternal recumbency, with the elbow joint in full extension. If the elbow cannot be completely extended, the x-ray beam is angled 10° to 20°, craniodistal to caudoproximal.
- Mediolateral. The animal is in lateral recumbency, with the elbow slightly flexed. The opposite leg is pulled caudally. Center the beam on the palpable medial epicondyle. The elbow is in extreme flexion, if visualization of the anconeal process is of importance.
- Craniolateral caudomedial oblique. This aids in visualization of the lateral aspect of the medial coronoid.

Antebrachium

- Craniocaudal. Place the animal in sternal recumbency. Extend the leg and position the elbow for a true craniocaudal projection. The film includes both elbow and carpus.
- Mediolateral. The animal is in lateral recumbency, with the leg in the neutral position. Move the opposite limb caudally; center the beam on the midshaft radius. It may be easier to obtain the radiograph if the elbow is slightly flexed. The elbow and carpal joint are included on film.

Carpus/Metacarpus

- Dorsopalmar (DP). By convention, positional terms change from cranial and caudal to dorsal and palmar distal to the radius. The animal is placed in sternal recumbency, with the extremity extended. Allow the elbow to abduct slightly so that the carpus is in true DP view. The x-ray beam is centered on the carpus or metacarpus.
- Mediolateral. The animal is placed in lateral recumbency, with the affected leg down. The carpus is slightly flexed; the x-ray beam is centered on the carpus. A lateral view of the metacarpus is often unrewarding.
- Oblique views. The animal is placed in sternal recumbency, with the carpus/metacarpus in DP. Rotate the extremity 45° in both directions for the two oblique views (dorsolateral to palmar medial oblique and dorsomedial to palmar lateral oblique).

Digits

- DP. The paw is placed flat against the cassette.
- ML. The animal is in lateral recumbency. The specific digit to be examined is pulled dorsally with tape.

Pelvis

Tranquilization may be necessary for routine VD and lateral radiographs. General anesthesia is necessary for Orthopedic Foundation for Animals (OFA) hip dysplasia films.

- Ventrodorsal extended hip. The animal is in dorsal recumbency, with the legs extended. The pelvis is straight; the femurs are parallel and as close to the cassette as possible. Patellas are superimposed over the distal femurs. The x-ray beam is centered on the hip joints. Stifles are included on the radiographs. Legs are the same distance apart as the acetabula.
- Lateral. The animal is in lateral recumbency, with the dependent leg pulled cranially. The nondependent leg is elevated with a foam block parallel to the table top.
- Lateral oblique. The animal is placed in lateral recumbency. A foam wedge is placed to elevate the dorsal aspect of the pelvis approximately 20°. Push the upper leg proximally to rotate.
- Ventrodorsal flexed hip (frog-legged position). The animal is in dorsal recumbency, and the femurs are flexed and abducted so that the stifles are lateral to the abdomen. The femurs are placed at an angle of 45° to the spine.

Femur

- Craniocaudal. The animal is in dorsal recumbency or in erect sitting position, and the leg is extended. The x-ray beam is centered at mid femur. Hip and stifle are included on the radiograph. Measurement is made at the proximal femur.
- Mediolateral. The animal is in lateral recumbency with the leg to be examined on the cassette. The opposite leg is abducted and rotated out of the x-ray beam's path. The x-ray beam is centered mid femur. Hip and stifle are included on the film.

Stifle

- Caudocranial. The animal is in ventral recumbency with the leg to be examined pulled caudally into maximum extension. In large dogs, the x-ray beam is angled 15° caudodistal to cranioproximal. The x-ray beam is centered at the joint space.

■ Mediolateral. Position is like that for the lateral femur, with the x-ray beam centered on the joint space. Usually, the tarsus is away from the cassette so you need to place a foam wedge under the hip and femur.

Tibia/Fibula

■ Caudocranial. Position is like that for a caudocranial stifle. The x-ray beam remains vertical and centered mid tibia. Stifle and tarsus are included on the film.

■ Mediolateral. The patient is in lateral recumbency with the tibia and fibula on film.

Tarsus

■ Dorsoplantar. The animal is placed in dorsal recumbency. The leg is extended, and the x-ray beam is centered at the proximal intertarsal joint.

■ Mediolateral. The patient is placed in lateral recumbency. The tarsocrural joint is slightly flexed. The x-ray beam is centered at the proximal intertarsal joint.

■ Oblique (45°). Dorsolateral to palmar medial oblique (DLPMO) and dorsomedial to palmar lateral (DMPLO) oblique. The animal is positioned in dorsal recumbency then rotated 45° in each direction (lateral and medial) for the two obliques.

Metatarsus/Digits

Position is just like that for metacarpus and digits of forelimbs.

Spinal Positioning and Technique

■ Materials needed include sandbags, foam wedges, markers (right and left), and Plexiglas trough to aid in positioning the animal without anyone in the room.

Technique

1. Use general anesthesia or heavy sedation in all but the most subdued animals. Exceptions are suspected fracture, congenital malformation with instability, and other diseases in which the animal's condition or protective mechanisms that have maintained stability will be compromised.

2. Short-scale, high-contrast (high mAs, low kVp) technique provides good detail. Use a grid and collimate to include only the spine.

3. *Positioning cervical spine, lateral view.* For radiography, the spine must be parallel to the cassette. In many cases, it is necessary to support the center of the neck with radiolucent positioning blocks (sponges). Place the head in a normal position (neither flexed nor extended) relative to the neck. The head must be lateral because it controls the position of the proximal neck. Pull the front legs back over the thorax to allow a thinning of the tissues over the caudal neck. The thorax must be in the accurate lateral position because it controls the position of the caudal neck. Extending the entire

neck may help open up the caudal cervical disc spaces. Both occipital and cervicothoracic areas are included on the radiograph.

Ventrodorsal view. The spine is not parallel to the cassette because of the anatomic variation between the head and thorax. The spine inclines away from the cassette at the thorax. The head is in a normal position (hard palate and dorsal nose at 60° angle to the cassette). If the head is in a true VD position, an undesirable arch is produced in the cervical spine. The mid plane of the head and thorax must be perpendicular to the cassette. Tilting the x-ray tube ventrocaudal to dorsocranial at approximately 10 to 20° permits visualization of the intervertebral disc spaces.

4. *Thoracolumbar spine, lateral view.* The mid plane of the entire body must be parallel to the cassette. Most animals must have the sternum elevated for good lateral views of the spine. Straightness may be accomplished by placing tension on the spine by pulling the front legs cranially and the rear legs caudally. Extending the entire neck may help open up the cranial thoracic disc spaces.

Ventrodorsal view. The mid plane of the entire spine must be perpendicular to the cassette. When the dorsal spines are prominent as in thin animals, radiolucent positioning blocks may be beneficial. The body may be held by placing tension on the legs.

■ Survey Spinal Radiography—general principles
  • At least two radiographic views of the area of interest are needed: lateral and ventrodorsal. Specific situations occur in which the VD projection in the noncontrast study provides the most useful view for the diagnosis. These include (1) a productive or destructive lesion that involves the transverse vertebral process of the lumbar segments or the costovertebral articulations; (2) a destructive process that involves the dorsal articular processes caudal to the anticlinal vertebral segment; (3) a malalignment characterized by lateral shifting of the vertebral segments; and (4) a rotation of the vertebral segments that is easier to detect on the VD view because of the abnormal appearance of the prominent oval shadow cast by the dorsal spinous process.
  • In the average-size dog, five vertebral segments can be adequately evaluated per film. Because of the divergence of the x-ray beam, all areas of interest have to be centered to evaluate intervertebral disc spaces.
  • Poor patient positioning and radiographic quality commonly occur when animals are not anesthetized or heavily sedated. Many radiographic lesions can be obscured by poor technique. Conversely, a normal structure can be falsely identified as a lesion.
  • Ideal spinal survey studies are listed in Table 5.

Skull Radiograph

Technique

1. General anesthesia or deep tranquilization of the patient is essential, if not specifically contraindicated

TABLE 5. Spinal Survey Studies

| | Centering | |
Study	Lateral	Ventrodorsal
Cervical spine	C3–4	C3–4
	C6–T1	(X-ray beam angled 15° ventrocaudal to dorsocranial)
Occipitoatlantoaxial (Rostrocaudal open mouth to visualize the dens)	C1	C1
	C1 flexion	
	C1 oblique	
Thoracic spine	T6–7	T6–7
Thoracolumbar spine	T6–7	T6–7
	T12–13	T12–13
	L3–4	L3–4
Lumbar spine	L3–4	L3–4
	L-S	
Lumbosacral spine	L-S flexion	L-S
	L-S extension	
Post-trauma	Center on area of suspected lesion.	Cross table-horizontal beam Center on area of suspected lesion.

by the patient's physical condition, in order to obtain radiographs of good diagnostic quality. The lack of proper patient restraint is the most common cause of skull radiographs of nondiagnostic quality.

2. The highest resolution (detail) radiographic image of the skull is produced with a nonscreen film or an ultradetail film/screen combination. Nonscreen film necessitates a 10- to 20-fold increase in mAs compared with film in par speed screen cassettes.

3. The positioning of the patient and the numbers of projections needed for a complete study depend upon the area of the skull being evaluated. A minimum of two views is necessary.

- Routine skull: Lateral, DV
- Nasal cavity and paranasal sinuses: Lateral, occlusal DV (Fig. 10); VD open mouth (Fig. 11) (extraoral film); frontal (primary beam parallel to the hard palate) (Fig. 12); lateral oblique (Fig. 13) (right and left) to evaluate small frontal sinuses
- Dental arches: Maxillary—Right and left lateral obliques (20° to 30°) (Fig. 14); VD open mouth (extraoral film); DV occlusal. Mandibular—right

and left lateral obliques (20° to 30°) open mouth (Fig. 15); VD occlusal (Fig. 16).
- Bisecting angle technique: Central beam is projected perpendicular to an imaginary plane that bisects the angle formed by the long axis of the tooth (or teeth) and the plane of the film (Fig. 17).
- Tympanic bullae (ears): DV, open mouth frontal. The primary beam bisects the angle of the opened temporomandibular joint (TMJ) (Fig. 18); lateral oblique (Fig. 19)(30° by 30°) right and left. Palpate the jugular processes; when these processes are oblique, the bullae will also be properly oblique.
- Foramen magnum: Rostrodorsal-caudoventral oblique (fronto-occipital). The central beam passes between the eyes and exits through the foramen magnum (Fig. 20).
- Temporomandibular joint: DV, open mouth frontal (see Fig. 18). Primary beam bisects the angle of the opened TMJ; lateral oblique (20° to 30°) right and left (see Fig. 13).
- Mandible: DV, lateral, lateral oblique (right and left)
- Maxilla: DV occlusal, VD open mouth; lateral, lateral oblique (right and left)

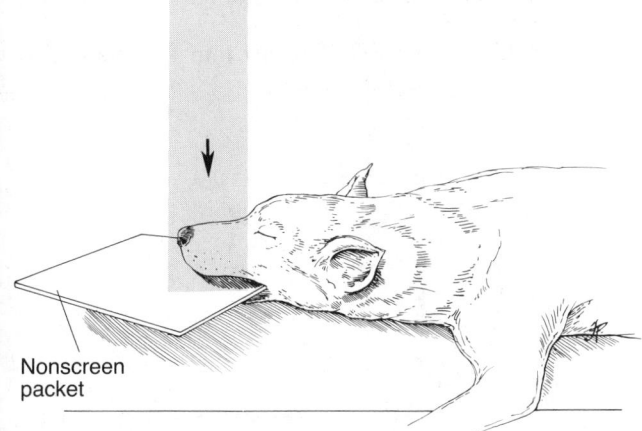

Nonscreen packet

Figure 10. Positioning for dorsoventral (DV) occlusal (intraoral) radiograph of the skull.

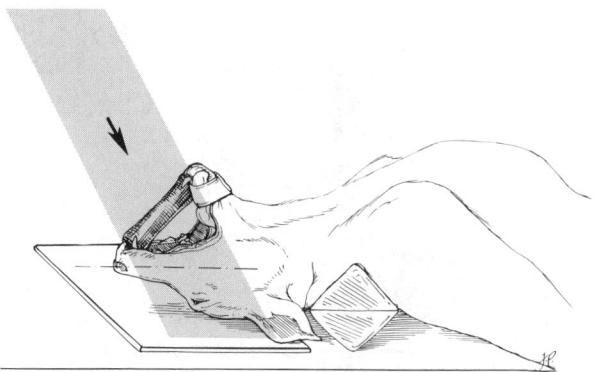

Figure 11. Positioning for the ventrodorsal (20 to 30° tube angle), open-mouth view of the skull.

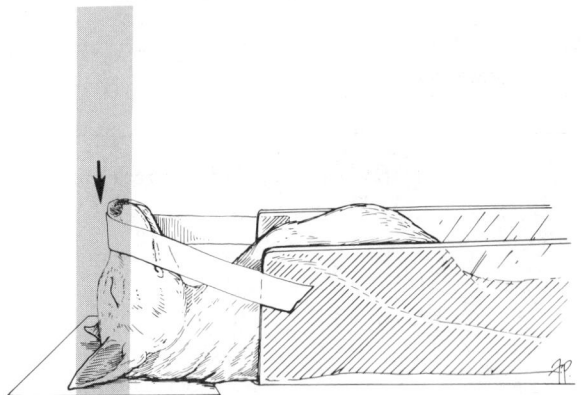

Figure 12. Positioning for the rostrocaudal (frontal) view of the skull.

- Zygomatic bone and orbit: DV, lateral, lateral obliques (right and left), frontal, VD open mouth

CONTRAST STUDIES

Contrast Medium

- Positive contrast medium—iodine (ionic, nonionic); barium (liquid, paste) (Table 6).
- Negative contrast medium—room air, CO_2

Contrast Procedures

- Excretory urography (EU), intravenous pyelogram (IVP), intravenous urogram (IVU)
  - A well-prepared animal is important for this contrast study. Withhold food for 12 to 24 hours. Give enemas the night before and at least 2 hours prior to the study. Determine renal function (blood urea nitrogen and creatinine values) prior to initiating study.

KEY POINT ▶ Always take scout films before the initiation of contrast studies of the urinary tract.

- Contraindications include dehydration. Contrast medium is hypertonic and will compromise an already unstable patient. Make sure the patient is properly hydrated prior to EU. Contraindicated in people with diabetes mellitus, multiple myeloma, heart failure, and known hypersensitivity to the contrast medium.

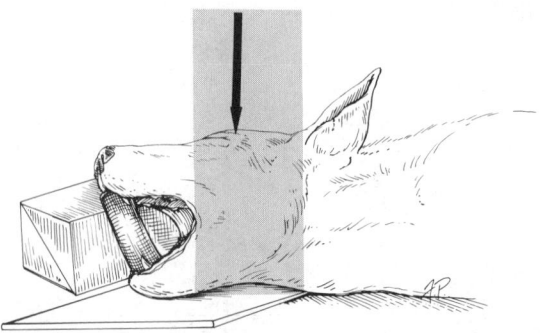

Figure 13. Positioning for the open-mouth lateral oblique (20° to 30°) view of the frontal sinuses.

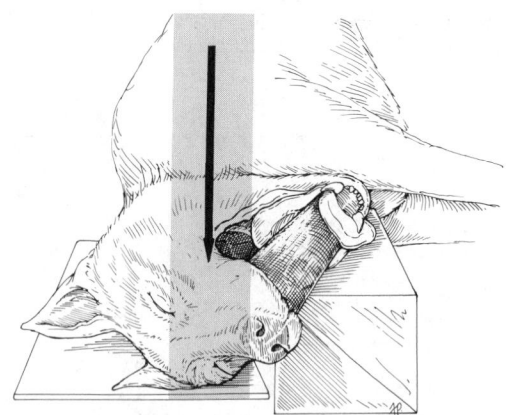

Figure 14. Positioning for the open-mouth lateral oblique (20 to 30°) view of the maxilla.

- Water-soluble, iodinated ionic contrast mediums (Renografin, Conray, Hypaque, Renovist). Dosage is 2 ml/kg IV (approximately 300 to 400 mg/ml iodine); not to exceed 90 ml or 35 gm of iodine. For animals with impaired renal function may need to double the dosage (4 ml/kg). Place an indwelling catheter, to help avoid perivascular injections, and allow IV access if complications occur. Give bolus as fast as possible.

Technique

1. Increase kVp 5 to 10% over scout films.
2. Keep the kVp at approximately 70 to produce better contrast between kidney and contrast medium.

- Radiographic sequence
  - (1) Immediate postinjection VD film demonstrates nephrographic phase.
  - (2) 5-minute VD and lateral films
  - (3) A wrap at 10 to 20 minutes after seeing contrast medium in the renal pelvis is placed between the bladder and kidney to compress the ureters causing the pelvis and diverticula of the kidney to completely distend for better evaluation.

    Contraindicated in cases of severely diseased bladder walls or mass lesions in which it may cause rupture.
  - (4) A 15-minute VD (lateral) film for evaluation of the pyelographic stage

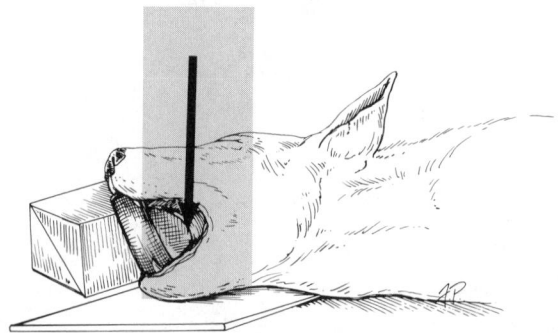

Figure 15. Positioning for the open-mouth lateral oblique (20 to 30°) view of the mandible.

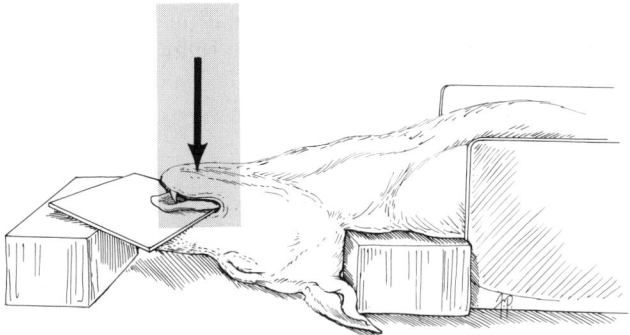

Figure 16. Positioning for the ventrodorsal (VD) occlusal (intraoral) view of the mandible.

(5) A 30-minute VD (lateral) film
(6) Remove the compression wrap and take lateral and VD radiographs.
(7) Modify this technique as needed for the suspected disease entity. For example, to evaluate for ectopic ureters oblique films at 15- to 20-minutes and pneumocystograms may be helpful in visualizing the distal ureters and vesicoureteral junctions.

• Complications include perivascular injection, which can be treated with instillation of saline into tissues to dilute; nausea/vomiting; adverse systemic (anaphylactoid) reaction; contrast-induced renal failure; kidneys become bright (contrast enhanced) and remain that way. Be careful when positioning in VD to avoid aspiration.

Cystography

■ Equipment
 • Contrast medium. For negative effects, use room air or CO_2; for positive effects, use water-soluble ionic iodinated contrast medium (not barium).
 • Catheters. Foley, tom cat, male dog, metal female catheters
 • Sterile lubricant gel
 • Three-way stopcock
■ Contrast studies
 • Negative contrast cystogram (pneumocystogram)
 • Positive contrast cystogram (technique of choice for identifying urinary bladder location and tears)
 • Double contrast cystogram (superior for demonstrating lesions involving the urinary bladder wall and intraluminal filling defects)

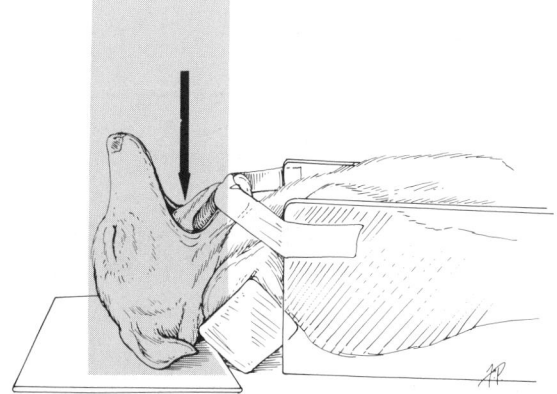

Figure 18. Positioning for the open-mouth rostrocaudal (basilar) view.

Technique

1. Withhold food for 12 to 24 hours
2. Warm water cleansing enemas the night before and 3 to 4 hours before the procedure
3. Sedation or tranquilization may be necessary, especially in cats and female dogs for catheterization.
4. A small amount of lidocaine (1 ml mixed with 2 ml of sterile saline) infused into the urinary bladder before the contrast agent may reduce urinary bladder spasm.
5. Catheter tip is placed within the bladder neck.
6. Empty the urinary bladder.
7. Infuse the contrast medium (1 to 7 ml, dependent upon animal's size), rotate the patient, and massage the bladder to distribute contrast medium and coat entire mucosal surface.
8. Slowly infuse negative contrast material. Complete distension equals adequately distended—judged by palpation, back pressure felt on syringe plunger, or reflux of gas around catheter.
9. Use scout film technique for negative contrast, and increase kVp 4 to 6 for positive contrast study.

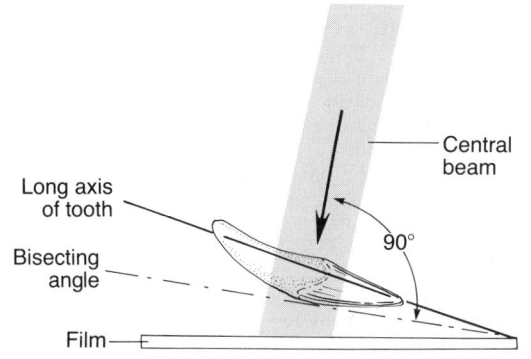

Figure 17. Bisecting angle technique for radiographing the teeth.

Central beam

Long axis of tooth

Bisecting angle

90°

Film

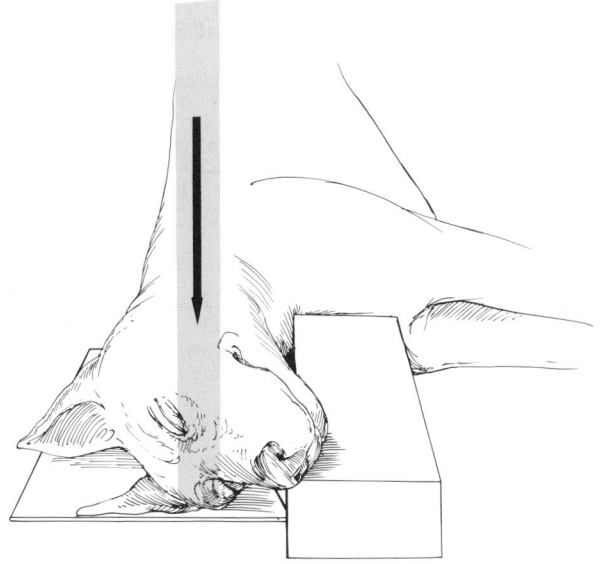

Figure 19. Positioning for the lateral oblique (30° nose elevated, then 30° oblique) view of tympanic bullae.

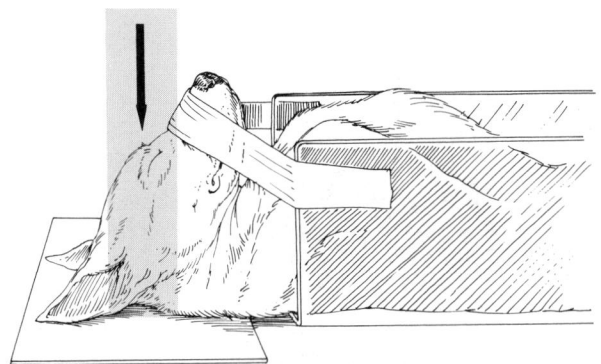

Figure 20. Positioning for the rostrodorsal-caudoventral (fronto-occipital) view of the skull.

10. Take at least two views (lateral and a lateral oblique); ideally, take three views (lateral and two lateral obliques).
11. Remove contrast material after study.

- Complications

  Fatal air embolism (rare cases). An increased risk exists with ulcerative or erosive cystitis. CO_2 is more soluble than room air in blood and thus less likely to cause this problem. Air embolism occurs immediately after the administration of negative contrast medium. Place the animal in the left lateral recumbency, and lower the head to maintain normal blood circulation through the heart. The air is trapped in the right ventricle.

  Iatrogenic trauma (hematuria, bacterial contamination, cystitis, rupture)

Urethrography

Retrograde with positive contrast, iodine

■ Equipment includes catheter (Foley, metal, male dog), sterile gel, lidocaine, water-soluble iodinated contrast medium.

Technique

1. Enema as needed to evacuate the colon prior to the study; scout films prior to the study to evaluate technique and preparation.
2. Pass a urinary catheter into the distal urethra. Balloon is inflated if the Foley catheter is used (in distal urethra for female dogs or cats and just proximal to the os penis in male dogs).
3. Administer 2 to 5 ml of lidocaine before injecting contrast material may reduce urethral spasm.
4. Male dogs are positioned with their legs drawn cranially.
5. Administer 10 to 20 ml contrast medium for male dogs and 5 to 10 ml for female dogs and cats, injected as a bolus. Radiographs are taken during the last few milliliters of injection.
6. Lateral radiograph may be sufficient, but subsequent lateral and VD oblique views may be helpful.

TABLE 6. Radiographic Contrast Agents

Barium Product	
Brand Names	***Manufacturers***
Esophotrast (Barium paste)	Barnes-Hind Barium Products Sunnyvale, CA 94086
E-Z-Paste (Esophageal cream)	E-Z-EM, Inc. Westbury, NY 11590
Barosperse (Esophageal cream)	Mallinckrodt St. Louis, MO 63160
Liqui-Jug (Barium suspension)	E-Z-EM, Inc. Westbury, NY 11590
Liquid Polibar (Barium suspension)	E-Z-EM, Inc. Westbury, NY 11590
E-Z-Jug (Barium suspension)	E-Z-EM, Inc. Westbury, NY 11590
Novopaque	Lafayette Pharmacal Lafayette, IN 47903
Iodinated Gastrointestinal Contrast Agent	
Gastrografin	Squibb Diagnostics New Bruswick, NJ 08903
Iodinated Contrast Agent	
Renovist, Renovist II, Renografin 60 or 76	Squibb Diagnostics New Brunswick, NJ 08903
Hypaque-M 75% or 90%	Winthrop Labs New York, NY 10016
Conray, Conray 30 or 400	Mallinckrodt St Louis, MO 63134
Myelographic Contrast Agent	
Omnipaque (Iohexol)	Winthrop Labs New York, NY 10016
Isovue (Iopamidol)	Squibb Diagnostics New Brunswick, NJ 08903

- Complications include iatrogenic trauma and bacterial contamination.

Esophagram

Technique

1. Survey cervical and thoracic radiographs.
2. Position animal in lateral recumbency.
3. Administer contrast medium (Table 6) (barium sulfate suspension, Esophotrast, barium burger) slowly into the buccal pouch.
4. Dose is variable (5 to 20 ml); need enough to induce swallowing and coat esophagus.
5. Obtain radiographs following swallows. Lateral view is most informative; right ventral oblique view may be helpful. Follow-up radiographs may be helpful if a bolus of contrast material is retained within the esophagus.

- Complications
  Aspiration
  Leakage of barium into mediastinum. Low osmolality, nonionic iodinated contrast medium may be indicated if perforation is suspected.

Gastrography

Technique

KEY POINT ▶ Prior to contrast studies of the gastrointestinal tract, discontinue all drugs that may influence motility.

1. Fast patient 12 to 24 hours prior to study.
2. Give cleansing enema the night before and 3 to 4 hours prior to the study, especially if complete upper gastrointestinal study may follow.
3. Take plain films prior to the study.
4. Obtain negative contrast gastrogram (pneumogastrogram) consisting of 6 to 16 ml of room air per kg body weight via stomach tube. Immediately take four views (right and left lateral, VD/DV). Valuable in the diagnosis of some radiolucent foreign bodies.
5. Obtain positive contrast gastrogram; barium (suspension), 30% weight/volume at a dose of 6 to 12 ml/kg (see Table 6). Administer via a stomach tube, and take films immediately (right and left lateral, VD/DV). Use to document gastric displacement, certain gastric foreign bodies, and gastric perforations. Barium begins leaving the stomach within 5 to 15 minutes. The stomach is emptied by 30 to 60 minutes in cats and 1 to 2 hours in dogs.
6. Double contrast gastrogram can be done as a separate study or during an upper gastrointestinal study. Give barium, 60% weight/volume at a dose of 1.5 to 3 ml/kg, and insufflate with room air at 10 ml/kg. These procedures are all done with a gastric tube in place. Immediately take DV/VD and right and left lateral films. The study is indicated in cases of suspected gastric wall and mucosal lesions.

Upper Gastrointestinal Study

- Contrast medium
  - Barium (suspension) 30 to 60% weight/volume (see Table 9). Dose is 8 to 16 ml/kg.

- Iodinated contrast (ionic and nonionic) agents (see Table 9) indicated with suspected perforation and quick determination of small intestine patency and location.
▪ For restraint in canines use acepromazine and in felines use ketamine/acepromazine preparations. See section 1, chapter 2 for dosages. These sedatives have less effect on motility than do many others.
▪ Preparation requires a 12 to 24 hour fast and an enema the night before and 3 to 4 hours prior to study.

Technique

1. Survey radiographs (right lateral (RL) and VD)
2. Immediately after administration of barium: Right and left laterals and DV and VD. At 15, 30, and 60 minutes, RL and VD radiographs are done. Be consistent unless a lesion is visualized that is better evaluated by repositioning the animal. Then, proceed at hourly intervals until the contrast material reaches the colon.
3. Modify this protocol for each individual depending upon the suspected disease entity or the lesions visualized during the procedure.
4. Expected transit time: Canine, 3–4 hours; feline, 1 hour

- Complications
  Aspiration of barium with or without gastric contents
  Barium peritonitis. If perforation is suspected, consider doing a contrast study with nonionic iodinated contrast medium.

▪ Myelography is the radiographic evaluation of the spinal cord by injection of a positive contrast agent into the subarachnoid space.
- Indications
  To evaluate transverse myelopathy
  To determine nature, location, and extent of a lesion prior to surgery
  To identify multiple lesions when one lesion might be masked by another lesion and therefore not detected clinically.
- Contraindications
  Diffuse myelopathy that is not amenable to surgery.
  Meningitis may be aggravated by contrast medium.
  Myelography is not indicated if survey radiographs and clinical signs are adequate for diagnosis.
- Contrast medium (see Table 6).
  Dose for cisternal tap—cervical study (0.2 to 0.3 ml/kg), thoracolumbar study (0.45 ml/kg); for lumbar tap—cervical study (0.45 ml/kg); thoracolumbar study (0.3 ml/kg).

Technique

1. General anesthesia

KEY POINT ▶ Always obtain survey spinal radiographs prior to myelogram.

2. Sterile preparation of the puncture site
3. Cerebral spinal fluid (CSF) collection and analysis if deemed necessary

4. Cisternal tap procedure

- Position the animal in lateral recumbency.
- Position the nose parallel to the table top and perpendicular to the spine.
- Use a 20- or 22-gauge, 1.5- to 2.5-inch spinal needle with the bevel directed caudally.
- Insert on the dorsal midline, between the occipital protuberance and wings of the atlas.
- Direct needle towards the mandible.
- If needle hits bone, move the needle cranially or caudally until it falls into the atlanto-occipital (AO) space.
- Remove the stylet and check for CSF flow often while advancing the needle.
- Inject contrast material slowly after seeing CSF in the needle.
- Elevate the head for 5 minutes before taking radiographs.
- Take lateral, VD (VD oblique if necessary) radiographs. Remove the endotracheal tube, if necessary, for VD radiograph.

5. Lumbar tap procedure

- Position the animal in lateral or sternal recumbency, and flex the rear legs to help open the interarcuate spaces.
- Use a 20- or 22-gauge, 1.5- to 3.5-inch spinal needle.
- Insert the needle through L_{5-6} interarcuate space for small dogs and cats and L_{4-5} for large dogs, on the dorsal midline just lateral to the dorsal spinous processes of L_6 at a 50 to 60° angle, in a cranioventral direction towards the interarcuate space at L_{5-6}. In cats, insert the needle off the cranial edge of L_6 dorsal spinous process perpendicular to the long axis of the spine. Direct the needle ventrally through the interarcuate space.
- The injection can be made in either the dorsal or ventral subarachnoid space. Always check for CSF flow prior to injection; however, it is not always obtained. Increase likelihood of obtaining CSF by elevating the head and shoulders prior to placing the needle.
- Small test injection followed by a radiograph (0.25 to 0.50 ml) is recommended to check the needle placement.
- Slowly inject total dosage. Take radiographs based on localization of neurologic examination.

6. Complications

- Seizures (reduced incidence with new contrast agents, e.g., iohexol)
- Exacerbation of clinical signs
- Hyperesthesia
- Apnea during injection
- Epidural injection will not have a negative impact on the health of the animal but will negatively affect the quality of the myelogram.
- Central canal filling occurs when the needle is placed through the center of the cord. It usually appears thin and sharply defined in the normal animal.

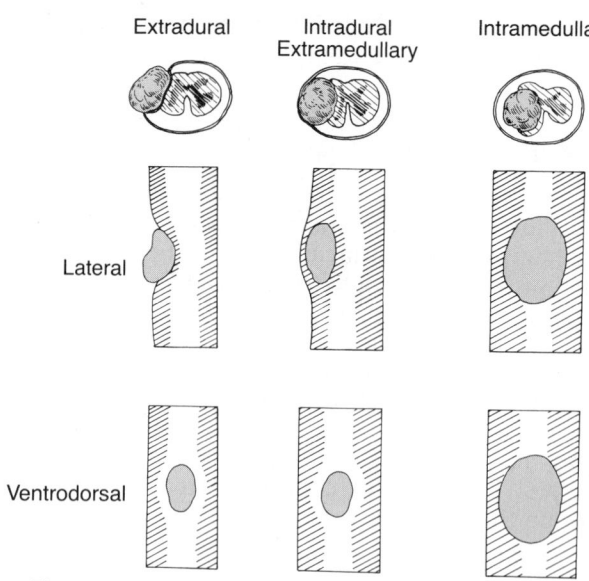

Figure 21. Radiographic patterns of myelographic lesions.

7. Interpretation

Lesions are divided into three categories (Fig. 21).

- 1. Extradural characterized by
  - Displacement of the spinal cord
  - Narrowing or compression of the subarachnoid space
  - Deviation of the subarachnoid space
  - Spinal cord may appear wide on opposite view.
- 2. Intradural extramedullary characterized by
  - Filling defect within the subarachnoid space ("Tee" sign)
  - Extradural or intramedullary component may be associated.
- 3. Intramedullary characterized by spinal cord widening in all views.

RADIATION SAFETY

Basic Radiation Safety

The objectives of radiation safety are obtaining the maximum amount of diagnostic information while at the same time keeping the radiation exposure to personnel and animals to a minimum.

KEY POINT ▶ The responsibility for radiation safety lies solely with the owners of the practice.

Radiation protection in veterinary medicine is the subject of the National Council on Radiation Protection and Measurements (NCRP) Report No. 36 entitled *Radiation Protection in Veterinary Medicine.** This report specifically outlines when radiation protection surveys are made. The report makes recommendations concerning tube housing, aluminum filtration, collimation types, and centering devices. A special section discusses radiography with portable and mobile diag-

---

*A copy of this report may be obtained from NCRP Publications, P.O. Box 30175, Washington, D.C. 20014.

nostic equipment. All practices need a copy of this report. Other NCRP reports that may be pertinent are No. 34 that discusses protection devices, No. 35 that discusses dental applications of diagnostic x-rays, and No. 17 that provides recommendations for the maximum permissible dose (MPD).

The MPD was established to keep the radiation exposure of workers below a level at which adverse effects might be observed during a lifetime and to minimize the incidence of genetic effects in the entire population. The MPD does not apply to animal patients, to radiation emitted from natural background sources, or to radiation therapy. The actual risk to an individual exposed to MPD is small, but the risk is directly proportional to received dosage. Therefore, radiation exposure must be keep as low as possible. Radiation can cause both tissue and genetic damage. The effects of radiation can be demonstrated in a short time, or they can be cumulative and not observed for a long time.

Individual states publish radiation control regulations that are reprinted from the states codes. These regulations include information concerning the licensing of x-ray machines, the licensing fee, and the procedure to be followed in obtaining licensing. The goal in diagnostic radiology is to obtain radiographs with minimum exposure to both patient and personnel.

Maximum Permissible Dose (MPD)

The maximum amount of radiation that, in light of current knowledge, will not produce injury. The maximum occupational dose is currently 5 rem per year.

KEY POINT ▶ There should be no occupational radiation exposure of anyone under 18 years of age.

Reducing Exposure

Three methods reduce radiation exposure: (1) increased distance between the individual and the radiation source, (2) decreased duration of exposure, (3) protective barriers between the individual and the radiation source.

- Limiting radiation exposure
  - Limit the number of individuals within the room where the procedure is taking place. Use positioning devices: sandbags, sponges, tape, Plexiglas trough. Chemical restraint is used whenever possible.

KEY POINT ▶ When you must be present within the radiographic room during film taking always wear protective clothing.

This may include lead apparel (apron, gloves, thyroid shield, protective goggles). Lead apparel is 0.5-mm lead equivalent. Hang aprons up to prevent the lead from cracking. Store gloves so that liners can dry. All protective clothing is checked at least twice a year for cracks and tears. This includes placing the items on a film cassette and radiographing them at an exposure of approximately 85 kVp.

KEY POINT ▶ Never permit any portion of the body to be within the primary beam.

This is not permitted even with the wearing of protective clothing.

- Never handhold any x-ray tube. All x-ray tubes leak radiation from the housing.
- Use a shielding device whenever possible to protect all or part of your body. Lead glass may be part of this shield so that you may continue to see the patient. Lead-impregnated acrylic or plastic panels may be hung from the ceiling to give added protection.*
- When using a horizontal x-ray beam never position any part of your body behind the cassette.
- Use collimation. An unexposed border on the radiograph demonstrates that the primary beam did not exceed the size of the cassette (film). This practice helps reduce scatter radiation by decreasing the interaction between the primary beam and tissue, therefore increasing radiographic quality. Check the collimator light for accuracy; replace the bulb as needed.
- Use fast film, fast rare earth screens, and high kVp techniques to lower the exposure factors and the amount of radiation produced.
- Use a 2.0-mm aluminum filter installed at the tube housing port to remove the softer (less energetic) radiation portion of the x-ray beam. This practice aids in the reduction of scatter radiation and exposure to the patient.
- Individuals within the room always stand as far away from the radiation source as possible. If you double the distance from the source of radiation, you decrease your exposure level by a factor of 4 (inverse square law).
- All personnel working with radiation are required to wear a film badge or some other method of monitoring the amount of exposure, if they have the potential to receive greater than ¼ MPD. Remember that wearing the device does not protect the individual, but it serves as a reminder of working in a potentially hazardous environment. For a monitoring device to be most helpful in determining exposure to radiation, it is worn consistently in the same location on the body outside the apron at the neck. Film badges register when exposed to heat, light, water, or pressure. They can be purchased through companies listed in Table 7.
- Never permit anyone under the age of 18 or a pregnant woman in the room during a diagnostic procedure.
- Rotate personnel, thus reducing the amount of exposure to each.
- Do not direct the x-ray beam into adjacent rooms that may be occupied.
- Use a gonadal shield for the patient.
- Always plan radiographic procedures (e.g., proper position and technique), thus reducing the number

---

*Available through Nuclear Associates, 100 Voice Rd., Carle Place, NY 11514.

TABLE 7. Sources of Film Badges

ICN Dosimetry Service 26201 Miles Rd. Cleveland, OH 44128 216/831-3000	Searle Analytic, Inc. 2000 Nuclear Drive Des Plaines, IL 60018 312/298-6001
R.S. Landauer, Jr. & Co. Glenwood Science Park Glenwood, IL 60425 312/755-1100	Teledyne Isotopes 50 Van Buren Ave. Westwood, NJ 07675 201/664-7070

of films needed, which ultimately reduces the exposure to patient and personnel.

Clinic Construction

- Check with your state's health department (radiation protection division) for the latest laws on radiation safety and clinic construction.
- Register your x-ray machine with the state.
- Many states are now conducting "surprise spot checks" of x-ray machines and radiographic records. Maintain film and technique logs for complete records (Figs. 22 and 23).
- If constructing a new clinic, a drawing of the layout must be sent to the state radiation protection department. This drawing indicates the location of the x-ray machine and demonstrates how the space in the room where the x-ray machine is located will be used. The use of the adjoining rooms and an estimate of the degree of traffic in these areas are determined. The radiation safety department then sends a computerized layout of wall, ceiling, and floor materials to be utilized in certain areas of your clinic. The average small animal practice radiology area needs at least three layers of ⅝-inch type-X gypsum board for all walls and ceilings. In 1993, new laws may take effect requiring solid cinder block walls in the radi-

ology area and ceiling to reduce exposure to personnel working outside the radiology area.

RADIOGRAPHIC INTERPRETATION

Radiology is a valuable adjunctive diagnostic tool. Do not interpret radiographs without considering the history, clinical signs, physical examination findings, and laboratory data. Radiographic signs are rarely pathognomonic; therefore, a specific diagnosis is seldom possible.

$$\begin{array}{c}\text{Roentgen}\\ \text{signs}\end{array} + \begin{array}{c}\text{History}\\ \text{Physical Examination}\\ \text{Laboratory}\\ \text{Findings}\end{array} = \begin{array}{c}\text{Differential}\\ \text{list}\end{array}$$

From the differential list additional tests can be done to help formulate a definitive diagnosis.

$$\begin{array}{c}\text{Differential}\\ \text{list}\end{array} + \begin{array}{c}\text{Contrast studies}\\ \text{Ultrasound}\\ \text{Laboratory data}\\ \text{Biopsy or}\\ \text{surgery}\end{array} = \begin{array}{c}\text{Definitive}\\ \text{diagnosis}\end{array}$$

Technique

1. Successful interpretation of radiographs depends upon many factors.

KEY POINT ▶ The most important factor in the successful interpretation of radiographs is the quality of the radiographs being examined.

2. At least two views at right angles to each other are needed. The use of right or left lateral radiographs is based upon the preference of the individual reading the radiographs. The same holds true for VD and DV but be consistent.

Radiology Log and Film Inventory

Date	Client Name	Type of Study Performed	Film Size and Number of Films			
			8×10	10×12 24×30	11×14 30×35	14×17 35×43

Figure 22. Radiology technique log.

Name _____

Clinic Number _____

Species _____ Breed _____   Radiology Technique Log

Sex _____ Date of Birth _____

Date	Exam	Views Taken	mAs	kVp	Grid	Table Top	Film Size	Screen	Notes

Figure 23. Film usage and inventory log.

3. Viewing conditions

   - Dark, quiet room
   - At least two view boxes to evaluate both simultaneously
   - Always place the film on the view boxes such that the anatomic structures are in the same position and direction: DV/VD with the animal's right to your left; lateral radiograph with the head to your left.
   - Use a shielded high-intensity (hot) lamp.
   - Read films slowly and thoroughly.
   - Always have radiology and anatomy texts within reach of the view boxes.

4. Evaluate the radiographs employing a systematic approach. Evaluate the entire film before concentrating on obvious lesions.

   - Use an area method, either peripheral to center or central to periphery evaluation.
   - Use an organ system method. Evaluate all parts of a system prior to examining the next system.
   - However you choose to evaluate films, be consistent from case to case.

5. Knowledge of normal radiographic anatomy is needed.

6. Descriptions of radiographic pathology involve the following:

   - Knowledge of normal topographic anatomy is a priority. An understanding that, particularly in the abdomen, some organs are nearly always seen, some organs are almost never seen or seen only when abnormal, and some organs are typically only partially seen. Because these organs are not always seen, one is still aware of where they are normally located. You must always be able to describe the location of the lesion based on what it is near or adjacent to or what is ventral, dorsal, lateral, medial, axial, abaxial, cranial, caudal, or rostral. Describe the effect the lesion is having on surrounding structures.
   - Roentgen (radiographic) signs

Radiopacity—Various radiographic opacities are due to the differential absorption of x-rays. The opacity of surrounding material also influences the observed opacity of a structure. The five radiopacities in decreasing order are those of metal, bone, soft tissue (fluid), fat, and gas. Metal is the only one that is not a biologic opacity.

Geometry—Size, shape, position, margination, and number.

Function—Excretion (intravenous urography), motility (upper gastrointestinal), patency, and integrity. Evaluation of function often requires contrast medium and multiple films.

ULTRASOUND

Ultrasound is rapidly becoming an accepted imaging modality in small animal practice. New and used equipment are available at reasonable prices, and usefulness has increased to include ophthalmic, cardiac, abdominal, and reproductive disease diagnosis. It is a safe, noninvasive diagnostic technique that provides information about the internal architecture of organs within the abdomen and thorax. Functional information can also be obtained with echocardiography. Ultrasound is not meant to replace diagnostic radiology but to complement it. Ultrasound is operator-dependent. The quality of the image and the information gained are directly related to the ability of the person doing the study.

Equipment

The major components of the diagnostic ultrasound imaging system are pulser, transducer, receiver, memory, and display. Electrical pulses are produced by the pulser and these drive the transducer. The transducer produces ultrasound pulses for each electrical pulse it receives. The transducer also produces electrical pulses for each ultrasound pulse (reflection) it receives from tissues. The electrical pulses go to the receiver, where they are converted to information that the memory can utilize. Information from the memory drives the display, which produces an image.

Suppliers of ultrasound equipment are listed in Table 8.

Machines

- Questions to consider prior to purchasing (leasing) ultrasound equipment.
  - What kind of scanning will I be doing (e.g., heart, abdomen, real-time, B mode, M mode)?
  - How large or small are my patients?
  - Is someone in the practice willing to accept primary responsibility for learning and doing the procedures?
  - How much money can I invest?
- Two types of real-time scanners
  - Linear array produces a rectangular image and can be utilized to evaluate broad areas, where no bony or gas-filled structures interfere. These scanners are usually less expensive. New machines start at $7500 to $10,000; used, $2000 to $3000). The major drawback is the transducer contact zone, which makes intercostal and subcostal (heart, liver, biliary tract, and right kidney) imaging difficult.
  - Sector scanner produces a pie-shaped image. Smaller contact zone is used, which makes intercostal and subcostal imaging less difficult.

Mechanical—The sound wave is focused a certain distance from the transducer (focal point). The sound wave is within focus for some distance on both sides of the focal point (focal zone). Resolution is best within this fixed focal zone. Scanner contains moving parts.

Phased (annular) array—No moving parts, therefore, more durable than mechanical scanners. The beam is formed by adding together many small beams from an array of small crystals. Scanner has variable (dynamic) focusing. The focal zone therefore can be placed anywhere in the image depth.

- Image display
  - M-Mode (Motion-Mode): Documents motion, especially that of the heart (echocardiography). A thin ultrasound beam is directed into the heart, is reflected back, and then is shown on the screen as numerous moving lines. Motion is indicated along the side, and time along the bottom of the screen.
  - B-Mode (Brightness-Mode): Echoes are displayed as dots. The brightness of the dot changes with the amplitude of reflection. The larger the reflection, the brighter the dot—no reflection, black dot. The location of the dot corresponds to the location of the reflector in the body.
  - Real time: The image is continually updated during the entire examination. This permits direct observation of moving structures (heart, bowel peristalsis).
- New vs. used equipment

New equipment purchase is ideal because some companies offer training (in-house or continuing education course) and a year-long warranty with service and parts (in-house service or another unit is made available while your unit is serviced by the company). Manufacturer-reconditioned units may provide a year-long or shorter warranty. The major disadvantage of new equipment obviously is the higher cost.

A great deal of used equipment is available owing to the advent of newer technology. Older, used, outdated equipment is being replaced with new equipment based on new technology. The price of old equipment is very attractive, sometimes as low as $1000. Although initial cost is low, some significant expense may be required, including service, maintenance, transducers, and accessories. If the appropriate frequency transducers do not come with the unit (often only 2 and 3 mHz transducers come with units that were used on human patients), the cost can increase three to four times to purchase 5 and 7.5 mHz transducers.

Transducers

- Transducers are available in a variety of frequencies (2 to 10 mHz). Low-frequency transducers

TABLE 8. Ultrasound Companies

Advanced Technology Laboratories 22100 Bothell Highway S.E. Bothell, WA 98041-3003 800/982-2011	Products Group International 2805 Wilderness Place Boulder, CO 80301 303/939-9380
Corometrics Medical Systems, Inc. 61 Barnes Park Rd. North Wallingford, CT 06492-0333 800/624-7265	E. I. Medical P.O. Box 5375 Loveland, CO 80538 303/669-1793
Classic Medical Supply, Inc. 815 S. US Hwy. 1 Jupiter, FL 33477 800/722-6838	Del Mar Avionics 1601 Alton Ave. Irvine, CA 92714 714/250-3200
Shimadzu Medical Systems 101 W. Walnut St. Gardena, CA 90248-3130 213/217-8855	Hewlett-Packard Medical 1200 E. Diehl Rd. P.O. Box 3068 Naperville, IL 60566-7068 708/505-8800
Ausonics Universal Medical Systems, Inc. 51 Smart Ave. Yonkers, NY 10704 914/423-1597	Interspec Medical 110 W. Butler Ave. Ambler, PA 19002 800/332-3246
Echo Ultrasound R.D. 2, Box 118 Reedsville, PA 17084-9772 800/233-0261	Parker Laboratories, Inc. 307 Washington St. Orange, NJ 07050 800/631-8888

TABLE 9. Transducer Selection

Transducer Type	Use
7.5 mHz	Eye, feline heart and abdomen, small canine abdomen (<25 lb), testicles
5.0 mHz	Medium-size dogs (<55 lb) heart and abdomen
3.5 mHZ	Very large breed dogs heart and abdomen

provide greater depth of penetration, but because of large wavelength, resolution is poorer. High-frequency transducers provide excellent resolution, but the beam is rapidly attenuated in tissue. They are therefore utilized to evaluate superficial tissues.

- Use as high a frequency transducer as possible to maximize resolution but still allow penetration to the depth needed.
- For transducer uses, see Table 9.

Ancillary Equipment

A guided biopsy attachment for the transducer, calipers, screen-labeling device, ECG, and M-mode/B-mode split screen. Portability of the machine must also be considered.

Ultrasonographic Accessories

- Positioners
  - V-trough is easily constructed from wood or Plexiglas).
  - Surgical table can be formed into a V.
  - Cardiac table (wood or Plexiglas) with holes so that the transducers may be brought up under the recumbent patient. Lateral recumbency causes the heart to lay against the chest wall, providing an ultrasonographic window to the heart.
- Standoff Pad
  - Commercially available pad. A water balloon or breast implant can also be employed.
  - Place between the transducer and the skin.
  - This pad provides an offset that serves to back the transducer away from the skin, moving the superficial structure to be imaged within the focal zone of the transducer.
- Couplant Gel is necessary to transmit sound from the transducer through the skin.
  - Numerous brands are commercially available
  - Water soluble, hypoallergenic available

Image Storing

Preserving the image to be included in the animal's medical record.

- Polaroid camera
- Heat-sensitive, thermal-paper recorder (Sony, Mitsubishi) costs start at $1200.
- Multiformat camera can record multiple images on x-ray film. These are very expensive, however.
- Video tape in which the images are recorded allowing evaluation by others at a later time.

Technique

1. Patient preparation

- Tranquilization is usually not required, but the patient must always be adequately restrained.
- The most common problem in obtaining good quality images is poor transducer skin contact. Clip the hair over the area to be imaged with a #40 blade. Hair tends to trap air that acts as a barrier to the ultrasound. Clean the exposed skin to remove dirt, oil, and debris prior to applying the coupling gel to help achieve the best image.

2. Patient positioning

- Most abdominal imaging is done from the ventral surface. Alternate scanning planes from lateral and lateral intercostal can be chosen to avoid gas. When gas is a problem, gentle abdominal pressure from the transducer usually displaces it.
- The heart is imaged through the intercostal spaces, usually while the animal is in lateral recumbency.

3. Ultrasound image

- It is a two-dimensional representation of a three-dimensional object.
- Ultrasound reflects the anatomy tomographically (cross sectionally).
- Ultrasound permits identification of internal organ architecture.

4. Image viewing

- Abdomen (Figs. 24 and 25)
- Cardiac (see sec. 6 for more discussion of echocardiography).
- Longitudinal scan—cardiac base to the left.
- Transverse scan—pulmonary valve (outflow tract) on the right of the screen.

Principles of Interpretation

Ultrasound Terminology

Anechoic—area void of echoes (seen as black).

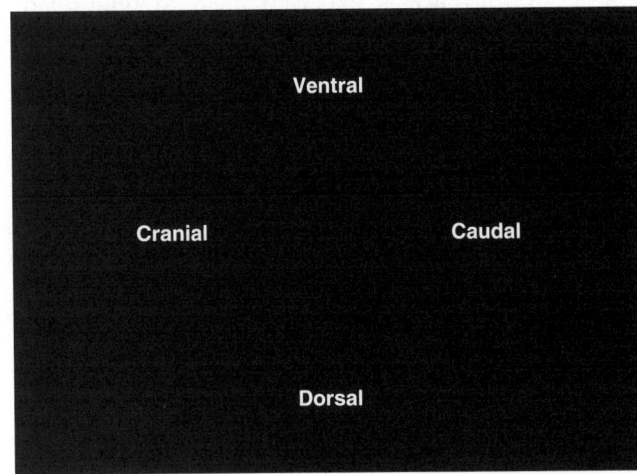

Figure 24. Viewing of a longitudinal (sagittal) ultrasound image.

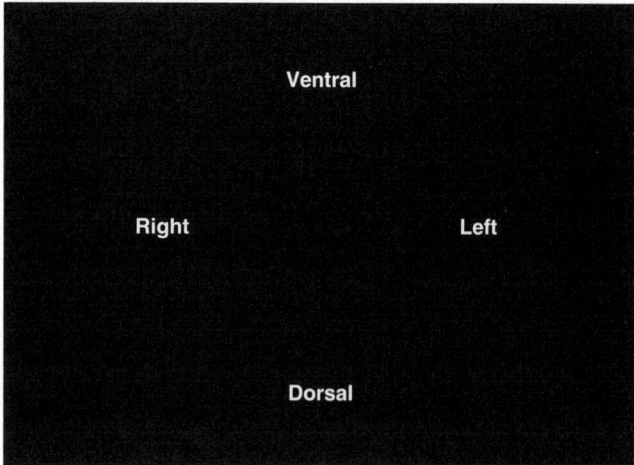

Figure 25. Viewing of a transverse (axial) ultrasound image.

Hypoechoic—lower level of echogenicity (darker) than adjacent structures.

Hyperechoic—higher level of echogenicity (brighter) than adjacent structures.

Isoechoic—level of echogenicity similar to adjacent structures.

Complexly echogenic—area of multiple echogenicities.

Ultrasonographic barriers—highly reflective or absorptive interfaces within the body that cause an almost complete attenuation of the sound beam. Examples include bone, mineral, and air. This barrier results in an absence of echoes deep to the interface (acoustic shadow).

Ultrasonographic windows—soft tissue organs adjacent to the body wall used to help avoid gas or bone and to facilitate deeper imaging. Examples include imaging through the spleen on the left lateral abdominal wall to visualize the left kidney and imaging through the urinary bladder to visualize the area where sublumbar lymph nodes are found.

Acoustic enhancement (through transmission)—sound passes through an anechoic structure with little attenuation and emerges with more intensity than expected in surrounding echogenic areas. This occurrence is expected deep to fluid-filled structures (e.g., gallbladder, hepatic cyst).

Organ Echogenicity

Rank of abdominal parenchymal organs from least to most echogenic:
- Renal medulla
- Renal cortex
- Liver
- Spleen
- Prostate
- Renal sinus

Ultrasound Use

See respective chapters for ultrasound use in specific diseases. See Table 10 for an overview of ultrasound in various organs.

TABLE 10. Ultrasound Uses

	Pathology	Usefulness
Heart	Wall thickness	+ + +
	Wall motion	+ + +
	Valve morphology	+ + +
	Valve motion	+ + +
	Mass lesion	+ + +
	Pericardial disease	+ + +
Thoracic area (extracardiac)	Pleural effusion	+ + +
	Pleural masses	+ + +
	Pulmonary masses*	+ + +
	Diaphragmatic hernia	+ +
	Mediastinal disease	+
Peritoneal cavity	Effusion	+ + +
	Carcinomatosis	+
	Lymphadenopathy	+ + +
Liver	Diffuse disease†	+/+ +
	Neoplasia	+ +/+ + +
	Abscess	+ +/+ + +
	Biliary disease	+ +/+ + +
	Portocaval shunt	+/+ +
	Nodular hyperplasia	+/+ +
Kidney	Hydronephrosis	+ + +
	Pyelonephritis	+/+ +
	Parenchymal disease‡	+ +
	Calculi	+ +/+ + +
	Perirenal disease	+ + +
	Neoplasia	+ + +
Urinary bladder	Calculi	+ + +
	Cystitis	+/+ +
	Neoplasia	+ + +
Adrenal gland	Hyperplasia	+/+ +
	Neoplasia	+ + +
Gastrointestinal system	Enteritis	+
	Obstruction	+ +/+ + +
	Intussusception	+ + +
	Foreign body	+ +/+ + +
	Neoplasia	+ +/+ + +
Pancreas	Pancreatitis	+/+ +
	Pseudocyst	+ +
	Neoplasia	+ +/+ + +
Reproductive tract	Ovary	+
	Testicular neoplasia	+ + +
	Peritesticular	+ + +
	Pregnancy	+ + +
Prostate	Infection	+ +
	Paraprostatic cyst	+ + +
	Neoplasia	+ +
Eye	Detached retina	+ + +
	Retrobulbar mass	+/+ +

*If mass contacts thoracic wall.
†Lipidosis, steroid hepatopathy, suppurative hepatitis (dependent upon severity of disease).
‡Glomerulonephritis, amyloidosis, ethylene glycol toxicity, renal dysplasia (dependent upon severity of disease).
+ + +: good; + +: fair, +: poor.

Intervention Ultrasound

- Uses
  - Ultrasound-guided needle biopsy for histopathology and culture
  - Ultrasound-guided fine needle aspirate (FNA) for cytology and culture
  - Cystocentesis (small bladder, difficult animals)

- Gallbladder aspirate for culture and cholangiography
- Abscess diagnosis and drainage
- Cyst diagnosis and drainage
- Renal pyelocentesis
■ Equipment
- Real-time B-mode scanner
- Transducer biopsy guide
- Needles, syringe, slides, culture medium, formalin containers
- Sterile glove or transducer cover
- Sterile ultrasound gel
- Sedatives, lidocaine
■ Patient preparation
- Complete abdominal ultrasound examination
- Choose site for FNA biopsy
- FNA—Rarely need sedation; sterile preparation of skin and transducer sterile glove cover
- Tissue biopsy—Sedation and/or local anesthesia; surgical preparation of skin and transducer
- Sterile glove cover
- Pack cell volume (PCV); total protein, activated clotting time
- (+/− prothrombin time, partial thromboplastin time)
- Check the PCV 3 to 4 hours post biopsy.
■ Methods
- Guided—Transducer has an attachable biopsy guide. Ultrasound machine has biopsy capabilities (software). Biopsy guide maintains needle in the scanning plane so that the entire procedure can be visualized.
- Directed—Organ or lesion of interest is imaged. The location, entrance angle, and depth are determined. Biopsy or aspirate is obtained blindly without ultrasound observation. More dependent on sonographer's experience. Biopsy guide and biopsy capable machine are not necessary.
- Free Hand—Biopsy site localized with transducer perpendicular to the skin. Needle is placed with the other hand into the scanning plane to the desired depth. Biopsy procedure can be observed with real time and is more dependent on sonographer's experience. Biopsy guide and biopsy capable machine are not necessary.
■ Complications—Very low incidence with all procedures.
- Peritonitis
- Hemorrhage
- Tumor spread

Supplemental Readings

Barber DL, Lewis RE: *Guidelines for Radiology Service in Veterinary Medicine.* American Veterinary Medical Association, 1982.

Kleine LJ, Warren RG: *Mosby's Fundamentals of Animal Health Technology Small Animal Radiology.* St. Louis: C.V. Mosby, 1983.

Morgan JP, Silverman S: *Techniques of Veterinary Radiography,* third edition. Davis, CA: Veterinary Radiology Associates, 1984.

NCRP Report No. 36 Radiation Protection in Veterinary Medicine. Recommendations of the National Council on Radiation Protection and Measurements. NCRP Publications, P.O. Box 30175, Washington, D.C. 20014.

Ticer JW: *Radiographic Technique in Veterinary Practice,* second edition. Philadelphia: W.B. Saunders, 1984.

Fluid Therapy for Dogs and Cats

Dennis J. Chew

Fluid therapy is one of the most important therapeutic measures in seriously ill animals. The effective administration of fluids requires an understanding of fluid and electrolyte dynamics in both healthy and sick animals.

Answer these questions in order to decide when fluid therapy is needed:

- Does a serious deficit or excess of water exist?
- Are there serious electrolyte disturbances (excesses or deficits)?
- Is there a serious disturbance in acid-base balance?
- Is there an immediate need for full nutritional support with calories and protein?

Answer these questions in order to provide appropriate fluid therapy:

- What route will fluids be given?
- How fast will fluids be given?
- What volume of fluids will be given?
- What quality (type) of fluids will be given?
- What, if any, supplements will be added to commercially available fluids?

Indications for Fluid Therapy

- Most commonly for the correction of dehydration, hypokalemia, and metabolic acidosis.
- Less commonly for the specific correction of hypernatremia, hyponatremia, hyperkalemia, metabolic alkalosis, hypocalcemia, and hypercalcemia.
- For parenteral nutrition (see sec. 1, ch. 3).

DISTRIBUTION OF BODY WATER AND ELECTROLYTES

Total body water (TBW) represents 50 to 70% of body weight in adults. Usually 60% is arbitrarily chosen as an average figure.

Two thirds of TBW is within cells (intracellular) or 40% of body weight.

One third of TBW is extracellular fluid (ECF) or 20% of body weight.

- Interstitial water composes 15% of body weight.
- Intravascular water composes 5% of body weight.

Sodium and chloride exist in high concentration in serum (ECF) and in low concentration within cells.

Potassium and phosphorus exist in high concentration within cells and low concentration in serum (ECF).

MAINTENANCE REQUIREMENTS

Maintenance is defined as the volume of fluid (ml) and amount of electrolyte (mEq or mg) that must be taken in on a daily basis to keep the volume of TBW and electrolyte content normal. Obligate losses of water and electrolytes occur daily as a consequence of normal metabolism. Water taken into the body in all of its forms equals water loss in normal animals. See Figure 1 for the specific maintenance requirements of electrolytes and water in caged dogs and cats. For daily maintenance water requirements for dogs, based on body weight, see Table 1.

- Water can be taken in by drinking, combined mechanically with food, or derived from food metabolism or tissue breakdown (see Table 1). Water is lost from the body through evaporation during breathing, from feces, and from urine. Obligatory loss of electrolytes occurs in fecal water and in urine, but the overall loss of electrolytes is less in proportion than is the loss of water.

Normal losses of water contain sodium and osmole concentrations less than those of extracellular fluid; consequently, they are hypotonic (hypo-osmolal).

Normal daily losses of water contain relatively more potassium than does the concentration of extracellular fluid.

Maintenance volume is chosen near 30 ml/lb/day (66 ml/kg/day) for cats and small dogs, whereas 20 ml/lb/day (44 ml/kg/day) is more appropriate for very large dogs.

- Maintenance volume is composed of two subcomponents:
  - Insensible loss (not readily measured losses from respiratory evaporation, passage of normal feces, and sweat, which is negligible in dogs and cats).
    Estimated at 10 ml/lb/day (22 ml/kg/day) in normal animals. Can increase during febrile states, panting, and high environmental temperatures.
  - Sensible loss (readily measured as urine production).
    Approximately 10 to 20 ml/lb/day (22 to 44 ml/kg/day) in normal animals.

Urine output can dramatically decrease in acute intrinsic renal failure (oliguria/anuria); during urinary obstruction (anuria); during severe dehydration (oliguria).

Urine output can dramatically increase in polyuric renal failure and postobstructive diuresis.

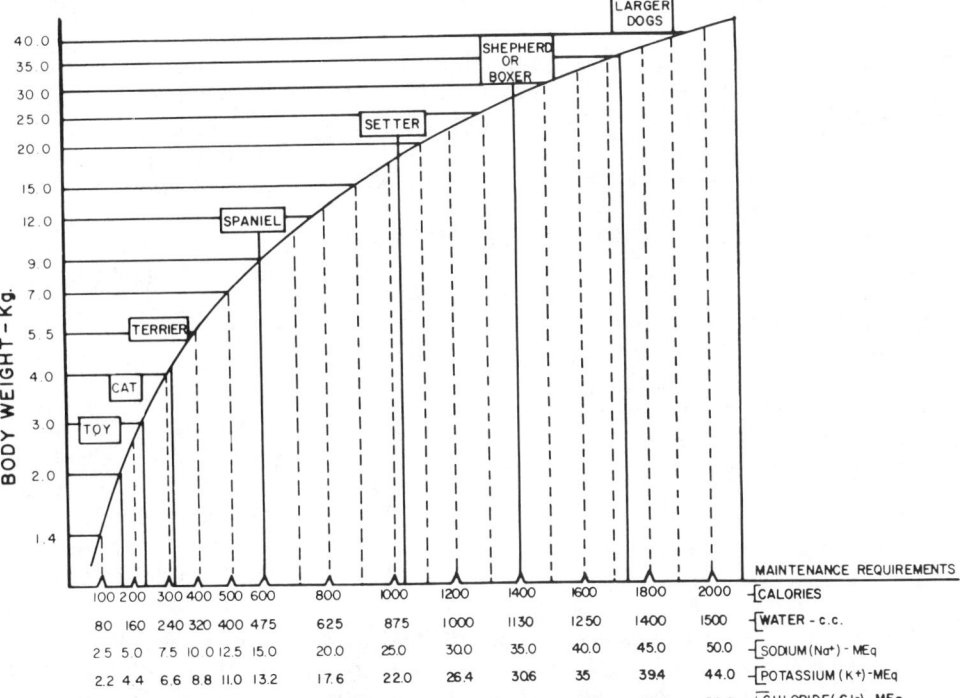

Figure 1. Maintenance fluid and electrolyte requirements of caged normal dogs and cats. (Finco, after Harrison JB: J Am Anim Hosp Assoc 8:179, 1972.)

TABLE 1. Daily Water Requirements for Dogs

Body Weight (kg)	Total Water/Day (mL)	Milliliters per Kg
1	140	140
2	232	116
3	312	104
4	385	96
5	453	91
6	518	86
7	580	83
8	639	80
9	696	77
10	752	75
11	806	73
12	859	71
13	911	70
14	961	68
15	1011	67
16	1060	66
17	1108	65
18	1155	64
19	1201	63
20	1247	62
25	1468	59
30	1677	56
35	1876	54
40	2068	52
45	2254	50
50	2434	49
60	2781	46
70	3112	44
80	3431	43
90	3739	41
100	4038	40

From Ross L: Fluid therapy for acute and chronic renal failure. Vet Clin North Am 19:343–359, 1989.

KEY POINT ▶ Lactated Ringer's and 0.9% sodium chloride solutions are *not* maintenance solutions because they contain far too much sodium and chloride, are too high in osmolality, and do not contain enough potassium.

■ 0.45% Sodium chloride in water or in 2.5% dextrose better approximates a maintenance solution for sodium and chloride content as well as for osmolality but does not contain adequate potassium. This does become an adequate maintenance solution when potassium is added to result in 20 to 30 mEq/L of potassium.

KEY POINT ▶ Maintenance fluids are low in sodium, chloride, and osmolality and high in potassium compared with normal plasma.

DEHYDRATION (REPLACEMENT NEEDS)

Dehydration exists when TBW decreases to less than normal.

■ Technically, dehydration refers to loss of pure water. Clinical fluid loss is usually accompanied by some loss of electrolytes.
■ Acute fluid and electrolyte loss in a disease process is initially from intravascular fluid.
 • Compensatory shifts of water and electrolytes from intracellular and interstitial compartments subsequently occur. The magnitude of these shifts depends on the tonicity and hydrostatic pressure of the remaining extracellular fluid. Consequently, dehydration can occur to different degrees in the various compartments.

Causes of Dehydration

- Decreased water intake (hypodipsia, adipsia)
  - Lack of food intake also decreases available water (water from oxidation and that which is physically present within the food).
  - Appetite and thirst centers may be depressed in systemically ill animals.
  - Accidental or deliberate deprivation of adequate water and food.
- Increased loss
  - Urinary (polyuria)—*common*
  - Gastrointestinal (vomiting, diarrhea)—*common*
  - Respiratory (fever, panting)
  - Skin (burns, large wounds)
  - Excessive salivation
  - Peritoneal dialysis

KEY POINT ▶ Fluid losses from the urinary and gastrointestinal tracts most frequently result in dehydration.

Disease processes can display a range of fluid and electrolyte loss combinations, from mostly water loss (hypotonic loss) to water loss with significant quantities of accompanying electrolytes (isotonic or hypertonic). Evaluate the tonicity and sodium concentration of the extracellular fluid in a dehydrated patient because this information gives clues to the nature of the fluid that was lost and helps determine the type of fluid to be given as replacement during treatment.

Characterization of Dehydration (Type)

The type of dehydration is defined based on the serum sodium concentration at the time of dehydration.

- *Isotonic dehydration* is the type that occurs most commonly and is defined by finding a normal serum sodium concentration (145 to 157 mEq/L) in the presence of dehydration. Isotonic dehydration occurs owing to the loss of water and electrolytes in proportion to those found in normal serum (isotonic loss).
- *Hypertonic dehydration* is the next most common type and is defined by an elevated serum sodium concentration (158 mEq/L or greater) in the presence of dehydration. Hypertonic dehydration occurs as a consequence of predominantly water loss—or water lost in excess of solute found in normal serum (hypotonic loss).
- *Hypotonic dehydration* is the least common type and is defined by a low serum sodium concentration (143 mEq/L or less) at the time of dehydration. Hypotonic dehydration theoretically occurs as solute is lost in excess of the concentration in normal serum (hypertonic loss). This is probably not the most significant mechanism, however. More likely is the loss of isotonic fluid. With continued intake and absorption of hypotonic fluids (such as drinking of water), the remaining extracellular sodium concentration is diluted to below normal.

Detection of Dehydration

Clinical tools to detect dehydration are limited in both sensitivity and specificity. No single test or procedure accurately assesses the magnitude of dehydration. Integration of historical findings, physical examination abnormalities and laboratory measurements is necessary to determine dehydration. Dehydration is not detectable by clinical means until at least 4 to 5% of body weight in water has been lost. An acute loss of greater than 12% body weight in water is considered life-threatening (Table 2).

History often leads the clinician to suspect dehydration and to assess its magnitude more accurately. Question the owner about volume of water intake (adipsia, hypodipsia, polydipsia, or normal). Because the volume of water intake may, in part, be a function stimulated by food intake, note also the presence or absence of anorexia. Abnormal losses of body fluid may be determined from the owner's answers to questions about vomiting, diarrhea, polyuria, panting, excessive salivation, and other bodily discharge. The duration of these historical signs and the magnitude of losses affect the magnitude of clinically detectable dehydration.

Physical examination provides general guidelines for detecting dehydration but is subjective (see Table 2.). Signs of listlessness and depression may occur from dehydration but may be partially attributable to underlying disease or concomitant electrolyte and acid-base abnormalities. As dehydration becomes more severe, decreased skin turgor, sunken eyes, dryness of mucous membranes, tachycardia, diminished capillary refill, and signs of shock may occur. An accurate recent body weight, when available, can be used as a baseline in order to compare the change in body weight as an indicator of change in body water.

KEY POINT ▶ An acute increase or decrease in an animal's body weight often reflects acute gain or loss of body water. This change is the most sensitive clinical tool for assessment of dehydration and rehydration. An acute loss or gain of 1 lb is the equivalent of 500 ml of fluid (1 kg = 1000 ml).

TABLE 2. Percentages of Detectable Dehydration

Dehydration	Signs
<5%	Not detectable; history may suggest dehydration.
5%	Subtle loss of skin elasticity
6–8%	Definite delay in return of skin to normal position, eyes may be sunken in orbits, slightly prolonged capillary refill time, mucous membranes may be dry.
10–12%	Tented skin stands in place, prolonged capillary refill time, eyes sunken in orbits, dry mucous membranes, signs of shock (increased heart rate, weak pulses) may be observed.
12–15%	Signs of shock, collapse, and severe depression; death imminent.

- Skin turgor assessment during physical examination is important for estimating the percentage of body weight loss due to dehydration. Skin turgor is evaluated by determining the time required for skin, gently lifted away from the body, to return to its original position. This is referred to as the skin pinch. Normal skin pliability (turgor) depends on hydration of the tissues in the area tested. Choose skin from the trunk as a test area. Avoid dependent areas and skin from the neck. Normal skin returns immediately to its initial position when lifted a short distance and released. Dehydrated skin shows varying degrees of slow return to the original position. As dehydration becomes progressive, the time required for return of the pinched skin to its initial position becomes greater. The clinician assigns increasing percentages of dehydration to abnormal skin turgor of increasing severity (see Table 2).

- Skin turgor is largely determined by hydration status of the interstitial tissues, although vascular and intracellular hydration also contribute. Elastin and adipose within skin and subcutaneous tissues also influence the apparent skin turgor.

- Many artifacts confuse interpretation of skin turgor. Skin turgor of obese animals may appear normal despite dehydration, owing to the large amounts of subcutaneous fat. The skin of an emaciated animal with normal hydration may fail to return to its normal position owing to a lack of subcutaneous fat and elastic tissue. Consequently, underestimating dehydration in obese animals and overestimating dehydration in emaciated animals occurs. Avoid cervical skin as a test area because redundant skin in this area confuses the results. Skin turgor changes in long-haired animals are more difficult to detect than those in short-haired animals. Differences in turgor assessment can occur in the same animal when standing and when recumbent.

KEY POINT ▶ Dehydration may be as little as 5% of body weight loss in lean dogs and as much as 10% or more in obese dogs before loss of skin turgor is detected.

- Other physical examination artifacts include dry mucous membranes that may occur in animals that pant continually and in those given anticholinergics. Sunken eyes may be seen in catabolic diseases in which tissue behind the globe is reduced or atrophy of the muscles of mastication has occurred.

KEY POINT ▶ Assessment of fluid, electrolyte, and acid-base status frequently is in error if the history and physical examination only are available for interpretation. The more seriously ill an animal, the more important the evaluation of laboratory data.

Laboratory

Simple laboratory testing. This is helpful in evaluation of intravascular hydration. Packed cell volume (PCV) recorded in % and total plasma protein (TPP) in gm/dl can be rapidly and inexpensively determined using a refractometer and microhematocrit. These two tests require only a few drops of blood that can be taken by capillary action from a 25-gauge venipuncture. Total plasma protein concentration may be more helpful in the detection of dehydration than is PCV. Increased TPP and PCV provide documentation for intravascular dehydration. Simultaneous evaluation of PCV and TPP is recommended in order to minimize interpretation errors due to pre-existing anemia or hypoproteinemia. Additional data are obtained when PCV and TPP are followed serially because increasing values identify progressive dehydration.

Urinalysis. UA is important in all cases of suspected dehydration. An elevated specific gravity (SG) represents the healthy kidney's response to decreased perfusion. The finding of dilute urine (< 1.030 SG) from a dehydrated animal immediately incriminates the kidneys as a major cause of, or contributor to, the dehydration.

Serum biochemistry. No test accurately documents the volume of fluid loss, but serum electrolyte evaluation helps to characterize the nature of the fluid that was lost.

Blood gases. Abnormalities in blood gas values may appear in dehydrated animals because of the loss or gain of certain body fluids, the activity of the underlying disease process itself, or the decreased perfusion of major organ systems.

KEY POINT ▶ Animals may be severely dehydrated, yet exhibit little or no changes within the serum biochemical test results. Likewise, the PCV/TPP findings can also be normal in the presence of dehydration.

Natural History of Specific Disease

Dehydration is anticipated in sick animals with certain disease syndromes known to predispose them to dehydration, regardless of physical examination or laboratory findings. For example, a collapsed diabetic animal is very likely to be dehydrated, as is the animal with advanced chronic renal failure or upper bowel obstruction.

Correction (Replacement) of Dehydration

- *Volume of fluid* to be replaced is calculated as follows, based on assessed % of dehydration and the patient's present body weight.
  - % dehydration × weight (kg) = liters of fluid to be replaced
  - % dehydration × weight (lb) × 500 = ml of fluid to be replaced
  - Alternatively, if a known recent body weight is available for comparison, replace 500 ml of fluid for every pound of acute body weight loss.
- *Type of fluid* that is chosen to accomplish this rehydration is based primarily on the serum sodium, chloride, and potassium concentrations.

KEY POINT ▶ Initial replacement with adequate fluid volume is usually more important than specific therapy for the electrolyte disorders.

- Return to the patient both the volume and quality (type) of fluid that has been lost or continues to be lost from the body. Base volume on measurement of the losses or, more commonly, on estimates. Base the quality of the fluid on the actual measurements of the losses or, more commonly, on the known biologic behavior of fluid losses associated with a specific disease.

KEY POINT ▶ Choose a fluid type or add supplements to stock fluids so that electrolytes deficient in the plasma or body are administered and those that are excessive in the plasma are avoided.

CONTEMPORARY LOSSES

These are fluid losses above the normal loss from insensible and sensible mechanisms. Usually volumes of fluid loss from vomitus and diarrhea are estimated. When the ongoing losses are excessive urinary losses, temporary urethral catheter collection may give the clinician a better idea as to their magnitude.

The total volume for 24-hour infusion (replacement plus maintenance) can be individually calculated (Figure 2), or it can be derived more generally from a multiple of maintenance needs (Table 3).

TYPES AND SELECTION OF FLUIDS

Table 4 lists a variety of available fluids and their composition.

Characterization of Fluids

- *Osmolality.* Parenteral fluids can be classified according to osmolality by comparison to the animal's normal serum osmolality of approximately 300 mOsm/kg. Osmolality of commercial fluids is largely determined by sodium and glucose concentrations. Fluids with osmolality less than 300 are hypotonic (e.g., 0.45% saline in water), those greater than 300

TABLE 3. Alternative Method to Calculate Maintenance Plus Dehydration Needs Using a Multiple of Maintenance*

Maintenance (M) plus Percent Dehydration†	ml/lb/day	Factor X Maintenance
M + 1	35	1.16
M + 2	40	1.33
M + 3	45	1.50
M + 4	50	1.67
M + 5	55	1.80
M + 6	60	2.00
M + 7	65	2.17
M + 8	70	2.33
M + 9	75	2.50
M + 10	80	2.70

*Maintenance is defined as 30 ml/lb/day.
†M is maintenance volume; + 1,2,3 . . . 10 refers to percent dehydration. Most animals with clinical dehydration (up to 10% dehydration) can be managed by infusion of between two and three times maintenance volume. Contemporary fluid losses are not considered in these calculations. Maintenance rate of infusion is started if the contemporary fluid loss is not excessive.

are hypertonic (e.g., 5.0% dextrose in 0.9% NaCl), whereas those near 300 (e.g., Ringer's solution, Normosol-R) are isotonic. Physiologic saline (0.9% NaCl) at 308 mOsm/kg is also within the isotonic range. Lactated Ringer's solution is often referred to as an isotonic solution in some species, but at 272 mOsm/kg it is mildly hypotonic for small animals.

KEY POINT ▶ Evaluation of serum sodium concentration as an indicator of tonicity provides the basis for initial choice of fluid treatment. If no laboratory measurements are available, correct dehydration using isotonic balanced solutions.

- Fluids can also be classified by their intended function for maintenance or replacement.
  - *Maintenance fluids* are polyelectrolyte solutions that differ greatly from serum because they are lower in sodium, contain additional potassium, and are hypotonic. Plasma-Lyte M in 5% dextrose (Travenol Laboratories, Deerfield, Illinois) and Normosol-M in 5% dextrose (CEVA Laboratories, Overland Park, Kansas) are commercially available products intended for this purpose. In both these products, the osmolality is increased owing

Figure 2. Summation of individual components of fluid need. Individual calculation of fluid volume needs, as listed, increases the likelihood of a more accurate fluid volume administration as needed by the patient.

_____ ml = **Rehydration** = % dehydration × weight (lb) × 500

+

_____ ml = **Sensible** = 10 to 20 ml/lb/day or measured

+

_____ ml = **Insensible** = 10 ml/lb/day

+

_____ ml = **Contemporary losses** = estimated or measured

_____ ml = **Total 24-hour needs**

TABLE 4. Composition of Solutions Used in Fluid Therapy

	Glucose[a] (g/L)	Na⁺ (mEq/L)	Cl⁻ (mEq/L)	K⁺ (mEq/L)	Ca²⁺ (mEq/L)	Mg²⁺ (mEq/L)	Buffer[b] (mEq/L)	Osmolarity (mOsm/L)	Cal/L	pH
			Dextrose Electrolyte Solution Composition							
5% dextrose	50	0	0	0	0	0	0	252	170	4.0
10% dextrose	100	0	0	0	0	0	0	505	340	4.0
2.5% dextrose in 0.45% NaCl	25	77	77	0	0	0	0	280	85	4.5
5% dextrose in 0.45% NaCl	50	77	77	0	0	0	0	406	170	4.0
5% dextrose and 0.9% NaCl	50	154	154	0	0	0	0	560	170	4.0
0.45% NaCl	0	77	77	0	0	0	0	154	0	5.0
0.85% NaCl (normal saline)	0	145	145	0	0	0	0	290	0	5.0
0.9% NaCl	0	154	154	0	0	0	0	308	0	5.0
3% NaCl	0	513	513	0	0	0	0	1026	0	5.0
Ringer's solution	0	147.5	156	4	4.5	0	0	310	0	5.5
Ringer's lactated solution	0	130	109	4	3	0	23(L)	272	9	6.5
2.5% dextrose in Ringer's lactated solution	25	130	109	4	3	0	28(L)	398	94	5.0
5% dextrose in Ringer's lactated solution	50	130	109	4	3	0	28(L)	524	179	5.0
2.5% dextrose in half-strength Ringer's lactated solution	25	65.5	55	2	1.5	0	14(L)	263	89	5.0
Normosol-M in 5% dextrose[c]	50	40	40	13	0	3	16(A)	364	175	5.5
Normosol-R[c]	0	140	98	5	0	3	27(A) 23(G)	296	18	6.4
Plasma-Lyte[d]	0	140	103	10	5	3	47(A) 8(L)	312	17	5.5
Plasma-Lyte M in 5% dextrose[c]	50	40	40	16	5	3	12(A) 12(L)	376	178	5.5
Plasma	1	145	105	5	5	3	24(B)	300	—	7.4
			Additives and Solutions							
20% mannitol	200(M)	0	0	0	0	0	0	1099	—	
7.5% NaHCO₃	0	893(B)	0	0	0	0	893(B)	1786	0	
8.4% NaHCO₃	0	1000(B)	0	0	0	0	1000(B)	2000	0	
10% CaCl₂	0	0	2720	0	1360	0	0	4080	0	
14.9% KCl	0	0	2000	2000	0	0	0	4000	0	
50% dextrose	500	0	0	0	0	0	0	2780	1700	4.2

[a]All glucose, with one exception: M, mannitol.
[b]Buffers used: A, acetate; B, bicarbonate; G, gluconate; L, lactate.
[c]CEVA Laboratories.
[d]Baxter Healthcare.
From Chew DJ, DiBartola SP: *Manual of Small Animal Nephrology and Urology.* New York, Churchill Livingstone, 1986, pp 308-309.

to the glucose but becomes hypotonic in the body when glucose is metabolized. Maintenance fluids can be made by mixing one part salt-rich solution (lactated Ringer's, 0.9% NaCl, or Ringer's solution) with two parts 5% dextrose in water and the addition of 15 to 20 milliequivalents of potassium chloride to each liter of final solution. Salt and sugar solutions can be physically combined before infusion, or they can be administered alternately to the patient.

- *Replacement fluids* must be formulated for specific electrolyte or alkali deficits. Additives such as potassium chloride, calcium chloride, or sodium bicarbonate are often added to commercially available solutions. This practice varies greatly according to the disease process and the laboratory measurements.

Fluids to be Kept on Hand

■ Clinical correction of most fluid problems can be accomplished by maintaining only a few stock solutions, usually lactated Ringer's solution, 0.9% sodium chloride, and 5% dextrose in water.

■ It is convenient, although not essential, to have 0.45% dextrose in 2.5% sodium chloride available.

- Alternatively, mix equal portions of 0.9% sodium chloride with 5% dextrose in water to provide the same solution.

■ These stock solutions are modified as needed with potassium, glucose, or bicarbonate supplements (see subsequent discussion).

■ Lactated Ringer's solution is most often chosen as a "physiologic" solution that is similar in composition to normal animal plasma with the exception of protein. This solution is usually the fluid of choice in the absence of laboratory data until more data about electrolyte, osmolality, and acid-base status are available.

■ The 0.9% sodium chloride or Ringer's solution is chosen when "extra" sodium or chloride is needed to maintain volume expansion or when the correction of metabolic alkalosis is needed.

■ The 5% dextrose in water is chosen when "extra" water is needed during a rehydrating process or when maintenance is indicated.

Supplementation of Parenteral Fluids

After sodium, potassium considerations are most important. Hypokalemia is commonly noted in hospi-

talized animals, particularly those with prolonged anorexia and on potassium-deficient fluids. Other supplements can include alkali, dextrose, phosphate, calcium, and vitamins.

■ *Potassium supplementation.* Potassium supplementation is usually provided as potassium chloride, although potassium phosphate is given under unusual conditions. It is most common to use commercially available sterile vials with 2 mEq/ml of potassium for addition to fluids. Potassium supplementation to fluids is indicated when the serum potassium concentration is less than 3.5 mEq/L.

- The modified Sliding Scale of Scott (Table 5) recommends adding potassium chloride to maintenance fluid volumes proportional to the degree of hypokalemia—the lower the potassium concentration, the greater the amount of potassium added to the fluids. Supplemented fluids provide 28, 40, 60, or 80 mEq/L of potassium. An exact number of milliequivalents for supplementation is not calculated using this method. Potassium supplementation employing this scale can be started during correction of dehydration if fluids are distributed evenly throughout the day.

- Alternatively, a fixed concentration of potassium from 20 to 30 mEq/L can be given in maintenance fluids and is particularly helpful when frequent monitoring of serum potassium concentration is not possible. This concentration corresponds to the lower end of the Sliding Scale of Scott. Potassium to 35 mEq/L can be given in subcutaneous fluids without irritation to local tissues.

- Potassium supplementation may still be indicated when the concentration is from 3.5 to 4.5 mEq/L. This supplementation can prevent the development of hypokalemia during fluid treatment and also can help replenish the total body potassium deficit that is not yet reflected by the serum potassium concentration. Maintenance needs for potassium in healthy dogs and cats are shown in Figure 1, but enhanced loss through urination during fluid administration can be expected.

KEY POINT ▶ Potassium is added at approximately 20 mEq/L for maintenance fluids when serum potassium concentration is from 3.5 to 4.5 mEq/L.

TABLE 5. Modified Sliding Scale of Scott

Serum K+ (mEq/L)	mEq K+ (To Add to 250 ml Fluid)	mEq K+ (To Add to 1 L Fluid)	Maximum Infusion Rate of IV Fluids (0.5 mEq/kg/hr)
<2.0	20	80	6
2.1–2.5	15	60	8
2.6–3.0	10	40	12
3.1–3.5	7	28	18
>3.5–<5.0	5	20	25

For dogs or cats with hypokalemia or for those with potassium depletion and normal serum potassium levels. This regimen is designed to be infused in maintenance volume of fluids.

- Caution is used whenever potassium-enriched fluids are infused.

The rate of potassium infusion is usually more important than the total number of milliequivalents. Do not exceed 0.5 mEq/kg/hr to reduce any possibility of development of hyperkalemia and cardiotoxicity.

Animals with alkalosis and potassium translocation may not require vigorous potassium supplementation, if the alkalosis can be corrected rapidly. Potassium can rapidly return from the cells to the extracellular water.

Animals with severe emaciation have reduced lean body mass available for potassium uptake and are less vigorously supplemented with potassium in the fluid.

Reduced renal function and azotemia can lead to potassium retention and hyperkalemia during infusion of potassium-supplemented fluids, particularly if oliguria is present. Less vigorous potassium supplementation and careful monitoring are indicated in this situation.

Potassium chloride supplementation increases the osmolality of fluids, particularly when high concentrations are provided. For example, potassium supplementation at 40 mEq/L increases the osmolality of the fluid by 80 mOsm/kg, 40 osmoles each from potassium and chloride. If the infused potassium and chloride enter the cells or are excreted, the transient increase in serum osmolality is of little concern.

KEY POINT ▶ Although potassium supplementation is often beneficial, too much can result in death due to hyperkalemia. Potassium supplementation at higher concentrations is not to be undertaken unless the serum concentration can be measured at least once daily. Electrocardiographic monitoring may be needed during supplementation of fluids with potassium in animals that are at risk for development of hyperkalemia.

■ *Alkali Supplementation*
- Addition of alkali to fluids is sometimes needed for partial correction of metabolic acidosis. It is not usually necessary or desirable to correct metabolic acidosis to normal by supplementation alone.
- Add sodium bicarbonate to fluids when alkali replacement is needed quickly.

Do not rely on acetate or lactate at concentrations in commercially available solutions to correct severe metabolic acidosis. Lactate and acetate require metabolic conversion to bicarbonate before they can contribute to the correction of acidosis.

KEY POINT ▶ Do not add sodium bicarbonate to fluids that contain calcium because calcium precipitate may occur.

- Calculate the alkali replacement from either the bicarbonate value reported on the blood gas analysis or the total CO_2 value on the serum biochemical profile. Total CO_2 (mEq/L) can be substituted for

bicarbonate in these calculations because it is usually only 1 to 2 mEq/L different.

Assume that normal HCO_3 is 24 mEq/L.

Subtract the patient's HCO_3 value from 24. This equals the HCO_3 deficit in mEq/L.

HCO_3 deficit × 0.6 × body weight (kg) = "missing" mEq bicarbonate from total body water at the time of sampling.

Administer total replacement mEq over several hours of the day. It may take as long as 18 hours for administered bicarbonate to equilibrate inside cells. It is sometimes desirable, in the presence of severe metabolic acidosis, to administer 1/4 to 1/2 of the calculated dose as a slow IV bolus injection and to add the remainder to fluids for 24-hour infusion.

HCO_3 deficit × 0.3 × body weight (kg) = "missing" mEq bicarbonate from extracellular water at the time of sampling.

Use this formula when (1) multiple injections of bicarbonate are likely to be needed during severe metabolic acidosis, (2) ongoing addition of acid or loss of alkali is anticipated, and (3) access to multiple HCO_3 measurements is possible.

- Without access to blood gas analysis or total CO_2, it is difficult to ascertain the magnitude of need.

If the suspicion and clinical diagnosis for metabolic acidosis is high, bicarbonate may be administered empirically. Estimated at mild acidosis, give 3 mEq/kg bicarbonate in fluids for 24 hours. Estimated at moderate acidosis, give 6 mEq/kg bicarbonate in fluids for 24 hours. Estimated at severe acidosis, give 9 mEq/kg bicarbonate in fluids for 24 hours.
- In crisis situations that require bicarbonate, administer 1 to 2 mEq/kg of sodium bicarbonate as an IV slow bolus injection and re-evaluate.
- Along with the bicarbonate, sodium is administered that can result in hypernatremia, hyperosmolality, hypertension, overhydration, and volume overload if not excreted.
- Overtreatment with alkali can also result in alkalosis, paradoxical cerebrospinal fluid (CSF) acidosis, ionized calcium shifts, and seizures.
■ *Dextrose supplementation.* If supplementation with dextrose is necessary, use 50% dextrose to vary the % dextrose in the final solution.
  - To increase the dextrose concentration by 2.5%, add 25 gm of dextrose, or 50 ml of 50% dextrose, to each liter.
  - Indications include hypoglycemia due to sepsis, insulin overdose, insulinoma, liver disease, and so forth. Dextrose supplementation at less than 10% concentration is not, however, effective as a source of calories in anorectic animals.
■ *Vitamin supplementation.* The need for vitamins during parenteral fluid therapy in cats or dogs is not proved. It is plausible, however, that vitamins may be beneficial.
  - Water-soluble vitamins can be conservatively added to parenteral fluids without known harm and may replenish rapidly depleted stores.

Dogs or cats in polyuric renal failure may benefit from water-soluble vitamins in parenteral fluids to replenish the urinary losses of these vitamins.

Thiamine deficiency can be of clinical concern in cats and can develop during anorexia while on fluids, as thiamine is not stored for long periods.

Initial signs of thiamine deficiency include anorexia, vomiting, and ataxia that can progress to dilated pupils and tonic ventroflexion of the neck, which is often confused with seizures. True seizures can also occur. Death is usually within 24 hours of convulsions, if the pet is not treated.

It is common practice to add 0.5 to 1.0 ml of water-soluble multi-vitamins to each liter of fluids to provide needed vitamins and to prevent thiamine deficiency.

- Water-soluble vitamins impart a yellow color to the fluids and makes them more easily visualized. This color facilitates the monitoring of the fluid bag to ensure that the rate of fluid administration is appropriate.

■ *Calcium supplementation*

- Calcium gluconate and calcium chloride can be supplemented in replacement and maintenance fluids for the correction of symptomatic hypocalcemia. This is discussed in detail in sec. 4, ch. 2. Calcium is not added to fluids containing lactate or acetate because precipitates may occur.

■ *Phosphorus supplementation*

- Hypophosphatemia is present when the serum concentration is < 2.5 mg/dL. Mild hypophosphatemia (2.0 to 2.5 mg/dL) is common and often transient. Mild-to-moderate hypophosphatemia often resolves quickly during the therapy directed at the underlying cause, without the need for phosphate supplementation.
- Severe hypophosphatemia (< 1.5 mg/dL) is uncommon but can be life-threatening, particularly when less than 1.0 mg/dL. Thus, it should be treated with supplementation with phosphate salts.

KEY POINT ▶ Clinically significant hypophosphatemia is most likely to be observed in patients with diabetes mellitus and may require specific treatment with phosphate salts.

- When necessary, add supplemental sodium phosphate and potassium phosphate to replacement and maintenance fluids for the correction of symptomatic or severe hypophosphatemia. Phosphate salts are not added to fluids that contain calcium.
- Treat only when the hypophosphatemia is severe and persistent. Oversupplementation can cause hyperphosphatemia, hypocalcemia, tetany/seizures, soft-tissue mineralization, hyperkalemia if from potassium phosphate, and hypernatremia if from sodium phosphate supplementation. Discontinue supplementation once the serum phosphorus concentration rises to > 2.0 mg/dL.
- The intravenous dosage for phosphate supplementation has been recommended at 0.01 to 0.03 mmol phosphate/kg/hr for 3 to 6 hours. A dosage of 2.5 mg/kg phosphate over 6 hours has also been suggested as a starting point. The most commonly used phosphate preparations provide 3.0 mmol/ml. For example, sodium phosphate provides 3.0 mmol/ml and 93.0 mg/ml phosphorus and 4.0 mEq/ml sodium.

General Guidelines for Fluid Selection

- If the serum sodium concentration is elevated, the animal has hypertonic dehydration and needs more water than salt for replacement (hypotonic fluid). Fluids that are effectively hypotonic (5% dextrose in water, 0.45% NaCl in 2.5% dextrose) are chosen. Dextrose solutions in a 2.5 to 5% concentration are considered to be effectively hypotonic because of the rapid dextrose metabolism that removes its contribution to osmolality. The magnitude of the elevation in serum sodium and the patient's clinical status determine whether dextrose in water or dextrose in some concentration of saline is administered. Lowering of severe hyperosmolality and hypernatremia too rapidly can be detrimental, particularly to the brain. Pure water without some electrolyte or glucose to add osmolality is not given as severe problems with hemolysis and rapid change in serum osmolality can occur.
- If the serum sodium concentration is normal, the animal has isotonic dehydration and needs replacement fluids that are near-normal in serum sodium concentration and osmolality. Ringer's solution or 0.9% sodium chloride are appropriate selections.
- If the serum sodium concentration is low, the animal has hypotonic dehydration and needs additional sodium relative to water. Hypertonic fluid infusion is theoretically indicated but clinically is not chosen, unless the hyponatremia and hypo-osmolality are very severe and symptomatic. Isotonic fluids are usually chosen for replacement because the kidneys must excrete unnecessary water and reclaim needed sodium.
- Choose 0.9% saline or lactated Ringer's solution for rapid infusion to animals in shock until vascular volume is stabilized. For a complete discussion of shock therapy, see sec. 6, ch. 14. Evaluate serum sodium to decide whether to continue this fluid or whether hypotonic fluids would be superior.
- Further selection of fluid type requires laboratory measurement of potassium, chloride, calcium, phosphorus, and blood gas values. When the serum concentration of an electrolyte is elevated, choose a fluid for infusion that lacks or is low in that electrolyte concentration. When the serum concentration of an electrolyte is low, choose a fluid for infusion that contains a high concentration of that electrolyte or provide supplementation of that electrolyte to the fluid. In some instances, supplemental electrolyte can be given to prevent deficits, as previously mentioned for potassium. Final osmolality of fluids for infusion is evaluated following supplementation of base solutions to ensure that they are appropriate because supplementation of base solutions often results in unappreciated hyperosmolality.
- *Preservatives.* Fluids containing preservatives of any kind are never used for administration to cats, puppies, or small dogs because of the likelihood of severe toxic reactions.
  - Benzoic acid derivatives are commonly found in

fluids for their antibacterial and antifungal effects, but cats are extremely susceptible to the toxic effects from these compounds even at low doses. Benzyl alcohol at 0.9% is commonly added to multiple dose vials of sodium chloride for injection.

Clinical signs of toxicity are mostly neurologic and include changes in behavior: apprehension; aggression; hyperexcitability (to light and sound); salivation; marked ataxia; fasciculations of the muscles of the head and ears; widely dilated, nonresponsive pupils; convulsions; and coma. Death follows. Immature animals may be at increased risk.

ROUTES OF ADMINISTRATION FOR PARENTERAL FLUIDS

The route of fluid therapy depends on the nature of the clinical disorder, its severity, and its onset (acute or chronic); the nature and magnitude of ongoing losses; and the composition of fluids to be given. The availability of personnel and equipment for monitoring required during IV therapy also influences the decision to choose the parenteral route.

Subcutaneous Route

Subcutaneous administration of fluids is common in dogs and cats. Choose either isotonic or mildly hypotonic fluids to enhance absorption.

KEY POINT ▶ Do not give 5% dextrose in water as an isotonic solution subcutaneously in cases of severe dehydration. Delayed absorption, with consequent equilibration of ECF electrolytes into the pocket of pooled, nonabsorbed subcutaneous fluid may occur.

Absorption of subcutaneous fluid is unreliable in conditions characterized by peripheral vasoconstriction (e.g., shock, severe dehydration, hypothermia). Never rely on this route for the emergency replacement of fluid in critically ill or severely dehydrated patients. Minimal dehydration may be corrected by this route, or dehydration in the anorexic animal may be prevented. In general, treat the critically ill or massively dehydrated animal initially with IV fluids and then SC fluids as the problems resolve.

The volume of fluid that can be administered subcutaneously is limited by the individual's skin elasticity. Animals differ in their abilities to tolerate the infused load comfortably. Choose the site of the SC infusions somewhere on the trunk so that the fluid does not gravitate into the limbs. Avoid areas with surgical wounds because fluid may dissect the healing tissues. Subcutaneous infusions may be given under gravitational forces through IV administration tubing or direct injection from a large-volume hypodermic syringe.

KEY POINT ▶ Use intravenous fluid administration whenever accurate delivery of fluid volume and potent pharmacotherapeutic agents are required.

Intravenous Route

Give hypotonic, isotonic, and hypertonic fluids by the IV route as the need arises. Rapid infusions of fluid volume may be readily accomplished by this route.

Vein Selection

- The jugular vein and cephalic vein are most commonly chosen for indwelling IV catheterization. The lateral saphenous and femoral veins also may be used.
- The jugular vein in cats and small dogs is preferred for mechanical reasons.
- The jugular vein is preferred in serious diseases regardless of patient size.
  - Advantages of the jugular vein include the ability to measure central venous pressure (CVP), to use large-bore catheters for more rapid infusions, to administer hypertonic solutions and other irritating drugs owing to greater dilutional effects from greater blood flow, and to obtain serial blood samples easily from the IV line. Use care to avoid clotting within the line.
  - The prime disadvantage of using peripheral veins is that the limb position often changes the rate of fluid infusion owing to partial or complete occlusion of the indwelling catheter.
  - In cats and small dogs, 19-gauge catheters are often used; 17-gauge catheters are generally used in larger animals. Larger-bore catheters may be of value in emergency situations. Clinician preference determines the type of catheter.

Intravenous Catheter Care

- Always perform aseptic catheter placement. This includes wide clipping of hair surrounding the vein and surgical scrub. After securing the catheter in the vein, place a gauze sponge with an antimicrobial cream over the puncture site.
- Catheter complications include thrombophlebitis, thromboembolism, bacteremia, and bacterial endocarditis, and catheter-fragment foreign body.
- To minimize problems
  - Place the catheter aseptically.
  - Do not allow the catheter to remain in a given vein longer than 48 to 72 hours.
  - Monitor the patient for fever, leukocytosis, and heart murmurs.
  - Keep the catheter site clean.
  - When the catheter is not in use, avoid clotting with heparinized saline (0.9% saline with 3 to 5 U heparin/ml).

Intraperitoneal Fluid Administration

- Severely anemic puppies and kittens may be transfused by this route when a vein cannot be catheterized (see sec. 3, ch. 1 for details of blood transfusion).
- This route may be considered for rewarming very hypothermic animals.
- Use isotonic to mildly hypotonic fluids for rehydration. Intravenous route is preferred when possible.

Intraosseous Route

- Rarely used until recently. Consider more often.
- Blood and crystalloid solutions can be infused safely.
- Bone marrow of femur, tibia, or humerus is catheterized with a bone-marrow needle and secured in place.
- Provides rapid access to circulation when venous catheterization is not successful or possible.

RATE OF FLUID INFUSION

- The rate of fluid administration depends on the extent and rapidity of the fluid loss, as well as on the composition of the fluid to be infused. Rapid or extensive fluid losses demand rapid replacement. In chronic disorders, it is not always necessary to replace the dehydration deficit rapidly. Some clinicians prefer to calculate the dehydration deficit, add it to the daily maintenance requirements, and distribute this fluid load over 24 hours. Others prefer to replace the dehydration deficit over the first few hours (referred to as "front-end loading"). The decision depends on the status of the individual animal. Deficit replacement of 75 to 80% on the first day and the remaining 25% deficit the second day is recommended by some clinicians. However, dehydration usually can be corrected safely within 24 hours in most cases.
- Maximal infusion rates may be necessary in the treatment of shock or severe dehydration. Isotonic fluid of 1 blood volume/hr (40 ml/lb/hr or 90 ml/kg/hr for a dog; 30 ml/lb/hr or 66 ml/kg/hr for a cat) is recommended as the maximal rate of IV fluid infusion without CVP monitoring.
- Measure urine output during rapid fluid infusion as a guide to organ perfusion. In the case of persistent oliguria, be careful about maximal fluid infusion and monitor CVP to avoid overhydration.
- In less critical conditions, distribute fluids evenly throughout the day. Physiologically, this technique may be advantageous because it allows more time for adequate equilibration of water and electrolytes between the body compartments. Ideally, a constant or continuous infusion of IV fluids over a 24-hour period accomplishes this. This ideal situation may not be possible if very small volumes of fluid are being infused or if 24-hour monitoring of the IV lines is unavailable.
  - Front-end loading of fluids to correct dehydration can be given over a 4- to 8-hour period when an animal's clinical condition dictates a more rapid correction of dehydration. Maintenance and contemporary losses can then be accomplished by infusion evenly over the remaining hours of the day.
  - When fluid infusion can be observed for only part of the day, 24-hour needs are distributed over the number of hours that someone can watch the drip. The catheter is then flushed with heparinized saline to maintain patency until the infusion resumes.

   If severe dehydration has been corrected, additional fluids can be given subcutaneously until the IV drip can be restarted the next day.
- The rate of infusion for the total 24-hour volume of fluid is specified as to the required number of milliliters per hour and the number of drops per minute to ensure accurate delivery of prescribed fluids.
- Intravenous administration sets are available in standard "macrodrip" volume of 10, 15, or 20 drops/ml. Pediatric administration sets also are available in the "minidrip" volume of 60 drops/ml. Patient size and volume of fluid to be infused determine the choice between the minidrip and macrodrip systems.
  - The minidrip administration set is most suitable for cats and small dogs because it allows a simpler quantitation of small volumes of fluid for infusion.
  - In cats and small dogs, use small (125 or 250 ml) bags or bottles to infuse fluids by gravity. This lessens the chance that too large a volume of fluid can accidentally be infused from a large reservoir.
- Once the drip set has been adjusted to the desired rate, mark the IV bottle or bag with adhesive tape as subsequently indicated to monitor the hourly volume of fluids received. This practice allows adjustment for individual variations (e.g., animal changing position of limb that contains the catheter).
- In dehydrated animals with either severe oliguria or diuresis, measurement of urine output may be helpful for accurately matching the needs of the animal with the fluid therapy ("ins and outs"). Without this system, a tendency exists to overestimate the actual fluid needs in an oliguric animal, resulting in overhydration, and to underestimate the fluid needs in a diuretic animal, resulting in failure to correct the dehydration.

   Replace previously calculated dehydration needs first and then proceed with the "ins and outs." In this technique, divide the day into six 4-hour intervals. The hour interval can vary and is chosen based on the severity of the condition (i.e., every hour or every 6 or 8 hours, as the need dictates). Determine the fluid needs for this interval, summating both calculated insensible (10 ml/lb or 22 ml/kg divided by 6, if 4-hour intervals are used), losses and measured sensible (urine-volume) losses. The measured volume of sensible losses from the previous 4-hour period is given back to the patient in the next 4-hour period.
  - Carry this procedure out in identical fashion for an additional three or more time periods. This type of close attention to fluid volume administration is of benefit in the initial management of critically ill animals, particularly when CVP and renal status are uncertain.
- The rate of IV fluid infusion is important when considering potassium-rich fluids and those containing a large quantity of alkali. See previous discussion, Supplementation of Parenteral Fluids.
- For small dogs and cats, consider the use of a Buretrol (Baxter Healthcare) or a similar device to accurately premeasure the fluids to be administered over the next few hours.
  1. Fluids from the reservoir bag are periodically used to reload the Buretrol device.
  2. This method minimizes the chance of overhydra-

tion because it allows more accurate delivery of small volumes.

- Infusion pumps provide an extremely accurate means of administering IV fluids.
  - Enter ml/hr or drops/min depending on the type of machine.
  - Electronic drip counter ensures accurate delivery.
  - Most pumps are equipped with alarm systems if fluid flow is interrupted.
  - A disadvantage is that new pumps are expensive. Refurbished used machines may be surprisingly affordable, however.
  - Especially useful for small dogs, cats, and animals receiving fluids supplemented with potassium or other agents.
- Table 6 lists the components of a complete prescription for fluid therapy.

MONITORING EFFICACY OF FLUID THERAPY

- Perform a physical examination several times daily during the initial fluid management to document rehydration, prevent overhydration, and detect contemporary fluid loss. The indicators of successful fluid therapy are normalization of skin turgor, moistening of mucous membranes, strengthening of pulses, increasing of perfusion (decreasing of refill time), and increasing of alertness. Table 7 provides guidelines for the data base required to adequately assess the success of fluid therapy. Table 8 lists the possible reasons why dehydration has not been adequately corrected.
- Increased body weight occurs during successful rehydration. An acute gain or loss of 1 lb suggests an increase or a decrease of 500 mL body water (or a 1 kg change in body weight is equivalent to 1000 ml). An anorexic animal, however, loses 0.1 to 0.3 kg body weight/day/1000 calories of the daily requirement, owing to tissue catabolism. Determine and record body weight accurately at least once daily.
- Follow packed cell volume (PCV) and total plasma

TABLE 6. Total Fluid Prescription

1. Type of fluid to be infused (choose one):
   _____ Lactated Ringer's solution
   _____ 0.9% Sodium chloride in water
   _____ 0.45% sodium chloride in 2.5% dextrose in water
   _____ 5% dextrose in water
2. Supplements and amounts to be added to the fluid:
   Sodium chloride _____
   Potassium chloride _____
   Sodium bicarbonate _____
   Glucose (dextrose) _____
   Calcium (gluconate) _____
   Phosphate _____
   Other (specify _____) _____
3. 24-Hour fluid volume: _____ ml
4. Route of infusion: _____
5. Rate of fluid administration: _____ ml/24 hr
   _____ ml/hr
   _____ ml/min
   _____ drops/sec

TABLE 7. Data Bases Before and During Fluid Administration

Minimum Data Base (mild illness and dehydration)
  Body Weight
  Packed cell volume (PCV); total plasma protein (TPP)
  Urine specific gravity
Extended Data Base (severe dehydration with collapse)
  All of the above, plus the following values:
    Serum sodium, potassium, and chloride
    Blood urea nitrogen (BUN) or serum creatinine
    Bicarbonate (total CO_2 from profile)
    Electrocardiogram
Advanced Data Base (shock, oliguria, heart failure)
  All of the above, plus the following values:
    Central venous pressure (CVP)
    Blood gas analysis (venous and arterial)

protein (TPP) serially during fluid therapy. Decreases in both PCV and TPP suggest successful intravascular rehydration.

- In difficult cases, particularly those animals with renal or heart failure, monitor the CVP to minimize the chances of overloading the heart and causing pulmonary edema when administering fluids rapidly (see sec. 1, ch. 3 for CVP measurement technique).
  - Monitor the CVP with a jugular catheter—the tip of which is level with the right atrium. Normal CVP is 0 to 10 cm H_2O.

    A sudden increase in CVP during fluid therapy indicates the inability of the cardiovascular system to accommodate the rate of fluid administration. Reduce the rate of administration accordingly.

    Signs of overhydration, unfortunately, can still occur even without a change in CVP.
- Closely monitor all animals receiving fluid therapy. Determine the serial serum electrolyte values in severely dehydrated animals receiving fluid therapy. Ideally, animals that had serum electrolyte deficiency or excess show improvement toward normal values after appropriate therapy. Follow the electrolyte determinations in those cases that had initially normal values to detect the possible consequences of volume expansion and changes in the underlying disease process.

KEY POINT ▶ Successful fluid therapy ultimately depends on the clinician's ability to detect and correct the underlying cause for the loss of fluid and loss or retention of electrolytes. Identifying and stopping the ongoing fluid losses are particularly important.

TABLE 8. Possible Causes of Failure to Correct Dehydration Adequately

Error in mathematic calculations
Error in assessment of initial degree of dehydration
Larger contemporary losses than expected
Too-rapid infusion resulting in diuresis and loss of fluid from body
Mechanical dysfunction of IV catheter or infusion system; calculated volume not infused
Increased sensible loss not appreciated (fever, panting)
Increased sensible loss not appreciated (polyuria)

OVERHYDRATION

Overhydration rarely occurs as a spontaneous disorder—it usually is iatrogenic following fluid treatments. Inability to excrete free water, as can occur in a variety of renal diseases and in congestive heart failure, predisposes the patient to overhydration.

Body weight continues to increase above and beyond that expected to accomplish rehydration. CVP progressively increases during advanced overhydration.

Physical Examination

Decreased volume of urinations may be noticed, or the bladder may remain small during fluid administration. A gelatinous feel to the SC tissues may precede the development of obvious peripheral edema. Pulmonary edema, manifested as lung crackles and tachypnea, may be detected. Vomiting, diarrhea, serous discharge from the nose and eyes, and chemosis can develop during overhydration. Venous overdistension may also be noted.

Laboratory

Progressive decreases in PCV and total protein may be found.

- Radiographs may reveal increased lung density indicating pulmonary edema. Cardiac enlargement may be noted, if congestive heart failure is imminent.
- Immediate correction may be difficult when renal and cardiac function are impaired. Stop all IV infusions and give furosemide at 2 to 4 mg/kg IV. Give another dose of furosemide but double the dose, if no diuresis occurs within 15 minutes. Morphine is considered as a treatment to increase compliance of pulmonary vessels. Peritoneal dialysis with hypertonic dialysate can be considered for acute volume overload rescue as can therapeutic phlebotomy.

6 Care of the Grieving Client

Susan Phillips Cohen

For many people, companion animals are important members of their social network. As a result, the death of a special pet may be upsetting, even devastating. Veterinarians and their staffs can help clients cope with loss before, during, and after the death of their loved one. As in the treatment of illness, effective intervention depends upon a sensitive assessment of the total situation.

ASSESSMENT OF SITUATION

Active Listening

- Careful, responsive listening allows us to understand another's point of view. Feeling understood helps one to listen and take action.
- While listening, encourage the speaker to continue by leaning forward, nodding, maintaining eye contact, and adding neutral comments, like "Umm hmm," "Yes," "Go on."
- In general, ask open-ended questions that do not limit answers. If the speaker seems confused or off target, ask closed questions that require specific information or short answers, like "Yes," or "No."
- Every so often, repeat the gist of the speaker's thoughts.
- When summarizing, try to capture both words and feelings.
- Once the other's beliefs are clear, offer new information and ideas in a way that relates to that person's interests and concerns.

Intuition and Analysis

- Develop and learn to trust hunches, feelings, mental pictures, and analogies, as a starting point in assessing clients.
- Test these by seeking information that supports or refutes your ideas.

Dynamic Assessment

- New information or a change in the client can alter an assessment.
- Many conditions can affect how a person appears, such as shock, exhaustion, illness, surprise, intoxication, and embarrassment.
- To remain open to change, observe carefully and listen actively.

Monitoring Intervention

- To test the effectiveness of your actions (interventions), consider the following:

- Does the person seem to understand?
- Can the person repeat what you have said?
- Do you seem to be reaching true agreement on what to do?
- Does the person seem to be feeling better, clearer, and calmer?
- If the answer is no, change your approach.
  - Explain the situation in different words.
  - Use handouts, models, and pictures.
  - In a nonjudgmental tone, acknowledge that understanding is still lacking and ask for the other person's input.

Stages of Grief

- The first response to loss, threatened loss, or other bad news is usually shock. Shock (numbness, denial) protects the emotional system from overloading. People may have a fixed expression and may not absorb information well. They may return to this stage several times.
- The middle stage of grief consists of painful feelings, such as anger, depression, longing, and guilt. Accept the client's behavior as normal and try not to take it personally.
- The final stage is resolution. People accept their loss as permanent and create a new life without the loved one.

ASSESSMENT OF THE CLIENT

Assessment of the client may help the veterinarian to predict the response to a difficult situation, such as the death of the pet.

Nonverbal Communication

Body language reveals how a client is feeling from moment to moment.

- Crossed arms or legs suggest defensiveness; open arms suggest confidence.
- Foot tapping, rapid breathing, or arms clutching the torso indicate nervousness or anxiety.
- A glassy-eyed look or fixed smile may mean the client has been stunned or confused by your words and may not be taking in your information.
- In standard American culture maintaining eye contact shows interest, trustworthiness. In other cultures, for example many Asian ones, polite people avoid eye contact with those who are older or higher in status.
- Watch how people position themselves in relation to

77

objects and each other. Standing behind a table puts a barrier between two people. Closing the distance between two people increases intimacy.

■ To help experience life as others do or to put people at ease, match their body position.

Appearance can reveal mood, socioeconomic status, and cultural differences.

■ People who appear neat, clean, and well-groomed usually feel good about themselves.
■ People who often appear unkempt or dirty may be severely depressed, disturbed, or homeless.
■ Wearing bright or dark colors can reflect both mood and social custom.
■ Be alert to disabilities. These may affect the ability to read instructions or to medicate a pet at home or to lift anything heavy.

Verbal Communication

Voice Quality

■ A very high-pitched voice suggests anxiety. Speech that varies little in pitch may mean the person is depressed.
■ Voices convey emotion, but shock, shame, or strong self-control can mask depth of feeling.

Speed

■ Rate of speed depends upon cultural difference (northeasterners speak faster than southerners) as well as mood.
■ Halting speech indicates embarrassment or lack of confidence, as well as some speech problems.

Language

■ Be alert to accents or other indications that English is not the client's first language. In communities where many people speak another language, have bilingual staff and handouts.
■ Pay attention to the type of words the client uses and match them. Although word choice often indicates educational level, a client's use of technical terms can also reflect a desire to equalize the relationship between you.
■ Some theorists believe word choice indicates a person's preferred way of taking in information. Someone who says, "I *see* what you mean," is visually oriented and should be given pictures and handouts. A person who says, "I *hear* what you're saying," relies on auditory sources and wants things explained. One who says, "I *feel* nervous," may be kinesthetic and may need models and hands-on demonstrations.

Information

■ Thorough, complete information indicates the person spends a great deal of time with the companion animal, is a good observer, and organizes thoughts well.
■ Extremely detailed information, such as an hour-by-hour journal containing exact amounts of food and

water consumed, is the mark of an anxious person, who has a strong need for precision and control.
■ Note who in the family seems to have the most information. This may be the person who is the most attached to the pet.
■ The kind of information a client offers shows beliefs about and experience with illness and treatment. Even in traditional American culture, people have widely varying notions about causes of disease. In addition, personal experience with diet, medication, surgery, or radiation therapy affect the willingness to proceed with the proposed treatment.

Social Situation

■ Although veterinarians may feel uncomfortable at first seeking information on a client's living situation, this may be critical to understanding how a client is reacting, what options a client has, and what a client will decide.
■ The first step is to be observant and to listen carefully to what a client volunteers.
■ If it becomes important to know more than the client has offered, begin by making observations or leading statements. For example, to an older woman wearing no wedding ring who has never mentioned family, a practitioner might say, "So it's just you and Brandy these days." Allow the client the opportunity to correct the impression.
■ If making observations does not provide needed information, ask specific questions. Make sure to let the client know why the answers are important.
■ The following elements affect the place of a companion animal in the client's life and the ability to care for a sick pet:
  • Who lives with the client?
  • Does the client have family, friends, neighbors, or others who provide companionship or assistance?
  • Have there been any recent events, such as change or loss, which might increase the importance of the human-animal bond?
  • What other aspects of the client's life might affect the ability to either care for the companion animal or make social connections, such as travel requirements, hours spent away from home, and disabilities that interfere with normal activities?

Philosophic and Religious Views

■ Religious views
  • People who hope to be reunited with loved ones in an afterlife may approach the experience of loss differently from those who do not have such a belief. Some faiths teach that companion animals do not have souls in the human sense.
  • Some religious people feel euthanasia is inappropriate and prefer to leave the moment of death to God.
  • Based on religious custom, some find cremation unacceptable.
■ Philosophic views
  • For those who make little distinction between humans and other animals, the question of who

has the right to make life-and-death decisions becomes more difficult.

- Many people who have close relationships with companion animals are uncomfortable weighing the quality of life for one family member against that of another. Such people may make enormous sacrifices to maintain the life and comfort of a sick or impaired pet.
- Death itself may carry significant symbolic meaning. Does it convey peace, that one is a loser, that one has achieved enough spiritual growth to move on to the next life? A highly negative view may cause a person to resist death for a loved one at any cost.

Role of Pet

- Level of attachment
  - Surveys indicate a high percentage of people with pets consider them to be members of the family.
  - For some, companion animals are equivalent to human beings and provide even more positive relationships.
  - In addition to statements of affection, many behaviors indicate attachment, such as having the pet sleep with the family, celebrating birthdays, and displaying the pet's photograph.
  - Different family members have different levels of attachment. The person who brings the pet to the veterinarian may not be the one who is most attached.
- Activities
  - Clients who share most routine activities with companion animals, such as eating and watching television, have more to lose when the pet dies.
  - For some people, companion animals are a primary source of play and laughter.
  - Pets are an important bridge to other people and vastly increase the amount of one's social contact. Loss of the companion animal severs other relationships and routines.

CARE BEFORE DEATH

Education

- From the first meeting with a client provide information about good health care and normal life span of the companion animal. When the pet finally does become ill, the client can take comfort in the knowledge he or she has done everything possible to care for the loved one.
- Grief begins with the fear of bad news. Once serious illness is diagnosed, tell the client what to expect about the following:
  - Cause
  - Course
  - Treatment options
  - Prognosis
- Tailor communications and general approach to the client.
  - Evaluate the client's social, emotional, and educational situation, as outlined in the previous section on assessment.

- Consider the effect of shock. Repeat and clarify as needed.
- Present information in more than one way. Multiple methods reinforce one another and increase the chances of reaching the client's preferred way of learning.
- Keep brochures about pet loss in public areas, so that clients can read or share them as they choose.
- Keep books and tapes about pet loss in your library to lend.

Preparation for Loss

Sudden Death vs. Long-Term Conditions

- Considerations in sudden illness or loss
  - Shock affects the ability to take action and slows recovery.
  - Little chance exists to build trust between veterinarian and client.
  - Client cannot save money to pay for treatment.
  - Other resources, such as time off from work or help from others may be intact.
  - Client has less time to consider or develop options.
- Considerations in long-term illness
  - Client has chance to absorb the situation, prepare for the end, and begin to grieve.
  - Veterinarian and client have time to develop a stable, trusting relationship.
  - Client has opportunity to do more for the companion animal—fewer regrets but resources may be exhausted.

Decision Making

- Review course of illness.

KEY POINT ▶ Encourage a visit with hospitalized pet to help client grasp the animal's current condition.

- Show test results.
- Demonstrate with models if possible.
- Discuss options.
  - Adults need choices.
    Reaching agreement is more effective than imposing plans.
    Making choices strengthens people emotionally.
  - Many options exist.
    Treat aggressively, moderately, or not at all.
    Euthanize or not.
      Who decides?
      What are the deciding factors?
      When and where is it performed?
      Who is present?
      Who performs the procedure?
    Care for the body in a special way; plan some other memorial. Discuss option for post-mortem examination to help determine cause of illness. Be sure to thank owners if they agree to a post-mortem examination.
    Cremate, bury, or freeze-dry according to the individual's preference.
    Plant tree, make collage, write letter, frame photo.

■ Work for consensus among veterinarian, client, and others.
  • Veterinarian's contributions
    Knows facts about illness, treatment alternatives, and prognosis.
    Knows how animals behave when in discomfort.
    Knows how companion animal has behaved in the hospital.
  • Client's contributions
    Knows how companion animal usually behaves.
    Knows own values, like "quality of life."
    Knows own social and emotional situation.
  • Others' contributions
    Friends and family offer help.
    Outside observers offer opinions, moral judgments.
    Veterinary team offers views about suffering and the emotional involvement of the client and clinician.

KEY POINT ▶ The final decision to euthanize a pet rests with the owner. Applying pressure to an owner can lead to resentment and prolongation of the grief period.

Client Resists Decision Making

■ State observations, including feelings.
■ If the client does not elaborate, acknowledge the silence: "This must be difficult to talk about."
■ If the client still does not elaborate, make tentative statements or ask questions. The questions will show support for any response the client might make.
■ Sometimes, the veterinarian strongly disagrees with a client's decision or lack of it. The veterinarian states honestly what he or she observes, believes, and values. For example, say "Mrs. Brown, I know this has been a difficult process for you. I wish Brandy didn't have the disease. I truly believe Brandy is suffering. We need to make a decision in the next 12 hours. Is there anything I can do to help you decide?"
■ If the client is still unable to decide, refer the person for counseling.

Counseling

■ Why seek professional counseling?
  • Professionals are trained to offer support, develop deep understanding of total situation, work with negative emotion, and reframe problem to make it more solvable.
  • They are perceived as neutral regarding a medical decision or family matters. Therefore, counseling is effective in reaching agreement.
  • The counselor is able to help facilitate interactions between client and veterinary team.
■ Who counsels?
  • Those with advanced training (masters degree) in mental health field.
  • Those with experience working with loss.
  • Those with an understanding of the relationship between people and companion animals.
■ When does the veterinarian refer a client for counseling?

  • Client requests it.
  • Client seems unable to make a decision and resists medically sound approach.
  • Client is at risk for severe grief reaction.
    Lives alone, seems isolated.
    Spends most of time with companion animal.
    Identifies strongly with pet.
    Has shared significant life events with pet.
    Rescued or was rescued by companion animal.
    Has extreme guilt about pet's condition.
    Has suffered other recent losses.
■ How should the practitioner make the referral?
  • Use a low key approach.
  • Focus on the client's feelings and experience.
  • Avoid judgmental, negative, and angry remarks.
  • Convey confidence in counselor's ability to help.
  • Leave follow-up to the client.
  • For example, say "Mrs. Miller, I can see this is a very painful decision for you. As you mentioned, it reminds you of your husband's death from cancer last year. Our practice works with a counselor, Pat Field. She really understands people who love companion animals and has helped a lot of people through tough times. Here's her card. Why don't you give her a call?"

CARE DURING DYING

Death Expected, Unassisted

Prepare client.

■ Suggest the last activities client may wish to share with companion animal, e.g., food treats, activities the animal enjoys doing, making a video.
■ Explain signs that death is imminent.
■ Tell client of the action to be taken before or during death.
■ Make sure the client knows what action to take if the process goes badly, e.g., location of emergency clinic.
■ Tell the client how to care for a pet's remains.
■ Routinely tell clients about emotional support services.

Death Unexpected

■ Prepare for a strong reaction, e.g., disbelief, dropped phone, cries.
■ Offer to call again, answer further questions.
■ Prepare for future anger, accusations. Allow the client to vent before offering new information or an alternative explanation.
■ With nondefensive, cooperative stance expect most clients to resolve shock, anger, and guilt.

Euthanasia Procedure

1. Review what brought everyone to this decision.
2. Make sure all parties agree—ask everyone, never push.
3. Set time, place, circumstances; have client sign a permission form.
4. Discuss disposition of the animal's body.

5. Explain the procedure—how medication works, that it is painless.

6. If the client is to be present, describe what will be seen, e.g., catheter, number of injections, possible gasps or twitches, nonclosing of the eyes. Place an IV catheter to avoid extravascular injection of the euthanasia solution. Consider anesthetizing the animal (e.g., with an ultrashort-acting barbiturate) prior to injecting the euthanasia solution.

7. Suggest the client sit near the head, stroke the pet, and talk to it during the procedure.

8. Some practitioners also speak quietly to the companion animal or client about what is happening.

9. Listen for heartbeat, pronounce death, e.g., "He's gone, Mr. Cummings." If the client seems not to understand, point out the pet is not breathing.

10. Allow time for tears and reminiscing with you or others.

11. Before the client departs, make a personalized positive statement about the companion animal, care, or relationship, e.g., "Fred was a good pet, we all loved him," or "You two had a special relationship. You did more than most to keep him healthy." "You made the right decision to have Fred euthanized."

12. Remind the client to call with any questions.

CARE AFTER DEATH

General Care

- Call the client within 24 hours; listen carefully before commenting.
- Reassure the client the decision was humane.
- Avoid exhortations to "look on the bright side," e.g., the pet lived to a normal age, the client is now free to pursue other interests, life goes on.
- Be prepared to return personal items, like leashes, or to provide a copy of the record. For some people having everything connected to the loved one helps the healing process.

KEY POINT ▶ Send a condolence card with a personal note signed by the clinician and staff.

- Understand the death of a pet may mean the loss of the relationship with the veterinarian and others. Assure the client he or she is still important.

Special Care

- Some clients need repeated or detailed information about their pet's death. Some may wish to review the record with you or to see where their loved one died. This is a normal part of grieving, unless the requests persist steadily for months or contain threats.
- Refer for counseling those clients who seem to remain in one phase of the grief process or who are at risk. Especially refer clients who seem seriously depressed or who are contemplating suicide.
- Learn to recognize signs of serious depression.
  - Significant weight loss or gain.
  - Sleep disturbance.
  - Seriously impaired ability to do or enjoy normal activities.
- Be alert to signs the client may be considering suicide. Though rare, immediate intervention is required if the client speaks in any way about ending life or wishing to die.

Supplemental Readings

Cohen SP, Fudin CE: *Animal Illness and Human Emotion*, vol. 3, number 1. *In* Kay WJ, Brown NJ, eds. *Problems in Veterinary Medicine*. Philadelphia: J. B. Lippincott Company, 1991.

Kay WJ, et al.: *Euthanasia of the Companion Animal: The Impact on Pet Owners, Veterinarians, and Society*. Philadelphia: The Charles Press, 1988.

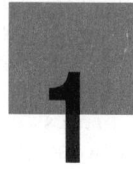

S E C T I O N 2

Infectious Diseases

Robert G. Sherding

1 Feline Leukemia Virus

Robert G. Sherding

ETIOLOGY AND PATHOBIOLOGY

Feline leukemia virus (FeLV) is a horizontally transmitted retrovirus that is a major cause of morbidity and mortality in domestic cats. In a nationwide survey of 27,976 cats in 1990–1991, 13.3% of cats were positive for FeLV. Mostly high-risk cats were surveyed, such as sick cats or healthy cats exposed to other cats outdoors. Other surveys have found the incidence to be 30 to 50% in healthy cats living in an infected household or cattery, 1 to 3% in healthy free-roaming cats, and less than 1% in healthy indoor cats and cats in purebred catteries.

Structure of the Virus

Certain structural components of the FeLV virion have clinical implications.

- Core—contains RNA and reverse transcriptase, an enzyme that allows insertion of FeLV into the DNA genetic code of an infected cell.
- Internal Proteins—the protein designated p27 is detected as FeLV antigen by conventional FeLV diagnostic tests.
- Envelope Glycoproteins (gp70)—consist of subgroup antigens A, B, C, or combinations of these. They determine infectivity, host range, and pathogenicity. They also elicit the protective host neutralizing antibody response that occurs upon natural exposure or vaccination.
- Envelope Protein (p15E)—a mediator of FeLV-related immunodeficiency.

Sequential Phases of FeLV Infection

An understanding of the pathogenesis of FeLV infection is a prerequisite for accurate interpretation of FeLV test results.

- Transmission
  - Primarily through intimate oronasal contact with infectious saliva
  - Transplacental and milkborne transmission are important sources of infection in kittens.
- After the initial stages of replication within oronasal and then systemic lymphoid tissues, FeLV infects bone marrow cells. This appears to be a pivotal phase in the pathogenesis and outcome of infection, insofar as persistent viremia subsequently develops if FeLV overwhelms the host immune response, whereas transient infection and recovery occur if the immune response is successful.
- Cats that develop persistent viremia shed virus in most body secretions, especially saliva, and thus they are contagious to other cats.

Host Immune Response

Immunity to FeLV is the collective result of humoral antibody, cell-mediated immune mechanisms, complement, and interferon. Humoral antibody responses have been the best characterized and include:

- Antiviral response is mediated by neutralizing antibody directed against FeLV envelope antigens.
- Antitumor response is mediated by anti-FOCMA (*f*eline *o*ncornavirus *c*ell *m*embrane–associated *anti*gen) antibody directed against FeLV-associated antigen (FOCMA) on the surface of FeLV-induced neoplastic cells.

Outcome of FeLV Exposure and Categories of Infection

The outcome of FeLV exposure is variable and can be categorized into three groups (Table 1):

Group 1 (Uninfected)

Group 1 contains 28% of exposed cats that do not get infected, either because of an inherent resistance to infection or because of insufficient exposure.

Group 2 (Persistently Infected)

Group 2 contains 30% of exposed cats that develop progressive infection with persistent viremia. This leads to FeLV-related disease after a variable disease-free interval. In a study that followed healthy FeLV-positive cats, the mortality rate was 33% at 6 months, 63% at 2 years, and 83% at 3.5 years.

Group 3 (Transiently Infected)

Group 3 contains 42% of exposed cats that develop a transient replicating infection that is subsequently rejected by the immune system.

- Replicating FeLV is usually eliminated 4 to 6 weeks after exposure, sometimes after a transient viremia lasting 1 to 5 weeks.
- These nonviremic cats that have "recovered" from transient infection usually become latent carriers of FeLV for a variable period of time. In latent FeLV infection, nonreplicating FeLV provirus remains dormant within the DNA genetic code of certain bone marrow and lymphoid cells. Latency can be detected only by specialized cell culture techniques or polymerase chain reaction assay in research labs.

TABLE 1. Categories of Infection Following FeLV Exposure

Category of Infection	Percent (%) of Exposed Cats	Consequences
Noninfected	28	Uninfected due to insufficient exposure (may or may not be susceptible)
Persistent infection	30	High risk of mortality due to immunosuppression, anemia, lymphoma, and other FeLV-related diseases
Transient infection Extinguished	30–35	Transient latency followed by recovery; immune to FeLV infection
Sustained latent infection	5–10	Usually asymptomatic and noncontagious; rarely, any one of the following can occur: recrudescence, in utero transmission to unborn kittens, milkborne transmission to kittens

KEY POINT ▶ Latent FeLV infection can not be detected by conventional FeLV diagnostic tests.

- In most transiently infected cats, all latent FeLV is eventually eliminated uneventfully as part of the normal recovery process. This usually occurs within 6 to 9 months of exposure, but can sometimes take a year or more.
- In some cats with latent FeLV (less than 10% of exposed cats), latency will persist indefinitely.
- Clinical significance of latency
  - Minimal risk of developing FeLV-related disease
  - Minimal risk of contagiousness to other cats by contact transmission
  - Rare possibility of recrudescence (e.g., steroid-induced) of active replicating FeLV and viremia
  - Occasional infection by latent FeLV-infected queens of kittens in utero or during nursing through local mammary excretion of FeLV

MANIFESTATIONS AND CLINICAL SIGNS

The clinical manifestations of FeLV are attributable to the oncogenic, cytopathic, and immunosuppressive effects of the virus. FeLV-induced neoplasia can be lymphoid or myeloid. Degenerative and cytopathic effects on various cells include bone marrow cells (anemia, neutropenia, thrombocytopenia), lymphocytes (T-lymphocyte depletion, lymphoid atrophy, lymphoid hyperplasia), intestinal cells (enteritis), and the fetus and placenta (abortion, stillbirth). The immunosuppressive effects of FeLV cause profound immunodeficiency, resulting in susceptibility to a wide variety of opportunistic infections. In addition, FeLV-related immune dysfunction can cause immune-mediated and autoimmune diseases.

Lymphoproliferative Neoplasms

Both lymphoma and lymphoid leukemias are associated with FeLV infection. For general information regarding lymphoma, see sec. 3, ch. 6; for treatment of lymphoma (i.e., chemotherapy) see sec. 3, ch. 5.

- Alimentary lymphoma
  - Mesenteric lymph nodes—palpable enlargement
  - Stomach—vomiting, anorexia, and weight loss
  - Intestine—diffuse infiltration of the intestinal wall (diarrhea and weight loss) or nodular mass in the intestinal wall (obstruction)
  - Liver—diffuse hepatomegaly or nodular tumor masses within the liver (icterus, weight loss, vomiting, abnormal liver tests)
  - Spleen—diffuse splenomegaly

KEY POINT ▶ Cats with gastrointestinal lymphoma are much older (mean age, 8 years) than cats with other forms of lymphoma, and up to 75% have negative results on FeLV blood tests.

- Mediastinal lymphoma (cranial mediastinal mass due to lymphoma of thymus or mediastinal nodes)

- Pleural effusion (dyspnea)
- Tracheal compression (dyspnea, cough)
- Esophageal compression (dysphagia, regurgitation)
- Sympathetic trunk impingement (Horner syndrome)
- Decreased cranial thoracic compressibility
- Mass palpable at thoracic inlet (rare)
■ Multicentric lymphoma
  - Generalized involvement of external and internal lymph nodes
  - Liver, spleen, kidneys, and other visceral organs
■ Renal lymphoma
  - Signs—nonspecific (early), renal failure, and uremia (late)
  - Kidneys palpably enlarged and nodular
■ Ocular lymphoma
  - Retrobulbar mass—mimics retrobulbar abscess
  - Third eyelid mass—mimics "cherry eye"
  - Corneal infiltration—mimics eosinophilic keratitis
  - Uveal infiltration and hemorrhage—mimics anterior uveitis or choroiditis
■ Nervous system lymphoma
  - Brain: seizures, ataxia, blindness, behavior aberrations, motor deficits, etc.
  - Spinal cord: paresis or paralysis
■ Cutaneous lymphoma: multiple firm, nonpainful cutaneous nodules
■ Lymphoid leukemia—primary bone marrow involvement with circulating neoplastic cells
■ Others: lung, heart, urinary bladder, nasal, etc.

Myeloproliferative Disorders

This is a group of neoplastic or neoplastic-like diseases characterized by the proliferation of one or more cell lines in the bone marrow at the expense and to the eventual exclusion of other marrow cells. The abnormal cells are often found in the peripheral blood as well as in the bone marrow, and their identification provides the diagnosis. These disorders are classified on the basis of the cellular origin of the abnormal cells.

■ Nonspecific signs—anorexia, depression, and weight loss
■ Progressive, unresponsive anemia and thrombocytopenia
■ Diffuse hepatomegaly (icterus), splenomegaly, and lymphadenopathy from extramedullary hematopoiesis and/or neoplastic infiltration

FeLV-Related Anemia

Anemia may occur as the sole primary manifestation of FeLV as well as being present with many other FeLV-related diseases.

■ Nonregenerative anemia: usually resulting from destruction, suppression, or abnormal maturation of RBC precursors in bone marrow
■ Other mechanisms: immune-mediated hemolysis, opportunistic *Hemobartonella felis* infection, bleeding from thrombocytopenia, and neoplastic or myelodysplastic bone marrow

■ Clinical signs: listlessness, weakness, mucous membrane pallor, anemic murmur, splenomegaly, retinal hemorrhages, and pica
■ Laboratory signs
  - Severe nonregenerative anemia (hematocrit may be <10%)
  - Erythrocyte macrocytosis
  - Leukopenia or thrombocytopenia—may accompany anemia
  - Bone marrow cytology—normal, hypocellular, aplastic, hypercellular, neoplastic, or disorderly
■ Treatment: blood transfusions and general supportive care (median survival in 49 treated cases was 4 months)

FeLV-Related Neutrophil Disorders

Neutrophils and myeloid precursors are usually infected in FeLV viremia.

■ FeLV-induced neutropenia can be transient (for first 3–5 weeks of bone marrow infection with FeLV), persistent, or cyclic (10–14 days). Signs include chronic or recurrent bacterial infections and fulminant sepsis.
■ Neutropenia can be a preneoplastic change that eventually develops into a myeloproliferative disorder.
■ Myeloblastopenia (panleukopenia-like syndrome) is characterized by profound panleukopenia (WBC = 300–3000/μl) and acute enterocolitis with fever, vomiting, and bloody diarrhea. Intestinal epithelial cells are heavily infected with FeLV.

FeLV-Related Platelet Disorders

Platelets and megakaryocytes are usually infected in FeLV viremia. Disorders include:

■ Thrombocytopenia
■ Macroplatelets—abnormally large platelets with bizzare shapes occurring commonly in viremic cats, especially those with severe anemia (may be miscounted as RBCs by electronic counters)
■ Platelet dysfunction (subclinical)

FeLV-Induced Immunodeficiency

FeLV causes profound lymphoid atrophy and suppression of the cat's immune system (especially T-lymphocytes), thereby increasing susceptibility to all types of infections, especially chronic or recurrent ones. This is the most important overall consequence of FeLV infection in many cats. Fever is often a presenting sign along with signs of any type of opportunistic infection. Some examples follow.

■ Viral—feline infectious peritonitis, herpesvirus
■ Fungal—*Cryptococcus, Aspergillus, Candida*
■ Rickettsial—*Hemobartonella*
■ Protozoal—*Toxoplasma, Cryptosporidium*
■ Bacterial
  - Oral—gingivitis, periodontitis, stomatitis
  - Respiratory infections—rhinitis, sinusitis, pneumonia, pyothorax

- Enteritis—*Salmonella, Campylobacter,* diarrhea of undetermined cause
- Cutaneous—pyoderma, nonhealing sores, abscesses, draining fistulas
- Septicemia

Distinctive Peripheral Lymph Node Hyperplasia

- There is marked symmetric enlargement of peripheral and visceral lymph nodes (especially mandibulars), up to three times normal size.
- Primarily affects young adult cats (6 months to 2 years of age): 50% are asymptomatic and 50% have fever, anorexia, and depression.
- Outcome: some cases resolve in 2 to 4 weeks (with corticosteroids, cyclophosphamide, vincristine); some recur; and some evolve into lymphoma months to years later.

Immune-Mediated Disorders

Several immune-mediated disorders have been associated with FeLV infection:

- Immune complex glomerulonephritis
- Chronic progressive polyarthritis
- Immune-mediated hemolytic anemia
- Immune-mediated thrombocytopenia
- Ulcerative mucocutaneous disorders (pemphigus-like)
- Systemic lupus erythematosus–like syndrome

The exact role of FeLV in these disorders is not fully understood, but it presumably involves viral antigen-antibody complexes or FeLV-induced disruption of immune regulation.

Infertility, Stillbirths, Abortions, and "Fading Kittens"

In FeLV-infected female cats, any of the following can occur: infertility, fetal resorption, abortion, stillbirth, "fading kitten syndrome" (viremic kittens), or milkborne transmission to nursing kittens.

Miscellaneous

A role for FeLV in the following list of disorders has been suggested but unproved: chronic enteritis, seborrheic dermatitis, eosinophilic granuloma complex, cutaneous horns, multicentric osteochondromas, urinary incontinence, persistent cystitis, anisocoria, and degenerative myelopathy.

DIAGNOSIS

Diagnostic testing for FeLV infection has become one of the most frequently performed procedures in veterinary practice. FeLV tests are used to diagnose FeLV-related illnesses, to screen for subclinical infection in cats presented for FeLV vaccination, and to identify and eliminate FeLV infections in catteries. FeLV tests are available on a mail-in basis through commercial laboratories; however, simple diagnostic kits that allow the rapid in-office testing of blood, saliva, or tears for the presence of FeLV are routinely used by most veterinarians.

Overview of Diagnostic Tests for FeLV

Two tests available for routine clinical diagnosis of FeLV infection are the immunofluorescent antibody (IFA) test and the enzyme-linked immunosorbent assay (ELISA). Both tests detect FeLV group-specific core antigens (p27). The IFA test requires a specialized commercial or university laboratory and uses a smear of peripheral blood or bone marrow. The ELISA test can be performed on blood, saliva, or tears using any of several in-office test kits or an outside commercial laboratory. Guidelines for interpretation of IFA and ELISA test results are presented in Table 2.

In addition to the IFA and ELISA tests, some research laboratories can assay tissues and body fluids for FeLV by virus isolation (VI) as the "gold standard" for detection of FeLV infection. This assay is not, however, routinely available for clinical use. The bone marrow reactivation test detects latent (dormant, nonreplicating) FeLV infection in cultured bone marrow cells but also is available only for research applications.

IFA Test

The IFA test indicates cell-associated viremia by detecting FeLV antigen in circulating neutrophils and platelets on smears of peripheral blood or in bone

TABLE 2. Interpretation of FeLV Test Results

Test	Result	Interpretations to Be Considered
IFA	Positive	Persistent viremia (95%)
		Transient viremia (5%)
		False-positive (rare in experienced laboratories): due to thick smear, clumped platelets, eosinophilia
IFA	Negative	Nonexposed/noninfected
		Prior transient infection; now recovered (uninfected/immune)
		Prior transient infection; now latent (nonreplicating) infection
		Early infection too soon to detect (may be ELISA-positive)
		Compartmentalized ELISA-positive infection
		ELISA-positive infection with replication of antigens but not whole virus
		False-negative: due to inadequate neutrophils and platelets on the slide (neutropenia/thrombocytopenia)
ELISA	Positive	Persistent viremia (also IFA-positive)
		Transient viremia (also IFA-positive)
		Antigenemia without cell-associated viremia (IFA-negative)
		False-positive due to laboratory error (IFA-negative) (see Table 4)
ELISA	Negative	Nonexposed/noninfected
		Prior transient infection; now recovered (uninfected/immune)
		Prior transient infection; now latent (nonreplicating) infection
		Very early subclinical infection, too early to detect

marrow cells. The IFA test is very specific for FeLV and regarded by some as the best test for confirming FeLV viremia. See Table 2 for IFA test interpretation.

■ Positive IFA indicates an advanced stage of FeLV infection and is highly correlated (98%) with virus isolation assays. It is also correlated with persistent viremia, in that 90 to 96% of IFA-positive cats remain persistently infected. Healthy IFA-positive cats can be retested monthly for 3 months to differentiate transient and persistent infection with reasonable certainty. This is because transient FeLV-positive infections can sometimes last for up to, but very rarely longer than, 3 months. Thus, if a positive IFA test remains positive for greater than 3 months, the infection is considered to be persistent, whereas if the test becomes negative within 3 months, the infection was transient.

■ False-positive IFA is very rare but can occur from improperly made blood smears that are too thick and cause nonspecific binding of the conjugate. Platelet clumping and eosinophilia can also cause rare false positives.

■ False-negative IFA may occur in neutropenia/thrombocytopenia and in early infections because the test does not usually become positive until FeLV infects and replicates in the bone marrow. A false-negative IFA test rarely may occur in low-level infections because the test is slightly less sensitive than the ELISA test.

ELISA Test

The ELISA test is used most commonly for routine screening for FeLV infection and can be performed on serum, plasma, whole blood, saliva, or tears. There are two formats for the ELISA test: the microwell ELISA and the membrane filter ELISA. Modifications of these are also available for testing saliva and tears. Each of these formats is available in test kit form for in-office testing (Table 3), and most provide results in less than 10 minutes. In addition, many commercial laboratories offer FeLV ELISA testing on mail-in specimens. See Table 2 for ELISA interpretation.

Microwell ELISA Format

The antibody-antigen-antibody sandwich ELISA reaction takes place on the inner surface of antibody-coated microwells. The microwell units are grouped for batch testing. Microwell-type ELISA test systems are the most susceptible to the various technical errors and pitfalls that cause false-positive results (see section on Discordancy).

Membrane Filter ELISA Format

The ELISA reaction takes place on antibody-coated dots on a flow-through membrane. The membrane filter-type ELISA systems (e.g., CITE and CITE Probe; IDEXX) are designed to reduce the risk of nonspecific false-positive reactions by providing flow-through design to facilitate thorough washing, individualization of test units to prevent splashing of reagents

TABLE 3. ELISA Test Kits for In-Office FeLV Diagnosis

Test Kit	Manufacturer	Format
Leukassay F-II*	Pitman Moore	Microwell
UNI-TEC FeLV	Pitman Moore	Membrane filter
DiaSystems FeLV-FLEX-II*	Fermenta	Microwell (also tests saliva and tears)
VIRACHEK/FeLV*	Synbiotics	Microwell
ASSURE/FeLV	Synbiotics	Tube (also tests saliva)
Leukotest (formerly ClinEase)*	Cambridge BioScience	Microwell
CITE-FeLV*	IDEXX	Membrane filter (also tests saliva and tears)
CITE-Combo	IDEXX	Membrane filter (also tests for FIV)
CITE-Probe FeLV	IDEXX	Programmed, self-contained membrane filter device
CITE-Probe-Combo	IDEXX	Programmed, self-contained filter device (also tests for FIV)

FeLV = feline leukemia virus; FIV = feline immunodeficiency virus.
*In a comparison study of five kits (Lopez NA, et al: J Am Vet Med Assoc 195:747, 1989), all kits had excellent sensitivity (100% for CITE, VIRACHEK, and ClinEase; 95% for Leukassay and DiaSystems). Specificity (based on elimination of false-positive results caused by anti-mouse antibodies) was excellent (100%) for CITE, VIRACHEK, and Leukassay, but ClinEase and DiaSystems recorded false-positive results for sera containing anti-mouse antibodies.

between specimens, a prefilter to filter out interfering biologic debris, and easy-to-interpret blue results on a white background. Also, positive and negative controls are built in for each patient specimen so that false-positive and false-negative reactions can be readily detected as such.

Positive ELISA

A positive ELISA indicates viremia (or antigenemia). In general, serum ELISA tests tend to become positive earlier following exposure to FeLV than the IFA test, and they tend to be more sensitive than the IFA test. After recent FeLV exposure, serum ELISA tests become positive 1 to 2 weeks earlier than saliva or tear ELISA tests. For other reasons as well, ELISA tests on saliva and tears will not detect as many FeLV infections as serum ELISA tests. Healthy ELISA-positive cats should be retested at monthly intervals for 3 months to determine whether the infection is transient or persistent.

False-positive ELISA

False-positive ELISA titers sometimes occur, especially with the microwell format, primarily because of technical errors discussed in the next section.

False-negative ELISA

False-negative ELISA results are unlikely because of the inherently high sensitivity of this test.

Interpretation of Discordant Test Results

KEY POINT ▶ The ELISA for FeLV is more sensitive and can detect infection earlier than the IFA test; however, false-positive results are more frequent with the ELISA. False-positive results are rare with the IFA test, and it has better correlation with persistent infection.

A major issue in FeLV testing is the fact that there is a considerable problem of discrepancy between ELISA and IFA test results. The agreement between a negative ELISA and IFA test is nearly 100%. The problem of discordancy primarily involves cats that test ELISA-positive but IFA-negative. Some reports suggest a discordant rate of 30% or higher; however, in recent years technical improvements in the ELISA systems have reduced this to about 10%. There are legitimate biologic explanations for a small degree of discordancy, but the principal cause of discordancy is false-positive ELISA results due to technical laboratory errors, especially with microwell test systems.

Biologic Factors That Cause Discordancy

Biologic factors can cause discordancy, but collectively these should not cause more than 5 to 10% of ELISA-positive cats to test IFA-negative.

- There is a brief period of a few weeks during early infection when FeLV antigens are detectable in the serum (ELISA-positive) but FeLV is not yet replicating in the bone marrow, so that blood cells do not yet contain virus (IFA-negative).
- The ELISA is also more sensitive and thus may detect low-level infections that the IFA test may miss; however, this is probably uncommon because there is 98% correlation between IFA test and virus isolation results.
- Persistent antigenemia (ELISA-positive) with a negative IFA test may occur when there is sequestration of FeLV infection with replication in sites other than bone marrow, or when there is replication of FeLV antigens but not whole virus. These cats have persistent discordancy even on repeat testing, but they do not usually shed virus and are not likely to be contagious to other cats.

Technical Pitfalls and Laboratory Errors That Cause Discordancy

The most frequent cause of discordancy is false-positive ELISA results due to technical error in the performance of the ELISA procedures, especially as performed using the microwell ELISA kits by inexperienced or improperly trained personnel (Table 4).

- The most common problem is false-positive reactions owing to the presence of residual conjugate in the microwell after washing. This can be caused by insufficient washing, splashing of conjugate between wells during the procedure, or nonspecific binding of conjugate to microdefects in the plastic microwells

TABLE 4. Causes of False-Positive Results on FeLV Microwell ELISA Tests

Residual conjugate remaining in the wells due to inadequate washing.
Splashing of conjugate between wells.
Nonspecific binding of conjugate to plastic defects.
Cell debris (e.g., saliva, hemolyzed serum) or fibrin that sticks to the well and traps conjugate.
Presence of enzymes or other bioactive materials in the sample.
Presence of cross-reacting anti-mouse antibodies in the sample.
Interfering antibodies in patient serum induced by recent vaccination (e.g., Bio-Rab, ImRab).
Misinterpretation of a weak positive reaction as a true positive result.

(or binding of conjugate to chew marks in the plastic device used for saliva testing).
- Biologic material in the sample may cause false-positive reactions. Cell debris and fibrin in the sample may stick to the microwell and trap conjugate. This is more likely to occur with saliva, tears, whole blood, or hemolyzed sera. Also, enzymes or other bioactive materials may react nonspecifically with the conjugate to produce the color change reaction.
- A false-positive ELISA reaction occasionally may be caused by anti-mouse antibodies in the patient specimen that cross-react with the murine-derived monoclonal antibody used as a reagent in the test system. Less than 1% of the cat population has interfering anti-mouse antibodies, and most test kits correct for this.

Recommendations for FeLV Testing

KEY POINT ▶ To reduce false-positive ELISA test results, analyze nonhemolyzed serum rather than whole blood, saliva, or tears, and use a membrane filter test rather than a microwell test.

- Because saliva and tear ELISA tests will only detect 80 to 90% of infected cats, do not use these to determine infection in individual cats. These tests can be used for mass screening of a group of cats to determine if FeLV is endemic and for detection of cats that are actively shedding virus.
- Use only ELISA antibody reagents that are monoclonal to provide optimal specificity and to reduce nonspecific false-positive reactions. All the currently available ELISA test kits now use monoclonal antibody reagents.
- Experience and meticulous technique are required to obtain accurate results with in-office microwell ELISA tests. Only under these circumstances is a microwell ELISA test kit an acceptable choice for routine FeLV screening. For most in-office testing situations, use the CITE or CITE Probe membrane filter ELISA rather than a microwell system, because they are less susceptible to technical error and have built-in positive and negative controls for each test. Alternatively, send specimens to a commercial laboratory for FeLV testing.

- To reduce false-positive results with microwell ELISA tests, perform thorough washing steps and avoid splashing of reagents between microwells.
- For diagnosis of a clinically ill cat, use the CITE-Combo or Probe-Combo ELISA test, because the clinical manifestations of FeLV and feline immuno-deficiency virus (FIV) are often indistinguishable and these kits test for both of these viruses simultaneously.
- Interpret weak positive ELISA reactions as suspicious rather than definitive and repeat the test (consider repeating using a different ELISA method, an IFA test, or an outside laboratory).
- In a healthy cat, always confirm an ELISA-positive test result by retesting in 4 to 6 weeks and perhaps again at 3 months to distinguish transient from persistent infection and to rule out laboratory error. For retesting, consider an IFA test because it correlates better with persistent infection and is less susceptible to false-postive results.

Antibody Tests

Serum antibody assays are of limited usefulness in the diagnosis or clinical evaluation of FeLV infection. They merely indicate prior exposure to FeLV through infection or vaccination but do not confirm current active infection. Vaccine-induced antibody titers have not correlated well with level of protection.

TREATMENT

There is as yet no proven effective treatment for FeLV, but research and therapeutic trials are in progress using various immune modulator and antiviral drugs.

Supportive care such as antibiotics for secondary bacterial infections, fluid therapy, and nutritional support may prolong survival in selected patients. Untreated lymphoma is usually fatal within 1 to 2 months, but anticancer chemotherapy (see sec. 3, ch. 5) can induce remission in many cats. The prognosis for cats with FeLV-related nonregenerative anemia and myeloproliferative disease is poor, although blood transfusions may prolong survival.

- Biologic response modifiers include nonspecific immune modulators and stimulants.
  - The following agents have generally been ineffective: promodulin, BCG, levamisole, and mixed bacterial toxins.
  - Preliminary results in limited trials with the following agents have been encouraging, with increased duration of survival and improved clinical signs (however, treated cats usually remain FeLV-positive): staphylococcal protein A (SPA), *Propionibacterium acnes* (ImmunoRegulin, ImmunoVet), low-dose oral human alpha-interferon (Roferon; Hoffman LaRoche), and Acemannan (derived from aloe vera).
- Antiviral drugs, such as suramin, zidovudine (AZT), and dideoxycytidine (DDC), have not yet been shown to be efficacious in treating FeLV infection, but therapeutic trials are in progress. Future prototypes developed for treatment of human AIDS retrovirus will likely be explored in cats with FeLV.
- Extracorporeal immunoadsorption for removal of immune complexes has been limited to research only.
- Bone marrow transplantation following whole-body irradiation also has been done only experimentally in cats.

PREVENTION AND CONTROL

Because of the devastating consequences of FeLV infection and its prevalence in the cat population, prevention is of vital importance. Preventative measures include vaccination of individual cats to reduce susceptibility, restriction of free roaming outdoors to reduce exposure, and control measures to reduce spread of FeLV in catteries.

Prevention in the Individual Cat: Vaccination

The effectiveness of FeLV vaccination and the methods used to demonstrate efficacy are controversial and unresolved issues, in part because most of the available efficacy data has been generated by manufacturers rather than by unbiased researchers. The currently available FeLV vaccine products and their various features are summarized in Table 5.

Administration

- All FeLV vaccines are given by subcutaneous or intramuscular injection beginning at 8 to 10 weeks of age or older; a second dose is given 2 to 4 weeks later, followed by an annual booster.
- FeLV testing at or before first vaccination is recommended by some but does not need to be strictly mandatory. There is no proven beneficial or detrimental effect from vaccinating a cat for FeLV that is already infected.

Safety

Safety is not a significant problem with any of the currently available vaccines.

Effectiveness

There is no consensus on the measure of effectiveness of an FeLV vaccine. Each vaccine is different, and to assess manufacturer advertising claims veterinarians must consider the following questions.

- Should effectiveness be judged on ability to protect against persistent infection, or on ability to protect against transient infection and latency as well?
- Must a vaccine contain all three subgroup envelope antigens A, B, and C, or is only type A needed because natural infections usually involve this subgroup (alone or in combination with B or C)?
- Does it make a difference whether a vaccine contains viral subunits as opposed to whole virus?
- Should an effective vaccine elicit anti-FOCMA tumor immunity as well as antivirus protection?
- How do vaccines with and without adjuvants com-

TABLE 5. Features of Commercially Available Feline Leukemia Virus Vaccines

	Leukocell 2 (SmithKline Beecham)	VacSyn/FeLV (Synbiotics)	Fel-O-Vax Lv-K (Fort Dodge)	GenetiVac FeLV (Pitman-Moore)	Fevaxyn-FeLV (Solvay)	Covenant (Haver)
Released	1989 (1985)	1989	1989	1990	1991	1993 (?)
Type[a]	Inactivated subunits	Inactivated whole virus	Inactivated whole virus	Recombinant gp70 subunit	Inactivated whole virus	Inactivated whole virus
Adjuvant[b]	Yes	No (High Ag)	Yes	Yes	Yes	Yes
Subgroups[c]	A, B, C	A, B, C	A	A subunit	A, B	A, B, C
Anti-FOCMA[d]	Yes	Yes	No	No	No	No
First Dose[e]	Age ≥9 wk	Age ≥9 wk	Age ≥10 wk	Age ≥8 wk	Age ≥9 wk	Age ≥10 wk
Second Dose	3–4 wk later	2–3 wk later	3–4 wk later	2–3 wk later	3–4 wk later	3–4 wk later
Booster	Annually	Annually	Annually	Annually	Annually	Annually
Reactions[f]	2.0%	0.01%	6.0%	6.2%	1.4%	—
Resist infection[g]						
Vaccinates	72% (18/25)	91% (40/44)	91% (82/90)	85% (17/20)	91% (80/88)	—
Controls	40% (4/10)	15% (3/20)	7% (4/58)	30% (6/20)	18% (4/22)	—
Efficacy[h]	53%	89%	90%	79%	89%	—

[a]Leukocell 2 is derived from Leukocell, which was released in 1985 as the first FeLV vaccine. Covenant was originally released in 1988 but was removed due to adverse reactions in 1989, and it has been reformulated for re-release in 1993.

[b]All FeLV vaccines use one or two adjuvants for enhanced immunogenicity, with the exception of VacSyn/FeLV, which contains a high antigenic mass. Most vaccine reactions are attributable to the adjuvants.

[c]Natural FeLV infections usually involve subgroup A envelope glycoprotein alone or in combination with B or C. Immunity elicited by a vaccine containing type A envelope antigen should be sufficient, but some vaccines also contain types B and C.

[d]Only Leukocell 2, as labeled, has demonstrated that it induces protective levels of anti-FOCMA antibody that protect against lymphoma.

[e]For all vaccines, dosages of 1 ml are given subcutaneously as scheduled. FeLV vaccine can be given simultaneously with other multivalent cat vaccines without interference.

[f]Side effects are usually mild and consist of transient listlessness, fever, or injection site pain. Acute hypersensitivity reactions (facial and paw edema, vomiting, diarrhea, acute collapse) are seen rarely. GenetiVac has been associated with occasional nodules and soreness at the injection site.

[g]Challenge data cannot be compared because of differences in age of cats, strain of FeLV, route of infection, dose of inoculum, and protocol for post-challenge testing as related to definition of protection and persistence.

[h]Efficacy is a calculation that takes into account the infection rate in vaccinates versus unvaccinated controls as follows:

$$\text{efficacy} = \frac{[\text{incidence of infection in controls as \%}] - [\text{incidence of infection in vaccinates as \%}]}{[\text{incidence of infection in controls as \%}]}$$

pare, considering that adjuvants enhance the immunizing capacity of antigens in vaccines, but that they also are the principal cause of adverse side effects?

KEY POINT ▶ Based on currently available information, there is insufficient evidence for recommending one vaccine product rather than another. Therefore, it is not justified to switch from one vaccine to another solely on the basis of manufacturers' claims.

Efficacy

- In general, vaccinated cats that are exposed to FeLV often develop transient viremia and sometimes latent infection despite vaccination; however, most vaccinated cats are apparently protected against persistent viremia and therefore against FeLV-related disease.
- Latent infections in exposed vaccinated cats are less frequent and usually do not persist, compared to unvaccinated cats. However, this benefit of vaccination may be overemphasized, as the clinical significance of latent infections is probably minimal anyway, as discussed in the beginning of this chapter.
- One vaccine (Leukocell 2) is also claimed by the manufacturer to protect against lymphoma because it elicits an anti-FOCMA antibody response.
- The major difficulty with comparing manufacturer efficacy data (i.e., percentage of cats protected after

laboratory challenge) is the variation in challenge methods used for each vaccine:
- Different routes ("natural" oronasal challenge vs. injection)
- Different FeLV strains (various field isolates vs. vaccine-derived strains)
- Different definitions of "persistent" infection in postchallenge follow-up (e.g., positive by ELISA vs. IFA testing vs. VI, and positive at time intervals after challenge that vary from 4 to 12 weeks or more)
- As a general guideline for discussing vaccination expectations with animal owners, expect 70 to 90% of vaccinated cats to be protected against persistent FeLV infection. This may need to be modified as further efficacy data becomes available.

KEY POINT ▶ All available vaccines produce less than 100% protection against FeLV; therefore, even though vaccination may reduce the risk of FeLV infection, effective prevention also requires measures that reduce the risk of exposure.

Control in the Cattery or Multicat Household

Control in FeLV-Positive Catteries

The following "test and removal program" is recommended.

- Test all cats on the premises for FeLV (expect to

find up to 30% persistently infected) and remove all confirmed FeLV-positive cats.

- Quarantine the cattery so that there is no movement of new cats into the cattery.
- Vaccinate the remaining FeLV-negative cats.
- Clean and disinfect (especially food and water dishes)—FeLV is susceptible to most detergents and disinfectants and survives only a few hours outside the host when allowed to dry.
- Retest all cats every 1 to 3 months and continue to remove any confirmed FeLV-positive cats.
- Once all cats on the premises have been negative on two successive testings 3 months apart, the cattery is considered "FeLV free."
- Then isolate all new incoming cats and test as described below.

Control in FeLV-Negative Catteries

The following precautions should be taken for incoming cats.

- Obtain incoming cats from a source with a negative FeLV history.
- Screen incoming cats with ELISA; if negative, vaccinate cats and then hold them in isolation for 3 months (in case they are incubating FeLV).
- After a second negative ELISA at the end of the 3-month quarantine, the cat can join the cattery.
- ELISA-positive titers should generally be confirmed by IFA testing or by a repeat ELISA; however, in cattery situations ideally the safest course is to reject the ELISA-positive cat from the cattery as "suspicious."

Supplemental Readings

Cotter SM: Anemia associated with feline leukemia virus. J Am Vet Med Assoc 175:1191, 1979.

Essex M, Sliski AH, Cotter SM, et al: Immunosurveillance of naturally occurring feline leukemia. Science 190:790, 1975.

Hardy WD Jr, Hess PW, MacEwen EG, et al: Biology of feline leukemia virus in the natural environment. Cancer Res 36:582, 1976.

Hawkins EC, Johnson L, Pedersen NC, Winston S: Use of tears for diagnosis of feline leukemia virus infection. J Am Vet Med Assoc 188:1031, 1986.

Jarrett O, Golder MC, Stewart MF: Detection of transient and persistent feline leukaemia virus infections. Vet Rec 110:225, 1982.

Jarrett O, Golder MC, Weijer K: A comparison of three methods of feline leukaemia virus diagnosis. Vet Rec 110:325, 1982.

Lewis MG, Wright KA, Lafrado LJ, et al: Saliva as a source of FeLV antigen for diagnosis of disease. J Clin Microbiol 25:1320, 1987.

Lopez NA, Jacobson RH, Scarlett JM, et al: Sensitivity and specificity of blood test kits for feline leukemia virus antigen. J Am Vet Med Assoc 195:747, 1989.

Lutz H, Jarrett O: Detection of feline leukemia virus infection in saliva. J Clin Microbiol 25:827, 1987.

Lutz H, Pedersen NC, Harris CW, et al: Detection of feline leukemia virus infection. Feline Pract 10:13, 1980.

McClelland AJ, Hardy WD Jr, Zuckerman EE: Prognosis of healthy feline leukemia virus infected cats. Dev Cancer Res 4:121, 1980.

Pacitti AM: The risk of transmission of FeLV from latently infected cats. In Kirk RW, ed.: Current Veterinary Therapy X. Philadelphia: W. B. Saunders, 1989, p 526.

Pedersen NC: The clinical significance of latent feline leukemia virus infection in cats. Feline Pract 14:32, 1984.

Rojko JL, Hardy WD Jr: Feline leukemia virus and other retroviruses. In Sherding RG, ed.: The Cat: Diseases and Clinical Management. New York: Churchill Livingstone, 1989, p 229.

Rojko JL, Hoover EA, Mathes LE, et al: Pathogenesis of experimental feline leukemia virus infection. J Natl Cancer Inst 63:759, 1979.

Rojko JL, Hoover EA, Quakenbush SL, Olsen RG: Reactivation of latent feline leukaemia virus infection. Nature (Lond) 198:385, 1982.

2 Feline Immunodeficiency Virus

Robert G. Sherding

ETIOLOGY

Feline immunodeficiency virus (FIV) is a member of the lentivirus subfamily of retroviruses.

- FIV primarily infects and gradually destroys selected populations of T-lymphocytes. After a prolonged, asymptomatic latent period that extends for years, the progressive loss of T-lymphocytes results in an immunodeficiency syndrome characterized by chronic and recurrent infections. Infection is life-long and eventually fatal.
- FIV was originally isolated in 1986 from a cattery in northern California; however, retrospective assay of stored cat sera has shown that FIV has been widespread in the world's cat population since at least the 1960's.
- Susceptible species include the domestic cat, lion, tiger, jaguar, snow leopard, panther, and bobcat.

Epidemiology

- Geographic distribution: FIV has been found worldwide and throughout North America. In a 1991 nationwide survey of 27,976 high-risk cats presenting to veterinarians, 7.4% overall were infected with FIV, compared with 13.3% infected with feline leukemia virus (FeLV) and 1.5% coinfected with both (data from IDEXX Inc.).
  - Of symptomatic cats, 11.6% were infected.
  - Of asymptomatic cats, 4.0% were infected.
  - Of low-risk cats living indoors in single-cat households, 1.4% were infected.
  - Of cats in purebred catteries, less than 1% were infected.
- High-risk/high-incidence situations
  - Free-roaming outdoor pet or stray cats or cats exposed to outdoor cats
  - Cats living in large multicat households that frequently introduce new cats
- Low-risk/low incidence situations
  - Indoor pet cats in single-cat households
  - Cats in closed, well-controlled catteries (incidence in purebred cats is low)
- Sex distribution: male cats outnumber females 3 to 1 (see section on transmission).
- Age distribution: FIV affects cats of all ages (reported range is 2 months to 18 years); however, the incidence increases with age, and FIV is most prevalent in cats 5 years of age and older.

KEY POINT ▶ Because of an extended aymptomatic latent period that is typical for lentiviruses, most FIV-infected cats that have clinical signs are older than 6 years of age.

Transmission

- FIV is shed in saliva and transmitted primarily through direct bitewound inoculation during territorial fights (hence the higher incidence in males). Experimentally, a single tooth puncture from an FIV-infected cat is a very efficient method of transmitting FIV.

KEY POINT ▶ Biting is the principal mode of FIV transmission. The highest risk for FIV is found in intact male cats that are allowed to roam freely outdoors, such that bitewound transmission can occur during territorial disputes.

- Transmission can occur through transfusion of contaminated blood.
- Transmission by fomites or by venereal, *in utero,* or lactogenic routes appears to be rare or nonexistent.
- Transmission through intimate contact during cohabitation is unlikely but not impossible. In a study that confined FIV-positive and -negative cats together in the same cages for 2 years, only one of the 20 negative sentinel cats became infected. Contact transmission has occurred on rare occasions in catteries, but the route or mechanism is unknown.

Public Health Risks

FIV appears to grow only in feline cells (lentiviruses in general are very species specific).

KEY POINT ▶ Sera from cat owners, veterinarians, animal health technicians, and researchers in contact with infected cats or materials were negative for antibodies to FIV.

CLINICAL SIGNS

Stage 1: Acute Primary Phase of Infection

This stage begins 4 to 6 weeks post-exposure; effects are transient and usually go unnoticed.

- Transient fever (occurs in 33% of infected cats; lasts 3–14 days)
- Neutropenia (lasts 1–9 weeks)
- Generalized lymphadenopathy (occurs in 100% of infections; lasts 2–9 months); lesion: follicular hyperplasia and plasmacytic infiltration
- Occasional complications: sepsis, cellulitis, pustular facial dermatitis, anemia, diarrhea, myeloproliferative disease

Stage 2: Asymptomatic Latent Phase of Infection

There is a prolonged latency of variable duration up to years before signs of immunodeficiency occur.

Stage 3: Chronic Terminal Phase of Infection

Stage 3 is characterized by an acquired immunodeficiency syndrome of chronic, recurrent opportunistic infections with waxing and waning signs that progressively worsen over months to years and may involve any one or a combination of the following manifestations.

- General manifestations
  - Progressive weight loss and debilitation ("chronic wasting")
  - Chronic recurrent bacterial infections that may partially resolve with antibiotics but recur
  - Recurrent fevers of unknown origin
  - Generalized lymphadenopathy
  - Persistent or recurrent anemia or leukopenia (neutropenia, lymphopenia)
- Chronic or recurrent bacterial infections (most consistent feature of FIV; percentages below refer to approximate incidence in symptomatic FIV-infected cats).
  - Oral cavity (>50%)—stomatitis, gingivitis, periodontitis (suppurative or plasmacytic)
  - Respiratory (30%)—purulent rhinitis and conjunctivitis; pneumonia
  - Intestinal (20%)—acute or chronic diarrhea due to severe enterocolitis that can be ulcerative, necrotizing, or pyogranulomatous
  - Cutaneous (15%)—pustular dermatitis, abscesses, purulent otitis
  - Urinary—recurrent urinary tract infections (cystitis, pyelonephritis)

KEY POINT ▶ The majority of cats clinically ill with FIV have abnormal physical findings in the oral cavity or around the face and ears, such as stomatitis, naso-ocular discharge, otitis externa, and dermatitis.

- Specific opportunistic infections
  - Viruses—calicivirus, herpesvirus
  - Chlamydia
  - Bacteria—*Staphylococcus, Pseudomonas,* mycobacteria, *Yersinia, Mycoplasma*
  - Fungi—*Candida, Cryptococcus, Aspergillus*
  - Rickettsia—*Hemobartonella*
  - Protozoa—*Toxoplasma, Giardia,* cryptosporidia, coccidia
  - Parasites—generalized *Demodex, Notoedres*
- Encephalopathy
  - Signs—behavioral changes, dementia, compulsive wandering, licking motions, facial twitching, seizures
  - Pathogenesis—possibly direct effect of FIV on the central nervous system
- Neoplasia
  - FIV-infected cats have a higher than expected incidence (5.6 times) of lymphoid and myeloproliferative neoplasia.
  - Other neoplasms have been found sporadically in FIV-positive cats.
  - This is likely the result of impaired immune surveillance function rather than being a direct cause and effect of FIV.

DIAGNOSIS

The diagnosis of FIV is usually based on the demonstration of anti-FIV serum antibodies using one of three formats: ELISA, IFA, or Western blot. Tests for detection of FIV antigen have been used, but they are not yet reliable enough to recommend. Virus isolation is used in research but is not available for clinical use.

KEY POINT ▶ Since FIV antibodies indicate prior exposure and infection, and since FIV infection is lifelong, a positive FIV antibody test means that the virus is present in the cat and will remain so for life.

ELISA Test for FIV Antibody

- The ELISA test is used as in-office screening for serum antibodies against FIV.
  - CITE-FIV (IDEXX)
  - CITE-Combo and Probe-Combo (IDEXX)—tests for both FeLV and FIV
  - Also available from many commercial laboratories on a mail-in basis
- Seroconversion occurs 2 to 4 weeks post-exposure.
- Accuracy is >99%; thus, it is the first choice for testing ill high-risk cats.
  - False-positives—0.5% nonspecific reactions (can be higher because of operator error); because of this, in low-risk asymptomatic cats, confirm ELISA positives with an IFA test or Western blot.
  - False-negative results can occur in the early stages of acute infection before seroconversion has occurred or rarely in the terminal stages of immunodeficiency when antibody levels may be depressed.

IFA Test for FIV Antibody

- Available on a mail-in basis from a few commercial laboratories
- Accuracy comparable to in-office ELISA tests

Western Blot Test

- Detects antibodies against specific viral proteins; considered to be the "gold standard" for confirming ELISA-positive results.

- Available in research and commercial laboratories.

Assays to Detect Viral Antigens

- Advantages of an antigen test—enables detection of cats in the early pre-seroconversion stage of infection and of cats in the terminal stages of infection when antigen levels may be high and antibody levels are depressed.
- Disadvantages—because of the low level of virus produced in lentivirus infections, assays for detection of viral proteins must be very sensitive. The antigen assays currently available for FIV are not as reliable as the antibody tests and thus cannot be recommended for routine clinical use.

Virus Isolation

- Researchers can isolate FIV from blood or body fluids of infected cats.

TREATMENT

KEY POINT ▶ Even though FIV is incurable, asymptomatic cats can live for years before developing clinical signs, and symptomatic cats can often be sustained for many months with the judicious use of antibiotics combined with supportive care.

Specific Antiviral Therapy

- No specific treatment for FIV is currently available; once a cat is infected with FIV it is infected for life.
- Future anti-retroviral therapies developed for human immunodeficiency virus (HIV) may or may not be applicable to FIV. Some of the current anti-HIV drugs (e.g., AZT) have been tried and are too toxic in cats. Others are being evaluated.

General Supportive Therapy

- Cats ill with FIV-related bacterial infections may sometimes respond dramatically to antibiotics. Treat each infection episode as it arises, using culture and sensitivity guidance whenever possible.
- Use fluid therapy and nutritional support as indicated by the patient's needs.
- Prevent exposure to other infectious diseases because of lowered resistance.
- Continue vaccinations (in early phases, FIV-positive cats will respond), but killed products are preferred.

- Avoid use of griseofulvin (dermatophyte drug), as FIV-seropositive cats have an increased risk of griseofulvin-induced neutropenia.
- In the terminal stages of FIV, the prognosis for response to treatment is poor, as indicated by persistent anemia or leukopenia, severe weight loss, or central nervous system signs.
- In one study, the mortality rate for FIV-positive cats at 6 months post-diagnosis was 15%.

PREVENTION

Isolate Infected Cats

Isolation is recommended until more is known about cat-to-cat contact transmission (non-bite transmission is considered very rare; see section on Transmission).

Prevent Exposure

- Advise owners not to allow cats to roam free.
- Recommend neutering of male cats (to reduce roaming/fighting).

KEY POINT ▶ The best prevention for FIV is not to allow cats to roam freely outdoors.

Vaccination

Vaccination against FIV is not yet available; vaccines are difficult to develop for lentiviruses.

- Lentiviruses hide from the host immune system in latent form in target cells.
- Lentiviruses exhibit considerable strain variation.
- Host immune responses to natural FIV infection are not yet understood.

Supplemental Readings

IDEXX Corporation: Report of The National FeLV/FIV Awareness Project, 1991.

Ishida T, et al.: Feline immunodeficiency virus infection in cats of Japan. J Am Vet Med Assoc 194:221, 1989.

Pedersen NC: Feline immunodeficiency virus infection. *In Feline Infectious Diseases.* Goleta, CA: American Veterinary Publications, 1988, p 115.

Pedersen NC, Ho EW, Brown ML, Yamamoto JK: Isolation of a T-lymphotropic virus from domestic cats with an immunodeficiency-like syndrome. Science 235:790, 1987.

Yamamoto JK, Hansen H, Ho EW, et al: Epidemiologic and clinical aspects of feline immunodeficiency virus infection in cats from the continental United States and Canada and possible mode of transmission. J Am Vet Med Assoc 194:213, 1989.

Yamamoto JK, Sparger E, Ho EW, et al.: Pathogenesis of experimentally induced feline immunodeficiency virus infection in cats. Am J Vet Res 49:1246, 1988.

3 Feline Infectious Peritonitis

Robert G. Sherding

Feline infectious peritonitis (FIP) is a progressive and fatal systemic immune-mediated disease of cats caused by a coronavirus. Despite its name, the lesions of FIP are not restricted to the peritoneum, and there are effusive and noneffusive forms of the disease.

ETIOLOGY

FIP Coronavirus

- FIP virus (FIPV) causes systemic infection of the macrophage system and induces severe, widespread immune complex–mediated vasculitis with necrosis and pyogranulomatous inflammation.
- Antibodies to FIPV or to the related feline enteric coronavirus (see sec. 2, ch. 7) sensitize cats to FIP, and humoral antibodies play a major role in pathogenesis of the disease.
- Closely related coronaviruses (feline enteric coronavirus, canine coronavirus, transmissible gastroenteritis virus of swine) can infect cats, but they do not cause systemic infection or FIP. The antibodies they elicit cross-react with FIPV antibodies and are thus indistinguishable by conventional serologic tests.

Epidemiology

- FIPV is distributed worldwide in domestic cats.
- FIPV affects exotic Felidae, including the lion, cougar, cheetah, jaguar, leopard, bobcat, sand cat, caracal, serval, and lynx.

Transmission

- FIPV is excreted in oral and respiratory secretions, feces, and possibly urine.
- Infection occurs by ingestion or inhalation under conditions of close contact.
- Recent evidence suggests that FIPV may survive in the environment for several days in dried form; thus, fomite transmission is also a possibility.

Risk Factors

- Young age (FIP most often occurs in cats between 6 months and 5 years of age, but cats of any age can be affected)
- Group confinement (multicat households, purebred catteries)
- Concurrent viral infection with feline leukemia virus (FeLV) or feline immunodeficiency virus (FIV)

CLINICAL SIGNS

Cats with FIP often present initially with nonspecific and nonlocalizing signs, such as fever, anorexia, inactivity, weight loss, vomiting, diarrhea, dehydration, and pallor (anemia). As the disease advances, nonspecific signs progress and the clinical signs are dominated by body cavity effusions in the "wet" form of the disease or by organ-specific findings in the noneffusive, or "dry," form (Table 1). Some cats manifest features of both forms of the disease.

KEY POINT ▶ Chronic fluctuating fever that is unresponsive to antibiotics is the most frequent early sign of FIP.

Incubation and Clinical Course

- The natural incubation period is extremely variable, usually ranging from a few days to a few weeks, but in some cats it extends for several months.
- The onset of clinical signs is often insidious, although FIP can sometimes develop very suddenly, especially in young kittens.

TABLE 1. Clinical Situations in Which the Diagnosis of FIP Should be Considered

Nonspecific Signs
Chronic unresponsive fever of unknown origin
Unexplained anorexia, depression, and weight loss
Reproductive failure or neonatal kitten mortality

Effusion Signs
Fluid distension of the abdomen
Scrotal swelling
Dyspnea due to pleural effusion

Organ-Specific Signs
Enlarged, firm, irregular kidneys
Icterus or hepatomegaly
Neurologic signs (multifocal and progressive)
Uveitis (iridocyclitis; chorioretinitis)
Splenomegaly
Mesenteric lymphadenopathy

Laboratory Findings
Nonregenerative anemia
Neutrophilic leukocytosis or leukopenia
Elevated serum protein (hyperglobulinemia)
Elevated serum liver enzymes and bilirubin (also bilirubinuria)
Azotemia of primary renal origin
Proteinuria of renal origin
Pyogranulomatous or fibrinous body cavity fluid (nonseptic exudate)
Elevated CSF protein and leukocytes (neutrophils)

■ Once viral dissemination occurs and clinical illness develops, the disease is almost always progressive and fatal. However, there is considerable variation in the duration of clinical illness prior to death; 3 to 6 weeks is typical, but prolonged illness exceeding 6 months can occur, as can intermittent illness punctuated by periods of remission.
  • For effusive FIP the clinical course is usually acute.
  • For noneffusive FIP the course is often slow, insidious, and smoldering.
  • Cats with only ocular involvement sometimes survive for a year or more.

Effusive (Wet) Form of FIP

KEY POINT ▶ In the effusive, or wet, form of FIP, 85% of infected cats have inflammatory effusion in the abdominal cavity and 35% have effusion in the thoracic cavity.

Abdominal Effusion (Peritonitis)

■ There is progressive, nonpainful distension of the abdomen with fluid.
■ Effusion is detected by palpation and percussion of a fluid wave. In the early stages, a small amount of abdominal fluid may be detected by palpation of intestinal loops that feel excessively slippery, as though the serosal surfaces are highly lubricated. Pain on palpation is rare.
■ Scrotal swelling may occur in intact males as a direct extension of the abdominal effusive process into the testicular tunics.
■ Extension of the peritoneal inflammation may involve the gastrointestinal tract (vomiting, diarrhea), hepatobiliary system (jaundice), or pancreas (vomiting due to pancreatitis).
■ Adhesions may organize the mesentery and omentum into an irregular, firm mass that is palpable in the cranioventral abdomen.
■ Abdominal effusion is confirmed by radiography or abdominocentesis and fluid analysis is usually strongly indicative of FIP (see section on Diagnosis).

Thoracic Effusion (Pleuritis)

■ Dyspnea and exercise intolerance are the major presenting signs because lung expansion is restricted by compression from fluid in the pleural space.
■ The animal may prefer a sitting or sternal recumbent posture to facilitate breathing. Increased respiratory distress may occur with exercise, with stressful handling in the hospital, or with repositioning in lateral recumbency (orthopnea).
■ Muffled heart and lung sounds may be found on auscultation, and dullness and a horizontal fluid line may be found on thoracic percussion.
■ Pericardial effusion (fibrinous pericarditis) may accompany pleural FIP and is detectable by echocardiography, but only rarely is this extensive enough to cause cardiac tamponade.
■ Thoracic effusion is confirmed by radiography or thoracocentesis (see sec. 6, ch. 22). Fluid analysis is usually strongly indicative of FIP (see section on Diagnosis).

Noneffusive (Dry) Form of FIP

KEY POINT ▶ The noneffusive, or dry, form of FIP is characterized by pyogranulomatous inflammation and necrotizing vasculitis in various organs, such as the abdominal viscera (liver, spleen, kidneys), eyes, central nervous system (CNS), and lungs.

Pyogranulomas may be seen as multiple, gray-white nodular masses of variable size on the surface and within the parenchyma of affected organs. Effusion is usually minimal or absent. The specific organs affected and the degree of resulting organ failure determine the presenting clinical signs.

Kidney Involvement

■ Pyogranulomatous nephritis—kidneys become palpably enlarged, firm, and irregular owing to the presence of granulomas scattered over the surface and extending into the renal cortex.
■ Occasionally, when renal involvement is extensive, signs of renal failure (e.g., polyuria-polydipsia) and azotemia (elevated BUN and serum creatinine) may develop.
■ Proteinuria is probably the most consistent laboratory finding in renal FIP. In addition, immune complex glomerulonephritis may develop in cats with any of the other effusive and noneffusive forms of FIP, although this is usually subclinical.

Liver Involvement

■ Pyogranulomatous hepatitis (hepatomegaly, jaundice, and nonspecific signs of hepatic failure) may occur.
■ The most consistent laboratory abnormalities are bilirubinuria and hyperbilirubinemia. Mild to moderate elevations of serum liver enzymes (alanine aminotransferase, alkaline phosphatase) and serum bile acids may also occur.

Involvement of Other Abdominal Organs

■ Granulomatous lesions may cause palpable enlargement of the visceral lymph nodes or spleen or thickening of the intestinal tract and omentum.
■ Pancreatic involvement, although uncommon, has been associated with diabetes mellitus.

Eye Involvement

■ Ocular lesions of FIP are usually bilateral and affect the vascular tunic or uvea (uveitis). Lesions may or may not impair vision.
■ Manifestations of exudative anterior uveitis (iridocyclitis) may include miosis, aqueous flare, hypopyon ("mutton-fat" deposits of cells and fibrin), hyphema, keratic fibrinocellular precipitates, anterior chamber adhesions (synechia), and edema and deep neovascularization of the cornea.
■ Chorioretinitis from posterior uveal involvement is detected by ophthalmoscopic examination and may include perivascular cuffing, exudative retinal detachment, and retinal hemorrhages.

Nervous System Involvement

- Multifocal pyogranulomatous meningoencephalitis may occur. In one report, 29% of all cats with FIP developed neurologic signs. The relentless progression and multifocal nature of the signs are characteristic features of neural FIP.
- The neuroanatomic distribution of the lesions determines clinical signs; some of the most common are posterior paresis, ataxia, tremors, vestibular dysfunction, seizures, hyperesthesia, and personality changes.
- Neuropathies occasionally involve the cranial nerves (e.g., trigeminal or facial) or peripheral nerves (e.g., brachial or sciatic).
- Some cats with neural FIP develop secondary hydrocephalus when the inflammatory process obstructs the flow of cerebrospinal fluid.
- The diagnosis of neural FIP depends on cerebrospinal fluid (CSF) analysis (see section on Diagnosis). Electroencephalography may show nonspecific changes.

Lung Involvement

- Granulomatous pneumonia usually is clinically silent and discovered at necropsy, although occasionally a persistent cough is manifested.
- On thoracic radiographs, pyogranulomatous pneumonia may be detected as diffuse, poorly-defined, patchy nodular densities within the pulmonary interstitium.

Reproductive Involvement

- FIP virus is a suspected but unconfirmed factor in cattery reproductive problems such as infertility, fetal resorptions, abortions, stillbirths, congenital malformations, and birth of weak or "fading kittens."

DIAGNOSIS

The diagnosis of FIP is usually suspected and diagnosed on the basis of clinical signs (see Table 1) and potential for exposure in conjunction with supportive findings on various laboratory evaluations (hematology, serum chemistry, cytology, serology), radiography, and biopsy (summarized in Table 2).

KEY POINT ▶ Clinical signs and results of laboratory evaluations in cats with FIP generally are not specific for the disease; however, collectively these may provide strong circumstantial evidence for a diagnosis of FIP.

Hematology and Serum Protein Electrophoresis

Hematology and serum protein electrophoresis assays are abnormal in most cats with FIP, reflecting the inflammatory and immune responses (see Table 2).

TABLE 2. Diagnosis of FIP

Parameter or Procedure	Findings Suggestive of FIP
Age	6 mo to 5 yr; or >10 yr
Habitat	Cattery or multicat household
Signs (see Table 1)	Fever (unresponsive)
	Effusion (abdominal; thoracic)
	Liver disease
	Renal disease (with renomegaly)
	Ocular disease (uveitis)
	CNS disease (multifocal)
Clinical course	Progressive
Complete blood count	Nonregenerative anemia
	Neutrophilia or neutropenia; left shift
	Lymphopenia
	Neutrophil inclusions (immune complexes?)
Plasma proteins	Hyperglobulinemia (polyclonal: gamma, alpha$_2$, beta)
	Hyperfibrinogenemia (400–700 mg/dl)
Serum chemistries	Abnormal liver tests (increased ALT, ALP, bile acids, bilirubin)
	Azotemia (increased BUN, creatinine)
Urinalysis	Proteinuria; bilirubinuria
Radiography	Effusions (abdominal, thoracic)
	Organomegaly (liver, kidney)
	Organ infiltration (lung)
Fluid analysis of effusion	
Appearance	Yellow, clear, sticky, foamy, fibrinous
Protein	4–10 g/dl (gamma globulin >32%, albumin <48%, A/G ratio <0.81)
Leukocytes	1000–20,000 cells/μl
Cytology	Pyogranulomatous exudate
Cerebrospinal fluid analysis	
Protein	90–2000 mg/dl (usually >200 mg/dl)
Leukocytes	90–9250 cells/μl (neutrophils >mononuclear)
Serology	High CV-Ab titer or fourfold rise (see text)
Histopathology	Vasculitis and pyogranulomatous inflammation

Serum Chemistry Profile and Urinalysis

These tests are useful in noneffusive FIP involving abdominal viscera to indicate liver, kidney, or pancreatic involvement (see Table 2).

Radiography

Radiography is useful mostly to confirm the presence of body cavity effusion (abdominal, pleural), organ enlargement (kidney, liver), or organ infiltration (lung). Affected abdominal organs can also be imaged by ultrasonography.

Fluid Analysis of Abdominal or Thoracic Effusions

The distinctive characteristics of the fluid strongly support a diagnosis of effusive FIP.

- The fluid appears pale yellow to golden in color and nearly translucent because of its relatively low cell count (usually 1000 to 20,000 nucleated cells/μl).
- The fluid may seem tenacious or sticky and may contain flecks, strands, or clots of fibrin.
- The fluid is foamy because of its high protein concentration, which can approach that of plasma, usually ranging from 4 to 10 g/dl. Considering the high

protein content of FIP fluid, the nucleated cell count is disproportionately low relative to that found in other types of exudate.

■ When necessary, protein electrophoresis of the fluid may help to establish the diagnosis of FIP based on the following criteria: a gamma globulin content that is at least 32% of the fluid protein, an albumin that is less than 48% of the fluid protein, and an albumin-to-globulin ratio (A/G) that is less than 0.81.

■ The cytologic pattern of FIP fluid is a nonseptic exudate, often called pyogranulomatous, because it is characterized by a predominance of well-preserved (nondegenerate) neutrophils and macrophages, but it also includes variable numbers of plasma cells and lymphocytes.

Analysis of CSF or Aqueous Humor of the Eye

These laboratory tests are valuable in evaluating cats with neural or ocular FIP. Both the protein concentration and leukocyte count (especially neutrophils) are consistently increased in CSF of cats with neural FIP and in aqueous humor of cats with intraocular FIP. (see Table 2).

Coronaviral Serology

Detection of coronaviral antibody (Ab) is informative, but the conventional methodology does not provide a definitive diagnosis because it does not differentiate FIP from non-FIP coronaviral (CV) infections or distinguish between carrier and active infection. Antibodies to all the related coronaviruses cross-react on this test, creating a problem in interpretation. Consider the following when interpreting a conventional CV-Ab titer.

Causes of a Positive Conventional CV-Ab Titer

(This test is not sufficiently *specific* to be used as a definitive diagnostic test.)

■ Seroconversion to FIPV
  • Active FIPV infection causing disease (especially if titer is ≥1:3200 in a test system that uses FIPV antigen (Ag), or if titer is ≥1:400 in a non–FIPV-Ag test system, or if titer rises fourfold)
  • Asymptomatic carrier of FIPV
  • Recovery from prior exposure to FIPV
  • Antibody response to FIP vaccination (postvaccinal titers in most cases will be negative or low)
■ Seroconversion to other coronaviruses
  • Feline enteric coronavirus (FECV)
  • Canine coronavirus (CCV)
  • Transmissible gastroenteritis virus (TGEV) of swine
■ False-positive as a result of recent vaccination (cross-reactivity to bovine serum)

Causes of a False-Negative Conventional CV-Ab Titer

(This test is not sufficiently *sensitive* to be used as a definitive diagnostic test.)

■ Laboratory error or insensitive assay system

■ Low antibody level resulting from:
  • Peracute infection
  • Drop in level in terminal stages of infection
  • Consumption of antibody in immune complexes

KEY POINT ▶ Use the conventional CV-Ab titer as a diagnostic aid for FIP rather than as a definitive diagnostic test. Interpret a positive titer to indicate that FIP is *possible* (low titer) or *probable* (high or rising titer), and interpret a negative titer to indicate that FIP is *unlikely*.

New Test for Anti-idiotypic FIPV-Ab

■ Microwell ELISA for detection of specific antibodies to disease-producing strains of FIPV is currently under development. (Virachek/FIP; Synbiotics).
■ This test is designed to detect FIPV antibodies but not antibodies to non-FIP coronaviruses (such as FECV), thereby eliminating the problem of false-positive titers occurring with the conventional test. However, reliability and specificity remain to be established.
■ Titer becomes positive within 2 weeks following experimental infection.
■ Antibodies elicited by FIP vaccine may confuse interpretation.

Other New Tests for FIP (in Development)

■ Immunofluorescent antibody (IFA) test for FIPV in conjunctival scrapings
■ Serologic test for FIPV antigen-antibody complexes
■ Test for FIPV antigen using DNA probes

Histopathology

Biopsy of affected tissues is a valuable diagnostic procedure in some cats, because the FIP lesions of vasculitis and pyogranulomatous inflammation are fairly distinctive.

TREATMENT

There is currently no known cure for FIP, nor has any treatment protocol been effective in prolonging life or consistently inducing remission in cats with the disease. Palliative treatment seems beneficial in some cats, but the response rate is low. Although there are occasional spontaneous remissions in cats that are only mildly affected or in those with only ocular involvement, these are rare.

KEY POINT ▶ Once a cat develops clinical illness due to FIP, the disease is nearly always fatal regardless of treatment.

Palliative Chemotherapy

Temporary remissions occasionally occur with chemotherapy protocols combined with intensive supportive and nursing care. Unfortunately, even with aggressive therapy in well-selected cases, a beneficial response occurs in less than 10% of treated cats.

- Cats most likely to respond are those with mild FIP that are in good physical condition with good appetite and an absence of neurologic signs, anemia, or concurrent retroviral infection (FeLV, FIV).
- Chemotherapy protocols combine a high dosage of corticosteroid with a cytotoxic alkylating agent such as chlorambucil, cyclophosphamide, or mephalan (Table 3).
- Corticosteroids and cytotoxic drugs have no effect on the virus itself, but by virtue of their anti-inflammatory and immunosuppressive effects, they are aimed at controlling the secondary immune-mediated inflammatory reactions that play a major role in the pathogenesis of the disease.
- Corticosteroids and cytotoxic drugs may adversely affect cellular immunity mediated by T-lymphocytes and macrophages and thereby have the potential to promote the viral infection.
- The principal side effects of cytotoxic drugs are anorexia and bone marrow suppression; thus, hemograms should be monitored periodically (see sec. 3, ch. 5 for more details on effects of these drugs).

TABLE 3. Treatment of FIP

Mode of Therapy	Specific Treatment Measures*
Supportive treatment	Parenteral fluid therapy to maintain hydration
	Nutritional therapy via tube feeding—nasogastric, gastrostomy, or pharyngostomy (see sec. 1, Ch. 3)
	Body cavity drainage as needed—especially thoracentesis to relieve dyspnea
	Blood transfusions—as needed for severe nonregenerative anemia
	Antibiotics—for control of complicating bacterial infections
Anti-inflammatory-immunosupppressive†	Prednisone—50–100 mg/M²/day, PO, q 24 h
	plus‡
	Chlorambucil (Leukeran)—20 mg/M², PO, q 2–3 wk
	or
	Cyclophosphamide (Cytoxan)—50 mg/M² q 48 h, or 200–300 mg/M² q 2–3 wk; PO
	or
	Melphalan (Alkeran)—2 mg/M² (¼ of 2-mg tablet), PO, q 48 h
Topical ophthalmic (for uveitis)	Prednisone acetate 1%—2–3 drops/eye q 6 h
	Atropine 1%—1–3 drops/eye up to q 6 h to maintain mydriasis
Experimental treatments	Antiviral drugs (generally too toxic to use in cats)—e.g., ribavirin, azidothymidine (AZT), acyclovir
	Immune modulators (efficacy not established)—e.g., interferon (Roferon), *Propionibacterium acnes* (ImmunoRegulin), thioproline (Promodulin)

*Cats most likely to respond are in good physical condition and have good appetite, with absence of CNS signs, anemia, and FeLV infection.

†For conversion of body weight to body surface area (M²), refer to conversion tables.

‡Choose only *one* of the three.

- Most published protocols recommend administration of cytotoxic agents daily, every other day, or for 4 consecutive days each week. Persistent drug-induced anorexia is a frequent problem with these schedules; an alternative is pulse administration, using a large dose of the drug once every 2 to 3 weeks. In this way, a few days after each dose the appetite usually rebounds and is maintained between treatment cycles. Also, the larger size of pulse dosages better matches the commercially available tablet sizes of some of the cytotoxic drugs.
- Regardless of the regimen chosen, if no response is noted within the first 2 to 4 weeks, consider the chemotherapy ineffective, and either modify or discontinue it. If a positive response does occur, continue the treatment for a minimum of 3 months and possibly indefinitely.

Treatment of Ocular FIP

- Use topical ophthalmic corticosteroids and topical atropine for mydriasis (see Table 3).
- Subconjunctival or retrobulbar injections of long-acting corticosteroids are recommended by some clinicians; however, it is unlikely that these methods of administration will result in any higher intraocular level of steroid than systemic administration.

Supportive Treatment

These measures may improve quality of life and possibly survival time.

- Intermittent body cavity drainage (in effusive cases)
- Parenteral fluid therapy
- Nutritional support (via nasogastric or gastrostomy tube feeding techniques; see sec. 1, ch. 3) (there is no evidence that megadoses of vitamins are beneficial in FIP)
- Blood transfusion (for severe nonregenerative anemia)
- Antibiotics (if secondary bacterial infections are suspected)

Experimental Treatments

Experimental protocols involve antiviral drugs that have a direct effect against FIPV and immune modulating drugs that promote a protective immune response through T-cell stimulation and macrophage activation. Further study is required before these can be recommended.

- Antiviral drugs include interferon, ribavirin (Virazole), azidothymidine (AZT; Retrovir), and acyclovir (Zovirax). Except for interferon, the therapeutic indices are unacceptably low, such that toxicity is likely at dosage levels required for antiviral effect.
- Immune modulating agents include interferon (Roferon), *Propionibacterium acnes* (ImmunoRegulin), thioproline (Promodulin), thymosin, isoprinosine, lentinan, and levamisole (Levisole)

PREVENTION

Vaccination

Description of FIP Vaccine

A modified-live, temperature-sensitive strain of FIPV became available in 1991 as an intranasal (IN) vaccine (Primucell FIP; SmithKline Beecham).

- It replicates locally in the nasopharynx, but not systemically because of temperature sensitivity.
- It stimulates local nasal and gut mucosal immunity, salivary immunoglobulin A antibody (IgA), and cell-mediated immunity (CMI).
- It does not sensitize animals to FIP disease because it elicits minimal humoral antibody response.
- It cross-protects against multiple strains of FIPV.

Recommendations for Use of FIP Vaccine

- Give 2 doses of 0.5 ml each, intranasally, 3 to 4 weeks apart, at 16 weeks of age or older.
- Revaccinate annually (or perhaps every 6 to 9 months in high-risk situations).

Vaccine Efficacy

- Survival in various trials conducted by the manufacturer was 71 to 85% in vaccinates versus 17 to 20% in nonvaccinates when challenged within 6 months or less of vaccination.
- Survival after challenge 12 months postvaccination was 60% (six of ten cats).
- Survival after a second challenge in 17 cats that had survived a previous challenge was 94%.
- Survival or protection against challenge correlates with prechallenge IgA antibody levels in saliva.

Vaccine Safety

- Based on data from the manufacturer, no serious adverse effects or sensitization (enhanced susceptibility to FIP) were noted:
  - In 16 cats vaccinated by the wrong route (SC twice)
  - In a few kittens vaccinated earlier than recommended at 3 to 4 weeks of age and again at 6 to 8 weeks
  - In 21 cats vaccinated during pregnancy, followed by vaccination of 11 of their kittens

  - In two cats vaccinated after receiving dexamethasone (1 mg/kg) on the 7th, 4th, and 2nd day before and on the day of vaccination
  - In ten cats vaccinated 4 months after feline leukemia virus (FeLV) exposure (at which time five were FeLV-positive and five were FeLV-negative)
  - In four cats vaccinated following survival from previous FIPV exposure
  - In 26 cats vaccinated following exposure to FECV
  - In 349 cats from ten FIP-endemic catteries
- There was no interference with simultaneous vaccination with FeLV, panleukopenia, and respiratory agents.
- Side effects in field trials included sneezing and sniffling in a small percentage of cats.

Recommendations for Control of FIP in Cattery Situations

- Isolate cats with signs of FIP.
- Control FeLV in the cattery by vaccination, testing, and removal (see sec. 2, ch. 1).
- Only allow entry of incoming cats that have negative FIPV-Ab titers.
- Use only proven queens in breeding programs; do not breed queens that have a previous history of producing sick or FIP-infected kittens.
- Use good husbandry (e.g., good hygiene and feeding practices, avoid overcrowding).

Supplemental Readings

Barlough JE, Stoddart CA: Feline coronaviral infections. *In* Greene CE, ed.: *Infectious Diseases of the Dog and Cat.* Philadelphia: W. B. Saunders, 1990, p 300.

Pedersen NC: Feline infectious peritonitis: Something old, something new. Feline Pract 6:42, 1976.

Pedersen NC: Feline infectious peritonitis. *In* Pedersen NC: *Feline Infectious Diseases.* Goleta, CA: American Veterinary Publications, 1988, p 45.

Shelley SM, Scarlett-Kranz J, Blue JT: Protein electrophoresis on effusions from cats as a diagnostic test for feline infectious peritonitis. J Am Anim Hosp Assoc 24:495, 1988.

Sherding RG: Feline infectious peritonitis. Compend Contin Educ 1:95, 1979.

Weiss RC: Feline infectious peritonitis and other coronaviruses. *In* Sherding RG, ed.: *The Cat. Diseases and Clinical Management.* New York: Churchill Livingstone, 1989, p 333.

Weiss RC: The diagnosis and clinical management of feline infectious peritonitis. Vet Med 86:14, 1991.

4

Feline Infectious Respiratory Disease Complex: Herpesvirus, Calicivirus, and Chlamydia

Robert G. Sherding

ETIOLOGY

The major causes of infectious upper respiratory disease of cats are two highly contagious viruses: feline herpesvirus-1 (FHV-1), also known as feline viral rhinotracheitis (FVR), and feline calicivirus (FCV). The clinical signs of infection with these two viruses overlap and are often indistinguishable; thus, they are often grouped together and referred to as the infectious respiratory disease complex or upper respiratory infection (URI) of cats. A feline strain of *Chlamydia psittaci* is a nonviral cause of mild upper respiratory signs in cats that is often grouped in this disease complex with FHV and FCV; however, its predominant manifestation is persistent conjunctivitis. Other potential respiratory pathogens, such as reovirus, *Mycoplasma* spp, and *Bordetella bronchiseptica,* are of minor significance and are not discussed here.

Transmission

Young kittens, unvaccinated cats, and cats confined in catteries or multicat households have the greatest risk of infection. Direct contact and fomites are the most important means of infection.

- Direct contact: oral, nasal, and ocular discharges are infective.
- Fomites: contaminated cages, examination tables, food and water dishes, and human hands and clothing can transmit the virus.
  - FHV—susceptible to drying and most disinfectants; survives 18–24 hours outside the host.
  - FCV—very resistant virus; average survival outside the cat is 8–10 days; preferred disinfectant is 1:32 solution of hypochlorite (bleach).
- Aerosol: sneezing and coughing can propel virus up to 4 feet into the air.

Subclinical Carriers as Reservoirs of Infection

Most cats (up to 80%) that recover from FHV and FCV infection remain subclinical carriers for months to years. Persistently infected or latent subclinical carriers perpetuate these viruses within the cat population and serve as the principal source for outbreaks in catteries, multicat households, research colonies, veterinary hospitals, and shelters.

- FHV: recovered carriers shed virus intermittently coinciding with reactivation of latent virus infection by stress. Episodes of shedding generally persist for 2 weeks and can be accompanied by recrudescence of mild clinical signs.

KEY POINT ▶ Shedding of FHV is often triggered by lactation in carrier queens at the time when kittens are losing passive maternal immunity (5–7 weeks) and becoming susceptible. This is an important source of upper respiratory infection in young kittens.

- FCV: recovered carriers shed virus from the oropharynx continuously for many months, or even years, and can infect other cats.

CLINICAL SIGNS

Typical signs of feline URI include anorexia, depression, fever, and naso-ocular discharge. Other signs specific to each etiologic agent are detailed below. The onset is often acute and the signs are more severe in young kittens. Clinical disease is usually self-limiting within 5 to 7 days. (See Table 1 for a summary of the clinical manifestations of FHV and FCV.)

Feline Herpesvirus

- Herpesvirus has an affinity for conjunctival, nasal, and upper airway (laryngotracheal) epithelium. Necrosis at these sites causes rhinitis, tracheitis, laryngitis, and conjunctivitis.
- Signs include sneezing, serous to mucopurulent naso-ocular discharge, cough, hypersalivation, and loss of voice.
- Corneal involvement causes keratitis or herpetic ulcers. Ulcers can have a punctate, oval, or branching (dendritic) pattern (see sec. 11, ch. 4).
- Infection during pregnancy may result in abortion or in a severe generalized form of infection in newborn kittens, characterized by fatal encephalitis or focal necrotizing hepatitis.
- Secondary bacterial complication of the lesions may worsen and prolong FHV disease. Bacterial pneumonia is a serious complication in young kittens.

Feline Calicivirus

■ Calicivirus has an affinity for oropharyngeal epithelium and alveolar pneumocytes of the lung.
■ Infection is manifested most often as oral ulceration, mild rhinitis (sneezing), and conjunctivitis, or viral interstitial pneumonia, depending on the strain of FCV. In some cats the tip of the nose may be ulcerated and crusted.
■ One FCV isolate reportedly causes consistent foot-pad and interdigital ulcers along with oral ulcers ("paw and mouth disease").
■ FCV was isolated from eight of ten cats with chronic ulcerative or proliferative gingivitis/stomatitis, but its role in chronic oral disease is uncertain.
■ A strain of FCV has been described that causes generalized pain (myalgia and arthralgia) without noticeable respiratory signs.
■ FCV has been isolated from the intestines and feces of cats with acute and chronic enteritis.

Feline Chlamydiosis

■ Ocular signs predominate, such as acute or chronic mucopurulent conjunctivitis that can begin unilaterally and later become bilateral (see sec. 11, ch. 3).
■ Mild nasal discharge, sneezing, and coughing can occur.
■ Very mild subclinical pneumonia can occur but usually is only detectable histologically.

DIAGNOSIS

For individually infected cats, a diagnosis of "viral respiratory disease" or URI based on clinical signs and likelihood of exposure is adequate for patient management. Virology is the only means of definitive diagnosis, and its availability is limited to selected reference and research laboratories (such as state animal diagnostic laboratories and colleges of veterinary medicine). Virology should, however, be considered for evaluation of disease outbreaks in groups of cats.

KEY POINT ▶ Severe naso-ocular signs are most consistent with FHV infection. Corneal ulceration is indicative of FHV while oral ulceration is more likely with FCV. Persistent conjunctivitis is the predominant sign in chlamydiosis.

Routine Laboratory Diagnostics

Complete blood count (CBC), serum chemistries, and urinalysis are usually normal except in severe infections complicated by bacteria, in which a neutrophilic leukocytosis may be found on the CBC.

Tests for Immunodeficiency Syndromes

Immunodeficient cats often develop persistent or recurrent signs of upper respiratory infection. Evaluate cats for underlying infections of feline immunodeficiency virus (FIV antibody test; see sec. 2, ch. 2) and feline leukemia virus (FeLV antigen test; see sec. 2, ch. 1) in the following situations:

TABLE 1. Clinical Manifestations of Feline Viral Respiratory Disease

Manifestation	Feline Herpesvirus (FHV-1)	Feline Calicivirus (FCV)
Incubation	3–5 days	1–3 days
Duration	5–10 days (or more)	5–7 days
Anorexia and depression	Severe and frequent	Mild and inconsistent
Fever	Frequent	Inconsistent (diphasic)
Nasal signs	Sneezing—severe Discharge—marked Ulcerated nares Turbinate necrosis Sequela—chronic rhinosinusitis	Sneezing—mild Discharge—mild or absent Ulcerated tip of nose
Ocular signs	Conjunctivitis—severe (serous to mucopurulent discharge, chemosis, photophobia) Ulcerative keratitis Panophthalmitis (neonates) Sequela—sicca ("dry eye")	Conjunctivitis—mild
Oral signs	Hypersalivation; rare ulcers	Frequent oral ulcers (tongue, palate) Sequela—chronic gingivitis
Pulmonary signs	Rare bacterial pneumonia	Occasional viral pneumonia
Other signs	Abortion Peracute neonatal death (hepatic necrosis)	Limping syndrome (arthritis, arthralgia, myalgia) Interdigital paw ulcers Enteritis (diarrhea and vomiting)
Postrecovery shedding	Intermittent (after stress)	Persistent

■ Cats with recurrent episodes of infectious respiratory disease
■ Vaccinated adult cats with unusually severe signs
■ Cats that have signs that linger beyond 2 weeks in duration.

Detection of Inclusion Bodies

■ FHV: intranuclear inclusions in conjunctival biopsies (H&E stain)
■ Chlamydia: intracytoplasmic inclusions in scrapings of conjunctival epithelium (Diff-Quik stain); mostly during the first 2 weeks of infection (see sec. 11, ch. 3)

Direct Immunofluorescence

■ Uses smears of nasal mucosa or conjunctiva to detect virus-infected cells
■ Best test for FHV

Virus Isolation

■ Uses cell culture of swabs from oropharynx, nasal cavity, or conjunctiva

■ Best test for FCV; acceptable test for FHV

Serology

■ Uses rising neutralizing antibody titer in serum from convalescent animal
■ Acceptable for presumptive diagnosis of FCV

TREATMENT

Viral respiratory disease is self-limiting in most cats within 5 to 7 days. Treatment is mainly supportive in nature, although in the future effective antiviral drugs may be developed. Hospitalize only cats that require parenteral fluid therapy, oxygen therapy, or enteral hyperalimentation.

KEY POINT ▶ Treat infectious respiratory disease in cats on an outpatient basis whenever possible in order to prevent cross-infection of other hospitalized cats.

Outpatient Treatment

Select the combination of treatments from the following list that are most applicable to the patient's manifestations.

■ Clean discharge from eyes and nares as needed.
■ Support nutrition and fluid intake:
  • Advise owners to offer a variety of flavorful, aromatic foods and broths to encourage continued intake of food and fluids.
  • Teach owners coax-feeding, force-feeding, and syringe feeding techniques.
  • Supplement diet with potassium (Tumil-K; Kaon) (see sec. 1, ch. 5) and vitamin B complex.
  • Diazepam (Valium) (0.1–0.2 mg/kg, IV, every 12–24 hours) or oxazepam (Serax; Wyeth) (2.5 mg total dose, PO, every 12 hours) as appetite stimulants just prior to feeding may overcome anorexia.
■ Provide rest and warmth (inhibits FHV replication).
■ Prevent inspissation of respiratory secretions:
  • Promote airway humidification (humidifier or vaporizer).
  • Prevent dehydration (prescribe oral fluids or subcutaneous administration of isotonic electrolyte solution).
■ Promote nasal decongestion:
  • Prevent inspissation of secretions (see above).
  • Oxymetazoline 0.25% nasal spray (Afrin; Schering), every 12 hours, may be used but is not well tolerated by most cats.
■ Irrigate necrotic oral lesions with 0.2% chlorhexidine solution (Nolvasan).
■ Control secondary infections with antibiotics:
  • For secondary bacterial infection—amoxicillin, ampicillin, cephalosporins
  • For chlamydia—tetracycline
■ Treat ocular lesions with topical eye medications (see sec. 11, chs. 3 and 4):
  • Antibiotics for bacterial complications

• Tetracycline ointments for chlamydia (continue for 4 weeks)
• Antivirals applied topically every 6 hours for herpetic ulcers (expensive): idoxuridine (Stoxil, Smith Kline; Dendrid, Alcon; Herplex, Allergan); trifluridine (Viroptic, Burroughs Wellcome); vidarabine (Vira-A, Parke Davis)

In-Hospital Treatment

In severe cases, hospitalization may be required for additional therapy.

■ For prolonged anorexia: enteral hyperalimentation for nutritional support (via pharyngostomy, gastrostomy, or nasogastric intubation; see sec. 1, ch. 3)
■ For moderate to severe dehydration: parenteral fluid therapy
■ For pneumonia and hypoxemia: oxygen via nasal catheter (see sec. 1, ch. 3) or oxygen cage

Sequelae

■ Subclinical viral carriers (see section on Etiology)
  • Cattery problem
  • FHV recrudescence
■ Chronic rhinitis/sinusitis following FHV infection (sometimes called "chronic snuffler"; see sec. 6, ch. 18 for discussion of medical and surgical approaches to treatment of chronic rhinitis and sinusitis)
  • Turbinate necrosis, ulceration, and osteolysis
  • Bacterial sinusitis
  • Persistent local FHV infection
■ Chronic ocular discharge (see sec. 11, ch. 3)
  • Bacterial or chlamydial follicular conjunctivitis
  • Tear duct blockage/infection (dacryocystitis)
  • Keratoconjunctivitis sicca (FHV)

PREVENTION

For prevention of infectious respiratory disease in the individual cat, vaccination is available for FHV, FCV, and chlamydia. For prevention of spread of disease in groups of cats confined together, additional control measures are indicated.

Vaccination

General Considerations

■ Local immunity plays an important role in protection.
■ FCV vaccine strains do not cross-protect against all isolates.
■ Protocol: incorporate FHV and FCV (chlamydia optional) into routine feline vaccination program; initially give two doses 3 weeks apart (starting at 9 weeks of age in kittens) and give booster annually.

KEY POINT ▶ Immunization protects against clinical illness but not infection. It does not prevent or eliminate chronic viral carrier states or virus shedding.

Injectable Vaccine

Two types are available: modified live virus (MLV) and inactivated virus.

- Advantages: less side effects and less chance of producing carriers
- Disadvantages: slow onset of protection; humoral immunity not as effective as local immunity
- Caution: oronasal exposure to injectable MLV vaccine by inadvertent aerosolization or spilling on the haircoat can occasionally cause sneezing and oronasal ulcers.

Intranasal Vaccine (MLV)

- Advantage: more rapid (1–4 days) and possibly more reliable protection through local immunity
- Disadvantage: mild postvaccinal sneezing and nasoocular discharge in some cats

Control Measures in Catteries

General Considerations

- FHV and FCV are perpetuated in catteries by virus that is shed from subclinical carriers and spread by aerosol, contact, and fomite transmission.
- When introducing a new cat, there is always a risk that the incoming cat is a subclinical carrier that can be the source for an outbreak.
- In endemic catteries, kittens lose their maternal immunity at 5 to 7 weeks and often become infected by virus shed from their own lactating dam.

KEY POINT ▶ Subclinical shedders of respiratory viruses are prevalent. Cats that are free of signs of disease are not necessarily free of infection, even if they have been well vaccinated.

Recommendations

- Vaccinate all cats routinely.
- Avoid incoming cats from infected sources.
- Vaccinate and then quarantine all incoming cats for 3 weeks:

- To protect the incoming cat from viruses in the cattery
- To protect the cattery from a new cat that might be in a state of virus incubation or stress-induced shedding of FHV
- For rapid onset of immunity in outbreak situations, use intranasal vaccine.
- In endemic catteries with infection problems in kittens at 5 to 7 weeks of age:
  - Vaccinate queens prior to breeding (and possibly during pregnancy 3 to 4 weeks prior to queening, but only with inactivated vaccine (e.g., Fel-O-Vax PCT, Fort Dodge), to enhance passive maternal antibody levels in kittens.
  - Wean kittens early at 4 to 5 weeks of age and raise them in isolation.
  - Use intranasal vaccine in kittens because it can induce local protection rapidly despite the presence of interfering maternal antibody.
- Identify and treat cats with chronic chlamydial conjunctivitis.
- In housing facilities for cats, avoid overcrowding, provide adequate ventilation (10 or more air changes per hour), maintain a warm nonfluctuating temperature, control humidity at about 50%, and provide separate cages with solid partitions and separate food and water dishes.
- Prevent fomite transmission by disinfecting cages (1:32 hypochlorite solution) and by minimizing crosscontamination by personnel.

Supplemental Readings

Ford RB: Infectious diseases of the respiratory tract. *In* Sherding RG, ed.: *The Cat: Diseases and Clinical Management.* New York: Churchill Livingstone, 1989, p 367.

Knowles JO, Gaskell RM: Control of upper respiratory diseases in multiple cat households and catteries. *In:* August JR, ed.: *Consultations in Feline Internal Medicine.* Philadelphia: W. B. Saunders, 1991, p 563.

Povey RC: Feline respiratory diseases. *In* Greene CE, ed.: *Infectious Diseases of the Dog and Cat.* Philadelphia: W. B. Saunders, 1990, p 346.

Scott FW: Feline respiratory viral infections. *In* Scott FW, ed.: *Infectious Diseases.* New York: Churchill Livingstone, 1986, p 155.

5 Canine Infectious Tracheobronchitis (Kennel Cough Complex)

Robert G. Sherding

Kennel cough complex (KCC) refers to a collection of highly contagious infectious diseases of the canine respiratory tract that cause tracheobronchitis and acute onset of a paroxysmal hacking cough lasting several days to a few weeks.

ETIOLOGY

Incriminated Etiologic Agents

- *Bordetella bronchiseptica*
- Canine parainfluenza virus (CPIV)
- Canine adenovirus, types 1 and 2 (CAV-1, CAV-2)
- Canine herpesvirus
- Canine reoviruses, types 1, 2, and 3
- Mycoplasmas and ureaplasmas

Transmission

KEY POINT ▶ Kennel cough is highly contagious via aerosol spread (cough, sneezing); therefore, it is common wherever dogs are housed or confined together (e.g., boarding kennels, animal shelters, pet shops, veterinary hospitals, and research facilities).

- These agents can also be transmitted by fomites (e.g., personnel, cages, food and water bowls).
- Incubation period is usually 5 to 7 days (range of 3–10 days).

Pathogenesis

- Mixed infections are common and have a synergistic effect in producing clinical disease. Individually, these infectious agents cause very mild disease or are harbored in the airways of asymptomatic carriers. The most frequent isolates in KCC are parainfluenza virus and *Bordetella bronchiseptica*.
- The primary target of these agents is the upper airway epithelium. The result is epithelial injury, acute inflammation, and dysfunction of the airway cilia.

KEY POINT ▶ In puppies and immunocompromised animals, secondary bacterial invasion of the lower respiratory tract may cause life-threatening pneumonia.

CLINICAL SIGNS

Mild Form

- The mild form of KCC is the most common.
- There is an acute onset of a dry-sounding, hacking cough due to tracheobronchitis. (Note: even though the cough is often described as dry, KCC is characterized by production of increased mucus.)

KEY POINT ▶ Cough is often followed by gagging or retching motions that may be mistaken for vomiting or choking by the owner.

- Cough may be high-pitched because of laryngitis and swollen vocal folds.
- Cough may be more frequent during exercise, excitement, or changes in temperature and humidity of inspired air.
- Cough is easily elicited on tracheal palpation or by pulling on the collar.
- Mild, serous naso-ocular discharge is seen occasionally.
- Typically the dog continues to eat, remains active and alert, and is nonfebrile.
- Clinical course is usually 7 to 14 days.

Severe Form

- The severe form of KCC is less common and is usually the result of mixed infections in unvaccinated puppies, especially from pet shop and animal shelter environments. Complicating bacterial bronchopneumonia seems to be the determinant of severity.
- Productive cough may be present due to tracheobronchitis plus bronchopneumonia.
- Anorexia, depression, and fever may be present.
- Naso-ocular discharge may be present (serous or mucopurulent rhinitis and conjunctivitis).
- The severe form is difficult to distinguish from canine distemper and can sometimes be fatal.

DIAGNOSIS

KCC is usually diagnosed on circumstantial evidence of clinical signs and exposure history. Hemograms, radiographs, and airway cytologies are usually unremarkable or reveal nonspecific findings.

Hemogram

- Mild form: usually normal or stress response (mature neutrophilia, lymphopenia)
- Severe form: neutrophilic leukocytosis with left shift in some cases

Thoracic Radiography

- Mild form: usually normal; a mild increase in interstitial lung density occasionally seen
- Severe form: interstitial density and alveolar pattern (bronchopneumonia)

Airway Cytology

- Evaluation of airway cytology is optional in mild cases. Specimens can be obtained by transtracheal washing or bronchoscopy (see sec. 6, ch. 16).
- Findings include increased mucus, mucopurulent exudate, and sometimes bacteria.

Cultures

- Nasal swabs or transtracheal or bronchial washings can be cultured for *Bordetella* and mycoplasma; evaluate cytology also.

KEY POINT ▶ Nasal swabs for isolation of *Bordetella* are as effective as lower airway culture.

- Isolation of *Bordetella* or mycoplasma allows only presumptive diagnosis because many aysmptomatic dogs harbor these organisms in the respiratory tract.

Virology

- Virus isolation (impractical for clinical use)
- Serology (paired acute and convalescent titers)

TREATMENT

Because many of the principles of treatment for bronchitis and bacterial pneumonia can be applied to dogs with KCC, refer to sec. 6, chs. 20 and 21.

General Guidelines

- For mild form: because this form is typically self-limiting in 7 to 14 days, dogs with mild signs do not necessarily require specific therapy.
- For severe form: because lower respiratory tract involvement can be fatal, treat aggressively for bacterial bronchopneumonia (see sec. 6, ch. 21). Avoid antitussives.
- For cough that persists for more than 14 days: Consider etiologies other than KCC and evaluate further with thoracic radiographs, hemogram, airway cytology and culture, and other diagnostics as appropriate.
- Whenever possible, treat KCC on an outpatient basis to prevent transmission to other hospitalized animals.

Antibiotics

- *B. bronchiseptica* usually is susceptible to chloramphenicol, tetracyclines, gentamycin, kanamycin, and novobiocin. Mycoplasmas are usually susceptible to tetracyclines. However, susceptibility can vary; therefore, when possible use culture and sensitivity testing to guide antibiotic choices, especially in the severe form or chronic cases.

KEY POINT ▶ Nebulization of antibiotics may be more effective than systemic use against *Bordetella* because the bacteria attach to the cilia on the mucosal surface and are hard to reach with systemic antibiotics.

- Nebulize gentamycin (Gentocin; Schering), 50 mg diluted in 2–3 ml saline, by Devilbiss jet nebulizer for 10 minutes, every 12 hours for 3 to 5 days.

Bronchodilators

- Rationale: to reverse reflex bronchoconstriction triggered by airway irritation, thereby reducing discomfort and cough
- Examples: theophylline, aminophylline, oxtriphylline, ephedrine, terbutaline (see sec. 6, ch. 20 for dosages)

Antitussives

- Rationale: in diseases with a productive cough, it is usually recommended to avoid antitussives, but in mild KCC (no fever or evidence of bronchopneumonia), the cough can be such a nuisance and source of discomfort for owner and patient that antitussives may be required for relief.
- Examples include dextromethorphan, codeine, hydrocodone, and butorphanol (see sec. 6, ch. 20 for dosages).

Supportive Care

- Adequate fluid intake, airway humidification, and rest

PREVENTION

Polyvalent vaccines are routinely used for puppy and annual booster vaccination programs by most veterinarians. These usually incorporate adenovirus and parainfluenza virus. In areas where KCC is common and in dogs exposed frequently to other dogs, a *Bordetella* vaccine is also indicated.

In the Animal: Immunization

- Adenovirus (injectable)
  - Vaccines containing either CAV-1 or CAV-2 will cross-protect for both.
- Parainfluenza Virus
  - Injectable—protects against disease but not infection (therefore, this may not curtail spread from carriers to susceptible dogs in a kennel outbreak).
  - Intranasal—protects against disease and infection.

- *Bordetella*
  - Injectable (bacterin)
  - Intranasal (live avirulent *Bordetella*)—more consistent protection than injectable (probably stimulates local IgA)

In the Kennel

- Isolate infected (coughing) animals.
- Use caretaker hygiene to prevent fomite spread.
- Ensure proper kennel ventilation (at least 12 air changes per hour; 15 to 20 is best).
- Use disinfectants such as sodium hypochlorite (Clorox), chlorhexidine (Nolvasan), and benzalkonium-Cl (Roccal-D).

Supplemental Readings

Appel MJG: Canine infectious tracheobronchitis (kennel cough): A status report. Compend Contin Educ Pract Vet 3:70, 1981.

Bemis DA, Appel MJG: Aerosol, parenteral, and oral antibiotic treatment of *Bordetella bronchiseptica* infections in dogs. J Am Vet Med Assoc 170:1082, 1977.

Dhein CR, Gorham JR: Canine respiratory infections. *In:* Scott FW, ed.: *Contemporary Issues in Small Animal Practice. Infectious Diseases.* New York: Churchill Livingstone, 1986, p 177.

Ford RB, Vaden SL: Canine infectious tracheobronchitis. *In:* Greene CE, ed.: *Infectious Diseases of the Dog and Cat.* Philadelphia: W. B. Saunders, 1990, p 259.

Roudebush P, Fales W: Antibacterial susceptibility of *Bordetella bronchiseptica* isolates from small companion animals with respiratory disease. J Am Anim Hosp Assoc 17:793, 1981.

6 Canine Distemper

Robert G. Sherding

Canine distemper is a severe, highly contagious multisystemic viral disease of dogs and other carnivores, seen worldwide.

ETIOLOGY

Canine distemper virus (CDV) is a morbillivirus of the family Paramyxoviridae. It is closely related to measles virus.

Epidemiology

- Distribution: Enzootic worldwide
- Incidence: All ages affected; however, incidence highest in unvaccinated puppies after loss of maternal immunity (6 to 12 weeks of age)
- Host range: Domestic dogs and many wild carnivores, including
  - Canidae family—fox, dingoe, coyote, wolf, jackal
  - Mustalidae family—ferret, mink, weasel, marten, skunk, badger, otter
  - Procyonidae family—raccoon, panda, kinkajou, coati
  - Possibly exotic Felidae, but not domestic cats

Transmission

- Infected animals shed virus in all body secretions and excretions.
- The primary source of exposure is aerosol.
- The greatest opportunity for spread occurs where dogs are kept in groups (e.g., pet shops, kennels, animal shelters, research colonies).
- Transplacental transmission is a rare source of distemper in young pups.
- Viral shedding usually ceases 1 to 2 weeks after recovery; therefore, "carrier state" transmission is not a big problem.
- The virus is labile in the environment, usually surviving only a few hours and no more than a few days outside of the host. It is readily destroyed by drying and by most disinfectants.

Pathogenesis

- Chronologic stages of infection
  - Airborne exposure leads to infection of tonsils and bronchial lymph nodes.
  - Systemic lymphoid tissues are infected next (day 2–5).
  - Viremia (day 6–9): a transient fever spike occurs, the first of two.
  - There is dissemination to epithelial tissues (epithe-liotropism) and the central nervous system (CNS); outcome varies depending on the host's immune response.
- If the immune response is rapid and effective, complete recovery and elimination of the virus (by day 14) occur with absent or mild clinical signs (i.e., subclinical infection in 50%).
- If the immune response fails to develop, the outcome is rapid, widespread dissemination of the virus to the epithelial tissues such as the respiratory and gastrointestinal tracts and to the CNS (acute encephalomyelitis), resulting in multisystemic signs (2–3 week postexposure), a second fever spike, and high mortality rate.
- If the immune response is sluggish or weak, multisystemic signs are prevented, but CNS localization can result in chronic encephalomyelitis with delayed onset of neurologic signs.
- Role of immunosuppression: CDV causes marked suppression of B- and T-cell–mediated immunity, lymphoid depletion, peripheral lymphopenia, and thymic atrophy.

KEY POINT ▶ Many of the clinical signs of distemper are attributable to secondary bacterial infections that are caused by the immunosuppressive effects of the virus.

CLINICAL SIGNS

Clinical signs are multisystemic and extremely variable. The mortality rate can vary from 0 to 100% depending on the virulence of the CDV strain and the age and resistance of the host.

General (Systemic)

- Malaise: anorexia, depression
- Fever of 103° to 105°F (39.5° to 41°C): diphasic (signs usually coincide with the second fever spike)

Respiratory System

- Rhinitis and conjunctivitis—serous to mucopurulent naso-ocular discharge
- Pneumonia
  - Initially—interstitial pneumonia (primary viral effect)
  - Later—bronchopneumonia (secondary bacterial infection)
  - Signs—cough, dyspnea, auscultable crackles

Gastrointestinal System

- Vomiting and diarrhea

Eye

- Keratoconjunctivitis (serous to mucopurulent ocular discharge)
- Chorioretinitis (ophthalmoscopic lesions)
- Optic neuritis (blindness)

Nervous System

KEY POINT ▶ Any region of the CNS can be affected by CDV. Diffuse or multifocal CNS involvement is typical. CNS signs can occur during, after, or in the absence of multisystemic signs.

Acute encephalomyelitis predominantly destroys gray matter (neurons), whereas subacute or chronic nonsuppurative encephalomyelitis predominantly affects white matter (demyelination). CNS signs can occur simultaneously with other multisystemic signs or can be delayed in onset until after apparent recovery. In some dogs, CNS involvement can occur as the only apparent manifestation of infection. (For additional details concerning the neurologic manifestations of CDV, see sec. 10, ch. 2.)

- Acute encephalitis: generalized seizures, so-called chewing-gum seizures, pacing, circling, behavior changes
- Midbrain, cerebellar, and vestibular: ataxia and other disturbances of gait
- Spinal cord: disturbances of gait, abnormal spinal reflexes, paresis, and abnormal proprioception
- Peripheral and cranial neuropathies (including optic neuritis)
- Myoclonus: rhythmic, repetitive, motor movements or muscle twitches

Miscellaneous

- Dental enamel hypoplasia (pitted teeth from infection prior to eruption of the permanent teeth)
- Hyperkeratosis of foot pads (hard pad disease)
- Abdominal pustules

DIAGNOSIS

KEY POINT ▶ The diagnosis of distemper is usually based on typical clinical signs in a young dog (2 to 6 months) that has a history of inadequate vaccinations and possibility of exposure to the virus.

In suspected cases of distemper, a complete blood count to assess leukocyte responses and thoracic radiographs to assess pneumonia are useful. In dogs presenting with neurologic disease suspected to be due to CDV, routine cerebrospinal fluid (CSF) analysis helps to distinguish CDV infection from other diseases. The presence of CDV-specific antibody in CSF can confirm the diagnosis but requires a special laboratory. Virology techniques can help to substantiate a diagnosis of distemper; however, this is usually not practical or necessary in most clinical situations, and false-negative results are common.

Hematology

- Lymphopenia
- Early leukopenia (associated with the initial temperature rise); later, neutrophilic leukocytosis

Thoracic Radiography

- Interstitial or alveolar pneumonia

CSF Analysis

- Elevated CSF protein and cell count (mostly lymphocytes) (see sec. 10, ch. 1)
- Presence of CDV-specific antibody: diagnostic of CDV but not present in all cases

Virology

- Detection of intracytoplasmic viral inclusion bodies in peripheral blood cells (lymphocytes), epithelial cells (cytology specimens), or biopsies
- Demonstration of viral antigen by immunofluorescence in cells from blood, CSF, cytology specimens, or frozen tissue specimens
- Virus isolation (difficult and expensive; best done on postmortem tissues)
- Negative test results do not rule out CDV.

Serology

- A single positive immunoglobulin G (IgG) titer is worthless because it does not distinguish current infection from past vaccination or exposure.
- The demonstration of a rising serum neutralizing antibody titer or a CDV-specific IgM titer is suggestive but not diagnostic of recent CDV infection.

TREATMENT

There is no effective antiviral treatment for CDV; therefore, treatment is symptomatic. Whenever possible, treat distemper on an outpatient basis to prevent aerosol exposure of other hospitalized animals.

Symptomatic Treatment

- Broad-spectrum antibiotics for secondary bacterial infection, especially pneumonia (see sec. 6, ch. 21)
- Humidification of airways
- For pneumonia: expectorants, bronchodilators (see sec. 6, ch. 20)
- For vomiting and diarrhea: antiemetics (see sec. 7, ch. 4) and antidiarrheals (see sec. 7, ch. 6)
- For seizures: anticonvulsants such as phenobarbital (see sec. 10, ch. 3)
- Good nursing care is important: eyes and nose kept clear of discharges; nutritional support; adequate fluid intake or fluid therapy

Intravenous Modified Live CDV Vaccine

■ This has no effect once clinical signs have started.
■ If given to an animal within 4 days of exposure (prior to signs), there is evidence that this may reduce the severity of the disease; however, vaccines that contain other agents (e.g., *Leptospira* or adenovirus) should not be given by the IV route.

Prognosis: Guarded

■ Mortality rate varies but is highest in young puppies and when there is severe fulminant multisystemic disease or progressive neurologic disease.
■ It is justified to recommend euthanasia for patients with progressive neurologic signs that are severe and incapacitating.

KEY POINT ▶ Do not be too optimistic with the owner, even with mild cases of distemper. The disease is often progressive in spite of therapy; some animals will seem to recover, and then the symptoms will exacerbate or incapacitating neurologic disease will develop.

Client Education

■ Discuss the multiplicity of signs that the owner may observe.
■ Advise owners to isolate their animal from others to prevent contagion.
■ Educate client as to proper immunization procedures for future reference.
■ Recommend at least a 1-week waiting period before bringing another dog onto the premises.

PREVENTION

Passive Maternal Antibody (Ab)

■ The neonatal pup acquires passive immunity against CDV from its dam; most of this maternal-derived Ab comes from colostrum absorbed during nursing in the first few hours after birth.
■ Maternal Ab will gradually disappear, but it protects most pups until after weaning. Maternal Ab in the pup generally falls below protective levels sometime between 8 and 14 weeks of age.
■ While present, maternal Ab also interferes with the response to vaccination; therefore, a series of vac-cinations are given at 3- to 4-week intervals between 6 and 16 weeks of age.

Vaccination

■ Modified live CDV vaccine is nearly 100% protective.
■ Measles virus vaccine is not as protective as CDV vaccine, but it partially protects pups in the face of interfering maternal Ab so long as the level of Ab is not too high.

KEY POINT ▶ For puppies 6 to 10 weeks of age, when a combined distemper-measles vaccine is given, the measles fraction can overcome maternal antibody interference if present and induce partial protection; however, if maternal Ab is no longer present, the distemper fraction can induce complete protection.

■ Recommendations
  • For puppies that received colostrum: vaccinate initially at 6 to 8 weeks of age and repeat every 3 to 4 weeks until 14 to 16 weeks of age. For the first vaccination in this series, consider using a combined distemper-measles vaccine.
  • For colostrum-deprived puppies: vaccinate initially at 4 weeks of age and give a second dose 2 to 4 weeks later. Do not use modified live virus (MLV) distemper vaccine in pups less than 3 to 4 weeks of age.
  • For dogs over 16 weeks of age: vaccinate twice, 2 to 4 weeks apart.
  • Postvaccinal encephalitis has occurred occasionally after MLV distemper vaccination, primarily when used simultaneously with MLV parvovirus vaccine in pups less than 6 to 8 weeks of age.

KEY POINT ▶ Immunity from distemper vaccination is solid and prolonged, but not necessarily lifelong. Annual vaccination boosters are recommended.

Supplemental Readings

Appel MJG: Canine distemper. *In* Barlough JE, ed.: *Manual of Small Animal Infectious Diseases.* New York: Churchill Livingstone, 1988, p 49.

Dhein CR, Gorham JR: Canine respiratory infections. *In* Scott FW, ed.: *Infectious Diseases.* New York: Churchill Livingstone, 1986, p. 177.

Greene CE, Appel MJ: Canine distemper. *In* Greene CE, ed.: *Infectious Diseases of the Dog and Cat.* Philadelphia: W. B. Saunders, 1990, p. 226.

7 Intestinal Viruses

Robert G. Sherding

Parvoviruses, coronaviruses, rotaviruses, and possibly astroviruses have been established as causes of viral enteritis and diarrhea in dogs and cats and are discussed in this chapter. In addition to these, numerous other viruses of uncertain enteropathogenicity have been discovered in canine and feline feces by virus isolation or electron microscopy. Examples in dogs are astrovirus, herpesvirus, enteroviruses, calicivirus, parainfluenza viruses, adenovirus, and picornavirus; viruses isolated in cats include astrovirus, calicivirus, picornalike virus, reovirus, and toga-like virus. In addition, the intestine may be involved as part of generalized viral infections in disorders such as canine distemper (see sec. 2, ch. 6), feline leukemia virus (see sec. 2, ch. 1), feline immunodeficiency virus (see sec. 2, ch. 2), and feline infectious peritonitis (see sec. 2, ch. 3).

CANINE PARVOVIRUS

Etiology

Canine parvovirus type 2 (CPV-2) is an acute, highly contagious enteritis of dogs that has been prevalent worldwide since the late 1970's.

KEY POINT ▶ CPV has an affinity for the rapidly dividing cells of the intestine, bone marrow, and lymphoid tissues and thus causes intestinal crypt necrosis, severe diarrhea, leukopenia, and lymphoid depletion.

Transmission

CPV infection occurs by the feco-oral route. During acute illness, and for about 1 to 2 weeks thereafter, massive amounts of parvovirus (over one billion virions per gram of feces) are shed in feces of infected dogs. Because the virus can survive and remain infectious for many months in the environment, fomites and environmental contamination play a major role in transmission.

Incubation

Signs of enteric disease usually occur 5 days after exposure, coincident with localization of virus in the mitotically active zones of intestinal crypt epithelia.

Age Incidence

Dogs of any age can be infected, but the incidence of clinical disease is almost entirely in puppies between weaning and 6 months of age. Puppies younger than 6 weeks are generally protected by passive maternal immunity, whereas most mature animals have been immunized or have seroconverted from subclinical infection.

Breed Incidence

Certain breeds appear to be at higher risk for parvovirus infection and susceptible to a more severe form of the disease. These include rottweilers, Doberman pinschers, and possibly pit bull terriers and black Labrador retrievers. The biologic basis for these breed susceptibilities is unknown.

Clinical Signs

- Parvovirus causes anorexia, depression, fever, vomiting, intractable fluid diarrhea (can be profuse and hemorrhagic), and rapidly progressive dehydration.
- Hypothermia, icterus, or hemorrhagic diathesis (disseminated intravascular coagulation) may develop terminally in those with bacterial sepsis or endotoxemia.
- Death may occur in severe cases, particularly in very young puppies and in the highly susceptible breeds, and is usually attributable to dehydration, electrolyte imbalances, endotoxic shock, or overwhelming bacterial sepsis related to leukopenia.
- The severity of clinical illness may be increased by factors such as stress, overcrowded or unsanitary kennel conditions, secondary bacterial infection, and concurrent diseases such as canine distemper, coronavirus, salmonellosis, campylobacteriosis, and intestinal parasitism.
- In nonimmunized mature dogs, mild or inapparent infections that result in seroconversion without clinical signs are probably common.
- In utero or postnatal infection can cause acute neonatal myocarditis. Since most dams are now immune and passively transfer immunity to their puppies, this form of perinatal parvoviral infection is practically nonexistent. Signs of parvoviral myocarditis include dyspnea due to acute heart failure, sudden death due to arrhythmias, and sometimes delayed-onset chronic congestive heart failure due to chronic myocardial fibrosis.

Diagnosis

Suspect parvovirus infection in young dogs that have an abrupt onset of vomiting and diarrhea, especially if associated with severe depression, fever, or leukopenia, or if these signs follow potential exposure to infected dogs or fomites.

KEY POINT ▶ Because of the difficulty in breaking through maternal antibody interference with vaccination in young puppies, prior vaccination does not necessarily exclude parvoviral infection, especially in puppies 6 to 20 weeks of age.

Hematology

- A complete blood count (CBC) is particularly useful because most dogs with parvoviral enteritis develop severe leukopenia due to lymphopenia and granulocytopenia, often with a total of only 500 to 2000 white blood cells/μl, and occasionally even less. Depletion of circulating mature neutrophils is caused by extensive loss of neutrophils through the damaged intestinal mucosa coupled with impaired myelopoiesis caused by bone marrow disruption from the virus. The severity of the leukopenia is generally proportional to the severity of the clinical illness, and a rebound neutrophilia is a useful indicator of impending recovery.
- The hematocrit is variable. The PCV is often normal but can be moderately decreased in some dogs because of intestinal hemorrhage (especially noticeable following rehydration), whereas in other dogs PCV can be elevated because of dehydration (hemoconcentration).

Serum Chemistries

Abnormal serum chemistries are variable and nonspecific, such as electrolyte imbalances (most frequently hypokalemia), prerenal azotemia, and increased bilirubin and liver enzymes (ALT and ALP).

Abdominal Radiography

Gas and fluid distension of the gastrointestinal tract due to ileus are frequent radiographic findings in parvoviral enteritis and must be differentiated from small intestinal obstruction (e.g., foreign body or intussusception). Carefully palpate the abdomen to help rule out mechanical obstruction. Barium contrast radiography often reveals mucosal irregularity (corrugation or scalloping) and prolonged transit time.

Serology

- Determination of an anti-CPV antibody in serum is not sufficient for diagnosis because up to 95% of dogs in the population have seroconverted from prior vaccination or exposure.
- Specific IgM analysis by indirect fluorescent antibody (IFA) test or a 2-mercaptoethanol procedure provides serologic evidence of recent infection, as IgM is found only in the first few weeks after infection.

Virology

KEY POINT ▶ Definitive diagnosis of parvoviral enteritis requires demonstration of active excretion of virus or viral antigen in the feces, because massive quantities of virus are shed during the acute illness.

- The most practical method for detecting parvovirus in the feces is the in-office membrane filter enzyme-linked immunosorbent assay (ELISA) (CITE-Parvo Test; IDEXX). Positive results are a reliable indicator of active fecal excretion of CPV-2. Occasionally false-negative results occur.
- Other methods for detecting fecal excretion of parvovirus, such as hemagglutination, latex agglutination, electron microscopy, and virus isolation, are less practical for routine clinical use because they require an outside diagnostic laboratory.

Necropsy

Necropsy diagnosis of parvovirus is based on identification of the characteristic intestinal lesions: necrosis of the rapidly proliferating intestinal crypt cells with secondary villous collapse and dilatation of the crypts with necrotic debris. Myeloid degeneration and widespread lymphoid depletion are also seen. Parvovirus can be demonstrated in frozen tissue samples by fluorescent antibody methods.

Treatment

Because the treatment of parvovirus is mainly supportive and similar to what would be used in most animals with severe gastroenteritis, institute therapy whether or not definitive tests are done or while awaiting the return of results.

Fluid Therapy

KEY POINT ▶ The cornerstone of treatment of CPV infection is rehydration and correction of electrolyte imbalances.

See sec. 1, ch. 5 for specific guidelines and procedures for fluid and electrolyte therapy. Continue fluid therapy until vomiting ceases and oral intake resumes.

- In severe cases, intravenous fluid and electrolyte replacement is preferred (e.g., lactated Ringer's supplemented with potassium).
- Dextrose may also be added to IV fluids at a 2.5% solution to control complicating hypoglycemia of sepsis.
- Avoid administration of fluids by the subcutaneous route in dogs with severe leukopenia, because there is a high incidence of secondary infection, cellulitis, and skin necrosis at administration sites.

Antibiotics

Antibiotics are indicated to control potentially life-threatening bacterial sepsis. Initially, administer antibiotics parenterally (such as cephalothin or ampicillin combined with gentamycin or amikacin), especially in dogs that are severely leukopenic or vomiting.

Dietary Restriction

Give nothing per os (fluid needs are met by IV infusion) until vomiting has ceased for at least 24 hours and diarrhea has subsided and is free of gross hemorrhage. This can take 3 to 5 days in severe cases. When feeding is resumed, give small frequent feedings of a bland digestible diet, such as Prescription Diet i/d (Hill's Pet Foods) or cooked skinless chicken and rice, until gastrointestinal function appears to have recovered. The transition back to regular feeding should be gradual.

Antiemetics

For frequent or persistent vomiting associated with delayed gastric emptying that sometimes occurs in parvoviral infection, administer metoclopramide (Reglan; A.H. Robins) at 0.5 mg/kg, every 8 hours, SC, or most effectively as a continuous infusion of 1–2 mg/kg every 24 hours diluted in IV fluids. For gastritis, control of gastric acid secretion with an H_2 receptor blocker (see sec. 7, ch. 4 for products and dosages) is often helpful as well. If these are unsuccessful in controlling vomiting, consider using a broad-spectrum phenothiazine antiemetic (see sec. 7, ch. 4), but not until dehydration has been corrected, because phenothiazines have a hypotensive effect.

Antidiarrheals

Parvoviral diarrhea is usually self-limiting and treatment to control diarrhea is not usually needed as long as fluid needs are met; however, when diarrhea is profuse and persistent, administer oral bismuth subsalicylate or loperamide (see sec. 7, ch. 6).

Infusion of Whole Blood or Plasma

Occasionally infusion of blood or plasma is necessary for treatment of severe blood loss anemia or hypoproteinemia.

Immunotherapy

Despite lack of availability and limited clinical experience with their use, there is some preliminary evidence of therapeutic benefit from treatment with high-titered anti-parvovirus serum or antiendotoxin hyperimmune plasma.

Prognosis and Complications

KEY POINT ▶ Most dogs with CPV enteritis recover if treated appropriately to control dehydration and sepsis.

Once an animal survives the first 3 to 4 days of illness, recovery usually occurs rapidly.

- Some animals, however, succumb to bacterial sepsis and endotoxemia resulting from the leukopenia, immunosuppression, and breakdown of the intestinal mucosal barrier caused by CPV. In general, the younger the animal, the higher the mortality rate.
- Other complications may include hypoglycemia (probably secondary to sepsis), hypoproteinemia, anemia, intussusception, liver disease, central nervous system signs (likely due to concomitant canine distemper), and numerous secondary bacterial infections, such as endocarditis, thrombophlebitis, pneumonia (caused by aspiration in some dogs), urinary tract infection, injection site abscesses, and intestinal salmonellosis and campylobacteriosis.

Prevention: Reducing Exposure

- Dogs with CPV infection shed massive amounts of virus in the feces during their illness. These, as well as the fomites and premises they contaminate, are highly infectious for other dogs. Thus, instruct the owner of a CPV-infected dog to keep the dog isolated from other dogs until at least 1 week after full recovery.

KEY POINT ▶ Elimination of CPV from infected premises is difficult because the virus is so resistant; however, disinfection with a 1:32 dilution of sodium hypochlorite bleach is effective.

- CPV is ubiquitous, and because it is so stable outside of the animal and easily transmitted by fomites, prevention of exposure is almost impossible. Nevertheless, until vaccinations are complete, keep young puppies isolated as much as possible from other animals and from potentially infected premises.

Prevention: Vaccination

Vaccination is the only realistic and effective means of prevention and control of this disease.

Maternal Antibody Interference

Although widespread vaccination against parvovirus has markedly reduced the incidence of the disease in North America, parvoviral enteritis continues to be a problem in puppies as they are nearing the end of their maternal antibody protection between 6 and 20 weeks of age. This is so despite vaccination because of a period of susceptibility when maternal antibodies are too low to protect but at the same time high enough to interfere with the response to vaccination.

KEY POINT ▶ In puppies from dams with high CPV titers, maternally derived antibody can persist at interfering levels for up to 18 weeks; thus, vaccination may not be able to break through this maternal antibody interference until as late as 18 weeks of age.

- In the first weeks of life, maternal antibody protects the puppy from infection, but at the same time it also interferes with active immunization.
- As the level of this maternal antibody gradually declines, there is a period of 2 to 4 weeks in which all puppies are refractory to vaccination but susceptible to infection if exposed.
- Almost all apparent "vaccination failures" in puppies probably result from exposure to infection during this critical period of susceptibility.
- Because the age at which pups can respond to vaccination for CPV is unpredictable, the most effective protocols use a series of vaccinations.

Recommendations for Routine Vaccination

- Advantages of attenuated, or modified live virus (MLV), CPV-2 vaccines over inactivated (killed) vaccines:
  - Better magnitude of protection
  - More rapid onset of protection (as early as 1–3 days)
  - Longer duration of protection ($\geq$20 months)
  - Better able to break through maternal antibody interference
  - Prevention of shedding of virulent CPV if exposed (killed vaccines protect only against clinical disease but do not prevent subclinical infection or shedding)

KEY POINT ▶ Commercially available CPV-2 vaccines effectively cross-protect against all known field strains of CPV, including the newer, so-called variant strains.

- In puppies, begin vaccination series at 6 to 8 weeks of age and vaccinate every 3 to 4 weeks until at least 16 and preferably 18 weeks of age. Do not space vaccinations less than 2 weeks apart, because interference from shorter intervals can impair vaccine efficacy.
- In unvaccinated dogs 16 weeks of age or older, give two doses of vaccine 2 to 4 weeks apart.
- Concurrent administration of MLV CPV and distemper vaccines is considered to be safe; however, some have recommended in puppies less than 9 weeks of age the use of measles instead of MLV distemper vaccine (see sec. 2, ch. 6) to prevent the rare occurrence of distemper vaccine–induced encephalitis.
- Revaccinate ("booster") animals annually; ideally, females should be revaccinated 2 weeks prior to breeding so that high maternal antibody titers are transferred to puppies.
- Use inactivated instead of MLV CPV vaccine in pregnant animals and in puppies less than 5 weeks of age (e.g., early vaccination in colostrum-deprived pups).

CANINE CORONAVIRUS

Etiology

Canine coronaviral enteritis is an acute contagious disease of dogs caused by an epitheliotropic virus that preferentially invades the enterocytes of the villous tips. The resulting villous destruction, atrophy, and fusion cause diarrhea of variable severity.

- The clinical importance of canine coronavirus (CCV) as a cause of enteritis is considered relatively minor.

KEY POINT ▶ Most CCV infections are subclinical, although occasional epizootics of severe enteritis have occurred, primarily associated with kennels and dog shows.

- CCV is shed subclinically for months postinfection from dogs and spreads rapidly by feco-oral transmission.

Clinical Signs

- Most dogs infected with CCV are asymptomatic, but some manifest an acute onset of anorexia and depression followed by vomiting and diarrhea. The character of the diarrhea varies from soft to watery and sometimes contains mucus and fresh red blood.
- Most dogs infected with CCV are afebrile. The signs are mild and easily confused with various other nonspecific causes of mild diarrhea of brief duration.

Diagnosis

Consider coronaviral enteritis in dogs with an acute onset of signs of gastroenteritis, especially if other dogs on the premises are affected. Since coronaviral enteritis is usually nonfatal and the only treatment is supportive, definitive laboratory confirmation is not needed for effective case management except to document an epizootic outbreak. Coronaviral enteritis should, however, be distinguished from the more severe multisystemic parvoviral infection.

KEY POINT ▶ In contrast to CPV infection, fever, leukopenia, hematochezia, and fatalities are not typical of coronaviral enteritis.

- Routine hematology, serum chemistries, and abdominal radiography are usually normal.
- Definitive diagnosis requires laboratory detection of CCV in feces by electron microscopy (EM) or by virus isolation during the acute illness. Fecal examination by EM requires fresh feces (specimens can be kept refrigerated but not frozen). Both false-positive and false-negative titers are a problem with EM because of misidentification of fecal particles. Virus isolation is not readily available to the clinician.

KEY POINT ▶ The mere identification of CCV in a dog's feces is not proof that it is the cause of diarrhea or illness, because CCV is shed in the feces of many healthy dogs.

- Serology can provide only a retrospective diagnosis via demonstration of a fourfold or greater rise in serum antibody titer in paired sera (at the time of illness and 2 to 6 weeks later).

Treatment

Coronaviral enteritis is treated like any other acute diarrhea with fluid therapy and symptomatic treatment such as dietary restriction (see sec. 7, ch. 6). Most dogs recover rapidly, although some have persistent diarrhea for 3 to 4 weeks. Fatalities have been reported, especially in neonates, but are considered rare.

Prevention

Vaccination for CCV is an optional part of the routine vaccination program for most dogs. Consider vaccinating dogs with a high risk of exposure, such as show and field trial dogs and kenneled (boarded) dogs.

- Killed (inactivated) CCV vaccine is commercially available; however, its efficacy (completeness and duration of immunity) and justification for use are controversial. In general, immunity to coronaviruses is brief and is mediated by local (IgA) immunity rather than the serum antibodies that would result from a parenteral vaccine. Parenteral vaccination does not prevent CCV infection, but it may reduce intestinal replication of virus and minimize clinical signs.

■ An attenuated (MLV) vaccine for CCV was briefly marketed but was withdrawn because of serious and sometimes fatal adverse reactions.

CANINE ROTAVIRUS

Etiology

Rotaviruses have been recognized as one of the most important causes of neonatal diarrhea in man and many other species of mammals and birds, but canine isolates appear to be rarely involved in causing diarrhea or clinical illness in dogs.

KEY POINT ▶ Rotavirus has not been shown to be an enteropathogen of major clinical importance in the dog.

■ The high incidence of antirotavirus antibodies in surveys of normal dogs (as high as 79%) indicates that most dogs experience rotavirus infection without showing signs.
■ Transmission is by the feco-oral route.
■ Rotaviruses replicate exclusively in the mature enterocytes of the villous tip, causing blunted villi that are populated mainly with immature secretory cells from the crypts.

Clinical Signs

In adult dogs, rotaviral infection is usually subclinical, but clinical signs of acute enteritis are occasionally seen in young puppies.

■ The diarrhea, which may be watery to mucoid, is usually self-limiting and of brief duration, although rare fatalities attributable to dehydration have been reported.
■ Experimental inoculation of neonatal (2 days old) gnotobiotic puppies with canine rotavirus results in diarrhea and mild to moderate villous atrophy; however, deprivation of colostrum predisposes to much more severe diarrhea.
■ It has been almost impossible to produce signs of rotavirus infection experimentally in dogs over 6 months of age.

Diagnosis

Active rotavirus infection can be established by detection of virus in feces by a commercial enzyme-linked immunosorbent assay (ELISA) (Rotazyme; Abbott Laboratories), electron microscopy, or virus isolation.

Treatment

Rotaviral enteritis is treated like other types of acute dirarrhea (see sec. 7, ch. 6), with emphasis on supportive measures such as fluid therapy and dietary restriction. Most animals recover uneventfully with minimal treatment.

Prevention

There is currently no vaccine available for canine rotavirus. In neonates, the only group significantly threatened by rotavirus infection, the best protection is to ensure nursing of colostral antibodies in the first hours after birth.

FELINE PANLEUKOPENIA VIRUS

Etiology

Feline panleukopenia virus (FPV) is a severe, highly contagious parvoviral infection of cats. Panleukopenia is relatively rare now because of effective control with vaccinations. Occasional infections are seen in unvaccinated kittens, especially those from shelters, farms, and urban stray populations.

■ FPV can infect all species of Felidae as well as raccoon, coatimundi, and mink.
■ FPV is shed in all body excretions for up to 6 weeks, especially feces.
■ FPV is very resistant to inactivation but can be inactivated with a 1:32 dilution of sodium hypochlorite bleach.
■ FPV is ubiquitous in the environment, where it can readily survive for more than 1 year and can be transmitted by oropharyngeal contact with contaminated fomites.
■ FPV has a predilection for rapidly dividing cells, particularly the following:
  • Intestinal crypt epithelium, resulting in acute enteritis
  • Hemopoietic tissue, resulting in panleukopenia
  • Lymphoid tissues, resulting in lymphoid depletion
  • In utero fetus, resulting in fetal death or cerebellar hypoplasia

Clinical Signs

Subclinical Infection of Adult Cats

Infection in susceptible adult cats is usually subclinical. The generalized form can rarely occur.

Generalized Infection of Kittens

The incidence and mortality rate are highest in young kittens. Clinical features are similar to those of canine parvoviral enteritis: anorexia, depression, high fever 104°–106°F (40° to 41°C), persistent vomiting, diarrhea, and progressive dehydration. Vomitus is usually a bile-stained fluid, and feces may be watery, mucoid, or bloody. Intestinal loops may be palpably thickened and firm (rope-like), fluid-filled, and painful. There is increased susceptibility to bacterial sepsis and endotoxemia.

Perinatal Infection of Neonates

In utero infection of the fetus at the end of gestation or of the neonate in the first 2 weeks after birth may permanently damage the central nervous system and cause cerebellar hypoplasia. Affected kittens show nonprogressive signs of ataxia, hypermetria, falling to the side, broad-based stance, and intention tremors (see sec. 10, chs. 1 and 2). At the same time, FPV may also invade the thymus of neonates, causing thymic atrophy and early neonatal mortality (fading kitten syndrome), and it may invade the retina, causing retinal dysplasia.

In Utero Infection of the Fetus

The only manifestation of infection in the pregnant cat may be transplacental infection of the developing embryo or fetus, leading to early embryonic resorption (infertility), fetal death, fetal mummification, abortion, and stillbirth.

Diagnosis

Feline panleukopenia is usually diagnosed presumptively on the basis of clinical signs of acute gastroenteritis in a young, susceptible (unvaccinated) cat with systemic involvement and profound panleukopenia.

KEY POINT ▶ Profound leukopenia (total white blood count often <500/µl) is a consistent feature of feline panleukopenia and usually lasts 2 to 4 days before rebounding as recovery occurs. The degree of leukopenia is proportional to the severity of clinical illness.

- Serum chemistry abnormalities are nonspecific and occur inconsistently, but can include electrolyte imbalances (especially hypokalemia), prerenal azotemia, and increased bilirubin and liver enzymes.
- If leukopenia persists for more than 5 days or is accompanied by severe nonregenerative anemia, consider the panleukopenia-like syndrome that is associated with feline leukemia virus infection (see sec. 2, ch. 1). Other panleukopenia "look-alike" diseases include acute salmonellosis, acute bacterial sepsis with endotoxemia, and gastrointestinal foreign body with perforation and peritonitis (e.g., linear foreign body).
- Serologic diagnosis (paired neutralizing antibody titers) and virus isolation have been used in research but are rarely applicable to clinical practice.
- Necropsy diagnosis is based on lesions of severe necrosis of intestinal crypts.

Treatment

- The treatment for feline panleukopenia is similar to that for canine parvoviral enteritis, mainly nonspecific supportive treatment such as rehydration, parenteral antibiotics, antiemetics, good nursing care, and restriction of dietary intake. Correction of severe dehydration is most important, and the parenteral route is best (see sec. 1, ch. 5).
- In young kittens with panleukopenia, the mortality rate is high (50–90%). A guarded prognosis is justified until impending recovery is indicated by cessation of vomiting and diarrhea, return of appetite to normal, return of body temperature to normal,

and rebound leukocytosis. On the other hand, complications such as hypothermia and shock (endotoxemia), jaundice, secondary bacterial or mycotic infection, and disseminated intravascular coagulation, usually indicate a fatal outcome.

Prevention

KEY POINT ▶ Vaccination is highly effective for prevention of feline panleukopenia.

- Both attenuated (MLV) and inactivated (killed) vaccines are effective, but MLV vaccination elicits a more rapid onset of protection. This can be an important consideration in high-risk environments such as shelters where cats are housed in groups.
- In kittens, vaccination can usually overcome maternal antibody interference by about 12 weeks of age.
- For routine vaccination: vaccinate at 8 to 9 weeks of age, then repeat every 2 to 4 weeks until 12 to 14 weeks of age (for a total of at least two doses for MLV and at least 3 for killed vaccines); then booster annually.

KEY POINT ▶ Use only inactivated panleukopenia vaccine in pregnant cats and in kittens under 4 weeks of age. MLV vaccine given perinatally can infect the unborn fetus or the neonatal cerebellum.

FELINE ENTERIC CORONAVIRUS

Etiology

Feline enteric coronavirus (FECV), a virus antigenically related to but distinct from the coronavirus that causes feline infectious peritonitis (FIP), appears to be ubiquitous in the cat population. Like enteric coronaviruses of other species, FECV invades the epithelium of the villous tip, resulting in villous atrophy.

KEY POINT ▶ FECV is shed in the feces of many normal cats, and a high percentage of cats are seropositive, indicating that inapparent infection is extremely prevalent.

Clinical Signs

- In young kittens, especially those 4 to 12 weeks of age, FECV can cause an acute but mild enteritis with diarrhea. Feces are soft to fluid and sometimes contain excess mucus and fresh red blood.
- Diarrhea may be accompanied by vomiting, low-grade fever, anorexia, and lethargy.
- Clinical signs are usually mild and self-limiting within 2 to 4 days. Fatalities are rare but have been reported.

Diagnosis

Serology can identify a convalescent rise in coronaviral antibody titer. This is more important because of the confusion it causes in interpretation of tests for FIP (see sec. 2, ch. 3) than as a diagnostic aid for enteric disease. Research facilities can use electron microscopy to identify coronaviral particles in fresh feces (specimens can be refrigerated but not frozen), but misidentification causes false-positive and false-negative results.

Treatment

Coronaviral enteritis is treated like any other acute dirarrhea (see sec. 7, ch. 6), with emphasis on supportive measures such as fluid therapy and dietary restriction. Most animals recover uneventfully.

Prevention

This virus appears to be practically ubiquitous and spreads very efficiently through catteries; thus, prevention may not be practical. Although vaccination specifically for enteric coronavirus is not available, an intranasal vaccine for the strains of coronavirus that produce FIP is now in use that probably cross-protects for the enteritis-producing strains (see sec. 2, ch. 3).

FELINE ROTAVIRUS

Etiology

As in the canine, rotavirus has been isolated from both normal and diarrheic feces of cats, especially kittens, but its enteropathogenic significance currently is unclear. Infection is restricted to the gastrointestinal mucosa. Subclinical infection in mature animals is probably frequent, as indicated by surveys that found antibodies to rotavirus in 26 of 94 clinically healthy British cats and 23 of 50 cats in Louisiana.

Clinical Signs

Subclinical infection is probably the rule; the exceptions are neonates and occasional cats that develop mild, nonspecific diarrhea of brief (1–2 days) duration.

Diagnosis

As in dogs, feline rotavirus can be detected in feces by EM or ELISA (Rotazyme).

Treatment

Rotaviral enteritis is treated like any other acute dirarrhea (see sec. 7, ch. 6), with emphasis on supportive measures such as fluid therapy and dietary restriction. Most animals recover uneventfully with minimal or no treatment.

Prevention

Vaccines are unavailable for rotavirus. Because natural immunity is short-lived, vaccination is unlikely to be warranted.

FELINE ASTROVIRUS

Etiology

Very little is known concerning this viral agent, but a few reports have identified astroviruses in the feces of cats with diarrhea, and mild diarrhea was reproduced experimentally in kittens. A survey of British cats determined a seroprevalence of less than 10%. Astrovirus infections in other species are limited to infection of the mature villous epithelial cells of the intestinal mucosa. Transmission is by the feco-oral route.

Clinical Signs

Feline astrovirus appears to cause mild, nonspecific diarrhea 4 to 14 days in duration. Transient low-grade fever, depression, and inappetance may also occur, but affected cats remain otherwise well. Astrovirus was implicated in a diarrhea outbreak in a cattery. As with other enteropathogenic viruses, kittens are most likely to be affected.

Diagnosis

Feline astrovirus is detected in feces by EM. Some cats shed the virus asymptomatically. Serum antibody to astrovirus has been identified in cats, but its significance is unknown.

Treatment

Diarrhea caused by astrovirus is treated like any other acute dirarrhea (see sec. 7, ch. 6), with emphasis on supportive measures such as fluid therapy and dietary restriction. Most animals recover uneventfully with minimal or no treatment.

Prevention

No preventive measures are available.

Supplemental Reading

Greene CE: Immunoprophylaxis and immunotherapy. *In* Greene CE, ed.: *Infectious Diseases of the Dog and Cat.* Philadelphia: W. B. Saunders, 1990, p 21.

Greene CE, Scott FW: Feline panleukopenia. *In* Greene CE, ed.: *Infectious Diseases of the Dog and Cat.* Philadelphia: W. B. Saunders, 1990, p 291.

Harbour DA, Greene CE: Feline astroviral and rotaviral infections. *In* Greene CE, ed.: *Infectious Diseases of the Dog and Cat.* Philadelphia: W. B. Saunders, 1990, p 313.

Pollock RVH: Feline panleukopenia and other enteric viral diseases. *In* Sherding RG, ed.: *The Cat: Diseases and Clinical Management.* New York: Churchill Livingstone, 1989, p 357.

Pollock RVH, Carmichael LE: Canine viral enteritis. *In* Greene, CE, ed.: *Infectious Diseases of the Dog and Cat.* Philadelphia: W. B. Saunders, 1990, p 268.

8 Rabies and Pseudorabies

Robert G. Sherding

RABIES

Etiology

- Rabies virus is a rhabdovirus that can infect virtually all warm-blooded animals. It primarily attacks the nervous system and is shed in saliva.
- Rabies is most important as a cause of a highly fatal encephalitis in humans. The incidence of human rabies in the United States is very low, and several countries are now classified as rabies-free.
- Rabies is transmitted in saliva from the bite of an infected animal. For both humans and domestic animals, the usual source is the bite of a rabid wild animal, most commonly a skunk, raccoon, bat, or fox. Some animals can shed rabies virus for prolonged periods in their saliva without evidence of clinical signs.
- Rabies virus is very labile outside the host; it is inactivated by many disinfectants.

KEY POINT ▶ Rabies is rare in dogs and cats in the United States; however, cats are more susceptible, and the incidence in cats is higher than in dogs. Wild animals are the principal reservoir of infection.

Pathogenesis

Rabies virus is transmitted in saliva into a deep bite wound, where it enters the peripheral nervous tissue and spreads centripetally along peripheral nerves to the spinal cord and brain. Centrifugal spread then occurs along peripheral nerves from the brain to other tissues such as the salivary glands. The incubation period before central nervous system (CNS) signs occur is extremely variable, but is usually 2 to 8 weeks. Virus shedding in saliva begins a short time (usually less than 10 days) before clinical signs appear.

Clinical Signs

The clinical course of rabies, although variable, is classically divided into 3 phases: the prodromal, furious, and paralytic phases. Death usually occurs within 3 to 7 days from the onset of signs.

Prodromal Phase (2–3 Days)

This phase often passes unnoticed, but there may be subtle signs of behavior change, fever, slow corneal and palpebral reflexes, and chewing at the bite site.

Furious Phase (2–4 Days)

Initially the limbic system of the CNS is invaded, resulting in signs of erratic behavior such as irritability, restlessness, barking, episodic aggression, vicious attacks on inanimate objects, pica, unexplained roaming, and abnormal sexual behavior. Ataxia, disorientation, and seizures may develop.

Paralytic Phase (2–4 Days)

Progressive lower motor neuron paralysis develops, causing signs of ascending paresis or paralysis of the limbs (often affecting a bitten extremity first), laryngeal paralysis (change in bark, dyspnea), pharyngeal paralysis (drooling, dysphagia), and masticatory paralysis (dropped jaw). These are followed by depression, coma, and death from respiratory paralysis.

Diagnosis

KEY POINT ▶ Early laboratory confirmation of animal rabies is essential so exposed humans can receive proper prophylaxis as early as possible.

For laboratory analysis of brain and salivary tissue for the presence of rabies virus or antigen, submit the animal's head chilled on wet ice in a leakproof container, along with appropriate information and hazard labeling. Specimens can be stored by refrigeration but not freezing, because thawing will ruin the specimen for subsequent virus detection.

Direct Fluorescent Antibody (DFA) Test. This is the test of choice used by most laboratories for rapid, reliable confirmation of rabies antigen in tissues. Brain tissue is used for routine postmortem testing. The DFA procedure can also be used for antemortem detection of rabies antigen in skin biopsies; however, a percentage of false-negative titers limits its usefulness.

Histopathology. This older, less sensitive test detects neuronal inclusions (Negri bodies), which are found in 75% of rabid dogs but rarely in cats.

Mouse Inoculation Test. This is a confirmatory test in which DFA-positive brain suspensions are inoculated intracerebrally into mice; the mice are then sacrificed and their brains examined by DFA testing 5 to 6 days postinoculation.

Tissue Culture Inoculation Test. This test is similar to the mouse inoculation test, except that cell cultures are inoculated and are examined by DFA testing 24 to 72 hours later.

Monoclonal Antibody Techniques. These techniques are used to differentiate vaccine virus strains from wild-type strains in DFA-positive brains.

Treatment

Rabies is almost always fatal in domestic animals. Because of the extreme public health danger, all animals suspected of rabies are either quarantined or euthanized, and local health department authorities must be notified.

Prevention in Dogs and Cats

KEY POINT ▶ For rabies prevention and vaccination, follow the guidelines in the Compendium of Animal Rabies Control, published annually by the National Association of State Public Health Veterinarians.

- Vaccinate and booster all dogs and cats against rabies.
  - Vaccinate at 3 months of age, 1 year later, and then every 1 or 3 years, depending on the product recommendations.
  - Side effects: local soreness, lameness, fever, and depression. These are due to the adjuvants; the neurologic complications of earlier attenuated, modified live virus (MLV) vaccines are no longer a problem.
- Do not vaccinate wild animals against rabies, even if they are kept as pets.
- Prevent pets from having contact with wild animals.
- Report all human and animal exposures to the local health department. Recommendations for dogs and cats exposed to rabies (bitten by a known rabid animal or a wild animal that is unavailable for testing) are as follows:
  - In a previously vaccinated dog or cat, revaccinate immediately and observe under quarantine conditions (leash confinement at home) for 90 days.
  - In an unvaccinated dog or cat, euthanize immediately for examination of tissues. If euthanasia is refused by the owner, strict quarantine without human or animal contact is required for 6 months, with vaccination 1 month prior to release.

Prevention in Humans

Approximately 15% of humans untreated after a bite from a known rabid animal become infected. Once signs develop in a human, rabies is almost always fatal.

- For pre-exposure prevention in high-risk situations (e.g., veterinarians and their employees), immunization with human diploid cell vaccine (HDCV) or another approved vaccine is recommended.

KEY POINT ▶ Immediately notify local health department authorities when an animal bite to a human has occurred or whenever there is the possibility of contact with a rabid animal.

- Recommendations for humans bitten by animals:
  - Instruct owners that they must quarantine and observe healthy pets that have bitten a human for 10 days. During quarantine conditions, such ani-

mals must be isolated from contact with other animals and confined in an escape-proof enclosure or building except for leash walking under owner control.
- Regard wild animals and stray or unwanted dogs and cats that have bitten a human as potentially rabid and euthanize for examination of tissues.
- Vigorously cleanse the wounds of an exposed human with copious amounts of soap and water to reduce virus in the wound. Ethanol (70%) or benzalkonium chloride (1–4%) are rabicidal. Depending on the circumstances, health authorities will decide immediately whether postexposure prophylaxis is indicated. Previously immunized humans receive two doses of vaccine (on days 0 and 3), whereas nonimmunized humans are given rabies immune globulin and five doses of vaccine (on days 0, 3, 7, 14, and 28).

PSEUDORABIES

Etiology

Pseudorabies is a herpesvirus that predominantly infects pigs (also called Aujeszky disease and mad itch). Most mammals are susceptible (but not humans) and infections are seen sporadically in dogs and cats in areas where the disease is enzootic in pigs. Pseudorabies in dogs and cats is almost always a direct result of ingestion of contaminated raw pork. The virus invades nerve endings in the pharynx and travels by way of nerve fibers to the brain where it causes fulminant panencephalitis.

Clinical Signs

Pseudorabies in dogs and cats causes an acute disease that is almost always fatal within 3 to 5 days of exposure. Initial signs may include depression and inactivity or anxiety and restlessness. The most characteristic sign (but not seen in every case) is intense pruritus that leads to excoriation and self-mutilation. Other signs may include fever, diarrhea, vomiting, copious hypersalivation, various cranial neuropathies, ataxia, and seizures. Progressive depression, dyspnea, coma, and death follow shortly thereafter; the duration of signs before death usually is only 36 to 48 hours.

KEY POINT ▶ Suspect pseudorabies in a dog or cat with acute onset of violent, frantic scratching and self-mutilation around the face, head, neck, and ears, especially if there is a history of exposure to pigs or of ingestion of raw pork in an endemic area.

Diagnosis

- It is virtually impossible to make a definitive antemortem diagnosis of pseudorabies in dogs and cats. Routine hematologic and serum chemistry evaluations are normal. Cerebrospinal fluid may show nonspecific increases in protein and mononuclear cells suggestive of viral encephalitis. Serologic tests used in pigs are not diagnostically useful in dogs and cats.

- Postmortem diagnosis is based on specialized virologic testing of brain tissue by immunofluorescent, virus isolation, or animal inoculation studies.

Treatment

No effective treatment is known.

Prevention

Pseudorabies can be prevented effectively in endemic areas by avoiding contact with pigs and never feeding raw pork. An effective vaccine is not yet available.

Supplemental Readings

August JR: Rabies. *In* Barlough JE, ed.: *Manual of Small Animal Infectious Diseases.* New York: Churchill Livingstone, 1988, p 39.

Greene CE, Dreesen DW: Rabies. *In* Greene CE, ed.: *Infectious Diseases of the Dog and Cat.* Philadelphia: W. B. Saunders, 1990, p 365.

Hand PJ: Rabies and other viral diseases of the nervous system. *In* Sherding RG, ed.: *The Cat: Diseases and Clinical Management.* New York: Churchill Livingstone, 1989, p 379.

Vandevelde M: Pseudorabies. *In* Greene CE, ed.: *Infectious Diseases of the Dog and Cat.* Philadelphia: W. B. Saunders, 1990, p 384.

9

Miscellaneous Viral Diseases

Robert G. Sherding

INFECTIOUS CANINE HEPATITIS

Etiology

Infectious canine hepatitis (ICH) is caused by canine adenovirus type 1 (CAV-1), a virus related to but distinct from CAV-2 that causes infectious tracheobronchitis (kennel cough).

Incidence

Dogs, foxes, and other canids are susceptible to CAV-1. Because of widespread use of vaccination, canine ICH is now rare and seen almost exclusively in unvaccinated dogs. Wild canids remain a reservoir of infection.

Transmission

CAV-1 is acquired through oronasal exposure. It is found in all tissues and is shed in all secretions during acute infection. It is also shed for at least 6 to 9 months in the urine after recovery. It is highly resistant to inactivation and disinfection, thus enabling spread by fomites and ectoparasites.

Pathogenesis

Following oronasal exposure, CAV-1 causes viremia and disseminates to all tissues, especially targeting hepatocytes and endothelial cells. Hepatocyte injury results in acute hepatic necrosis or chronic active hepatitis (see sec. 7, ch. 8).

Endothelial injury can affect any tissue, but CAV-1 is particularly noted for its effects on corneal endothelium (corneal edema, anterior uveitis), renal glomeruli (glomerulonephritis), and vascular endothelium (disseminated intravascular coagulopathy [DIC]).

Clinical Signs

Peracute Infection

Acutely ill dogs become moribund and die within hours.

Acute Infection

A 5- to 7-day course is characterized by fever 103°–106°F (39.5°–41°C), vomiting, diarrhea, abdominal pain, tonsillitis-pharyngitis, cervical lymphadenopathy and edema, and hemorrhagic diathesis (petechiae and ecchymoses, epistaxis, melena). Central nervous system (CNS) signs (disorientation, depression, stupor, coma, and seizures) may occur as a result of hepatic encephalopathy, hypoglycemia, or nonsuppurative encephalitis.

Ocular Infection

Ocular symptoms, occurring with acute infection or following recovery from inapparent infection, include corneal edema (cloudy cornea, also called "hepatitis blue eye") and anterior uveitis (blepharospasm, flare, miosis, and complicating glaucoma) (see sec. 11, chs. 4 and 6).

Chronic Active Hepatitis

Infected dogs with partial immunity may develop a persistent hepatic infection that causes chronic active hepatitis (see sec. 7, ch. 8).

Diagnosis

Suspect ICH based on clinical signs in an unvaccinated dog, especially if less than 1 year old.

Routine Laboratory Evaluations

ICH may cause neutropenia/lymphopenia (early), neutrophilic leukocytosis (later), increased ALT and ALP, hemostatic abnormalities typical of DIC (see sec. 3, ch. 2), and occasionally hypoglycemia.

Definitive Diagnosis

Although definitive diagnosis is not essential for successful treatment, ICH can be confirmed by serologic testing, virus isolation, immunofluorescent studies, or histopathology (centrolobular hepatic necrosis with intranuclear viral inclusions).

Treatment

Treatment is supportive until recovery from the acute stage of infection and hepatocellular regeneration can occur. This usually requires parenteral fluid therapy using potassium and dextrose-supplemented solutions (see sec. 1, ch. 5), treatment for DIC (see sec. 3, ch. 2), treatment for hepatic encephalopathy (see sec. 7, ch. 8), and antibiotics for secondary bacterial complications such as pneumonia or pyelonephritis.

Prevention

Vaccination has been highly effective for preventing CAV-1 infection.

■ Modified live virus (MLV) CAV-1 or CAV-2 vaccines (see sec. 2, ch. 5) can induce effective immunity against ICH. Unlike CAV-2, CAV-1 vaccine viruses can localize in the kidney and produce mild nephritis and urine shedding of virus or they may localize in the eyes and produce anterior uveitis (in approximately 0.4% of vaccinates; the cloudy cornea usually is transient but sometimes is irreversible.)

- Administer at least two doses, 3 to 4 weeks apart at 8 to 10 weeks and at 12 to 14 weeks of age. This is usually combined with canine distemper vaccinations (see sec. 2, ch. 6). Annual revaccination is recommended, although initial immunization likely persists for life.

CANINE ACIDOPHIL CELL HEPATITIS

Etiology

A transmissible form of hepatitis has been described in dogs in Great Britain. Although the etiologic agent has not been identified, evidence strongly suggests it is a virus and that it is distinct from CAV-1 and CAV-2.

Clinical Signs

Clinical forms of the disease, which may represent stages of progression, include acute hepatitis, chronic persistent hepatitis, cirrhosis, and occasionally hepatocellular carcinoma. Early signs, such as anorexia, vomiting, and occasional fever, are nonspecific. Later signs reflect progressive hepatic failure (ascites, hepatic encephalopathy).

Diagnosis

Laboratory findings are nonspecific and typical of those found in other types of acute and chronic liver disease (see sec. 7, ch. 8). Increased serum ALT and ALP activities are the most consistent abnormalities. Diagnosis depends on liver biopsy to identify hepatitis associated with characteristic acidophil cells.

Treatment and Prevention

Specific measures for treatment and prevention are unknown; however, supportive treatment for liver failure in general and specific treatment used in other forms of hepatitis and cirrhosis may be applicable (refer to sec. 7, ch. 8).

CANINE HERPESVIRUS

Etiology

Canine herpesvirus (CHV) infects only canids. Its biologic behavior is similar to herpesviruses of other species, and it is relatively easily inactivated outside the host.

Incidence

CHV is widespread in the canine population; however, it causes clinical disease almost exclusively in newborn puppies during the first month of life.

Transmission

Perinatal infection can be acquired before, at, or soon after birth via in utero transmission; during passage through the birth canal; or by direct oronasal contact with infected littermates, the dam's infectious oronasal secretions, or fomites. Respiratory and venereal transmission may be important in adults.

Clinical Signs

Whether signs occur and what they are depend on the animal's age at exposure.

Prenatal Infection

Fetal resorption, abortion, or stillbirth occur rarely.

Neonatal Infection

Infection before 1 to 2 weeks of age leads to viremia and virus dissemination to all tissues, resulting in a fatal generalized form of disease. The susceptibility to this form of CHV is related to the narrow temperature range of 35° to 36°C needed for optimal growth of CHV, which coincides with the body temperature often found in neonates in the first week of life.

- Neonatal infection is characterized by multifocal lesions of necrosis and hemorrhage (DIC) in many organs, including kidneys, adrenals, liver, spleen, gastrointestinal (GI) tract, lung, and CNS.
- Signs include depression, refusal to nurse, incessant crying, subnormal body temperature, yellow-green diarrhea, abdominal pain, nasal discharge, petechial hemorrhages on mucosal surfaces, skin papules, and CNS signs (coma, opisthotonus, and seizures). Death usually occurs within 24 to 48 hours.
- This form occurs in puppies born to a seronegative dam. Subsequent litters produced by the dam are rarely infected because of protective maternal immunity.

Adult and Older Puppy Infections

Marked resistance to CHV develops abruptly in animals after 1 to 2 weeks of age due to effects of higher body temperature and better immune function; thus, infection beyond 2 weeks of age results only in mild or inapparent infection that is confined to the respiratory and genital tracts.

- Transient, mild respiratory and conjunctival signs with episodic shedding can occur.
- A possible manifestation is vaginitis/balanoposthitis. This is characterized by lymphofollicular lesions of the genital mucosa with or without mild hyperemia and discharge (see sec. 8, chs. 12 and 16). Local genital infection may be a source of venereal transmission between adult animals and of vaginal transmission to neonates during birth.

Diagnosis

- For infected neonates: the age of onset and clinical signs are fairly characteristic. Positive serologic titers

(virus neutralizing antibody) in the dam and surviving pups provides additional presumptive evidence. Necropsy lesions are usually diagnostic.
- For adult carriers: virus isolation from the oropharynx or genital lesions confirms the diagnosis.

Treatment

There is no effective treatment for CHV. Treatment of the neonatal form is probably not warranted because it is almost always fatal, and the few puppies that do recover often have irreversible neurologic sequelae (e.g., cerebellar dysfunction).

Prevention

An effective vaccine for CHV is unavailable.

- In breeding kennels, promote proper husbandry practices and maintain warm ambient temperatures for neonates.
- In kennels with CHV problems:
  - Isolate infected bitches and their litters.
  - Disinfect the premises (CHV is susceptible to most detergents and disinfectants).
  - Administer hyperimmune antiserum (harvested from bitches that have recently produced CHV-infected litters), 1–2 ml, intraperitoneally, for prophylaxis in unaffected newborn puppies, including healthy-appearing members of an infected litter.

CANINE VIRAL PAPILLOMATOSIS

Etiology

The canine papillomavirus causes mucocutaneous tumors that are benign and self-limiting. Virus-induced papillomas are multiple (often 50–100 separate tumor nodules) and occur in young dogs, in contrast to noninfectious papillomas, which are solitary and usually affect older dogs. Transmission appears to be by direct viral contact with oral mucosa. The incubation period is 1 to 2 months.

Clinical Signs

The three forms of infectious papillomatosis in dogs are oral, ocular, and cutaneous.

- Oral papillomatosis is by far the most common form and usually affects dogs under 2 years of age. Lesions begin as smooth, white mucosal elevations that develop into cauliflower-like warts on the lip margins, oral mucosa, tongue, palate, pharynx, and epiglottis. They usually increase in number and size for 4 to 6 weeks and then begin to regress. Common presenting signs are halitosis, ptyalism, reluctance to eat, and oral bleeding.
- Ocular papillomatosis is uncommon; it affects dogs 6 months to 4 years of age and is characterized by papillomas on conjunctiva, cornea, and eyelid margins.
- Cutaneous papillomatosis is rare (see sec. 3, ch. 9).

Diagnosis

The history and physical appearance of the lesions are adequate for diagnosis of oral and cutaneous papillomatosis. In the ocular form of the disease, confirmatory excisional biopsy is advisable to exclude other ocular tumors that may have a similar physical appearance.

Treatment

- For the oral form, treatment is not necessary, because viral oral papillomas usually regress spontaneously within 3 months once immunity develops. There have been rare reports of failure to regress for over 2 years.
- Removal by surgical excision, cryosurgery, or electrosurgery is indicated for ocular papillomas and for oral lesions that interfere with eating or that bleed and discharge excessively. Submit tissues for biopsy to confirm the diagnosis. Removal of some of the tumors often triggers regression of the remaining ones.
- When regression fails to occur, remission can be induced in some dogs with weekly administration of vincristine or cyclophosphamide at the usual antitumor doses (see sec. 3, ch. 5).

FELINE POXVIRUS

Etiology

Cowpox virus causes disease in cats more often than in any other species, including cows, but has been recognized only in Europe. The disease is characterized by widespread skin lesions with occasional systemic involvement. The source of infection is contact with rodents, mainly through contaminated skin wounds.

Clinical Signs

- The initial inoculation site or skin wound (usually a bitewound on the head, neck, or forelimb) is called the primary lesion.
- Then, 1 to 3 weeks later, after a period of viremia and sometimes mild systemic signs (low fever, anorexia, depression, and mild upper respiratory signs), widespread secondary pox lesions develop. These lesions begin as multiple, small (1 mm) skin nodules that progress and increase in number over 2 to 4 days to become well-circumscribed ulcers covered with scabs. Most cats have more than ten of these pox lesions. Buccal ulcers are seen occasionally.
- The scabs dry and fall off in 4 to 6 weeks, revealing underlying healing skin. Some lesions result in permanent bald patches.
- The disease is worsened by immunosuppressive conditions, such as feline leukemia or feline immunodeficiency virus infection or glucocorticoid therapy. Rarely, fatalities occur due to secondary bacterial infection.

Diagnosis

■ Suspect feline poxvirus in a cat with typical secondary pox lesions following a recent history of a primary skin wound lesion.

■ Confirm by detection of virus (preferred method) in the scabs by electron microscopy or by virus isolation, detection of poxvirus-specific antibody by serologic methods, or detection of the characteristic histopathologic abnormalities in skin biopsies.

Treatment

There is no specific treatment for poxvirus infection, but the disease is self-limiting and skin lesions regress in 4 to 6 weeks. Antibiotics and topical cleansing help to control secondary bacterial infection of skin lesions, but take proper precautions (e.g., wear rubber gloves when handling cats) because cowpox virus is potentially transmissible to humans. Corticosteroids are contraindicated.

Supplemental Readings

INFECTIOUS CANINE HEPATITIS

Greene CE: Infectious canine hepatitis and canine acidophil cell hepatitis. *In* Greene CE, ed.: *Infectious Diseases of the Dog and Cat.* Philadelphia: W. B. Saunders, 1990, p 242.
Polzin DJ: Infectious canine hepatitis. *In* Barlough JE, ed.: *Manual of Small Animal Infectious Diseases.* New York: Churchill Livingstone, 1988, p 11.

CANINE HERPESVIRUS

Barlough JE, Carmichael LE: Canine herpesvirus. *In* Barlough JE, ed.: *Manual of Small Animal Infectious Diseases.* New York: Churchill Livingstone, 1988, p 19.
Carmichael LE, Greene CE: Canine herpesvirus infection. *In* Greene CE, ed.: *Infectious Diseases of the Dog and Cat.* Philadelphia: W. B. Saunders, 1990, p 252.

CANINE VIRAL PAPILLOMATOSIS

Calvert CA: Canine viral papillomatosis. *In* Greene CE, ed.: *Infectious Diseases of the Dog and Cat.* Philadelphia: W. B. Saunders, 1990, p 288.
Rosenthal RC: Canine viral papillomatosis. *In* Barlough JE, ed.: *Manual of Small Animal Infectious Diseases.* New York: Churchill Livingstone, 1988, p 7.

FELINE POXVIRUS

Bennett M, Gaskell RM, Baxby D: Feline cowpox virus infection. *In* Greene CE, ed.: *Infectious Diseases of the Dog and Cat.* Philadelphia: W. B. Saunders, 1990, p 362.

10

Rickettsial Diseases

C. Guillermo Couto

GENERAL FEATURES OF RICKETTSIAL DISEASES IN DOGS AND CATS

Rickettsial diseases are quite common in dogs but are extremely rare in cats (with the exception of hemobartonellosis). Most rickettsial diseases in dogs are tick-borne, with the exception of salmon poisoning (discussed later in this chapter). The mode of transmission of hemobartonellosis has not yet been elucidated. Because these diseases are acute in endemic areas, there is a higher prevalence during (or after) warm weather, when ticks are more prevalent.

The clinical course of rickettsial diseases can be acute (e.g., Rocky Mountain spotted fever, hemobartonellosis, ehrlichiosis) or subacute to chronic (e.g., ehrlichiosis, salmon poisoning). Most rickettsial infections respond to tetracycline, doxycylcine, or chloramphenicol. Multisystemic rickettsial diseases are described here. For a discussion of the hemotropic rickettsial agent *Hemobartonella,* see sec. 3, ch. 1.

CANINE EHRLICHIOSIS

Canine ehrlichiosis is a relatively common rickettsial disease of dogs, which has recently been confirmed as a zoonosis. Synonyms used in the literature for this disorder include tracker dog disease, tropical canine pancytopenia, canine hemorrhagic fever, and canine typhus. It is distributed worldwide and achieved prominence in the media and among veterinarians during the Vietnam war, when a large proportion of military dogs contracted this disease. Because of its chronic and insidious nature, ehrlichiosis is prevalent year-round rather than only during the warm months of the year.

Etiology

Agents

- *Ehrlichia canis* (mononuclear strain)
- *Ehrlichia equi* (neutrophilic strain)
- *Ehrlichia platys* (platelet strain)
- Two new species of *Ehrlichia* have been recognized (but not yet named) in the dog.
- Experimentally, inoculation of *Ehrlichia risticii* (Potomac horse fever agent) has induced mild clinical or subclinical disease in dogs and cats.

Transmission

- The vector and reservoir is the common brown dog tick (*Rhipicephalus sanguineus*), which can transmit organisms for at least 5 months postengorgement. Ehrlichiosis, as well as other rickettsial diseases, can also be transmitted iatrogenically through contaminated blood transfusions.
- The incubation period is 7 to 21 days.
- The organism is transmitted through tick bites. Ticks ingest the organism from an infected host.

Pathogenesis

- The acute phase of ehrlichiosis is variable in duration (2 to 4 weeks) and severity (mild to severe). The organism replicates in mononuclear cells, mainly in the mononuclear phagocytic system (MPS) in lymph nodes, spleen, liver, and bone marrow, resulting in hyperplasia of this cell line and organomegaly (lymphadenopathy, splenomegaly, and hepatomegaly). Thrombocytopenia (due to peripheral destruction of platelets) with or without anemia and leukopenia (or leukocytosis) is common during this phase (see below).
- The subclinical phase is characterized by persistence of the organism following apparent recovery from the acute phase. Dogs may eliminate the organism during this phase, or infection may progress to the chronic phase.
- The chronic phase occurs when the immune system is ineffective and the organism cannot be eliminated.

KEY POINT ▶ In nonendemic areas canine ehrlichiosis is usually chronic.

Clinical Signs and Laboratory Abnormalities

Clinical signs vary in the different phases of the disease.

Acute Phase

- Clinical signs and physical examination findings mainly are the result of widespread MPS (lymphoreticular) hyperplasia and hematologic abnormalities. Therefore, pyrexia, generalized lymphadenopathy, splenomegaly, hepatomegaly, dyspnea or exercise intolerance due to pneumonitis, neurologic signs caused by meningoencephalitis, and petechiae and ecchymoses due to thrombocytopenia dominate the clinical presentation. Antibody titers may be negative during this phase, as it takes up to 3 weeks to develop a significant titer.
- Hematologic and biochemical abnormalities include thrombocytopenia, mild to severe anemia, leukopenia or leukocytosis, hypercellular bone marrow

cytology, mild hyperglobulinemia, and mild elevation in liver enzyme activities.

Subclinical Phase

- Patients are asymptomatic. Mild hematologic and biochemical changes may be identified.

Chronic Phase

- Clinical signs can be mild or severe, develop 1 to 4 months after inoculation of the organism, and reflect the MPS hyperplasia and hematologic abnormalities. Any of the following may be observed: weight loss, pyrexia, spontaneous bleeding, pallor due to anemia, generalized lymphadenopathy, hepatosplenomegaly, anterior and/or posterior uveitis, neurologic signs caused by meningoencephalomyelitis, and intermittent limb edema.
- Hematologic and biochemical abnormalities are usually pronounced and include mono-, bi-, or pancytopenia due to bone marrow hypoplasia; bone marrow and splenic plasmacytosis; lymphocytosis occasionally composed of large granular lymphocytes; hyperglobulinemia caused by polyclonal (or less often a monoclonal) gammopathy; hypoalbuminemia; and proteinuria.

KEY POINT ▶ Clinical signs, physical findings, and laboratory abnormalities in dogs with chronic ehrlichiosis may resemble multiple myeloma or chronic lymphocytic leukemia.

Diagnosis

- Identification of the organism in fine needle aspiration cytology of the spleen, lymph nodes, and lungs is possible, but extremely unlikely. Plasmacytosis is frequently present in these cytologic specimens.
- The indirect fluorescent antibody (IFA) test for *E. canis* is highly sensitive. Although mild cross-reactivity with other rickettsial organisms is possible, titers greater than 1:10 are considered diagnostic. Diagnostic titers may not be detected until 2 to 3 weeks postinoculation. As with other infectious diseases, high titers do not confer protection against reinfection. Titers may persist for up to 9 to 12 months.

Treatment

- Tetracycline and its derivative doxycycline are the drugs of choice for dogs with ehrlichiosis. Chloramphenicol is also effective, but its advisability is questionable in dogs with cytopenias. Doxycycline is my drug of choice, at a dose of 2.5 to 5 mg/kg, PO, every 12 to 24 hours for 10 to 14 days. Tetracycline is used at a dose of 22 mg/kg, PO, every 8 hours for 14 to 21 days, and should be administered on an empty stomach. Recent evidence suggests that enrofloxacin (Baytril), at therapeutic doses, may be effective in dogs with erlichiosis.
- Imidocarb dipropionate (Imzol), an anticholinesterase parasympathomimetic, administered at a dosage of 5 mg/kg, SC and repeated in 14 days, has been highly effective in dogs with refractory ehrlichiosis and in dogs with *E. canis* and *Babesia canis* mixed infections. However, this drug is not yet available in the United States.
- Institute supportive therapy (blood or blood products, fluids, etc.) as deemed necessary (see discussions of tranfusions elsewhere in text).

Prognosis and Prevention

- The prognosis for canine erlichiosis is excellent with appropriate treatment, unless the bone marrow is severely hypoplastic. Clinical response in the chronic forms may take 3 to 4 weeks. The chronic form of the disease appears to be more severe in German shepherd dogs and Doberman pinschers.
- Tick control constitutes the mainstay of prevention for ehrlichiosis. Low doses of tetracycline or doxycycline may be used in endemic areas during tick season (tetracycline, 3 mg/kg, PO, every 24 hours; or doxycycline, 1–2 mg/kg, PO, every 24 hours).

INFECTIOUS CYCLIC THROMBOCYTOPENIA

Ehrlichia platys causes infectious cyclic thrombocytopenia, in which fairly asymptomatic dogs develop thrombocytopenia at 1- to 2-week intervals. It is confined mainly to the Gulf Coast and is diagnosed on the basis of serology for *E. platys* (by IFA testing), or by identification of this organism within platelets in a Giemsa-stained blood smear. (For a discussion of the differential diagnosis of thrombocytopenia, see sec. 3, chs. 1 and 2.) Treatment is as for other rickettsial diseases.

ROCKY MOUNTAIN SPOTTED FEVER

This tick-borne disease is most prevalent in the east coast, midwest, and plains regions, and it represents the most important rickettsial disease in humans. Because of its acute nature, most cases occur during tick season, between April 1 and September 1.

Etiology

Agent

- Rocky Mountain spotted fever (RMSF) is caused by *Rickettsia rickettsii*.

Transmission

- The recognized vectors for *R. rickettsii* are the American dog tick *(Dermacentor variabilis)*, found primarily east of the Great Plains and in parts of the west coast, and the wood tick *(Dermacentor andersoni)*, found in one area ranging from the Rocky Mountains to the Cascades. These are three-host ticks; the permanent hosts are humans, dogs, and cats, and the reservoirs are rodents and dogs. Ticks do not usually infect the hosts until they have been attached for a minimum of 5 to 20 hours. This disease can also be transmitted iatrogenically through blood transfusions.

■ The incubation period varies from 2 to 14 days.

Pathogenesis

■ Ticks usually acquire the organism through feeding on infected animals, although vertical tick transmission can also occur.
■ Once inoculated into the host via a bite, the organism quickly invades and replicates in vascular endothelial cells, resulting in widespread vasculitis, platelet aggregation, and activation of disseminated intravascular coagulation (DIC).

Clinical Signs and Laboratory Abnormalities

Natural and experimental infection can lead to *subclinical* or *acute* manifestations of RMSF.

Subclinical Stage

In the subclinical stages, dogs are usually asymptomatic, but laboratory abnormalities such as mild thrombocytopenia may be detected.

Acute Stage

Most dogs with acute RMSF present between April and September. The clinical signs and laboratory abnormalities are variable in severity, and, if the disorder is untreated, last from 2 to 4 weeks. Because of the acute course, ticks are commonly found on the dog (or were recently removed by the owner).

■ Common clinical signs and physical examination findings in dogs with acute RMSF include anorexia, pyrexia, neurologic signs (altered mental status, vestibular signs), myalgia/arthralgia, generalized lymphadenopathy, edema of the face and limbs, and dyspnea or exercise intolerance due to pneumonitis. The rash, petechiae, and ecchymoses commonly seen in humans (which confer the name to this disease) are seen in only less than 20% of affected dogs. Cardiac arrhythmias (due to myocarditis) can also occur and may result in sudden death.
■ Hematologic and biochemical abnormalities in dogs with RMSF include leukocytosis with left shift and monocytosis, mild anemia, thrombocytopenia, evidence of DIC (see sec. 3, ch. 2), increased liver enzyme activities, azotemia, hypercholesterolemia, hyponatremia, hypochloremia, and metabolic acidosis.

Diagnosis

■ Serum titers usually do not rise until after 2 to 3 weeks following inoculation. Therefore, obtain paired serum samples in patients with acute signs of disease.
■ Several serologic tests are available for the diagnosis of RMSF, including micro-indirect fluorescence antibody (micro-IFA), immunofluorescence, and enzyme-linked immunosorbent assay (ELISA) tests. Of these, the micro-IFA test is most commonly used in dogs.
■ In the micro-IFA test, titers greater than 1:128 are usually considered diagnostic; however, a fourfold rise in titer (in comparison of a sample obtained during acute disease with a convalescent sample) is preferred in order to establish a definitive diagnosis.
■ IgM titers (indicative of acute infection) can also be detected by a modified micro-IFA technique. High titers can be detected for up to 1 year following successful treatment of the disease.
■ The direct immunofluorescence test to detect rickettsial antigens can be performed in fresh or paraffin-embedded tissues. This test is diagnostic as early as 3 to 4 days postinoculation and can be performed on skin biopsies obtained with a local anesthetic and biopsy punch.

Treatment

■ Tetracycline and its derivative doxycycline are the drugs of choice for dogs with RMSF. Chloramphenicol is also effective, at a dose of 15 to 25 mg/kg, PO, IM, or IV, every 8 hours. Doxycycline is my drug of choice, at a dose of 2.5 to 5 mg/kg, PO or IV, every 12 to 24 hours for 7 to 10 days. Tetracycline is used at a dose of 22 mg/kg, PO, every 8 hours for 10 to 14 days, and should be administered on an empty stomach.
■ Recently, enrofloxacin at a dose of 3 mg/kg, PO, every 12 hours was shown to be effective in dogs with experimentally induced RMSF.
■ Institute supportive therapy as needed.

KEY POINT ▶ Dogs with acute onset of neurologic signs, pyrexia, and other systemic signs in areas endemic for RMSF should be treated with intravenous doxycycline until a definitive diagnosis can be established

Prognosis and Prevention

■ The prognosis for dogs with the acute form of the disease is good when treatment is promptly instituted. Responses occur within hours of initiating appropriate drug administration. Mortality is high if the diagnosis and treatment are delayed until the later stages of the disease.
■ Dogs with severe central nervous system (CNS) signs may die within hours of instituting treatment.
■ Prevention involves strict tick and rodent control.

SALMON POISONING

Salmon poisoning is a rickettsial disease of dogs in the Pacific Northwest, which has a high morbidity and mortality. It is not a tick-borne disease.

Etiology

Agent

■ *Neorickettsia helminthoeca*
■ Elokomin fluke fever agent

Transmission

Dogs acquire the disease after ingesting raw salmon (or related fish) that contain the metacercariae of the fluke *Nanophyetus salmincola* infected with *Neorickettsia helminthoeca* or the Elokomin fluke fever agent. These flukes require three hosts to complete a life cycle: snail, fish (salmonid), and dog (or bird).

Pathogenesis

- Five to 7 days after a dog ingests contaminated fish, the fluke matures and attaches to the intestinal epithelium of the dog, inoculating the organism. After infecting the intestinal epithelium, the organisms disseminate to the MPS organs (lymph nodes, spleen, and liver) and to other organs such as the CNS and the lungs.
- The incubation period ranges from 5 to 21 days.

Clinical Signs and Laboratory Abnormalities

- Clinical signs and physical findings in dogs with acute salmon poisoning include pyrexia followed by hypothermia, diarrhea (usually hemorrhagic), vomiting, profound weight loss, mild serous naso-ocular discharge, and generalized lymphadenopathy, which can be marked.
- Laboratory abnormalities are nonspecific.

Diagnosis

- Operculated fluke eggs are found on direct fecal smears or by fecal washing-sedimentation techniques.
- Giemsa-stained fine needle aspirates of enlarged lymph nodes usually reveal a reactive lymph node hyperplasia with intracytoplasmic rickettsial bodies in macrophages.

Treatment

- Give tetracycline or doxycycline as described for canine erlichiosis or RMSF. Because of the severe vomiting and diarrhea, give IV antibiotics (e.g., doxycycline) when possible.
- Praziquantel (Droncit; Haver), 10–30 mg/kg, PO or SC, given once, or mebendazole (Telmintic; Pitman Moore), 50 mg/kg/day, PO for 10 to 14 days, eliminates the fluke.
- Use supportive treatment as needed.

Prognosis and Prevention

- The prognosis is good with appropriate treatment.
- To prevent the disease, keep dogs from feeding on raw infected fish.
- Freezing or thoroughly cooking fish destroys the metacercariae and rickettsiae.

Supplemental Readings

CANINE EHRLICHIOSIS

Breitschwerdt EB: Tick-transmitted diseases. Proc Ninth Annual Vet Med Forum, ACVIM. New Orleans, 1991, p 137.
Greene CE, Burgdorfer W, Cavagnolo R, et al: Rocky Mountain spotted fever in dogs and its differentiation from canine ehrlichiosis. J Am Vet Med Assoc 186:465, 1985.
Troy GC, Forrester SD: Canine ehrlichiosis. *In* Greene CE, ed.: *Infectious Diseases of the Dog and Cat.* Philadelphia: W. B. Saunders, 1990, p 404.
Troy GC, Vulgamott JC, Turnwald GH: Canine ehrlichiosis: A retrospective study of 30 naturally occurring cases. J Am Anim Hosp Assoc 16:181, 1980.

ROCKY MOUNTAIN SPOTTED FEVER

Greene CE, Burgdorfer W, Cavagnolo R, et al: Rocky Mountain spotted fever in dogs and its differentiation from canine ehrlichiosis. J Am Vet Med Assoc 186:465, 1985.
Greene CE, Breitschwerdt EB: Rocky Mountain spotted fever and Q fever. *In* Greene CE, ed.: *Infectious Diseases of the Dog and Cat.* Philadelphia: W. B. Saunders, 1990, p 419.

SALMON POISONING

Gorham JR, Foreyt WJ: Salmon poisoning disease. *In* Greene CE, ed.: *Infectious Diseases of the Dog and Cat.* Philadelphia: W. B. Saunders, 1990, p 397.

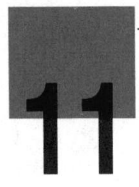

Leptospirosis, Brucellosis, and Other Bacterial Infectious Diseases

Robert G. Sherding

A large diversity of bacteria can infect dogs and cats. This discussion focuses on leptospirosis and brucellosis. Other infectious diseases caused by bacteria are summarized in Table 1, and most are described in the respective organ-system chapters. Borreliosis (Lyme disease) is mainly a joint disease (see sec. 9, ch. 31); brucellosis is mainly a cause of impaired reproductive function (see sec. 8, ch. 18). *Bordetella bronchiseptica* is associated with the canine infectious tracheobronchitis complex (see sec. 2, ch. 5), and tetanus causes severe neuromuscular dysfunction (see sec. 10, ch. 6). Salmonellosis, campylobacteriosis, yersiniosis, and Tyzzer disease primarily involve the intestinal tract (see sec. 7, ch. 6). Actinomycosis and nocardiosis are causes of pyothorax (see sec. 6, ch. 22) and chronic skin disease (see sec. 5, ch. 1). Mycobacterial infections are associated with chronic skin disease (see sec. 5, ch. 2).

LEPTOSPIROSIS

Etiology

Leptospirosis is caused by serovars of *Leptospira interrogans,* a filamentous, motile spirochete that infects most wild and domestic animals including humans. Several serovars infect dogs and cats, but clinical disease occurs only in dogs. The serovars that are associated with canine leptospirosis include *L. icterohaemorrhagiae, L. canicola,* and *L. grippotyphosa.*

Transmission

Infection is spread by recovered animals that shed organisms in their urine for months to years following infection. Exposure usually occurs by mucocutaneous contact with leptospires in the environment (contaminated water, food, bedding, soil, vegetation, or fomites). The organisms penetrate mucosa or abraded skin. In addition, transplacental, venereal, and bite-wound transmission can occur. Wild animal and rodent populations are reservoirs for leptospirosis.

Pathogenesis

Leptospiremia occurs 4 to 12 days postinfection. The primary targets in leptospirosis are the kidneys and the liver. Fever and disseminated vascular coagulation (DIC) may occur.

- *Leptospira* replicates in renal tubule epithelium and can cause acute injury and renal failure (especially *L. canicola*). Renal colonization and urine shedding are prolonged, even for months following recovery.
- *Leptospira* can injure hepatocytes, resulting in acute hepatic necrosis (especially *L. icterohaemorrhagiae*), icterus, hepatic fibrosis, and occasionally chronic active hepatitis (reported with *L. grippotyphosa*).
- Infection typically is subclinical in vaccinated (immune) and adult dogs and in all cats.

Clinical Signs

- Systemic signs of illness: fever, depression, anorexia, vomiting, reluctance to move (due to generalized muscle pain, renal pain, or meningitis), dehydration, and congested mucous membranes; vascular collapse and peracute death in some animals
- Acute renal failure, usually with oliguria or anuria (see sec. 8, ch. 1)
- Acute hepatic failure, usually with icterus and DIC (see sec. 7, ch. 8)
- Signs of DIC: widespread petechial and ecchymotic hemorrhages, melena, hematemesis, and epistaxis
- Occasional manifestations: abortion or stillbirths, uveitis, and meningitis

Diagnosis

Complete Blood Count (CBC)

- Leukopenia (early)
- Neutrophilia with left shift (at usual time of presentation)
- Thrombocytopenia and abnormal hemostasis reflecting DIC (see sec. 3, ch. 2)

Urinalysis

- Proteinuria, pyuria, cylindruria, bilirubinuria, and isosthenuria

Serum Chemistries

- Azotemia—increased blood-urea nitrogen (BUN), creatinine

TABLE 1. Bacterial Infectious Diseases of Dogs and Cats

Disease	Etiology (Source)	Clinical Signs	Diagnosis	Treatment
Leptospirosis	*Leptospira interrogans* (serovars: *L. canicola, L. icterohaemorrhagiae, L. grippotyphosa*) (urine shedding)	Acute renal failure, acute hepatic failure, anorexia, depression, fever, myalgia, DIC	Serology (MA, ELISA)	Penicillin, dihydrostreptomycin
Borreliosis (Lyme disease)	*Borrelia burgdorferi* (tick-borne)	Fever, polyarthritis (shifting lameness)	Serology (IFA, ELISA)	Tetracycline or doxycycline
Brucellosis	*Brucella canis* (semen, vaginal discharges, urine)	Male: infertility, orchiepididymitis, scrotitis Female: infertility, abortion Male & Female: lymphadenopathy	Serology (slide test, tube test, AGID) Blood culture	Minocycline or doxycycline plus dihydrostreptomycin; spay/castrate
Bordetellosis (kennel cough)	*Bordetella bronchiseptica* (respiratory secretions)	Acute tracheobronchitis (cough)	Culture (airways)	Gentamycin aerosol
Tetanus	*Clostridium tetani* (wound contamination)	Muscle rigidity, stiffness, tetanic spasms (neurotoxin-induced)	Clinical signs	Tetanus antitoxin; penicillin G or metronidazole; sedatives
Campylobacteriosis	*Campylobacter jejuni* (feces)	Watery mucoid diarrhea or subclinical carrier	Fecal culture, fecal microscopy	Erythromycin, neomycin, clindamycin, or chloramphenicol
Salmonellosis	*Salmonella typhimurium, S. enteritidis* (feces)	Acute gastroenteritis: fever, vomiting, diarrhea, bacteremia; subclinical carrier	Fecal culture	Enrofloxacin, trimethoprim-sulfa, or chloramphenicol
Yersiniosis	*Yersinia enterocolitica* (human feces)	Diarrhea (rare) or subclinical carrier	Fecal culture	Chloramphenicol, tetracyclines, etc.
Tyzzer disease	*Bacillus piliformis* (rodent feces)	Acute hepatic necrosis, necrotizing ileocolitis	Necropsy lesions, cell culture isolation	None (100% fatality)
Plague	*Yersinia pestis* (rodent fleas and rodent ingestion)	Cat: lymph node abscess, high fever, fatal septicemia Dog: mild fever or no signs	Lymph node cytology, culture, and IFA; serology	Streptomycin, chloramphenicol, or tetracycline; flea control
Tularemia	*Francisella tularensis* (tick-borne; ingestion of rabbits or rodents)	Fever, lymphadenopathy, draining abscesses, fatal bacteremia	Serology (agglutinating antibody titer), culture	Streptomycin or gentamycin
Actinomycosis	*Actinomyces* spp (oral flora migration, bitewounds)	Subcutaneous abscesses, draining fistulous tracts, pyothorax, osteomyelitis	Cytology (gram-positive filamentous rods), culture of exudate	Penicillin; debride wounds; drain and lavage pyothorax
Nocardiosis	*Nocardia* spp (soil via wounds, plant awns, inhalation)	Subcutaneous abscesses, draining fistulous tracts, pyothorax, pneumonia	Cytology (gram-positive filamentous rods), histopathology, culture of exudate	Sulfa drugs; debride wounds; drain and lavage pyothorax
Tuberculosis	*Mycobacterium tuberculosis, M. bovis, M. avium* (Dog: inhalation) (Cat: ingestion, eg. milk)	Dog: granulomatous pneumonia, hilar lymphadenopathy Cat: granulomatous enteritis, mesenteric lymphadenopathy	Cytology (acid-fast bacteria); intradermal skin test (dogs only); culture (difficult)	Not recommended because of public health concerns and refractoriness
Feline leprosy	*M. lepraemurium* (contact with rats)	Ulcerating cutaneous nodules	Cytology or biopsy (acid-fast bacteria)	Surgical excision; dapsone (toxic)
Atypical mycobacteriosis	*M. fortuitum-chelonei* (skin contact with contaminated soil and water)	Spreading subcutaneous fistulous tracts	Cytology or biopsy (acid-fast bacteria)	Gentamycin, doxycycline, trimethoprim sulfa, or enrofloxacin

DIC = disseminated intravascular coagulation; MA = microscopic agglutination; ELISA = enzyme-linked immunosorbent assay; IFA = indirect fluorescent antibody; AGID = agar-gel immunodiffusion.

■ Elevated liver enzymes (ALT, AST, ALP) and bilirubin
■ Electrolyte imbalances reflecting renal and gastrointestinal effects

Serology

■ Microscopic agglutination (MA) test
  • Titer becomes positive after 1 week, peaks at 3 to 4 weeks, and remains positive for months after both natural infection and after vaccination.
  • To confirm current infection (versus previous infection or vaccination), a rising titer must be demonstrated. The titer during acute illness should increase fourfold when repeated during convalescence.
  • Because the timing of the titer peak varies, take a convalescent titer 2 to 3 weeks postinfection, and another 1 to 2 weeks later.
  • Although single titers are never diagnostic of current infection, titers ≥1:300 are suggestive, and titers ≥1:1000 are highly indicative of leptospirosis. However, booster vaccines given in the preceding 2 to 3 months can produce titers that overlap with these values.
■ Combined IgM-IgG enzyme-linked immunosorbent assay (ELISA) titers
  • IgM titer becomes positive within the first week of infection (before MA) and persists for 2 weeks.
  • IgG titer becomes positive 2 to 3 weeks after infection and persists for months.
  • Although not as available as the MA test, these help to differentiate current infection from previous infection or vaccination.

KEY POINT ▶ *Leptospira* organisms are fastidious, slow-growing, and difficult to culture, and they are difficult to identify in fluids or tissues; thus, serology in conjunction with clinical signs is the most practical means of diagnosis.

Treatment

■ Institute general therapy for dehydration (see sec. 1, ch. 5), acute renal failure (see sec. 8, ch. 1), acute hepatic failure (see sec. 7, ch. 8), and DIC (see sec. 3, ch. 2), as described in the appropriate chapters of this book. Anuria and fulminant DIC are life-threatening complications of leptospirosis that need immediate attention.
■ Antibiotics:

KEY POINT ▶ The antibiotic of choice for eliminating leptospiremia is penicillin and for eliminating leptospiruria is dihydrostreptomycin.

  • For leptospiremia: penicillin G (25,000–40,000 units/kg, IM or IV, every 12 hours for 2 weeks)
  • For leptospiruria: dihydrostreptomycin (once azotemia resolves): 15 mg/kg, IM, every 12 hours for 2 weeks).
  • Alternatives (lower efficacy): doxycycline, tetracycline, ampicillin, and amoxicillin
■ Leptospirosis is zoonotic; thus, recommend precautions and proper hygiene, especially regarding exposure to contaminated urine. Use iodine disinfectants such as povidone-iodine (Betadine).

Prevention

Because prevention of exposure is not a realistic expectation, routine vaccination for leptospirosis is recommended. Vaccination helps reduce the incidence and severity of leptospirosis, but it does not prevent subclinical infection or urine shedding.

■ Bivalent *Leptospira* bacterin (*L. canicola* and *L. icterohaemorrhagiae*) is a component of most polyvalent canine vaccines (included with canine distemper virus, parvovirus, adenovirus, etc.) used for routine vaccination programs.
■ Vaccinate dogs at 9, 12, and 15 weeks of age. At least three doses are required for primary immunization. Annual revaccination is recommended, but since the duration of immunity averages 6 to 8 months, dogs in endemic areas or high-risk situations should be vaccinated more frequently (every 4 to 6 months).
■ Newer, improved vaccines derived from *Leptospira* outer membrane antigens may become available, with the following advantages over existing bacterins:
  • Protection against subclinical infection and shedding
  • More rapid onset of protection
  • Fewer doses required for primary immunization
  • Fewer allergic reactions

CANINE BRUCELLOSIS

Etiology

Canine brucellosis is caused by *Brucella canis,* a gram-negative coccobacillus.

Transmission

B. canis is found in semen (venereal), vaginal discharges (at estrus, breeding, and postabortion), aborted fetal tissues, and urine. Infection occurs by penetration of oronasal, conjunctival, and genital mucous membranes by the organisms.

Pathogenesis

Brucellosis is characterized by a prolonged leukocyte-associated bacteremia that lasts 6 to 64 months.

■ *Brucella* organisms most often localize in:
  • The lymphoid and mononuclear phagocyte systems (lymphoreticular hyperplasia)
  • The prostate and testes of the male (orchiepididymitis, infertility)
  • The gravid uterus of the female (infertility, abortion)
■ Rarely, the eye (anterior uveitis), kidney (glomerulonephritis), or intervertebral discs (discospondylitis) are involved.

Clinical Signs

Generalized lymphadenopathy, splenomegaly, and poor reproductive performance are the principal manifestations. Fever and systemic illness are rare.

- In males: infertility and physical findings of scrotal swelling, scrotal dermatitis, enlarged epididymus (epididymitis), and testicular atrophy
- In females: abortion of dead, partially autolyzed fetuses at 45 to 59 days of gestation without any other signs of being ill, persistent discharge for 1 to 6 weeks following abortion, and failure to conceive (due to early fetal resorption)

Diagnosis

KEY POINT ▶ Suspect brucellosis in any bitch that aborts 2 weeks prior to term.

- Routine CBC, urinalysis, and serum chemistries are normal except for occasional hyperglobulinemia.
- Lymph node cytology reveals nonspecific reactive hyperplasia.
- Semen abnormalities—more than 80% of sperm are morphologically abnormal, with increased leukocytes, and aspermia in the chronic stages.

Serology

Because other bacteria elicit antibodies that cross-react with *B. canis,* false-positive results are a problem. Hemolysis (hemoglobin) also causes false-positive results. False-negative titers can result from sequestration of infection or recent antibiotics. It can take 4 weeks to seroconvert; thus, when screening dogs for entry into to breeding kennel, a negative test on day 1 and again after 4 weeks is required.

- Rapid slide agglutination test (D-Tec CB; Pitman Moore) is an in-office screening test to detect suspects that need further testing. This test has accurate negative predictive value but false-positive titers are common. Some 99% of negatives are true negatives, whereas only one half to two thirds of positives are confirmed to be truly infected.
- Tube agglutination and agar gel immunodiffusion tests are available at commercial and state diagnostic laboratories. These titers are more specific for brucellosis but are not definitive (titers 1:50 to 1:100 are suspicious; titers ≥1:200 are highly suggestive).
- A positive blood culture is based on the characteristically prolonged bacteremia of brucellosis. Urine, semen, vaginal discharges, and aborted fetal tissues can also be cultured for *Brucella* organisms

KEY POINT ▶ Although a single high titer usually is indicative of active brucellosis, a positive blood culture is the gold standard for definitive diagnosis and should be used whenever possible for confirmation.

Treatment

- *Brucella* organisms are refractory to antibiotics and very difficult to eradicate (because of intracellular location and, in males, inaccessibility of blood-pros-

tate barrier). Bacteremia can recur months after cessation of treatment.
- The recommended antibiotic regimen is very expensive: minocycline (25 mg/kg, PO, every 12 hours for ≥3 weeks) combined with dihydrostreptomycin (10 mg/kg, IM, every 12 hours for 1 week). Gentamycin can be substituted for the dihydrostreptomycin. Efficacy is estimated to be about 80%.
- Less effective alternatives are doxycycline (5–10 mg/kg, PO, every 12 hours) or tetracycline (22–25 mg/kg, PO, every 8 hours) combined with dihydro-streptomycin.
- Recommend no further breeding and castration or ovariohysterectomy of infected animals
- Recommend caution for people in contact with *Brucella*-positive dogs because there have been rare instances of human infection. Canine brucellosis is regarded as a low-level public health risk.

Prevention

- Test all breeding stock for *Brucella* before entry into a breeding program and, ideally, prior to each breeding in females and once or twice yearly in males.
- Eliminate infected dogs from breeding kennels.

Supplemental Readings

LEPTOSPIROSIS

Boothe DM, Lees GE: Leptospirosis. *In* Barlough JE, ed.: *Manual of Small Animal Infectious Diseases.* New York: Churchill Livingstone, 1988, p 143.
Greene CE, Shotts EB: Leptospirosis. *In* Greene CE, ed.: *Infectious Diseases of the Dog and Cat.* Philadelphia: W. B. Saunders, 1990, p 498.

CANINE BRUCELLOSIS

Carmichael LE, Greene CE: Canine brucellosis. *In* Greene CE, ed.: *Infectious Diseases of the Dog and Cat.* Philadelphia: W. B. Saunders, 1990, p 573.
Pollock RVH, Carmichael LE: Canine brucellosis. *In* Barlough JE, ed.: *Manual of Small Animal Infectious Diseases.* New York: Churchill Livingstone, 1988, p 183.

BORRELIOSIS

Greene LT: Lyme borreliosis. *In* Greene CE, ed.: *Infectious Diseases of the Dog and Cat.* Philadelphia: W. B. Saunders, 1990, p 508.

TETANUS

Greene CE: Tetanus. *In* Greene CE, ed.: *Infectious Diseases of the Dog and Cat.* Philadelphia: W. B. Saunders, 1990, p 521.

SALMONELLOSIS, CAMPYLOBACTERIOSIS, YERSINIOSIS, TYZZER DISEASE

Fox JG, Greene CE, Jones BR: Enteric and other bacterial infections. *In* Greene CE, ed.: *Infectious Diseases of the Dog and Cat.* Philadelphia: W. B. Saunders, 1990, p 538.

FELINE PLAGUE

Macy DW, Gasper PW: Plague. *In* Greene CE, ed.: *Infectious Diseases of the Dog and Cat.* Philadelphia: W. B. Saunders, 1990, p 621.

TULAREMIA

Kaufman AF: Tularemia. *In* Greene CE, ed.: *Infectious Diseases of the Dog and Cat.* Philadelphia: W. B. Saunders, 1990, p 628.

MYCOBACTERIAL INFECTIONS

Greene CE, Kunkle GA: Mycobacterial infections. *In* Greene CE, ed.: *Infectious Diseases of the Dog and Cat.* Philadelphia: W. B. Saunders, 1990, p 558.
Wilkinson GT: Mycobacterial infections. *In* Barlough JE, ed.: *Manual of Small Animal Infectious Diseases.* New York: Churchill Livingstone, 1988, p 213.

ACTINOMYCOSIS AND NOCARDIOSIS

Hardie EM: Actinomycosis and nocardiosis. *In* Greene CE, ed.: *Infectious Diseases of the Dog and Cat.* Philadelphia: W. B. Saunders, 1990, p 585.
Love DN: Actinomycosis and nocardiosis. *In* Barlough JE, ed.: *Manual of Small Animal Infectious Diseases.* New York: Churchill Livingstone, 1988, p 203.

12 Systemic Mycoses

Robert G. Sherding

The four major deep systemic mycoses of dogs and cats are histoplasmosis, blastomycosis, coccidioidomycosis, and cryptococcosis. These are discussed in this chapter. Other fungi that usually affect individual organs are discussed in the appropriate organ-system chapters; for example, phycomycosis (oomycosis, zygomycosis) is described in sec. 7, ch. 6; nasal aspergillosis is described in sec. 6, ch. 21; and several cutaneous fungi are discussed in sec. 5, chs. 1 and 3.

KEY POINT ▶ Histoplasmosis, blastomycosis, and coccidioidomycosis are endemic to defined regions of North America (Fig. 1).

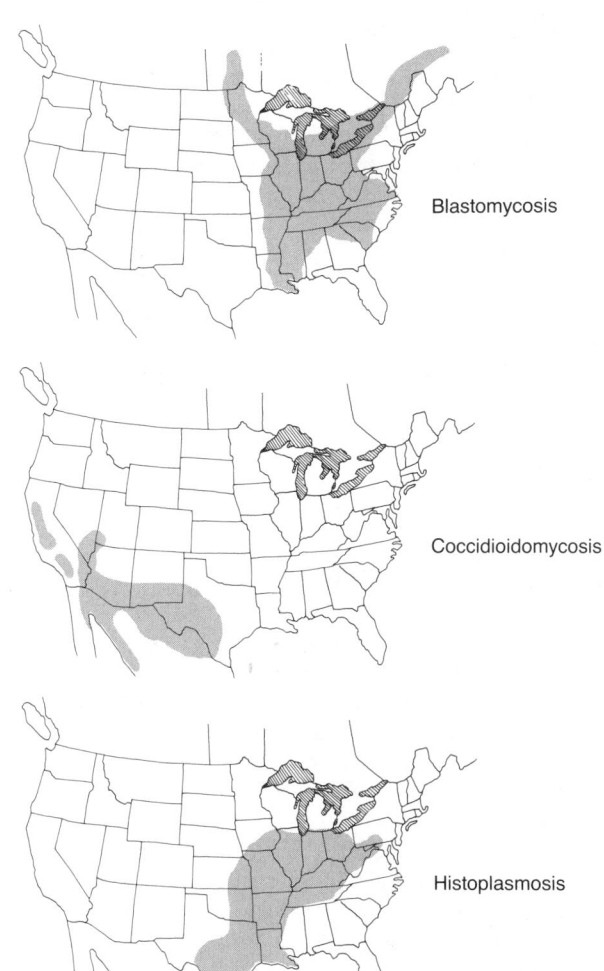

Figure 1. Geographic distribution of blastomycosis, coccidioidomycosis, and histoplasmosis in North America.

HISTOPLASMOSIS

Etiology

- The cause of histoplasmosis, *Histoplasma capsulatum,* is a dimorphic soilborne fungus found in many temperate and subtropical regions of the world. In North America, the disease is most prevalent in the river valley regions of the central United States, especially in areas bordering the Mississippi River and its tributaries (see Fig. 1).
- At ambient temperatures, soil enriched by decomposing nitrogenous matter (eg., feces of birds or bats) provides an ideal growth media for the mycelial phase of *Histoplasma.* The principal route of infection is by inhalation of airborne spores and mycelial fragments in windblown soil; however, intestinal infection via ingestion also may occur. At body temperature (37°C), *Histoplasma* organisms transform into a yeast phase that causes intracellular infection of macrophages.
- Histoplasmosis primarily invades the lung and cells of the mononuclear phagocyte system, but widespread hemolymphatic dissemination to virtually any tissue or organ system can occur.
- The outcome of exposure is influenced by level of exposure, age (clinical disease is most common in young animals less than 5 years of age), breed (highest incidence in sporting and hound breeds, perhaps due to higher exposure risk), immunosuppressive factors (steroids may enhance dissemination), and host cell–mediated immunity. Inapparent infections without evidence of clinical disease are common.

Clinical Signs

Benign Asymptomatic Pulmonary Form

The benign form is an inapparent, self-limiting infection confined to the respiratory tract and is the most common outcome of natural infection. It is recognized radiographically as multiple, discrete, calcified interstitial foci (inactive encapsulated or healed lesions) and sometimes as calcified tracheobronchial lymph nodes.

Acute Pulmonary Form

The acute pulmonary form of histoplasmosis is characterized by severe fulminant granulomatous pneumonia with signs of cough, dyspnea, fever, and severe malaise. The radiographic findings are pronounced diffuse linear or nodular interstitial infiltrates, often with patchy alveolar infiltrates and moderately enlarged tracheobronchial lymph nodes.

Chronic Pulmonary Form

Chronic histoplasmosis is more common than the acute form and is characterized by chronic granulomatous pneumonia (diffuse or multifocal) with marked tracheobronchial lymphadenopathy that causes extrinsic airway compression. Clinical signs include chronic cough and mild dyspnea with variable weight loss and fever. Radiographically, massive enlargement of the tracheobronchial lymph nodes and variable linear or interstitial infiltrates are seen.

Intestinal Form

Intestinal histoplasmosis is the most common extrapulmonary form in dogs and may represent dissemination or primary infection by ingestion. The colon, small intestine, or a combination of both can be affected by extensive granulomatous thickening of the bowel wall and mucosal ulceration, often accompanied by mesenteric and visceral lymphadenopathy. Intractable diarrhea and progressive weight loss are the most consistent clinical signs.

- Granulomatous colitis—bloody-mucoid large bowel diarrhea and tenesmus (when the rectum is involved, mucosal proliferations may be detected by digital palpation of the rectum)
- Granulomatous enteritis—voluminous watery small bowel diarrhea, malabsorption, cachexia, protein-losing enteropathy, and palpably thickened intestines
- Other signs—fever, pallor, inappetance, vomiting, lethargy, and abdominal effusion

Other Extrapulmonary Disseminated Forms

Extrapulmonary dissemination may produce a diversity of acute or chronic manifestations, with or without clinical evidence of accompanying pulmonary involvement. The macrophage-monocyte system is a common site of dissemination.

- Liver—hepatomegaly, icterus, ascites
- Spleen—splenomegaly
- Lymph nodes—peripheral or abdominal lymphadenopathy
- Bone marrow—anemia
- Peritoneum—omental masses, mesenteric adhesions, nodular or granular serosal surfaces
- Eyes—exudative anterior uveitis, multifocal granulomatous chorioretinitis, optic neuritis
- Central nervous system—ataxia, seizures, etc.
- Skin—fistulous tracts that drain pus or subcutaneous nodules
- Bone—lameness associated with proliferative or lytic bony lesions
- Oral cavity—ulcers

Diagnosis

Histoplasmosis should be suspected on the basis of clinical signs in animals from endemic areas. The results of routine laboratory evaluations are variable and nonspecific. Radiographic findings in the pulmonary form are often highly suggestive of histoplasmosis. Serology provides a presumptive diagnosis, but identification of the *Histoplasma* organisms is necessary for definitive diagnosis.

Hematology

- Normochromic-normocytic nonregenerative anemia
  - Can be the result of chronic inflammation, dissemination of *Histoplasma* into the bone marrow, intestinal blood loss, or hemolysis
- Neutrophilic leukocytosis or neutropenia with left shift, monocytosis
  - *Histoplasma* organisms may be seen within circulating monocytes or neutrophils on routine blood smears, especially if 1000 cells are examined in differential cell counts or if buffy coat smears are examined.
- Thrombocytopenia
  - Usually mild and subclinical; however, platelet counts of less than 50,000/µl are occasionally seen in association with macroplatelets in the circulation and increased megakaryocytes in the bone marrow, suggesting platelet consumption or destruction.

Chemistry Evaluations

- Hypoalbuminemia, with or without concomitant hyperglobulinemia
  - Usually mild, but may be pronounced in dogs with severe protein-losing enteropathy.
- Elevated serum liver enzymes and bilirubin (with hepatic dissemination)
- Abnormal absorption tests in diffuse small intestinal disease
  - Impaired xylose absorption
  - Increased fecal fat
  - Decreased serum levels of folate and cobalamin (see sec. 7, ch. 6)

Radiography

- Thoracic radiography (in the pulmonary form of histoplasmosis)
  - Linear or nodular (''miliary'') interstitial pulmonary infiltrates
  - Hilar density around the tracheal bifurcation due to tracheobronchial lymphadenopathy
  - Patchy alveolar infiltrates, calcified pulmonary interstitial nodules (healed lesions), and calcified tracheobronchial lymph nodes
- Contrast barium radiography (in the intestinal form of histoplasmosis)
  - Irregularity of the intestinal mucosa and thickening of the bowel wall, which are nonspecific indicators of a diffuse infiltrative lesion
- Other radiographic findings (depending on sites of dissemination)
  - Hepatosplenomegaly
  - Abdominal or thoracic effusions
  - Lytic-proliferative bone lesions

Serology

- Tests that detect anti-*Histoplasma* antibodies are not sufficiently reliable for definitive diagnosis; thus, every effort should be made to confirm infections through identification of the *Histoplasma* organisms.
- A complement fixation titer of 1:16 or greater or a positive agar-gel immunodiffusion (AGID) (precipitin) test is considered strongly suggestive of histoplasmosis.
- Unfortunately, these tests often yield false-negative results in animals with histoplasmosis. In addition, other mycotic infections (e.g., blastomycosis) may cross-react on serodiagnostic tests for histoplasmosis, and anticomplementary sera may make complement fixation unusable in some animals.

KEY POINT ▶ Definitive diagnosis of histoplasmosis requires identification of *Histoplasma* organisms in cytology, biopsy, or culture specimens.

Cytology

Exfoliative cytology and fine-needle aspiration generally are the most practical and high-yield methods for definitive diagnosis of histoplasmosis. Wright, Giemsa, or Diff-Quik stains (American Scientific Products, McGraw Park, IL) are ideal for identification of *Histoplasma* in cytology preparations. The organisms are found most often intracellularly within the cytoplasm of macrophages as round to oval bodies, 2 to 4 μm in size, surrounded by a characteristic clear halo or "pseudocapsule" that results from shrinkage during staining. Sources of cytologic specimens with potential diagnostic benefit depend on sites of involvement.

- Respiratory tract—bronchoscopic alveolar lavage, transtracheal washing, fine-needle lung aspirate
- Intestinal tract—smears of rectal mucosal scrapings, impression smears of endoscopic biopsies, and fine-needle aspirates of abdominal lymph nodes or intestinal masses
  - Consider endoscopy of the colon and duodenum for the collection of diagnostic cytology or biopsy specimens. Histoplasmosis lesions appear endoscopically as areas of irregular mucosal thickening and proliferation that produce a corrugated or cobblestone appearance, with or without mucosal hemorrhage and ulceration.
- Liver, spleen, or lymph node aspirates
- Abdominal or thoracic effusions
- Bone marrow aspirates and buffy coat smears of peripheral blood
- Skin lesion impression smears
- Oculocentesis

Histopathology

Biopsies of affected tissues reveal granulomatous inflammation, but organisms are usually sparse and difficult to see with H&E stain. Detection of organisms in biopsies may be facilitated by use of special fungal stains such as periodic acid–Schiff (PAS), Grocott-Gomori methenamine silver nitrate, or Gridley.

Culture

Any of the specimens mentioned above for cytologic or biopsy identification of *Histoplasma* also can be used to culture the fungi in Sabouraud's media; however, these fungi are difficult to isolate in culture and require 10 to 14 days for growth.

Treatment

Treat histoplasmosis with ketoconazole, amphotericin B, or a combination of these. Treatment regimens and prevention are discussed at the end of this chapter.

BLASTOMYCOSIS

Etiology

- *Blastomyces dermatitidis* is a dimorphic soilborne fungus with a geographic distribution (see Fig. 1) similar to that of *Histoplasma*.
- Inhalation of soilborne spores is the primary route of infection and leads to mycotic pneumonia. In addition, primary skin infection sometimes occurs from direct cutaneous inoculation. Extrapulmonary dissemination is very common in blastomycosis.
- Dogs are considered highly susceptible to blastomycosis, and the canine infection rate in endemic areas is ten times the human infection rate.

Clinical Signs

Young (<5 years) male large-breed dogs are most frequently infected. Blastomycosis is relatively rare in cats. Nonspecific signs of fever, anorexia, weight loss, and depression are common.

Pulmonary Form

Cough and dyspnea are typical presenting signs. Respiratory manifestations may include (in decreasing order of frequency):

- Acute or chronic interstitial pyogranulomatous pneumonia, usually involving all lung lobes diffusely, sometimes focally
- Tracheobronchial lymphadenopathy
- Pleural effusion

Extrapulmonary Disseminated Form

Blastomycosis very commonly disseminates, especially to the skin (40% of cases) and eyes (40% of cases), and to a lesser extent to the peripheral lymph nodes, bone, central nervous system (CNS), male genitalia, oral cavity, and nasal cavity.

- Cutaneous blastomycosis may be manifested as fistulas that drain pus or bloody fluid, circumscribed raised ulcerating pyogranulomas, deep abscesses, paronychia, and regional lymphadenopathy.
- Ocular involvement may include anterior uveitis, chorioretinitis, or panophthalmitis.
- Fungal osteomyelitis is manifested as lameness and swelling.

- CNS involvement may cause seizures, dementia, blindness, or ataxia.
- Granulomatous orchitis and prostatitis occur in 11% of infected male dogs.

Diagnosis

Hematology

Typical findings are a regenerative neutrophilic leukocytosis, mild nonregenerative anemia, and monocytosis.

Thoracic Radiography

Radiography generally reveals a nodular (usually miliary) or diffuse pulmonary interstitial infiltrate and moderate tracheobronchial lymphadenopathy. Less frequent findings include alveolar infiltrates, lobar consolidation, focal solitary nodules, pleural effusion, and cavitary lesions.

Serology

Serology provides a presumptive diagnosis of blastomycosis based on a positive AGID test (90% reliable) or a complement fixation titer of 1:32 or greater.

Cytology, Biopsy, and Sabouraud's Culture

Identification of *Blastomyces* organisms by one of these methods is required for definitive diagnosis. The source of specimens and method of procurement depend on sites of involvement.

- *Blastomyces* in tissues appears as an extracellular yeast (5–20 μ) with broad-based budding and a prominent, double-refractile cell wall. The stains mentioned for histoplasmosis can be used.
- Cytologies most often diagnostic for blastomycosis include pulmonary cytology (transtracheal washing, bronchoalveolar lavage, fine-needle lung aspirate), skin impression smears, and lymph node aspirates; however, any affected tissue can be sampled. Specimens for culture can be collected in a similar manner as for histoplasmosis.

KEY POINT ▶ Since *Blastomyces* yeast bodies are usually plentiful and easily identified in lesions, cytologies are the initial diagnostic tests of choice because of ease and rapidity of results.

- In blastomycosis lesions, fungal organisms are generally more prevalent and easily identified than in histoplasmosis lesions, and the inflammation is more pyogranulomatous than granulomatous.

Treatment

Blastomycosis can be treated with either ketoconazole or amphotericin B as individual drugs, but a combination of these is probably better. Treatment regimens and prevention are discussed at the end of this chapter.

COCCIDIOIDOMYCOSIS

Etiology

- *Coccidioides immitis* is a soilborne fungus distributed geographically to the dry, desert-like regions of the southwestern United States (see Fig. 1). In the soil, *Coccidioides* grow as mycelia that form arthrospores.
- Infection occurs by inhalation of these soilborne and windblown arthrospores. Cutaneous inoculation may occur, but rarely. In body tissues, *Coccidioides* form large spherules (20–100 μ) that release hundreds of endospores.

Clinical Signs

Self-limiting Inapparent Form

This subclinical form of coccidioidomycosis is common.

Pulmonary Form

Pulmonary coccidioidomycosis is characterized by acute or chronic granulomatous pneumonia and tracheobronchial lymphadenopathy with signs of cough, fever, malaise, and occasionally dyspnea.

Extrapulmonary Disseminated Form

This form is usually chronic and may involve the bones and joints (mostly osteoproliferative bone reaction), abdominal viscera (spleen, liver, lymph nodes, omentum, kidneys), heart and pericardium, eyes, CNS, male genitalia, and skin (usually fistulas over bone lesions).

Diagnosis

Hematology

Findings may include a variable leukocytosis, monocytosis, and anemia.

Radiography

Granulomatous pneumonia and hilar lymphadenopathy are similar to that described for histoplasmosis. Dissemination to bone is common, especially to the long bones, and it results in multifocal osteoproliferative lesions on radiographs.

Serology

A fairly reliable presumptive diagnosis can be made on the basis of the precipitin test, which detects the early IgM response, and the complement fixation test, which detects the later and sustained IgG response.

Cytology, Biopsy, and Sabouraud's Culture

Definitive diagnosis depends on identifying the organisms (spherules) in affected tissues, using cytology, biopsy, or culturing on Sabouraud's media as described for histoplasmosis and blastomycosis.

Treatment

Coccidioidomycosis usually is treated with oral ketoconazole for a minimum of 8 to 12 months, and sometimes indefinitely, using the regimens described in the last section of this chapter. Amphotericin B is not quite as effective but can be used in animals that do not tolerate ketoconazole.

CRYPTOCOCCOSIS

Etiology

- *Cryptococcus neoformans* is found in many geographic regions. Infection is acquired from inhalation of soilborne organisms or, usually in urban areas, from inhalation of organisms found in pigeon excreta.
- The organisms are budding yeasts (4–7 μ) that possess a prominent polysaccharide capsule. This thick capsule is essential to the pathogenicity of this fungus, in that it inhibits plasma cell function, phagocytosis, leukocyte migration, and complement. The capsule also allows the organisms to stand out in stained cytology preparations for easy identification and is the basis for the cryptococcal capsular antigen diagnostic test.

Clinical Signs

KEY POINT ▶ In cats, *Cryptococcus* has a predilection for the nasal cavity, where the airborne organisms initially deposit, accounting for the chronic granulomatous rhinitis and sinusitis seen in at least 50% of cats with the disease.

In contrast to cats, clinically evident nasal disease is rare in dogs with cryptococcosis; instead, CNS and eye involvement are the predominant findings. Surprisingly, lung involvement is evident clinically only rarely; yet 50% of dogs and cats have lung lesions at necropsy. Fever occurs in less than 25% of the cases; in fact, temperatures exceeding 37°C inhibit *Cryptococcus*.

Nasal Form

The principal signs of nasal involvement are unilateral or bilateral mucopurulent or bloody nasal discharge, sneezing, sniffling, deformity of overlying nasal bones, and mucinous nasal granulomas at the nostril.

Extra-respiratory Disseminated Form

The preferred sites for dissemination are the CNS (cats, 25%; dogs, over 50%), eyes (cats, 25%; dogs, over 50%), and skin (cats and dogs, 25–30%).

- CNS involvement is mostly from local extension through the cribiform plate that results in diffuse or mass-like granulomatous meningoencephalitis or myelitis. Signs may include seizures, circling, head-pressing, blindness, dementia, ataxia, paresis, and cranial nerve (CN) deficits (eg., CN II, VII, VIII).
- Eye involvement may include granulomatous (exu-

dative) chorioretinitis, anterior uveitis, and optic neuritis.
- Skin involvement usually manifests as firm nodules that rapidly enlarge and then ulcerate and ooze, mostly in the head area, and often near the nostrils.
- Other dissemination sites may include peripheral lymph nodes (especially the submandibulars), pharynx and oral cavity, kidneys (30% of animals have granulomas at necropsy), liver, spleen, heart, and skeletal muscle.

Diagnosis

Hematology

Findings are often normal, except for occasional neutrophilia or eosinophilia.

Radiography

Nasal radiographs may indicate nasal bone lysis or expansion or an abnormal soft tissue density within the nasal cavity or frontal sinus.

Serology

Serologic testing provides a presumptive diagnosis based on detection of capsular antigen in serum, cerebrospinal fluid (CSF), or urine using latex agglutination or complement fixation. False-negative results may occur, especially in nondisseminated disease.

Cytology, Biopsy, and Sabouraud's Culture

Definitive diagnosis requires identification of the organisms in cytologies (eg., nasal exudate, CSF, skin exudate or impressions, lymph node aspirates, urine, oculocentesis) using Gram's, PAS, new methylene blue, or India ink stains or in biopsies using mucicarmine, H&E, PAS, or silver stains. *Cryptococcus* can also be cultured from similar specimens on Sabouraud's media.

Treatment

Treat cryptococcosis with ketoconazole, amphotericin B, or flucytosine combined with amphotericin B, as discussed in the following section.

TREATMENT OF SYSTEMIC MYCOSES

Systemic mycoses are generally progressive without treatment. Effective treatment regimens have included:

- An azole derivative, such as either ketoconazole (Nizoral, Janssen) or itraconazole (Janssen), as single drugs
- Amphoteracin B (Fungizone, Squibb) as a single drug
- Dual therapy using a combination of amphotericin B and ketoconazole or amphoteracin B and 5-flucytosine

General Principles of Treatment

- The oral azoles, such as ketoconazole and itraconazole, are currently the first-choice antifungal drugs for single-agent treatment if the disease is not fulminating or life-threatening. The newer generation azole, itraconazole, appears to be particularly promising and should be commercially available in the near future. Preliminary results suggest that itraconazole may be more effective than ketoconazole because it has better absorption, greater potency, quicker onset of action, longer duration of action, and less toxicity.

■ The major disadvantages of amphotericin B are that it must be given intravenously and is frequently nephrotoxic. Nevertheless, amphotericin B can be combined with ketoconazole or itraconazole for the initial treatment of advanced or rapidly progressing infections because of its more rapid onset of antifungal activity and because clinical experience suggests combination antifungal therapy may be more effective than either drug alone.

KEY POINT ▶ Regardless of the treatment regimen, the unpredictable response in the disseminated forms of the disease should dictate a guarded prognosis, especially if the CNS is involved.

Ketoconazole

Ketoconazole is the initial drug of choice for treatment of histoplasmosis and coccidioidomycosis. It is effective in most cats and some dogs with cryptococcosis. For blastomycosis, it is most effective after initial treatment with amphoteracin B.

Pharmacology

■ The advantages of ketoconazole, a synthetic imidazole, as a first-choice drug for treatment of the systemic mycoses are the convenience of oral administration and the absence of nephrotoxicity.

■ Ketoconazole depends on hepatobiliary metabolism and excretion, and it is distributed widely except in the CNS, eye, and testes.

■ Acidity is required for optimal absorption of ketoconazole; thus, avoid concurrent use of antacids or drugs such as H_2 blockers that inhibit gastric acid secretion. There is conflicting evidence concerning whether the drug is absorbed better in fasted or fed animals; however, because nausea and vomiting seem to be less of a problem if the daily dosage is divided and given with food, I prefer this approach.

KEY POINT ▶ Ketoconazole inhibits the biosynthesis of ergosterol in the fungal cell membrane. Because the onset of this fungistatic effect may be delayed for 1 to 2 weeks after therapy is initiated, the clinical response to ketoconazole may be slow.

Induction Therapy

The usual oral dosage of ketoconazole for induction therapy in both dogs and cats ranges from 10 to 30 mg/kg/day. Divide this total daily dose into two or three doses for better gastrointestinal tolerance.

■ For dogs—use the higher end of this range (20–30 mg/kg).

■ For cats—start at the lower end of this dosage range (10–20 mg/kg/day, or a total dose of 50 mg once daily) because cats generally are more susceptible to the side effects of ketoconazole. If tolerance is still a problem in a cat, administer a dosage of 20 mg/kg on alternate days.

Maintenance Therapy

■ Once remission is achieved, ketoconazole is continued at a maintenance dosage of at least 10 mg/kg/day for an additional 3 to 4 months (6–8 months in coccidioidomycosis). The total duration of therapy is usually at least 4 to 6 months (8–12 months or longer in coccidioidomycosis).

■ Because ketoconazole is a fungistatic drug, the duration of therapy is variable and relapses have occurred up to 1 year after therapy was discontinued. If recrudescence occurs, a full course of ketoconazole is reinstituted for at least another 6 to 8 months.

Combination Therapy

For initial treatment of advanced or rapidly progressing disseminated infections, use amphotericin B (see below) in combination with ketoconazole for the first few weeks. This regimen provides faster antifungal action and may increase the remission rate.

KEY POINT ▶ If there is CNS, ocular, or genital involvement, the initial daily dosage of ketoconazole may need to be 40 mg/kg to reach effective tissue concentrations, although this dosage will increase the risk of side effects. Recommend castration of dogs with mycotic orchitis or prostatitis, such as occurs in blastomycosis.

Side Effects

■ The most common immediate side effects of ketoconazole are anorexia, vomiting, and diarrhea. These can usually be minimized by dividing the daily doses and administering them with food.

■ Longer-term side effects may include hepatotoxicity (hepatomegaly, elevated serum liver enzymes, icterus), weight loss, and haircoat changes (lightening of color, alopecia). Because of hepatic effects it is advisable to monitor serum liver enzymes monthly during treatment. The liver, gastrointestinal and haircoat reactions are usually reversible with reduction in dosage.

■ Ketoconazole inhibits adrenal and testicular steroidogenesis. In dogs, but not cats, ketoconazole diminishes serum testosterone and cortisol while increasing serum progesterone. Ketoconazole is embryotoxic and teratogenic and thus should not be used in pregnant animals.

Itraconazole and Other Newer Azoles
Itraconazole

Itraconazole is a newer generation azole derivative that should soon be available commercially as an oral antifungal drug.

- Dosage: Administer in both dogs and cats at 5 mg/kg, PO, once or twice daily. As with ketoconazole, consider combining amphotericin B with itraconazole as initial therapy in animals with rapidly progressive, life-threatening systemic mycotic infection.
- Side effects: Although itraconazole may cause anorexia and hepatotoxicity, it has fewer liver and gastrointestinal side effects than ketoconazole, especially in cats, and it does not appear to inhibit adrenal and testicular steroidogenesis. Experimentally, dogs have received daily dosages of 40 mg/kg for 3 months without toxicity. An occasional side effect noted in treated animals is vasculitis, which produces ulcerative skin lesions and limb edema. This adverse reaction appears to be dose-dependent and reversible.

Fluconazole and Other Azoles

Fluconazole and other azoles are currently in development or under investigation. They may be found effective for treatment of intestinal or disseminated histoplasmosis. Documented reports of successful use of these agents in animals are lacking, but these drugs generally have improved potency and a broader spectrum of antifungal activity with less toxicity than ketoconazole. The major advantage of fluconazole over other azoles is its much better penetration of the CNS in fungal meningitis; a disadvantage is that it is expensive.

Amphotericin B

As a single drug, amphotericin B is most effective for treatment of blastomycosis and histoplasmosis. It is moderately effective for cryptococcosis and coccidioidomycosis. In severe cases of blastomycosis and histoplasmosis, combine amphotericin B with ketoconazole for an initial 2- to 4-week induction phase of therapy, and then follow up with ketoconazole for several months of maintenance.

Pharmacology

- Amphotericin B (Fungizone; Squibb) is a polyene antibiotic for IV use that has both fungicidal and fungistatic actions. It binds to ergosterol of fungal cell membranes, thereby causing cell membrane damage and leakage of cell contents.
- Amphotericin B distributes well into most tissues, except for the CNS and eye. It is metabolized locally in the tissues; thus, its elimination is not impaired in situations of nephrotoxicity.
- Amphotericin B is available as a powder in a 50-mg vial that is first reconstituted with 10 ml of sterile water that does not contain any preservatives. Because amphotericin B forms a precipitate in acidic or electrolyte solutions, only 5% dextrose-in-water solution should be used for the final dilution. The drug is light-sensitive and should be protected from prolonged exposure to direct light. The reconstituted product has stable potency for 1 day at room temperature and 7 days at refrigerator temperature (4° C).

Dosage and Administration

- In dogs, administer amphotericin B at a dose of 0.5 mg/kg, IV, on alternate days for 3 days per week, such as a Monday-Wednesday-Friday schedule.
- In cats, use a lower dosage of 0.15–0.25 mg/kg, IV, because of greater sensitivity to the toxic effects of the drug.
- There are two basic methods of administration: rapid and slow IV infusion techniques.
  - In the rapid infusion technique, dilute the dose of amphotericin B in 20–60 ml of 5% dextrose solution and give as an IV injection over 3 to 5 minutes.
  - In the slow infusion technique, dilute the dosage in 250–500 ml of 5% dextrose solution and give as a constant-rate IV infusion over a period of 4 to 6 hours or more. This slower, more diluted drip method of delivery is preferred because it may reduce the nephrotoxicity of amphotericin B, although this is unproven.
- In advanced, life-threatening fungal disease, use either a high-dose protocol of 1.0 mg/kg every other day or an accelerated protocol of 0.5 mg/kg daily. Both of these methods increase the risk of nephrotoxicity, although less so with the high-dose alternate-day protocol.

Renoprotective Measures

These measures are aimed at enhancing renal blood flow and glomerular filtration rate to reduce nephrotoxicity (see section on Side Effects), although efficacy has not been well documented.

- Hydration of the patient prior to treatment is an important consideration for preventing nephrotoxicity.
- Dilution of amphotericin in 5% dextrose solution and administration by the slow IV infusion method over a period of 4 to 6 hours or more seems to lower the risk of nephrotoxicity.
- One or more of the following proposed renal-sparing treatments may be given with each amphotericin treatment:
  - Concurrent administration of mannitol (Vedco), 0.5–1.0 g/kg, IV
  - Saline loading to promote a sodium diuresis— 0.9% sodium chloride solution, 50 ml/kg, IV, given over a period of 1 to 3 hours before amphotericin or concurrently using a different vein to avoid amphotericin precipitation
  - Furosemide (Lasix), 2 mg/kg, IV
  - Aminophylline, 6–10 mg/kg

Duration of Therapy

- If amphotericin B is used as a single drug, continue treatment for 6 to 12 weeks until a minimum total cumulative dosage of 9–12 mg/kg is achieved or for at least 1 month beyond clinical remission.
- If amphotericin B is used in combination with ketoconazole, give amphotericin for the first 3 to 4 weeks to induce remission until the total cumulative dosage reaches 4–6 mg/kg, at which time continue ketoconazole alone for maintenance.

Side Effects

The major side effect of amphotericin B is nephrotoxicity. Other side effects in dogs and cats include transient fever of 24 to 36 hours in duration after the first dose, anorexia, nausea/vomiting, thrombophlebitis (local irritant effect), and perivascular irritation if extravasated.

■ Nephrotoxicity is due to a combination of reduced renal blood flow (arteriolar vasoconstriction) and direct renal tubular injury. Although there is considerable individual variation in susceptibility to nephrotoxicity, most animals treated with amphotericin B show some degree of renal dysfunction.

■ Urinalysis and renal function (serum creatinine, BUN) should be evaluated before initiating amphotericin therapy and should be monitored frequently during treatment. In general, the earliest evidence of a renal effect is decreased urine specific gravity. This is followed by abnormal numbers of renal cells and casts in the urine sediment, and eventually azotemia may develop.

KEY POINT ▶ If BUN exceeds 50 mg/dl or serum creatinine exceeds 2.5 mg/dl during amphotericin therapy, treatment should be suspended until BUN/creatinine levels return to normal. Azotemia in most cases is reversible when the drug is discontinued.

Flucytosine

Flucytosine (5-FC) (Ancobon; Roche) is an antimitotic, antifungal drug used in conjunction with amphotericin B for treatment of cryptococcosis. It is especially useful when there is CNS involvement, because 5-FC attains 60–80% of serum concentration in CSF.

■ Use 5-FC only in combination with amphotericin B, because fungal resistance develops rapidly if it is used alone.

Dosage

Give 25–50 mg/kg, PO, q6–8h, or 125–250 mg total dose/day for cats.

Side Effects

The toxicity of 5-FC is hepatic and hematologic (leukopenia, thrombocytopenia).

PREVENTION

Because the principal source of systemic mycotic infection is windblown fungal elements from the soil, there is no practical means of prevention in endemic areas. High concentrations of *Histoplasma* can be found in chicken excreta, and of *Cryptococcus* in pigeon excreta; thus, exposure to these sources should be avoided. Animal-to-animal transmission of these mycotic infections is not likely. Although humans can be infected from the same environmental sources as animals, animal-to-human transmission is very rare. Vaccination for these mycoses is not available.

Supplemental Reading

Armstrong PJ, DiBartola SP: Canine coccidioidomycosis: A literature review and report of 8 cases. J Am Anim Hosp Assoc 19:937, 1983.

Barsanti JA, Jeffery KL: Coccidioidomycosis. *In* Green CE, ed.: *Infectious Diseases of the Dog and Cat*. Philadelphia: W. B. Saunders, 1990, p 696.

Clinkenbeard KD, Wolf AM, Cowell RL, Tyler RL: Canine disseminated histoplasmosis. Comp Cont Educ 11:1347, 1989.

Ford, RB: Canine histoplasmosis. Comp Cont Educ 2:637, 1980.

Grant SM, Clissold SP: Itraconazole: A review of its pharmacodynamic and pharmacokinetic properties, and therapeutic use in superficial and systemic mycoses. Drugs 37:310, 1989.

Greene CE: Antifungal chemotherapy. *In* Green CE, ed.: *Infectious Diseases of the Dog and Cat*. Philadelphia: W. B. Saunders, 1990, p 649.

Legendre AM: Systemic mycotic infections. *In* Sherding RG, ed.: *The Cat: Diseases and Clinical Management*. New York: Churchill Livingstone, 1989, p 427.

Legendre AM: Blastomycosis. *In* Green CE, ed.: *Infectious Diseases of the Dog and Cat*. Philadelphia: W. B. Saunders, 1990, p 669.

Medleau L: Imidazoles and triazoles. *In* Kirk RW, ed.: *Current Veterinary Therapy X*. Philadelphia: W. B. Saunders, 1989, p 577.

Medleau L, Barsanti JA: Cryptococcosis. *In* Green CE, ed.: *Infectious Diseases of the Dog and Cat*. Philadelphia: W. B. Saunders, 1990, p 687.

Mitchell M, Stark DR: Disseminated canine histoplasmosis: A clinical survey of 24 cases in Texas. Can Vet J 21:95, 1980.

Moriello, KA: Ketoconazole: Clinical pharmacology and therapeutic recommendations. J Am Vet Med Assoc 188:303, 1986.

Noxon JO: Systemic antifungal chemotherapy. *In* Kirk RW, ed.: *Current Veterinary Therapy X*. Philadelphia: W. B. Saunders, 1989, p 1101.

Stickle JE, Hribernik TN: Clinicopathological observations in disseminated histoplasmosis in dogs. J Am Anim Hosp Assoc 14:105, 1978.

Willard MD: Treatment of fungal and endocrine disorders with imidazole derivatives. *In* Kirk RW, ed.: *Current Veterinary Therapy X*. Philadelphia: W. B. Saunders, 1989, p 82.

Wolf AM, Belden MN: Feline histoplasmosis: A literature review and retrospective review of 20 new cases. J Am Anim Hosp Assoc 20:995, 1984.

Wolf AM, Troy GC: Deep mycotic diseases. *In* Ettinger SJ, ed.: *Textbook of Veterinary Internal Medicine*. Philadelphia: W. B. Saunders, 1989, p 341.

Toxoplasmosis, Neosporosis, and Other Multisystemic Protozoal Infections

Robert G. Sherding

The protozoa that infect dogs and cats can be broadly classified into two categories: those that primarily live in the intestinal tract and those that disseminate and cause multisystemic disease. Enteric protozoal infections include intestinal coccidiosis, giardiasis, trichomoniasis, amebiasis, and balantidiasis (see sec. 7, ch. 6).

Toxoplasmosis, the most important multisystemic protozoal infectious disease in North America, is described in detail in this chapter, along with neosporosis. Several other multisystemic protozoal infections are important in tropical and subtropical regions of the world but are relatively uncommon in the United States. These are summarized in Table 1 and include diseases transmitted by insect vectors, such as leishmaniasis, trypanosomiasis (Chagas disease), hepatozoonosis, babesiosis, and cytauxzoonosis, and others that are transmitted without vectors, including encephalitozoonosis, acanthamebiasis, and pneumocystosis. Protozoa that parasitize erythrocytes, such as *Babesia* spp and *Cytauxzoon felis,* are discussed in sec. 3, ch. 1.

TOXOPLASMOSIS

Etiology

Toxoplasma gondii is an obligate intracellular protozoan parasite. The feline species is the definitive host for this coccidia, but most warm-blooded animals can be infected as intermediate hosts, including dogs and humans. Serologic surveys in the United States estimate that 30% of cats and 25 to 50% of humans have been infected.

Routes of Transmission

Ingestion of Infected Animal Tissues. The ingestion of meat (carnivorism) that contains *Toxoplasma* cysts is the primary source of infection in cats. This includes uncooked meat (or meat scraps scavenged from garbage) or hunted prey (mice, birds, etc). Ingestion of raw or undercooked meat also is an important source of toxoplasmosis in dogs and humans. Ingestion of tachyzoites in raw milk, especially from goats, can be a source of infection.

Ingestion of Oocysts Shed in Cat Feces. Food, water, and soil contaminated with sporulated *Toxoplasma* oocysts are potentially important sources of infection for intermediate hosts such as humans, dogs, food-producing animals, and rodents. This is a relatively minor source of infection in the primary host, the cat. Oocysts can be transported by cockroaches, flies, and earthworms.

Congenital (Transplacental) Infection. When a pregnant animal or human becomes infected during gestation, *Toxoplasma* can cross the placenta and infect the unborn fetus. For this reason, toxoplasmosis has major public health significance in humans. In dogs and cats, congenital toxoplasmosis is uncommon, but it can be a cause of abortion, stillbirth, or neonatal mortality.

Stages of Infection

Fecal Oocyst Stage of Infection (Sporozoite Stage). In cats that ingest infected meat from an intermediate host, the encysted *Toxoplasma* are liberated by the digestive enzymes and invade the intestinal epithelial cells. Multiplication within the intestinal epithelium results in fecal excretion of millions of oocysts beginning 3 to 10 days after exposure and continuing for 1 to 2 weeks. Infection by oocyst ingestion is a less important source in cats, but when it does occur, subsequent shedding of oocysts is delayed for 3 weeks or more and is much less pronounced. As excreted, oocysts are oval-shaped, 10×12 μm in size, and unsporulated. To become infectious, excreted oocysts must first sporulate, which takes at least 24 hours and as long as 3 weeks. These sporulated oocysts can remain infectious in the environment for months, and in soil for longer than 1 year. Clinical signs, if they occur at all, usually do not develop until the period of oocyst shedding is over.

KEY POINT ▶ Fecal excretion of *Toxoplasma* oocysts, which can contaminate soil, water, and food and infect other animals, occurs only in the definitive host, the cat.

Acute Tissue Stage of Infection (Tachyzoite Stage). Simultaneous with intestinal multiplication in cats or following infection by ingestion or transplacental transfer in any species, *Toxoplasma* invades extraintestinal tissues via blood and lymph. Almost any cell in any tissue can be parasitized by these rapidly-multiplying tachyzoite forms. The tachyzoites eventu-

TABLE 1. Systemic Protozoan Infections of the Dog and Cat

Diseases	Etiology (Source)	Endemic Locations	Clinical Signs	Diagnosis	Treatment
Leishmaniasis	*Leishmania* spp (sandfly vector; bloodborne)	Southwest U.S. (rarely; Texas, Oklahoma), Mediterranean region, Central and South America, Asia, Africa	*Disease in dogs only:* chronic diffuse skin hyperkeratosis (dry scaling), dry brittle haircoat, skin nodules, mucocutaneous ulcers, fever, muscle atrophy, weakness, cachexia, anorexia, inactivity, vomiting, diarrhea, lymphadenopathy, splenomegaly, uveitis, conjunctivitis, bleeding (epistaxis, melena), immune disease (glomerulonephritis, systemic lupus, hemolytic anemia, polyarthritis).	*General:* Endemic region, hyperglobulinemia, hypoalbuminemia, proteinuria, azotemia, elevated serum liver enzymes, anemia, positive autoimmune tests (Coomb test, antinuclear antibody, LE cell test). *Specific:* —Identify organisms by cytology (lymph node, bone marrow, spleen, liver). —Serology: not as sensitive or specific.	*Caution:* Zoonotic with public health risks. *Investigational per CDC:* —Meglumine antimonate (Glucantime; Specia): 100 mg/kg; IV, SC, q24h for 1 mo. —Sodium stibogluconate (Pentostam; Wellcome): 30–50 mg/kg; IV, SC, q24h for 1 mo. *Prognosis:* Fair to good for remission but guarded to poor for cure.
American trypanosomiasis (Chagas disease)	*Trypanosoma cruzi* (reduviid "kissing" bug vector; bloodborne)	Southern U.S. (rarely), Central and South America	*Disease in dogs only:* Acute myocarditis (fever, weakness, sudden collapse, fatal tachyarrhythmias); chronic cardiomyopathy (after 1–3 years—heart failure, ascites, pleural effusion, edema); lymphadenopathy, splenomegaly, meningoencephalitis.	*General:* Endemic region, abnormal cardiac evaluations (radiographic, electrocardiographic, echocardiographic). *Specific:* —Identify organisms in blood (direct or buffy coat smear) or lymph node aspirates. —Serology: positive in active or past infection.	*Caution:* Zoonotic with public health risks. *Investigational per CDC:* —Nifurtimox (Lampit; Bayer): 2–7 mg/kg, PO, q6h for 3–5 mo. —Benznidazole: 5 mg/kg, PO, q24h for >2 mo. *Prognosis:* Poor.
Hepatozoonosis	*Hepatozoon canis* (tickborne)	U.S. (Texas, Oklahoma, Louisiana), Brazil, Europe, Asia, Africa	*Disease in dogs only:* Episodic fever, cachexia, chronic myositis and periosteal bone proliferation (reluctance to move, generalized muscle pain and atrophy), bloody diarrhea, naso-ocular discharge.	*General:* Endemic region, mild anemia, neutrophilic leukocytosis, wide-spread periosteal bone proliferation. *Specific:* Identify organisms in blood smear (in WBC) or in muscle biopsy (most reliable test).	*Palliative:* aspirin. *Efficacy unproven:* —Diminazene aceturate (Berenil 10%; Ganaseg), 3.5 mg/kg, IM, once. —Imidocarb dipropionate, (Imizol; Wellcome), 5–6 mg/kg, SC/IM, once. —Primaquine phosphate, 0.5 mg/kg, SC, once. *Prognosis:* Poor (response but no cure).
Babesiosis	*Babesia* spp. (tick vector; bloodborne)	*Dog: B. canis, B. gibsoni* (U.S. and worldwide) *Cat: B. felis,* etc. (Africa, Asia, South America)	Hemolytic anemia (pallor, depression, weakness, jaundice, hemoglobinuria, fever, splenomegaly), weight loss, subclinical carrier.	*General:* Regenerative anemia (often Coomb positive), thrombocytopenia. *Specific:* —Identify organisms in Giemsa-stained smears of capillary blood (from ear or toenail) or splenic aspirate. —Serology: IFA titer >1:40 is positive.	*Dogs:* —Diminazene aceturate (Berenil 10%; Ganaseg), 3.5 mg/kg, IM, once. —Phenamidine isethionate (Lomidine; May & Baker), 15 mg/kg, SC, q24h × 2 days. —Imidocarb dipropionate (Imizol; Wellcome), 5 mg/kg, SC or IM, once. *Cats:* —Primaquine phosphate, 0.5 mg/kg, IM, once. *Prognosis:* Good but relapses are common.
Cytauxzoonosis	*Cytauxzoon felis* (tick vector; bloodborne)	U.S. (south central and southeastern states)	*Disease in cats only:* Anorexia, depression, high fever, anemia, jaundice, congestion and edema of lungs, spleen, liver, shock, death in less than 1 week.	*General:* free-roaming in a wooded area. *Specific:* Indentify organism in blood smear (ring-shaped RBC inclusions) or cytology of bone marrow, lymph node, or spleen.	*Efficacy unproven:* —Parvaquone (Clexon; Coopers or Wellcome), 10–30 mg/kg, IM or SC, q24h for 2–3 days. *Prognosis:* Poor.

TABLE 1. Systemic Protozoan Infections of the Dog and Cat *Continued*

Diseases	Etiology (Source)	Endemic Locations	Clinical Signs	Diagnosis	Treatment
Encephalitozoonosis	*Encephalitozoon cuniculi* (oronasal exposure to urine spores or ingestion of infected tissues)	U.S. (rarely), Europe, South Africa	*Neonatal disease in kennels:* stunted growth, acute nephritis (renal failure) and encephalitis (depression, muscle spasms, ataxia, seizures, blindness, aggression, paralysis).	*General:* Nonregenerative anemia, azotemia, pyuria, hematuria, elevated CSF protein and mononuclear cells. *Specific:* —Identify spores in gram-stained urine sediment. —Serology: IFA or ELISA titer ≥1:20 is suggestive and >1:40 is confirmatory.	No treatment known.
Acanthamebiasis	*Acanthamoeba* spp (water, sewage, soil)	U.S. (very rare; epizootics seen in greyhounds)	*Disease in dogs only:* Pneumonia (fever, cough, dyspnea, naso-ocular discharge), encephalitis (ataxia, seizures); mimics canine distemper.	Leukopenia; no diagnostic test available (identify organisms in lung biopsies).	No treatment known.
Pneumocystosis	*Pneumocystis carinii* (airborne)	Worldwide (very rare)	*Disease in dogs only:* Acute or chronic pneumonia in immunocompromised dogs (nonfebrile, exercise intolerance, dyspnea, mild cough, weight loss).	*General:* Neutrophilic leukocytosis, diffuse radiographic alveolar and interstitial lung densities. *Specific:* Identify organisms in lung cytology or biopsies (Giemsa and methenamine silver stains).	Trimethoprim-sulfa (Tribrissen), 15 mg/kg, PO, q6h for 2 wks. *Prognosis:* Fair to guarded.

LE = lupus erythematosus; IFA = indirect fluorescent antibody; ELISA = enzyme-linked immunosorbent assay.

ally rupture and destroy the cell, releasing organisms to infect new cells and thereby producing foci of necrosis and inflammation. In a small percentage of animals, these lesions become extensive enough to cause overt clinical disease, the signs being dependent on which tissues are most severely affected. In the majority of animals, however, the rapid multiplication stage is brief, and, as immunity develops and before signs occur, aggregates of these organisms encyst and become dormant.

Chronic Tissue Encystment Stage of Infection (Bradyzoite Stage). Coincident with the onset of immunity, slowly multiplying bradyzoite forms develop and form large (10–50 μm) tissue cysts, especially in muscle, brain, and visceral tissues. There is minimal host response to these cysts, and they can persist in this dormant form for the life of the chronic carrier animal. They usually do not cause any clinical signs except in the rare instances when they rupture within the central nervous system (CNS) or eye or when the infection reactivates to an acute stage because of immunosuppression.

KEY POINT ▶ In carnivores such as the cat, the principal source of infection is ingestion of *Toxoplasma* in the cyst stage, which is found in the meat of chronically infected food-producing animals, small mammals, and birds.

Clinical Signs

Clinical toxoplasmosis is recognized more frequently in cats than in dogs, but the spectrum of signs is similar for both species.

■ Nonspecific signs of anorexia, depression, and fever (often >104°F and unresponsive to antibiotics) are common.
■ Other signs are mostly determined by the site and extent of injury from extraintestinal dissemination.
■ Clinical signs can occur at the time of initial infection (acute or primary toxoplasmosis) or from reactivation of encysted infection (chronic or secondary toxoplasmosis) caused by an underlying immunosuppressive condition.

KEY POINT ▶ Most animals with toxoplasmosis are asymptomatic and have only serologic evidence of infection. It is estimated that up to 30% of cats in the United States have *Toxoplasma* antibodies, with the highest prevalence in free-roaming and feral cats that hunt for their food.

Ocular Signs

Uveitis (iridocyclitis, chorioretinitis) is one of the most common forms and can cause aqueous flare, keratic precipitates, hypopyon, or fundic lesions (see sec. 11, chs. 6 and 8).

Respiratory Signs

Acute necrotizing pneumonia is common and can cause progressive dyspnea.

Neuromuscular Signs

- Encephalomyelitis can cause seizures, ataxia, tremors, paresis/paralysis, and cranial nerve deficits, depending on location of the lesions within the CNS.
- Myositis can cause hyperesthesia, stiff gait, and muscle atrophy.

Digestive Tract Signs

- Hepatitis and cholangiohepatitis can cause anorexia, vomiting, diarrhea, jaundice, and ascites.
- Pancreatitis can cause anorexia, vomiting, abdominal pain, and jaundice.
- Enterocolitis can cause vomiting and diarrhea.
- Mesenteric lymphadenitis can cause palpable abdominal lymph nodes.

Cardiac Signs

- Myocarditis can cause cardiac arrhythmias or heart failure.

Reproductive Signs

- Transplacental infection can cause birth of stillborn kittens or kittens that die of neonatal toxoplasmosis of the lung, liver, and CNS.

Diagnosis

KEY POINT ▶ Because toxoplasmosis often is an opportunistic disease associated with immunosuppression, consider underlying factors such as feline immunodeficiency virus, feline leukemia virus, feline infectious peritonitis, hemobartonellosis, canine distemper, and glucocorticoid or antitumor therapy.

Hematology and Serum Chemistries

- Any of the forms can cause leukopenia with degenerative left shift (in acute disease) or neutrophilic leukocytosis; nonregenerative anemia can also occur.
- Hepatitis can cause elevated serum bilirubin, liver enzymes, and bile acids.
- Pancreatitis can cause elevated serum amylase or lipase.
- Myositis can cause elevated muscle enzymes (e.g., CPK, SGOT).

Radiography

- The pulmonary form can cause generalized coalescing, patchy alveolar and interstitial pulmonary infiltrates, and mild pleural effusion.
- Abdominal forms can cause abdominal effusion and hepatomegaly.

Serology

For the most complete assessment of disease activity, evaluate immunoglobulin (Ig) M, IgG, and antigen simultaneously on a single serum sample.*

IgM Titer. IGM titers are determined by enzyme-linked immunosorbent assay (ELISA).

- IgM titer rises initially at 1 to 2 weeks after exposure (coincides with usual onset of signs) and persists for less than 12 weeks in most cats, thereby paralleling disease activity.
- Interpretation: IgM titer ≥1:64 suggests active or recent infection.
- A prolonged positive IgM titer may be associated with reactivation of chronic infection or delayed antibody class shift from IgM to IgG caused by concurrent feline immunodeficiency virus infection or glucocorticoid therapy.

KEY POINT ▶ The serum IgM *Toxoplasma* antibody titer is the serologic test of choice for diagnosis of active or recent infection.

IgG Titer. Various serologic methods may be used to measure IgG titers.

- IgG titer rises initially at 2 to 4 weeks after exposure and usually persists for more than 1 year; thus, a single positive IgG titer does not distinguish previous infection from current active infection.
- Interpretation: A fourfold rise in the IgG titer in paired specimens over a 2- to 3-week period is indicative of active infection. Both must be measured together in the same test run on the same day.

KEY POINT ▶ A single high serum IgG *Toxoplasma* antibody titer is NOT diagnostic of active infection, no matter how high the titer level.

Toxoplasma Antigen Titer. This measurement can be done using ELISA.

- Becomes positive initially 1 to 4 weeks after exposure and then remains intermittently positive for up to 1 year.
- Does not distinguish active from past infection and thus has no advantage over antibody titers.

Identification of Toxoplasma Organisms

Detection of Tachyzoites

- Characteristic intracellular inclusions can be identified in aspirate and impression smear cytologies stained routinely or in biopsies.
- Specimens to consider include lung, liver, lymph nodes, body cavity fluids, and cerebrospinal fluid.
- Disadvantage: Tachyzoites are often sparse and difficult to find.

---

*Available at Veterinary Diagnostic Laboratory, College of Veterinary Medicine, Colorado State University, Fort Collins, CO 80523.

Detection of Oocysts in Feces

- The best method for detection is Sheather's sugar centrifugation-flotation:
  - Sheather's solution: 500 g table sugar, 320 ml distilled water, and 6.5 g phenol crystals melted in hot water bath.
- Disadvantages: Oocysts are small, easily overlooked, and morphologically indistinguishable from certain other coccidia (*Hammondia* spp, *Besnoitia* spp) without specialized animal inoculation studies.
- Nevertheless, assume coccidian oocysts 10×12 μm in size in feline feces to be *Toxoplasma* until proved otherwise.

KEY POINT ▶ Detection of fecal oocysts is not a reliable diagnostic test for toxoplasmosis because oocyst shedding occurs only briefly and usually ends before clinical signs begin.

Treatment

Although it is estimated that about 60% of animals with clinical illness due to toxoplasmosis recover with treatment, no therapy is consistently effective; thus, the prognosis is guarded. Mortality rate is highest in neonates and in animals that are severely immunosuppressed. Antitoxoplasma drugs include clindamycin, sulfonamides, pyrimethamine, trimethoprim-sulfa, doxycycline, and various experimental agents currently under investigation.

KEY POINT ▶ Clindamycin is the treatment of choice for toxoplasmosis.

Clindamycin

- Dosage: Antirobe (Upjohn), 25–50 mg/kg per day, divided into two or three doses, PO or IM, for at least 2 weeks beyond remission.
- Actions: inhibits replication of *Toxoplasma;* effective for treatment of clinical disease and for reducing oocyst shedding; penetrates the blood-brain and blood-eye barriers.
- Side effects: anorexia, vomiting, and diarrhea; these are dose-dependent.

Adjunct Therapy for Uveitis

- 1% prednisone drops, topically, every 6 to 8 hours for 2 weeks

Prevention

KEY POINT ▶ The question often is raised, how dangerous is a healthy pet cat with a positive *Toxoplasma* antibody titer? Because oocyst shedding is usually over by the time the titer rises, and because reinfection of an immune cat usually results in little or no shedding, a cat with a positive titer poses less of a danger to its owner than an antibody-negative (nonimmune) cat.

Prevention in Cats

Do not feed cats raw meat, viscera, or bones, nor allow them to scavenge these from garbage.

- Do not allow cats to
  - Ingest raw (unpasteurized) milk, especially from goats
  - Roam free where they can hunt prey (mice, birds) for food
  - Eat mechanical vectors (cockroaches, flies, earthworms)

Prevention in Humans

KEY POINT ▶ Pregnant women should avoid contact with soil, cat litter, and raw meat.

- Do not eat raw or undercooked meat (cook meat to 150°F to kill *Toxoplasma*).
- Wash hands and all materials (e.g., cutting boards, sink tops, knives) that come in contact with raw meat.
- Boil water before drinking if source is questionable.
- Empty litter box daily (24 hours or more are required for fecal oocysts to sporulate and become infectious) and disinfect with boiling or scalding water.
- Wear gloves when gardening; wash garden vegetables thoroughly before eating in case soil is contaminated with *Toxoplasma* oocysts.
- Keep sandboxes covered when not in use so that cats cannot defecate in them.
- Control the stray cat population to reduce oocyst contamination of the environment (cats that defecate in the soil are likely to be the same cats that must hunt for their food and thereby have a high risk of infection).
- To reduce entry of *Toxoplasma* into the food chain, prevent cats from roaming where food-producing animals and their food are kept.

KEY POINT ▶ Because of the way in which cats defecate, bury their feces, and keep their haircoats clean, transmission of *Toxoplasma* oocysts to humans by touching and caring for a pet cat is unlikely.

NEOSPOROSIS

Etiology

Neospora caninum is a coccidian parasite that resembles *Toxoplasma* in tissues and only recently has been recognized as a distinct species. Its full life cycle is not known. Natural infections have been seen in dogs, and cats have been infected experimentally.

Clinical Signs

Multifocal, progressive neuromuscular signs predominate as a result of nonsuppurative encephalomyelitis, polyradiculoneuritis, and fibrosing polymyositis. These signs can include ascending paralysis, stiffness, muscle atrophy and contracture, and dysphagia. Phlebitis and dermatitis have also been seen.

Diagnosis

- Muscle involvement may cause increased serum levels of muscle enzymes (CPK, AST) and abnormal electromyographic findings (see sec. 10, ch. 6).
- Cerebrospinal fluid (CSF) shows a mildly increased protein (20–50 mg/dl) and increased leukocytes (10–50 cells/µl) composed of a mixture of small and large mononuclear cells and neutrophils.
- *Neospora* does not cross-react on serologic tests for *Toxoplasma*.
- *Neospora* organisms may be detected in CSF or biopsies of infected tissues.

Treatment and Prevention

Information on effective treatment or prevention is not yet available.

Supplemental Readings

TOXOPLASMOSIS AND NEOSPOROSIS

Dubey JP: Toxoplasmosis and other coccidial infections. *In* Sherding RG, ed.: *The Cat: Diseases and Clinical Management.* New York: Churchill Livingstone, 1989, p 439.

Dubey JP, Greene CE, Lappin MR: Toxoplasmosis and neosporosis. *In* Greene CE, ed.: *Infectious Diseases of the Dog and Cat.* Philadelphia: W. B. Saunders, 1990, p 818.

Lappin MR: Feline toxoplasmosis. *In* Kirk RW, ed.: *Current Veterinary Therapy X.* Philadelphia: W. B. Saunders, 1989, p 1112.

Lappin MR, Greene CE, Prestwood AK, et al: Diagnosis of recent *Toxoplasma gondii* infection in cats by the use of an enzyme-linked immunosorbent assay for immunoglobulin M. Am J Vet Res 50:1580, 1989.

Lappin MR, Greene CE, Winston S, et al: Clinical feline toxoplasmosis: Serologic diagnosis and therapeutic management of 15 cases. J Vet Intern Med 3:139, 1989.

LEISHMANIASIS

Buckner RG: Leishmaniasis. *In* Barlough JE, ed.: *Manual of Small Animal Infectious Diseases.* New York: Churchill Livingstone, 1988, p 343.

Slappendel RJ, Greene CE: Leishmaniasis. *In* Greene CE, ed.: *Infectious Diseases of the Dog and Cat.* Philadelphia: W. B. Saunders, 1990, p 769.

TRYPANOSOMIASIS (CHAGAS DISEASE)

Barlough JE: American trypanosomiasis (Chagas Disease). *In* Barlough JE, ed.: *Manual of Small Animal Infectious Diseases.* New York: Churchill Livingstone, 1988, p 349.

Barr SC: American trypanosomiasis. *In* Greene CE, ed.: *Infectious Diseases of the Dog and Cat.* Philadelphia: W. B. Saunders, 1990, p 763.

HEPATOZOONOSIS

Craig TM: Hepatozoonosis. *In* Greene CE, ed.: *Infectious Diseases of the Dog and Cat.* Philadelphia: W. B. Saunders, 1990, p 778.

Craig TM: Hepatozoonosis. *In* Barlough JE, ed.: *Manual of Small Animal Infectious Diseases.* New York: Churchill Livingstone, 1988, p 369.

BABESIOSIS

Breitschwerdt EB: Babesiosis. *In* Greene CE, ed.: *Infectious Diseases of the Dog and Cat.* Philadelphia: W. B. Saunders, 1990, p 796.

Huxsoll DL: Babesiosis. *In* Barlough JE, ed.: *Manual of Small Animal Infectious Diseases.* New York: Churchill Livingstone, 1988, p 383.

CYTAUXZOONOSIS

Kier AB: Cytauxzoonosis. *In* Greene CE, ed.: *Infectious Diseases of the Dog and Cat.* Philadelphia: W. B. Saunders, 1990, p 792.

Wagner JE, Kier AB: Cytauxzoonosis. *In* Barlough JE, ed.: *Manual of Small Animal Infectious Diseases.* New York: Churchill Livingstone, 1988, p 391.

ENCEPHALITOZOONOSIS

Regan K, Shadduck JA, Botha WS: Encephalitozoonosis. *In* Barlough JE, ed.: *Manual of Small Animal Infectious Diseases.* New York: Churchill Livingstone, 1988, p 399.

Szabo JR, Pang V, Shadduck JA: Encephalitozoonosis. *In* Greene CE, ed.: *Infectious Diseases of the Dog and Cat.* Philadelphia: W. B. Saunders, 1990, p 786.

ACANTHAMEBIASIS

Harrison LR, Bauer RW: Acanthamebiasis. *In* Greene CE, ed.: *Infectious Diseases of the Dog and Cat.* Philadelphia: W. B. Saunders, 1990, p 815.

PNEUMOCYSTOSIS

Farrow BRH: Pneumocystosis. *In* Barlough JE, ed.: *Manual of Small Animal Infectious Diseases.* New York: Churchill Livingstone, 1988, p 407.

Greene CE, Chandler FW: Pneumocystosis. *In* Greene CE, ed.: *Infectious Diseases of the Dog and Cat.* Philadelphia: W. B. Saunders, 1990, p 854.

Hematology/Oncology

Rodney L. Page

1 Erythrocytes, Leukocytes, and Platelets

Rose E. Raskin

ERYTHROCYTE DISORDERS

Anemia—Overview

Anemia is characterized by a reduction in the number of red blood cells or hemoglobin content or both. It is one of the most frequent hematologic abnormalities encountered in practice. Anemia is not a disease, but rather the reflection of a disease state. Therefore the cause of the anemia is determined to best treat the condition. Causes of anemia may be divided into three general categories: blood loss, hemolysis, and decreased red blood cell production.

Clinical Signs

- The patient may present with lethargy, weakness, anorexia, heart murmur, dyspnea, and pale or icteric mucous membranes.
- Occasionally the animal may appear normal, but routine blood evaluation prior to an elective surgical procedure may uncover the abnormality.
- Sedentary animals, especially cats, often have moderate degrees of anemia that go unnoticed for long periods.
- Splenomegaly frequently accompanies anemia as a response to increased extravascular hemolysis or extramedullary hematopoiesis.

General Diagnostic Considerations

Several tests can be used to document and characterize the anemia morphologically or by etiology.

History and Physical Examination. These should determine the following:

- Occurrence of trauma or surgery
- Drug, chemical, or toxin exposure
- Concurrence of infectious, parasitic, or neoplastic disease
- Duration of disease, sites of blood loss, and presence of organomegaly.

Complete Blood Count (CBC) (Table 1)
- Packed cell volume (PCV) is the most accurate and least expensive method of documenting anemia. Spin hematocrit tubes 5 minutes at 12,000–15,000 × G. Evaluate plasma color following centrifugation.
- Determine plasma protein or total solids by refractometer.
- Red blood cell (RBC) count is usually performed by an automated cell counter. This value is necessary for calculation of RBC indices.
- Hemoglobin concentration (Hgb) is determined most accurately by the cyanmethemoglobin method, using a colorimeter or spectrophotometer. Artifactual increases may occur with gross lipemia or excessive number of Heinz bodies, both of which produce light interference.
- Mean corpuscular volume (MCV) may be determined directly by the automated cell counters or calculated.

$$\text{MCV (femtoliters)} = \frac{\text{PCV} \times 10}{\text{RBC}(10^6/\mu l)}$$

The MCV reflects RBC size and may be categorized

TABLE 1. Hematology Reference Ranges*
for Dogs and Cats

Parameter	Canine	Feline
PCV (%)	37–54	30–47
Hgb (g/dl)	13–19	9–15
RBC ($\times 10^6/\mu l$)	5.4–8.5	5.8–10.7
MCV (fl)	64–74	41–51
MCH (pg)	22–27	13–18
MCHC (g/dl)	34–36	31–35
Reticulocytes ($\times 10^3/\mu l$)	<60	<40 Aggregate
		<500 Punctate
Platelets ($\times 10^3/\mu l$)	160–430	300–800
WBC (/μl)	6000–17,000	5500–19,500
Segmented Neutrophils (/μl)	3000–11,500	2500–12,500
Banded Neutrophils (/μl)	0–300	0–300
Lymphocytes (/μl)	1000–4800	1500–7500
Monocytes (/μl)	150–1350	0–850
Eosinophils (/μl)	100–1250	0–1500
Basophils (/μl)	<100	<100
Plasma Protein (g/dl)	6.0–7.8	6.2–8.0
Fibrinogen (mg/dl)	100–400	100–300

Source: University of Florida, Veterinary Clinical Pathology Laboratory.
*These values are only meant as a guide; individual laboratories may vary in their ranges, depending on instrumentation and regional differences.

as macrocytic suggesting increased RBC turnover, microcytic suggesting defective cell growth, or normocytic (unchanging cell size). Note that the Japanese Akita normally has microcytic erythrocytes.

■ Other erythrocyte indices (mean corpuscular hemoglobin—MCH; mean corpuscular hemoglobin concentration—MCHC) help to classify the types of anemia into normochromic and hypochromic, which will reflect the presence of reticulocytes or abnormal hemoglobinization.

■ The most important part of the CBC involves an evaluation of the blood smear for morphologic abnormalities. Report and quantitate changes in size (anisocytosis), shape (poikilocytosis), and color (polychromasia). The presence of immature nucleated forms and basophilic stippling often signal abnormal erythropoiesis or defective circulation of red cell precursors. Infectious parasites and Heinz bodies may be found upon careful examination.

Reticulocyte Counts. This is the most accurate method to evaluate regeneration. Counts are recommended when PCV falls below 30% in dogs and 20% in cats. Incubate equal volumes of blood and 0.5% new methylene blue stain together for 15 to 20 minutes; then make a routine blood smear and count the number of aggregate and punctate forms per 1000 erythrocytes. Absolute numbers of reticulocytes per μl are calculated by the following formula:

$$\text{Absolute reticulocytes per } \mu l = \frac{\% \text{ reticulocyte percentage} \times \text{RBC}/\mu l}{100}$$

Dogs normally have 0 to 1% reticulocytes (0–60,000/μl). In normal cats, aggregated reticulocytes range from 0 to 0.4% (0–40,000/μl) and punctate reticulocytes are less than 5% (< 500,000/μl). Aggregate reticulocytes represent the most active or recent form of regeneration in the dog and cat. Punctate

reticulocytes in cats, which do not stain as polychromatophilic cells, represent regenerative attempts that occurred 2 to 4 weeks previously. By using the PCV instead of the RBC count, a corrected reticulocyte percentage may be calculated as:

$$\text{Corrected \% reticulocytes} = \% \text{ reticulocytes} \times \frac{\text{patient's PCV}}{\text{normal PCV}}$$

Normal PCV is considered 45% for dogs and 35% for cats. A corrected percent reticulocyte value greater than 1% indicates increased RBC regeneration. Once initiated at the bone marrow level, regeneration may take at least 3 days before reticulocytes appear in the circulation.

Fecal Examination and Urinalysis. These tests are performed to determine sources of blood loss and function of the kidney.

Biochemical Profiles. Biochemical profiles may reveal organic disease that can affect the ability to regenerate erythrocytes.

Bone Marrow Evaluation. This is necessary whenever regenerative attempts appear diminished. Hemolytic conditions do not warrant marrow examination unless the response is less than normally expected. Results must always be compared with a recent CBC to determine the current status of regeneration.

■ This is a sterile procedure often performed with only local anesthesia; however, mild tranquilization or general anesthesia may be used if necessary.

■ Sites frequently used in dogs include the dorsal ilium, humerus (best for obese animals), and femur (small dogs or puppies). Sites frequently used in cats include the femur, transilial and dorsal ilium.

■ Aspiration biopsy (special needles required*) is performed as follows:
  • Pass the needle with the stylet a few millimeters into the bone until it is firmly embedded.
  • Place a 12-ml syringe coated with 5% EDTA solution onto the biopsy needle and collect 1–2 ml of bloody material.
  • Place the marrow material on a plastic Petri dish and pick up the glistening particles with a microhematocrit tube.
  • Gently blow this material out of the tube onto a glass slide.
  • Make a squash preparation by laying a second slide on the first and drawing them apart.

■ Core biopsy (special needle required†) is performed using the following procedure:

■ Pass the needle with stylet through the skin and subcutaneous tissues.

■ Remove the stylet while advancing the needle 0.5–1.5 cm into the bone, depending on the size of the animal.

■ Twist the instrument sharply to cut the sample and withdraw the needle slowly.

■ Remove the core sample and roll it onto a glass slide

*Illinois sternal disposable needle, 15–18 ga, 1–2″ long; Baxter Healthcare Corp., Valencia, CA.
†Jamshidi aspiration/biopsy disposable needle, 11–13 ga, 2–4″ long; Baxter Healthcare Corp., Valencia, CA.

for cytologic examination; following this, place sample in 10% buffered formalin for histologic fixation.

Principles of Transfusion Therapy

Therapy depends on the etiology of the anemia. Rapid decreases in PCV warrant replacement of whole blood. However, slow daily decreases in PCV of 1 to 3% may not cause clinical signs of dyspnea or weakness.

Crossmatching. Perform crossmatching prior to transfusion. The procedure, which involves collection of red blood cells and serum or plasma from the donor and the patient, is as follows:

- Wash erythrocytes and pellet three times in 0.9% saline.
- Make a 4% cell suspension by adding 4.8 ml of saline to 0.2 ml of cells.
- Measure compatibility between donor and patient at three temperatures: 37°C, 20°C, and 4°C.

Donors are incompatible if any agglutination or hemolysis occurs in the major crossmatch. The types of crossmatch are defined as:

Major: 100 μl donor cells + 100 μl patient serum/plasma
Minor: 100 μl patient cells + 100 μl donor serum/plasma
Controls: 100 μl of donor/patient cells to 100 μl of donor/patient serum or plasma

Under emergency conditions, donors may be used if mild agglutination occurs in the minor crossmatch. The crossmatching procedure is as follows:

- Following 15 minutes of incubation, centrifuge tubes at 280 G for 1 minute.
- Note any hemolysis in supernatant and gross agglutination of resuspended cells.
- Place a small drop on glass slide and examine for microscopic agglutination.

Whole Blood Transfusion. In dogs, this procedure is best performed using animals negative for DEA-1 and DEA-7 blood types. Although most cats have Type A blood, it is best to crossmatch blood, because only 1 ml of mismatched blood can cause a fatal transfusion reaction in cats.

Estimated dosage is 10–20 ml/kg in dogs and cats, with a maximum of 40 ml in an adult cat. A more specific guideline for the amount of donor blood in anticoagulant (ml) is:

$$\text{kg} \times 80 \text{ (dog) or } 60 \text{ (cat)} \times \frac{[\text{desired PCV} - \text{patient PCV}]}{\text{donor PVC}}$$

When performing whole blood transfusion:

- Use appropriate filters and administration sets to retain clotted blood or debris.
- Warm blood prior to administration.
- For the first 30 minutes, keep initial rate of administration slow (0.25 ml/Kg) to observe any incompatibility reactions (recommended rate of whole blood infusion in general is 10 ml/kg/hour). The rate of infusion depends upon the hydration status of the patient.
- Evaluate hematocrit before and after transfusion:
  • To document relative improvement.
  • To screen for hemolysis as an indicator of incompatibility.

Blood component therapy is described more fully in sec. 3, ch. 2.

Blood Loss Anemia

Large volumes of blood must be lost before appreciable changes occur in the numbers of erythrocytes or PCV. The immediate loss of blood results in little or no change in the PCV, owing to the concurrent loss of RBCs and plasma fluids. Over the course of several hours to days, redistribution of fluids occurs, resulting in a lowered PCV and plasma protein. Depending upon the amount of blood lost and the time period over which it is lost, regenerative responses may range from moderate to extremely weak. Chronic blood loss causes decreased iron stores, resulting in decreased RBC production.

Etiology

Causes of blood loss include:

- Trauma
- Surgery
- External and internal parasitism
- Tumors of the gastrointestinal (GI) and urinary systems
- Coagulation abnormalities

Treatment

Administer crossmatched whole blood for *acute* hemorrhage when the PCV drops to 20 to 25% in the dog or cat. Also consider autotransfusion if hemorrhage has recently occurred in a body cavity, and the blood is not contaminated with bacteria or neoplastic cells.

Hemolytic Anemia

A variety of causes are associated with hemolytic loss of RBCs. The net effect often is a very strong to moderate regenerative response (Fig. 1). However, in some cases, the anemia may occur so rapidly that the animal may have too little time to mount a regenerative response by the time the condition is recognized. A period of 2 to 3 days is necessary for RBC maturation, once the stimulation from hypoxia or severe RBC depletion has occurred. Depending on the severity or acuteness of the destruction and the conjugating ability of the liver, icterus may or may not be present. Plasma protein concentrations usually are normal.

Etiology

Causes of hemolytic anemia include:

- Congenital abnormalities
- Immune-mediated destruction

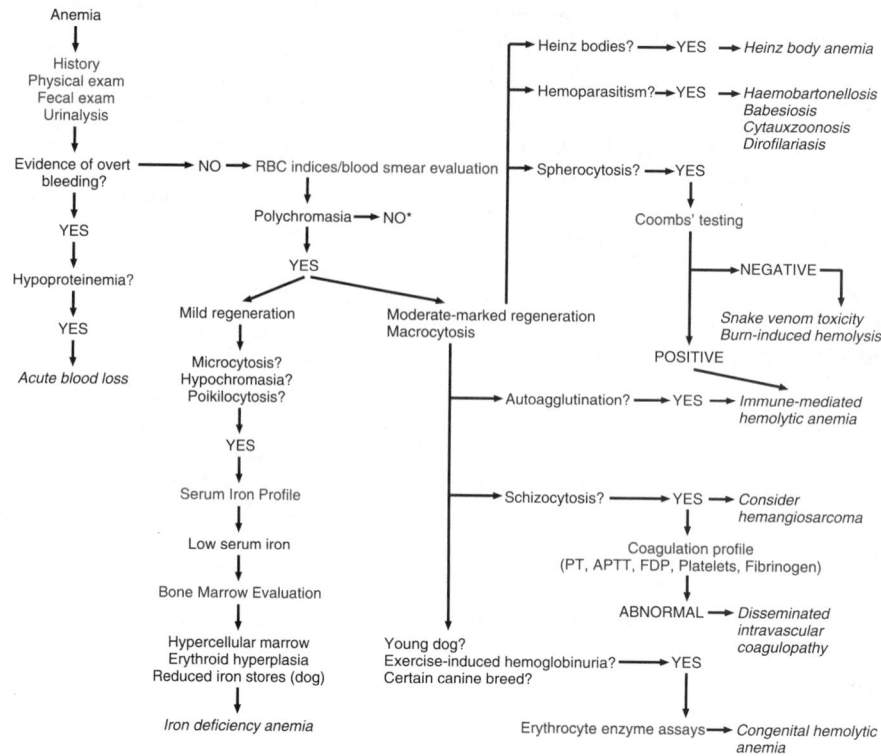

Figure 1. Diagnostic approach to common regenerative anemias in dogs and cats *See Figures 2 and 3. (PT, prothrombin time; APTT, activated partial thromboplastin time; FeLV, feline leukemia virus; FDP, fibrin degradation products.)

- Infections
- Chemical or toxic agents
- Mechanical fragmentation
- Hypophosphatemia.

Congenital Erythrocyte Abnormalities

Pyruvate kinase deficiency is an erythrocyte enzyme deficiency associated with an autosomal recessive inheritance. During anerobic glycolysis, pyruvate kinase is necessary for the production of ATP, which erythrocytes need to maintain their integrity and viability. The condition has been recognized in several breeds, including the basenji, beagle and West Highland White terrier. Young animals usually present with anemia at 2 months to 1 year of age. The outcome of the disease is usually death by 3 years of age. Myelofibrosis and osteosclerosis may occur resulting in reduced hematopoiesis. Frequent RBC destruction may lead to hemosiderosis and failure of organs such as the liver. Diagnosis of the disease is suggested clinically by the presence of an intense reticulocytosis (15–70%) in a young dog. Echinocytosis, or erythrocytes with sharp projections unrelated to crenation, may be seen in the circulation. Definitive diagnosis requires a special erythrocyte assay for the enzyme.

Phosphofructokinase deficiency has been identified in English Springer spaniels as an autosomal recessive inheritance. This glycolytic enzyme deficiency causes a decrease in 2,3-diphosphoglycerate (2,3-DPG) concentration, resulting in an increase in intracellular pH. Erythrocytes from affected animals are especially fragile under alkaline conditions. Intravascular hemolysis may occur during hyperventilation-induced alkalemia,

resulting in periodic bouts of hemoglobinuria and sometimes bilirubinuria. A constant state of hypoxia is produced by the low levels of 2,3-DPG, with subsequent increased oxygen binding to hemoglobin. The result is persistent reticulocytosis (7–23%) even though the PCV is normal or mildly decreased. The enzyme deficiency is diagnosed by specialized erythrocyte assays.

Hereditary stomatocytosis is an autosomal recessive trait in Alaskan malamutes associated with chondrodysplasia. The defect may involve abnormalities of the cell membrane or of ion transport leading to increased water content and a larger cell size (96 fl). Dwarfism is recognized clinically, and there is a mild hemolytic anemia and slight reticulocytosis (2%). RBC numbers are reduced, but the PCV remains normal because of enlarged erythrocytes. Morphologically, some RBCs appear to have a slit or mouth-like area of central pallor.

Feline porphyria is an infrequent inheritable trait that results in an enzyme deficiency affecting heme synthesis. Clinical signs include pink urine, pinkish-brown teeth, and severe anemia resulting from the deposition of red non-heme pigments and the lysis of erythrocytes when exposed to sunlight. Discolored teeth often fluoresce red under ultraviolet light. Skin photosensitization can occur; therefore, exposure to sunlight should be avoided. The disease can be prevented by not breeding carrier animals.

Hereditary nonspherocytic hemolytic anemia is recognized in two breeds: poodles and beagles. Poodles develop an autosomal dominant condition that resembles pyruvate kinase deficiency, but decreases in this enzyme are not demonstrable. Affected animals have a persistent macrocytic hypochromic anemia (PCV of 13–31%) with moderate reticulocytosis. It is clinically evident by 1 year of age and fatal by age 3. Myelofibrosis, osteosclerosis, and hemosiderosis are present at death. In beagles, the condition presents with chronic anemia and moderate reticulocytosis. The mode of inheritance is likely autosomal recessive. The disease is less severe in beagles than in poodles, and the disorder can remain subclinical for up to 4 years in affected dogs. In both breeds, RBCs are morphologically normal and enzyme activities are not affected. The short RBC life span in beagles may be caused by an unidentified membrane abnormality.

Immune-Mediated Hemolytic Anemia

See section on systemic immune-mediated disease (sec. 3, ch. 3).

Infectious Causes of Hemolysis

Haemobartonellosis is caused by a rickettsial organism that infects the RBCs of dogs (*Haemobartonella canis*) and cats (*H. felis*). It can be transmitted by ticks and fleas, or by queens to their newborn kittens in the absence of blood-sucking arthropods. Splenectomy (especially in the dog), immunosuppression caused by glucocorticoid therapy, or stress in cats with latent *H. felis* infection will predispose the development of clinical disease in the animal infected by the organism. Clinical signs include those generally observed with anemia. Weight loss may occur if the anemia develops slowly while acute, severe anemia produces sudden depression and icterus. Splenomegaly is often noted. Laboratory findings generally reflect a strong regenerative response in the CBC. The absence of marked anisocytosis or polychromasia in confirmed cases of feline haemobartonellosis may suggest peracute infections with too little time to respond or concurrent infection with feline leukemia virus (FeLV) or feline immunodeficiency virus (FIV). Thin smears, made directly without anticoagulant, will assist in finding the epicellular organisms. Blood films should be well stained without precipitate to minimize any confusion in identifying the parasite. Cats often have coccoid or ring shapes, whereas dogs mostly have linear chain forms. A positive Coombs' test may be associated with feline haemobartonellosis, presumably due to RBC membrane alteration. Treatment involves blood transfusion if the anemia is severe. Prednisolone (2 mg/kg, PO, every 12 hours) may be necessary initially to suppress the severe immune-mediated destruction of red cells. Tetracyclines should be given at a dose of 20 mg/kg orally every 8 hours for 3 weeks. Cats who recover may become latent carriers.

Babesiosis is a tick-borne protozoal disease affecting erythrocytes of mostly dogs (*Babesia canis, B. gibsoni*). Clinical signs of the acute disease include splenomegaly, icterus, anemia, thrombocytopenia, hemoglobinuria and fever. It is common in kennel conditions and is especially associated with greyhounds. Diagnosis is made by examination of a blood smear. A clear, teardrop-shaped organism in erythrocytes, sometimes seen in pairs, is the most common form that occurs in the United States. An indirect fluorescent antibody (IFA) serum test is available. Concurrent infections with *Ehrlichia canis* may occur. Treatment involves

diaminazene aceturate (Berenil, Hoechst-Roussel) (3.5 mg/kg IM given once), imidocarb dipropionate (Imizol, Coopers Animal Health) (2–6 mg/kg IM given once), or pentamidine isethionate (Lomadine, Lyphomed) (10–15 mg/kg SC twice daily (q12h) for 2 days). These drugs are not approved for use in the United States and are difficult to obtain.

Cytauxzoonosis is a highly fatal protozoal disease caused by *Cytauxzoon felis*. It is a tick-borne infection, most prevalent in the wooded areas of the southern United States. Initial clinical signs include anorexia, dehydration, and lethargy, with gradual development of fever. This progresses rapidly to icterus, moderate anemia, thrombocytopenia, and splenomegaly. Cats usually die within a week after clinical signs are recognized. Diagnosis is generally made post mortem by histologic identification of large schizonts in endothelial cells of the lungs, liver, bone marrow, or spleen. Terminally, blood films may contain small (1–2 μm in diameter) ring or "safety pin" structures within erythrocytes. Treatment has not been successful despite the use of antibiotics and supportive care. All reported cases have been fatal.

Leptospirosis usually is associated with kidney disease (*Leptospira canicola*) or hemolysis, icterus and coagulopathies (*L. icterohaemorrhagiae*). Toxins released from proliferating organisms interfere with cellular metabolism and damage cells. Clinical signs involve fever, anorexia, vomiting, and depression initially, followed by icterus, mucosal hemorrhages, hemoglobinuria, and urinary inflammation. Diagnosis is based on demonstration of leptospires in the urine by darkfield microscopy or in the liver and kidney by histologic examination. Serologic testing of paired samples is also available. Treatment requires supportive care and antibiotics (see sec. 2, ch. 11).

Chemical or Toxic Injury of Erythrocytes

Heinz body anemia is produced by oxidant agents that cause precipitation of hemoglobin. Accelerated red cell destruction involves intravascular fragmentation or extravascular phagocytosis by the spleen. Chemicals, drugs, or plants associated with Heinz body formation include acetaminophen, methylene blue, onions, vitamin K_3, DL-methionine, topical benzocaine (e.g., Cetacaine) sprayed on the larynx to aid intubation, and propylene glycol. Cats are predisposed to oxidant damage because of their hemoglobin structure. Clinical signs occur acutely, such as depression, hemoglobinemia, hemoglobinuria, moderate to severe anemia, and occasional icterus. Diagnosis is made by observation of a single, large, pale staining area in erythrocytes of Romanowsky-stained blood smears. They may also appear as a single blunt projection caused by the Heinz body bulging from the membrane surface. These structures appear as dark blue spots when stained with new methylene blue in a direct wet mount procedure or following incubation of the stain with the blood. Erythrocyte refractile bodies are similar to Heinz bodies but are smaller, infrequent, and present in normal cats. Contrast these to many large Heinz bodies with signs of a regenerative response. Treatment primarily involves removal of the source of oxidant. Emetics can be used if recent ingestion has

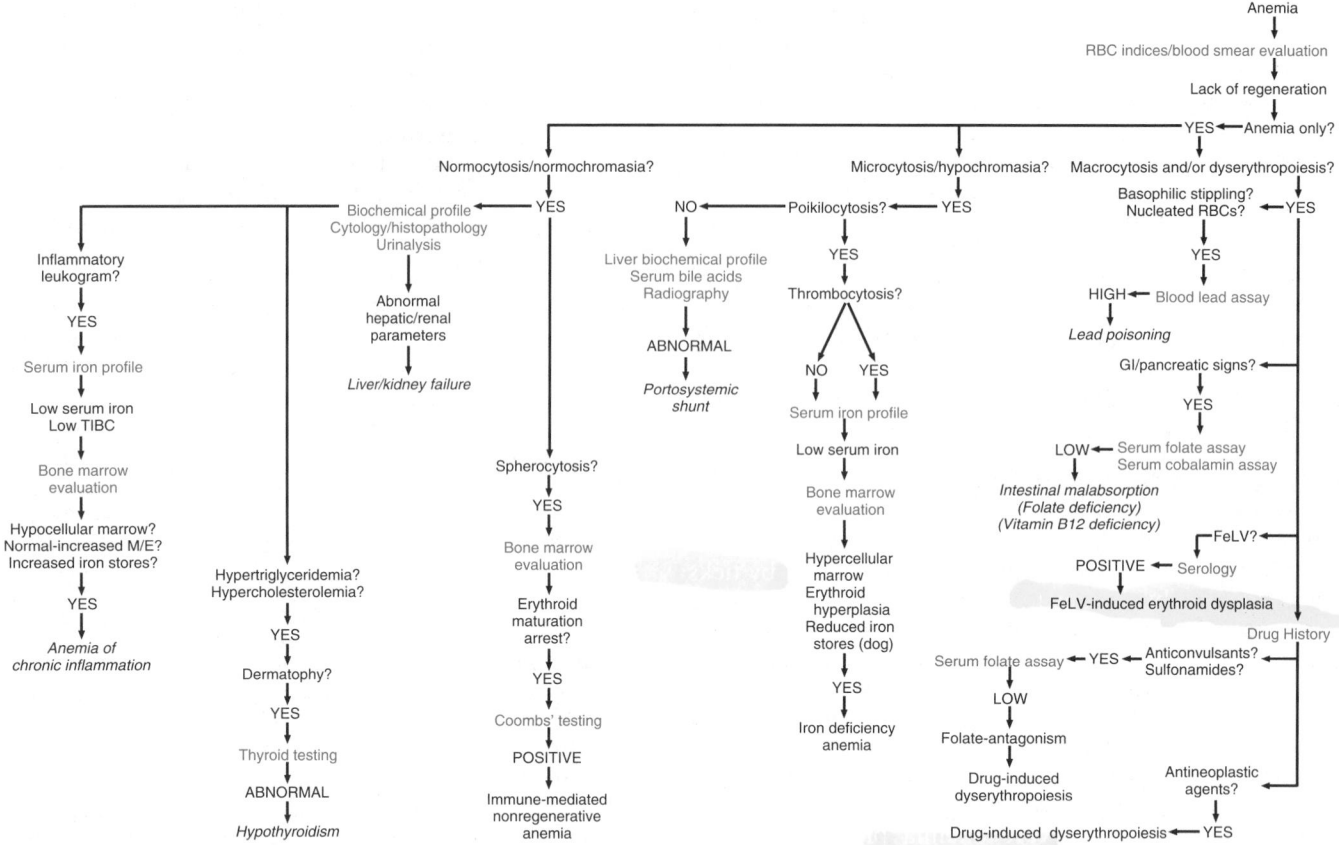

Figure 2. Diagnostic approach to common nonregenerative anemias in dogs and cats. *Anemia.* (TIBC, total iron-binding capacity; M/E, myeloid-to-erythroid ratio).

occurred. Give blood transfusions or other forms of supportive care, as indicated. For acetaminophen-induced toxicity, give acetylcysteine (Mucomyst, Mead Johnson), 140 mg/kg, PO, initially; then give 70 mg/kg every 4 hours for 4 to 5 treatments.

Methemoglobinemia occurs from the oxidation of iron in hemoglobin. This form of oxidized hemoglobin is unable to bind oxygen that is present, producing a state of relative hypoxia. Agents causing methemoglobinemia are similar to those mentioned under Heinz body formation. Both conditions can be present together, but methemoglobinemia tends to occur before Heinz bodies appear. Dogs with a rare enzyme (NADH-methemoglobin reductase) deficiency, may develop a mild to moderate form of the disease. Clinically, the mucous membranes appear blue-gray or cyanotic if methemoglobin levels exceed 30%. The patient is often dyspneic, weak, and ataxic. The appearance of dark red or chocolate-colored blood, even after exposure to air, is diagnostic for the condition. The color change, from dark to bright red in normal blood, is readily visible by a spot test on filter paper. The blood of affected animals will show no such color change. Quantitative measurement is performed by spectrophotometry at specialized laboratories. Treatment is similar to Heinz body anemia. In addition, methylene blue, if carefully administered, has been used to treat the condition. A dose of 1 mg/kg IV given as a 1% solution is recommended for small animals. Caution is necessary to avoid potentiating a hemolytic crisis. Therapy is usually not required for dogs with the reductase enzyme deficiency.

Snake venom toxicity has been recognized as a cause of hemolysis. Toxins, such as those produced from coral snakes, may be associated with spherocyte formation, in addition to neurologic and coagulation abnormalities. Diagnosis is based upon the presence of a regenerative anemia and a bite wound with a history supporting recent exposure to a snake. Treatment involves use of a specific venom antidote and supportive care.

Zinc toxicity can produce intravascular hemolysis in dogs. Sources of the zinc include ingestion of galvanized wire or kennel cage nuts, and pennies produced since 1983. Diagnosis involves presence of a regenerative anemia and proof of zinc exposure. Radiograph the abdomen to identify metallic foreign bodies in the GI tract and remove the source of zinc via surgery or endoscopy.

Mechanical Fragmentation of Erythrocytes

Dirofilariasis may produce anemia following intravascular hemolysis as large numbers of adult heartworms (*Dirofilaria immitis*) obstruct blood flow, causing turbulence that mechanically disrupts erythrocytes. Clinical signs reflect the organs affected, such as the lungs, liver, and kidneys. A postcaval syndrome results from obstruction of the caudal vena cava causing, in addition to hepatic failure, erythrocyte fragmentation

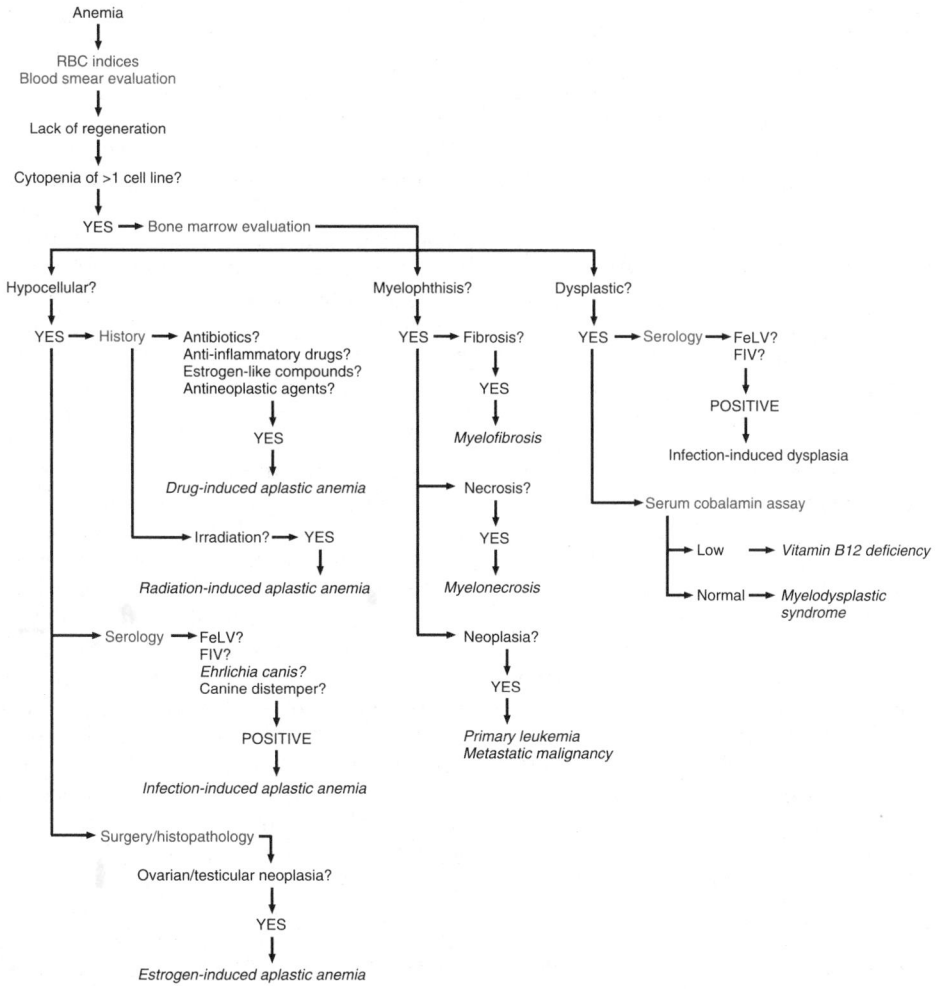

Figure 3. Diagnostic approach to common nonregenerative anemias in dogs and cats. *Pancytopenia.* (FeLV, feline leukemia virus; FIV, feline immunodeficiency virus).

(schizocytosis), hemoglobinemia, and hemoglobinuria. Definitive diagnosis is based on detection of circulating microfilaria in the blood or on serologic detection of circulating antigens or antibodies (see sec. 6, ch. 10).

Disseminated intravascular coagulopathy may cause a microangiopathic hemolytic anemia due to fibrin deposition that results from damage to small blood vessels. Mechanical fragmentation of erythrocytes appears in blood smears as schizocytes or spherocytes. The etiology involves a variety of conditions, such as neoplasia, infections, necrosis, toxins, and immune complex formation. These can lead to massive tissue destruction and activation of clotting pathways. Diagnosis is based on consumption of platelets (thrombocytopenia), reductions in clotting factors (prolonged PT and APTT, hypofibrinogenemia), and increased amounts of fibrin degradation products. Treatment is aimed at the inciting condition (see sec. 3, ch. 2).

Nonregenerative Anemia

Nonregenerative anemia is generally related to direct toxicity of erythroid precursors in the bone marrow or secondary suppression of erythropoiesis (Fig. 2). Often neutrophils and platelets are also affected (Fig. 3).

Reduction in erythrocytes, leukocytes, and platelets in circulation is termed pancytopenia. Aplastic anemia is used to describe bone marrow failure involving the three cell lines that leads to peripheral pancytopenia. The bone marrow in this condition is severely hypoplastic, with total or near complete replacement of hematopoietic elements by adipose tissue. In contrast, crowding from abnormal cellular infiltrates can suppress hematopoiesis, producing myelophthisis. Chronic, nonregenerative anemias may not require blood transfusion until the PCV falls below 15% in the dog and 12% in the cat.

Etiology

Causes of nonregenerative anemia include:

- Infectious agents
- Nutritional disturbances
- Organic disease
- Endocrine abnormalities
- Toxic agents
- Myelophthisis
- Irradiation
- Immune-mediated destruction

Infectious Agents

FeLV-associated anemia is usually normochromic and normocytic to macrocytic. The majority of cases are nonregenerative and related to suppression or destruction of erythroid progenitor cells. In addition, the virus affects the stromal microenvironment of the bone marrow coincidental with the development of anemia. About 10% of the cases are hemolytic with regeneration related to immune destruction of erythrocytes. Diagnosis is based on positive ELISA or IFA tests. Bone marrow aspirate smears or core biopsy sections indicate decreased cellularity with increased fat infiltration when the infection is not associated with a proliferative leukemia. Treatment will vary depending upon concurrent conditions such as neoplasia, haemobartonellosis, FIV, or FIP. Supportive care, in the form of blood transfusions, antibiotics, appetite stimulants and anabolic steroids, are often necessary (see sec. 2, ch. 1).

Other viruses, such as FIP, FIV, feline panleukopenia, canine parvovirus, and canine distemper, have been associated with suppression of erythropoiesis. The anemia is often mild to moderate and nonresponsive. Other cell lines, such as granulocytes or lymphocytes, are more severely affected. Diagnosis is usually determined by exposure history, clinical signs, virologic/serologic tests, characteristic histopathologic lesions, and identification of viral particles or inclusions within affected cells. In canine distemper, erythrocytes or leukocytes may contain one or more pale blue spots in the cytoplasm with Romanowsky-type stains. However, these inclusions stain a deep purple color with Diff-Quik.

Ehrlichiosis is a rickettsial disease caused by *Ehrlichia canis* and transmitted by ticks. It produces thrombocytopenia and a mild to moderate anemia as the most frequent hematologic abnormalities. Leukopenia and pancytopenia are less frequent findings and often occur late in the disease. Diagnosis is based upon positive or rising serum titers. Intracytoplasmic morulae are infrequently found in mononuclear cells or granulocytes, during the acute stage of the disease. Bone marrow, at this time, is often normocellular to hypercellular with increased numbers of megakaryocytes and plasma cells. Hyperglobulinemia as a polyclonal gammopathy is often noted. In the chronic or late stages of the disease, bone marrow cellularity decreases severely, with fat replacing hematopoietic elements (see sec. 2, ch. 10).

Leishmaniasis is an infrequent protozoal disease in dogs caused by *Leishmania* spp. The parasite, transmitted by sandflies, produces visceral or cutaneous manisfestations. History usually indicates travel outside the United States to Greece, Spain, or Italy. An endemic focus in Oklahoma has been reported. Clinical signs, which develop over months, include anorexia, weight loss, lymphadenopathy, and ulcerative dermatitis. Diagnosis is often made by cytology or histopathology. Organisms are present in macrophages of the bone marrow, lymph nodes, spleen, and liver. Serology and tissue culture are additional diagnostic aids. A mild to moderate normocytic, normochromic anemia may occur. Hyperglobulinemia accompanies the plasmacytosis found in tissues. The disease is zoonotic and infected dogs can serve as a reservoir to people. Euthanasia should be considered. Treatment involves antimony compounds (as listed in Table 1, sec. 2, ch. 13), although these drugs may be difficult to obtain.

Nutritional Deficiencies

Iron deficiency produces a poorly regenerative anemia due to deficient hemoglobin synthesis. It occurs with increased iron utilization, such as during growth or pregnancy, from decreased intestinal absorption of iron, and most commonly, when iron stores are reduced through hemorrhage or blood loss. Etiologies for this include neoplasia with tissue necrosis, trauma, internal or external parasites (hookworms, fleas), coagulopathies, and various gastrointestinal diseases that cause hematemesis, melena, or hematochezia. Diagnosis is based on history and low serum iron levels. Erythrocytes in blood smears may appear normal in size but lighter in color, with increased central pallor (hypochromasia). Electronic cell counters report an MCV <60 fl (microcytosis) in dogs. Poikilocytosis may be prominent in the form of schizocytes, keratocytes, codocytes, and elliptocytes. Thrombocytosis occurs in 50% of canine cases. Iron profiles have normal to increased levels of transferrin (total iron-binding capacity) and decreased serum iron levels (in cats < 60 μg/dl; in dogs <80 μg/dl). Percent saturation of transferrin in iron deficient animals is often <19% (normal is about 33%). Bone marrow examination is necessary to determine iron storage amounts, especially in the dog. It is less helpful in the cat, which normally lacks stainable iron in the bone marrow. Aspirate and core biopsies of the bone marrow indicate hypercellularity with marked erythroid proliferation. Treatment involves iron supplementation following correction of the inciting cause. Ferrous sulfate is given at a rate of 4–6 mg of iron/kg/day orally in divided doses. Therapy is continued for several weeks to months until the PCV and MCV return to normal.

Cobalamin (vitamin B_{12}) deficiency may occur through acquired disorders, such as, small intestinal disease, exocrine pancreatic insufficiency, or bacterial overgrowth in dogs. Selective malabsorption of vitamin B_{12} has been described in giant schnauzers having an autosomal mode of inheritance. Clinical signs include weight loss, decreased appetite, and failure to thrive at 3 months of age. Laboratory findings include chronic normocytic, normochromic, nonregenerative anemia with occasional erythroid dysplasia in peripheral blood or bone marrow. Serum cobalamin levels can be measured to determine affected animals (see sec. 7, ch. 6). Resolution of clinical and hematologic effects occurs with parenteral administration of cobalamin (initially 1 mg IM daily).

Folate deficiency may produce macrocytic anemia in animals with neoplasia, intestinal malabsorption, liver disease, and severe anorexia or starvation. Drugs such as anticonvulsants (phenobarbital, primidone), sulfonamides (sulfasalazine, trimethoprim-sulfadiazine) and antineoplastic agents (methotrexate) may act as folate antagonists by impairing its absorption or production. Diagnosis is based on a history of drug exposure or concurrent disease. Serum folate levels can be measured (see sec. 7, ch. 6) to confirm the deficiency. The hemogram may indicate a normochromic anemia with macrocytosis and megaloblastic changes in erythroid precursors. Treatment is aimed at the inciting cause along with oral folate supplementation (5 mg/day in dogs; 2.5 mg/day in cats).

Organic Disease

Anemia of chronic inflammation is a frequent cause of nonregenerative anemia. The mechanism may involve increased macrophage activity, reduced iron availability for erythropoiesis through sequestration in macrophages, and decreased RBC survival. Primary infections and neoplasia are most often responsible for chronic inflammation. The animal may present with prolonged anorexia, weight loss, and weakness. Other clinical signs reflect the actual source of chronic inflammation or organ systems affected. Laboratory findings include a normocytic, normochromic anemia, inflammatory leukogram, low serum iron, low total iron-binding capacity, and increased bone marrow stores of iron. The bone marrow is usually hypocellular with a normal to increased myeloid-to-erythroid ratio. Treatment will depend upon the original cause. Iron supplementation does not effectively reverse this form of anemia.

Chronic kidney disease may be associated with normocytic, normochromic nonregenerative anemia. The mechanisms involved include reduced erythropoiesis, decreased red cell survival, and blood loss. Diagnosis of renal failure involves the presence of azotemia and an abnormal urinalysis. For pathogenesis, diagnosis, and treatment see sec. 8, ch. 1.

Chronic liver disease may be associated with normocytic, nonregenerative anemia. Pathogenetic mechanisms include concurrent inflammation with iron sequestration, reduced erythropoiesis, and decreased RBC survival. Blood loss may occur from coagulopathies related to decreased synthesis of clotting factors. Portosystemic shunts may develop erythrocyte microcytosis, with or without anemia, possibly related to a relative decrease in iron availability. Laboratory findings suggestive of hepatic disease include elevated serum liver enzymes (ALT, SAP, GGT), increased serum bile acid levels, hypoalbuminemia, and hyperbilirubinemia. Blood smears often reveal poikilocytosis (acanthocytes, budding fragmentation) (see sec. 7, ch. 8).

Endocrine Disease

Hypothyroidism may present with mild anemia in one third of the cases. Pathogenetic mechanisms include reduced tissue oxygen demand and depressed erythropoiesis at the stem cell level. Diagnosis is based on history, dermatologic signs and hormone assay results (see sec. 4, ch. 1).

Hyperestrogenism is associated with endogenous production by tumors (e.g., testicular Sertoli cell or ovarian granulosa cell) or exogenous administration of estrogenic compounds. The mechanism of reduced erythropoiesis is thought to occur at the level of DNA transcription. Moderate to severe anemia may be accompanied by thrombocytopenia and leukopenia. Diagnosis of an estrogen- producing tumor may be confirmed by surgical removal with subsequent recovery of the cell lines. Supportive care, such as blood transfusion and anabolic steroids, may be necessary.

Hypoadrenocorticism may be a cause of nonregenerative anemia in a small percentage of cases. The anemia is usually discovered following fluid replacement for volume deficits associated with the disease (see sec. 4, ch. 3).

Drug and Toxin-Induced Disease

Drugs (e.g., estrogens, phenylbutazone, antineoplastic agents, thiacetarsamide, quinidine, meclofenamic acid, and trimethoprim-sulfadiazine) are associated with reduced erythropoiesis and aplastic anemia in dogs. Exogenous estrogens are toxic in the dog, depending on the dose given and age of the animal (worse in older dogs). Initially, anemia and thrombocytopenia occur along with leukocytosis, which is an inflammatory neutrophilia. Later, pancytopenia develops. After drug cessation, recovery begins in 1 month, starting with leukocytosis and followed by the return of the other cell lines. Chloramphenicol administration in cats causes a dose-dependent, reversible marrow suppression involving the erythroid series primarily. Dogs are much less sensitive to chloramphenicol. Treatment for drug-induced aplastic anemia often includes supportive care, such as blood transfusions, anabolic steroids, and antibiotics in severe cases, once the drug has been stopped.

Lead poisoning causes a mild anemia in some cases, possibly due to increased RBC fragility and abnormal erythropoiesis. Lead primarily affects heme synthesis, causing defective maturation. Other clinical signs involve GI and neurologic disturbances. Diagnosis is often based on a history of exposure to lead in paint or automobile batteries. Heparinized blood samples are used to determine lead levels. Affected animals have levels greater than 0.06 mg/dl. The hemogram strongly suggests lead poisoning when large numbers of nucleated RBCs are present with a normal or slightly decreased PCV. The anemia is often normocytic and normochromic but may be microcytic and hypochromic. Basophilic stippling is best seen with Romanowsky-stained blood films prepared without EDTA anticoagulant. Polychromasia generally is rare. Bone marrow aspirates or core biopsies are characterized by maturation arrest at the metarubricyte stage. Treatment in dogs and cats involves calcium EDTA (100 mg/kg) diluted to 10 mg/ml in 5% dextrose and given SC, in four divided doses, daily for 5 days.

Myelophthisis

Neoplasia of the bone marrow can occur with primary hemolymphatic tumors or metastatic tumors. Mild infiltrates or focal lesions within the bone marrow produce minimal peripheral blood changes. Cytopenias occur if the involvement is diffuse and severe. Approximately 57% of dogs with multicentric lymphoma have metastasis to the bone marrow at the time of diagnosis. Only half of these have evidence of abnormal cells in circulation. Diagnosis requires bone marrow examination by both aspirate and core biopsies (see discussion of Leukemic Disorders).

Myelofibrosis usually occurs as a result of marrow damage produced by inflammation, necrosis, neoplasia, and toxic agents and may be seen in the terminal stages of pyruvate kinase deficiency. Pancytopenia is observed in severe cases along with poikilocytosis in the form of dacryocytes and schizocytes. Bone marrow aspiration attempts usually produce "dry taps" (i.e., blood alone without marrow particles). Bone marrow core biopsy is diagnostic. Myelofibrosis is also associated with myelodysplastic syndrome and acute myelogenous leukemia in cats (see discussion of Dysplastic Disorders and Leukemic Disorders). Supportive care, including antibiotics, blood transfusions, anabolic steroids, and glucocorticoids, is often required in severe cases. Myelofibrosis may be reversible under some conditions.

Myelonecrosis is an uncommon cause of nonregenerative anemia. It is often associated with neoplasia, but may be related to infections or toxic agents. The mechanism likely involves occlusion of microcirculation or direct injury to endothelium. Diagnosis is based on bone marrow examination. Aspirate biopsies may contain peripheral blood, degenerative cells, increased macrophage activity, and amorphous stringy material representing necrotic bone marrow particles. Focal to diffuse regions of necrosis appear on histologic sections of bone marrow. Treatment includes removal of the inciting cause along with supportive care. Prognosis is often poor.

Osteopetrosis is an uncommon inheritable condition affecting the normal development of bone. It causes obliteration of the marrow cavities by bone and may be associated with refractory anemia or pancytopenia in immature or young adult dogs. Clinical signs are usually related to anemia. Diagnosis is established by the inability to obtain bone marrow material on aspiration and by distinctive radiographic findings. Increased bone density is present and cortices are thickened, leaving a narrow medullary region. Histologic examination of medullary bone reveals thickened trabeculae, reduced marrow cavities, and an absence of osteoclasts. Despite supportive care, the prognosis is poor.

Irradiation acts as a local cytotoxic agent for cancer therapy. It is also used to treat hemolymphatic malignancies and genetic defects prior to bone marrow transplantation. High doses produce irreversible pancytopenia and aplastic bone marrow. Supportive care e.g., blood transfusions, antibiotics, and immunosuppressive drugs are often given following transplantation.

Immune-Mediated Destruction (Pure RBC Aplasia)

This uncommon condition is characterized by severe reduction of erythroid stem cells without affecting granulocytic or megakaryocytic lines. The myeloid-to-erythroid ratio is usually 10:1 to 20:1. Coombs' testing has been positive in a few dogs. The mechanism is considered to be immune-mediated since the disease often responds to prednisolone and/or cyclophosphamide therapy.

Polycythemia

Relative Polycythemia

Increase in RBCs (erythrocytosis) in relative polycythemia is generally related to fluid depletion (e.g., dehydration or hemoconcentration). However, excitement or fear may cause splenic contraction and a transient rise in PCV. Greyhounds normally have a high PCV of 60%. Clinical signs include dark red mucous membranes with slow capillary refill time. Diagnosis is based on a history of stress or fluid loss, elevated PCV, and increased RBC and plasma protein concentrations. The erythrogram returns to normal following fluid replacement. If splenic contraction is suspected, the PCV should be retaken after the patient has relaxed.

Absolute Polycythemia

The erythrocytosis in absolute polycythemia may be primary or secondary, with a sustained increase in the circulating RBC mass, based on erythropoietin production. Primary erythrocytosis, or polycythemia vera, has low serum erythropoietin that suggests that the increased RBC numbers are derived from an intrinsic stem cell defect (see section on Leukemic Disorders). Secondary erythrocytosis involves overproduction of erythropoietin. Causes of secondary erythrocytosis include hypoxia (e.g., caused by high altitude, chronic pulmonary disease, or cardiac disease with right-to-left shunting), tumors that produce erythropoietin (e.g., renal lymphoma, renal carcinoma, and renal fibrosarcoma), and renal disease (e.g., pyelonephritis). Diagnosis of hypoxia is based on history and evidence of lung disease or right-to-left shunting heart disease (see section 6). Renal disease, benign or malignant, can be excluded by urinalysis, radiography, ultrasonography, or biopsy. Erythropoietin levels are useful, but the assays are not yet readily available. Treatment of secondary erythrocytosis often involves removal of the inciting cause (e.g., nephrectomy).

LEUKOCYTE DISORDERS

Congenital Disorders

Pelger-Huet Anomaly

Pelger-Huet anomaly is an inherited disorder in dogs and cats involving granulocyte maturation. Leukocyte function in dogs is not impaired and there is no predisposition to infection or immunodeficiency. Chondrodysplasia has been recognized in a cat with a homozygous form of this disorder. Diagnosis is based on the appearance of mature leukocytes in blood that have nuclei with condensed, coarse, and patchy chromatin lacking segmentation. The nuclear shapes often resemble those of bands, metamyelocytes, and myelocytes. The cytoplasm undergoes normal maturation. Abnormalities frequently are found during routine preoperative screening and may be mistaken as a severe left shift. Inflammatory conditions should be ruled out. No treatment is necessary.

Feline Chediak-Higashi Syndrome

This is a rare, inheritable disorder seen in blue-smoke Persian cats with yellow eye color. Pathogenesis involves abnormal and enlarged lysosomal granule formation in granulocytes and monocytes. Affected cats may be photophobic with cataract formation. There is increased bleeding time due to platelet granule defects. On Romanowsky stains, neutrophils contain characteristic large, pink to magenta cytoplasmic inclusions that stain positive with peroxidase and Sudan black B. These cats do not exhibit an increased susceptibility to infection.

Mucopolysaccharidosis

Mucopolysaccharidosis is an inheritable lysosomal storage disease reported in Siamese cats, dachshunds, and Plott hounds. The enzyme deficiency leads to skeletal and facial deformities as well as to neurologic deficits. Neutrophils contain coarse, reddish granules that stain metachromatically with toluidine blue. Cells must be distinguished from toxic neutrophils. Experimentally, bone marrow transplantation has been used to treat the condition. Affected animals should not be bred.

Abnormal Granulation Syndrome in Birman Cats

This is a genetic anomaly recognized in Birman cats without associated clinical disease. Diagnosis is based on the presence of fine, pinkish-purple granules within the cytoplasm of neutrophils. These lysosomal granules have normal morphology, and neutrophil function is unaffected.

Neutrophilia

Neutrophilia is defined as >11,500 neutrophils/μl in the dog and >12,500 neutrophils/μl in the cat.

Physiologic

Epinephrine release as the result of stress, fear, or strenuous muscular exertion causes demargination of leukocytes, producing a rapid rise in neutrophils and lymphocytes. Within 20 minutes the cell counts return to normal. The effect is more common and greater in cats than in dogs.

Corticosteroid-Induced

Neutrophilia may be related to exogenous administration or endogenous release of glucocorticoids. Cells are released from marginating pools and bone marrow storage pools. The magnitude and duration of the effect depends on the type of corticosteroid given. Diagnosis is determined by the history and by the presence of concurrent lymphopenia, eosinopenia or monocytosis, without a left shift. Neutrophil hypersegmentation is common due to a prolonged life span.

Inflammatory

Evidence of inflammation is an increase in nonsegmented forms of neutrophils, termed a left shift. Etiology involves infectious and noninfectious sources. Infectious agents include bacteria, systemic fungi, protozoa, or rickettsiae (see section 2). Noninfectious conditions involve tissue necrosis, such as necrotizing pancreatitis, neoplasia, thrombosis, and burns. Certain malignancies (e.g., metastatic fibrosarcoma or renal tubular carcinoma) are reported to induce a leukemoid response, presumably as a paraneoplastic disorder, rather than from tissue necrosis alone. Leukemoid counts range from 50,000 to 100,000 WBC/μl with a left shift back to bands, metamyelocytes, and myelocytes. This extreme degree of leukocytosis is also observed with severe abscessation (e.g., pyometra). Immune-mediated reactions, such as systemic lupus erythematosus, can result in a left shift with neutrophilia. A granulocytopathy syndrome involving Irish setters is a congenital cause of inflammatory neutrophilia. Neutrophils appear morphologically normal, but have impaired bactericidal activity related to a deficiency of adhesion proteins. Affected dogs have recurrent bacterial infections with extreme leukocytosis that can mimic chronic granulocytic leukemia (see section on Leukemic Disorders). Diagnosis of inflammatory neutrophilia is based on a careful history and CBC evaluation. A regenerative left shift requires a simultaneous neutrophilia. A left shift without neutrophilia is considered degenerative, especially if there is neutropenia or if more nonsegmented forms are present compared with mature neutrophils. In addition to a significant shift toward immaturity (bands >1000/μl), neutrophils may exhibit toxicity. Toxins released from bacteria are mostly responsible for the focal or diffuse cytoplasmic basophilia and vacuolation found in mature or immature neutrophils. Antibiotic responsiveness suggests a bacterial cause. Tests for specific infectious agents and immune-mediated disorders may be indicated. Treatment will depend upon the inciting cause.

Neoplastic

See discussion of Leukemic Disorders.

Neutropenia

Neutropenia is defined as <3000 neutrophils/μl in the dog and <2500 neutrophils/μl in the cat.

Congenital

Cyclic neutropenia or cyclic hematopoiesis is an inherited disorder of gray collies. It is characterized by periodic fluctuations in neutrophils and to a lesser extent in monocytes, platelets, and reticulocytes as a result of the intrinsic bone marrow stem cell defect. Neutropenic cycles recur at 12-day intervals. Clinical signs during neutropenic episodes include lethargy, pyrexia, anorexia, arthritis, keratitis, and respiratory or GI infections. Diagnosis is based on history, clinical signs, and cyclic decreases in cell counts. Carrier animals can be determined only by test mating. Antibiotics and supportive care are necessary during neutropenic cycles. Most affected dogs die within 6 months following chronic recurrent infections. Experimental treatments involve bone marrow transplantation and administration of lithium carbonate (21–26 mg/kg/day) or granulocyte-colony stimulating factor.

Infectious

Consumption of neutrophils during severe systemic inflammation often produces neutropenia with an increase of immature forms, termed a degenerative left shift. Gram-negative bacteria are usually involved, as with septicemia, severe enteritis, and other severe bacterial infections. Systemic mycoses and protozoal infections (e.g., *Toxoplasma*) can also cause neutropenia. Reduced granulopoiesis may be associated with viruses such as FeLV, FIV, feline panleukopenia virus, and canine parvovirus. FeLV is associated with a cyclic neutropenia that may respond to lithium and prednisone. *Ehrlichia canis* may also cause bone marrow suppression (see sec. 2, ch. 10). Diagnosis is based on the history, CBC, and bone marrow findings, in addition to specific serologic or bacterial culture results. Neutropenia without a marked left shift may indicate peracute consumption without adequate time for bone marrow response. The lack of a left shift, if persistent, suggests an absolute reduction of neutrophilic precursors or myeloid hypoplasia of the bone marrow. Treatment is directed at the inciting cause.

Toxic

Drugs that cause neutropenia due to myelotoxicity include estrogens, chloramphenicol, and cancer chemotherapeutic agents (see discussion of Nonregenerative Anemia). Antineoplastic agents that can cause neutropenia include cyclophosphamide, chlorambucil, busulfan, melphalan, cisplatin, cytosine arabinoside, methotrexate, vincristine, doxorubicin, and hydroxyurea. Cephalosporins occasionally have been associated with myelotoxicity, as well as those drugs listed previously (see discussion of Nonregenerative Anemia). Endotoxins resulting from gram-negative sepsis produce a transient neutropenia. Mechanisms involve a shift of neutrophils from the circulation to the marginating pools and a shortened circulating half-life (normal is approximately 5.5 to 7.5 hours). Treatment requires cessation of the drug and supportive care, particularly antibiotics.

Immune-Mediated

Destruction of antibody-coated neutrophils by macrophages is a mechanism of neutropenia considered to occur in animals, but this has not been well documented. As in immune-mediated hemolysis, the disorder may involve antibody directed against surface antigens of the cell itself, or antibody toward drug antigens attached to neutrophils. Definitive diagnosis requires detection of antineutrophil antibodies on the cells or in serum; however, such assays are not currently available for clinical usage. The bone marrow is expected to show myeloid hyperplasia, with a marked decrease in late stage forms. One suspected case in a dog was responsive to immunosuppressive doses of prednisone.

Myelophthisis

See discussion of Nonregenerative Anemia.

Irradiation

See discussion of Nonregenerative Anemia.

Monocytosis
Corticosteroid-Induced

Monocytosis, particularly in the dog, can be induced by glucocorticoid administration. Diagnosis is based on the history, but when this is unavailable, the presence of concurrent lymphopenia, eosinopenia, and mature neutrophilia should suggest the effects of corticosteroids.

Inflammatory

Acute and chronic inflammatory diseases that cause a high demand for macrophages may produce monocytosis. These include immune-mediated disorders, tissue necrosis, foreign body reactions, and mycobacterial and fungal infections. Diagnosis is based on the history, physical examination, immunologic testing, cytology, and histopathology.

Neoplastic

See discussion of Leukemic Disorders.

Eosinophilia
Parasitic

Peripheral eosinophilia may result from infiltration of the skin, respiratory tract, and alimentary tract by such parasites as *Ancylostoma* spp., *Trichuris vulpis*, *Toxocara canis*, *Dirofilaria immitis*, *Dipetalonema reconditum*, lungworms (*Aelurostrongylus abstrusus*, *Capillaria* spp, *Filaroides* spp), and *Paragonimus kellicotti*. Definitive diagnosis of parasitism is determined by positive fecal examinations, tracheobronchial washes, thoracic radiographs, and heartworm serologic or concentration techniques.

Allergic/Inflammatory

Hypersensitivity reactions can occur owing to the effects of fleas, food, grasses, and nonspecific allergens. The production of IgE causes mast cell degranulation and release of chemical mediators that attract eosinophils. The skin, respiratory, GI, and genitourinary systems often are infected. Eosinophilic granuloma is a localized infiltration of the dermis by eosinophils that occurs in the oral cavity or skin of dogs and cats (see sec. 5, ch. 14). The history, physical examination, skin or food testing, and tracheobronchial lavage help to locate the type of allergen and the system most affected. In the case of eosinophilic granuloma, impression smears and histopathology may be diagnostic. Peripheral eosinophilia is commonly found in these conditions. Treatment usually involves elimination of the allergen, along with antihistamine and glucocorticoid administration.

Paraneoplastic Syndrome

Tumor-associated eosinophilia has been reported in dogs with fibrosarcoma, anaplastic mammary carcinoma, and mast cell tumors. In cats, mast cell tumors and lymphoma are the neoplasms most commonly associated with eosinophilia. Diagnosis depends on normalization or reduction of the eosinophil count in response to removal of the tumor.

Hypereosinophilic Syndrome in Cats

Hypereosinophilic syndrome is an uncommon form of peripheral eosinophilia accompanied by severe infiltration of eosinophils into many organs, often including the gastrointestinal tract, liver, spleen, lymph nodes, and lung. It resembles a leukemia of well-differentiated eosinophils resulting from an apparent involvement of the bone marrow. The cause is idiopathic and difficult to separate from eosinophilic leukemia. Clinical signs may include anorexia, weight loss, fever, vomiting, diarrhea, and lymphadenopathy. Death results from organ dysfunction caused by tissue infiltration.

Neoplastic

See discussion of Leukemic Disorders.

Eosinopenia

Endogenous release or exogenous administration of corticosteroids produces eosinopenia within a few hours. Levels normalize in 1 day after a single dose is given. Mechanisms implicated are enhanced margination, decreased bone marrow release, and reduced bone marrow production. Absolute reductions in eosinophils or relative decreases from a previous eosinophilia suggest the effects of glucocorticoids. Elevated cortisol levels and an endocrine dermatopathy support hyperadrenocorticism (see sec. 4, ch. 3).

Basophilia

Parasitic

Heartworm infection, including occult disease, is a frequent cause of basophilia in dogs and cats. Dogs with hookworms may also have basophilia. Diagnosis often involves concurrent eosinophilia and positive proof of parasitic infestation. Basophil granules in dogs and cats normally stain poorly. The cells are frequently mistaken for toxic neutrophils in dogs or for faded eosinophils in cats.

Allergic

Hypersensitivity reactions cause IgE production in such organs as the skin and lungs. The immune response leads to increased numbers of mast cells and basophils.

Lipid Metabolism

An association between basophilia without eosinophilia, and lipemia is thought to be related to deficiency of heparin, which is found in basophils and is needed to activate lipoprotein lipase. This enzyme is necessary to clear lipemia. However, this is observed infrequently.

Systemic Mastocytosis

Basophilia was found in five of 16 dogs with systemic mastocytosis. It also occurs in cats with splenic mastocytoma (see sec. 3, ch. 7).

Neoplastic

See discussion of Leukemic Disorders.

Lymphocytosis

Epinephrine-Induced

A transient rise in lymphocytes occurs with severe exertion or physiologic stress. This is especially significant in the young cat. Transient lymphocytosis that normalizes after a short time suggests epinephrine effects on the leukogram.

Infectious

Lymphocytosis may be due to antigen stimulation caused by FeLV, *Ehrlichia canis, Rickettsia rickettsii*, and systemic fungi (see sec. 2, chs. 1, 10, and 12). Modified live vaccines may also produce lymphocytosis, along with the morphologic appearance of reactivity, about 1 week postimmunization. Slightly enlarged lymphocytes with deeply basophilic cytoplasm resembling plasma cells support the diagnosis of reactivity from antigen stimulation. Hyperglobulinemia due to a polyclonal gammopathy and plasma cell infiltration of tissues also may occur.

Neoplastic

Lymphocytosis resulting from metastatic lymphoma occurs in 20% of dogs and cats with lymphoma. Acute or chronic lymphoid leukemia often is characterized by lymphocytosis and atypical or immature lymphoid cells. However, rare blast cells may be found in nonneoplastic conditions such as immune-mediated hemolytic anemia and canine ehrlichiosis. Persistent hematologic abnormalities must be present to consider neoplasia and should be evaluated further with bone marrow aspiration and core biopsies (see sec. 3, ch. 6).

Lymphopenia

Corticosteroid-Induced

Endogenous or exogenous corticosteroids produce an absolute lymphopenia or a normal value reduced from a previous lymphocytosis. It is transient, as cell counts return to normal within 1 to 3 days following drug withdrawal. Lymphopenia may also relate to redistribution of lymphocytes to other tissues. (see discussion of Neutrophilia). Lymphopenia often accompanies the stress of many acute diseases.

Infectious

Viral agents, such as canine distemper virus, FeLV, FIV, and canine or feline parvoviruses, cause lymphopenia due to direct lymphoid tissue injury.

Lymphatic Damage

Rupture or malformation of lymphatic vessels (e.g., chylothorax or protein-losing enteropathy from lymphangiectasia) can cause lymphopenia due to a loss of lymph fluid into the chest or gut lumen (see sec. 6, ch. 22 and sec. 7, ch. 6). Destruction of normal lymph node architecture or blockage of lymph drainage, as in lymphoma, may also lead to lymphopenia (see sec. 3, ch. 6).

Congenital

Combined immunodeficiency of T- and B-lymphocytes occurs in bassett hounds. It is associated with severe bacterial infections within the first few weeks of life. Diagnosis is based on the presence of low immunoglobulin levels, depressed T-cell function, and histologic evidence of lymphoid cell depletion, as well as peripheral lymphopenia. Supportive therapy with antibiotics is suggested, but death may occur in severe cases.

Mastocytosis or Mastocythemia

See sec. 3, ch. 7.

PLATELET DISORDERS

Thrombocytopenia

Platelets may be decreased in number through:

- Immune-mediated injury
- Increased consumption
- Sequestration
- Decreased production

Overview

Clinical Signs
- Petechial or ecchymotic hemorrhages involving the mucous membranes or skin are common manifestations of thrombocytopenia.
- Epistaxis, melena, hematuria, hyphema, or prolonged bleeding from venipuncture sites or wounds often occur.
- Evidence of inciting conditions such as infection, neoplasia, or splenomegaly may be present.

General Diagnostic Considerations
- The history should determine the occurrence of trauma, surgery, drug or toxin exposure, and neoplasia as well as the time period involved.
- Physical examination will disclose sites of hemorrhage, presence of hepatosplenomegaly, and concurrent infections or neoplasia.
- Use CBC to screen for hematologic abnormalities including the adequacy of the platelet numbers.
- Perform platelet counts on fresh samples (within 1–2 hours). Thrombocytopenia is considered to be <100,000 platelets/μl. However, clinical signs of bleeding are not expected until there are <20,000 platelets/μl.
- Include both aspirate and core biopsies in bone

marrow evaluation to check for megakaryocyte numbers.
- Perform clotting profile, including fibrinogen, prothrombin time (PT), activated partial thromboplastin time (APTT), or activated coagulation time (ACT), to help rule out other coagulopathies (as described in sec. 3. ch. 2). Note that ACT may be slightly prolonged if platelet counts are <10,000/μl.
- Perform a von Willebrand factor assay if the breed and clinical signs suggest a deficiency (see sec. 3, ch. 2).
- Bleeding time, a platelet function test, may be prolonged owing to low platelet numbers.

Treatment. Supportive therapy may include fresh blood transfusions (administered within 8 hours of collection) if both platelets and RBC numbers are low. If only platelets are needed, administer platelet-rich plasma (see sec 3, ch. 2).

Immune-Mediated Platelet Injury

This is one of the most frequent and important causes of thrombocytopenia manifested by clinically significant bleeding (see sec. 3, ch. 3).

Increased Platelet Consumption or Sequestration

Infectious Agents. Thrombocytopenia produced by such agents as *Ehrlichia canis*, *E. platys*, and *E. equi* presumably is due to increased platelet activation and consumption. Bone marrow evaluation during the acute course of the disease indicates megakaryocytic hyperplasia. The diagnosis of ehrlichiosis is based on a history of tick exposure and positive serologic testing (see sec. 2, ch. 10).

Modified Live Virus Vaccination. Canine distemper virus vaccine may induce thrombocytopenia within 1 week postvaccination. The effect is transient but may persist for as long as 3 weeks. It is rarely of clinical significance unless surgery is performed during the platelet count nadir.

Hemorrhage. Bleeding can consume platelets. Consumption of platelets may occur through hemorrhage alone or in association with bacterial or viral infections that produce inflammation. Endotoxemia from gram-negative bacteria leads to endothelial damage and platelet activation. Diagnosis is based on history, physical examination, cytology, histopathology, and culture techniques. Treatment is aimed at the inciting agent. Whole blood or platelet transfusions may be necessary if thrombocytopenia is severe.

Disseminated Intravascular Coagulation. This condition leads to increased consumption of platelets as well as clotting factors. It is most often associated with infections, neoplasia, heartworm disease, pancreatitis, and shock. Clinical signs involve petechial and ecchymotic hemorrhages. Organ dysfunction usually reflects the effects of the primary disease. Diagnosis is based on the findings in tests of coagulation, including hypofibrinogenemia, prolonged PT and APTT, increased fibrin degradation products, and decreased antithrombin III activity. Microthrombi formation is found on histopathology. Treatment is aimed at the inciting or underlying cause when possible. Supportive care, including fluids, is necessary to prevent shock. Replacement of platelets and coagulation factors using fresh plasma is usually indicated. Heparin is rarely indicated, especially if the hemorrhagic stage has already occurred (see sec. 3, ch. 2).

Splenomegaly. The spleen normally stores approximately one third of the body's platelets. With enlargement of the spleen from any cause, there will be an increase in blood volume that will sequester more platelets within endothelial passages, resulting in thrombocytopenia. Physical examination of an enlarged spleen without evidence of other conditions that induce thrombocytopenia supports the diagnosis. It is usually of little clinical significance if associated with benign enlargements of the spleen (see sec. 3, ch. 4).

Decreased Platelet Production

Congenital Thrombocytopenia. Cyclic hematopoiesis in gray collie dogs may exhibit thrombocytopenia of a cyclic nature (see discussion of Neutropenia).

Infectious Agents. Canine distemper virus, parvoviruses, FeLV, and *Ehrlichia canis* are associated with reduced thrombopoiesis. About 20% of animals with ehrlichiosis have megakaryocytic hypoplasia of the bone marrow, especially in the late stages of the disease (see sec. 2, chs. 1, 6, 7, and 10).

Drug-Induced. Causes of drug-induced thrombocytopenia are similar to those that produce aplastic anemia (see section on Nonregenerative Anemia). Antineoplastic agents such as cisplatin, cyclophosphamide, chlorambucil, doxorubicin, and hydroxyurea produce significant thrombocytopenia.

Myelophthistic Thrombocytopenia. See discussion on Nonregenerative Anemia.

Thrombocytosis

Physiologic

Increased numbers of platelets are released from the spleen due to epinephrine release or during heavy exercise. Pulmonary stores of platelets may also be released during exercise. This is transient and of no clinical significance.

Reactive

Conditions associated with reactive or regenerative thrombocytosis include acute blood loss, iron deficiency anemia, trauma, surgery, inflammation, splenectomy, hyperadrenocorticism, and neoplasia. Tumors that may cause thrombocytosis include mast cell tumors, hemangiosarcoma, osteosarcoma, some carcinomas, and lymphocytic leukemia. Vincristine administration produces increased production and cytoplasmic fragmentation of megakaryocytes because of a reduced maturation time. There are no clinical signs directly related to transiently elevated platelet counts. Diagnosis is supported by history, physical examination, platelet count >600,000/µl (dog) or >800,000/µl (cat), and mild to moderate megakaryocytic bone marrow hyperplasia without evidence of circulating megakaryoblasts. Pseudohyperkalemia can occur owing to leakage of potassium from clotted platelets. Therefore, plasma is preferred for measurement of potassium levels in thrombocytotic samples. Treatment depends on the inciting cause.

Neoplastic

See discussion of Leukemic Disorders.

DYSPLASTIC DISORDERS

Congenital

An inherited disorder of toy and miniature poodles is associated with abnormal morphology of erythrocytes and their precursors. Affected animals present with no clinical signs of anemia, and the dysplastic findings are usually incidental. Diagnosis is based on the breed and on findings of a normal hematocrit, presence of macrocytosis (MCV >80 fl), megaloblastosis in the blood and bone marrow, and absence of polychromasia or reticulocytosis. An asynchrony in maturation between the nucleus and cytoplasm characterizes RBC abnormalities. Neutrophil hypersegmentation and giantism may also occur but is less common. The condition persists and is not responsive to folate or cobalamin.

Infectious

Abnormal morphology of erythroid, granulocytic, and megakaryocytic lines occurs in cats infected with either FeLV or FIV (see sec. 2, chs. 1 and 2). Macrocytosis, megaloblastosis, neutrophil giantism, hypersegmentation, and dwarf megakaryocyte formation characterize the dysplastic changes found as a result of viral effects on nuclear development. Peripheral cytopenias arise from abnormal maturation of affected cell lines. Clinical signs often include concurrent bacterial or protozoal infections, neoplasia, and chronic wasting. Definitive diagnosis requires serologic testing. Treatment is supportive in nature.

Drug-Induced

Dyserythropoiesis characterized by macrocytosis, megaloblastoid changes, nuclear fragmentation, sideroblastosis, and siderocytosis may occur in animals treated with azathioprine, cyclophosphamide, cytosine arabinoside, vincristine, or chloramphenicol. Diagnosis is based on blood and bone marrow samples taken during routine post-treatment hematologic evaluations. These changes are not associated with folate deficiency. Normal morphology of hematopoietic cells occurs several days following cessation of drug therapy.

Nutritional

Erythroid dysplastic changes and neutrophil hypersegmentation may occur in giant schnauzers with an inherited selective malabsorption of vitamin B_{12} (in this chapter under Nonregenerative Anemia). A macrocytic nonregenerative anemia is found in acquired folate deficiencies such as intestinal malabsorption, neoplasia, liver disease, or severe starvation. In addition, drugs such as anticonvulsants, antibiotics, and antineoplastic agents that inhibit folate metabolism produce megaloblastic changes in erythroid precursors (see Nonregenerative Anemia).

Myelodysplastic Syndrome

Myelodysplasia is characterized by persistent peripheral cytopenias in two or three hematopoietic cell lines together with features of abnormal maturation. This condition often precedes an overt leukemia by several weeks to months. Cats affected usually are seropositive for FeLV. Clinical signs involve chronic infections, lethargy due to anemia, and hemorrhage. Despite the cytopenias, the bone marrow is usually hypercellular, with a mild increase in numbers of myeloblasts. Dysplastic changes in the blood or bone marrow include macrocytosis, megaloblastosis, nuclear fragmentation, abnormal cytoplasmic granulation, neutrophil hypersegmentation or hyposegmentation, cell giantism, and micromegakaryocyte and macrothrombocyte formation. As the condition may persist for long periods of time without major clinical disease, treatment is usually supportive, including antibiotics and blood transfusions as needed. Antineoplastic agents, such as low-dose cytosine arabinoside, have been used to induce normal maturation and prevent conversion to a malignant state. Results with these agents have been mixed and therefore cannot be recommended as treatment.

LEUKEMIC DISORDERS

Lymphoid Leukemia

See sec. 3, ch. 6 on Lymphoproliferative Diseases.

Myeloid (Nonlymphoid) Leukemia

The etiology for this group of leukemias is generally unknown, although they are often associated with viral infection (e.g., FeLV), immunologic dysfunction, and irradiation. Clinical signs include pale mucous membranes (except in polycythemia vera), fever, lethargy, weight loss, chronic infections, hepatosplenomegaly, mild lymphadenopathy, and hemorrhagic tendencies. Myeloid leukemias are suggested by the history (e.g., FeLV infection), clinical signs of unexplained or frequent infections, and hematologic abnormalities that affect multiple cell lines. Definitive diagnosis is made from bone marrow aspirate and core examinations. Cytochemical staining of blast cells from blood and bone marrow smears may be performed on unfixed slides submitted to special laboratories to determine the cell type primarily involved. Treatment generally consists of supportive care (e.g., antibiotics, blood transfusions, and fluids). Antineoplastic agents, including corticosteroids, cytosine arabinoside, chlorambucil, busulfan, and hydroxyurea, have been used with limited success. Bone marrow transplantation has been attempted in the cat, but is cost-prohibitive for clinical application.

Acute Myelogenous Leukemia

Acute myelogenous leukemia (AML) is relatively common among leukemias and often associated with FeLV in cats. It is characterized by a high percentage of myeloblasts in the bone marrow (>30% of nonerythroid cells). These cells have pale basophilic cytoplasm that may contain several small red granules. Nuclei are round with prominent nucleoli. Intermediate- and late-stage forms of neutrophils are present to a variable degree. The CBC often indicates a severe nonregenerative anemia and thrombocytopenia. Total leukocyte counts are usually elevated. Cytochemical staining of blast cells is variably positive for peroxidase, Sudan black B, chloroacetate esterase, leukocyte alkaline phosphatase, and acid phosphatase. Rebounding from neutropenia, such as that following feline panleukopenia infection, can cause the blood to appear neoplastic owing to the presence of large numbers of myeloblasts. Persistent hematologic abnormalities must occur to confirm leukemia.

Chronic Granulocytic (Neutrophilic) Leukemia

This disorder is characterized by a low percentage of myeloblasts in the bone marrow, with increased numbers of early forms such as progranulocytes to metamyelocytes in the blood and bone marrow. WBCs are markedly elevated (40,000–200,000/μl). Anemia is mild to moderate and platelet counts are variable. Marrow myeloid-to-erythroid ratio is 4:1 to 25:1. This form of leukemia must be differentiated from leukemoid reactions caused by highly suppurative infections such as pyometra (see section on Neutrophilia). Death often occurs months after detection and may be associated with a blast cell crisis, severe anemia, and thrombocytopenia.

Eosinophilic Leukemia

This type of leukemia is rare, but has been documented in the cat and is associated with FeLV infection. It is characterized by a high eosinophil count (>50,000/μl) with a shift toward immaturity. A moderate anemia may be present. It may be difficult to differentiate this malignancy from reactive hypereosinophilic conditions, e.g., allergies, parasitism, eosinophilic inflammatory diseases, mast cell tumors, and certain lymphomas (see discussion of Eosinophilia). Leukemic eosinophils will spread from the bone marrow and infiltrate other tissues, such as the lymph nodes, liver, and spleen.

Basophilic Leukemia

This disorder is very rare and most cases have been reported in the dog. Mature and immature basophils are increased in the blood or bone marrow, and tissue infiltration may occur. Basophilic leukemia must be differentiated from mast cell leukemia (see sec. 3, ch. 7).

Monocytic Leukemia

This condition has been reported in both dogs and cats. It is characterized by moderate to marked increases of blast cells in the bone marrow. These cells have basophilic cytoplasm that lacks any obvious granulation. Nuclei exhibit extreme irregularity, which gives the cell a folded appearance. Nucleoli are usually prominent. Cytochemical staining of the blast cells is generally positive for nonspecific esterases and acid phosphatase.

Myelomonocytic Leukemia

This is a common form of myeloid leukemia in dogs and cats. It involves the common stem cell for both granulocytes and monocytes. Cytochemical staining suggests the presence of both monoblasts and myeloblasts.

Erythroleukemia

Erythroleukemia incorporates the varied manifestations of erythroid leukemic cells. Rubriblasts may predominate or may be combined with neoplastic myeloblasts. Dysplastic changes are frequently prominent, such as megaloblastosis, neutrophil giantism, or hypersegmentation. Normochromic macrocytes and nucleated RBCs are found in the blood, without regenerative signs of polychromasia or reticulocytosis. Over time, this form of leukemia may change in appearance and progress to involve predominantly granulocytic precursors. It is frequently associated with FeLV infection in cats.

Polycythemia Vera

Polycythemia vera occurs rarely in dogs and cats. Clinical signs differ from other myeloid leukemias in that they relate to increased RBC mass and blood hyperviscosity. Mucous membranes are dark red because of hematocrits of 65 to 82%. Splenomegaly is usually not present. Polyuria, polydipsia, hemorrhage, and neurologic disorders occur in 50% of canine cases. Diagnosis requires ruling out other causes of erythrocytosis (see discussion of Polycythemia). Arterial blood gas evaluations are normal with no evidence of hypoxia. Erythropoietin levels are absent or reduced when measured by an exhypoxic polycythemic mouse or rabbit bone marrow bioassay, which must be performed at specialized laboratories. WBC and platelet counts are normal to mildly elevated. Bone marrow examination indicates hyperplasia of the erythroid line, with normal morphology and maturation. Treatment consists of phlebotomy for immediate relief (10–20 ml/kg/day). Survival of at least 1.5 years is possible with hydroxyurea (Hydrea, Squibb) given at 30 mg/kg/day for 1 week, then 15 mg/kg once daily until

remission; then taper to lowest effective frequency of administration based on monitoring hematocrit. Monitor cats more closely because of greater risk of myelotoxicity. Radiophosphorus ^{32}P (2.4–3.3 mCi/m^2) has been used with encouraging results.

Megakaryocytic Leukemia

This is the rarest type of leukemia reported in dogs and cats. It is associated with irradiation in the dog. Laboratory findings indicate severe nonregenerative anemia, leukopenia, and often thrombocytopenia, although platelet counts are variable. Megakaryoblasts may appear in the circulation, and platelet morphology is often bizarre, characterized by giantism and abnormal granulation. Hemolymphatic organs usually are infiltrated by the neoplastic population, which rules out a benign proliferation.

Primary Thrombocythemia

Primary, or essential, thrombocythemia is a neoplastic proliferation of platelets reported in the dog and cat. It is not related to transient or reactive increases (see section on Thrombocytosis). Clinical signs include splenomegaly and platelet function abnormalities such as spontaneous bleeding and thromboembolism. Platelet counts are persistently above 600,000/μl. Neutrophilia may also be present. Treatment may include mephalan (2–4 mg/m^2), hydroxyurea (500 mg/m^2), or radiophosphorus ^{32}P (2.4–3.5 mCi/m^2). Therapy produces a survival of 1 to 14 months.

Supplemental Readings

Blue JT, French TW, Kranz JS: Non-lymphoid hematopoietic neoplasia in cats: A retrospective study of 60 cases. Cornell Vet 78:21, 1988.

Center SA, Randolph JF, Erb HN, Reiter S: Eosinophilia in the cat: A retrospective study of 312 cases (1975–1986). J Am Anim Hosp Assoc 26:349, 1990.

Green CE: *Infectious Diseases of the Dog and Cat.* Philadelphia: W. B. Saunders, 1990.

Harvey JW, French TW, Meyer DJ: Chronic iron deficiency anemia in dogs. J Am Anim Hosp Assoc 18:946, 1982.

Helfand SC, Couto CG, Madewell BR: Immune-mediated thrombocytopenia associated with solid tumors in dogs. J Am Anim Hosp Assoc 21:787, 1985.

Hoenig M: Six dogs with features compatible with myelonecrosis and myelofibrosis. J Am Anim Hosp Assoc 25:335, 1989.

Jain NC: *Schalm's Veterinary Hematology.* 4th ed. Philadelphia: Lea & Febiger, 1986.

Latimer KS, Rakich PM: Clinical interpretation of leukocyte responses. Vet Clin North Am 19:637, 1989.

Weiss DJ, Armstrong PJ: Non-regenerative anemias in the dog. Compend Contin Educ Pract Vet 6:452, 1984.

Weiss DJ, Raskin R, Zerbe C: Myelodysplastic syndrome in two dogs. J Am Vet Med Assoc 187:1038, 1985.

2 Coagulation Disorders

Marjory Brooks

Coagulation disorders are a group of bleeding diatheses caused by dysfunction of the clotting cascade and subsequent failure of fibrin clot formation. Included in this discussion of coagulation disorders are von Willebrand's disease and disseminated intravascular coagulation. Common bleeding diatheses that are not coagulation disorders include thrombocytopenia and acquired platelet dysfunction (platelet disorders are discussed in sec. 3, ch. 1). Patients affected with coagulation disorders must be differentiated from those with bleeding that results from damaged or diseased blood vessels.

ETIOLOGY

Categories of bleeding disorders are listed in Table 1 and include coagulation factor deficiencies, von Willebrand's disease, and disseminated intravascular coagulation.

Coagulation Factor Deficiencies

Acquired Deficiencies

Acquired deficiencies of functional coagulation factors are common disorders and are caused by decreased production of coagulation factors or inactivation of existing factors.

Production Defect. Most coagulation factors are proteins, synthesized in the liver. Clinically significant reduction in these factors most often accompanies acute fulminant necrosis, chronic cirrhosis, and portosystemic shunting diseases; each of these can cause severe liver failure and marked reduction in functional hepatic mass (see sec. 7, ch. 8).

Inactive Factors
- The prothrombin group of coagulation factors (factors II, VII, IX, and X) requires vitamin K for activation.
  - The most common vitamin K deficiency state in small animal medicine occurs after ingestion of anticoagulant rodenticides, which deplete body stores of vitamin K. Potency and duration of effect vary for different poisons.
  - Posthepatic biliary obstruction and infiltrative bowel disease can cause vitamin K deficiency by reducing its intestinal absorption.
  - Occasionally bleeding due to vitamin K deficiency

is seen in neonates born prematurely or delivered by cesarean section.
- Heparin inhibits coagulation factor function by greatly enhancing activity of antithrombin III, a natural plasma anticoagulant.
  - Bleeding due to iatrogenic factor inactivation results from overdose of heparin for treatment of thrombotic disorders or from excessive heparinization of transfused blood products.
  - Release of heparin from mast cell tumor granules often causes local tissue hemorrhage and edema. In rare cases, massive degranulation of disseminated tumor causes systemic anticoagulation.

Inherited Factor Deficiencies

Inherited factor deficiencies are caused by mutations in genes coding for specific individual coagulation proteins. These defects are most common in certain lines of purebred dogs and cats and are usually perpetuated when asymptomatic carriers are bred. They also may arise by new, spontaneous mutations in previously unaffected pedigrees. Inheritance patterns vary for different individual factor deficiencies.

X-linked Traits. Hemophilia is the most common severe coagulation factor deficiency and is inherited as an X-linked recessive trait.

- Males inheriting one abnormal gene from their mother express the trait, whereas females inheriting one abnormal gene from either parent are asymptomatic carriers.
- Spontaneous mutations in the factor VIII gene cause hemophilia A and arise about three times as often as those in the factor IX gene. Hemophilia B is the specific deficiency of factor IX.
- German shepherds, especially those with European dogs in their pedigree, have the highest prevalence of canine hemophilia A.

Autosomal Traits. Males and females express these traits with equal frequency.

- Clinically significant bleeding disorders due to inherited deficiencies of factors XI, X, VII, and II and fibrinogen have been described.
- Factor XII deficiency is common in cats but does not cause abnormal hemostasis.

Von Willebrand's Disease

Von Willebrand's disease (vWD) is the most common inherited bleeding disorder in dogs. Bleeding in affected individuals is caused by deficiency or dysfunction of von Willebrand factor (vWF), a plasma protein

Supported in part by NIH grant HL 09902 from the NHLBI PHS/DHHS.

TABLE 1. Classification and Causes of Coagulation Disorders

Category	Cause
Coagulation factor deficiency	

Acquired (multiple) factor deficiencies	Decreased factor production
	    Liver failure (acute necrosis, chronic cirrhosis, portosystemic shunts)
	
	Decreased factor activation
	    Vitamin K deficiency (anticoagulant rodenticide toxicity, biliary obstruction, malabsorption, neonatal)
	    Heparin excess (iatrogenic, mast cell tumor)

Inherited (single) factor deficiency	X-linked traits—males affected
	    Hemophilia A—factor VIII deficiency (most common defect in dogs and cats; German shepherd breed has highest prevalence)
	    Hemophilia B—Factor IX deficiency (Airedale, Bichon, cats)
	
	Autosomal traits—males and females affected
	    Dysfibrinogenemia—uncommon (borzoi, French bulldog)
	    Prothrombin deficiency—uncommon (boxer, English cocker)
	    Factor VII deficiency—mild bleeding (beagle)
	    Factor X deficiency—severe bleeding (American cocker)
	    Factor XI deficiency—severe bleeding (English springer spaniel, Kerry blue terrier)
	    Factor XII deficiency—no abnormal bleeding (common in DSH cats)

von Willebrand's disease	Inherited form—autosomal trait
	    Variable severity in affected dogs, high prevalence (Doberman pinscher, golden retriever, standard poodle, Corgi, Akita, others)
	    Severe bleeding in affected dogs (Scottie, Sheltie, German shorthaired pointer, Chesapeake retriever)
	
	Acquired form—bleeding associated with systemic disease
	    Endocrinopathy (thyroid insufficiency, cortisol insufficiency, estrus, parturition)
	    Infection (viral, bacterial, postvaccinal)
	    Drug therapy (sulfa-trimethoprim, nonsteroidal anti-inflammatory drugs)

Disseminated intravascular coagulation	Factor depletion and systemic fibrinolysis
	    Neoplasia (hemangiosarcoma, prostatic and mammary carcinoma, lymphoid tumors)
	    Sepsis
	    Intravascular hemolysis
	    Severe tissue injury (burns, crush wounds)

critical for normal platelet function in the primary phase of hemostasis.

- The trait is autosomal; both males and females can transmit and/or express vWD.
- Apparent acquired forms of vWD are seen in which individuals first exhibit signs of abnormal hemostasis as adults. In these cases concurrent infection, hormonal fluctuation, or endocrinopathy (especially thyroid insufficiency) is often present when bleeding diathesis is expressed.
- Breeds with the highest prevalence of the vWD trait include the Doberman pinscher, Scottish terrier, Shetland sheepdog, golden retriever, Pembroke Welsh corgi, and standard poodle.

Disseminated Intravascular Coagulation

Disseminated intravascular coagulation (DIC) is a disease process that results from loss of localized clot formation and secondary diffuse activation of the fibrinolytic system.

- Disorders that trigger the DIC process cause widespread damage to vascular tissue, or platelet aggregation and consumption, or intravascular release of tissue phospholipid.
- Clinically, DIC most often accompanies severe systemic diseases such as sepsis, neoplasia (especially hemangiosarcoma, prostatic and mammary carci-

noma, lymphosarcoma), burn or crush wounds, and intravascular hemolysis.

- Bleeding occurs in association with DIC when coagulation factors are depleted and systemic fibrinolysis degrades clots before vessel repair is complete. Thrombocytopenia and platelet dysfunction often accompany DIC and exacerbate bleeding.

CLINICAL SIGNS

Coagulation disorders are characterized by spontaneous hemorrhage and/or excessive bleeding after surgery or trauma. Hemorrhage into CNS may cause acute onset of neurologic dysfunction or sudden death. Thrombocytopenia (see sec. 3, ch. 1), not coagulation disorders, is by far the most common cause of petechiae in small animals. Hemorrhagic macules, papules, and ecchymoses are lesions most characteristic of primary or secondary vasculitic disorders.

- Coagulation factor deficiencies tend to cause spontaneous bleeding into chest, abdomen, or muscles, and subcutaneous hematoma formation.
- vWD is most often associated with spontaneous hemorrhage from mucosal surfaces of oral and nasal cavities, or intestinal and genitourinary tracts.
- Bleeding in association with DIC is usually severe and occurs from mucosal surfaces and into body

TABLE 2. Diagnostic Checklists Based on Results of Quick Assessment Tests (QATs)

QAT	Result/Interpretation	Checklist
Platelet estimate	Low/thrombocytopenia	See sec. 3, ch. 1
Bleeding time	Prolonged/defect of primary hemostasis	History (drug exposure, familial bleeding) CBC/metabolic profile Radiography vWF:Ag Thyroid function Fibrin split product titer Platelet aggregometry
Activated clotting time	Prolonged/defect of intrinsic coagulation system	History (toxin exposure, familial bleeding) Coagulation screening assays Coagulation factor analysis CBC/metabolic profile Liver function Radiography Fibrin split product titer Response to vitamin K therapy

cavities; in addition, signs of the underlying disease are usually present.

■ Bleeding from venipuncture sites most often accompanies severe deficiencies of multiple coagulation factors or fulminant DIC. Absence of this sign does not rule out a clinically significant coagulation disorder.

DIAGNOSIS

KEY POINT ▶ The first consideration when evaluating bleeding patients is to differentiate blood loss due to injury of a single or local group of blood vessels from a systemic bleeding diathesis. This distinction is usually apparent after thorough history, physical examination, and evaluation of quick assessment tests.

History

The history should include specific questions to identify previous episodes of spontaneous bleeding or excessive hemorrhage after surgery or trauma.

■ Gingival bleeding from tooth eruption and bleeding from docking or dewclaw removal are common signs of inherited coagulation factor deficiency and vWD. Conversely, history of severe trauma or invasive surgical procedure without excessive hemorrhage rules out an inherited hemostatic defect.

■ Patients with histories of hepatic disease or disorders associated with DIC are at risk for acquired coagulation defects and should be further evaluated prior to invasive procedures.

Physical Examination

Physical examination should define as thoroughly as possible the nature, severity, and precise anatomic source of hemorrhage. In patients with a single obvious site of external blood loss, ophthalmoscopy, digital anorectal examination, careful auscultation, and joint palpation may identify additional sites of hemorrhage that would be suggestive of coagulation disorder.

Radiographic Examination

Radiography of the chest and abdomen can detect fluid densities indicative of bleeding in pleural, peritoneal, or retroperitoneal spaces. Intrapulmonary hemorrhage causes an alveolar pattern on thoracic films. Epistaxis, hematuria, and gastrointestinal hemorrhage may be difficult to differentiate as signs of local vessel trauma versus signs of systemic coagulation disorder. Contrast radiography, ultrasonography, and computed tomography (CT) can noninvasively identify erosive, infiltrative, or mass lesions causing vessel damage.

Quick Assessment Tests

Quick Assessment Tests (QATs) are useful for identifying hemostatic defects and evaluating hemostatic function prior to performing invasive procedures. Table 2 presents additional diagnostic considerations, based on the results of QATs, for differentiating coagulation disorders from other hemostatic defects. Table 3 lists expected results of the following QATs for categories of common coagulation disorders.

Slide Estimate of Platelet Number. Thrombocytopenia can be ruled out if examination of a stained blood film under oil immersion reveals at least 7-10 platelets per field for dogs, and 10-15 platelets per field for cats.

Activated Clotting Time (ACT). Most common acquired and inherited coagulation factor deficiencies can be detected by prolongation of ACT, a functional test of the intrinsic clotting system.

■ Procedure for ACT Test:
  • Collect 2 ml of whole blood directly into a test tube, maintain the needle (Vacutainer; Becton-Dickinson) in the vein, remove the first tube and replace it with a second evacuated tube containing siliceous earth (Vacutainer, Becton-Dickinson) to withdraw a second 2-ml sample.
  • Warm the evacuated tube to 37°C prior to sampling.

TABLE 3. Expected Results of Quick Assessment Tests (QATs) for Coagulation Disorders

Category	Tests			
	Platelet Count	ACT	TBT	BMBT
Coagulation factor deficiency				
Acquired deficiencies	N	A	A	N
Inherited deficiencies				
Hemophilia (A and B)	N	A	A	N
Dysfibrinogenemia, prothrombin				
Factor X, XI deficiencies	N	A	A	N
Factor VII deficiency	N	N	N	N
Factor XII deficiency	N	A	N	N
vWD (Inherited and acquired)	N	N	A	A
DIC (hemorrhagic phase)	A	A	A	N/A

ACT = activated clotting time; TBT = toenail bleeding time; BMBT = buccal mucosal bleeding time; vWD = von Willebrand's disease; DIC = disseminated intravascular coagulation; N = normal; A = abnormal.

- Immediately after blood collection, gently invert the second tube several times to mix blood with activator, and then place it in a heating block calibrated at 37°C.
  - After incubation for 45 sec, remove the tube from the block at 5- to 10-sec intervals, gently tilt it, and evaluate for clot formation.
- ACT is the time elapsed from sampling to clot formation.
- Normal range of canine ACT is 60–120 sec; feline range is 60–70 sec.
- ACT may be technically difficult to perform in cats and small dogs.
- Sampling from the jugular vein is not recommended in patients with severe hemorrhagic disorders, because iatrogenic hematoma formation and subsequent upper respiratory obstruction may occur.

Bleeding Time Tests

Bleeding time tests are *in vivo* measures of hemostatic function performed by making a standard wound and timing the interval to cessation of blood flow. These tests should be performed only on patients with platelet counts >100,000/μl, because significant thrombocytopenia prolongs bleeding time.

Buccal Mucosa Bleeding Time (BMBT) Test
- Procedure:
  - Evert the lip and then hold it in place with gauze that encircles the muzzle and causes the buccal veins to engorge slightly.
  - Using a template device (Simplate II; Organon Teknika) make two incisions in mucosa of the upper lip.
  - Collect hemorrhage from the wounds on filter paper applied underneath, but not directly to, bleeding sites.
- BMBT is the average time elapsed from triggering

the device until blood stops flowing from both incisions.
- Normal BMBT is 2–3 minutes for dogs and cats.
- BMBT is prolonged in patients with acquired and inherited platelet dysfunction and vWD but is normal in patients with coagulation factor deficiencies and in some patients with DIC.
- Cats usually require sedation for BMBT testing, but most dogs will tolerate this procedure without chemical restraint.

Toenail Bleeding Time (TBT) Test
- Procedure:
  - Using a guillotine-type toenail clipper, make a clean transection at the tip of the nail cuticle.
  - Allow blood to flow freely from the injury.
- The time from transection until blood ceases to flow is the TBT.
- Normal TBT is 5 to 6 minutes; accuracy depends on technique and immobilization of the patient's digit during the procedure.
- TBT is less specific than BMBT and is prolonged for patients with clinically significant coagulation factor deficiencies, vWD, platelet dysfunction, and bleeding due to DIC.
- The TBT test is best performed on sedated or anesthetized patients.

Definitive Tests

Definitive tests to diagnose coagulation disorders depend on correct sampling technique and test systems that are specifically validated for evaluating canine and feline patients. Table 4 lists coagulation factors of the intrinsic, extrinsic, and common pathways, a classification system that is useful for *in vitro* diagnosis of bleeding disorders. Table 5 presents expected results of diagnostic tests for categories of common coagulation disorders.

Coagulation Screening Assays. These tests measure the time, in seconds, for *in vitro* fibrin clot formation. Prolongation of screening assay times beyond laboratory normal range, or greater than 5–7 sec from control of same species is indicative of coagulation factor deficiency or inhibition.

- Activated partial thromboplastin time (aPTT) is sensitive to deficiencies of intrinsic and common coagulation pathways.
- Prothrombin time (PT) detects deficiencies in extrinsic and common pathways.

TABLE 4. Coagulation Factors of the Intrinsic, Extrinsic, and Common Pathways

Intrinsic	Extrinsic	Common
High molecular weight kininogen	Tissue thromboplastin	Factor X
Prekallikrein	Factor VII	Factor V
Factor XII		Factor II (prothrombin)
Factor XI		Factor I (fibrinogen)
Factor IX		
Factor VIII		

TABLE 5. Definitive Diagnostic Tests for Coagulation Disorders

Category	Tests	Results
Coagulation factor deficiency		
Acquired deficiencies		
Liver failure	APTT, PT, TCT	Prolonged
	Fibrinogen*	Low
	Factor analysis	Low activity most factors, variable activity—factor VIII
Vitamin K deficiency	APTT, PT	Prolonged
	TCT, fibrinogen	Normal
	Factor analysis	Low activity—factors II, VII, IX, X
Heparin excess	APTT, PT	Prolonged
	TCT	Marked prolongation
	Fibrinogen	Normal
Inherited deficiencies		
Hemophilia	APTT	Prolonged
	PT, TCT, fibrinogen	Normal
	Factor analysis	Low activity—factor VIII (hemophilia A) or factor IX (hemophilia B)
Dysfibrinogenemia	APTT, PT, TCT	Prolonged
	Fibrinogen	Low
Prothrombin deficiency or factor X deficiency	APTT, PT	Prolonged
	TCT, fibrinogen	Normal
	Factor analysis	Low activity—factor II or X
Factor VII deficiency	PT	Prolonged
	APTT, TCT, fibrinogen	Normal
	Factor analysis	Low activity—factor VII
Factor XI or XII deficiency	APTT	Marked prolongation
	PT, TCT, fibrinogen	Normal
	Factor analysis	Low activity—factor XI or XII
vWD (acquired and inherited)	Bleeding time	Prolonged
	vWF:Ag	Low
	vWF cofactor, multimers	Abnormal
DIC (hemorrhagic phase)	APTT, PT, TCT	Prolonged
	Fibrinogen, ATIII	Low
	Platelet count	Progressive decrease
	Fibrin split products†	Positive titer
	Red cell morphology	Schistocytes

APTT = activated partial thromboplastin time; PT = prothrombin time; TCT = thrombin clotting time; vWF:Ag = von Willebrand factor antigen; vWD = von Willebrand's disease; DIC = disseminated vascular coagulation.
*Normal fibrinogen concentration is 300–600 mg/dl.
†Normal fibrin split product concentration is <10 μg/ml.

- Fibrinogen concentration (mg/dl) is a quantitative measure of plasma fibrinogen.
- Thrombin clotting time (TCT) detects both deficiency and dysfunction of fibrinogen.
- Based on abnormalities detected in screening assays, specific single or multiple coagulation factor deficiencies are identified using individual factor analysis.

Specific vWF Assays. Specific tests must be performed to establish diagnosis of vWD. Clotting time tests, coagulation assays, and platelet counts do not detect abnormal vWF.

- Measurement of vWF antigen (vWF:Ag) is the most commonly used quantitative vWF assay.
- Patients with vWF below normal range (established at each testing laboratory) are considered at risk for carrying and/or expressing the vWD trait.
- In addition to low plasma vWF, severely affected individuals have abnormal *in vivo* bleeding time.

Diagnosis of DIC. Definitive diagnosis of DIC cannot be based on any one test, but depends on a combination of clinical signs and laboratory abnormalities.

- The presence of serum fibrin degradation products (FDP) or fibrin split products (FSP), especially in increasing titers, is compatible with ongoing systemic fibrinolysis usually caused by DIC.
- Additional findings, characteristic of the hemorrhagic phase of DIC, include:
  • Falling platelet count
  • Low plasma fibrinogen and antithrombin III
  • Prolongation of all coagulation screening assays
  • Presence of schistocytes on stained peripheral blood smears

TREATMENT

KEY POINT ▶ Successful management of patients with coagulation disorders requires establishing an accurate diagnosis and then administering appropriate transfusion and nontransfusion support. Pretreatment samples are invaluable for establishing definitive diagnosis early in the course of disease.

Transfusion Therapy

Transfusion therapy to supply active factors is required for patients with severe, inherited coagulation factor deficiencies and vWD and for patients with acquired disorders that are not responsive to correction of an underlying disease process. Table 6 lists blood products and dosages for treating specific coagulation disorders (see sec. 3, ch. 1 for description of cross-matching protocol).

- Transfusion of whole blood, administered within 4 to 6 hours of collection, supplies active coagulation factors and vWF, as well as red blood cells (RBCs).
- Transfusion of plasma products (fresh plasma, fresh frozen plasma, plasma concentrate), rather than whole blood, reduces the risk of immunologic transfusion reactions, most importantly RBC sensitization. Plasma components can also be transfused preoperatively and repeatedly in 1 day without causing volume overload.
- Cross-species transfusions of any blood product are contraindicated because anaphylaxis can result.

Nursing Care

Nursing care practices that reduce hemorrhage include:

- Confinement to limit activity
- Feeding soft food
- Avoidance of neck leads and intramuscular injections
- Use of peripheral veins for blood sampling and intravenous catheter placement

Do not give platelet inhibitory drugs, including sulfa and nonsteroidal anti-inflammatory agents.

Wound Management

Good management reduces the need for transfusion in some patients with coagulation disorders and mucosal or cutaneous hemorrhage. The best treatment, for even small wounds, usually is suture and/or pressure bandages. Application of tissue adhesive (Vetbond; 3M) to focal areas of bleeding also can limit local blood loss.

Drug Therapy

Vitamin K Therapy

Vitamin K therapy improves hemostasis only in vitamin K deficiency states. It often is initiated pending test results, but its maintenance is not indicated when diagnosis of inherited factor deficiency, nonobstructive liver disease, vWD, or DIC is made.

Anticoagulant rodenticide toxicities are the most common cause of vitamin K deficiency in dogs and cats. Vitamin K reverses the anticoagulant effect of

rodenticides over a period of 24–48 hours from initiation of therapy.

Warfarin is a relatively short-acting poison, and treatment for a total of 1 week usually is adequate. Standard treatment is as follows:

- Administer an initial dose of vitamin K_1 (Aquamephyton; Merck, Sharpe and Dohme), 2.2 mg/kg SC.
- Follow with the same dose divided into two doses given q12h until active bleeding subsides.
- Then substitute an oral preparation (Mephyton) at the same twice-daily dosage.

To treat toxicity from second-generation, or long-acting, rodenticides (diphacinone, pindone, bromadiolone, and brodifacoum):

- Transfusion is indicated for patients having severe anemia or pulmonary hemorrhage at presentation (see Table 6).
- Initiate parenteral vitamin K_1 as for warfarin (2.2 mg/kg SQ).
- Administer vitamin K_1 at 1.1 mg/kg SQ, q12h until hematocrit value stabilizes and active bleeding subsides.
- Maintain oral vitamin K_1 at 1.1 mg/kg PO, q12h for a total of 2 weeks.
- Taper the initial dose by one-half every 2 weeks during treatment.
- To prevent relapse, continue therapy for 4 to 6 weeks.

Subcutaneous injection of vitamin K is the preferred parenteral route because intravenous vitamin K can cause anaphylaxis, and hematomas may form at intramuscular injection sites. Vitamin K_3 (Synkayvite; Roche) is not effective in the treatment of rodenticide toxicity because of its delayed onset of action.

Hormonal Therapy

Hormonal therapy may reverse bleeding resulting from acquired vWd in association with endocrine disorders.

Thyroid insufficiency (see sec. 4, ch. 1) is common in many of the breeds that have a high prevalence of the vWD trait.

- To treat responsive animals:
  - Supplement with L-thyroxine at a dose of 0.02 mg/kg q12h.

TABLE 6. Guidelines for Transfusion

Product	Volume	Interval
Fresh whole blood*	12–20 ml/kg	q 24 h
Fresh plasma*	6–10 ml/kg	q 8–12 h
Fresh frozen plasma (FFP)**		
Plasma cryoprecipitate†	1 unit/5 kg‡	q 8–12 h
Cryosupernatant¶	6–10 ml/kg	q 8–12 h

*Collected in citrate-based anticoagulant and administered within 4 hours of collection.
**Frozen within 4–6 hours of collection; stored below −20°C.
†Prepared from FFP for treatment of vWD, factor VIII, and fibrinogen deficiency.
‡1 unit of precipitate is produced from 75 ml of FFP.
¶Prepared from FFP for treatment of prothrombin group (factors II, VII, IX, X) and factor XI deficiencies.

- Hemostasis improves within 24 to 48 hours of initiating therapy.
- Maintenance of thyroid hormone therapy may prevent subsequent bleeding episodes.

■ Because not all patients respond, bleeding time and clinical status are assessed after thyroid hormone supplementation to determine whether hemostasis has improved.

Desmopressin acetate (DDAVP; USV Pharmaceutical), a vasopressin analog, has shown efficacy in transiently improving hemostasis in some dogs affected with vWD.

■ DDAVP's activity is probably due to release of vWF from intracellular stores, and its effectiveness depends on the patient's ability to produce functional vWF protein.
■ Duration of action, after a dose of 1 μg/kg SC, is 3–4 h; repeated dosage within 24 h does not prolong response time.
■ Correction of abnormal bleeding time is demonstrated before undertaking invasive procedures, because many patients do not respond.

Heparin Therapy

Heparin (100 U/kg q6–8h SC) is useful in managing certain cases of DIC in which ongoing systemic coagulation is causing signs of vessel thrombosis or embolism.

■ Remember that heparin can exacerbate bleeding by inhibiting platelet and coagulation factor function.

■ Transfusion therapy with fresh blood or blood products to replace active coagulation factors, antithrombin III, and platelets, is more likely than heparin therapy to benefit patients presenting with severe hemorrhage in association with DIC.

KEY POINT ▶ The critical factor for successfully managing all patients with DIC is identification and correction of the underlying disorder.

Supplemental Readings

Brooks M: Transfusion medicine. Parts I and II. Proc Am Coll Vet Intern Med 1990, 77–84.

Dodds WJ: Acquired von Willebrand's disease. Proc Am Anim Hosp Assoc 1989, 614.

Dodds WJ: Bleeding disorders. *In* Morgan RV, ed: *Handbook of Small Animal Practice*. New York: Churchill Livingstone, 1988, p 773.

Forsythe LE, Willis SE: Evaluating oral mucosa bleeding times in healthy dogs using a spring-loaded device. Can Vet J 30:344, 1989.

Madewell BR: Sample preparation for the laboratory. *In* Kirk RW, ed.: *Current Veterinary Therapy X*, Philadelphia: W. B. Saunders, 1989, p 410.

Mount ME: Diagnosis and therapy of anticoagulant rodenticide intoxications. Vet Clin North Am 18:115, 1988.

Slappendel RJ: Disseminated intravascular coagulation. *In* Kirk RW, ed.: *Current Veterinary Therapy X*. Philadelphia: W. B. Saunders, 1989, p 451.

Wingfield WE, Van Pelt D: Abnormal bleeding. Vet Clin North Am 19:1275, 1989.

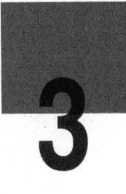

3 Systemic Immune-Mediated Diseases

James P. Thompson

Numerous immune-mediated or immune-associated diseases have been identified in dogs and cats. Management of these diseases focuses mainly on the recognition of the disease and appropriate immunosuppressive chemotherapy. This chapter focuses on the recognition and management of immune-mediated hemolytic anemia, immune-mediated thrombocytopenia, and systemic lupus erythematosus as frequently observed systemic abnormalities of the immune system. Organ-specific immune-mediated diseases are discussed in the respective organ system sections of this book; notably, pemphigus and other cutaneous immune disorders are discussed in sec. 5, ch. 9, rheumatoid and immune polyarthropathies in the Orthopedic section, and immune-mediated neuromuscular disorders in the Neurology section.

IMMUNE-MEDIATED HEMOLYTIC ANEMIA

The major clinical concern in immune-mediated hemolytic anemia (IMHA) is accelerated erythrocyte destruction resulting from antibodies attached to the erythrocyte surface. Antibody-coated erythrocytes are destroyed by one of two basic mechanisms: extravascular phagocytosis or intravascular hemolysis.

Extravascular phagocytosis is the most common form of IMHA. Phagocytosis occurs primarily in the spleen and liver. Typically, IgG-coated erythrocytes are removed by the spleen, and IgM-coated erythrocytes are trapped by the liver; erythrocytes initially trapped by the liver can be released and subsequently removed by the spleen. For additional description of the spleen's role in this process, see sec. 3, ch. 4.

Intravascular hemolysis is the result of antibody-induced complement activation. This class of IMHA is generally associated with IgM antibodies or very high concentrations of serum IgG.

Etiology

KEY POINT ▶ IMHA is caused by a type II hypersensitivity (cytotoxic) immune response characterized by antibody molecules directed against red blood cell surface antigens.

- Antibody may be directed against unaltered endogenous erythrocyte membrane antigens (primary autoimmune hemolytic anemia) or to exogenous antigens (secondary IMHA).

- The specific etiology of IMHA usually goes unrecognized. Occasionally the clinician can associate a drug with the onset of clinical and hematologic signs. Most cases of IMHA will be classified as idiopathic until detailed studies of erythrocyte membrane antigens and antibody against these antigens are performed.

- A familial predisposition exists in dogs that implies a potential underlying genetic predilection. All breeds of dogs are susceptible, but poodles, Old English sheepdogs, Irish setters, and cocker spaniels are predisposed. Affected dogs usually are between 2 and 8 years of age. Female dogs appeared to be affected three to four times more frequently than male dogs.

KEY POINT ▶ Approximately one-half to three-fourths of IMHA in cats is associated with feline leukemia virus infection. Other feline diseases associated with IMHA include hemobartonellosis and lymphoma. No breed or sex predilection has been observed.

Clinical Signs

- Patients usually are presented for vague primary complaints that may include sensitivity to cold, anorexia, listlessness, weakness, and depression.
- Gastrointestinal disturbances manifested by pica, vomiting, and diarrhea may be observed in some pets.
- Patients occasionally are presented with the primary complaint of icterus.

Diagnosis

Physical Examination

The physical examination typically reveals pale mucous membranes, tachycardia, and tachypnea. A systolic heart murmur may be auscultated because of decreased blood viscosity. If extravascular hemolysis is the prominent mechanism of erythrocyte destruction, hepatomegaly or splenomegaly may be present. If the major mechanism of erythrocyte destruction is intravascular hemolysis, icterus and fever may be observed. Peripheral lymphadenopathy also may be noted.

Complete Blood Count, Serum Biochemistry Profile and Urinalysis

Complete Blood Count (CBC). The most important aspect of the hemogram is the erythron response, which typically indicates a regenerative anemia that is characterized by macrocytosis. The presence of spherocytes (small globular erythrocytes without central pallor) in the absence of schistocytes (erythrocyte fragments) is nearly pathognomonic for IMHA. The CBC frequently demonstrates a leukocytosis characterized by an absolute neutrophilia and left shift; total leukocyte counts as high as 60,000/μl blood with 4000 metamyelocytes have been observed. The plasma fibrinogen concentration usually is elevated. If hemolysis is present in the patient's blood specimen, consider a diagnosis of intravascular lysis; be careful, however, to rule out lipemia-induced or sampling technique–induced *in vitro* hemolysis.

Serum Biochemistry Profile. This assay generally is unrewarding. Serum lactic dehydrogenase activity usually is elevated as a result of enzyme release from damaged erythrocytes. Serum alanine and aspartate aminotransferase and alkaline phosphatase activities may be elevated. In extensive extravascular and intravascular hemolysis, hyperbilirubinemia is present, but the clinician probably already knows this, based on the presence of icterus.

Urinalysis. Urinalysis is useful to document the presence of hemoglobinuria or bilirubinuria; remember that any amount of bilirubinuria in cats is abnormal, whereas dogs may exhibit detectable levels in the absence of disease. Excessive proteinuria may indicate extensive glomerular damage resulting from immune-complex deposition associated with intravascular lysis of circulating erythrocytes. Cylindruria (the presence of excessive numbers of casts in the urine) suggests tubular damage. If an active urine sediment is present, as evidenced by an excessive number of casts and inflammatory cells, adequate fluid intake is critical to ensure appropriate blood flow to the damaged kidney.

Anti-Erythrocyte Antibody Detection

KEY POINT ▶ Definitive diagnosis is made by detecting antibody molecules or complement on the surface of circulating erythrocytes.

Direct Agglutination Test. The clinician should attempt to demonstrate the presence of antibody-coated erythrocytes by performing the direct agglutination test.

■ Place a drop of anticoagulated whole blood on a microscope slide and mix with the blood one drop of physiologic saline. The one drop of added saline is to reduce the plasma protein concentration by half and prevent rouleau formation; the reduction of antibody concentration by half generally does not reduce the concentration of antibody significantly to prevent agglutination of erythrocytes. If sufficient antibody molecules are present, agglutination will be observed.

Direct Coombs Test. This test is used to identify antibodies bound to circulating erythrocytes when the concentration of antibody molecules is too low to cause direct agglutination. It should be performed in cases

that demonstrate anemia in the absence of direct agglutination.

KEY POINT ▶ It is important to draw blood for Coombs testing prior to transfusion.

The Coombs reagents must be species specific. These reagents usually recognize IgG, IgM, and C3b; C3b is the membrane-bound protein-split product deposited on the erythrocyte surface from the third component of the complement cascade. Antibody or complement bound to the erythrocyte surface is then detected by cross-linking these molecules with species-specific reagents directed at these molecules.

In the interpretation of Coombs test results, it is important to understand the causes of false-positive and false negative results.

■ A false-positive test can be seen most frequently in cases in which:
  • Patients have received a prior erythrocyte transfusion
  • There is nonspecific adsorption of serum immunoglobulins onto the surface of damaged erythrocytes, such as occurs in disseminated intravascular coagulation (DIC).
■ A false negative test is caused most frequently by:
  • Poor laboratory technique
  • Insufficient antibody on the red blood cell (RBC) membrane to permit detection with the Coombs test.

In the absence of a positive Coombs test result, the clinician is justified in making a diagnosis of immune-mediated hemolytic anemia only when underlying infection, neoplasia, and erythrocyte enzyme deficiencies have been eliminated.

Concurrent Diseases

Disorders that may accompany IMHA include immune-mediated thrombocytopenia and/or systemic lupus erythematosus; both of these are discussed later in this chapter. In all cases of IMHA, perform an absolute platelet count and submit serum for an indirect fluorescent antinuclear antibody (IFAA) test. In patients with a reduced platelet count and hypofibrinogenemia, rule out disseminated intravascular coagulation as an underlying etiology for the thrombocytopenia (see sec. 3, ch. 1).

Treatment

The therapeutic goal is to prevent further destruction of erythrocytes and to maintain tissue oxygenation. The erythron mass will ideally return to normal, although a mildly decreased packed cell volume (PCV) can still be compatible with a good quality of life.

Control of Erythrocyte Destruction

Treatment to reduce erythrocyte destruction focuses on:

■ Reducing Fc receptors (immunoglobulin-binding receptors) on neutrophils, monocytes, and macrophages to prevent phagocytosis of antibody-coated erythrocytes.

■ Blocking remaining Fc receptors on neutrophils, monocytes, and macrophages, thereby further reducing erythrocyte phagocytosis.

■ Preventing continued formation of anti-erythrocyte antibody.

Reduce Fc Receptors. To reduce Fc receptors on phagocytic cells, treat with glucocorticoids.

■ Parenterally administered dexamethasone (0.1–0.2 mg/kg q12h IV) is preferred by many clinicians for initial in-hospital treatment.

■ Then use oral prednisone or prednisolone (1 mg/kg q12h PO) for follow-up maintenance; 3 to 6 months usually is required.

■ To prevent glucocorticoid-induced gastric ulceration, consider using concomitant cimetidine (Tagamet; SmithKline); (5–10 mg/kg q6–12h IV or PO) or other measures described in sec. 7, ch. 4 to control gastric acid and its effects.

Block Remaining Fc Receptors. Block remaining Fc receptors on neutrophils, monocytes, and macrophages by treatment with danazol (Danocrine; Winthrop) (5 mg/kg q12h PO). Danazol is a pituitary gonadotropin suppressant used to treat women with endometriosis. It blocks the Fc receptors, reducing the capacity of phagocytic cells to destroy the erythrocyte. It is generally used for the initial 2 weeks of therapy in conjunction with corticosteroids. The drug is expensive and has been associated with liver enzyme elevation and vaginitis in women.

Prevent Anti-erythrocyte Antibody Formation. This is accomplished to some degree through the use of glucocorticoids; however, consider using a more potent humoral immune suppressive agent such as cyclophosphamide (Cytoxan; Bristol-Myers) along with glucocorticoids and danazol in patients that exhibit direct autoagglutination of blood or in patients with intravascular erythrocyte lysis. These patients generally have high concentrations of serum antibody and a poorer prognosis; thus, more aggressive attempts to prevent antibody formation are indicated. As a side effect, cyclophosphamide can decrease the peripheral platelet count, which potentially can lead to a bleeding diathesis. The presence of pre-existing thrombocytopenia should be noted, and consideration should be given to the risk-benefit ratio of using cyclophosphamide; do not give cyclophosphamide if the platelet count is <30,000/μl. Patients with severe gastrointestinal irritation manifested by vomiting and/or diarrhea also probably should not receive cyclophosphamide, because it can inhibit epithelialization of the gastrointestinal tract and predispose to bleeding.

Cyclophosphamide is given by one of two methods:

■ Single IV bolus at a dosage of 200 mg/m² (see Table 4 in sec. 3, ch. 5, for conversion of body weight in lb or kg to surface area in m²)

■ Oral dosage:
 • For dogs—50 mg/m² every other day.
 • For cats—200 mg/m² q2wk.

IV administration is generally used in dogs and cats that require a blood transfusion and have direct autoagglutination or intravascular erythrocyte lysis. The drug will inhibit an immune response to the transfused blood as well as to the patient's own erythrocytes. Do not give this more frequently than once every 2 weeks.

Oral administration is used in dogs that are refractory to glucocorticoid and danazol therapy or in dogs that have direct agglutination or intravascular hemolysis but do not require immediate blood transfusion.

KEY POINT ▶ Cyclophosphamide may suppress reticulocytosis and may cause thrombocytopenia, although its greatest effect is on lymphocytes and the immune function. If reticulocytopenia or severe thrombocytopenia develops, discontinue cyclophosphamide therapy. Patients with nonregenerative immune-mediated hemolytic anemia present a therapeutic dilemma.

Antibody serum levels are not immediately reduced following the administration of cyclophosphamide. Circulating antibodies must decline by normal antibody catabolism of roughly 3 weeks according to serum half-life clearance. In immune-mediated erythrocyte destruction, it is possible that the half-life of antibody with specificity for circulating erythrocytes will be shorter because of adsorption onto circulating erythrocytes. Nevertheless, it will likely require one to two weeks before any significant benefit from cyclophosphamide will be appreciated.

Blood Transfusions

Transfusions should be given only if necessary, as the procedure may accelerate or precipitate a hemolytic crisis. When transfusion is necessary, use crossmatched blood. In addition, consider administering cyclophosphamide to decrease the potential for an antibody response to the transfusion. If a second blood transfusion is required within 7 days and the initial transfusion was not rejected, it probably is unnecessary to repeat a blood crossmatch if a compatible donor has been previously identified. If more than 7 days has elapsed, a primary immune response to the previously transfused blood may have occurred and reevaluation of a blood crossmatch is imperative.

Other Therapies

Plasmapheresis. Plasmapheresis is the removal of plasma (and antibodies) from withdrawn blood and retransfusion of the blood cells. It is performed to decrease the amount of circulating antibody with erythrocyte specificity. This results in a decreased rate of autologous destruction.

Splenectomy. This procedure must be approached with caution because an enlarged spleen may represent a source of significant extramedullary hematopoiesis. Prior to recommending splenectomy, a bone marrow aspirate should document significant erythroid hyperplasia. Also, consider performing fine needle aspiration cytology of the enlarged spleen to document significant erythrophagocytosis. If significant erythrophagocytosis is present, splenectomy not only prevents this phenomenon, but also removes a likely source of significant antibody production. (See also sec. 3, ch. 4 for a discussion of the spleen's role in this disease and for a description of splenectomy.)

Prognosis

The prognosis is guarded in the presence of severe hepatic disease or renal disease and when IMHA is associated with immune-mediated thrombocytopenia and/or systemic lupus erythematosus. Patients with intravascular hemolysis and direct agglutination have the poorest prognosis and highest death rate. Mortality occurs in approximately 30 to 40% of all patients despite appropriate clinical management. Complications can include DIC, acute thromboembolism, sepsis, renal failure, and persistent hemolysis despite therapy.

IMMUNE-MEDIATED THROMBOCYTOPENIA

Decreased circulating platelets are presumed the result of increased antibody-mediated and complement-mediated thrombocyte phagocytosis within the spleen, liver, and bone marrow or secondary to decreased platelet production following destruction of megakaryocytes within the bone marrow. Immune-mediated thrombocytopenia (IMT) may occur as a single disease entity or may occur in association with other immune-mediated disease. The simultaneous occurrence of IMT and hemolytic anemia is known as Evan's syndrome. Other immune-mediated diseases that may occur concurrently with IMT include systemic lupus erythematosus and rheumatoid arthritis.

Etiology

KEY POINT ▶ Similar to IMHA, IMT is an example of a type II or cytotoxic hypersensitivity.

- Antibody may be directed against endogenous or exogenous thrombocyte surface antigens. The specific etiology is usually unidentified. However, certain drugs have been shown to create a hapten-platelet antigen complex and induce an antibody response; sulfadiazine and propylthiouracil, a drug used to treat hyperthyroidism in cats, have been associated with acquired IMT.
- The disease is observed commonly in dogs and rarely in cats. The average age of afflicted dogs is 5 to 6 years. Female dogs are affected nearly twice as frequently as males. Miniature poodles, toy poodles and Old English sheepdogs may be predisposed.

Clinical Signs

Patients are usually presented for the primary complaint of bleeding. Bleeding most often is manifested by mucous membrane petechiation, dermal ecchymosis, and melena. Epistaxis, hyphema, hematemesis, and hematuria are observed less frequently. Lethargy and weakness also may be reported.

KEY POINT ▶ Bleeding may be related not only to the absolute platelet numbers but also to the rate of platelet decline, the stability of capillary endothelial membranes, and the incidence of traumatic events.

Diagnosis

KEY POINT ▶ The diagnosis of IMT generally is made by eliminating other causes of thrombocytopenia. Diagnostic tests exist that demonstrate platelet-specific antibody or antibody-coated megakaryocytes, but clinical signs and patient response to treatment generally are considered diagnostic.

Physical Examination

The physical examination most commonly reveals signs related to bleeding, especially mucous membrane petechiation, dermal ecchymosis and petechiation, and melena. Fundoscopic examination may show retinal hemorrhage. Splenomegaly and/or hepatomegaly may be found on abdominal palpation. Tachycardia, tachypnea, and physiologic heart murmur may be noted, depending on the extent of blood loss. Some animals are febrile.

Complete Blood Count, Serum Biochemistry Profile, and Urinalysis

The CBC must, by definition, demonstrate a thrombocytopenia, which in most animals with IMT is severe. Often there are <30,000 platelets/µl in patients with overt bleeding. Blood films typically exhibit very few platelets; however, both microthrombocytes and macrothrombocytes usually are seen. Many animals will demonstrate anemia and hypoproteinemia if bleeding has occurred. If the bleeding episode has been recent, the anemia will be normocytic and normochromic and lack signs of regeneration. If an episode of significant bleeding occurred more than 3 or 4 days prior to analysis, then a macrocytic, hypochromic anemia with reticulocytosis may be observed. Prolonged bleeding can cause an iron-deficient, microcytic hypochromic anemia.

Serum Biochemistry Profile. This typically is normal.

Urinalysis. Urinalysis may demonstrate proteinuria as the result of antigen-antibody complex deposition within the glomerulus and complement-induced glomerulitis. Hematuria is only rarely observed.

Coagulography

A coagulogram will rule out intrinsic and extrinsic coagulation system defects (see sec. 3, ch. 2) as a cause of excessive bleeding with secondary platelet consumption.

Bone Marrow Cytology

Perform this procedure to document megakaryocytic response to the peripheral thrombocytopenia. In IMT, the megakaryocytes generally are increased with a predominance of immature forms. Only occasionally, when antibodies are directed against the megakaryocytes themselves, are the megakaryocytes decreased; ehrlichiosis and hyperestrogenemia are other differential diagnoses associated with megakaryocytic hypoplasia.

Platelet Factor-3 Test

This test has been used to detect serum antibody with specificity against platelets. However, 30 to 70% of animals suspected of having IMT do not exhibit a positive test result. The major pitfall associated with the platelet factor-3 test is that it uses platelets collected from a healthy dog rather than platelets collected from the patient. When patient serum is mixed with normal platelets, the assumption is made that the specific platelet antigen to which the serum antibody is directed will be present on the platelets collected from the healthy dog. This assumption may not necessarily be true and probably explains many of the observed false-negative test results.

Bone Marrow Direct Fluorescent Antibody (DFA) Test

The DFA test may be used to detect antibody bound to megakaryocytes; however, this test is technically demanding, subjective, and not routinely performed. There must be adequate megakaryocytes in the bone marrow in order to locate these cells for immunofluorescent microscopic examination, and in the presence of adequate megakaryocytes, an immune-mediated disease directed at megakaryocytes is unlikely.

Treatment

KEY POINT ▶ Treatment objectives are to resolve and prevent bleeding, reduce platelet destruction, and increase platelet release from megakaryocytes in selected patients.

Reduce Platelet Destruction

This is accomplished by the combined use of glucocorticoids and danazol (Danocrine). Glucocorticoids are the mainstay of therapy. Dexamethasone may be more effective than prednisone or prednisolone.

- Give dexamethasone (0.1–0.2 mg/kg q12h IV) for the first day followed by prednisone or prednisolone (1 mg/kg q12h PO).
- It is strongly advised that patients also receive cimetidine (5–10 mg/kg q6–12h IV or PO) in an attempt to prevent glucocorticoid-associated gastric ulceration.
- Danazol (5 mg/kg q12h PO) is used concurrently with the glucocorticoids as an additional aid to prevent platelet phagocytosis (see Immune-Mediated Hemolytic Anemia).

Increase Platelet Release

Platelet release from the bone marrow is increased by administration of vincristine (Oncovin; Lilly) (0.025 mg/kg IV) not more frequently than once weekly.

Adequate bone marrow megakaryocytes must be present in order for vincristine to induce platelet release.

Blood and Plasma Transfusion

Use blood and platelet-rich plasma transfusions to support tissue oxygenation and to assist hemostasis, respectively. These transfusions will not restore the platelet count to normal; however, one clinical study suggests that dogs that receive a platelet-rich transfusion may be less likely to exhibit relapsing thrombocytopenia. Compatible erythrocytes as determined by major crossmatch analysis should be used for whole blood transfusions (see sec. 3, ch. 1).

Other Therapies

Splenectomy. Reserve splenectomy for patients that exhibit refractory IMT.

- This therapy is based on the assumption that the spleen is responsible for persistent platelet destruction and that removal of the spleen will:
  - Remove macrophages responsible for platelet ingestion
  - Remove a large source of plasma cells manufacturing platelet-specific antibody.
- Perform splenectomy when splenomegaly is present and is not due to significant extramedullary hematopoiesis.
- Evaluate the bone marrow cytology and document the presence of bone marrow megakaryocytic hyperplasia.

Following splenectomy, up to 50% of dogs exhibit platelet counts >200,000/μl and do not require medical therapy to maintain a normal platelet count. The remaining dogs may exhibit recurring thrombocytopenia (details of splenectomy are described in sec. 3, ch. 4).

Vincristine-Loaded Platelet Transfusion. This complicated procedure is reserved for patients with refractory IMT. The rationale is that *in vitro* incubation of platelets with vincristine results in the binding of vincristine to tubulin within the platelet cytoplasm. Following IV injection, macrophages of the reticuloendothelial system ingest the vincristine-loaded platelets and are destroyed. The major pitfall of this technique may be related to natural macrophage turnover. Repetitive treatment may be necessary and is technically difficult.

Prognosis

The prognosis for IMT is good. Approximately 40 to 50% of dogs will experience only a single thrombocytopenic episode that responds to treatment within 2 to 7 days. Patient signalment, severity of initial thrombocytopenia, and the time required to achieve a platelet count of >50,000/μl cannot identify dogs that will exhibit relapsing thrombocytopenia. Therefore, periodic monitoring is essential. Environmental stress and/or hormonal imbalance may precipitate relapses. Consider ovariohysterectomy for intact females following correction of the thrombocytopenia and bleeding abnormalities. Approximately 20% of patients will die, usually as the result of severe intestinal hemorrhage.

SYSTEMIC LUPUS ERYTHEMATOSUS

Systemic lupus erythematosus (SLE) is characterized by its ability to affect numerous organ systems. SLE has been called "the great imitator." A wide variety of clinical presentations occur. Tissue inflammation is induced by circulating, soluble antigen-antibody complexes that diffuse into vascular endothelial spaces, activate the complement cascade, and facilitate the perivascular accumulation of inflammatory cells. The inflammation may result in acute necrotizing vasculitis with progressive fibrinoid deposition and sclerosis. Deposition of immune complexes within the renal glomerulus leads to membranous glomerulitis; diffusion of immune complexes into joints results in polyarthritis.

Etiology

KEY POINT ▶ SLE is an example of type III hypersensitivity caused by circulating antigen-antibody complexes. Occasional concurrent type II hypersensitivity occurs due to antibodies that bind surface antigens on erythrocytes, thrombocytes, and leukocytes.

- The etiology is unknown.
- A familial tendency exists; however, no defined inheritance pattern has been documented. Shetland sheepdogs, collies, Afghan hounds, beagles, Irish setters, Old English sheepdogs, poodles, and German shepherds may be overrepresented.
- The mean age of afflicted dogs is approximately 6 years. There is no sex predilection.

Clinical Signs

- The onset of signs may be acute or insidious. Signs may wax and wane for a considerable time before presentation.
- The most common reason for clinical presentation is a gait abnormality manifested by stilted movement or shifting leg lameness. This abnormality may be the result of polyarthritis (see sec. 9, ch. 30) or polymyositis (see sec. 10, ch. 6). Approximately 75% of dogs will exhibit polyarthritis at some time during the progression of the disease.
- The animal may be presented for the complaint of focal or diffuse skin lesions that can affect virtually any body area (see sec. 5, ch. 9).
- Nonspecific complaints include malaise, anorexia, and weakness.

Diagnosis

The diagnosis of SLE is based on clinical assessment and evaluation of laboratory tests.

KEY POINT ▶ One specific diagnostic test for SLE does not exist. The diagnosis of SLE is based on documentation of (1) two major signs and a positive serologic test or (2) one major sign, two minor signs, and a positive serologic test. SLE is considered probable when there are (1) one major sign and positive serology or (2) two major signs and negative serology.

Clinical findings are separated into major and minor signs:

- Major signs include nonerosive polyarthritis, polymyositis, bullous dermatitis, proteinuria, and immune-mediated hemolytic anemia, thrombocytopenia, and leukopenia.
- Minor signs consist of fever of unknown origin, oral ulceration, pleuritis, myocarditis, pericarditis, peripheral lymphadenopathy, dementia, and seizures.

Physical Examination

Identify major and minor signs in the physical examination. The joints may be distended and painful; muscle pain and/or diffuse muscle wasting may be evident; and cutaneous lesions may be noted. Cutaneous manifestations, seen in nearly 50% of dogs, may include a symmetric or focal distribution of lesions affecting any body part. Mucocutaneous junctions and the oral cavity commonly are affected. The lesions may exhibit ulceration, erythema, crusting, oozing, and alopecia. Cellulitis, furunculosis, scarring, and leukoderma may be observed. Pyrexia and peripheral lymphadenopathy may be noted.

Complete Blood Count, Serum Biochemistry Profile, and Urinalysis

Complete Blood Count. The CBC may exhibit evidence of immune-mediated hemolytic anemia, thrombocytopenia, or leukopenia if a concurrent type II hypersensitivity to these cells exists. If a regenerative anemia is present without evidence of detectable blood loss or autoagglutination, perform a direct Coombs test. The PCV may be below 20%.

- If a nonregenerative anemia exists, evaluate bone marrow cytology.
- If the hemogram demonstrates thrombocytopenia and/or leukopenia, follow up with bone marrow evaluation.
- If the hemogram demonstrates a nonregenerative anemia, thrombocytopenia, and leukopenia, and the bone marrow is nonregenerative:
  - Submit a serum sample for *Ehrlichia canis* titer (see sec. 2, ch. 10).
  - Treat the patient with tetracycline (20 mg/kg q8h PO) or doxycycline (10 mg/kg q12h PO) pending serology results.
- In the absence of immune-mediated anemia, thrombocytopenia, or leukopenia, the hemogram usually demonstrates:
  - Leukocytosis characterized by neutrophilia and monocytosis.
  - Increased plasma fibrinogen
  - Elevated plasma proteins compatible with chronic inflammation.

Serum Biochemistry Profile. Results are not specific for SLE; however, assessment of serum albumin, globulin, urea nitrogen, creatinine, and muscle enzyme concentrations is important.

- If hypoalbuminemia, azotemia, or creatinemia exist, evaluate with urinalysis.
- If serum aspartate aminotransferase activity is elevated above alanine aminotransferase activity:
  - Suspect muscle inflammation
  - Assess serum creatine phosphokinase activity

  or
  - Obtain a muscle biopsy, particularly if muscle pain and/or atrophy exists.
- If serum globulin levels are significantly increased, perform serum electrophoresis to document polyclonal gammapathy compatible with lupus erythematosus.

Urinalysis. Urinalysis may reveal proteinuria with or without casts. As many as 50% of cases will exhibit evidence of glomerulitis as detected by the presence of proteinuria. Proteinuria can be quantitated in a 24-hour urine collection or assessed as the ratio of urine protein concentration to urine creatinine concentration (see sec. 8, ch. 1).

KEY POINT ▶ Absence of proteinuria does not rule out SLE.

Arthrocentesis

Perform *arthrocentesis* in patients that exhibit distended joints or lameness potentially related to arthritis. Cytologic analysis should reveal an increased cell count composed predominantly of nondegenerated neutrophils and some mononuclear cells and characterized by decreased synovial fluid viscosity, and absence of bacteria.

Radiography

Radiograph affected joints to document a nonerosive arthropathy.

Serologic Tests

Serologic tests that aid in the diagnosis of SLE include the indirect fluorescent antinuclear antibody (IFAA) test and the lupus erythematosus (LE) cell test. False-negative results may occur following recent glucocorticoid therapy, and false-positive titers may occur in other chronic inflammatory diseases, such as bacterial endocarditis.

IFAA Test. This indirect immunofluorescent test documents the presence of serum antibodies with specificity for nuclear antigens. It may be more sensitive than the LE cell test.

LE Cell Test. This test detects the presence of antinuclear antibodies in plasma by documenting phagocytized antibody-coated nuclear material within neutrophils and macrophages. Neutrophils or macrophages with phagocytized antibody-coated nuclear material are referred to as LE cells. This is a cytologic test that requires documentation of the number of LE cells seen on a buffy coat smear.

Treatment

The goal of treatment is to reduce tissue inflammation. It also is important to manage associated organ failure, avoid bacterial infections, and treat any identified infections specifically and aggressively.

The *reduction of tissue inflammation* usually is achieved through the use of prednisone or prednisolone (1–3 mg/kg q12h PO) until clinical improvement is observed. If improvement is not noted within 10 days, then concurrently administer:

- For dogs—azathioprine (Imuran; Burroughs Wellcome) (2 mg/kg q24h PO) for 10 days
- For cats—chlorambucil (Leukeran; Burroughs Wellcome) (0.25–0.5 mg/kg q48–72h PO).

Once clinical remission has been achieved, decrease drug dosage to the lowest possible amount that clinically controls the disease. Aspirin (dogs, 10–25 mg/kg q8h PO; cats, 10–40 mg/kg q72h PO) may provide additional analgesic, antipyretic, and anti-inflammatory relief. Remember that aspirin therapy is contraindicated in the presence of thrombocytopenia and gastrointestinal ulceration. Treatment will likely need to be continued indefinitely; however, following remission for 6 to 8 weeks, a trial period without treatment can be tried.

KEY POINT ▶ SLE is associated with excess production of a wide variety of anticytoplasmic and antinuclear antibodies. Therapy with immunosuppressive agents such as glucocorticoids, azathioprine, and chlorambucil may reduce serum concentrations of these antibodies; however, serum antinuclear antibody titers usually remain high during periods of clinical disease remission.

Prognosis

The prognosis is guarded. Approximately 40% of dogs die within 1 year of diagnosis. Severe organ dysfunction makes the prognosis worse. The presence of severe infection warrants a grave prognosis. Patients often die of bronchopneumonia, septicemia, and steroid-induced pancreatitis.

Supplemental Readings

Jans HE, Armstrong PJ, Price GS: Therapy of immune-mediated thrombocytopenia: A retrospective study of 15 dogs. J Vet Intern Med 4:4, 1990.

Lewis RM, Picut CA: *Veterinary Clinical Immunology: From Classroom to Clinics.* Philadelphia: Lea & Febiger, 1989.

Thompson JP: Immunologic diseases. *In* Ettinger S, ed.: *Textbook of Veterinary Internal Medicine.* 3rd ed. Philadelphia: W. B. Saunders, 1989, p 2297.

Werner LL, Gorman NT: Immune-mediated disorders of cats. Vet Clin North Am 14:1039, 1984.

Williams DA, Maggio-Price L: Canine idiopathic thrombocytopenia: Clinical observations and long-term follow-up in 54 cases. J Am Vet Med Assoc 185:660, 1984.

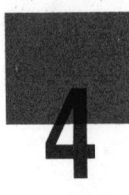

4 Diseases of the Spleen

Margaret C. McEntee
Rodney L. Page

The spleen has many important functions, and is commonly an active or passive participant in a number of disease processes. As a part of the mononuclear phagocyte (reticuloendothelial) system, the spleen functions to filter and phagocytize cells (e.g., senescent red blood cells) and particles (e.g., bacteria). The spleen has an important role in a number of infectious diseases through phagocytosis, antibody production, and modulation of hemoparasitic infections. The spleen has a significant storage capacity. Splenic contraction occurs in response to stress (exercise, blood loss, excitement, etc.) with a resultant rise in blood volume.

Splenic disorders usually are identified as a result of change in shape, size, and function of the spleen. Symmetric or asymmetric enlargement of the spleen can generally be detected on physical examination or radiographic evaluation. Other signs (weakness, pallor, coagulation abnormalities) are related to, or are a function of, the underlying disease process.

Therapeutic decisions must be based on accurate clinical diagnosis. Splenectomy, for instance, may result in increased morbidity and mortality, and therefore should be performed only when necessary.

ANATOMY/HISTOLOGY

There are four main components to the spleen: the fibromuscular capsule, white pulp, marginal zone, and red pulp.

Fibromuscular Capsule. The capsule surrounds the spleen and branches to form trabeculae. The smooth muscle component allows for contraction and distention of the spleen.

White Pulp. The white pulp consists of lymphocytes and reticuloendothelial (RE) cells distributed along arterial vessels that form cylindrical structures called periarterial lymphatic sheaths rich in T-lymphocytes. B-lymphocytes are located in nodules along these sheaths and represent areas of B-lymphocyte proliferation and antibody production. As a result of blood flow dynamics, plasma is delivered to the white pulp while erythrocytes continue into the marginal zone. Soluble antigens are delivered to the white pulp for immune recognition and processing.

Marginal Zone. The marginal zone is not well developed in the dog and cat. It separates the white pulp from the red pulp. In other species, macrophages that have a phagocytic function are present as blood is filtered through this region.

Red Pulp. The red pulp consists primarily of venous sinuses, a reticulum filled with macrophages, and blood. As the arteries enter the red pulp, they lose the periarterial lymphatic sheath, and are surrounded by a dense sheath of reticulum and macrophages called the periarteriolar macrophage sheath (also known as ellipsoids). Endothelial cells in the terminal arterial capillaries are separated by gaps. Particles, cells, and plasma pass through the gaps into the periarteriolar macrophage sheath, which is the major site for clearance of blood-borne particles. The red pulp is the site for culling abnormal blood cells and processing of particulate antigens for presentation to the white pulp, where an immune response is mounted.

PHYSIOLOGY/FUNCTIONS

Hematopoiesis

The spleen is a hematopoietic organ during fetal development, but the *normal* adult spleen in the dog and cat has no hematopoietic activity. The red pulp retains the ability for extramedullary hematopoiesis upon demand.

Reservoir Function

Normally 90% of the red cells pass quickly through the spleen while the remaining red cells take 7 to 8 minutes to move through the red pulp, which constitutes the splenic reservoir. In anesthetized dogs the distended spleen may contain up to 30% of the red cell mass. With contraction the packed cell volume (PCV) may rise 10 to 20% in dogs and cats. The blood storage capacity of the feline spleen is less than that of the canine spleen.

Filtering Functions

Within the red pulp, active phagocytic cells deplete oxygen and glucose, which stresses erythrocyte metabolism and results in decreased red blood cell (RBC) deformability. These events, coupled with the slow blood flow, aid in removal of abnormal or senescent RBCs. Reticulocytes (immature erythrocytes that contain RNA) normally are sequestered in the spleen for remodeling and then released as mature erythrocytes.

Pitting is the removal of cytoplasmic inclusions that occurs because inclusions cause the RBCs to be less deformable. This occurs within the spleen, resulting in the removal of mitochondria, Howell-Jolly bodies, Heinz bodies, intracellular organisms, and nuclei. Pit-

TABLE 1. Localized Splenomegaly

Non-Neoplastic	Neoplastic
Nodular hyperplasia	Primary
Hematoma	Hemangiosarcoma
Abscess	Hemangioma
	Sarcoma
	Secondary

ting does not occur in the cat because of larger apertures in the walls of the pulp venule.

Immunologic Functions

Phagocytosis. The slow circulation in the spleen enhances contact time, and hence phagocytosis of microorganisms. The liver is more effective at removing blood-borne bacteria in the presence of specific antibacterial antibody, because of its larger size and greater blood flow. In the absence of a significant amount of specific antibody, the spleen becomes crucial for removal of bacteria.

RBCs acquire surface immunoglobulins as part of the aging process. Splenic macrophages remove the portion of the erythrocyte membrane coated with IgG, resulting in formation of a spherocyte. Spherocytes are less deformable and hence are culled.

The spleen plays an important role in protection against RBC parasites such as *Hemobartonella* and *Babesia*, because of its pitting function.

Antibody Synthesis. Antigen processing occurs as a result of contact between splenic macrophages and blood. The splenic macrophages present the antigens to the immunocompetent cells of the spleen resulting in B-lymphocyte proliferation and humoral antibody production. Evidence suggests that in asplenic patients, early events in antibody production are normal but the role of the spleen in augmenting stimulated lymphocyte subpopulations is compromised.

Cellular Immunity. Studies suggest that the spleen may play a role in T-cell activities and in providing host defense against solid tumor cells.

Miscellaneous Functions

Other functions of the spleen include:

- Storage and activation of factor VIII coagulant activity and factor VIII antigen
- Regulation of the formation, liberation, and degradation of angiotensin-converting enzyme
- Modulation of plasma norepinephrine levels and/or renal PGE2 activity
- Iron storage and recycling of iron to the bone marrow

ETIOLOGY/PATHOGENESIS

Splenic disorders can be separated into two categories: localized or asymmetric splenomegaly (e.g., discrete splenic mass) and generalized or symmetrical splenomegaly.

Causes of localized splenomegaly (Table 1) include:

- Primary or metastatic neoplasia
- Nodular hyperplasia
- Hematoma
- Abscess

Generalized splenomegaly (Table 2) may result from:

- Inflammatory/infectious diseases
- Hyperplastic splenomegaly
- Congestive splenomegaly
- Infiltrative diseases including both neoplastic and non-neoplastic diseases

Splenic masses are more common in dogs, whereas generalized splenomegaly is more common in cats.

TABLE 2. Generalized Splenomegaly

Infectious	Hyperplastic	Congestive	Infiltrative
Bacterial	Immune-mediated	Pharmacologic	Neoplastic
Septicemia	AIHA		Lymphoma
Toxoplasmosis	IMT	Portal Hypertension	Leukemia
Salmonellosis	SLE	Splenic Torsion	Mastocytosis
			Malignant histiocytosis
Viral	Hypersplenism		Multiple myeloma
ICH	Primary (idiopathic)		
FIP	Secondary		Non-neoplastic
			Extra-medullary hematopoiesis
Mycotic			Hypereosinophilic syndrome
Blastomycosis			Amyloidosis
Histoplasmosis			
Parasitic			
Hemo-bartonellosis			
Rickettsial			
Ehrlichiosis			
RMSF			

ICH = infectious canine hepatitis; FIP = feline infectious peritonitis; RMSF = Rocky Mountain spotted fever; AIHA = autoimmune hemolytic anemia; IMT = immune-mediated thrombocytopenia; SLE = systemic lupus erythematosus.

Localized Splenomegaly

Neoplasia

Hemangiomas and hemangiosarcomas are the most common neoplastic splenic masses and are very common in the dog but rare in the cat. Other primary neoplastic splenic masses include fibrosarcoma, leiomyosarcoma, leiomyoma, osteosarcoma, undifferentiated sarcoma, chondrosarcoma, rhabdomyosarcoma, myxosarcoma, liposarcoma, myelolipoma, and occasionally lymphoma. Metastasis to the spleen may occur from a number of sites.

Nodular Hyperplasia

Splenic nodular hyperplasia can be single or multiple nodules that are benign accumulations of lymphoid cells.

Trauma

Trauma can result in subcapsular hematoma formation, causing a mass effect in the spleen. Commonly no underlying cause can be identified. Splenic hematomas cannot be distinguished from hemangioma/hemangiosarcoma on the basis of size or shape, and histopathology is required to make the diagnosis. Trauma may result in splenic rupture potentially requiring surgical intervention.

Splenic trauma can also lead to splenosis, which is the dissemination of splenic tissue into the abdominal cavity (and potentially into the thoracic cavity if there is also a diaphragmatic tear) and the subsequent development of daughter spleens.

Abscess

Splenic abscesses can form from hematogenous spread of microorganisms but are very rare in the dog and cat.

Generalized Splenomegaly

Inflammatory/Infectious Disease

A wide range of infectious diseases can result in diffuse splenomegaly. A partial list of the disorders that may be associated with splenomegaly is provided in Table 2 (please refer to the various chapters in this book on infectious diseases for details concerning these). The various types can be classified upon the basis of the primary type of cellular infiltrate.

Hyperplastic Splenomegaly

This type of splenomegaly occurs as a result of hyperplasia of the REs and lymphoid components of the spleen in response to blood-borne antigens and to RBC destruction (e.g., immune-mediated hemolytic anemia).

Congestive Splenomegaly

Splenic enlargement resulting from congestion can occur through a number of different mechanisms. Splenic distension occurs as a result of smooth muscle relaxation in the splenic capsule and trabeculae with the use of tranquilizers (e.g., phenothiazine) and barbiturates. Portal hypertension secondary to right-sided congestive heart failure, caudal vena cava obstruction, and intrahepatic obstruction may cause splenic congestion. Splenic torsion alone or in conjunction with gastric dilatation-volvulus can cause splenomegaly.

Infiltrative Diseases

Neoplastic Infiltration. This is one of the most common causes of splenomegaly. Splenomegaly is common in patients with acute and chronic leukemias (more common in the acute form). In leukemic patients, splenic enlargement primarily is due to the presence of neoplastic lymphocytes of hematogenous origin, but extramedullary hematopoiesis (EMH) may also play a role. Other neoplastic conditions that result in diffuse splenomegaly in dogs and cats include systemic mastocytosis, lymphoma, multiple myeloma, and malignant histiocytosis (dogs).

Non-neoplastic Infiltration

EMH is relatively common in dogs. RBC destruction, severe splenic or extrasplenic inflammation, immune-mediated thrombocytopenia, neoplastic infiltration of the spleen, bone marrow hypoplasia, and splenic congestion can stimulate EMH.

Hypereosinophilic syndrome of cats can lead to infiltration of the spleen with mature eosinophils (see sec. 3, ch. 1). This syndrome is characterized by a peripheral blood eosinophilia, bone marrow hyperplasia of the eosinophil precursors, and multiple organ infiltration by mature eosinophils. Splenic amyloidosis can cause splenomegaly but is relatively rare.

Hypersplenism

Hypersplenism, strictly defined, is characterized by:

- Cytopenia(s)
- Bone marrow hyperplasia of the affected cell line or a normocellular bone marrow
- Splenomegaly
- Resolution of the cytopenia in response to splenectomy

Hypersplenism results mainly from the filtering and phagocytic functions of the spleen.

- *Primary hypersplenism* occurs when the splenic dysfunction is idiopathic.
- In *secondary hypersplenism*, an underlying disease process is identified that has resulted in splenomegaly.

Hyposplenism

Hyposplenism, or decreased splenic function, can occur secondary to a wide range of disease processes. A number of hematologic changes are recognized in association with hyposplenism, including reticulocytosis, acanthocytes, and Howell-Jolly bodies. These changes are the same as those seen in splenectomized animals.

CLINICAL SIGNS

Clinical signs of splenic disease typically are nonspecific and are more likely to be related to the underlying disease process than to enlargement of the spleen. Clinical signs include anorexia, weight loss, weakness, abdominal distension, vomiting, diarrhea, and polyuria/polydipsia.

DIAGNOSIS

History

The history can aid in identifying patients with certain types of splenic disease. For example, patients presenting with a relatively acute onset of abdominal distension and retching may have splenic torsion in conjunction with gastric dilatation-volvulus. Periodic weakness or collapse, particularly in certain breeds (e.g., German shepherds), raises the suspicion of splenic hemangiosarcoma with intermittent hemorrhage. A history of tick exposure in patients with splenomegaly can aid in the diagnosis of Rocky Mountain spotted fever and erhlichiosis. Owners may report enlarged lymph nodes in patients with lymphoma. A history of drug exposure in a patient with a bleeding disorder may indicate drug-induced immune-mediated thrombocytopenia.

Physical Examination

The spleen is located in the left cranial abdominal quadrant and is oriented dorsoventrally. The normal spleen is palpable in many dogs and cats.

Splenomegaly (diffuse or localized) often can be detected with careful abdominal palpation. Raising the animal's front quarters during abdominal palpation can aid in identification of an enlarged spleen by shifting the abdominal contents caudally. Position of the spleen and ease of identification can vary, depending on such factors as breed conformation, presence of ingesta in the stomach, and whether the patient is overweight. If splenic enlargement has been identified, exercise caution because it is possible to rupture the spleen, especially in the case of splenic hemangiosarcoma.

Splenomegaly is not always evident on physical examination. Additional tools such as abdominal radiography or ultrasound may be necessary to identify an enlarged spleen.

Other physical examination findings may include abdominal distension, peritoneal effusion, pain upon palpation of the abdomen, petechiae, ecchymoses, pale mucous membranes, and fever.

Minimum Data Base

The hemogram is the most helpful in diagnosing splenic disorders. Changes in the hemogram essentially are a result of either hyposplenism or hypersplenism. A biochemical profile and urinalysis as well as a complete blood cell count (CBC) should be performed on all patients with splenic disease.

Hypersplenism is not as common as hyposplenism.

Changes seen with hypersplenism include regenerative anemia, neutropenia, thrombocytopenia, and other cytopenias. Abnormalities associated with hyposplenism include target cells, acanthocytes, Howell-Jolly bodies, nucleated RBCs, an increased percentage of reticulocytes, and thrombocytosis. Similar changes can be seen in splenectomized patients.

Spherocytes commonly are found in patients with autoimmune hemolytic anemia. If thrombocytopenia is the only hematologic abnormality detected, consider immune-mediated thrombocytopenia (see sec. 3, ch. 3).

Biochemical abnormalities are more likely to reflect the primary disease process than to result from splenic enlargement. Hemoglobinemia and resultant hemoglobinuria are commonly identified in dogs with splenic torsion.

Abdominal Radiography

Abdominal radiography, ultrasonography, and other imaging modalities such as computed tomography and magnetic resonance imaging provide information about splenic anatomy but not about function. Radiographs should be taken prior to tranquilization or anesthesia, because these can cause splenomegaly.

In dorsoventral (or ventrodorsal) radiographic views of the abdomen, the spleen normally is seen between the gastric fundus and the left kidney. It is more variable in position and size in lateral radiographs.

Abdominal radiographs may be useful:

- To confirm splenic enlargement and indicate whether the enlargement is localized or generalized
- To identify concurrent problems such as gastric dilatation-volvulus (GDV), hepatomegaly, abdominal lymph node enlargement, and peritoneal effusion

Abdominal Ultrasonography

Ultrasound procedures (see sec. 1, ch. 4 for a general description) can be helpful in many situations, including:

- Identification of a focal mass, multiple masses, or diffuse splenomegaly
- Evaluation of patients with ascites due to congestion or peritoneal effusion due to splenic rupture, when there is a loss of abdominal detail on survey radiographs
- Evaluation of the parenchyma of the spleen
- Assessment of the splenic vasculature, especially in dogs with splenic torsion
- Aid in guiding fine-needle aspiration and biopsy of the spleen

Fine-Needle Aspiration Cytology

Fine-needle aspiration cytology is a valuable tool that can aid in the selection of patients for exploratory surgery, splenic biopsy, and splenectomy. Conversely, it can help identify those patients that would not benefit from splenectomy.

The procedure includes the following steps:

- Place the patient in right lateral or dorsal recumbency.
- Restraint or mild sedation usually is sufficient. Avoid general anesthesia, because splenic congestion can result in hemodiluted samples.
- Clip and prepare the site sterilely. Manually localize and stabilize the spleen.
- Use a 22- or 25-gauge needle 1 to 1½ inches long.
- Following the procedure, observe the patient for 3–6 hours for evidence of hemorrhage.

KEY POINT ▶ Fine-needle aspiration cytology is an easy and safe procedure that can aid in the diagnosis of splenic disease in more than 50% of animals.

Aspiration cytology is contraindicated in patients with large cavitary lesions, which may rupture during aspiration. In patients with splenic hemangiosarcoma, aspiration can result in seeding of the tumor along the tract, as well as splenic rupture and seeding of the abdominal cavity. Thrombocytopenia is *not* considered a contraindication for this procedure.

Potential complications include splenic rupture, hemorrhage, damage to other abdominal organs, peritonitis, and abdominal seeding of a splenic neoplasm. In two reports describing the use of this technique in a total of 63 patients, no complications were encountered.

Splenic Function Studies

Nuclear imaging studies employ ^{51}Cr-labeled heat-damaged red cells or 99mTc sulfur colloid, which are cleared by the spleen and provide a measure of splenic function. The procedure has limited availability for veterinary patients.

Hematologic changes evident on a routine hemogram, such as Howell-Jolly bodies, nucleated RBCs, and acanthocytes may be indicative of functional hyposplenism. Hematology is the primary means of evaluating splenic function in cats and dogs with splenic disorders.

Miscellaneous Tests

Bone Marrow Aspiration Cytology. Bone marrow aspiration cytology or a core bone marrow biopsy is indicated in patients with splenomegaly and cytopenia(s) (see sec. 3, ch. 1 for details on bone marrow biopsy technique). Splenic enlargement may reflect an underlying bone marrow hypoplasia or aplasia. The spleen is capable of supplementing the hematopoietic function of the bone marrow when necessary.

Lymph Node Aspiration Cytology. Lymph node aspiration cytology or biopsy is indicated in patients with peripheral lymphadenopathy. Marked peripheral lymphadenopathy typically is associated with lymphosarcoma. Mild or moderate peripheral lymph node enlargement can be seen in a number of different diseases, including infectious and immune-mediated disorders.

Serologic Tests. Serologic tests for specific infectious and immune diseases can be performed. Rickettsial titers for ehrlichiosis, Coombs test for immune-mediated hemolytic anemia, and antinuclear antibody testing for systemic lupus erythematosus, may be indicated for some patients. The diagnosis of immune-mediated thrombocytopenia usually is made by elimination of other causes of thrombocytopenia (see sec. 3, ch. 3). There are specific tests for immune-mediated thrombocytopenia, but they are not readily available. Blood cultures as well as cultures of other fluids (e.g., urine) or sites may be indicated in patients suspected of having diseases such as bacterial endocarditis, diskospondylitis, or septicemia.

TREATMENT

Splenectomy

Splenectomy is indicated for patients with splenic rupture, splenic torsion, or splenic masses, and in symptomatic patients.

Splenectomy in cats with systemic mastocytosis can significantly prolong life expectancy even if mast cells are present in the peripheral circulation.

Because of the potential for splenic rupture and death in patients with hemangiosarcoma, splenectomy is recommended. These patients typically are not cured by surgery and usually have evidence of recurrence within 4 months. Adjuvant therapy (chemotherapy) is indicated but has been shown to be beneficial only in dogs with no or minimal gross evidence of spread at the time of splenectomy (Table 3).

Splenectomy is contraindicated in patients with immune-mediated hemolytic anemia or thrombocytopenia, unless other forms of treatment have failed; in most patients with lymphoma or leukemia when there is splenic involvement (splenomegaly); and in patients with bone marrow hypoplasia or aplasia, because the spleen is the major hematopoietic organ in these patients.

Comment: Splenectomy may be a therapeutic option in selected patients with lymphoma and leukemia.

In human patients with non-Hodgkin's lymphoma, the indications for splenectomy are massive splenomegaly, hypersplenism syndrome, and autoimmune complications.

KEY POINT ▶ Generalized splenomegaly often is not a surgical disease. Attempt to diagnose and treat the underlying disorder prior to performing a splenectomy.

Technique

1. Prepare the ventral abdomen for aseptic surgery.
2. Make a ventral midline abdominal incision from the xyphoid to 2–4 cm cranial to the pubis, or more caudally if necessary.
3. Place a Balfour retractor to expose the abdominal viscera.
4. Examine the spleen and other abdominal organs for evidence of abnormalities.
5. Gently pull the spleen out of the abdominal cavity.

Partial Splenectomy

6. Doubly ligate the splenic branches of the splenic artery and vein to the affected area of the spleen

TABLE 3. Treatment Protocols for Hemangiosarcoma in the Dog

VAC Protocol 1

Day 1: doxorubicin,* 30 mg/m² IV; premedication-diphenhydramine, 0.5 mg/lb IV (maximum of 40 mg); cyclophosphamide† (CTX), 100–150 mg/m² IV
Day 7: vincristine‡, 0.7 mg/m² IV
Day 15: vincristine, 0.7 mg/m² IV
Day 21: repeat protocol

Prophylactic oral antibiotic therapy is recommended, such as Tribrissen, 15 mg/lb q12h for 14 days starting on day 1.

VAC Protocol 2

Day 1: doxorubicin and diphenhydramine, as above; vincristine 0.7 mg/m² IV
Day 7: CTX, 50 mg/m² PO SID for 4 days
Day 15: CTX, 50 mg/m² PO SID for 4 days
Day 21: repeat protocol

This protocol can be used for patients that are unable to visit the veterinarian weekly for treatment.

VAC = vincristine-Adriamycin-cyclophosphamide.
*Doxorubicin (Adriamycin; Adria Labs., Columbus, OH) is potentially cardiotoxic. Evaluate an ECG and echocardiography (m-mode) prior to therapy. Repeat the cardiac evaluation at treatment number 4 or 5. The maximum amount of doxorubicin that should be administered over a course of treatment is 180 mg/m² or six dosages. If the patient develops a murmur or, more importantly, an arrhythmia, discontinue therapy.
†Cyclophosphamide (Cytoxan; Mead-Johnson, Evansville, IN) can cause hemorrhagic cystitis. If it occurs, discontinue cyclophosphamide immediately and usually limit therapy to oral antibiotics and corticosteroids. Resolution of signs occurs within days to 8 weeks later.
‡Oncovin (Eli Lilly, Indianapolis, IN) Evaluate a CBC prior to each chemotherapy treatment to check for bone marrow suppression, and periodically evaluate a metabolic panel to monitor for evidence of nephrotoxicity secondary to the doxorubicin.
Monitor patient progress monthly (radiographic evaluation as well as abdominal ultrasonography). Allow completion of 2 to 3 courses of treatment prior to making a decision about response to therapy.

with absorbable suture. Divide the vessels between the ligatures.

7. Place two non-crushing clamps (e.g., Doyen) on the spleen between the healthy and diseased areas.
8. Divide between the clamps and remove the splenic tissue.
9. Oversew the splenic capsule on the remaining spleen (3–0 or 4–0 polydioxanone (PDS), simple continuous suture).

Total Splenectomy

6. Doubly ligate all of the splenic branches of the splenic artery and vein with absorbable suture. Ligate the vessels close to the hilus of the spleen. Usually, two or three vessels can be included in each ligature. If possible, preserve the left gastroepiploic artery and vein (Fig. 1) (this may not be possible when removing large splenic tumors).
7. Divide each vessel between the ligatures and remove the spleen.
8. An alternative and more rapid procedure for total splenectomy is to place vascular clamps across the vessels prior to ligation. Include two or three of the vessels in each clamp. Divide the vessels between each pair of clamps and then place the next pair of clamps (see Fig. 1). After all vessels have been clamped and divided, remove the spleen. Ligate all vessels with absorbable sutures.

9. When splenic torsion is present, do not untwist the spleen, because release of tissue breakdown products and bacteria may result. Ligate the entire vascular pedicle with two or three absorbable ligatures. Consider placing a transfixing ligature in large dogs. Place two clamps across the vascular pedicle, divide between them, and remove the spleen. Remove the remaining clamp and check the pedicle for hemorrhage.
10. Check the vessels for hemorrhage. Close the abdomen in a routine fashion.

The gross appearance of the spleen cannot be used to differentiate hematoma, hemangioma, and hemangiosarcoma. A histopathologic diagnosis is crucial for determining postoperative treatment and prognosis.

Post-splenectomy sepsis is a serious complication in humans and can be fatal. Therefore, partial splenectomy or splenic biopsy may be advisable in certain animals. Partial splenectomy is a viable option for those animals with localized masses unless malignancy is suspected.

Other possible complications of splenectomy include exacerbation of certain diseases such as hemobartonellosis and babesiosis in animals that are latent carriers, and cytopenia(s) in patients with EMH secondary to a primary bone marrow disorder.

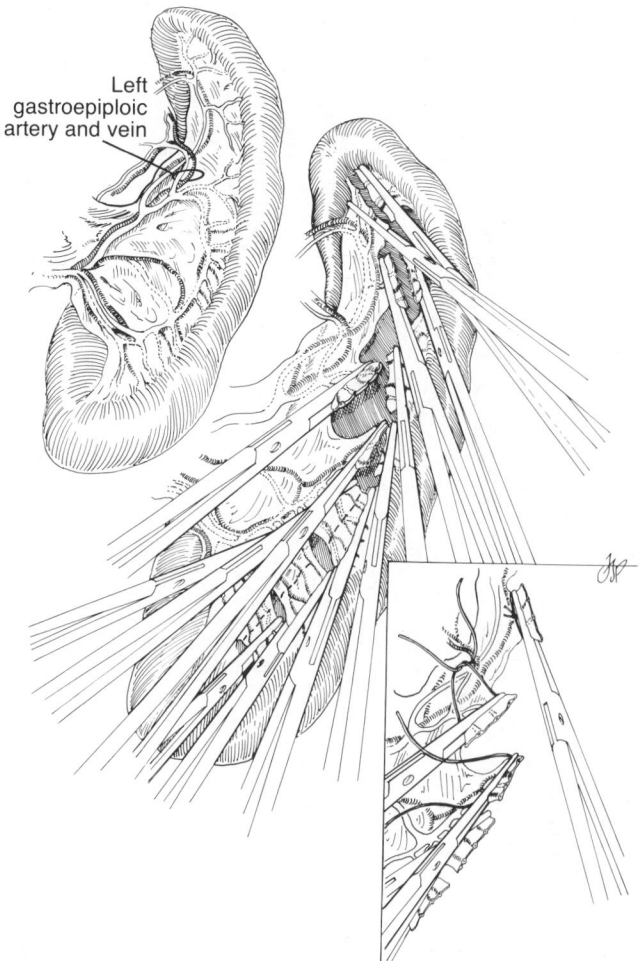

Figure 1. General procedure for total splenectomy. See text for details.

Treatment of the Underlying Disease Process

■ Treat infectious diseases with appropriate antibiotic therapy and supportive care.
■ Treat immune-mediated diseases (immune-mediated hemolytic anemia, immune-mediated thrombocytopenia) with:
  • Immunosuppressive doses of corticosteroids and other drugs as necessary (e.g., cyclophosphamide)
  • Blood component therapy, if indicated (as described in sec. 3, chs. 1 and 2).

Additional Therapy

Chemotherapy alone or in conjunction with the necessary supportive care is recommended for patients with acute and chronic leukemia and lymphosarcoma (see sec. 3, ch. 6); and for dogs with systemic mastocytosis (see sec. 3, ch. 7) and hemangiosarcoma.

Treatment of Dogs with Hemangiosarcoma

For general recommendations, see Table 3. Evaluation should include a complete blood count (CBC), including a coagulation panel, if indicated, thoracic and abdominal radiographs, and cardiac and abdominal ultrasonography if available.

Dogs with splenic hemangiosarcoma should be splenectomized. Splenectomy decreases the tumor burden and eliminates the risk of splenic rupture. Splenic rupture can occur as part of the natural progression of the disease, as a result of trauma (including abdominal palpation), or after initiation of chemotherapy in those tumors that respond to chemotherapy.

Supplemental Readings

Couto CG: Diseases of the lymph nodes and spleen. *In* Ettinger SJ, ed.: *Textbook of Veterinary Internal Medicine*. Philadelphia; W. B. Saunders, 1989, p 2225.

Greene CE: *Clinical Microbiology and Infectious Diseases of the Dog and Cat*. Philadelphia; W. B. Saunders, 1984.

Hosgood G. Splenectomy in the dog: A retrospective study of 31 cases. J Am Anim Hosp Assoc 23:275, 1987.

Johnson KA, Powers BE, Withrow SJ, et al: Predictors of neoplasia and survival after splenectomy. J Vet Intern Med 3:160, 1989.

Konde LJ, Wrigley RH, Lebel JL, et al: Sonographic and radiographic changes associated with splenic torsion in the dog. Vet Radiol 30:41, 1989.

O'Keefe DA, Couto CG: Fine-needle aspiration of the spleen as an aid in the diagnosis of splenomegaly. J Vet Intern Med 1:102, 1987.

Sills RH: Splenic function: Physiology and splenic hypofunction. Crit Rev Oncol Hematol 7:1, 1987.

Spangler WL, Culbertson MR: Prevalence, type and importance of splenic diseases in dogs: 1,480 cases (1985–1989). J Am Vet Med Assoc 200:829, 1992.

Wrigley RH, Konde LJ, Park RD, Lebel JL: Ultrasonographic features of splenic lymphosarcoma in dogs. J Am Vet Med Assoc 193:1565, 1988.

5 Principles of Oncology

Stephen D. Gilson
Rodney L. Page

Cancer management in companion animals has evolved considerably over the past two decades as the result of several significant factors. Improved health care of animals has increased the age distribution of dogs and cats, which increases the likelihood of cancer in this population. Clients are more aware of treatment options for their pets with cancer and are often willing to make the emotional and financial commitment to pursue therapy. There have been significant improvements in the treatment of certain types of cancer that encourage continued investigation. Aggressive surgical procedures have provided prolonged survival for many oro facial tumors (see sec. 9, ch. 4) and permit limb-sparing techniques for dogs with primary bone tumors (see sec. 9, ch. 22). Radiation therapy has been refined in both technological and clinical application and has become an essential tool for optimal management of cancer in companion animals. The use of chemotherapy in combination with surgery or radiation therapy has resulted in better management of hemangiosarcoma and osteosarcoma in dogs as well as mammary carcinoma in cats.

Finally, exciting results using biologic response modifiers (immunotherapy) in dogs with osteosarcoma and lymphosarcoma has re-established the importance of this modality. Veterinarians engaged in any type of small animal practice now manage pets with cancer on a weekly or daily basis and must be familiar with current trends in diagnosis and treatment. Many chapters in this section as well as in other sections of this book provide current useful information for the management of patients with cancer. This chapter provides the background, principles, rationale, and applications of cancer diagnosis and treatment.

INITIAL CLINICAL CONSIDERATIONS

Signalment. Many neoplasms more commonly affect animals of a certain age, sex, or breed, and such knowledge often aids diagnosis. Table 1 is a partial list of specific breeds and characteristics of dogs and cats predisposed to certain types of neoplasia.

History. The onset and duration of the mass, growth rate, and prior treatment may narrow the diagnostic evaluation and treatment options as well as help define behavioral characteristics of the neoplasm.

Physical Examination. The goal of examination is to characterize concurrent diseases that may limit treatment or survival and to define the extent of the tumor burden. Actual measurements of the lesion(s) using calipers is useful for discussions with clients and to document tumor response. It is essential to determine the invasiveness of the tumor to plan adequately the surgical biopsy and/or resection of a lesion. Regional lymph nodes must be evaluated for size, consistency, and fixation to adjacent tissues. Physical examination findings also help in selection of ancillary diagnostic procedures necessary to define tumor extent (specific imaging techniques, bone marrow aspiration/biopsy, endoscopy).

Client Counseling. Cancer treatment in companion animals evokes considerable emotion and ethical deliberation for both owners and veterinarians. It is helpful to first determine the goals and expectations of clients for their pets prior to discussing diagnosis and treatment. Once the diagnosis and staging is completed, treatment options can be considered. Treatment recommendations and prognostic factors evolve rapidly for many types of cancer. Therefore, consultation with a specialist regarding specific treatment options will often assist with decision making. Treatment availability and financial considerations must also be considered.

DIAGNOSTIC EVALUATION
Clinical Evaluation

General health status is assessed to identify disease that may affect adversely the prognosis and limit or alter therapy. After a thorough physical examination, the screening laboratory evaluation generally includes a complete blood cell count (CBC), serum biochemistry panel, and urinalysis. Other diagnostic tests are performed as indicated.

Survey radiographs are indicated to:

- Detect metastasis
- Determine potential bone involvement
- Evaluate orthopedic soundness prior to amputation or limb-sparing surgery in dogs with osteosarcoma
- Localize oral or nasal masses

Contrast radiographic studies can determine the extent of gastrointestinal and genitourinary neoplasia (For description of these procedures, see sec. 1, ch. 4.) Computed axial tomographic (CAT) scanning is becoming more available and defines the invasive characteristics of deep-seated tumors much more clearly than survey radiographs. CAT scanning procedures are particularly helpful when planning involved surgical procedures.

TABLE 1. Some Factors Predisposing Dogs and Cats to Specific Neoplasms

Factor	Predilection for
Age	
Histiocytoma	Young dogs
Viral papilloma	Young dogs
Sex	
Malignant melanoma	Males
Perianal adenoma	Males
Adrenal tumors	Females
Meningiomas	Females (dog), Males (cat)
Color	
Squamous cell carcinoma	Nonpigmented regions
Malignant melanoma	Darkly pigmented regions
Breed	
Skin tumors	Basset, boxer, Bull mastiff, Scottish terrier, weimaraner
Mast cell tumors	Brachycephalic breeds
Bone tumors	Large/giant breeds
Thyroid tumors	Boxer, beagle, golden retriever
Hemangiosarcomas	Golden retriever, German shepherd

Ultrasonography can be used to:

- Determine the proximity of a tumor to large blood vessels
- Determine the cavitary or cystic nature of masses
- Evaluate possible intra-abdominal metastases to lymph nodes or organs
- Assess the initial and post-treatment tumor volume (see sec. 1, ch. 4).

Important diagnostic procedures include cytologic examinations of bone marrow aspirates, buffy coat preparations of peripheral blood samples and fine-needle aspiration biopsies of accessible tumors and regional lymph nodes. (See sec. 3, ch. 1 for description of the technique for bone marrow aspiration.) Fine-needle aspiration can be accomplished on any accessible mass. Often, a rapid inexpensive diagnosis, using fine needle aspiration, can be made for certain tumor types (lipomas, sebaceous adenomas, and mast cell tumors). Do not over-interpret cytologic evaluation of fine needle aspirates or bone marrow specimens. Base treatment decisions on cytologic diagnosis only when a definitive diagnosis can be made, as with lymphosarcoma and mast cell tumors.

Tumor Biopsy

Many techniques are available for tissue biopsy. The method selected should safely and simply procure adequate tissue samples to provide an accurate diagnosis without compromising treatment. Biopsies can be excisional (complete removal of the tumor) or nonexcisional (removal of only a portion of the tumor). Nonexcisional techniques include:

- Cytology from a fine-needle aspirate, brush samples, impression smears or effusions
- Histopathology of cutting forceps biopsies, cutting needle biopsies, punch biopsies, and incisional biopsies.

Principles of Tumor Biopsy

In general, excisional biopsy is preferable if the mass is small (<3 cm in diameter), freely movable, and without adjacent tissue invasion. The specimen must contain a complete margin of normal tissue (preferably 2–3 cm in all directions). Specific indications for excisional biopsy include:

- Lymph node involvement
- Small cutaneous nodules with ample surrounding normal tissue
- Mammary gland tumors
- Tumors of the central nervous system (to provide decompression)
- Masses found during a laparotomy or thoracotomy

KEY POINT ▶ Excisional biopsies are considered a therapeutic procedure only when complete tumor removal is histologically verified *and* when the tumor is benign or of low-grade malignancy. In other situations, excisional biopsy should be used to consider a more definitive treatment recommendation.

Incisional biopsy is recommended if a definitive diagnosis or histologic grade would influence the treatment decision. For example, the histologic grade of soft tissue sarcomas and mast cell tumors (see sec. 3, ch. 7) are prognostic factors that can be helpful in treatment planning. Biopsy results may suggest the degree of surgical resection necessary for definitive control or indicate that additional types of therapy may be beneficial.

Ideal histologic samples contain the neoplastic tissue and some adjacent normal tissue to evaluate the tumor boundary. Superficial tumors should be sampled at the tumor/normal tissue interface away from regions of ulceration, necrosis, or inflammation. Deep biopsies (>1 cm) may be necessary to avoid sampling only overlying tissue. Biopsy at the tumor margin can be undesirable in certain deep-seated tumors if it disrupts and thereby extends the tumor margin. This can necessitate wider resection or a larger radiation field for adequate treatment. Biopsy needles are preferred for deep-seated tumors. The biopsy incision or needle tract for *every* biopsy should be preplanned because it is a potentially contaminated region and should be removed at the time of the definitive procedure or included in the radiation treatment field. Recommended procedures for processing biopsy samples include:

- Fix tissue samples for routine histopathologic evaluation in 10% buffered formalin (10:1 formalin to tissue ratio).
- For electron microscopy, fix samples in glutaraldehyde solution.
- Obtain samples for culture or other special analyses at the same time to avoid a second biopsy procedure if histologic analysis identifies an inflammatory or other non-neoplastic process.
- Include a complete history and description of the clinical and surgical findings with the laboratory submission.

- Use suture tags to identify areas of possible inadequate resection.

A pathologist should assign a histologic grade to each tumor specimen. A histologic grade represents the degree of malignancy and is based on tissue differentiation, mitotic activity, and extent of necrosis within the tumor. The grade often has prognostic significance and can suggest treatment alternatives. If the histologic diagnosis is questionable or does not seem to match your clinical judgment, discuss the results with the pathologist.

Tumor Staging

Accurate staging requires an understanding of the biologic behavior of different tumor types and a thorough diagnostic evaluation. Staging, ideally, is utilized to:

- Determine the extent of neoplastic disease
- Provide a framework for rational treatment planning
- Facilitate communication between clinicians
- Allow for uniform comparison and evaluation of treatment results
- Aid in prognostication

Several staging systems are available. Most are based on assessment of local, regional, and distant disease involvement. Some systems include other factors such as presence or absence of clinical signs (e.g., lymphomas), histologic grade (e.g., mast cell tumors), and site (e.g., squamous cell carcinoma of the mouth, tonsil, pinna, digit). The TNM (tumor-node-metastasis) system devised by the World Health Organization is the standard system for staging most tumors in veterinary medicine. Table 2 describes this staging scheme and gives several examples. Staging schemes are reviewed often because new prognostic information is constantly being acquired.

GENERAL THERAPEUTIC CONSIDERATIONS
Tumor Biology and Natural History

Rational treatment planning involves basic knowledge of the potential for local recurrence and metastasis of the neoplasm. Tumors predisposed to local recurrence should be managed aggressively from the time of initial diagnosis. The probability of long term tumor control is greatest when the tumor is undisturbed by previous therapeutic intervention. The risks and benefits of aggressive management must be carefully explained. However, most owners will recognize the obvious benefit of prolonged tumor response with reduced overall expense if the tumor can be managed with a single, albeit initially more costly, procedure compared with multiple, suboptimal attempts at tumor control.

Treatment Options

Many options exist for cancer management. In addition to single-treatment modalities for cancer management, multi-modality therapy can be considered (e.g., surgery and radiation therapy). It is important

TABLE 2. World Health Organization TNM Classification of Tumors

T = Tumor Size or Extent
T_1–T_4 represent specific size categories designated for each tumor type.

N = Lymph Node Involvement
N_1–N_3 ($\pm$ a, b) describes regional lymph node characteristics such as number of nodes enlarged, tissue adhesion, and presence or absence of neoplasia.

M = Metastasis
M_0 or M_1 indicates absence or presence of distant metastasis.

Example—TNM Classification of tumors of the oral cavity in dogs or cats:

T: Primary Tumor
T_{is} = Preinvasive tumor (in situ)
T_0 = No evidence of tumor
T_1 = Tumor < 2 cm diameter
T_2 = Tumor 2–4 cm diameter
T_3 = Tumor 3 cm diameter
    subclassification of a (no bone invasion) or b (bone invasion) can be added.

N: Nodes
N_0 = No evidence of LN enlargement
N_1 = Movable ipsilateral nodes enlarged
N_2 = Movable contralateral/bilateral nodes enlarged
N_3 = Fixed nodes

M: Metastasis
M_0 = No metastasis
M_1 = Metastasis detected

Example of Stage Grouping for Oral Tumors:

Stage	T	N	M
I	T_1	N_0, N_{1a}, N_{2a}	M_0
II	T_2	N_0, N_{1a}, N_{2a}	M_0
III	T_3	N_0, N_{1a}, N_{2a}	M_0
	Any T	N_{1b}	M_0
IV	Any T	Any N_{2b}, N_3	M_0
	Any T	Any N	M_1

From Owen, L.N. Classification of Tumours in Domestic Animals. Geneva: WHO, 1980.

to remember, however, that only those treatment modalities that are effective alone should be considered for combined therapy. For resistant forms of cancer such as soft tissue sarcomas and melanomas, multimodality therapy offers the greatest potential.

Goals of Treatment

Maintaining the highest quality of life for the longest period of time is always the goal of cancer management in companion animals. This goal must be considered within the context of client emotional and financial restrictions. Decisions are often difficult. The greatest service that can be provided to a client with a pet that has cancer is a knowledgeable *unbiased* assessment of the condition and a frank discussion of options sufficient to allow the client to make an informed decision. This may involve consultation with or referral to a specialist or a comprehensive cancer center.

PRINCIPLES OF THERAPY
Surgery

Surgery is primarily useful for localized or regional neoplasms. *En bloc* dissection of regional lymph nodes may also be appropriate (e.g., as part of a radical mastectomy in cats; see sec. 3, ch. 8). Surgery may be useful for treatment of metastatic disease if the tumor is slow-growing or is causing functional impairment or morbidity.

Applications

Surgery has been and will remain the most widely applied modality for cancer control. Surgery can be used for prevention of certain neoplasms; for example, ovariohysterectomy before an animal is 2.5 years of age reduces the risk of mammary neoplasia. For many types of cancer, surgery is essential for diagnosis, staging, and treatment (cure or palliation). Surgery may also be necessary in management of oncologic emergencies (obstruction or perforation) and complications related to chemotherapy or radiotherapy (drug extravasation or osteoradionecrosis).

Principles

Decide the extent of resection prior to the surgical procedure. This decision must be based on biopsy results, knowledge of tumor behavior and size, and the physical constraints or limitations provided by surrounding tissues (Fig. 1). In tumors that are highly malignant or are extensive in size (>3 cm in diameter), marginal resection is insufficient for prolonged tumor control.

KEY POINT ▶ Aggressive *initial* surgical management of neoplasia may be the most important principle for improved cancer control. Complete resection of malignant neoplasms is less likely with subsequent surgeries.

■ Protect normal tissue from tumor cell contamination by use of barrier drapes and laparotomy sponges. Changes in gloves, instruments, and drapes may be necessary to prevent contamination. Copious lavage

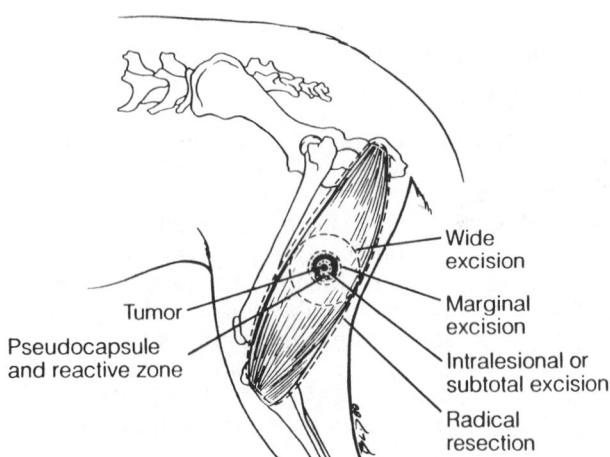

Figure 1. Surgical options for removal of a neoplasm. Wide excision or a more radical, compartmental resection is recommended for tumors that are not superficial or are infiltrative. Additional therapy may be indicated from histologic evaluation of tumor specimen. (Reprinted with permission from Gilson SD, Stone EA: Compend Cont Educ Pract Vet 12:1047–1058, 1990.)

of surface wounds also reduces the likelihood of residual tumor.
■ Minimize manipulation of tumor by placing stay sutures in marginal tissue.
■ Ligate vascular and lymphatic vessels early and always before severing, to prevent shedding of tumor emboli.
■ Fulgurate or electrocoagulate exposed surfaces if tumor margins are disrupted.

KEY POINT ▶ A pseudocapsule often surrounds many deep tumors. This is not a true capsule and provides no barrier to tumor invasion. Adequate normal tissue margins are necessary despite the presence of a pseudocapsule.

■ When *en bloc* resection (i.e., removal of the mass and all surrounding tissue) is performed, maintain adequate margins and make the dissection from the most peripheral lymph node toward the primary mass.
■ When using postoperative radiotherapy, irradiate all surgically exposed tissues plus a margin of normal tissue. Consider the treatment field when developing tissue grafts, flaps, and placing drains.
■ Resect all neoplastic tissue, leaving the wound open to heal by second intention if necessary.
■ Submit all resected specimens for histologic analysis and evaluation of surgical margins.

Sources of Failure

Proper presurgical evaluation and technique will minimize treatment failure, which can result from:

■ Surgery-related morbidity and mortality
■ Local or regional tumor recurrence
■ Tumor seeding or metastatic disease

Chemotherapy

Few types of cancer are chemosensitive. Lymphoid neoplasia is the most chemosensitive form of cancer (see sec. 3, ch. 6). Most nonlymphoid tumors are only moderately chemosensitive, and survival times have been extended infrequently with chemotherapy alone. However, improvement in tumor response may be possible with further refinements in chemotherapy protocols.

Table 3 lists the most common antineoplastic agents used in veterinary medicine. Indications and major toxicity are also listed. Table 4 is a conversion schedule for estimating body surface area for dogs and cats based on body weight. The use of cytotoxic agents must be done safely and with appropriate precautions to avoid exposure to health care workers. General guidelines for the safe handling of cytotoxic agents are given in Table 5.

Application

Most chemotherapeutic agents are administered intravenously. This is convenient and relatively noninvasive. Chemotherapy can also be given by intraarterial or intracavitary routes to increase the tu-

TABLE 3. Common Chemotherapeutic Agents Used in Veterinary Medicine

	Indication	Recommended Dosages	Toxicity
Alkylating Agents			
Cyclophosphamide (Cytoxan; Mead-Johnson)	Lymphoproliferative disorders, mast cell tumors, hemangiosarcoma, miscellaneous carcinomas	50 mg/m² PO q48 hr 50 mg/m² PO q24h for 4d weekly 100–300 mg/m² IV q3wk	BM, GI, Hemorrhagic cystitis
Chlorambucil (Leukeran; Burroughs-Wellcome)	Lymphoproliferative disease, macroglobulinemia	2–4 mg/m² q24–48h	BM
Melphalan (Alkeran; Burroughs-Wellcome)	Multiple myeloma	2–4 mg/m² PO q24–48h	BM
Cisplatin (Platinol; Bristol)	Osteosarcoma, transitional cell carcinoma, squamous cell carcinoma	50–70 mg/m² IV q3wk (vigorous hydration)	BM, GI, renal; Do not use in cats
Carboplatin (Paraplatin; Bristol)	Similar to cisplatin	250–300 mg/m² IV q3wk	BM, GI
Antimetabolites			
Methotrexate (Lederle)	Lymphoproliferative disorders	2.5 mg/m² PO q24h 15–20 mg/m² IV q3wk	BM, GI, renal
5-Fluorouracil (Roche)	Gastrointestinal and hepatic carcinoma	150–200 mg/m² IV q7d	BM, GI, CNS; Do not use in cats
Cytosine Arabinoside (Cytosar-U; Upjohn)	Lymphoproliferative disorders, myeloproliferative disorders	100 mg/m² IV or SC for 4 days q3–4wk	BM, GI
Plant Alkaloids			
Vincristine (Oncovin; Eli Lilly)	Lymphoproliferative disorders, mast cell tumors, sarcomas, carcinomas	0.5–0.7 mg/m² IV q7d	GI, peripheral neuropathy; vesicant
Antibiotics			
Doxorubicin (Adriamycin; Adria Labs.)	Lymphoproliferative disorders, soft tissue sarcoma, carcinomas	30 mg/m² IV q3wk (maximum cumulative dose = 180–240 mg/m²)	BM, GI, cardiac; severe vesicant; urticaria, alopecia
Mitoxantrone (Novantrone; Lederle)	Lymphoproliferative disorders	5–6 mg/m² q3wk	BM
Hormones			
Prednisone	Lymphoproliferative disorders, mast cell tumors, brain tumors	20–50 mg/m² q24–48h as needed	Iatrogenic Cushing's syndrome, GI
Miscellaneous			
L-Asparaginase (Elspar; Merck, Sharp & Dohme)	Lymphoproliferative disorders	10,000–30,000 IU/m² IM, SC, or IP as needed (pretreat with antihistamines, steroids)	Anaphylaxis, pancreatitis, coagulopathy

m² = body surface area in square meters (see Table 4); PO = per os; IV = intravenously; IM = intramuscular; SC = subcutaneously; IP = intraperitoneal; BM = bone marrow; GI = gastrointestinal; CNS = central nervous system.

mor/drug exposure. Antineoplastic agents can be given alone or in combination with other drugs or treatment types. Drugs can be given prior to surgery (neoadjuvant) or following cytoreductive surgery (adjuvant). The optimal sequence of combination therapy is controversial.

- Advantages of neoadjuvant chemotherapy include:
  - Potential reduction of tumor burden, necessitating less radical surgery
  - Tumor vasculature not altered by surgery, permitting undisturbed delivery of drug.
- Advantages of surgery followed by chemotherapy include:
  - Treatment of the primary mass
  - Recruitment of adjacent dormant tumor cells into a chemosensitive cell cycle phase
  - Smaller tumor burden.

A preplanned protocol, regardless of sequence, is important for management of tumors that are likely to recur following single-modality treatment such as medium or large infiltrative masses with an intermediate or high grade of malignancy.

Principles of Chemotherapy

- In general, chemotherapy is most effective against a small tumor burden and against tumors with a high growth fraction.
- Use only drugs with documented activity against the specific tumor type. Administer all drugs at maximum tolerated doses and intervals.
- Some protocols are designed in two phases: an initial phase of intensive therapy (induction), followed by a maintenance period using different antineoplastic agents.
- Combination chemotherapy using agents with different mechanisms of action and no overlap in toxicity

TABLE 4. Conversion from Body Weight (kg) to Body Surface Area in Square Meters (m²) for Dogs*

kg	m²	kg	m²
0.5	0.06	29.0	0.94
1.0	0.10	30.0	0.96
2.0	0.15	31.0	0.99
3.0	0.20	32.0	1.01
4.0	0.25	33.0	1.03
5.0	0.29	34.0	1.05
6.0	0.33	35.0	1.07
7.0	0.36	36.0	1.09
8.0	0.40	37.0	1.11
9.0	0.43	38.0	1.13
10.0	0.46	39.0	1.15
11.0	0.49	40.0	1.17
12.0	0.52	41.0	1.19
13.0	0.55	42.0	1.21
14.0	0.58	43.0	1.23
15.0	0.60	44.0	1.25
16.0	0.63	45.0	1.26
17.0	0.66	46.0	1.28
18.0	0.69	47.0	1.30
19.0	0.71	48.0	1.32
20.0	0.74	49.0	1.34
21.0	0.76	50.0	1.36
22.0	0.78	51.0	1.38
23.0	0.81	52.0	1.40
24.0	0.83	53.0	1.41
25.0	0.85	54.0	1.43
26.0	0.88	55.0	1.45
27.0	0.90	56.0	1.47
28.0	0.92	57.0	1.48

*Specific values can be calculated using the following formula:

$$\text{Body surface area (m}^2) = \frac{(k) \times (Wt)^{2/3}}{10^4}$$

where (k) = 10.1 for dogs and 10.0 for cats.

results in enhanced cell destruction, reduced induction of drug resistance, and minimal toxicity.
■ Continue chemotherapy past the time of complete remission because microscopic tumor remains after clinically detectable tumor has resolved.

Sources of Failure

Treatment failures result from excessive chemotherapy-related side effects or from progressive tumor

TABLE 5. Practical Recommendations for Safe Handling of Cytotoxic Antineoplastic Agents

1. Designate a specific hospital location for drug handling (reconstitution, preparation, disposal, etc.).
2. Use an absorbent, disposable, plastic-backed sheet to cover work surface; change regularly.
3. Wear latex nonpermeable gloves when handling all cytotoxic agents.
4. Reduce exposed skin surfaces by wearing lab coats, gowns, etc. Wear particulate respiratory filtration masks to prevent inhalation of aerosolized drug particles.
5. Reconstitute all materials carefully and safely, avoiding potential contamination of materials or aerosolization.
6. Clean reconstituted material of any contamination and properly mark and date it.
7. Dispose of contaminated materials in leak-proof, puncture-resistant containers. Proper disposal by health regulatory officials is necessary.
8. Wash hands thoroughly after removing gloves.

growth because of intrinsic or acquired drug resistance. Intrinsic resistance results from genetic mutations within cancer cells that provide mechanisms for circumventing drug effects. The larger a tumor is, the more likely is the existence of resistant cells. Clinically detectable tumors are apt to have several drug-resistant clones. Other causes of intrinsic resistance include:

■ Sites where cells may be protected (sanctuary sites such as the central nervous system)
■ Tumor cell dormancy or insensitivity to specific actions of the drugs
■ Insufficient drug delivery.

Acquired resistance arises from continued exposure to drugs at sublethal doses. Cancer cells may survive long enough to:

■ Develop alternate metabolic pathways
■ Change transport mechanisms
■ Initiate cellular repair
■ Inhibit drug activation

Resistance can develop to a single drug, a group of drugs, or many classes of drugs (pleiotropic resistance). Pleiotropic resistance is most commonly associated with the anthracyclines and vinca alkaloids.

Radiation Therapy

Radiation therapy is primarily useful for local and regional neoplasia. In selected cases it is used for palliation of painful, inoperable, and metastatic tumors.

Applications

Radiation therapy is administered as a single modality or combined with surgery, chemotherapy, or hyperthermia. It can be administered:

■ As the initial form of therapy (neoadjuvant radiotherapy)
■ Concurrent with other therapies such as surgery (intraoperative radiation therapy) or chemotherapy
■ As postoperative therapy (adjuvant radiotherapy).

Timing of various modalities of treatment is important:

■ If surgery follows radiation therapy, allow 3 to 4 weeks for the acute response of normal tissue to be repaired.
■ Delay radiation therapy approximately 7 to 10 days following most surgical procedures to prevent wound healing complications. However, when extensive surgery has been completed, more time may be necessary prior to initiating radiation therapy.

Relative radiation sensitivity of selected common neoplasms in dogs and cats is summarized in Table 6.

Principles of Radiotherapy

■ Radiation is more effective against a small tumor burden.
■ All potentially affected tissues (such as regional lymph nodes as well as the tumor itself) and a margin of normal tissue should be irradiated.

TABLE 6. Relative Radiation Sensitivity of Selected Canine Tumors

Tumor Type	Site	Radiation Response
Squamous carcinoma	Gingiva	Good
	External nose	Poor
	Tonsil	Fair–poor
	Nasal cavity	Poor
Malignant melanoma	Oral	Fair
Acanthomatous epulis	Gingiva	Excellent
Fibrosarcoma	Nasal cavity	Fair–good
Chondrosarcoma	Nasal cavity	Fair–good
Adenocarcinoma	Nasal cavity	Fair–good
Transmissible venereal tumor	Variable (usually penis and vulva)	Excellent
Soft tissue sarcoma	Peripheral	Poor–good
Mast cell tumor	Cutaneous	Fair–excellent
Perianal adenoma	Perianal	Good
Meningioma	Brain	Fair
Osteosarcoma	Any site	Fair (palliation only)
Solitary lymphoproliferative disease	Any site	Excellent

■ The radiation dose administered should be the maximum dose tolerated by adjacent normal tissues.
■ Frequent, small doses of radiation (e.g., ≤3 Gy/fraction) are preferable to decrease side effects of radiation in tissues that cannot repair radiation damage (e.g., bone, nerves).
■ Tumor volume after radiation therapy may not change quickly. The rate of change does not necessarily correlate with long-term response.

Minimize damage to normal tissue by accurate treatment planning. CAT scans of the affected region may be necessary to obtain the optimal treatment plan, which generally involves multiple, overlapping treatment fields from different directions. Toxicity from radiation can be acute, occurring during therapy or in the first few weeks after irradiation (mucous membrane inflammation, moist desquamation, hair loss, tissue inflammation), or late, occurring many months or years after treatment (e.g., contraction and fibrosis, tissue necrosis, cataract formation, etc.).

Sources of Failure

Treatment failures result from radiation-related toxicity to normal tissue and tumor- or treatment-related factors.

■ Tumor-related factors include:
  • histologic tumor type (some tumor cells are inherently more radioresistant)

  • tumor volume (larger volume increases the likelihood of radioresistant cells and hypoxia)
■ Treatment-related factors include:
  • inadequate radiation dose
  • geographic miss (i.e., portion of tumor outside the treatment field)

Meticulous technique and utilization of advanced radiotherapy planning technology will minimize these factors.

Miscellaneous Therapy

Hyperthermia

Heat may be an effective adjunct to other therapy because heat enhances the cytotoxic effect of radiation and many chemotherapy agents. Hyperthermia may be induced locally by ultrasound or microwaves or can be utilized as whole-body hyperthermia induced by a humidified chamber or radiant heat device.

Immunotherapy

Immunotherapy has emerged with renewed potential. Selective or nonselective induction of the host immune response by administration of various biologic response modifiers (such as bacterial agents, interferons, monoclonal antibodies, and lymphokines) may enhance the elimination of tumor cells. Immunotherapy appears to have the greatest potential as an adjunct to other therapies when it is used to eliminate microscopic residual disease.

Photodynamic Therapy

Many tumor cells selectively accumulate certain systemically administered photoactive chemicals. Tumors are then exposed to light of selected wavelengths (laser light) and the photoactive substances are activated, thereby becoming cytotoxic. Various photoactive drugs and light sources are currently being tested. Early results indicate that photodynamic therapy may be useful for treatment of localized and superficial solid tumors.

Nutritional Management

Many animals with cancer have alterations of metabolism that result in malnutrition. When severe, these alterations result in the clinical syndrome of cancer cachexia. Malnutrition impairs the immune system, inhibits wound healing and normal cell repair, and increases treatment morbidity and mortality.

■ Factors contributing to malnutrition include:
  • Anorexia
  • Decreased nutrient intake
  • Metabolic or digestive abnormalities that cause inefficient or inappropriate use of nutrients
  • Treatment-related factors such as nausea and vomiting

■ Proposed mechanisms of cachexia include:
  • Tumor-produced anorexigenic substances
  • Alterations in brain neurotransmitter and anabolic hormone function.

Treatment is directed toward early elimination of the cachexia syndrome (by elimination of neoplasia) and supportive care to minimize its effects during the interim. Nutritional support is provided by enteral or parenteral feeding, (see sec. 1, ch. 3) and is provided when patients do not eat for more than 5 days or have greater than 10% acute loss of body weight. Laboratory parameters indicative of malnutrition include hypoalbuminemia, lymphopenia, and anemia.

Post-Treatment Monitoring

Patient monitoring after therapy is important to assess toxicity, adjust subsequent treatment, and monitor tumor response.

- Evaluate animals at regular intervals (e.g., 1, 2, 3, 5, 7, 9, and 12 months).
- Tailor the diagnostic tests to each patient and to the particular stage and expected behavior of the tumor.
- Remember that the goal of follow-up evaluation is to detect tumor recurrence or metastasis at the earliest possible time, to maximize the response to alternative therapy.

Supplemental Readings

Gilson SD, Stone EA: Management of the surgical oncology patient. Compend Cont Educ Pract Vet 12:1047, 1990.

Gilson SD, Stone EA: Principles of oncologic surgery. Compend Contin Educ Pract Vet. 12:827, 1990.

Helfand SC: Principles and applications of chemotherapy. Vet Clin North Am 20:987, 1990.

MacEwen EG: Current concepts in cancer therapy: Biologic therapy and chemotherapy. Sem Vet Med Surg (Small Anim). 1:5, 1986.

McLeod DA, Thrall DE: The combination of radiation and surgery in the treatment of cancer: A review. Vet Surg 18:1, 1989.

Page RL, Thrall DE, Dewhirst MW, Meyer RE: Whole-body hyperthermia. Rationale and potential use for cancer treatment. J Vet Intern Med. 1:110, 1987.

Swanson LV: Potential hazards associated with low-dose exposure to antineoplastic agents Parts I/II. Compend Cont Educ 10:293 and 615, 1988.

Thoma RE: Phototherapy. In Kirk RW, ed.: Current Veterinary Therapy VII: Small Animal Practice. Philadelphia: W. B. Saunders, 1983, p 438.

Thrall DE: Radiation therapy. 10th Kal Kan Symposium, Columbus, OH. 1986, p 53.

Thrall DE, McLeod DA, Bentel GC, Dewhirst MW: A review of treatment planning and dose calculation in veterinary radiation oncology. Vet Radiol 30:194, 1989.

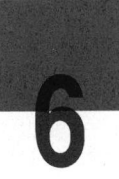

6 Lymphoid Neoplasia

David M. Vail
Gregory K. Ogilvie

Lymphoproliferative disorders are characterized by neoplasia involving cells or cell lines of lymphoid origin, including lymphoma, lymphoid leukemia, and multiple myeloma/plasmacytoma. Because of differences in diagnosis, therapy, and prognosis among these conditions, they are discussed here as separate entities.

LYMPHOMA

Lymphoma (lymphosarcoma) is defined as a lymphoid neoplasm primarily affecting lymph nodes or other solid visceral organs such as the liver or spleen. It is the most common of the lymphoproliferative disorders in small animals. Middle-aged to older dogs are primarily affected, without sex predilection. Although lymphoma can occur in any purebred or mixed breed dog, it may be more prevalent in German shepherds, boxers, poodles, bassets and St. Bernards.

No breed or sex predilection exists for cats. The median age is 3 years for feline leukemia virus (FeLV)-positive and 7 years for FeLV-negative cats.

Etiology

Retroviral. A retroviral etiology for certain forms of lymphoma has been demonstrated in a variety of species including cats, chickens, and humans. In the cat, direct evidence exists for FeLV-induced lymphoma and indirect evidence for feline immunodeficiency virus (FIV) induced lymphoma. Conclusive evidence of a viral etiology is not yet established in the dog.

Genetic. A genetic predisposition for the development of certain forms of lymphoma may exist.

Carcinogenic Agents. Exposure to chemical, physical, and viral carcinogens may play a role in the development of many tumor types.

Classification and Clinical Signs

Traditionally, lymphoma is classified based on anatomic site. Clinical signs vary with the sites involved. The frequency of occurrence of the different anatomic forms in the cat population varies in different regions of the world. Overall, the mediastinal form is most common in the cat, followed by alimentary, renal, multicentric, leukemic, and miscellaneous extranodal forms.

World Health Organization (WHO) clinical staging of lymphoma can also be used to classify the extent of the disease (Table 1).

Multicentric Lymphoma. This is the most common form in the dog. It usually manifests as increased lymph node size with nonspecific signs such as inappetence, weight loss, polyuria/polydypsia, and lethargy. Hepatic and splenic involvement, manifested as diffuse organ enlargement, also are common in multicentric lymphoma (some oncologists prefer to classify liver and spleen involvement as the alimentary form).

Alimentary Lymphoma. This type of lymphoma often is associated with vomiting, diarrhea, and nonspecific signs such as weight loss and lethargy. In addition to the gastrointestinal tract (GI), some oncologists include liver, spleen, and kidney forms in this category.

Mediastinal Lymphoma. This form of lymphoma often causes respiratory signs secondary to pleural effusion, the mass effect of the tumor, or the precaval syndrome (i.e., facial and forelimb edema caused by reduced venous and/or lymphatic drainage). About 40 to 50% of mediastinal lymphomas in the dog are associated with hypercalcemia, which can cause polyuria/polydypsia, anorexia, and weakness. Mediastinal lymphoma is much more common than the cutaneous form.

Cutaneous Lymphoma. Cutaneous lymphoma involves single or multiple skin lesions that can vary greatly in appearance. It may mimic other skin disorders such as seborrhea, pemphigus, and pyoderma. The cutaneous lesions can begin as a mild eczematous pruritic plaque and progress to nodular tumors. Ap-

TABLE 1. World Health Organization Clinical Staging for Lymphoma*

Stage†	Criteria
I	Involvement limited to single lymph node or lymphoid tissue in a single organ (excluding bone marrow)
II	Involvement of many lymph nodes in regional area (with or without tonsils)
III	Generalized lymph node involvement
IV	Liver and/or spleen involvement (with or without stage III)
V	Manifestations in blood and involvement of bone marrow and/or other organ systems (with or without stages I to IV)

*Reprinted with permission from World Health Organization: Owen LN: *TNM Classification of Tumors in Domestic Animals*. Geneva: WHO, 1980.
†Each stage is subclassified into: (a) without systemic signs and (b) with systemic signs.

193

proximately half of the reported cases of cutaneous lymphoma are pruritic.

Extranodal Forms. Miscellaneous extranodal forms of lymphoma include lymphoma of the eyes, central nervous system (CNS), bones, heart, kidneys, urinary bladder, and nasal cavity. Their presentations vary with respect to the site of involvement.

Diagnosis

The diagnosis of lymphoma is based on a complete history, physical examination, tissue diagnosis, and clinical staging. Clinical staging should include a complete blood count (CBC), platelet count, bone marrow aspiration or core biopsy, biochemistry profile, and thoracic and abdominal radiographs.

History

The history should include an evaluation of past and present water intake and urination frequency because they may reflect hypercalcemia and subsequent renal disease.

Physical Examination

Perform a complete physical examination for all animals with lymphoma.

- Palpate all lymph nodes (including rectal palpation of sublumbar nodes) and abdominal viscera.
- Because bone marrow involvement can result in hematologic abnormalities, closely examine mucous membranes for signs of pallor or petechiae.
- Visceral involvement can lead to organ failure; therefore, look for any physical signs that may be indicative of liver or kidney disease (e.g., icterus, uremic ulcers).
- Ophthalmic abnormalities are present in more than one-third of dogs with lymphoma and include uveitis, hemorrhage, and ocular infiltration.

KEY POINT ▶ Canine lymphoma usually is a disease of middle-aged and older animals; thus, it is essential to perform a complete examination to identify concomitant problems in other systems.

Laboratory Studies

Hematologic Abnormalities. Hematologic abnormalities occur in the majority of dogs and cats with multicentric lymphoma. Common abnormalities, in decreasing frequency, include atypical immature lymphocytes in the circulation, thrombocytopenia, eosinopenia, anemia, and nucleated erythrocytes.

The anemia is usually that of chronic disease (normocytic, normochromic, and nonregenerative); however, a small percentage of animals have indices compatible with blood loss or hemolysis. FeLV-positive cats are more likely to be anemic then cats who are not infected.

Bone marrow aspirate/core biopsy may reveal an altered bone marrow myeloid:erythroid ratio and bone marrow infiltration with neoplastic lymphocytes.

Biochemical Abnormalities

KEY POINT ▶ Serum calcium will be elevated in 15 to 20% of dogs with lymphoma. The likelihood of hypercalcemia is greatest in dogs with the mediastinal form.

- Paraneoplastic hypercalcemia (i.e., elevated serum calcium) may serve as a marker for response to therapy; however, it is more clinically significant as a cause of hypercalcemic nephropathy, a potentially irreversible cause of renal failure (see sec. 8, ch. 1).
- Elevations in blood urea nitrogen and serum creatinine may result from neoplastic infiltration of the kidneys, hypercalcemic nephrosis, or dehydration.
- Increased serum concentration of liver enzymes or bilirubin may indicate neoplastic infiltration of the liver.
- Abnormally elevated serum globulins may be noted in some B-cell lymphomas.

FeLV Status. Approximately 80% of cats with mediastinal and multicentric lymphoma are FeLV-positive, in contrast to 50% with renal lymphoma, 30% with alimentary lymphoma, and a minority with cutaneous forms.

Imaging Studies

Radiography and ultrasonography (see sec. 1, ch. 4), while not diagnostic for lymphoma, are often useful for staging or determining the extent of disease.

- Half of all dogs with lymphoma have evidence of enlarged sternal and sublumbar lymph nodes, spleen, and liver.
- Thoracic radiographs are important for identification of thoracic masses that are due to mediastinal lymphoma and are recommended in any dog with hypercalcemia of unknown etiology.
- Contrast studies of the upper GI tract are abnormal in most animals with GI lymphoma.

Histopathology and Cytology

Histopathologic and cytologic evaluation of affected tissues is necessary for confirmation of lymphoma.

- Fine-needle aspiration cytology of lymph nodes, visceral organs, and other involved sites can be suggestive of neoplastic disease; however, conclusive histologic diagnosis is recommended.

KEY POINT ▶ In the cytologic evaluation of lymph nodes in cats, neoplastic involvement is difficult to distinguish from benign lymphadenopathy syndromes. For this reason, only histopathologic examination is definitive.

- Avoid sampling lymph nodes draining reactive areas of the body (e.g., submandibular lymph nodes in the presence of periodontal disease) because reactive lymphoid hyperplasia can mask (or mimic) the true neoplastic condition.

Additional Diagnostic Tests

Additional tests may be necessary to confirm the diagnosis of the extranodal forms of lymphoma.

Stage the disease by performing a CBC, bone marrow evaluation, and thoracic and abdominal radiography. Staging is important in animals with extranodal lymphoma to ensure that the disease is not a sequela of the more common multicentric forms and to determine if the disease is indeed localized to the extranodal site.

Perform exploratory laparotomy and full-thickness biopsy or fine-needle aspiration to diagnose most cases of alimentary lymphoma. Endoscopic biopsies of the mucosa may be too superficial to diagnose GI lymphoma, because lymphoma usually originates in the submucosa. In addition, GI lymphoma is often accompanied by lymphocytic/plasmacytic mucosal infiltrations that may be misdiagnosed as a benign condition.

Cytological evaluation of cerebrospinal fluid (CSF) may be helpful in the diagnosis of CNS lymphoma in the dog, but CSF is rarely abnormal in feline spinal lymphoma because the tumor is usually extradural. Computed tomography and myelography may be helpful.

Differential Diagnosis

The differential diagnosis (DDx) varies with the anatomic form of the disease.

- DDx for lymphadenopathies includes infectious diseases (e.g., bacterial, viral, rickettsial, parasitic, and fungal; see sec. 2), immune-mediated diseases (e.g., systemic lupus erythematosus; see sec. 3, ch. 3), and other types of metastatic neoplasia.
- DDx for alimentary lymphoma includes lymphocytic-plasmacytic enteritis, other types of intestinal neoplasia, granulomatous bowel disease, and hypereosinophilic syndrome (see sec. 7, ch. 6).
- DDx for mediastinal lymphoma includes ectopic thyroid tumors, heart base tumors, thymoma, and pulmonary lymphomatoid granulomatosis.
- DDx for cutaneous lymphoma includes infections, immune-mediated and parasitic skin disorders, and other neoplastic dermatopathies.

Treatment

Chemotherapy

Systemic chemotherapeutic protocols are the mainstay of therapy for multicentric and systemic lymphomas. Without treatment, most animals with lymphoma succumb to their disease in 4 to 6 weeks. Treatment can be quite gratifying, with a high percentage of complete remissions and good quality of life that is generally maintained throughout remissions.

Single-agent chemotherapy is less expensive and less toxic than combination chemotherapy. However, with the notable exception of doxorubicin (Adriamycin; Adria Labs.), it is not as effective as combination chemotherapy (see sec. 3, ch. 5).

Published chemotherapeutic protocols for canine lymphoma with reported remission and survival data are presented in Table 2. Regardless of the protocol used, remission rates and durations of remission and survival are comparable in the majority of cases. We prefer the University of Wisconsin-Madison canine lymphoma protocol presented in Table 3. Complete remission rate (84%), median remission time (252 days), and median survival time (357 days) are the best reported to date. However, cures are still rare in canine and feline lymphoma.

Drug therapy for multicentric lymphoma may have to be altered in the presence of thrombocytopenia ($<75,000/\mu$l) and neutropenia ($<2500/\mu$l). Chemotherapeutic regimens that tend to spare bone marrow that are usually safe in the presence of low white blood cell (WBC) and platelet counts include prednisone, L-asparaginase, and vincristine. If myelosuppression is attributed to chemotherapy, discontinue treatment for 5 to 7 days, repeat the CBC and platelet count; when the platelet and WBC counts have rebounded, reinstitute therapy at a decreased dose or frequency.

In the cat, protocols based on *c*ytoxan, *o*ncovin, *p*rednisone (COP) are the gold standard against which new protocols are measured. Overall, remission rates for feline lymphoma are about 65%, with a 7-month median survival, although median survival can approach 18 months in FeLV-negative stage I or II cats.

Extranodal Lymphoma Therapy

Therapy unique to extranodal lymphoma depends on the site of involvement and the extent of disease. Extranodal lymphoma that is determined, following thorough staging, to be a local disease can be treated locally (e.g., excisional surgery, radiotherapy) without the necessity for systemic chemotherapy. Diligent reevaluation schedules should be followed to identify recurrence or spread of disease.

Therapy for CNS lymphoma is dependent on location, the capacity of drugs to cross the blood-brain barrier, and the presence of disease outside the CNS. Surgical intervention can be used for diagnosis or removal of accessible CNS tumors, but usually this is not feasible or practical. More commonly surgery is combined with adjuvant chemotherapy or radiotherapy. Of the chemotherapeutic agents commonly utilized in veterinary medicine, only prednisone and cytosine arabinoside consistently cross the blood-brain barrier in therapeutic concentrations. Radiotherapy has also been used successfully for the treatment of CNS lymphoma.

Rescue Therapy

Rescue therapy, defined as an attempt to re-establish remission when an animal's disease returns following a successful remission, has not been carefully studied in the veterinary literature. However, some guidelines apply:

- If disease returns while the animal is on chemotherapy, discontinue the drug regimen. However, if a drug used in the past was not currently being used when the disease returned, it may still be an effective choice and can be reinstated if superior alternatives do not exist.

TABLE 2. Published Chemotherapeutic Protocols for Canine Lymphoma*

Protocol†		Case Numbers	Complete Remission Rate (%)	Median (Mean) Remission Time (days)	Median (Mean) Survival Time (days)
No.	Drug(s)				
1	CTX 50 mg/m² PO daily for 4 days/wk × 8 courses Ara-C 100 mg/m² IV daily for 4 days VCR 0.5 mg/m²/wk IV × 8 courses Prednisone 40 mg/m² for 7 days, then 20 mg/m² every 2 days thereafter Maintenance: CTX 50 mg/m²/day PO for 4 days/wk Prednisone 10 mg/m² BID q 48 h *or* 6-MP 50 mg/m²/day PO *or* MTX 2.5 mg/m² PO BID weekly	20	65	66	186
2	CTX 300 mg/m² PO every 3 wk VCR 0.75 mg/m²/wk IV for 4 wk; then every 3 wk Prednisone 1 mg/kg/day PO for 21 days, then every 2 days	77	75	180	N/R
3	Protocol No. 2 above for 7 wk; then DOX 30 mg/m² replaces every third CTX treatment; all therapy stopped at 78 wk	46	83	210	N/R
4	VCR 0.7 mg/m² IV day 1 and 14 L-ASP 400 IU/kg IP or IM day 1 CTX 200–250 mg/m² IV day 7 MTX 0.6–0.8 mg/kg IV day 7 Repeat procedure above; *except* use L-ASP, for rescue only; substitute CHLOR 1.4 mg/kg PO for CTX if dog is in remission	147	77	140	265
5	Doxorubicin 30 mg/m² IV q21 days × 5 courses	37	59	131	230
	Rescue with CTX, VCR, Prednisone, L-ASP	21	76	206(189)	270(265)

CTX = cyclophosphamide (Cytoxan; Bristol-Myers); Ara-C = cytosine arabinoside (Cytosar; Upjohn); VCR = vincristine (Oncovin; Lilly); MP = 6-mercaptopurine (Purinethol; Burroughs Wellcome); MTX = methotrexate (Lederle); DOX = doxorubicin (Adriamycin; Adria Labs.); L-ASP = L-asparaginase (Elspar; Merck, Sharp & Dohme); CHLOR = chlorambucil (Leukeran; Burroughs Wellcome).

*Modified with permission from MacEwen EG, Young KM: Canine lymphoma and lymphoid leukemias. *In* Withrow SJ, MacEwen EG, eds.: *Clinical Veterinary Oncology*. Philadelphia: J. B. Lippincott, 1989.

†See Table 4 in sec. 3, ch. 5 for conversion of body weight to body surface area (m²) for calculating dosages recommended here.

TABLE 3. University of Wisconsin-Madison Canine Lymphoma Protocol

Cycle 1 Induction
Week 1: Vincristine 0.7, mg/m2 IV; L-asparaginase 400 IU/kg IM; and once daily prednisone, 2 mg/kg PO
Week 2: Cyclophosphamide, 200 mg/m² IV, and once daily prednisone, 1.5 mg/kg PO.
Week 3: Vincristine, 0.7 mg/m² IV, and once daily prednisone, 1.0 mg/kg PO
Week 4: Doxorubicin, 30 mg/m² IV, and once daily prednisone, 0.5 mg/kg PO
Week 6: Vincristine, 0.7 mg/m² IV
Week 7: Cyclophosphamide, 200 mg/m² IV
Week 8: Vincristine, 0.7 mg/m² IV
Week 9: Doxorubicin, 30 mg/m² IV
Cycle 2
If in complete remission at week 9, continue treatment at 2-week intervals alternating vincristine 0.7 mg/m² IV chlorambucil (Leukeran) 1.4 mg/kg PO, vincristine 0.7 mg/m², and methotrexate 0.8 mg/kg IV. Doxorubicin 30 mg/m² is substituted for every second methotrexate treatment. This cycle continues through week 25.
Cycle 3
If in complete remission at week 25, continue treatment sequence outlined in Cycle 2, but now at 3-week intervals. This cycle continues through week 51.
Cycle 4
If in complete remission at week 51, continue with treatment sequence outlined in Cycle 2, but now at 4-week intervals. Doxorubicin is no longer substituted for methotrexate. All treatment is discontinued at week 156.

- Favorable rescue rates have been reported using doxorubicin, actinomycin D (Cosmegen; Merck Sharp and Dohme), mitoxantrone (Novantrone; Lederle Labs.), or dacarbazine (DTIC-Dome; Miles).
- The probability of attaining a new remission and the length of the subsequent remission are usually half those of the previous treatment.

Experimental Therapies

Experimental therapies for lymphoma that are being evaluated include:

- Immunotherapy in combination with traditional chemotherapy
  - Nonspecific immunostimulants, such as levamisole, and various bacterial extracts have not been efficacious
  - Tumor cell vaccines derived from the host's own tumor and the use of specific monoclonal antibodies are presently undergoing evaluation.
- Total body irradiation (TBI) in combination with bone marrow transplant (BMT) techniques; these procedures may become available to the practitioner on a referral basis in the near future.

Therapy for Hypercalcemia

Treatment of hypercalcemia secondary to lymphoma is best accomplished by attaining tumor remission. If necessary, diuresis with high sodium crystalloids (0.9% NaCl) delivered at twice maintenance rate (see sec. 4, ch. 2) alone or in combination with furosemide (Lasix) (2 mg/kg IV) is usually successful. The addition of prednisone will also decrease serum calcium levels, however, this should only be initiated following a histologic or cytologic diagnosis.

Prognosis

Prognostic Indicators

- Age, body weight, and breed do not appear to affect the length or success of remission or the overall survival for lymphoma.
- Most studies fail to reveal a relationship between the WHO clinical stage (see Table 1) and response to therapy in the dog; however, bone marrow involvement (especially with associated cytopenias) is associated with decreased survival.
- In cats, the higher the clinical stage, the lower the remission rate and survival time (approximately 90% complete remission rate in stage I versus 50% in stage III or higher).
- Female dogs enjoy significantly longer remission and survival times: for example, the median survival time in female dogs who undergo chemotherapy is 375 days, compared with 214 for male dogs.
- Leukemia, anemia, neutropenia, sepsis, and widely disseminated tumors all have a negative impact on response to therapy and on survival times in the cat.
- Anatomic site of involvement affects outcome. Alimentary, cutaneous, and leukemic forms of lymphoma have a poorer prognosis than multicentric forms.

- FeLV status, while it may not affect remission rates, is associated with significantly shorter survival times in affected cats.

LYMPHOID LEUKEMIA

Leukemia is defined as the proliferation of neoplastic cells in the bone marrow; such cells may or may not be circulating in the peripheral blood. There are two major categories of lymphoid leukemia: acute lymphoblastic leukemia and chronic lymphocytic leukemia. Both forms are relatively rare in dogs; however, they may constitute up to one-third of feline lymphoid neoplasms.

Acute Lymphoblastic Leukemia

Acute lymphoblastic leukemia (ALL) is defined as an abnormal proliferation of morphologically immature lymphoblasts in the bone marrow or peripheral blood. This form of leukemia is rapidly progressive and responds poorly to therapy.

Epidemiology and Clinical Signs

- No sex, breed, or weight predilection exists. Most affected dogs are of late middle age; the mean age in cats with ALL tends to be younger, owing to an association with FeLV.
- Clinical signs can include fever, generalized or abdominal pain, anorexia, splenomegaly, and pale mucous membranes.
- Anemia occurs in nearly half of ALL patients, and one-fourth are thrombocytopenic.
- The majority of cats with ALL are FeLV-positive.

Diagnosis

- Diagnosis depends on documentation of abnormal lymphocytes in the bone marrow or peripheral blood.
- The presence of 30% or more abnormal cells in the bone marrow is diagnostic.
- Most patients have absolute leukocytosis with circulating abnormal lymphocytes; 10% are classified as having aleukemic leukemia (bone marrow involvement without peripheral blood involvement).
- In some forms, the neoplastic lymphoid cells are very undifferentiated, making special histochemical stains necessary to differentiate them from other forms of leukemia and myeloproliferative conditions.
- ALL may be clinically differentiated from late stages of lymphoma by:
  - The more acute progression of ALL
  - Less likelihood of lymphadenopathy (<50%)
  - Poor response to therapy
  - Shorter survival times.

Treatment and Prognosis

- A poor prognosis resulting from a meager response to therapy generally is the rule.
- Because of severe bone marrow disruption in ALL, chemotherapeutic agents that have a relatively low degree of bone marrow toxicity may be necessary in

cases of severe neutropenia (<2500/μl) or thrombocytopenia (<50,000/μl). A myelosuppressive drug like cyclophosphamide or doxorubicin is added to the treatment protocol when neutrophil and platelet numbers are adequate.

■ A combination of vincristine, prednisone, and L-asparaginase can be used in those cases with severe neutropenia and thrombocytopenia. The dosage regimes are the same as those described in Table 2 for lymphoma.

Chronic Lymphocytic Leukemia

Chronic lymphocytic leukemia (CLL) is defined as an abnormal proliferation of morphologically mature lymphocytes in the bone marrow or peripheral blood. It occurs primarily in older dogs and cats.

Clinical Signs

■ Presenting complaints for the most part are nonspecific and include lethargy, inappetence, polyuria/polydipsia, bleeding diathesis, intermittent lameness, and episodes of collapse.

■ Two-thirds of dogs have lymphadenopathy and splenomegaly; pale mucous membranes and fever are common.

Hematologic Abnormalities

■ The majority of animals are anemic (normocytic, normochromic, and nonregenerative) and approximately half are thrombocytopenic.

■ One-third of dogs are hyperproteinemic, and 50% have monoclonal gammopathies on serum electrophoresis, often with Bence Jones proteins in the urine, indicative of a B-cell origin.

■ All reported cases in cats are FeLV-negative.

Treatment and Prognosis

■ Therapy for CLL is recommended only if the patient is symptomatic or if anemia, hyperglobulinemia, splenomegaly, or lymphadenopathy are present.

■ The prognosis for CLL greatly exceeds that for ALL.

■ Prednisone and chlorambucil are the drugs most commonly used, and nearly 75% of animals respond, with median survivals of nearly 1 year.

■ Chlorambucil (Leukeran), 20 mg/m² PO, given every 1 to 2 weeks, or 6 mg/m² daily, has provided excellent results.

PLASMA CELL NEOPLASMS

There are three primary clinical forms of plasma cell neoplasms: multiple myeloma (MM), solitary plasmacytoma of bone, and extramedullary plasmacytoma. MM is the most common form; the other two occur rarely. Plasma cell neoplasms are extremely rare in cats.

Multiple Myeloma
Epidemiology and Clinical Signs

■ MM occurs primarily in aged dogs with no sex predilection. German shepherd dogs may be at greater risk.

■ Clinical signs include nonspecific anorexia, listlessness, and polyuria/polydipsia.

■ Most dogs present with lameness secondary to paresis or pain.

■ About 50% of affected dogs develop bleeding diathesis (epistaxis or gingival bleeding) secondary to hyperviscosity syndrome or thrombocytopenia.

Hematologic Abnormalities

■ Three-fourths of animals with MM have associated monoclonal gammopathy, either the IgG or IgA subtype. A rare IgM-secreting primary macroglobulinemia (Waldenström's disease) also exists.

■ Light-chain (Bence Jones) proteins may be detectable in the urine. These proteins cannot be detected by routine urine dipstick analysis and require phoretic technique to be identified.

■ Dogs with MM often have nonregenerative, normocytic/normochromic anemia. Approximately 30% are thrombocytopenic, and 10% have circulating abnormal plasmacytes.

■ About 15 to 20% of MM patients are hypercalcemic secondary to bone resorption caused by osteoclast-activating factors or other substances released by the tumor.

Diagnosis

Diagnosis involves identification of the following triad of abnormalities:

■ Bone marrow plasmacytosis (>20 to 30% plasma cells).

■ Radiographic evidence of osteolytic bone lesions; often observed in dorsal spinous vertebral processes.

■ Serum or urine myeloma proteins, as revealed by immunoelectrophoresis.

Histological confirmation may be necessary to those cases which do not meet all three criteria.

Differential Diagnosis (DDx)

■ DDx for monoclonal gammopathy includes ehrlichiosis (see sec. 2, ch. 10) and benign hypergammaglobulinemia syndrome, which has been described in the dog.

■ DDx for plasmacytosis includes carcinomas, connective tissue disorders, liver disease, hypersensitivity states, and infections, especially ehrlichiosis (see sec. 2, ch. 10).

Treatment and Prognosis

■ The short-term prognosis for MM is normally good, and long-term remissions are the rule.

■ Extensive bone lesions, light chain proteinuria, hypercalcemia, and anemia have been reported to be negative prognostic indicators.

■ Combination chemotherapy using melphalan (Alkeran; Burroughs Wellcome) (0.1 mg/kg daily for 10 days; then every other day) has resulted in published remission rates of 90% and median survival times of 540 days.

- Serum protein levels should normalize within 2 to 3 months.
- Fractures accompanying MM can be treated by surgical reduction in combination with chemotherapy or radiotherapy. Healing will normally accompany remission of the MM.
- Rescue therapy is not well documented once remission is lost. Doxorubicin, vincristine, and dexamethasone combinations appear to work well in humans and may be of benefit in dogs.

Solitary Plasmacytoma of Bone

Solitary plasmacytoma of bone is rare. It usually is not accompanied by a secretory protein but tends to progress to systemic MM. Localized lesions can be treated with surgery or radiotherapy; however, careful clinical staging and a strict re-evaluation schedule should be established because to the propensity for the development of systemic disease.

Extramedullary Plasmacytoma

Extramedullary plasmacytoma occurs equally in both sexes. It occurs most often in older dogs (mean 9.7 years). It appears primarily as a solitary mucocutaneous lesion of the mouth but also may affect the feet, trunk, and ears. The prognosis appears to be very good for solitary extramedullary plasmacytoma in the dog, with only a small percentage going on to develop MM. Cure can be obtained with localized surgical resection or radiotherapy.

Supplemental Readings

Couto CG: Hemolymphatic neoplasms. *In* Sherding RG, ed.: *The Cat: Diseases and Clinical Management.* New York: Churchill Livingston, 1989, p 606.

Hardy WD, MacEwen EG: Feline retroviruses. *In* Withrow SJ, MacEwen EG, eds.: *Clinical Veterinary Oncology.* Philadelphia: J. B. Lippincott, 1989, p 362.

Keller ET, MacEwen EG, Rosenthal RC, et al: Evaluation of prognostic factors and sequential combination chemotherapy for canine lymphoma. J Vet Int Med (In press).

MacEwen EG, Young KM: Canine lymphoma and lymphoid leukemias. *In* Withrow SJ, MacEwen EG, eds.: *Clinical Veterinary Oncology.* Philadelphia: J. B. Lippincott, 1989, p 380.

Matus RE, Leifer CE, MacEwen EG, et al.: Prognostic factors for multiple myeloma in the dog. J Am Vet Med Assoc 188:1288, 1986.

Mooney SC, Hayes AA, MacEwen EG, et al.: Treatment and prognostic factors in lymphoma in cats: 103 cases (1977–1981). J Am Vet Med Assoc 194:696, 1989.

Rojko JL, Hardy WD: Feline leukemia virus and other retroviruses. *In* Sherding RG, ed.: *The Cat: Diseases and Clinical Management.* New York: Churchill Livingstone, 1989, p 229.

Theilen GH, Madewell BR: *Veterinary Cancer Medicine.* 2nd Ed. Philadelphia: Lea & Febiger, 1987, p 392.

7 Soft Tissue Sarcomas and Mast Cell Tumors

Joanne C. Graham
Deborah A. O'Keefe

SOFT TISSUE SARCOMAS

Soft tissue sarcomas are tumors that arise from mesodermal tissue, they compose 14 to 17% of all malignancies in the dog and approximately 7 to 9% in the cat. These tumors are nonepithelial and extraskeletal and may arise from fibrous tissue, adipose tissue, muscle, and synovial tissue, as well as from blood and lymph vessels. Schwannomas, or neurofibrosarcomas, arise from primitive ectodermal tissues but are included in the soft tissue sarcoma category because of similarities in location, clinical presentation, and clinical behavior. Soft tissue sarcomas are classified histologically according to the specific tissue of origin. However, some tumors are so undifferentiated that this classification is difficult. These tumors are appropriately named undifferentiated sarcomas.

Etiology

The etiology of the majority of soft tissue sarcomas remains unknown. Several causes and predisposing factors have been suggested. These include: genetic predisposition, viral agents, chemical carcinogens, ionizing radiation, foreign body implantation, and trauma.

Genetic Predisposition. This is suspected to play a role in tumor development because certain breeds of dogs have a higher incidence of sarcomas. These breeds include boxers, German shepherds, Great Danes, Saint Bernards, golden retrievers, and basset hounds.

Viral Agents. Viruses have been implicated as causes of sarcoma development in rodents, poultry, nonhuman primates, and cats. Feline sarcoma viruses (FeSVs) are replication-defective variants of the feline leukemia virus (FeLV) (see sec. 2, ch. 1). These retroviruses induce formation of multicentric fibrosarcomas in young cats. In contrast, solitary fibrosarcomas found in older cats are not usually associated with FeSV.

Chemical Carcinogens. Chemical carcinogens and environmental contaminants have been shown to induce sarcomas in rodents and humans. Although this has not been documented in dogs and cats, it is likely that it occurs.

Ionizing Radiation. X-rays, gamma rays, and particulate radiation have been shown to cause sarcoma development. In dogs, sarcomas have been reported

following orthovoltage radiotherapy of acanthomatous epulides.

Foreign Implants. Implants, particularly metallic orthopedic implants, are known to cause sarcoma development at the implant site. It is believed that this is the result of a foreign body reaction in the tissues rather than a direct carcinogenic effect of the implant. The majority of these tumors are osteosarcomas, although fibrosarcomas and undifferentiated sarcomas have been reported.

Trauma. Both single and chronic traumatic episodes have been associated with intraocular sarcomas in the cat.

Biologic Behavior

In general, soft tissue sarcomas are locally invasive and infiltrative along fascial planes, resulting in poorly defined tumor margins. They are often slow to metastasize, but when they do it is via hematogenous spread to the lungs and liver. A brief description of the various soft tissue sarcomas follows.

Liposarcoma—Malignant tumor of adipocytes
- Rare in dogs and cats
- Invasive and aggressive
- Commonly occurring on the ventrum
- Metastasis uncommon
- "Infiltrative lipomas," believed by some to be well differentiated liposarcomas, frequently occurring on extremities

Hemangiopericytoma—tumor of pericytes, spindle-shaped, contractile cells that surround precapillary arterioles
- Common in dogs (German shepherds at risk)
- Slow-growing
- Encapsulated appearance but quite infiltrative and recurrence following excision common
- Frequently occurring on extremities
- Metastasis rare and slow-growing

Fibrosarcoma—tumor of fibrocytes
- Common in dogs and cats
- Locally invasive, slow-growing
- No site predilection
- Metastasis rare

KEY POINT ▶ Multicentric fibrosarcomas of young cats (less than 5 years) are caused

200

by FeSV. These cats are always FeLV-positive.

Hemangiosarcoma—tumor of blood vessel endothelium (see also sec. 3, ch. 4)
- Common in dogs (German shepherds at risk); rare in cats
- Very invasive, rapid-growing
- Spleen, heart, skin common sites
- Metastasis common

Schwannoma/neurofibrosarcoma—tumor of the nerve sheath or Schwann cell
- Relatively uncommon in dogs and cats
- Invasive, slow-growing
- Frequently occurring in the brachial or lumbosacral plexuses
- Progressive lameness possible
- Metastasis rare

Myxosarcoma—fibrosarcoma-like tumor with a mucinous matrix
- Rare in dogs and cats
- Infiltrative
- No site predilection
- Metastasis uncommon

Rhabdomyosarcoma—tumor of striated muscle
- Uncommon in dogs and cats
- Infiltrative
- Heart, bladder, appendicular muscles possible sites
- Metastasis possible
- Botryoid rhabdomyosarcomas (grapelike appearance) found in the bladders of young large-breed dogs

Leiomyosarcoma—tumor of smooth muscle
- Rare in dogs and cats
- Solitary, infiltrative, slow-growing
- Gastrointestinal or genitourinary tracts most common sites
- Metastasis possible
- Obstructive signs or perforation possible effects

Synovial cell sarcoma—tumor of periarticular mesenchymal tissue, *not* the synovial membrane (see sec. 9, ch. 22)
- Uncommon in dogs, few reports in cats
- Large-breed male dogs at risk
- Aggressive tumor
- Bones on both sides of major joints commonly involved
- Metastasis possible (up to 50%)

Lymphangiosarcoma—tumor of lymphatic endothelial vessels
- Rare in dogs and cats
- May be invasive
- Metastasis rare
- Draining tracts on skin possible sign

Malignant fibrous histiocytoma—tumor containing a mixture of fibroblast-like cells and histiocyte-like cells
- Uncommon in dogs and cats
- Invasive (may cause bone lysis)
- Usually found in subcutaneous tissue

- Metastasis rare

Clinical Signs

Clinical signs depend on the location, size, and degree of invasiveness of the tumor as well as on the presence and degree of metastatic disease.

- Soft tissue sarcomas are more common in older animals (mean age 9 years).
- Because of the widespread distribution of mesodermal tissues in the body, soft tissue sarcomas may occur in almost any anatomic location, including the abdomen.
- Tumors may become quite large before any clinical signs are apparent. They are often first noticed by the owner, either by observation or while handling the animal.
- Certain types of sarcoma may invade bone, causing lameness, or may obstruct lymphatics, causing edema.
- Gastrointestinal leiomyosarcomas may cause signs of obstruction (vomiting) or melena.
- Smooth muscle sarcomas of the bladder may cause hematuria or dysuria.
- Hemangiosarcomas may cause a variety of clinical signs, including collapse due to tumor rupture and hemorrhage.

Diagnosis

The goals of diagnosis are to identify the histologic type of the primary tumor, to delineate the extent of the tumor, and to determine if metastatic disease is present. Although history, physical examination, laboratory evaluation, and diagnostic imaging provide valuable information, the only way to obtain a definitive diagnosis is through biopsy and histopathologic evaluation of the tumor.

History

The history helps to determine how long the mass has been present and the rate of growth. Also important is information regarding exposure to carcinogens and past traumatic incidents. Concurrent systemic disturbances provide insight as to the possible presence of metastatic disease or paraneoplastic syndromes.

Physical Examination

Perform a thorough examination to determine the number of masses and their physical characteristics. In general, benign neoplasms are well delineated, slow-growing, and freely movable. They are seldom ulcerated or inflamed. Malignant tumors are often rapid-growing, fixed masses with ill-defined borders. However, some sarcomas are slow-growing and appear well demarcated. The appearance of these masses can be misleading and should not preclude biopsy.

A careful search may reveal evidence of metastasis. Palpate the regional lymph nodes for size and mobility. Look for hepatomegaly and increased respiratory sounds or dyspnea as a sign of systemic involvement.

Clinical Pathology

Studies such as a complete blood count (CBC), platelet count, serum biochemical profile, and urinalysis often are unremarkable; however, they should be evaluated in animals with soft tissue sarcomas because they may suggest the presence of metastatic disease, paraneoplastic syndromes, or other concurrent disease. The values obtained also provide a baseline for future therapy. Abnormalities may include:

- Anemia of chronic inflammatory disease
- Leukocytosis
- Thrombocytopenia (may be associated with disseminated intravascular coagulation)
- Hypoglycemia
- Increased serum concentrations of alanine transferase (ALT), alkaline phosphatase (ALP), and gamma-glutamyl transpeptidase (GGT)

Diagnostic Imaging

Radiography
- Radiograph the mass to aid in determining the extent of the sarcoma.
- Radiograph the thorax and abdomen to help identify metastatic disease.
- Dystrophic calcification caused by some anaplastic sarcomas may be seen on the radiograph.

Ultrasonography. Use this technique to help determine the character, consistency, and extent of the mass. Ultrasound procedures are especially useful in the examination of abdominal masses.

Computed Tomography (CT). This modality, when available, is particularly useful in precise localization of a mass.

Biopsy

Biopsy is essential to obtain a definitive diagnosis. (See sec. 3, ch. 5 for details on the principles of tumor biopsy.)

- Plan carefully to ensure that a representative sample of the mass is obtained.
- Submit all biopsies for histopathologic evaluation.

Several methods for biopsy are available:

- Fine-needle aspiration (FNA) using a 22- or 25-gauge needle and a 12-ml syringe
  - Because soft tissue sarcomas do not exfoliate well, FNA is limited in value.
  - FNA, however, is useful in the diagnosis of lipomas, lymphomas, and inflammatory masses that may appear similar to soft tissue sarcomas.
- Needle punch biopsy (NPB) using Franklin modified Vim-Silverman needles (V. Mueller Co., Chicago, IL) or Tru-Cut biopsy needles (Travenol Labs., Deerfield, IL)
  - NPB is useful for externally palpable masses.
  - A larger sample of tissue can be obtained than with FNA.
  - NPB usually can be performed under local anesthesia.

- Incisional biopsies yield an even larger sample than NBP biopsies.
  - Plan the biopsy site so that it can be excised later when definitive resection is done.
  - Include some normal tissue in the sample when possible.
- Excisional biopsies are indicated when:
  - Knowledge of the histologic type of the tumor does not change the treatment
  - Total excision is no more invasive than other types of biopsy.

Clinical Staging

An attempt should be made to stage all soft tissue sarcomas. Clinical staging is based on the classification system developed by the World Health Organization (WHO) (Table 1).

Treatment

The goal of treatment is to remove the primary tumor in its entirety, when possible, and to treat microscopic disease and metastasis. In the case of benign and some malignant tumors, surgical resection can be curative. In animals with nonresectable malignant tumors, attempts are made to prolong survival time while providing a good quality of life.

Surgery

Surgical excision remains the mainstay of therapy for soft tissue sarcomas. However, many of these tumors recur because of inadequate resection. Well-planned, aggressive initial surgery has the greatest likelihood of success.

KEY POINT ▶ Excise soft tissue sarcomas with 2- to 3-cm margins in all planes.

- Remove overlying subcutaneous tissues and skin as well as underlying tissues to which the mass is fixed. (In some cases limb amputation is indicated.)
- Include all previous biopsy sites in the excision.

TABLE 1. World Health Organization (WHO) Clinical Staging System for Canine Soft Tissue Sarcomas

T: Primary Tumor	N: Regional Lymph Node	M: Distant Metastasis
T_0—no evidence	N_0—no evidence	M_0—no evidence
T_1—tumor < 2 cm	N_1—movable ipsilateral	M_1—metastasis present
T_2—2 cm > tumor < 5 cm; minimal invasion	N_2—movable contralateral	
T_3—tumor >5 cm	N_3—fixed a—metastasis absent b—metastasis present	
T_4—very invasive		

Stage	
I	$T_1N_0M_0$, $T_2N_0M_0$
II	$T_1N_1M_0$, $T_2N_1M_0$
III	$T_1N_{2,3}M_0$, $T_2N_{2,3}M_0$, $T_3N_{0-3}M_0$, $T_4N_{0-3}M_0$, any N_b
IV	any M_1

From Owen, LN: Classification of Tumours in Domestic Animals. World Health Organization, Geneva, Switzerland.

TABLE 2. Chemotherapeutic Protocols for Soft Tissue Sarcomas*

Drug (Trade Name)	Manufacturer	Dosage	Route	Day
1. Adriamycin				
Doxorubicin (Adriamycin)	Adria Labs.	30 mg/m²	IV	1
Repeat cycle every 21 days.				
2. VAC Protocol (Dogs Only)				
Vincristine (Oncovin)	Eli Lilly	0.7 mg/m²	IV	8 and 15
Doxorubicin (Adriamycin)	Adria Labs.	30 mg/m²	IV	1
Cyclophosphamide (Cytoxan)	Bristol-Myers	100–150 mg/m²	IV	1
		or		
		50 mg/m²	PO	3–6

Repeat cycle on day 22; usual number of cycles is 4–5. Do not exceed a cumulative dose of Adriamycin of 240 mg/m². Because this protocol is myelosuppressive, the prophylactic use of trimethoprim-sulfa is recommended (30 mg/kg PO q12h).

Drug (Trade Name)	Manufacturer	Dosage	Route	Day
3. ADIC Protocol (Dogs Only)				
Doxorubicin (Adriamycin)	Adria Labs.	30 mg/m²	IV	1
Dacarbazine (DTIC)	Miles Lab.	200 mg/m²	IV	1–5
		or		
		800–1000 mg/m²	IV	1

Repeat cycle on day 22; usual number of cycles is 4–5.

Drug (Trade Name)	Manufacturer	Dosage	Route	Day
4. VCM Protocol (Dogs and Cats)				
Vincristine (Oncovin)	Eli Lilly	0.5 mg/m²	IV	1
Cyclophosphamide (Cytoxan)	Bristol-Myers	50 mg/m²	PO	2–5
Methotrexate†	Lederle Labs.	15 mg/m²	IV	1

Repeat cycle every 14 days for six treatments, then every 21 days for four treatments.

*Caution: The use of chemotherapeutics requires careful handling and knowledge of potential toxicities. See sec. 3, ch. 5 for discussion of chemotherapy. Also, see Table 4, sec. 3, ch. 5 for conversion of body weight to body surface area (m²).
†Pretreat with NaHCO₃, 2 mEq/kg, in 250–500 ml D5W IV over a period of 1 h; give methotrexate 30 min after vincristine.

- Remove the tumor intact in order to prevent seeding of normal tissue with malignant cells.
- Have the specimen margins histologically evaluated for completeness of excision.
- Do not remove regional lymph nodes unless they are involved.
- Also resect any solitary metastatic pulmonary nodules.

Radiation Therapy

Soft tissue sarcomas are reported to be less radioresponsive than carcinomas. However, radiation therapy alone has been reported to achieve up to 67% tumor control for approximately 1 year. Long-term control rates are poor. Radiation therapy is used more frequently to reduce tumor volume preoperatively or to irradiate incompletely excised tumor fields.

Repeat irradiation of previously irradiated tumors is possible. A 38% local control rate at 1 year following repeat irradiation has been reported. Unfortunately, if the regrowth of tumors is within 4 to 5 months of the first treatment, the chance of complications resulting from additional radiation therapy is much higher.

Hyperthermia

Hyperthermia involves the use of electromagnetic radiation or ultrasound to heat tissues. Hyperthermia is cytotoxic when used alone; however, the best results are seen when it is used as a combined modality with radiation or chemotherapy. A 91% response rate has been reported in dogs with hemangiopericytomas treated using orthovoltage irradiation in combination with hyperthermia.

Chemotherapy

Chemotherapy has been used with variable success to treat soft tissue sarcomas. Agents most often used are vincristine, doxorubicin, cyclophosphamide, and dacarbazine. Commonly used protocols are outlined in Table 2. Combination protocols that include doxorubicin are most effective. In dogs, response rates vary from 35 to 75%, depending on the tumor type and protocol used. One study of 13 cats with various tumors including sarcomas reported a 61% partial response rate using vincristine, cyclophosphamide, and methotrexate.

MAST CELL TUMORS

Mast cell tumors (MCTs) compose approximately 7 to 20% of cutaneous neoplasms in the dog and 15% in the cat. MCTs may develop in almost any location but are found most commonly in the skin and subcutaneous tissues of the dog, and in the skin, spleen, liver, and visceral lymphatics of the cat. Mast cells are a normal component of the immune system and are important in the inflammatory response to tissue trauma. Cytoplasmic granules found in mast cells contain biologically active substances such as heparin, histamine, platelet-activating factor, and eosinophilic chemotactic factor. The quantity and type of granules in MCTs depends on the degree of differentiation. Well-differentiated tumors contain more heparin than undifferentiated tumors, which have a higher histamine content.

Etiology

The cause of MCTs is unknown; however, breed predisposition, chronic inflammation, and viruses may play a role.

Breed Predisposition. Boxers, Boston terriers, English bulldogs, and English bull terriers are at risk. However, MCTs in boxers are more likely to be well-differentiated and may have a more favorable prognosis. Siamese cats under 4 years of age have been reported to have a higher incidence of cutaneous histiocytic-like MCTs.

Chronic Inflammation. Chronic inflammatory sites in the dog have been reported to give rise to MCTs.

Viruses. The speculation that viruses may have a role in MCTs stems from experimental studies in which dogs developed MCTs after being given injections of cell-free tumor extracts.

Biologic Behavior

KEY POINT ▶ Because it is often difficult to histologically differentiate benign from malignant tumors, all MCTs should be considered potentially malignant.

In the Dog

- Approximately 50% of MCTs are malignant.
- Tumor location and rate of growth may help predict biologic behavior:
  - Tumors in preputial, inguinal, and perineal areas may be more malignant.
  - Slow-growing localized MCTs may have a better prognosis. (In one study, tumors that were present for 28 weeks or longer prior to removal had a more favorable prognosis.)
- Regional lymph nodes, spleen, and liver are the most common sites of metastasis.
- Bone marrow involvement can occur.
- Pulmonary metastasis is uncommon.

In the Cat. Controversy exists about location and biologic behavior of MCTs in cats.

Older literature suggests that:

- Half of all MCTs arise from the skin and half from viscera.
- The majority of MCTs in cats are malignant.

Recent literature reports that:

- A higher percentage of MCTs may arise from the skin.
- The majority of MCTs do not display malignant behavior.
  - In particular, histiocytic MCTs seen in young Siamese cats have a benign course, often regressing spontaneously.

Clinical Signs

Clinical signs depend on the location and size of the tumor as well as on secondary systemic complications caused by the MCT.

- In the dog, most MCTs are observed as solitary masses in the skin of the trunk and perineal area (50%), followed by the extremities (40%), and the head and neck (10%).
- In the cat:
  - 40 to 60% of cutaneous MCTs are solitary masses on the head and neck.
  - Visceral MCTs arise in the spleen, small intestine, liver, and visceral lymphatics.
  - Cats with visceral MCTs may present with anorexia, vomiting, or diarrhea.
- Dermal MCTs are usually well-defined, raised masses which can be hairless, ulcerated, and erythematous.
  - Dermal MTCs may be diffuse, erythematous thickenings in the skin.
  - Subcutaneous MCTs may resemble lipomas.
- Mechanical manipulation of MCTs may cause degranulation, resulting in erythema and wheal formation (Darier's sign).

KEY POINT ▶ Gastroduodenal ulcers have been reported in up to 80% of dogs with MCTs and are thought to be related to histamine release. These animals may have anorexia, vomiting, diarrhea, and melena.

- Heparin and proteolytic enzyme release by MCTs at the time of surgery may prolong coagulation times and delay wound healing.

Diagnosis

History, physical examination, clinical pathology, tumor and bone marrow cytology, and radiography are useful in the diagnosis and staging of MCTs. An attempt should be made to stage all MCTs because the stage affects prognosis and therapeutic decisions. A classification system for staging has been developed by WHO (Table 3).

History

The history can determine the length of time the mass has been present and the rate of growth.

TABLE 3. World Health Organization (WHO) Clinical Staging System for Canine Mast Cell Tumors

Stage:

I	One dermal tumor without regional lymph node involvement
II	One dermal tumor with regional lymph node involvement
III	Multiple dermal tumors or a large infiltrative tumor with or without regional lymph node involvement
IV	Any tumor with distant metastasis, or recurrence with metastasis

Stages are subdivided into:
   (a) Without systemic signs
   (b) With systemic signs

Physical Examination

A thorough examination can detect the location and number of masses. Palpate carefully for hepatomegaly, splenomegaly, and lymph node enlargement as a sign of metastasis.

Clinical Pathology

The clinical pathology may be unremarkable. Examine a CBC and a buffy coat smear for evidence of systemic dissemination. Circulating mast cells, eosinophilia, and basophilia are more common in the dog than in the cat. Microcytic-hypochromic anemia may suggest gastrointestinal hemorrhage.

Bone Marrow Aspiration

This is a more sensitive indicator of bone marrow involvement than a buffy coat smear. The presence of greater than 10 mast cells per 1000 nucleated cells is abnormal.

Radiography

Perform abdominal radiography to detect hepatomegaly, splenomegaly, and sublumbar lymph node enlargement. Thoracic radiographs are seldom helpful.

Biopsy

Fine-Needle Aspiration. MCTs usually can be diagnosed by fine-needle aspiration. Aspirates generally contain mast cells, eosinophils, and fibroblasts.

Histopathology. Histopathology is important to evaluate completeness of excision and histologic grade.

Grading of Tumors. The most widely used grading system (Patnaik, et al., 1984) assigns grades I, II, and III to well-, moderately, and poorly differentiated tumors, respectively (based on histopathologic appearance).

The histologic grade affects prognosis:

- Low-grade tumors are less likely to recur or metastasize.
- Dogs with low-grade tumors have increased survival times.

Treatment of Canine Cutaneous Mast Cell Tumors

Treatment of MCTs may include surgery, radiation therapy, chemotherapy, or some combination of the three. The type of treatment instituted depends primarily on the histologic grade and clinical stage of the tumor. A summary of current treatment recommendations for dogs is given in Table 4.

Surgery

Wide surgical excision is the treatment of choice for canine MCTs; however, approximately 50% of tumors may recur.

KEY POINT ▶ Although they appear to be discrete masses, MCTs usually extend deep into surrounding tissues, making wide surgical excision imperative.

TABLE 4. Therapy of Canine Mast Cell Tumors

WHO Stage	Patnaik Grade	Recommended Therapy
I	I and II	Surgical excision Complete: observation Incomplete: wider excision or radiation therapy
I	III	Surgical excision Complete: prednisone* Incomplete: wider excision and prednisone* or radiation and prednisone*
II	I–III	Surgical excision Complete: prednisone* Incomplete: Wider excision and prednisone* or radiation and prednisone* or prednisone* alone
III and IV		Local therapy if possible plus one of the following: Prednisone* CVP† chemotherapy Vincristine 0.5–0.75 mg/m²/IV weekly

*Prednisone: 40 mg/m², PO, SID for 1 week; then 20 mg/m² SID for 3 weeks; then 20 mg/m² every other day for 3 weeks; then reduce the dose by 50% every 3 weeks.

†CVP: Cyclophosphamide (Cytoxan; Bristol-Myers) 50 mg/m² PO every other day or 4 days a week; vinblastine (Velban; Eli Lilly) 2 mg/m² IV once a week; prednisone 20–40 mg/m² PO every other day.

- Administer an antihistamine (e.g., Benadryl, Parke-Davis; 2 mg/kg IV) just prior to surgery to decrease the effects of histamine release from the tumor.
- Excise the mass with 3-cm margins on all sides.
- Have the specimen margins histologically evaluated for completeness of excision.
- If the tumor extends to the margins, plan a second, wider excision (if possible).
- Remove regional lymph nodes if tumor is present.
- If tumors are incompletely excised or nonresectable, proceed with radiation therapy and/or chemotherapy.

Radiation Therapy

Radiation therapy alone or in combination with other treatment modalities may be used to treat incompletely excised or nonresectable MCTs.

- Give a total dosage of 40–48 Gy over a period of 3 to 4 weeks.
- One-year control rates range from 48 to 78%.
- Irradiate involved regional lymph nodes, if necessary.

Chemotherapy

Chemotherapy is recommended for systemic mastocytosis and nonresectable or incompletely excised tumors. Glucocorticoids are commonly used to produce partial or complete remissions in dogs.

- Prednisone and prednisolone are most commonly used for oral therapy (see Table 4 for dosage).
- Intralesional triamcinolone (1 mg/cm of tumor diameter once every 14 days) may be used; however, side effects are more common with this route.
- Combination therapy using cyclophosphamide, vin-

blastine, and prednisone has been reported to cause remissions in dogs refractory to glucocorticoids.

■ Discontinue therapy in animals that remain tumor-free after 6 months.

Ancillary Drug Therapy

Dogs and cats with systemic mastocytosis or gastro-duodenal hemorrhage should receive ancillary drug therapy.

■ Use H2-antagonists to reduce gastric acid secretion and help decrease the incidence and severity of gastrointestinal ulcers in MCT patients. Administer:
 • Cimetidine (Tagamet, SmithKline; 5–10 mg/kg PO q8h)
 or
 • Ranitidine (Zantac, Glaxo, Inc.; 1–2 mg/kg PO q12h) (see sec. 7, ch. 4)
■ When an active gastrointestinal ulcer is suspected in an animal with MCT, also administer:
 • Sucralfate (Carafate, Marion Labs., 250–1000 mg PO q6–8h) (see sec. 7, ch. 4 for use and actions)

Treatment of Feline Mast Cell Tumors

Cutaneous

■ Wide surgical excision is the treatment of choice.
■ Chemotherapy and radiotherapy have not been well evaluated but may be helpful in recurrent or metastatic tumors.

Visceral

■ Splenectomy may ameliorate clinical signs in cats with splenic MCTs even when other organs are involved.
■ Treat intestinal MCTs by wide surgical excision (5- to 10-cm margins).
■ Chemotherapy has not been critically evaluated; however, prednisone alone or in combination with vincristine and cyclophosphamide does not appear to prolong survival times.

Supplemental Readings

SOFT TISSUE SARCOMAS

Brown NO, Hayes AA, Mooney S: Combined modality therapy in the treatment of solid tumors in cats. J Am Anim Hosp Assoc 16:719, 1980.

Dubielzig RR: Ocular sarcoma following trauma in three cats. J Am Vet Med Assoc 184:578, 1984.

Helfand SC: Chemotherapy for nonresectable and metastatic soft tissue tumors. Columbus, OH; Proceedings Kal Kan Symposium, 1986.

Madewell BR, Theilen GH: Tumors of the skin and subcutaneous tissues. *In* Theilen GH, Madewell BR, eds.: *Veterinary Cancer Medicine.* Philadelphia: Lea & Febiger, 1987, p 233.

McChesney SL, Withrow SJ, Gillette EL, et al.: Radiotherapy of soft tissue sarcomas in dogs. J Am Vet Med Assoc 194:60, 1989.

Owen LN, ed.: TNM Classification of Tumors in Domestic Animals. 1st Ed. Geneva: World Health Organization, 1980.

Priester WA, McKay FA: *The Occurrence of Tumors in Domestic Animals.* National Cancer Institute Monograph 54. Bethesda: U.S. Dept. of Health and Human Services, 1980.

Richardson RC, Anderson VL, Voorhees WD, et al.: Irradiation-hyperthermia in canine hemangiopericytomas: Large animal model for therapeutic response. J Natl Cancer Inst 73:1187, 1984.

Thrall DE, Goldschmidt MH, Biery DN: Malignant tumor formation at the site of previously irradiated acanthomatous epulides in four dogs. J Am Vet Med Assoc 178:127, 1981.

Turrel JM, Theon AP: Re-irradiation of tumors in cats and dogs. J Am Vet Med Assoc 193:465, 1988.

White AS: Clinical Diagnosis and Management of Soft Tissue Sarcomas. *In* Gorman ND, ed.: *Oncology: Contemporary Issues in Small Animal Practice.* New York: Churchill Livingstone, 1986, p 243.

Withrow SJ, MacEwen EG: *Clinical Veterinary Oncology.* Philadelphia: J. B. Lippincott, 1989.

Mast Cell Tumors

Bostock DE: The prognosis following surgical removal of mastocytomas in dogs. J Small Anim Pract 14:27, 1973.

Buerger RG, Scott DW: Cutaneous mast cell neoplasia in cats: 14 cases (1975–1985). J Am Vet Med Assoc 190:1440, 1987.

Guerre R, Millet P, Groulade P: Systemic mastocytosis in a cat: Remission after splenectomy. J Small Anim Pract 20:769, 1979.

Holzinger EA: Feline cutaneous mastocytomas. Cornell Vet 63:87, 1973.

Macy DW: Canine and feline mast cell tumors: Biologic behavior, diagnosis, and therapy. Semin Vet Med Surg (Small Anim) 1:72, 1986.

Macy DW, MacEwen EG: Mast cell tumors. *In* Withrow SJ, MacEwen EG, eds.: *Clinical Veterinary Oncology.* Philadelphia: J. B. Lippincott, 1989, p 156.

Madewell BR, Theilen GH: Tumors of the skin and subcutaneous tissues. *In* Theilen GH, Madewell BR, eds.: *Veterinary Cancer Medicine.* Philadelphia: Lea & Febiger, 1987, p 233.

O'Keefe DA: Canine mast cell tumors. Vet Clin of North Am: 20:4, 1990.

Owen LN, ed.: TNM Classification of Tumors in Domestic Animals. 1st Ed. Geneva: World Health Organization, 1980.

Patnaik AK, Ehler WJ, MacEwen EG: Canine cutaneous mast cell tumor: Morphologic grading and survival time in 83 dogs. Vet Pathol 21:469, 1984.

Turrel JM, Kitchell BE, Miller LM, Theon A: Prognostic factors for radiation treatment of mast cell tumor in 85 dogs. J Am Vet Med Assoc 193:936, 1988.

Wilcock BP, Yager JA, Zink MC: The morphology and behavior of feline cutaneous mastocytomas. Vet. Pathol. 23:320, 1986.

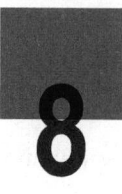

Mammary Gland Neoplasia

Elizabeth Arnold Stone

Mammary gland neoplasia is a disease of older female dogs and cats. Canine mammary gland tumors (MGTs) are the most common tumors in the bitch. In female cats, only cutaneous tumors and lymphomas are more common than MGTs. Mammary gland tumors are very rare in male dogs and cats.

ETIOLOGY

- The cause of mammary gland neoplasia is unknown.
- Although virus-like particles have been identified in feline and canine MGTs, their role as a causative agent is unlikely.
- About 50% of canine mammary carcinomas have estrogen receptors.
- Progesterone administration may be associated with the development of MGTs in cats, but a cause-and-effect relationship has not been established. Feline MGTs very commonly are progesterone receptor–positive.
- Dogs with benign MGTs have more than a threefold risk of subsequently developing a mammary malignancy of a different cell type.

KEY POINT ▶ Approximately 50% of MGTs in dogs are malignant. In cats, 86% of MGTs are malignant.

CLINICAL SIGNS

- A mass or swelling develops in the ventral thoracic or abdominal region. The mass is usually part of the mammae, but may appear distant to the mammary gland.

  Metastatic lesions in the lungs may cause dyspnea.

DIAGNOSIS

The diagnostic plan is directed toward determining the extent of the disease and establishing the stage.

History

- Owner may have noticed the tumor, or it may have been an incidental finding during a routine physical examination.
- Owner may have delayed seeking veterinary assistance. Average time from owner observation of mammary masses in cats to presentation to a veterinarian is 5 months.

- Signalment
  - In dogs, the risk of developing MGTs increases markedly after about 6 years of age.
  - Greatest frequency of canine MGT is reported in sporting breeds (pointers, retrievers, English setters, spaniels), poodles, Boston terriers, and dachshunds.
  - Feline carcinomas occur most often in cats 8 to 12 years of age.
  - In cats, 99% of MGTs occur in intact females.
  - Siamese cats are reported to have twice the risk of developing mammary carcinoma as all other breeds combined.

Physical Examination

- In dogs, MGTs develop most frequently in the caudal mammary glands.
- Depending on the time of recognition, the tumors may be small and movable, lobular and firm, fixed to the body wall, and ulcerated.
- Dogs with inflammatory carcinoma will have diffusely swollen glands with poor demarcation between normal and abnormal tissue, which may be confused with mastitis.
- However, in mastitis the swelling is more localized and occurs after estrus, whelping, or false pregnancy.
- In young intact female cats, mammary hypertrophy can be mistaken for MGT.
- Mammary hypertrophy resulting from either endogenous or exogenous progesterone stimulation can be readily differentiated by the case history, and if necessary, histologic examination.
- In cats, infiltrated lymphatics may look like linear beads.
- Axillary and inguinal lymph nodes may be enlarged.
- Carefully examine dogs for evidence of lameness and bony swelling.
- If these signs are present, radiograph the affected area and obtain a nuclear bone scan, if possible.
- However, do not routinely have bone surveys done in asymptomatic dogs because the incidence of bony metastasis is small (only 3.3% in one study even when tumors were clinically large and aggressive or histologically anaplastic).

Radiography

- Radiograph the thorax to look for metastasis; 25 to 50% of malignant MGTs in dogs have metastasized before surgery.
- If caudal glands are involved, radiograph the abdomen to evaluate the iliac lymph nodes.

- Consider using ultrasonography for evaluating the size and consistency of the iliac lymph nodes.

Histologic Evaluation

- Do not routinely perform aspiration or biopsy of mammary masses if surgical excision is contemplated. Most MGTs are difficult to classify based on cytologic diagnosis. Cytologic examination may be useful, however, to differentiate inflammatory carcinoma from mastitis in dogs, and mammary hypertrophy from mammary carcinoma in cats.
- Aspirate skin masses on the ventral abdomen that are not associated with the mammary glands to determine if they are mast cell tumors. Enlarged inguinal or axillary lymph nodes are aspirated. Presence of carcinoma cells within the lymph node indicates malignancy and invasiveness and worsens the prognosis.
- The histopathologic diagnosis does not alter current treatment recommendations for MGTs (except for inflammatory carcinoma as explained below). Although about 50% of MGTs are benign, many dogs have multiple tumors, often of different histologic types, both benign and malignant.
- The definitive diagnosis of MGT is based on histologic examination of each mass. Thus, surgical excision is performed for both diagnostic and therapeutic purposes. A wide excision is essential to ensure complete removal of the tumor cells (see sec. 3, ch. 5).

Other Diagnostic Tests

If the animal is to be operated on, perform a CBC, biochemical profile, and urinalysis. These animals are usually older and may have concurrent diseases that require further evaluation.

If there is evidence of pleural fluid on thoracic radiographs, aspirate the thorax and examine the fluid microscopically.

SURGICAL THERAPY

The primary treatment objective is to destroy the cancerous tissue while maintaining the animal's quality of life.

Indications. Surgical excision of noninvasive mammary gland carcinoma is beneficial in dogs. Surgical excision:

- Allows a histologic diagnosis
- Can modify disease progression
- Can improve quality of life
- Can be curative

Contraindications. Dogs with inflammatory carcinomas usually die soon after the diagnosis is made because the tumor is extremely aggressive and readily metastasizes. Treatment should be palliative, using anti-inflammatory drugs and antibiotics. Surgery is not recommended for these animals because:

- It is impossible to remove all affected tissues.

- Disseminated intravascular coagulation is often induced.

The following discussion excludes inflammatory carcinoma.

KEY POINT ▶ No particular surgical procedure (i.e., radical vs. simple mastectomy) has been shown to be more effective than others for dogs with MGTs.

Resection Margins. Resection margins should be determined before surgery. Dissect only normal tissues during surgery; do not disrupt the tumor itself. The margins should be at least 1 cm from the neoplastic tissue.

Gland Excision in Dogs. Past recommendations have suggested regional mastectomy for MGTs in dogs (i.e., remove glands 4 and 5 for tumors in 4 or 5; remove glands 1, 2, and 3 for tumors in 1, 2, and 3). These recommendations were based on the lymphatic drainage in normal dogs. However, space-occupying masses will disrupt normal drainage and open new channels between other glands.

Thus, in dogs the number of excised glands is based on having adequate resection margins of normal tissue around the tumor.

Gland Excision in Cats. In cats, removal of all glands on an affected side decreases local recurrence compared with a lumpectomy. However, this may not prolong survival time.

Other Recommendations

- If the tumor has invaded the subcutaneous tissue beneath the gland, include the ventral fascia of the underlying muscle in the excision.
- If the tumor has invaded the body wall, remove a wide section of body wall *en bloc* with the tumor.
- Remove the inguinal lymph nodes routinely during mastectomy of gland 5.
- Axillary nodes are usually not removed with the gland 1 unless there is palpable or cytologic evidence of abnormality.

Surgical Strategy

Lumpectomy. Removal of tumor and 1 cm of normal tissue, without removal of surrounding gland (*lumpectomy*) is adequate if the tumor is small (<5 mm), circumscribed, and noninvasive.

Simple Mastectomy. In many instances, it is easier to remove the entire mammary gland (*simple mastectomy*) and avoid the problems of milk and lymph leakage into the wound.

Regional Mastectomy. When the incision must extend into the adjacent gland or glands in order to obtain adequate margins, the adjacent gland or glands are also removed (*regional mastectomy*). Consider the blood supply to individual mammary glands when planning and executing the mastectomy (Fig. 1). When 2 or more glands are neoplastic, the clinician must choose the most efficient approach. Involvement of two or three adjacent glands necessitates a regional mastectomy.

Complete Unilateral Mastectomy. When multiple glands contain tumors, all of the ipsilateral glands and

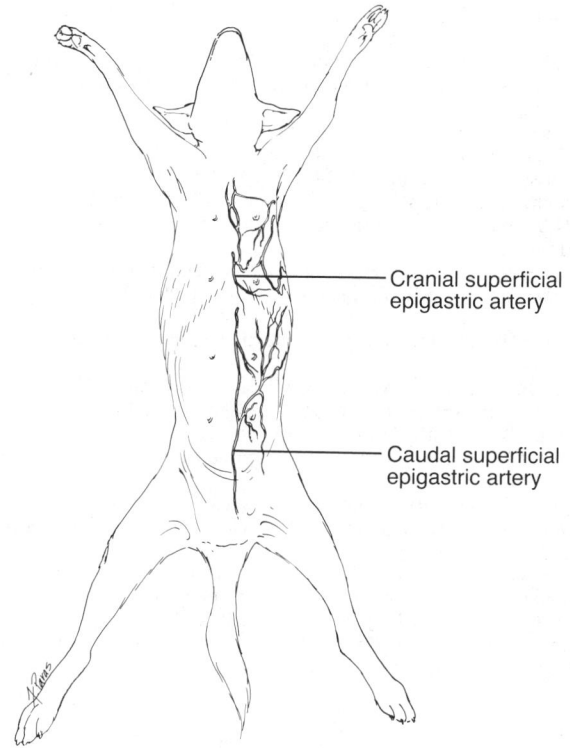

Figure 1. The blood supply to the individual mammary glands is considered in the planning and during the execution of the mastectomy.

intervening tissue are removed *(complete unilateral mastectomy)*, rather than excising each gland separately and leaving tissue between glands.

Tumors in Contralateral Glands

Tumors in contralateral glands may be excised by bilateral simple, regional, or complete mastectomy. The limiting factor is the amount of skin that will be available after excision for closure. In relatively flat-chested dogs, such as Yorkshire terriers or Pekingese, and in cats, bilateral complete mastectomy is possible.

In a deep-chested dog, such as an Irish setter or a pointer, often it is not possible to excise contralateral cranial glands with adequate margins and still be able to close the skin. In this type of dog, perform a staged bilateral mastectomy. Operate on one side and then, after 2 to 4 weeks, operate on the other side.

Skin and Subcutaneous Tissue

After incision of skin and subcutaneous tissues are incised:

- Suture drapes or towels to the normal wound edges to protect the skin from tumor implantation.
- Do not handle tumor with tissue forceps or fingers.
- Place stay sutures in the margin tissues.

After excision:

- Rinse the wound with 0.5–1 liter of warm saline solution to remove exfoliated tumor cells.
- Replace contaminated gloves and surgical instruments before beginning skin closure.

Meticulous closure of the subcutaneous tissues helps relieve tension across the incision and prevents problems associated with surgical dead space.

Ovariohysterectomy. Ovariohysterectomy performed at the time of tumor excision has not been shown to alter prognosis. If an ovariohysterectomy is planned for other reasons during the same surgery, it should be done before the mastectomy to avoid seeding the abdomen with tumor cells. If the MGT extends across the midline perform the mastectomy first, lavage the area and use new gloves and instruments for the ovariohysterectomy.

Biopsy Evaluation

Because multiple tumor types can be present within one mass and each mass may be different, submit all excised tissue for histopathologic examination. Mark the edges of the tissue with suture material or India ink so that the pathologist can maintain proper orientation.

MEDICAL THERAPY

Chemotherapy. Successful chemotherapy for canine mammary carcinoma has not been reported. Cyclophosphamide and doxorubicin induced short-term partial and complete response in 50% of cats with metastatic or nonresectable local disease. However, these drugs cause severe anorexia and mild myelosuppression. The value of these drugs as an adjunct to surgical excision is not known.

Anti-Estrogen Therapy. In the future, anti-estrogen therapy may prove beneficial in some dogs because about 50% of mammary carcinomas have estrogen receptors.

Biologic Response Modifiers. Biologic response modifiers such as levamisole and bacille Calmette-Guérin (BCG), have not been proven successful.

PROGNOSIS

Client education regarding therapy for MGTs is complicated by the variable prognoses reported in the literature. Early reports suggested that overall mean survival times after diagnosis of mammary gland carcinoma in dogs ranged from 4 to 11 months; 75% of dogs died or were euthanized for tumor-related problems within 2 years of surgery.

Recently, cancer mortality following excision of nonmetastatic carcinomas was reported as 27%. Most cancer deaths occurred within the first postoperative year. Cancer mortality for dogs with invasive carcinomas or carcinomas with distant metastasis was 80%. The recurrence rate was higher in dogs with grossly invasive carcinomas (44%) than in dogs with benign and noninvasive carcinomas (12%).

Other studies have shown that:

- Dogs with tumors <3 cm in diameter have better prognosis than dogs with tumors >3 cm in diameter.
- The presence of multiple tumors does not seem to change the prognosis in dogs.

- Mammary gland sarcoma and inflammatory carcinoma have a very poor prognosis.
- Cats with mammary carcinoma treated by surgical excision have an average survival of 7.7 months.
- Cats with tumors <2 cm have less local recurrence and increased survival times than cats with tumors >2–3 cm.
- Survival may be decreased in cats with multiple tumors.

PREVENTION

KEY POINT ▶ The risk of MGT is almost completely eliminated in dogs that are spayed before their first estrus.

Ovariohysterectomy has a sparing effect on the development of MGT in dogs if done before the fourth estrus or before 2.5 years of age.

Ovariectomized cats have 0.6% the risk for developing mammary carcinoma compared with intact cats.

Supplemental Readings

Allen SW, Mahaffey EA: Canine mammary neoplasia: Prognostic indicators and response to surgical therapy. J Am Anim Hosp Assoc 25:540, 1989.

Gilbertson SR, Kurzman ID, Zachrau RE, et al.: Canine mammary epithelial neoplasms: Biologic implications of morphologic characteristics assessed in 232 dogs. Vet Pathol 20:127, 1983.

Hellmen E, Lindgren A: The accuracy of cytology in diagnosis and DNA analysis of canine mammary tumours. J Comp Pathol 101:443, 1989.

Jeglum KA, deGuzman E, Young KM: Chemotherapy of advanced mammary adenocarcinoma in 14 cats. J Am Vet Med Assoc 187:157, 1985.

Kurzman ID, Gilbertson SR: Prognostic factors in canine mammary tumors. Semin Vet Med Surg 1:25, 1986.

MacEwen EG, Hayes AA, Harvey HJ, et al.: Prognostic factors for feline mammary tumors. J Am Vet Med Assoc 185:201, 1984.

Mollermark G, Kangstrom LE, Eliasson I, et al.: Distribution of nuclear DNA-content in canine mammary tumours. J Small Anim Pract 29:309, 1988.

Moulton JE: Tumors of the mammary gland. In Moulton JE, ed.: Tumors in Domestic Animals. Berkeley: University of California Press, 1990, p 518.

Ogilvie GK, Allhands RV, Reynolds HA: Use of radionuclide imaging to identify malignant mammary tumor bone metastases in dogs. J Am Vet Med Assoc 195:220, 1989.

Weijer K, Hart AAM: Prognostic factors in feline mammary carcinoma. J Nat Cancer Inst 70:709, 1983.

9 Tumors of the Skin and Subcutaneous Tissues

Janet L. Peterson
C. Guillermo Couto

The skin and subcutis are the most common sites of neoplasia in the dog, accounting for approximately 30–40% of all tumors. In the cat, 20% of all tumors originate in the skin and subcutis, making it the second most common site of origin. Most canine skin tumors are benign, whereas most feline skin tumors are malignant.

KEY POINT ▶ Skin tumors are not to be ignored. Advising owners to "watch the tumor," rather than to seek a diagnosis, is potentially life-threatening to their dogs or cats.

The most common skin tumors in the dog include lipomas, mast cell tumors, histiocytomas, and sebaceous gland hyperplasia/adenomas. In comparison, the most common skin neoplasms in the cat are basal cell tumors, squamous cell carcinomas, fibrosarcomas, and mast cell tumors. Breeds at increased risk for skin tumors include bassett hound, boxer, bullmastiff, Scottish terrier, and Weimaraner. No apparent breed predilection exists in the cat. In general, skin and subcutaneous tumors are more common in older dogs and cats. Common tumors in younger dogs include histiocytomas, transmissible venereal tumors, and viral papillomas. The etiology of most canine and feline tumors is unknown; however, some tumors have been associated with defined etiologic agents, such as those listed in Table 1.

Physical examination may assist the clinician in formulating a list of potential tumors in the small animal patient. A basic working knowledge of the anatomic location and tissue of origin of various tumors can assist one in making educated decisions. Additionally, fine needle aspiration usually allows the clinician to make a definitive diagnosis without requiring an incisional or excisional biopsy.

CLASSIFICATION

Skin tumors can be classified by tissue of origin (Table 2), anatomic location (Table 3), or stratum of origin (Table 4). Miscellaneous tumors affecting the skin are listed in Table 5.

DIAGNOSIS

General Principles

- Diagnosis and characterization of a skin mass are important for several reasons. Knowledge of the tumor type prior to surgical excision allows the clinician (1) to plan an appropriate surgical approach (e.g., in a mast cell tumor that requires 3-cm margins beyond the tumor edges), (2) to consider radiation therapy (e.g., in a nonresectable mast cell tumor), and (3) to institute medical treatment (e.g., in a transmissible venereal tumor, vincristine chemotherapy is usually curative).

- To detect the presence of metastatic disease prior to surgery, evaluate every enlarged regional lymph node cytologically (fine needle aspiration) or histologically. Additionally, consider lymph node excisional biopsy at surgery for more accurate staging.

- Perform thoracic radiography (three views) on all animals with suspected (or confirmed) malignant tumors with potential for pulmonary metastases. Perform abdominal radiography and/or abdominal ultrasonography in those cases in which dissemination to the abdominal organs or cavity or multicentricity is suspected (e.g., mast cell tumor, hemangiosarcoma). Evaluate skeletal structures on thoracic and abdominal radiographs for the presence of metastatic disease.

KEY POINT ▶ Diagnosis and staging of a skin tumor prior to surgery are critical to insure

TABLE 1. Etiologic Agents

Viruses
    Canine squamous papillomas, warts, feline sarcoma virus–associated multiple fibrosarcomas
Solar and ionizing radiation
    Squamous cell carcinoma
Hormones
    Perianal adenoma
Thermal injuries
    Squamous cell carcinomas, mast cell tumors
Genetic factors
Immunologic compromise
    Feline lymphomas
Age
    Several tumors

TABLE 2. Classification of Skin Tumors by Tissue of Origin

Epithelial Neoplasia
Papilloma
Sebaceous adenoma/hyperplasia/adenocarcinoma
Perianal adenoma/hyperplasia/adenocarcinoma
Basal cell tumor
Ceruminous gland adenoma/adenocarcinoma
Squamous cell carcinoma
Apocrine gland adenocarcinoma
Intracutaneous cornifying epithelioma (keratoacanthoma)
Dermoid/epidermal inclusion cyst
Mesenchymal Neoplasia
Lipoma/infiltrative lipoma/liposarcoma
Fibrosarcoma
Nerve sheath tumor
Hemangiosarcoma
Hermangiopericytoma
Histiocytoma
Mast cell tumor
Extramedullary plasmacytoma
Melanoma

complete excision and to determine appropriate additional treatment.

Fine Needle Aspiration Cytology

Supplies

- Aspiration gun (Aspir Gun; The Everest Co., Linden, NJ)
- 12- or 20-cc syringe
- 22- or 25-gauge needle

TABLE 3. Classification of Skin Tumors by Anatomic Location

Head and Neck
Basal cell tumor
Squamous cell carcinoma
Sebaceous adenoma
Papilloma
Histiocytoma
Mast cell tumor (primarily in cats)
Ceruminous gland adenoma/adenocarcinoma
Hemangiosarcoma
Extremities
Mast cell tumor
Hemangiopericytoma
Squamous cell carcinoma (nail bed)
Malignant melanoma (nail bed)
Nerve sheath tumor
Synovial cell sarcoma
Hemangiosarcoma
Trunk
Mast cell tumor
Lipoma
Sebaceous gland adenoma
Fibrosarcoma
Nerve sheath tumor
Hemangiosarcoma
Perineum/Genitals
Mast cell tumor
Perianal adenoma
Transmissible venereal tumor
Perianal adenocarcinoma
Anal sac (apocrine gland) adenocarcinoma

TABLE 4. Classification of Skin Tumors by Stratum of Origin

Dermoepidermal
Basal cell tumor
Squamous cell carcinoma
Sebaceous adenoma/hyperplasia
Mast cell tumor
Perianal adenoma
Malignant melanoma
Ceruminous gland adenocarcinoma
Lymphoma
Transmissible venereal tumor
Hemangioma/hemangiosarcoma
Cysts
Subcutaneous
Mast cell tumor
Hemangiopericytoma
Lipoma
Hemangiosarcoma
Nerve sheath tumor
Fiobrosarcoma

- Glass cover slips or glass slides
- Diff-Quik or Wright-Giemsa stain

Technique

1. Isolate and hold the mass firmly while inserting the needle into it.
2. Apply negative pressure (10–20 cc) to the syringe to obtain cells.
3. Release the negative pressure prior to withdrawing the needle from the mass.
4. Remove the needle from the syringe and fill the syringe with air.
5. Replace the needle and expel the contents (in the hub of the needle) onto the glass slide or cover slip.
6. Prepare the smear by placing a clean slide or cover slip over the slide with cells and pulling them apart in a parallel motion ("horizontal pull apart" technique).

Cytologic Classification of Neoplasia

Cytology can be utilized to classify masses. First, determine if the mass is neoplastic or non-neoplastic. If it is non-neoplastic, the decision must be made as to whether it is inflammatory or noninflammatory. Masses can also be classified as mixed, as in the case of a neoplastic mass with a necrotic center and associated inflammation. Infectious agents (e.g., bacteria, fungi, protozoa) may also be identified cytologically.

Cytologic examination may allow classification of tumors into one of three categories: epithelial, mes-

TABLE 5. Miscellaneous Tumors Affecting the Skin

Intracutaneous cornifying epitheliomas (keratoacanthomas)
Trichoepitheliomas and pilomatrixomas (tumors of the hair follicles)
Epidermal inclusion cysts (epidermoids, epidermoid cysts)
Dermoid cysts

enchymal, and round cell neoplasm (includes epithelial, mesenchymal, and melanocytic tumors).

Epithelial Tumors

Epithelial cells cluster owing to the presence of desmosomes. Aspiration cytology reveals round to polygonal cells with distinct cell membranes, basophilic cytoplasm (with and without vacuoles), and cell-to-cell association. Cell-to-cell association may be absent in squamous cell carcinomas.

Mesenchymal Tumors

Mesenchymal tumors arise from connective tissue, including fibrous tissue; muscle; fat; and blood vessels. Mesenchymal tumors do not exfoliate well upon fine needle aspiration; however, when they do exfoliate, they appear as individual cells or small groups of cells, with a spindle to polygonal shape and indistinct cell membranes.

Round Cell Tumors

On a fine needle aspirate, round cell tumors tend to exfoliate as single cells. Transmissible venereal tumor cells usually clump, however. Round cells have distinct cell membranes like those of epithelial cells. Some cells may have cytoplasmic granules (mast cells, melanoma cells, large granular lymphocytes).

Round cell tumors include lymphomas, melanomas, histiocytomas, transmissible venereal tumors, mast cell tumors, and plasma cell tumors. Additionally, squamous cell carcinomas and basal cell tumors can cytologically resemble round cell tumors.

Incisional Biopsy

Baker Biopsy Punch

■ The skin punch biopsy is a relatively simple technique for obtaining a sample of superficial masses. The advantage of skin punch biopsies is that they require only local anesthetic and can be accomplished in a short time.

Tru-Cut Needle Biopsy (Travenol Laboratories)

■ Tru-Cut needle biopsies can be utilized to obtain representative samples of larger or subcutaneous masses. Local anesthesia only is required.

Wedge Biopsy

■ A routine surgical procedure is used to obtain a "wedge" biopsy.

Excisional Biopsy

Excisional biopsy implies that all or most of the tumor or mass is removed and submitted for histopathologic examination. This approach is indicated for small, easily excisable masses. Margins of excised tissue are at least 1 cm from the tumor's edge in all cases. All excised tumors must be properly fixed. Label each tumor by location, if there are multiple tumors, and send all samples to a qualified veterinary pathologist for examination.

KEY POINT ▶ Perform histopathologic examinations on all excised skin masses, no matter how "benign" they appear. Appropriate

treatment necessitates a definitive diagnosis.

Staging

Clinical staging is helpful to characterize the extent of the disease. Obtain thoracic radiographs (left and right lateral and ventrodorsal views) when malignancy is suspected. Perform abdominal radiography or ultrasonography for tumors such as cutaneous hemangiosarcomas and mast cell tumors to evaluate for splenic and hepatic involvement (metastases or primary tumor).

BRIEF DESCRIPTIONS OF SELECTED TUMORS OF THE SKIN AND SUBCUTANEOUS TISSUE

Epithelial Neoplasia

Papillomas (Squamous Papillomas, Squamous Cell Papillomatosis, Warts, Cutaneous Papillomatosis)

Origin and Etiology. These tumors originate from the squamous epithelium. Papillomas have a viral DNA etiology in puppies, but the etiology is unknown in older dogs.

Description. Papillomas may appear as cauliflower- or wart-like growths that are usually well-encapsulated. They can be sessile or pedunculated and may bleed, if traumatized. They can occur as a single tumor (usually nonviral etiology) or multiple tumors (usually viral etiology) in the skin, mucous membranes, or mucocutaneous regions.

Epidemiology and Biologic Behavior. Papillomas are common in dogs but rare in cats. The viral-induced papillomas in young dogs often appear as multiple or occasionally single masses on the head, eyelids, feet, or mouth. In older dogs, nonviral papillomas tend to appear as solitary dermoepidermal masses. Some papillomas can transform into squamous cell carcinomas.

Treatment. Papillomas tend to regress spontaneously in younger dogs (usually within 1 to 2 months) and therefore do not require treatment. Surgically remove viral papillomas that do not regress and papillomas of nonviral etiology, if they pose a clinical problem.

Sebaceous Gland Adenoma/Hyperplasia

Origin and Etiology. These tumors originate from the epithelium of the sebaceous glands.

Description. These tumors are common in dogs and rare in cats. Hyperplasia usually appears as pink, smooth, lobulated wart-like growths that are firm, dermoepidermal, well-circumscribed masses with an alopecic surface. They may or may not be pigmented and can occur anywhere on the body. These tumors are frequently multiple. They often appear as bleeding and ulcerated masses. Sebaceous gland adenocarcinoma is poorly circumscribed, large, invasive, and frequently ulcerated. These are extremely rare.

Cytology. Cytologic examination of sebaceous gland

hyperplasia reveals mature secretory epithelial cells, frequently with a "signet-ring appearance" due to the accumulation of secretions within the cell. Sebaceous adenocarcinoma cells exhibit the typical features of malignancy.

Epidemiology and Biologic Behavior. Sebaceous gland hyperplasia can occur as single tumors; however, they frequently tend to occur in multiple sites. They occur in older female dogs, especially poodles and cocker spaniels. When metastases from sebaceous gland adenocarcinoma occur, they are generally to the regional lymph nodes and subsequently to the lungs.

Treatment. Surgical excision of sebaceous gland hyperplasia may not be necessary unless in an area that is easily traumatized. Perform wide surgical excision on all sebaceous adenocarcinomas. Adjunct treatment with radiotherapy and/or FAC protocol (5-fluorouracil, doxorubicin, and cyclophosphamide) (Appendix I) may be beneficial.

Perianal Adenoma/Hyperplasia/Adenocarcinomas

Origin and Etiology. Perianal adenoma, hyperplasia, and adenocarcinoma originate from the perianal (hepatoid) glands that encircle the anus of the dog. These glands are also located in the skin of the tail, prepuce, and thigh, and over the dorsum of the back. The growth and maintenance of these cells are dependent upon the presence of testosterone.

Description. Perianal adenoma and hyperplasia can occur as solitary or multiple nodules. These are most common in intact male dogs. The behavior of both is usually benign. They can be found wherever perianal glands are located (see Origin and Etiology), but they are most common in the perineal region. Perianal adenocarcinomas are frequently larger, ulcerative, and more invasive than adenomas.

Cytology. Cytologic examination usually reveals large hepatoid cells. It is impossible to differentiate perianal adenoma from hyperplasia. Malignancy can be difficult to assess solely on the basis of cytology.

Epidemiology and Biologic Behavior. Perianal adenocarcinomas metastasize to the local lymph nodes, especially the iliac lymph nodes, and to the lungs. These tumors occur primarily in male dogs.

Treatment. Perianal adenomas usually regress with castration because of their testosterone dependency. Castration is therefore recommended in all dogs in which perianal adenomas constitute a problem. Aggressive surgical excision is performed on all resectable perianal adenocarcinomas and those perianal adenomas that fail to respond to castration. Radiation therapy or chemotherapy is an option using the VAC (vincristine, doxorubicin, and cyclophosphamide) or FAC protocol (see Appendix I).

Basal Cell Tumors (Basal Cell Carcinoma, Basal Cell Epithelioma)

Origin and Etiology. Basal cell tumors originate from the basal cells of the epidermis and adnexa.

Description. Basal cell tumors commonly occur as solitary nodules. They can be sessile or pedunculated, firm, and well-demarcated from the underlying tissues. These tumors are frequently pigmented, contain cystic spaces, and occasionally are ulcerated (in cats). Basal cell tumors tend to be found more frequently on the head, neck, and shoulder of the dog. They are commonly found almost anywhere in the cat, in which they represent the most common skin tumor.

Cytology. Cells may be arranged in cords or palisades. Palisading clusters and uniform nuclei are generally seen on cytologic examination. The cells usually appear malignant on cytologic and histopathologic examination.

Epidemiology and Biologic Behavior. These tumors are common in older dogs and cats. Poodles and cocker spaniels may be at an increased risk for these tumors. They are usually benign and may have been present from months to years prior to diagnosis. When these tumors are histologically identified as basal cell carcinomas, this finding is generally a reliable diagnosis and their behavior must be considered to be very aggressive.

Treatment. Wide surgical excision is the treatment of choice for basal cell tumors. Complete excision is curative. Nonresectable or invasive tumors can be successfully treated with radiation therapy.

Ceruminous Gland Adenomas/Adenocarcinomas

Origin and Etiology. Ceruminous gland adenomas and ceruminous gland adenocarcinomas originate from the epithelium of the ceruminous glands in the ear canal.

Description. They are usually brown tumors associated with cerumen production, which may resemble chronic otitis. Ceruminous gland adenomas are small, pedunculated masses, which are frequently located near the tympanic membrane and extend exteriorly. Adenocarcinomas are similar to adenomas; however, they are frequently invasive.

Cytology. Cytologic examination reveals mature or immature (ceruminous gland adenocarcinoma) secretory cells with epithelial characteristics.

Epidemiology/Biologic Behavior. This is the most common external ear tumor in older dogs and cats but appears to be more common in cats.

Treatment. Total ear canal resection may be necessary to completely excise this tumor (see sec. 5, ch. 22). Surgical removal may be sufficient in animals with ceruminous gland adenomas; however, external beam irradiation is strongly recommended for ceruminous gland adenocarcinomas and recurrent or nonexcisable adenomas.

Squamous Cell Carcinomas

Origin and Etiology. Squamous cell carcinomas are induced by ultraviolet light exposure in cats and dogs with hypopigmented areas. They originate from stratified squamous epithelium. The cell of origin is the keratinocyte.

Description. These tumors frequently appear as ulcerated, necrotic, nonhealing lesions. Common sites in dogs include the ventral abdomen, digits, limbs, scrotum, lips, and nose. In the cat, they include the pinnae, lips, nose, and eyelids. Proliferative tumors may resemble a red firm plaque or a cauliflower-like lesion. Digital squamous cell carcinoma can be proliferative, ulcerative, and erosive. It can appear as a nonhealing wound. Multiple, nailbed squamous cell carcinomas have been observed in black dogs.

Cytology. These epithelial cells are polygonal and may keratinize as they mature. Typical epithelial cells mixed with keratinizing cells are frequently noted. Aging squamous epithelial cells tend to be more angular or polyhedral, with a pyknotic nucleus and bluer cytoplasm. Abundant neutrophils and other inflammatory cells are frequently observed.

Epidemiology and Biologic Behavior. These tumors occur more frequently in cats, especially in white cats, or in hypopigmented areas that are more likely to be exposed to sunlight (ear tips and nose). Dogs have an increased frequency of these tumors in the ventral abdomen, especially; trunk; scrotum; and lips. They are locally invasive with late metastases to the lymph nodes and to the lungs.

Treatment. Complete surgical excision is recommended for squamous cell carcinomas if they are in an accessible location. Complete pinnae resection is advised for tumors of the ear and amputation for squamous cell carcinoma of digit (see sec. 9, ch. 20). Radiation therapy is utilized for dogs and cats with nonresectable or incompletely excised squamous cell carcinomas.

Anal Sac or Apocrine Gland Adenocarcinomas

Origin and Etiology. Apocrine gland adenocarcinomas are derived from the apocrine glands that empty into the anal sac.

Description. These tumors can vary from very small masses that can be located only after careful rectal and perirectal palpation to large masses protruding from the rectum. They may cause ulceration of the overlying skin.

Cytology. Cytologic examination reveals large cells with abundant cytoplasm and eccentric, round nuclei.

Epidemiology/Biologic Behavior. Apocrine gland adenocarcinomas are most commonly found in older female dogs. Hypercalcemia is frequently associated with these tumors. Metastases are common (90%) and most frequently to the regional lymph nodes.

Treatment. Surgical excision offers the best option for a cure. Chemotherapy may also be considered (melphalan, FAC; see Appendix I). Hypercalcemia generally resolves following remission of this tumor.

Intracutaneous Cornifying Epithelioma (Keratoacanthoma)

Origin and Etiology. This tumor is derived from the superficial epithelium between hair follicles.

Description. Intracutaneous cornifying epitheliomas may be located on the skin of the neck, dorsal thorax, legs, and occasionally on the ventral abdomen. A toothpaste-like material may be expressed from these masses.

Cytology. Cytologic evaluation may reveal keratin associated with inflammatory cells.

Epidemiology/Biologic Behavior. These are benign tumors that can occur in a solitary form in many breeds and in a multicentric form in Norwegian elkhound and keeshond dogs.

Treatment. Surgical excision is the treatment of choice, although it may not be required.

Dermoid/Epidermal Inclusion Cyst

Origin and Etiology. Dermoid and epidermal inclusion cysts originate from the dermis and epidermis. Epidermal inclusion cysts are frequently secondary to an occluded hair follicle, whereas dermoid cysts may be developmental defects.

Description. Dermoid cysts contain epidermal appendages, hair, and sebaceous and sweat gland secretions in addition to the keratin that is in the epidermal inclusion cysts. A semisolid material is frequently contained within these cysts.

Cytology. A clear-to-brown fluid is frequently obtained for cytologic examination.

Epidemiology/Biologic Behavior. These are benign tumors.

Treatment. Surgical excision is the treatment of choice, although it is not always required.

Mesenchymal Neoplasia

Lipomas/Infiltrative Lipomas/Liposarcomas

Origin and Etiology. Lipomas, infiltrative lipomas, and liposarcomas originate from adipocytes or fat cells.

Description. Lipomas can occur as either single or multiple masses and are located over the thorax, sternum, abdomen, and proximal limbs of dogs. These masses are usually subcutaneous; well-circumscribed, although not necessarily well-encapsulated; fluctuant; soft; and sometimes multilobulated. Infiltrative lipomas infiltrate the deep tissue and are extremely difficult to excise. Liposarcomas are uncommon and usually solitary tumors, which tend to be very infiltrative, firm, and poorly circumscribed.

Cytology. Fatty-appearing material is usually present on the slide prior to staining. Most cells from aspirates of lipomas are "washed off" by the methanol in the fixative. Occasionally, oily material with few intact adipocytes or fatty cells remains on the slide or cover slip. Cytology of liposarcoma reveals immature mesenchymal cells with vacuoles and round, indented nuclei. Variation in cell size is common, and occasionally multinucleation is noted.

KEY POINT ▶ It is important to evaluate all "lipomas" cytologically because they are indistinguishable from mast cell tumors in physical appearance and clinical presentation.

Epidemiology/Biologic Behavior. Lipomas are benign tumors that appear to be more common in older spayed female dogs. They are the most common mesenchymal tumor in the dog but are extremely rare in the cat. Infiltrative lipomas are also benign; however, because of their highly infiltrative nature, they may require extensive surgical excision, including amputation of the affected limb. Liposarcomas are extremely rare in both dogs and cats but are found most often in dogs over 10 years of age. They are locally invasive and may metastasize to the lungs and/or liver.

Treatment. Complete surgical excision is recommended for all liposarcomas. It may or may not be necessary to remove lipomas, depending on their size and location and the owner's preference. If surgery is considered, remove these lipomas while they are small and before they become too large and difficult to resect.

Fibrosarcomas

See section 3, chapter 7.

Response to chemotherapy is variable. Histologically, poorly differentiated fibrosarcomas and fibrosarcomas with giant cells in cats appear to be more responsive to chemotherapy. Chemotherapy protocols include VAC (cats, dogs; see Appendix I) and ADIC (doxorubicin and dacarbazine)(dogs; see Appendix I). Other treatment options include radiation therapy and hyperthermia.

Nerve Sheath Tumors (Neurofibromas/ Neurofibrosarcomas, Schwannomas, Neurolemmomas)

See section 3, chapter 7.

Hemangiosarcomas (Malignant Hemangioendotheliomas and Angiosarcomas)

Origin and Etiology. These tumors originate from the vascular endothelium.

Description. Hemangiosarcomas are generally solitary masses found on the limbs, flank, or neck. They can occur in the skin and/or subcutaneous tissue. Those in the subcutaneous tissue may also infiltrate into the underlying muscle. Hemangiosarcoma must be differentiated from hemangioma.

Cytology. Cytology reveals spindle-shaped or polygonal cells with large nuclei and a lacy chromatin pattern; one or more nucleoli; and a bluish, usually vacuolated cytoplasm. Hemangiosarcomas can also exfoliate cells in sheets similar to those of epithelial cells.

Epidemiology/Biologic Behavior. Hemangiosarcomas of the skin may be either primary or metastatic. Hemangiosarcomas are much more common in dogs, especially German shepherds, than cats. The prognoses of these tumors are variable, depending upon location. The patient in which the tumor is confined to the dermis has an excellent prognosis. If the tumor involves the subcutaneous tissue, the prognosis is poor. Muscular involvement warrants a guarded prognosis.

Treatment. Complete surgical excision is recommended, when feasible. Chemotherapy is probably not necessary for those tumors involving only the dermis, whereas those involving the subcutaneous tissue with or without muscular involvement probably require chemotherapy (for VAC protocol, See Appendix I).

Hemangiopericytomas

See section 3, chapter 7.

Histiocytomas

Origin and Etiology. The origin of canine cutaneous histiocytomas is the monocyte-macrophage cells in the skin.

Description. This is a dermoepidermal tumor frequently located on the head and neck and less commonly on the extremities. They are round, alopecic, sometimes pink or erythematous, and they occasionally ulcerate. Because of their gross appearance, they are also referred to as "button tumors."

Cytology. Cytology reveals a round cell tumor with a moderate amount of cytoplasm and, possibly, an eccentrically located nucleus. Histiocytomas also tend to be highly pleomorphic and moderately vacuolated. Lymphocytes are abundant. These tumors can appear inflammatory.

Epidemiology/Biologic Behavior. These tumors generally exhibit benign behavior and are found mostly in young dogs (approximately 1 to 3 years). Histiocytomas usually regress spontaneously within 4 to 8 weeks of diagnosis. This tumor does not occur in cats.

Treatment. Observation may be appropriate in most of these tumors, because the majority regress with age. Surgical excision is recommended if this tumor does not regress in a reasonable period of time, in older dogs, for cosmetic reasons, and to avoid erroneous diagnosis and further growth of the tumor.

Mast Cell Tumor (Mastocytoma, Mast Cell Sarcoma, and Mastocytosis)

See section 3, chapter 7.

Extramedullary Plasmacytoma

See section 3, chapter 6.

Transmissible Venereal Tumor

See also section 8, chapter 12.

Origin and Etiology. Transmissible venereal tumors are frequently transmitted at coitus or through close contact. The cell of origin is considered to be from the monocyte macrophage system.

Description. Transmissible venereal tumors tend to occur on the face and the external genitalia and are frequently presented as ulcerated, cauliflower-like masses.

Cytology. Cytology reveals round-to-ovoid cells, with round nuclei and numerous mitotic figures. The cytoplasm is blue or transparent, contains distinct clear vacuoles, and is surrounded by a distinct cell membrane.

Epidemiology/Biologic Behavior. This tumor tends to be transmitted by coitus, licking, biting, and scratching. Transmissible venereal tumor occurs more frequently in areas where dogs are free roaming. No breed or sex predilection has been observed. These tumors have a low metastatic potential.

Treatment. Transmissible venereal tumors may be cured with vincristine chemotherapy (see Appendix I) or with radiation therapy.

Malignant Fibrous Histiocytoma (Extraskeletal Giant Cell Tumors)

See section 3, chapter 7.

Melanocytic Tumors (Melanomas)

Origin and Etiology. Melanomas originate from melanocytes (melanin-producing cells) or melanoblasts—cells of neuroectodermal origin.

Description. These are typical brown-to-black pigmented nodules (although they may be nonpigmented), and occur more frequently on the face, trunk, feet, scrotum, mucocutaneous regions, and nailbeds.

Cytology. Cytologic examination may reveal cells that vary from round to spindle-shaped. They frequently contain brown-to-black granules.

Epidemiology/Biologic Behavior. Melanomas are considerably more common in dogs than in cats. Tumors originating in the skin tend to be benign, whereas tumors of the mucocutaneous regions (e.g., oral cavity, nailbeds) tend to be malignant.

Treatment. Local recurrence and distant metastases are very common. Other than surgery, most therapy does not seem to work. Results of chemotherapy have been unrewarding; however, DTIC is the drug of choice.

APPENDIX I

Chemotherapy Protocols

See section 3, chapter 5 for principles of chemotherapy.

Cutaneous Lymphoma

See section 3, chapter 6.

Mast Cell Tumors (Systemic)

See section 3, chapter 7.

Soft Tissue Sarcomas

See also section 3, chapter 7.

- ■ ADIC protocol (dogs)
  - • Doxorubicin (Adriamycin): 30 mg/m² body surface area (BSA), IV, q/3 weeks

- • DTIC (Dacarbazine): 1000 mg/m² BSA, IV drip for 6–8 hours; repeat q/3 weeks
- • Trimethoprim-sulfadiazine: 15 mg/kg, PO, q12h
- ■ VAC protocol (21 day cycle) (dogs)
  - • Vincristine (Oncovin): 0.75 mg/m² BSA, IV, days 8, 15
  - • Doxorubicin (Adriamycin): 30 mg/m² BSA, IV, day 1
  - • Cyclophosphamide (Cytoxan): 100–200 mg/m² BSA, IV, day 1
  - • Trimethoprim-sulfadiazine: 15 mg/kg, PO, q12h
- ■ VAC protocol (21 day cycle) (cats)
  - • Vincristine (Oncovin): 0.5 mg/m² BSA, IV, days 8, 15
  - • Doxorubicin (Adriamycin): 20 mg/m² BSA, IV, day 1
  - • Cyclophosphamide (Cytoxan): 100–200 mg/m² BSA, IV, day 1
  - • As above

Carcinomas

- ■ FAC protocol
  - • 5-Fluoruracil (5-FU): 150 mg/m² BSA, IV, days 8, 15
  - • Doxorubicin (Adriamycin): 30 mg/m² BSA, IV, day 1
  - • Cyclophosphamide (Cytoxan): 100–200 mg/m² BSA, IV, day 1
  - • Trimethoprim-sulfadiazine: 15 mg/kg, PO, q12h

Transmissible Venereal Tumors

- ■ Vincristine (Oncovin): 0.5 mg/m² BSA, IV, once weekly until resolution of the tumor and at least 1 week beyond resolution of the tumor.

Anal Sac or Apocrine Gland Adenocarcinomas

- ■ FAC protocol
- ■ Melphalan (Alkeran)
  - • Melphalan (Alkeran): 2 mg/m² BSA, PO, q24h × 1 week; then every other day (QOD)

Supplemental Readings

Holzworth J: *Diseases of the Dog and Cat.* Philadelphia: W.B. Saunders, 1987.
Theilen GH, Madewell BR: *Veterinary Cancer Medicine.* Philadelphia: Lea & Febiger, 1987.
Withrow SJ, MacEwen EG: *Clinical Veterinary Oncology.* Philadelphia: J.B. Lippincott, 1989.

Endocrine and Metabolic Disorders

Mark E. Peterson

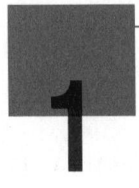

1 Thyroid Gland

Thomas K. Graves
Mark E. Peterson
Stephen J. Birchard

HYPOTHYROIDISM IN DOGS

In dogs, hypothyroidism is a multisystemic disorder. The clinical signs reflect the generalized effects of decreased cellular metabolic functions caused by thyroid hormone deficiency. The disease occurs most frequently in middle-aged dogs of mid- to large-sized breeds. Breeds reported to be predisposed to hypothyroidism include the Golden retriever, Doberman pinscher, Irish setter, miniature schnauzer, dachshund, cocker spaniel, and Airedale terrier. There is no sex predilection. The disease is more common in spayed than in intact bitches.

Etiology

Primary (thyroidal) hypothyroidism is caused by destruction of the thyroid gland itself and accounts for more than 95% of clinical cases of the disease.

- Lymphocytic thyroiditis
  - Diffuse infiltration of the thyroid gland by lymphocytes
  - Clinical signs develop when more than 75% of the thyroid gland has been destroyed.
  - Probably an immune-mediated disease
- Idiopathic thyroid gland atrophy
  - Replacement of thyroid parenchyma by adipose tissue and absence of inflammatory cells
  - Probably a primary degenerative disorder

- Uncommon causes of primary hypothyroidism in dogs include congenital or juvenile-onset hypothyroidism (e.g., dyshormonogenesis, thyroid gland dysgenesis), replacement of thyroid gland parenchyma by nonfunctional neoplastic tissue (e.g., thyroid carcinoma), iatrogenic surgical thyroidectomy, and radioactive iodine therapy. The use of antithyroid drugs in the treatment of hyperthyroidism is another extremely rare cause.

Secondary (pituitary) hypothyroidism is caused by impaired secretion of thyroid-stimulating hormone (TSH) by the pituitary gland. This etiology accounts for less than 5% of cases of canine hypothyroidism.

- Pituitary tumors. Destruction of normal pituitary thyrotrophic cells by neoplastic invasion can result in TSH deficiency.
- Cystic Rathke's pouch. This form of secondary congenital hypothyroidism has been documented in German shepherd pituitary dwarfs (see sec. 4, ch. 6).

Tertiary (hypothalamic) hypothyroidism is deficient production and/or release of thyrotropin-releasing hormone (TRH) and is believed to be an extremely rare cause of hypothyroidism in dogs.

"Poor converters" have defects in the peripheral conversion of T_4 to T_3 (the more active form of thyroid hormone), and these are thought to be the cause of rare cases of hypothyroidism in dogs, but this has yet to be documented.

Clinical Signs

The clinical signs of hypothyroidism are due to decreased cellular metabolic rate caused by decreased circulating thyroid hormone concentrations (Table 1). Clinical signs are often vague and can range from mild to severe.

Generalized Appearance and Behavior

- Weight gain (mild to marked obesity) without increase in appetite
- Lethargy, dullness, exercise intolerance
- Cold intolerance and hypothermia—"heat-seeking"

Integument

- Alopecia, haircoat dryness, excessive shedding, retarded hair regrowth
  - Usually bilaterally symmetric
  - Ventral and lateral trunk, caudal thighs, dorsal tail, dorsal nose, and ventral neck are common sites.
- Cutaneous hyperpigmentation
- Myxedema. Thickening of skin, especially facial, due to glycosaminoglycan accumulation, "tragic" facial expression.
- Secondary pyoderma can lead to pruritus, but most dogs with hypothyroidism do not have pruritus.

Nervous System and Muscle

- Weakness and exercise intolerance
- Peripheral neuropathy (rare)
  - Vestibular neuropathy (head tilt)
  - Facial nerve palsy
  - Dragging of front feet (exact cause unclear)

Cardiovascular System

- Bradycardia, weak apex beat
- Impaired myocardial contractility, decreased QRS amplitude

TABLE 1. Frequency of Common Clinical Signs and Routine Laboratory Findings in Dogs with Hypothyroidism

	Percent (%) of Dogs
Clinical Signs	
Lethargy/mental dullness	70
Alopecia/hair loss	65
Weight gain/obesity	60
Dry haircoat/excessive shedding	60
Anestrus (15 intact females)	40
Hyperpigmentation	25
Cold intolerance/hypothermia	15
Bradycardia	10
Laboratory Findings	
Hypercholesterolemia	80
Normocytic, normochromic anemia	50

Reproductive System

- Anestrus, infertility, abortion in female
- Inappropriate galactorrhea in female
- Loss of libido in male
- Testicular atrophy, hypospermia, infertility in male

Eyes

Ocular manifestations of canine hypothyroidism are rare and appear to be associated with hyperlipidemia.

- Corneal lipid deposits
- Chronic uveitis, secondary glaucoma
- Keratoconjunctivitis sicca

Bleeding Disorders

A suggested relationship exists between canine hypothyroidism and von Willebrand's disease. Thyroxine is known to increase factor VIII coagulant activity in both euthyroid and hypothyroid patients. A dog with mild factor VIII or factor VIII–related antigen deficiency could have an exacerbation of bleeding tendencies upon development of hypothyroidism.

Diagnosis

Canine hypothyroidism is probably one of the most overdiagnosed diseases in small animal practice. Many diseases and conditions can mimic the clinical signs of hypothyroidism. Some of these clinical signs, even in dogs with normal thyroid function, can improve following administration of exogenous thyroid hormone. Obesity, exercise intolerance, and dermatopathy are common in the middle-aged dog population. A variety of nonthyroidal factors can lead to low serum thyroid hormone measurements in euthyroid dogs. Definitive diagnosis of canine hypothyroidism requires careful attention to clinical signs and to the thyroid gland biopsy findings or the demonstration of low serum concentrations of thyroid hormones, which are unresponsive to TSH administration.

Screening Laboratory Tests

- Complete blood count. Normocytic, normochromic, nonregenerative anemia may be present with hypothyroidism.
- Serum biochemical analysis
  - Hypercholesterolemia is the biochemical hallmark of hypothyroidism.
  - Hypertriglyceridemia is a less common finding.

Basal Thyroid Hormone Determination

- Serum T_3 concentrations are of less diagnostic value.
- The finding of a low serum T_4 concentration does not confirm a diagnosis of hypothyroidism.
  - Concurrent nonthyroidal disease commonly causes low serum thyroid hormone concentrations (e.g., renal failure, diabetes mellitus, hyperadrenocorticism, hepatic disease).
  - Many agents (e.g., glucocorticoids, anticonvulsants, radiographic contrast agents, nonsteroidal anti-inflammatory drugs) can alter thyroid hormone metabolism and plasma or tissue binding of thyroid hormones, leading to falsely low serum concentrations.

KEY POINT ▶ The finding of low resting serum T_4 and T_3 concentrations is consistent with hypothyroidism but is not absolutely diagnostic. Low values are also found in dogs with a variety of nonthyroidal diseases and in dogs treated with glucocorticoids and other drugs.

TSH Stimulation Test

Low (often undetectable) serum T_4 concentration that fails to increase adequately following administration of exogenous, bovine TSH confirms a diagnosis of hypothyroidism in the dog.

- Test protocol. Protocols for this test vary widely, and the laboratory performing the hormone assays needs to be consulted.
  - Collect blood for basal serum T_4 determination.
  - Administer TSH (e.g., Thytropar, Rhône-Poulenc Rorer) intravenously at a dose of 0.1 U/kg, up to a maximum dose of 5 U/dog.
  - Collect blood sample 6 hours post-TSH administration for serum T_4 determination.
- Criteria for interpreting the test is established by each individual diagnostic laboratory. In general, however, the finding of a low basal serum T_4 concentration that fails to increase by approximately 15 nmol/L (1.5 µg/dl) is highly suggestive of hypothyroidism.
  - Do not use ratios or "fold" increases in T_4 concentration to evaluate test results.
  - In cases of equivocal results, the following equation may prove helpful:

k = 0.5 × basal T_4 concentration (nmol/L)
  + difference between post-TSH and pre-TSH T_4 concentration (nmol/L)

or

k = 6.4 × basal T_4 concentration (µg/dl)
  + 12.8 × difference between post-TSH and pre-TSH T_4 concentration (µg/dl)

Dogs with k values <15 are considered hypothyroid; those with values >30 are considered euthyroid. Alternative diagnostic tests are used in dogs with k values between 15 and 30.

Thyroid Gland Biopsy

Histologic examination of thyroid gland tissue is a reliable means of diagnosing primary hypothyroidism in dogs. It is the best means to confirm lymphocytic thyroiditis. The major disadvantage of this diagnostic test is the anesthetic and surgical risk involved.

KEY POINT ▶ The TSH stimulation test is currently the best means of confirming hypothyroidism in dogs.

Treatment

Treatment of canine hypothyroidism involves daily thyroid hormone supplementation. Clinical signs of the disease usually resolve completely within a few months of initiation of thyroid hormone replacement. Care is taken to confirm the diagnosis before initiating therapy, because lifelong thyroid hormone replacement therapy is required in dogs with hypothyroidism.

Synthetic L-Thyroxine (L-T₄)

L-T_4 is the hormone replacement compound of choice for treatment of dogs with hypothyroidism. Various inexpensive commercial preparations are available, and their use is widespread.

- Dosage of L-T_4 is 0.01 to 0.02 mg/kg, PO, q12h.
- In large dogs, it is advisable to calculate the dosage of L-T_4 based on body surface area, which is proportional to metabolic rate, rather than on body weight. In these cases, the dose of L-T_4 is 0.5 mg/m², PO, q12h. (See sec. 3, ch. 5 for estimation of surface area.)
- Monitor for signs of hyperthyroidism (e.g., polyuria, polydipsia, tachycardia, restlessness, diarrhea, very high serum T_4 and T_3 concentrations).
- Adjust the dose of L-T_4 based on clinical signs and measurement of serum T_4 concentrations, usually 2 weeks after beginning therapy. Serum T_4 concentrations should be high-normal to slightly high when checked at expected "peak" concentrations (4 to 8 hours "post-pill").

Synthetic L-Triiodothyronine (L-T₃)

This is not recommended for treatment.

Synthetic L-T₃ and L-T₄

These combinations are not recommended for treatment.

KEY POINT ▶ The thyroid hormone supplementation of choice for treating dogs with hypothyroidism is L-thyroxine (L-T_4).

FELINE HYPOTHYROIDISM

Naturally occurring hypothyroidism is extremely rare in the cat. Most clinical cases of feline hypothyroidism occur as a result of treatment for hyperthyroidism—also a rare occurrence. Noniatrogenic feline hypothyroidism has been reported only in kittens that are presented for dwarfism. Cretinism is the most common cause of endocrine congenital dwarfism in cats (growth hormone deficiency has not been reported in cats).

KEY POINT ▶ Spontaneous hypothyroidism is extremely uncommon in cats.

Etiology

Congenital hypothyroidism is associated with thyroid gland atrophy or defective thyroid hormone biosynthesis. In many kittens, this condition may go undetected and result in early death.

Primary iatrogenic hypothyroidism results from surgical removal of thyroid glands or destruction by radioactive iodine in the treatment of feline hyperthyroidism.

Clinical Signs

Congenital Hypothyroidism

- Disproportionate dwarfism (stunted growth of long bones, enlarged head)
- Lethargy and mental dullness
- Hypothermia
- Bradycardia
- Bilaterally symmetric alopecia does *not* occur.

Primary Iatrogenic Hypothyroidism

- History of treatment for hyperthyroidism
- Lethargy
- Seborrhea sicca, dry haircoat
- Obesity is common
- Bilaterally symmetric alopecia does *not* occur.

Diagnosis

- Strong index of suspicion based on history and clinical signs.
- Confirmed by finding subnormal resting serum T_4 concentration that fails to increase 4 to 6 hours after IV administration of TSH (see Hypothyroidism in Dogs).

Treatment

- Treatment for congenital cretinism is not total because growth abnormalities and mental deficiencies may not be alleviated.
- Treatment for iatrogenic hypothyroidism involves daily T_4 supplementation.
  - Initial dosage of T_4 is 0.01 to 0.02 mg/kg (10 to 20 μg/kg) per day, PO.
  - Dosage is adjusted based on resolution of clinical signs and on post-pill serum T_4 concentrations.

FELINE HYPERTHYROIDISM

Feline hyperthyroidism, a multisystemic metabolic disorder resulting from excessive circulating concentrations of thyroid hormone, is the most common endocrinopathy of middle-aged and old cats. There is no breed or sex predilection. The clinical signs of the disease are the result of increased basal metabolic rate and the inability to meet excessive metabolic demands.

Etiology

- *Functional adenomatous hyperplasia of one or both lobes of the thyroid gland,* causing high circulating concentrations of T_4 and T_3, is the most common cause. Both lobes are enlarged in approximately 70% of cases. The pathogenesis of this adenomatous hyperplasia is unknown.
- *Thyroid carcinoma* occurs in only 1 to 2% of cats with hyperthyroidism. Feline hyperthyroidism most closely resembles the toxic nodular goiter in human patients that is also caused by hyperfunctioning adenomatous thyroid nodules.

Clinical Signs

All of the clinical manifestations of hyperthyroidism are due to the effects of excessive thyroid hormones. These effects are generally stimulatory. They cause increased heat production and heightened protein, carbohydrate, and lipid metabolism in virtually all body systems and tissues. Clinical signs can range from mild to severe (Table 2).

KEY POINT ▶ The classic clinical signs of feline hyperthyroidism include weight loss despite an increase in appetite.

General Appearance and Behavior

- Weight loss
- Restlessness, hyperexcitability, difficult to examine
- Impaired stress tolerance. The feline patient is prone to respiratory distress and weakness when stressed. Cardiac arrhythmias or arrest can occur in extreme cases.
- Unkempt haircoat, excessive shedding and matting of hair, especially in long-haired cats, are seen.

Thyroid Gland

- Enlargement of one or both lobes of the thyroid gland is palpable in more than 90% of cats with hyperthyroidism. To palpate the thyroid gland, extend the cat's neck and tilt the head back slightly. Using the thumb and forefinger, gently palpate the tissue on either side of the trachea, starting at the

TABLE 2. Frequency of Historical and Clinical Signs in Cats with Hyperthyroidism

Clinical Findings	Percent (%) of Cats
Weight loss	95–98
Hyperactivity/difficult to examine	70–80
Polyphagia	65–75
Tachycardia	55–65
Polyuria/polydipsia	45–55
Cardiac murmur	20–55
Vomiting	33–50
Diarrhea	30–45
Increased fecal volume	10–30
Decreased appetite	20–30
Lethargy	15–25
Polypnea (panting)	15–30
Muscle weakness	15–20
Muscle tremor	15–30
Congestive heart failure	10–15
Dyspnea	10–15

larynx and moving caudally to the thoracic inlet (see sec. 1, ch. 1).

■ A small percentage of cats have intrathoracic thyroid nodules that evade palpation.

Nervous System and Muscle

■ Hyperactivity
■ Weakness and increased fatigability

Gastrointestinal System

■ Increased appetite is due to increased energy utilization and high metabolic demands. The increased caloric intake observed in most cats is, however, inadequate to compensate for increased demand.
■ Decreased appetite. Approximately 10% of cats with hyperthyroidism experience periods of decreased appetite. The cause is unclear.
■ Vomiting, often secondary to polyphagia, occurs shortly after eating.
■ Diarrhea and increased volume and frequency of defecation are due to polyphagia, intestinal hypermotility, and decreased fat absorption.

Renal System

■ Polyuria/polydipsia. Thyroid hormones may have a diuretic action. Alternatively, a hypothalamic disturbance associated with hyperthyroidism might cause primary polydipsia, with secondary renal medullary solute washout.

Respiratory System

■ Dyspnea, panting, and hyperventilation at rest are attributable to any of the following: respiratory muscle weakness, increased tissue carbon dioxide production, inability to meet tissue oxygen demand, and congestive heart failure (see subsequent discussion).

Cardiovascular System

■ Tachycardia, systolic murmurs, gallop rhythm, and other arrhythmias. These signs can be attributable to the catecholamine-like effects of thyroid hormone and increased tissue oxygen demand, or they may be associated with other signs of congestive heart failure (CHF) secondary to hyperthyroidism.
■ Signs of CHF (e.g., dyspnea, muffled heart sounds, tachycardia, ascites) may develop, especially in cats with severe or advanced hyperthyroidism. Electrocardiographic and echocardiographic findings are often suggestive of hypertrophic or, much less commonly, dilative cardiomyopathy. Hyperthyroidism results in a high-output cardiac state in which vascular resistance is low and cardiac output is high due to increased tissue metabolism and oxygen requirements. The cardiac compensatory mechanisms are dilation (in response to volume overload) and hypertrophy (in response to dilation). There also appears to be a direct myopathic effect of thyroid hormones on cardiac muscle.

Apathetic Hyperthyroidism

■ In about 10% of cats with hyperthyroidism, the predominant clinical signs are depression, lethargy, anorexia, and weakness rather than hyperexcitability, restlessness, and polyphagia observed in 90% of cases.
■ Weight loss and cardiac abnormalities are common findings in these cats.

Diagnosis

The diagnosis of feline hyperthyroidism is made on the bases of clinical signs; palpable goiter (thyroid enlargement); and, except in cases of occult hyperthyroidism (see subsequent discussion), high serum T_4 concentrations. Serum T_3 concentrations are less useful in diagnosis of feline hyperthyroidism. The differential diagnosis for cats with clinical signs of hyperthyroidism includes diabetes mellitus, renal disease, gastrointestinal lymphoma, and chronic inflammatory bowel disease. Cardiac manifestations of hyperthyroidism can be confused with cardiomyopathy. Cats with elevated serum liver enzyme levels can be difficult to distinguish from cats with primary liver disease.

Screening Laboratory Tests

■ Complete blood count
  • Mature leukocytosis and eosinopenia are common findings.
  • A slight elevation in packed cell volume (PCV) is found in more than half of cats with hyperthyroidism. Macrocytic erythrocytes may cause an elevated mean corpuscular volume (MCV).
■ Serum biochemical analysis
  • High alanine aminotransferase (ALT), aspartate aminotransferase (AST), and serum alkaline phosphatase (SAP) activity occur singly or in combination in 50 to 75% of cats with hyperthyroidism.

Thyroid Hormone Measurement

■ Increase resting serum concentrations of T_4 and, less reliably, T_3 are the biochemical hallmarks of hyperthyroidism in the majority of cats with the disease.
■ Some cats (5 to 10%) maintain normal serum T_3 concentrations despite elevations in T_4. These cats generally have milder disease. Serum T_3 concentrations in these cats is expected to increase eventually.
■ Thyroid hormone concentrations in some cats are subject to a degree of fluctuation. In cats with mild disease, serum T_4 concentrations have been shown to fluctuate in and out of the normal range. The finding of a single normal serum T_4 concentration, along with the clinical signs of hyperthyroidism, does not rule out the diagnosis of this disease, especially if the thyroid enlargement can be palpated.
■ Severe concurrent systemic nonthyroidal illnesses (e.g., renal disease, primary hepatic disease, diabetes mellitus) can cause serum thyroid hormone concentrations to decrease. Because nonthyroidal illness is expected to reduce the serum thyroid hormone concentration into the subnormal range in an euthyroid cat, concomitant hyperthyroidism is suspected in any

middle-aged to old cat with high-normal serum T_4 concentration associated with severe, nonthyroidal illness, especially if the clinical signs of hyperthyroidism are also present.

KEY POINT ▶ In most cats with hyperthyroidism, the diagnosis can be confirmed by the finding of a high serum T_4 concentration alone.

Thyroid Radionuclide Uptake and Imaging

- Increased thyroidal uptake of radioiodine after the administration of a small tracer dose of radionuclide is a characteristic finding in hyperthyroidism in cats. However, the relative lack of nuclear medicine facilities available to small animal practitioners limits the usefulness of this diagnostic modality.
- Thyroid imaging (scanning) can be performed with either radioiodine or pertechnetate and is useful in delineating hyperfunctioning thyroid tissue. This technique is a helpful adjunct in the diagnosis of feline hyperthyroidism and provides valuable preoperative information. The disadvantage is that nuclear medicine facilities are required.

Diagnosis of Occult Hyperthyroidism

Some cats with early or mild hyperthyroidism have high-normal resting serum T_4 concentrations despite the presence of clinical signs of thyrotoxicosis. This condition is referred to as occult hyperthyroidism.

Basal Thyroid Hormone Determinations. If a high-normal serum T_4 concentration is found in a cat suspected of having hyperthyroidism, the measurement is repeated a few weeks later. Fluctuation of thyroid hormone concentrations in and out of the normal range has been documented in cats with early, mild hyperthyroidism.

T_3 Suppression Test. Administration of exogenous T_3 causes suppression of pituitary TSH secretion and a subsequent drop in thyroidal T_4 secretion in the normal cat. In cats with autonomously hyperfunctioning thyroid adenomas, TSH secretion has been chronically suppressed and exogenous T_3 administration does not appreciably affect the pituitary-thyroid axis. The protocol for the T_3 suppression test is as follows:

- Collect a blood sample for T_4 and T_3 measurement.
- Administer oral T_3 (liothyronine: Cytomel; Smith Kline) starting the next morning at a dosage of 25 μg/cat, q8h, for 2 days.
- On the morning of the 3rd day, the cat is given a final 25 μg dose of T_3 before being returned to the veterinarian within 6 hours for blood sampling.
- Serum T_4 and T_3 levels are measured by the same assay on both pre-exogenous and postexogenous T_3 blood samples.
- In cats with hyperthyroidism, minimal, if any, suppression of serum T_4 occurs. A rise in serum T_3 concentrations confirms the owner's compliance in administering the drug to the cat.

Thyrotropin-Releasing Hormone (TRH) Response Test. Administration of TRH at a dose of 0.1 mg/kg causes a two-fold or greater increase in serum T_4 concentrations over basal values at 4 hours. In contrast, serum T_4 concentrations in cats with mild hyperthyroidism generally increase little, if at all, after administration of TRH. The reason for the lack of response is the fact that TSH secretion is chronically suppressed to a great extent in cats with hyperthyroidism. Although the effects are transient, TRH administration causes hypersalivation, tachypnea, and vomiting in most cats. However, this test is less time-consuming than the T_3 suppression test and does not rely on owner compliance.

KEY POINT ▶ In cats with early, mild hyperthyroidism, resting serum T_4 concentrations may be normal. Provocative tests can confirm occult hyperthyroidism.

Treatment

Treatment of hyperthyroidism is usually rewarding and is aimed at reducing circulating concentrations of thyroid hormone. This is accomplished by blocking production of thyroid hormone from the thyroid gland or by destruction or removal of hyperfunctioning adenomatous thyroid tissue. Antithyroid drugs can be administered effectively to block thyroid hormone synthesis but are not curative. The adenomatous thyroid tissue can be removed by surgical thyroidectomy or destroyed by radioiodine therapy. Upon return to euthyroidism, the clinical manifestations of thyrotoxicosis, including cardiac abnormalities, generally resolve completely.

Antithyroid Drugs

- Methimazole (Tapazole; Lilly) and propylthiouracil (PTU) are the two thiourylene antithyroid drugs available in the United States. Both are supplied in tablet form and act by inhibiting synthesis of thyroid hormones.
- PTU is not recommended for cats. This drug produces a high incidence of mild to serious adverse effects, including anorexia, vomiting, lethargy, immune-mediated hemolytic anemia, thrombocytopenia, and development of serum antinuclear antibodies in both normal and hyperthyroid cats.
- Methimazole is better tolerated and safer than PTU in the cat and can be considered the antithyroid drug of choice for hyperthyroidism.
- Initially, methimazole is administered at a dosage of 5 to 15 mg/day, depending on the severity of the hyperthyroid state. Ideally, the methimazole dose is divided q8h to q12h. Some cats have been effectively managed by giving methimazole once a day.
- Complete blood counts, including platelets, and serum T_4 determinations are performed every 2 weeks during the first 3 months of drug therapy.
- The daily drug dosage is increased or decreased by 2.5 to 5 mg. Further testing is continued at 2- to 3-week intervals until the lowest daily dose is found that effectively maintains serum T_4 concentrations within the low-normal range.
- Mild clinical side effects associated with methimazole treatment are relatively common (approximately

15% of cats) and include anorexia, vomiting, and lethargy. Self-induced excoriations of the face and neck also may develop in a few cats within the first few weeks of therapy.

■ A variety of hematologic abnormalities may develop in cats during treatment with methimazole. Those abnormalities that do not appear to be associated with any adverse effects include eosinophilia, lymphocytosis, and transient leukopenia with a normal differential count. More serious hematologic reactions that develop in a few cats treated with methimazole include severe thrombocytopenia and agranulocytosis (panleukopenia).

■ If serious hematologic reactions develop during methimazole therapy, the drug is stopped and supportive care given. These adverse reactions should resolve within 5 days after the methimazole is withdrawn. Most life-threatening side effects usually develop quickly after beginning the drug again. Alternative therapy with surgery or radioiodine is then considered.

■ Long-term antithyroid drug treatment has advantages over surgery and radioiodine treatment, including the absence of certain complications such as postsurgical hypoparathyroidism. Unlike surgery and radioiodine, antithyroid drug therapy requires no advanced skills, training, or special licensing, and is a practical choice for most practitioners.

KEY POINT ▶ Daily antithyroid drugs can block T_4 secretion and control hyperthyroidism, but surgery or radioiodine can cure the disorder.

Surgical Thyroidectomy

See section on thyroidectomy.

■ Usually successful
■ Preoperative thyroid imaging is useful if available.
■ Modified extracapsular method is more effective for removal of all diseased tissue.

KEY POINT ▶ Methimazole is used for 2 to 4 weeks preoperatively (if possible) to restore euthyroidism and to reduce anesthetic and surgical risks.

■ Monitor for postoperative hypocalcemia secondary to removal or damage of the parathyroid glands (only a risk following bilateral thyroidectomy).
■ Postoperative laryngeal paralysis due to recurrent laryngeal nerve damage occurs uncommonly.
■ After bilateral thyroidectomy, serum T_4 concentrations are often below normal, but thyroid hormone supplementation is rarely needed for periods of longer than 2 to 3 months. Permanent, surgically induced hypothyroidism in cats is rare. Long-term thyroxine replacement is needed only in those cats that develop clinical signs of hypothyroidism (e.g., lethargy, weight gain, dermatopathy) together with persistently low serum T_4 concentrations.

Radioactive Iodine Therapy

■ Usually successful
■ No preoperative medication or anesthesia needed.

■ Lowest incidence of side effects of any treatment modality
■ Radioiodine therapy is not widely available and is not accessible in many areas.
■ Requires adherence to strict radiation safety regulations
■ Treatment protocols vary depending on the facility and the severity of disease.
■ Often expensive

CANINE THYROID NEOPLASIA

Unlike thyroid tumors in cats, the majority of thyroid neoplasms in dogs do not secrete excessive thyroid hormone. Less than 20% of these tumors are associated with hyperthyroidism. Because these tumors can destroy normal thyroid parenchyma, hypothyroidism sometimes occurs.

KEY POINT ▶ Most canine thyroid tumors, unlike feline thyroid tumors, are large invasive carcinomas.

About 90% of canine thyroid tumors are malignant. Local invasion into the larynx; trachea; cervical muscles, vessels, and nerves; and esophagus occurs with great frequency. Distant metastasis, especially to the lungs, is noted in 60 to 80% of cases. The prognosis associated with most of these tumors is poor.

Clinical Signs

See Table 3.

Nonthyrotoxic Thyroid Tumors

Clinical signs are related to the structural damage to the cervical area and metastatic disease.

■ Goiter, palpable cervical mass is often hard and

TABLE 3. Incidence of Clinical Signs in Dogs with Thyroid Tumor

Signs	Percent (%) of Cases
Nontoxic (Euthyroid or Hypothyroid) Thyroid Tumor	
Goiter	100
Respiratory distress/cough	30
Vomiting	10
Dysphagia	10
Anorexia	10
Weight loss	5
Hyperfunctional (Hyperthyroid) Thyroid Tumor	
Goiter	100
Polydipsia/polyuria	95
Weight loss	80
Weakness/fatigue	75
Polyphagia	70
Heat intolerance	60
Nervousness	50
Hyperdefecation/diarrhea	30
Tremor	20

attached to surrounding soft tissues and irregular in shape.
- Respiratory distress, cough
- Vomiting
- Dysphagia
- Anorexia
- Weight loss

Hyperfunctional Thyroid Tumors

See Feline Hyperthyroidism for explanation of similar signs.

- Goiter, palpable cervical mass is often hard and attached to surrounding soft tissues and irregular in shape.
- Polydipsia, polyuria (common)
- Weight loss
- Polyphagia
- Heat and stress intolerance
- Nervousness, hyperexcitability
- Diarrhea, increased volume of feces
- Tremors

KEY POINT ▶ In dogs, most thyroid tumors that result in hyperthyroidism are malignant (carcinoma). Polydipsia and polyuria are very prominent clinical signs.

Diagnosis

Thyroid carcinoma is suspected in any dog with a ventral cervical mass.

- *Thyroid gland biopsy* is mandatory for the diagnosis of thyroid carcinoma.
- *Screening laboratory tests* are performed. Thoracic radiography is an essential part of the diagnostic workup because pulmonary metastasis occurs commonly.
- Unless clinical signs are suggestive of hyperthyroidism or hypothyroidism, *determination of serum thyroid hormone concentrations* is unnecessary.
- *Thyroid imaging (thyroid scan)* can be useful in determining the size and location of neoplastic thyroid tissue.

Treatment

The prognosis for the animal with thyroid carcinoma depends upon the developmental stage and size of the tumor. Small tumors that have not metastasized can sometimes be cured by surgical excision. For patients with more extensive tumors or tumors that have metastasized, the prognosis is usually poor and treatment is rarely curative regardless of the modality.

Surgery

See section on thyroidectomy.
- Can be a difficult procedure
- Successful removal of all thyroid carcinoma tissue is very rare.

Chemotherapy

See also sec. 3, ch. 5, Oncology.
- Doxyrubicin 30 mg/m² body surface area (for con-

version table, see sec. 3, ch. 5), IV, every 3 weeks for five treatments.
- This drug's most limiting chronic toxicosis is congestive cardiomyopathy.
- Combination treatment with doxyrubicin and cyclophosphamide has been used with varying degrees of success and with less cardiac toxicity.

External Beam (Cobalt) Irradiation

- Useful adjunct therapy for thyroid carcinoma
- Combination of surgical debulking followed by external irradiation may be considered in those rare cases in which most of the tumor was resected.

Radioactive Iodine

- Administration of large doses of ¹³¹I (10 to 100 mCi) can temporarily control hyperfunctional thyroid carcinomas and can lead to palliation of clinical signs of hyperthyroidism. However, this treatment will most likely fail to control metastatic growth.
- Radioiodine will not work well in dogs with nontoxic thyroid tumors that have a low degree of radioiodine uptake.

THYROIDECTOMY

Thyroidectomy in dogs and cats is usually performed to treat neoplasia of the gland. Biopsy is occasionally performed but not as commonly as the complete removal of one or both lobes. A thorough understanding of thyroid anatomy and physiology is necessary prior to performing surgery.

Anatomy

Thyroid

- The thyroid gland consists of two lobes located just caudal to the larynx.
- The normal gland is pale tan and approximately 1 to 1.5 cm in length.
- Blood supply is via the cranial thyroid artery (branch of the common carotid artery (Fig. 1). The caudal

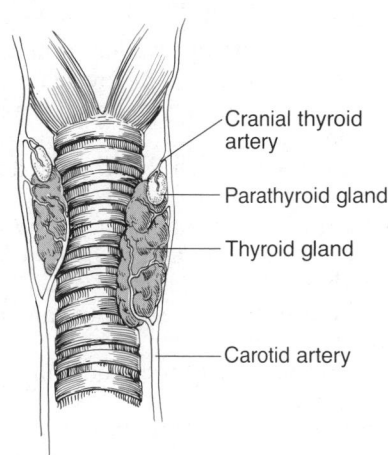

Figure 1. Gross appearance of bilateral thyroid tumors in a cat.

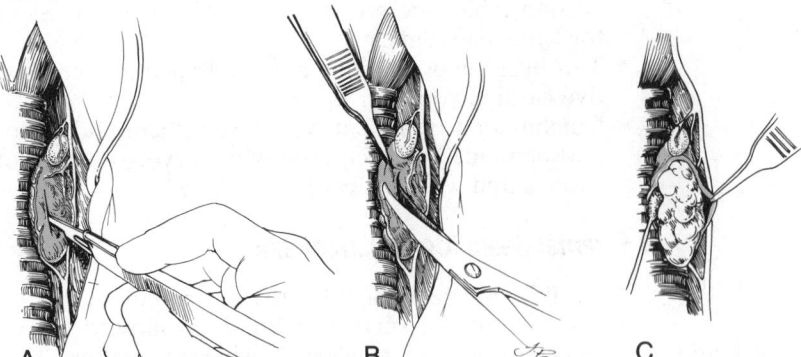

Figure 2. Intracapsular dissection for removal of a thyroid tumor in a cat. Make a nick incision (A) in a relatively avascular area of the thyroid capsule and extend the incision with scissors (B). Bluntly remove the gland from the capsule using a sterile cotton-tipped applicator (C). Ligate or cauterize blood vessels as necessary.

thyroid artery is absent in cats. Venous drainage is via cranial and caudal thyroid veins.
■ The thyroid gland has a distinct but thin capsule.

Parathyroid

■ Two parathyroid glands are associated with each thyroid lobe: one intracapsular (internal) and one extracapsular (external). The extracapsular parathyroid gland is usually located at the cranial pole of the thyroid.
■ The parathyroid is usually off-white and can be confused with fat; the gland is usually 2 to 5 mm in length.
■ Blood supply to the parathyroid glands is also from the cranial thyroid artery.
■ Only one functional parathyroid gland is required for normocalcemia.

Thyroidectomy in the Cat

Preoperative Considerations

■ If available, review the thyroid radionuclide scan to determine the extent of the disease (e.g., Is the tumor unilateral or bilateral? Are ectopic tumors present?).
■ Hyperthyroidism is a multisystemic disease that can be associated with anesthetic and surgical complications.
■ In addition to establishing euthyroidism with antithyroid drugs (see earlier section in this chapter), correct dehydration preoperatively if necessary.
■ Obtain thoracic radiographs to evaluate the heart's size and the presence of any pulmonary problems or mediastinal masses.
■ Anesthesia (see sec. 1, ch 2 for drug dosages and other specifics).
   • Premedicate with acepromazine. Avoid anticholinergics, such as atropine and glycopyrrolate.
   • Induce with a thiobarbiturate IV.
   • Maintain anesthesia with isoflurane and oxygen via a cuffed endotracheal tube.
   • Closely monitor the electrocardiogram for arrhythmias.
   • Have propranolol (Inderal; Wyeth-Ayerst) ready in the event that premature ventricular contractions develop. Dilute to make a solution of 0.1

mg/ml and give 0.01 mg IV slowly (over 3 to 5 minutes).

Surgical Procedure

Objectives
1. Remove all abnormal thyroid tissue.
2. Maintain meticulous hemostasis.
3. Preserve at least one of the parathyroid glands.

Equipment
1. Standard surgical pack
2. Bipolar cautery
3. Tenotomy scissors
4. Sterile cotton-tipped applicators
5. Gelfoam

Technique

1. Place the cat in dorsal recumbancy with the front legs tied caudally and the neck slightly hyperextended with a rolled towel.
2. Prepare the ventral cervical region from caudal mandibles to manubrium for aseptic surgery.
3. Incise the skin on the ventral cervical midline from larynx to manubrium.
4. Separate the paired sternohyoideus and sternothyroideus muscles and retract the muscles with self-retaining retractors.
5. Carefully examine both thyroid lobes. Remove the affected lobes. If doubt exists as to involvement of a lobe, remove it because microscopic adenomatous hyperplasia may be present.
6. Attempt to identify the parathyroid glands.
7. Ligate the caudal thyroid vein and grasp the caudal aspect of capsule.
8. Dissection as in Figures 2 and 3.
   Use the intracapsular technique if the parathyroid glands are not visible (see Fig. 2). When implementing the intracapsular technique, be sure to remove all remnants of thyroid tissue that may remain attached to the capsule. Employ the extracapsular technique if the parathyroid glands are visible and can be easily separated from the thyroid (see Fig. 3).
   Maintain meticulous hemostasis with judicious use of bipolar cautery and small pieces of Gelfoam.
9. Routinely close muscle, subcutaneous tissue, and

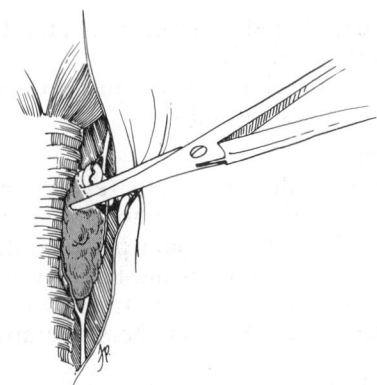

Figure 3. Extracapsular dissection for removal of a thyroid lobe in a cat. Incise the thyroid capsule immediately adjacent to the parathyroid gland. Carefully cauterize capsular blood vessels, if necessary. Bluntly separate the thyroid gland from the parathyroid gland using a sterile cotton-tipped applicator. After ligating or cauterizing blood vessels as necessary, remove the thyroid gland and its capsule.

skin. This is the same as that in the dog, as discussed in the section that follows.

Postoperative Care and Complications

■ Monitor for hypothermia, hemorrhage at the incision site, and hypocalcemia.
■ Hypoparathyroidism
  • Rare with careful surgical technique (5% incidence of hypocalcemic tetany)
  • Check serum calcium concentrations for 48 hours postoperatively or longer if the concentration is dropping.
  • Monitor for tetany if calcium concentration is dropping.
  • Treatment of hypoparathyroidism is described in sec. 4, ch 2.
■ Thyroid hormone replacement (see previous discussion on iatrogenic feline hypothyroidism).
■ Relapse of hyperthyroidism is rare (10% incidence, 2 to 3 years postoperatively) but does occur, probably because of the incomplete removal of adenomatous tissue. Treat by surgical removal of remaining thyroid tissue. The incidence of hypoparathyroidism is higher than with the first surgery.

Thyroidectomy in the Dog
Preoperative Considerations

■ Accurate preoperative diagnosis is important. Fine needle aspirate or tissue biopsy of the thyroid tumor helps establish the type of tumor.

KEY POINT ▶ Biopsy of thyroid tumors in the dog can result in significant hemorrhage. Observe the patient closely after biopsy.

■ Cervical radiographs may be helpful to determine the presence of tracheal displacement or tumor calcification. Thoracic radiographs are mandatory to rule out the diagnosis of pulmonary metastasis or other cardiopulmonary disorder.

Surgical Procedure
Objectives
1. Completely remove or debulk the thyroid mass.

2. Preserve at least one parathyroid gland.
3. Minimize blood loss.
4. Preserve recurrent laryngeal nerves.

Equipment
1. Standard general surgical pack and sutures
2. Gelpi or Weitlaner retractors
3. Army-Navy retractors
4. Penrose drains

Technique

1. Patient preparation and surgical approach are same as those described for the cat.
2. Dissection
   a. These tumors are very vascular, and dissection is difficult.
   b. Avoid injury to the esophagus, carotid artery, jugular vein, vagosympathetic trunk, and recurrent laryngeal nerve (Fig. 4).
   c. A stomach tube or small endotracheal tube in the esophagus helps identify this structure.
   d. Ligate or cauterize the extensive vascular network and carefully dissect out the tumor (Fig. 5).
   e. If possible, identify and preserve the parathyroid glands. With large malignant tumors, this step may be impossible.
   f. If complete removal is impossible, debulk the mass, leaving the portion closest to the larynx intact to preserve the parathyroid glands.
3. Closure
   a. Place Penrose drains if significant dead space results from tumor removal.
   b. Close the muscle routinely with simple continuous, absorbable suture; the subcutaneous tissue

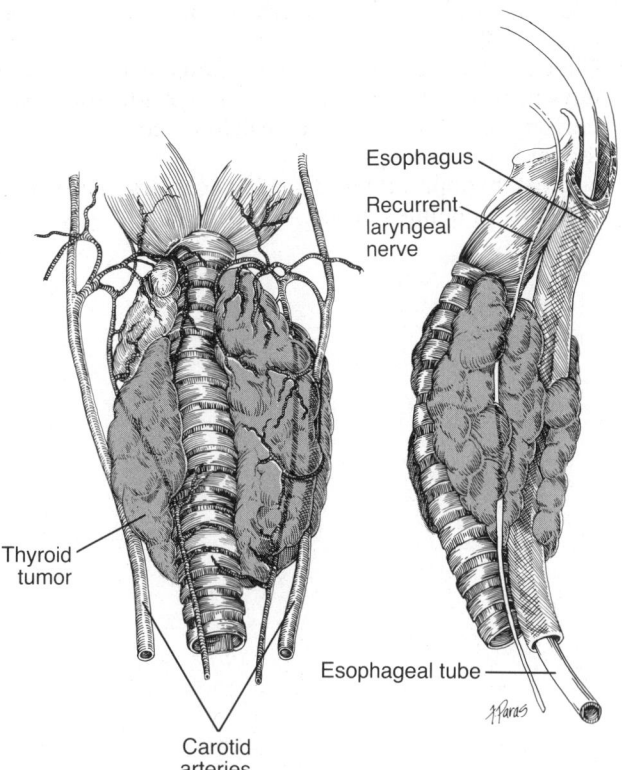

Figure 4. Gross appearance of a thyroid carcinoma in a dog.

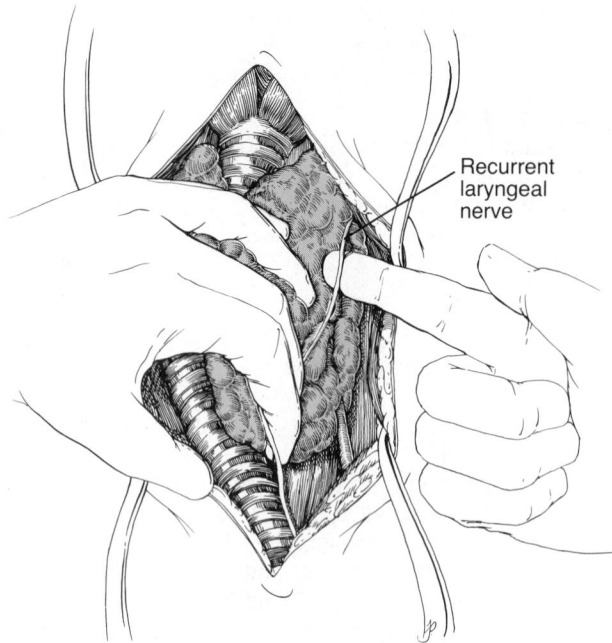

Recurrent
laryngeal
nerve

Figure 5. Remove canine thyroid tumors with a combination of blunt and sharp dissection. Finger dissection of the tumor and surrounding structures may be necessary for large invasive tumors. Be careful when handling the recurrent laryngeal nerve to avoid the possibility of postoperative laryngeal paralysis.

with simple continuous, absorbable suture; and the skin with simple interrupted, nonabsorbable suture.

Postoperative Care and Complications

Short-term

- Closely monitor for hemorrhage or seroma formation.
- Check serum calcium concentrations at least 2 to 4 days postoperatively if a bilateral thyroidectomy was performed. Monitor the calcium concentrations longer if decreasing.
  - Treat hypoparathyroidism if necessary, according to the guidelines in sec. 4, ch. 2.

- Check serum T_3 and T_4 levels if bilateral thyroidectomy is performed.
  - Treat hypothyroidism if present (see previous discussion of hypothyroidism).

Long-term

- Re-evaluate the dog frequently (every 3 months) for recurrence of the primary tumor and metastasis.
- Adjunctive therapy. Consider postoperative chemotherapy or radiotherapy if the tumor was malignant (see previous discussion on treatment of thyroid tumors and sec. 3, ch. 5 on chemotherapy).

Supplemental Readings

Birchard SJ, Peterson ME, Jacobson A: Surgical treatment of feline hyperthyroidism: Results of 85 cases. J Am Anim Hosp Assoc 20:705, 1984.

Evans HE, Christensen GC: *Miller's Anatomy of the Dog*, Philadelphia: WB Saunders, 1979, p 611.

Harari J, Patterson JS, Rosenthal RC: Clinical and pathologic features of thyroid tumors in 26 dogs. J Am Vet Med Assoc 188:1160, 1986.

Leav I, Shiller AC, Rijnberk A, et al.: Adenomas and carcinomas of the canine and feline thyroid. Am J Pathol 83:61, 1976.

Peterson ME, Kintzer PP, Cavanagh PG, Fox PR, et al.: Feline hyperthyroidism: Pretreatment clinical and laboratory evaluation of 131 cases. J Am Vet Med Assoc 183:103, 1983.

Peterson ME, Kintzer PP, Hurvitz AI: Methimazole treatment of 262 cats with hyperthyroidism. J Vet Intern Med 2:150, 1988.

Peterson ME, Kintzer PP, Becker DV, Hurley JM: Radioactive iodine treatment of a functional thyroid carcinoma producing hyperthyroidism in a dog. J Vet Intern Med 3:20, 1989.

Peterson ME: Treatment of feline hyperthyroidism. *In* Kirk RW, Bonagura JD, eds.: *Current Veterinary Therapy X*. Philadelphia: W. B. Saunders, 1989, p 1002.

Peterson ME: Feline hypothyroidism. *In* Kirk RW, Bonagura JD, eds.: *Current Veterinary Therapy X*. Philadelphia: W. B. Saunders, 1989, p 1000.

Peterson ME, Ferguson DC: Thyroid diseases. *In* Ettinger SJ, ed.: *Textbook of Veterinary Internal Medicine: Diseases of the Dog and Cat*. Philadelphia: W. B. Saunders, 1989, p 1632.

Peterson ME, Graves TK, Gamble DA: Triiodothyronine (T_3) suppression test. An aid in the diagnosis of mild hyperthyroidism in cats. J Vet Intern Med 4:233, 1990.

Rijnberk A, Leav I: Thyroid tumors. *In* Kirk RW, ed.: *Current Veterinary Therapy X*. Philadelphia: W. B. Saunders, 1977, p 1020.

Welches CD, Scavelli TD, Matthiesen DT, Peterson ME: Occurrence of problems after three techniques of bilateral thyroidectomy in cats. Vet Surg 18:392, 1989.

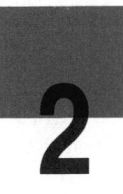

2

Disorders of the Parathyroid Gland and Calcium Metabolism

Marcia Carothers
Dennis Chew
Tom Van Gundy

NORMAL CALCIUM METABOLISM

The calcium ion is a major component of bone and is very important in many biologic processes such as muscle contraction, blood coagulation, neural excitability, membrane permeability, and enzyme activity. Although calcium is the most abundant electrolyte in the body, most of this ion is present in the skeleton and is not available for immediate use.

Distribution

There are three major fractions of serum calcium: protein-bound, ionized (or free), and complex-bound calcium.

Protein-Bound Calcium. This fraction accounts for approximately 40% of the total serum calcium concentration. Albumin is the primary protein bound to calcium; this binding increases as the pH increases and decreases as the pH decreases.

Ionized or Free Calcium. This is the biologically active form of calcium and makes up approximately 50% of the total serum calcium concentration.

Complex-Bound Calcium. Complex-bound calcium composes approximately 10% of the total serum calcium concentration. This form is bound to anions such as lactates, bicarbonates, citrates, and sulfates.

KEY POINT ▶ The partitioning of calcium is influenced by the amount of calcium entering and leaving the extracellular fluid, the quantity of protein available for binding, and the acid-base status.

Measurement of Serum Calcium

Colorimetric Methods. Colorimetric measurements of serum calcium are subject to spurious results if lipemia or hemolysis is present.

Potentiometry. This ion-selective method has the advantage of measuring total and ionized calcium concentrations. However, this technique requires special handling of the sample (i.e., anaerobically maintained) and is not readily available at most laboratories.

Corrected Total Calcium Values. These are calculated to adjust for abnormalities in serum protein or albumin concentrations. The following formulas are helpful guidelines for interpreting serum calcium under conditions of hypoproteinemia or hypoalbuminemia.

Corrected total calcium (mg/dl) =
  Serum total calcium (mg/dl)
  − serum albumin (gm/dl) + 3.5
      or
Serum total calcium (mg/dl)
  − 0.4 [serum total protein (gm/dl)] + 3.3

Regulation of Calcium

Calcium levels are regulated primarily through the actions of three hormones: parathyroid hormone (PTH), calcitonin, and vitamin D.

Parathyroid Hormone. PTH is produced by the chief cells of the parathyroid glands and is the principal hormone that controls minute-to-minute regulation of serum calcium concentration. Secretion of this hormone is stimulated by hypocalcemia. Hydroxylation of 25-hydroxycholecalciferol to 1,25-dihydroxycholecalciferol and other vitamin D metabolites is partially regulated by PTH. The major target organs are bone and kidneys.

- Bone—PTH mobilizes calcium from the skeletal reserves to the extracellular fluid (ECF).
- Kidney—PTH has a direct effect on renal tubular function, leading to decreased phosphate resorption and phosphaturia and increased absorption of calcium.

KEY POINT ▶ The net effect of PTH is to increase serum calcium and decrease serum phosphorus concentrations.

Calcitonin. This polypeptide is secreted by the C (parafollicular) cells of the thyroid glands. The rate of secretion increases with increased calcium concentration. Bone and kidneys are the major target organs.

- Bone—Calcitonin blocks bone resorption by inhibiting the release of calcium and phosphorus from bone.
- Kidney—Calcitonin decreases the resorption of phosphorus and calcium.

KEY POINT ▶ The net effect of calcitonin is to decrease the serum calcium and phosphorus concentrations.

Vitamin D. Vitamin D (ergosterol and cholecalciferol) primarily affects bone, intestines, and kidneys. Small amounts of 1,25-dihydroxycholecalciferol (the active metabolite of vitamin D) are necessary for the PTH effect on bone (permissive effect).

- Bone—Vitamin D metabolites stimulate osteoclastic calcium mobilization and resorption of bone.
- Intestine—Vitamin D increases calcium, phosphorus, and magnesium absorption.
- Kidney—Vitamin D increases renal tubular resorption of calcium and phosphorus.

KEY POINT ▶ The net effect of vitamin D is to increase both serum calcium and phosphorus concentrations.

HYPERCALCEMIA

The definition of hypercalcemia is a fasting serum total calcium concentration >12.0 mg/dl in dogs and >11.0 mg/dl in cats. Young dogs may have a mild hypercalcemia (usually <13.0 mg/dl) related to skeletal growth. Lipemic and/or hemolyzed blood samples may result in spurious elevations of calcium and should be interpreted with caution.

Etiology

See Table 1 for list of etiologies of hypercalcemia.

Clinical Signs

The development of clinical signs from hypercalcemia depends on the magnitude of the calcium elevation, how quickly the hypercalcemia developed, and the duration of the hypercalcemia. Serum total calcium concentrations of <15 mg/dl may not be associated with systemic signs; however, serum concentrations of >18 mg/dl are often associated with severe life-threatening signs. Abnormalities in sodium and potassium may magnify clinical signs of hypercalcemia because of their effects on cell membrane permeability, particularly in nerve and muscle. Soft tissue mineralization may occur with prolonged hypercalcemia when the product of calcium (mg/dl) times phosphorus (mg/dl) equals 70.

- Polydipsia and polyuria are the most common signs of hypercalcemia, owing to direct stimulation of the thirst center and a decreased ability of the kidneys to concentrate the urine.
- Anorexia, vomiting, and constipation can result from decreased excitability of gastrointestinal smooth muscle.
- Generalized weakness may develop from decreased muscle excitability.
- Depression, muscle twitching, and seizures can occur as neurologic manifestations.
- Cardiac arrhythmias can develop from direct effects on the myocardium or secondary to cardiac mineralization.

Diagnostic Evaluation

Abnormalities depend on the underlying cause, severity, and duration of the hypercalcemia (see Conditions Associated with Hypercalcemia).

History and Physical Examination. A complete history and thorough examination are essential to the diagnosis of the cause of the hypercalcemia.

Laboratory Tests. Tests such as serum calcium assay, complete blood count (CBC), and serum chemistry profile can aid in the diagnosis.

Radiography. Soft tissue mineralization of the kidneys, heart, lungs, stomach, and other tissues may be present radiographically.

Electrocardiography. Prolongation of the PR interval, shortening of the QT interval, and cardiac arrhythmias (ventricular fibrillation) may develop with severe hypercalcemia.

Principles of Treatment of Hypercalcemia

The definitive treatment of hypercalcemia is treating or removing the underlying cause. Unfortunately, the etiology may not be apparent, and supportive measures must be taken to decrease the serum calcium concentration (see Table 2 for specific drugs and dosage recommendations). Supportive measures may include the following.

Volume Expansion. Volume expansion with intravenous 0.9% NaCl solution decreases hemoconcentration and encourages renal calcium loss by improving glomerular filtration rate and sodium excretion, which results in less calcium resorption.

Loop Diuretics. Diuretics such as furosemide increase calcium excretion; however, high doses may be needed (see Table 2). The use of diuretics in a dehy-

---

TABLE 1. Conditions Associated with Hypercalcemia

Nonpathologic Conditions
Lipemia
Non-fasted serum samples
Young growing dogs
Laboratory error or improper handling of sample

Transient Conditions
Hemoconcentration
Hyperproteinemia

Pathologic Conditions
Malignancy-associated hypercalcemia
  Lymphoma
  Adenocarcinoma of the apocrine glands of the anal sac
  Multiple myeloma
  Metastatic bone tumors
  Miscellaneous tumors (lymphocytic leukemia, mammary carcinoma, fibrosarcoma, pancreatic adenocarcinoma, testicular interstitial cell tumor, lung carcinoma, squamous cell carcinoma, thyroid adenocarcinoma, and osteosarcoma)
Hypoadrenocorticism
Renal failure
Hypervitaminosis D
  Cholecalciferol (rodenticide) toxicity
  Iatrogenic—dietary supplementation
  Houseplants (*Cestrus diurnum*, day-blooming jessamine, *Solanum malocoxylon, Triestum flavescens*)
  Granulomatous disease—blastomycosis
Primary hyperparathyroidism
Bone lesions—sepsis, disuse osteoporosis
Severe hypothermia

TABLE 2. Treatment of Hypercalcemia

Treatment	Dose	Indications	Comments
Volume Expansion			
SC saline (0.9%)*	75–100 ml/kg/day	Mild hypercalcemia	Contraindicated if peripheral edema is present
IV saline (0.9%)*	100–125 ml/kg/day	Moderate to severe hypercalcemia	Contraindicated in congestive heart failure and hypertension
Diuretics			
Furosemide (Lasix; Hoechst)	2–4 mg/kg q12h to q8h IV, SC, or PO	Moderate to severe hypercalcemia	Volume expansion necessary prior to use of this drug
Alkalinizing Agent			
Sodium bicarbonate	1 mEq/kg IV slow bolus; may continue at 0.3 × base deficit × kg per day	Severe hypercalcemia	Requires close monitoring
Glucocorticoids			
Prednisone	1–2.2 mg/kg q12h PO, SC, or IV	Moderate to severe hypercalcemia	Do not use these drugs prior to identification of etiology
Dexamethasone (Azium; Schering)	0.1–0.22 mg/kg q12h IV or SC		May make definitive diagnosis difficult
Bone Resorption Inhibitors			
Calcitonin (Calcimar; Rhone-Poulenc-Rorer)	4–6 IU/kg SC q12h to q8h	Hypervitaminosis D toxicity	Response may be short-lived; vomiting may occur
Diphosphonates, EHDP (Didronel; Norwich Eaton)	5 mg/kg daily to q12h	Moderate to severe hypercalcemia	Expensive; use in dogs limited
Mithramycin (plicamycin) (Mithracin; Miles)	25 μg/kg IV in D5W over 2–4 h q2–4 wk	Severe, refractory hypercalcemia	Limited use in dogs and cats; nephrotoxicity, hepatotoxicity
Miscellaneous			
EDTA	25–75 mg/kg/h	Severe, refractory hypercalcemia	Nephrotoxic
Peritoneal dialysis	Low calcium dialysate	Severe, refractory hypercalcemia	Short duration of response; use in hypercalcemia not reported

*Potassium supplementation is necessary. Add 5–40 mEq KCl/liter, depending on serum potassium concentration (see sec. 1, ch. 5).

drated patient is contraindicated because volume contraction and further hemoconcentration may worsen the hypercalcemia. Thiazide diuretics, which will decrease calcium excretion by the kidneys, are contraindicated.

Sodium Bicarbonate. Sodium bicarbonate given as an IV bolus or as a continuous infusion has been shown to decrease serum total calcium concentrations. Although the magnitude of calcium reduction is mild, alkalosis also favors the shift of ionized calcium to protein-bound calcium. Sodium bicarbonate therapy is more beneficial when combined with other treatments.

Glucocorticoids. Glucocorticoids decrease bone resorption of calcium, decrease intestinal calcium absorption, and increase renal calcium excretion, leading to substantial decrease in serum calcium concentration in animals with hypercalcemia secondary to lymphoma, myeloma, hypervitaminosis D, and hypoadrenocorticism.

KEY POINT ▶ The use of glucocorticoids prior to the establishment of the etiology of hypercalcemia may make definitive diagnosis difficult.

Calcitonin. Calcitonin has been reported as an antidote to cholecalciferol toxicity by the manufacturer of a cholecalciferol-based rodenticide. However, decreasing the serum calcium may be a short-term (hours) effect requiring multiple treatments.

Diphosphonates. These compounds inhibit osteoclastic bone resorption, but reports of their use in veterinary medicine have been limited.

Mithramycin. This drug is a potent inhibitor of osteoclastic bone resorption; however, mithramycin has been associated with many serious side effects, such as thrombocytopenia, hepatic necrosis, renal necrosis, and hypocalcemia.

EDTA. Ethylene diaminetetra-acetic acid (EDTA) reduces the ionized fraction of calcium by chelating calcium, which is then excreted by the kidneys. Since EDTA is nephrotoxic, this therapy should be used only for severe refractory hypercalcemia.

Peritoneal Dialysis. This procedure, using a calcium-free dialysate, may be considered as a last resort when other methods fail to decrease serum calcium concentration.

CONDITIONS ASSOCIATED WITH HYPERCALCEMIA

Important conditions are discussed here. For a complete list of hypercalcemia-related conditions, see Table 2.

Hypercalcemia Associated with Malignancy

KEY POINT ▶ Malignancy-associated hypercalcemia is the most common cause of persistent hypercalcemia in dogs and cats.

Hypercalcemia primarily results from increased osteoclastic bone resorption; however, increased renal tubular resorption and increased intestinal absorption also may play a role. Factors that may be produced by tumors and result in humoral hypercalcemia of malignancy (pseudohyperparathyroidism) include PTH, PTH-related protein, transforming growth factor, 1,25-dihydroxycholecalciferol, prostaglandin E_2, osteoclast-activating factor, and other cytokines (interleukin-1, interleukin-2, and gamma interferon).

KEY POINT ▶ In dogs, lymphoma, adenocarcinoma of the apocrine glands of the anal sac, and multiple myeloma are the most common tumors associated with hypercalcemia.

Lymphoma

Lymphoma is the most common tumor associated with hypercalcemia in the dog. (see sec. 3, ch. 6). Of dogs with lymphoma, 10 to 40% have been reported to have concurrent hypercalcemia, and a large number of these have the mediastinal form of lymphoma. Although detectable lymphadenopathy usually is present, hypercalcemia may be the first abnormality noted.

A thorough physical examination, together with thoracic and abdominal radiography, abdominal ultrasonography, multiple lymph node aspirates or biopsies, and multiple bone marrow aspirates may be necessary to make the diagnosis.

Treatment with corticosteroids will decrease the serum calcium; however, their lymphocytic effect makes subsequent identification of lymphoma very difficult. Hypercalcemia lymphomas have a shorter survival time with chemotherapy than normocalcemic lymphomas. The return of hypercalcemia may precede clinical evidence of tumor regrowth in animals undergoing chemotherapy.

Apocrine Gland Adenocarcinoma of the Anal Sac

This tumor usually occurs in older female dogs, with hypercalcemia developing in approximately 90% of cases. Humoral mechanisms are most likely responsible for the hypercalcemia, as a PTH-like protein has been identified from tumor tissue in dogs. The tumor is usually malignant and has metastasized to regional lymph nodes at the time of diagnosis.

Surgical resection is associated with reduction of serum calcium (see sec. 7, ch. 12 for description of surgery). Failure to remove all of the tumor or recurrence of the tumor usually results in the return of hypercalcemia. Despite surgical excision, radiation, and various chemotherapy protocols, the tumor usually recurs, and reported survival times range from 2 to 21 months.

Multiple Myeloma

Multiple myeloma in dogs has been associated with hypercalcemia in 10 to 15% of cases. Humoral factors as well as direct lysis of bone may account for the increased serum calcium. Long-time survival has been reported following treatment of multiple myeloma with chemotherapy (see sec. 3, ch. 6), but the presence of associated hypercalcemia, light chain proteinuria, and extensive bony lesions is associated with a shorter survival time.

Hyperadrenocorticism

Hyperadrenocorticism (Addison's disease) has been associated with mild hypercalcemia (<15 mg/dl) in approximately 20% of dogs with the disease. Multiple factors that may result in the hypercalcemia include increase in calcium citrate (complex calcium), hemoconcentration (relative increase), increase in renal resorption of calcium, and increased affinity of serum proteins for calcium. Although total serum calcium concentrations may be increased, the ionized fraction usually is normal. Resolution of the hypercalcemia occurs quickly with therapy for hypoadrenocorticism (see sec. 4, ch. 3).

Renal Failure

Renal failure occasionally is associated with hypercalcemia of unknown pathogenesis. Familial renal disease is associated more often with hypercalcemia than with other forms of chronic renal failure. Hypercalcemia may be present in acute renal failure during the polyuric phase.

KEY POINT ▶ In renal failure, hypercalcemia is associated with hyperphosphatemia. If hypophosphatemia or normophosphatemia is present, look for another cause of the hypercalcemia.

Hypervitaminosis D

KEY POINT ▶ Hypercalcemia usually is associated with hyperphosphatemia in hypervitaminosis D.

Rodenticides Containing Cholecalciferol

Cholecalciferol-based rodenticides (Quintox Bell Labs; Rampage, CEVA; Rat-Be-Gone, Ortho) have gained popularity over anticoagulant rodenticides because, unlike anticoagulant rodenticides, there is no rodenticide resistance, and there is no secondary toxicity to species that ingest poisoned rodents. Although one manufacturer (Bell Labs) reports the LD_{50} to be 88 mg/kg, toxicity has been seen with much lower doses (<10 mg/kg). Duration of the effect may last for weeks.

Clinical signs are vague and related to the development of hypercalcemia (see previous discussion of Clinical Signs). Hypercalcemia is often severe (serum calcium 15–20 mg/dl) and accompanied by hyperphosphatemia at initial presentation. Azotemia may occur several days after ingestion, secondary to renal damage from hypercalcemia.

The goals of treatment are to:

- Decrease the absorption of cholecalciferol in the gastrointestinal tract.
- Correct the fluid and electrolyte imbalances.
- Reduce the hypercalcemia.

- Treat miscellaneous complications such as seizures and cardiac arrhythmias.

  Corrective measures include:

- A low calcium diet (e.g., Hill's Prescription Diets k/d, u/d, and s/d) and restriction of milk products
- Phosphate binders that do not contain calcium (e.g., aluminum hydroxide, Amphojel, Wyeth; 10–30 mg/kg q8h, PO with meals), which may be helpful in decreasing the calcium:phosphorus product.
- Avoidance of exposure to sunlight to decrease the conversion of 7-dehydroxycholesterol to vitamin D in the skin.

In severe cases of hypercalcemia, aggressive treatment with IV fluids, furosemide, prednisone, and/or calcitonin (see Table 2) may be necessary for several weeks. Because of the prolonged half-life of 25-hydroxycholecalciferol, monitor serum calcium, phosphorus, and creatinine weekly for 4 to 6 weeks. If aggressive therapy is maintained for several weeks, complete recovery is usually achieved.

Iatrogenic Vitamin D Intoxication

Iatrogenic (excessive dietary supplementation, post–vitamin D therapy) vitamin D intoxication has been reported following the administration of vitamin D products. Use of ergocalciferol (vitamin D_2) may cause hypercalcemia because its slow onset of action and prolonged duration make it difficult to dose correctly.

Treatment is directed at discontinuing the supplement or decreasing the dose of vitamin D (see discussion of Hypoparathyroidism, Surgery of the Parathyroid Gland, in this chapter).

Houseplants

Houseplants such as *Cestrus diurnum* (the day-blooming jessamine), *Solanum malacoxylon*, and *Triestum flavescens* contain a substance similar to calcitriol that may cause hypercalcemia when ingested.

Granulomatous Diseases

Granulomatous disorders such as systemic fungal diseases and tuberculosis are rare causes of hypercalcemia in dogs. Serum calcium concentrations return to normal with treatment (e.g., antifungal drugs, surgical removal).

Primary Hyperparathyroidism

Primary hyperparathyroidism results from excessive secretion of PTH by one or more abnormal parathyroid glands. This disease has been reported infrequently in dogs and cats. Persistent hypercalcemia is characteristic of this disease.

Etiology

Primary hyperparathyroidism may be caused by:

- Solitary parathyroid adenoma
- Parathyroid carcinoma (infrequent)
- Parathyroid hyperplasia of one or all four glands (rare)

- Gross enlargement may not be present.
- The diagnosis is made based on microscopic abnormalities.
- Hereditary neonatal parathyroid hyperplasia has been reported in two German shepherd puppies.

Signalment

- Middle-aged or older animals are at risk:
  - Dogs—5 to 13 years, mean age 10 years
  - Cats—8 to 15 years, mean 12.9 years
- There is no sex predilection in dogs; however, of seven reported cats, five were female.
- No breed predilection has been noted, but the keeshond, German shepherd, and Norwegian elkhounds are overrepresented, and five of the seven reported cats were Siamese.

Clinical Signs

- Anorexia, lethargy, and depression are the most common signs, but many animals may be asymptomatic.
- Polydypsia and polyuria are usually present.
- Constipation, weakness, shivering, twitching, vomiting, stiff gait, and facial swelling are less often reported.

Physical Examination

- In dogs, the physical examination is usually normal.
- In cats, 50% may have palpable cervical masses.

Diagnosis

Laboratory Tests. Hypercalcemia, normal to low serum phosphorus, and decreased urine specific gravity are the most consistent findings. Azotemia and increased serum alkaline phosphatase and alanine aminotransferase activity may be present in some patients with moderate hypercalcemia. If renal failure is present, the serum phosphorus may be increased above normal. A high normal or increased PTH concentration (based on comparison with normal values for a validated immunoassay) in hypercalcemic animals with normal renal function is suggestive of primary hyperparathyroidism.

Hemology. The hemogram is usually unremarkable.

Radiography. The radiogram generally is normal but may reveal generalized osteopenia, increased bone resorption typically at the subperiosteal surfaces, and cyst-like areas in bone.

Exploratory Surgery. Exploratory surgery of the cervical region is a diagnostic alternative if no other cause of hypercalcemia can be determined.

- If a parathyroid nodule is not identified, give an IV infusion of methylene blue (3 mg/kg) to aid in the identification of parathyroid tumors.
  - Although complications are uncommon with this technique, hemolysis, acute renal failure, and death have been reported.
- Negative findings may be due to ectopic PTH production (e.g., parathyroid adenoma in the cranial mediastinum or a nonparathyroid tumor producing PTH).

Treatment

Treatment of primary hyperparathyroidism is surgical excision of the parathyroid adenoma. Prior to surgery, attempt to decrease the hypercalcemia with IV fluids (saline) and furosemide (see Table 2; see also discussion of Parathyroidectomy).

HYPOCALCEMIA

Hypocalcemia is defined as a serum total calcium concentration < 8.5–9.0 mg/dl. Normal serum calcium concentration in older dogs may be slightly lower than that in middle-aged dogs.

Etiology

Various causes of hypocalcemia are listed in Table 3. Hypoalbuminemia is the most common cause of a low serum total calcium; however, it is of no clinical consequence because only the protein-bound fraction is affected. A mildly decreased serum calcium without signs of hypocalcemia also is seen in various systemic conditions such as renal failure, pancreatitis, and intestinal malabsorption. In the section that follows, conditions associated with symptomatic hypocalcemia are discussed.

Clinical Signs

The severity of clinical signs may not always be commensurate with the degree of hypocalcemia. Concurrent acid-base disorders, other electrolyte imbalances, and ionized calcium concentration play a role in the development of clinical signs that are often episodic.

■ Tremors, twitching, tetany, muscle spasms, and gait changes (stiffness and ataxia) result from increased

---

TABLE 3. Conditions Associated with Hypocalcemia

Causes of Severe Symptomatic Hypocalcemia
Puerperal tetany/eclampsia
Hypoparathyroidism
   Spontaneous (lymphocytic parathyroiditis)
   Iatrogenic secondary to bilateral thyroidectomy
   Postoperative secondary to removal of parathyroid adenoma/
     carcinoma
   Phosphate enemas (acute hyperphosphatemia causes reciprocal
     calcium decrease)
Causes of Mild Asymptomatic Hypocalcemia
Hypoalbuminemia (most frequent cause of hypocalcemia)
Primary renal disease (see sec. 8, ch. 1)
   Chronic renal failure
   Acute renal failure (urethral obstruction, ethylene glycol
     toxicity)
Pancreatitis (see sec. 7, ch. 10)
Intestinal malabsorption syndromes (see sec. 7, ch. 6)
Chelating agents that bind calcium (EDTA, citrates, oxalates,
   phosphates)
Rhabdomyolysis due to soft tissue trauma
Nutritional secondary hyperparathyroidism
Dilutional with infusion of calcium-free fluids
Laboratory error/artifact
Idiopathic (unexplained)

---

neuromuscular excitability. Occasionally generalized seizure activity may be seen.
■ Behavior changes (restlessness, aggression, panting, hypersensitivity to stimuli, and disorientation) are frequent.
■ Bradycardia, hyperthermia, polyuria, polydipsia, and vomiting are sometimes seen.

Diagnostic Evaluation

History and Physical Examination. A complete history and a thorough physical examination can aid in the diagnosis of the underlying cause of the hypocalcemia.

Routine Laboratory Tests. Tests should include a serum calcium (total and ionized if possible) assay, CBC, and serum chemistry profile.

Electrocardiography. Prolongation of QT interval and ventricular premature contractions may be seen on electrocardiogram (ECG).

See specific diseases discussed below for other diagnostic tests.

Principles of Treatment of Hypocalcemia

The definitive treatment for hypocalcemia is to eliminate the underlying cause. Supportive measures, including the following, to restore normocalcemia can be administered pending the diagnosis (Table 4).

Parenteral Calcium. This may be necessary in patients with active tetany, hyperthermia, and seizures.

■ Calcium gluconate and calcium chloride usually are given by slow IV administration.
■ Signs of toxicity from injection of too much calcium too fast include bradycardia and shortening of the QT interval.
■ Calcium can also be diluted in saline and given as a continuous IV drip to maintain normal serum calcium concentrations (see Table 4).
■ Calcium gluconate (diluted 1:1 with saline) may be given SC.

Oral Calcium. Oral calcium supplementation may be beneficial.

■ The daily requirements are 1–4 g for dogs and 0.5–1 g for cats.
■ Base the dose of calcium on the amount of elemental calcium in the product.

Vitamin D. Vitamin D supplementation usually is necessary to increase calcium absorption in the intestines.

■ Several forms of vitamin D are available, and the response and duration of these drugs depend on the form used.
■ Iatrogenic hypercalcemia is a common complication of treatment.

CONDITIONS ASSOCIATED WITH HYPOCALCEMIA

Puerperal Tetany or Eclampsia

Puerperal tetany or eclampsia occurs in lactating bitches and queens as a result of calcium loss into the

TABLE 4. Treatment of Hypocalcemia

Parenteral Calcium*				
Drug	**Preparation**	**Available Calcium**	**Dose**	**Comment**
Calcium gluconate	10% solution	9.3 mg Ca/ml	Slow IV to effect (0.5–1.5 ml/kg IV) 5–15 mg/kg/h IV 1–2 ml/kg diluted 1:1 with saline SC q8h	Stop if bradycardia or shortened QT interval occurs; infusion to maintain normal Ca may be given SC
Calcium chloride	10% solution	27.2 mg Ca/ml	5–15 mg/kg/h IV	Give only IV, as extremely caustic perivascularly

Oral Calcium†				
Drug	**Preparation**	**Available Calcium (%)**	**Dose**	**Comment**
Calcium carbonate	Many sizes	40% (tab.)	25–50 mg/kg/day	Most common calcium supplement
Calcium lactate	325-, 650-mg (tab.)	13%	25–50 mg/kg/day	
Calcium chloride	Powder	27.2%	25–50 mg/kg/day	
Calcium gluconate	Many sizes (tab.)	10%	25–50 mg/kg/day	May cause gastric irritation

Vitamin D				
Preparation	**Daily Dose**	**Time for Maximal Effect to Occur**	**Time for Toxicity Effect to Resolve**
Vitamin D₂ (ergocalciferol)	Initial: 4000–6000 U/kg/day Maintenance: 1000–2000 U/kg once daily to once weekly	5–21 days	1–18 weeks
Dihydrotachysterol	Initial: 0.02–0.03 mg/kg/day Maintenance: 0.01–0.02 mg/kg q 24–48 h	1–7 days	1–3 weeks
1,25-Dihydroxyvitamin D₃ (calcitriol)	0.03–0.06 μg/kg/day	1–4 days	2–14 days

*Do not mix calcium solution with bicarbonate-containing fluids because precipitation may occur.
†Calculate dose based on elemental calcium content.

milk and poor dietary calcium intake (see Table 3). In nonlactating animals, this condition may be associated with high calcium supplementation resulting in suppression of PTH secretion and increasing calcitonin secretion. These changes decrease the osteoclast pool and availability of bone calcium.

Clinical Signs

- Small bitches with large litters are most often affected; puerperal tetany is rare in large dogs and cats.
- Onset of signs is acute, occurring most often 2 to 4 weeks post partum.
- Tetany, tremors, twitches, and seizures are common.
- Hyperthermia may occur in severe cases.
- Panting and restlessness may be early signs.

Diagnosis

Diagnosis is made based on history, clinical signs, hypocalcemia (total serum calcium usually < 7 mg/dl), and response to treatment.

Treatment

- Immediately give an IV infusion of calcium (slow IV administration to effect; then 5–15 mg/kg/h of elemental calcium).
- Supplement oral calcium (25–50 mg/kg/day of elemental calcium) for the remainder of lactation.

- Supplement vitamin D if serum calcium concentration remains low.
- If tetany recurs during the same lactation, wean the litter from the bitch.

Hypoparathyroidism

The marked hypocalcemia seen in hyperparathyroidism results from a deficiency in PTH. Hypoparathyroidism in dogs and cats may be spontaneous, iatrogenic, or postoperative.

Spontaneous Hypoparathyroidism. Spontaneous hypoparathyroidism occurs uncommonly in dogs and cats.

Iatrogenic Hypoparathyroidism. This form may occur after bilateral thyroidectomy (see sec. 4, ch. 1).

Postoperative Hypoparathyroidism. Hypoparathyroidism secondary to parathyroidectomy for parathyroid adenoma/carcinoma and hyperplasia may occur as a result of atrophy of the remaining glands. Normal function of the glands usually returns in 4 to 6 weeks.

Etiology

- Lymphocytic parathyroiditis and atrophy are the most common causes and presumably are autoimmune.
- Other causes include parathyroid gland destruction (postoperative) ischemia, and agenesis.

Signalment

- In dogs the mean age is 6 years, although a wide age range (6 weeks to 12 years) has been reported. In cats, young to middle-aged patients are reported.
- Females are more commonly reported in dogs, but four of the five reported feline cases were males.
- Canine breeds predisposed to developing hypoparathyroidism include toy poodles, miniature schnauzers, Labrador retrievers, German shepherds, and terriers.

Clinical Signs

- Signs are usually episodic and most often include:
  - Nervousness, tremor, and twitching
  - Rigid limb extension, stiff gait, and muscle spasms
- Other signs include:
  - Ataxia, panting, and episodic weakness
  - Facial rubbing, biting at feet, and aggression
  - Polydipsia and polyuria
  - Vomiting and diarrhea
  - Weight loss, anorexia, depression, and listlessness

Physical Examination

- Neuromuscular findings—extensor rigidity, muscle fasciculations, and seizures
- Cardiac findings—tachycardia, paroxysmal tachyarrhythmias, and weak pulses
- Cataracts—small punctate to linear (reported in a few dogs and cats)

Diagnosis

- Hypocalcemia is severe usually <6 mg/dl.
- Hyperphosphatemia is usually present.
- ECG findings include prolongation of QT and ST segments, deep wide T waves, and tachyarrhythmias.
- PTH concentrations are low compared with normal values for validated immunoassay.
- Parathyroid biopsy confirms lymphocytic parathyroiditis.

Treatment

Treatment of hypoparathyroidism is directed at restoring serum calcium level to the low end of the normal range. Avoid elevating calcium levels above this in order to prevent calcium-induced renal damage due to the lack of PTH (see Table 4 for dosages).

- If hypocalcemic tetany or seizures are present, immediately administer calcium intravenously.
- For maintenance of normocalcemia, supplement oral calcium and vitamin D.

Hypercalcemia. Hypercalcemia is a common complication of vitamin D therapy and may be delayed and prolonged depending on the type of vitamin D supplementation used. Monitor serum calcium concentrations weekly at first, and then monthly when serum calcium has stabilized at the desired level. If hypercalcemia does occur as a complication of treatment, manage as discussed in the Hypercalcemia section of this chapter. Discontinue calcium supplementation and use vitamin D alone at a lower dosage for maintenance.

Postoperative Hypoparathyroidism. Supplement calcium and vitamin D postoperatively (see Table 4). If serum calcium concentrations remain normal, discontinue calcium supplementation and then gradually decrease and finally discontinue vitamin D. Evaluate serum calcium weekly for 1 month. If hypocalcemia returns, reinstitute vitamin D and calcium supplementation. Occasionally, permanent supplementation is necessary.

PARATHYROIDECTOMY

Parathyroidectomy is the treatment of choice for primary hyperparathyroidism caused by benign functional adenomas of the parathyroid gland in dogs. Functional adenocarcinomas are very rare. Parathyroidectomy is an infrequent procedure because primary hyperparathyroidism is uncommon in dogs and extremely rare in cats.

Anatomy. Familiarity with normal thyroid and parathyroid anatomy is essential prior to surgery (see sec 4, ch. 1).

Preoperative Considerations

- Always submit all excised parathyroid gland tissue for histopathology to confirm the diagnosis.
- Ectopic parathyroid gland adenomas are uncommon but may be present in the cranial mediastinum or near the base of the heart.
- Visualization of parathyroid adenomas can be enhanced with preoperative intravenous infusion of methylene blue (3 mg/kg). However, this has been associated with severe hemolysis and fatal acute renal failure in some cases.
- If the animal is hypercalcemic, decrease serum calcium levels (see Table 2) preoperatively to reduce risks of anesthesia and surgery.

Surgical Procedure

Objectives

- Explore the thyroid and parathyroid region.
- Remove the parathyroid adenoma.
- Maintain meticulous hemostasis.

Equipment

- Standard general surgical pack and suture
- Self-retaining retractors (e.g., Gelpi)
- Magnifying loop (optional)

Technique

1. Place the dog in dorsal recumbency with the forelimbs tied caudally and the neck hyperextended with a rolled towel.
2. Prepare the ventral cervical region from caudal mandible to manubrium for aseptic surgery.
3. Incise the skin on the ventral midline from larynx to manubrium.
4. Separate the paired sternohyoideus and sternothyroideus muscles.

5. Exploration
   a. Identify all four parathyroid glands if possible. The nonadenomatous glands are often atrophied and difficult to identify.
   b. Parathyroid adenomas are firm, whitish solid structures 4 to 20 mm in diameter.
   c. If an enlarged parathyroid gland is cystic, it is probably not a neoplasm but an incidental congenital cyst.
   d. If a readily identifiable mass is not found in the thyroid area, explore the accessible region along the trachea to the base of the neck and cranial mediastinum.
   e. Avoid injury to the carotid sheath structures and recurrent laryngeal nerves.
6. Dissection of the mass
   a. Perform complete excision of the mass, utilizing appropriate blunt and sharp dissection. Remove the associated thyroid lobe if necessary.
   b. Carefully examine the surgical field for evidence of residual hemorrhage prior to closure.
7. Closure
   a. Routinely close the muscle (simple continuous absorbable suture), subcutaneous tissue (simple continuous absorbable suture), and skin (simple interrupted nonabsorbable monofilament suture).

Postoperative Care and Complications

■ Monitor for hypothermia, hemorrhage at the incision site, and hypocalcemia.
■ Postoperative hypocalcemia
   • Return of serum calcium concentrations to normal or subnormal values indicates successful parathyroidectomy.

KEY POINT ▶ Most dogs will exhibit hypocalcemia within 48 hours of tumor removal.

   • Check serum calcium concentrations 1 and 2 days postoperatively. Frequent evaluation of calcium concentration is indicated if a hypocalcemic trend is noted.
   • Monitor for muscle tremors, excitement, and tetany if calcium concentrations are decreasing.
   • Treat hypocalcemia according to previously described guidelines.
   • Hypocalcemia without clinical signs usually does not require treatment unless the total serum calcium is <6 mg/dl.
■ Weekly evaluation of serum calcium concentrations allows modification of Vitamin D and calcium therapy.
   • Gradually decrease dosages to maintain low-normal serum calcium levels until the atrophied parathyroid glands begin to function normally.
■ Hypercalcemia may result from replacement therapy and should be avoided if possible.

Prognosis

The prognosis is good if the tumor is found and excised. Pre-existing hypercalcemia-mediated renal dysfunction may be irreversible.

Supplemental Readings

Berger B, Feldman EC: Primary hyperparathyroidism in dogs: 21 cases (1976–1986). J Am Vet Med Assoc 191:350, 1987.

Capen CC, Martin SL: Calcium-regulating hormones and diseases of the parathyroid glands. *In* Ettinger SJ, ed.: *Textbook of Veterinary Internal Medicine—Diseases of the Dog and Cat.* Philadelphia: W. B. Saunders, 1983, p 1523.

Chew DJ, Carothers MA: Hypercalcemia. Vet Clin North Am [Small Anim Pract]19:265, 1989.

Chew DJ, Meuten DJ: Disorders of calcium and phosphorus metabolism. Vet Clin North Am 12:411, 1982.

Feldman EC, Nelson RW: Hypocalcemia—hypoparathyroidism. *In* Feldman EC, Nelson R, eds.: *Canine and Feline Endocrinology and Reproduction.* Philadelphia: W. B. Saunders, 1987, p 357.

Feldman EC, Nelson RW: The parathyroid gland—primary hyperparathyroidism. *In* Feldman EC, Nelson R, eds.: *Canine and Feline Endocrinology and Reproduction.* Philadelphia: W. B. Saunders, 1987, p 328.

Kruger JM, Osborne CA, Polzin DJ: Treatment of hypercalcemia. *In* Kirk, RW, ed.: *Current Veterinary Therapy IX: Small Animal Practice.* Philadelphia: W. B. Saunders, 1986, p 75.

Meuten DJ, Armstrong PJ: Parathyroid disease and calcium metabolism. *In* Ettinger SJ, ed.: *Textbook of Veterinary Internal Medicine: Diseases of the Dog and Cat.* Philadelphia: W. B. Saunders, 1989, p 1610.

Nesbitt T, Crowe SW, Aronsohn M: The parathyroid. *In* Slatter DH, ed.: *Textbook of Small Animal Surgery.* Philadelphia: W. B. Saunders, 1985, p 1874.

3

Adrenal Gland

Rhett Nichols

Mark E. Peterson

Holly S. Mullen

HYPOADRENOCORTICISM

Hypoadrenocorticism is a syndrome resulting from a deficiency of glucocorticoid and/or mineralocorticoid secretion from the adrenal cortex. In dogs, spontaneous hypoadrenocorticism is uncommon but well recognized; the disease is rare in cats.

Etiology

Primary Adrenocortical Insufficiency

Primary adrenocortical insufficiency (Addison's disease) is the result of atrophy or destruction of all layers of the adrenal cortex. This usually causes a deficiency of both classes of corticosteroids. In dogs and cats, causative factors include:

- Idiopathic (probably immune-mediated)
- Iatrogenic—may be caused by mitotane therapy for canine hyperadrenocorticism. Mineralocorticoid concentrations usually remain normal.
- Granulomatous (fungal) adrenalitis, neoplasia, hemorrhage

Secondary Hypoadrenocorticism

This condition results from insufficient pituitary ACTH secretion with resultant glucocorticoid deficiency. Mineralocorticoid concentrations usually remain normal. It can be caused by:

- Abrupt withdrawal of long-term and/or high-dose exogenous corticosteroid therapy
- Megestrol acetate (Ovaban; Schering) therapy in cats
- Lesions of the hypothalamus or pituitary gland (e.g., tumors)
- Idiopathic adrenocorticotropic hormone (ACTH) deficiency (rare)

Signalment

- Age: Most dogs and cats are less than 7 years; range 6 months to 10 years.
- Breed: In dogs, any breed can be affected, but Black Standard poodles are predisposed. No breed predilection has been reported in cats.
- Sex: Female predilection is reported in dogs (70% females in one study). No sex predilection has been observed in cats.

Clinical Signs

Hypoadrenocorticism has been referred to as the "great pretender" because most clinical signs can mimic those seen in other disorders.

Acute or End-Stage Adrenocortical Insufficiency

- Weakness and depression progressing to collapse
- Bradycardia and other hyperkalemia-associated arrhythmias
- Shock caused by hypovolemia, poor vascular tone, and reduced cardiac output

Subacute or Chronic Adrenocortical Insufficiency

- Intermittent anorexia, vomiting, and diarrhea
- Muscle weakness, lethargy, and depression (result of poor tissue perfusion, metabolic acidosis, and hyperkalemia)
- Transient response of clinical symptoms to fluid and/or corticosteroid administration
- Exacerbations of clinical signs associated with stress

Diagnosis

History and Clinical Signs

A high index of suspicion is necessary because history and clinical signs are nonspecific and easily confused with common disorders such as:

- Gastrointestinal disease
- Primary renal failure
- Other causes of acute collapse or episodic weakness (cardiovascular disease, neuromuscular disease, metabolic disorders)

Hemogram

- Absolute eosinophilia and lymphocytosis may occur.
- Increased packed cell volume (PCV) and total plasma protein may result from dehydration.
- Mild anemia is present in some cases.

Serum Biochemical and Electrolyte Abnormalities

KEY POINT ▶ Hyperkalemia and hyponatremia are seen in the majority of cases of primary hypoadrenocorticism.

- Serum electrolyte concentrations
  - Early primary hypoadrenocorticism may be asso-

ciated with normal serum electrolyte concentrations.

- Iatrogenic hypoadrenocorticism caused by mitotane or ketoconazole therapy usually is associated with normal serum electrolyte concentrations.
- Secondary hypoadrenocorticism is always associated with normal serum electrolyte concentrations.

■ Azotemia due to renal or prerenal causes may be seen.

■ Hypercalcemia is seen in 25% of affected dogs and cats, possibly due to decreased renal calcium excretion.

■ Hypoglycemia (rare) may result from decreased gluconeogenesis and glycogenolysis.

■ Metabolic acidosis may occur.

Urine Specific Gravity

Urine specific gravity is often below 1.030. This urine concentrating defect probably results from medullary washout secondary to renal sodium wasting.

Electrocardiographic Abnormalities

■ ECG changes are primarily dependent on the degree of hyperkalemia. Acid-base balance and serum sodium and calcium concentrations also play a role.

■ Widening and flattening of P waves, increased duration of the PR interval

■ Increased T wave amplitude

■ Decreased amplitude and prolongation of QRS complexes

■ Bradycardia

■ Sinoventricular rhythm and atrial standstill (absence of P waves)

Radiographic Findings

■ Microcardia and hypoperfusion of lungs (as manifestations of hypovolemia)

■ Megaesophagus (rare)

ACTH Simulation Test

This test is necessary for definitive diagnosis of hypoadrenocorticism. This test measures the relative "thickness" of the adrenal cortex.

■ *Protocol*
  • In dogs, obtain a plasma or serum sample for cortisol analysis before and 2 hours after IM injection of 2.2 U/kg of ACTH gel.
  • Alternatively, obtain samples before and 1 hour after IV injection of 0.25 mg of synthetic ACTH (Cortrosyn; Organon Pharmaceuticals, West Orange, NJ) (disregard body weight).
  • In cats, obtain a plasma or serum sample for cortisol analysis before and 1 and 2 hours after IV administration of 0.125 mg of Cortrosyn.
■ Dogs and cats with hypoadrenocorticism will show a "blunted" or absent cortisol response to ACTH administration.
  • *Primary hypoadrenocorticism*: Basal and post-ACTH concentrations of cortisol usually are <1 μg/dl (<30 nmol/liter).

  • *Secondary hypoadrenocorticism*: The serum cortisol response to exogenous ACTH is blunted; however, post-ACTH concentrations of cortisol usually are >2.5 μg/dl (>70 nmol/liter).
■ False elevations of cortisol concentrations may occur after administration of prednisone, prednisolone, cortisone, or fludrocortisone because these cross-react on the cortisol radioimmunoassay.
  • Discontinue these drugs 24 to 48 hours prior to the test.
■ Dexamethasone and desoxycorticosterone pivalate (DOCP) will not interfere with the cortisol assay; however, dexamethasone is a potent steroid and will suppress the pituitary adrenal axis.

Plasma Concentration of ACTH

Plasma concentration of ACTH is high (>500 pg/ml) in dogs and cats with primary hypoadrenocorticism and very low (<20 pg/ml) or undetectable with secondary hypoadrenocorticism.

Treatment

KEY POINT ▶ Collect proper blood samples and perform necessary diagnostic testing prior to instituting therapy.

The ACTH stimulation test (preferably using synthetic ACTH administered IV) can be performed simultaneously with initial therapy if dexamethasone is used for glucocorticoid replacement because it will not influence the cortisol assay.

Acute Hypoadrenocorticism

Treatment in acute adrenal insufficiency is directed toward:

■ Correcting hypotension and hypovolemia
■ Improving vascular integrity
■ Providing an immediate source of glucocorticoids
■ Correcting electrolyte imbalances and acidosis

Hypovolemia and Hyponatremia

■ Rapidly infuse 0.9% NaCl solution, 40–80 ml/kg/h IV, over the first 1–2 hours; then gradually reduce rate to maintenance requirements, depending upon patient response.

■ Administer dexamethasone (Azium), 0.5–2.0 mg/kg IV, or dexamethasone sodium phosphate (Azium-SP), 2–4 mg/kg IV. Repeat in 2–6 hours if needed.

■ Convert to maintenance with prednisone, prednisolone, or cortisone acetate (see below) over the following 3–5 days.

Hyperkalemia

■ Hyperkalemia associated with hypoadrenocorticism usually can be successfully treated with parenteral fluid therapy (0.9 NaCl solution) only.

■ For severe hyperkalemia causing life-threatening bradyarrhythmias and atrial standstill, consider agressive therapy (e.g., administration of sodium bicarbonate or calcium salts or insulin and dextrose IV).

Acidosis

- Consider sodium bicarbonate therapy if severe acidosis is present (pH < 7.1) (see sec. 1, ch. 5).
- Give 25% of calculated dose IV during the first 6 hours of therapy if serum bicarbonate concentration is <12 mEq/liter.
- Correction of acidosis also drives extracellular potassium into cells, thereby reducing hypercalcemia.

Other Supportive Care as Needed

- Correct hypothermia.
- If hypoglycemia is present, give 50% dextrose (0.5–1.5 ml/kg IV slowly.)

Chronic or Subacute Adrenocortical Insufficiency

Dogs and cats with primary hypoadrenocorticism require chronic glucocorticoids and mineralocorticoid supplementation and sometimes the addition of salt to the diet. Animals with secondary hypoadrenocorticism can be managed with glucocorticoid supplementation only.

Hypovolemia

- Give 0.9% NaCl solution, 60–80 ml/kg/day IV, for correction of hypovolemia.
- Decrease fluid volume over 48–96 hours, based on return to normal clinical and laboratory parameters.

Mineralocorticoid Supplementation
Use one of the following:

- Flurocortisone acetate (Florinef; Squibb), 0.02 mg/kg/day PO
  - Initially monitor serum electrolytes, BUN, and creatinine every 1–2 weeks until stabilized in the normal range; then re-evaluate every 3–4 months. Adjust mineralocorticoid dosage based on these results; serum potassium concentrations frequently remain at 4.5–5.2 mEq/liter.
  - Increase or decrease the total dose by 0.05–0.10 mg/day; the average dose to control disease is 0.02 mg/kg/day.
- Desoxycorticosterone pivalate (DOCP; Ciba-Geigy), 1–2 mg/kg IM every 3–4 weeks, controls the disease in most dogs, but up to 3 mg/kg may be needed.
  - DOCP is a long-acting injectable mineralocorticoid.
  - DOCP is currently not approved by FDA for use in small animals; client waiver forms may be obtained from manufacturer.

Glucocorticoid Supplementation
- Many patients require glucocorticoid supplementation in addition to mineralocorticoid therapy to prevent signs of glucocorticoid deficiency or to control persistent mild azotemia. Give one of the following:
  - Prednisone or prednisolone, 0.2–0.4 mg/kg/day PO, usually given in the morning to simulate diurnal rhythm of endogenous cortisol secretion.
  - Cortisone acetate, 1 mg/kg/day PO, given in the morning
  - Give 2- to 10-fold higher glucocorticoid doses for brief periods of stress or illness.

CANINE HYPERADRENOCORTICISM

Spontaneous canine hyperadrenocorticism (Cushing's syndrome) refers to the clinical signs and biochemical abnormalities that result from chronic exposure to glucocorticoid excess.

Etiology

Causes include pituitary-dependent hyperadrenocorticism, adrenocortical neoplasia, and iatrogenic hyperadrenocorticism.

Pituitary-Dependent Hyperadrenocorticism. This is the most common cause of the naturally occurring disorder, accounting for 85% of cases. Excessive secretion of ACTH, usually from a pituitary microadenoma, causes bilateral adrenocortical hyperplasia and leads to cortisol excess.

Functional Adrenocortical Tumors. These tumors are seen in approximately 15% of dogs with spontaneous Cushing's syndrome. About 50% of the adrenocortical tumors are benign.

Iatrogenic Hyperadrenocorticism. Excessive or prolonged administration of corticosteroids can cause iatrogenic hyperadrenocorticism.

- Clinical signs and physical examination findings are similar to those seen in the natural disease.
- The adrenal cortex in this condition is atrophied.

Signalment

- Age: Spontaneous hyperadrenocorticism is primarily a disease of middle-aged and older dogs; however, the age ranges from 6 months to 20 years.
- Breed: Poodles, dachshunds, Boston terriers, and boxers are predisposed, although all breeds can be affected.
- Sex: No sex predilection is seen in dogs with pituitary-dependent hyperadrenocorticism. In contrast, 70% of dogs with adrenal tumors are female.

Clinical Signs

KEY POINT ▶ Dogs with hyperadrenocorticism usually develop clinical signs that reflect dysfunction of many organ systems, although in some dogs only one clinical sign may predominate.

General Appearance

- Pendulous, distended, or "pot-bellied" abdomen
- Bilaterally symmetric alopecia with dull, dry haircoat
- Thin skin
- Hyperpigmentation
- Muscle atrophy
- Testicular atrophy

Urinary System

- Polyuria and polydipsia are seen in the majority of dogs with hyperadrenocorticism. Glucocorticoids decrease the renal tubular reabsorption of water by increasing glomerular filtration rate and renal blood flow and by inhibiting the action of antidiuretic hormone (ADH) at the tubular levels.

■ Lower urinary tract infection from cortisol excess and its associated signs of pollakiuria, hematuria, and stranguria are sometimes seen.

Respiratory System

■ Excessive panting is quite common and may be due to decreased pulmonary compliance, pulmonary hypertension, or the direct effects of cortisol on the respiratory center.
■ Severe respiratory distress can be caused by pulmonary thromboembolic disease, a relatively uncommon complication of hyperadrenocorticism.

Endocrine System

■ Some dogs with hyperadrenocorticism develop diabetes mellitus and the associated clinical signs of polyuria, polydipsia, weight loss, and polyphagia.
■ The hallmark of steroid-induced diabetes is the development of insulin resistance, defined clinically as persistent hyperglycemia despite insulin doses of >2.5 U/kg/administration.
■ Cortisol antagonizes the actions of insulin by interfering with its action at the cellular level.

Central Nervous System (CNS): Neuromuscular System

■ Lethargy is the most common CNS disturbance. Lethargy may be associated with high concentrations of ACTH or the effects of excessive cortisol on cerebral enzymes and on neurotransmitter synthesis.
■ CNS signs of circling, seizures, and behavior change may be caused by the compressive effects of a large expanding pituitary tumor.
■ Muscle weakness is common and results from muscle wasting secondary to the catabolic effects of glucocorticoid excess.

Reproductive System

Testicular atrophy and female infertility are related to low concentrations of pituitary follicle-stimulating hormone (FSH) and luteinizing hormone (LH) caused by negative feedback from high circulating cortisol concentrations.

Diagnosis

History

Determine from the history if there has been recent treatment with exogenous glucocorticoids. Common owner complaints include polyuria and polydipsia, polyphagia, and hair loss.

Physical Examination

Look for evidence of the clinical signs listed above when performing the physical examination.

Routine Laboratory Testing

■ High serum alkaline phosphatase activity (composed of steroid-induced isoenzyme) is seen in up to 85% of dogs with hyperadrenocorticism.
■ High serum cholesterol concentrations and alanine transferase (SGPT) activity are common.
■ Mild elevations in blood glucose are commonly seen. Overt diabetes mellitus (glucose >250 mg/dl) occurs in 10% of dogs with hyperadrenocorticism.
■ The urinalysis often reveals urine of low specific gravity (<1.020).
  • Proteinuria is not uncommon. Severe proteinuria (urine protein:creatinine ratio >3) is usually related to glomerular disease or urinary tract infection.
■ The hemogram may reveal a stress leukogram and mild erythrocytosis.

Radiography

■ Hepatomegaly is often seen.
■ Approximately one third of adrenal tumors are mineralized and therefore are radiopaque.
■ Mineralization of bronchial walls is not uncommon.

Computed Tomography (CT)

■ Pituitary tumors >1 cm in diameter (macroadenomas or macroadenocarcinomas) are relatively easy to define on CT.
■ Pituitary microadenomas may be identified if they are ideally positioned or approach 1 cm in diameter.
■ CT is the most accurate and reliable method to image adrenal glands, followed by diagnostic ultrasonography and plain radiography. With CT, the location of the adrenal tumor and evidence of metastasis can be identified in most cases.

Pituitary-Adrenal Function Tests

Basal Serum Cortisol Concentrations. Basal serum (or plasma) cortisol concentrations are not useful in diagnosing hyperadrenocorticism because of constant fluctuation throughout the day.

ACTH Stimulation Test. This is the most commonly used adrenal function test. Because the ACTH stimulation test measures the relative "thickness" of the adrenal cortex, it is the best test to differentiate spontaneous from iatrogenic hyperadrenocorticism.

■ *Protocol*
  • Obtain a plasma or serum sample for cortisol analysis before and 2 hours after intramuscular injection (IM) of 2.2 U/kg ACTH gel (Vedco).
  • Alternatively, obtain plasma samples before and 1 hour after IV or IM injection of 0.25 mg of synthetic ACTH (Cortrosyn; Organon Pharmaceuticals, West Orange, NJ), regardless of body weight.
■ Of dogs with pituitary-dependent hyperadrenocorticism, 85% show an exaggerated cortisol response to exogenous ACTH. A poststimulation cortisol >20 μg/dl is consistent with a diagnosis of hyperadrenocorticism, whereas normal usually is 6–17 mg/dl.

- Dogs with iatrogenic hyperadrenocorticism have a "blunted" response or no response to ACTH administration.
- Of dogs with adrenocortical tumors, 50% show exaggerated cortisol responses, whereas the remainder have normal responses. Some dogs with adrenal carcinoma have extremely marked cortisol responses to ACTH (post-ACTH cortisol concentrations >50 μg/dl or 1500 nmol/liter).

Low-Dose Dexamethasone Suppression Test.

This test is useful to confirm the diagnosis of hyperadrenocorticism. The overall sensitivity for diagnosing hyperadrenocorticism approaches 90%; however, in most cases this test will not differentiate pituitary-dependent hyperadrenocorticism from cortisol-secreting adrenal neoplasia.

- *Protocol*
  - Collect plasma or serum samples for cortisol determination before and 4 and 8 hours after IV or IM administration of 0.015 mg/kg of dexamethasone (Azium; Schering).
- In general, serum cortisol concentrations of normal dogs fall below 1 μg/dl (30 nmol/L) by 4 hours after administration of dexamethasone and remain suppressed for the entire 8-hour period of the test. In contrast, cortisol concentrations in most dogs with hyperadrenocorticism remain above 1 μg/dl (30 nmol/liter) during the 8-hour test period.
- A third of dogs with pituitary-dependent hyperadrenocorticism show a pattern of "escape" from suppression; serum cortisol concentrations fall below 1 μg/dl (30 nmol/liter) by 4 hours after administration of dexamethasone and rise above 1 μg/dl (30 nmol/liter) by hour 8 of the test. Virtually all dogs with this test pattern have pituitary-dependent hyperadrenocorticism.

Urinary Cortisol:Creatinine Ratio.

This screening test for hyperadrenocorticism is convenient. We recommend its use with one of the other screening tests.

- *Protocol*
  - Submit a morning urine sample to the laboratory for urine cortisol (by routine radioimmunoassay technique) and urine creatinine determinations.
  - With urine cortisol expressed as nmol/L and creatinine expressed as mmol/L, a ratio of >35 is considered suggestive of hyperadrenocorticism.

Endogenous Plasma ACTH Concentration.

This test reliably distinguishes pituitary-dependent hyperadrenocorticism from adrenocortical tumors.

- In theory, dogs with pituitary-dependent hyperadrenocorticism have normal to high ACTH concentrations (usually >40 pg/ml), whereas those with adrenal tumors have low or undetectable plasma concentrations of ACTH (usually <20 pg/ml).
- This test is expensive, and the specifics of sample handling are difficult for most practitioners. Plasma collected in EDTA must be centrifuged and frozen immediately in plastic or polypropylene tubes and sent by overnight delivery packed in dry ice. Validated ACTH assays are not yet widely available.

High-Dose Dexamethasone Suppression Test.

This is useful to differentiate pituitary-dependent hyperadrenocorticism from adrenocortical neoplasia.

- *Protocol*
  - Obtain a serum or plasma sample for cortisol determination before and 4 and 8 hours after IV or IM injection of 0.1–1.0 mg/kg of dexamethasone.
  - In dogs with pituitary-dependent hyperadrenocorticism, the degree of cortisol suppression tends to be greater after administration of the dose of 1.0 mg/kg.
- Dogs with adrenal tumors secrete autonomously and do not show feedback suppression of cortisol after administration of a high dose of dexamethasone, with serum cortisol concentrations remaining >1.5 μg/dl (>40 nmol/liter) during the testing period.
- Of dogs with pituitary-dependent hyperadrenocorticism, 85% show adequate feedback suppression of cortisol (<1.5 μg/dl or <40 nmol/liter) after administration of a high dose of dexamethasone.
- The remaining 15% fail to show adequate cortisol suppression (i.e., all cortisol values remain >1.5 μg/dl (>40 nmol/liter). In these dogs, the results of high-dose dexamethasone suppression testing cannot be distinguished from the results in dogs with adrenal tumors. Many of these dogs with nonsuppressible pituitary-dependent hyperadrenocorticism have large pituitary tumors.

Treatment

Medical Management of Pituitary-Dependent Hyperadrenocorticism Using Mitotane

Mitotane (*o,p'*DDD, Lysodren; Bristol-Meyers) is the drug most frequently used in the treatment of hyperadrenocorticism in dogs. Mitotane causes selective necrosis of the zona fasciculata and zona reticularis of the adrenal cortex. The administration protocol involves an initial induction phase that uses a daily dosage for induction of remission, followed by a maintenance phase that uses a dosage once or twice weekly.

Induction Phase

- The *initial loading dosage* is 30–50 mg/kg/day divided and given twice a day for 7 to 10 days.
- Administer a glucocorticoid (e.g., prednisone or prednisolone, 0.2 mg/kg/day) during the induction phase to help prevent the development of adverse effects secondary to hypoadrenocorticism.
  - Common side effects during the induction phase include lethargy, vomiting, anorexia, weakness, and diarrhea.
  - If adverse effects occur during initial therapy, stop the drug and give glucocorticoids until the dog can be evaluated.
- The effectiveness of therapy is best monitored using the ACTH stimulation test.

KEY POINT ▶ The goal of therapy is to achieve subclinical hypoadrenocorticism whereby both basal and post-ACTH cortisol concentrations are within the normal basal cortisol range (1–5 µg/dl or 30–150 nmol/liter for most laboratories).

- If basal and post-ACTH cortisol concentrations fall below the normal range (<1 µg/dl or 30 nmol/liter), temporarily suspend the mitotane and supplement glucocorticoids as needed until circulating cortisol concentrations normalize. Cortisol levels generally return to the normal range in 2 to 4 weeks, at which time resume mitotane therapy.
- If basal or post-ACTH cortisol concentrations are above the normal resting range, continue daily mitotane treatment and repeat ACTH stimulation tests at intervals of 5–10 days until serum cortisol concentrations fall within the normal resting range.

Maintenance Phase

■ When normal cortisol concentrations are documented by ACTH stimulation testing, continue mitotane at a *maintenance dosage* of 30–50 mg/kg weekly in 2–3 divided doses. Life-long maintenance therapy is necessary to maintain remission of the disease.
■ If adverse side effects occur during maintenance therapy, stop the drug and supplement glucocorticoids. In most cases, maintenance mitotane can be resumed 2–6 weeks later, once serum cortisol concentrations have returned to the normal resting range.
■ About 5% of dogs develop iatrogenic hypoadrenocorticism with associated electrolyte changes of hyponatremia and hyperkalemia. These dogs generally require life-long supplementation with mineralocorticoids (i.e., fludrocortisone acetate or DOCP) (see discussion on hypoadrenocorticism in this chapter).
  - Nearly 50% of dogs with hyperadrenocorticism have a relapse of disease within 12 months while on maintenance therapy; these cases require re-induction with daily dosages of mitotane for 7–10 days, followed by a higher or more frequent dosage than before for maintenance.

Medical Management of Pituitary-Dependent Hyperadrenocorticism and Concurrent Diabetes Mellitus Using Mitotane

KEY POINT ▶ In diabetics with Cushing's syndrome, treatment with mitotane removes the cause for the insulin resistance (the cortisol excess) and reduces the daily insulin requirements in most cases.

■ For induction, give mitotane at 25–35 mg/kg daily for 7 to 10 days.
■ Monitor urine glucose twice daily; with each negative urine glucose measurement, decrease insulin dosage by 10% (see sec. 4, ch. 4 on Diabetes Mellitus). These dogs are susceptible to hypoglycemia.
■ For ACTH stimulation and maintenance therapy, follow the same guidelines given above for the management of the nondiabetic dog with pituitary-dependent hyperadrenocorticism.

Medical Management of Hyperadrenocorticism Using Ketoconazole

■ Ketoconazole (Nizoral; Janssen Pharmaceutical, Piscataway, NJ) reversibly inhibits adrenal steroidogenesis.
■ The initial dosage is 10 mg/kg given twice daily.
■ Assess adrenal reserve with an ACTH stimulation test after 7–10 days of therapy.
■ The goal of therapy is to achieve subclinical hypoadrenocorticism whereby both basal and post-ACTH cortisol concentrations are within the normal basal cortisol range (1–5 µg/dl or 25–150 nmol/liter for most laboratories).
■ Once adequate control is achieved, life-long twice-daily therapy must be maintained for proper management of the hyperadrenocorticism.
■ The major drawbacks of ketoconazole compared with mitotane include its high cost, the necessity for life-long twice-daily administration, and a reported lack of efficacy in some cases, probably from poor gastrointestinal absorption.

Radiation Therapy in the Treatment of Pituitary-Dependent Hyperadrenocorticism

■ Radiation therapy may be useful in those cases of hyperadrenocorticism caused by a pituitary macroadenoma or macrocarcinoma.
■ In general, the total dose of radiation is delivered in fractions over a period of 4–6 weeks. Complications appear to be minimal.
■ Dogs with a pituitary macroadenoma and severe neurologic signs have a grave prognosis.
■ The disadvantages of radiation therapy include its high cost and limited availability.

KEY POINT ▶ Advances in diagnostic imaging (CT and magnetic resonance imaging) have allowed the antemortem diagnosis of pituitary macroadenomas. Treatment of pituitary tumors may be attempted with radiotherapy, especially if a diagnosis of macroadenomas can be made before the onset of profound neurologic signs.

Surgical Management of Adrenocortical Tumors

See the discussion of adrenalectomy later in this chapter.

Medical Management of Adrenocortical Tumors Using Mitotane

Therapy using mitotane has been successful for over 24 months in some dogs with adrenocortical adenomas and carcinomas.

■ *Protocol*
  - Administer mitotane initially at a daily dosage of 50–75 mg/kg/day.
  - Repeat ACTH stimulation testing every 2 weeks to evaluate adrenal reserve.
  - Administer a glucocorticoid (e.g., prednisone or prednisolone, 0.2 mg/kg/day) to help prevent the

development of adverse effects secondary to hypoadrenocorticism.

KEY POINT ▶ The goal of therapy is to destroy all functional, neoplastic adrenocortical tissue. Therefore, both the serum basal and post-ACTH cortisol concentrations should be low to undetectable (<1 μg/dl or <30 nmol/liter).

- Maintenance dosages of mitotane as high as 200 to 300 mg/kg weekly may be necessary.
- Common side effects include anorexia, weakness, and lethargy. If adverse reactions occur, stop the drug and start therapy again later at a lower dosage.

Patient Monitoring

The prognosis for hyperadrenocorticism is always guarded because of the many complications associated with the disease. The average life span after diagnosis is 2 years. Complications include:

- Thromboembolism
- Infection
- Hypertension
- Congestive heart failure
- Recurrence of symptoms
- Progression of CNS signs

Mitotane overdosage and underdosage can complicate therapy; long-term monitoring is therefore necessary.

- Instruct owners to observe for recurrence of symptoms, especially polyuria and polydipsia.
- Perform the ACTH response test every 3–6 months to assess adrenal reserve and to guide mitotane dosage adjustments.

FELINE HYPERADRENOCORTICISM

Etiology

The causes of hyperadrenocorticism in cats, as in the dog, are pituitary-dependent hyperadrenocorticism, adrenocortical neoplasia, and iatrogenic hyperadrenocorticism.

- *Pituitary-dependent hyperadrenocorticism* is the most common cause of the naturally occurring disorder in cats, accounting for 85% of the cases.
- *Functional cortisol-secreting neoplasms of the adrenal cortex* are present in approximately 15% of cats with spontaneous hyperadrenocorticism.
- *Iatrogenic hyperadrenocorticism* is a well-recognized disorder in the cat, despite the relative resistance to the effects of glucocorticoids when compared to dogs.

Signalment

- Age: Spontaneous hyperadrenocorticism is a disease of middle-aged and older cats.
- Breed: There is no breed predilection.
- Sex: Female cats are primarily affected.

Clinical Signs

General Appearance

- Pendulous, distended, or "pot-bellied" abdomen
- Bilaterally symmetric alopecia with dull, dry hair coat.
- Thin skin
- Muscle atrophy

Endocrine and Urinary System

- *Polyuria, polydipsia,* and *polyphagia.* In contrast to dogs with the disease, the cause of polyuria and polydipsia in cats appears to be primarily the result of a hyperglycemic osmotic diuresis secondary to diabetes mellitus.
- *Glucose intolerance* and *insulin resistance.*

KEY POINT ▶ The majority of cats (almost 80%) with hyperadrenocorticism have concurrent diabetes mellitus.

Diagnosis

History

Look for a history of recent treatment with exogenous glucocorticoids. Common owner complaints include polyuria and polydipsia, pot-bellied appearance, thin skin, bilateral alopecia, and the development of insulin-resistant diabetes mellitus.

Physical Examination

Many of the clinical signs listed above will be present in the physical examination.

Routine Laboratory Testing

- Severe hyperglycemia and glycosuria are seen in up to 80% of cases.
- Hypercholesterolemia is common.
- The hemogram may show leukocytosis, eosinopenia, and lymphopenia, but these findings are inconsistent.

KEY POINT ▶ In contrast to the situation in dogs with the disease, high serum alkaline phosphatase is *not* a consistent finding in cats with hyperadrenocorticism.

Pituitary-Adrenal Function Tests

ACTH Stimulation Test. This is a valuable screening test for hyperadrenocorticism in cats.

- *Protocol*
  - Collect a plasma or serum sample for cortisol analysis before and at 60 and 120 minutes after intramuscular injection of 2.2 U/kg ACTH gel (the greatest rise in cortisol occurs at 2 hours in 60% of normal cats; the remaining 40% have peak cortisol concentrations at 1 hour post-ACTH injection).
  - Alternatively, obtain plasma or serum samples before and 60 minutes after IV administration of 0.125 mg of synthetic ACTH (Cortrosyn).
- Approximately 70% of cats with naturally occurring

hyperadrenocorticism show an exaggerated cortisol response (>15 μg/dl or 400 nmol/liter) to exogenous ACTH.
■ Cats with iatrogenic hyperadrenocorticism show a "blunted" or no response to ACTH.
■ Exogenous administration of ACTH cannot differentiate pituitary-dependent hyperadrenocorticism from a functional adrenal tumor.

Low-Dose Dexamethasone Suppression Test. This test has not been standardized for diagnosis of hyperadrenocorticism in cats and is not recommended for cats.

High-Dose Dexamethasone Suppression Test. This test is useful for discriminating normal cats or cats with nonadrenal disease from cats with spontaneous hyperadrenocorticism. In contrast to most dogs with pituitary-dependent hyperadrenocorticism, the majority of cats with pituitary-dependent disease fail to show adequate cortisol suppression after high-dose dexamethasone suppression testing. Therefore, this test cannot readily differentiate pituitary-dependent hyperadrenocorticism from adrenal tumor in cats.

■ *Protocol*
  • Collect plasma or serum samples for cortisol analysis before and at 4 and 8 hours after intravenous administration of 0.1 mg/kg dexamethasone.

Plasma ACTH Concentrations. Endogenous plasma ACTH concentrations can be used to distinguish pituitary-dependent hyperadrenocorticism from adrenocortical tumors in cats.

■ Cats with pituitary-dependent hyperadrenocorticism will have normal to high plasma ACTH concentrations (>40 pg/ml).
■ Cats with adrenal tumors will have low concentrations (<20 pg/ml; often too low to be detectable).

KEY POINT ▶ Low-dose dexamethasone suppression tests have not been well-standardized in the cat. The high-dose dexamethasone suppression test (0.1 mg/kg IV) is the preferred method of screening for hyperadrenocorticism in cats.

Imaging Techniques

These modalities, especially abdominal ultrasonography and CT, can sometimes identify adrenal tumors.

Treatment

Medical Treatment

■ The use of *mitotane* is not recommended in cats because of poor tolerance and lack of efficacy.
■ *Ketoconazole* does not appear to block adrenocortical steroid production in normal cats (in contrast to dogs) and does not appear to be very useful in the treatment of feline hyperadrenocorticism.
■ *Metyrapone,* an enzyme inhibitor that blocks adrenal synthesis of glucocorticoids, has been used with mixed results in treating cats with hyperadrenocorticism. Some cats treated with this agent have showed

clinical improvement at dosages ranging from 200 to 250 mg without development of side effects.

Surgical Treatment

In cats with adrenal tumors, unilateral adrenalectomy should be performed. Bilateral adrenalectomy is indicated for treatment of pituitary-dependent hyperadrenocorticism (see discussion of adrenalectomy later in this chapter).

KEY POINT ▶ Surgical adrenalectomy is the most successful means of treating hyperadrenocorticism in cats. Medical therapy has been disappointing.

PHEOCHROMOCYTOMA

Etiology

Pheochromocytoma is a catecholamine-producing tumor derived from endocrine cells of the adrenal medulla. It is rare in dogs and has not been reported in the cat. In fact, most pheochromocytomas are unexpected findings at necropsy.

Signalment

■ Pheochromocytoma generally occurs in older dogs.
■ There is no breed or sex predilection.

Clinical Signs

KEY POINT ▶ Pheochromocytoma is rarely diagnosed ante mortem. Clinical signs of pheochromocytoma are vague and episodic.

Clinical signs develop either as a result of the space-occupying nature of the adrenal tumor and its metastasis or as a result of excessive secretion of catecholamines and resulting systemic hypertension.

Weakness, anorexia, vomiting, weight loss, and excessive panting are the most frequent signs, but these occur in less than 50% of affected dogs.

Diagnosis

History, Physical Examination, and Routine Laboratory Testing

■ History, physical examination findings generally are vague (e.g., lethargy and tachypnea) and do not help to diagnose pheochromocytoma.
■ An abdominal mass can be palpated in about 10% of dogs with pheochromocytoma.
■ Routine laboratory evaluations typically are normal.

Radiology and Other Imaging Techniques

■ Abdominal radiographs reveal a cranial abdominal mass in the region of the adrenal gland in up to one third of dogs with pheochromocytoma.
■ Specialized imaging techniques such as abdominal ultrasonography and CT are extremely useful for detecting and characterizing adrenal masses.

Arterial Blood Pressure

Up to 50% of dogs with pheochromocytoma are hypertensive. Catecholamine secretion, and therefore hypertension, tends to be episodic.

Biochemical and Pharmacologic Tests

Measurement of urinary catecholamines and resting plasma catecholamine concentrations and clonidine suppression and phentolamine tests can be used to demonstrate excessive production of catecholamines (epinephrine and norepinephrine) or their metabolites. Unfortunately, the limited availability, technical difficulty, and expense of these tests and assays severely limit their use in veterinary medicine.

KEY POINT ▶ The antemortem diagnosis of pheochromocytoma in dogs must usually rely on surgical exploration.

Treatment

- Adrenalectomy is the treatment of choice for pheochromocytoma (see the following discussion of adrenalectomy).
- Control catecholamine-induced cardiac arrhythmias and severe hypertension before and during surgery (see discussion of adrenalectomy).

ADRENALECTOMY

Adrenalectomy usually is performed for treatment of hyperadrenocorticism in the dog and cat. Unilateral adrenalectomy is done primarily for removal of adrenal neoplasia (adenoma, adenocarcinoma, or pheochromocytoma). Bilateral adrenalectomy is less commonly used for bilateral adrenocortical hyperplasia. The anatomy and surgical and medical management for adrenalectomy is the same in the dog and cat. Adrenalectomy is performed infrequently in cats owing to the low incidence of hyperadrenocorticism and adrenal neoplasia.

Surgical Anatomy of the Adrenal Gland

- The adrenal glands are paired, flattened bilobed glands located retroperitoneal and craniomedial to the kidneys (Fig. 1).
- The right adrenal gland lies about the level of the last thoracic to the first lumbar vertebrae.
- The capsule of the right adrenal gland may be contiguous with the tunica externa of the caudal vena cava.
- The left adrenal gland is slightly caudal to the right and is separated from the caudal vena cava by a layer of fat.
- Adrenal size is breed-dependent. In dogs, the average size is 22 mm long, 10 mm wide, and 4 mm thick.
- The adrenal glands are well vascularized by branches of the renal, accessory renal, phrenic, cranial abdominal, phrenicoabdominal, and lumbar arteries.
- Venous drainage is through the left and right adrenal and the phrenicoabdominal veins.

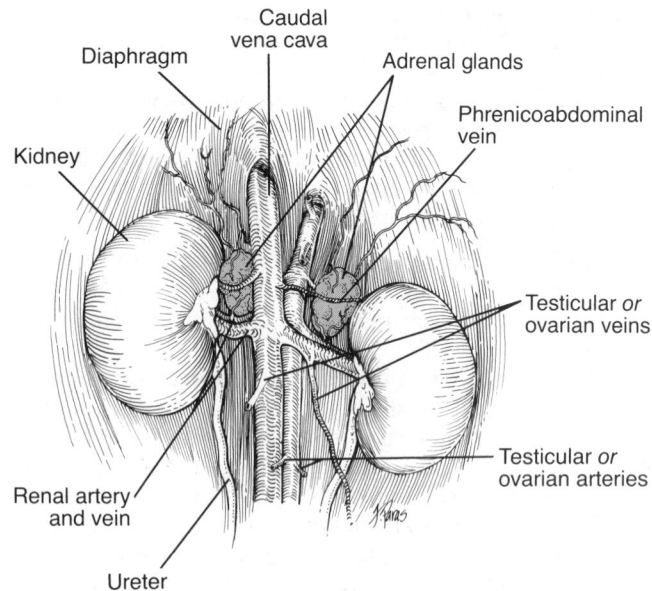

Figure 1. Anatomy of the adrenal glands from the ventral midline approach.

- The phrenicoabdominal artery crosses the dorsal surface of the adrenal glands; the phrenicoabdominal vein courses across the ventral surface. These paired vessels are the largest supplying the adrenal glands.

Preoperative Considerations

- Obtain a minimum data base consisting of CBC, serum chemistry profile, and thoracic radiographs.
- Abdominal radiographs may help localize a unilateral adrenal mass, especially if the tumor is mineralized.
- Ultrasonography may also be helpful to identify a mass and determine if invasion of the vena cava has occurred.
- Correct any fluid and electrolyte abnormalities.

Anesthesia and Perioperative Care for Patient with Hyperadrenocorticism

- Induce and maintain anesthesia following standard procedures (see sec. 1, ch. 2).
- Isoflurane is preferred over halothane, as it does not sensitize the myocardium to catecholamines.
- Administer a broad-spectrum bactericidal antibiotic by IV bolus 30 minutes before surgery.
- Supplement corticosteroids in the form of dexamethasone (0.1–0.2 mg/kg IV) immediately prior to the onset of surgery and again at the completion of the surgical procedure.

Anesthesia for Pheochromocytoma

- Avoid premedication with atropine because of potential for severe tachycardia.

KEY POINT ▶ Dogs with pheochromocytoma produce high circulating concentrations of the catecholamines 1-epinephrine and 1-norepinephrine, which may cause profound dysrhythmias.

- Induce anesthesia with sodium thiamylal (3–6 mg/kg, IV) or oxymorphone (0.1–0.3 mg/kg IV) and glyco-pyrrolate.
- Isoflurane is the inhalant agent of choice for dogs with pheochromocytoma.
- Administer methoxyflurane (rather than halothane) if isoflurane is not available.
- Administer fluids and antibiotics as for hyperadre-nocorticism.
- Closely monitor blood pressure and ECG.
- To manage ventricular arrhythmias give either lido-caine (1 mg/kg IV) or propranolol (0.1–0.3 mg/kg IV).
- Treat hypertensive episodes with phentolamine (al-pha blocker) (0.02–0.1 mg/kg IV), repeated as needed.
- Manage hypotension with vigorous fluid administra-tion.

Surgical Procedure

Objectives

- Handle tissue gently, especially tumor tissue.

KEY POINT ▶ Surgical handling of a pheochromocytoma may precipitate catecholamine release and hypertension. Profound hypotension may rapidly occur following tumor removal.

- Use meticulous hemostasis to minimize blood loss.
- Avoid trauma to the caudal vena cava.
- Close the linea with a nonabsorbable suture material.

KEY POINT ▶ Animals with hyperadrenocorticism are prone to delayed healing and incisional infection because of cortisol inhibition of fibroblast proliferation and collagen synthesis.

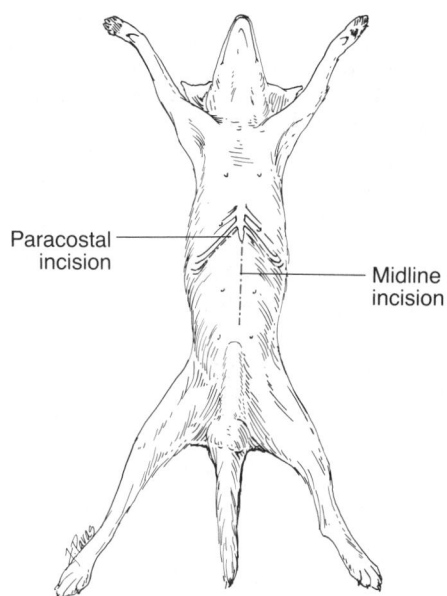

Figure 2. Incision for the ventral midline approach may be extended paracostal for better exposure of the adrenal gland.

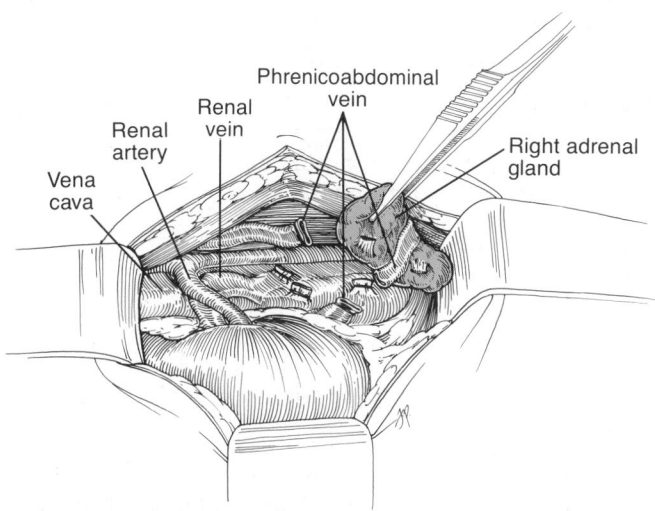

Figure 3. Surgical anatomy of the right adrenal gland and its associated vascular structures as viewed from the retroperitoneal approach.

Equipment

- Standard general surgical pack and suture
- Balfour retractors
- Bipolar cautery
- Sterile cotton-tipped applicator sticks
- Hemostatic clips
- Gelfoam

Technique

1. Make a ventral midline abdominal incision, extend-ing from the xiphoid to about 2 cm caudal to the umbilicus. This may be combined with a paracostal incision (Fig. 2).
   a. Alternatively, use a retroperitoneal approach (Fig. 3). This provides good exposure of the ipsilateral gland but must be performed bilater-ally if bilateral adrenalectomy is required.
2. Expose the affected gland(s) and isolate with mois-tened laparotomy sponges.
3. Facilitate gentle dissection by the use of cotton-tipped applicator sticks, especially when separating the gland from the vena cava.
4. Ligate the phrenicoabdominal artery and vein and any other vascular structures serving the adrenal gland. Hemostatic vascular clips are very helpful for this.

KEY POINT ▶ Identify and preserve the renal artery and vein, which may lie close to the adrenal glands.

5. Completely resect all abnormal tissue, including tumor thrombus in the vena cava, if possible.
6. Prior to closure, carefully check the surgical field for hemorrhage.
7. Inspect the abdominal viscera, especially the liver, for metastatic disease.
8. Perform a routine, three-layer abdominal closure using nonabsorbable suture material to close the linea alba.

Complications

Complications may include:

■ Hemorrhage
■ Cardiac arrest and/or dysrhythmias
■ Fluid and electrolyte abnormalities
■ Pulmonary artery thrombosis
■ Pancreatitis
■ Acute renal failure
■ Pneumonia
■ Adrenal insufficiency

Postoperative Care

Unilateral Adrenalectomy for Adrenocortical Tumor

■ Supplement glucocorticoids with prednisone (0.5 mg/kg PO q12h for 3 days, then taper over 10–14 days to 0.2 mg/kg PO q24h) until the contralateral adrenal gland is functioning normally.
■ Perform an ACTH stimulation test on the first postoperative day and at 2- to 4-week intervals following surgery until adrenal function is normal.
■ The remaining adrenal gland usually functions normally within 2 months following surgery.

Unilateral Adrenalectomy for Pheochromocytoma

Function of the contralateral gland is not suppressed; therefore, there is no need for postoperative glucocorticoid or mineralocorticoid supplementation.

Bilateral Adrenalectomy

■ Supplement glucocorticoids with prednisone, 0.2 mg/kg/day.
■ Mineralocorticoid supplementation (fludrocortisone acetate and DOCP) is necessary (see the preceding discussion of hypoadrenocorticism).
■ Check serum electrolytes periodically to adjust the dosages of mineralocorticoid replacement therapy.

Prognosis

Unilateral Adrenocortical Tumor

■ Good if the tumor is benign.
■ Fair if the tumor is malignant but completely resected.

■ Extremely poor for invasive adenocarcinomas.

Unilateral Pheochromocytoma

■ Excellent prognosis for benign tumor.
■ About 50% pheochromocytomas are malignant and metastatic at the time of surgery, carrying a grave prognosis.

Bilateral Adrenal Hyperplasia

■ Fair to good prognosis; however, medical therapy is preferred over surgery for this lesion.
■ Metastatic disease is not a problem; however, regulating the iatrogenic hypoadrenocorticism created by bilateral adrenalectomy may be difficult.

Supplemental Readings

Bouriad H, Feeney DA, Caywood DD, Hayden DW: Pheochromocytoma in dogs: 13 cases (1980–1985). J Am Vet Med Assoc 191:1610, 1987.
Enns SG, Johnston DE, Eigenmann JE, Goldschmidt MH: Adrenalectomy in the management of canine hyperadrenocorticism. J Am Anim Hosp Assoc 23:557, 1987.
Feldman EC, Peterson ME: Hypoadrenocorticism. Vet Clin North Am [Small Anim Pract] 14:751, 1984.
Kintzer PP, Peterson ME: Use of o,p'-DDD in treatment of canine hyperadrenocorticism caused by hyperfunctional adrenal neoplasia. In Kirk RW, Bonagura JD, eds.: Current Veterinary Therapy X. Philadelphia: W. B. Saunders, 1989, p 1034.
Kintzer PP, Peterson ME: Mitotane (o,p'-DDD) treatment of 200 dogs with pituitary-dependent hyperadrenocorticism. J Vet Intern Med 5:182, 1991.
Peterson ME, Nesbitt GH, Shaer M: Diagnosis and management of concurrent diabetes mellitus and hyperadrenocorticism in 30 dogs. J Am Vet Med Assoc 178:66, 1981.
Peterson ME: Considerations and complications in anesthesia with pathophysiologic changes in the endocrine system. In Short CE, ed.: Principles and Practice of Veterinary Anesthesiology. Philadelphia: Williams & Wilkins, 1987, p 251.
Peterson ME, Greco DS, Orth DN: Primary hypoadrenocorticism in ten cats. J Vet Intern Med 3:55, 1989.
Scavelli TD, Peterson ME, Matthiesen DT: Results of adrenalectomy for hyperadrenocorticism caused by adrenocortical neoplasia in 26 dogs. Vet Surg 15:133, 1986.
Twedt DC, Wheeler SL: Pheochromocytoma in the dog. Vet Clin North Am [Small Anim Pract] 14:767, 1984.

4 Diabetes Mellitus

Richard W. Nelson

Diabetes mellitus is a complex disorder resulting from inability of the pancreatic islets to secrete insulin and/or from impaired insulin action in tissues. These abnormalities ultimately cause hyperglycemia, glucosuria, and the classic clinical signs of polyuria, polydipsia, polyphagia, and weight loss. Diabetes mellitus is one of the most common endocrinopathies of dogs and cats and can be fatal if incorrectly diagnosed or inappropriately treated.

ETIOLOGY

Insulin-Dependent Diabetes Mellitus (IDDM)

- IDDM is the most common clinically recognized form of diabetes mellitus in the dog and cat.
- IDDM is characterized by hypoinsulinemia and a minimal to no increase in endogenous insulin following administration of an insulin secretagogue (e.g., glucose).
- The etiology is undoubtedly multifactorial. Inciting factors in the development of IDDM include:
  - Genetic predispositon
  - Infection
  - Insulin antagonistic diseases and drugs (e.g., hyperadrenocorticism, growth hormone in acromegaly, and progesterone; these are discussed elsewhere in sec. 4)
  - Immune-mediated ileitis and pancreatitis in dogs
  - Islet-specific amyloidosis in cats
- Loss of beta cell function is irreversible in IDDM, and life-long insulin therapy is mandatory to maintain glycemic control of the diabetic state.

Non–Insulin-Dependent Diabetes Mellitus (NIDDM)

- Clinically evident NIDDM is rare in dogs; however, approximately 20% of diabetic cats have NIDDM at the time of initial diagnosis.
- Destruction of the beta cells is not the predominant pathologic alteration. Rather, carbohydrate intolerance is due to:
  - Impaired insulin secretion by the beta cells
  - Insulin resistance in insulin-responsive tissues
  - Accelerated hepatic glucose production
- Because the beta cells maintain some insulin-secretory function, hyperglycemia tends to be mild, ketoacidosis is uncommon, and the necessity for insulin therapy is variable.
- The etiopathogenesis of feline NIDDM is unknown.

Obesity and islet-specific amyloid deposition plays a role in some cats.

Diabetic Ketoacidosis (DKA)

- Dogs and cats with DKA have a relative or absolute insulin deficiency as a result of:
  - Hypoinsulinemia in undiagnosed IDDM
  - Inappropriately low insulin dosages in a treated diabetic dog or cat
  - Impaired insulin action and/or insulin resistance caused by concurrent illness or drugs
- Insulin deficiency has several effects:
  - It initiates lipolysis. The nonesterified fatty acids released from adipose tissue are ultimately converted to ketone bodies (i.e., acetoacetic acid, beta-hydroxybutyric acid, acetone), which cause the ketosis and acidosis of ketoacidosis.
  - It impairs the utilization of ketone bodies by peripheral tissues.
- An excess of diabetogenic hormones (i.e., glucagon, catecholamines, cortisol, and growth hormone), fasting, and dehydration also contribute to the increase in gluconeogenesis and ketogenesis of DKA.
- Increased production and decreased utilization of ketone bodies results in accumulation of ketones in the blood, spillage of ketones into the urine, and development of metabolic acidosis.

CLINICAL SIGNS

- Clinical signs of IDDM and NIDDM do not develop until hyperglycemia results in glucosuria.
- The history in virtually all diabetic patients includes polydipsia, polyuria, polyphagia, and weight loss. These may be accompanied by clinical signs associated with any one of several potential diabetic complications (see Table 1).
- Occasionally the owner will present a dog because of sudden blindness caused by cataract formation.
- Many diabetic dogs and cats are obese but are otherwise in good physical condition. However, dogs and cats with prolonged untreated diabetes may have lost weight.
- Diabetic cats may develop a plantigrade posture with the hocks touching the ground when the cat walks. This posture is believed to be caused by diabetic neuropathy.
- In dogs and cats with DKA, additional clinical signs may include depression, weakness, tachypnea, vomiting, and a strong odor of acetone on the breath.

TABLE 1. Complications of Diabetes Mellitus

Complication	Principal Manifestation
Ketoacidosis	Vomiting; depression; Kussmaul's respirations; collapse
Cataracts	Blindness
Retinopathy	Ophthalmoscopic lesions
Neuropathy	Weakness
Pancreatitis	Vomiting; abdominal pain
Exocrine pancreatic insufficiency	Diarrhea; weight loss
Hepatic lipidosis	Hepatomegaly
Glomerulonephropathy	Oliguric renal failure
Bacterial infections	
Urinary	Cystitis; pyelonephritis
Respiratory	Pneumonia (cough, dyspnea, fever)
Cutaneous	Pyoderma

- In animals with severe metabolic acidosis, slow, deep breathing (Kussmaul respiration) may be observed.

DIAGNOSIS

KEY POINT ▶ Diagnosis of diabetes mellitus requires documentation of appropriate clinical signs (polyuria, polydipsia, polyphagia, and weight loss) in association with hyperglycemia and glucosuria. In the cat, determine whether the diabetes is IDDM or NIDDM.

- Measure blood glucose and urine glucose with appropriate blood (Chemstrip bG) and urine (Keto-Diastix) reagent test strips to allow rapid confirmation of diabetes mellitus in both dogs and cats. Concurrent documentation of ketonuria establishes DKA.
- Document both hyperglycemia and glycosuria when establishing a diagnosis of diabetes mellitus.
  - Hyperglycemia differentiates diabetes mellitus from primary renal glycosuria.
  - Glucosuria differentiates diabetes mellitus from transient, epinephrine-induced stress hyperglycemia.
- Diabetes mellitus in the dog is almost always IDDM.
- In the cat measure baseline serum insulin concentration, perform an insulin response test (e.g., intravenous glucose tolerance test, glucagon tolerance test), or evaluate response to therapy to differentiate between IDDM and NIDDM.
  - A baseline insulin concentration >120 pM/liter or one or more serum insulin concentrations >120 pM/liter at any time during an insulin response test suggests either NIDDM or carbohydrate intolerance induced by an insulin antagonistic disorder (e.g., hyperadrenocorticism) or drug (e.g., megestrol acetate).
  - Some cats subsequently shown to have NIDDM have initial test results suggestive of IDDM. The ultimate differentiation often is made retrospectively, after the clinician has had several weeks to

assess the animal's response to therapy and need for insulin.
- When the diagnosis of diabetes mellitus has been established, obtain a thorough laboratory evaluation, including a complete blood count (CBC), serum biochemical panel, serum lipase assay, and urinalysis with bacterial culture (Table 2).

TREATMENT
Therapy for DKA

The *goals of initial therapy* for DKA are:

- Provide adequate amounts of insulin to normalize intermediary metabolism.
- Restore water and electrolyte losses.
- Correct acidosis.
- Identify precipitating factors.
- Provide a carbohydrate substrate when required by the insulin treatment.

To guide therapy, evaluate the following:

- Urinalysis, hematocrit, and blood glucose
- Venous total carbon dioxide or arterial acid-base parameters
- Blood urea nitrogen (BUN) or serum creatinine
- Serum electrolytes
- Electrocardiogram

For a complete discussion of the clinical use of fluid, electrolyte, and bicarbonate therapy, see sec. 1, ch. 5.

Fluid Therapy

During fluid therapy:

- Monitor the patient's alertness, heart rate, mucous membrane moisture, capillary refill time, pulse pressure, and skin turgor.
- Serially evaluate the central venous pressure, urine output, body weight, and pulmonary and cardiac auscultation.

The type of fluids used depends on the animal's

TABLE 2. Common Clinicopathologic Alterations Associated with Diabetes Mellitus

Hemogram
  Neutrophilic leukocytosis

Biochemistry profile
  Hyperglycemia
  Hypercholesterolemia
  Increased ALT
  Increased SAP
  Hyperamylasemia
  Hyperlipasemia

Urinalysis
  Urine specific gravity usually >1.020
  Glycosuria
  Ketonuria
  Proteinuria
  Bacteriuria
  Hematuria
  Pyuria

ALT = alanine aminotransferase; SAP = serum alkaline phosphatase.

electrolyte status, blood glucose concentration, and osmolality.

Osmolality

- Unless serum electrolytes dictate otherwise, initially give 0.9% saline supplemented with potassium (see below).
- If the osmolality is >350 mOsm/kg, consider giving hypotonic fluids (0.45% saline); however, use hypotonic fluids with extreme caution in dogs and cats with DKA. This avoids cerebral edema caused by the differences in osmolality of blood versus central nervous tissue, which develops with insulin and hypotonic fluid therapy.
- Estimate osmolality using the following formula:

$$\begin{array}{ccccc} \text{Osmolality} & = & 2(\text{Na} + \text{K}) & + & 0.05(\text{glucose}) & + & 0.33(\text{BUN}) \\ (\text{mOsm/kg}) & & (\text{mEq/liter}) & & (\text{mg/dl}) & & (\text{mg/dl}) \end{array}$$

Volume and Rate of Administration

- Determine the initial volume and rate of fluid administration by assessing the degree of shock, the dehydration deficit, the patient's maintenance requirements, the plasma protein concentration, and the presence or absence of cardiac disease.
- Direct fluid administration at gradually replacing all deficits over a period of 24–48 hours.
- Initially, give fluids at 1.5 to 2 times maintenance (60–100 ml/kg/day); base subsequent adjustments on frequent assessment of hydration status, urine output, severity of azotemia, and persistence of vomiting and diarrhea.

Serum Electrolytes. Monitor serum electrolytes frequently (at least twice a day) and make necessary adjustments. After the initial 4–6 hours of fluid therapy:

- If the serum sodium concentration is 140–155 mEq/liter, change the IV fluids to Ringer's solution.
- If the serum sodium concentration is 140 mEq/liter, maintain the patient on 0.9% sodium chloride solution.
- If the serum sodium concentration is >155 mEq/liter, give 0.45% saline solution.

Potassium Therapy

- During therapy for DKA, the serum potassium concentration will fall because of:
  - Rehydration (dilution)
  - Correction of acidemia (shift of hydrogen ions out of cells in exchange for potassium)
  - Insulin-mediated cellular uptake of potassium
  - Continued urinary losses
- Most dogs and cats with DKA initially have normal or decreased serum potassium concentration.
- Dogs and cats with hypokalemia require aggressive potassium replacement therapy to replace deficits and to prevent worsening hypokalemia after initiation of insulin therapy.
- Base the amount of potassium required on actual measurement of serum potassium concentration (Table 3).
- If an accurate measurement of serum potassium is not available, add 40 mEq of potassium to each liter of IV fluids.

TABLE 3. Guidelines for Potassium Supplementation in IV Fluids*

Blood Potassium (mEq/liter)	K⁺ Supplement/liter of fluids (mEq)
>3.5	20
3.0–3.5	30
2.5–3.0	40
2.0–2.5	60
<2.0	80

*The rate of potassium administration should not exceed 1 mEq/kg body weight/hour.

- Of the added potassium, 5% should be as potassium chloride and 50% as potassium phosphate. In addition to controlling hypokalemia, this will help prevent hypophosphatemia following initiation of insulin therapy (see below).
- Base subsequent adjustments in potassium supplementation on measurement of serum potassium, preferably done twice a day until serum electrolytes are stable and in the normal range.

Phosphate Therapy

- Phosphorus shifts from tissues to the extracellular compartment in a manner similar to that of potassium.
- The metabolic acidosis of DKA results in a shift of phosphorus from the intracellular to the extracellular compartment. Consequently, hypophosphatemia is not commonly identified at initial presentation, even though total body phosphorus levels may be severely deficient.
- Initiation of insulin therapy and correction of metabolic acidosis may result in a dramatic shift in extracellular phosphorus into the intracellular compartment, causing hypophosphatemia.
- The primary clinical manifestations of hypophosphatemia are hemolysis and anemia.
- Phosphorus is usually supplemented by adding potassium phosphate solution to IV fluids (preferably using a calcium-free solution such as 0.9% saline).
  - In the dog, supplement phosphate at 0.01–0.03 mMol/kg/hour for 3–6 hours, and then recheck the blood phosphorus concentration.
  - Alternatively, determine the amount of potassium required and then supplement with 50% potassium chloride and 50% potassium phosphate. This method is also used for cats.

Adverse Effects. Adverse effects from overzealous phosphate administration include:

- Iatrogenic hypocalcemia and its associated neuromuscular signs
- Hypernatremia
- Hypotension
- Metastatic calcification

Contraindications. Phosphorus supplementation is not indicated for dogs or cats with hypercalcemia, hyperphosphatemia, oliguria, or suspected tissue necrosis.

Bicarbonate Therapy

- Determine the need for bicarbonate therapy on the basis of clinical signs and measurement of bicarbonate or total venous CO_2 concentration.
- Bicarbonate therapy usually is unnecessary when plasma bicarbonate (or total venous CO_2) is 12 Eq/liter or greater, especially if the patient is alert. Correct acidosis in these patients with insulin and fluid therapy.
- Initiate therapy when the plasma bicarbonate concentration (or total venous CO_2) is 11 mEq/liter or less.

KEY POINT ▶ Correct metabolic acidosis slowly in the peripheral circulation, thereby avoiding major alterations in the pH of the cerebrospinal fluid (CSF). *Never* give bicarbonate by bolus infusion.

- Calculate the bicarbonate deficit (i.e., milliequivalents of bicarbonate initially needed to correct acidosis to the critical level of 12 mEq/liter) using the formula:

mEq HCO_3^- =
body weight (kg) $\times$ 0.4 $\times$ (12 $-$ patient's HCO_3^-) $\times$ 0.5

  - The difference between the patient's serum bicarbonate concentration and the critical value of 12 mEq/liter represents the treatable base deficit in DKA.
  - The factor 0.5 provides one half of the required dose of bicarbonate in the IV infusion. In this manner, a conservative dose is given over 6 hours.
- After 6 hours of therapy, re-evaluate the acid-base status and repeat the calculations.
- When the plasma bicarbonate level is >12 mEq/liter, further bicarbonate supplementation is not needed.

Insulin Therapy

KEY POINT ▶ The *goal* of initial insulin therapy, using only rapid-acting regular or Semilente insulin, is to slowly lower the blood glucose concentration to 200–250 mg/dl, preferably over an 8–10 hour time period. An hourly decline of approximately 75 mg/dl is ideal.

Regular or Semilente Insulin. The intermittent IM insulin regimen works well for the initial management of dogs or cats with DKA.

- In dogs and cats with severe DKA, administer an initial regular insulin loading dose of 0.2 U/kg followed by 0.1 U/kg every hour thereafter until blood glucose concentration is lowered to <250 mg/dl.
  - Administer the insulin into the muscles of the rear legs to ensure that the injections are not inadvertently being deposited in fat or subcutaneous tissue.
- Measure the blood glucose concentration every 1–2 hours with Chemstrip bG reagent strips.

- Once blood glucose concentration is <250 mg/dl, discontinue this regimen and initiate regular insulin, given every 4–6 hours IM or, if hydration status is good, every 6–8 hours SC.
  - The initial dose usually is 0.1–0.4 U/kg, with subsequent adjustments based on blood glucose concentrations.
- When the blood glucose concentration is <250 mg/dl, add enough 50% dextrose to the IV infusion solution to create a 5% dextrose solution.
  - Maintain the blood glucose concentration at 150–250 mg/dl until the patient is stable and eating.

Longer-Acting Insulin. Do not change to longer-acting insulin (e.g., Lente, Ultralente) until the patient is stable, eating, and not vomiting, maintaining fluid balance without any IV infusions, and no longer acidotic, azotemic, or electrolyte-deficient.

- Make the initial dose of longer-acting insulin the same as the last dose of regular insulin.
- Initiate dietary therapy and base subsequent adjustments in the longer-acting insulin dosage on measurement of serial blood glucose concentrations, as discussed below for nonketotic diabetes.

Therapy for Nonketotic Diabetes Mellitus

The primary goals of therapy for both IDDM and NIDDM are to have a satisfied owner with a healthy, interactive pet and to maintain the blood glucose concentration as close to normal (100 mg/dl) as possible.

- These goals can be accomplished through:
  - Proper insulin administration
  - Diet and exercise
  - Oral hypoglycemic medications; avoidance or control of concurrent illness
- Which therapeutic regime is ultimately successful depends, in part, on the number of functional beta cells in the pancreas.
- In addition, manage concurrent diabetogenic conditions such as hyperadrenocorticism, acromegaly, or megestrol acetate treatment as discussed elsewhere in this book.
- Provide a relatively consistent level of daily exercise.
- Recommend ovariohysterectomy in nonbreeding females to prevent destabilization of glycemic control with fluctuations in reproductive hormones.

Dietary Therapy

- Dietary therapy is indicated for all cats and dogs with diabetes mellitus.
- The goal of dietary therapy is to:
  - Correct obesity
  - Maintain consistency in the timing and caloric content of meals
  - Furnish a diet that minimizes postprandial fluctuations in blood glucose

Type of Food. To minimize fluctuations in postprandial blood glucose concentration, feed canned and dry kibble foods that contain a predominance of complex carbohydrates; avoid soft moist foods.

KEY POINT ▶ Diets containing increased amounts of fiber help promote weight loss, slow glucose absorption from the intestinal tract, reduce postprandial fluctuations in blood glucose, and enhance control of hyperglycemia.

- The most effective diets in the management of excess body weight and both IDDM and NIDDM are those that contain the most fiber and digestible complex carbohydrates on a dry matter basis (Tables 4 and 5).
- Use caution when feeding diets with high-fiber content to thin diabetic dogs and cats because high-fiber diets have a low caloric density that can interfere with weight gain and may result in further weight loss.
- Initially feed a low-fiber diet with high caloric density to thin diabetic animals. Once normal body weight is attained, gradually substitute a diet containing increased fiber content.

Caloric Intake. Calculate caloric intake to maintain the dog or cat near its normal body weight (for further information see sec. 1, ch. 3)

- The daily caloric requirement for the mature dog and cat is 60–85 kcal of metabolizable energy per kilogram of ideal body weight (higher for smaller dogs).
- Because the amount required by an animal may be as much as 50% above or below the calculated requirement, adjust the amount fed on an individual basis.
- When an animal is overweight, reduce weight grad-

TABLE 4. Fiber and Digestible Complex Carbohydrate Content of Some Commercially Available High-Fiber Dog Foods*

	Crude Fiber*	Digestible Complex Carbohydrates*
Prescription Diet r/d		
Canned	25	36
Dry	22	39
Prescription Diet w/d†		
Canned	16	54
Dry	13	56
Science Diet Maintenance Light†		
Canned	14	57
Dry	8	61
Fit and Trim		
Dry	9	61
Gaines Cycle 3 Light		
Canned	8	37
Dry	5	53
Prescription Diet g/d		
Canned	7	57
Dry	6	54
Alpo Light		
Canned	5	39
Iams Less Active		
Dry	3	50

*Values are listed as % dry matter.
†Recommended by the author.

TABLE 5. Fiber and Digestible Complex Carbohydrate Content of Some Commercially Available High-Fiber Cat Foods

	Crude Fiber*	Digestible Complex Carbohydrates*
Prescription Diet r/d		
Canned	28	24
Dry	19	30
Prescription Diet w/d†		
Canned	12	22
Dry	10	37
Science Diet Maintenance Light		
Canned	7	25
Dry	7	39
Iams Less Active		
Dry	2	41

*Values are listed as % dry matter.
†Recommended by author.

ually over a period of 2–4 months until targeted body weight is reached.

Feeding Schedule. The feeding schedule should enhance the actions of insulin and minimize postprandial hyperglycemia.

- The daily caloric intake should be ingested when insulin is still present in the circulation and capable of handling glucose absorbed from the meal.
- Feeding the diabetic dog or cat after insulin action has waned will result in increasing blood glucose concentration beginning 1–2 hours postprandial. If this occurs, adjust one or more of these factors:
  - The type of insulin
  - The frequency of insulin administration
  - The timing of the meals

KEY POINT ▶ Within the time frame of insulin action, feed multiple small meals rather than one large meal to minimize the hyperglycemic effect of each meal.

- For dogs and cats that are "nibblers" throughout the day, allow free access to food. For "gluttonous" dogs and cats, feed two or three meals daily, depending on the frequency of insulin administration and owner compliance.

Oral Hypoglycemic Drugs

Sulfonylureas. Sulfonylureas (Table 6) stimulate insulin secretion, decrease hepatic glucose production, partially reverse the postbinding defect in insulin action, and increase the number of cellular insulin receptors. Functional beta cells must exist for sulfonylureas to be effective.

- Sulfonylureas are relatively ineffective in improving glycemic control in dogs with diabetes mellitus but are useful in some diabetic cats.

Glipizide. Glipizide (Glucotrol; Pfizer, New York, NY), at a dose of 5 mg/cat q8–12h, has been efficacious

TABLE 6. Oral Sulfonylurea Drugs Currently Available in the United States

Generic Name	Trade Name	Relative Potency
Tolbutamide	Orinase	1
Acetohexamide	Dymelor	2.5
Tolazamide	Tolinase	5
Chlorpropamide	Diabinase	6
Glipizide*	Glucotrol	100
Glyburide	Micronase	150
	Diabeta	150

*Glipizide has been effective in some cats at a total dose of 5 mg q 8–12 h in conjunction with correction of obesity and dietary therapy.

in some diabetic cats with NIDDM when used in conjunction with dietary therapy and correction of obesity.

- Adverse reactions to glipizide in cats include vomiting, hypoglycemia, icterus, and increased hepatic enzyme concentrations.
- In humans, bone marrow depression and blood dyscrasias can occur, but these have not been observed in diabetic cats.
- Nevertheless, periodic evaluation of a hemogram and serum biochemical panel is indicated for cats on long-term glipizide therapy.

Insulin Therapy

The properties of beef/pork insulin preparations are described in Table 7.

KEY POINT ▶ The initial insulin of choice for the diabetic dog is Lente insulin given as a single morning injection. For small dogs (<15 kg) give approximately 1.0 U/kg of body weight. For large dogs (>25 kg) give 0.5 U/kg.

KEY POINT ▶ The initial insulin of choice for the diabetic cat is Ultralente insulin. For the average-sized cat give a total dose of 1 to 3 U as a single morning injection.

TABLE 7. Properties of Beef/Pork Insulin Preparations Used in Dogs and Cats*

Type of Insulin	Route of Administration	Duration of Effect (Hours)	
		Dog	Cat
Regular crystalline,	IV	1–4	
Semilente	IM	3–8	
	SC	4–10	
NPH (Isophane)	SC	6–24	4–12
PZI	SC	6–28	6–24
Lente†	SC	8–24	6–18
Ultralente‡	SC	8–28	8–24

*Purified pork and recombinant human insulins appear to be more potent, act faster, and have a shorter duration of effect than beef/pork insulins. Major manufacturers of insulin include Eli Lilly Co., E.R. Squibb and Sons, and Novo Nordisk.
†Initial insulin of choice for the diabetic dog.
‡Initial insulin of choice for the diabetic cat.

Combination beef/pork insulin is recommended initially. Purified pork insulin and recombinant human insulin (Humulin; Eli Lilly, Indianapolis, IN) are less antigenic but have a shorter duration of effect than combination beef/pork insulin. As such, they are generally reserved for animals that have problems with insulin activity (insulin resistance).

Adjustments in Insulin Therapy Using the Serial Blood Glucose Curve

- Assessment of insulin therapy is necessary:
  - To initially regulate the diabetic patient
  - To check periodically on the status of glycemic control in the patient who is doing well in the home environment
  - To re-establish glycemic control in the patient in which clinical manifestations of hyperglycemia or hypoglycemia have developed
- To assess insulin therapy:
  - Follow the daily insulin and feeding routine.
  - Measure blood glucose concentrations, ideally beginning at the time of the AM insulin injection, every 1–2 hours for 12–24 hours.

KEY POINT ▶ The goal of insulin therapy in the diabetic dog without cataracts is to maintain the blood glucose concentration at 100–180 mg/dl; in the diabetic dog that is blind because of cataract formation and in the diabetic cat, the goal is 100–250 mg/dl. (If utilizing glucose test strips, maintain the blood glucose concentration at >80 mg/dl.)

Insulin Effectiveness. The first parameter to be assessed is the effectiveness of the insulin at lowering the blood glucose concentration.

- To make this assessment, consider:
  - The insulin dosage
  - The highest blood glucose concentration
  - The difference between the highest and lowest blood glucose concentration
- If the insulin is not effective in lowering the blood glucose concentration, then consider any of the following:
  - Inappropriate insulin administration technique
  - Insulin underdosage
  - Insulin overdosage (Somogyi phenomenon)
  - Very short duration of action of insulin
  - Falsely increased blood glucose concentrations associated with severe stress during the blood sampling procedure
  - Insulin resistance

Insulin Resistance

- There is no insulin dosage that clearly differentiates insulin resistance from insulin underdosage. In the author's experience, glycemic control can be established:
  - In most diabetic dogs, with a dosage of 1.0 U/kg or less of intermediate or long-acting insulin administered once or twice daily
  - In most diabetic cats, with a total dose of 5 U or

less of long-acting insulin administered once or twice a day

- Therefore, suspect insulin resistance when insulin dosages exceed these amounts, especially when the insulin dosage exceeds 2.2 U of insulin/kg with minimal improvement in glycemic control.

■ If insulin resistance is suspected, a diagnostic evaluation is warranted to identify the underlying etiology (Table 8). Some dogs and cats, however, require large amounts of insulin with no obvious cause of the relative insulin ineffectiveness.

Glucose Nadir. If insulin is effective in lowering the blood glucose concentration, the next parameter to assess is the lowest blood glucose concentration, or the glucose nadir.

■ The glucose nadir should be ≥100 mg/dl (≥80 mg/dl if using glucose test strips).
■ If the glucose nadir is <80 mg/dl, decrease the insulin dosage according to the following guidelines:
  - If the diabetic dog or cat is receiving an "acceptable" dose of insulin (≤1.0 U/kg), decrease the insulin dosage by approximately 25%.
  - If a large amount of insulin is being given (e.g., >2.2 U/kg), reinstitute glycemic regulation utilizing the insulin dosage recommended for the initial regulation of the diabetic dog or cat.
■ Evaluate blood glucose concentrations 4 to 7 days after changing the insulin dose and make further adjustments in the insulin dose after reviewing these results.

Duration of Effect. When the glucose nadir is ≥100 mg/dl (≥80 mg/dl if using glucose test strips), the duration of effect of the insulin can be assessed.

■ The duration of effect is roughly defined as the time from the insulin injection until the blood glucose concentration exceeds 200–250 mg/dl. Ideally, insulin action should last 22–24 hours.
■ To determine duration of insulin effect from an abbreviated (8–12 hours) serial glucose curve, it is important to obtain at least one blood glucose concentration 2–3 hours after the early evening meal.
  - Classically, the abbreviated glucose curve in a dog or cat with short duration of insulin action has the highest blood glucose first thing in the morning; subsequent blood glucose concentrations decline throughout the day; the glucose nadir occurs at the time of the early evening meal; and subsequent

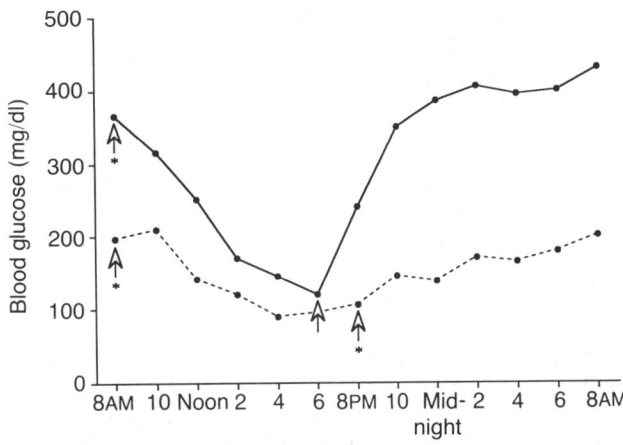

Figure 1. Serial blood glucose concentrations in a dog with a short duration of Lente insulin action (top line) and subsequent improvement in glycemic control following initiation of Lente insulin twice daily (broken line). Notice the marked morning hyperglycemia, acceptable glucose nadir, and increase in blood glucose concentration following the evening meal when the dog received Lente insulin only once daily. Insulin administration (asterisks); food (arrows).

postprandial blood glucose concentrations increase (Fig. 1).
  - The severity of clinical signs, morning hyperglycemia, and glucose nadir allow assumptions to be made concerning the duration of effect of the insulin.

Use the duration of effect as a guide to adjustments needed to establish glycemic control.
For the diabetic dog:

■ If NPH or Lente insulin has a duration of effect of 16–20 hours and clinical signs of hyperglycemia are present, consider changing to Ultralente insulin.
■ If a diabetic dog is already receiving Ultralente insulin once a day, if its duration of effect is 16–20 hours, and if clinical signs of hyperglycemia are present, consider a supplemental dose of regular or Semilente insulin administered in the late evening.
  - Alternatively, discontinue Ultralente insulin and replace it with Lente or NPH insulin given q12h.
■ If the duration of effect of NPH Lente, or Ultralente insulin is 10–14 hours, administer the insulin twice a day.
■ If the duration of effect of NPH or Lente insulin is <10 hours, administer Ultralente insulin once or, more likely, twice a day.

For the diabetic cat:

■ If the duration of effect of Ultralente insulin is ≤12 hours, administer Ultralente insulin q12h.
■ If the duration of effect of Ultralente insulin is >12 hours and the cat is doing well at home, a change in frequency of administration may not be warranted.
■ If the duration of effect of Ultralente insulin is >12 hours and the owner reports clinical signs of hyperglycemia, administer Ultralente insulin q12h and adjust the insulin dosage correspondingly to prevent hypoglycemia, especially if the duration of effect is 12–15 hours.
  - Alternatively, administer Lente insulin q12h.

TABLE 8. Possible Causes of Apparent Insulin Resistance in the Dog and Cat

Problems in insulin administration
Inactive or outdated insulin
Diestrus or pregnancy
Hyperadrenocorticism
Acromegaly
Infection
Administration of diabetogenic medications
Anti-insulin antibodies
Impaired insulin absorption from subcutaneous sites
Somogyi phenomenon

Before deciding to alter the insulin dosage, consider the glucose nadir and the difference between the blood glucose concentrations measured at the time of each anticipated insulin injection.

- If the blood glucose concentration is approximately the same at the time of each anticipated insulin injection, adjust the insulin dose based on the glucose nadir and administer the same dosage at each injection.
- If there is a marked difference in blood glucose concentration (e.g., >100 mg/dl) between the anticipated AM and PM injection times and the PM blood glucose concentration is less than the AM glucose concentration, administer a conservative dose of insulin (sufficient to maintain the glucose nadir at about 120 mg/dl) initially at each injection.
- Monitor the blood glucose concentration at the time of each insulin injection, as well as during the middle of the day, for the initial 5–7 days to identify hypoglycemia.

Home Management

- The most important parameter to assess in the home is the owner's subjective opinion of the pet's water intake, urine output, and body weight. If these factors are normal, the diabetes usually is well controlled.
- Encourage owners of diabetic dogs to check the animal's urine daily for glucose and ketones. Have them check the urine prior to the evening meal and not in the morning.
  - If the animal is responding properly to the injections, the urine will be negative for glucose prior to feeding.
  - Encourage owners to check the urine once a week (e.g., during weekend), as many times during the day as possible. The urine of the well-controlled diabetic pet will be free of glucose for most of a 24-hour period.
  - Do not adjust the insulin dosage based on morning urine glucose concentrations. Instead, administer a fixed dosage of insulin based on the results of in-hospital serial blood glucose testing.
- Urine monitoring is not mandatory for diabetic cats; however, it can be utilized to identify problems with insulin therapy. As in the dog, persistent glycosuria suggests a problem that requires evaluation via in-hospital serial blood glucose determinations.
- In the healthy diabetic dog or cat, evaluate a serial blood glucose curve every 2–4 months.
  - Evaluate serial blood glucose curves early if glycosuria becomes persistent or clinical signs recur.

- Make adjustments in insulin therapy on the basis of these results.

Management in Perioperative Period

Elective major surgery should be delayed until the patient's clinical condition is stable.

The goal of therapy during the perioperative period is to prevent hypoglycemia, severe hyperglycemia (>400 mg/dl), and ketosis.

Suggested Protocol

- Follow the normal insulin and feeding schedule the day prior to surgery.
- Give no food after midnight.
- On the morning of surgery, give half the calculated daily morning dose of insulin. For the remainder of the day, administer regular crystalline insulin SC, as needed to control hyperglycemia (usually every 4–8 hours).
- During and following surgery, maintain the patient on IV infusion of 5% dextrose in water until oral intake of food is re-established. Adjust the rate of dextrose infusion needed to prevent hypoglycemia (<80 mg/dl).
- Monitor blood glucose concentration with reagent strips hourly and adjust dextrose infusion and regular insulin administration appropriately (ideal blood glucose concentration is 100–300 mg/dl during the perioperative period).

On the day after surgery, the diabetic dog or cat usually can be returned to the routine schedule of insulin administration and feeding. Maintain a patient that is not eating on IV dextrose infusion and regular crystalline insulin until appetite returns.

Supplemental Readings

Alejandro R, Feldman EC, Shienvold FL, et al.: Advances in canine diabetes mellitus research: etiopathology and results of islet transplantation. J Am Vet Med Assoc 193:1050, 1988.

Chastain CB, Nichols CE: Low-dose intramuscular insulin therapy for diabetic ketoacidosis in dogs. J Am Vet Med Assoc 178:561, 1981.

Gerich JE: Oral hypoglycemic agents. N Engl J Med 321:1231, 1989.

Johnson KH, O'Brien TD, Betsholtz C, et al.: Islet amyloid, islet-amyloid polypeptide, and diabetes mellitus. N Engl J Med 321:513, 1989.

Nelson RW: Feline diabetes mellitus. Veterinary Medical Report, 3:4, 1991.

Nelson RW: *Textbook of Veterinary Internal Medicine*. Philadelphia: W. B. Saunders, 1989, p 1676.

Nelson RW, Lewis LD: Nutritional management of diabetes mellitus. Semin Vet Med Surg 5:178, 1990.

Nelson RW, Himsel CA, Feldman EC, et al.: Glucose tolerance and insulin response in normal-weight and obese cats. Am J Vet Res 51:1357, 1990.

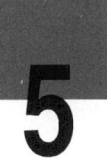

5 Pancreatic Beta Cell Neoplasia

Richard W. Nelson
S. Kathleen Salisbury

Tumors of the beta cells of the pancreatic islets are functional tumors that secrete excessive amounts of insulin independent of normal regulatory mechanisms. Hyperinsulinism causes hypoglycemia and corresponding clinical signs. It is important to consider beta cell neoplasia in the differential diagnosis of hypoglycemia in middle-aged and older dogs.

ETIOLOGY

- Insulin-secreting tumors almost always are malignant.
- Metastatic sites include the lymphatics and lymph nodes (duodenal, mesenteric, hepatic, splenic), liver, mesentery, and omentum.
- The hyperinsulinemia caused by beta cell tumors interferes with glucose homeostasis by decreasing the rate of glucose release from the liver and by increasing the uptake of glucose by insulin-sensitive tissues.
  - The net effect is promotion of hypoglycemia and secretion of the diabetogenic hormones (most notably glucagon and epinephrine).
  - The clinical signs of hypoglycemia result from neuroglycopenia and stimulation of the sympathoadrenal system.

CLINICAL SIGNS

- The most common clinical signs include seizures, weakness, collapse, and ataxia (Table 1).
- Clinical signs are usually present for 1 to 6 months prior to presentation to the veterinarian.
- Clinical signs tend to be episodic and often develop during fasting, exercise, excitement, and eating.

DIAGNOSIS

KEY POINT ▶ The diagnosis of an insulin-secreting beta cell tumor requires initial confirmation of hypoglycemia and then documentation of inappropriate insulin secretion.

Signalment

The signalment (i.e., older dog), normal physical examination, and lack of abnormalities other than hypoglycemia on hemogram, biochemical panel, and urinalysis strongly suggest beta cell neoplasia as the cause of the hypoglycemia (Table 2).

- Insulin-secreting tumors typically occur in the middle-aged or older dog, with an age range of 6–14 years.
- There is no apparent sex or breed predilection, although the Standard poodle, boxer, fox terrier, German shepherd, and Irish setter are commonly affected in our hospital.
- Islet cell neoplasia is a rare diagnosis in cats.

Physical Examination

The physical examination of dogs with insulin-secreting tumors is surprisingly unremarkable.

- Weight gain is evident in some dogs and is probably a result of the potent anabolic effects of insulin.
- Peripheral neuropathies have been reported in dogs with insulin-secreting tumors and may be manifested as proprioception deficits, depressed reflexes, and muscle atrophy.

Laboratory Studies

- The only consistent abnormality found on the hemogram, biochemical panel, and urinalysis is hypoglycemia.
- Hypoalbuminemia, hypophosphatemia, hypokalemia, and an increase in alkaline phosphatase and alanine aminotransferase have been reported, but these findings are considered nonspecific and not helpful in achieving a definitive diagnosis.
- A correlation has not been found between liver enzyme elevations and the presence of metastasis of the pancreatic tumor to the liver.

Blood Glucose Assay
- Dogs with insulin-secreting tumors occasionally may have a normal blood glucose concentration on random testing. Such a finding does not eliminate inter-

TABLE 1. Clinical Signs Associated with Beta Cell Neoplasia in the Dog

Seizures	Muscle fasciculations
Weakness	Bizarre behavior
Collapse	Lethargy
Ataxia	Weight gain
Posterior paresis	Polyphagia

TABLE 2. Differential Diagnoses for Hypoglycemia

Beta cell neoplasia
Nonpancreatic neoplasia
   Hepatocellular carcinoma
   Leiomyosarcoma
Hepatopathy
Sepsis
Hypoadrenocorticism
Toy breed puppy
Chronic renal failure
Glycogen storage disorder
Starvation

mittent hypoglycemia as a cause of episodic weakness or seizure activity.

- To identify hypoglycemia, fast the animal and evaluate the blood glucose hourly.
- A fast of 8 hours or less is successful in demonstrating hypoglycemia in most dogs with insulin-secreting tumors; occasionally longer fasts are required.

Ultrasonography

Abdominal ultrasonography can be used to identify a mass in the region of the pancreas and to assess for potential metastatic lesions in the liver and surrounding structures; however, negative findings do not rule out the possibility of an insulin-secreting tumor.

Insulin Secretion Measurement

Confirmation of an insulin-secreting neoplasm requires documentation of inappropriate insulin secretion during hypoglycemia. Measuring a serum insulin concentration when the blood glucose is <60 mg/dl will usually establish the diagnosis. A 4- to 10-hour fast may be required to obtain this level of hypoglycemia, but when the blood glucose concentration falls to <60 mg/dl, the simultaneous blood insulin concentration is interpreted as follows:

- The blood insulin is above normal (>120 pM/liter); the presence of an insulin-secreting neoplasm is likely.
- The blood insulin is in the high normal range (60–120 pM/liter); the presence of an insulin-secreting tumor remains possible.
- The blood insulin is in the low normal range (30–60 pM/liter); an insulin-secreting tumor has not been confirmed.
  - Low normal blood insulin may be found with hypoglycemia associated with non-islet cell tumors as well as insulin-secreting tumors.
  - Blood insulin in the low normal range in a dog with hypoglycemia is an indication for further diagnostics, including repeating the blood glucose and insulin determinations.
- The blood insulin is below the normal range (<30 pM/liter); insulinopenia has been documented, and an insulin-secreting tumor has been ruled out.

MEDICAL TREATMENT FOR ACUTE HYPOGLYCEMIC CRISIS

The acute onset of clinical signs of hypoglycemia (see Table 1) typically occurs in the dog in the home environment or immediately postoperatively in the dog with an inoperable tumor or metastases. Therapy depends on the severity of clinical signs and the location of the dog or cat (i.e., home or hospital).

- In the hospital, administer 50% dextrose solution (2–15 ml) slowly IV until clinical signs are controlled.
- If the dog is home, instruct the owner to rub a sugar-containing solution (e.g., Karo syrup) on the buccal mucosa until clinical signs are controlled.
- Dogs and cats with hypoglycemia should respond to the administration of glucose in 30–120 seconds.

KEY POINT ▶ It is imperative to avoid overstimulation of the tumor when administering dextrose IV. Overstimulation of the tumor can result in excessive release of insulin into the circulation and cause severe rebound hypoglycemia. A vicious cycle that is difficult to break may ultimately result in persistent seizures and eventual death.

- The goal of therapy is to control the clinical signs, not correct hypoglycemia, through the judicious administration of dextrose.
- Administer small amounts of dextrose slowly rather than large boluses rapidly to minimize stimulation of the tumor.
- Avoid administering excessive amounts of dextrose.

Seizures. If intractable seizures due to hypoglycemia develop:

- Discontinue bolus injections of dextrose.
- Begin continuous IV infusion of 2.5–5.0% dextrose solution at one and one-half to two times the maintenance rate (90–120 ml/kg/24hr).
- Add dexamethasone, 0.5–1.0 mg/kg, to the intravenous fluids and administer over a period of 6 hours.
- Administer the somatostatin analogue SMS 201-995 (Octreotide; Sandoz, Inc.), 10 to 40 μg, SC, q8–12h, to decrease insulin secretion by the tumor.
- Aggressive anticonvulsant therapy or pentobarbital anesthesia, as described in sec. 10, ch. 3, for control of intractable seizures may be necessary to gain time until the aforementioned therapy becomes effective.

SURGICAL TREATMENT

Surgical Anatomy

The pancreas consists of the right and left lobes, and the body.

Right Lobe. The right lobe is located in the mesoduodenum adjacent to the descending duodenum. The proximal portion of the right lobe is intimately associated with the duodenum (Fig. 1). The cranial and caudal pancreaticoduodenal arteries supply the right lobe of the pancreas and the duodenum. Damage to the pancreaticoduodenal vessels may result in avascular necrosis of the duodenum.

Left Lobe. The left lobe is located caudodorsal to the stomach in the deep leaf of the greater omentum. It is exposed by reflecting the greater omentum, spleen, and stomach cranially and retracting the transverse

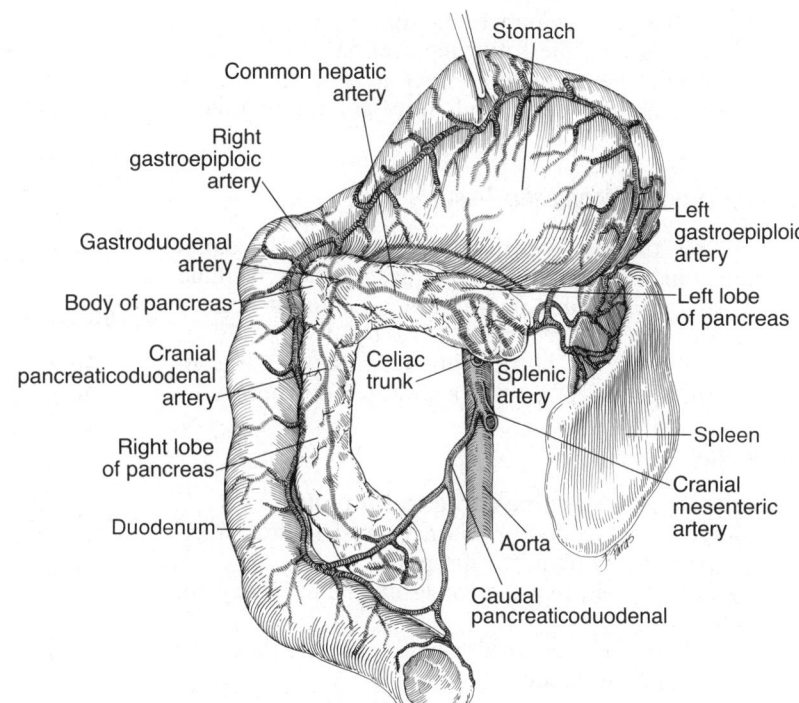

Figure 1. Schematic of anatomic location and blood supply of the right and left lobes of the pancreas.

colon caudally. This lobe of the pancreas is supplied by branches of the gastroduodenal, common hepatic, and splenic arteries.

Body of the Pancreas. The body of the pancreas is located at the cranial duodenal flexure and is in close proximity to the pylorus and common bile duct. The portal vein crosses the dorsal portion of the body.

Lymphatics. Lymphatics from the pancreas drain into the duodenal, hepatic, splenic, and mesenteric lymph nodes.

Pancreatic Ducts. Excretory ducts of the pancreas exit the pancreatic parenchyma in the area of the body to enter the duodenum. There are usually two, which intercommunicate within the gland. There are several variations in the anatomy of the pancreatic ducts:

- In the dog, most commonly the pancreatic duct enters the duodenum with the common bile duct at the major duodenal papilla approximately 5 cm distal to the pylorus. The accessory pancreatic duct, which is the main pancreatic duct, enters the duodenum at the minor duodenal papilla approximately 8 cm distal to the pylorus (Fig. 2).
- In the cat, the pancreatic duct is the main excretory duct; the accessory duct often is absent.

Preoperative Considerations

- To minimize hypoglycemia during the preoperative period, feed the animal frequent small meals and, if necessary, give prednisone, 0.25–0.5 mg/kg orally q12h.
- Fluid therapy prior to and during surgery is important to maintain systemic blood pressure and pancreatic perfusion, thereby minimizing the development of pancreatitis.

KEY POINT ▶ On the *day of surgery*, administer a balanced electrolyte solution containing 5% dextrose intravenously at one and one-half to two times daily maintenance requirements. *Intraoperatively*, administer this same solution at a rate of 8–16 ml/kg/hr.

Surgical Procedure

The objectives of exploratory celiotomy are to:

- Confirm the presence of neoplasia.
- Define the clinical stage of the tumor.

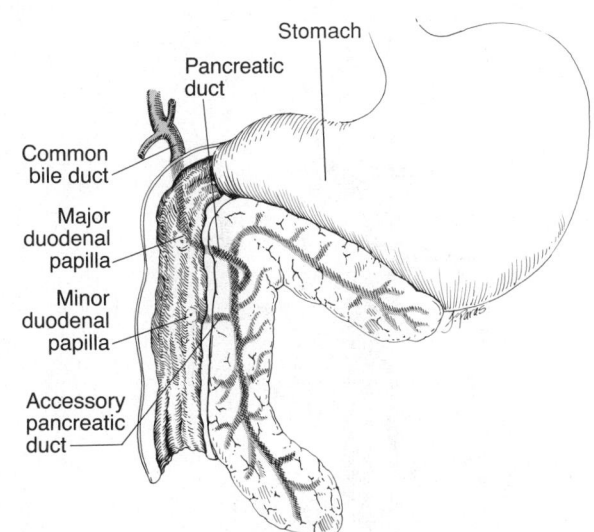

Figure 2. Schematic of the anatomic location of the pancreatic ducts in relationship to the duodenum.

■ Remove the primary pancreatic tumor and any meta-static lesions (see the following section).
  • Although this may not effect a cure, it usually reduces clinical signs and may facilitate medical management.

Identification of Neoplastic Tissue

Islet cell tumors occur with approximately equal frequency in all areas of the pancreas. Although single lesions are most common, multiple lesions in nonadjacent areas of the pancreas have been reported in about 15% of cases. Diffuse involvement of the pancreas without a discrete mass also has been reported.

Technique

Using Visual Examination and Palpation

1. Approach the abdomen via a ventral midline incision from the xiphoid to the pubis.
2. Examine the entire pancreas visually and by careful palpation.
   a. Islet cell tumors are usually firmer than the surrounding tissue.
   b. Islet cell tumors may be small and sandwiched between pancreatic lobules so that they are not readily apparent on visual examination.

Technique

Using Methylene Blue IV Infusion

The following technique to facilitate tumor identification utilizes intravenous infusion of methylene blue.

1. Surgically expose the pancreas as described previously.
2. Administer methylene blue as an intravenous infusion in normal isotonic saline solution to a total dose of 3 mg/kg body weight. Begin the infusion 30 minutes before the pancreas is exposed.

3. Methylene blue is concentrated by the endocrine pancreas and will intensely stain hyperfunctional areas.
   a. Normal pancreatic endocrine tissue is stained a dusky slate blue.
   b. Hyperfunctional tissue is stained more intensely (often a reddish blue).
4. Potential complications include hemolytic anemia and acute renal failure postoperatively.

Technique

Removal of Neoplastic Tissue

1. Remove abnormal pancreatic masses by partial pancreatectomy or by local excision. Make a wide excision and handle the pancreas very gently to avoid inducing pancreatitis.
2. Remove tumors located in the left lobe or the distal portion of the right lobe by partial pancreatectomy (Fig. 3).
   a. Divide the mesentery surrounding the affected lobe and ligate and divide the appropriate vessels.
   b. Incise the mesentery covering both surfaces of the pancreas at the level of transection of the lobe.
   c. Remove the lobe at least 1 to 2 cm proximal to the tumor.
   d. Bluntly separate the lobules using a mosquito hemostat, dissecting alternately from each side of the gland.
   e. Isolate the main duct, ligate with a monofilament synthetic suture material, and transect it.
3. When the tumor is located in the proximal portion of the right lobe or the body, local excision of the tumor, including at least 1- to 2-cm margins of normal-appearing pancreatic tissue, is the preferred technique because of the vascular and ductal anatomy of the area.

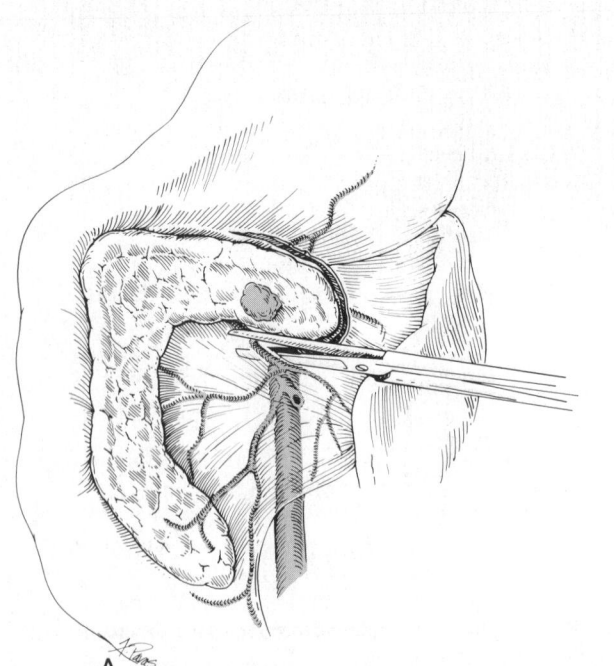
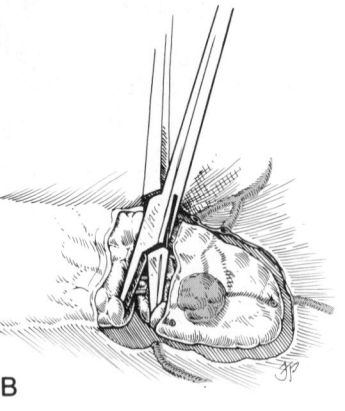
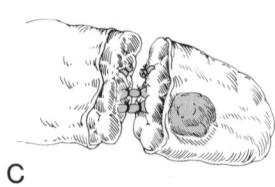

Figure 3. *A* to *C*, Schematic of partial pancreatectomy procedure.

a. Gently separate the pancreatic lobules by blunt dissection with a mosquito hemostat. Cauterize small vessels and ligate and divide larger vessels.
b. Preserve the pancreaticoduodenal vessels supplying the duodenum. Avoid damaging the pancreatic ducts and the common bile duct.
4. Explore the entire abdomen for evidence of metastatic disease. The most common sites of metastasis are the liver and regional lymph nodes (duodenal, hepatic, splenic, greater mesenteric).

KEY POINT ▶ Metastatic disease is common; approximately 45% of cases have identifiable metastasis to the liver or regional lymph nodes at the time of surgery.

a. Resect all enlarged lymph nodes and suspicious hepatic lesions if possible and submit them for histopathologic examination.
b. Biopsy lesions that cannot be completely excised.

KEY POINT ▶ Many dogs with metastases of islet cell neoplasms can be managed medically for longer than a year.

5. Thoroughly lavage the abdomen prior to closure with warm, sterile isotonic saline to dilute any pancreatic secretions that may have been released during surgical manipulation of the pancreas.
6. Close the abdomen routinely.

Postoperative Care and Complications

Postoperative Care

- Give nothing per os for 48 hours.
- Administer IV a balanced electrolyte solution containing 5% dextrose at one and one-half to two times daily maintenance requirements (90–120 ml/kg/24 hr).
  - Monitor the blood glucose concentration twice daily.
  - Discontinue the dextrose infusion if hyperglycemia (>150 mg/dl) develops.
- If vomiting does not occur, offer small amounts of water after 48 hours and then small amounts of a bland easily digestible diet (e.g., rice and cottage cheese) after 72 hours.
- If the dog tolerates a bland diet well, resume the normal diet in 5 to 7 days.

Complications

- Hyperglycemia may occur following surgery due to inadequate insulin secretion by atrophied nonneoplastic beta cells. This often resolves within a few days.
  - If hyperglycemia and glycosuria persist for several days following surgery, initiate insulin therapy (see sec. 4, ch. 4).
  - Diabetes mellitus is usually transient and resolves within a few weeks to several months.
  - Periodically, discontinue insulin therapy on a trial basis to determine if endogenous insulin production is resuming.

- If hypoglycemia does not resolve postoperatively or if it recurs following resection of an islet cell tumor, assume metastatic disease to be present and institute medical therapy for chronic hypoglycemia, as described in the following section.
- Other potential postoperative complications include pancreatitis, duodenal (from vascular compromise) necrosis, and central nervous system dysfunction secondary to prolonged hypoglycemia.

MEDICAL TREATMENT FOR CHRONIC HYPOGLYCEMIA

Initiate palliative medical management for chronic hypoglycemia when an exploratory celiotomy is refused by the owner or when an inoperable tumor or metastases result in recurrence of clinical signs.

The goals of chronic palliative therapy are to:

- Reduce the frequency and severity of clinical signs.
- Prevent an acute hypoglycemic crisis through dietary management and the use of nonspecific antihormonal therapy.

Antihormonal therapy minimizes hypoglycemia by:
- Increasing absorption of glucose from the intestinal tract
- Increasing hepatic gluconeogenesis and glycogenolysis
- Inhibiting the synthesis, secretion, or peripheral cellular actions of insulin

Diet and Exercise Recommendations

- Feed frequent small meals to provide a constant source of calories, which may prevent or reduce the number of hypoglycemic episodes.
- Use a diet that is high in proteins, fats, and complex carbohydrates.
- If commercial pet food is used, recommend a combination of canned and dry food, fed in 3 to 6 small meals daily.
- Avoid simple sugars (including soft moist foods) except as needed to treat signs of hypoglycemia.
- Limit exercise to short walks on a leash.

Glucocorticoid Therapy

Goal of Therapy. Initiate glucocorticoids when dietary manipulations are no longer effective in preventing signs of hypoglycemia.
Mechanisms. Glucocorticoids antagonize the actions of insulin at the cellular level, stimulate hepatic glycogenolysis, and provide the necessary substrates for hepatic gluconeogenesis.

Dosage
- Administer prednisone at an initial dosage of 0.5 mg/kg/day given in divided doses.
- Increase the dosage as needed to control clinical signs of hypoglycemia up to a maximal daily dose of 4 to 6 mg/kg/day.
  - Signs of iatrogenic hypercortisolism ultimately limit the amount of prednisone that is administered.

Diazoxide Therapy

Mechanism. Diazoxide (Proglycem, Schering Corp.) is a benzothiadiazide diuretic that inhibits insulin secretion, stimulates hepatic gluconeogenesis and glycogenolysis, and inhibits tissue use of glucose. The net effect is the development of hyperglycemia.

Goal of Therapy. The goal of diazoxide therapy is to establish a dosage in which hypoglycemia and its clinical signs are reduced or absent, while avoiding hyperglycemia (>180 mg/dl) and its associated clinical signs.

Dosage

- Administer diazoxide at an initial dosage of 10 mg/kg q12h PO.
- Gradually increase the dose as needed to control signs of hypoglycemia, but do not exceed 60 mg/kg/day.

Side Effects

- The most common adverse reactions to diazoxide are anorexia and vomiting.
  - Minimize these by administering diazoxide with a meal or temporarily decreasing dosage.
- Other potential complications include diarrhea, tachycardia, bone marrow suppression, aplastic anemia, thrombocytopenia, diabetes mellitus, sodium and fluid retention, and cataracts.

SMS 201-995 Therapy

- SMS 201-995 (Octreotide, Sandoz, Inc.) is an analogue of somatostatin that inhibits the secretion of insulin by normal and neoplastic beta cells.
- The responsiveness of insulin-secreting tumors to the suppressive effects of SMS 201-995 is variable, being dependent on the presence of membrane receptors for somatostatin on the tumor cells.
- The dosage is 10 to 40 μg SC, q8–12h.
- Adverse reactions have not been seen at these dosages.

PROGNOSIS

The long-term prognosis for survival is guarded to poor owing to the malignant nature of insulin-secreting tumors and the often extended period of time (months) before a diagnosis is established.

- The mean survival time for dogs treated medically is approximately 12 months from the onset of clinical signs of hypoglycemia.
- The ability of surgery to improve the prognosis depends on the clinical stage of the disease, most notably the presence or absence of metastasis.

A multi-university study (Caywood et al., 1988) involving a total of 73 dogs with insulin-secreting neoplasia found:

- 50% of dogs with a solitary tumor and no visible metastases at the time of surgery were free of hypoglycemia 14 months following surgery.
- Less than 20% of dogs with visible metastasis were disease-free at 14 months.
- 80% of dogs with a solitary mass were dead 24 months from the time of diagnosis.
- Approximately 50% of dogs with metastasis to the liver (the most common site) were dead by 6 months and all were dead by 18 months from the time of diagnosis.

Supplemental Readings

Breitschwerdt EB, Loar AS, Hribernik TN, et al: Hypoglycemia in four dogs with sepsis. J Am Vet Med Assoc 178:1072, 1981.

Caywood DD, Klausner JS, O'Leary TP, et al.: Pancreatic insulin-secreting neoplasms: Clinical, diagnostic, and prognostic features in 73 dogs. J Am Anim Hosp 24:577, 1988.

Feldman EC, Nelson RW: *Canine and Feline Endocrinology and Reproduction.* Philadelphia: W. B. Saunders, 1987, p 304.

Fingeroth JM, Smeak DD: Intravenous methylene blue infusion for intraoperative identification of pancreatic islet-cell tumors in dogs. Part II: Clinical trial and results in four dogs. J Am Anim Hosp Assoc 24:175, 1988.

Leifer CE, Peterson ME, Matus RE: Insulin-secreting tumor: Diagnosis and medical and surgical management in 55 dogs. J Am Vet Med Assoc 188:60, 1986.

Leifer CE, Peterson ME, Matus RE, et al.: Hypoglycemia associated with nonislet cell tumor in 13 dogs. J Am Vet Med Assoc 186:53, 1985.

Mehlhaff CJ, Peterson ME, Patnaik AK, et al.: Insulin-producing islet cell neoplasms: Surgical considerations and general management in 35 dogs. J Am Anim Hosp Assoc 21:607, 1985.

Nelson RW: *Textbook of Veterinary Internal Medicine.* Philadelphia: W. B. Saunders, 1989, p 1676.

6 Hypothalamus and Pituitary Gland

John F. Randolph
Mark E. Peterson

NORMAL ANATOMY AND PHYSIOLOGY

The *pituitary* gland (hypophysis) consists of the neurohypophysis surrounded by the adenohypophysis.

Neurohypophysis

The neurohypophysis, also called the *pars nervosa* and *infundibulum* (Fig. 1), extends ventrally from the hypothalamus.

- It is composed of nerve tracts terminating from nuclei within the hypothalamus.
- Antidiuretic hormone (ADH, vasopressin) and oxytocin, produced by the supraoptic and paraventricular hypothalamic nuclei, travel down the axons to be stored in and secreted from the neurohypophysis.

Adenohypophysis

The adenohypophysis is an embryonic outgrowth of the pharynx connected to the hypothalamus by a vascular network that allows humoral control of adenohypophyseal secretions by the hypothalamus.

- In response to neurotransmitters, specialized neurosecretory cells within the hypothalamus release factors that control production and secretion of hormones from the adenohypophysis (Table 1).
- Hormones produced by target endocrine organs in response to specific adenohypophyseal hormones exert a negative feedback (or feedback inhibition) on further elaboration of the hypothalamohypophyseal hormones.
  - Because growth hormone (GH), prolactin, and melanocyte-stimulating hormone (MSH) do not have target endocrine organs to participate in negative feedback controls, releasing and inhibiting factors from the hypothalamus control production of these hormones (see Table 1).
- The adenohypophysis is subdivided into the pars distalis, pars tuberalis, and pars intermedia (see Fig. 1).
  - The pars intermedia, unlike the pars distalis, does not have an extensive blood supply contiguous with the hypothalamus.
  - Rather, the cells of the pars intermedia appear to release their hormones in response to dopaminergic and serotonergic innervation.

Adenohypophyseal Cells. These are classified by staining properties of their secretory granules.

- Immunohistochemical staining identifies the specific hormone content of the cells.
- Hematoxylin and eosin staining identifies adenohypophyseal cells as:
  - Acidophils: Somatotrophs and luteotrophs
  - Basophils: Gonadotrophs, corticotrophs and thyrotrophs
  - Chromophobes (cells that do not stain selectively): Degranulated, undifferentiated, or actively synthesizing cells (some investigators consider chromophobes to include corticotrophs).

Alternative Nomenclature

Alternatively, the pituitary gland is composed of the anterior lobe and posterior lobe, with the two lobes separated by the hypophyseal cleft (the residual lumen of Rathke's pouch) (see Fig. 1). The terms anterior and posterior, although anatomically correct for the human pituitary, are not accurate when used to describe the lobes of the feline or canine pituitary gland.

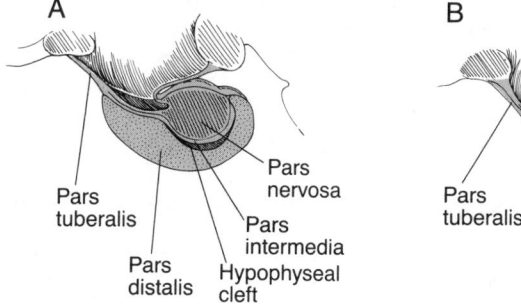 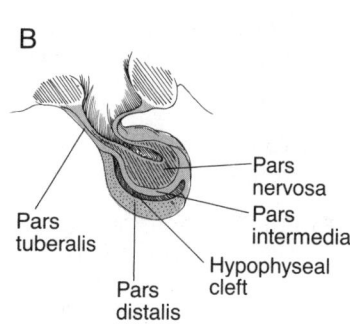

Figure 1. Schematic diagram of a mid-sagittal section through the pituitary gland of a normal dog *(A)* and cat *(B)*. (Modified from Dellman HD, Brown DM: *Textbook of Veterinary Histology*, 3rd ed. Philadelphia: Lea & Febiger, 1987.)

TABLE 1. Adenohypophyseal Hormones and Their Regulatory Hypothalamic Hormones

Adenohypophyseal Hormone	Hypothalamic Hormone
Thyroid-stimulating hormone (TSH)	Thyrotropin-releasing hormone (TRH)
Adrenocorticotropic hormone (ACTH)	Corticotropin-releasing hormone (CRH)
Growth hormone (GH, somatotropin)	GH-releasing hormone (GHRH, somatocrinin)
	GH-inhibiting hormone (somatostatin)
Follicle-stimulating hormone (FSH)	Gonadotropin-releasing hormone (GnRH)
Luteinizing hormone (LH)	Gonadotropin-releasing hormone (GnRH)
Prolactin (luteotropic hormone [LTH])	Prolactin-releasing factor Prolactin inhibitor (dopamine)
Melanocyte-stimulating hormone (MSH)	MSH-releasing hormone (MSH-RH)
	MSH release–inhibiting hormone (MSH-RIH)

- Anterior lobe: Pars tuberalis (glandular pituitary stalk) and the pars distalis
- Posterior lobe: Pars nervosa and pars intermedia

DISEASES OF PITUITARY HORMONE EXCESS

GH-Secreting Pituitary Hyperplasia/Neoplasia: Acromegaly

Excess production of GH causes overgrowth of bone, connective tissue, and viscera. If GH oversecretion (hypersomatotropism) occurs after closure of the epiphyses, acromegaly develops. In acromegaly, only the membranous bones (e.g., nose, mandible, and portions of the vertebrae) increase in length, because the long bones cannot grow longitudinally once the epiphyses close.

Growth hormone exerts both direct and indirect effects on the body. The indirect actions of GH, mediated by somatomedin C (also known as insulin-like growth factor I [IGF-I]), are anabolic and include increased protein synthesis and soft tissue and skeletal growth. In contrast, the direct effects of GH are predominantly catabolic (e.g., lipolysis and restricted cellular glucose transport).

Etiology

- In dogs: Endogenous (diestrus) or exogenous progestogens cause acromegaly by inducing hyperplasia and hypertrophy of the GH-secreting somatotrophs of the pituitary.
- In cats: The major cause of acromegaly is a GH-secreting tumor of the pituitary gland.

KEY POINT ▶ Acromegaly in dogs is caused by progestogens. Feline acromegaly develops from a GH-secreting pituitary tumor.

Clinical Signs

Signalment
- Age: Middle to old age
- Breed: No breed predilection
- Sex: Most acromegalic cats are male, whereas acromegalic dogs are female.

General Appearance

KEY POINT ▶ The clinical features of acromegaly develop so insidiously that they are frequently overlooked.

- Large paws
- Soft tissue swelling of the head and neck with prominent skin folds
- Prognathism due to mandibular enlargement
- Widened interdental spaces
- Macroglossia
- Increase in body size and weight
- Pot-bellied appearance
- Long, thick, or coarse haircoat
- Rapid growth of toenails

Respiratory System
In dogs: Excessive panting, exercise intolerance, and inspiratory stridor because oropharyngeal soft tissue proliferation compresses the upper airway.

In cats: Dyspnea as a result of pulmonary edema or pleural effusion from GH-induced cardiac failure

Cardiovascular System
In cats, cardiac involvement includes:

- Systolic murmur (64%)
- Cardiomegaly (86%)
- Congestive heart failure (43%) characterized by pulmonary edema, pleural effusion, or ascites

Endocrine System

KEY POINT ▶ Some dogs and all cats with acromegaly have insulin-resistant diabetes mellitus.

- Diabetes mellitus and its accompanying clinical signs of polyuria, polydipsia, and polyphagia develop because GH restricts cellular glucose transport.
  - Insulin resistance results, and large doses of insulin (> 2.2 U/kg/day) are frequently needed to control the hyperglycemia.
- In acromegalic cats, the growth-promoting effects of GH lead to enlargement of endocrine glands (thyroid, parathyroid, adrenal), but the function of these glands remains normal.
- In contrast, dogs in which acromegaly is created by chronic administration of progestogens have subnormal basal cortisol concentrations.
  - The glucocorticoid-like activity of these progestogens probably suppresses ACTH secretion and causes secondary hypoadrenocorticism.

Skeletal System
- Spondylosis deformans
- Hyperostosis of the skull
- Mandibular enlargement (prognathism)
- Arthritis: Excess GH causes proliferation of cartilage

and soft tissue, resulting in widening of the joint space.

- In some cats, degenerative arthropathy develops with time.
- Acromegalic dogs seem less likely to develop joint problems.

Nervous System. Growth of the pituitary tumor in feline acromegaly may impinge on brain tissue, causing circling, seizures, or behavioral changes.

Urinary System

- GH excess causes renal hypertrophy and increased glomerular filtration rate and renal plasma flow.
- Renal failure develops in about 50% of acromegalic cats. The kidneys of these cats have mesangial thickening of the glomeruli that may result from the glomerulosclerosis associated with unregulated diabetes mellitus and GH-mediated glomerular hyperfiltration.

Reproductive System. Dogs with progesterone-induced acromegaly may develop pyometra, mucometra, and mammary gland nodules.

Diagnosis

KEY POINT ▶ Suspect acromegaly in bitches receiving progestogens and in intact female dogs that develop diabetes mellitus or laryngeal stridor due to soft tissue overgrowth. Suspect acromegaly in all cats with insulin-resistant diabetes mellitus.

Physical Examination. Look for the clinical signs listed above. To confirm enlargement of the head and paws, redundant skin folds, and prognathism, compare the animal's appearance with earlier photographs of the animal, if possible.

Routine Laboratory Tests

- Severe hyperglycemia and glucosuria are found in all cats and some dogs with acromegaly. Despite the poorly regulated diabetic state of most acromegalic cats and the usual promotion of ketogenesis by GH, ketosis rarely develops.
- Less frequently, increases in cholesterol, alanine aminotransferase (ALT), and serum alkaline phosphatase (ALP) may be caused by the diabetic state. However, in many acromegalic dogs without diabetes, ALP activity is increased.
- Mild to moderate hyperproteinemia occurs in 50% of acromegalic cats, but the serum protein electrophoretic pattern is normal.
- Hyperphosphatemia may occur secondary to increased renal tubular reabsorption of phosphorus by GH.
- There may be stress leukogram, anemia (in dogs, cause uncertain), or mild erythrocytosis (in cats, due to GH-stimulated erythropoiesis).
- Acromegalic cats that develop renal failure have persistent proteinuria (100–300 mg/dl) with dilute urine specific gravity (1.015–1.025).

Radiography

Examine for:

- Visceral enlargement (cardiomegaly, hepatomegaly, renomegaly)
- Soft tissue proliferation (oropharyngeal region, head, limbs)
- Bony changes (spondylosis, hyperostosis of the calvarium, periarticular periosteal reaction)
- Left ventricular and septal hypertrophy in acromegalic cats with cardiomegaly (by echocardiogram)

Nuclear Imaging and Computed Tomography (CT). These modalities are helpful in identifying a possible pituitary tumor.

GH Determination. Increased circulating GH concentrations confirm a diagnosis of acromegaly. However, GH concentrations may be normal in some acromegalic patients and may be increased in a variety of other diseases.

- Increased GH concentration in the presence of profound hyperglycemia supports a diagnosis of acromegaly because hyperglycemia would normally be expected to suppress GH secretion.
- A glucose suppression test may be helpful diagnostically in nonhyperglycemic animals suspected of having acromegaly.
- Alternatively, an integrated 24-hour GH concentration determined by frequent sampling throughout the day may be more indicative of GH hypersecretion than solitary determinations.
- Validated GH radioimmunoassays are not widely available for the dog or cat. Until such assays are routinely obtainable, to diagnose *feline acromegaly*, rely on:
  - Clinical and laboratory features characteristic of acromegaly
  - Radiologic documentation of a pituitary mass
  - Normal results on thyroid and adrenal testing
- Base a presumptive diagnosis of *canine acromegaly* on:
  - Characteristic clinical and laboratory findings
  - Exposure to a progestogen source and improvement in clinical signs following removal of that progestogen source
  - No evidence of spontaneous hyperadrenocorticism on adrenal testing
- Determination of somatomedin C (IGF-I) gives an indirect indication of GH concentration. Acromegalic dogs have increased somatomedin C (IGF-I) concentrations, but similar measurements in cats have not been reported.

Treatment

Progesterone-Induced Acromegaly. Treat progesterone-induced acromegaly by ovariohysterectomy or discontinuation of progestogen drugs. The soft tissue overgrowth and respiratory stridor resolve; however, the skeletal changes persist. The insulin requirement for GH-induced diabetes mellitus also declines, but the reversibility of the diabetes depends on the insulin reserve of the pancreatic beta islet cells.

Growth Hormone–Secreting Pituitary Tumors. Manage these tumors by surgery, radiation, or drug therapy.

Surgery. Acromegaly attributable to a GH-secreting pituitary tumor has not yet been corrected by surgery.

- Because surgical excision of the tumor probably will necessitate hypophysectomy, expect deficiencies of pituitary hormones postoperatively.
- Before surgery, precisely localize the pituitary tumor by CT because neoplastic extension into the hypothalamus precludes surgery.

Radiation. The results of *cobalt irradiation* (total dose of 4800 cGy divided equally in 12 treatments during 4 weeks) in two acromegalic cats were variable. In one cat, no effect was seen on tumor size or GH concentration; in the other cat, the tumor shrunk with subsequent reduction in GH concentration. These changes developed within 2 months of radiation treatment but lasted for only 6 months before relapse.

Pharmacologic management includes dopamine agonists and long-acting somatostatin analogues.

- Dopamine agonists. Bromocriptine lowers GH concentrations in many acromegalic humans, but its effect on GH concentrations in acromegalic cats is unknown.
- Long-acting somatostatin analogues. Analogues such as SMS 201–995 (Octreotide) inhibit GH secretion in most humans with acromegaly. However, subcutaneous doses of Octreotide, ranging from 10 to 200 μg/day, did not reduce GH concentrations in four acromegalic cats.

Management of Concurrent GH-Induced Conditions. Provide symptomatic treatment of GH-related disorders in the initial management of acromegalic dogs and the long-term care of acromegalic cats.

- Congestive heart failure in some acromegalic cats initially responds to furosemide treatment (1.0–2.5 mg/kg q12–24 h) (see sec. 6, ch. 6, for more details on treatment of congestive heart failure).
- Inspiratory stridor in acromegalic dogs partially responds to cage rest, cooling, and oxygen therapy.
- The diabetes mellitus of feline acromegaly generally is refractory and requires insulin (NPH, PZI, or ultralente) twice daily. In some cats, combinations of short-acting insulin (regular insulin) with NPH insulin may help control hyperglycemia (see sec. 4, ch. 4 for more details on management of diabetes mellitus).

Prevention

- No preventive measures currently are known to avoid the development of GH-secreting pituitary tumors in cats.
- Prevent acromegaly in dogs by ovariohysterectomy of nonbreeding bitches and judicious use of progestogen drugs.

ACTH-Secreting Pituitary Hyperplasia/Neoplasia: Cushing's Disease

Hyperplasia or neoplasia of the pituitary corticotrophs with resultant oversecretion of adrenocorticotropic hormone (ACTH) is the major cause of hyper-adrenocorticism (Cushing's disease) in the dog and cat. Excess ACTH may originate from the corticotrophs in either the pars distalis or the pars intermedia. Clinical signs, diagnostic testing, and treatment of Cushing's disease are discussed in sec. 4, ch. 3.

DISEASES OF PITUITARY HORMONE DEFICIENCY

Hypopituitary Dwarfism: GH Deficiency

Etiology

- In German shepherds and Carelian bear dogs, hypopituitary dwarfism is inherited as an autosomal recessive trait, and is associated with cystic distension of the craniopharyngeal duct (Rathke's pouch).
- It is not known whether expansion of the pituitary cyst destroys adjacent adenohypophyseal tissue or whether a primary defect in differentiation and secretory capability of the adenohypophyseal cells creates the cyst.
- Weimaraners develop GH deficiency in association with thymic abnormalities.

Clinical Signs

Signalment
- Age: Young animals are affected. Discrepancies in growth compared with littermates are apparent at 6–8 weeks of age.
- Breed: This is an autosomal recessive trait in the German shepherd and Carelian bear dog.
- Sex: There is no sex predilection.

General Appearance
- Growth retardation is characterized by proportionately stunted short stature. Affected German shepherd dogs usually fail to exceed 13.5 kg in body weight or 47.5 cm in shoulder height by 1 year of age.
- The hair is soft and woolly, with retention of secondary (lanugo) hairs and lack of primary (guard) hairs. Progressive, bilaterally symmetric truncal alopecia develops with age.
- Dental eruption is delayed.

Concurrent Deficiencies of Other Pituitary Hormones
- Thyroid-stimulating hormone (TSH) deficiency (secondary hypothyroidism; see sec. 4, ch. 1)
- ACTH deficiency (secondary hypoadrenocorticism; see sec. 4, ch. 3)
- Follicle-stimulating hormone/luteinizing hormone (FSH/LH) hormone (secondary hypogonadism; see sec. 8, ch. 14)

Diagnosis

Differentiate hypopituitary dwarfism from other causes of growth retardation (Fig. 2).

History. Identify breed predisposition and postnatal onset of growth problems (see Fig. 2).

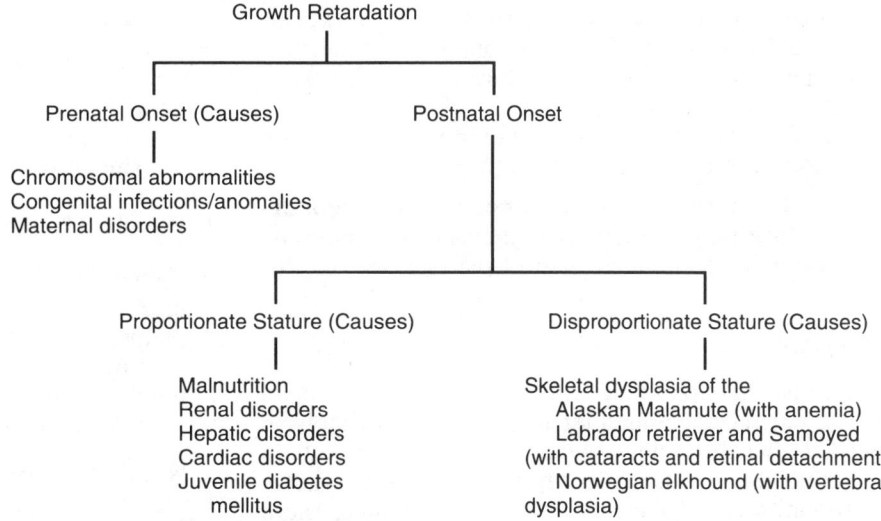

Figure 2. Classification of growth retardation by onset of growth problems and stature of dog.

Physical Examination
- The puppy is proportionately stunted.
- The haircoat initially remains as the animal matures, but truncal alopecia eventually develops.
- Additional clinical features characteristic of hypothyroidism, hypoadrenocorticism, or hypogonadism depend on the extent of hypophyseal involvement.

Routine Laboratory Tests. Hematologic, serum biochemical, and urinalysis results usually are normal for immature dogs. Hypophosphatemia may result from lack of GH-mediated renal tubular reabsorption of phosphorus.

Radiographic Abnormalities
- Delayed closure of the epiphyses
- Delayed dental eruption
- Delayed or incomplete calcification of the os penis

Growth Hormone Determination
- Basal GH concentrations do not differentiate normal dogs from dogs with GH deficiency.
- GH stimulation tests classically have been used to evaluate pituitary GH secretory capability.
- Measure circulating GH concentrations in fasted dogs before and 15, 30, 45, 60, and 90 minutes after IV administration of:
  - 0.1 or 0.3 mg of xylazine/kg (Rompun; Haver) or
  - 3, 10, 16.5, or 30 μg of clonidine/kg (Catapres; Boehringer Ingelheim)
- Interpretation:
  - In normal dogs, circulating GH concentrations increase within 30 minutes of xylazine or clonidine administration and then decline by 60 to 90 minutes.
  - In dogs with hypopituitary dwarfism, no substantial increase in GH concentration develops after pharmacologic stimulation.

In some children with GH neurosecretory dysfunction, GH response to pharmacologic stimulation is normal; nevertheless, spontaneous physiologic pulsatile GH secretion is decreased, as determined by 24-hour blood sample monitoring. A similar disorder may account for the delayed growth recently reported in a litter of German shepherds.

Somatomedin C-IGF-I Measurement. Currently, validated GH radioimmunoassays are not routinely available for the dog. However, measurement of serum somatomedin C(IGF-I), produced in response to GH, gives an indirect indication of GH concentration.

- In GH-deficient German shepherds with pituitary dwarfism, somatomedin C(IGF-I) concentrations are subnormal.
- Somatomedin C(IGF-I) concentrations in related but clinically unaffected dogs that are presumably heterozygous for the dwarf trait are intermediate between the IGF-I concentrations found in normal German shepherds and those obtained in dwarf German shepherds.

Other Tests

- To investigate for secondary hypothyroidism associated with hypopituitary dwarfism, perform a thyrotropin-releasing hormone (TRH) or thyroid-stimulating hormone (TSH) stimulation test (sec. 4, ch. 1).
- To investigate for secondary hypoadrenocorticism associated with hypopituitary dwarfism, perform corticotropin-releasing hormone (CRH) or ACTH stimulation test (sec. 4, ch. 3).

Skin Biopsy
- In canine GH deficiency, nonspecific histologic skin changes (atrophy of hair follicles, epidermis, and sebaceous glands) are similar to those seen in other canine endocrinopathies; however, a decreased number of elastin fibers are present in the dermis.

Treatment

Growth Hormone Replacement Therapy
- Administer bovine, human, or porcine GH preparations subcutaneously at *0.3 IU/kg weekly* divided

into two or three doses for 6 to 8 weeks; however, GH replacement is difficult to obtain and expensive.

- No increase in size occurs if dogs present for treatment after epiphyseal closure.
- Because GH is diabetogenic, monitor blood glucose concentrations during treatment.

Thyroid Hormone or Glucocorticoid Replacement Therapy. Initiate therapy if concurrent hypothyroidism or hypoadrenocorticism exist (see sec. 4, chs. 1, 3).

Prevention

Because hypopituitary dwarfism is inherited in an autosomal recessive manner in the German shepherd and Carelian bear dogs, genetic counseling may help eliminate this disease. Identify possible heterozygotes by somatomedin C(IGF-I) assay, and eliminate these carrier animals from the breeding programs.

Diabetes Insipidus:
Antidiuretic Hormone Deficiency

Diabetes insipidus (DI) is an uncommon condition characterized by marked polyuria and secondary polydipsia. The disorder may be classifed as neurogenic or nephrogenic in origin. Neurogenic (central) DI is a complete or partial failure of the neurohypophysis to release antidiuretic hormone (ADH), whereas nephrogenic DI indicates a lack of renal responsiveness to ADH.

Etiology

Neurogenic DI develops from disorders that disrupt the ADH-producing hypothalamic neurohypophyseal neurons.

- Idiopathic
- Central nervous system (CNS) trauma
- CNS neoplasia
- CNS inflammation
- Congenital anomalies

Clinical Signs

Signalment
- Age is variable, depending on cause.
  - Idiopathic DI has no specific age predilection.
  - Animals with suspected congenital DI are less than 1 year of age.
  - Animals with DI caused by CNS neoplasia are older.
- Breed: No predilection
- Sex: No predisposition

Polyuria and Polydipsia
- ADH acts on the distal tubules and collecting ducts of the kidneys to allow increased water reabsorption.
- With a deficiency of ADH, water diuresis ensues.
- This primary polyuria results in volume contraction and subsequent compensatory polydipsia.

Diagnosis

The diagnosis of DI requires its differentiation from other, more common causes of polyuria and polydipsia

such as primary renal disease, diabetes mellitus, pyometra, feline hyperthyroidism, and canine hyperadrenocorticism.

History. The history usually identifies profound polyuria and polydipsia (>100 ml/kg/day; normal is approximately 40–70 ml/kg/day) findings usually are normal.

Physical Examination. Findings usually are normal.

- Weight loss (if the animal is preoccupied with drinking)
- Dehydration (if water is withheld)
- Neurologic signs (e.g., disorientation, seizures, blindness) may develop in animals with pituitary or hypothalamic neoplasia or trauma.

Routine Laboratory Tests. Hematologic and serum biochemical results are usually normal, or consistent with mild dehydration (mild increases in packed cell volume and serum concentrations of total protein and sodium).

KEY POINT ▶ Urine dipstick and sediment evaluations are normal, but urine specific gravity (USG) is persistently 1.000–1.007 in the dog, and 1.008–1.012 in the cat.

Animals with partial deficiencies in ADH may produce more concentrated urine. Urine culture is negative.

Radiography. Findings usually are normal.

Nuclear Imaging and CT. These can aid in identifying a pituitary or hypothalamic lesion.

Water Deprivation Tests. Perform these tests to determine whether ADH is released from the neurohypophysis in response to subclinical to mild dehydration, and whether the kidneys can respond to the released ADH. Minimal increases in plasma osmolality should stimulate release of ADH.

KEY POINT ▶ Water deprivation tests are contraindicated in animals that are already dehydrated (since the stimulus to ADH release already exists) or in the presence of other laboratory abnormalities (e.g., azotemia, hypercalcemia).

Because water deprivation provokes dehydration, these tests are potentially dangerous and can result in acute renal failure, neurologic complications, and death. For this reason, even if routine laboratory test results are normal, screening for renal insufficiency and hyperadrenocorticism may be advisable prior to subjecting an animal to water deprivation.

Abrupt Water Deprivation Test
- Procedure: See Table 2.
- Interpretation: When deprived of water, normal animals can concentrate the USG to 1.075 in cats and 1.045 in dogs. Nevertheless, a USG of 1.025 (or a corresponding urine osmolality of 900 mOsm/kg) is generally considered an adequate response to water deprivation. Failure to concentrate to this degree in the absence of renal disease or other laboratory abnormalities indicates that the animal

has neurogenic or nephrogenic DI and/or renal medullary washout (Fig. 3).

Gradual Water Deprivation Test
Patients with renal medullary washout will not concentrate their urine on an abrupt water deprivation test. Gradual reduction in water intake, however, does allow them to re-establish the medullary gradient.

■ Procedure: See Table 2.
■ Interpretation: Failure to concentrate urine in the absence of renal disease or other laboratory abnormalities indicates that the animal has neurogenic or nephrogenic DI (see Fig. 3).

ADH Response Test. If the animal fails to concentrate urine adequately following water deprivation, perform an ADH response test. The test evaluates the effect of exogenous ADH on the renal tubular ability to concentrate urine in the face of dehydration.

■ Procedure:
  • Immediately following either water deprivation test, administer aqueous vasopressin (Pitressin; Parke-Davis) 0.5 U/kg (maximum dose, 10 U) IM.
  • Withhold all water and food during the test.
  • Empty the urinary bladder and measure USG (and osmolality if possible) at 30, 60, 90, and 120 minutes after vasopressin injection.
  • The animal may drink once the test is completed.
■ Interpretation: Failure to concentrate urine with water deprivation followed by a rise in urine specific gravity to >1.025 after ADH administration is di-

TABLE 2. Procedures for Abrupt and Gradual Water Deprivation Tests

Abrupt Water Deprivation Test	Gradual Water Deprivation Test
Empty urinary bladder and measure urine specific gravity (and urine osmolality if possible). Weigh animal. Withhold food and water. Every 2–4 hours, reweigh animal, empty urinary bladder, and measure urine specific gravity (and urine osmolality if possible). Use the criteria below as end points.	Quantitate daily unrestricted water consumption. Measure urine specific gravity and weigh animal. Reduce water intake by 5% daily (to not less than 66 ml/kg/day). Feed normally. Weigh animal and measure urine specific gravity daily. Use the criteria below as end points.

Stop the test when any of the following occur:
1. The animal loses more than 5% of its body weight.
2. The animal is clinically dehydrated or ill.
3. The urine specific gravity exceeds 1.025.

agnostic of neurogenic DI (see Fig. 3); an inability to concentrate urine by the ADH response test is indicative of nephrogenic DI or uncorrected renal medullary washout (see Fig. 3).

Treatment

ADH Replacement
To provide ADH replacement use one of the following:

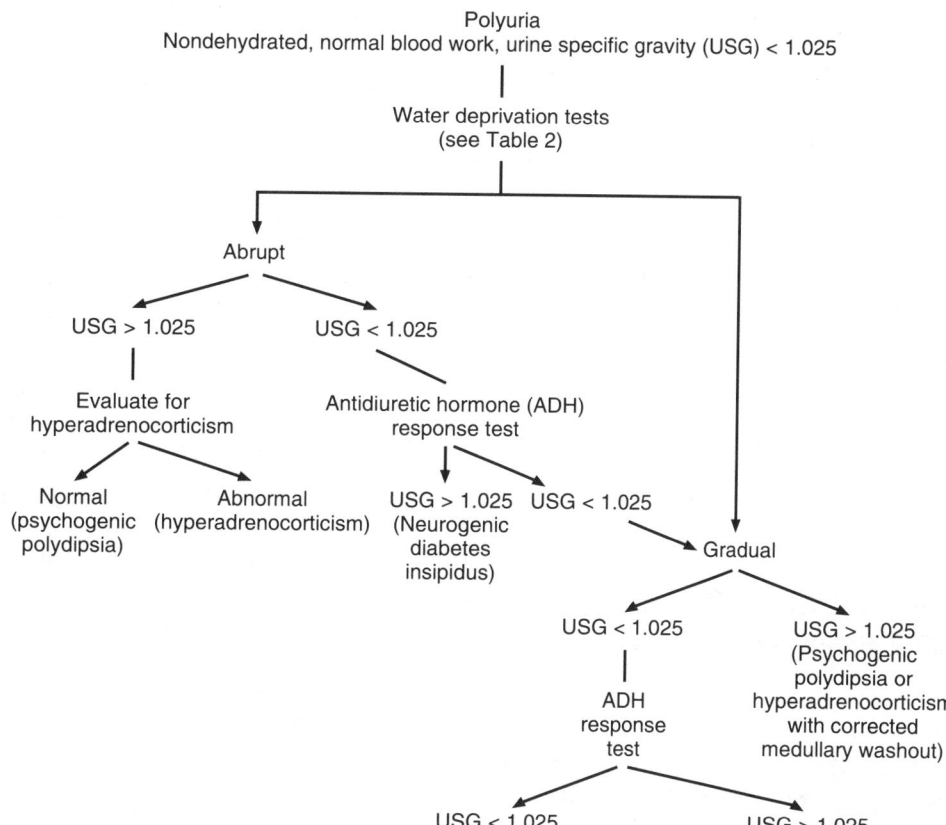

Figure 3. Algorithm for evaluation of an animal with polyuria/polydipsia.

■ Vasopressin tannate in oil
■ 1-Desamino-8-D-arginine vasopressin (dDAVP) (Desmopressin; Rorer)
■ Lysine vasopressin (Diapid; Sandoz)

Vasopressin tannate in oil is an extract of ADH prepared from bovine and porcine pituitaries. Production of this repositol form of ADH has been discontinued by the manufacturer.

dDAVP is a synthetic analogue of vasopressin.

■ It is available as an aqueous solution (100 μg/ml) intended for intranasal use.
■ It also is effective when applied topically in the conjunctival sac (1 to 4 drops q12–24h).
■ Adjust the daily dose to control polyuria and polydipsia.
■ The major disadvantage is its expense.

Lysine vasopressin also is an aqueous solution of synthetic vasopressin intended for intranasal use.

■ Unlike dDAVP, which has a duration of 10–27 hours, lysine vasopressin has an antidiuretic effect of only 4–6 hours.

Hydrochlorothiazide (Hydrodiuril; Merck, Sharp, and Dohme) may reduce the polyuria of DI, but it is never as effective as ADH replacement. Chlorothiazide diuretics reduce total body sodium by an initial natriuresis, resulting in decreased extracellular fluid volume and reduced glomerular filtration rate (GFR). These changes cause increased fluid reabsorption in the proximal renal tubule and reduced urine output.

■ Administer hydrochlorothiazide at a dose of 2–4 mg/kg q12h PO.
■ Restrict salt intake, as this potentiates the drug's effectiveness.
■ Because hypokalemia may develop with thiazide diuretic therapy, monitor serum electrolyte concentrations during treatment.

Chlorpropamide (Diabinese; Pfizer) is an oral hypoglycemic agent that potentiates the action of ADH on the renal distal tubules and collecting ducts. Because chlorpropamide requires the presence of some ADH in order to be effective, it will reduce only the polyuria in animals with partial ADH deficiency.

■ Administer chlorpropamide at a dose of 10–40 mg/kg/day.
■ Monitor blood glucose concentrations during treatment.

Secondary (Pituitary) or Tertiary (Hypothalamic) Hypoadrenocorticism: ACTH or CRH Deficiency

(See sec. 4, ch. 3)

Secondary (Pituitary) or Tertiary (Hypothalamic) Hypothyroidism: TSH or TRH Deficiency

(See sec. 4, ch. 1)

MISCELLANEOUS DISORDERS

Adipsia/Hypodipsia

Adipsia/hypodipsia is absent or reduced thirst. Normally, with water loss, mild increases in plasma osmolality stimulate osmoreceptors in the hypothalamus to increase water consumption and ADH secretion. However, even with maximal ADH secretion, hyperosmolality (specifically hypernatremia) escalates unless the thirst mechanism is intact. With adipsia or hypodipsia, hypernatremia develops with resultant dehydrating effects on the cells of the CNS. It is usually unclear whether the defect in thirst in these animals is due to an increased osmoreceptor threshold (reset set point) or to structural lesions in the thirst center of the hypothalamus.

Etiology

■ Idiopathic
■ Hypothalamic dysplasia/congenital anomalies
■ Hypothalamic degeneration
■ Hypothalamic inflammation, neoplasia, or trauma

Clinical Signs

■ Signalment
  • Age: Young (usually <1 year) in idiopathic and congenital forms of the disorder
  • Sex: Female predisposition in the miniature schnauzer
  • Breed: Miniature schnauzer
■ Depression/stupor/coma
■ Personality change
■ Disorientation
■ Anorexia
■ Weakness/lethargy
■ Irritability/seizures

Because hypothalamic conditions associated with adipsia/hypodipsia may cause neurologic signs regardless of the sodium concentration, the relative contribution of hypernatremia to the development of clinical signs can be assessed once a normal sodium concentration is restored.

Diagnosis

History. Adipsia/hypodipsia has occured despite free access to water, and the clinical signs listed above are present.

Physical Examination. There is evidence of dehydration and signs of altered mentation.

Routine Laboratory Tests. Hematologic, serum biochemical, and urinalysis results are consistent with dehydration:

■ Hypernatremia (profound)
■ Hyperosmolality (profound)
■ Hyperchloremia
■ Azotemia (mild)
■ Hyperalbuminemia (mild)
■ Hypersthenuria

Radiography. Findings usually are normal.

Nuclear Imaging and CT. These techniques can sometimes identify a hypothalamic lesion; however, studies have been normal in adipsic miniature schnauzers.

Treatment

The brain attempts to adapt to the hyperosmolar state by increasing its cellular osmolality with sodium, potassium, amino acids, and unidentified solutes (idiogenic osmoles). If plasma hyperosmolality is corrected too rapidly, the brain cells will continue to be hyperosmolar relative to the plasma, and cerebral edema may develop.

KEY POINT ▶ Rapid correction of chronic hyperosmolar states may lead to cerebral edema.

- For *initial management* of the normotensive animal to correct hypernatremia without lowering serum osmolality too rapidly, administer a sodium-restricted isotonic fluid, IV (5% dextrose in water or 0.45% NaCl with 2.5% dextrose) to correct the animal's water deficit.
- Calculate the animal's water deficit based on the serum sodium concentration or osmolality and a normal total body weight of water of 60%:

Water deficit (liters) =
0.6 × body weight (kg)

$$\times \left(1 - \frac{\text{normal sodium (mEq/liter)}}{\text{patient sodium (mEq/liter)}} \right)$$

OR

$$\left(1 - \frac{\text{normal osmolality (mOsm/kg)}}{\text{patient osmolality (mOsm/kg)}} \right)$$

- Replace the water deficit so as not to lower serum sodium concentration by more than 2 mEq/liter/hour. Generally, this rule translates to replacing the calculated water deficit during a period of 2–3 days.
- Add maintenance fluid requirement (60 ml/kg/day) with isotonic polyionic solution to the daily infusion.
- If the animal is hypotensive, re-establish tissue perfusion with isotonic saline or Ringer's solution before using sodium-restricted fluids. The osmolality of these solutions is still less than the patient's serum osmolality, so some reduction in serum sodium concentration and osmolality may occur.
- For *chronic management* once the animal is eating, mix maintenance daily water intake (50 to 60 ml/kg/day) with food.

Supplemental Readings

Crawford MA, Kittleson MD, Fink GD: Hypernatremia and adipsia in a dog. J Am Vet Med Assoc 284:818, 1984.

Eigenmann JE: Pituitary-hypothalamic diseases. *In* Ettinger SJ, ed.: *Textbook of Veterinary Internal Medicine.* Philadelphia: W. B. Saunders, 1989, p 1579.

Feldman EC, Nelson RW, eds.: *Canine and Feline Endocrinology and Reproduction.* Philadelphia: W. B. Saunders, 1987.

Peterson ME, Taylor RS, Greco DS, et al.: Acromegaly in fourteen cats. J Vet Intern Med 4:192, 1990.

Peterson ME, Randolph JF: Endocrine diseases. *In* Sherding RG, ed.: *The Cat: Diseases and Clinical Management.* New York: Churchill Livingstone, 1989, p 1095.

Skin and Ear Disorders

Kenneth Kwochka

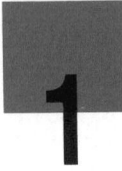

Pyoderma

Edmund J. Rosser Jr.

Pyoderma refers to any pyogenic infection of the skin, particularly bacterial. Pyoderma is a very common problem in clinical practice. The bacterial skin infection may be primary, in which case appropriate treatment often resolves the problem. However, much more commonly, the pyoderma is secondary to another underlying problem, which alters the skin's resistance to infection. Until the underlying problem is identified, the infection usually responds only temporarily to therapy and subsequently recurs.

Pyodermas are caused by bacterial colonization or invasion of the skin by coagulase-positive staphylococci, usually *Staphylococcus intermedius*. Invariably this is the initiating organism. In chronic, recurrent, or deep pyodermas, secondary bacterial invaders may be present, especially *Pseudomonas* spp., *Proteus* spp., and *Escherichia coli*.

SURFACE PYODERMAS

A surface pyoderma is a bacterial colonization of the surface of the epidermis only, without invasion into the stratum corneum or hair follicles.

Etiology

- *Self-trauma* to the skin, due to an underlying pruritic or painful process, can result in a focal surface pyoderma referred to as *acute moist dermatitis* ("hot spot"). Underlying conditions that may be associated with the development of hot spots are listed in Table 1.
- *Deep skin folds*, where the skin rubs against itself causing irritation, can result in a surface pyoderma

referred to as a *skin fold pyoderma* (intertrigo). These skin folds create a moist, dark, and warm environment with poor air circulation and subsequent bacterial growth and inflammation. These can occur in any skin fold in any breed of dog, but intertrigo is most commonly associated with the skin folds in certain breeds of dogs. Table 2 lists the anatomic sites of the more common skin fold pyodermas and their breed predispositions and includes

TABLE 1. Conditions That May Be Associated With the Development of Hot Spots*

Disease Category	Examples
Allergic skin diseases	Flea allergy dermatitis Atopy Food allergy Allergic contact dermatitis Staphylococcal hypersensitivity
Ectoparasites	Canine scabies Cheyletiellosis
Otitis externa	Allergic otitis externa Ceruminous otitis externa
Environmental causes	Irritant contact dermatitis Poor grooming Burs or plant awns in the skin or hair coat
Musculoskeletal disorders	Hip dysplasia Degenerative joint disease Arthritis and other arthropathies
Anal sac problems	Impacted anal sacs Anal sacculitis

*From Rosser EJ, Sams A: Pruritus. *In* Allen DG, ed.: *Small Animal Medicine*. Philadelphia: J. B. Lippincott, 1991, p 704.

TABLE 2. Skin Fold Pyodermas

Anatomic Site	Breed Predisposition	Comments
Lip fold	Cocker spaniel Springer spaniel Saint Bernard Irish setter	Lower lip fold Halitosis
Facial fold	Brachycephalic types Shar Pei	Between nose and eyes Lateral facial region
Body fold	Shar Pei	Also any breed with pendulous mammary glands Obese patients
Vulvar fold	None	Obese females Juvenile vulva Spayed early in life
Leg fold	Chondrodystrophic types (Basset, Dachshund)	Obese patients
Tail fold	Bulldog Boston terrier Pug	"Corkscrew tails" Anal odor

lip fold, facial fold, vulvar fold, tail fold, body fold, and leg fold pyodermas.

Clinical Signs

- *Acute moist dermatitis* (hot spot) is usually a single alopecic lesion that is circumscribed, erythematous, thickened, and erosive. A thin exudative film occurs over the surface, and peripheral hairs are matted onto the lesion. The lesion develops subsequent to the dog's chewing and licking at a focal area of pruritus or pain and develops within a matter of hours. The lesion is usually painful.
- *Skin folds* that develop surface pyoderma are characterized by inflammation and mild exudation. This pyoderma is best identified by simply widening the skin fold. The area is often noted to be malodorous. The animal is usually rubbing, licking, or biting excessively at the area. Evidence may exist of excoriation, alopecia, and erythema around the skin fold region. Table 2, as mentioned, lists the various skin fold pyodermas, some of the breed predispositions, and other comments.

Diagnosis

Acute Moist Dermatitis (Hot Spot)

KEY POINT ▶ Acute moist dermatitis is usually diagnosed by the history of the dog's traumatizing the skin, acute onset, rapid development of the lesion (within hours), and the typical appearance of the lesion on physical examination.

- *History* includes questioning the owner about the presence of any pruritic skin disease, painful process, or environmental irritant that might indicate the reason for the dog's self-trauma of the area (see Table 1). In instances of recurrent hot spot forma-

tion, identify the underlying problem to prevent any further recurrences.
- *Physical examination*
See the discussion of the clinical signs for acute moist dermatitis.

Skin Fold Pyodermas

KEY POINT ▶ Skin fold pyodermas are usually diagnosed by close inspection of the skin fold and demonstration of inflammation, mild exudation, and malodor from within the fold.

Treatment

Acute Moist Dermatitis

Whenever an underlying disease process can be identified, it is important to institute the specific treatment recommended for that disease as well as the treatment for the hot spot. One objective of treatment is to clip and clean the lesion to facilitate aeration and to allow better contact and penetration of topical agents.

- *Topical therapy.* First gently clip and thoroughly cleanse the area with an antiseptic shampoo, such as povidone-iodine (Betadine; Purdue Frederick Co.) or chlorhexidine (Nolvasan; Fort Dodge Labs). Because the lesion is often very painful, this step may require sedation or general anesthesia. Dry the lesion by applying an astringent, such as Burow's solution (Domeboro powder and water; Dome Labs) or hamamelis extract (DermaCool, Allerderm Inc.). Apply an antibiotic/steroid, such as Panolog Cream (Solvay Inc.), q12h, for 5 to 10 days.
- *Systemic therapy.* Corticosteroids are indicated in the treatment of hot spots because the lesion is often painful or pruritic and because the most common underlying causes are allergic skin diseases. Treatment is initiated with a short-acting, injectable form of prednisolone, such as prednisolone phosphate in aqueous suspension at a dose of 0.5 mg/kg, IM. It is followed the next day by oral prednisolone at a dose of 0.5 mg/kg q12h for 5 to 7 days—then, 0.5 mg/kg q24h for 5 to 7 days.

Skin Fold Pyodermas

- The *objectives of treatment* are to cleanse and disinfect the skin fold region using agents that will dry the area and prevent recurrence of pyoderma.
- *Topical therapy.* First gently expose and cleanse the skin fold with a benzoyl peroxide shampoo (OxyDex Shampoo, DVM Pharmaceuticals; Pyoben Shampoo, Allerderm Inc.). Dry the area manually or with a mild astringent, such as Burow's solution (Domeboro powder and water; Dome Labs) or hamamelis extract (DermaCool, Allerderm Inc.). Follow with a twice-daily application of a benzoyl peroxide gel (OxyDex Gel, DVM Pharmaceuticals; Pyoben Gel, Allerderm Inc.) into the skin fold region for 10 to 14 days.

In cases involving a more severe inflammatory response, the first 2 to 3 days of treatment consists of the twice-daily application of an antibiotic/steroid cream (Panolog Cream; Solvay Inc.) into the skin fold region. Once the inflammation has subsided, institute the benzoyl peroxide gel.

Prevention

Skin Fold Pyodermas

- *Topical therapy.* Because the skin folds that develop pyoderma are usually deep, owing to a given breed characteristic, this condition tends to be a low-grade, recurrent problem (see Table 2). Once the infection has been treated as recommended, use the benzoyl peroxide gel as needed to prevent recurrence. This measure may require application ranging from daily to once or twice weekly.
- *Corrective surgery.* When a more permanent solution to the problem is desired, remove the skin fold using cosmetic surgery techniques. These include cheiloplasty for lip fold pyodermas, V/Y plasty for facial fold pyodermas, episioplasty for vulvar fold pyodermas, and amputation for tail fold pyodermas (see sec. 5, ch. 16).

SUPERFICIAL PYODERMAS

A superficial pyoderma is a bacterial invasion of the epidermis that can manifest itself in one of two ways. The bacteria can penetrate the stratum corneum with the subsequent formation of subcorneal pustules and is referred to as *impetigo* (puppy pyoderma). Second, the bacteria can invade the opening of the hair follicle causing inflammation and is referred to as *folliculitis.*

Etiology

- *Coagulase-positive staphylococci* are the most common pathogens involved in a superficial pyoderma. *S. intermedius* is most frequently isolated.
  - *Impetigo* is most often observed in young dogs before puberty. The condition can result from certain contributing factors, such as poor nutrition, dirty environment, and ectoparasitic or endoparasitic infection.
  - *Superficial folliculitis* is occasionally a primary problem induced by coagulase-positive staphylococci. However, folliculitis secondary to another disease is much more common. Identify the underlying disease in cases of recurrent superficial folliculitis. See the discussions of recurrent superficial and deep pyodermas.

Clinical Signs

- *Impetigo* occurs as pustules in the inguinal and ventral abdominal regions. Occasionally, pustules are noted in the axillary region. The pustules do not involve hair follicles (i.e., no hair shafts protrude through the center of the pustule). Minimal erythema is noted, and the patient is usually nonpruritic. Impetigo is often an incidental finding during the physical examination of a recently acquired puppy.
- *Superficial folliculitis* initially appears similarly to impetigo, with pustules in the inguinal and ventral

abdominal region. However, pustules often extend to the axillary region and the ventrolateral thorax. The pustules are oriented around the hair follicle (i.e., hair shafts protrude through the center of the pustule). The base of the pustule is often erythematous, and the patient is usually pruritic. Other lesions may include papules, crusts, and epidermal collarettes. When the truncal skin is affected, the hair coat often takes on a "moth-eaten" appearance.

Diagnosis

Impetigo

KEY POINT ▶ Impetigo is usually diagnosed in young dogs before puberty by observing nonfollicular pustules in the inguinal and ventral abdominal region with minimal erythema and absence of pruritus.

- *History* includes questioning the owner about the animal's previous and current nutrition and housing environment.
- *Physical examination*
  See clinical signs for impetigo.
- *Cytologic examination* of the contents of an intact pustule most often reveals neutrophils and cocci.
- *Skin scrapings* are routinely examined for the presence of ectoparasites, such as *Demodex canis, Sarcoptes scabiei,* and *Cheyletiella* spp.
- *Bacterial culture* is rarely necessary. When cultures are done, however, *S. intermedius* is usually isolated.
- *Skin biopsy* is rarely necessary to establish the diagnosis of impetigo. Histopathology indicates subcorneal pustules containing neutrophils and cocci.
- Check the puppy for intestinal parasites.

Superficial Folliculitis

KEY POINT ▶ Superficial folliculitis is usually diagnosed by observing pustules around hair follicles in the inguinal, ventral abdominal, and axillary regions. The base of the pustule is erythematous, and the patient is usually pruritic.

- *History.* Superficial folliculitis is often secondary to an underlying disease. Question the owner about the affect of antibiotic therapy alone on the disease problem. This is a very important diagnostic tool in the systematic approach to a patient with recurrent pyoderma. See also the discussions of recurrent superficial and deep pyodermas.
- *Physical examination*
  See the discussion of the clinical signs for superficial folliculitis.
- Upon staining, *cytologic examination* of the contents of an intact pustule usually reveals neutrophils and cocci.
- *Skin scrapings* are routinely examined for the presence of ectoparasites, such as *D. canis, S. scabiei,* and *Cheyletiella* spp.
- *Bacterial culture and sensitivity* tests are indicated in cases of recurrent superficial folliculitis to evaluate

for resistant bacteria. Cultures usually indicate the presence of *Staphylococcus intermedius*. The sensitivity results are used as guidelines for antibiotic selection.

■ *Skin biopsy* findings indicate the presence of folliculitis or perifolliculitis, and coccoid bacteria are usually observed within the hair follicle.

Treatment

Impetigo

KEY POINT ▶ Objectives include identifying contributing factors for superficial pyoderma and correcting these as an adjunct to specific treatment. Improve the nutritional status and the housing environment and treat any endoparasitic or ectoparasitic infection.

■ *Topical therapy* is usually all that is required for this superficial staphylococcal infection, once any predisposing factors have been eliminated. Bathe the dog with a benzoyl peroxide shampoo (OxyDex Shampoo, DVM Pharmaceuticals; Pyoben Shampoo, Allerderm Inc.) two to three times weekly for 2 to 3 weeks.

■ *Systemic antibiotic therapy* is rarely indicated. However, when topical therapy fails to resolve the pyoderma, add a systemic antibiotic to the topical therapy protocol. Table 3 lists the most commonly provided antibiotics and their recommended dosages for staphylococcal pyodermas in the dog.

Superficial Folliculitis

KEY POINT ▶ A treatment objective is to be certain that an appropriate antibiotic for staphylococci has been selected (see Table 3) and that the duration of therapy has been adequate. The treatment required for folliculitis is generally more vigorous than that required for impetigo. In recurrent cases, define the underlying disease process and initiate a systematic approach to the disease. See the discussions of recurrent superficial and deep pyodermas.

■ *Topical therapy* includes twice weekly bathing of the pet with a benzoyl peroxide shampoo (OxyDex

Shampoo, DVM Pharmaceuticals; Pyoben Shampoo, Allerderm Inc.) for 3 weeks.

■ *Systemic antibiotic therapy* can be initially selected on an empirical basis, choosing an antibiotic effective against coagulase-positive staphylococci (see Table 3). The recommended duration of treatment is a minimum of 21 consecutive days.

DEEP PYODERMAS (DEEP FOLLICULITIS AND FURUNCULOSIS)

A deep pyoderma is a bacterial skin infection that extends beyond the epidermis and into the dermis and occasionally into the subcutaneous tissues. Although there are many possible forms of deep pyoderma, this discussion is limited to the most common form, deep folliculitis and furunculosis. Furunculosis is defined as an inflammation of the hair follicle that breaks through the hair follicle wall and extends into the dermis and occasionally into the subcutaneous tissues.

Etiology

■ Coagulase-positive staphylococci are the most common pathogens involved in the initiation of a deep pyoderma. *S. intermedius* is the most frequently isolated.

■ In contrast to a superficial pyoderma, secondary invasion with other bacteria often occurs with *Pseudomonas* spp., *Proteus* spp., or *E. coli*.

■ The development of a deep pyoderma is rarely a primary disease process and is invariably related to some other underlying problem. See the discussions of recurrent superficial and deep pyodermas.

Clinical Signs

■ Deep folliculitis and furunculosis initially begin as superficial folliculitis. See discussion of the superficial pyoderma, the clinical signs, and superficial folliculitis.

■ When deep folliculitis and furunculosis develop, the papules and pustules become larger and nodular upon palpation. Exudation and crust formation follow. Draining tracts may develop. Hemorrhagic bullae may also be noted.

■ In addition to the inguinal, ventral abdominal, and axillary regions, the pressure and wear areas of the body can be affected. The disease may then become generalized.

■ The lesions are painful and/or pruritic.

■ Peripheral lymphadenopathy is a common finding. Signs of systemic illness may be present (anorexia, depression, weight loss). The patient may also be febrile, a possible indication of bacteremia and/or septicemia.

Diagnosis

KEY POINT ▶ Deep folliculitis and furunculosis are usually diagnosed by observing papules and pustules that become nodular upon palpation, with exudation, crust formation, and draining tracts.

TABLE 3. Systemic Antibiotics Recommended in the Treatment of Staphylococcal Pyodermas

Antibiotic	Recommended Dosage	Route Administered
Oxacillin	22 mg/kg q8h	Oral
Erythromycin	11 mg/kg q8h	Oral
Chloramphenicol	33–55 mg/kg q8h	Oral, IM, SQ, IV
Cefadroxil	22 mg/kg q8h	Oral
Cephalexin	22 mg/kg q8h	Oral
Amoxicillin/Clavulanate	14 mg/kg q12h	Oral
Trimethoprim-sulfadiazine	30 mg/kg q12h	Oral

■ *History*. Deep folliculitis and furunculosis are invariably secondary to an underlying disease process. Question the owner about the affect of antibiotics alone on the disease, as this a very important diagnostic tool in the systematic approach to a patient with recurrent pyoderma. See discussions of recurrent superficial and deep pyodermas.

■ *Physical examination*
See the clinical signs for deep folliculitis and furunculosis.

■ *Cytologic examination* of pustules, exudates, and draining tracts usually reveals neutrophils, macrophages, cocci, and rods.

■ Obtain *skin scrapings* to evaluate for *D. canis* mites—a common ectoparasitic cause of deep pyoderma.

■ Perform *bacterial culture and sensitivity* tests in all cases of deep pyoderma. This form of pyoderma is capable of causing bacteremia and/or septicemia, resulting in a life-threatening situation.

■ *Fungal cultures* are recommended in cases of deep pyodermas that are refractory to antibiotic therapy. Fungi are another possible cause of deep folliculitis and furunculosis. Fungal diseases to consider include sporotrichosis, blastomycosis, coccidioidomycosis, aspergillosis, histoplasmosis, and cryptococcosis.

■ *Skin biopsy findings* indicate the presence of deep folliculitis, perifolliculitis, and furunculosis. Bacterial or fungal organisms may or may not be identified upon special staining.

■ Perform *blood cultures* for bacteria in a patient with a fever and evidence of systemic illness.

Treatment

KEY POINT ▶ Be certain that an appropriate antibiotic has been selected to eliminate the organism causing the deep pyoderma. Choose the antibiotic based on the results of the bacterial culture and sensitivity tests. In general, treatment is more vigorous than that for superficial folliculitis. In recurrent cases, define the underlying disease process and initiate a systematic approach.

■ *Topical therapy*
• Clip the hair around the affected areas. In cases of generalized deep pyoderma in long-coated breeds of dogs, clip the entire body.
• Initially bathe the patient twice daily (preferably in a whirlpool bath) using a povidone-iodine preparation (Weladol Shampoo, Pittman Moore Inc.; Betadine Whirlpool Concentrate, Purdue Frederick Co.) for the first 1 to 2 weeks of treatment. As the patient responds to treatment and the lesions have dried and begun to heal, change the treatment to once to twice weekly bathing with a benzoyl peroxide shampoo (OxyDex Shampoo, DVM Pharmaceuticals; Pyoben Shampoo, Allerderm Inc.) for the next 4 to 8 weeks.

■ *Systemic antibiotic* selection is always based on the results of bacterial culture and sensitivity tests in cases of deep pyoderma. Use the appropriate dosage

(see Table 3). Treat for approximately 6 to 8 consecutive weeks. Severe cases of deep pyoderma may require a longer treatment regimen. Treat for at least 2 weeks beyond the complete clinical remission of the infection.

RECURRENT SUPERFICIAL AND DEEP PYODERMAS

Antibiotic-responsive but recurrent pyoderma is often a very frustrating problem in clinical practice. This section stresses the need to evaluate the patient with this problem for some of the more common, underlying diseases associated with recurrent pyoderma.

Etiologic and Predisposing Conditions

■ *Inappropriate selection* of the antibiotic or inadequate duration of the therapy can be a simple reason for the development of recurrent pyoderma. For recommendations on treatment see the discussions of superficial pyoderma treatment and superficial folliculitis, deep pyoderma treatment and Table 3.

■ *Long-term glucocorticoid* use can predispose the patient to recurrent pyoderma and cause varying degrees of iatrogenic Cushing disease. Most patients with pyoderma are pruritic; therefore, glucocorticoids are often used as adjuncts to the antibiotic therapy. This treatment is acceptable on a first time basis. Discontinue glucocorticoids once it becomes apparent that the pyoderma is a recurrent problem. By treating the pruritic patient that has pyoderma with antibiotics only, very important information can be learned. This can then help guide the clinician as to which underlying disease condition to suspect. See the section on diagnosis and the use of antibiotics and response to therapy as a guideline for the type of underlying disease to suspect.

KEY POINT ▶ The following discussion of common underlying diseases resulting in recurrent pyoderma requires that the patient has first been placed on a prolonged antibiotic treatment protocol, as discussed under the section on diagnosis! Therefore, the observations being made are those that are noted after the pyoderma has been symptomatically in remission.

■ *Allergic skin diseases*
• Patients with *flea allergy dermatitis* have pruritus that persists after resolution of the pyoderma that primarily affects the caudal third of the body. Most patients initially have this problem in warmer weather only. For further discussion, see sec. 5, ch. 6, on flea allergy dermatitis.
• Patients with *atopy* have pruritus that persists after the resolution of the pyoderma that affects various combinations of the following areas of the body: face, ears, axillae, inguinal region, proximal cranial foreleg region, and feet. Most patients initially

have the problem in warmer weather only. For further discussion, see sec. 5, ch. 7 on atopy.

- Patients with *food allergy* have pruritus that persists after resolution of the pyoderma that affects various combinations of the following areas of the body: face, ears, axillae, inguinal region, proximal cranial foreleg region, and feet. All patients have a nonseasonal (i.e., year-round) problem from the onset. For further discussion, see sec. 5, ch. 8, on food allergy.

■ *Parasitic skin diseases*
- Patients with *demodicosis* may be pruritic, once the pyoderma has resolved. As previously stated, all patients with pyoderma require that several deep skin scrapings be performed, because demodicosis is a common cause of recurrent pyoderma that can be easily diagnosed. For further discussion, see sec. 5, ch. 4 on demodicosis.
- Patients with *scabies* have pruritus that persists after resolution of the pyoderma that initially affects the ear, elbow, and hock regions. All patients have a nonseasonal (i.e., year-round) problem from the onset. For further discussion, see sec. 5, ch. 5, on scabies.

■ Patients with *keratinization abnormalities* may be pruritic, once the pyoderma has resolved. The lesions that persist are suggestive of keratinization (seborrheic) abnormality. For further discussion, see sec. 5, ch. 10, on keratinization defects.

■ *Endocrine skin diseases*
- Patients with *hypothyroidism* and *Cushing's disease* are nonpruritic, once the pyoderma has resolved. The patient is evaluated by history and physical examination for evidence suggestive of these metabolic diseases. For further discussion see sec. 4, chs. 1 and 3.

■ Patients with *staphylococcal hypersensitivity* exhibit a temporary resolution of both the pyoderma and the pruritus on antibiotic treatment alone. Staphylococcal hypersensitivity as a primary disease is one of the more controversial topics in veterinary dermatology. In this disease the staphylococcal infection alone, without any underlying disease, is the cause of the pruritus (i.e., primary pruritic pyoderma). This disease is best diagnosed by exclusion of other underlying causes for recurrent pyoderma. Therefore, all of the underlying diseases discussed to this point must first be systematically ruled out before one can establish the diagnosis of primary staphylococcal hypersensitivity.

■ *Immunodeficiency disorders* as the primary cause for recurrent pyoderma are rare. Disorders to consider are cell-mediated immunity disorders, such as T-lymphocyte deficiency, and humoral immunity disorders, such as IgA deficiency.

Clinical Signs

See discussions of the clinical signs of superficial pyoderma, superficial folliculitis, and deep pyoderma.

Diagnosis

■ First see the procedures discussed for the diagnoses of superficial pyoderma, superficial folliculitis, and deep pyoderma.

■ Use antibiotics as a diagnostic tool. The antibiotic along with antibacterial shampoo therapy is provided without any antipruritic drugs, especially glucocorticoids. The patient is treated in this manner for 3 weeks and then re-examined. If the patient is still pruritic, note the distribution pattern and question the owner as to whether the condition was initially a predominantly warm weather seasonal problem or a nonseasonal problem. For common underlying pruritic skin diseases, see the discussion of etiology. If the lesions and pruritus have both resolved on antibiotic treatment alone, continue the antibiotic treatment for 8 consecutive weeks. In some instances, this treatment results in a permanent resolution of the pyoderma. If the pyoderma recurs after stopping antibiotic therapy, evaluate the animal for underlying endocrine disease, staphylococcal hypersensitivity, and immunodeficiency disorder (see the discussion of etiology).

■ For specific testing procedures to diagnose the various underlying disease problems, please refer to the appropriate chapters as recommended under etiology of recurrent pyodermas.

■ Tests for the evaluation of primary immunodeficiency disorders are not readily available and are usually offered only by veterinary university laboratory services. Testing procedures to consider are the mitogen stimulation test for the evaluation of lymphocyte function and the measurement of serum IgA levels for the indirect evaluation of a secretory IgA disorder.

Treatment

■ *Specific treatment of the identified underlying disease* is the most important component in the resolution of an antibiotic responsive but recurrent pyoderma. Refer to the appropriate chapters as recommended under the section on etiology of recurrent pyodermas.

■ *Topical therapy* (see discussions of the treatment and topical therapy of superficial pyoderma, superficial folliculitis, and deep pyoderma).

TABLE 4. Staphage Lysate Injection Protocol*

Week	Volume (ml)
1	0.25
2	0.50
3	0.75
4	1.00

*Follow this protocol with 1 to 2 ml every 3 to 21 days as needed to prevent recurrence of the pyoderma. Injections are given subcutaneously.

From Rosser EJ, Sams A: Papular/pustular, vesicular/bullous, and erosive/ulcerative dermatoses. *In* Allen DG, ed.: *Small Animal Medicine*. Philadelphia: J.B. Lippincott, 1991, p. 719.

■ *Systemic therapy* is discussed under treatment for superficial pyoderma, superficial folliculitis, and deep pyoderma.

■ *Immunomodulating drug therapy* is indicated in cases of primary staphylococcal hypersensitivity and primary immunodeficiency disorders. Many treatment alternatives are available, but my preference is to use a staphylococcal bacterin (Staphage Lysate, Delmont Labs). See Table 4 for the recommended Staphage Lysate injection protocol. Remember that the patient is also placed on an appropriate systemic antibiotic for the first 4 to 8 weeks of treatment.

Supplemental Readings

Kwochka KW: Recurrent pyoderma. *In* Griffin CE, Kwochka KW, MacDonald JM, eds.: *Current Veterinary Dermatology.* St. Louis: C.V. Mosby Co., in press.

Muller GH, Kirk RW, Scott DW: *Small Animal Dermatology.* Philadelphia: W.B. Saunders, 1989, p 244.

Rosser EJ, Sams A: Papular/pustular, vesicular/bullous, erosive/ulcerative dermatoses. *In* Allen DG, ed.: *Small Animal Medicine.* Philadelphia: J.B. Lippincott Co., 1991, p 711.

Rosser EJ, Sams A: Pruritus. *In* Allen DG, ed.: *Small Animal Medicine.* Philadelphia: J.B. Lippincott Co., p 689.

2 Mycobacteriosis

Alan C. Mundell

Although a variety of mycobacterial organisms can cause sporadic disease in human beings and in animals, feline leprosy and atypical mycobacteria are the principal mycobacterial organisms seen in small animal practice that produce skin lesions. All mycobacterial organisms contain a lipid-rich cell wall that inhibits host defense mechanisms and imparts a characteristic staining property in the laboratory. This staining property involves the retention of carbolfuchsin after acid and alcohol decolorization. Thus, mycobacteria are classified as acid-fast staining organisms.

FELINE LEPROSY

Feline leprosy is a mycobacterial disease of cats that was first recognized in Australia during the early 1960's. The condition has since been identified in New Zealand, Great Britain, France, the Netherlands, and the west coast of the United States and Canada. The disease is usually confined to cats living in port cities and coastal areas. Feline leprosy has no breed or sex predilection. However, age of onset is usually 2 to 5 years.

Etiology

- The cause of feline leprosy is *Mycobacterium lepraemurium,* the rat leprosy organism. Although the rat leprosy organism had been suspected for many years, it was only in the 1980's that sophisticated culture techniques and biochemical analysis could identify *M. lepraemurium* as the etiologic agent.
- The mode of transmission is unknown. However, rat bites, insect vectors, and aerosolization of contaminated nasal secretions are proposed methods of transmission.
- In experimental infections, the incubation period is 2 to 18 months.

Clinical Signs

- These consist of skin lesions that range from solitary to multiple, intradermal to subcutaneous, nodular to plaque-like, and haired to ulcerated. Fistulation and exudation are uncommon.
- Although skin lesions may occur anywhere on the body, head and limbs are frequent sites. Additionally, lesions may occur on the lips, gums, tongue, and nasal mucosa. Regional lymph nodes may be enlarged with lymphoid hyperplasia and infiltration of epithelioid cells and macrophages. The feline

leprosy organism is occasionally isolated from these lymph nodes.
- Rarely will the condition disseminate to spleen, bone marrow, liver, kidney, lung, or adjacent muscle. The cats (unlike those cats with localized infection) are usually ill.

Diagnosis

- The diagnosis is achieved primarily through histologic evaluation in conjunction with compatible history, physical examination, cytology, culture, and laboratory animal inoculation findings.
- The differential diagnosis for feline leprosy includes atypical mycobacteriosis, tuberculosis, foreign body dermatitis, deep mycotic infections, mycetomas, dermatophyte pseudomycetomas, chronic bacterial infections, eosinophilic granuloma complex, and neoplasia.
- *History* must be compatible with feline leprosy. The cat will typically be young to middle-aged, allowed to roam, living in a cool, moist, coastal climate.
- *Physical examination* findings usually reveal lesions that are firm and indolent and lack exudation or fistulation. Lesions are frequently solitary or regionally grouped. Affected cats appear clinically healthy and oblivious to the disease. However, all cats are evaluated for underlying immunosuppressive diseases, including feline leukemia and feline immunodeficiency viruses (see sec. 2, chs. 1 and 2).
- *Cytology* of lesional impression smears consists of mixed inflammatory cells with macrophages and histiocytes containing variable numbers of acid-fast bacilli. Ziehl-Neelsen and a modified Fite's stain are the acid-fast stains most commonly used.
- *Biopsy* specimens of lesions are fixed in 10% buffered formalin and evaluated histologically, using both hematoxylin-eosin and acid-fast stains (Ziehl-Neelsen and modified Fite's). The histology is somewhat analogous to that of human leprosy with the presence of both tuberculoid and lepromatous forms. The tuberculoid form consists of primarily nonencapsulated epithelioid granulomas that are interspersed with neutrophils and surrounded by a zone of lymphocytes. Low numbers of organisms are associated with this tuberculoid pattern. The lepromatous form is composed of sheets of large foamy macrophages that contain large numbers of acid-fast bacilli. In human beings, the lepromatous form indicates a more immunocompromised host and thus imparts a poorer prognosis. In cats, however, this correlation remains to be demonstrated. One major

histologic difference between human and feline leprosy is the lack of consistent cutaneous nerve infiltration by the feline leprosy organism.

KEY POINT ▶ *Culture of the feline leprosy mycobacterium is difficult to obtain because the organism fails to grow on blood agar and standard mycobacterial media (Lowenstein-Jensen and Stonebrink).*

A 1% Ogawa egg yolk medium can be used to grow the organism when incubated under precise temperature and CO_2 conditions. Most commercial laboratories do not perform Ogawa egg yolk medium cultures. However, tissue maceration cultures (obtained via sterile biopsies) incubated on blood agar and routine mycobacterial media can help differentiate the feline leprosy organism from the atypical or tuberculosis-causing mycobacterium.

- *Laboratory animal inoculation* is used primarily in research to propagate and investigate the feline leprosy organism. This procedure is of greatest value when differentiating feline leprosy from tuberculosis. Only the tuberculosis-producing mycobacteria will routinely kill guinea pigs within 6 to 8 weeks after inoculation.

Treatment

- *Treatment* may not be necessary when lesions are small, unobtrusive, and likely to be self-limiting. However, this strategy is seldom effective and is recommended only for lesions that appear to be resolving spontaneously at the time of diagnosis.

KEY POINT ▶ *Surgical excision is the treatment of choice when lesions are limited in number and wide surgical margins can be used. However, disease recurrence is common and may require additional surgical intervention and/or medical management.*

- *Medical management* has been attempted utilizing a variety of drugs that have shown efficacy in treating human leprosy. Dapsone and rifampin were the first human antileprosy drugs investigated. Unfortunately, in the cat, toxicity to these drugs is common and efficacy is variable. An evaluation of another common human antileprosy drug, clofazimine (Lamprene, Ciba-Geigy), was more encouraging. Clofazimine is an iminophenazine dye with antimycobacterial properties that is suspended in olive oil and packaged in 50- and 100-mg capsules. Although the pharmacokinetics of clofazimine in the cat are unknown, a dosage of 2 to 3 mg/kg, q24h, PO, for 6 to 12 weeks past complete clinical resolution appears to be very effective. At this dosage minimal side effects are noted. Higher dosages may produce transient elevations in liver enzyme levels. In order to obtain the proper feline dose, the capsule is punctured and the contents proportioned. Latex gloves are worn to prevent staining of hands. Clofazimine is not approved by the United States Food and Drug Administration (FDA) for animal use.

Prevention

- This is probably best achieved by confining cats to an exclusively indoor environment. Because of the rare and sporadic nature of the disease, it is unlikely that this measure is necessary.
- Avoidance of immunosuppressive drugs while disease is active may help prevent exacerbation.

ATYPICAL MYCOBACTERIOSIS

Nontuberculous, nonlepromatous mycobacteria are classified as atypical or opportunistic. Runyon placed these mycobacteria into four groups, depending on laboratory culture properties. Almost all dog and cat atypical mycobacterial skin infections belong to the rapid-growing group IV. These saprophytic, facultative pathogens are ubiquitous in nature and are typically isolated from water and moist soil. Atypical mycobacteriosis is more prevalent in cats than in dogs, with no apparent age, breed, or sex predilection.

Etiology

Mycobacterium fortuitum-chelonei complex, M. phlei, M. thermoresistible, M. xenopi, and *M. smegmatis* have produced skin lesions in dogs and cats. In the United States, *M. fortuitum-chelonei* is responsible for most atypical mycobacterial infections. Skin infection follows contamination of traumatized skin, especially bite wounds and deep scratches.

Clinical Signs

- These consist of dermal to subcutaneous soft nodules that tend to ulcerate and drain a serous to seropurulent discharge. Tissue grains are not present. Unlike feline leprosy, fistulation and exudation are classically observed. Lesions can occur anywhere on the body; however, flank and inguinal regions are common locations.
- Except for regionalized lymphadenopathy, clinical signs of systemic disease are uncommon, even when lesions are extensive.

Diagnosis

- The diagnosis is achieved primarily through bacterial culture findings and histologic evaluation. The differential diagnosis for cutaneous atypical mycobacteriosis is extensive and includes feline leprosy (in cats only), tuberculosis, foreign body dermatitis, deep mycotic infections, mycetomas, dermatophyte pseudomycetomas, chronic bacterial infections, generalized demodicosis (in dogs primarily), sterile nodular panniculitis, pansteatitis, eosinophilic granuloma complex, and neoplasia.

KEY POINT ▶ Atypical mycobacterial organisms are difficult to isolate. All suspected cases are cultured. Biopsies are performed, and lesional exudates are collected for cytologic examination.

■ *History* must be compatible with cutaneous atypical mycobacteriosis. A history of trauma to the involved area weeks to months prior to the onset of lesions is not uncommon.

■ *Physical examination* findings reveal soft nodules that fistulate and drain. Lesions are typically nonpainful, and the animal otherwise appears healthy.

■ *Cytology* of lesional impression smears and smears of biopsy tissue consists of mixed inflammatory cells and, occasionally, an acid-fast bacillus. Cytologic evaluation frequently fails to confirm the presence of acid-fast organisms. Ziehl-Neelsen and modified Fite's stain are the acid-fast stains most commonly used.

■ *Biopsy* samples of lesions are handled in a manner similar to that in feline leprosy except that special techniques, such as snap (instant) freezing the formalin-fixed tissue prior to staining or rapid Ziehl-Neelsen staining, may be necessary to reveal the organism. Characteristically, fewer acid-fast bacilli are observed in atypical mycobacteriosis than in feline leprosy. Nodular pyogranulomatous dermatitis along with panniculitis is the common histologic pattern. If organisms are found they are usually located within extracellular lipid vacuoles that are ringed by neutrophils. Besides the paucity of organisms, atypically mycobacteriosis also differs from feline leprosy by the extracellular location of the organisms.

■ *Culture* consists of growing the organism on standard mycobacterial media (Lowenstein-Jensen and Stonebrink) as well as on blood agar. Sterile swab and biopsy techniques are employed to obtain cultures. The laboratory is notified that atypical mycobacteriosis is suspected so that appropriate cultures are performed. Runyon group IV mycobacteria are called rapid growers because colonies appear within 7 days after media inoculation. In contrast, most other mycobacteria are either difficult to culture or require weeks to months to grow.

■ *Laboratory animal inoculation* is seldom performed. If cultures fail to identify the mycobacterial organism and the possibility of tuberculosis exists, guinea pig inoculation is performed.

Treatment

These options vary greatly because reported cases are too infrequent to establish a preferred therapeutic protocol.

KEY POINT ▶ Most reports of successful disease management are anecdotal or involve low numbers of cases. Because the condition naturally waxes and wanes with occasional prolonged periods of remission, the success of all treatment options must be carefully assessed. Clinical remission may be more easily achieved in the dog than in the cat.

■ An approach of no therapy may be taken if the disease involves a reasonably small area and the condition does not bother the animal or owner. When owners are unwilling to commit to a prolonged course of therapy, allowing the disease to naturally undergo its cycle may be a viable alternative. In time, the skin lesions may become more extensive; however, the disease rarely becomes systemic.

■ *Surgical excision* is most successful when dealing with small, simply excised lesions. Wide surgical margins must be made. Unfortunately, surgical site dehiscence is common.

KEY POINT ▶ Surgically debulking the lesions while treating the animal with a prolonged course of an appropriate antibiotic may provide a prolonged remission. Surgical excision may be more effective when managing canine lesions.

■ *Medical management* has been attempted using a variety of drugs. Table 1 contains the dosages of the more effective agents. Most of these drugs are not approved by the FDA for use in dogs or cats. *In vitro* sensitivity testing may be helpful when selecting a therapeutic agent. However, the clinical response is frequently less than what the sensitivity test suggests. In general, medication is administered for 2 to 6 months past clinical cure. If the medication is effective in achieving clinical remission but the lesions return after discontinuing the medication, prolonged or indefinite therapy may be needed. It is imperative that all therapy be closely monitored for development of adverse side effects. This monitoring typically requires periodic blood and urine laboratory evaluation, especially for drugs with known potential toxicities (e.g., aminoglycosides with nephrotoxicity, ototoxicity). It is beyond the scope of this chapter to discuss drug toxicities and the monitoring procedures. However, this information is available in current human and veterinary pharmacology text-

TABLE 1. Selected Drugs for Treatment of Cutaneous Atypical Mycobacteriosis

Treatment	Product (Manufacturer)	Dosage
Clofazimine	Lamprene (Ciba-Geigy)	8–12 mg/kg, q24h, PO
Enrofloxacin*	Baytril (Mobay)	2.5–5 mg/kg, q12h, PO
Doxycycline	Vibramycin (Pfizer)	2.5–5 mg/kg, q12h, PO
Amikacin	Amiglyde-V (Fort Dodge)	5–7 mg/kg, q12h, SC, IM
Kanamycin	Kantrim (Fort Dodge)	5–7 mg/kg, q12h SC, IM
Gentamicin	Gentocin (Schering-Plough)	2 mg/kg, q12h, SC, IM

*An adjunctive transdermal route of drug delivery has also been used by mixing a 1:1 solution of 2.27% enrofloxacin in 90% dimethyl sulfoxide. A dose of 1 ml is applied to affected areas.

books. A thorough understanding of all drugs administered increases the safety of the therapeutic protocol.

Prevention

■ This is best achieved by decreasing the likelihood of traumatic injury to the skin and subcutaneous tissue. If animals are allowed to roam freely, confining them to house or yard may decrease the likelihood of trauma. However, because of the rare and sporadic nature of the disease, these measures are probably unnecessary.

■ Avoidance of immunosuppressive drugs may help prevent exacerbation or recurrence of atypical mycobacteriosis.

Supplemental Readings

Kunkle GA: Feline leprosy. *In* Greene CE, ed.: *Infectious Diseases of the Dog and Cat.* Philadelphia: W.B. Saunders, 1990, p 567.

Kunkle GA: Atypical mycobacterial infections. *In* Greene CE, ed.: *Infectious Diseases of the Dog and Cat.* Philadelphia: W.B. Saunders, 1990, p 569.

Muller GH, Kirk RW, Scott DW: *Small Animal Dermatology.* Philadelphia: W.B. Saunders, 1989, p 274.

Mundell AC: New therapeutic agents in veterinary dermatology. Vet Clin North Am Sm Anim Pract 20:1544, 1990.

White PD: Enrofloxacin-responsive cutaneous atypical mycobacterial infection in two cats. Proceedings of the Annual Meeting of the American Academy of Veterinary Dermatology. 7th Annual Meeting, Phoenix, AZ: 95, 1991.

White SD: Cutaneous mycobacteriosis. *In* Kirk RW, ed.: *Current Veterinary Therapy IX Small Animal Practice.* Philadelphia: W.B. Saunders, 1986, p 529.

3 Dermatophytosis

Karin Muth Beale

Dermatophytosis is an infection of keratinized tissues usually caused by one of three species of dermatophytes: *Microsporum, Trichophyton,* and *Epidermophyton.* These organisms are keratinophilic and invade and live within the keratinized hair, nail, or skin. The majority of infections in dogs and cats are caused by three species of dermatophytes: *M. canis, M. gypseum,* and *T. mentagrophytes.* Other fungi are uncommon causes of dermatophytosis in pets. Dermatophytes are classified into groups based on their natural habitat as geophilic, zoophilic, or anthropophilic. Geophilic dermatophytes naturally inhabit the soil, zoophilic species are adapted to animals, and humans are the hosts for anthropophilic species. As a general rule, geophilic and anthropophilic dermatophytes tend to produce much more inflammatory lesions in animals than do the more host-adapted species.

ETIOLOGY

Microsporum gypseum

M. gypseum is a geophilic dermatophyte that normally inhabits the soil and decomposes keratinaceous debris. However, this organism is the second most common cause of dermatophytosis in dogs in the United States, and it occasionally infects cats. *M. gypseum* is most commonly isolated from animals that spend much time outdoors. Because the organism is not specifically adapted to living on animals, it tends to incite inflammation. Lesions are commonly seen in areas with significant soil contact, such as the feet and muzzle.

Microsporum canis

This zoophilic dermatophyte is responsible for the majority of the clinical cases of dermatophytosis in dogs. *M. canis* is the cause of approximately 98% of the cases of feline dermatophytosis. It was previously thought that cats served as the reservoir for *M. canis;* however, recent studies show that it is rarely isolated from healthy cats. The isolation of *M. canis* from a dog or cat is a significant finding and requires treatment.

Trichophyton mentagrophytes

This zoophilic dermatophyte is the third most common cause of dermatophytosis in dogs and less commonly affects cats. *T. mentagrophytes* is the most common cause of dermatophytosis in rodents and rabbits. Pet rodents or rabbits should be considered as possible reservoirs of infection. Wild rodents are commonly infected, and the infections may be clinically inapparent. Cats that hunt may be predisposed to acquiring infection with this type of dermatophyte.

Anthropophilic Dermatophytes

Anthropophilic dermatophytes such as *Microsporum audouini* rarely affect pets but can cause intensely inflamed lesions in animals. Zoophilic species of dermatophytes other than *M. canis* and *T. mentagrophytes,* such as *T. equinum, T. verrucosum,* and *M. nanum,* may cause dermatophytosis in dogs or cats; however, such animals usually are in contact with livestock that are natural reservoirs or hosts for those organisms.

CLINICAL SIGNS

Canine Dermatophytosis

- Canine dermatophytosis is characterized by alopecia and scaling. Usually there are focal to multifocal circumscribed affected patches of skin.
- Hair loss, broken hairs, scaling, pustules, papules, exudation, crusting, and hyperpigmentation may be seen. Pruritus is variable.
- The classic lesion is a circular area of alopecia and scaling with central healing; however, the lesions may be irregular in appearance.
- Several factors influence the severity of the lesions. Young and immunocompromised animals tend to develop more extensive lesions that take longer to resolve than do those of healthy adult animals. This is because the ability to mount an effective inflammatory response is necessary to eliminate the infection. Additionally, the pathogenicity and the species of dermatophyte affect the amount of inflammatory response.

Kerion

A kerion is a round, raised, nodular lesion that results when follicular rupture, furunculosis, and pyogranulomatous inflammation occur with a dermatophyte infection.

- Kerions are most commonly seen in dogs on the limbs and face.
- The etiology usually is *M. gypseum.*
- These lesions often are secondarily infected with *Staphylococcus intermedius.*

283

Generalized Dermatophytosis

Generalized dermatophytosis is uncommon in the dog and is usually caused by *M. gypseum* or *T. mentagrophytes*.

- Characteristic findings are widespread alopecia and seborrhea with or without pruritus.
- Other lesions, similar to those of focal dermatophytosis, may be present as well.
- Generalized dermatophytosis in adult dogs is often associated with immunosuppression or systemic disease.

Feline Dermatophytosis

KEY POINT ▶ Feline dermatophytosis can present in many different clinical forms. Consider dermatophytosis in the differential diagnosis of most feline dermatoses.

Classic "Ringworm"

Ringworm lesions may be present in cats; however, the circular lesions of alopecia and scaling with central healing are much less common in cats than in dogs. Cats may have what appears to be a localized infection, when in reality the infection is generalized. This is especially true of long-haired cats.

Subclinical Infection

Adult cats may have subclinical dermatophyte infections. These cats may have minimal (e.g., a minor degree of scaling or a few broken hairs) to no apparent clinical lesions. These cats are important in the spread of dermatophytosis, and culture is necessary to identify affected cats.

Miliary Dermatitis

In cats, dermatophytosis may occur as a *miliary dermatitis* that may or may not be pruritic (see sec. 5, ch. 14).

Symmetric Alopecia

Symmetric alopecia may be caused by dermatophytosis in cats. Excessive grooming as a result of pruritus, combined with follicular inflammation, can lead to excessive hair loss in some cats.

Pseudomycetoma

- Pseudomycetoma (Majocchi's granuloma) is a form of granulomatous dermatitis in the cat caused by a dermatophyte, usually *M. canis*.
- This type of lesion is most common in Persian cats.
- In this lesion the fungus is sequestered in the dermis but does not proliferate; a nodular, ulcerating dermatitis is the result.
- Affected cats usually have generalized dermatophytosis.

Onychomycosis

- This dermatophyte infection of the nails is seen in both dogs and cats.
- The lesions usually are caused by *T. mentagrophytes*.
- The nails are dry, cracked, brittle, and frequently deformed.
- Often there is a concurrent infection with inflammation of the nail fold, and the pads may be affected as well.

DIAGNOSIS

KEY POINT ▶ False-positive diagnosis of dermatophytosis in animals with circular lesions of alopecia is common. Follicular infections with *Demodex* and *Staphylococcus* organisms produce similar lesions.

- Dermatophytosis should not be diagnosed solely on the basis of clinical signs. Because of the numerous clinical conditions in dogs and cats that can mimic dermatophytosis, it is necessary to perform specific diagnostic procedures to obtain a definitive diagnosis.
- Canine dermatophytosis
  - In the dog, the most common cause of circular alopecia is staphylococcal folliculitis (see sec. 5, ch. 1), followed by localized demodicosis (see sec. 5, ch. 4).
  - Follicular infections with different organisms share common reaction patterns of papules, pustules, alopecia, scaling, and crusting.
  - Use diagnostic tests such as skin scrapings, bacterial cultures, and skin biopsies to rule out some of the more common causes of focal alopecia in dogs.
  - Consider dermatophytosis in the differential diagnosis of a generalized scaling, crusting alopecic dermatosis. A number of different conditions can cause a generalized dermatitis similar to that seen in generalized dermatophytosis in the dog (Table 1).
  - The differential diagnosis for kerions and pseudomycetomas includes the various causes of nodular dermatitides, such as cutaneous neoplasms, staphylococcal furunculosis, and acral lick dermatitis (see Table 1). Kerions are generally found as raised, pink, solitary lesions with a predilection for the face, mimicking histiocytomas.
- Feline Dermatophytosis
  - The list of disorders to be considered in the differential diagnosis of feline dermatophytosis is extensive and includes all causes of miliary dermatitis and symmetric alopecia (see sec. 5, ch. 14 and ch. 13).

History

An accurate history can provide useful information regarding the possible source of infection.

- Obtain an accurate drug history.

TABLE 1. Differential Diagnosis for Dermatophytosis in Dogs

Focal to Multifocal Dermatophytosis
Demodicosis
Staphylococcal folliculitis
Dermatophilosis
Abrasions
Pemphigus foliaceus/erythematosus
Zinc-responsive dermatosis

Generalized Dermatophytosis
Demodicosis
Staphylococcal folliculitis
Dermatophilosis
Pemphigus foliaceus
Cheyletiellosis
Sebaceous adenitis
Primary keratinization defects
Secondary keratinization abnormalities (allergic dermatoses, endocrinopathies, nutritional deficiencies, etc.)
Mycosis fungoides (epidermotropic lymphoma)

Kerions
Histiocytoma, mast cell tumor, other neoplasms
Staphylococcal furunculosis
Demodicosis and furunculosis
Acral lick dermatitis
Foreign bodies
Subcutaneous mycoses
Actinomycotic infections
Mycobacterial infections

Onychomycosis/Nail Fold Dermatophytosis
Staphylococcal onychitis
Demodicosis
Zinc-responsive dermatosis
Pemphigus vulgaris/foliaceus

■ Try to determine whether the animal has had any abnormalities suggestive of systemic disease, particularly older animals.

Physical Examination

■ Look for symptoms suggestive of dermatophytosis.
■ Thoroughly examine adult animals with widespread lesions, especially dogs, for signs of systemic disease such as hyperadrenocorticism.

Wood's Light Examination

■ Use the Wood's light to screen for dermatophytosis. The light emitted may cause fluorescence of hairs infected with *M. canis.*

■ Be wary of false-positive results. Scale, ointments, creams, and bacterial folliculitis may all fluoresce under the light; however, they do not give the typical apple-green fluorescence of the hair shaft seen with *M. canis* infection.

KEY POINT ▶ Hairs infected with *M. gypseum* and *T. mentagrophytes* do not fluoresce an apple-green color under Wood's light, and less than 50% of *M. canis*–infected hairs fluoresce. Use the Wood's light only as a screening tool, not as a confirmatory diagnostic test.

Direct Microscopic Examination of Hair

Direct microscopic examination can provide a diagnosis of dermatophytosis within minutes if affected hairs are properly examined.
■ Selection of the sample to be examined is critical.
  • Pluck hair from areas of active inflammation.
  • Broken or frayed hairs are ideal.
  • If there was fluorescence with Wood's light examination, select those individual hairs that fluoresced.
■ Place the hairs to be examined on a glass slide.
  • Clear the sample to facilitate observation of spores and hyphae (Table 2).
  • When the specimen has been cleared, scan the slide using low magnification (10 ×) for abnormal hairs. Look for hairs that are frayed, swollen, and pale.
  • When you have located the hair, examine it at a higher magnification (20–40 ×).
■ The presence of ectothrix spores surrounding the hair and of hyphae within the hair shaft is diagnostic for dermatophytosis.
  • Ectothrix spores appear as round-to-oval, greenish, translucent beads (Fig. 1).
This technique requires some practice. A negative direct microscopic examination does not rule out dermatophytosis.

KEY POINT ▶ Avoid false-positive diagnoses based on direct examination. Dermatophytes do not produce macroconidia in the tissue. Nonpathogenic fungal conidia and plant

TABLE 2. Clearing Agents for Specimens of Hair to Be Examined Microscopically

Agent	Instructions
10–20% KOH	Place several drops on the slide, apply a coverslip, and allow the slide to clear for 30 minutes before examining.
10–20% KOH	Follow the same procedure as above, but gently heat the slide for 15 seconds, allow it to cool, and then examine it.
2 parts KOH, 1 part DMSO	Place several drops on the slide, apply a coverslip, and allow it to clear for 5 minutes before examining.
Chlorphenolac (50 g chloral hydrate, 25 ml liquid phenol, and 25 ml liquid lactic acid)	Place several drops on the slide, apply a coverslip, and examine immediately.

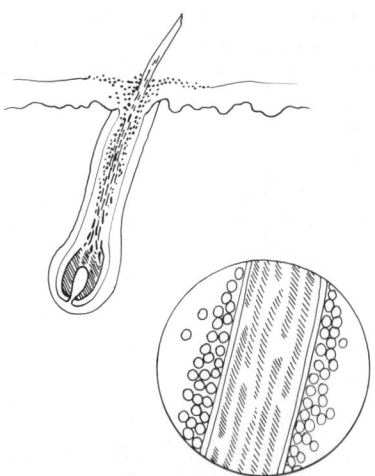

Figure 1. Arthrospores can be visualized outside infected hair shafts (ectothrix) in animals. Fungal hyphae may be seen within infected hair shafts.

pollen are frequently mistaken for dermatophytes; these structures are darkly pigmented whereas dermatophytes are not.

Fungal Culture

KEY POINT ▶ *Fungal culture is the most reliable and definitive method of identifying infected animals; it is the only method of species identification and should be performed in all suspected cases of dermatophytosis.*

The ideal culture media for dermatophytes is dermatophyte test media (DTM), which is composed of Sabouraud's agar, antimicrobials to inhibit bacterial and fungal saprophyte growth, and phenol red as a pH indicator. DTM is available in screw-cap containers or in plates with DTM on one side and plain Sabouraud's agar on the other. The plates are preferred over the tubes because it is easier to obtain samples from the plates for species identification. Plain Sabouraud's agar is better for evaluating colony morphology because DTM may suppress the formation of conidia and alter colony coloration.

Technique

1. Specimen collection of hair involves three steps:
   a. Clip hairs to 0.5 cm in an area of active inflammation; areas of broken, stubbly hairs of positive Wood's light fluorescence are ideal.
   b. Lightly swab the area with alcohol and allow to air-dry.
   c. Gently remove the clipped hairs from the follicles; hemostats are ideal for this purpose.
2. Place hairs on the media (not deeply embedded).
3. In cases of onychomycosis, clip the proximal nail into small pieces for culture.

4. Place the sample (hairs or nail particles) in a dark environment, protected from UV light and desiccation. Do not close the container tightly.
5. Observe the sample daily for colony growth and for a color change in the media.
6. As a general rule, dermatophytes turn DTM red simultaneously with colony growth, whereas saprophytes generally do not turn the media red until after a week or so of growth.
7. Fungal colonies that are darkly pigmented (blue, green black or a combination) are *not* dermatophytes.

KEY POINT ▶ Some species of fungi other than dermatophytes may turn the DTM media red within the first 7–10 days; therefore, microscopic examination of the mycelia is necessary to identify the fungus definitively as a dermatophyte.

Identification of Subclinically Infected Cats

■ Identification of the dermatophytosis in the asymptomatic cat can be accomplished using a toothbrush technique. Vigorously brush the cat over the entire body with a new toothbrush.
■ Gently place the collected hairs and scale onto the fungal culture media.

Identification of Dermatophyte Species from a Fungal Colony

The colony morphology in combination with the characteristic microscopic morphology allows identification of the dermatophyte species causing the infection (Table 3). The easiest and most practical method of observing microscopic morphology is the "acetate tape" method.

■ Gently touch a 2-cm strip of clear acetate tape to the surface of a mature culture colony (>5 days). A colony on plain Sabouraud's agar is preferable, if available.
■ Then place the tape over a glass slide with a drop of lactophenol cotton blue or new methylene blue stain.
■ Observe the slide microscopically for identification of dermatophyte species by conidia formation (Fig. 2).

Biopsy and Histopathology

Generally it is not necessary to biopsy skin for identification of a dermatophyte infection. However, dermatophytes may be visible in hematoxylin and eosin (H & E)-stained sections and are readily detected with periodic acid–Schiff (PAS) and GMS stains. In cases of suspected dermatophyte onychomycosis, the nail itself may be submitted in 10% formalin for histopathologic evaluation.

TABLE 3. Colony and Microscopic Morphology of Dermatophyte Cultures on Sabouraud's Dextrose Agar

Organism	Colony Morphology	Microscopic Morphology*
Microsporum canis	The surface is cottony to woolly and white. The reverse side is yellow-orange.	Abundant spindle-shaped macroconidia with thick, spiny walls and a terminal knob are present. Six or more cells are found in the macroconidia. One-celled microconidia are uncommon.
Microsporum gypseum	The surface is flat, granular, and light tan to cinnamon in color with white mycelia. The reverse side is pale yellow to tan.	Abundant spindle-shaped macroconidia with no terminal knobs are present. Macroconidia contain up to six cells. Microconidia are uncommon.
Trichophyton mentagrophytes	The surface usually is cream-colored and powdery. The reverse side is tan to brown, or red.	Some strains produce spiral hyphae. Microconidia are numerous and often are arranged in grapelike clusters along the hyphae. Macroconidia are uncommon; if present, they are slender and cigar-shaped with smooth thin walls.

*See Figure 2.

TREATMENT

KEY POINT ▶ Dermatophytosis is a zoonotic disease, and children and immunocompromised individuals are at increased risk; therefore, minimize exposure of people and other animals to the affected animal.

Dermatophyte infections are usually self-limiting; however, plan treatment with the goals of eliminating the infection in the animal and preventing the spread of infectious materials to other pets or people in the household (Table 4). Systemic therapy is not indicated in all cases, and often appropriate topical therapy is all that is needed.

Topical Therapy

- Use topical therapy in all cases, regardless of whether systemic antifungal drugs are being used. Table 5 lists products for topical treatment of dermatophytosis in dogs and cats.
- Shave or clip the affected area of skin to prevent dissemination of infected hairs into the environment.
- Perform a complete body clip and generalized topical therapy with whole-body dips or shampoos on all animals with multifocal or generalized infections.
- Chlorhexidine shampoos or dips, lime sulfur dips, and captan dips are the most frequently recommended treatments and are associated with minimal side effects.
- Treat dogs with one or a few focal lesions with creams, lotions, or sprays (see Table 5).
- Use whole-body therapy in all cases of feline dermatophytosis.
- Continue treatment for 1–2 weeks after resolution of clinical signs or until obtaining a negative culture finding.

Systemic Antifungal Therapy

Systemic therapy is indicated when dermatophytosis does not respond to topical therapy alone or when lesions are widespread.

- Use topical therapy such as antifungal dips or shampoos in conjunction with systemic antifungal therapy in all cases.
- Continue treatment until a negative culture is obtained and clinical signs have resolved.
  - In cases of onychomycosis, this can take up to 1 year.

Currently two systemic antifungal drugs are commonly used in the United States for the treatment of dermatophytosis (see Table 5).

Griseofulvin

This fungistatic antimicrobial is the most frequently used drug for the treatment of dermatophytosis. Absorption of the drug is enhanced when it is given with a fatty meal. Griseofulvin is available in microsize and ultramicrosize formulations in polyethylene glycol to enhance absorption so that lower doses can be used.

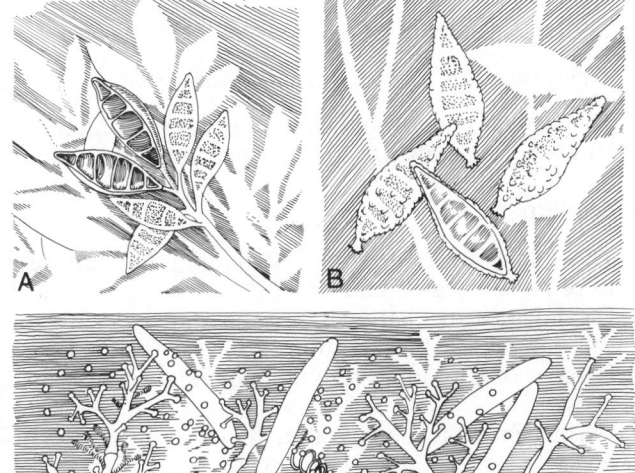

Figure 2. Identification of dermatophyte species from mature fungal colonies is possible by microscopically examining the conidia morphology. (*A, Microsporum gypseum; B, M. canis; C, Trichophyton mentagrophytes.*)

TABLE 4. Summary of Approach to Therapy in Dogs and Cats with Dermatophytosis*

Extent and Type of Lesion	Recommended Therapy†
In Dogs	
One to several small focal areas of alopecia, crusting, and scaling	Clip affected and surrounding areas and apply topical therapy in the form of creams, ointments, or lotions.
Multifocal areas of alopecia, crusting, and scaling	Clip affected and surrounding areas. Apply antifungal creams, ointments, or lotions to affected sites and/or treat the whole body with antifungal dips or shampoos.
Multifocal areas of alopecia, crusting, and scaling with extensive body involvement, or generalized dermatophytosis	Clip the entire hair coat. Treat the whole body with antifungal dips or shampoos and treat with systemic antifungal drugs.
Kerions	Combine systemic antifungal therapy with topical therapy on the lesion and on other affected areas. Surgical removal of a lesion is curative; however, the animal should be treated for the dermatophytosis that is likely to be present in other areas. Systemic antibiotics may be necessary if a secondary bacterial folliculitis/furunculosis also is present.
In Cats	
Dermatophytosis	Clip the entire haircoat, especially of long-haired cats. Apply whole body topical therapy with shampoos or dips. Use systemic antifungal drugs initially or if topical therapy alone fails.
Pseudomycetomas	If the lesion is solitary, surgical removal is best. If the lesions are multiple, use systemic antifungal therapy. Use whole-body topical therapy in either case.

*See Table 5 for specific agents.
†Antifungal therapy should be continued for 1–2 weeks after an apparent clinical cure or until the animal has a negative fungal culture.

- Never administer griseofulvin, which is a teratogen, to pregnant animals.
- Common side effects include anorexia, vomiting, and diarrhea.
- Less common side effects, which appear to be idiosyncratic, include pyrexia, icterus, ataxia, angioedema, and myelosuppression.
- During therapy, monitor purebred cats, which may be predisposed to developing myelosuppression.
- Do not treat cats infected with feline immunodeficiency virus (FIV) with griseofulvin, as they are very susceptible to toxicity with this drug.

Ketoconazole

Ketoconazole is a fungistatic imidazole derivative with broad-spectrum antifungal activity against both superficial and deep mycotic infections. It is recommended in the treatment of animals with griseofulvin-resistant dermatophytosis and of animals that cannot tolerate griseofulvin therapy. For further information concerning usage and side effects of ketoconazole, see sec. 2, ch. 12).

Itraconazole

Itraconazole is a new antifungal drug that has been used experimentally in the United States in the treatment of various mycotic diseases in the dog and cat (see sec. 2, ch. 12). This drug has been successful in the treatment of generalized dermatophytosis unresponsive to ketoconazole and griseofulvin. Itraconazole shows excellent *in vitro* antifungal activity against dermatophytes. Eventually it may be available for clinical treatment of dermatophytosis in the United States.

PREVENTION

When planning and carrying out preventive measures, remember that dermatophyte spores can remain viable in the environment for over 1 year.

Control of Dissemination of Infective Materials

This procedure is necessary to ensure that:

- The animal is not reinfected after being treated.
- Household members and other pets are not infected.

Procedure

- Thoroughly vacuum floors, carpeting, and furniture to remove infected hairs.
- Clean surfaces that will not be damaged by the solution with a 1:10 dilution of bleach (NaOCl).
- Dispose of grooming equipment or clean as described above.
- Wash hands thoroughly after handling infected animals.

Identification of the Source of Exposure

- Examine other animals in the household.
- Specific dermatophyte species that are cultured can provide helpful clues. For example, if *T. mentagrophytes* is isolated from a dog that spends most of the time indoors and there is a pet rodent in the house-

TABLE 5. Therapeutic Agents Available for Pets with Dermatophytosis

Agent	Brand Name (Manufacturer)	Application	Comments	Side Effects
Shampoos				
Chlorhexidine	Nolvasan (Ft. Dodge) ChlorhexiDerm (DVM)	every 3–5 days	Few side effects; antibacterial	Occasional irritation; corneal ulcers
Povidone-iodine	Weladol (Pitman-Moore)	every 5 days	Not recommended for cats or light-haired animals	Iodine toxicity may occur; stains white or light coats
Ketoconazole	Nizoral Shampoo (Janssen)	3 times weekly	Bathe first with a keratolytic shampoo if necessary	
Dips				
Chlorhexidine	Nolvasan Solution (Ft. Dodge)	0.5–1% solution every 3–5 days	Few side effects; antibacterial	Occasional irritation; corneal ulcers
Captan	Orthocide spray (Chevron Chemicals)	2% (2 Tbs/gal) every 3–5 days	Contact sensitizer in people	Vomiting in cats
Lime-sulfur	Lym Dyp (DVM)	2 oz/gal every 3–5 days	Antipruritic, antiparasitic, malodorous	Stains light coats; occasional irritation
Povidone-iodine	Betadine Solution (Purdue Frederick)	1:4 dilution in water every 5 days	Staining common	Iodine toxicity (especially in cats); occasional irritation
Sodium hypochlorite (bleach)		1:20 dilution in water every 5 days		Occasional irritation; will bleach dark haircoats
Products for Local Therapy				
Miconazole	Conofite (Pitman-Moore)	q12h	Available as cream, lotion, and spray	Occasional local irritation
Clotrimazole	Veltrim (Haver)	q12h	Available as cream	Occasional local irritation
Ketoconazole	Nizoral (Janssen)	q12h	Cream with few side effects	
Thiabendazole	Tresaderm (MSD Agvet)	q12h	Should be refrigerated; antipruritic, antibacterial	Occasional contact allergic reactions
Econazole	Spectazole (Ortho)	q12h	Available as cream	
Systemic Antifungal Drugs				
Griseofulvin			Divide the dose q12h; administer with a fatty meal	Nausea, vomiting, diarrhea; idiosyncratic myelotoxicity (especially in cats); ataxia, pyrexia, icterus, angioedema
Microsize	Fulvicin-U/F (Schering) Grifulvin V (Ortho)	20–50 mg/kg 20–50 mg/kg	Tablets Pediatric suspension	Nausea, vomiting, diarrhea; idiosyncratic myelotoxicity; ataxia
Ultramicrosize	Gris-PEG (Dorsey)	5–10 mg/kg		
Ketoconazole	Nizoral (Janssen)	10 mg/kg q24h	Administer the dose divided q12h if nausea or anorexia occurs	Gastric irritation, anorexia, hepatotoxicity; idiosyncratic lightening of haircoat

hold, brush culture the rodent for the presence of dermatophytes.
■ Treat all infected animals in the household.

Preventive Measures in Cattery

■ Identify all infected animals. For best results, use the toothbrush technique described previously.
■ Separate infected from culture-negative animals.
■ Treat infected cats until tests are culture-negative before reintroducing them to the general cat population.
■ Disinfect cages on a regular basis and vacuum and disinfect air vents.
■ Never use the same grooming equipment on infected and culture-negative cats.

■ Place all new animals brought into a cattery in isolation until culture-negative results have been obtained.

Supplemental Readings

Elewski BE, Hazen PG: The superficial mycoses and the dermatophytes. J Am Acad Dermatol 21:655, 1989.
Foil CS: Dermatophytosis. *In* Greene CE, ed.: *Clinical Microbiology and Infectious Diseases of the Dog and Cat.* Philadelphia: W. B. Saunders, 1990, p 659.
Foil CS: Cutaneous fungal diseases. *In* Nesbitt GH, ed.: *Dermatology.* New York: Churchill Livingstone, 1987, p 123.
Moriello KA: Management of dermatophyte infections in catteries and multiple-cat households. Vet Clin North Am [Small Anim Pract] 20:1457, 1990.
Muller GH, Kirk RW, Scott DW: Fungal diseases. *In Small Animal Dermatology.* Philadelphia: W. B. Saunders, 1989, p 295.

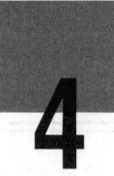

4 Demodicosis

Alan C. Mundell

Demodicosis refers to the inflammatory parasitic skin disease of dogs and cats caused by an abnormal proliferation of a mite from the genus *Demodex*. The mites are considered part of the normal skin fauna when present in low numbers. The disease state, demodicosis, is most frequently recognized in the dog. When generalized and chronic, demodicosis is a frustrating and difficult condition to treat.

ETIOLOGY
Canine Demodicosis

Canine demodicosis occurs when there is an overpopulation of the mite, *Demodex canis* (Fig. 1), on the skin. The mite is a normal inhabitant of the hair follicle and occasionally of the sebaceous gland. Although it is not known what allows the mites to proliferate by the thousands, genetic and/or immunologic abnormalities are suspected.

- The entire *life cycle* of the mite is spent on the host and consists of four major stages: egg, larva, nymph (several stages), and adult. The life cycle is believed to take between 20 and 35 days to complete.
- *Transmission* occurs during the first few days of life by direct contact from dam to pup.
- The mites are not considered to be contagious to normal healthy adult dogs. Thus, demodicosis is most likely a dysfunction of the dog, not an increase in virulence of the mite.

Feline Demodicosis

In the cat, the disease state is induced by the excessive proliferation of one of two *Demodex* mite species.

- *Demodex cati* was the mite species first recognized. *D. cati* resembles *D. canis* in appearance, cutaneous habitat, and life cycle. The life cycle of this mite is believed to be completed in 18 to 24 days.
- The second type of *Demodex* mite is unnamed. This mite has a shorter and wider abdomen than *D. cati* and resembles the hamster mite, *D. criceti*. Little is known about its life cycle. This unnamed *Demodex* species resides in pits in the stratum corneum, not in hair follicles or sebaceous glands.

CLINICAL SIGNS
Localized Demodicosis
Canine

- Canine localized demodicosis typically occurs in dogs less than 1 year of age. There is no breed or sex predilection.
- The lesions are commonly observed on the head and extremities.
- Alopecia is the most consistent finding with variable degrees of erythema, scale, hyperpigmentation, comedo formation, pyoderma, and pruritus.
- It is estimated that in approximately 10% of dogs with localized demodicosis, the condition becomes generalized.

Feline

- Feline demodicosis (localized or generalized) has no breed or sex predilection. However, most cases occur in older cats.
- Localized demodicosis in the cat usually appears as a focal area of alopecia on the face or ears.
- As with canine localized demodicosis, the degree of erythema, scale, hyperpigmentation, comedo formation, and pruritus is variable. Secondary pyodermas are rare.

Generalized Demodicosis
Canine

- Generalized demodicosis in the dog frequently is categorized according to the age of initial disease onset (juvenile or adult). Although both types have identical clinical signs, the distinction is the result of differences in predisposing factors and prognosis.
  - Adult-onset generalized demodicosis has a more guarded prognosis because of the increased probability of serious predisposing conditions.
  - The prognosis for dogs less than 1 year of age with

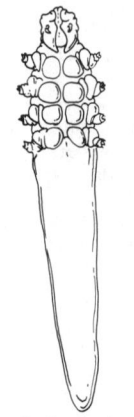

Figure 1. *Demodex canis.*

generalized demodicosis is more favorable because spontaneous cures are not uncommon.

■ Clinical signs of generalized demodicosis consist of large, multifocal to regional areas of alopecia. These areas typically have scaling, crusting, erythema, comedo formation, hyperpigmentation, and pyoderma.
  • If the pyoderma is deep, lymphadenopathy and cutaneous drainage tracts with hemorrhagic to purulent exudates may be present.
■ Occasionally, cellulitis occurs in dogs with generalized demodicosis.

Feline

Generalized demodicosis in the cat may present with a variety of clinical signs.
■ Lesions range from large areas of patchy alopecia with variable amounts of erythema, scale, crusts, and hyperpigmentation to regional miliary dermatitis.
■ Secondary pyodermas are rare.
■ When pruritic, the intensity of the itch is usually mild. Intense pruritus is rarely observed.

Pododemodicosis/Otodemodicosis

Canine

In the dog, pododemodicosis may be exclusively confined to the feet or may be present in conjunction with more generalized disease. A similar situation exists with otodemodicosis in the external ear canal. The reason for addressing these areas separately is because of the increased treatment difficulty and the more guarded prognosis when these areas are involved.

■ Pododemodicosis
  • This may manifest as mild erythematous alopecia of the paws with variable degrees of scaling and crusting.
  • However, in chronic and/or severe infestations the interdigital, nail fold, and palmar areas frequently are swollen with crusted papules, nodules, pustules, vesicles, drainage tracts, and scar tissue formation.
■ Otodemodicosis
  • The usual clinical signs are ceruminous otitis externa with erythema and swelling.
  • When untreated, the otitis externa may become purulent and/or proliferative.
  • Canine otodemodicosis as a solitary condition is rarely identified.

Feline

■ Pododemodicosis in the cat is not usually a distinct clinical entity but a manifestation of a more generalized condition.
  • The lesions are not as severe as typically seen in canine pododemodicosis.
  • Partial alopecia with variable degrees of erythema, scale, crusts, and pruritus are the usual clinical signs.
■ In feline otodemodicosis, a ceruminous otitis externa is the most common clinical sign. The external ear infestation may be the only indication of demodicosis or it may be a part of a more generalized disease.

DIAGNOSIS

KEY POINT ▶ Demodicosis usually is diagnosed from skin scrapings. Take skin scrapings of all alopecias, pyodermas, and keratinization disorders.

History

The history can help to identify possible predisposing causes.

■ Suspect canine demodicosis if there is a familial history of demodicosis and the clinical signs are compatible.
■ Question owners about potentially taxing events or conditions that could decompensate the animal's ability to control the proliferation of the mite. Purported events or conditions that may predispose to developing demodicosis include:
  • Stress, poor nutrition, trauma, separation anxiety, and chronic fatigue.
  • Estrus, parturition, and lactation.
  • Parasitism, rapid growth, vaccinations, adverse environmental temperatures, and debilitating disease.
■ Older dogs and cats frequently have an underlying internal disease or neoplastic condition that predisposes them to develop demodicosis. The underlying conditions may be incipient at the time of demodicosis diagnosis and may require months, possibly years, to be recognized.
■ The use of immunosuppressive agents such as corticosteroids, antineoplastic drugs, or antilymphocyte antibodies can induce or exacerbate localized or generalized demodicosis.

Physical Examination

Perform a thorough physical examination to identify predisposing factors and/or diseases.

Laboratory Tests

Use laboratory tests to screen for predisposing diseases, especially when canine generalized demodicosis and feline demodicosis (localized or generalized) are present.

■ Serum biochemical profile, urinalysis, and complete blood cell count (CBC) are the basic screening tests.
■ Additionally, test all cats for feline leukemia virus (FeLV) and feline immunodeficiency virus (FIV) (see sec. 2, chs. 1 and 2).
■ If the history, physical examination, and screening laboratory tests indicate endocrine or possible internal organ dysfunction, perform more specific tests (e.g., low-dose dexamethasone suppression test to rule out hyperadrenocorticism [see sec. 4, ch. 3]).

Skin Scrapings

This is the primary method for diagnosing demodicosis.

Procedure

- Clip hair over area to be scraped.
- Squeeze skin gently to facilitate mite collection.
- Scrape skin using a dull #10 surgical blade moistened with mineral oil.
  - Stroke the skin in the direction of hair growth until capillary bleeding occurs.
  - Place debris on a glass slide containing one drop of mineral oil.

KEY POINT ▶ Obtain multiple scrapings!

Examination of Scrapings

Examine slide under low-power magnification (40 × and 100 ×).

- Because *Demodex* mites are normal skin inhabitants, finding one mite does not confirm the diagnosis of demodicosis; however, it does increase the suspicion of demodicosis. Therefore, following such a finding, perform multiple deep-skin scrapings.
- Use skin scrapings to monitor the response to therapy, the ratio of live to dead mites, and the ratio of adult to immature forms.
  - If there is an increase in live mites or immature forms, mite resistance to therapy may be occurring.

Skin Biopsies

- Use skin biopsies when demodicosis is suspected but mites cannot be identified (see sec. 5, ch. 15 for skin biopsy technique). This occasionally occurs in chronically affected areas (especially feet) where scar tissue impedes proper scraping.
- Biopsies may be necessary to diagnosis demodicosis in Chinese Shar Pei dogs.

Ear Swabs and Ear Curettes

Use ear swabs and curettes to obtain otic debris for mite evaluation.

TREATMENT

KEY POINT ▶ *Never* use corticosteroids in dogs or cats with demodicosis. If possible, avoid the use of all immunosuppressive agents.

The ideal therapeutic agent for the treatment of canine and feline demodicosis should be safe, highly effective, easy to administer, reasonably priced, and approved by the United States Food and Drug Administration (FDA). Unfortunately such a drug does not exist.

The only FDA-approved agent for the treatment of canine generalized demodicosis is amitraz (Mitaban; Upjohn). (This drug, which can be moderately effective when used as labeled, is discussed in detail in a

separate section below.) No FDA-approved treatment is available for feline demodicosis. Therefore:

- Consider the risk-to-benefit ratio when recommending therapies not approved by the FDA.
- Advise clients of all treatment options and success and risks of each.
- Obtain written client consent when using treatments not approved by the FDA.

Localized Demodicosis

Canine

- Localized demodicosis in the dog usually is a self-limiting condition, especially in dogs less than 18 months of age. Thus, the primary goal is to identify and eliminate predisposing causes.
- Spontaneous remission typically occurs within 2 months. If lesions persist or if owners insist on treatment, use topical agents.
- Frequently used products are 1% rotenone ointment (Goodwinol; Goodwinol Products) and benzoyl peroxide shampoos or gels (Oxydex, DVM or Pyoben, Allerderm).
- Treat lesions once daily until skin scrapings are negative.
- Rotenone ointments and benzoyl peroxide gels can be irritating, especially because they are not rinsed off. Use these agents with caution when treating periocular lesions; ocular irritation can be severe.
- Although therapies designed to treat generalized demodicosis (e.g., amitraz) are effective for localized demodicosis, they are best reserved for the generalized condition.
- Limiting the use of more potent acaricidal agents helps decrease the potential for developing acaricide resistance. This ensures peak acaricidal performance for when the agent is needed most.

Feline

Treat localized demodicosis in the cat in a manner similar to that for canine localized demodicosis. Although localized lesions can spontaneously regress, many progress and become generalized. In cats, the rotenone and benzoyl peroxide agents used to treat canine localized demodicosis are less effective and more irritating. Although feline localized demodicosis, like canine localized demodicosis, has been treated successfully with the drug amitraz (see below), its use is discouraged for the reasons previously stated.

Canine Generalized Demodicosis

Besides the FDA-approved protocol for using amitraz (see below) for canine generalized demodicosis, several moderately effective treatments are available.

- Common to all protocols is the need to identify and correct predisposing factors.
- Additionally, treat all secondary pyodermas with appropriate antibiotic and topical therapy (see sec. 5, ch. 1). If a deep pyoderma is present, base antibiotic selection on bacterial culture and sensitivity results (see sec. 5, ch. 1).

Amitraz—FDA-Approved Protocol

This drug is a formamidine acaricidal compound that inhibits monoamine oxidase. However, the precise acaricidal mechanism of action is unknown.

Procedure

- Closely clip all medium- to long-haired dogs. Repeat monthly or as necessary.
- Bathe animal with a benzoyl peroxide shampoo.
- Allow shampoo to remain on dog for 10 minutes prior to rinsing.
- Completely dry dog before proceeding with amitraz rinses.

KEY POINT ▶ Do not apply amitraz to dogs with extensive open lesions (deep pyodermas with drainage tracts). Postpone application until antibiotics and shampoo therapy improve lesions.

- Prepare a fresh 0.025% amitraz solution (1 vial of Mitaban per 2 gallons of water) and sponge on dog. Sponging procedure should last at least 10 minutes.
  - While dog is being sponged, soak the feet in mixture.
- Apply amitraz solution in well-ventilated areas, taking strict protective measures to avoid human exposure.
- Keep animal dry (including feet) until next amitraz application (2 weeks later).
- Continue amitraz applications every 2 weeks until no viable mites are found after at least 2 successive treatments.

Results

- Reported long-term cure rates (no mites identified for more than 1 year) are variable (20–99%). However, a well-controlled study found only a 53% long-term cure rate.
- The percentage of dogs in which mite populations are adequately controlled is much higher. These dogs remain asymptomatic while receiving maintenance applications.

Side Effects

- A variety of adverse side effects have been reported; the most common are mild transient sedation, pruritus, and/or gastrointestinal disturbances.
- The manufacturer (Upjohn) believes that the drug temporarily alters the dog's homeostatic maintenance abilities. Therefore, avoid placing the dog in stressful situations for at least 24 hours after dipping.
- Many side effects have been associated with the amitraz's alpha$_2$-adrenergic stimulatory property.
- Experimentally, these side effects have been reversed using xylazine reversal doses of yohimbine (0.11 mg/kg) (Yobine; Lloyd Labs). In the dog, yohimbine is FDA-approved only as an intravenous xylazine reversing agent.

Amitraz Weekly Rinses (Protocol Not Approved by FDA)

- Apply amitraz as previously outlined, except at a once-weekly rate.

- Continue acaricidal rinses for 2 to 6 weeks after multiple negative skin scrapings.
- Long-term cure rates for this protocol are believed to be 60–70%.

Amitraz Daily Half-Body (Alternating) Rinses
(Protocol Not Approved by FDA)

This protocol was devised by Dr. Ton Willemse, State University of Utrecht, and Dr. Linda Medleau, University of Georgia.

Procedure

- Prepare 0.125% amitraz solution from a 12.5% amitraz solution (1 ml of Taktic [Coopers], in 100 ml of water).
- Clip dog and treat pyodermas as previously discussed. Bathe dogs with concurrent keratinization disorders once weekly with appropriate shampoos.
- Using a sponge, rub 0.125% amitraz solution daily onto one-half of the dog's body. Alternate the treated and untreated halves daily. Air-dry the dog.
- During the first week of therapy hospitalize and monitor the dog for adverse side effects.
- Continue therapy for 2 weeks after multiple skin scrapings are negative.

Additionally, Dr. Medleau treats all dogs with pododermatitis with daily foot soaks using the 0.125% amitraz solution. All dogs receive otic treatments (1.5 ml Taktic in 8.5 ml of mineral oil q3–7d) unless otic irritation develops.

Results

As of this writing, this study has not been in effect long enough to obtain precise long-term cure rates. However, all dogs have completed the clinical trial for at least 4 months with an 81% rate of resolution. This includes a 75% resolution rate in dogs previously found to be unresponsive to standard whole-body biweekly, weekly, or twice-weekly amitraz dips.

Side Effects

- Dr. Willemse reported no adverse side effects. Dr. Medleau reported a low incidence of adverse side effects (<6%). Only one dog displayed mild transient sedation that spontaneously resolved without a change in therapy.
- Extreme caution must be used with this procedure in order to prevent adverse side effects in human beings.

KEY POINT ▶ Conventional amitraz protocols are tried first before resorting to daily applications.

Daily Oral Milbemycin Oxime (Protocol Not Approved by FDA)

Milbemycin (Interceptor; Ciba-Geigy) is a macrolide antibiotic derived from the fermentation of *Streptomyces hygroscopicus*. The drug is presently approved by the FDA as a once-monthly heartworm preventive agent for dogs. The precise mechanism of action against the *Demodex* mite currently is unknown.

The protocol reviewed here is based on the research conducted by Dr. William Miller and Dr. Danny Scott at Cornell University. Dogs treated in their study were heartworm-negative adult dogs with generalized demodicosis. All dogs were in reasonably good health with no identifiable predisposing factors. Concurrent pyodermas were treated with oral antibiotics; benzoyl peroxide shampoo baths and amitraz rinses were not used during the clinical trial.

- A variety of dosages were tested; the dosage of 1 mg/kg q24h for 1 month past the point of negative skin scrapings appeared to be the most effective.
- The only adverse side effect was ataxia in small dogs receiving daily milbemycin doses of >2.5 mg/kg. The ataxia disappeared quickly following discontinuation of the medication.
- The study has not been in effect long enough to draw accurate conclusions about long-term cure rates. However, the data suggest a cure rate of approximately 60% with a control rate of >80%.

Feline Generalized Demodicosis

- Identify and treat any underlying abnormalities. Generalized demodicosis in the cat is a potential marker for internal disease.
- Clip all medium- to long-haired cats prior to topical therapy.
- Because there are no FDA-approved treatments for generalized (and localized) demodicosis in cats and because cats are very sensitive to many insecticides, always try the most benign therapy first.
  - Presently, this consists of topical 2–3% lime sulfur (Lym Dyp, DVM) applied once weekly for 2–4 weeks past the point of negative skin scrapings.

Amitraz Rinse (Protocol Not Approved by FDA)

- A potentially more effective, but also potentially more hazardous, treatment involves a weekly topical application of a 0.0125% amitraz solution.
- Continue the rinses for at least 2 weeks past the point of negative skin scrapings.
- Common side effects include mild sedation, anorexia, diarrhea, ptyalism, and abnormal behavior. These side effects are usually mild and transient.
  - However, if side effects are severe, an experimental (not approved by FDA) dose of yohimbine (0.11 mg/kg IV) may resolve the clinical signs.

Pododemodicosis/Otodemodicosis

Canine

In the dog, pododemodicosis and otodemodicosis are usually associated with more generalized disease; therefore, treat these demodicoses as previously discussed. However, because of the difficulty in treating these areas, the following additional measures (not approved by FDA) often are required.

- Treat affected feet daily or q48h using either standard aqueous dilutions of amitraz (0.025%) or amitraz mixed with mineral oil (1 ml of Mitaban/15–30 ml of mineral oil). (*Caution:* amitraz/mineral oil treatments can be messy!)
- Treat otodemodicosis with either daily topical rotenone therapy (Canex; Pitman-Moore) or amitraz in mineral oil (as described above) administered q2–7d (see also previous discussion of amitraz daily half-body rinses under Canine General Demodicosis).
- If irritation develops, discontinue medication or increase the treatment interval.

Feline

Pododemodicosis and otodemodicosis in the cat, like their canine counterparts, usually are associated with more regional or generalized conditions.

- Feline pododemodicosis usually is not a distinct entity and does not require special management.
- Feline otodemodicosis may appear as a distinct condition and may be treated similarly to canine otodemodicosis.
- Discontinue therapy when no mites are found upon ear swabbing or when it is no longer necessary to treat the more generalized condition. Additionally, discontinue if irritation develops.

KEY POINT ▶ Check with current state and federal laws when using insecticides in an extra-labeled manner.

PREVENTION

KEY POINT ▶ Advise all owners of dogs with generalized demodicosis to have them neutered. This prevents the stresses associated with breeding and the transmission of a heritable trait.

A key to prevention of demodicosis in pets is to identify and eliminate all potential predisposing factors. If possible, avoid all future use of any immunosuppressive agent.

Supplemental Readings

Kwochka KW: Canine Demodicosis. *In* Kirk RW, ed.: *Current Veterinary Therapy IX: Small Animal Practice.* Philadelphia: W. B. Saunders, 1986, p 531.

Medleau L: Recently described feline dermatoses. Vet Clin North Am [Small Anim Pract] 20:1626, 1990.

Medleau L, Willemse T: Efficacy of daily Amitraz therapy for generalized demodicosis in dogs: Two independent studies. Proceedings of the Annual Meeting of the American Academy of Veterinary Dermatology 7th, 1991, p 41.

Miller WH, Scott DW: Milbemycin in the treatment of generalized demodicosis in the dog. Proceedings of the Annual Meeting of the American Academy of Veterinary Dermatology 7th, 1991, p 44.

Muller GH, Kirk RW, Scott DW: *Small Animal Dermatology.* Philadelphia: W. B. Saunders, 1989, p 395.

Scabies, Notoedric Mange, and Cheyletiellosis

Richard K. Anderson

Scabies, notoedric mange, and cheyletiellosis are parasitic dermatoses caused by acarine mites living on or within the skin of the host animal. The resultant lesions may be due to mechanical damage from the burrowing mite, pruritogenic substances secreted by the mite, or a hypersensitivity reaction developed against one or more extracellular products of the mite. Variability of clinical manifestations of these parasitic dermatoses probably reflects variations in the duration and intensity of the hypersensitivity reaction and in the capacity of the host to limit parasite multiplication.

Exposure to these mites and the corresponding incidence of parasitic dermatoses are closely related to environmental factors, especially animal contact and the presence of endemic areas. Although the causative mites are not completely host-specific, they do exhibit host preference. They also have zoonotic potential for causing dermatoses in humans.

SCABIES

Etiology

- Scabies (sarcoptic mange) is an intensely pruritic papulocrustous dermatosis of dogs caused by the epidermal mite *Sarcoptes scabiei* var. *canis* (Fig. 1).

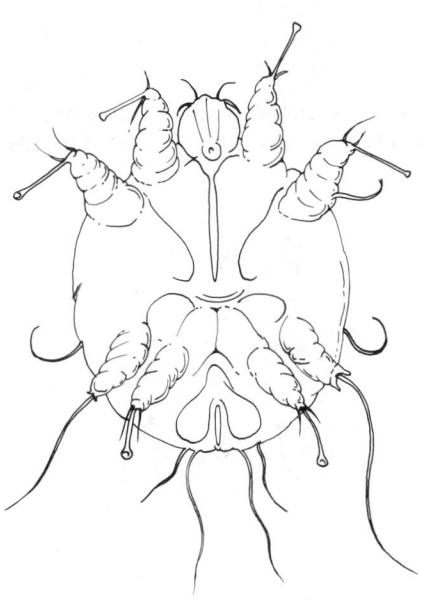

Figure 1. *Sarcoptes scabiei.*

Although fairly host-specific, the mite can affect cats, foxes, and humans for variable periods of time.

- The adult mite is microscopic (200–400 μ), roughly circular in shape, and characterized by two pairs of short legs cranially, which bear long unjointed stalks with suckers, and two pairs of rudimentary legs caudally that do not extend beyond the border of the body.
- The parasite completes its life cycle (egg-larva-nymph-adult) in 17–21 days in tunnels in the stratum corneum.
  - Adult mites live approximately 4 weeks, but they are susceptible to drying and can live only a few days off the host.
- Scabies is highly contagious and is primarily transmitted by direct contact, but grooming instruments and kennels may harbor mites.
- The rather long incubation period (2–8 weeks) makes it difficult to trace the source of the infestation.
- Occasionally within a group of dogs in the same kennel, only one dog will have clinical signs of scabies.
- The fact that only small mite populations are typically found in most dogs with scabies suggests that hypersensitivity plays an important role in the course of the disease.

Clinical Signs

KEY POINT ▶ Scabies is manifested primarily by intense pruritus that usually is minimally responsive to corticosteroids. Even during the physical examination, the dog will scratch and chew at itself.

- Pruritus and lesions are most severe on the ventral aspects of the body and the face. Areas classically affected include the elbows, hocks, ventral thorax, and margins of the pinna. Advanced lesions may be more generalized.
- Early lesions are characterized by a polymorphous eruption with erythematous macules and papules, patchy alopecia, and small hemorrhagic crusts. Chronic lesions include marked alopecia, accumulation of scale and crusts, and lichenification.

Diagnosis

- Suspect scabies based on:
  - History of rapid onset of intense pruritus with inconsistent response to corticosteroids

- Exposure of the affected dog to other animals
- Pruritic dermatitis involving dogs and humans in contact with affected dog
- Nature and distribution of cutaneous lesions as described

■ Perform superficial skin scrapings from nonexcoriated areas, with emphasis on the ears, elbows, hocks, and ventral thorax.
  - Even with multiple scrapings the mite is often difficult to find; often only the large oval eggs or small foci of brown fecal pellets can be found, but these are of diagnostic significance.

KEY POINT ▶ Failure to find the mite should not eliminate the diagnosis of scabies. Always utilize trial therapy if the diagnosis remains in question and the degree of suspicion is high enough to justify its use.

■ Differential diagnosis includes any pruritic skin disease, especially allergic and other parasitic dermatoses.

Treatment

KEY POINT ▶ The emergence of resistant strains of the *Sarcoptes* organism and the array of commercial products available makes selection of parasiticides difficult. Products highly efficaceous in one geographic location may be ineffective in another.

■ When scale and crusts are present, bathe with keratolytic shampoos prior to dipping.
■ Dips known to be effective include:
  - Amitraz (Mitaban; Upjohn), applied three times at 2-week intervals; (not approved for this use by the United States Food and Drug Administration [FDA])
  - Lime sulfur, 4% solution, applied weekly for six treatments or for 2 weeks past clinical remission; the safest dip for young animals or sick and debilitated patients
■ Ivermectin (Ivomec injection for cattle; MSD Agvet) is very effective at 0.3 mg/kg three times at 2 week intervals, PO or SC.
  - It is not approved by the FDA for usage in dogs at this dosage and should not be administered to collies, collie crosses, Shetland sheepdogs, or Australian shepherds.
  - Evaluate the animal's heartworm status prior to drug administration.
■ Treat all dogs in contact with the patient or on the premises.
■ Although the mites die after a few days when off the host, clean up the environment and use a parasiticide such as malathion once when there are a number of animals affected (as in a kennel or pet shop).

NOTOEDRIC MANGE
Etiology

■ Notoedric mange (feline scabies) is an intensely pruritic, crusting dermatosis of cats caused by the sarcoptiform mite, *Notoedres cati* (Fig. 2). The mite may also infest dogs, foxes, and rabbits and may cause transient lesions in humans in contact with infested animals.
■ Although rarely seen today, notoedric mange may be endemic in a few localities, especially inner city areas.
■ *N. cati* is a burrowing mite very similar to *Sarcoptes scabiei* in both morphology and life cycle. *N. cati* is smaller than *S. scabiei* and has a dorsal anus in contrast to the terminal anus of *S. scabei*.
■ Notoedric mange is highly contagious, usually by direct contact. The mite can survive off the host for only a few days.
■ Although characteristically a disease of adult cats, notoedric mange may present as a fulminating dermatitis in kittens.
■ Usually, large numbers of mites are found on affected animals; however, allergic disease associated with the presence of very few mites may be more frequent than realized.

Clinical Signs

■ Lesions appear first on the margin of the pinna but spread rapidly to the face and neck. Occasionally, lesions can be found on the feet and perineum.
■ Initially there is a papular eruption, but the skin soon becomes thickened with dry, adherent crusts.
■ Intense pruritus results in self-induced alopecia, erythema, and excorations.

Diagnosis

■ The intense pruritus and distribution of lesions are diagnostic features.

KEY POINT ▶ As opposed to dogs with canine scabies, cats with feline scabies have large numbers of mites that are easily found on skin scrapings. The best areas to scrape are the ears and face. Utilize trial therapy only if the diagnosis remains in question and the degree of suspicion is high enough to justify its use.

Differential diagnoses include food hypersensitivity, *Otodectes* infestation, atopy, dermatophytosis, cheyle-

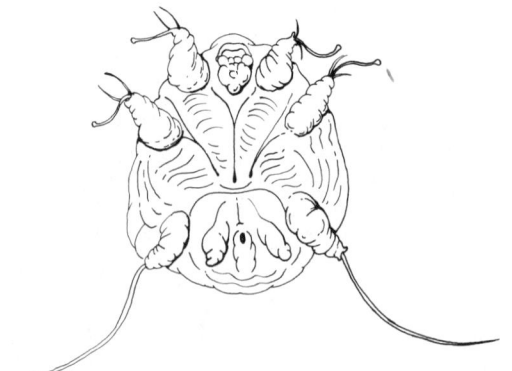

Figure 2. *Notoedres cati.*

tiellosis, pemphigus foliaceus or erythematosus, systemic lupus erythematosus, and fight wounds.

Treatment

- Bathe the cat with a keratolytic shampoo before dipping.
- Dips that may be effective include:
  - Lime sulfur, 2% solution, applied weekly for 6 weeks; the safest dip for young kittens or sick and debilitated animals
  - Amitraz (Mitaban; Upjohn), 0.025%, applied once and repeated in 2 weeks (not approved for cats by FDA)
- Ivermectin (Ivomec injection for cattle, MSD Agvet) is effective at 0.3 mg/kg, given three times at 2-week intervals, PO or SC (not approved for cats by FDA).
- Treat other animals in the household concurrently.
- Because the mite does not persist for long off the host, a single thorough cleaning of the environment suffices. Use residual insecticide in a cattery where multiple animals are infested with the mite. A residual insecticide for adult fleas can be used.

CHEYLETIELLOSIS

Etiology

- Cheyletiellosis (*Cheyletiella* dermatitis) is a dorsally distributed papulocrustous or scaling dermatosis caused by the surface mite, *Cheyletiella yasguri* (dog, Fig. 3); *C. blakei* (cat), and *C. parasitovorax* (rabbit).
- The three species of mites may go freely to various host species including humans. The disease may not be as uncommon as previously thought.
- *Cheyletiella* species are comparatively large (500 μ), saddle-shaped mites that can be identified by their prominent hooklike accessory mouth parts. All four pairs of legs extend beyond the body margin and bear combs terminally.
- The life cycle (egg-larva-nymph-adult) is spent en-

tirely on the host and is completed in approximately 5 weeks.
- The mites are surface dwellers that feed on skin surface debris and tissue fluids. Female mites can live off the host for as long as 10 days.
- Cheyletiellosis is highly contagious. Indirect transmission via fomites may be as important as direct transmission.
- The pathogenicity of Cheyletiella infestation is highly variable. Presence of the mite on some hosts induces hyperkeratosis that may or may not be associated with pruritus; other hosts, possibly because of acquired immunity, may have asymptomatic infestations.

Clinical Signs

- The lesions elicited by the mite are characterized primarily by a scaling and crusting exfoliative or papular dermatitis with dandruff-like flakes in the haircoat.
- Dorsal trunkal distribution is typical, although generalized distribution may occur.
- Pruritus is highly variable, ranging from completely absent to intense.
- Asymptomatic carriers may occur.

KEY POINT ▶ The most common clinical presentation is a puppy or kitten recently acquired from a petshop, kennel, or cattery with a variably pruritic, dorsal scaling dermatosis.

Diagnosis

The variability in clinical presentation along with the difficulty in finding the mite can make cheyletiellosis a challenging condition to diagnose.

- Suspect cheyletiellosis based on:
  - Nature and distribution of the cutaneous lesions as previously described
  - Exposure of the patient to other animals
  - Involvement of in-contact animals and humans; clinical signs in human contacts are often characteristic (pruritic papules with central necrosis) and may be the only evidence that the animal in the household is infested.
- Techniques used to demonstrate the mite or its eggs include:
  - Examination of the surface of the skin and haircoat for "crawling white scales" with a magnifying lens
  - Superficial skin scrapings
  - Acetate (Scotch) tape impression smears of the affected areas
  - Collection of epidermal debris with a flea comb followed by 10% KOH digestion and centrifugation with a saturated sugar solution
  - Fecal flotation

KEY POINT ▶ The most effective diagnostic techniques are the acetate tape impression smears and the collection of epidermal debris with a flea comb.

- In some cases, the mite or its eggs cannot be dem-

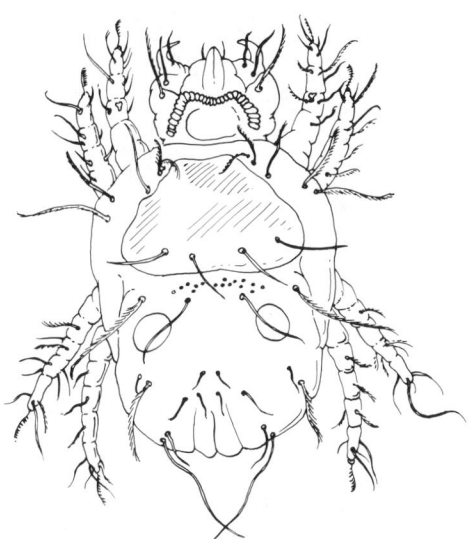

Figure 3. *Cheyletiella yasguri.*

onstrated, and diagnosis thus depends on the response to therapy.

- Differential diagnoses include other mite infestations, pediculosis, flea allergy dermatitis, all of the causes of seborrhea, and all of the causes of miliary dermatitis in the cat.

Treatment

KEY POINT ▶ Although *Cheyletiella* mites appear to be susceptible to most insecticides, they may be extremely difficult to eradicate. Treatment of the patient, all in-contact animals, and the premises is mandatory!

- Bathe animal with an antiseborrheic shampoo to remove crusts and scales prior to dipping.

- Treat cats or rabbits with pyrethrin shampoos or 2% lime sulfur dips. Organophosphates, carbamates, or lindane are effective for use on dogs. Repeat treatment weekly for 6–8 weeks.
- Ivermectin (Ivomec injection for cattle; MSD Agvet), 0.3 mg/kg given three times at 2-week intervals, PO or SC, is effective in dogs, cats, and rabbits (not approved for this use by FDA).
  - Evaluate the dog's heartworm status prior to administration.
  - Do not administer to collies, collie crosses, Shetland sheepdogs, or Australian shepherds.
- Clean and spray animal's quarters and bedding with a residual insecticide appropriate for killing adult fleas. Professional exterminators may be required.

6 Flea Allergy Dermatitis

Craig E. Griffin

Flea allergy dermatitis (FAD) is a hypersensitivity reaction to one or more components of flea saliva. Several types of hypersensitivities, such as cutaneous basophil hypersensitivity, immunoglobulin E (IgE)-mediated immediate hypersensitivity, late-onset IgE reaction, and delayed-type hypersensitivity, can occur alone or in combination. The hypersensitivity reactions cause inflammation and pruritus, which induce most of the lesions.

In most geographic areas, FAD is the most common cause of skin disease. During the summer often it is the most common disease seen by the small animal practitioner.

ETIOLOGY

- *Ctenocephalides felis* is the species that usually infests both dogs and cats.
- *Pulex irritans* and less commonly *Ctenocephalides canis* may be responsible in some areas.

CLINICAL SIGNS

- *Primary lesions*
  - *Pruritus* is the primary clinical sign observed by the owner and can be manifested as chewing (as if eating corn on the cob), rubbing, rolling, or scratching. Cats may groom excessively or pull out their hair. Severe chewing may lead to excessive wear of the incisors and canines.
  - *Papules* and *erythematous macules* also usually are present.
- *Secondary lesions* result from the chronic inflammation and pruritus-induced trauma. Alopecia, broken hairs, dry hair, scaling, hyperpigmentation, and lichenification may occur.
- *Pattern of involvement* most often includes tail base and dorsal lumbar region. The caudal thighs, groin, and abdomen frequently are affected, although less severely than the dorsal lumbar region. In chronic and severe cases, there will be extension of the lesions cranially.

KEY POINT ▶ Pinnal or facial involvement in the dog is not typical of FAD and suggests the presence of other concurrent allergic diseases.

- *Cats with FAD* commonly have miliary crusts in the cervical region as well as dorsal lumbar. Lesions may be limited to the abdomen and groin or cervical area.

- *Secondary problems* that may occur often represent focal sites of infection, foci of severe trauma possibly from the itch-scratch cycle, or a different pathologic reaction. Acute moist dermatitis (hot spots), acral pruritic nodules, eosinophilic plaques, and eosinophilic granulomas may be seen in dogs and cats.
- *Superficial or deep pyoderma* may develop, especially in animals repeatedly treated with corticosteroids. Animals with superficial pyoderma will present with pustules, crusted papules, or circular spreading rings of crust over erythematous erosions, lichenified plaques, or papules.

DIAGNOSIS

KEY POINT ▶ Flea allergy dermatitis is diagnosed in pruritic animals with typical patterns of involvement and evidence of fleas. Always consider the presence of coexistent allergies. Frequently they are overlooked.

History

Identify typical patterns of involvement and seasonality compatible with presence of fleas. Obtain information regarding the number and type of pets, housing and type of floor covering, possible sources of exposure to fleas, current pesticide use, and client concerns regarding the use of pesticides.

Physical Examination

The following procedures may be useful:

- Examine for fleas or flea dirt in long-haired animals by brushing the pet over white paper; in short-haired animals flea combing may be helpful.
- Closely examine areas of involvement typical for other allergies (see sec. 5, chs. 7 and 8) for evidence of coexisting disease.
- Closely examine the dorsal lumbar area for papules, which are the primary lesions seen in canine FAD.
- Carefully palpate the skin in cats, this is important because the typical small crusted papules (miliary crusts) often are more easily felt than seen.
- Shave the haircoat to allow closer observation of the lesions.
- Look for lymphadenopathy in cats, a common finding in chronic FAD.

Dermatopathology

- Dermatopathology is not specific but may be suggestive of or compatible with FAD.
- A superficial mixed perivascular dermatitis with eosinophils is typical in FAD.

Intradermal Testing

Intradermal testing with 1/1,000 w/v flea antigen (Greer) has been documented as a reliable test for diagnosing FAD.

- Positive reactions may occur in 15 minutes (immediate), 6–8 hours (late onset), or 24–48 hours (delayed).
- A positive test indicates that flea hypersensitivity is present, but it does not document that all clinical signs are related to fleas.
- A negative test at all observation times usually indicates (>90%) that flea allergy is not present.
- False-negative results may occur if glucocorticoids and antihistamines are not properly withdrawn prior to testing.

In Vitro Testing

The radioallergosorbent test (RAST) and the enzyme-linked immunosorbent assay (ELISA) have not been documented to be as accurate as intradermal testing (sec. 5, chs. 7 and 8).

False-negative results are the most common problem, and false-positive results may also occur in RAST and ELISA.

Response to Therapy

A favorable response following parasiticidal therapy directed against fleas is helpful in making a diagnosis of FAD. It does not eliminate the diagnosis of coexisting diseases.

KEY POINT ▶ The most definitive diagnosis requires a positive intradermal test, the presence of fleas, and a complete response to effective flea control.

TREATMENT

FAD is best treated by eliminating exposure to the flea allergen (effective flea control). When a complete flea control program is utilized, more than 90% of cases can be controlled without additional treatment. Raising the allergic and pruritic thresholds by treating coexistent problems also may be helpful. In cases in which adequate flea control cannot be achieved, blocking the allergic reaction with systemic therapy is required.

Decrease Allergic Load (Flea Control)

Complete flea control requires treating the affected pet, other pets in the same environment, and the pet's environment. In severely infested environments, effective control may take 4 to 8 weeks to achieve. Client compliance and proper application of insecticides is required. Once flea control is achieved, clients may find that only one or two aspects of flea control are required for maintenance.

KEY POINT ▶ Failure to obtain client compliance and improper application of parasiticidal agents are the major reasons for poor response of FAD patients to flea control.

Environmental Treatment

Because the majority of flea eggs, larvae, and pupae are located in the environment, it is essential to treat environmental areas.

Indoors. Treatment of indoor areas is critical when the affected animal spends most of the time indoors. This is the habitat that can be controlled most effectively.

- In houses in which floors are primarily carpeted, electrostatically charged sodium polyborate powder (Rx for Fleas) is most effective, lasting up to 1 year. It is also safe, with no reported toxicity.
- Monthly spraying of all floor surfaces and furniture that pets have access to with chlorpyrifos, permethrin, or pyrethrin in conjunction with a growth hormone regulator (methoprene, fenoxycarb) is advisable. Effective products include Siphotrol Plus II House Treatment (Vet-Kem), Ectogard House and Carpet Spray (Tech America), and Impass Complete Premise Spray (Coopers).
  - If pyrethrin alone is utilized, weekly spraying for the first 3 weeks is necessary.

KEY POINT ▶ Be careful when using organophosphates in an environment in which cats are present. Some cats are very sensitive and may have problems with toxicity even after a single application.

- Microencapsulation technology makes possible less frequent application of parasiticides without utilizing a growth hormone regulator (Sectrol Pet and House Flea Spray and Duratrol Premise Spray, 3M).
- Treat linoleum and tile floors by frequent mopping with routine disinfectants.

Outdoors. Treat outdoor pens and similar enclosures weekly for 3 weeks and then monthly. A liquid application of chlorpyrifos, permethrin, or diazinon is preferred. Although helpful in long-term control, granular and microencapsulated insecticides have been less beneficial for obtaining initial control.

Unaffected Pets

Treat unaffected animals in the same environment with adulticidal flea products that lack flea repellent effects.

- Weekly or bimonthly dips with chlorpyrifos (Duratrol Dip, 3M) or permethrin (Expar Dip, Coopers; Permectrin, Bioceutic) products are effective.

KEY POINT ▶ Do not use permethrin dips on cats because toxicity may result. Also, use only permethrin sprays that are approved for cats on this species.

- In cases in which dips cannot be utilized, use sprays or foams containing pyrethrins and/or permethrin at the maximum approved frequency.
- Use an approved flea collar on cats that cannot be treated with dips, sprays, or foams.

Affected Pets

Treat affected animals with an adulticidal product and repellents as frequently as allowed for these products.

- Do not apply alcohol-containing products frequently because of their drying effect.
- Combination of weekly dips (see above) and sprays (DuoCide L.A., Allerderm/Virbac; Synerkyl Spray, DVM; Sectrol Pet and Household Spray and Sectrol Flea Foam, 3M) between dips is most effective.
- Use water-based pyrethrin and/or permethrin sprays (DuoCide L.A., Allerderm/Virbac) that contain a repellent. Apply daily if approved for such use.
  - If used in conjunction with a dip, a light mist on the surface of the coat is all that is required.
  - If used alone, apply the spray to the skin surface (not just the hair).
- Avoid using systemic parasiticidal agents because flea bites are required for their effectiveness; however, their use is preferable to no treatment.

Increase Allergic/Pruritic Threshold

- Control *concurrent allergic diseases* such as atopy and food allergy.
- Treat *secondary pyoderma,* which often increases pruritus, with systemic antibiotics (see sec. 5, ch. 1).
- Eliminate *dry skin* by use of baths, moisturizing sprays or rinses, and fatty acid supplements.
- Remove other *irritants or allergens on the skin surface,* which may aggravate inflamed skin, by frequently bathing the animal.

Block Allergic Reactions

A variety of systemic drugs may be used to alter the allergic reaction. This approach is often utilized at the beginning of the flea control program and to break the itch-scratch cycle. Resort to long-term use of systemic drugs only when clients cannot effectively control fleas. This most often occurs with outdoor/roaming pets, especially cats.

Systemic Glucocorticoids

Systemic glucocorticoids usually are required. Prednisone or prednisolone, 1.0–2.0 mg/kg, q12–24h PO, is initially utilized to stop the pruritus associated with FAD.

- Use oral triamcinolone acetonide (Vetalog, Solvay), 0.25–0.5 mg/kg, q12–24h PO, if PD/PU or polyphagia associated with prednisone/prednisolone is unacceptable to the client.
- When pruritus is controlled, change to an alternate-day program and then taper to the lowest effective dose.

Antihistamines

Antihistamines are infrequently effective for FAD. They may be used in conjunction with glucocorticoids and have a synergistic effect that makes possible a reduction in the glucocorticoid dose.

- Diphenhydramine HCl (2 mg/kg, q8h PO), hydroxyzine HCl (2 mg/kg, q8h PO), and doxepin HCl (1–2 mg/kg, q12h PO) may be useful.
- Chlorpheniramine may be helpful in dogs at a total dose of 2–6 mg, q8–12h PO. It is especially useful in cats at a total dose of 2mg, q12h PO.

Fatty Acid Supplements

Fatty acid supplements (DVM Derm Caps, DVM) alone rarely control FAD. However, they may be helpful in controlling concurrent atopy, alleviating dry skin, and modulating the production of inflammatory mediators. These effects may raise the pruritic/allergic threshold and have a synergistic effect with other treatments, allowing a reduction in the glucocorticoid dose.

Hyposensitization

Hyposensitization used with standard protocols has not been shown to be efficacious. However, hyposensitization used alone has been reported to be an effective control in individual cases. It is not considered cost effective for most clients, considering the low percentage of efficacy.

PREVENTION

- Prevention is achieved by long-term continuation of a flea control program. Long-term treatment may not have to be as complete or as frequent as the initial treatment program.
- Prevention works best by anticipating increases in flea population and increasing the use of parasiticidal therapy just prior to the onset of environmental conditions favoring these increases.
- When pets are primarily indoors and do not roam loose, environment control is preferred as the major method of flea control.
- Outdoor/roaming animals require both pet and environmental therapy when the weather is conducive to flea activity.

Supplemental Readings

Bevier-Tournay DE: Fleas and flea control. *In* Kirk RW, ed.: *Current Veterinary Therapy X*. Philadelphia: W. B. Saunders, 1989, p 586.

Kwochka KW: Fleas and related disease. Vet Clin North Am 17:1235, 1987.

MacDonald JM, Miller TA: Parasiticide therapy in small animal dermatology. *In* Kirk RW, ed: *Current Veterinary Therapy IX*. Philadelphia: W. B. Saunders, 1986, p 571.

Schick MP, Schick RO: Understanding and implementing safe and effective flea control. J Am Anim Hosp Assoc 22:421, 1986.

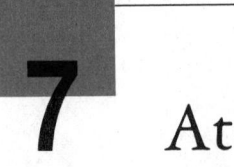

7 Atopy

Patricia D. White

Canine atopy is considered to be due to an inherited tendency to develop IgE antibodies to environmental allergens (molds; grass, tree, and weed pollens; epidermal agents; house dust; house dust mites). Although popular theory states that canine atopy develops subsequent to sensitization to environmental allergens via the respiratory tract, the ventral, pedal, and facial distribution of cutaneous lesions strongly suggests that percutaneous exposure may also play a role in the development of clinical signs. This disease comprises a significant proportion of canine dermatologic complaints and has been estimated to involve 3–15% of the canine population.

Feline atopy is believed to be a type I hypersensitivity reaction to environmental allergens. There are ample examples of cutaneous and respiratory allergic diseases in cats caused by exposure to aeroallergens in support of this theory, but there is no evidence to support an inherited predisposition to the development of atopy in this species. Feline atopy may present with a variety of focal and diffuse clinical signs including miliary dermatitis, eosinophilic granuloma, eosinophilic ulcer, eosinophilic plaque, and symmetric alopecia.

ETIOLOGY

Pathogenesis

- Atopy classically is described as an *IgE-mediated type I hypersensitivity reaction.* Once contact is made, the allergen is processed by tissue macrophages into a form which can be presented with the assistance of T helper lymphocytes to B lymphocytes. The B cells then produce allergen-specific IgE antibodies and memory cells. The IgE antibodies affix to tissue mast cells and basophils. Upon re-exposure, allergens bind the surface IgE molecules. Cross-linking of two IgE antibodies results in degranulation of the mast cell and the release of preformed inflammatory mediators and stimulation of the arachidonic acid cascade. The combination of preformed and arachidonic acid–derived (leukotrienes, prostaglandins, and hydroxy fatty acids) inflammatory mediators results in the development of signs of inflammation (erythema, edema, pruritus).
- A reaginic antibody similar to canine IgE has been identified in cats, but its relationship to atopy is unknown.

Incidence

KEY POINT ▶ Atopy is the second most common allergic skin disorder in dogs and cats, second only to flea allergy dermatitis.

- Age of onset is between 1 and 3 years. The disease usually starts as a seasonally pruritic dermatosis with the signs peaking in the summer and fall. The problem may become perennial.
- Both sexes are represented, although female dogs may have a slightly higher incidence of occurrence.
- Breeds predisposed to developing atopy include Cairn, West Highland white, and wire-haired fox terriers; Lhasa apsos; golden and Labrador retrievers; boxers; bulldogs; dalmatians; English and Irish setters; and Chinese Shar peis. The disease also occurs in mixed-breed dogs.
- Because atopy in cats is diagnosed less frequently than in dogs, age, breed, and sex trends are not appreciated.

CLINICAL SIGNS

Pruritus

Pruritus is the hallmark of atopy in both dogs and cats.

- Pruritus is the only sign early in the process, with no observable skin lesions. An itch-scratch-itch cycle is established leading to self-trauma that may be severe.
- In dogs, as the disease progresses, face rubbing, foot chewing, and scratching lead to erythema, alopecia, edema, lichenification, and hyperpigmentation of the periocular, perilabial, interdigital, ventral, axillary, and antebrachial regions of the body.
- Acral lick granulomas are commonly seen is some breeds, such as the Doberman pinscher and dalmatian, and reflect focally intense pruritus and severe self-trauma.

Other Signs in Dogs

Otitis Externa. This disorder may accompany the other clinical signs or may be the sole presenting complaint.

- A pruritic and erythematous pinna and ear canal in the early stages of the disease eventually leads to a secondary yeast or bacterial infection that presents as a brown waxy or purulent exudate.

Pyoderma. *Superficial bacterial infection* is the most common but frequently overlooked problem accompanying canine atopy.

- The self-trauma caused by pruritus encourages the

302

establishment of pathogenic bacteria, leading to pyoderma.

■ Staphylococcal antigens are capable of eliciting a toxic, inflammatory, or antigenic effect on epidermal and dermal tissues, resulting in cutaneous damage with the release of proteolytic enzymes and inflammatory mediators. Because pyoderma may be intensely pruritic, the presence of this condition in an animal with atopy worsens the existing pruritus (sec. 5, ch. 1.).

Seborrheic Dermatitis. Dermatitis characterized by flaky skin and a dry or greasy haircoat often occurs in conjunction with the pruritus and pyoderma.

Other Signs in Cats

■ Cats commonly present with a *head and neck pruritus* or *ventral abdominal dermatitis with alopecia.*

■ Clinical signs also include one or a combination of the following:
  • Mild to severe symmetric alopecia without dermatitis
  • Focal or diffuse miliary dermatitis (see sec. 5, ch. 14)
  • Eosinophilic plaques, ulcers, and granulomas (see sec. 5, ch. 14)
  • Generalized seborrhea

DIAGNOSIS

KEY POINT ▶ The diagnosis of atopy is based on history, clinical signs, elimination or control of other causes of pruritic dermatitis, and results of appropriate diagnostic tests. Age of onset, season of occurrence, breed, and response to therapy provide adequate information to make a tentative diagnosis.

History

A thorough and complete history is mandatory; look for seasonal pattern of occurrence that may progress to a nonseasonal problem.

Physical Examination

The typical distribution of skin lesions corresponds to the severity of pruritus.

■ Of affected animals, 60–70% have visible skin lesions including erythema, papules, scale, alopecia, hyperpigmentation, and lichenification involving the face, ears, feet, axilla, flexor and extensor surfaces of joints, groin, and abdomen.

■ Reddish brown discoloration of the hair in dogs and bilaterally symmetric or ventral abdominal alopecia in cats are changes associated with licking and chewing.

Differential Diagnosis

■ In the differential diagnosis, consider:*
  • Demodicosis

*Consult the appropriate chapters for details regarding diagnosis of these conditions.

• Dermatophytosis
• Food, contact, and flea allergies
• Scabies
• Intestinal parasite hypersensitivity
• Superficial pyoderma

■ In every case:
  • Take skin scrapings for sarcoptic and demodectic mange mites. Perform a dermatophyte culture and a fecal examination for parasites.

■ In nonseasonally pruritic animals, institute a hypoallergenic food trial.

■ A serum biochemistry profile and complete blood count (CBC) help to identify metabolic or endocrine causes of the dermatosis.

■ Screen for flea infestation because about 80% of atopic dogs also are allergic to fleas.
  • Use a flea comb to check for the presence of fleas, flea eggs, and flea feces.
  • If there is evidence of fleas, treat both the animal and its environment.

KEY POINT ▶ Eliminate or control fleas prior to evaluating and treating atopy, which can be time-consuming and expensive.

Specific Diagnostic Tests

Intradermal Allergy Testing

■ Select intradermal allergy testing (IDST) in cases in which:
  • The animal's allergy season lasts longer than 3 months.
  • Medical therapy no longer controls the symptoms.
  • Avoidance of the allergen is not possible.

■ Consider the *cost* of allergens and supplies and the time involved in test kit preparation before choosing to perform the IDST. This test must be performed an average of 2–3 times weekly to ensure accuracy and consistency of test results.

To maximize the information gained from the IDST, take the following precautionary measures prior to skin testing:

■ Withdraw anti-inflammatory drugs, which are the most common cause of false-negative results, for an appropriate period before performing the IDST. Withdrawal time depends on the drug, carrier vehicle, route of administration, and duration of therapy.
  • Discontinue topical (including otic and ophthalmic) and short-acting systemic glucocorticoids (prednisone and prednisolone) for a *minimum* of 3 weeks before an IDST. Longer-acting corticosteroids require a withdrawal time of 6 weeks (dexamethasone, triamcinolone acetonide) to 12 weeks (methylprednisolone acetate).
  • Discontinue antihistamines for at least 2 weeks.
  • Although other nonsteroidal anti-inflammatory drugs (NSAIDs) and essential fatty acid (EFA) supplements have not been critically evaluated, these products theoretically may depress the response to intradermal allergens by affecting the production of inflammatory mediators. Therefore, discontinue these drugs for 2 weeks before skin testing for maximum results.

■ Other causes of false-negative results include outdated allergens, too little allergen, subcutaneous injections, off-season testing, and anergy.

KEY POINT ▶ The best time of year to test a dog or cat with seasonal allergies is at the end of the season when clinical signs have declined. Animals with nonseasonal allergies may need to be tested twice a year.

■ Perform histamine response test prior to testing or prior to referring for intradermal allergy testing
  • As a pre-test, inject 0.1 ml of 1:100,000 histamine phosphate as the positive control and 0.1 ml of saline as the negative control intradermally prior to performing the full skin test.
  • Read the test 15 minutes after making the injections.
  • A red, firm wheal approximately 15 mm in diameter or four times the size of the saline control bleb is an adequate positive response for histamine.
■ Many dogs may be tested with manual restraint, but endogenous glucocorticoid release may affect the results. If chemical restraint is necessary, xylazine HCl (Rompun, Haver) is the sedative of choice and will not interfere with the results
  • Give atropine sulfate at 0.02–0.04 mg/kg IM or SC, 15 minutes before administering the xylazine (0.1–0.2 mg/kg IV). The two drugs may also be mixed in the same syringe and given together IV.
  • Other anesthetics and tranquilizers may cause false-negative results.
■ Cats may be tested with manual restraint in lateral recumbency or with the use of a cat bag. Ketamine HCl (Ketaset, Fort Dodge; 5–10 mg/kg IM) is the sedative of choice for cats.
■ Cats may be skin tested using the same antigens as in the canine test. Read test sites within 10 minutes because the reactions are less indurated, are less erythematous, and dissipate more quickly than in dogs.
■ Results of the IDST should correlate with clinical history in order to be diagnostic. The reader is referred to the report by Halliwell and Gorman (1989) for a complete discussion of interpretation of test results.

In Vitro Allergy Tests

In vitro allergy tests may be helpful when intradermal allergy testing is not an option because of lack of availability, drug interference, or poor condition of the skin. The radioallergosorbent test (RAST) (Spectrum Laboratories; Mesa, AZ) and the enzyme-linked immunosorbent assay (ELISA) (AREST; Bioproducts DVM, Tempe, AZ) are commercially available *in vitro* diagnostic tests.

These tests detect *circulating group-specific IgE antibodies*. The benefit of a test based on identifying allergen group-specific IgE is of questionable value in cats.

Mechanism. The RAST and ELISA are based on incubation of the patient's antibody-laden serum with a substrate containing antigen.

■ After incubation, the substrate is rinsed to remove unbound antibody.
■ Anti-canine IgE labeled with a radioisotope (RAST) or an enzyme (ELISA) is then added to detect the antigen-antibody complexes formed during the incubation period.
■ After several additional washings, the number of complexes is evaluated by a gamma counter to measure the amount of radioactivity (RAST) or a spectrophotometer to measure the degree of color change (ELISA).
■ These values are compared with a standard curve from positive control counts to arrive at a semiquantitative measurement of group specific IgE antibodies.

Advantages

■ The RAST and ELISA have the following reported benefits:
  • Only 3–5 ml of serum are necessary.
  • Antihistamines and other NSAIDs need not be discontinued.
  • Dogs with severely affected skin may be evaluated.
  • Whether residual effects from long-term or concurrent use of corticosteroids can affect test results is controversial.

Accuracy

■ Agreement between these tests and IDST results varies with the allergen (ragweed, 82%; dandelion, 12%).
■ Reproducibility has been shown to be 79.3% for the RAST and 93.1% for the ELISA.
■ Both tests have been linked with frequent false-positive results (i.e., normal dogs identified as atopic). False-positive results are thought to be due to high levels of circulating endoparasitic or ectoparasitic IgE antibodies.
■ Results of serologic testing and formulation of an allergy vaccine should correlate with the clinical history. Response to hyposensitization based on serologic test results is reportedly comparable to that seen with IDST results. However, a well-controlled study has not been performed to substantiate these reports.

TREATMENT
General Treatment Principles

KEY POINT ▶ When planning management of atopy, consider the presence of concurrent dermatologic abnormalities, length of allergy season, severity of clinical signs, and response to medical therapy. Strict avoidance or elimination of the allergen is the most effective long-term therapeutic approach but is seldom practical or feasible. Consequently, use immunotherapy and medical management to develop a protocol that is tailor-made to fit the individual animal's specific needs.

Pruritic Threshold and Summation of Effects

The understanding and control of these two conceptual phenomena that occur with clinical atopy determine the degree of success of medical therapy.

- The *pruritic threshold* is an individually determined point at which pruritic stimuli will cause an individual to scratch.
- *A summation of effects* occurs when a single stimulus is not sufficient to push the patient over its pruritic threshold, but when a second or third pruritic stimulus is added, pruritus occurs.
  - For example, a dog with atopy remains asymptomatic until xerosis or pyoderma (each potentially pruritic alone) provides the additional stimulus to exceed the pruritic threshold.
  - Treating the pyoderma or xerosis makes the animal asymptomatic again.

One goal of therapy is to eliminate all factors that lower the pruritic threshold and result in clinical disease. Other dermatologic conditions such as xerosis, pyoderma, and external parasites should be controlled before attempting to treat the allergy.

Concurrent Pyoderma

Concurrent *superficial pyoderma* is the most commonly overlooked cause of pruritus in allergic dogs.

- Pyoderma typically is characterized clinically by follicular papular and pustular eruptions, serous crusts, epidermal collarettes, and patchy alopecia (for a detailed discussion of pyoderma, see sec. 5, ch. 1).
- An impression smear of a pustule stained with Diff-Quik (Baxter Healthcare Corp.) reveals degenerating polymorphonuclear leukocytes that often have phagocytized cocci.

Canine Pyodermas

Most canine pyodermas are caused by *Staphylococcus intermedius*. Choose antibiotics based on the most likely sensitivity of this organism; penicillins and tetracyclines are never an appropriate choice.

- Give antibiotics for a *minimum* of 3 weeks and continue for 1 week beyond clinical remission.
- *Erythromycin and lincomycin.* Erythromycin (11–18 mg/kg, q8h PO) and lincomycin (22 mg/kg, q12h PO) are first-choice bacteriostatic antibiotics. Their spectrum of activity is narrow and specific for beta-lactamase–resistant bacteria.
  - Erythromycin is inexpensive but must be given three times a day and tends to make animals vomit. To avoid this side effect, administer the antibiotic with food at half the dose, q12h, for the first 2 days.
  - Lincomycin has the advantage of requiring only twice-daily administration, but it is expensive.
- *Oxacillin.* Oxacillin (Oxacillin Capsules Rx, Biocraft; Prostaphlin, Squibb) (22 mg/kg, q8h PO) is an ex-

cellent narrow-spectrum antibiotic for treatment of superficial pyoderma; however, it is very expensive.
- *Amoxicillin-clavulanate.* Amoxicillin-clavulanic acid (Clavamox, SmithKline Beecham) (22 mg/kg, q12h PO).
- *Sulfa-containing antibiotics.* Potentiated sulfa-containing antibiotics such as trimethoprim/sulfadiazine (Tribrissen, Coopers; Di-Trim, Syntex) and trimethoprim-sulfamethoxazole (22 mg/kg, q12h PO) are broad-spectrum antibiotics used to treat cases of pyoderma that have responded poorly to narrow-spectrum agents. Ormetoprim-sulfadimethoxine (Primor, Hoffmann–La Roche), a newer potentiated sulfa-containing agent, has the advantage of requiring only once-daily administration (25 mg/kg given PO on day 1; then 12.5 mg/kg, q24h PO).
  - Keratoconjunctivitis sicca is a common side effect of sulfa-containing antibiotics. In addition, a polysystemic hypersensitivity reaction characterized by myalgia, joint swelling, and neurologic abnormalities has been noted in some dogs, especially Doberman pinschers.
  - These problems are reversible upon discontinuation of the antibiotic; however keratoconjunctivitis sicca may be permanent.
- *Cephalexin.* Reserve cephalexin (22mg/kg, q8h PO, or 33mg/kg, q12h PO) for chronic, resistant bacterial infections.
- *Quinolone antibiotics.* These are the newest group of antibiotics to be used for pyodermas. Although resistance is seldom seen with these drugs, mutations can develop with prolonged use. Therefore, consider quinolones "last resort" antibiotics to be used cautiously and infrequently.
  - Enrofloxacin (Baytril, Haver; 2.5–5.0 mg/kg, q12h PO) is currently the only quinolone antibiotic approved for use in both dogs and cats.
- A focal or generalized, dry or greasy seborrheic dermatitis may also occur secondarily and can be treated topically with an antibacterial or antiseborrheic shampoo.

Feline Pyodermas

- Feline pyodermas are rare, are most commonly caused by *Staphylococcus* organisms and are usually responsive to a 2-week course of amoxicillin (22 mg/kg, q12h PO).

Immunotherapy with Hyposensitization

KEY POINT ▶ This is the treatment of choice for animals that exhibit signs for longer than 3–4 months, remain uncomfortable with symptomatic therapy, or cannot tolerate corticosteroids.

Medical management generally provides immediate relief and is best for short-term use. However, because of the potential for long-term negative systemic effects as well as the need for higher dosages over time, consider hyposensitization for better optimal management of the disease in both dogs and cats. Ideally, the goal of therapy is to increase the patient's ability to tolerate environmental allergens without clinical signs.

Realistically, immunotherapy allows a significant reduction in symptomatic medical therapy and, occasionally, its elimination.

- Of treated dogs, 40–85% are reported to show 50% improvement or better with hyposensitization. Response to therapy may be equivalent with either IDST or serologic test–based vaccines.
- Most allergy vaccines are made from alum-precipitated or aqueous extracts. Response to both types of vaccines has been similar. Aqueous extracts are the most popular and are widely available in veterinary medicine.
  - Alum-precipitated extracts are more expensive than aqueous but are associated with fewer adverse reactions and allow longer intervals between injections.
  - Aqueous extracts are less expensive but must be administered more frequently.
- An allergy vaccine is made for the individual patient based on either serologic or intradermal test results. In addition, selection of antigens is based on the presence of allergens in the environment and a strong correlation of clinical signs with the pollination season.
- No more than 10 antigens are placed in one vaccine, and the maximum amount of antigen should not exceed 20,000 protein nitrogen units (PNU) per milliliter. Although there is no single standard vaccine protocol, all require an initial loading period followed by a maintenance dosage. Once the maintenance dosage is reached, it is repeated every 3 weeks and continued year-round.
- Side effects associated with the vaccine include post-injection pruritus, pain, and urticaria and occasionally vomiting or diarrhea. Severe anaphylaxis is rare.
- Response to therapy varies with each animal and usually takes several months. Approximately 25% show some improvement in 3 months, another 50% in 6 months, and the remaining 25% in 6–12 months.
  - Continue therapy for at least 9–12 months before deciding on efficacy.
  - Make sure that other causes of pruritus or dermatitis (fleas, pyoderma, dry skin) are not the cause of a perceived failure.
- One goal of therapy is to control signs with the minimum amount of medication.
- Signs may return or worsen during the allergy season. The frequency of allergen injections may need to be increased during this period.
  - Antihistamines or alternate-day short-acting glucocorticoids may be added to the immunotherapy and may be required early in the allergy season before the increased allergen dosage can take effect.
- Animals that show an initial response but relapse should be evaluated for other causes (summation of effects).
  - A second test may be required to identify allergens that were missed because of the time of year when the first test was performed or because the animal has developed sensitivity to new allergens.

Medical Therapy

Medical therapy is the most common approach to management of atopy in both dogs and cats. Choose this protocol when an owner does not wish a full diagnostic work-up, when the allergy season is short, or an animal is too old to fully benefit from hyposensitization.

Medical therapy may also be adjunctive to hyposensitization. Use antihistamines, glucocorticoids, NSAIDs, essential fatty acid (EFA) supplements, and topical shampoo therapy to help control the signs of atopy with the therapeutic protocol designed to fit the animal's specific needs.

Antihistamines

Antihistamines control pruritus in approximately 40% of purely atopic dogs and is the drug of choice for symptomatic therapy. The magnitude of response varies individually. If antihistamines are unable to control all the signs, they are at least "steroid-sparing," allowing a lower dosage of glucocorticoids to be used.

KEY POINT ▶ Identify and control other cutaneous diseases such as flea allergy, food allergy, xerosis, and superficial pyoderma because antihistamines are rarely effective when these conditions are present.

- Six classes of antihistamines are used to provide anti-inflammatory and antipruritic benefit through blockage of H_1 receptors. Some antihistamines also have antianxiety, analgesic, or sedative effects that add to patient comfort.
- Antihistamines used commonly with canine atopy include chlorpheniramine maleate (2 mg/dog <5.5 kg, q12h PO; 4 mg/dog 5.5–27 kg, q12h; and 8 mg/dog >27 kg, q12h PO); diphenhydramine HCl (2.2 mg/kg, q8–12h PO); doxepin HCl (Adapin, Pennwalt; Sinequan, Roenig; 0.5–1.0 mg/kg, q12h PO); hydroxyzine HCl (2.2 mg/kg, q8–12h PO).
- Side effects include sedation, hyperexcitability, and anticholinergic reactions.
- Some of the newer antihistamines such as terfenadine (Seldane, Merrell Dow) (5–10 mg/kg, q12h PO) and clemastine fumarate (Tavist, Sandoz) 0.05 mg/kg q12h PO) have shown some benefit in a limited number of cases but are expensive.
- It is helpful to prescribe a 2-week course for each of three different antihistamines representing different classes, and then choose the one most effective for maintenance therapy.
- Chlorpheniramine HCl (2–4 mg/cat, q12h PO) is the antihistamine of choice for pruritus and self-induced alopecia in cats.
- Approximately 20–40% of atopic dogs can be adequately controlled with antihistamines alone. Antihistamines in combination with avoidance, immunotherapy, EFA supplements, or NSAIDs may render the animal asymptomatic.

Glucocorticoids

Systemic Glucocorticoids

- These drugs are very effective in controlling pruritus; however, use them as exclusive therapy only in seasonally (less than 3 months in duration) allergic animals.

■ Glucocorticoids are valuable as adjunctive therapy; their use along with antihistamines, EFA supplements, or immunotherapy allows smaller quantities to be given less frequently.

■ Although they are the most rapidly effective of anti-inflammatory drugs, they are also associated with the worst side effects.

■ Principles for the use of systemic glucocorticoids include
  • The cause of pruritus has been well established.
  • Contributory processes have been appropriately eliminated.
  • The risks to the patient have been minimized.
  • Alternative therapy has been explored and exhausted.
  • The appropriate class, formulation, and dosage have been chosen.

■ Never use glucocorticoids when a pyoderma is present concurrently.

Mechanism of Action

■ Glucocorticoids decrease inflammation and pruritus by:
  • Inhibiting chemotaxis of inflammatory cells,
  • Inhibiting normal function of lymphocytes and macrophages,
  • Stabilizing cellular membranes and thereby preventing mast cell degranulation and the release of intracellular and membrane associated inflammatory mediators.
  • Inhibiting vasodilation and the resulting erythema and edema.

■ Once the corticosteroid is discontinued, these processes proceed uninhibited. Symptoms return and are often more severe than before therapy.

■ Anti-inflammatory dosages do not interfere with antibody production or antigen-antibody interaction.

■ Low-dose alternate-day therapy provides the antipruritic effects without interfering significantly with the hypothalamic-pituitary-adrenal axis (HPAA) or the normal immune response.

Side Effects

Side effects are numerous and reflect individual sensitivity as well as formulation, dosage, and duration of therapy.

■ *A stress leukogram* (leukocytosis with neutropenia, eosinopenia, monocytosis) and increased serum alkaline phosphatase is seen in almost every case. Some animals also show an increase in serum alanine aminotransferase, glucose, and cholesterol.

■ *Polyuria, polydypsia, polyphagia, and weight gain* are commonly observed with the short-acting oral glucocorticoids (prednisolone and prednisone) and reflect the mineralocorticoid activity of these drugs. Changing to a glucocorticoid with minimal mineralocorticoid activity such as methylprednisolone (Medrol, Upjohn) will eliminate these effects.

■ Occasionally an animal will become *anorectic*, with evidence of *weight loss and muscle wasting*. Panting,

muscle weakness, exercise intolerance, hepatomegaly, and pancreatitis also may occur.

■ All glucocorticoids *suppress the HPAA*. With repositol glucocorticoids, this suppression lasts longer than the anti-inflammatory effects. Slowly withdraw long-acting glucocorticoids that have been administered for an extended period of time, because treated animals are functionally addisonian and will not have the reserve necessary to respond to stress. Alternate-day prednisone and prednisolone will prevent this phenomenon.

■ Some animals demonstrate bizarre *behavior changes* on minor dosages of glucocorticoids; these are eliminated on discontinuance of the drug.

■ *Dermatologic changes* observed in both dogs and cats that are associated with glucocorticoids include xerosis, comedone formation (dogs), loss of skin tone and elasticity, epidermal and dermal atrophy, bruising, and calcinosis cutis (dogs).

■ *Suppression of immune and inflammatory responses* may result in the development of a pyoderma, demodicosis, or dermatophyte infection.

KEY POINT ▶ When previously well-controlled animals become acutely pruritic or develop a nonpruritic pustular dermatosis, take skin scrapings, fungal culture, and culture of an intact pustule for bacteria. Positive results dictate weaning from the corticosteroid, appropriate treatment of the infection, and the use of an alternate symptomatic therapeutic protocol designed for these patients.

Dosage and Formulation

■ The dosage and formulation of a glucocorticoid determines whether it will have antipruritic, anti-inflammatory, or immunosuppressive effects.
  • Classified as *short-acting glucocorticoids*, prednisone and prednisolone are anti-inflammatory when given at an initial dosage of 2.2 mg/kg, q12h PO to cats, and 0.5 mg/kg, q12h PO to dogs. Antipruritic effects are seen with 0.1–0.25 mg/kg, q12h PO in the dog and with 0.5 mg/kg, q12h PO in the cat.
  • An anti-inflammatory dosage of the *intermediate-acting glucocorticoids* such as triamcinolone (Vetalog, Solvay) and methylprednisolone sodium phosphate (Medrol, Upjohn) is 0.25 mg/kg, q24h for 5 days, then q48h, PO. These corticosteroids are ideal for managing the seasonally atopic animal with a limited season.
  • Anti-inflammatory dosages of dexamethasone are 0.2–0.4 mg/kg, q24h IM. These *long-acting glucocorticoids* continue to suppress the HPAA long after the antipruritic effects have waned and are not to be used for maintenance therapy.

■ *Course of therapy*. Initiate therapy at an anti-inflammatory dose q12h for 5 days, reduce to q24h for 5 days, and then administer q48h for 2 weeks.

■ If the animal remains asymptomatic, further reduce the dosage to the lowest possible level that will control pruritus. Continue this dose throughout the allergy season.

- Methylprednisolone acetate (Depo Medrol, Upjohn) is a potent *ultra-long-acting glucocorticoid.*
  - The use of this glucocorticoid is of questionable value in canine atopy and is restricted to dogs with very short (less than 3 months) allergy seasons whose symptoms can be managed with one or two injections. Never administer it more frequently than every 6–8 weeks.
  - Methylprednisolone acetate (4.4 mg/kg, q6w IM) is frequently the corticosteroid of choice for the pruritic cat. Do not administer it more frequently than q6–8 weeks.

Topical Glucocorticoids

Use these agents to treat focal areas of inflammation. The potency of the preparation is determined by the specific steroid and its concentration, the carrier vehicle (lotion, cream, or ointment), and the method of application. The more occlusive the vehicle, the more potent the product.

- Remember that dry lesions should be moistened so that a more occlusive dressing can be used, whereas moist lesions must be allowed to dry.
- Side effects may be local (poor wound healing, cutaneous atrophy, or pigmentary changes) or systemic (iatrogenic hyperadrenocorticism, folliculitis), depending on the potency of the product and how much is systemically absorbed.
- Control the dermatitis using a potent fluorinated steroid such as amcinonide (Cyclocort, Lederle) for the first several days. Then switch to the lowest-potency topical steroid that will control the dermatitis over the long term (0.5–1.0% hydrocortisone cream).

Essential Fatty Acids

The essential fatty acids (EFAs), which comprise linoleic acid (LA), alpha linolenic acid (ALA), and arachidonic acid (AA), are long-chain omega-3 (ALA) and omega-6 (LA and AA) polyunsaturated fatty acids that are incorporated into all cellular membranes. They are required for all cellular membrane structure and function, cannot be synthesized *de novo*, and therefore must be provided in the diet. EFAs also exhibit anti-inflammatory properties.

- EFA supplements marketed for used in cutaneous inflammatory skin disease contain a combination of gamma linolenic acid (GLA, from evening primrose oil), eicosapentaenoic acid (EPA, from fish oil), and linoleic acid (LA, from vegetable oil).
- Administration of GLA alone and in combination with EPA has resulted in improvement in redness, scale, and pruritus associated with human inflammatory skin diseases. Clinical improvement is associated with simultaneous changes in tissue eicosanoids and fatty acids. Studies indicate that optimal biochemical effects are not seen until 6 weeks of therapy. Comparable studies have not been performed in dogs.
- EFA veterinary products (Derm Caps, DVM; EFA-Z Plus, Allerderm/Virbac) have demonstrated variable and modest improvement in pruritus, erythema, and coat condition when used alone.
  - The amount and ratio of specific fatty acids in veterinary products vary considerably. It is unknown whether the type or quantity is appropriate to achieve the desired results in any product.
  - Because a variety of proteolytic enzymes and inflammatory mediators are involved in the pathogenesis of allergic dermatitis in dogs and cats, results range from zero to marked improvement. Realistically expect a mild to moderate improvement in clinical signs when administering EFA supplements alone.
  - Synergistic effects are achieved when used with antihistamines or glucocorticoids. Administer at twice the manufacturer's recommended dosage q12h for a minimum of 6 weeks before assessing response.

Non-Steroidal Anti-Inflammatory Agents

- Aspirin (10 mg/kg, q12h PO with food) is occasionally beneficial and provides temporary relief from pruritus and inflammation, especially during periods of glucocorticoid withdrawal (usually 1–2 weeks) prior to skin testing.
- Anorexia, vomiting, melena, or evidence of abnormal bleeding signals the need to discontinue the drug.
- Do not use NSAIDs in cats.

Supportive Topical Therapy

This is one of the most beneficial forms of adjunctive therapy.

- The broad range of products available allows the therapy to be fairly specific for the dermatologic problem.
- As the condition improves, modify topical therapy accordingly.
- Disadvantages are:
  - It is time-consuming for the owner.
  - The patient must be fairly cooperative.
  - The immediate benefits (reduction in pruritus) are usually short-lived.

Shampoo Therapy. Shampoo therapy is helpful in the atopic animal to remove dirt and antigenic debris, to rehydrate a dry stratum corneum, and to provide the soothing effects of hydrotherapy.

KEY POINT ▶ Contact time for shampoo therapy is at least 10 minutes. Less time results in the removal of surface oils without the benefit of rehydrating the stratum corneum.

- *Cool water soaks* are excellent for managing acute exacerbations of local and generalized pruritus.
  - An astringent such as aluminum acetate (Domeboro, Miles Lab.) may be added to the water (one tablet or packet per pint of water) and will decrease the redness and swelling associated with inflammation.
  - Colloidal oatmeal products (Aveeno, Rydelle Labs.) added to the cool water or used in a

shampoo (Epi-Soothe, Allerderm/Virbac) will reduce the redness, swelling, and pruritus for several hours after application.

■ *Humectants* (Humilac, Allerderm/Virbac; Micro Pearls Humectant Spray, Evsco) and *bath oils* (HyLyt*efa, DVM; Sesame Oil Rinse, Veterinary Prescription; Alpha Keri Bath Oil, Westwood) help raise the pruritic threshold by eliminating dry skin conditions.
  • The most beneficial effects are seen when applied after the stratum corneum has been hydrated.
  • The most even distribution is achieved when the product (2–5 capfuls) is added to one-half gallon of water and used as a rinse after the bath.

■ *Antibacterial shampoos* include benzoyl peroxide (Pyoben, Allerderm/Virbac; OxyDex and Sulf-Oxydex, DVM) and chlorhexidine (Nolvasan, Fort Dodge; ChlorhexiDerm, DVM). Benzoyl peroxide shampoos have the added benefit of follicular flushing and antipruritic activity but can be very drying. Follow the bath with a humectant or bath oil rinse to cancel this side effect.

■ *Antiseborrheic shampoos* containing 2% sulfur and 2% salicylic acid (SebaLyt, DVM; Sebolux, Allerderm/Virbac) have mild antipruritic and antibacterial properties in addition to their ability to reduce the production of epidermal scale.
  • Tar shampoos, which usually are formulated with sulfur and salicylic acid, provide the additional benefit of strong degreasing activity but tend to be irritating.
  • Do not use tar products on cats.

Supplemental Readings

Bevier D: Long-term management of atopic disease in the dog. Vet Clin North Am 20:1487, 1990.

Griffin C: RAST and ELISA testing in canine atopy. *In* Kirk RW, ed.: *Current Veterinary Therapy X*. Philadelphia: W. B. Saunders, 1989, p 592.

Halliwell REW, Gorman NT: *Veterinary Clinical Immunology*. Philadelphia: W. B. Saunders, 1989, p 232.

Halliwell REW, Kunkle GA: The radioallergosorbent test in the diagnosis of canine atopic disease. J Allergy Clin Immunol 62:236, 1978.

Nesbitt GH: Canine allergic inhalant dermatitis: A review of 230 cases. J Am Vet Med Assoc 172:55, 1978.

Willemse TA. Atopic dermatitis. *In* Nesbitt GH, ed.: *Contemporary Issues in Small Animal Practice: Dermatology*. New York: Churchill Livingstone, 1987, p 57.

Willemse TA, Van Den Brom WE, Rijnberk A: Effect of hyposensitization on atopic dermatitis in dogs. J Am Vet Med Assoc 184:1277, 1984.

8 Food Hypersensitivity

Stephen D. White

Adverse reactions to foods have been well documented in small animals. The terms "food allergy" and "food hypersensitivity" have been used interchangeably in the human and veterinary medical literature to describe symptoms induced by food ingestion in which there are demonstrable or highly suspected immunologic reactions. The terms "food intolerance" and occasionally "food sensitivity" have been used when immunologic etiology is unlikely or has not been established. Although the etiology of abnormal reactions to ingested foods has not always been well established in small animals, common usage dictates the use of the terms food hypersensitivity and food allergy. The author prefers the former as being more accurate in describing an abnormal response of the immune system. For discussion of inhalant allergies, see sec. 5, ch. 7.

ETIOLOGY

The exact mechanisms of food hypersensitivity have not been delineated in dogs and cats. Reactions to food have been noted in dogs and cats that could be termed immediate (i.e., hypersensitivity type I, occurring within minutes to hours after ingestion) and delayed (i.e., type IV, occurring within hours to days of ingestion).

- Food contaminants such as pathogenic bacteria, toxins, food additives such as tartrazines, and vasoactive amines such as tyramine in cheese have all been implicated or suspected as mimicking food hypersensitivity in humans. Their importance in small animals is unknown.
- Suspected or confirmed dietary allergens are numerous in the literature and include beef, pork, chicken, cow's milk, horse meat, eggs, wheat, oats, fish, whale meat, soy products, and fungal contaminants in drinking water.
  - The author has identified fish as an offending allergen in 50% of cats with food hypersensitivity.
  - The vast array of foodstuffs used in commercial pet foods, as well as variable processing methods, probably accounts for the large numbers of allergens reported.

CLINICAL SIGNS

KEY POINT ▶ Age of onset of food hypersensitivity is variable, most animals having been fed the offending diet for at least 2 years. Owners seldom relate the onset of clinical signs to any recent change in diet.

No age, breed, or sex predilections have been noted in dogs or cats with food hypersensitivity. Clinical signs are variable.

- Pruritus is the most common sign in dogs; rarely, nonpruritic animals are reported. The pruritus is often distributed similar to that in inhalant allergies (i.e., feet, ears, face, and axillae). Cutaneous lesions noted in dogs include papules, erythema, epidermal collarettes, pododermatitis, seborrhea, and otitis externa.
- In cats with food hypersensitivity, clinical signs include generalized pruritus, miliary dermatitis, facial and head pruritus, pruritic angioedema-urticaria, eosinophilic plaque, eosinophilic ulcers, and erythema.
- Gastrointestinal signs (vomiting, diarrhea) have also been noted (see sec. 7, chs. 4 and 6). In cats, food hypersensitivity has been manifested as lymphocytic-plasmacytic colitis; there is little evidence to support dietary allergy as a cause of lymphocytic-plasmacytic enteritis in dogs.
- Neurologic signs (epileptiform seizures, malaise) and respiratory distress (asthma-like syndromes) occasionally have been reported.
- Multiple organ involvement is uncommon.

DIAGNOSIS

- The following situations may lead the clinician to an increased suspicion of food hypersensitivity:
  - Nonseasonal occurrence of pruritic skin lesions
  - Lack of response to steroidal or other anti-inflammatory drugs in dogs and cats
  - Lack of response to progestational drugs in cats.

Laboratory Findings

There are no consistent laboratory findings in small animals with food hypersensitivity. Peripheral eosinophilia may or not be present. Histopathologic findings are nondiagnostic, usually characterized by a perivascular dermatitis, with neutrophils or mononuclear cells predominating and variable secondary suppurative changes. Tissue eosinophilia is uncommon but has been reported.

Intradermal Skin Testing

Intradermal skin testing with food extracts usually has been unrewarding in humans and small animals, possibly owing to changes in composition of the allergen with digestion or to improper dilution of the test allergen.

Serologic Diagnostic Tests

Serologic diagnostics utilizing the radioallergosorbent test (RAST) or the enzyme-linked immunosorbent assay (ELISA) for reaginic antibodies have been used in human beings and correlate with history and provocative exposure tests in over 50% of cases reported. However, the data from two recent studies, one utilizing RAST (White and Mason, 1990) and one utilizing the ELISA test (Jeffers et al., 1991), have shown that these tests are of no value in small animals.

KEY POINT ▶ The most valid and most often used method for diagnosis of food hypersensitivity is the restricted ("hypoallergenic") test diet.

Hypoallergenic Test Diet

- Place the animal on a diet with a very limited number of foodstuffs, preferably those to which the animal has had little or no previous exposure. The author generally uses a diet limited to (non-instant) rice and lamb in a 1:1 mix for dogs, and a lamb-based baby food (Strained Lamb Baby Food, Gerber) for cats, simply because most small animals are not exposed to lamb on a routine basis. However, individualize the test diet on the basis of a careful dietary history.
- Hypoallergenic diets should be free of colorings, preservatives, and flavorings. Do not give palatable medications, such as certain heartworm preventatives (substitute another type of heartworm preventative for the duration of the diet), and omit all vitamin and mineral supplements.
- Commercially prepared pet foods, including prescription diets, diets containing no preservatives, and diets marketed as "natural," are *not* adequate test diets. These products do not meet the criteria for a true restricted test diet because of the many foodstuffs they contain and the processing of these ingredients.
- Clinical signs may recur when animals are switched from the home-prepared test diet to the aforementioned prescription or "natural" foods.
- Occasionally, an animal may be presented to the clinician with pruritus so severe that administration of oral corticosteroids is justified while the diet is in progress.
  - Administer prednisone or prednisolone, 0.5–1.0 mg/kg, q24h PO, for 10 days, and then stop.
  - Continue the diet for a minimum of 2 weeks beyond discontinuation of the medication in order to properly evaluate response to diet.
  - Apply the same guidelines when giving antibiotics to animals with secondary pyoderma.

Results

- Clinical improvement has been reported to occur from 24 hours to 3 weeks after starting the diet.

Recommended duration of the diet varies from 3 days to 8 weeks.
- In the author's experience, 4–6 weeks is a reasonable length of time in which to expect some improvement. Improvement is best defined as a reduction of pruritus (or other clinical signs if pruritus is absent).
- If only partial improvement is noted, the diet may not have been given long enough for full effectiveness.
- Alternatively, evaluate the restricted diet's content and consider a change (e.g., substitute potatoes for rice).
- Consider other, concurrent hypersensitivities, such as fleas and inhalant allergens.

TREATMENT

Once improvement is noted, several alternatives are open to the clinician.

- Ideally, challenge the animal with its original diet in order to substantiate the diagnosis. A relapse in the condition will usually be seen within 72 hours but may take as long as 10 days. The literature usually recommends adding individual foodstuffs to the restricted diet at 5- to 10-day intervals until a balanced diet is achieved or the offending allergen(s) is discovered.
- Many owners are unwilling to exacerbate a clinically improved animal or separate out various components of foods to determine potential allergens and are more interested in achieving a balanced, less expensive diet as soon as possible.
- When maximum improvement is noted on the test diet, the author usually changes the diet to a lamb-based (Prescription Diet d/d [dry], Hill's Pet Products, Topeka, KS) prescription diet, or one of several commercial diets without commercial additives (Cornucopia Natural Pet Foods, Huntington, NY; Nutro Max, Nutro Products, Inc., City of Industry, CA). If the new diet is not tolerated, most animals show a recurrence of clinical signs within 72 hours, although a few pets may take longer.
- If the animal cannot tolerate a commercial diet, use a home-prepared diet consisting of a protein and carbohydrate source supplemented with vitamins, minerals, and, for cats, sufficient taurine (60–100 mg of taurine daily). Supplementation with 0.5 teaspoons of clam juice per day, recommended by some, is *not* adequate taurine supplementation.

Supplemental Readings

Carlotti DN, Remy I, Prost C: Food allergy in dogs and cats: A review and report of 43 cases. Vet Derm 1:55, 1990.

Jeffers JG, Shanley KJ, Meyer EK: Diagnostic testing for canine food hypersensitivity. J Am Vet Med Assoc, 198:245, 1991.

Pion PD, Power HT, Rogers QR, Kittleson MD: Taurine for cats [letter]. J Am Vet Med Assoc 194:1005, 1989.

Prelaud P: The basophil degranulation test in the diagnosis of canine allergic skin disease. *In* Von Tscharner C, Halliwell REW, eds.: *Advances in Veterinary Dermatology, Vol I.* London: Baillière Tindall, 1990, p 117.

Rosser EJ: Food allergy in the dog: A prospective study of 51 dogs. Proceedings, American Academy of Veterinary Dermatology and American College of Veterinary Dermatology, 1990.

White SD: Food hypersensitivity in 30 dogs. J Am Vet Med Assoc 188:695, 1986.

White SD, Mason IS: Proceedings of the Dietary Allergy Workshop. *In* Von Tscharner C, Halliwell REW, eds.: *Advances in Veterinary Dermatology, Vol. I.* London: Baillière Tindall, 1990, p 404.

White SD, Sequoia D: Food hypersensitivity in cats: 14 cases (1982–1987). J Am Vet Med Assoc 194:692, 1989.

Immune-Mediated Dermatoses

Karen Helton-Rhodes

Immune-mediated dermatoses are a relatively uncommon group of diseases in domestic animals. This group may be divided into autoimmune and immune-mediated according to immunopathogenesis.

- Autoimmune diseases, which include the pemphigus complex, bullous pemphigoid, and Vogt-Koyanagi-Harada syndrome, are characterized by a specific antibody or cell-mediated immune response produced and directed against a normal component of the skin or body.
- Systemic lupus erythematosus and cutaneous (discoid) lupus erythematosus are examples of immune-mediated dermatoses in which antigen:antibody complexes are formed and then deposited in various locations (vessel walls, glomeruli of the kidney, or basement membrane zone of the skin) (see sec. 3, ch. 3). This deposition of immune complexes may then trigger an inflammatory response that results in tissue destruction.
- Vasculitis may be placed in the autoimmune or the immune-mediated category, depending upon the underlying etiology (see sec. 5, ch. 12).

PEMPHIGUS COMPLEX

The pemphigus complex of diseases includes pemphigus foliaceus (the most common of this group), pemphigus erythematosus, pemphigus vulgaris, and pemphigus vegetans.

KEY POINT ▶ Pemphigus foliaceus is the most common autoimmune skin disorder in dogs and cats.

- Pemphigus erythematosus is considered a variant of pemphigus foliaceus. It may have clinical and histopathologic features of lupus erythematosus and is therefore considered a "cross-over" between the pemphigus and lupus erythematosus complexes.
- Pemphigus vegetans is an extremely rare variant of pemphigus vulgaris that is distinguished clinically from the other autoimmune diseases by the production of lesions that are vegetative (i.e., proliferative) rather than pustular or ulcerative.

Etiology

The exact cause or stimulant of the production of the pemphigus antibody is unknown.

- Some investigators believe that a virus spread by an insect vector may be the initial stimulus. This theory gains support from the observation of an endemic form of pemphigus (fogo selvagem) in humans in South America.
- Genetic factors may be equally important.
- In humans, once formed, the antibody binds with components found in the core of the desmosome (desmoglein I or plakoglobin). Desmosomes function as attachment areas between keratinocytes of the skin. This binding stimulates plasminogen activators, serine proteases, which subsequently cause the conversion of plasminogen to plasmin.
  - The production of plasmin causes the disruption of the desmosome attachments and therefore a loss of keratinocyte adhesion. This loss of adhesion between adjacent cells is called acantholysis and the individual cells are termed acantholytic cells.
- All of the diseases in the pemphigus complex appear to have the same immunopathogenesis, but the location of the bulla or separation within the epidermis differs (e.g., pemphigus foliaceus has a more superficial bulla than pemphigus vulgaris).

Clinical Signs

Pemphigus Foliaceus

- Breeds that are predisposed include akitas, chow chows, bearded collies, dachshunds, Doberman pinschers, schipperkes, and rottweilers.
- Lesions consist of erythematous macules that progress rapidly to a pustular phase and then appear as a dry, yellow crust. These lesions may be limited to the pinnal, perioral, periocular, dorsal muzzle, nasal planum, and/or nail bed regions or they may be generalized.
- Animals may present with marked hyperkeratosis (scaling) of the foot pads with or without nail bed involvement. The nails usually are normal.
- Cats commonly exhibit a marked paronychia that appears as a thick "cheesy" core of exudate when the nails are extruded manually.
- Mucocutaneous and oral lesions are rare.
- Pruritus is variable.

Pemphigus Erythematosus

- Pemphigus erythematosus is a rarely recognized variant of pemphigus foliaceus.
- Collies appear to be at risk.
- Lesions are similar to those of pemphigus foliaceus but are limited to the face.
- Some animals may show depigmentation of the planum nasale.

Pemphigus Vulgaris

- Lesions are characterized as vesicobullous eruptions that rapidly ulcerate, leaving thick crusts.
- Lesions may be primarily mucocutaneous in location or generalized.
- Onychomadesis (loss or shedding of the nails) and foot pad ulcerations are common.
- Ulceration of the oral cavity may be an initial presenting sign in over 50% of cases.
- Pruritus and pain are variable.

Pemphigus Vegetans

- Pemphigus vegetans is an extremely rare variant of pemphigus vulgaris.
- Lesions usually are generalized rather than mucocutaneous.
- Lesions are vegetative (proliferative) or verrucous (wartlike).

Diagnosis

KEY POINT ▶ Histopathologic examination of skin biopsies gives the most valuable diagnostic information. Obtain at least three biopsies of the freshest pustules, vesicles, or bullae or from the edge of an ulcerated lesion.

Pemphigus Foliaceus

- Direct smear of an intact pustule or surface beneath a thick crust reveals numerous acantholytic cells.
- Complete blood count (CBC), serum biochemical profile, and urinalysis are nondiagnostic.
- Antinuclear antibody (ANA) tests are negative.

KEY POINT ▶ False-positive ANA titers may be seen in animals with pemphigus, rheumatoid arthritis, idiopathic thrombocytopenia, autoimmune hemolytic anemia, thyroiditis, endocarditis, cancer, hepatotoxicity, feline leukemia, feline infectious peritonitis, dirofilariasis, demodicosis, and flea allergy dermatitis, and even may be seen in clinically normal animals.

- Histopathologic findings include subcorneal and/or intragranular pustules with acantholytic cells.
- Direct immunofluorescent antibody (IFA) tests and direct immunoperoxidase staining (IPS) tests are positive, with intercellular staining of immunoglobulin and/or complement in the upper one third of the epidermis.

KEY POINT ▶ Indirect pemphigus titers using serum are unreliable in dogs and cats.

KEY POINT ▶ IFA is positive in only 50% of autoimmune cases, whereas IPS is very sensitive and is positive in 95% of confirmed cases. However, IPS is not very specific; positive results are obtained in 73% of animals with pyoderma, 67% with dermatophytes, 50% with demodicosis, and 100% with scabies. Also, IPS is

positive with the immunoreactant IgG in an intercellular pattern in biopsies obtained from normal canine planum nasale and foot pads. IFA is positive with the immunoreactant IgM in a basement membrane zone pattern in 75% of normal canine nasal biopsies and 45% of biopsies of normal foot pads, thus yielding false-positive results.

Pemphigus Erythematosus

- Direct smears are similar to those of pemphigus foliaceus.
- CBC, serum biochemical profile, and urinalysis are nondiagnostic.
- Antinuclear antibody (ANA) tests are positive, with low titers, in 50% of cases.
- Histopathologic findings include subcorneal and/or intragranular pustules, hydropic degeneration of the basal cell layer, and dyskeratotic cells.
- IFA and IPS are positive, with staining in the intercellular pattern with or without concurrent staining in the basement membrane zone.

Pemphigus Vulgaris

- Direct smears are similar to those of pemphigus foliaceus.
- CBC, serum biochemical profile, and urinalysis are nondiagnostic.
- ANA tests are negative.
- Histopathologic findings include suprabasilar pustules with acantholysis.
- IFA and IPS are positive, with intercellular deposition of immunoglubulin or complement in the lower one third of the epidermis.

Pemphigus Vegetans

- Direct smears are similar to those of pemphigus foliaceus.
- CBC, serum biochemical profile, and urinalysis are nondiagnostic.
- ANA tests are negative.
- Histopathologic findings include intraepidermal acantholytic eosinophilic microabscesses with significant surface crusting and verrucous vegetations and papillomatous proliferations.
- IFA and IPS are positive, with an intercellular staining pattern.

Treatment

General Considerations

Management is similar for each of the diseases in the pemphigus complex.

KEY POINT ▶ The goal in treating autoimmune skin diseases is to keep the condition in satisfactory remission on "safe" dose medication. It is better for the animal to have a few lesions present on low-dose alternate-day steroids than for the animal to have normal skin on high doses of daily steroids.

- For initial therapy choose prednisolone. If the response is poor, add a chemotherapeutic agent such as azathioprine to the protocol.
- For more rapid and complete resolution of clinical signs with less resistance to therapy, start with a regimen of prednisone and an adjunctive chemotherapeutic drug.
- Maintain medications at a high dose until clinical signs have resolved at least 75–85%, then gradually decrease dosages while monitoring the animal for exacerbation of disease.
- Taper either the prednisone or the chemotherapeutic agent first, depending on side effects noted.
- Another option is to alternate the dosage decreases of the two medications until there is complete remission and therapy is no longer necessary or until the minimal dosage of drug needed to control the disease is found.
- Initially, monitor CBC and platelet count every 2 weeks. After the disease is controlled and the level of medication is being tapered, gradually decrease the frequency of monitoring to every 1–2 months.

Therapeutic Protocols

Prednisone as a Single Therapeutic Agent

- Prednisone, 2–4 mg/kg, divided q12h PO (dogs) or 2–6 mg/kg, divided q12h PO (cats)
- Use in conjunction with sun blocks and topical steroids.
- Treatment of choice for pemphigus erythematosus

Prednisone with Azathioprine

- Prednisone, 2–4 kg, divided q12h PO, in combination with azathioprine (Imuran, Burroughs-Wellcome), 1–2 mg/kg q24–48h PO (dogs)
- Treatment of choice for pemphigus foliaceus, pemphigus vulgaris, and pemphigus vegetans
- Side effects of azathioprine include vomiting, diarrhea, pancreatitis, dermatitis, anemia, bone marrow suppression, and hepatotoxicity.
- Monitor CBC and platelet count every 2 weeks.

KEY POINT ▶ Do not use azathioprine in cats because of idiosyncratic reactions characterized by severe, nonresponsive leukopenia and thrombocytopenia.

Prednisone with Chlorambucil

- Prednisone, 2–4 kg, divided q12h PO, in combination with chlorambucil (Leukeran, Burroughs-Wellcome), 0.2 mg/kg, q24–48h PO
- Treatment of choice for pemphigus complex in small dogs and all cats
- Toxicity from this protocol is mild and includes vomiting, anorexia, and diarrhea (usually resolves when the dose is changed from a daily to an alternate-day regimen) and a mild, gradual, and rapidly reversible myelosuppressive effect.
- Monitor CBC and platelet count every 2 weeks.

Gold Therapy

- Aurothioglucose (gold salts) (Solganal, Schering) 1 mg/kg, q1wk IM, until remission is achieved (usually 6–8 weeks); then every 2 weeks for 6 months; then monthly as a maintenance regimen
- Prednisone, 2 mg/kg, divided q12h PO, also may be needed until remission is achieved.
- Gold therapy is suitable for both dogs and cats; however results appear to be much better in cats.
- Auranofin (Ridaura, SmithKline Beecham), an oral form of gold salts, has been tried in a limited number of cases but needs further investigation for use in dogs and cats.
- Side effects include thrombocytopenia, aplastic anemia, toxic epidermal necrolysis, stomatitis, nephrotic syndrome, hepatoxicity, dermatitis, and pancreatitis. Eosinophilia may herald toxicity.
- Monitor CBC, platelet count, and urinalysis every 2 weeks during the first 3 months of treatment and serum chemistry values monthly.

BULLOUS PEMPHIGOID

Etiology

The immunopathogenesis of bullous pemphigoid involves antibody production directed against the hemidesmosomes located in the lamina lucida region of the basement membrane zone of the skin. The complement cascade is then activated, causing the release of components C3a and C5a, which triggers mast cell degranulation. Mast cell mediators attract inflammatory cells that release lysosomal enzymes, resulting in tissue destruction and the production of a subepidermal blister.

Clinical Signs

- Bullous pemphigoid is a relatively uncommon autoimmune dermatosis.
- Collies, Doberman pinschers, and Shetland sheepdogs may be predisposed.
- Clinical signs and lesions mimic those of pemphigus vulgaris.
- Vesicles and bullae of bullous pemphigoid are more stable than those seen with pemphigus; this is most likely due to the depth of the lesion.
- Oral cavity lesions are common and occur in 80% of cases, but they are not usually the initial presenting clinical sign. Cutaneous or mucocutaneous vesicobullous lesions generally precede oral cavity involvement.
- Pruritus and pain are variable.

Diagnosis

- Direct smears are negative for acantholytic cells because this disease does not affect intercellular adhesion.
- CBC, serum biochemical profile, and urinalysis are nondiagnostic.
- ANA is negative.
- Histopathologic findings include a subepidermal cleft

or bulla with a lichenoid infiltrate of neutrophils and/ or eosinophils.
- IFA and IPS are positive, with a linear band of staining along the basement membrane zone.

Treatment

Therapeutic options are the same for bullous pemphigoid as those available for the pemphigus complex.

VOGT-KOYANAGI-HARADA SYNDROME
Etiology

The exact immunopathogenesis of Vogt-Koyanagi-Harada (VKH) syndrome is unknown. In humans, circulating lymphocytes from patients with VKH syndrome show significant cytotoxic activity against P-36 human melanoma cells. The factors responsible for the development of cellular hyperactivity against melanin-containing cells have not been determined. A deficiency of T suppressor cells, viral inducement of immunologic abnormality, and genetic factors have all been implicated.

Clinical Signs

- Akitas, samoyeds, and Siberian huskies appear to be predisposed.
- In humans, three phases have been recognized:
  - Meningoencephalitic phase—fever, malaise, headache, nausea, vomiting, and tinnitus
  - Ophthalmic phase—photophobia, uveitis, blindness
  - Dermatologic phase—leukoderma (acquired lack of skin pigment) and leukotrichia (acquired lack of hair pigment)
- Dogs appear to exhibit primarily the ophthalmic and dermatologic phases.
- Dermatologic lesions (leukoderma, leukotrichia) affect primarily the nose, lips, footpads, eyelids, and anus.
- Erosions and ulcerations may or may not be present in conjunction with leukoderma.

Diagnosis

- Direct smears are negative.
- CBC, serum biochemical profile, and urinalysis are nondiagnostic.
- ANA is negative.
- Histopathologic findings include a histiocytic interface dermatitis with pigmentary incontinence (histiocytes contain fine melanin granules).
- IFA and IP are negative.

Treatment

- Treatment is similar to that for the pemphigus complex.
- VKH syndrome is very difficult to control and usually requires high levels of prednisone and azathioprine.
- Ocular changes usually dictate the therapeutic course. For treatment of uveitis, see sec. 11, ch. 6.

LUPUS ERYTHEMATOSUS COMPLEX
Etiology

The exact immunopathogenesis of systemic lupus erythematosus (SLE) and discoid (cutaneous) lupus erythematosus (DLE) is unknown. Antigen:antibody complexes are produced and subsequently lodge in small vessels and the basement membrane zone of the skin (SLE and DLE) and in various organ systems (SLE). Genetic factors, T cell defects, B cell hyperactivity, hormonal alterations, and viral inducement of antigen:antibody complex formation have all been implicated. (See sec. 3, ch. 3 for more information about SLE.)

Clinical Signs
Discoid Lupus Erythematosus

- Collies, Shetland sheepdogs, German shepherds, and Siberian huskies are predisposed.
- There are no internal manifestations of disease except in very rare "potential" cross-over cases that, in time, become more consistent with SLE.
- The initial lesion is an area of depigmentation or erythema that slowly progresses to erosions, ulcers, and crusts.
- The planum nasale is the area most commonly affected although lesions have been noted on the eyelids, lips, foot pads, and concave surface of the pinnae and in the oral cavity.
- Profuse hemorrhage may occur following minor trauma to the planum nasale.
- Sunlight exacerbates the lesions and may play a role in the pathogenesis of DLE.

Systemic Lupus Erythematosus

- Collies and Shetland sheepdogs are predisposed.
- SLE is a multiorgan disease with dermatologic manifestations in 32–54% of cases.
- Cutaneous signs associated with SLE include ulcerative stomatitis, seborrhea, mucocutaneous ulceration, foot pad ulceration, panniculitis (lupus profundus), urticaria, and purpura.
- Noncutaneous signs of SLE (see sec. 3, ch. 3) include polyarthritis, fever, glomerulonephritis, hemolytic anemia, thrombocytopenia, polymyositis, neurologic signs, pleuritis, myocarditis, and lymphadenopathy.

Diagnosis
Discoid Lupus Erythematosus

- Direct smears are nondiagnostic.
- CBC, serum biochemical profile, and urinalysis are nondiagnostic.
- ANA is positive in 5% of cases of DLE (may indicate those animals with the potential for conversion to SLE that therefore should be closely monitored).
- Histopathologic findings include a lichenoid interface dermatitis composed primarily of lymphocytes and plasma cells, thickened basement membrane zone, hydropic degeneration of the basal cell layer, apop-

totic keratinocytes in the lower layers of the epidermis, pigmentary incontinence, and an excess of dermal mucin.
- IFA and IPS are positive, with a granular or rough band of immunoglobulin and/or complement deposited at the basement membrane zone.

Systemic Lupus Erythematosus

- Direct smears are nondiagnostic.
- CBC, serum biochemical profile, and urinalysis may show a variety of abnormalities, depending on the noncutaneous organs involved (see sec. 3, ch. 3).
- ANA is positive in 85–90% of cases.
  - The negative titers in 10–15% of ANA tests may be a laboratory "fault" because of the current inability of most laboratories to test for extractable nuclear antigens.
- The LE cell preparation is unreliable and not routinely used in veterinary medicine.
- Histopathologic findings include epidermal and dermal lesions similar to those seen in DLE and also may include leukocytoclastic vasculitis and mononuclear panniculitis.
- IFA and IP are positive, with a band of staining at the basement membrane zone of the skin and involved dermal and subcutaneous vessels.

Treatment

Discoid Lupus Erythematosus

- Administer *prednisone*: 2 mg/kg, divided 12h PO.
- *Topical corticosteroids* may be applied to the planum nasale and may be the only form of corticosteroid needed to treat and control mild cases.
- Apply *topical sunscreens* to the planum nasale during periods of sun exposure.
- Vitamin E 400 IU, q12h PO, may be helpful. Give vitamin E 2 hours before or after a meal.
  - Vitamin E has a 30–60 day lag phase, and therapy usually is maintained for the life of the dog.
  - No side effects have been reported in the dogs. Problems noted in humans include thrombophlebitis, hypertension, fatigue, cardiac disease, and diabetes mellitus.
- Severe cases of DLE may require the use of *azathioprine,* as described in the treatment of the pemphigus complex.

Systemic Lupus Erythematosus

- *Prednisone* and *azathioprine* combination therapy are recommended, as described for the treatment of pemphigus.
- *Gold salts are contraindicated* because of the potential for both the drug and the disease to produce glomerulonephritis.
- In severe cases of anemia and thrombocytopenia, *splenectomy* may be indicated.

VASCULITIS
Etiology

Most of the recognized vasculitic syndromes are caused by deposition of immune complexes within vessel walls. Complement components are then activated and act as chemoattractants for neutrophils. Neutrophils infiltrate the vessel wall and release lysosomal enzymes such as elastase and collagenase, which damage the vessel wall. Thrombosis, occlusion, hemorrhage, and necrosis may develop. Blood flow turbulence and hydrostatic tension may also play a role in the immunopathogenesis of vasculitis.

Inciting causes of vasculitis are varied and include allergic diseases, bacterial and viral infections, drug reactions, chemicals, neoplasia, SLE, rickettsial diseases, polyarteritis nodosa, rheumatoid arthritis, and cold hemagglutinin disease. (See sec. 3, ch. 3 for more information on vasculitis.)

Clinical Signs

- Vasculitis is a polysystemic disease.
- Dermatologic signs include petechia, ecchymoses, hemorrhagic bullae, ulcerations, urticaria, and edema.
- Noncutaneous signs are similar to those described for SLE.

Diagnosis

- Direct smears are nondiagnostic.
- Diascopy, the application of a glass slide pressed to an erythematous lesion, may help rule out vascular fragility. The lesion clears if the erythema is due to vascular dilatation but remains if hemorrhage or vascular leakage has occurred.
- CBC, serum biochemical profile, and urinalysis changes are dependent on the underlying etiology and on the target organ system.
- ANA is negative unless SLE is the underlying cause of the vasculitis.
- Histopathologic findings include leukocytoclastic vasculitis, fibrinoid degeneration of vessel walls, thrombosis, and endothelial swelling.
- IFA and IPS may be positive in early lesions, with immunoglobulin and complement detected in and around vessel walls. Affected animals will have high levels of circulating immune complexes and low levels of complement.

Treatment

- Treatment is similar to that described for pemphigus.
- Do not use steroids if there is an infectious etiology.
- Sulfone therapy (Dapsone, Jacobus), 1 mg/kg, q24h PO, may be used in cases of idiopathic neutrophilic vasculitis.

Supplemental Readings

Crawford MA, Foil CS: Vasculitis: Clinical syndromes in small animals. Compend Contin Educ 11:400, 1989.
Muller GH, Kirk RW, Scott DW: *Small Animal Dermatology,* 4th Ed. Philadelphia: W. B. Saunders, 1989, p 497.
Rosenkrantz W: Immunomodulating drugs in dermatology. *In* Kirk RW, ed.: *Current Veterinary Therapy X.* Philadelphia: W. B. Saunders, 1989, p 570.

10 Keratinization Defects

Kenneth W. Kwochka

Primary defects of keratinization are dermatoses that are manifested clinically by localized or generalized excess scale formation. The scale may be formed from the interfollicular epidermis or may emanate from hair follicles as comedones and follicular casts. Histologically, the most striking abnormalities involve the keratinizing structures of the body including the epidermis, hair follicle outer root sheath, and hair cuticle.

KEY POINT ▶ Cutaneous scaling of dogs is a very common clinical sign. In most cases, it is not due to a primary keratinization defect but is secondary to other dermatologic diseases. Conditions causing secondary scaling include demodicosis, scabies, cheyletiellosis, atopy, food allergy, flea allergy, pyoderma, dermatophytosis, hypothyroidism, hyperadrenocorticism, sex hormone abnormalities, pemphigus foliaceus, mycosis fungoides, and environmental influences. A primary keratinization defect is never diagnosed until the secondary causes of scaling have first been considered.

ETIOLOGY

For most of the diseases classified as primary keratinization defects, the pathophysiology is unknown. For others, the cause is known and the primary pathophysiology involves a defect in the keratinizing epithelium or the cutaneous glandular function.

- *Primary idiopathic seborrhea* is the most common chronic keratinization disorder in dogs. Predisposed breeds include cocker spaniels, English springer spaniels, West Highland white terriers, basset hounds, Irish setters, German shepherds, dachshunds, Doberman pinschers, Chinese Shar Peis, and Labrador retrievers. In cocker spaniels and Irish setters, at least part of the pathophysiology of scale formation involves hyperproliferation of basal epidermal keratinocytes.
- *Vitamin A–responsive dermatosis* is a rare, nutritionally responsive scaling disorder primarily in cocker spaniels. Similar syndromes have been reported in other breeds, including miniature schnauzers, Labrador retrievers, and Chinese Shar Peis in Europe. This condition is not a systemic vitamin A–deficiency but probably represents a local deficiency in the epidermis, a problem with uptake in the skin, a disorder of cutaneous utilization, or a positive pharmacologic effect of high doses on the epidermis.
- *Zinc-responsive dermatosis* is a rare nutritionally responsive scaling disease of several breeds of dogs, especially Alaskan malamutes and Siberian huskies. The incidence of this disease seems to be decreasing.
- *Epidermal dysplasia* is an extremely severe keratinization disorder reported only in West Highland white terriers. It appears to be a genetic keratinization abnormality, although the actual mode of inheritance and pathophysiology are unknown.
- *Lichenoid-psoriasiform dermatosis* is an extremely rare, probably inherited, keratinization defect. It has been reported only in English springer spaniels.
- *Schnauzer comedo syndrome* is a follicular keratinization defect of miniature schnauzers characterized clinically by multiple comedones along the dorsal midline of the back. It is probably genetic because of the exclusive occurrence in miniature schnauzers. There may be a developmental defect in the hair follicle leading to abnormal keratinization, comedo formation, follicular plugging and dilation, and secondary bacterial folliculitis.
- *Ichthyosis* is an extremely rare congenital keratinization defect of dogs, especially terriers, characterized by very severe scaling of the skin and footpads. The canine disease seems to most closely resemble lamellar ichthyosis seen in children. Ichthyosis may be an autosomal recessive trait in dogs, as it is in humans, although the exact genetics have not been studied.
- *Sebaceous adenitis* is an inflammatory disease process directed against the sebaceous glands of the skin. Predisposed breeds include standard poodles, Akitas, Samoyeds, and Vizslas. The pathophysiology is unknown but may include an inherited defect of sebaceous gland development; an immune-mediated sebaceous gland destruction; a primary follicular keratinization defect, with obstruction of sebaceous ducts and inflammation; and an abnormality in lipid metabolism, affecting sebaceous secretions and keratinization.
- *Idiopathic nasodigital hyperkeratosis* is a primary keratinization disorder characterized by excess keratin accumulation on the planum nasale, footpads, or both. It is most commonly seen in cocker spaniels and English springer spaniels, although any breed may be affected.
- *Canine ear margin dermatosis* is a rare idiopathic keratinization defect, which affects only the pinnae of the ears in a bilaterally symmetric pattern. This dermatosis occurs primarily in dachshunds.
- *Canine acne* is a fairly common disorder of follicular

keratinization resulting in comedones and secondary bacterial folliculitis and furunculosis. It is seen most commonly in short-coated breeds, especially English bulldogs, boxers, Doberman pinschers, and Great Danes. Canine acne may be due to abnormalities in sebaceous secretions, resulting in altered follicular keratinization, comedo formation, and secondary bacterial folliculitis. The organisms most commonly isolated are *Staphylococcus intermedius* and *Staphylococcus aureus*.

CLINICAL SIGNS

Disorders of keratinization are characterized clinically by mild-to-severe dry, waxy, or greasy scales. Some degree of "seborrheic odor" is associated with the skin condition. Because hair follicles and glandular structures may also be involved, it is not unusual to see comedones and follicular casts. *Comedones* are blackheads resulting from dilation of hair follicles with keratin plugs. *Follicular casts* are tightly adherent scale around hair shafts. Common secondary findings include alopecia, inflammation, crusts, pruritus with secondary excoriations, and pyoderma.

KEY POINT ▶ Primary keratinization defects are usually hereditary and appear during the first 2 to 3 years of life. A breed incidence for these disorders is known. An observant owner will usually indicate that the scaling was present prior to the development of secondary signs.

■ *Primary idiopathic seborrhea* has clinical signs ranging from dry scaling to greasy scaling, to scaling and greasiness with inflammation and pruritus, and any combination of these abnormalities on the same animal.
  • *Seborrhea sicca* describes the dry scaling of several breeds with primary idiopathic seborrhea. These animals have dull dry hair coats with focal to diffuse accumulations of white to gray nonadherent scales. Breeds affected with this form of idiopathic seborrhea include Doberman pinschers, Irish setters, German shepherds, and dachshunds.
  • *Seborrhea oleosa* is reserved for primary idiopathic seborrheic breeds with greasy skin and haircoat. These dogs have greasy, brownish-yellow clumps of lipid material that adhere to the skin and hair. The material on the hair shafts has been described as "nit-like." Concurrent ceruminous otitis is common. One of the most common owner complaints with this form is a severe rancid odor. The breeds most predisposed to this form include cocker spaniels, English springer spaniels, basset hounds, West Highland white terriers, Chinese Shar Peis, and Labrador retrievers.
  • *Seborrheic dermatitis* is a more severe variant of seborrhea oleosa. The clinical lesions are as described for seborrhea oleosa but additionally there is significant cutaneous inflammation, bacterial folliculitis, pruritus, and multifocal plaques of hyperkeratotic material with inflammation. The most common areas of the body involved are the external ear canals, ear pinnae, ventral neck, chest, axillae, and inguinal and perineal areas.

■ *Vitamin A–responsive dermatosis* has clinical signs consisting of refractory generalized scaling, dry haircoat with easy epilation, prominent comedones, and hyperkeratotic plaques with large "fronds" of keratinous material protruding from the follicular ostia. The plaques are usually on the ventral and lateral thorax and abdomen, but the neck and face may also be involved. Other clinical features include a rancid odor from the skin, ceruminous otitis externa, and varying degrees of pruritus.

■ *Zinc-responsive dermatosis* is typically divided into the following two clinical syndromes:
  • *Zinc-responsive dermatosis of Siberian huskies and Alaskan malamutes* is the first syndrome. It is also reported in Doberman pinschers and Great Danes.

    Alaskan malamutes have a genetic defect affecting zinc absorption from the intestines. Thus, the condition may occur even while the dog is on a well-balanced commercial diet.

    Zinc-responsive dermatosis may be precipitated by stress, estrus, and gastrointestinal disorders affecting absorption.

    Diets high in calcium and phytate (plant derived protein) may also precipitate the disorder by binding zinc in the gastrointestinal tract.

    Lesions usually develop in dogs before puberty or in young adulthood. They include alopecia, erythema, scaling, and crusting involving the face, head, scrotum, and legs. Lesions often encircle the mouth, chin, eyes, ears, prepuce, and vulva. Thick crusts may be found on the elbows and other pressure points of the body. The footpads may be hyperkeratotic. The haircoat is generally dull and dry.
  • *Zinc-responsive dermatosis of rapidly growing puppies* on zinc-deficient diets or oversupplemented vitamins and minerals, especially calcium, is the second syndrome. It is also seen with diets high in phytate.

    Commonly affected breeds include Great Danes, Doberman pinschers, beagles, German shepherds, German shorthaired pointers, Labrador retrievers, and Rhodesian ridgebacks.

    In addition to the scaling and crusting, the dogs have secondary infections, lymphadenopathy, depression, and anorexia. The most obvious cutaneous lesions involve the head, elbows, other joints, and footpads.

■ *Epidermal dysplasia* of West Highland white terriers develops in either sex, usually during the first year of life.
  • Clinical signs begin with erythema and pruritus of the ventrum and extremities. These rapidly progress to a generalized disorder ("armadillo disease") with severe erythema and pruritus, alopecia, hyperpigmentation, lichenification, lymphadenopathy, greasy skin and hair coat, rancid odor, ceruminous otitis, and secondary bacterial infection.
  • Some of the dogs have secondary *Malassezia pachydermatis* colonization of the surface and in-

fundibular keratin, which may contribute to the severity of the disease.

KEY POINT ▶ Secondary *Malassezia* colonization may be associated with any of the primary and secondary causes of scaling. Always look for the presence of this yeast with skin swabs, cytologic examination, and skin biopsies.

- *Lichenoid-psoriasiform dermatosis* of English springer spaniels has clinical signs including nonpruritic, erythematous, lichenoid papules and plaques, involving the pinnae, external ear canal, preauricular and periorbital skin, lips, prepuce, and inguinal region. Chronic cases have papillomatous-type lesions, which may involve the face, ventral trunk, and perineum. A more generalized distribution of greasy scales and crusts may also be present.
- *Schnauzer comedo syndrome* usually develops in young adult dogs. Clinical signs include crusted, papular comedones (blackheads) along the dorsal midline of the back, from the neck to the tail.
  - In the early stages and in mild cases, the lesions are difficult to visualize through the haircoat but are more easily palpated as "bumps" down the back.
  - Animals with advanced cases frequently have secondary bacterial folliculitis and, rarely, furunculosis. The lesions may be accompanied by pruritus and pain. The infection leads to alopecia, with a "moth-eaten" appearance to the coat. The condition is chronic—for the life of the dog.
- *Ichthyosis* is reported most commonly in terriers and terrier crosses. In most cases, the entire body is covered with tightly adherent fine white scales. Some may appear as feathered keratinous projections. Extensive alopecia, hyperpigmentation, and lichenification may occur. Large quantities of waxy adherent scales may also be produced, especially in the flexural creases and intertriginous regions. Severe footpad hyperkeratosis may be present with the margins more severely involved.
- *Sebaceous adenitis* has two different clinical presentations related to coat length as follows:
  - Long-coated breeds, such as standard poodles, Akitas, and Samoyeds, have *nonpruritic patchy or symmetric alopecia* with excess scale formation and dull brittle hairs. Specific areas include the dorsal planum of the nose, top of the head, dorsal neck and trunk, tail, and pinnae. Advanced lesions include tightly adherent silver-white scales, follicular casts, matted hair, and secondary bacterial folliculitis.
  - Short-coated breeds, such as Vizslas, have *circular areas of alopecia and scaling* of the head, ears, trunk, and extremities. These areas may enlarge and eventually coalesce into serpiginous patterns or diffuse alopecia.
- *Idiopathic nasodigital hyperkeratosis* may have focal or diffuse lesions characterized by tightly adherent, thick accumulations of keratin on the nasal planum, footpads, or both. This material is usually extremely dry and may be accompanied by cracks, fissures, erosions, and ulcers. Severe footpad involvement may result in pain and lameness.
- *Canine ear margin dermatosis* has greasy plugs adhering tightly to the skin surface and hair shafts on the pinnal margins. Alopecia may develop with time. Pruritus is usually absent. In severe, untreated cases a progression to ulceration and necrosis has been reported due to thrombosis of capillaries that supply blood to the pinnal margins. This condition may result in severe scarring and fissures.
- *Acne* lesions include comedones, papules, pustules, and furuncles of the chin, lips, and muzzle. In some cases, lesions are mild and inapparent to the owner. In others, severe cellulitis with multiple draining tracts and pain occurs. In most dogs, spontaneous resolution takes place after sexual maturity. However, in the short-coated breeds, it may be a recurrent problem for the life of the animal, especially if not treated correctly when young.

DIAGNOSIS

KEY POINT ▶ No specific laboratory test exists for a definitive diagnosis of a primary keratinization disorder. A combination of factors is used, including age of onset, breed, history, diagnostic elimination of the more common secondary causes of scaling, findings on histologic examination of skin biopsies, and response to therapy.

KEY POINT ▶ Skin biopsy (see sec. 5, ch. 15) is the most important diagnostic tool for primary keratinization defects. Biopsy results not only help to make a definitive diagnosis but also help to rule out dermatoses associated with secondary scaling. Take several biopsies from lesions of various ages. Send samples to a veterinary pathologist who specializes in dermatopathology.

- A definitive diagnosis of *primary idiopathic seborrhea* requires a number of different supporting factors, including age of onset, breed, history, diagnostic elimination of secondary causes of scaling, and findings on histopathologic examination of skin biopsy specimens.
  - The most important aspect of the diagnostic plan is a full investigation for secondary causes of scaling. The primary differentials are allergic dermatitis, scabies, dermatophytosis, demodicosis, bacterial folliculitis, hypothyroidism, and vitamin A–responsive dermatosis.
  - Biopsy samples are usually characterized by orthokeratotic and parakeratotic hyperkeratosis, follicular hyperkeratosis, and dyskeratosis. Often, the follicular abnormalities are more impressive than are the changes in the surface epidermis.
- *Vitamin A–responsive dermatosis* is characterized clinically by an early age of onset of refractory generalized scaling with hyperkeratotic plaques in cocker spaniels.

- A firmer diagnosis can be made with skin biopsy findings consisting of marked follicular hyperkeratosis and very distended follicular ostia, mild orthokeratotic hyperkeratosis of the epidermis, and mild irregular epidermal hyperplasia.
- Even with classic clinical and histologic findings, a definitive diagnosis can be confirmed only by response to supplementation with vitamin A alcohol-retinol.
- The major diagnostic differentials for this condition include primary idiopathic seborrhea, zinc-responsive dermatosis, generic dog food dermatosis, sebaceous adenitis, and superficial necrolytic dermatitis.

■ *Zinc-responsive dermatosis* is characterized clinically by early age of onset, dietary history, breed, and physical examination findings.
  - A firmer diagnosis is made with skin biopsy findings consisting of a marked diffuse surface and follicular parakeratotic hyperkeratosis and a hyperplastic superficial dermatitis.
  - A definitive diagnosis can be confirmed only by response to dietary zinc supplementation.
  - Important diagnostic differentials for this syndrome include demodicosis, dermatophytosis, pemphigus foliaceus, generic dog food dermatosis, and superficial necrolytic dermatitis.

■ *Epidermal dysplasia* is characterized clinically by early age of onset of severe ventral erythema and pruritus rapidly progressing to chronic lesions in a West Highland white terrier.
  - A firmer diagnosis is made with skin biopsy findings consisting of a hyperplastic perivascular dermatitis with epidermal abnormalities, including hyperchromasia, excessive keratinocyte mitosis, crowding of basilar keratinocytes, epidermal "buds," loss of epidermal cell polarity, and parakeratosis. Budding yeast organisms and gram-positive cocci may also be found in surface and infundibular keratin.
  - The principal diagnostic challenge in these dogs is to determine if the condition is caused by epidermal dysplasia, some other pruritic skin disease, or their combination.

    Primary diagnostic differentials that must be considered include atopy, food allergy dermatitis, scabies, and primary idiopathic seborrhea. These should all be evaluated by appropriate testing or response to therapy in the diagnostic workup.

    A definitive diagnosis of epidermal dysplasia can be made only with characteristic clinical and histologic findings and after these other diagnostic differentials have been eliminated.
  - Another challenge is to determine how much the secondary bacterial infection or the *Malassezia* colonization is contributing to the severity of the clinical condition. This can be assessed only by evaluating response after treatment with appropriate topical and systemic antimicrobial agents.

■ *Lichenoid-psoriasiform dermatosis* is characterized clinically by the early age of onset of refractory plaque-like lesions involving the face, ears, and ventrum in an English springer spaniel.
  - Perform skin scrapings and fungal culture to rule out the diagnoses of demodicosis and dermatophytosis.
  - The definitive diagnosis is made with skin biopsy findings. Histologic examination reveals a lichenoid dermatitis (i.e., a band of mononuclear cells in the superficial dermis) with psoriasiform epidermal hyperplasia, intraepidermal microabscesses, and Munro's microabscesses. Advanced lesions may show papillated epidermal hyperplasia and papillomatosis.

■ *Schnauzer comedo syndrome* is characterized clinically by dorsal follicular comedones in a miniature schnauzer.
  - A firmer diagnosis is confirmed by skin biopsy with dilated hair follicles filled with keratinous debris. Dilated or cystic sebaceous or apocrine glands, folliculitis, perifolliculitis, or furunculosis may be found.
  - Diagnostic differentials include demodicosis, dermatophytosis, and bacterial folliculitis.
  - Obtain a complete drug history in miniature schnauzers with comedo syndrome. Glucocorticoids are comedogenic, and long-term administration may precipitate or worsen the condition. I have also seen older miniature schnauzers with endogenous Cushing's disease develop dorsal comedones.

■ *Canine ichthyosis* is characterized clinically by congenital, severe cutaneous scaling and footpad hyperkeratosis in terriers.
  - Histologic findings confirm the definitive diagnosis. They include increased mitotic activity in the basal keratinocytes, a prominent stratum granulosum, a severe laminated orthokeratotic hyperkeratosis, vacuolated keratinocytes in the superficial epidermis, and a follicular hyperkeratosis and plugging.
  - Because of the congenital nature of this disorder, it is rarely confused diagnostically with other keratinization defects. However, if its presence at birth cannot be firmly established, the diagnostic differentials include zinc-responsive dermatosis, nasodigital hyperkeratosis, primary idiopathic seborrhea, canine distemper virus, pemphigus foliaceus, lupus erythematosus, hypothyroidism, generic dog food dermatosis, and superficial necrolytic dermatitis.

■ A tentative clinical diagnosis of *sebaceous adenitis* is made based on breed, history, and clinical findings.
  - A definitive diagnosis is made with the biopsy findings, including nodular granulomatous to pyogranulomatous inflammation at the level of the sebaceous glands.
  - Ask the pathologist to perform special stains for bacteria and fungi. Perform cultures for bacteria and fungi.
  - Advanced lesions are characterized histologically by a complete loss of sebaceous glands with periadnexal fibrosis.

■ *Idiopathic nasodigital hyperkeratosis* is diagnosed by finding nasal and/or digital hyperkeratosis without evidence of other concurrent diseases.
  - All diseases that may cause the lesions must be considered. Unfortunately, the list is long, including canine distemper virus, pemphigus foliaceus,

pemphigus erythematosus, lupus erythematosus, nasal solar dermatitis, hypothyroidism, zinc-responsive dermatosis, generic dog food dermatosis, and superficial necrolytic dermatitis. Pemphigus foliaceus and lupus erythematosus are the most common causes of nasal and digital hyperkeratosis.

- I recommend extensive diagnostic tests only when the condition is severe or when the clinical signs lead me to believe that one of the other more serious diseases listed previously is present. Idiopathic nasodigital hyperkeratosis is merely cosmetic for most dogs and requires neither extensive diagnostic workup nor treatment.
- When warranted, a complete diagnostic evaluation requires a good history; complete blood count; serum biochemical profile; thyroid evaluation with baseline T_4 and possibly a TSH stimulation test; biopsy for histologic evaluation; and antinuclear antibody test.
- Biopsy for direct immunofluorescence testing is valuable but taken from fresh lesions on other parts of the body. Skin from the nose and footpads commonly shows false-positive reactions.
- Histopathologic findings are most helpful in ruling out the diagnostic differentials. Abnormalities for idiopathic nasodigital hyperkeratosis are nonspecific and consist of irregular epidermal hyperplasia with severe orthokeratotic and parakeratotic hyperkeratosis.

■ In the early stages of the disease when scale only is present, the tentative clinical diagnosis of *canine ear margin dermatosis* is made by breed and clinical signs alone.

- Perform skin scrapings and fungal culture to rule out the diagnoses of scabies (a consideration only if pruritus is present), demodicosis, and dermatophytosis.
- Skin biopsy findings reveal prominent orthokeratotic and parakeratotic hyperkeratosis. However, biopsy is unnecessary and the ear margin is a difficult part of the body from which to remove tissue.
- The differential diagnoses are more extensive when the condition has progressed to ulceration and necrosis and include lupus erythematosus, pemphigus complex, cutaneous vasculitis, dermatomyositis, cold agglutinin disease, frostbite, drug reactions, and lymphoreticular neoplasms.

  Diagnostic procedures to differentiate these diseases include complete blood count, serum biochemical profile, urinalysis, skin biopsy for routine histologic examination and direct immunofluorescence, Coombs' testing, and antinuclear antibody testing.

  Skin biopsy specimens reveal necrosis and ulceration. Some sections may demonstrate vascular thrombosis. However, the changes are rather nonspecific and may be seen with many of the diagnostic differentials. Therefore, all of the aforementioned diagnostic tests are recommended to eliminate the differentials and to establish a definitive diagnosis of canine ear margin dermatosis.

■ A tentative clinical diagnosis of *canine acne* is made

by the history, age, and breed and the clinical appearance of the lesions.

- Differential diagnoses include demodicosis, dermatophytosis, and bacterial folliculitis.
- Perform skin scrapings and fungal culture in all cases.
- Cytologic examination of pustular contents or exudate from furuncles will confirm the presence or absence of suppurative inflammation and cocci. Consider culture and susceptibility testing in cases of deep infection, when a systemic antibiotic is to be selected.
- Skin biopsy findings provide a definitive diagnosis but are rarely needed.

TREATMENT

KEY POINT ▶ After a definitive diagnosis of a primary keratinization defect is established, warn owners that the condition is most likely controllable but not curable. Some type of topical and systemic treatment will probably be needed for the remainder of the patient's life.

Most of the primary keratinization disorders are treated with various combinations of topical antiseborrheic agents in shampoo formulations and systemic retinoids (i.e., vitamin A or its metabolites).

■ As in most primary keratinization disorders, the treatment goal in *primary idiopathic seborrhea* is to control scale formation, not cure the disease.

- Moisturize the skin and haircoat when dry scaling is present. This task is accomplished with twice weekly moisturizing hypoallergenic shampoos (HyLyt*efa, DVM Pharmaceuticals; Allergroom, Allerderm/Virbac) and frequent moisturizing rinses (HyLyt*efa Bath Oil Coat Conditioner, DVM Pharmaceuticals; Humilac, Allerderm/Virbac).
- When dry scaling is severe and some keratolytic activity is needed, the treatment usually consists of sulfur and salicylic acid shampoos (SebaLyt, DVM Pharmaceuticals; Sebolux, Allerderm/Virbac) followed by moisturizing rinses.
- Dietary supplementation with essential fatty acids (DVM DermCaps, DVM Pharmaceuticals) may also be beneficial.
- Use keratolytic and keratoplastic degreasing shampoos to control the scale and odor associated with seborrhea oleosa. Effective topical agents include coal tar (Clear Tar, Veterinary Prescription; NuSal-T, DVM Pharmaceuticals; T-Lux, Allerderm/Virbac; LyTar, DVM Pharmaceuticals; Allerseb-T, Allerderm/Virbac), benzoyl peroxide (OxyDex, DVM Pharmaceuticals; Sulf OxyDex, DVM Pharmaceuticals; Pyoben, Allerderm/Virbac), and selenium sulfide (Selsun Blue; Ross).
- The synthetic retinoid, etretinate (Tegison; Roche) has been effective for idiopathic seborrhea in cocker spaniels, springer spaniels, Irish setters, golden retrievers, and mixed-breed dogs at 1 mg/kg, q24h, PO. Response is seen within 2 months

and consists of decreased scale, odor, and pruritus, and softening and thinning of seborrheic plaques. Some dogs have been maintained without signs of toxicity over several months on alternate-day therapy.

KEY POINT ▶ The synthetic retinoids are associated with teratogenicity. Do not use in breeding animals, and warn clients about the serious potential risks from accidental human ingestion. Other potential side effects include keratoconjunctivitis sicca; pain in legs and joints; and mild elevations in cholesterol, triglycerides, and liver enzyme levels. These are usually reversible upon discontinuation of therapy or lowering the dosage.

- Use systemic antibiotics for patients with secondary bacterial folliculitis.
- A 7- to 10-day course of prednisone or prednisolone at an anti-inflammatory dose may occasionally be needed during periods of severe inflammation and pruritus in dogs with seborrheic dermatitis.

■ Treat patients with *vitamin A–responsive dermatosis* with 625 to 800 IU/kg, q24h, PO, of vitamin A alcohol (retinol).
- Improvement is seen within 4 to 6 weeks, complete remission is obtained by 10 weeks, and treatment is needed for life.
- Retinol at this dosage is well tolerated in dogs; therefore, no clinicopathologic monitoring is necessary.
- Keratolytic shampoos containing benzoyl peroxide have excellent follicular flushing activity. Twice weekly treatment helps remove keratinous debris from follicles and hastens recovery.

■ Treatment of *zinc-responsive dermatosis* depends upon the specific syndrome.
- The first syndrome of zinc-responsive dermatosis usually responds to zinc sulfate at 10 mg/kg, q24h or divided q12h, PO, with food. An alternative is zinc methionine (Zinpro; SmithKline Beecham) at 2 mg/kg, q24h, PO. Correct any dietary imbalances (e.g., high calcium and phytate). Symptoms resolve rapidly, but lifetime therapy is usually needed. Zinc may cause vomiting in which case lower the dose and give the medication with food.
- The second syndrome in puppies usually responds over time to dietary corrections alone. However, recovery may be hastened by supplementation as discussed for the first syndrome. Some puppies may need supplementation until maturity.

■ *Epidermal dysplasia* is generally nonresponsive to medical therapy. The prognosis is poor, especially if the condition is chronic and severe secondary changes have occurred.
- Two forms of therapy offer hope in at least some of these dogs. First, in patients with secondary *M. pachydermatis* colonization, there may be significant improvement in pruritus and skin condition with ketoconazole (Nizoral; Janssen) at 10 mg/kg, q24h, PO, and twice weekly application of topical ketoconazole (Nizoral Shampoo; Janssen) for 3 to 4 weeks.

Over time, the yeast colonization will return secondary to the keratinization defect. However, this problem can sometimes be controlled with periodic ketoconazole shampoos.

A sulfur and benzoyl peroxide shampoo (Sulf OxyDex; DVM Pharmaceuticals) has also been helpful in the long-term management of some cases.
- Second, in some cases seen very early in the course of the disease and before chronic cutaneous changes occur, a dramatic response may occur to immunosuppressive levels of short-acting glucocorticoids.

Administer prednisone or prednisolone at 1.1 to 2.2 mg/kg, q12h, PO, until the condition is controlled. Follow by a very gradual decrease in the dosage to alternate-day therapy for long-term maintenance.

Some patients experience relapse, whereas others remain in long-term remission.

Before such therapy is used, evaluate the patient for allergies and explain to the owner the side effects of long-term steroid administration.

■ *Lichenoid-psoriasiform dermatosis* is a waxing and waning dermatitis. Response is minimal to medical therapy.
- Antibiotics, especially erythromycin, may be helpful when secondary pyoderma is present.
- Prednisone at 2.2 mg/kg, q24h, PO, has improved lesions in some cases but has not resulted in complete remission.

■ The majority of cases of *schnauzer comedo syndrome* can be controlled with periodic application of benzoyl peroxide shampoos (OxyDex, DVM Pharmaceuticals; Pyoben, Allerderm/Virbac) to flush follicles and control secondary bacterial folliculitis.
- A combination benzoyl peroxide and sulfur shampoo (Sulf OxyDex; DVM Pharmaceuticals) is especially effective because of an enhanced keratolytic activity.
- Benzoyl peroxide gels (OxyDex Gel, DVM Pharmaceuticals; Pyoben Gel, Allerderm/Virbac) are helpful to remove tightly adherent comedones.
- Gentle agitation with a mildly abrasive sponge (Buff-Puff) helps to mechanically remove adherent comedones.
- Systemic antibiotics for a minimum of 3 weeks are indicated to control secondary staphylococcal folliculitis.
- If there is no response to topical therapy, the synthetic retinoid isotretinoin (Accutane; Roche) at 1 to 2 mg/kg, q24h, PO, has been very effective. Rapid response is seen within 3 to 4 weeks. After lesions resolve, most dogs can be maintained in remission without signs of toxicity on alternate-day therapy.

■ The long-term prognosis for *ichthyosis* is poor because of the severity of the scale formation and because of the continual therapy that will be needed for the entire life of the patient.
- Topical therapy is helpful, including warm water soaks to help remove scales, antiseborrheic shampoos (SebaLyt, DVM Pharmaceuticals; Sebolux, Allerderm/Virbac), antiseborrheic gels (KeraSolv, DVM Pharmaceuticals; Retin-A, Ortho) for lo-

cally severe lesions, lactic acid as a total body rinse or spray (Humilac, Allerderm/Virbac; Micro Pearls Humectant Spray, Evsco Pharmaceuticals), and a combination rinse of 75% propylene glycol and 25% humectants (Humilac, Allerderm/Virbac). Topical therapy, other than shampoos, is used twice daily until the scale and odor are controlled and then is used as often as necessary for maintenance.

- Excellent results have been obtained with isotretinoin (Accutane; Roche) at 1 to 2 mg/kg, q24h, PO, and etretinate (Tegison; Roche) at 1 to 2 mg/kg, q24h, PO. Remission is within 8 to 12 weeks. Some dogs can be maintained on alternate-day therapy.

■ Response to therapy for *sebaceous adenitis* depends upon the stage and severity of the disease.

- Immunosuppressive dosages of glucocorticoids may be effective very early in the course of the disease when severe inflammation is present.
- Isotretinoin (Accutane; Roche) at 1 mg/kg, q12–24h, PO, may be effective in refractory cases, especially in short-coated breeds. After remission is obtained, the goal is to gradually decrease the dosage to 1 mg/kg, q48h, PO.
- Etretinate (Tegison; Roche) at 1–2 mg/kg, PO, is effective and may be useful, especially in long-coated breeds.
- Cyclosporine (Sandimmune; Sandoz) has also been used in refractory cases at 5 mg/kg, q12h, PO.
- Topical therapy with sprays or rinses consisting of 75% propylene glycol and 25% humectants (Humilac; Allerderm/Virbac) are helpful when applied once daily.
- Other therapy consists of essential fatty acid dietary supplements, antiseborrheic shampoos and emollients, antibiotics, and antibacterial and follicular flushing shampoos.

■ Medical treatment of *idiopathic nasodigital hyperkeratosis* includes hydration of the hyperkeratotic tissue by water soakings or wet dressings followed by application of petrolatum jelly as an occlusive agent to help seal moisture into the stratum corneum.

- Although simple hydration may be adequate for mild lesions, more severe hyperkeratosis requires a topical agent with keratolytic activity. A gel containing salicylic acid, lactic acid, and urea (KeraSolv Gel; DVM Pharmaceuticals) is helpful as is topical 0.025 or 0.01% tretinoin gel (Retin-A; Ortho). The gel is used q12h until the condition is controlled, followed by application as needed for long-term maintenance. Irritation may be a problem, especially with tretinoin.
- Corticosteroid and antibiotic ointments, creams, or gels may be needed when severe inflammation or secondary infection is present.
- When very severe projections of keratin are present, especially on footpads and causing lameness, they may be surgically removed by trimming the dead tissue with scissors.

■ The mild scaling form of *ear margin dermatosis* is usually controllable but rarely curable with topical therapy.

- Periodic use with an antiseborrheic shampoo to remove the scales and waxy accumulations is all that is needed to control the mild form of the condition. Helpful agents include sulfur and salicylic acid (SebaLyt, DVM Pharmaceuticals; Sebolux, Allerderm/Virbac) and benzoyl peroxide (OxyDex, DVM Pharmaceuticals; Sulf OxyDex, DVM Pharmaceuticals; Pyoben, Allerderm/Virbac).
- A topical glucocorticoid cream, such as 1% hydrocortisone, may be needed in severe unresponsive cases or in those with severe inflammation.
- The advanced ulcerative and necrotic stage is resistant to medical therapy. However, the condition can usually be cured by surgical removal of the affected ear margin.

  Tissue is removed well into the normal portion of the pinna. This can be done to both pinnae, resulting in a symmetric and cosmetically acceptable outcome.

  The full list of differential diagnoses for this condition is considered before such aggressive surgery. The procedure will not be effective if the ulceration is due to autoimmune disease, vasculitis, or dermatomyositis.

■ Mild cases of *canine acne* need no treatment and spontaneously resolve with sexual maturity. Aggressive topical therapy may actually worsen the condition by mechanical trauma of inflamed hair follicles.

- For the more severely affected patient, treatment includes benzoyl peroxide shampoos (OxyDex, DVM Pharmaceuticals; Sulf OxyDex, DVM Pharmaceuticals; Pyoben, Allerderm/Virbac) and gels (OxyDex Gel, DVM Pharmaceuticals; Pyoben Gel, Allerderm/Virbac). These are applied twice daily until control is noted and then as needed for maintenance. Benzoyl peroxide is effective because of its follicular flushing and antimicrobial activity. It may cause cutaneous irritation in some animals.
- The most effective topical antibiotic for control of the secondary infection associated with canine acne is mupirocin (Bactoderm, SmithKline).

  This antibiotic has excellent activity against gram-positive cocci, is bactericidal, works well at an acid pH, is not systemically absorbed, and is not chemically related to other antibiotics. It penetrates well into granulomatous deep pyoderma lesions and, therefore, works well when furuncles and draining tracts have developed on the chin.

  Mupirocin is applied q12h. I often alternate it with benzoyl peroxide for the follicular flushing activity, which that agent offers.

- In recurrent cases or in those with deep infections, systemic antibiotics and warm water soaks are necessary.
- Short-term glucocorticoids, such as prednisone or prednisolone, at 1.1 mg/kg, q24h, PO, help reduce inflammation associated with foreign body granulomas secondary to ingrown hairs or keratin debris. This results in a more rapid response, but the steroids are administered for only 7 to 10 days, while the antibiotics are continued for much longer until the chin pyoderma has resolved.
- Cases refractory to more conventional therapy may

benefit from topical tretinoin (Retin-A; Ortho), q12h, or systemic isotretinoin (Accutane; Roche) at 1 to 2 mg/kg, q24h, PO.

Supplemental Readings

August JR, et al.: Congenital ichthyosis in a dog: Comparison with the human ichthyosiform dermatoses. Compend Contin Educ Pract Vet 10:40, 1988.

Gross TL, et al.: Psoriasiform lichenoid dermatitis in the springer spaniel. Vet Pathol 23:76, 1986.

Ihrke PJ, Goldschmidt MH: Vitamin A–responsive dermatosis in the dog. J Am Vet Med Assoc 182:687, 1983.

Kunkle GA: Zinc-responsive dermatoses in dogs. *In* Kirk RW, ed.: *Current Veterinary Therapy VII.* Philadelphia: W.B. Saunders, 1980, p 472.

Mason KV, et al.: Characterization of lichenoid-psoriasiform dermatosis of springer spaniels. J Am Vet Med Assoc 189:897, 1986.

Power HT, Ihrke PJ: Synthetic retinoids in veterinary dermatology. Vet Clin North Am 20:1525, 1990.

Scott DW, Miller WH: Epidermal dysplasia and *Malassezia pachydermatis* infection in West Highland white terriers. Vet Dermatol 1:25, 1989.

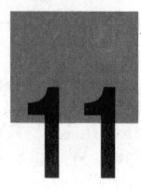

11 Growth Hormone–Responsive Alopecia and Sex Hormone–Associated Dermatoses

Lynn P. Schmeitzel

Growth hormone (GH)–responsive alopecia is an acquired symmetric alopecia of adult dogs that responds to growth hormone supplementation. The Pomeranian, poodle, chow chow, Samoyed, keeshond, and American water spaniel breeds are most frequently affected.

Sex hormone (SH)–associated dermatoses are skin diseases in any age, sex, or breed of dog that are caused by sex hormone imbalances or that respond to sex hormone treatment. A variety of organ systems including the skin may be clinically affected.

GH-responsive alopecia and SH–associated dermatoses are less common than dermatoses caused by hypothyroidism and hyperadrenocorticism (see sec. 4, chs. 1 and 3). However, these syndromes should be considered as differential diagnoses for suspected endocrine dermatoses of dogs.

ETIOLOGY

The cause of GH-responsive alopecia and of many of the naturally occurring suspected SH–associated dermatoses is unknown. Imbalances in growth hormone, estrogen, progesterone, and androgens often are suspected, although proof may be lacking. Imbalances in more than one of these hormones may be observed in the same dog.

Growth Hormone

- GH, also called somatotropin, is secreted by the pituitary gland.
- GH has anabolic effects on tissues that are directly mediated by the hormone and indirectly mediated by somatomedins, which are insulin-like growth factors produced in response to GH.
- In pituitary dwarfism, absolute GH deficiency causes alopecia and decreased elastin fiber content in the skin.
- Although some cases of GH-responsive alopecia are GH-deficient, a large number (up to 30%) have normal GH function tests, suggesting another etiology.
- Adrenal and gonadal sex hormone imbalances have also been observed in some dogs affected with GH-deficient alopecia. (See sec. 4, ch. 6 for further discussion of pituitary diseases.)

Estrogens

- Estrogens, including 17β-estradiol, estrone, and estriol, are produced by the ovaries, testes, and adrenal cortex and by peripheral conversion of androgens.
- Estrogens increase or decrease epidermal thickness, cause hyperpigmentation and sebaceous gland atrophy, decrease hair growth, increase dermal thickness, and decrease subcutaneous fat thickness.
- Hypoestrogenism and hyperestrogenism have been associated with clinical signs.
- Exogenous estrogen administration by any route may cause signs of hyperestrogenism in dogs.

Androgens

- Androgens, including dehydroepiandrosterone (and its sulfated conjugate), androstenedione, testosterone, and dihydrotestosterone, are produced by the ovaries, testes, and adrenal cortex and by peripheral conversion of weaker androgens to more potent androgens.
- Androgens increase epidermal thickness, pigmentation, sebum production, and dermal thickness and have variable effects on hair growth.
- In cases of GH-responsive alopecia, response to castration in the chow chow and other breeds and the presence of elevated serum androgen concentrations of adrenal origin in the pomeranian breed suggest that this syndrome may be associated with androgenic hormone imbalance.

Progesterone

- Progesterone is produced by the ovaries, testes, and adrenal cortex and is a precursor hormone for both androgens and estrogens.
- Progesterone has androgenic, synandrogenic, and antiandrogenic effects.
- Relatively little is known regarding the effects of progesterone on the skin, although hyperprogesteronemia has been observed in dogs with testicular tumors and GH-responsive alopecia.

Photoperiod

- Photoperiod regulates pineal gland hormone release.
- A reduction in photoperiod increases pineal hormone release, suppresses hypothalamic-pituitary go-

nadotropin release, and reduces sex hormone concentration.

■ Abnormal release of these hormones associated with changes in the photoperiod may cause seasonal flank alopecia.

Clinical Signs

Skin

■ *Alopecia* is bilateral and symmetric and involves the neck, trunk, caudal thighs, pinnae, and tail while sparing the head and distal legs.
- In SH-associated dermatoses the alopecia may begin in the perineum and flank regions.
- Bilateral flank alopecia may develop on a seasonal basis: fall/winter in males and spring/summer in spayed females.
- Some dogs develop complete alopecia of the affected areas; other dogs lose their guard (primary) hairs and retain their undercoat (secondary) hairs.
- Hair remaining in the affected areas is often dry and brittle, and epilates easily. Hair on the head and distal legs is usually normal in amount and texture.
- Presence of disease may not be known until the dog is clipped and the hair fails to regrow.
- In some dogs the first clinical sign is a failure to shed in the spring.
- Postpartum telogen defluxion is a "normal" generalized alopecia that develops about 6–8 weeks after whelping in certain bitches.

■ *Hyperpigmentation* usually develops after the alopecia and may be very intense, especially in GH-responsive alopecia.

■ *Coat color changes* are observed mostly in darker-haired dogs. Their coats may fade and develop a reddish tint.

■ *Skin* may be thinner, normal, or thicker.

■ *Linear preputial dermatosis* is a well-demarcated area of erythema or hyperpigmentation on the ventral aspect of the prepuce and may be observed in dogs with testicular neoplasms.

■ *Pruritus* is usually minimal or absent unless a secondary pyoderma or seborrhea is present also. Rarely, a hormonal "hypersensitivity" with intense pruritus may occur that disappears with neutering.

■ *Perianal adenomas* and *tail gland hyperplasia* have been associated with hyperandrogenism of gonadal or adrenal origin.

Reproductive Disorders

Reproductive abnormalities may or may not be observed in sex hormone–associated dermatoses. (See respective chapters for further discussion of these syndromes.)

■ *Gynecomastia* may be present in both sexes affected with SH-associated dermatosis. The nipples and/or mammary glands are enlarged, and a small amount of secretion may be expressed from the nipples.

■ *Feminization* is usually associated with hyperestrogenism. Affected males may lack libido, have a pendulous prepuce, and attract other male dogs.

Affected females often have an enlarged clitoris and vulva.

■ *Infantile vulva and mammary glands* may be observed in hypoestrogenism.

■ *Testicular abnormalities* often are observed in intact male dogs with sex hormone imbalances.
- A testicle may be enlarged because of a testicular tumor, and the opposite testicle will atrophy if the tumor is producing estrogen or estrogen-like hormone.
- Some dogs will have atrophy of both testicles.
- Some cases are unilateral or bilateral cryptorchid.

■ *Prostatic hyperplasia* may be associated with hyperandrogenism or hyperestrogenism (due to squamous metaplasia of the gland).

■ *Irregular heat cycles, pseudocyesis, and pyometra* may be associated with hair loss in the intact bitch.

■ *Libido* may be increased or decreased in the male dog. Some females may develop nymphomania or excessive mounting of other female dogs. Increased aggression may develop concurrently with increased libido, primarily when hyperandrogenism is present.

■ *Vaginal hyperplasia/prolapse* may be observed in hyperestrogenism.

Other Clinical Signs

■ Urinary incontinence in the spayed female may be associated with hypoestrogenism.

■ Bone marrow suppression may be associated with hyperestrogenism.

DIAGNOSIS

KEY POINT ▶ Before making a diagnosis of GH-responsive alopecia or SH-associated dermatosis, rule out hypothyroidism and hyperadrenocorticism with appropriate function tests (as described in sec. 4, chs. 1 and 3).

Signalment

GH-Responsive Alopecia. This syndrome usually develops in young adult dogs of the Pomeranian, chow chow, poodle, Samoyed, keeshond, and American water spaniel breeds near the onset of puberty, although any age may be affected.

SH-Associated Dermatoses. These may develop in any age, sex, or breed of dog.

■ Recently a castration-responsive dermatosis (Woolly syndrome) in Siberian huskies, Alaskan malamutes, and keeshonds has been described.

■ Seasonal flank alopecia occurs in intact and castrated male Airedale terriers, English bulldogs, and boxers; and in spayed female English bulldogs, boxers, miniature schnauzers, and miniature poodles.

History

Identify any reproductive abnormalities or behavior changes and their association with the development of skin lesions.

Physical Examination

- Evaluate the skin for secondary seborrhea and pyoderma and for perianal adenomas.
- Evaluate the testicles, vulva, nipples, and mammary glands for asymmetry, enlargement, or atrophy. Squeeze the nipples to determine if a secretion can be expressed.
- Palpate the abdomen for an enlarged uterus (pyometra) or abdominal mass (from ovarian tumor or from testicular tumor in a cryptorchid animal).
- Palpate the prostate for enlargement.
- Examine the mucous membranes for color (paleness) and petechiae.
- Palpate sublumbar lymph nodes for enlargement.

Laboratory Tests

Serum Biochemical Profile, Urinalysis, Complete Blood Count (CBC), and Platelet Count

- Perform these tests in dogs with bilateral symmetric alopecia to identify abnormalities indicating other differentials such as hypothyroidism (see sec. 4, ch. 1) and hyperadrenocorticism (see sec. 4, ch. 3), or to identify severe metabolic derangements causing telogen/anagen defluxion.
- A CBC and platelet count may reveal anemia, leukopenia, and thrombocytopenia in dogs with hyperestrogenism.

Skin Scrapings and Fungal Cultures

Use these tests to rule out demodicosis and dermatophytosis as causes of the alopecia.

Preputial or Vaginal Cytology

Cytologic examination can reveal cornified cells with pyknotic or absent nuclei in dogs with hyperestrogenism.

Skin Biopsy

- See sec. 5, ch. 15 for technique.
- Take skin biopsy to confirm presence of an endocrinopathy, such as orthokeratotic hyperkeratosis, follicular keratosis and dilatation, telogenization of hair follicles (follicular atrophy), epidermal melanosis, epidermal atrophy, and sebaceous gland atrophy.
- Histologically, some cases of hyperestrogenism may have a superficial perivascular dermatitis (spongiotic or hyperplastic) instead of an endocrinopathy.
- Skin biopsy can also identify a secondary pyoderma.

Radiography

- Abdominal radiography and ultrasonography identify intra-abdominal testicular and ovarian masses and sublumbar lymphadenopathy, indicating possible metastasis.
- Thoracic radiography identifies ovarian and testicular tumor metastases.

Endocrine Function Tests

- Perform thyroid function tests before evaluating sex hormones in most cases (see sec. 4, ch. 1).

- Adrenal function tests:
  - Perform a low-dose dexamethasone suppression test before evaluating sex hormones in most cases to determine if hypercortisolemia (see sec. 4, ch. 3) is present.
  - An adrenocorticotropic hormone (ACTH) stimulation test evaluates adrenal gland production of sex hormones and their precursor hormones. The samples can be sent to the University of Tennessee College of Veterinary Medicine (contact author for details) for testing.
- Baseline sex hormones
  - Most laboratories evaluate 17β-estradiol, progesterone, and testosterone.
  - Results may be "normal" in SH-associated dermatoses because many sex hormones are not being measured (e.g., dihydrotestosterone, estrone, estriol, biosynthetic precursors).
- GH function tests are not available commercially.

Laparoscopy or Exploratory Surgery

Surgery may be necessary to identify ovarian cysts and tumors in females and cryptorchid testicular tumors in males.

TREATMENT

GH-responsive alopecia may respond to neutering, sex hormone alterations, or GH supplementation. SH-associated dermatoses may respond to neutering or sex hormone alterations. If response is not observed with one therapeutic modality, switch to another modality.

KEY POINT ▶ *Neutering* is the treatment of choice in intact animals affected with GH-responsive alopecia or SH-associated dermatoses.

Sex Hormone Supplementation

Diethylstilbestrol (DES, Lilly)

- Give 0.1 mg up to 1.0 mg total dose, q24h PO, for 3 weeks; stop for 1 week; then repeat the 3-week treatment.
- Observe for response in 3 months.
- After response is achieved, continue the same dose once or twice weekly for maintenance.
- If estrogen therapy causes signs of estrus, reduce dose by one-half.

KEY POINT ▶ *Caution:* Estrogen therapy may cause fatal bone marrow suppression manifested by anemia, leukopenia, and thrombocytopenia. This is most likely after repositol injections of estradiol cyclopropionate. Perform weekly CBC and platelet counts while dogs are on daily DES therapy.

Methyltestosterone (Metandren; Ciba) or Fluoxymestrone (Halotestin; Upjohn).

- Give 0.5 mg/kg up to 30 mg total dose, q48h PO, for 3 months.

- After response is achieved, continue same dose once or twice weekly for maintenance.
- Possible side effects include aggressive behavior, hepatotoxicity, prostatic hypertrophy, and perianal gland hypertrophy.

Growth Hormone Supplementation

- Use only after neutering and sex hormone supplementation have been tried and shown to be ineffective.
- This product is available on a very limited basis, although bovine somatotropin may become readily available in the future.
- Give 0.1 IU/kg three times per week, SQ, for 4 to 6 weeks.
- Observe for response in 4–6 weeks after completion of therapy.
- Remission of clinical signs after discontinuing GH varies from 6 months to greater than 3 years.
- Review the effects of GH excess (acromegaly) in sec. 4, ch. 6.

KEY POINT ▶ Growth hormone is diabetogenic, and dogs treated with GH may develop transient or permanent diabetes mellitus.

Measure fasting blood glucose levels before and weekly during GH supplementation. Discontinue supplementation if hyperglycemia persists.

Other Therapies

Megestrol acetate (Ovaban; Schering) may be effective for its antiandrogen effects. Mitotane (Lysodren; Bristol-Myers) can be used in dogs with excessive adrenal gland production of sex hormones (see sec. 4, ch. 3).

Supplemental Readings

Lothrop CD, Jr: Pathophysiology of canine growth hormone-responsive alopecia. Compend Contin Educ 10:1346, 1988.

Miller WH, Jr: Sex hormone-related dermatoses in dogs. *In* Kirk RW, ed.: *Current Veterinary Therapy X*. Philadelphia: W. B. Saunders, 1989, p 595.

Schmeitzel LP: Sex hormone-related and growth hormone-related alopecias. Vet Clin North Am [Small Anim Pract] 20:1579, 1990.

Schmeitzel LP, Lothrop CD Jr: Hormonal abnormalities in Pomeranians with normal coat and in Pomeranians with growth hormone-responsive dermatosis. J Am Vet Med Assoc 197:1333, 1990.

Scott DW: Seasonal flank alopecia in ovariohysterectomized dogs. Cornell Vet 80:187, 1990.

Necrotizing Skin Diseases

Gail A. Kunkle

ETIOLOGY

Necrotizing dermatitis has many causes (Table 1). The etiology may be autoimmune, drug-induced, environmental, or infectious. Other causes include vasculitis, neoplasia, toxic epidermal necrolysis, erythema multiforme, vascular compromise, and necrolytic migratory erythema.

Autoimmune Diseases

Autoimmune diseases that affect the skin can be systemic or confined to the cutaneous tissues alone. These include the lupus erythematosus complex, bullous pemphigoid, the pemphigus complex, and cold agglutinin disease. Autoimmune skin diseases are discussed elsewhere (see sec. 5, ch. 9).

Vasculitis

Vasculitis is an inflammatory process that occurs in blood vessels and can result in necrosis of the vessels and subsequent death of the adjacent tissue. Several factors may initiate vasculitis. Necrotizing vasculitis can be seen with a variety of infections caused by bacteria (especially when infection is widespread), viruses, disseminated fungi, and tick-borne organisms such as *Rickettsia rickettsii.*

Systemic autoimmune disease can result in the deposition of immune complexes within vessel walls, leading to complement activation and influx of neutrophils. Subsequent release of enzymes from the neutrophils in the vessel walls can lead to vessel necrosis, thrombosis, and death of the surrounding tissue. Systemic diseases including neoplasia may similarly result in vessel wall necrosis through toxin production.

Specific drugs can induce lesions of vasculitis in animals; the antifungal drug, itraconazole, at dosage of 5 mg/kg, q12h PO, has been observed to cause vasculitides in some dogs. Allergic vasculitis that is leukocytoclastic has been noted in the skin of animals in association with drug administration, especially antibiotics. Focal cutaneous vasculitis has been reported at the site of rabies vaccination. Unfortunately, a specific cause of vasculitis cannot be elucidated in a significant number of cases.

Neoplasia

Neoplasia can lead to necrosis of the skin through a variety of mechanisms. As mentioned previously, neoplasia can cause vasculitis. Through release of necrosis factors generated by the tumor cells, there may be local death of tissues. Also, the encroaching growth of a rapidly advancing lesion may cause circulatory compromise leading to cutaneous tissue necrosis. A wide variety of neoplastic conditions may cause dermal necrosis, such as cutaneous lymphosarcoma.

Drug-Induced Necrosis

Necrotizing dermatosis is a rare side effect of various drugs. Drugs may induce hypersensitivity that is manifested in a variety of ways. Toxic epidermal necrolysis and erythema multiforme are commonly associated with drug administration (described subsequently). Other cutaneous lesions associated with drug administration in the dog and cat include vesiculobullous eruptions that may precede ulceration, and purpura that may subsequently appear necrotic. Mechanisms for necrosis and ulceration of the skin in drug reactions have not been clearly defined.

Toxic Epidermal Necrolysis and Erythema Multiforme

These disorders are considered together here because the causes of both are similar. The histology and clinical courses of the two, however, are quite separate. Drugs known to cause toxic epidermal necrolysis in the dog and cat and also implicated in erythema multiforme include levamisole, penicillins, cephalosporins, sulfonamides, gold salts, 5-fluorocytosine, and antiserum. Infections, toxins, malignancies, and systemic diseases such as cholanagiohepatitis, hepatic necrosis, and endocarditis have also been associated with these disorders. In some cases, initiating factors are not identified.

Environmental Factors

Environmental factors associated with necrosis and/or ulceration of the cutaneous tissues include not only chemicals but also agents found in the natural environment, such as spiders and snakes and heat (e.g., sunlight, burns), and cold (frostbite).

- *Contact irritant chemicals* can caustically burn or necrose the skin after topical exposure. The list of primary irritants is extensive and includes soaps, detergents, insecticidal sprays, fertilizers, and caustics such as strong acids or alkalies.
- *Snakes,* including pit vipers (copperhead, cottonmouth, and rattlesnake) and coral snakes, produce venoms that alter the integrity of blood vessels, blood cells, and coagulation; affect the nervous system; and result in necrosis at the site of envenomation.

TABLE 1. Classification and Causes of Necrotizing Dermatoses

Category	Cause

Autoimmune	Lupus erythematosus (see sec. 5, ch. 9)
	    Systemic
	    Discoid
	Bullous pemphigoid (see sec. 5, ch. 9)
	Pemphigus complex (see sec. 5, ch. 9)
	    Pemphigus vulgaris
	Cold agglutinin disease
	Vasculitis

Vasculitis	Sepsis Immune-mediated Systemic disease Drug-induced Hypersensitivity Idiopathic
Neoplasia	Squamous cell carcinoma (see sec. 3, ch. 9) Mast cell (see sec. 3, ch. 7) Lymphoma (see sec. 3, ch. 6) Other tumors (see sec. 3, ch. 9)
Drug-induced	Antibiotics Biologicals Barbiturates Phenylbutazone Gold salts
Toxic epidermal necrolysis/erythema multiforme	Drug-induced Systemic disease Neoplasia Idiopathic
Environmental	Contact irritant Snake bite Spider bite Radiation Burns Frostbite Decubitus ulcers
Infectious	Bacterial cellulitis (see sec. 5, ch. 1) Deep fungal infection (see sec. 2, ch. 12)
Vascular compromise	Thrombovascular necrosis Mechanical occlusion Diabetes mellitus (see sec. 4, ch. 4)
Necrolytic migratory erythema	Hepatopathy/cirrhosis (see sec. 7, ch. 8) Diabetes/glucagonoma

- *Spiders* (e.g., brown recluse) cause necrotizing skin lesions by injection of a potent dermonecrotic toxin into the tissue when they bite. The enzymes in the venom and the immunologic response of the host both play a role in dictating the clinical response.
- *Radiation injuries* may be acute or chronic, and necrosis and ulceration of the tissue can occur days to weeks after exposure.
- *Burn injuries* can result from heat, sun, flames, scalding liquids, friction, and electricity.
- *Frostbite* occurs when exposure to environmental cold results in vasoconstriction so severe that the effects are not totally reversible upon rewarming of the tissues.
- *Decubitus ulcers* are a form of vascular compromise related to environmental conditions, characterized by loss of soft tissue cushion over bony prominences.

Infection

Necrosis of the skin can result from local bacterial or fungal cellulitis. Another mechanism for necrosis in infections is vasculitis, as discussed previously.

Vascular Compromise

Vascular compromise can occur whenever there is interruption of the normal circulation to an area of tissue. This is involved in many of the aforementioned conditions and can be the result of a thrombus, vasculopathy, or mechanical or pressure constriction.

Necrolytic Migratory Erythema

This condition, also known as diabetic dermatopathy, can occur secondary to diabetes mellitus or cirrhosis. The exact metabolic etiology is unknown.

CLINICAL SIGNS

Autoimmune Diseases

- Animals usually present with an acute combination of dermatologic clinical signs, including vesicles, bullae, ulcers, hemorrhagic nodules, and erosive lesions.
- The mucocutaneous junctions sometimes are also involved.
- The animal is generally middle-aged or older and may have other systemic signs.
- See sec. 5, ch. 9 for discussion of autoimmune diseases.

Vasculitis

- The most common clinical signs are necrosis and ulceration, especially of the pressure points, the foot pads, the pinnae, and the extremities. Limb edema may also occur.
- Mucocutaneous ulcers may or may not be prominent.
- Fever, lymphadenopathy, anorexia, and depression may be present.
- Signs may be chronic or gradual in onset or may be acute.

Neoplasia

- Clinical signs depend on the type and location of the tumor as well as the stage of the disease.
- In epidermotropic lymphoma and in some cases of cutaneous lymphoma, ulceration and necrosis of the tissues at the mucocutaneous junctions may be seen with or without obvious tumors.
- In other cases of cutaneous lymphoma, multifocal cutaneous necrotic lesions may occur without mucocutaneous lesions.

Drug-Induced Necrosis

- Drug-induced cutaneous lesions have variable presentations and can mimic almost any condition.
- When due to a systemically administered drug, the cutaneous lesions frequently start out focally but rapidly become generalized.

- The exception to the above is the *fixed drug eruption,* which always occurs in the same local area on subsequent exposures. Fixed drug reactions can result in focal ulceration.
- Most drug eruptions begin either at the mucocutaneous junctions or on the trunk.
- Initially, there may be generalized erythroderma or erythematous macules, followed by vesiculation and then necrosis or ulcerated skin. Historically these may occur during the first exposure to a drug. They do not usually develop clinically until after 5–7 days of drug administration.
- Drug reactions to topically applied drugs can occur if the animal has an idiosyncratic reaction or more often if prior exposure has induced hypersensitivity.
- Contact allergic dermatitis can be the result of a topical drug, and extensive ulceration can occur, especially if the diagnosis is not made early.

Erythema Multiforme/Toxic Epidermal Necrolysis

Erythema Multiforme (EM)

- EM tends to be less severe than TEN.
- Multifocal lesions may appear papular, macular, vesicular, bullous, or target-like, with central areas of redness surrounded by an erythematous ring.
- The patient may show systemic signs of malaise and fever.
- Cutaneous lesions usually progress to multifocal ulceration.

Toxic Epidermal Necrolysis (TEN)

- The initial signs of TEN may be similar to those of EM, but it is a much more serious disease.
- Eventually full-thickness necrosis and sloughing of the skin occur, often involving large areas of skin and with the clinical appearance of burned skin.
- Skin that at first glance may look fully haired and normal will slide to one side and then can be totally lifted from the underlying dermis (Nikolsky sign).

KEY POINT ▶ Because of the extensiveness of TEN, it is crucial to pursue an early diagnosis and to eliminate the inciting cause as quickly as possible while providing aggressive supportive therapy.

Environmental Factors

Clinical signs of necrotizing dermatoses resulting from environmental causes depend on the specific etiology.

Contact Irritant Dermatitis

- This condition can occur wherever the skin was exposed to the irritant.
- The feet, scrotum, and ventral abdomen usually are involved if the animal had walked or lain on the causative agent.
- The muzzle or oral cavity may be involved if the animal tried to remove the caustic compound orally.
- Various other distributions can also occur.

Snake Bites

- Most snake bites occur during the spring and summer in rural regions with a large indigenous population of venomous snakes.
- The face and extremities are common sites of involvement.
- Cutaneous lesions begin with localized soft tissue swelling that spreads rapidly.
- Local hemorrhage occurs, followed by necrosis of tissue and sloughing.

Spider Bites

- Spider bites commonly occur on the face and extremities.
- The bite generally is accompanied by relatively little swelling. Pain, pruritus, erythema, and local discomfort usually follow much later than with snake bites.

Radiation

- Radiation injury occurs in the anatomic area where radiation has been previously administered.
- Clinical signs include erythema of the skin, moist desquamation, pigmentation or change in hair color, and loss of hair.

Burns

- Thermal burns can cause significant necrosis and loss of skin.
- The history usually identifies a potential source of injury such as heat, flames, scalding liquids, friction, sun, and electricity.
- Depending on the depth of the burn, necrosis may involve only the epidermis or may extend deeper into the tissues.
- Clinical signs usually include pain, erythema, and eschar formation on full-thickness burns.
- Deeper burns may result in shock, electrolyte and protein disturbances, and life-threatening secondary bacterial infection.

Frostbite

- Frostbite is most commonly seen as necrosis and sloughing of the tips of the ears or tail after exposure of the animal to intense cold.
- In the dog, the scrotum frequently is affected.
- Debilitated animals are more susceptible because of immobility and poor circulation.

Decubitus Ulcers

- Decubitus ulcers usually are secondary to pressure necrosis in recumbent animals.
- Stifles, elbows, hocks, and other pressure points are common sites.
- Lesions are well demarcated, with full-thickness necrosis usually extending to the underlying musculature.

Infection

- Necrosis due to infectious causes usually is seen as local areas of bacterial cellulitis or abscessation secondary to trauma or to embedded foreign bodies.

- Immunologic response to the infection or foreign body causes central necrosis of the tissue due to release of neutrophilic enzymes. The lesion ruptures and drains externally at the most necrotic site.

Vascular Compromise

- Sloughing or ulcerated lesions usually occur in the tissues in which the circulation has been disturbed.
- Thrombovascular necrosis often occurs in dachshunds on the most dependent portion of the aural pinnae.
- With mechanical occlusion of the circulation, the necrotic lesion will be distal or beneath the obstruction. For example, a rubber band tightened around the tail over time will cause underlying tissue death and sloughing of the distal tail.
- In diabetes mellitus, vasculopathies may rarely occur in the extremities of dogs and cats. Usually there is a chronic ulcerated lesion on an extremity that fails to heal even with treatment.

Necrolytic Migratory Erythema

- This condition generally involves ulceration of the mucocutaneous junctions, face, foot pads, and extremities.
- Often extensive crusts are present over the ulcerated areas.

DIAGNOSIS

The diagnostic approach to necrotizing skin disease must be quickly initiated. It should be as thorough as possible to increase the chance of a definitive diagnosis. Extensive necrosis of the skin is a dermatologic emergency and may result in death.

KEY POINT ▶ Diagnosis is best made by routine histopathology from representative primary cutaneous lesions and/or tissue samples adjacent to necrosis, in conjunction with a careful history and thorough physical examination.

History

- Identify or exclude several of the potential etiologies of necrotizing dermatoses.
- Record environmental factors and take a thorough drug history.
- Establish a careful timetable of events. The owner's description of the earliest cutaneous lesions and onset of any systemic signs are important aspects of the diagnosis.

Physical Examination

- Thoroughly examine all of the skin, including the inside of the ears, the oral cavity, and haired as well as nonhaired skin.
- Note any primary lesions.
- Look for secondary lesions and for evidence of how they may have developed.

- Palpate all peripheral lymph nodes for enlargement.
- Take the body temperature.
- Perform a general physical examination, including examination of the eyes, auscultation of the chest, and palpation of the abdomen, to evaluate the animal for systemic signs.

Serum Biochemical Profile, Urinalysis, and Complete Blood Count (CBC)

- Evaluate in animals with systemic signs such as anorexia, depression, and fever.
- Use as baseline information for any animal in which you expect early clinical signs to progress.

Hematologic Tests

- Rickettsial titers or other disease-specific hematologic tests are indicated in certain cases.

Tests for Systemic Immune-Mediated-Diseases

- Perform antinuclear antibody (ANA) testing of serum to confirm suspicion of an immune-mediated disorder and to assess the presence or absence of antibodies directed against multiple nuclear antigens.
- Other immune tests such as Coombs testing and cryoglobulin identification may be indicated in cases in which specific diseases are suspected.
- See sec. 3, ch. 3 for further discussion of testing for systemic immune-mediated diseases.

Skin Biopsy

- Skin biopsy is an important diagnostic tool in necrotizing skin diseases (see sec. 5, ch. 15).
- Collect lesions that are primary eruptions and/or skin immediately adjacent to necrotic skin.
- Use formalin as fixative for tissues collected early in the course of the disease. A pathologist familiar with dermatopathology often can determine if a systemic or topical disease is present. Many specific etiologies can be identified if representative tissues samples are collected.
- Tissues placed in Michel's fixative and processed for presence of antibody (immunofluorescence testing or immunoperoxidase) are helpful in confirming a suspected autoimmune disease. However, absence of positive immunofluorescence does not rule out autoimmunity as a cause.

Skin and Blood Cultures

- Evaluate the patient for infection by culturing the skin for bacterial and fungal agents.
- For systemic diseases, blood cultures may be indicated.

Other Diagnostic Methods

- Use *liver function tests* in the assessment of a suspected case of necrolytic migratory erythema.
- *Radiography* and *ultrasonography* are useful if cutaneous lesions are suspected to be secondary to malignancy or systemic disease.

■ In rare cases, *response to therapy, or to removal of a suspected inciting drug* confirms the diagnosis.

TREATMENT

KEY POINT ▶ Therapy is most effective when a specific etiology is identified; treatment can then be focused on the elimination or modification of the cause.

Cutaneous necrosis is best managed aggressively with treatment directed against a definitive cause.

■ If there is any possibility that drugs are implicated, discontinue all drugs until making a definitive or probable diagnosis.
■ If secondary infection is a concern, administer a broad-spectrum antibiotic (preferably one that the patient has not previously received).
■ Toxins associated with tissue necrosis can have systemic effects; therefore, debride tissues and flush frequently with sterile saline.
■ In cases in which identification is not possible, give supportive care.
■ Hydration and provision of a high-quality protein diet are important aspects of therapy.

Autoimmune Diseases

■ Treatment depends on the type of disease and the severity and extent of lesions.
■ Initially, give systemic corticosteroids at immunosuppressive dosages (prednisone or prednisolone, 2.2–4.4 mg/kg, q12–24h PO).
■ Other immunosuppressive drugs such as azathioprine (Imuran, Burroughs Wellcome), cyclophosphamide (Cytoxan; Bristol-Myers), and chlorambucil (Leukeran; Burroughs Wellcome) may be necessary in individual cases (see sec. 5, ch. 9).

Vasculitis

■ The goal of management is treatment of the underlying disease.
■ If immune complexes are being deposited in vessel walls, give immunosuppressive corticosteroids or other drugs.
■ If sepsis or generalized bacterial, fungal, or rickettsial disease is identified, treat the infectious agent.
■ If the vasculitis is drug-induced, discontinue the offending drug immediately.
  • Corticosteroids at anti-inflammatory doses (prednisone or prednisolone, 1.1 mg/kg, q12–24h PO) are advocated by some for the management of drug-induced vasculitis.
■ In cases of idiopathic and hypersensitivity-induced vasculitis, corticosteroids may be beneficial.
■ Some cases are self-limiting. In other instances, dapsone (Avlosulfone; Jacobus) has induced remission.
  • Initial dosage is 1 mg/kg, q8–12h PO; when the disease is controlled, gradually reduce the dosage.
  • Potential side effects include leukopenia, thrombocytopenia, and hepatotoxicity; use dapsone with caution.
  • Other sulfonamides such as sulfasalazine have been used successfully to treat vasculitis in a few dogs.

Neoplasia

■ Specific treatment depends on the type of tumor, its potential for metastasis, and its biologic behavior.
■ Surgical resection is indicated for solitary lesions.
■ Base treatment of other tumors on current recommendations for the individual type (see sec. 3, chs. 5, 6, 7, and 9).

Drug-Induced Necrosis

■ Discontinue the offending drug immediately.
■ If the adverse effects resolve and are known to be dosage-dependent, resume therapy at a much lower dosage if the primary disease mandates continuation of the drug.
■ In most instances, do not give the suspect drug to the animal in the future.
■ The effects of corticosteroids, both at immunosuppressive and at anti-inflammatory levels for drug reactions, are highly controversial. Assess each case individually for potential advantages and disadvantages.

Toxic Epidermal Necrolysis

■ A diagnosis of TEN represents a true dermatologic emergency. Immediately discontinue any suspect drugs and search for systemic disease or neoplasia.
■ Once full-thickness necrosis of the skin begins, start aggressive supportive care with intravenous fluids such as lactated Ringer's solution to replace estimated fluid loss.
■ Keep affected tissues clean and debrided; cover with a topical cream such as silver sulfadiazine (Silvadene; Marion) to decrease evaporation from large denuded areas.
■ Corticosteroids (prednisone or prednisolone, 2.2–4.4 mg/kg, q12h, PO, initially, and then reduce) are recommended, especially early in the course of the disease.
■ The prognosis is guarded, and in spite of removal of the causative agent or disease, TEN can continue to progress and may be fatal.

Erythema Multiforme

■ Discontinue any potential causative drugs as soon as possible and give supportive care.
■ Symptoms may continue for several days past withdrawal of the offending agent, and pain and scarring may occur.
■ The prognosis for survival is better if the primary causative condition is not life-threatening.

Environmental Factors

Contact Irritant Dermatitis

■ Remove the irritant and give supportive care.

Snake Bites

- Snake bite envenomation therapy varies with the severity of the clinical signs, location of the bite, and length of time since the bite.
- Initially, immobilize the lesion and keep the patient quiet.
- Application of tourniquets is controversial, as is glucocorticoid therapy.
- When polyvalent antivenom (Antivenin; Ft. Dodge) is indicated, give one vial slowly IV as soon as possible after the bite.
  - Repeated injections may be necessary.
  - Monitor closely for anaphylactic reactions.
- Broad-spectrum antibiotics are generally indicated because both anaerobes and aerobes are often involved in sequelae to the bite.
- Keep lesions clean and debride wounds regularly.

Spider Bites

- Arthropod bites caused by the brown spider and the brown recluse spider progress due to potent dermonecrotic toxins.
- Excise the bite wound if the lesion is identified early as a bite by one of the spiders named above.
- Corticosteroids and antivenom do not appear to affect local necrosis. However, when systemic signs are present, corticosteroids combined with supportive care are beneficial.
- Intravascular hemolysis and renal failure are possible sequelae.

Radiation

- Treat acute radiation damage with gentle topical cleansing, followed by topical creams. An Elizabethan collar restraint may be necessary.
  - Use medications to control pain if required.
- In chronic radiation injury, an area of cutaneous atropy caused by acute damage later necroses and sloughs. The condition usually is progressive.
  - Supportive care is the primary treatment.

Burns

- Treat burns according to their depth and extent over the body.
- Apply intensive and aggressive topical therapy in severe cases.
- Give medications such as morphine (0.2 mg/kg, SC or IM) to control pain.
- Cleanse, debride, and cover burns with an antibacterial cream (e.g., Silvadene).
- Fluid replacement and protein supplementation are important.
- Because secondary bacterial (e.g., *Pseudomonas*) infection is common, systemic broad-spectrum antimicrobial drug therapy is essential.
- Skin grafts may be necessary for extensive full-thickness burns (see sec. 5, ch. 19).
- The prognosis depends on the extent of surface area involved.

Frostbite

- Because animals with frostbite usually are presented long after the damage has occurred, supportive care and debridement are necessary.
- In early cases, rapidly rewarm the tissues in water heated to 40–42°C.
- Whirlpool therapy can be helpful.
- Manage pain with medications.
- Keep lesions uncovered if self-trauma can be minimized.
- Administer systemic antibiotics for secondary infection.

Decubitus Ulcers

- The goal of treatment is to make the patient ambulatory again. If this is not possible, then supportive care is optimal.
- Clean and rotate the patient often. Soft bedding or a water mattress is useful.
- Keep all ulcerated areas free of fecal and urine contamination.
- A wide variety of topical agents (with insulin, enzymes, and/or antibiotic and antibacterial agents) are available.
- Surgical debridement and reconstruction are useful in some cases.

Infection

- When infection results in necrosis of tissue, administer systemic antimicrobial therapy against the offending etiologic agent, based on culture and sensitivity testing.
- Establish and maintain appropriate drainage.

Vascular Compromise

- When vascular compromise occurs in thrombovascular necrosis of the ears, the therapy of choice is resection of all affected tissue.
- When mechanical occlusion causes incomplete circulation to the tissue, remove the mechanical device.
- In diabetes mellitus, the optimal approach to the vasculopathy is to carefully monitor and control the diabetes.

Necrolytic Migratory Erythema

- Treatment of necrolytic migratory erythema has been unsuccessful to date in most cases.
- Some cases have a tendency to wax and wane over months in spite of therapy.
- Supportive care is beneficial in certain instances.

Supplemental Readings

Fadok VA: Necrotizing skin diseases. *In* Kirk RW, ed.: *Current Veterinary Therapy VII.* Philadelphia: W. B. Saunders, 1983, p 473.

Kunkle GA: Ulceration. *In* Dermatology Proceedings 138, Post Graduate Committee in Veterinary Science. University of Sydney, 1990, p 113.

13 Feline Symmetric Alopecia

Vicki J. Scheidt

Alopecia is defined as the absence of hair from skin areas where it normally is present. In order to properly describe the clinical problem and formulate an appropriate differential diagnosis, it is helpful to further categorize alopecia based on the degree (partial or complete), duration (permanent or transient), and distribution (generalized, localized, or regional) of the hair loss. Alopecia in the cat, whether symmetric or asymmetric, may be associated with varying degrees of pruritus and skin reactivity, depending on the underlying disease. It is important to note the degree, distribution, and relationship of the pruritus and skin lesions associated with the alopecia.

In animals, the haircoat aids in thermal regulation and protects the skin, and it has important aesthetic qualities. Cats are fastidious and spend a great deal of time grooming their coats. Normal grooming behavior aids in hair removal and normal shedding. When grooming becomes excessive, however, it may accentuate hair damage and skin disease.

Hair follicles have specific cycles of growth (anagen) and rest (telogen) that are primarily stimulated by changes in photoperiod and, to a lesser extent, by temperature. From winter to late spring in temperate climates, hair growth is minimal and the thick winter coat is shed. Cats who live outside in colder climates, therefore, may shed excessively in late spring and develop a transient thinning of the coat (hypotrichosis). Secondary hairs undergo a growth phase in the fall and winter that results in the thick, heavy coat needed for the colder temperatures. Seasonal changes are less dramatic in tropical regions and in environments with artificial lighting (e.g., where cats are confined indoors). In these animals, a small amount of hair loss occurs continuously.

ETIOLOGY

Multiple factors play a role in normal hair follicle development and growth (Table 1). Absence or changes in one or more of these factors can alter the normal growth process and result in alopecia. The underlying causes of feline symmetric alopecia can vary, depending on the area or region of the body affected. This chapter reviews the causes of symmetric alopecia that are primarily confined to the trunk (dorsum, perineum, caudal thighs, flanks, ventral abdomen, and chest). The underlying causes of feline symmetric alopecia affecting the trunk region have been classified into those that are associated with self-trauma or pruritus (e.g., licking and scratching) and those that are nonpruritic (Table 2).

KEY POINT ▶ It is important to determine whether pruritus and concurrent skin inflammation are present when formulating a differential diagnosis for symmetric alopecia in the cat.

- *Psychogenic alopecia* is often an enigma. Alopecia develops because the cat excessively licks, bites, or pulls out hair from those areas normally groomed (e.g., perineum, ventral abdomen, and flank). The etiology or inciting factor may be due to a primary disease, such as impacted anal glands, or to a pruritic skin disease, such as atopy or allergy to food or fleas. However, in many cases, a stressful event, such as being moved to a new surrounding, hospitalized, or boarded and the loss of a favorite companion or the introduction of a new pet or person (baby) into the environment, will precipitate this condition. Psychogenic alopecia is most common in nervous or "high-strung" animals, such as Siamese, Abyssinian, or black cats. Typically, the areas affected are regions the cat can easily lick, such as the dorsal lumbosacral region, tail, medial and caudal thighs, ventral abdomen, flanks, and perineum. Partial to complete alopecia and stubbled hairs may be observed alone or with focal areas of erythema, erosion, exudation, and crusting.
- *Feline endocrine alopecia* is a disease of unknown cause. It is presumed to result from hormonal imbalances or deficiencies based on the positive response obtained following treatment with various hormones. This condition is characterized by nonpruritic, symmetric hair loss involving the perineum, ventral abdomen, and caudal or medial thighs. Although the alopecia may spread to the flanks, lateral thorax, and proximal tail, the dorsum is usually spared. A thinning of the hair, rather than complete baldness, with normal, unaffected skin is observed. Feline endocrine alopecia primarily affects neutered females and males. However, the syndrome has also been reported in intact cats. Significant controversy exists regarding the relationship of hypothyroidism with feline endocrine alopecia. Although affected cats usually have normal baseline serum thyroxine (T_4) levels, some have had lower serum T_4 levels at 6 hours following stimulation with thyroid-stimulating hormone (TSH) compared with normal cats. These findings suggest that some cats with feline endocrine alopecia may have a low thyroid reserve. Although feline hyperadrenocorticism is rare, both natural and iatrogenic Cushing's disease can produce symmetric alopecia of the trunk or pinnae and thin hypotonic skin.

TABLE 1. Internal and External Factors Influencing Hair Follicle Growth and Development

> **Internal Factors**
> Genetic
> Hormonal
> Immunologic
> Neoplastic
> Stress
> **External Factors**
> Nutritional
> Infectious
> Bacterial
> Fungal (dermatophytes)
> Parasitic
> Physical (traumatic)
> Chemical (toxins, drug therapy)

■ *Flea infestation* associated with mild pruritus and minimal dermatitis can cause symmetric alopecia of the dorsum, proximal tail, flanks, perineum, and ventral abdomen. Fleas and/or their feces are usually present on examination. Although a similar presentation can be seen in cats allergic to the flea bite, flea-allergic cats are much more pruritic and, typically, have concurrent skin lesions (miliary dermatitis), along the dorsum, tail base, and ventral abdomen (see sec. 5, ch. 6).

■ *Food allergy* in cats is associated with nonseasonal pruritus and with a variety of clinical presentations, including symmetric alopecia (see sec. 5, ch. 8). The skin lesions and severe pruritus may be generalized or confined to the face and ears. Alopecia, whether diffuse or symmetric, results from excessive scratching, licking, or chewing triggered by an allergic reaction to specific food items (see sec. 5, ch. 8). Stubbled or broken hairs, with or without concurrent focal erythema, papules, and crusting (miliary dermatitis), is usually present.

■ *Feline atopy* may be associated with seasonal or nonseasonal alopecia and pruritus (see sec. 5, ch. 7). Similar to feline food allergy, the alopecia is secondary to pruritus and associated with broken or stubbled hairs and concurrent skin lesions. The alopecia may be generalized or confined to the head and neck or dorsum.

TABLE 2. Underlying Causes of Feline Symmetric Alopecia of the Trunk

Pruritic or Self-Inflicted	Nonpruritic
Psychogenic alopecia	Feline endocrine alopecia
Allergic dermatoses	Sex hormonal
Food allergy	Hypothyroid
Atopy	Hyperadrenocorticism
Flea allergy	Systemic disease
Demodicosis	Diabetes mellitus
Dermatophytosis	Renal disease
Otodectic mange	FELV/FIV*
	Telogen effluvium
	Demodicosis
	Dermatophytosis

*Feline leukemia and feline immunodeficiency viruses.

■ *Dermatophytosis* is a common cause of localized or generalized alopecia in cats (see sec. 5, ch. 3). Fungal organisms invade the hair shaft and grow downward but do not penetrate the mitotic region. Alopecia is not permanent unless the follicle is destroyed by secondary inflammation. A wide spectrum of clinical presentations can be seen with dermatophytosis, including the asymptomatic carrier state in many long-haired cats. Classically, the alopecia is focal to diffuse and associated with small numbers of fractured or stubbled hairs and with mild epidermal erythema and scaling. The majority of dermatophyte infections (98%) in cats are caused by the zoophilic fungus, *Microsporum canis*.

■ *Demodicosis* is a rare cause of alopecia in cats (see sec. 5, ch. 4). The pathogenesis of feline demodicosis is reported to be similar to that described in the dog and caused by either *Demodex cati* or a recently described and unnamed *Demodex* species. *D. cati* is a normal inhabitant of feline skin, which under favorable conditions proliferates in hair follicles and causes patchy to diffuse alopecia. Lesions consist of focal to diffuse alopecia, erythema, scaling, and crusts, which may be localized and self-limiting or generalized. In some cases, these lesions mimic feline endocrine alopecia. Generalized demodicosis in the cat is usually associated with an underlying disease, such as feline leukemia, immunodeficiency viral infections, or diabetes mellitus. A pruritic, symmetric alopecia of the trunk caused by an unnamed *Demodex* species has been described in cats.

■ *Otodectic mange* is the most common cause of otitis externa in cats (see sec. 5, ch. 21). Otodectic mites can live on the skin surface and cause symmetric alopecia over the lower back and tail base. Concurrent otitis externa may or may not be present. The degree of pruritus is variable.

■ *Telogen effluvium* is a syndrome in which the anagen cycle is shortened and a wave of hair follicles simultaneously enters the resting phase. Conditions associated with physiologic stress (e.g., fever, shock, pregnancy and lactation, malnutrition, adverse drug reactions, and severe debilitating disease) can precipitate rapid shedding in animals. The resultant alopecia can be partial to complete and localized or generalized. Usually it is nonpruritic. Affected hairs are easily epilated by friction or grooming.

■ *Systemic disease* can produce diffuse, symmetric or asymmetric hair loss in the cat. Hair follicles are sensitive to pathologic and physiologic changes from systemic diseases, such as end-stage kidney disease, chronic hepatitis, diabetes mellitus, and viral infections (feline leukemia and feline immunodeficiency viruses). The degree of pruritus and skin lesions associated with the alopecia is variable.

CLINICAL SIGNS

■ Feline symmetric alopecia is either pruritic (a direct result of excessive licking or hair pulling) or nonpruritic (hair falls out independently). The finding of stubbled or broken hairs suggests self-trauma. However, invasion of organisms, such as dermatophytes, into the hair shafts can also produce fractured or stubbled hairs.

■ Excoriations, erosions, and/or ulcerations in conjunction with stubbled hairs usually imply that the hair and skin changes are self-inflicted. These lesions, however, may also be secondary manifestations of a primary vesicular or bullous disease.

■ Easy epilation of hair from the skin implies that the follicle is in the resting stage. However, hairs frequently epilate when a cat is stressed or debilitated.

■ Cats that are nervous, poorly adjusted, or high strung are more likely to develop excessive grooming behavior and subsequent alopecia.

■ Pruritic or self-inflicted alopecia that is responsive to systemic corticosteroid therapy suggests an underlying allergic or parasitic etiology. Alopecia that is responsive to systemic, progestational therapy, however, may have a hormonal, an allergic, or a psychogenic basis.

■ Systemic signs (e.g., anorexia, vomiting, weight loss, polydypsia, polyphagia, and polyuria) may be present, when the alopecia is associated with either primary systemic disease (e.g., renal disease and diabetes mellitus) or hormonal imbalance (e.g., iatrogenic Cushing's disease).

DIAGNOSIS

KEY POINT ▶ Feline symmetric alopecia can usually be classified as pruritic or nonpruritic based on the history and gross appearance of the haircoat and skin. In such a situation, the goal of the diagnosis is to identify the underlying disease. When self-induced alopecia is suspected but not supported by the history and physical findings, restricting the cat from licking the area, using an Elizabethan collar for 4 to 6 weeks, is often conclusive. In such a case, baseline diagnostic tests (e.g., skin scrapings and fungal culture) are always done first.

■ *Historical information* identifies the presence of excessive licking or hair pulling: the past and current hormonal status; the environmental changes, which might have been stressful and preceded alopecia; the general psychologic state; the concurrent systemic signs; and the nutrition- and therapy-related causes.

■ *Physical examination* is thorough and includes a thorough evaluation of the integument and all internal organ systems.

• Examine hair shafts and follicles from affected areas grossly and microscopically for structural abnormalities (e.g., fractures, bulges, and constrictions). Telogen hairs plucked from the skin have a fusiform appearance and a dry, white clubbed-shaped root upon gross or microscopic examination. In contrast, growing or anagen hairs have a blunt end that is glistening, pigmented, and surrounded by a root sheath.

• Examine the skin in both alopecic and nonaffected

areas for the presence of primary (erythema, papules) and secondary (crusts, scale, hyperpigmentation) lesions. Note the thickness and elasticity of the skin.

• Search for external parasites (fleas, flea dirt).

• Note abnormalities in other organ systems.

■ Perform *skin scrapings* to rule out the diagnosis of feline demodicosis, *Otodectes cynotis,* and other external mite infestations.

■ Perform *fungal culture* to confirm or rule out a possible dermatophyte infection. Examine the affected hairs with an ultraviolet light (Wood's lamp). Only about 50% of the cases of *Microsporum canis* fluoresce, however. Use hairs that fluoresce an apple-green color, both for culture and microscopic examination for fungal spores or hyphae, employing a clearing agent (KOH). Refer to sec. 5, ch. 3 for details concerning the diagnosis of dermatophytosis.

■ Collect *ear smears* from cats with concurrent otitis externa or with a history of recurrent otodectic mange (ear mites).

■ Institute an *elimination diet* trial, as described in sec. 5, ch. 8, using rice and lamb baby food or rabbit meat, in cats with a history of symmetric alopecia and nonseasonal, steroid-responsive licking or pruritus. The diagnosis of food allergy is confirmed with the amelioration of the pruritus and/or excessive licking during a 4- to 6-week diet trial and the recurrence of these signs following the provocative exposure to the original diet.

■ Perform *intradermal testing* for flea and environmental allergens in a cat with a history of seasonal (summer to fall) and nonseasonal pruritus that is responsive to systemic corticosteroid therapy. Correlate positive reactions with the history of allergen exposure and seasonality (see sec. 5, ch. 7).

■ *Skin biopsy* samples from affected and unaffected areas are helpful in evaluating the growing stages of the hair follicles and in identifying any concurrent follicular inflammation—whether infectious, parasitic, or allergic.

■ Obtain *baseline serum thyroid levels* or perform a *TSH stimulation test* in cats with nonpruritic alopecia and histopathologic findings consistent with an endocrine-based alopecia. TSH stimulation test results are superior to serum baseline thyroid level results for diagnosing hypothyroidism in the dog and cat and is the test of choice (see sec. 4, ch. 1).

■ Do an *adrenocorticotropic hormone (ACTH) stimulation test* in cats with nonpruritic alopecia and concurrent polyuria; polydipsia; polyphagia; lethargy; pendulous abdomen; and thin, easily torn skin—to identify iatrogenic or naturally occurring hyperadrenocorticism (see sec. 4, ch. 3).

■ Perform a *complete blood count, serum biochemical profile,* and *urinalysis* in cats with symmetric alopecia and systemic signs (e.g., fever, depression, and anorexia) to identify any underlying primary disease (diabetes mellitus) or adverse reaction to previous therapy (iatrogenic Cushing's disease from prolonged systemic corticosteroid or progestational therapy). The finding of peripheral eosinophilia in a cat with seasonal or nonseasonal pruritus and/or licking is supportive of allergic or parasitic dermatitis diagnosis. Abnormalities in the serum biochemical profile or the urinalysis can be helpful in identifying a primary organ dysfunction.

■ Do *feline leukemia* and *feline immunodeficiency viral tests* in cats with generalized demodicosis, nonhealing skin infections, or protracted systemic signs (see sec. 2, chs. 1 and 2).

TREATMENT

Feline symmetric alopecia is often managed with "scientific neglect" during the early stages when the hair loss is mild and pruritus is absent. However, if the alopecia progresses or is observed to be self-inflicted, the underlying cause is pursued, so that appropriate treatment can be prescribed. It is important to determine from the onset whether the hair loss is due to a self-inflicted behavior (licking, chewing, hair pulling) or to an underlying disease (hormonal, systemic). Many cats are "closet lickers," therefore, the owners may not observe excessive licking or chewing. In such a case, applying an Elizabethan collar on the animal for 3 to 4 weeks can be very helpful in identifying whether the cat is actually licking the hair out. Chronic cases of symmetric alopecia that are associated with secondary skin changes and pruritus often require symptomatic treatment with anti-inflammatory agents, such as systemic corticosteroids, during the initial stages of the diagnostic workup. Long-term or prolonged corticosteroid therapy is avoided, however, until the underlying cause has been identified and appropriately treated.

■ Use *anti-inflammatory therapy* in cats with symmetric alopecia and concurrent pruritus that are suspected of having an underlying allergic disease (e.g., food allergy, atopy, and flea allergy). Short-term treatment with systemic antihistamines or corticosteroids may be used during the initial stages, until the causative allergen is identified through a diet trial or an intradermal allergy testing and either eliminated or appropriately controlled through a hypoallergenic diet, hyposensitization, or flea control.
  • *Systemic antihistamines,* compared with systemic corticosteroids, are generally not as effective in controlling pruritus in cats. Chlorpheniramine maleate, given at 2 mg/cat, q12h, PO, has been shown by Miller in 1990 to be an effective treatment in cats with pruritus of an unknown or idiopathic nature.
  • *Fatty acid supplements,* such as DVM Derm Caps (DVM Pharmaceuticals) at 0.11 ml/kg, q24h, PO, are occasionally effective in controlling pruritus in cats when given alone or in combination with antihistamines (chlorpheniramine). However, 4 to 8 weeks may be required before improvement is noted.
  • *Systemic corticosteroids* are very effective in the management of pruritus in cats. Unlike dogs, cats require much higher doses of corticosteroids to suppress or control pruritus of an allergic nature. Compared with other species, cats appear to be more resistant to the harmful side effects (hyper-

adrenocorticisim) of systemic corticosteroid therapy. Administer prednisolone or prednisone at 2 mg/kg, q24h, PO, for 7 to 10 days—then administer on an alternate-day schedule and gradually taper to the lowest effective dose. Methylprednisolone acetate (Depo-Medrol; The Upjohn Co.) given at 4 to 5 mg/kg or 20 mg/cat, SC, is also effective when administered every 2 to 3 weeks. Do not repeat repositol injections at this dosage for longer than 2 to 3 months.
  • *Systemic progestational compounds* have been used for years to treat various feline skin diseases, including symmetric alopecia, both pruritic (e.g., atopy, psychogenic alopecia) and nonpruritic (e.g., endocrine alopecia). In cats, progestational compounds, such as megestrol acetate (Ovaban, Schering-Plough), are immunosuppressive and have potent anti-inflammatory activity. They exhibit a wide spectrum of actions and side effects. Serious side effects reported in cats include decreased spermatogenesis, development of pyometra, mammary gland fibroadenomatous hyperplasia in both male and female intact and neutered animals, permanent or transient diabetes mellitus, adrenocortical suppression, and numerous behavioral abnormalities (e.g., polyphagia with subsequent weight gain, polyuria, polydipsia, and lethargy). The dosage in cats is variable and ranges from an induction of 2.5 to 5.0 mg per cat, q24h, for 5 days, decreased to every other day and tapered to 2.5 to 5.0 mg every 5 to 7 days for 1 to 2 months.

KEY POINT ▶ Progestational compounds are not approved for use in cats. Because of this and the numerous side effects, they should be provided only as the last choice.

■ *Hormonal therapy* has been successfully used to treat nonpruritic, symmetric alopecia in the cat that is associated with normal-appearing skin and classified as endocrine in origin (see sec. 5, ch. 11). Although various hormones have been effective in the treatment of feline endocrine alopecia, relapses are common and intermittent life-long therapy is often necessary.
  • *Combined estrogen-testosterone* therapy has been successful in both neutered male and female cats with endocrine alopecia. Repositol testosterone (12.5 mg/cat) and repositol diethylstilbestrol (0.625 mg/cat) is given IM alone or in combination. Although hair regrowth is usually present by 6 weeks, relapses are common. Side effects, including signs of estrus in females, aggressive behavior or urine spraying in males, and hepatobiliary disease in both, have been reported following androgen and/or estrogen therapy.
  • *Thyroid hormone* therapy has been found to be effective in cats with endocrine alopecia, despite normal serum baseline thyroid levels. T_4 replacement therapy with sodium levothyroxine is effective at 0.05 to 0.1 mg, q12–24h, PO. Sodium liothyronine (Tertroxin; Glaxo Co.) given at 50 mcg, q12h, PO, has been reported to produce

complete hair regrowth in 73% of cats treated (Thoday, 1986).

- *Progestational compounds* can be effective in the management of feline endocrine alopecia. Megestrol acetate (2.5 to 5.0 mg/cat, once every other day, for 1 to 2 months) is preferred to repositol progesterone because of the potential side effects of the latter in cats.
- *Adrenalectomy,* either unilateral or bilateral, is the treatment of choice for naturally occurring hyperadrenocorticism in the cat (see sec. 4, ch. 3). Discontinuation and avoidance of systemic corticosteroids and progestational compounds are recommended in cats with iatrogenic hyperadrenocorticism.

■ *Antianxiety drugs or tranquilizers* may be necessary in conjunction with behavior modification for cats with psychogenic alopecia or stress-induced symmetric alopecia. Identification and removal (if possible) of the predisposing cause is extremely important, because response to systemic treatment is variable and requires much patience and effort on the part of the owner. Treatment with diazepam, phenobarbital, or megestrol acetate is given as adjunctive therapy to behavioral modification. The main goal is to relax the cat and eventually discontinue the antianxiety medication.

- *Diazepam* (Valium; Roche) given at 1 to 2 mg/cat, q24h, PO, for 4 to 8 weeks has a calming effect and is effective in some cases.
- *Phenobarbital* given at 2 to 5 mg/kg, q12h, PO, is effective. However, adjustment of the dosage may be required.
- *Progestational compounds* (megestrol acetate) act directly on the limbic system and behavior center transforming the "high-strung" cat into a very "euphoric," affectionate animal. The dosage is 2.5 to 5.0 mg/cat, q24h, PO, for 5 days—then, every other day for 2 weeks, tapered to twice a week for a total treatment period of 2 to 3 months.

■ *Specific therapy* for other causes of feline symmetric alopecia include the following:

- A *hypoallergenic diet* is fed to cats with symmetric alopecia caused by an underlying food allergy (see sec. 5, ch. 8). Home-cooked diets containing lamb, green vegetable baby food, rabbit meat, and cooked rice can be used. However, a vitamin-mineral supplement is added daily. Some cats allergic to food tolerate Prescription Diet c/d (Hill's Pet Foods) (canned and dry) or Feline Anergen (Wysong).
- *Hyposensitization* has been reported to be an effective treatment for feline atopy. The percent of atopic cats that are controlled following desensitization, however, is not well documented (sec. 5, ch. 7).
- *Flea control* is a critical part of the management of feline flea allergy and infestation (sec. 5, ch. 6). A successful flea control program includes (1) weekly treatment of the cat allergic to fleas and all contact pets and (2) concurrent treatment of both the indoor and outdoor environment. Flea powders and sprays containing synergized pyrethrins have quick flea kill but poor residual activity. The microencapsulated pyrethrins (Sectrol Flea Spray and Sectrol Flea Foam; 3M Animal Care Products) provide immediate flea kill and residual activity, and they are safe for use in cats. Hyposensitization has been shown to be ineffective as a treatment for flea allergy in the cat.
- *Clinical management of feline dermatophytosis* always includes clipping and cleansing of affected areas, generalized topical antifungal therapy, isolation and appropriate sanitation, and systemic antifungal therapy (griseofulvin) in severe generalized cases. Refer to sec. 5, ch. 3 for details concerning the treatment of feline dermatophytosis.
- *Miticidal solutions* containing 2% lime sulfur, 0.025% amitraz (Mitaban, The Upjohn Co.), or malathion may be effective when applied weekly for 4 to 6 weeks in cats with symmetric alopecia caused by *Demodex cati* or *Demodex* sp. However, neither amitraz nor malathion are approved for use in cats (sec. 5, ch. 4).
- *Clinical management of otodectic mange* in cats with symmetric alopecia includes weekly application of a parasiticidal powder or spray over the entire body. Both the affected cat and all contact animals are treated for 4 to 6 weeks with a miticidal otic preparation.

Supplemental Readings

Kirk RW: Feline alopecia. *In* Kirk RW, ed.: *Current Veterinary Therapy VII.* Philadelphia: W. B. Saunders, 1980, p 490.

Miller WH, Scott DW: Efficacy of chlorpheniramine maleate for management of pruritus in cats. J Am Vet Med Assoc 197:67, 1990.

Muller GH, Kirk RW, Scott DW: *Small Animal Dermatology,* 4th ed. Philadelphia: W. B. Saunders, 1989, p 701.

Scott DW: Feline dermatology 1900–1978: J Am Anim Hosp Assoc 16:334, 1980.

Scott DW: Feline dermatology 1979–1982: Introspective retrospections. J Am Anim Hosp Assoc 20:537, 1984.

Thoday KL: Differential diagnosis of symmetric alopecia in the cat. *In* Kirk RW ed.: *Current Veterinary Therapy IX.* Philadelphia: W. B. Saunders, 1986, p 545.

Thoday KL: Aspects of feline symmetric alopecia. *In* Von Tscharner C, Halliwell REW, eds.: *Advances in Veterinary Dermatology,* Volume 1. London: Baillière Tindall, 1990, p 47.

14 Miliary Dermatitis and Eosinophilic Granuloma Complex

Wayne S. Rosenkrantz

Miliary dermatitis (MD) and eosinophilic granuloma complex (EGC) are extremely common cutaneous reaction patterns in the cat. The term miliary is a descriptive one, and it implies that the papules and crusts characteristic of the syndrome resemble millet seeds. The term eosinophilic granuloma is also descriptive of a group of lesions affecting the skin and oral cavity of the cat. The three clinical histologic syndromes included in this complex are eosinophilic ulcer, eosinophilic plaque, and linear granuloma.

ETIOLOGY

KEY POINT ▶ Miliary dermatitis and eosinophilic granuloma complex are neither final diagnoses nor pathognomonic for any one disease. Many etiologies exist for both reaction patterns. The ability to control or cure chronic or recurrent cases is dependent upon pursuing an underlying diagnosis. The two conditions share similar etiologies and therefore are discussed together in this chapter.

Underlying causes or predisposing factors for MD and EGC (Table 1) include (1) allergies, (2) parasites, (3) infectious diseases, and (4) miscellaneous conditions.

- *Allergies* to fleas, biting insects (e.g., mosquitos and flies), foods, and inhaled and contact substances have been associated with MD in the cat. With the exception of contact allergies, all of these reactions have been associated with the EGC. In particular, flea and other biting insect hypersensitivities have been emphasized as etiologies in the EGC.
- *Parasites,* such as fleas, *Cheyletiella, Notoedres,* chiggers, *Otodectes,* lice, cat fur mites, and endoparasites, have been associated with MD. Fleas have also been implicated in EGC as a cause of a hypersensitivity reaction. These parasitic entities also produce lesions in MD by way of a hypersensitivity reaction. Refer to the respective chapters concerning these various parasites for additional information.
- *Infectious* causes for both entities include bacterial infections and dermatophytosis. In EGC, viral infections are an additional consideration.

- The most common bacteria isolated in both entities include *Staphylococcus,* β-hemolytic *Streptococcus, Pasteurella,* and *Bacteroides* species. Positive clinical response to a variety of antibiotics in both MD and EGC gives support to a bacterial etiology.
- The major dermatophyte species isolated from cats is *Microsporum canis* (sec. 5, ch. 3). This dermatophyte can produce MD, but it can also be found on cats without MD. The species is rarely isolated from EGC lesions, and its significance in this complex is questionable.
- *Miscellaneous* conditions causing MD include genetic factors, immune-mediated diseases, drug reactions, nutritional factors, epitheliotropic lymphoma, and idiopathic causes. Genetic factors, immune-mediated disease, and idiopathic causes have received attention as etiologies in EGG.
- Hereditary (genetic) factors have been implicated based on reports of offspring from affected cats, which have developed similar MD or EGC lesions.
- Immune-mediated disorders, such as pemphigus foliaceus, can produce MD-like lesions. Immune-mediated disease has not received much consideration in EGC, although antiepithelial antibodies (IgG) have been documented in cats with eosinophilic ulcers.
- Drug reactions can mimic any skin disease. Cases of MD drug-induced lesions have been seen but are rare. Drug-induced EGC lesions have not been reported.
- Nutritional deficiencies related to fatty acid or biotin deficiencies have been reported in the older literature as causes of MD. Such deficiencies are unlikely in cats on commercial well-balanced diets.
- Cutaneous epitheliotropic lymphoma (mycosis fungoides) in its initial phase can cause erythema, scaling, and occasionally papules. Therefore, this lymphoma can mimic MD.
- Idiopathic cases exist in both MD and EGC. Such cases most likely reflect the inability to identify one of the aforementioned diseases. Undefined allergic reactions are considered to account for a number of these idiopathic cases.

CLINICAL SIGNS

- The lesions of MD are usually erythematous small papules (1 to 2 mm) that develop into crusts. Secon-

TABLE 1. Etiologies of Miliary Dermatitis and Eosinophilic Granuloma Complex

	Miliary Dermatitis	Eosinophilic Granuloma Complex
Allergies		
Flea allergy	+ + + +	+ + + +
Mosquito and biting fly hypersensitivity	+	+ + +
Food allergy	+ + +	+ + +
Atopy	+ + +	+ + +
Contact allergy	+	
Parasitic		
Fleas	+ + +	+ +
Cheyletiella	+ +	
Notoedres	+ +	
Chiggers (trombiculiasis)	+ +	
Otodectes	+ +	
Lice (pediculosis)	+ +	
Demodicosis	+	
Cat fur mite	+	
Endoparasites	+	
Infectious Diseases		
Bacterial	+ + +	+ + +
Dermatophytosis	+ + +	+
Viral		+
Miscellaneous Conditions		
Genetic		+
Immune-mediated diseases	+	+
Drug reactions	+	
Nutritional	+	
Neoplasm (epitheliotropic lymphoma)	+	
Idiopathic causes	+ + +	+ + +

+ = Rare cause of syndrome.
+ + = Uncommon cause of syndrome.
+ + + = Frequent cause of syndrome.
+ + + + = Major cause of syndrome.

dary lesions result from self-trauma and produce alopecia, erosions, excoriations, and acute pyotraumatic dermatitis. The distribution can be localized to a specific area or generalized. The dorsal lumbosacral, cervical, and groin areas are the most common sites affected.

■ Additional physical signs that may be noted in MD include the following:
- Periperial lymphadenopathy of the inguinal lymph nodes
- Personality changes such as depression and hiding
- Pain or twitching over affected sites
- Concurrent lesions of EGC.

■ The lesions of the EGC are variable and tend to be classified based on three subclinical divisions.
- First, the eosinophilic ulcer (e.g., indolent, rodent, and lip ulcers) is a well-circumscribed, red-brown to yellow, ulcerated lesion most commonly found on the upper lip of the cat. The lesions are generally nonpainful and nonpruritic.
- Second, the eosinophilic plaque is a well-circumscribed, raised exudative lesion that is highly pruritic and generally found over the abdomen or groin. This lesion is the most common form of EGC in cats with concurrent MD.
- Third, the linear granulomas (i.e., eosinophilic collagenolytic granulomas) are seen primarily in young cats and are well-circumscribed, raised, er-

ythematous to yellow linear, papular, or nodular lesions. They most commonly are found in a linear pattern over the caudal thighs and in a nodular pattern in the oral cavity. Other sites include the bridge of the nose, chin, lips, pinnae, foot pads, and paws.

DIAGNOSIS

■ *History* helps identify seasonal allergies, such as flea and insect hypersensitivities, atopy, and chiggers. A history of pruritus with MD lesions is more typical of parasitic and allergic hypersensitivity disorders.

■ *Physical examination* can also help narrow the differential diagnosis in both MD and EGC.
- The distribution of MD lesions favors some etiologies over others:

   Dorsal distribution (especially the lumbosacral area) favors flea hypersensitivity. Cheyletiellosis can also have a dorsal distribution.

   When the head and neck are affected consider notoedric mange, otodectic mange, food allergy, atopy, pyoderma, or pemphigus.
- The distribution of EGC lesions is less helpful in limiting the differential diagnoses.

   Nasal and pinnal forms of eosinophilic collagenolytic granulomas tend to support the diagnosis of insect bite reactions.

   Eosinophilic plaques over the groin and abdomen tend to favor the diagnosis of flea hypersensitivity.

   Pruritic cervical EGC lesions are more commonly seen in food allergy, atopy, or bacterial infection.

■ *Minimum data base*
- *Skin scrapings, Scotch tape preparations,* and *combings of hair and dander* for fleas and mites are very important in the initial MD diagnostic evaluation.
- *Skin cytology* can be of value to determine the presence of infectious organisms and inflammatory cells. Skin cytology is obtained by fine needle aspirate of the lesion or by touching a glass slide to the lesion. Tissue eosinophilia favors the diagnosis of parasitic and allergic disorders.
- *Dermatophyte culture* is the best way to rule out a dermatophyte as the cause of MD (see sec. 5, ch. 3).

■ *Additional Diagnostic Testing*
- *Bacterial culture and sensitivity tests,* performed on a skin biopsy sample, can give additional information on etiology and choice of correct antibiotic for therapy.
- *Complete blood counts* may reveal peripheral eosinophilia associated with parasitic and allergy disorders, especially that of flea allergy. Peripheral eosinophilia tends to be seen in most cases of eosinophilic plaque and in many cases of eosinophilic collagenolytic granuloma regardless of the cause.
- *Serum biochemical analysis* helps rule out other concurrent medical problems. *Viral testing* for

FELV and FIV are recommended in recurrent cases of MD and EGC (see sec. 2, chs. 1 and 2). Results of both chemistry and viral screens will influence treatment and prognosis.

- *Dermatopathology* is one of the most important diagnostic tests performed. Findings may support the clinical assessment, suggest additional differentials, or provide a specific diagnosis. In regard to EGC, specific histologic patterns have been associated with the three clinical entities.

  Eosinophilic ulcer is usually characterized by a chronic ulcerative suppurative dermatitis. On occasion histologic observation may reveal an eosinophilic collagenolytic dermatitis with palisading granulomatous inflammation.

  Eosinophilic plaque is characterized by marked, intercellular (spongiotic dermatitis) edema and tissue eosinophilia.

  Eosinophilic granuloma is characterized by eosinophilic collagenolytic dermatitis with palisading granulomatous inflammation.

- A *food elimination diet* is the only way to accurately rule out food allergy. Such a diet consists of a protein source that the cat does not or has not eaten routinely. The common choice is lamb baby food, but ham baby food, home-cooked chicken, fish, rabbit, and other protein sources have been provided successfully (see sec. 5, ch. 8). The diet is fed strictly for 6 weeks. Long-term management is discussed under treatment.

- *Intradermal allergy testing* helps rule out the diagnoses of insect and inhaled allergies. Allergy testing in the cat is difficult to perform and interpret. Testing is, therefore, best done by an experienced veterinary allergist (see sec. 5, ch. 7).

TREATMENT

KEY POINT ▶ Many forms of therapy have been described for both MD and EGC. The best long-term management is achieved when a definitive diagnosis of the underlying cause has been established and specific therapy for that disease prescribed.

Corticosteroid Therapy

This therapy can be tried in first-time cases of MD and EGC. In chronic recurrent cases, alternative therapy is given, based on information from an appropriate workup. Even with proper workups, refractory allergies or idiopathic cases of both MD and EGC may require long-term corticosteroid therapy. A variety of corticosteroids can be tried.

- Methylprednisolone acetate (Depo-Medrol, Upjohn Co.) given at 4 mg/kg, IM, is a commonly utilized, and often efficacious, long-acting injectable corticosteroid. Cases of refractory EGC may need 3 injections at 2-week intervals. In general, after remission, do not use methylprednisolone acetate more often than every 3 months.

- As an alternative to methylprednisolone acetate, give anti-inflammatory doses of prednisone at 2.2 mg/kg, q24h, PO, for resolution of lesions. Decrease the dose to 1 to 2 mg/kg, q48h, PO, for maintenance.

- Some cases can be successfully managed with initial injections of methylprednisolone acetate and then maintained with oral prednisone at 1 to 2 mg/kg, q48h, PO.

Antihistamine Therapy

Two antihistamines can be tried in cases of atopy and flea allergy and idiopathic cases of MD and EGC: chlorpheniramine at 2 to 4 mg, q12h, PO, or hydroxyzine hydrochloride at 10 mg, q12h, PO. Of the two, chlorpheniramine appears more effective and has fewer sedative or excitatory side effects.

Food Allergy Management

After determining that a cat has a food allergy, manage with a balanced home-cooked diet or a commercial diet that is tolerated (see sec. 5, ch. 8). In general, cats require additional levels of the amino acid taurine and protein. Commercial taurine supplements are available. Commercial diets used with some success include Hill's canned Prescription Diet d/d, canned meats (e.g., Kal Kan Chicken), and Feline Wysong Anergen.

Hyposensitization Therapy

Hyposensitization has limited efficacy in the cat. However, some cases of EGC due to feline atopy have been successfully managed with antigen injections (see sec. 5, ch. 7). Flea hyposensitization has had little benefit in controlling flea allergy in the cat. Protocols are similar to those in dogs.

Parasiticidal Therapy

Because parasites directly or indirectly, via a hypersensitivity reaction, contribute to the lesions in MD and EGC, the control of parasites on the pet and in the environment is extremely important. Topical flea control is described in sec. 5, ch. 6. Parasites requiring environmental control include fleas, mosquitos, biting flies, *Cheyletiella,* chiggers, and *Otodectes* (see sec. 5, ch. 5). Ivermectin (Ivomec; Merck) therapy has been used successfully for *Notoedres, Otodectes,* and *Cheyletiella.* The dosage is 0.2 mg/kg, SC, weekly for a total of 3 treatments. Although ivermectin is not approved for parasite control in the cat, it has been used safely and without serious side effects. Injection site reactions are occasionally seen in the cat.

Infectious Therapy

Use antibiotic therapy for primary or secondary infections in both MD and EGC. Initially, select antibiotics empirically based on cytologic findings. In chronic cases, culture and sensitivity results are employed. Antibiotics for empirical therapy include trimethoprim-potentiated sulfas at 30 mg/kg, q12h, PO; cefadroxil (Cefa-Tabs; Fort Dodge) at 20 mg/kg, q12h,

PO; or amoxicillin-clavulanate (Clavamox; Smith-Kline Beecham) at 12 to 15 mg/kg, q12h, PO. Continue treatment for a minimum of 2 weeks and 10 days past clinical cure. Therapy for dermatophytosis is described in detail in sec. 5, ch. 3.

Progestational Therapy

Progestational compounds have been advocated for treating both MD and EGC. Most veterinary derma-tologists do not use or recommend these products because of their potential for severe side effects. They are not approved for use in cats. With the effectiveness of other forms of therapy, progestational drug therapy is undesirable.

Supplemental Reading

Rosenkrantz W: Eosinophilic granuloma confusion. *In* August JR (ed.): *Consultations in Feline Internal Medicine.* Philadelphia: W. B. Saunders, 1990, pp 121–124.

15 Skin Biopsy

Robert O. Schick
Mary P. Schick

BIOPSY SELECTION

- Properly selected, collected, and processed skin biopsies are likely to provide the definitive diagnosis and prognosis for many skin diseases. Skin biopsy samples are valuable in determining the malignancy of neoplastic skin lesions as well as their invasive nature.
- Biopsy "fresh" vesicles, bullae, or pustules that are less than 24 hours old. Skin lesions, such as non-healing wounds, pigmented lesions, and purpura, and those of infiltrative diseases, such as discoid or systemic lupus erythematosus and amyloidosis, are best biopsied within 1 month of detection.

KEY POINT ▶ Biopsy of primary and fresh skin lesions is most likely to yield a definitive diagnosis. Certain types of skin lesions yield less valuable information, because of altered histology, including chronic, traumatized, previously treated, or old lesions.

EQUIPMENT

- A cold sterilization tray filled with an appropriate antiseptic solution holding the various instruments is used for easy accessibility.
- Use the following instruments to handle the delicate skin specimens:
  - A pair of scissors (straight or curved iris)
  - Fine eye forceps
  - Curved hemostats
  - Needle holder
  - Suture scissors
  - Scalpel blades (# 11 or # 15)
  - Scalpel handle
  - Black indelible-ink pen (Sharpie; Sanford Corp.)
- Obtain disposable skin punch biopsies (Baker's Biopsy Punch; Key Pharmaceutical, Inc.) primarily of 4 and 6 mm (Fig. 1).

KEY POINT ▶ To obtain the best skin punch biopsy, do not reuse the disposable punches.

- Lidocaine 2% (Lidocaine 2%; Butler Company) or lidocaine HCl 1% solution with epinephrine 1:100,000 (Xylocaine 1%; Antra Pharmaceutical Products, Inc.) is the local anesthetic of choice.

BIOPSY PROCEDURES

Scalpel Wedge Biopsy

The scalpel is most commonly used to perform excisional biopsies, especially subcutaneous ones that are not amenable to punch biopsies.

- Indications
  - To obtain a large sample or an entire lesion
  - To provide lesional, transitional, and normal tissue for histopathologic viewing
  - To excise deep lesions or neoplasms: the lower dermis or subcutaneous fat provides characteristic histologic features.
  - To excise an entire neoplasm along with adjacent normal tissue to assess histologically for depth and width of neoplastic cell infiltration.

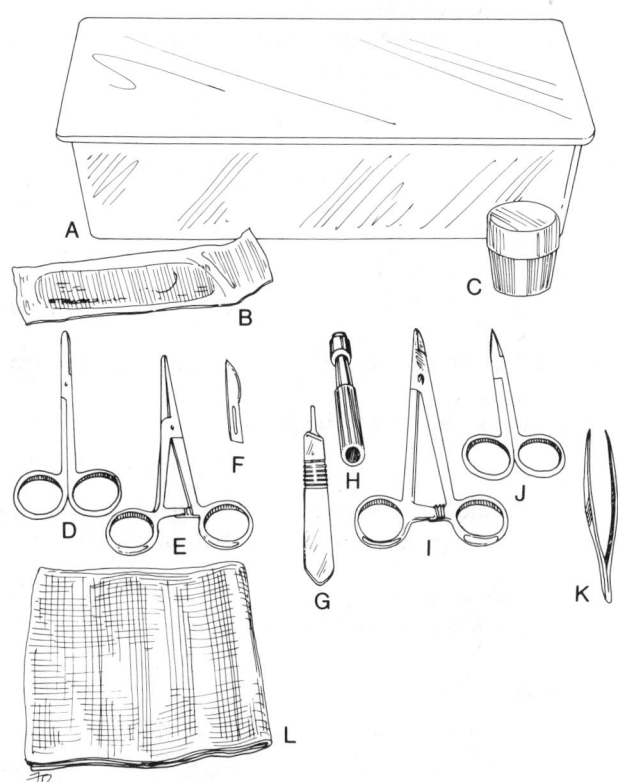

Figure 1. Skin punch biopsy instruments. *A,* Cold sterilization boat; *B,* suture material; *C,* formalin specimen container; *D,* suture scissors; *E,* straight hemostats; *F,* scalpel blades; *G,* scalpel blade handle; *H,* biopsy punch; *I,* needle holders; *J,* iris scissors; *K,* tissue forceps; and *L,* gauze sponges.

- Advantages
  - Total removal of solitary neoplasm may be possible.
  - Fragile bullous or vesicular lesions and subcutaneous fat are easily obtained intact.
  - Specimen preparation on the long axis may provide a microscopic histologic view of the abnormal issue, transitional zone, and normal tissue boundaries, so that a prognosis as well as a diagnosis may be obtained.
- Disadvantages
  - Pain to the animal and extensive time may be involved in removal.
  - General anesthesia may be required.
  - Large defects may not allow for cosmetic closure.

Technique

1. Use local or general anesthesia, depending on the size and location of the lesion.
2. The scalpel is held perpendicularly or slightly angled with respect to the lesion to allow for the best cosmetic closure. The adjacent subcutaneous tissues are undermined to loosen the skin for best closure.

Punch Biopsy

This is the most commonly used technique to obtain skin specimens for histologic examination.

- Indications
  - For collection of abnormal tissue for histologic examination
  - For biopsy of samples from neoplasms
  - For biopsy of samples from early bullous, vesicular, or pustular lesions

KEY POINT ▶ Take multiple biopsy samples to obtain optimal histologic examination of the various stages of a particular skin disease.

- Advantages
  - This relatively easy and fast procedure usually provides for the definitive diagnoses of skin diseases.
  - A minimal number of sutures is required to close the skin defect.
  - Minimal cosmetic defects are created by the procedure.
- Disadvantages
  - Subcutaneous fat may be lost during the biopsy procedure precluding its histopathologic examination.
  - Multiple skin biopsy samples may be necessary for adequate representation of the disease process.

Technique

Consider general anesthesia for the biopsy of skin lesions that have definite or suspected subcutaneous involvement as well as those in sensitive areas: pedicular, perioral, periauricular, perianal, and so forth.

1. Clip hair at the biopsy site. No cleansing or other topical preparations are advised.

2. To ensure accurate biopsy of anesthetized lesions, mark the biopsy site with an indelible ink pen.
3. Use a 25-gauge needle and 1 cc syringe to inject 0.50 to 1.0 cc of lidocaine or lidocaine with epinephrine SC at the site to be biopsied.
4. Biopsy the lesion skin approximately 5 minutes after anesthetizing.
5. Take the biopsy specimens entirely within lesion boundaries.
6. Rotate the 4-mm or 6-mm disposable biopsy punch (preferred size by most veterinary pathologists) in one direction through the skin and into the subcutis.
7. Gently remove the resultant core of skin with a pair of fine eye forceps and iris scissors.
8. The 25-gauge needle employed to inject local anesthesia can also elevate the biopsy sample.
9. Impale the subcutaneous fat with it, and lift for cutting from underneath.
10. Quickly transfer the specimens into the fixative solution.
11. Suture the biopsy sites if needed. This may not be necessary for 4-mm defects, but use one to two sutures for 6-mm defects.

Shave Biopsy

- Indications
  - The shave biopsy is used in human medicine when a skin disease process is suspected to be limited to the epidermis or upper dermis. In veterinary medicine, there are fewer applications.
- Advantages
  - A very fast procedure
  - Some superficial lesions (e.g., papillomas and skin tags) may be totally removed and submitted for histopathologic examination.
  - No suturing is needed.
  - Minimal to no scarring occurs afterwards, because the lower dermis is left intact.
- Disadvantages
  - Can be used to diagnose only benign and extremely superficial lesions.
  - Cannot be used to determine the depth of neoplastic infiltration. Only benign superficial neoplasms can be diagnosed.

Technique

1. Local anesthesia is optional, depending on the lesion's size and location.
2. The skin is raised as a fold. The scalpel blade is held parallel to the skin surface.
3. The scalpel is then used to cut across the lesion.
4. After the shave biopsy, use curettage or electrodesiccation to remove deeper aspects of the lesion.

Curettage

This is the least satisfactory method of collecting skin specimens for histopathologic examination. It is unavoidable that scanty, superficial, fragmented, and distorted skin specimens are collected. If this technique is attempted, make a single firm stroke across the lesion to obtain the best specimen.

HANDLING FORMALIN-FIXED SKIN BIOPSY SPECIMENS

- Bisect all nodules that might have an infectious etiology.
- Submit half the nodule for histopathology; submit the other half in a sterile container for bacterial and fungal cultures.
- After removing the skin specimen, quickly roll the core sample or blot the wedge sample on bibulous (absorbent lint-free) paper to remove excess blood. Gently press the skin specimen subcutaneous side down onto a piece of a wooden tongue depressor.
- The specimen is now in correct anatomic orientation and is floated upside-down or immersed in 10% phosphate–buffered formalin fixative for routine histologic examination.
- The fixative volume is ten times the sample volume to ensure proper fixation.
- Large specimens, such as wedge biopsy samples, are sliced to limit thickness to 2 cm regardless of area.
- Keep the freshly formalin-fixed specimens at room temperature for at least 6 hours before shipping in the extreme cold of winter.
- Avoid freezing of formalin-fixed biopsy tissue.
- Enclose a brief but detailed summary of the patient's clinical history and lesions with the specimens.

KEY POINT ▶ Decide upon any special histopathology studies before immersing tissue into formalin. Formalin may ruin the sample for these purposes.

KEY POINT ▶ Specimens are submitted to a veterinary pathologist with training in dermatopathology.

HANDLING MICHEL'S MEDIA-FIXED SKIN BIOPSY SPECIMENS

- Immunologic abnormalities of the skin, especially of connective tissue and in bullous diseases, may result in deposition of immunoglobulin, complement, and fibrin. These depositions in the skin may be detected by direct immunofluorescent microscopy.
- When submitting skin specimens for direct immunofluorescence, use the same biopsy procedures as those done for formalin fixation.

KEY POINT ▶ Take the Michel's media samples before the samples for routine histopathology. Formalin residue on the instruments can lead to false-negative direct immunofluorescence results.

- Michel's transport media and fixative maintain skin specimens indefinitely at room temperature.
- Skin punch biopsies of 4 mm allow for the best penetration of the fixative.
- Negative immunofluorescence test results do not eliminate the diagnosis of an autoimmune disease. This test is positive in only 50% of autoimmune skin diseases.
- Positive immunofluorescence test results do not always confirm autoimmune disease. The test results may be positive in many infectious and inflammatory dermatoses and in some normal dogs and cats.

KEY POINT ▶ Save the Michel's media-fixed specimens at the hospital. Do not submit them for direct immunofluorescence until the results of the routine histopathologic examination of the formalin-fixed specimens indicate changes consistent with autoimmune skin disease.

Supplemental Readings

Fitzpatrick TB, et al.: *Dermatology in General Medicine,* third edition. New York: McGraw-Hill, 1987, p 47.

Ihrke PJ, Gross TL: The skin biopsy: maximizing benefits. Scientific Proceedings of the American Animal Hospital Association, 1988, p 299.

Lever WF, Schaumburg-Lever G: Introduction. *In* Pedersen DD, ed.: *Histopathology of the Skin.* Philadelphia: J. B. Lippincott, 1983, p 1.

16 Surgery of Intertriginous Dermatoses

Jamie R. Bellah

Intertriginous dermatoses are surface pyodermas that are associated with skin folds. Chronic skin apposition results in friction, minor trauma, and poor air circulation along with a moist environment conducive to colonization and infection by bacteria.

KEY POINT ▶ Inflammation and exudate associated with pyoderma cause pain, pruritus, and malodor. Conservative treatment is only palliative. Resolution of these conditions can be accomplished only by surgery.

ETIOLOGY

Normal skin defense mechanisms are as follows:

- Intact epidermis and stratum corneum
- Sebum that contains antibacterial fatty acids
- Skin microflora that may secrete antibiotic-like substances

Skin fold pyoderma is classified as a surface pyoderma.

- Bacteria remain on top of the skin.
- Warm, moist environment within recess of the skin fold allows colonization by *Staphylococcus intermedius* or *S. aureus*.
- Other infecting bacteria include *Streptococcus, Escherichia coli, Pseudomonas, Proteus,* and *Candida.*
- Superficial skin erosions and inflammation result.
- Self-trauma and obesity tend to worsen the condition.

Locations, characteristics, and breeds associated with intertriginous dermatoses include the following:

- Facial or nasal fold
  - Frequently associated with secondary ulcerative keratitis
  - Brachycephalic breeds: Pekingese, English bulldog, pug, French bulldog, Boston terrier
  - Persian cats.
- Lip fold
  - Common in dogs with excessive mandibular labial tissue, such as spaniels, Saint Bernard, Irish setter, Newfoundland, Golden retriever, Labrador retriever
  - Redundant lip fold is usually located behind the mandibular canine tooth.
  - Can be bilateral.
  - Causes severe halitosis.

- May occur after partial mandibulectomy or maxillectomy if a skin fold is created during wound closure.
- Body fold
  - Usually affects obese or Chinese Shar Pei dogs.
  - With Shar Pei puppies, body folds become less redundant with growth but persist on the head and face.
  - May occur in female dogs or cats along the abdominal midline if mammary glands or body fat creates a skin fold.
  - Moist seborrhea predisposes the animal to body fold pyoderma.
- Vulvar fold
  - Most common in older, obese spayed female dogs and rarely cats.
  - Seen in younger dogs with infantile vulvas.
  - Accumulation of urine and vaginal secretions occur.
  - Animal may have a secondary urinary tract infection.
- Tail fold ("screw tail")
  - Common in English bulldog, pug, Boston terrier, and schipperke breeds
  - Also seen in Manx cats.
  - Caused by redundant skin around the tail and the corkscrew conformation of the terminal coccygeal vertebrae.
  - A full-thickness ulcer may be present in the skin under the ventrally deviating tail. Such a condition can be very painful and uncomfortable for affected dogs.
  - Contamination by fecal flora causes fulminating pyoderma.
  - Self-trauma and scooting exacerbate the condition.

PREOPERATIVE CONSIDERATIONS

- Conservative treatment, including clipping hair from the skin fold, cleansing with dilute antibacterial solutions, medicated soaps, antiseborrheic shampoos, astringents, and topical and systemic antibiotics, is palliative only.
- Medical treatment may be advisable prior to surgery in some animals to lessen the amount of wound exudate and to lower bacterial numbers at the time of surgery.
- In the presence of severe infection (i.e., tail fold

pyoderma), a preoperative antimicrobial is justified to prevent a postoperative wound infection.

■ When show animals are affected, counsel the owner with regard to the expected postoperative appearance and consult breed requirements for show.

SURGICAL PROCEDURES

Objectives

■ *En bloc* excision of the skin fold and associated pyoderma.
■ Resolution of wound infection.

Equipment

■ Standard general surgical pack.
■ Suture material appropriate for infected wounds.
■ Bone-holding forceps aid manipulation of the tail during caudectomy for screw tail.
■ Bone-cutting forceps or Gigli saw for caudectomy
■ Penrose drains

Technique

1. *Facial or nasal fold excision*
   a. Position the animal in ventral recumbency
   b. Protect the eyes with an ophthalmic ointment during preparation and surgery.
   c. Clip hair from the facial skin folds and ventral eyelids sufficient to drape an appropriate margin around the fold to be excised.
   d. Plan the boundaries of the incision so that removal of too much skin is avoided. Skin is needed for closure without tension (Fig. 1*A*).
   e. With two paired incisions, excise enough of the facial fold to alleviate the recess created by the

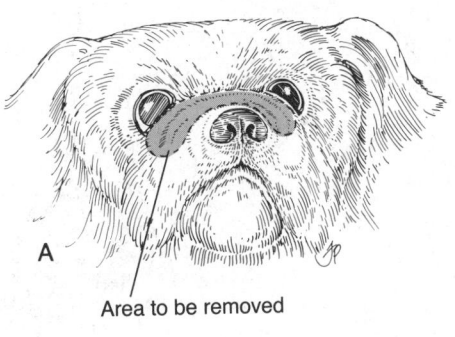

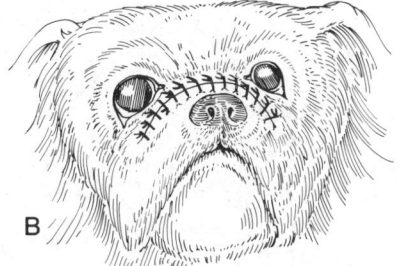

Area to be removed

Figure 1. Facial fold excision. *A,* Incision boundaries are planned so that enough skin for closure without tension remains. *B,* Final suture pattern.

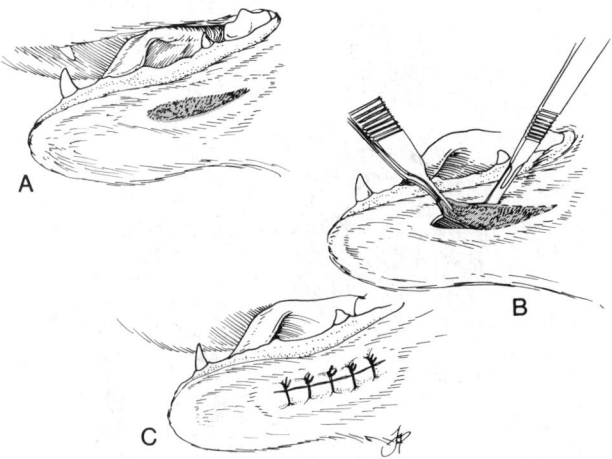

Figure 2. Lip fold excision (cheiloplasty). *A,* Preparation of skin. *B,* Excision of fold. *C,* Closure pattern.

fold and to eliminate any chance of hair contacting the eye.

KEY POINT ▶ Stay at least 1 cm from the medial canthus of the eye, and avoid lacrimal structures and large vessels in the region.

   f. Undermine skin edges gently and carefully, if required.
   g. Closure is done in two layers using fine (3-0 or 4-0) absorbable suture for subcutaneous tissue and fine monofilament suture for skin closure (Fig. 1*B*).
   h. Cut the suture ends short so that they do not contact the cornea.

2. *Lip fold excision* (cheiloplasty)
   a. Position the animal in dorsal recumbency.
   b. Clip and prepare the skin over the mandible from its rostral tip to the mandibular angle (Fig. 2*A*).
   c. Make an elliptical incision around the lip fold, and remove the entire fold and infected region (Fig. 2*B*).
   d. It is very rare that the mucosal surface of the lip needs to be incised.
   e. Try to avoid incising the underlying muscles of the lip.
   f. Close the incision in two layers using fine absorbable suture for subcutaneous tissue and fine nonabsorbable suture for skin (Fig. 2*C*).
   g. Closure of the buccal mucosa, if incised, is done with fine interrupted absorbable sutures.

3. *Body fold excision*
   a. Position the dog so that optimum access to the body fold to be removed is accomplished.
   b. Prepare the skin wide enough so the fold can be excised in its entirety.
   c. Make two incisions parallel to the fold near its base being certain to leave sufficient skin for closure.
   d. Closure is done in two layers using fine absorbable suture for subcutaneous tissues and interrupted nonabsorbable sutures for skin apposition.

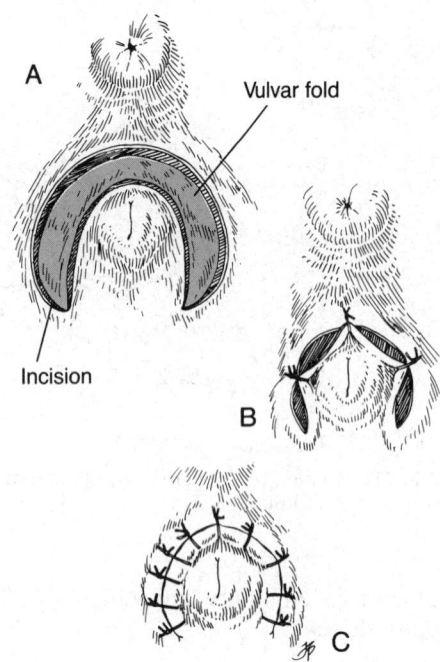

Figure 3. Vulvar fold excision (episioplasty). *A,* Incision pattern around base of vulvar fold. *B,* Simple sutures approximate wound margin. *C,* Suture pattern.

e. Mastectomy (see sec. 3, ch. 8) may be required to resolve body fold pyoderma that has resulted from rolls of abdominal fat or from pendulous mammary tissue.
4. *Vulvar fold excision* (episioplasty)
   a. Place the animal in ventral recumbency with the perineal region at the end of the table. If the rear legs are draped over the end of the table be sure to pad them sufficiently.
   b. Place a pursestring suture around the anus.
   c. Prepare the perivulvar region for aseptic surgery.
   d. Make an elliptical incision around the base of the vulvar fold, which is then undermined and removed (Fig. 3*A*).
   e. Place simple interrupted cuticular sutures equidistant from one another around the incision to approximate the wound margins (Fig. 3*B*). This step helps to determine if adequate skin and subcutaneous fat have been removed.
   f. Close the skin in two layers using fine absorbable suture for subcutaneous tissue and fine nonabsorbable sutures for skin (Fig. 3*C*).
   g. Remove the pursestring suture.
5. *Tail fold excision and caudectomy*
   a. Place the animal in ventral recumbency with the perineum facing the end of the table. A frogleg position is used for this procedure.
   b. Place a pursestring suture around the anus.
   c. Clip the entire perineum and tailhead region.
   d. It is difficult to clip hair from the fold region adequately, thus use a prophylactic antimicrobial drug given before and during surgery.
   e. Make an incision around the tail and tail fold. Skin dorsal to the tail may be preserved and aids in cosmetic skin closure (Fig. 4*A*).
   f. Attempt to dissect around the tail and skin fold without penetrating the fold.

g. Sometimes, because ventral deviation of the tail causes full-thickness erosion through the skin and *en bloc* excision cannot be performed, layered debridement must be done.
   h. Manipulate the tail using bone-holding forceps (Fig. 4*B*).
   i. Incise coccygeal and levator ani muscular attachments.
   j. Using a Gigli wire or bone-cutting forceps, transect the tail rostral to its ventral deviation.

KEY POINT ▶ Be careful during transection of the tail not to traumatize the rectum, which is just ventral to the tail base.

k. Use several interrupted absorbable sutures to close dead space.
   l. Place Penrose drains at this time, if necessary.
   m. Close the wound in two layers, utilizing fine absorbable sutures for subcutaneous tissues and fine nonabsorbable sutures for skin apposition (Fig. 4*C*).
   n. Remove the pursestring suture.

POSTOPERATIVE CARE AND COMPLICATIONS
Postoperative Care

■ Prevent self-trauma (Elizabethan collar).
■ Antimicrobial therapy may be based on culture and sensitivity testing if deemed necessary.

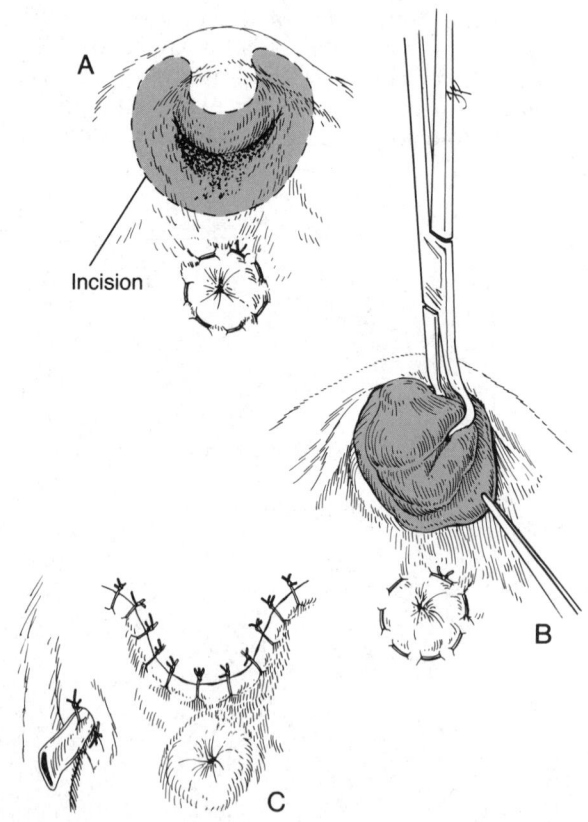

Figure 4. Tail fold excision and caudectomy. *A,* Make a pursestring suture around the anus, and incise the tail-fold region as shown. *B,* Tail is manipulated with tail-holding forceps. *C,* Wound closure pattern and drain.

- Keep oral incisions free of food and saliva.
- Keep perineal incisions clean, and remove fecal contamination.
- Remove Penrose drains in 3 to 5 days.

Complications

- Self-trauma
- Wound infection
- Dehiscence
- Ectropion (aggressive facial fold removal)
- Insufficient skin fold removal (relapse of pyoderma)

Supplemental Readings

Krahwinkel DJ, Bone DL: Surgical management of specific skin disorders. *In* Slatter DH, ed.: *Textbook of Small Animal Surgery.* Philadelphia: W. B. Saunders, 1985, p 501.

Krahwinkel DJ, Jr: Correction of specific skin defects. *In* Swaim SF, ed.: *Surgery of Traumatized Skin: Management and Reconstruction in the Dog and Cat.* Philadelphia: W. B. Saunders, 1980.

McLoughlin M: Surgical management of skin fold pyoderma. *In* Bojrab MJ, ed.: *Current Techniques in Small Animal Surgery, 2nd edition.* Philadelphia: W. B. Saunders, 1990, p 489.

Muller GH, Kirk RW, Scott DW: *Small Animal Dermatology.* Philadelphia: W. B. Saunders, 1989, p 792.

17 Closure of Traumatic Wounds Using Adjacent Skin

Steven F. Swaim

Following proper initial management of a traumatic wound by debridement and lavage, the wound may be closed. Sufficient viable tissue must be present to allow closure without excessive tension. Wounds may be closed by primary closure, delayed primary closure, or secondary closure. See sec. 5, ch. 18, for a discussion of open wound management.

ANATOMY

- Dogs and cats have abundant skin on the trunk and neck but a sparsity of skin on the distal limbs.
- Direct cutaneous vessels run parallel to the skin surface and supply the subdermal plexus of the skin. See sec. 5, ch. 19, for more details regarding blood supply to the skin.
- Some areas of the body have panniculus musculature underlying the skin. The skin's blood supply runs both superficial and deep to this musculature.
- Other areas of the body have loose areolar fascia deep to the dermis in which vasculature is located, and in other areas the skin is closely associated with underlying fascia.

PREOPERATIVE CONSIDERATIONS

KEY POINT ▶ If a traumatically induced wound is to be closed, it is imperative that the tissues be viable and clean enough that wound healing can progress uneventfully. Perform adequate debridement and lavage.

- Perform a thorough physical examination and appropriate diagnostic tests on all traumatized animals to rule out associated injuries.
- Perform primary closure when:
  - The animal is in good condition.
  - A short time (6 to 12 hours) has elapsed since injury.
  - Minimal contamination and tissue trauma have occurred.
  - Adequate debridement and lavage have been done.
- Perform delayed primary closure when:
  - Wounds show evidence of heavy contamination, purulent exudate, residual necrotic or questionable tissue, edema, erythema at the wound margins, lymphangitis, and skin tension.
  - Local infection has been controlled by debridement, lavage, topical and/or systemic antibiotics, and adherent bandages. This control is usually 3 to 5 days after infliction.
- Perform a secondary closure when:
  - The wound is in the reparative stage of healing at presentation, with a healthy bed of granulation tissue and evidence of epithelialization.
  - The wound has disrupted and has subsequently developed a healthy bed of granulation tissue.
  - It has been necessary to leave the wound open for longer than 5 days to control infection (see Preoperative Considerations, Delayed primary closure, Local infection control).

SURGICAL PROCEDURES

Primary or Delayed Primary Closure *Without* Tension

- Objectives
  - Close the wound
  - Provide drainage if necessary

Equipment

- Standard general surgical pack
- Undyed polyglactin 910, 3-0 (Vicryl; Ethicon, Inc.) and polypropylene or nylon, 3-0 (Prolene or Ethilon; Ethicon, Inc.)
- Wound lavage solution of 0.05% chlorhexidine (Nolvasan Solution; Ft. Dodge).
- Penrose drain

Technique

1. Pack the wound with sterile surgical sponges moistened with physiologic saline, or fill it with sterile water soluble lubricant (K-Y Jelly; Johnson & Johnson).
2. Prepare the area around the wound for aseptic surgery.
3. Remove the wound packing or sterile lubricant.
4. Lavage the wound frequently during surgery.
5. Use as few simple interrupted absorbable sutures as necessary to close dead space in deep layers of the wound.
6. Be careful not to include major vessels or nerves in the sutures.

7. Place a Penrose drain if there is any possibility of residual dead space and/or wound drainage.
8. Place a simple continuous suture in the subcutaneous tissue at the wound edge using absorbable suture material.
9. Employ nonabsorbable simple interrupted sutures to close the skin.

■ Postoperative care and complications
  • Postoperative care
    Place absorbent surgical sponges over the suture line, with extra sponges over the emergence of the drain.
    Apply an absorbent secondary wrap to the area, followed by an outer wrap of porous adhesive tape.
    Change the bandage daily, especially if a drain was placed, noting the amount and nature of drainage.
    Remove the drain and discontinue bandaging when the drainage becomes minimal.
    Remove the skin sutures 7 to 10 days postoperatively.
  • Complications
    Hematoma, seroma, or infection may result from improper wound evaluation, debridement, lavage, closure, and drain management.

Primary, Delayed Primary, or Secondary Closure *With* Tension

■ Objectives
  • Close the wound
  • Relieve tension on the wound closure
  • Provide drainage if necessary
■ Equipment
  • See Surgical Procedures, Primary or Delayed Primary Closure *Without* Tension, Equipment.

Technique

1. The general techniques for closure of wounds with tension are the same as those for primary or delayed primary closure without tension (see Surgical Procedures, *Primary or Delayed Primary Closure Without Tension,* Technique), with the exception of suture pattern (see tension-relieving suture patterns discussed subsequently).
2. Wounds that are in the reparative stage of healing with healthy granulation tissue and epithelialization.
    Excise epithelium from the edge of the wound, leaving healthy granulation tissue in the center.
  a. Gently clean the surface of the granulation tissue with 0.05% chlorhexidine solution (Fig. 1).
3. Gently undermine the skin surrounding the wound.
  a. Undermine bluntly, using Metzenbaum scissors, leaving some loose areolar connective tissue on the dermis or undermine beneath any panniculus musculature that is present.
  b. Undermine sharply with scissors or scalpel blade in areas where skin is closely associated with the underlying fascia.

KEY POINT ▶ Leave large identifiable blood vessels (i.e., direct cutaneous blood vessels)

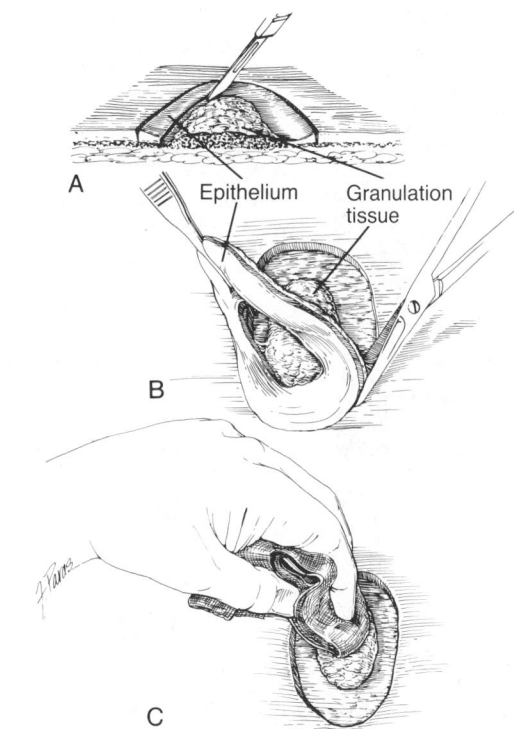

Figure 1. Preparation of a wound in the reparative stage of healing for secondary closure. *A,* Incising the epithelium. *B,* Removing the epithelium. *C,* Cleaning the surface of the healthy granulation tissue.

intact when undermining. Good judgment is needed when manipulating recently traumatized skin to avoid added insult to skin vasculature, which could result in skin slough.

4. One of several tension-relieving suture patterns may be used to close the wound.
  a. Place "walking" sutures (my choice for closing wounds under tension) with absorbable material in staggered parallel rows, beginning just in front of the plane where undermining stopped. Place a simple continuous subcuticular absorbable suture along the wound edge before skin closure with nonabsorbable simple interrupted sutures (Fig. 2).
  b. Place nonabsorbable vertical mattress sutures near the wound edge over segments of Penrose drain. Use simple interrupted nonabsorbable sutures to appose skin edges (Fig. 3).
  c. Place nonabsorbable "far-near-near-far" or "far-far-near-near" sutures in the order of their names to act as apposition and tension sutures (Fig. 4).
  d. Preplace nonabsorbable stent sutures deep to the wound tissues prior to closure of the wound. These sutures are then tied over a roll of surgical sponges or a rolled towel to act as a tension suture as well as to obliterate dead space (Fig. 5).
5. Use one of several relaxing incisions for additional tension release.
  a. Make unilateral or bilateral bipedicle flaps when undermining does not provide enough relaxation

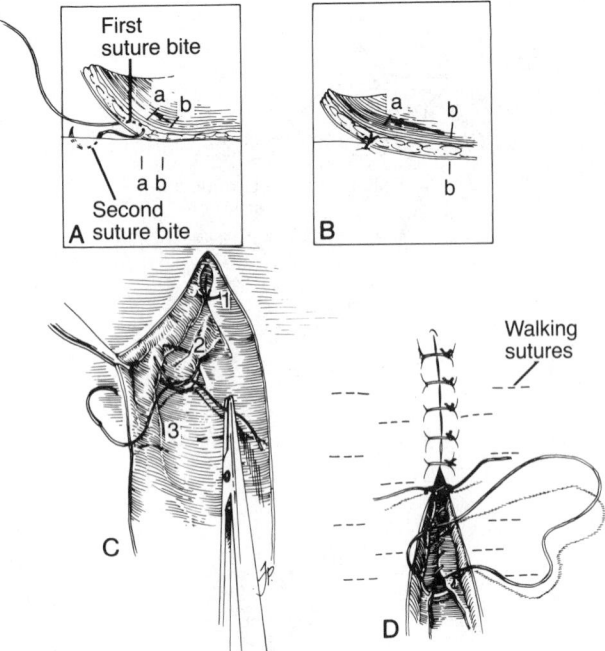

Figure 2. "Walking" sutures. *A,* Placing first and second suture bites. Segment of skin to be stretched (a to b). *B,* Tying a "walking" suture advances the skin towards the center of the wound (a to b increased). *C,* "Walking" sutures placed in rows. *1,* Walking suture tied; *2,* Placing a walking suture; *3,* Areas where bites will be taken for a walking suture (broken lines). *D,* Placing a simple continuous subcuticular suture along the wound edge, and simple interrupted skin apposition sutures. Broken lines are buried walking sutures. (After Swaim SF: The repair of the skin: Techniques of plastic and reconstructive surgery. *In* Bedford PGC, ed.: *Atlas of Canine Surgical Techniques.* Oxford: Blackwell Scientific Publications, 1984, p 49 and Swaim SF, Henderson RA: *Small Animal Wound Management.* Philadelphia: Lea & Febiger, 1990, p 92.)

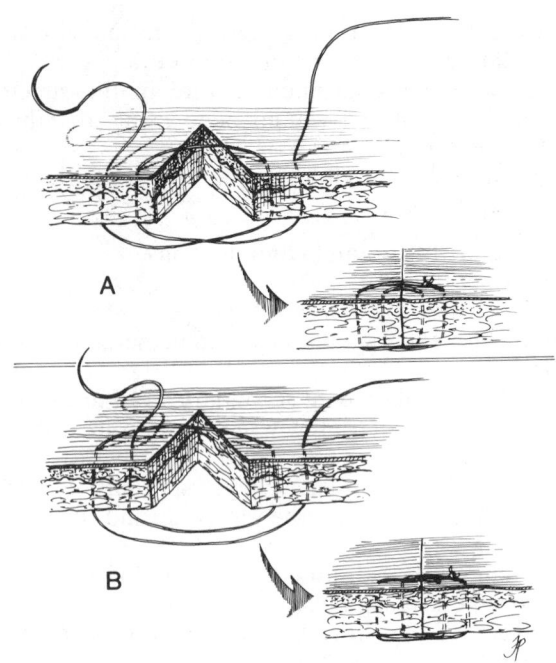

Figure 4. Combination apposition and tension sutures. *A,* "Far-near-near-far" sutures. *B,* "Far-far-near-near" sutures. (After Swaim SF, Henderson RA: *Small Animal Wound Management.* Philadelphia: Lea & Febiger, 1990, p 95.)

walking sutures to advance and tack the flaps in place and a regular or tension-relieving suture pattern to suture the skin. Close the defects left from moving the flaps (Fig. 6). Make unilateral or bilateral simple relaxing incisions as in creating a bipedicle flap. Move the flaps and suture in place as with bipedicle flaps. Do not close the defects that remain from moving the flaps but leave them to heal as open wounds (Fig. 7).

b. Make multiple, punctate, relaxing incisions 1-cm long and 0.5-cm apart in parallel, staggered rows

for wound closure. Make an incision parallel to the wound's long axis but slightly curved toward the wound, with the width of the created flaps being equal to the wound width. Use absorbable

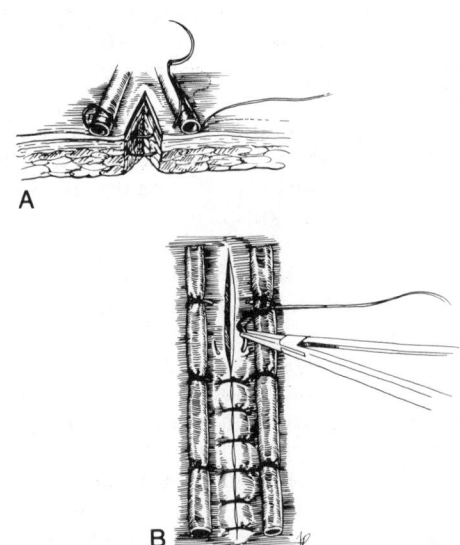

Figure 3. Vertical mattress tension sutures. *A,* Vertical mattress sutures placed over Penrose drains. *B,* Simple interrupted skin apposition sutures used with tension sutures.

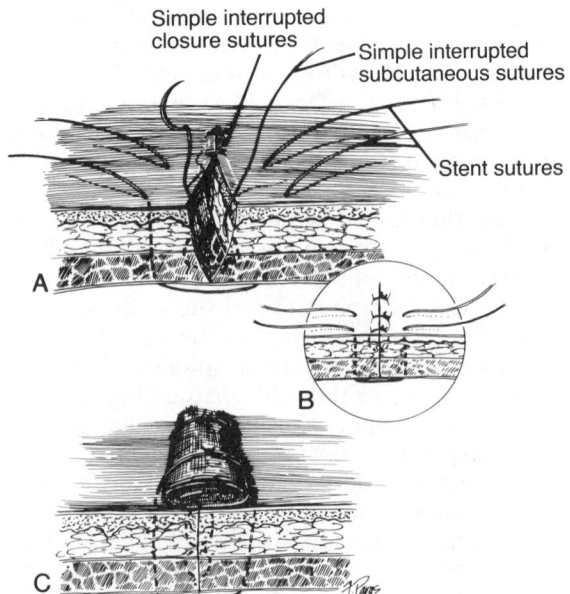

Figure 5. Stent sutures. *A,* Stent sutures are preplaced deep to the wound tissues. *B,* Wound tissues are closed. *C,* Stent sutures are tied over a roll of gauze or rolled towel.

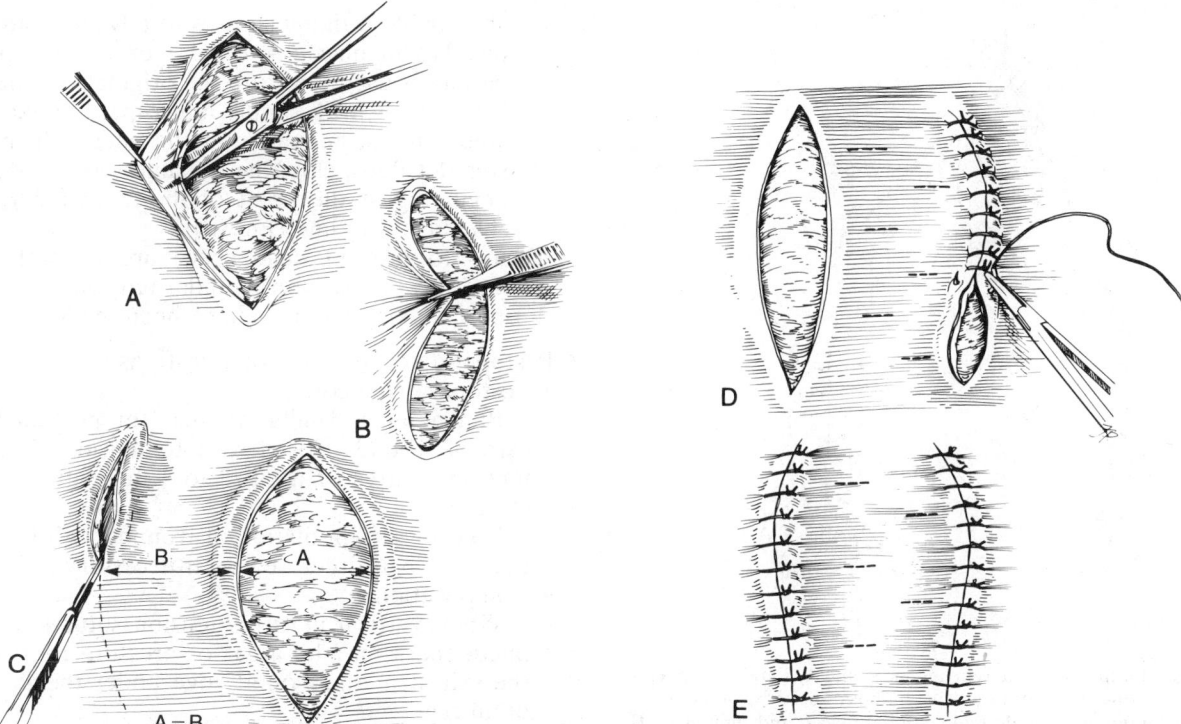

Figure 6. Unilateral bipedicle flap. *A,* Undermining the skin on the side of defect from which the flap will come. *B,* Checking to see if undermining provided sufficient skin for wound closure. *C,* Making an incision to create a bipedicle flap. Wound and flap width are equal (A = B). *D,* Flap being sutured into position after walking sutures have advanced it (broken lines). *E,* Donor site sutured. (After Swaim SF, Henderson RA: *Small Animal Wound Management.* Philadelphia: Lea & Febiger, 1990, p 100.)

bilaterally, as needed to allow wound closure as a simple continuous intradermal absorbable suture is placed and tightened. Final skin apposition is with simple interrupted, nonabsorbable sutures (Fig. 8).

c. Design and incise a 60° equal angle, equal limb-length Z-plasty adjacent to the wound with the central limb of the Z in the direction in which relaxation is needed. After undermining the skin edges and Z-plasty flaps, close the wound using

Figure 7. Bilateral simple relaxing incisions. *Top,* One bipedicle flap has been created on each side of the wound, with flaps equal in width to the defect width (A = B). *Bottom,* After undermining and moving the flaps with walking sutures (broken lines) to close the wound, the relaxing incision defects are left to heal as open wounds. (After Swaim SF, Henderson RA: *Small Animal Wound Management.* Philadelphia: Lea & Febiger, 1990, p 100.)

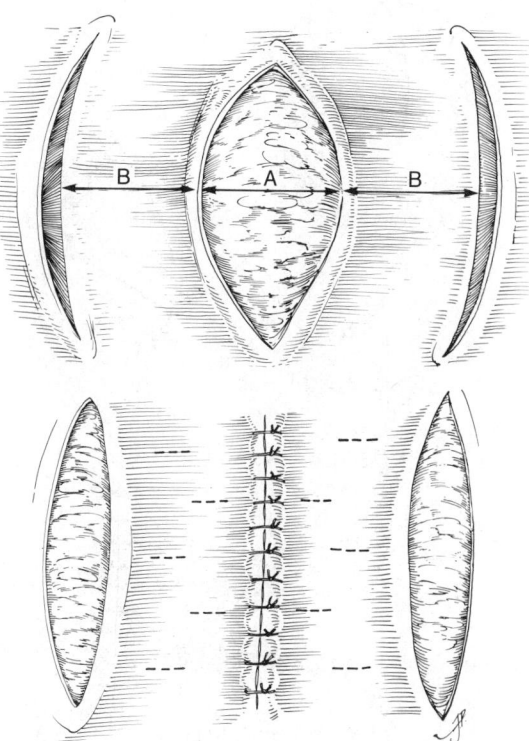

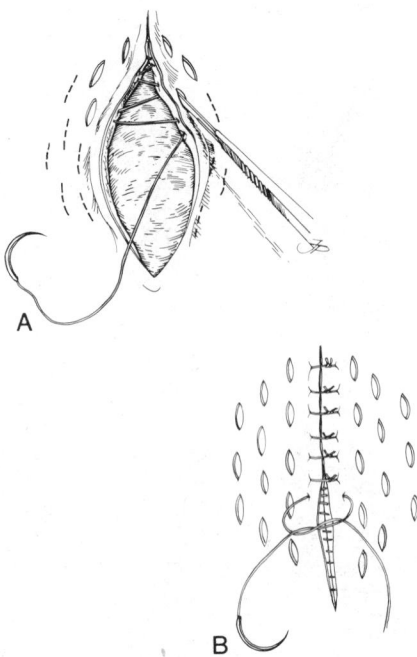

Figure 8. Multiple punctate relaxing incisions. *A,* Parallel staggered rows of incisions are made as needed on both sides of a wound while a simple continuous intradermal suture is placed and tightened. *B,* Final wound apposition with simple interrupted sutures. (After Swaim SF, Henderson RA: *Small Animal Wound Management.* Philadelphia: Lea & Febiger, 1990, p 105.)

regular or tension sutures. Suture the Z-plasty flaps into their new positions (Fig. 9).

d. Make a V-shaped incision adjacent to the wound with the point of the V away from the wound. After undermining the resulting skin flap, use absorbable walking sutures to advance and tack the flap in place. A regular or tension suture pattern is used to suture the original skin defect. Close the V with simple interrupted nonabsorbable sutures, beginning at the ends. When tension develops, close the remainder of the defect, beginning at the point of the V to form a Y-shaped suture line (Fig. 10).

6. Drains to prevent dead space are generally not needed in wounds sutured under tension, especially if open relaxing incisions have been made.

■ Postoperative care and complications
- Postoperative care

  Bandaging is similar to that for postoperative care of wounds closed without tension. Remove tension sutures (if used) 3 to 4 days after wound closure.

  Prevent self-mutilation of wounds with Elizabethan collar or other device, if necessary.

- Complications

  When vertical mattress tension sutures are applied, there may be areas of pressure necrosis of the skin near the wound edge under the Penrose drain segments.

  Simple relaxing incisions may result in a wound equal in size to the closed wound.

  Large and numerous multiple punctate relaxing incisions may result in good tension relief but may jeopardize the blood supply to the skin between incisions with a resultant slough.

  Skin closed too tightly around a limb may result in a "biologic tourniquet," with edema and hypothermia distal to the closure site. Skin closed too tightly around the thorax may result in impaired

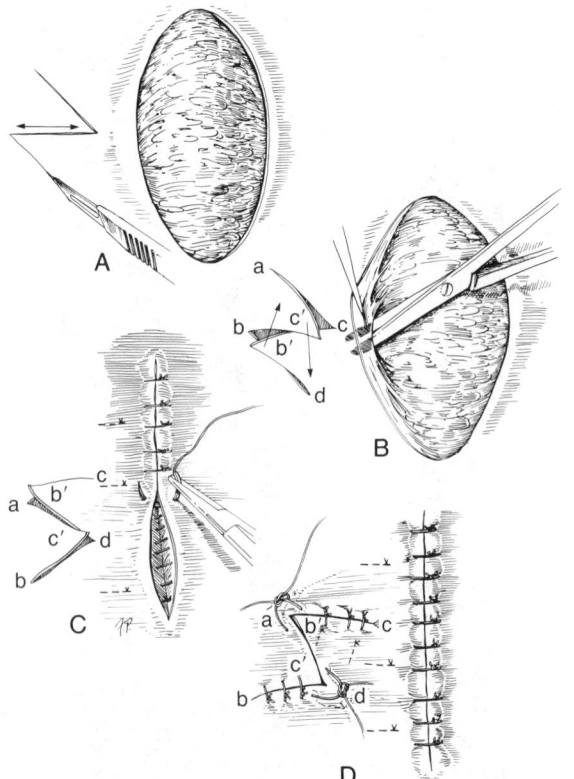

Figure 9. Z-plasty as a relaxing incision for wound closure. *A,* A 60° equal-angle, equal limb-length Z-plasty designed adjacent to a wound, with the central limb in the direction relaxation is needed. *B,* Z-plasty has been cut. Z-plasty flaps and adjacent skin are undermined (arrows indicate Z-plasty flap transposition). *C,* Closure of the defect with automatic transposition of Z-plasty flaps. *D,* Suturing the Z-plasty flaps into their new positions. (After Swaim SF, Henderson RA: *Small Animal Wound Management.* Philadelphia: Lea & Febiger, 1990, p 103.)

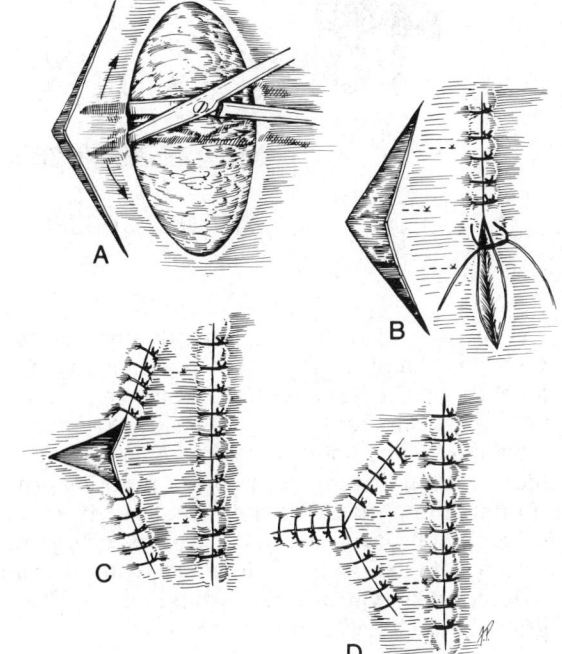

Figure 10. V-to-Y plasty relaxing incision. *A,* A V-shaped incision is made adjacent to the defect with point of the V away from the defect. Skin between the defect and incision is undermined. *B,* Closure of the defect with walking sutures holding the flap in position (broken lines). *C,* Closure of the V-shaped incision beginning at the ends. *D,* Closure of the stem of the Y. (After Swaim SF, Henderson RA: *Small Animal Wound Management.* Philadelphia: Lea & Febiger, 1990, p 101.)

respiration. Consider suture removal to release the tension in such cases.

Supplemental Readings

Lee AH, Swaim SF, Henderson RA: Surgical drainage. Compend Contin Educ 8:94, 1986.
Lee AH, Swaim SF: Granulation tissue and how to take advantage of it in management of open wounds. Compend Contin Educ Pract Vet 10:163, 1987.

Pavletic MM: Undermining for repair of large skin defects in small animals. Mod Vet Pract 67:13, 1986.
Swaim SF: Management of skin tension in dermal surgery. Compend Contin Educ 2:758, 1980.
Swaim SF, Henderson RA: *Small Animal Wound Management.* Philadelphia: Lea & Febiger, 1990, pp 9–51, 87–106.
Tobin GR: Closure of contaminated wounds: Biologic and technical considerations. Surg Clin North Am 64:639, 1984.
Vig MM: Management of integumentary wounds of extremities in dogs: An experimental study. J Am Anim Hosp Assoc 21:187, 1985.

18 Open Wound Management

Michael S. Bauer

The concept of leaving wounds open is not new—Guy de Chauliac advocated treatment by nonclosure as early as the 13th century. However, surgeons and veterinary surgeons have been slow to appreciate the advantages and indications of open wound management. The following information pertains primarily to traumatic wounds. Wounds resulting from tumor or other tissue excision usually can be closed or reconstructed immediately, if sufficient tissue is available.

Reconstruction of open wounds using skin flaps or grafts is discussed in sec. 5, ch. 19.

ADVANTAGES

- Results in optimal drainage compared with other drainage options.
- Allows daily inspection to assess progress and to adjust treatment plans.
- Allows continual debridement by surgical, chemical, or mechanical means.
- Allows daily lavage of the wound when indicated.

DISADVANTAGES

- Time-consuming and requires greater effort.
- Expense to the owner is often greater with open wound management, because the patient remains hospitalized in most instances.
- Wound must be protected.
- Nosocomial infection must be prevented.

INDICATIONS

- Wounds heavily contaminated
- Wounds with established infections
- Wounds with excessive tissue damage
- Wounds with recurrent closure failures
- Wounds with inadequate skin available for closure.

INITIAL MANAGEMENT

Patient Evaluation

- Evaluate and treat life-threatening disorders, such as hypovolemic shock, thoracic injuries, and abdominal injuries, before wound management.
- Evaluate the patient for concurrent orthopedic or neurologic injuries, e.g., fractures away from the wound and spinal cord injuries.

- If the wound involves an extremity, evaluate for concurrent neurologic, vascular, and orthopedic injuries.
  - *Neurologic.* Traumatic wounds of the extremities, even severe ones, rarely cause neurologic impairment at the level of the wound. However, neurologic damage may have occurred. Therefore, determine the neurologic status of the limb.
  - *Vascular.* Vascular compromise resulting in catastrophic necrosis is rare even in severe wounds of the extremities. However, evaluation of tissues distal to the wound for viability remains an important procedure when considering wound management.
  - *Orthopedic.* Concurrent orthopedic injuries occur commonly with wounds involving the extremities. Palpate the limb; test joints for stability; and obtain appropriate radiographs, if indicated.

Wound Evaluation

- Some form of analgesia or anesthesia may be required to examine the wound. Severe wounds that require debridement and massive cleaning may necessitate general anesthesia. Smaller wounds may be managed with IV narcotics or ultrashort-acting barbiturates for analgesia/anesthesia.
- During wound inspection, wear sterile gloves to prevent nosocomial infection.
- The following are determined:
  - The amount of tissue damage
  - The presence or likelihood of infection
  - The feasibility of salvaging the limb if an extremity is involved
  - If the limb is salvageable, whether the wound should be closed or treated by open wound management
  - The anticipated expense for the client
- Obtain bacterial cultures prior to cleaning.

Clipping and General Cleaning

Protect the wound during clipping by the use of towel clamps and temporary sutures or by placing sterile, water-soluble gel within the wound. If an extremity is involved, clip and clean the portion of the limb likely to be included within the bandage. Clean intact skin with an antiseptic soap.

Cleaning the Wound

KEY POINT ▶ Surgical debridement and lavage are excellent methods of removing debris and bacteria from the wound.

358

- *Lavage solution.* The ideal lavage solution is sterile, nonirritating, normothermic, and isotonic. Sterile saline meets all these criteria.
  - Although tap water does not meet all of the criteria, it has also been utilized successfully.
  - Antiseptics or antibiotics for wound lavage remain controversial. Some of these agents have been shown to be cytotoxic and interfere with local host defense mechanisms, especially in *in vitro* studies using cell culture techniques. Other *in vivo* studies, however, have not demonstrated adverse effects and in fact, wound healing was enhanced in some instances. This is an area of wound management that needs further investigation and is left to the discretion of the surgeon.
- *Lavage delivery systems.* Many delivery systems have been employed for wound lavage. From a practical standpoint, delivery systems can be classified into those that deliver high, medium, or low pressure.
  - High-pressure lavage systems (e.g., Water Pik) generate pressures near 60 psi and are superior at dislodging bacteria and debris. However, high-pressure lavage in areas of loose skin attachment has been shown to drive bacteria into tissues back from the wound edge. This may result in microabscess formation.
  - Medium pressure of 8 psi has been shown to dislodge bacteria and foreign debris. The most practical lavage system that is capable of generating this pressure is a large syringe and an 18-gauge needle attached to an IV fluid delivery system (Fig. 1). This is the system that I prefer.

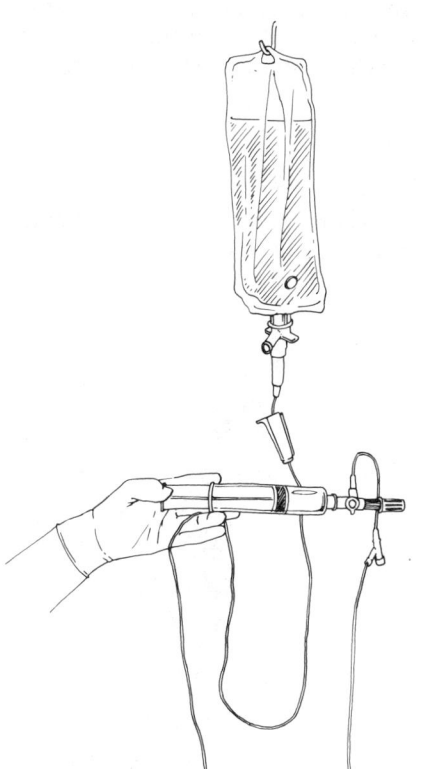

Figure 1. A bag of warm, isotonic fluids, an IV fluid administration set, a three-way stopcock, a large syringe, and an 18-gauge needle may be used to generate approximately 8 psi for wound lavage.

- Low-pressure lavage is ineffective at dislodging debris and bacteria. However, experiments designed to study low pressure have used a one-time lavage approach. Whether daily lavage with low pressure has any beneficial effect is unknown. Low-pressure lavage is obtainable using a bulb syringe, a large syringe without a needle, or tap water from a faucet.

Debridement

KEY POINT ▶ Surgical debridement is the most effective way to remove devitalized tissue.

- Avoid surgical debridement of critical tissues of questionable viability.
- Determine tissue viability by visual inspection and palpation.
- Signs suggesting nonviability include
  - Bluish-black, shiny black, or shiny white discoloration
  - Leathery texture
  - Thinness of skin
  - Easily epilated hair.
- Red discoloration or severe edema is not necessarily an indicator of nonviability.
- Chemical or enzymatic debridement is employed infrequently. It has the advantage of selectively debriding devitalized tissue while sparing viable structures but can be irritating to healing tissues.
- Mechanical debridement is an effective way of using the primary bandage layer to remove debris on a daily basis. This method is reviewed more completely in the bandaging section.

Bandaging

Bandages are composed of a primary layer which is in contact with the skin and wound, a secondary layer for absorption (e.g., cotton padding), and a tertiary layer to secure the bandage. Support rods, splints, and so forth are applied when necessary.

- The primary layer of the bandage may be adherent or nonadherent.
  - Adherent bandages may be further classified into wet-to-wet, dry-to-dry, and wet-to-dry. Wet dressings encourage the movement of viscous exudate away from the wound into the secondary layer. Dry dressings adhere to nonviable and necrotic tissues and act as a form of mechanical debridement when removed.

    Wet-to-dry dressings are the most commonly used adherent bandages because they have beneficial effects on wounds with exudate and necrotic material. For wet-to-dry dressings, soak sterile gauze sponges in sterile saline or other lavage solutions (e.g., chlorhexidine); hand squeeze as much liquid as possible from the sponge aseptically; place the sponge in contact with the wound; and apply the secondary and tertiary layers of the bandage. Pack the saline-soaked sponges into the deep recesses of the wound if present. After 12 or 24 hours, the damp gauze dries, adheres to necrotic tissues, and serves as a mechanical debridement tool when removed.

Dry-to-dry dressings are used on wounds that have little or no exudate but do have nonviable tissue present. Dry-to-dry dressings are simply dry gauze sponges placed in contact with the wound.

Wet-to-wet dressings are used on wounds with exudate but no necrotic material. For wet-to-wet dressings, soak gauze sponges in saline or another appropriate lavage solution and place them in contact with the wound. A layer of dry material is not used over the maintained sponges.

- Nonadherent dressings are composed of products with nonadherent properties (e.g., Telfa Pad). This type of bandage does not adhere to the wound, therefore, newly formed granulation tissue and epithelial are not disrupted. Use nonadherent primary layers when healthy-appearing granulation tissue or epithelium begins to form and when the wound is not producing fluid.
- The secondary layer of a bandage acts as an absorptive layer, which helps draw fluid away from the wound.
- The secondary layer of the bandage is usually made up of cotton.
- The tertiary layer is gauze and tape and acts to hold the bandage in place.
- Some wounds, especially those with concurrent orthopedic injuries, may require immobilization.
- To accomplish this incorporate support rods or splints into the tertiary layer of the bandage.
- Tie-over bandages hold the primary and secondary layers in place when the wound is in an area inaccessible to standard bandaging techniques, e.g., over the hip or shoulder and the axilla.

Technique

1. With a large suture, place several "eyelets" around the wound (Fig. 2).
2. Apply the primary and secondary layers of the bandage (Fig. 3).
3. Lace sterile gauze or umbilical tape through the eyelets to hold the bandage in place (Fig. 4).
4. If possible, cover the bandage with a tertiary layer.

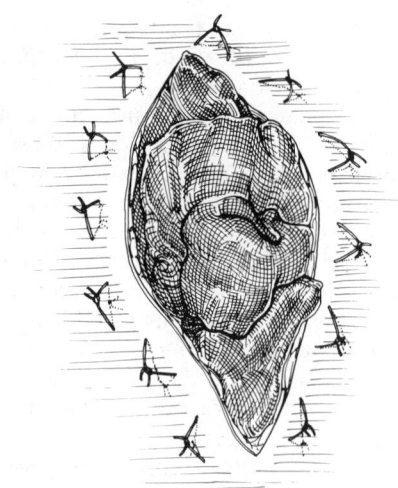

Figure 3. Appropriate primary and secondary bandage layers are placed over the wound.

Antibiotics

- Topical or systemic antibiotic therapy is controversial unless an established infection is present. Even so, antibiotic use is debatable. Infection is most effectively managed by good open wound management techniques. A few general guidelines may be followed if antibiotics are believed to be indicated.
  - Culture wounds with established infection and base antibiotic selection on culture and sensitivity results.
  - While awaiting results, broad-spectrum antibiotics, such as first generation cephalosporins, may be administered.
  - In animals with severe wounds that show signs of septicemia, consider the combination of an IV beta-lactam (cephalosporin or penicillin) and aminoglycoside antibiotic (gentamicin or amikacin).

DAILY MANAGEMENT
Frequency

- In most instances, wounds are unbandaged and inspected on a daily basis.

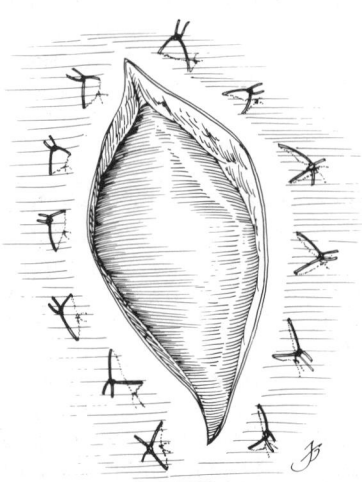

Figure 2. Eyelets for a tie-over dressing are placed around the wound using large suture material.

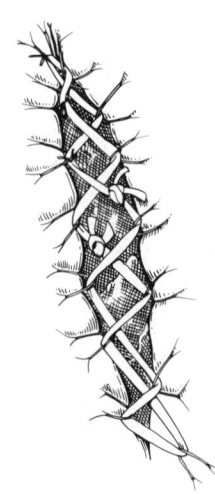

Figure 4. Sterile gauze or umbilical tape is laced over the layers.

- Wounds with excessive tissue damage or established infection may require rebandaging and inspection twice a day.
- Wounds with healthy granulation tissue and active epithelialization may need inspection only once every several days.

Analgesia

- Initially, animals with extensive wounds require analgesia or anesthesia at the time of bandage changing and daily wound management.
- Once granulation tissue begins to form (about 7 days), most animals tolerate bandage changes, wound lavage, and so forth.

Bacterial Cultures

- If at any point, the wound appears infected or the character of the discharge changes, obtain bacterial cultures by swabbing the wound or exudate or submitting tissue that has been debrided.

Debridement

- Intermittent surgical debridement is the best means for removing devitalized tissue (see previous discussion).
- Mechanical debridement is an excellent means of daily debridement by use of either wet-to-dry or dry-to-dry primary layers within the bandage.

Lavage

- Daily wound lavage helps dislodge bacteria, remove debris, dilute exudate, and promote drainage.
- Not all wounds require daily lavage.
- Lavage may be beneficial in wounds with moderate amounts of exudate or discharge, continuing necrosis, or remaining debris.
- Consider whirlpool baths for animals with extensive wounds over the thorax or abdomen.

Rebandaging

- During wound healing, the type of primary layer varies, depending on wound conditions.
- Use adherent dressings when exudate or necrotic material is present.
- Once the wound begins to form healthy-appearing granulation tissue and epithelialize, replace adherent bandages with nonadherent bandages (see previous discussion).

WOUND CLOSURE

In general, wounds can be closed safely once healthy-appearing granulation tissue begins to form or epithelium begins to appear. This is "mother nature's" signal that the wound is healthy, blood supply is adequate, and persistent infection is unlikely.

The wound may be left to heal by second intention or by one of various wound closure options.

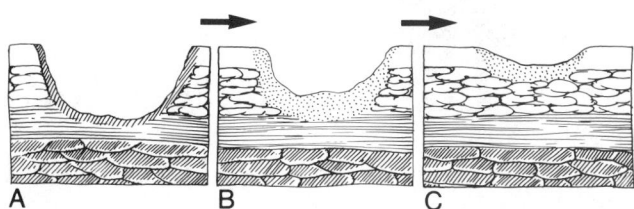

Figure 5. Second intention healing involves the formation of granulation tissue, wound contraction, and epithelialization. *A,* Unsuitable for closure; *B,* Formation of granulation tissue. *C,* Further healing through wound contraction and epithelialization. (Modified from Swaim, SF: Surgery of Traumatized Skin. Philadelphia: W. B. Saunders, 1980, p. 163.)

Second Intention Healing

Second intention healing involves the formation of granulation tissue, wound contraction, and epithelialization (Fig. 5).

Advantages

- Additional surgery is usually avoided.
- Less expense may be involved compared with other closure options.
- Wounds are covered with full-thickness, normal-appearing skin, if the wound completely contracts (i.e., no tension).

Disadvantages

- Contracture (excessive wound contraction and scar tissue) may result in disfigurement.
- Contracture may lead to decreased motion, if a joint is involved.
- If the wound does not contract adequately, epithelium may not completely cover the remaining defect.
- If a large defect is covered with epithelium, the epithelium is often fragile and easily disrupted.

Delayed Primary Closure

See sec. 5, ch. 17.

Secondary Closure

Secondary closure involves wound closure following the formation of healthy-appearing granulation tissue (see sec. 5, ch. 17).

Supplemental Readings

Bauer MS, Aiken S: The healing of open wounds. Sem Vet Med Surg 4:268–273, 1989.

Bauer MS, Remedios AM, Stanley BJ: Open wound management and treatment of postoperative infections in eight dogs. Can Vet J 30:46–49, 1989.

Lee AH, Swaim SF: Granulation tissue: How to take advantage of it in management of open wounds. Compend Contin Educ Pract Vet 10:163–171, 1988.

Peacock EE: Inflammation and the cellular response to injury. *In* Peacock EE, ed.: *Wound Repair*, 3rd edition. Philadelphia: W. B. Saunders, 1984, pp 1–14.

Swaim SF: *Surgery of Traumatized Skin: Management and Reconstruction in the Dog and Cat*. Philadelphia: W. B. Saunders, 1980.

Swaim SF, Wilhalf D: The physics, physiology, and chemistry of bandaging open wounds. Compend Contin Educ Pract Vet 7:146–156, 1985.

19 Selected Skin Graft and Reconstructive Techniques

Stephen J. Birchard
Daniel D. Smeak

Large skin wounds can occur (1) from trauma directly to the skin or to its blood supply; (2) secondary to necrotizing skin diseases (see sec. 5, ch. 12); and (3) after en bloc removal of large skin, subcutaneous, or body wall neoplasms. Most open wounds eventually heal by the formation of granulation tissue, wound contraction, and epithelialization. Skin flaps or grafts are indicated when wound healing is not progressing; full-thickness skin is necessary to prevent problems caused by repeated trauma (e.g., in the dorsum of the leg or paw); the open wound is so large it will cause significant patient morbidity; and wound contracture is likely to cause a significant problem (e.g., the wound is over a joint). Skin flaps are usually preferred over skin grafts because they are simpler to perform and have a higher success rate. However, if sufficient skin is not available adjacent to the wound, a skin graft may be necessary.

Consider several factors before deciding upon creation of skin flaps or skin grafts, such as viability of adjacent tissue, systemic illness that may affect wound healing, function of the affected area of the body, tolerance of the wound by the animal, feasibility of long-term bandaging of the affected part, desired cosmetic result, and cost to the owner. Thoroughly discuss these factors with the owner prior to performing any of these procedures.

In this chapter we discuss practical methods of reconstructing skin using skin flaps and grafts. More complicated methods of skin grafting that require specialized skill or equipment, such as using a dermatome for split-thickness skin grafts, or tube grafts, are not discussed in this chapter. Primary closure of skin wounds is reviewed in section 5, chapter 17, and open wound management in section 5, chapter 18.

SURGICAL ANATOMY

Skin

The skin is composed of the epidermis and dermis.

- Structures that compose the skin adnexa, hair follicles, sweat glands, and sebaceous glands are located in the dermis.
- Besides adnexa, the dermis is composed of fibroblasts; collagen fibers; and various other structures, such as blood vessels, nerves, tissue cells, and fluid.

Subcutaneous Tissue

The subcutaneous tissue is mainly comprised of loose connective tissue, including elastic fibers, fat, blood vessels, and nerves.

Cutaneous Muscles

- Thin, superficial muscles, collectively called the panniculus muscle, lie within the subcutis in both dogs and cats. Examples are the platysma muscle in the neck and the cutaneous truncus muscle in the trunk.
- Preservation of these muscles is a very important principle in the formation of skin flaps for reconstruction.

Blood Supply to the Skin

- Deep or subdermal plexus
  - This plexus is the major source of blood supply to the skin and of most importance to the surgeon.

KEY POINT ▶ When creating skin flaps in dogs and cats, preserve the deep vascular plexus.

  - In regions where cutaneous musculature is present, this vascular network is present on the superficial and deep layers of the muscle. Dissection beneath this thin muscle layer is critical to flap survival.
  - Direct cutaneous arteries are present in several areas of the body. They arise from deep vessels that course superficially and run parallel to the skin. These direct cutaneous arteries communicate with the deep vascular plexus.
- Middle and superficial plexuses complete the layers of vascular network to the skin.

SKIN FLAPS

Skin flaps are a means of reconstructing open wounds by using adjacent or regional skin that is advanced or rotated to the wound to allow closure. Local or regional blood vessels supplying these flaps are maintained. Therefore, skin flaps do not require a bed of granulation tissue for their blood supply and nutrition. Skin flaps can be classified according to their blood supply, such as random subdermal flaps versus axial pattern flaps, or according to their location with respect to the recipient bed, such as local flaps versus distant flaps.

Random Subdermal Flaps

Random subdermal skin flaps are those constructed with skin adjacent to the wound and are not based on a direct cutaneous artery. Viability of these skin flaps is dependent upon the availability of local blood vessels. To help prevent avascular necrosis of the flap, it has been recommended to make the flap base slightly wider than the flap body. Random subdermal skin flaps can be further classified as *advancement flaps* and *transposition flaps*, depending upon how the flap is moved to the defect; *single pedicle* and *bipedicle flaps*, depending on how the flap is attached to the body; and *direct distant flaps*, depending on use for extremity skin defects.

- Advancement refers to how the flap is moved to the wound. These are usually rectangular flaps. Simple advancement flaps are undermined and pulled (horizontally or vertically) directly to the wound (Fig. 1).
- Transposition flap is constructed immediately adjacent to the wound, and is rotated (clockwise or counterclockwise) to cover the wound (Fig. 2).
- Direct distant flaps include thoracic or abdominal single pedicle or bipedicle direct distant flaps that can be used as a method for transferring skin to the distal extremities.
  - Single pedicle: Attached to the body only at one end (Fig. 3*A, C*). The pedicle provides the vascular attachment to the flap.
  - Bipedicle: Attached to the body at both ends (Fig. 3*B*).
  - These flaps are transferred from a distance to the recipient defect. The lesion is advanced to the flap rather than the flap being transferred to the lesion as in construction of advancement flaps.
  - Forelimb defects are more often reconstructed using this technique than rear limb defects.

Indications

- Advancement and transposition flaps
  - For large skin wounds that are located in areas

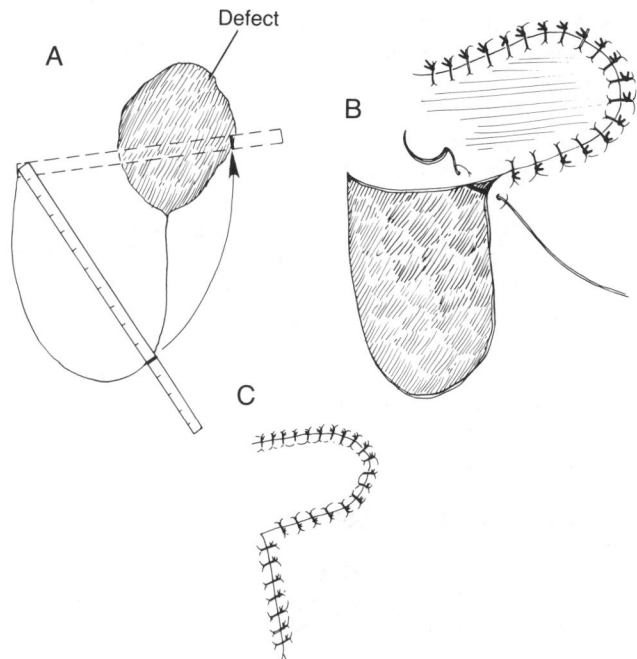

Figure 2. Transposition flap. After measuring the length of flap needed, make the incisions and rotate the flap to the defect. Suture the flap first and then close the remaining defect.

with adjacent loose, redundant skin (e.g., neck, flank, dorsal trunk) that allow formation and closure of defects remaining after flap transfer without tension.

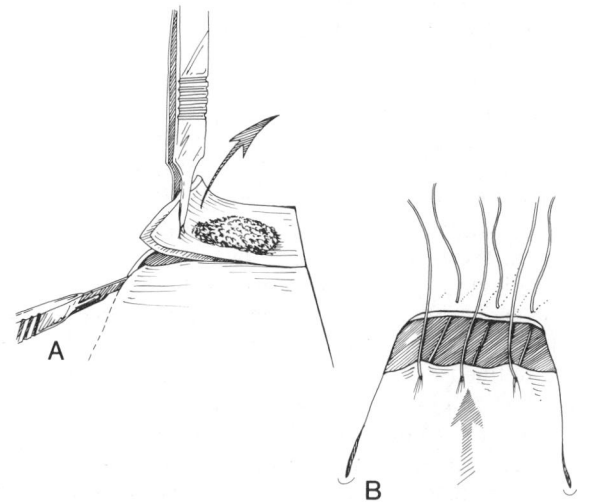

Figure 1. Simple advancement flap. Make the initial incisions (*A*), then deeply undermine the flap and advance to the defect (*B*).

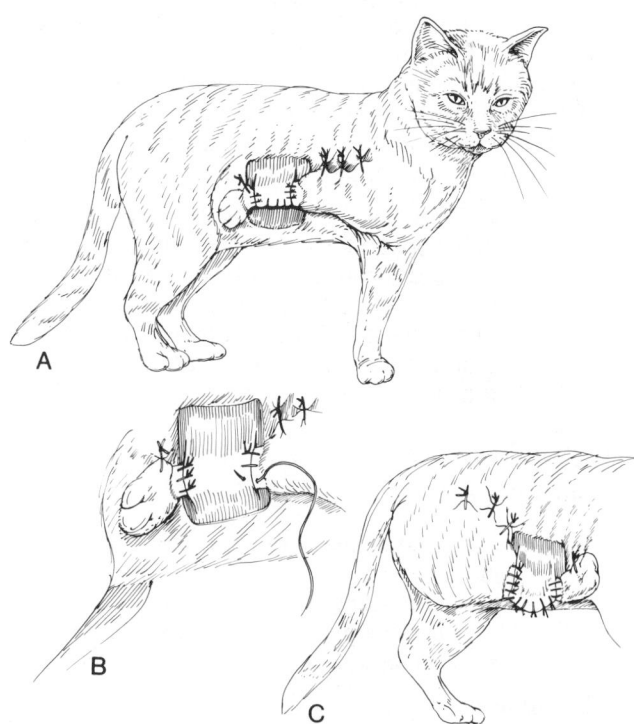

Figure 3. Direct distant flap. Make the skin flap using the lateral thoracic or abdominal skin. Suture the flap to the limb defect. This flap can have a single (*A*) or double (*B*) pedicle. Secure the limb to the lateral body wall with skin sutures placed between the leg and the body wall. Place a padded bandage around the body to help stabilize the elevated limb.

- As a general rule, do not consider these flaps for denuded areas distal to the stifle, elbow, or tail head.
- Direct distant pedicle flaps
  - For large wounds of the distal extremities in which local skin is not available or would be closed under excessive tension.
  - These flaps are usually made from skin over the lateral thoracic or abdominal wall. The leg is attached to the side of the animal's body for a period of time while healing of the pedicle to the extremity wound progresses. The pedicle is removed from the thorax or abdomen and the leg returned to its normal position.
  - These flaps are very successful, but patient tolerance is variable.

Preoperative Considerations

- Carefully plan the surgical procedure. Review vascular anatomy of the region. The size, location, shape, and condition of the wound dictates the type of flap.
- Check the looseness and pliability of the skin adjacent to the lesion or wound to determine feasibility of the intended skin flap.
- Consider administration of prophylactic antibiotics, given intravenously at induction of anesthesia, if significant contamination of the surgical site is possible.
- Prepare the recipient bed preoperatively to ensure that the area is free of infection, foreign material, and necrotic tissue.
- Distant flap technique requires two surgical procedures to complete. The owner is made fully aware of the costs involved, the inconvenience of bandage management, and the problems related to the prolonged immobilization period. Hair direction and cosmetic problems are more common with distant compared with local flap techniques.

KEY POINT ▶ Consider the mobility of the extremity that contains the defect when determining the location and type of direct distant flap. Evaluate the size and temperament of the patient. Smaller animals with calm dispositions seem to tolerate this technique best.

Surgical Procedure

Objectives

- To provide full-thickness reconstruction of a large skin wound.
- To avoid tension along the suture line.
- To create flaps that maintain viability and preserve satisfactory cosmesis.

Equipment

- Standard surgical pack and suture
- Measuring device to plan length and width of flaps
- Sterile marking pen to draw incisions (optional). Sterile methylene blue and a cotton-tipped applicator can be effective as a marker.

- A piece of sterile double-knit cloth can be used as a pattern for designing flaps intraoperatively.
- Penrose drains (¼–½ in)

Technique

Advancement or Transposition Flaps

1. Carefully position the patient to free up any available skin in the region and to reduce tension while the flap is being sutured.
2. Aseptically prepare a liberal amount of skin in the region of the proposed flap and donor sites.
3. Remove epithelialized portions of the granulation bed by sharp dissection. Attachments of skin at the margin of the granulation bed are undermined to free up the bordering skin.
4. Gently manipulate the skin margins surrounding the defect to ascertain the availability of adjacent local skin.
5. Optimally, the donor area has enough skin available to elevate a flap without leaving a secondary defect that cannot be closed primarily.
6. If possible, avoid choosing a donor area that may be subject to excessive motion or tension.
7. Choose the type of flap depending on the availability of skin, shape and location of the defect, and size of the area to be covered.
8. It is better to create two adjacent short flaps rather than one long flap, which has a greater risk of necrosis from inadequate blood supply.
9. Try to design the flap such that the base is slightly wider than the width to avoid inadvertently devascularizing the flap.
10. Design the flap to fill the defect without tension.
11. Create the flap by sharply incising along the preplanned donor skin margins.
12. Use stay sutures or fine skin hooks when elevating the flap to avoid causing excessive damage.

The depth of flap undermining is very important to preserve the deep vascular plexus under the panniculus muscle group. Be especially careful when undermining in the region of the base of the flap to avoid interrupting critical direct cutaneous vessel branches.

13. Transfer the skin flap to the defect (see Figs. 1 and 2).
14. Consider placing a Penrose drain in large dead space areas (under flaps and donor areas) if the condition of the tissues warrants it. Exit the drain in a ventral dependent area of the wound away from the primary suture line.
15. Meticulously close subcutaneous tissues with fine (4–0 to 5–0), simple interrupted, absorbable suture material to evenly distribute skin tension.
16. Use fine (4–0) monofilament nonabsorbable suture material placed in a simple interrupted pattern to close the skin. This allows for individual control of suture tension. If fluid accumulation develops in the dead space, simple removal of one or two skin sutures in a gravity-dependent area often allows adequate drainage.

Technique

Direct Distant Flap (Single or Double Pedicle)

1. The entire limb and lateral thoracic, for a forelimb defect, or abdominal wall, for a rearlimb defect, are aseptically prepared. When preparing a bipedicle flap, meticulously clip and clean the portion of paw or limb that will be in contact with the subcutaneous tissue.
2. Position the affected limb in the most comfortable angle possible to locate the donor area (see Fig. 3).
3. Construct the flap so that any movement of the limb will pull the flap onto the defect rather than away from it.
4. Create a bipedicle flap, if the defect is large or nearly circumferential (Fig. 3B), or a single pedicle flap, if the defect is less than 180° circumferential (Fig. 3A, C), using the principles described in the advancement flap technique section.
5. After creating a single pedicle flap, a skin defect remains that must be closed. Use advancement or rotation flaps to close this defect.
6. Place the limb through the bipedicle flap or adjacent to the single pedicle flap.
7. Suture as much of the flap to the defect margins as possible.
8. Small Penrose drains may be placed to drain fluids that may accumulate under the flap or limb.
9. Large (2–0 to 0) suture material can be selected to help tack the skin of the limb to the thoracic wall skin in several areas to help immobilize the limb.

KEY POINT ▶ Complete immobilization of the limb is mandatory for 14 days to ensure adequate vascularization of the flap from the wound bed.

10. Design a bandage for immobilization that will remain in place for the full 2 weeks but will still allow the flap area to be monitored and separately rebandaged.
11. If the flap appears healthy, the pedicles are sharply incised from the donor area. Remaining free skin margins are sutured to the defect to complete the transfer.

Axial Pattern Flaps

Axial pattern flaps are those skin flaps that are developed using a major direct cutaneous artery as the primary blood supply. Considerably more flexibility in the length and mobility of these flaps is possible compared with random skin flaps. These flaps can be made with long vascular pedicles to transfer skin to more remote areas of the body, because of the preservation of the direct cutaneous artery allowing an adequate perfusion of a large area of tissue. Axial pattern flaps are created in a one-step procedure, as compared with the direct distant flaps.

Axial pattern flaps can be based upon many direct cutaneous arteries, such as the caudal superficial epigastric; the cervical cutaneous branch of the omocer- vical, thoracodorsal, deep circumflex iliac, and the genicular branch of the saphenous artery. The caudal superficial axial pattern flap is commonly selected for large defects of the proximal thigh and flank. Only this technique is described here. However, other axial pattern flaps as listed previously can be created using similar principles and are described in veterinary surgical textbooks (see Pavletic, 1990).

Indications

■ Similar to those for random subdermal flaps except that axial pattern flaps are used when the skin defect is very large.
■ A major direct cutaneous artery and vein must be fairly close to the skin defect for this technique to be indicated.

Preoperative Considerations

■ Same as those for random subdermal flaps, plus:
 • Carefully plan the design of the flap.
 • Consider how the resultant defect of the donor area will be closed.
 • Be sure the skin and the direct cutaneous artery that will be used for the flap are viable.

Surgical Procedure

Objectives

■ Same as those for random skin flaps, plus:
 • Preserve viability of the direct cutaneous artery by avoiding excessive surgical trauma to the tissue.

Equipment

■ Same as that for random skin flaps.

Technique

Caudal Superficial Epigastric Axial Pattern Flap

1. Use preparation and tissue handling principles as described for advancement or rotation flaps.
2. Be particularly careful when positioning the patient such that the vascular pedicle will not become distorted before planning the incisions.
3. Incisions are created as shown in Figure 4.
4. The entire mammary chain up to the cranial thoracic gland can be included in this flap.
5. Deeply undermine the flap just superficial to the abdominal fascia.
6. Dissect very carefully around the origin of the direct cutaneous vessel to avoid inadvertent damage to this vessel that is vital to the survival of the flap.
7. Avoid creating a kink in the base of the flap, which could obstruct blood flow.
8. Drain the dead space if needed.
9. Suture the flap to the defect as described for the other flap techniques.

Postoperative Care and Complications

All Flap Types

■ Restrict exercise until suture removal.
■ Apply an Elizabethan collar before the patient is

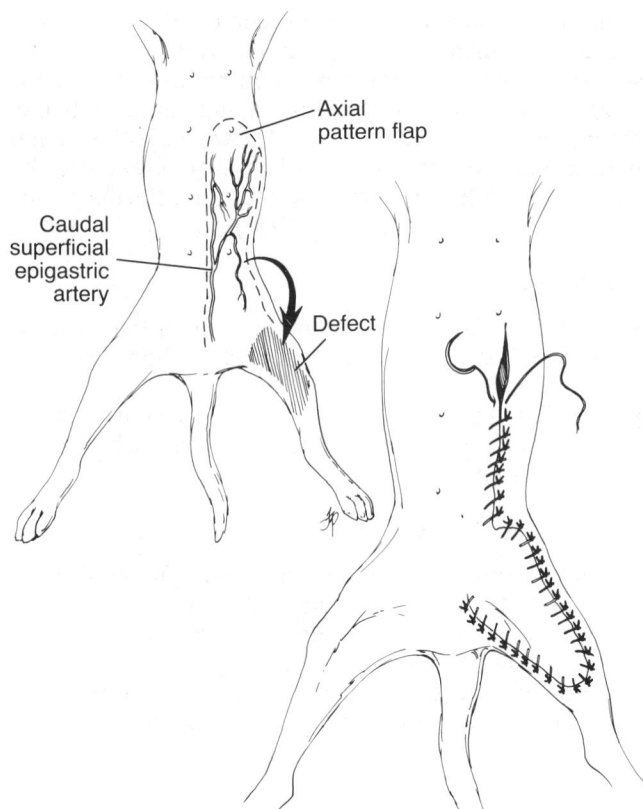

Figure 4. Example of an axial pattern flap. This flap is based upon a direct cutaneous artery—the caudal superficial epigastric artery. Design the flap around this artery and deeply undermine the skin and mammary tissue. Rotate the flap and suture to the defect.

recovered from anesthesia and leave on the animal until the flaps are completely healed.

■ Change wound dressings as necessary.

■ Immobilize the limb for at least 14 days for direct distant flap techniques.

■ Major complications resulting from skin flaps include local problems, such as partial or total ischemia of the flap, infection, seroma, and dehiscence of the flap or donor suture line.

■ Dehiscence of donor site incisions is usually due to excessive skin tension. If dehiscence occurs, allow these areas to heal by second intention.

FREE SKIN GRAFTS

Free skin grafts involve complete removal of skin from one area of the body and implantation to another. These grafts are completely separated from their blood supply, and they are dependent upon the wound bed for viability. For the first 3 or 4 days after grafting, the skin graft obtains its nutrition from the wound bed by diffusion, a process called imbibition. During this process, the graft acts like a sponge soaking up fluid and oxygen from the granulation tissue of the wound. This is a very delicate process that is easily disrupted by complicating factors, such as excessive movement of the wound, seroma formation, and infection. During this initial phase of healing, the graft usually looks its worst, appearing congested and sometimes purple.

After a few days, this appearance dramatically improves if the graft "takes."

After the first 3 to 4 days, the viability of the graft depends upon ingrowth of capillaries from the wound bed into the graft (i.e., inosculation). These are very fragile structures and are easily damaged by trauma, such as licking of the graft; excessive motion; and infection. Once this blood supply becomes well-established, viability of the graft is maintained.

Skin grafts vary in their final cosmetic result. The best cosmesis is obtained from the establishment of a full-thickness skin graft, because this allows hair to form over the area. However, full-thickness grafts are the most difficult to establish, because they are thicker than split-thickness grafts. This greater thickness makes the initial process of imbibition more difficult, resulting in a higher incidence of graft failure.

Pinch Skin Grafts

Pinch skin grafting is performed by simply harvesting small (2–3 mm) sections of full-thickness skin and placing them into the wound granulation bed. They are not difficult to perform and are highly successful. However, the major disadvantage of pinch grafts is the final cosmetic result. Uniform full-thickness skin does not form over the wound with pinch grafts; therefore, very little hair grows over the area.

Preoperative Considerations

■ Determine the desired result of the graft. If a high degree of success and rapid epithelialization of the wound are desired, consider pinch grafts. If complete regrowth of hair and excellent cosmesis are necessary, employ a different skin graft method, such as mesh graft. If the recipient site is over a joint or area that is frequently traumatized, full-thickness grafts may be needed and pinch grafts may not be satisfactory.

KEY POINT ▶ Maximize the chances of graft "take" by properly preparing the wound bed before grafting.

Use standard techniques of wound debridement, lavage, and bandaging (see sec. 5, ch. 18) for several days prior to grafting to establish a healthy bed of granulation tissue. Postpone the graft procedure if any evidence of infection is present.

Surgical Technique

Objectives

■ To establish epithelial coverage of an open wound.

■ To atraumatically harvest small plugs of skin from an area of redundant skin.

■ To implant these plugs of skin into an area of healthy granulation tissue to promote healing.

Equipment

■ Same as for skin flaps, plus:
 • Several # 15 scalpel blades
 • Skin biopsy punch (optional)

Technique

1. Aseptically prepare the wound bed and the harvest site.
2. Gently pick up the skin with thumb forceps or stay suture and excise a 1-mm piece of skin, using the # 15 scalpel blade. Be careful not to include subcutaneous tissue with the skin pinch.
3. Alternatively, harvest the skin using a skin biopsy punch. Place the punch at the same angle as the hair follicle during harvesting.
4. Trim subcutaneous tissue from the bottom of the pinch of skin.
5. Place the skin pinch or punch in a saline-moistened surgical sponge.
6. Make a "vest pocket" stab incision in the granulation tissue with a # 15 scalpel blade (Fig. 5).
7. Slide the skin pinch into the incision in the granulation tissue (Fig. 5). Be sure the epithelial side of the pinch is facing out.
8. Repeat this process as many times as necessary to have skin pinches covering the wound at about 1 to 2 cm apart.
9. Place a nonadherent dressing over the wound. The primary layer of the dressing can be a petrolatum-impregnated gauze or a gauze sponge with a thin layer of triple antibiotic ointment (Bacitracin-Neomycin-Polymyxin; Pharmaderm).
10. Let the donor sites heal by second intention.

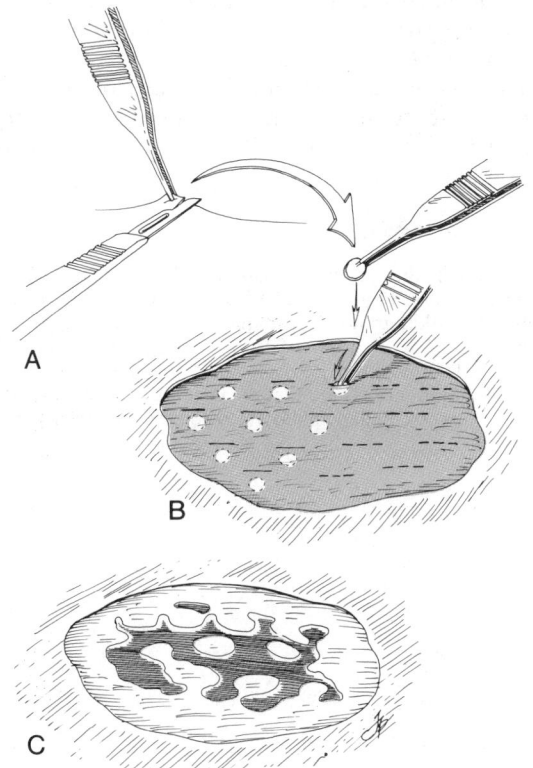

Figure 5. Pinch skin graft. Obtain small pinches of skin using a scalpel. (*A*) Make small "vest-pocket" incisions in the granulation bed, and slide skin pinches into these incisions with the epidermal side facing out. (*B*) Pinches can be approximately 1 to 2 cm apart. Wound will be filled in by epidermal growth from the pinch grafts (*C*).

Postoperative Care and Complications

- Restrict exercise to leash walking only.
- Change the wound dressing every day for the first 5 to 7 days, then every 2 to 3 days if wound healing is progressing normally.
- Keep the wound dressed until it is completely covered with epithelium.
- If necessary, place an Elizabethan collar on the animal to prevent licking of the wound.
- Potential complications include dislodgement of the pinch grafts due to self-trauma or excessive motion and poor cosmetic result due to sparsity of hair formation.

Mesh Skin Grafts

Mesh skin grafts are usually full-thickness skin grafts that are harvested, stripped of subcutaneous tissue, and "meshed" by making several scalpel cuts in them. The purposes of making the multiple holes in the graft are to increase coverage of the wound by the graft and to allow escape of fluid from underneath the graft. Mesh grafts provide better cosmesis than pinch grafts. The healed wound has some hair coverage although it may not be as much as on the surrounding skin, depending on how much the mesh is expanded.

Mesh grafts are fairly simple to perform and require no special equipment. Although reportedly effective in both dogs and cats, our results have been very good in cats (nearly 100% success), but only fair in dogs (approximately 50%).

Preoperative Considerations

- These are the same as those for pinch grafts.
- Consider the administration of prophylactic systemic antibiotics (beginning preoperatively) to prevent infection of the graft.
- Do not perform the procedure if any evidence of infection is present in either the donor or recipient sites.

Surgical Procedure

Objectives

- To establish epithelial and some full-thickness skin coverage of the wound.
- To atraumatically harvest the donor skin from an area of redundant skin.
- To meticulously prepare the graft for implantation by removing all subcutaneous fat and creating a mesh by making multiple small holes in the skin.

Equipment

- Same as for pinch grafts, plus:
  A sterile board (plastic, wood, or cardboard) for stretching out and preparing the graft.
  # 11 scalpel blade

Technique

1. Aseptically prepare the donor and recipient sites.
2. Estimate the size of the wound by measuring or cutting out a template using sterile drape material.

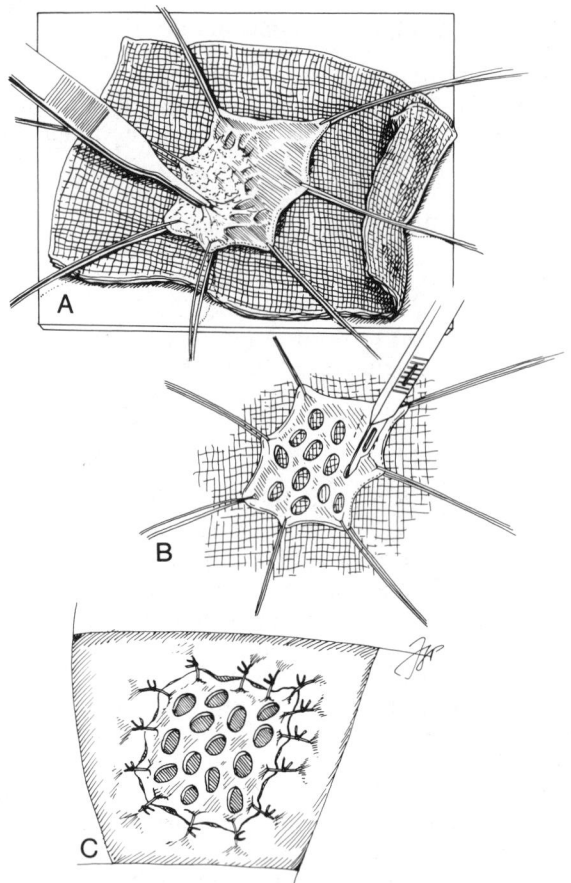

Figure 6. Mesh skin graft. Harvest skin and stretch it out on a sterile board using stay sutures (*A*). Meticulously remove all subcutaneous fat and make multiple slits in the graft using a scalpel (*B*). Suture the graft, with the epidermal side facing out, to the granulation bed (*C*).

3. Sharply excise the donor skin from an area of redundant skin (e.g., dorsum of the neck and lateral flank area).
4. Avoid excising the subcutaneous tissues.
5. Note the direction of hair growth in the harvested skin.
6. Place multiple stay sutures at the edge of the harvested skin.
7. Place the skin on a sterile board (epidermal side

down), and stretch it out using the stay sutures (Fig. 6).
8. Carefully dissect all remaining subcutaneous fat from the skin using sharp dissection (Fig. 6*A*).
9. Lavage the skin frequently with sterile saline.
10. Make multiple full-thickness holes, approximately ½ cm in length and ½ to 1 cm apart (Fig. 6*B*).
11. Place the mesh graft on the wound.
12. Position the graft such that the hair growth will be in the same direction as that of the adjacent hair.
13. Suture the graft to the surrounding skin (Fig. 6*C*).
14. Suture the graft under slight tension so that the mesh expands and the granulation tissue can be seen through the graft (Fig. 6*C*).
15. Place additional tacking sutures from the center of the graft to the granulation bed to prevent movement of the graft and separation of the graft from the wound bed.
16. Cover the wound with a nonadherent dressing (see the description under pinch grafts). Consider a wet-to-dry dressing, if wound exudation occurs.

Change the dressing frequently (2 to 3 times daily) to prevent desiccation of the primary layer and adherence to the graft.

Postoperative Care and Complications

■ Same as for pinch grafts, plus:
  • Prevent desiccation of the graft by applying small amounts of triple antibiotic ointment or sterile petrolatum directly on the skin graft.
  • Immobilize the limb if grafting over a joint (e.g., elbow, carpus, stifle, hock) to prevent excessive movement of the graft.
  • The major complication is failure of the graft to heal due to infection, excessive motion, or any interference with the adherence of the graft to the granulation tissue.

Supplemental Readings

Pavletic MM: Pedicle grafts. *In* Slatter DH, ed.: *Textbook of Small Animal Surgery.* Philadelphia: W. B. Saunders, 1985, p 458.
Pavletic MM: Skin-grafting techniques. *In* Bojrab MJ, ed.: *Current Techniques in Small Animal Surgery,* 3rd ed. Philadelphia: Lea & Febiger, 1990, p 460.
Swaim SF: Skin grafts. *In* Slatter DH, ed.: *Textbook of Small Animal Surgery.* Philadelphia: W. B. Saunders, 1985, p 486.

20 Pinnal Diseases

Mary P. Schick
Robert O. Schick

The ear's pinna is a relatively common site for numerous dermatologic diseases. Distinct underlying etiologies exist for most pinnal diseases, even though clinically they may appear similar (Table 1). Careful differentiation is paramount in obtaining a definitive diagnosis and successful treatment.

Pinnal dermatoses may be primary or secondary. Primary pinnal dermatoses are defined as those limited to or those that arise on the pinnae before affecting other body areas. Secondary pinnal dermatoses involve the pinnae along with other body lesions. Factors that must be considered in the diagnosis of either primary or secondary diseases include self-trauma, sun exposure, and age, breed, and sex of the animal.

In all patients with pinnal disease, definitive diagnosis, prognosis, and therapeutic protocol depend upon a thorough history of the disease, complete physical examination, and several routine baseline diagnostic aids. The patient history determines the duration and progression of the pinnal lesions, development of similar lesions on other body areas, and concurrent systemic signs. Previous medications and treatment response are also important factors. The physical examination assesses the site and extent of disease. It is important to determine whether the haired or non-haired areas of the pinnae are affected.

KEY POINT ▶ Certain diseases, such as demodectic mange, dermatophytosis, and bacterial pyoderma, are usually restricted to hair follicle invasion.

A routine minimum laboratory data base allows for a definitive diagnosis (Table 2). The data base may detect other organ system involvement and provides a baseline evaluation of organ system function for future reference, prior to initiation of medication.

Histopathologic examination of lesions provides valuable information in the diagnosis of pinnal disease. The pinnal biopsy specimen must be taken with extreme care. A permanent scarring defect may result as a complication of pinnal biopsy. For skin biopsy techniques, please refer to section 5, chapter 15.

KEY POINT ▶ Histopathologic examination and possibly immunofluorescence testing enable differentiation of pinnal diseases that are clinically similar.

Consider more specific laboratory evaluations, including hormonal assays, food restriction diets, intradermal allergy tests, and direct immunofluorescence

tests of skin biopsy specimens, to obtain a definitive diagnosis.

INFLAMMATORY PINNAL DISEASES

Most pinnal skin diseases are characterized by erythema. Pinnal erythema is frequently followed by secondary scaling and alopecia. In this discussion, the most common etiologies of pinnal erythema are presented.

Allergic Inhalant Dermatitis, Contact Dermatitis, and Food Allergy Dermatitis

Clinical Signs

These particular diseases may affect both pinnae solely or concurrently with other body areas. Refer to the respective chapters on each of these diseases for further information. Inhalant and food allergic dermatoses appear clinically as diffuse erythema and accompanying edema or urticarial lesions of the concave or convex or both surfaces of the pinna. Contact allergies usually occur nonseasonally on surfaces of the pinna that touch the offending agent. Initially, in any of these three allergic diseases, the animal may exhibit "flare-ups" of erythema and accompanying pruritus that may appear and remit spontaneously. With time, an initial seasonal pattern of erythema and pruritus may become year-long with allergic inhalant dermatitis. Chronic trauma of the pinna may cause excoriation, secondary infections, fibrosis, and alopecia.

Diagnosis

- The differential diagnoses of these allergic pinnal dermatoses include pruritic otitis externa secondary to mange mite infestation, foreign body embedment (e.g., grass awns), or bacterial folliculitis.
- Diagnosis of inhalant or food allergy is made by obtaining the minimum data base for pinnal dermatoses in addition to special food restriction diets and intradermal allergy tests (see sec. 5, chs. 7 and 8).

Treatment

- Ideally, identified offending allergens are eliminated from the animal's environment and signs of allergy disappear. Upon removal of the allergen in contact allergic animals, the improvement in clinical signs is dramatic. In most situations of inhalant allergic der-

TABLE 1. Differential Diagnoses of Pinnal Diseases Based on Clinical Presentation

Clinical Manifestation	Differential Diagnoses
Macules/papules	Parasitic dermatoses/ hypersensitivities Bacterial folliculitis Drug eruption Food allergy Dermatophytosis Lupus erythematosus
Nodules	Neoplasia Eosinophilic granuloma complex Mycoses
Vesicles	Pemphigus/pemphigoid Dermatomyositis Lupus erythematosus
Pustules	Pemphigus/pemphigoid Dermatomyositis Lupus erythematosus Demodectic mange Drug eruption Dermatophytosis Bacterial folliculitis Eosinophilic folliculitis
Alopecia (focal)	Bacterial folliculitis Drug eruption Dermatophytosis Demodectic mange Dermatomyositis Alopecia areata Sex hormone imbalance Notoedric mange (feline)
Hyperpigmentation	Hypothyroidism Sex hormone imbalance Hyperadrenocorticism Growth hormone responsive
Induration	Juvenile cellulitis Neoplasia Urticaria
Erosions/ulcers	Parasitic infestation Dermatomyositis Vasculitis Dermatophytosis Pemphigus/pemphigoid Toxic epidermal necrolysis
Exfoliation	Pemphigus Cutaneous lymphoma Icthyosis Hepatocutaneous syndrome
Plaques	Lichenoid psoriasiform dermatosis Lichenoid dermatosis Cutaneous lymphomas

matitis, the allergens (as identified by intradermal skin testing) are not easily removed. Hyposensitization of the animal to the various inhalant allergens is the treatment of choice (see sec. 5, ch. 7).

■ Pinnal pruritus secondary to inhalant allergic dermatitis may be controlled initially by topical and/or systemic corticosteroids. Administer anti-inflammatory doses of oral prednisone (0.5–1.0 mg/kg) on alternate days or as infrequently as possible. Oral antibiotic therapy may be instituted as necessary to control secondary bacterial infections.

KEY POINT ▶ Contact and food allergic animals respond unpredictably to systemic corticosteroid therapy. Inhalant allergic animals usually respond well, at least initially.

Feline Solar Dermatitis

Clinical Signs

■ Chronic sun exposure of white-haired pinnae and other white-haired facial areas of cats may cause feline solar dermatitis. This syndrome also occurs in dogs but less frequently.

■ The clinical signs of pinnal erythema and scaling (solar dermatitis) are considered precancerous and herald malignant transformation into carcinoma *in situ*. Squamous cell carcinoma is usually locally invasive. With time, the ear pinna becomes progressively edematous, ulcerated, hemorrhagic, and deformed (fissuring, curling, and finally obliteration).

Diagnosis

■ Differential diagnoses include feline scabies, frostbite, trauma, pemphigus complex, systemic lupus erythematosus, and other cutaneous neoplasias.

■ Definitive diagnosis requires skin biopsy. Extensive pinnal involvement necessitates submandibular lymph node biopsy to assess for metastasis.

Treatment

■ Solar dermatitis is responsive to supportive therapy. Reduce the animal's sun exposure as much as possible.

■ Apply topical sun screen cream on the ears as necessary. Do not use a PABA (para-aminobenzoic acid)–based product, because this is a contact sensitizing agent.

■ Treatment of squamous cell carcinoma is most amenable to pinnal resection or amputation depending upon the extent of neoplasia. The carbon dioxide laser has been used safely and effectively to resect pinnal and facial squamous cell carcinoma in cats. Laser surgery affords the most cosmetically favorable results when compared with conventional surgery.

TABLE 2. Minimum Data Base for Pinnal Dermatoses

Otoscopic examination
Microscopic examination
    Skin scrapings for mites and fungi
    Cytology (impression smears)
    Mineral oil ear swab for mites
Culture for bacteria and fungi
Skin biopsy
    Histopathologic examination
    Immunofluorescence testing (if indicated)
Blood analysis
    Complete blood count, serum biochemical profile, endocrine
      screen (if indicated)
Urinalysis

Dermatophytosis

Clinical Signs

Superficial fungal infections (see sec. 5, ch. 3) of the pinnae in dogs and cats are most commonly caused by *Microsporum canis*. Initially, minimal-to-marked erythema is present. Infected hair follicles and intrafollicular epidermis become inflamed, and focal to multiple areas of alopecia and scaling occur secondarily.

Diagnosis

Diagnostic aids include skin scrapings (to detect fungal arthrospores microscopically), fungal culture, and skin biopsy. Once the definitive diagnosis of dermatophytosis is made, the rest of the animal's body is brushed with a sterile toothbrush. This sample is submitted for fungal culture.

Treatment

■ Treatment includes clipping the pinna and whole body if necessary (depending upon the toothbrush sample's culture results), topical dips in lime sulfur (LymDyp, DVM Pharmaceuticals) weekly for a minimum of 8 weeks, and daily topical applications of antifungal creams (Conofite, Pitman-Moore). Institute an oral griseofulvin (Gris-Peg, Dorsey) regimen for 6 to 8 weeks for each infected and in-contact animal if the disease is extensive on the body, especially in Persian cats. For further information on treatment of generalized dermatophytosis, refer to section 5, chapter 3.

Demodicosis

Clinical Signs

Demodicosis of the ear pinna may occur in dogs and cats (see sec. 5, ch. 4). The clinical picture of infestation is similar to that of dermatophytosis because of the mite's predilection to inhabit hair follicles. Erythema, scaling, and alopecia are common clinical signs.

Diagnosis

Obtain multifocal skin scrapings of the pinnae and other body areas as well as skin biopsies to determine the extent of infestation. Perform laboratory testing of blood to detect underlying systemic abnormalities.

Treatment

Clip the pinnal and other body hair as necessary. Apply whole body dips or localized therapy using the appropriate agents as described in section 5, chapter 4.

Juvenile Cellulitis (Juvenile Moist Pyoderma, Puppy Strangles)

Clinical Signs

The pinnae are usually affected bilaterally. There is no breed predilection. Any number of puppies in a litter may be affected (see sec. 5, ch. 1); puppies between 4 and 16 weeks of age are most commonly affected. Diffuse erythema and edema of the pinna progress rapidly to pustular, erosive-to-ulcerative, exudative dermatitis. Other facial areas and submandibular lymph nodes may become involved and exude a purulent exudate. This disease is considered to be a sterile inflammatory process of unknown etiology.

Diagnosis

Obtain the minimum data base to make a definitive diagnosis.

Treatment

■ Treat the lesions topically with astringent soaks (Domeboro, Miles). Initiate a regimen of oral prednisone, usually 1.0 mg/kg, q12h, PO for 14 days and oral bactericidal antibiotic for 14 days as soon as possible. Refer to section 5, chapter 1, for additional information.

SCALING AND CRUSTING PINNAL DISEASES

Differential diagnoses of pinnal lesions of this type include fly strike and canine breed–specific epidermal keratinization defects.

Fly Strike

Clinical Signs

This is a summer-fall disease of dogs that are confined primarily outdoors. *Stomoxys calcitrans* is the most common species of biting blood-feeding flies. Others incriminated are *Culicoides* spp. and *Simulium* spp. that cause erythematous, papular pinnal lesions. Affected dogs exhibit head shaking and ear scratching in response to the extremely irritating fly bites. Secondary pinnal excoriation, exudation, and hemorrhage appear on the ear tips of erect-eared dogs and at the proximal fold of the pinna of pendulous-eared dogs. Other facial areas may be involved as well.

Diagnosis

■ Differential diagnoses include sarcoptic mange, otodectic mange, atopy, vasculitis, and systemic lupus erythematosus.
■ Obtain the minimum data base using appropriate diagnostic aids to make the definitive diagnosis (see Table 2).

Treatment

Treat the problem in a two-step approach.

■ First, eradicate the flies in the dog's immediate environment.
■ Second, apply topical fly repellent (Skin So Soft, Avon Products) and/or insecticides onto the entire body of the dog with more on the head areas.
■ Apply topical antibiotic-corticosteroid ointments (Panalog, Solvay) to the affected pinna to decrease inflammation and secondary bacterial infection and to provide a mechanical barrier against flies.

Ear Margin Seborrhea

Clinical Signs

Keratinization disorders of the pinna occur most commonly in pendulous-eared breeds of dogs, such as cocker spaniels and dachshunds (see sec. 5, ch. 10, for a complete discussion of seborrhea). Clinical signs include scaling, crusting, and alopecic areas on the margins, especially severe on the apex of the pinna. Pinnal hair becomes embedded with scale crusts in a waxy exudate.

Diagnosis

■ Differential diagnoses include zinc-responsive dermatosis, dermatophytosis, pemphigus complex, sarcoptic mange, systemic lupus erythematosus, ichthyosis, and vasculitis. Obtain the minimum data base to make the definitive diagnosis (see Table 2).

Treatment

■ While awaiting biopsy results, initiate supportive therapies: antiseborrheic shampoo and application of follicular flushing agents that contain benzoyl peroxide (Pyoben Gel, Allerderm).
■ Topical corticosteroid cream or synthetic vitamin A gel (Retin-A Gel, Ortho Pharmaceutical Corp.) may be effective long-term therapy for idiopathic keratinization defects. For additional information, refer to section 5, chapter 10.

Otodectic Mange

Clinical Signs

Initially, *Otodectes cyanotis* may infest the external ear canal and cause pruritic otitis externa in dogs and cats (see sec. 5, ch. 5). Hypersensitivity to these mange mites results in severe self-trauma to the pinna, even though the number of mites may be small. Erythema, papules, excoriations, and alopecia are initial signs that progress into edema, exudation, fissuring, crusting, and scabbing.

Diagnosis

■ Differential diagnoses include other mange mite infestations, other parasitic infestations, and so forth.
■ Obtain the minimum data base to make the definitive diagnosis (see Table 2).

Treatment

■ Treat all infested and in-contact animals with weekly pyrethrin-based shampoos for 4 weeks and/or weekly applications of pyrethrin-based flea powder to the entire body for 4 weeks.
■ Concurrently, initiate local therapy using one of the numerous mineral oil–based acaricidal ear preparations (Tresaderm, Merck; Mitox, SmithKline Beecham). Drops are applied daily to the external ear canal and pinna as directed by the manufacturer.

Sarcoptic and Notoedric Mange

Clinical Signs

These particular mange mites are primarily host specific (*Sarcoptes scabeii* var. *canis* in dogs; *Notoedres cati* in cats) (see also sec. 5, ch. 5). Dogs and cats that become infested with these mites develop similar clinical lesions of yellow crusting and intense pruritus. The pinnal margins as well as the ventrum, elbows, and hocks of dogs and the head and neck areas of cats are the most common areas of involvement. However, if the animal has been treated with topical or systemic corticosteroids, pruritus may be dampened.

Diagnosis

■ Diagnosis is made through identification of the mites by microscopic examination of skin scrapings.
■ If scabies is suspected but no mites are found, a diagnostic and therapeutic miticidal trial is performed. A good dramatic response is considered as evidence of a positive diagnosis.
■ Parasitic infestations, such as those caused by sticktight fleas or ticks, may cause similar clinical signs. Such parasites are readily identified on the pinnad. Other differential diagnoses include allergic dermatoses, seborrheic dermatitis, dermatophytosis, pemphigus foliaceus, and systemic lupus erythematosus.

Treatment

■ Treat sarcoptic or notoedric mange with weekly whole body lime sulfur dips of the affected animals and all in-contact animals for at least 6 to 8 weeks. This therapy is the safest and most effective treatment available.
■ Dipping dogs and cats with 0.025% amitraz (Mitaban, Upjohn) twice at 2-week intervals reportedly kills these mange mites. Mitaban is not approved for use to kill these types of mites in cats and dogs.
■ Oral and injectable ivermectin (Ivomec, MSD Agvet) at 200–300 µg/kg effectively treats both mange mite infestations. Either treatment mode is given twice at 2-week intervals to dogs and cats. Ivermectin is not approved for use to treat these particular mange mite infestations in dogs and cats in the United States. For further information, refer to section 5, chapter 5.

KEY POINT ▶ Never use ivermectin to treat a collie-type dog or a shetland sheepdog–type dog for sarcoptic mange mite infestation because of potential adverse drug reactions.

PUSTULAR PINNAL DISEASES

Clinical Signs

■ Primary pustular lesions may or may not be observed on the pinna owing to their fragility. Secondary crusting and scaling are usually seen.

Diagnosis

- Common differential diagnoses include pemphigus foliaceus and demodicosis.
- Rare pustular dermatoses include subcorneal pustular dermatosis, linear IgA dermatosis, and dermatitis herpetiformis.
- Primary bacterial pyodermas do not commonly affect solely the pinna.
- Obtain the minimum data base to rule in or out the various differential diagnoses.

Treatment

- The treatment protocol of choice must be made prudently and is predicated on the results of histopathologic examination of pustular pinnal lesions.

NODULAR PINNAL DISEASES

Clinical Signs

Most nodular diseases of the pinna are neoplastic (see sec. 3, ch. 9, for a complete discussion of cutaneous neoplasia). In addition to squamous cell carcinoma, as previously discussed, other neoplasms with predilections for the pinnae include basal cell carcinomas, histiocytomas, mast cell tumors, fibrosarcomas, and benign sebaceous adenomas (hyperplasia). Other papular-to-nodular lesions located on the concave aspect of the feline pinna may include linear granulomas (see sec. 5, ch. 14) and deep mycotic infections (see sec. 2, ch. 12).

Diagnosis

Perform a skin biopsy for histopathologic examination to make the definitive diagnosis.

Treatment

Surgical resection is the treatment of choice for most neoplasms. Carbon dioxide laser surgery allows for the most precise removal of nodular neoplasms with minimal to no cosmetic defects. If conventional surgery is used, care must be taken not to create undue cosmetic defects in this sensitive area. Other types of nodular diseases are treated according to their definitive diagnoses.

NONINFLAMMATORY PINNAL DISEASES

Pattern/Endocrine Alopecia

Male Dachshund

- The male dachshund may develop a nonpruritic bilateral noninflammatory pinnal alopecia at approximately 1 year of age. The condition is probably hereditary and slowly progresses to complete pinnal baldness within several years. Owners may not notice slowly progressing alopecia until the dog is of middle age.
- No specific treatment exists for alopecia of hereditary origin.

Female Dachshund

- Spayed female dachshunds may develop pinnal alopecia associated with hypoestrogenemia and concurrently involving the perineum, ventral abdomen, and ventral neck areas. Differential diagnoses include demodectic mange, dermatophytosis, and endocrine disease. The diagnosis is determined by obtaining the minimum data base for pinnal dermatoses along with special hormonal assays, if needed. Estrogen replacement is recommended for female dogs with hypoestrogenemia.

Cats

- In cats, hyperadrenocorticism can cause pinnal alopecia and fragile, atrophic skin. One of the hallmarks of iatrogenic hyperadrenocorticism in cats is an obvious medial curling of the tips of the pinnae.
- Obtaining the minimum data base for pinnal dermatoses and performing specific adrenal function tests are necessary to diagnose this disease.
- Treat pituitary-dependent hyperadrenocorticism in cats carefully with o,p'-DDD (Lysodren, Bristol-Myer Co.) as described in section 4, Chapter 3. Lysodren is a chlorinated hydrocarbon and a potential toxin to cats.

Some Siamese cats and some miniature poodles develop spontaneous, periodic, bilateral pinnal alopecia of unknown origin. In these specific breeds, alopecia may last for several months and hair then regrows without treatment.

For additional information regarding nonpruritic alopecia, refer to section 5, chapters 11 and 13 and other appropriate chapters in the endocrine section of this book.

Alopecia Areata

Clinical Signs

Alopecia areata is a rare condition that may occur with focal or multifocal areas of alopecia at the pinnal base and on the head of dogs and cats.

Diagnosis

The diagnosis is based on physical findings and histopathology.

Treatment

Although corticosteroids are recommended in treating human patients, the response in animals is variable. Some animals spontaneously regrow hair within 6 months to 2 years.

Melanoderma and Alopecia of Yorkshire Terriers

Clinical Signs

This dermatosis is of unknown etiology. The disease is seen primarily in young Yorkshire terriers and may be inherited. There is no sex predilection. Affected dogs develop symmetric alopecia and marked hyperpigmentation of the pinnae and bridge of the nose and, occasionally, of the feet and tail. The lesions are nonpruritic and nonpainful.

Diagnosis

Diagnosis is made based upon clinical signs and histopathology.

Treatment

Therapy is supportive and nonspecific.

MISCELLANEOUS PINNAL DISEASES

Ear Margin Necrosis

- A variety of etiologies may produce this lesion, including vasculitis, cold agglutinin disease, frostbite, and squamous cell carcinoma.
- Necrosis of the pinnae was reported to occur in cats that had ingested spoiled scallops and in cats with various severe systemic disorders such as disseminated intravascular coagulation.
- Treatment depends upon the definitive diagnosis obtained from the minimum data base for pinnal dermatoses (see Table 2).

Sterile Eosinophilic Pinnal Folliculitis

- This is an idiopathic, nonseasonal, bilaterally symmetric alopecia with follicular papules and pustules. Affected animals are otherwise healthy.
- Diagnosis is made by biopsy of the affected pinnae.
- This disorder is chronic and requires long-term topical and/or systemic corticosteroid maintenance therapy.
- We have diagnosed a similar condition in two young cats less than 1 year of age. In each cat, the cause was ruled idiopathic and remitted spontaneously within 1 month of diagnosis and without recrudescence.

Cold Agglutinin Disease

- This rare immune-mediated disorder occurs in animals when the IgM class of autoantibodies reacts with erythrocytes at temperatures below $32°C$.

- Exposure to cold temperature results in pinnal erythema of the apex margin which progresses to ulceration and necrosis. Usually, all body extremities are affected.
- A positive Coombs test result for IgM at $4°C$ confirms the diagnosis. Underlying neoplastic or infectious diseases must be identified and treated aggressively.
- Treatment of idiopathic cold agglutinin disease includes immunosuppressive dosages of corticosteroids and elimination of exposure to cold temperatures. See section 5, chapter 9 for more information on immune-mediated dermatoses and section 3, chapter 3 for information on systemic immune-mediated diseases.

Trauma

- Traumatic damage may affect the epidermis, dermal vasculature, and underlying cartilage of the pinna. Mange mite infestations of the pinna, puncture wounds, lacerations, and secondary bacterial infections may incite pinnal pruritus and subsequent self-trauma. Aural hematomas may appear as fluctuant-to-firm pinnal swellings as a result of trauma to pinnal vasculature.

  - *Ear fissures* are the result of chronic active trauma to the ears from scratching or shaking the head. These fissures usually enlarge and hemorrhage. Underlying factors include parasitic infestations and otitis (interna/externa). Treatment consists of surgical resection of the distal pinna just proximal to the edge of the fissures. Bandage the ear across the head to prevent the trauma caused by postoperative head shaking.
  - *Pinnal lacerations* are managed as described for other wounds in section 5, chapters 17 to 19. Principles of pinnal surgery are discussed in section 5, chapter 22.

Supplemental Readings

Griffin CE: Diseases of the pinnae. The 1986 Scientific Proceedings of the American Animal Hospital Association, 1988, p 198.
Muller GH, Kirk RW, Scott DW: *Small Animal Dermatology.* Philadelphia: WB Saunders, 1989, pp 698, 814.
Scheidt VJ: Dermatoses of the pinnae. *In* Kirk RW, ed.: *Current Veterinary Therapy X: Small Animal Practice.* Philadelphia: WB Saunders, 1989, pp 621.

21 Otitis Externa

James O. Noxon

Otitis externa is an inflammation of the soft tissue components of the external auditory meatus. This condition is one of the most common and frustrating problems encountered in small animal practice. Otitis externa can be a primary or secondary disease process.

KEY POINT ▶ Otitis externa is often a clinical manifestation of a generalized dermatologic condition.

The cause of otitis externa in a patient may be multifactorial, making the diagnosis and treatment difficult.

ETIOLOGY

Primary Factors

- Primary factors are those conditions or disorders that initiate the inflammatory process within the ear canal.
- Examples include parasites *(Otodectes cynotis);* allergies (food, atopy, contact); foreign bodies (grass awns, foxtails); keratinization disorders (seborrhea); and, less frequently, trauma, autoimmune disease, sebaceous adenitis, and zinc-responsive dermatosis.
- Primary factors may initially induce disease outside the external ear canal. Otitis externa may be an extension of a pinnal disorder (see sec. 5, ch. 20) otitis media, or otitis interna (see sec. 5, ch. 23).

Predisposing Factors

- Predisposing factors facilitate the inflammation by permitting an environment conducive to survival of perpetuating factors.
- Examples include conformation of the ear canal (long canal with a deep vertical component), moisture in the canal, hair in the ears (e.g., in poodles and terriers), breed predisposition (e.g., Chinese Shar Pei, stenotic canals), immunodeficiency syndromes, endocrine imbalances, iatrogenic ear trauma (e.g., hair removal and cleaning with cotton-tipped applicators), and obstructive disease (e.g., cancer, polyps, and hyperplasia).

Perpetuating Factors

- Perpetuating factors sustain and aggravate the inflammatory process.
- Mechanisms include occlusion of the canal, which prevents drying or proper application of medication; secretion of irritating factors; alterations in pH of the canal; and formation of a focus of infection (otitis media).

- Examples include bacterial infections (*Staphylococcus intermedius, Proteus mirabilis, Pseudomonas aeruginosa, Corynebacterium* spp., and *Escherichia coli*) and yeast infection *(Malassezia pachydermatis).* Otitis media serves as a source of infectious agents, and chronic hyperplastic changes of the ear canal may obstruct the canal.

KEY POINT ▶ Medication may also act as a perpetuating factor (or a primary factor) of otitis externa, by causing secondary contact irritation or allergy (e.g., neomycin and topical anesthetics) or by leaving residue in the canal (e.g., oil-based preparation).

CLINICAL SIGNS

Signs Directly Related to Ear Involvement

- Head shaking
- Scratching and rubbing of the ears
- Pain around the ears or head (manifested as crying or whining)
- Malodor
- Behavioral changes
  - Pets may become irritable and aggressive towards family members as a result of ear pain.
  - Licking of ears by *other* pets in the household may indicate malodor and an inflammatory process.
- The pet's loss of hearing, although difficult to document, is a common owner's complaint.

Signs Reflecting an Underlying (Predisposing) Dermatologic Disorder

- Face rubbing, sneezing, foot licking, anal scooting, and generalized scratching suggest underlying allergic disease.
- Severe pruritus may incriminate parasitic (scabies, *Notoedres* mange) or allergic (flea allergy dermatitis) causes.
- Scaling and crusting may indicate seborrheic disease or sebaceous adenitis as a primary disease.
- Recurrent bacterial dermatitis suggests an endocrine imbalance or immunologic insufficiency.
- Accompanying alopecia may reflect various factors.
  - Bilaterally symmetric alopecia with easily epilated hair is a feature of endocrine disease.
  - Focal alopecia or alopecia characterized by broken or fragmented hairs may indicate trauma (pruritus) or infectious (bacterial, fungal) disease.

Signs of Accompanying Otitis Media and Otitis Interna

(See sec. 5, ch. 23.)

DIAGNOSIS

Diagnostic procedures are directed towards identifying primary factors (initiating factors), predisposing factors, and perpetuating factors. All etiologic factors must be considered for successful long-term management of the patient.

- *History* is used to detect evidence of allergies (seasonality), parasites (possible exposure), and environmental factors of concern.
  - Determine the frequency of ear problems and the response to previous treatment, which may give important clues about the pathologic processes.
- *Physical evaluation* includes palpation of the external ear canals, smelling of the ears, and careful examination of the skin over the entire body for evidence of systemic disease.
  - Examination is needed for vestibular and cranial nerve abnormalities that could indicate otitis media and otitis interna (see sec. 5, ch. 23).
- *Otoscopic examination* (see sec. 1, ch. 1).
  - Evaluate for the size of the ear canals; the presence of parasites, exudate, hair, or foreign material; the color of the epithelium; the presence of ulcers or masses; and the appearance and integrity of the tympanic membrane.
  - Sedation of the animal may be necessary.
    Topical anesthesia with 1 to 2% lidocaine hydrochloride, 0.5% proparacaine, or other similar agents may be sufficient.
    General anesthesia is indicated for removal of most foreign objects; for biopsy; and for thorough evaluation of the horizontal ear canal, in some patients.
    Avoid trauma to the ear canal by advancing the otoscope cone only while directly visualizing the canal.
  - Otic changes
    Erythema (reddened epithelium)
    Exudation: dark, dry, granular exudate is found with ear mite infection; moist, yellow, odoriferous exudate is often a sign of bacterial infection; brown and waxy exudate is consistent with yeast infection and overgrowth; and yellow, waxy-to-oily exudate is found with keratinization disorders.
    Hyperplasia (lichenification, hyperpigmentation) is a sign associated with chronicity. Surgical management may be necessary in patients with severe hyperplasia (occlusion).
    Ulceration suggests more severe disease and indicates a need for aggressive treatment.

KEY POINT ▶ *Cytology* is a rapid, inexpensive diagnostic procedure that is indicated in all cases of otitis externa.

- *Cytology* often provides an indication for the best initial treatment plan.

- Use a cotton-tipped applicator to swab the external canal as deeply as possible without packing exudate farther into the ear canal. Remove and gently roll the applicator on a clean glass slide.
- Examine slides prior to staining or after adding mineral oil to look for external parasites. Stain with a modified Wright-Giemsa preparation (Diff-Quik; American Scientific Products).
- Examine for parasites, cellular components, and infectious agents (bacteria, yeast, fungi). Notice whether infectious agents are present within inflammatory cells or free in the exudate.
- *Culture and susceptibility testing*
  - Culture is indicated in recurrent otitis and in severe ulcerated otitis when bacteria are seen during the cytologic examination.
  - Culture from both ears if disease is bilateral, because flora may be different in each one.
- *Biopsy*
  - Indicated when abnormal growths are detected.
  - Biopsy instruments, designed for endoscopic procedures, are useful to collect a small tissue sample from the ear canal.
  - Excisional biopsy of lesions is preferred whenever possible.
- *Radiography* is occasionally indicated (especially in severe or chronic otitis) to evaluate the patency of the ear canal, to detect the presence of otitis media and otitis interna, and to determine the extent of involvement of surrounding structures.
- *Miscellaneous diagnostic tests* are helpful to identify predisposing and primary factors. See respective chapters for details on these tests. Tests frequently recommended include hematology, serum biochemistry profiles, urinalysis, thyroid function tests, adrenal function tests, intradermal skin tests, *in vitro* allergy tests, skin scrapings, fungal cultures, and dietary trials.

TREATMENT

The initial treatment of otitis externa is directed towards control of the active inflammatory process, because this aspect of the disease is of immediate concern to the client and patient. After the perpetuating factors are controlled, treatment is directed towards removing the underlying predisposing factors and the disease processes.

Successful long-term management of otitis externa requires identification and treatment of perpetuating factors, predisposing factors, and primary etiologic factors.

Principles of Medical Treatment

- Most commercial ear preparations contain multiple therapeutic agents. Select otic preparations carefully for the desired active agents (Table 1).

KEY POINT ▶ Do not apply cleansing agents, parasiticides, ceruminolytic/keratolytic agents, disinfectants, ototoxic antimicrobials, or oil-based medications

TABLE 1. Active Ingredients Commonly Present in Otic Preparations

Ceruminolytic
Hexamethyltetracosane
Docusate sodium (dioctyl sodium sulfosuccinate, DSS)
Squalane
Keratolytic
Carbamide peroxide
Benzoic acid
Salicylic acid
Sulfur
Resorcinol
Antifungal
Nystatin
Thiabendazole
Miconazole
Clotrimazole
Cuprimyxin
Antibacterial
Chloramphenicol
Colistin
Neomycin B sulfate
Gentamicin
Polymyxin B
Penicillin G
Bacitracin
Sulfacetamide
Sulfur
Anti-inflammatory
Glucocorticoids
Hydrocortisone
Prednisolone
Isoflupredone acetate
Triamcinolone acetonide
Dexamethasone
Fluocinolone acetonide
Dimethyl sulfoxide
Antiparasitic
Pyrethrins
Thiabendazole
Carbaryl
Rotenone
Topical anesthetic
Tetracaine
Lidocaine

into the ear canal of animals in which the tympanic membrane is ruptured.

- Choose the delivery vehicle for medication carefully.
  - Lotions and solutions are more easily applied deep in the external canal.
  - Oil-based medications are useful to treat dry, scaly lesions, such as those of seborrhea sicca.
  - Creams, pastes, and powders are difficult to apply deep in the external ear canal and may leave a residue. These formulations are rarely indicated in the treatment of otitis externa in dogs and cats.
- Apply topical otic medications liberally to ensure delivery of adequate amounts of medication to the deeper aspects of the canal.
- Gently massage the external canal to help to deliver medications deep into the horizontal canal.

Cleaning the External Canal

KEY POINT ▶ The initial objective of medical management of otitis externa is to clean and dry the external canal. This process

makes the environment less favorable for sustained microbiologic growth and reduces the inflammatory process in most patients.

- Supplies and equipment include ear-cleansing solutions, bulb or injection syringe, ear curette, and cotton balls. A water propulsion device may be helpful, if used on low settings.
- Several commercially available irrigating solutions are effective for cleansing the external ear canal (Table 2).
- A dilute chlorhexidine solution is effective for the initial cleansing of the ear canal (Table 3). This procedure can be performed in unsedated animals without causing discomfort.
  - If a foreign body is suspected, perform cleansing gently and follow by suction to dry the canal prior to otoscopic examination.
  - General anesthesia may be necessary.
- Ceruminolytic agents may be applied in cases of severe, exudative otitis to facilitate removal of the wax—they are most effective when applied to the external canal for 15 minutes prior to flushing. Ceruminolytic agents are contraindicated when the tympanic membrane is not intact.
- Use warm 0.9% saline to flush the ear canal when the integrity of the tympanic membrane is suspect.
- Employ the ear curette carefully to remove impacted debris and wax. General anesthesia is recommended.

Drying the External Canal

- Several commercial drying solutions are available. Active ingredients include acetic acid, sulfur, boric acid, alcohol, benzoic acid, and others.
- Infusion of solutions containing alcohol can result in severe discomfort (stinging sensation) to the patient and are avoided when the external ear canal is ulcerated.

Specific Topical Therapy

- Topical anti-inflammatory agents

KEY POINT ▶ Glucocorticoids applied to the external canal are significantly absorbed and will affect the hypothalamic-pituitary-adrenal axis.

- Otic glucocorticoid administration may interfere with diagnostic procedures, such as intradermal skin tests, adrenal function tests, thyroid function tests, and routine hematologic and biochemical tests (e.g., serum alkaline phosphatase activity).
- Use the least potent glucocorticoid necessary to accomplish the desired effect.
- Most preparations also contain antiparasitic and/or antimicrobial agents.
- Topical antibacterial agents
  - Base choice upon cytologic findings or culture and susceptibility results.
  - Medications include: aminoglycosides, chloramphenicol, chlorhexidine, iodophors, propylene glycol, and silver sulfadiazine cream (1%) (Silvadene;

TABLE 2. Commercial Preparations Useful in Cleaning and Drying the External Ear Canal*

Category	Product	Active Ingredients
Cleansing/flushing solutions	Oti-Clens (SmithKline)	Propylene glycol
		Malic acid
		Benzoic acid
	Epi-Otic Cleanser (Allerderm)	Lactic acid
		Salicylic acid
		Propylene glycol
		Docusate sodium
	Nolvasan Otic (Fort Dodge)	Chlorhexidine
	ChlorhexiDerm Otic (DVM Pharmaceuticals, Inc.)	Chlorhexidine
	BETADINE solution (Purdue Fredrick)	Povidone iodine
	Xenodine (Solvay)	Polyhydroxydine solution
Drying Solutions	ClearX Ear Treatment Drying Solution (DVM)	Acetic acid
		Sulfur
		Hydrocortisone acetate
	H/B101 (Maurry)	Hydrocortisone
		Burow's solution
	PANODRY (Solvay)	Boric acid
		Isopropyl alcohol

*Commercial otic medications generally have more than one function. Products listed are examples—many other effective medications are commercially available.

Marion). TRIS-EDTA alone or added to antimicrobials increases the sensitivity of resistant *Pseudomonas* spp. to several antibiotics. Other antibiotic preparations, available as otic or ophthalmic preparations for humans, may be applied to the external ear canal. Examples include colistin sulfate (Coly-mycin Otic; Parke-Davis) and tobramycin (Tobrex Ophthalmic Solution; Alcon).

- Topical antifungal agents
  - Clotrimazole (Lotrimin; Schering) is effective against *Malassezia* spp. yeast.
  - Miconazole lotion (Conofite; Pitman-Moore) may be used in the external canal to control yeast or

fungal infections (contains alcohol and may be irritating).
  - Chlorhexidine
  - Povidone iodine
  - Cuprimyxin cream
- Topical antiparasitic agents
  - Preparations containing pyrethrins, carbaryl, thiabendazole, and rotenone are effective against ear mites.
  - Apply these preparations to the external ear canal regularly (every day or every other day) for three weeks.
  - Apply a topical parasiticide (i.e., preparations used for adult fleas) to the skin over the remainder of the animal once weekly during the treatment period.
  - Acidifiers, such as acetic acid and benzoic acid, are somewhat helpful in controlling yeast and bacterial infections.

Systemic Therapy

- Systemic glucocorticoids may help alleviate the pain and inflammation of otitis externa.
  - Administer a single injection of short-acting glucocorticoid (Meticorten; Schering) or prednisone (1.1 mg/kg, q24h, PO) for 5 to 7 days.
  - Short-term glucocorticoid therapy is occasionally useful to reduce the inflammation in an ear. This allows a thorough otoscopic examination of the external canal. Administer the glucocorticoid as described previously, and perform the otic examination 24 to 48 hours later.
  - Long-term glucocorticoid therapy may be indicated in a patient with an allergic disease.
- Systemic antimicrobial therapy is indicated in a patient with bacterial otitis externa when the tympanic membrane is ruptured (see sec. 5, ch. 23), the

TABLE 3. Guidelines for Ear Cleaning

1. Prepare solution by mixing chlorhexidine solution (Nolvasan Skin and Wound Cleanser; Fort Dodge) with lukewarm water to form a 1:10 to 1:20 dilution. Other cleansing solutions may be substituted.
2. Infuse the solution to completely fill the external canal.
   a. If a bulb is used, do not form a tight seal with the canal and syringe tip.
   b. A 6-ml syringe (without needle) works well to fill the canal.
   c. Avoid directing a stream of solution on the tympanic membrane or forcing the solution into the canal under pressure.
3. Place a clean, dry, cotton ball at the entrance to the external canal.
4. Gently massage the external canal, working the solution from deep in the canal to the external opening.
5. Replace the cotton ball periodically to absorb the solution and exudate.
6. Repeat the process as needed (5 to 10 times), until the cotton ball is clean after massage.
7. The canal may be aspirated using a small-bore polypropylene catheter attached to a syringe, in order to remove fluid for better visualization of the canal.
8. If necessary, infuse a drying solution and repeat the process one or two times.

epithelium of the canal is ulcerated, or the inflammatory cells containing bacteria are found during cytologic examination.

• Systemic antifungal therapy is rarely necessary but is indicated in patients with severe recurrent yeast infections, in patients that are difficult to medicate topically, or in patients with otitis externa that is caused by a systemic mycotic agent (e.g., *Cryptococcus* spp.). Ketoconazole (10 mg/kg, q24h, PO) is effective against *Malassezia pachydermatis* infection or overgrowth in dogs and cats.

• Ivermectin (300 μg/kg, PO) is reported to be effective against ear mite infections in dogs and cats. Treatment may be necessary weekly for 3 to 4 doses to eliminate infection. Do not administer this to collies and collie-mix breed dogs or to known heartworm-infected animals, because treatment of these breeds or in these circumstances may result in profound adverse reactions.

PREVENTION

■ *Behavioral modification* is directed towards decreasing activities that predispose the animal to otitis, such as swimming, running through the woods and fields, and so forth.

■ *Regular medical care* may decrease the recurrence of otitis externa in predisposed patients.
• Thoroughly clean and dry ears after swimming.
• Regularly clean ears of pets with seborrheic disorders.

KEY POINT ▶ Remove hair only when indicated by the patient's history. Hair clipping or plucking is not recommended as part of routine ear care in most animals, because the irritation associated with these procedures may predispose them to otitis externa.

■ *Surgical management* of otitis externa is indicated to correct conformational defects that predispose an animal to inflammatory disease and to improve ventilation and drainage in affected ears (see sec. 5, ch. 22).

Supplemental Readings

August JR: Otitis externa: a disease of multifactorial etiology. Vet Clin North Am 18:731, 1988.

Chester DK: Medical management of otitis externa. Vet Clin North Am 18:799, 1988.

Macy DW: Diseases of the ear. *In* Ettinger SJ, ed.: *Textbook of Veterinary Internal Medicine.* Philadelphia: W. B. Saunders, 1989, p 246.

Wilke JR: Otopharmacology. Vet Clin North Am 18:783, 1988.

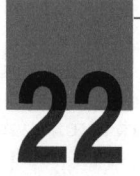

22 Surgery of the External Ear Canal and Pinna

Daniel D. Smeak

Surgery of the external ear canal in a small animal is usually performed to treat infection that is unresponsive to medical therapy. Generally, the aim of external ear canal surgery is to provide exposure and drainage for the vertical and horizontal ear canal or to remove irreversibly infected tissue or neoplasia.

Success of ear surgery relies on:

- Accurate diagnosis
- Appreciation of the severity and extent of the disease
- Appropriate postoperative medical treatment of the local disease and any underlying systemic skin disease.

KEY POINT ▶ As a general rule, surgical intervention is considered as soon as appropriate medical treatment for otitis externa fails.

As ear disease progresses, more extensive surgery is required to relieve clinical signs. Frequency and severity of complications, however, also increase as the surgery becomes more extensive.

Auricular hematoma is discussed later in this chapter.

GENERAL SURGICAL INDICATIONS

- For ear disease that fails to respond to appropriate medical treatment.
- For relapse of clinical signs after initial response to medical therapy.
- For extensive irreversible changes of cartilage and/or epithelium.
- For a predisposing factor causing the ear condition (congenital or acquired malformation, narrowing or aplasia of the ear canal, or neoplasia).

KEY POINT ▶ External ear surgery is rarely indicated in the cat except for traumatic or neoplastic conditions. Inflammatory ear polyps extending into the external ear canal do not require external ear surgery for removal. See middle ear surgery (see sec. 5, ch. 24) for further information.

ANATOMY

Understanding the anatomy of the ear and related structures is critical to successful ear surgery. The surgeon must identify and preserve several key structures, especially during horizontal canal dissection.

External Ear Canal (Figs. 1 and 2)

- The normal external ear canal is a pliable cartilaginous tube lined by glandular epithelium, extending from the base of the pinna to the tympanic membrane.
- The normal canal is between 5 and 10 cm long and narrows to between 4 and 7 mm in diameter, proximally.

Vertical Ear Canal

- From the external opening (aditus), the vertical canal (auricular cartilage) runs ventrally and slightly rostrally, before bending towards the skull to form the shorter horizontal canal.

Horizontal Ear Canal

- The horizontal canal consists of a circular (annular) cartilage, extending from the ligamentous attachment to the auricular cartilage medially to the short osseous ear canal (projection of the petrous temporal bone). The canal ends at the tympanic membrane.

Important Local Structures

Glands
- The V-shaped parotid salivary gland overlays the ventrolateral aspect of the vertical ear canal and extends ventral to the distal aspect of the horizontal ear canal.

Blood Vessels (Fig. 2B)
- Blood supply to the ear is via the great auricular artery, arising from the external carotid artery located medial to the parotid gland and ventral to the osseous bulla.
- Small branches of the great auricular and maxillary arteries run dorsally, parallel to the long axis of the pinna, and medial to the pinna cartilage.

Nerves (Fig. 2B)
- The facial nerve arises from the stylomastoid foramen located just caudal to the osseous ear canal.
- The nerve courses rostroventrally directly under the horizontal ear canal.
- Terminal branches of the facial and auriculotemporal branch of the mandibular portion of the trigeminal nerve are located just cranial to the ear canal.

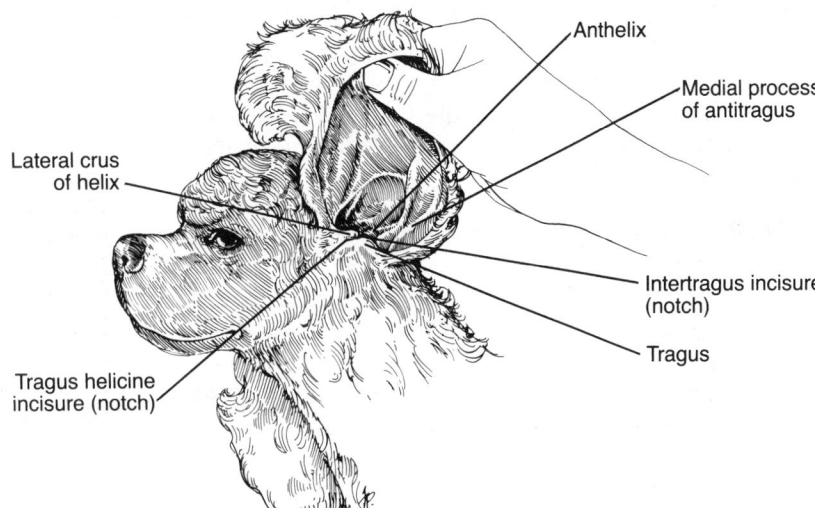

Figure 1. Anatomy of the external aditus of the ear.

Labels: Lateral crus of helix, Tragus helicine incisure (notch), Anthelix, Medial process of antitragus, Intertragus incisure (notch), Tragus

PREOPERATIVE CONSIDERATIONS

An accurate preoperative diagnosis along with determination of the extent of disease is important when choosing the surgical procedure.

The ear canal is difficult to prepare aseptically, and contamination is inevitable during surgery.

A broad-spectrum, bactericidal, IV antibiotic (optimally based on preoperative culture and susceptibility) is given before and during surgery so that adequate blood levels are maintained in tissues during dissection.

Ear Palpation

- Sharp pain elicited on deep palpation of the external ear canal usually indicates middle ear infection.
- Palpation of severely thickened and firm ear canal tissue indicates irreversible changes have occurred.

Dermatologic Examination

- Perform a complete dermatologic examination and obtain appropriate tests to determine if primary systemic skin disease (e.g., hypothyroidism and atopy) is present.

Neurologic Examination

- Perform a neurologic examination, especially in chronic cases of otitis externa, to evaluate for facial nerve involvement (e.g., hemifacial spasm and slow or absent palpebral reflex) and involvement of inner ear structures (e.g., nystagmus and circling).
- Evaluate the patient's ability to hear and bring the deficits to the owner's attention before contemplating bilateral ear ablation in the pet.

Radiographic Examination

- Ventrodorsal skull radiograph is the view of choice to evaluate horizontal canal diameter and to determine whether the walls of the canal have undergone irreversible changes (calcification).

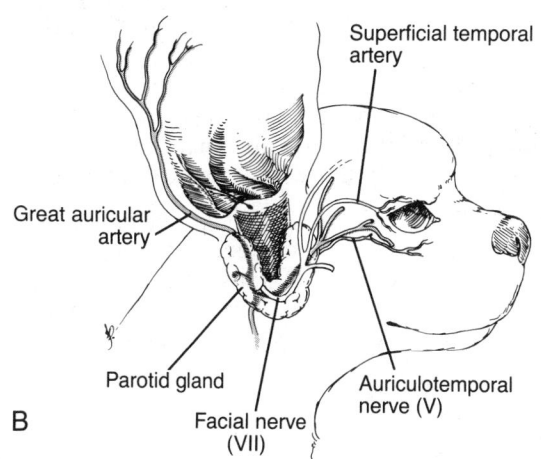

A — Labels: Vertical canal, Horizontal canal, Inner ear, Tympanic bulla, Osseous ear canal, Annular cartilage, Auricular cartilage

B — Labels: Superficial temporal artery, Great auricular artery, Parotid gland, Facial nerve (VII), Auriculotemporal nerve (V)

Figure 2. Lateral view of the head showing important anatomic structures of the external ear canal. *A,* Transverse section the head showing ear canal regions and middle ear and inner ear structures. *B,* Location of branches of the external carotid artery in relation to the ear canal and middle ear, and important neural structures in the external ear canal region.

KEY POINT ▶ Middle ear involvement (sec. 5, ch. 23) must be evaluated before deciding upon the surgical procedure.

■ Open-mouth radiography of the bulla is the view of choice to evaluate middle ear involvement (see sec. 5, ch. 23).

KEY POINT ▶ Lack of any osseous changes on bulla radiographs does not rule out otitis media.

■ Bulla osteitis takes months to form following deep-seated infection. Changes are often very subtle, and evaluation of fluid density within the bulla is also not an accurate method of diagnosis.

Otoscopic Examination

■ Perform a thorough ear cleansing after obtaining the appropriate diagnostic samples for culture and susceptibility, cytology, and biopsy (see sec. 5, ch. 21).
■ Otoscopic examination is the most important diagnostic modality to evaluate the severity and extent of disease and tympanic membrane rupture.

KEY POINT ▶ A thorough otoscopic examination usually cannot be accurately performed unless the animal is anesthetized.

Staging of Neoplastic Disease

■ Regional lymph node aspiration, cytology, biopsy, and thoracic radiographs are warranted if neoplasia is suspected in the underlying ear disease.

LATERAL EAR CANAL RESECTION—ZEPPS MODIFICATION (LECR)

Objectives

■ To expose the medial portion of the vertical canal and horizontal ear canal. Exposure enhances medical treatment of otitis externa and changes local ear conditions favoring drainage.
  • Ventilation of the area improves the local environment, decreasing moisture, humidity, and temperature.
■ To resect the lateral portion of the vertical ear canal to remove tumors or to relieve congenital or acquired nonproliferative vertical canal stenosis that is restricting ear drainage and medical treatment.

KEY POINT ▶ LECR is not performed if the horizontal or vertical ear canal is hyperplastic and filled with proliferative tissue. Likewise, LECR is contraindicated if medically uncontrolled primary skin disease (e.g., seborrhea) is present, because progressive ear disease would be expected in the remaining ear canal.

Equipment

■ Standard general surgical pack and suture
■ Heavy serrated straight Mayo scissors

Technique (Fig. 3)

1. Place the animal in lateral recumbency with the head positioned, aseptically prepared, and draped so that the ear region, including the pinna, exposed and all anatomic relationships are identifiable.
2. Use forceps to determine vertical canal depth and position of the horizontal canal.
3. Incise the lateral portion of the vertical ear canal and reflect ventrally.
4. Preserve the proximal portion of the lateral canal flap for a "drain board."
5. Begin closure at the base of the flap, then appose the distal flap to the skin. Appose the remaining ear epithelium and skin so that no cartilage is exposed.

Postoperative Care and Complications

■ Continue systemic antibiotics until the incisions are healed and the ear discharge has stopped.
■ Continue appropriate topical medical treatment and ear cleansing until no signs of ear infection are present.
■ Place an Elizabethan collar to prevent self-inflicted trauma to the wound until suture removal.
■ If wound dehiscence occurs, I prefer to let it heal by second intention closure.
■ Sutures are removed in 14 days.
■ Continue treatment of primary skin disorders as required.

Prognosis

■ Prognosis for control of ear disease is good provided that:
  • Surgery is performed correctly and for the right indication
  • No middle ear disease is present
  • Postoperative medical management of otitis externa is appropriate.
■ Up to 35% of LECRs fail because the aforementioned considerations are not met.

VERTICAL EAR CANAL ABLATION (VECA)

This technique combines some of the advantages of the LECR (maintenance of horizontal canal drainage) and total ear canal ablation (removal of chronically infected vertical canal tissue).

KEY POINT ▶ VECA is contraindicated if hyperplastic irreversible disease or neoplasia is present in the horizontal canal.

In my experience, if chronic hyperplastic tissue is present in the vertical canal it usually extends into the horizontal canal. Therefore, this procedure is not commonly indicated, but VECA may be an alternative method for those patients requiring LECR.

Objectives

■ To remove the vertical ear canal and preserve the horizontal canal.
■ To provide drainage for the horizontal canal.

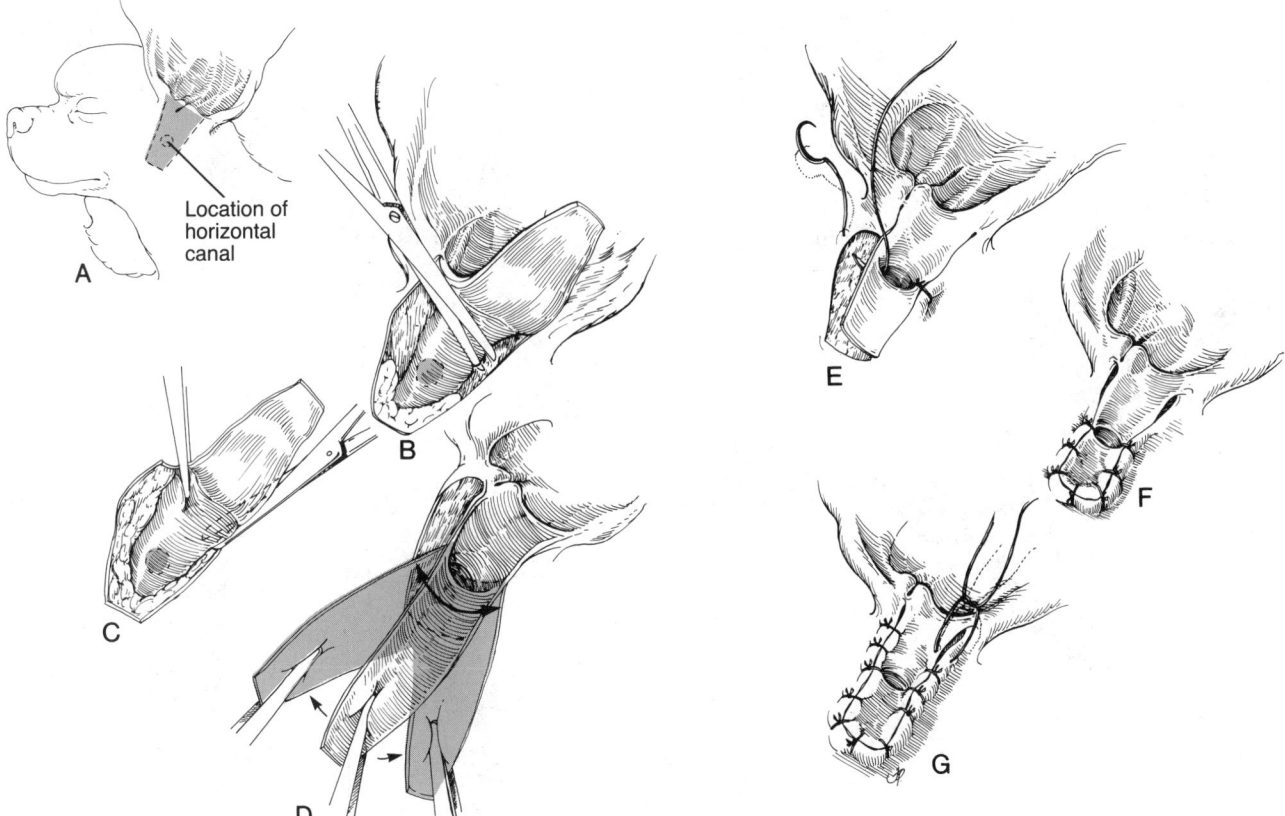

Figure 3. Lateral ear canal resection technique. *A,* Two skin incisions are extended parallel to each other from the intertragic notch and tragohelicine notch, tapering down to a distance of 1.5 to 2 cm between the incisions, about 1.5 to 2.5 cm (depending upon the size of the animal) ventral to the horizontal ear canal. A transverse incision joins the two vertical incisions, and the skin flap is undermined dorsally up to the margin of the aditus.

B, An incision is made through the subcutaneous tissue to the level of the vertical ear cartilage. The entire lateral aspect of the vertical ear canal is exposed by blunt and sharp dissection of the subcutaneous tissue in a rostral and caudal direction and parotid gland ventrally.

C, An Allis tissue forceps is placed on the tragus, and dorsal traction is applied so that the vertical ear canal can be seen from the dorsal aspect of the head. With scissors, two incisions are made through the vertical ear canal on the rostrolateral and caudolateral margins while maintaining dorsal traction. The rostral and caudal incisions are extended ventrally in an alternating fashion until the floor of the horizontal canal is reached. The vertical canal is essentially divided into lateral and medial halves.

D, Incisions are extended medially toward the head until the horizontal canal is fully exposed after the lateral wall is reflected ventrally. The base of the lateral wall flap should approximate the width of the horizontal canal. More cartilage can be removed from the remaining ear canal as necessary to fully expose the remaining vertical canal. The flap is manipulated rostrally and caudally until the horizontal canal is held open as wide as possible.

E, The skin flap and all but the proximal portion of the lateral wall are removed. The 1.5- to 2-cm cartilage (drain board) flap remaining is modified to lay flat and fit the skin defect ventral to the horizontal ear canal.

F, Closure begins by placing simple interrupted 3-0 to 4-0 monofilament nonabsorbable sutures from the caudal and rostral margins of the proximal most aspect of the drain board to the skin. Throughout closure, sutures are placed through ear canal epithelium and cartilage first and then to skin to aid in skin coverage of cartilage.

G, The remaining portion of the flap is then apposed to the skin with simple interrupted sutures so that the flap is flat against the head. Additional sutures are placed so that the skin and ear canal epithelium edges are apposed but not crushed.

Equipment

■ Same as that for LECR.

Technique (Fig. 4)

1. Patient positioning, skin preparation, and vertical ear canal exposure are the same as those described for LECR.
2. Isolate the entire vertical ear canal and resect distal to the annular cartilage.
3. Incise the remaining vertical ear canal to create a dorsal and ventral flap.
4. Appose the skin to ear epithelium.
5. The closure forms a T-shape.

Postoperative Care and Complications

■ Similar to those of lateral ear canal resection.
■ This procedure affects ear carriage; LECR rarely does.

Prognosis

Prognosis is good provided the procedure is performed for the correct indications. In a large retrospective study of 75 dogs undergoing VECA, 72 were asymptomatic within 12 weeks postoperatively.

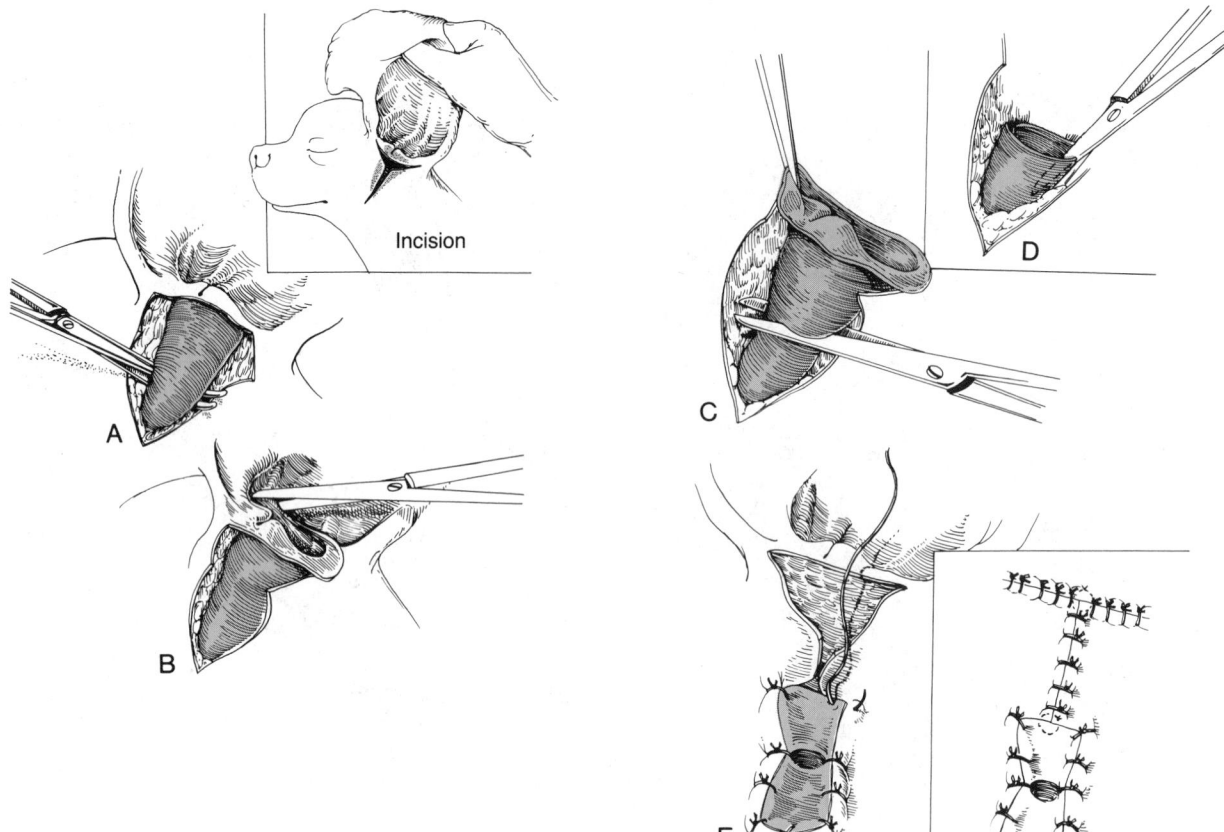

Figure 4. Vertical ear canal ablation technique. Use technique similar to LECR through Figure 3B.

A, Blunt dissection is continued medially until the entire vertical canal is isolated and freed up. Dissection is directed just underneath the cartilage to avoid damaging vascular supply to the pinna.

B, The auricular cartilage is cut with heavy straight Mayo scissors removing all affected tissue on the dorsal aspect of the medial vertical canal and pinna. This step allows complete mobilization of the vertical canal, which remains attached only at its proximal aspect.

C, The vertical canal is removed approximately 1 to 2 cm distal to the annular cartilage junction.

D, Remaining vertical canal is incised rostrally and caudally, if necessary, to fully expose the horizontal ear canal.

E, The ventral flap is sutured to the skin in a fashion similar to that in lateral ear resection.

F, The dorsal flap is sutured to appose the cut edges of the canal and skin with simple interrupted 3-0 to 4-0 monofilament nonabsorbable material. Remaining skin is apposed to form a T-shaped closure.

TOTAL EAR CANAL ABLATION (TECA)

Total ear canal ablation is a salvage procedure that involves removal of the entire vertical and horizontal ear canal cartilage and epithelium. If severe horizontal canal disease is present only TECA will be successful in eliminating the associated clinical signs.

KEY POINT ▶ Neglected chronic otitis externa results in extensive chronic inflammatory changes in periannular tissue. These greatly increase the risk of iatrogenic complications associated with difficult ear canal dissections.

Objective

- To remove the entire external ear canal without trauma to the facial nerve.

Indications

- Severe ear trauma that cannot be adequately managed with reconstruction.

- Congenital or acquired deformity affecting the horizontal ear canal.
- Irreversible hyperplastic and proliferative ear disease or neoplasia extending to the horizontal canal.
- Persistent otitis externa following LECR or VECA. If signs stem from middle ear infection, drainage of the middle ear is all that may be required provided the horizontal ear canal is not irreversibly affected.

KEY POINT ▶ TECA alone is contraindicated when middle ear infection is present, because it eliminates a drainage exit for the tympanic cavity. The auditory tube cannot be relied upon to drain thickened exudates within the middle ear. In these common instances, TECA can be successfully performed provided a means of tympanic bulla drainage is allowed.

Equipment

- Standard general surgical pack and suture
- Gelpi or Weitlaner self-retaining retractors

- Senn retractors
- Heavy, serrated Mayo scissors
- Suction apparatus and Frazier suction tip
- Electrocoagulation unit and sterile electrode
- Lempert and Cleveland bone rongeurs
- Straight Simon and Daubenspeck curettes
- Penrose drains (¼ inch)
- # 8 French Silastic feeding tube.

Technique (Fig. 5)

1. Use the same positioning, skin preparation, and draping as those in LECR.
2. Make a T-shaped incision to expose the ear canal.
3. Reflect loose connective tissue from the vertical ear canal.
4. Isolate the vertical and horizontal canal by blunt and sharp dissection. Maintain dissection immediately adjacent to the ear canal cartilage. Occasionally the facial nerve is found imbedded into the annular cartilage.
5. Careful dissection along the stylomastoid foramen isolates the origin of the nerve.
6. Sharply dissect the nerve out along its course within the horizontal canal.
7. In some patients with chronic proliferative otitis externa, a greenish-brown epithelial pouch forms between the tympanic bulla and annular cartilage. This epithelium extends lateral and ventral to the tympanic bulla. Removal of this tissue is critical to the success of the surgery, because chronic fistulation occurs if it is not fully removed. Use hemostatic forceps to grasp the edges of the pouch and, with traction, bluntly dissect the pouch out without injuring major local vessels and nerves.
8. Sharply amputate the annular cartilage from the petrous temporal bone, excise the ear canal, and submit it for biopsy.

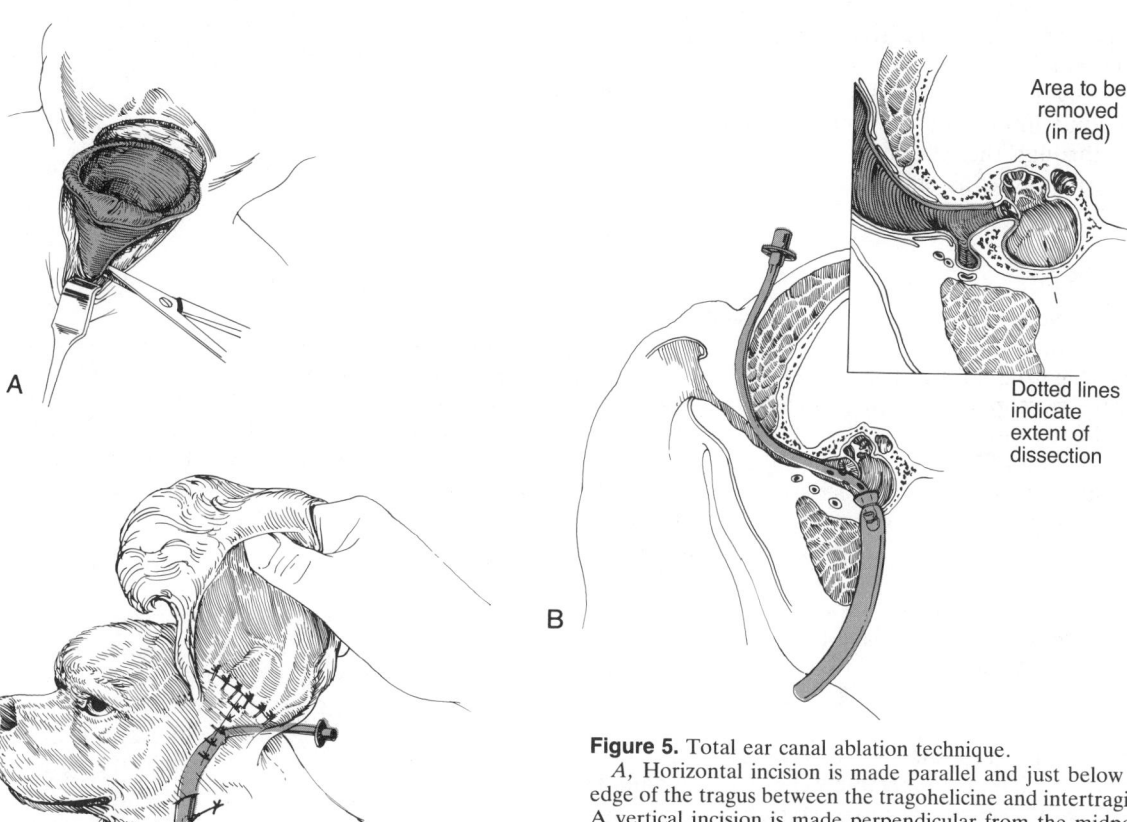

Figure 5. Total ear canal ablation technique.

A, Horizontal incision is made parallel and just below the upper edge of the tragus between the tragohelicine and intertragic notches. A vertical incision is made perpendicular from the midpoint of the horizontal incision to a point just ventral to the horizontal canal, forming a T-shaped incision. The two triangular skin flaps are undermined and retracted, exposing the lateral aspect of the ear canal. After hemostasis is achieved, the vertical canal is bluntly dissected free from the surrounding tissues, avoiding the auricular vessels located medial to the canal.

Heavy serrated Mayo scissors are used to cut the medial aspect of the proximal vertical ear canal connecting the ends of the original horizontal incision. Removal of wedge-shaped portions of skin from the rostral and caudal vertical skin margins and retention of as much of the normal medial vertical canal as possible encourages ear support in cats and dogs with erect ears.

The parotid gland is retracted ventrally. By a combination of blunt and sharp dissection, the horizontal canal is isolated to the level of the tympanic bulla. While maintaining meticulous hemostasis, dissection continues as close to the cartilage as possible, carefully exposing and retracting the facial nerve away from the line of dissection.

B, Transverse section of head shows common location of epithelial pouch between annular cartilage and petrous temporal bone. If otitis media is present, a lateral bulla osteotomy is performed to expose the bulla for curettage and to improve ventral drainage. Crosshatching indicates area of resection of the lateral and ventral osseous bulla. Modified ingress-egress system for irrigation and drainage of the tympanic cavity is in place.

C, Completed ear ablation showing placement of drainage system and skin closure.

9. Carefully remove the secretory epithelial lining of the short osseous external auditory canal by curettage. Submit this lining for culture and susceptibility.

10. Examine the middle ear for exudates and chronic thickened epithelium. If no changes are evident, place a Penrose drain within the dead space remaining where the ear canal was removed, exiting ventral to the T-shaped incision.

11. Place a percutaneous suture through the dorsal end of the Penrose tube to prevent premature dislodgement.

12. If middle ear infection is present, remove the ventral and lateral aspect of the bulla with rongeurs.

13. Remove all epithelium and debris with irrigation and curettage.

14. Avoid inner ear structures on the craniodorsal aspect of the bulla.

15. I prefer an ingress-egress irrigation/drainage system postoperatively to treat severe proliferative middle ear infection.

16. Alternatively, the entire skin incision is left to heal by second intention; the middle ear is then irrigated through the wound.

17. Place subcutaneous and skin sutures to form a T-shaped wound.

Postoperative Care

■ Examine wounds for evidence of fluid accumulation or ensuing infection.
  • Rebandage daily until drainage stops.
  • If acute postoperative infection occurs, open the wound for drainage.
  • Flush and bandage the wound daily.
■ Administer systemic antibiotics based on susceptibility testing and potential for causing ototoxicity for a minimum of 3 to 4 weeks, if otitis media is present (see sec. 5, ch. 23).
■ Remove skin sutures in 14 days.
■ Remove Penrose tubes placed in TECA without obvious signs of middle ear infection when drainage has significantly decreased. Generally, this is in 3 to 4 days.
■ Patients with established severe otitis media may require extensive postoperative wound management.
■ Perform irrigation of the ingress/egress system once or twice daily with 25 ml lukewarm 1:10 diluted povidone-iodine (BETADINE) solution and saline (or TRIS-EDTA if *Pseudomonas* sp. is isolated) for 5 to 10 days.

Complications

KEY POINT ▶ Owner education is critical before attempting TECA because the following serious and long-standing complications are possible.

■ Acute postoperative wound infection (up to 40% of patients).
■ Facial nerve damage (most are temporary; permanent paralysis occurs in <10% of patients).

■ Transient hypoglossal nerve dysfunction (rare and usually temporary).
■ Chronic fistulation from unresolved middle ear infection or persistent ear canal epithelium may occur up to 1 to 2 years following surgery (<10% of patients).
■ If inner ear signs are present before surgery, their exacerbation is common after surgery. Neurologic signs usually improve over time if otitis media is controlled but minor signs usually persist indefinitely.
■ Horner's syndrome (usually temporary) if middle ear surgery is also performed.
■ Dogs undergoing bilateral TECA generally hear about as well as they did before the surgery.
■ Like VECA, this procedure affects ear carriage.

Prognosis

Long-term follow-up for dogs undergoing TECA shows improvement in clinical signs in up to 90% of patients and shows the same or worse in 10%. Poor results usually are caused by persistent infection from unresolved middle ear infection or retained infected epithelial tissue. A total of 25 of 26 owners of dogs undergoing TECA with long-term follow-up indicated satisfaction with the procedure and improvement in their dogs' demeanor.

AURICULAR HEMATOMA

Auricular or aural hematoma is an accumulation of blood within the cartilage of the pinna caused by violent head shaking or scratching. The blood collection is usually confined to the concave surface of the pinna. This injury is most often seen in pendulous-eared dogs but is occasionally seen in erect-eared dogs and, less frequently, in cats.

KEY POINT ▶ Underlying causes of auricular hematomas are inflammatory conditions affecting the pinna or external ear canal such as those associated with foreign bodies, atopy, food allergy, bacterial infection, yeast infection, ear mites, and so forth. Because this condition is most often secondary to another, the underlying cause of the irritation must be identified, if possible, to avoid further injury and recurrence.

KEY POINT ▶ Auricular hematomas are drained as soon as possible, because delay often leads to enlargement and extension throughout the pinna. With time, fibrous organization of the hematomas eventually leads to a permanently thickened, cauliflower-like ear.

Anatomy

The major blood supply to the pinna is derived from branches of the external carotid artery and internal maxillary vein. The great auricular arteries and veins arborize and course longitudinally along the long axi on the convex side of the pinna. Mattress pattern sutures placed in the ear are oriented parallel to these vessels to avoid interrupting the blood supply to the pinna.

Preoperative Considerations

- The first objective for management of auricular hematomas is to identify the source of the ear irritation.
- Perform a thorough otoscopic examination to identify abnormalities within the ear canal.
- Complete history and dermatologic examination are recommended, particularly when no obvious cause of the irritation is uncovered during otoscopic examination.
- Rule out the diagnosis of atopy or other systemic manifestation of skin disease.
- If the cosmetic appearance of the pinna is of secondary importance to the owner, the incision and drainage technique is the most consistently successful. I prefer this technique for more chronic hematomas, because it allows for thorough debridement of organized clots.
- A more cosmetic and less time-consuming technique is the drainage-only procedure. Use this technique only in hematomas with fluid consistency (acute cases) and, preferably, those located towards the distal aspect of the pinna. Owners must understand that recurrence develops more often with drainage only compared with incision and suture. Simple aspiration alone is not a good option, because recurrence of the hematoma is unacceptably common.

Surgical Procedure

Objectives

- To treat the source of irritation
- To drain the hematoma
- To maintain apposition of cartilage surfaces for an adequate time to prevent recurrence

Equipment

- Standard general instrument pack

Technique

Incision, Drainage, and Bandage

1. Clip both sides of the pinna and prepare the ear for aseptic surgery
2. Incise the hematoma with a #10 blade in a linear fashion on the concave side.
3. Make this incision along the long axis of the pinna extending the length of the hematoma. Removal of a strip of skin to widen the incision and permit drainage is not necessary.
4. Explore the hematoma and remove any fibrin tags or blood clots.
5. Place 1-cm wide mattress sutures (3-0 or 4-0 monofilament nonabsorbable material) parallel to and no closer than 0.5 cm from the incision.

6. Hold the incised edges of the skin 2 to 3 mm apart when placing the first row of sutures. Sutures need not penetrate both skin surfaces because this creates another source of irritation and entry way for contamination.
7. Pass the needle carefully from the concave surface of the pinna, catching both cartilage planes.
8. Place the remaining mattress sutures in a staggered fashion 1 cm apart until the entire dead space area is obliterated.
9. Tie sutures with just enough tension to appose cartilage surfaces

Drainage Only

1. Aseptically prepare the skin on the concave surface of the pinna only. I do not clip the convex, haired surface because this creates more inflammation, which could lead to continual head shaking or scratching.
2. Make a small 0.5 to 1-cm incision extending into the hematoma at its most proximal and distal extent on the pinna.
3. Remove all fluid and fibrin tags with mosquito hemostats and digital expression.
4. Place a drain (1/4-inch Penrose or sterilized IV extension tubing) through the dead space and made to exit both stab wounds.
5. Suture the drain to the skin near the stab incisions with a loose nonabsorbable suture.

Postoperative Considerations

- Following treatment of the hematoma by the incision method, bandage the affected ear over the top of the head in pendulous-eared dogs. Bandage erect ears in an upright position.
  - Leave the ear canal exposed in each method to permit cleansing and medication as needed.
  - Leave the bandages on for at least 10 days and change as needed.
  - Remove sutures in 3 weeks.
- No bandages are used for the drainage-only method unless the patient continues violent or persistent head shaking.
  - Use an Elizabethan collar to reduce the incidence of self-trauma in all cases.
  - Leave drains in place for 3 to 4 weeks.
  - Instruct the owners to watch for signs of infection and to milk out any fluid that may accumulate within the hematoma during this time.
  - Instruct the owners about the proper treatment of the primary source of the ear irritation.
- The appearance of the ear following surgery is related to the drainage technique and to the chronicity of the hematoma.
  - Make no guarantees to the owners regarding the final cosmetic appearance of the ear and the impossibility of recurrence, because these are often unpredictable.
- Weekly re-evaluation of the patient before and after drainage determines the response to primary treatment and any problem related to wound management.

Supplemental Readings

Beckman SL, Henry WB, Cechner P: Total ear canal ablation combining bulla osteotomy and curettage in dogs with chronic otitis externa and media. J Am Vet Med Assoc 196:84, 1990.

Fraser G, Gregor WW, Mackenzie CP, et al.: Canine ear disease. J Sm Anim Pract 10:725, 1970

Gregory CR, Vasseur PB: Clinical results of lateral ear canal resection in dogs. J Am Vet Med Assoc 182:1087, 1983.

Grono LR: The external ear canal. *In* Slatter DH, ed.: *Textbook of Small Animal Surgery*. Philadelphia: W. B. Saunders, 1985, p 1906.

Harvey CE: Ear canal disease in the dog. J Am Vet Med Assoc 177:136, 1980.

Krahwinkel DJ, Pardo AD, Sims MH, Bubb WJ: Effect of ear ablation on auditory function as determined by brain stem auditory-evoked responses and subjective evaluation. (Abstract.) Vet Surg 1:70, 1989.

Siemering GH: Resection of the vertical ear canal for treatment of chronic otitis externa. J Am Anim Hosp Assoc 16:753, 1980.

Smeak DD: Total Ear Canal Ablation. *In* Bojrab MJ, ed.: *Current Techniques in Small Animal Surgery*. Philadelphia: Lea & Febiger, 1990, p 140.

Smeak DD, DeHoff WD: Total ear canal ablation. Clinical results in the dog and cat. Vet Surg 15:161, 1986.

Wooley RE, Jones MS, Gilbert JP, Shotts EB: *In vitro* action of combinations of antimicrobial agents and EDTA-tromethamine on *Pseudomonas aeruginosa*. Am J Vet Res 44:1521, 1983.

23 Otitis Media and Otitis Interna

Linda G. Shell

Otitis media—An inflammation of the middle ear structures, which include the tympanic membrane, tympanic cavity, auditory or eustachian tube, three auditory ossicles, and tympanic nerve (a small branch of the facial nerve).

Otitis media is most often a sequela to otitis externa, having an incidence rate of 16% in early cases of otitis externa to 50% in chronic cases. For a complete discussion of otitis externa, see sec. 5, ch. 21.

KEY POINT ▶ Otitis media is always suspected in cases of chronic or recurrent external ear canal disease.

Occasionally, otitis media may result from extension of a pharyngeal infection via the auditory tube or from hematogenous spread of pathogens to the middle ear.

Otitis interna—An inflammation of the inner ear structures, which include the cochlea, vestibule, and semicircular canals. The most likely route of infection to the inner ear is an extension of otitis media. Hematogenous extension has occasionally been observed.

ETIOLOGY

Causes of middle ear inflammation include (1) bacteria, (2) yeasts and fungi, (3) parasites, (4) foreign bodies, (5) trauma, (6) polyps, and (7) neoplasms.

- *Bacteria* are the most common causes of otitis media. *Staphylococcus* and *Streptococcus* spp. are among the most frequently isolated organisms, but they have also been isolated from the middle ears of healthy dogs. This makes their role as the primary inducers of inflammation questionable. Other bacteria that have been isolated from cases of otitis media include *Proteus*, *Pseudomonas*, *Escherichia coli*, and *Clostridium* spp. Although it is not known what organisms are most commonly involved in otitis interna, it is presumed that they are the same as those in otitis media.
- *Yeasts and fungi* are uncommon causes of otitis media and interna. *Malassezia canis*, *Aspergillus* spp., and *Candida* spp. are among those most frequently mentioned. *Paecilomyces* is a rare cause.
- *Parasites,* such as the mite *Otodectes cynotis*, occasionally contribute to the rupture of the tympanic membrane and the subsequent signs of otitis media and interna, especially in cats.
- *Foreign bodies,* such as plant awns, are more com-

mon in the western United States and are suspect when clinical signs are unilateral.
- *Trauma* is an uncommon cause of otitis media and interna.
- *Polyps* can occur in the middle ear cavity or auditory tube of cats. Some polyps push through the tympanic membrane and can be observed in the external ear canal.
- *Neoplasms* can initiate inflammation because of their expansive or invasive growth. Squamous cell carcinoma, fibrosarcoma, and lymphoma have been reported to occur in the middle ear, and neurofibrosarcoma, meningioma, and carcinoma have been reported to occur in the inner ear.

CLINICAL SIGNS

Otitis Media

- Many clinical signs of otitis externa (see sec. 5, ch. 21) are common with otitis media, because otitis media is frequently a sequela to chronic otitis externa. Unrecognized otitis media is an important cause of recurrent or chronic otitis externa.
- Signs include head shaking, pawing, or rubbing the affected ear, discharge from the external ear canal and increased sensitivity or pain when the head is touched or the mouth is opened.
- Depression, anorexia, and fever are uncommon signs.
- Injury to the facial nerve, as it courses near the middle ear, produces drooping of the upper lip or ear, drooling of saliva, and decreased or absent palpebral reflex.
- Horner's syndrome may be present if injury occurs to the sympathetic nerve fibers that course near the middle ear. Ipsilateral miosis, ptosis, enophthalmus, and protruding nictitans may be observed. Other causes of Horner's syndrome are discussed in section 11, chapter 11.
- Keratitis sicca, characterized by reduced tear production and mucopurulent ocular exudate, may occur if the parasympathetic nerves that innervate the tear glands are injured (see sec. 11, ch. 9). These nerve fibers course with the facial nerve.

Otitis Interna

- Head tilt, circling, leaning, or rolling to the affected side are observed with unilateral inner ear inflammation.
- Spontaneous horizontal or rotary nystagmus may be

TABLE 1. Characteristics of Normal and Abnormal Tympanic Membranes

Characteristic	Normal	Abnormal
Transparency	Translucent	Cloudy Opaque
Luster	Glistening	Dull
Color	Pearl-gray	Blue: intra-tympanic hemorrhage Red: acute otitis media White: purulent material Amber: serous exudate

Tension	Slightly concave	Bulging: material
		  accumulated behind
		  tympanum

Vessels	Radiating	Obscured or torn

prominent. The fast phase of the nystagmus is away from the side of the lesion.

- Ataxia of limbs is present, yet the animal can usually ambulate and perform postural reactions with no decrease in strength.
- Vomiting may occasionally occur because of the vestibular connections to the emetic center in the brain stem.
- Hearing loss is not usually detected clinically unless bilateral inflammation is present.
- Signs of bilateral otitis interna include wide head excursions, little or no spontaneous nystagmus, absent or poor oculocephalic response, and ataxia of all limbs. An erect tail and a crouched posture are frequently observed in cats.
- Occasionally, bacterial migration from the inner ear to the brain stem occurs, producing severe depression, loss of limb strength and conscious proprioception, and possibly other cranial nerve deficits.

DIAGNOSIS

- *History* identifies the clinical signs and any predispositions to external ear disease.
- *Physical examination* may detect systemic signs of disease or localized infections that suggest hematog-

enous spread of pathogens to the middle or inner ears.

- Palpate the temporomandibular joints for irregularities, swelling, or pain.
- Examine the pharynx for signs of inflammation or masses that could have spread to or from the middle ear via the auditory tube.
- *Otoscopic examination* (see sec. 1, ch. 1) detects signs of otitis externa; ruptured, bulging, or discolored tympanic membrane; or obstruction of the ear canal. The presence of ulcerations, masses, exudate, or hyperplastic tissue often hampers the visualization of the tympanic membrane (Table 1). Lavage of the ear canal with warm normal saline may help remove exudate and debris.

KEY POINT ▶ In many cases heavy sedation or general anesthesia is necessary to thoroughly examine the external ear canal and the tympanic membrane.

- *Neurologic examination* detects signs of Horner's syndrome and/or facial nerve dysfunction, which may be observed with middle ear disease. Signs of vestibular dysfunction support inner ear disease. See section 10, chapter 2, for a discussion of the differential diagnosis of vestibular and cranial nerve disorders.

KEY POINT ▶ Peripheral vestibular signs, which occur with otitis interna, must be distinguished from central vestibular signs, which occur with brain stem disease (Table 2).

- The *Schirmer tear test* evaluates the integrity of the parasympathetic nerve fibers to the eye.
- *Cytologic examination* of exudate may help to identify an etiologic agent. Take samples before flushing or cleaning of the ear canal.
- *Culture and sensitivity* are also helpful to identify an etiologic agent and appropriate antibiotic therapy. Take samples prior to cleaning of the ear canal.
- *Myringotomy* is done if the tympanic membrane is bulging or discolored (see sec. 5, ch. 24). Use a 20-gauge, 3.5-inch spinal needle or blunt probe and direct it through a clean otoscope cone to perforate the tympanic membrane caudal to the malleus.

TABLE 2. Vestibular Signs Associated with Inner Ear Versus Brain Stem Locations

Sign	Inner Ear	Brain Stem
Head tilt	Present	Present
Circling	Present	Present
Falling, rolling	Present	Present
Positional strabismus	Present	Present
Nystagmus	Usually spontaneous and type (horizontal, rotary) does not vary with position of head.	Usually not spontaneous but found with changes in head position; type (horizontal, rotary, vertical) varies with head position.
Conscious proprioception	Normal	Delayed or absent
Horner's syndrome	May be present	Absent
Cranial nerve deficits	VII	V, VI, VII
Gait changes	Mild to severe ataxia	Ataxia and weakness
Postural reactions (hopping, hemiwalking, wheelbarrowing, and so forth)	Normal if examined slowly	Weak or absent
Cerebellar signs (hypermetria, head intention tremors)	Absent	May be present.

- Using a syringe attached to the needle, aspirate fluid or material and evaluate by cytology and culture. The small hole in the tympanic membrane usually seals over rapidly.
- *Radiographs*
  - Ventrodorsal, oblique lateral, and open mouth views are recommended and necessitate general anesthesia for proper positioning.
  - A soft tissue density in the normally air-filled tympanic cavity suggests fluid, granulation tissue, or neoplasia.
  - Destruction of the bulla may be seen with osteomyelitis or neoplasia.
  - Changes may not be present for several weeks in acute cases of otitis media.
  - Chronic cases may show only sclerosis or thickening of the normally fine outline of the bulla.

KEY POINT ▶ Absence of radiographic signs of otitis media does not rule out the disease.

TREATMENT

Otitis Media

The goals of treatment of otitis media are to remove infected, inflammatory, or foreign material from the bulla and to provide ventilation and drainage. These goals are accomplished with medical and/or surgical intervention, depending upon the chronicity and results of otoscopic and radiologic evaluations. For details of treating the external ear canal (otitis externa) see section 5, chapter 22.

- *Flushing* the ear canal with warm normal saline helps eliminate debris and aids visualization of tympanic membrane. Use a water-propulsion dental device (Water Pik) very carefully, suction systems, or bulb syringes.
  - Always dry the ear canal after flushing by gentle aspiration, low-vacuum suction, or Otic Domeboro solution (Miles Pharmaceuticals).
- *Myringotomy* is indicated if the tympanic membrane is intact but discolored and bulging (see Diagnosis and sec. 5, ch. 24). A myringotomy allows for samples to be obtained for culture and cytology and allows for some drainage from the middle ear cavity to relieve pain and pressure.
  - Flush the middle ear cavity with warm normal saline through the same perforation if followed by aspiration of the saline. Use 12-gauge, 3.5-inch cannula to enlarge the opening.
- *Systemic antibiotics*
  - If there is no radiographic evidence of fluid or

material within the bulla, use systemic antibiotics for 3 to 6 weeks.
  - If a culture cannot be obtained, administer broad-spectrum antibiotics, such as chloramphenicol (25 to 50 mg/kg, q6 to 8h, PO), a cephalosporin (e.g., cefadroxil, 20 mg/kg, q12h, PO; cephalexin 10 to 30 mg/kg, q8h, PO, SQ, IM, or IV), or trimethoprim-sulfa (15 to 30 mg/kg, q12h, PO). Do not use trimethoprim-sulfa if keratitis sicca is present or if tear production is decreased.
  - If little or no response occurs with systemic antibiotic treatment, repeat radiographs of the bulla. Exploratory bulla surgery may be necessary (see sec. 5, ch. 24).
  - If otoscopic or radiographic evaluations support the presence of fluid or material within the middle ear cavity, systemic antibiotics are indicated. Surgery is frequently necessary to allow for proper drainage (see sec. 5, ch. 24).
- *Topical therapeutic agents*
  - Use cautiously if the tympanic membrane is not intact, because many drugs can cause ototoxicity characterized by acute deafness or vestibular signs.
  - Ototoxic agents include aminoglycosides (gentamicin, neomycin), chloramphenicol, iodine, iodophors, and chlorhexidine.
- Use *artificial tears* as described in section 11, chapter 9, if keratitis sicca is present.
- Consider *surgery* if there is radiographic evidence of fluid or material in the tympanic bulla or poor response to medical treatment (see sec. 5, ch. 24).

KEY POINT ▶ Re-evaluate the ear canal 1 week after beginning treatment and every 2 weeks afterwards, until the problem is resolved. Repeat flushing may be needed.

Otitis Interna

- Treat underlying otitis externa and media if present.
- If only otitis interna is present, use systemic antibiotics as outlined for otitis media.
- If the signs do not abate in 1 to 3 weeks, repeat the bulla radiographs to evaluate the possibility of otitis media acting as a nidus of infection that may require surgical intervention.

Supplemental Readings

Denny HR: The results of surgical treatment of otitis media and interna in the dog. J Small Animal Pract 14:585, 1973.
Shell LG: Otitis media and otitis interna. Vet Clin North Am: Small Anim Pract 18:885, 1988.
Spreull JSA: Tympanotomy, bulla osteotomy and vestibular osteotomy. *In* Bojrab MJ, ed.: *Current Techniques in Small Animal Surgery*. Philadelphia: Lea & Febiger, 1975, p 71.

24 Surgery of Otitis Media and Otitis Interna

Harry W. Boothe

Selection of a surgical procedure to treat otitis media and interna is based upon duration of clinical signs, response to previous treatment, status of external ear canal, and surgeon's familiarity with related anatomy and technique. Surgical options for treating otitis media and interna include myringotomy, lateral bulla osteotomy, and ventral bulla osteotomy. Nasopharyngeal polyps are most appropriately excised using a bulla osteotomy in combination with other excision techniques. Potential complications of bulla osteotomy surgery include facial nerve injury, Horner's syndrome (ptosis, miosis, enophthalmos, nictitating membrane protrusion, and vestibular signs. See sec. 5, ch. 23 for diagnosis and medical treatment of otitis media and interna.

ANATOMY

- The tympanic membrane slopes downwards, forwards, and inwards—towards the middle ear cavity. The membrane is composed of a larger, more peripherally located pars tensa and a smaller, triangular-shaped pars flaccida.
- The air-filled tympanic cavity constitutes the major portion of the middle ear and is connected to the nasopharynx by the auditory tube.
- Structures located within the dorsal aspect of the tympanic cavity include the three auditory ossicles, associated muscles and ligaments, and tympanic nerve.

KEY POINT ▶ The feline tympanic cavity is divided into a larger ventromedial and a smaller dorsolateral compartment by a nearly complete thin bony septum.

- Surgically important structures near the tympanic bulla are the facial nerve (ventrolaterally), the carotid artery (medially), and the hypoglossal nerve (ventrally).

MYRINGOTOMY

Preoperative Considerations

- Thorough cleansing of the external ear canal is indicated to enable the myringotomy to be performed under the guidance of otoscopic monitoring.
- Myringotomy can be performed alone or in a combination with bulla osteotomy.

Objectives

- Drain and flush material from within the tympanic cavity.
- Obtain specimens for microbiologic and cytologic sampling.
- Instill medication into the tympanic cavity.

Equipment

- 3/32-inch Steinmann pin.
- Closed-end 3.5 Fr. feline urethral catheter.
- Warm physiologic saline solution and 12-ml syringe.

Technique

1. Position the patient in lateral recumbency and clean the ear canal.
2. Incise the caudoventral aspect of the tympanic membrane under otoscopic guidance with the Steinmann pin.
3. Insert the end of the feline urethral catheter into the tympanic cavity and aspirate material from the middle ear cavity.
4. Collect samples for microbiologic and cytologic analysis.
5. Gently flush the tympanic cavity with saline until the washings are clear. Aspirate fluid from the middle ear cavity.
6. Instill a nonototoxic antibiotic (avoid aminoglycosides) into the tympanic cavity.

Postoperative Care and Complications

Short-term

- Administer systemic antibiotics based upon cultural and susceptibility results for at least 3 weeks.
- Potential short-term complications are usually limited to transient vestibular signs and/or Horner's syndrome.

Long-term

- Little long-term drainage results from myringotomy alone.
- With successful resolution of otitis media, healing of the tympanic membrane occurs in approximately 50% of the animals.
- Recurrence of otitis media is a potential long-term complication.

Prognosis

■ Myringotomy is more likely to resolve otitis media if it is performed early in the course of the disease.

LATERAL BULLA OSTEOTOMY

Preoperative Considerations

■ Determine the condition of the external ear canal.
■ Evaluate the radiologic appearance of the tympanic bulla and the microbiologic status of the middle ear prior to lateral bulla osteotomy.
■ Lateral bulla osteotomy is simplest when performed in conjunction with a total ear canal ablation. If the external ear canal is normal or only mildly affected by infection, bulla osteotomy can be performed via a lateral (without ear canal ablation) or ventral approach. The ventral approach technique is preferred by most surgeons.
■ Assess the integrity of the facial nerve preoperatively.

Objectives

■ Provide access to the tympanic cavity for diagnostic intervention.
■ Provide drainage and access to the middle ear cavity for therapeutic intervention (e.g., flush, curettage, and resection of abnormal tissue).

Equipment

■ Standard general surgery pack and suture
■ Periosteal elevator, Steinmann pin, hand chuck, and rongeurs
■ Warm saline solution and tubing for flushing the tympanic cavity

Technique for Lateral Bulla Osteotomy Without Total Ear Canal Ablation

1. Position the patient in lateral recumbency, and prepare the lateral aspect of the head and neck.
2. Incise the skin over the vertical ear canal to a point ventral to the horizontal ear canal (Fig. 1).
3. Bluntly dissect between the parotid salivary gland and the ventral aspect of the horizontal ear canal to reveal the facial nerve.
4. Retract the facial nerve ventrocaudally near its exit from the stylomastoid foramen.
5. Elevate the soft tissue overlying the lateral aspect of the osseous bulla using a periosteal elevator.
6. Enter the tympanic cavity ventral to the horizontal ear canal with the Steinmann pin and hand chuck.
7. Enlarge the osteotomy site ventrally with rongeurs.
8. Obtain microbiologic samples, and flush the middle ear cavity using warm saline solution. If curettage is performed, avoid traumatizing the inner ear structures on the dorsomedial aspect of the bulla.
9. Instill a nonototoxic antibiotic into the tympanic cavity.
10. Place and secure a drain tube into the tympanic cavity by suturing it to the adjacent soft tissue with fine absorbable suture material.

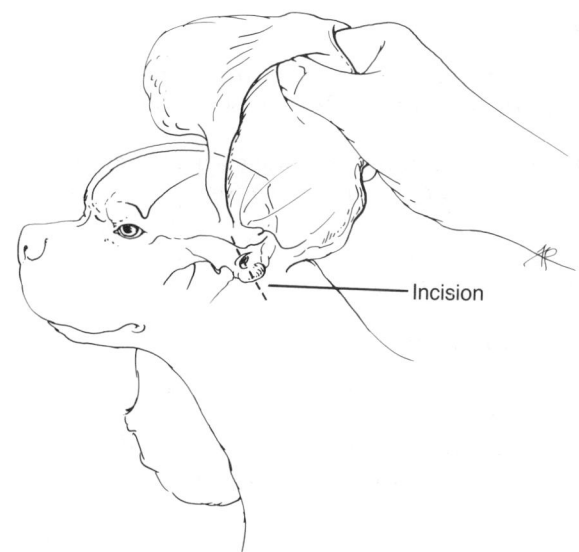

Figure 1. Skin incision for performing a lateral bulla osteotomy.

11. Routinely close the subcutaneous tissue (simple interrupted, absorbable suture) and the skin (simple interrupted, nonabsorbable suture).
12. Position the drain tube so that it exits the skin adjacent to the primary incision.

Technique for Lateral Bulla Osteotomy With Total Ear Canal Ablation

1. Position the patient in lateral recumbency, and prepare the lateral aspect of the head and neck, including the external ear canal.
2. Incise the skin over the vertical ear canal, and perform a total ear canal ablation.
3. Reflect the soft tissue from the lateral aspect of the tympanic bulla, insert the rongeur tips into the external auditory meatus, and remove the ventral aspect of the bony auditory meatus.
4. Extend the osteotomy site as far ventrally into the middle ear cavity as possible, and flush the cavity with warm saline solution.
5. Place a fenestrated drainage tube to exit the ventral aspect of the bulla osteotomy site and skin adjacent to the primary incision.

Postoperative Care and Complications

Short-term

■ Prevent self-inflicted trauma to the drain tube by using an Elizabethan collar or similar device.
■ Facial nerve damage, manifested by inability to close the eye and by drooping of the upper lip on the ipsilateral side, may be observed.

KEY POINT ▶ Administer eye lubricant (artificial tears) to animals with facial nerve damage to prevent corneal ulceration.

■ Continue local treatment (warm saline flushes) as long as the drain tube is in place.
■ Continue appropriate systemic antibiotic for at least 3 weeks.

Prognosis

- Extent of response to bulla osteotomy tends to be incomplete in long-standing cases of otitis media and interna.
- Immediate response following bulla osteotomy indicates a more favorable prognosis.

VENTRAL BULLA OSTEOTOMY

Preoperative Considerations

- See Preoperative Considerations under Lateral Bulla Osteotomy.
- Radiographically assess the density of the tympanic bulla to assist in the initial osteotomy procedure.

Objectives

- See Objectives under Lateral Bulla Osteotomy.
- To establish ventral drainage of the middle ear cavity.

Equipment

- See Equipment for Lateral Bulla Osteotomy Without Total Ear Canal Ablation.

Technique

1. Position the patient in dorsal recumbency, and prepare the ventral cervical region from the mid-mandibular area to the wings of the atlas.
2. Incise the skin just off the midline between the level of the angular process of the mandible and the wings of the atlas (Fig. 2).
3. Bluntly dissect between the digastric muscle and the hyoglossal and styloglossal muscles. The hypoglossal nerve on the lateral aspect of the hyoglossal muscle helps verify the proper dissection plane.

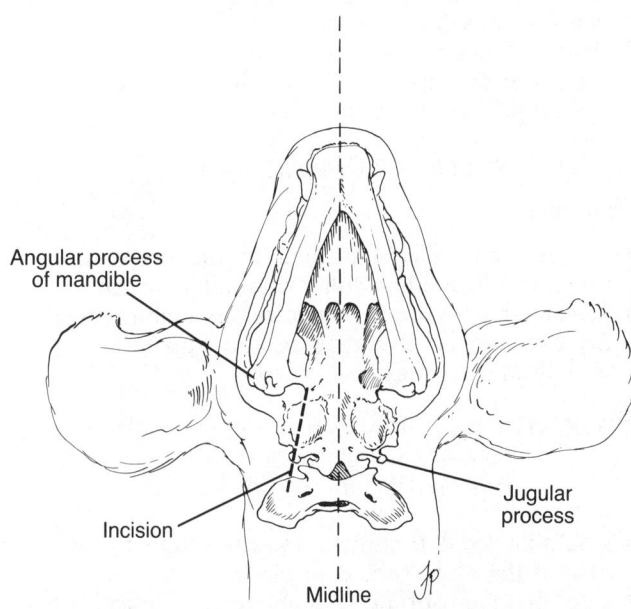

Figure 2. Incision for ventral bulla osteotomy.

Angular process of mandible

Incision

Midline

Jugular process

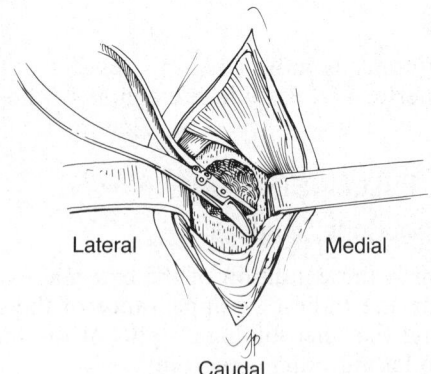

Figure 3. Osteotomy technique.

Lateral

Medial

Caudal

4. Carefully retract the adjacent musculature to reveal the rounded tympanic bulla between the more angular jugular process of the skull (caudal) and the angular process of the mandible (rostrolateral).
5. Reflect the thin muscle that covers the osseous bulla—in the dog.
6. Accurately locate the bulla before proceeding with the osteotomy. Penetrate the ventral aspect of the tympanic bulla with a Steinmann pin in a hand chuck, and enlarge the osteotomy site using rongeurs (Fig. 3).
   a. Fenestrate the septum in the cat to fully expose the tympanic cavity.
7. Flush the middle ear cavity, and place a drain to exit the ventral cervical skin through a separate skin incision. The dorsal aspect of the drain may also be positioned to exit the external ear canal.
8. Routinely close the subcutaneous tissue (simple interrupted, absorbable suture) and the skin (simple interrupted, nonabsorbable suture).

Postoperative Care and Complications

- See Postoperative Care and Complications under Lateral Bulla Osteotomy.

SURGICAL MANAGEMENT OF NASOPHARYNGEAL POLYPS

See also section 6, chapter 17.

Preoperative Considerations

- Carefully inspect the nasopharynx by rostrally displacing the soft palate to assess the size of the nasopharyngeal mass.
- Radiographically assess the tympanic bulla to determine the potential involvement of the middle ear cavity.

Objectives

- Excision of the mass using both an oral approach and a ventral bulla osteotomy.
- To remove the mass from the nasopharynx or ear canal utilizing a simple traction technique, while carefully excising polypoid tissue from the tympanic cavity.

Equipment

- See Equipment for Lateral Bulla Osteotomy Without Total Ear Canal Ablation.

Technique

1. Position the cat in dorsal recumbency with the mouth held open.
2. Rostrally displace the soft palate using a soft tissue retractor to provide adequate exposure of the mass.
3. Apply traction to the mass to remove the pharyngeal component of the polyp.
4. Perform a ventral bulla osteotomy, as previously described, and excise tissue proliferations within the tympanic cavity using careful curettage.
5. Examine the ipsilateral ear canal, and excise any polypoid tissue.

Postoperative Care and Complications

Short-Term

- Temporary (e.g., 1 to 2 weeks) Horner's syndrome is common following curettage of the middle ear cavity.
- See short-term complications following lateral bulla osteotomy.

Long-Term

- Recurrence of the polyp is possible, although less likely, following both excision by traction and bulla osteotomy than following excision by traction alone.

- Disruption of the otic ossicles from trauma to the dorsal aspect of the tympanic cavity results in hearing loss.

Prognosis

- The long-term outlook following removal of naso-pharyngeal polyps using both the traction excision and ventral bulla osteotomy techniques is good. Recurrence is uncommon.

Supplemental Readings

Beckman SL, Henry WB Jr, Cechner P: Total ear canal ablation combining bulla osteotomy and curettage in dogs with chronic otitis externa and media. J Am Vet Med Assoc 196:84, 1990.

Boothe HW Jr: Bulla osteotomy. In Bojrab MJ, ed.: Current Techniques in Small Animal Surgery. Philadelphia: Lea & Febiger, 1990, p 147.

Evans HE, Christensen GC: Miller's Anatomy of the Dog. Philadelphia: W. B. Saunders, 1979, p 1062.

Howard PE, Neer TM, Miller JS: Otitis media. Part II. Surgical considerations. Compend Contin Educ Pract Vet 5:18, 1983.

Kapatkin AS, Matthiesen DT, Noone KE, et al.: Results of surgery and long-term follow-up in 31 cats with nasopharyngeal polyps. J Am Anim Hosp Assoc 26:387, 1990.

Little CJL, Lane JG: The surgical anatomy of the feline bulla tympanica. J Small Anim Pract 27:371, 1986.

Sharp NJH: Chronic otitis externa and otitis media treated by total ear canal ablation and ventral bulla osteotomy in thirteen dogs. Vet Surg 19:162, 1990.

Cardiopulmonary System

John D. Bonagura

---

1 Physical Examination

Robert L. Hamlin

Physical examination follows the obtaining of a complete history and the consideration of the signalment. Diagnosis—or at the very least a number of plausible diagnoses—may be made in many instances by history and signalment; however, following a thorough physical examination, a single, "most likely" diagnosis can be made with reasonable assurance in most patients with cardiac problems. Physical examination is performed best in a systematic manner, initially conducting those portions that are least likely to aggravate or to cause discomfort to the patient. Physical examination of the cardiovascular system can be separated into four steps: *inspection, palpation percussion,* and *auscultation.* What separates the physical examination from the remainder of the cardiac examination is the close relationship between the veterinarian and the patient, and, with the exception of the stethoscope, the absence of elaborate instrumentation (e.g., radiography, echocardiography). (See Heart Failure, sec. 6, ch. 6.)

INSPECTION

Inspection of the patient is conducted as one obtains the history. It should be performed while the animal enters the room; while the pet stands, sits, or walks; while the owner supports the pet; and while the pet stands alone.

- *Condition* of the patient is classified according to the degree of fat.
  - Normal overweight animals *usually* are not ill from heart failure but may manifest signs and symptoms caused by pulmonary disease (e.g., chronic lung disease, pulmonary fibrosis).
  - Animals with moderate to longstanding heart failure are often thin to cachectic.
- *Attitude* of an animal with heart failure is *usually* depressed.
- *Posture* of animals with heart failure is often:
  - Standing—reluctant to lay down—with thoracic limbs abducted and neck extended to ease ventilation.
  - Swayback with the tail between the legs because of muscular weakness occasionally caused by digitalis toxicity from either too much drug or renal excretion

    electrolyte imbalance from aggressive use of diuretics along with reduced water and food consumption

    the diseases themselves; dogs with cardiomyopathy often have weakness of skeletal muscles and dogs with heart failure are often exhausted owing to the work of breathing.

- *Color of mucous membranes*
  - May be cyanotic in late stages of heart failure or in puppies or very young dogs with tetralogy of Fallot or other congenital heart defects with right to left intracardiac shunts (see sec. 6, ch. 12). (Note: Cyanosis occurs much more commonly in all stages of pulmonary diseases.)
  - May be dark red in stages just prior to frank cyanosis.
  - May be pale with concomitant anemia or low cardiac output but without pulmonary congestion (e.g., low output heart failure, aortic stenosis).
- *Swelling* of the torso may be a result of
  - gas in the gastrointestinal (GI) tract, often indicating

chronic obstructive pulmonary disease (COPD) or pulmonary failure (PF)
primary GI disease.
- enlargement of abdominal organs, indicating passive congestion due to right-sided heart failure
COPD/PF leading to pulmonary and systemic venous hypertension
primary disease of abdominal organs (e.g., neoplasia).
- pitting edema of the limbs, brisket, or prepuce due to right-sided heart failure.

KEY POINT ▶ Subcutaneous edema in the absence of ascites or jugular distension argues *against* a diagnosis of congestive heart failure.

■ *Pattern of ventilation* is extremely important. Characterize the
- *Rate* of breaths per minute. It should be between 15 and 50 but may increase from excitement, fever, anxiety, warm environment, COPD/PF, left-sided heart failure, or pulmonary injury.
- *Depth of ventilation* is difficult to quantify, but hyperpnea (increased depth) is often a symptom of a blood gas derangement as observed in diabetes mellitus; not often observed in heart disease except with severe pulmonary edema.
- *Dyspnea* (labored ventilation) may occur as increased rate and/or depth of ventilation or merely as increased effort. With dyspnea one observes
bulging eyes
flaring nares
outward motion of thoracic limbs
reluctance to lay down
abdominal "pumping"
extension of neck and open mouth breathing.
■ *Cough* is a sign of both heart and lung disease. It may be
- *hacking, honking, brassy cough,* indicating disease of the large airways, such as
tracheobronchial collapse (see sec. 6, ch. 19).
compression of the left mainstem bronchus due to mitral regurgitation or generalized cardiomegaly
tracheobronchitis
bronchopulmonary parasitism.
(Note: This type of cough is seldom due to injury of the parenchyma of the lung, e.g., edema, pneumonia.)
- subtle or "half-hearted" cough caused by
pulmonary edema
pneumonia
diaphragmatic hernia.
(Note: So-called moist or truly productive coughs usually indicate an exudative process; however, in *late stages of left-sided congestive heart failure* it is common to have serosanguineous pulmonary edema fluid gush from the nares and/or mouth.)
■ Analysis of the *jugular vein* (Fig. 1) is simpler if the hair is clipped from around the jugular furrow or if it is moistened with 70% alcohol.
- A hard, distended jugular vein that collapses

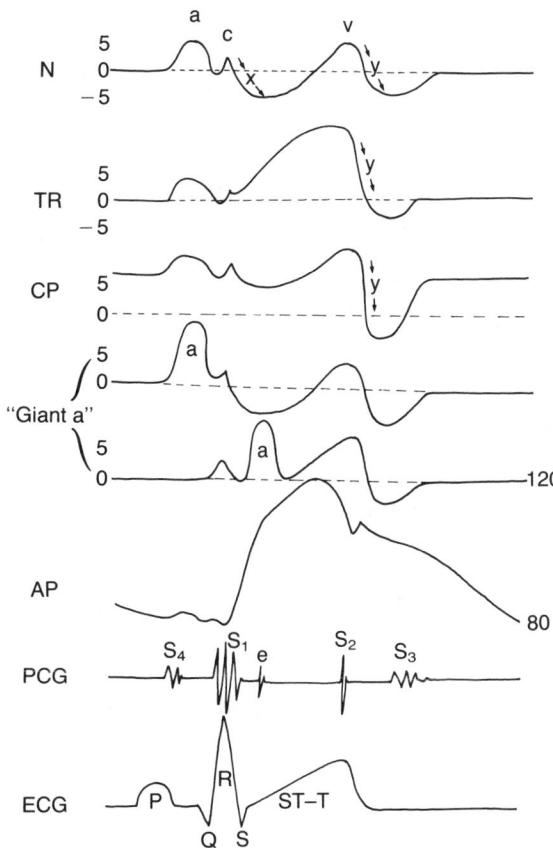

Figure 1. Analysis of venous pulses. A normal pulse is shown for reference (N), as are systemic arterial pressure (AP), phonocardiogram (PCG), and electrocardiogram (ECG). Abnormal pulses shown are those produced by tricuspid regurgitation (TR) and constrictive pericarditis (CP); also shown are two types of "cannon 'a' waves."

briefly immediately after the second heart sound is consistent with pericardial tamponade, such as that observed in dogs with hemorrhage in the pericardial sac due to a bleeding neoplasm or an idiopathic hemorrhage and a rupture of the left atrium with severe mitral regurgitation.
constrictive pericarditis (see sec. 6, ch. 9)
COPD/PF.
- Vigorous pulsation of the jugular vein
("Cannon 'a' waves") occurring more than 120 times/minute with the ventricular rate usually very slow: below 60/minute indicates third-degree (complete) or high-grade second-degree atrioventricular block.
occurring between the first and second heart sounds indicating regurgitation of blood from the right ventricle to right atrium during tricuspid regurgitation.
occurring just before the first heart sound in rare instances of tricuspid stenosis or possibly with stiffness of the ventricles (e.g., pulmonic stenosis)
- Hepatojugular reflux—pushing on the abdomen of a standing dog displaces the liver dorsad and "milks" blood from the liver to the right side of the heart. If the right ventricle cannot pump the

extra venous return through the lungs or if right ventricular filling is restricted owing to pericardial tamponade or constriction, the extra venous return "wells up" in the jugular vein, producing added distension.

- Jugular vein normally collapses totally when the long axis of the torso makes a head-up tilt at an angle of 45° with the horizontal.
- If it does not, the venous pressure may be elevated owing to heart failure, COPD/PF, or ventricular filling restriction due to pericardial disease.

    (Note: The jugular vein also normally collapses during inspiration and immediately after the second heart sound.)

■ Inspect the pharynx and mouth to identify
- tonsillitis
- pharyngitis
- soft palate redundancy
- neoplasia
- periodontal disease.

■ Watch the animal walk to identify and to quantify
- exercise tolerance of heart failure or COPD
- weakness due to heart failure or severe aortic stenosis
- neuromuscular or skeletal disease.

PALPATION

■ Technique performed best
- with the animal standing and being held by an assistant with the assistant's hands cupped around the neck.
- with the palpator at the side or back of the animal
- by the palpator placing his or her hands in the axilla and sliding them caudad stopping at
    the second to third intercostal space
    the fourth to sixth intercostal space
    just caudad to the rib cage
    all points on the abdomen
    the femoral arteries.

■ Determine where the heart "thumps" most vigorously on the thoracic wall. The point of maximal impulse (PMI) is normally at the fifth intercostal space two to three fingerbreadths from the left sternal border *and* at the right third intercostal space near the right sternal border (Fig. 2). Cardiomegaly or space-occupying intrathoracic masses may displace this impulse.

■ Classify heart sounds according to
- Intensity (see Auscultation).
- "Booming" S_1 indicates forceful contraction, short atrioventricular conduction (PQ interval), or skinny thorax.
- "Soft" S_1 indicates weak ventricle, long atrioventricular conduction (PQ interval), obesity, hyperinflation of lungs, pleural effusion, pneumothorax.
- Frequency—to assess autonomic tone and heart rhythm.
- Regularity—to detect arrhythmias.
- Presence or absence of thrill—palpable manifestation of murmur.

    (Note: This indicates a murmur of at least grade V of VI.)

■ Palpate for abnormal breath sounds
- "Snoring" of sonorous rhonchi (rattling sounds)
- "Honks" of tracheal wall vibrations due to collapse
- "Tight" crackles or rales.

■ Gently palpate under caudal ribs to identify hepatomegaly.

■ Palpate abdomen for organomegaly or neoplasia.

■ Palpate femoral arteries for rate that is relatively independent of body size.

Heart Rates	Dog	Cat
Quiet (asleep)	50 to 90	90 to 120
During examination	80 to 160	140 to 220
Exercise	230	230

- Force (Table 1)
- Rhythm

    Respiratory sinus arrhythmia—average rate is usually as described previously for sleep. Speeds up during inspiration but seldom more than three or, at most, four heartbeats during an inspiration.

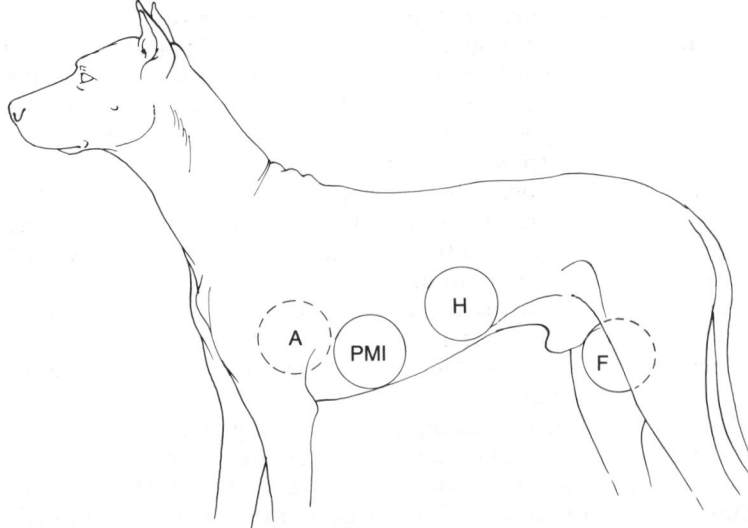

Figure 2. Schematic diagram of a dog from the left side showing regions of palpation. (Solid line circles represent left side, dotted line circles, right side.) A is the region where the second heart sound is palpated most forcefully and where the thrills of aortic or pulmonic stenosis are felt best (on both the right and left sides). PMI is the point of maximal cardiac impulse on the left hemithorax. H is the region just under the caudal ribs where the liver is best felt. F indicates the regions where femoral arterial pulsations are best felt.

TABLE 1. Typical Systemic Arterial* Pulses for Animals with Varying Physiologic and/or Pathologic States

	Character	Pressure Systolic/ Diastolic	Pressure Differentials	Rate	Pulse Force
Normal animal	Normal	120/80	40	Normal	N
Patent ductus arteriosus or aortic regurgitation	Bounding	160/40	120	Increased	PDA, AR
Aortic stenosis or early heart failure	Weak	90/60	30	Increased	AS, HF
Mitral regurgitation, ventricular septal defect, late heart failure, or hyperkinetic ventricle	Sharp, brief	120/80	40	Rapid	MR, VSD, HF, HK

*For example, femoral artery.

(Note: More than four beats during inspiration may indicate abnormal ventilation caused by chronic pulmonary disease.)

Pulse rate slows during exhalation, occasionally to rates as low as 30 beats per minute but only very briefly.

Atrial fibrillation or frequent short bursts of supraventricular or ventricular tachycardia: rapid pulse rate; irregularly irregular (i.e., *not* in sync with ventilation); variable intensity; and *pulse deficit*—fewer femoral pulses than heartbeats.

Occasionally supraventricular or ventricular premature beats occurring singly and characterized by apparent single skipped pulses followed by a pulse stronger than usual.

- Weak pulses found in
  - Heart failure
  - Aortic stenosis
- Extremely bounding (water hammer) pulses found in
  - Patent ductus arteriosus
  - Aortic regurgitation
  - Complete heart block with very slow ventricular rate.
- Regularly irregular pulses in sync with respirations with sinus arrhythmia.
- Show "skipped" beats (when combined with cardiac auscultation) with single premature depolarizations.
- Rapid and irregularly irregular pulses with atrial fibrillation or with supraventricular or ventricular tachycardias in brief bursts.
  (Note: They are not rapid in large breed dogs with hypothyroidism or dogs with relatively slow-conducting atrioventricular nodes approaching complete heart block.)
- Absent pulses in cats with aortic embolism due to cardiomyopathy or endocarditis.

PERCUSSION

This is the technique (Fig. 3) of thumping on the thorax and/or abdomen to determine the relative density of structures underneath the points of percussion (see sec. 6, ch. 24).

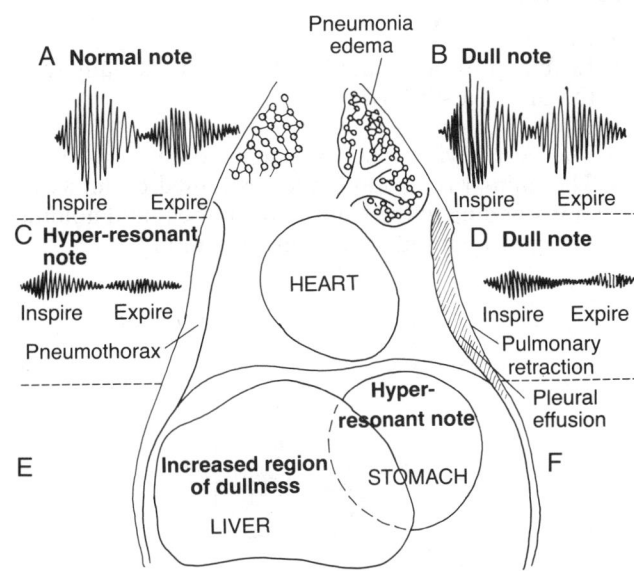

Figure 3. Schematic diagram of thorax and cranial portion of the abdomen viewed from the ventral aspect. A indicates the normal breath sounds and percussion. B shows a dull percussion note and louder than expected inspiratory and expiratory sounds due to pneumonia or edema. C represents the hyper-resonant percussion note and diminished breath sounds caused by pneumothorax, as illustrated by air between the thoracic wall and collapsed lung. D demonstrates a dull percussion note and diminished breath sounds due to pleural effusion, shown as density between thoracic wall and lungs. E indicates dull percussion notes because of an enlarged, dense liver. F is a hyper-resonant percussion note caused by gas in the stomach.

Types of percussion notes and their meanings are as follows:

■ *Hyper-resonant notes* sound like a tympany drum and indicate a normal lung or a gas-filled structure (e.g., pneumothorax, hyperinflated lung, gas-filled stomach) underneath.

(Note: Hyper-resonant sounds may be illustrated by drinking a can of carbonated beverage, jumping up and down for 15 seconds, and then thumping on the left side of your abdomen just over your stomach.)

■ *Dull notes* sound "dead," like thumping one's skull, and indicate a dense, usually water-filled structure (e.g., pneumonia, pleural effusion, pulmonary edema, consolidation) underneath.

(Note: The normal notes of percussion may be learned by percussing thoraces from many normal male and female animals of varying ages and body conformations. Regions of cardiac dullness are less obvious in quadrupeds than in primates, but pulmonary densities may be detected effectively by percussion.)

See Figure 3, which synthesizes the findings of percussion and auscultation for the differential diagnoses of
• Edema/pneumonia
• Pneumothorax
• Pleural effusion
• Consolidation/neoplasia
• COPD/pulmonary fibrosis.

AUSCULTATION

■ Definition
  • Listening to heart and breath sounds, usually with the aid of a stethoscope.
■ Methods
  • The best environment is a quiet room.
  • The animal is standing and restrained by an assistant standing to the front of the patient and holding the mouth closed to discourage panting.

• Instruments
  Stethoscope
    Preferably wooden ear pieces large enough to occlude most of the external acoustic meatus but not so large as to be airtight.
    (Note: The internal canal of the ear piece must be clean, and the outside sanitized if used by more than one person.)
    Two tubes of commercial stethoscope tubing extend from ear pieces to chest piece.
    Chest piece has a hard rubber or Bakelite diaphragm for characterizing high-pitched sounds and a deep trumpet bell for relatively low-pitched sounds.
• Musculator is to the back or side of patient and keeps a hand or arm between the pet's mouth and his or her face.
■ Areas of auscultation (Figs. 4 and 5)

ABNORMALITIES OF AUSCULTATION, PERCUSSION, AND PALPATION

■ Normal (see Fig. 3 for normal and abnormal breath sounds and percussion)
  • Normal vesicular breath sounds with sounds of inspiration being louder than sounds of expiration.
  • Percussion note of normal resonance—i.e., not too dull and not too resonant.
    (Note: In order to know what normal is, you must auscultate and percuss hundreds of normal animals of various ages, breeds, and conformations.)
■ Pulmonary edema and/or pneumonia (see sec. 6, ch. 20)
  • Breath sounds are termed bronchial or bronchovesicular—meaning that sounds are louder in both inspiration and expiration but are much louder and higher pitched during expiration. The increased intensity arises from these sounds being "made" normally at larger airways but being transmitted better than usual via water-logged parenchyma.

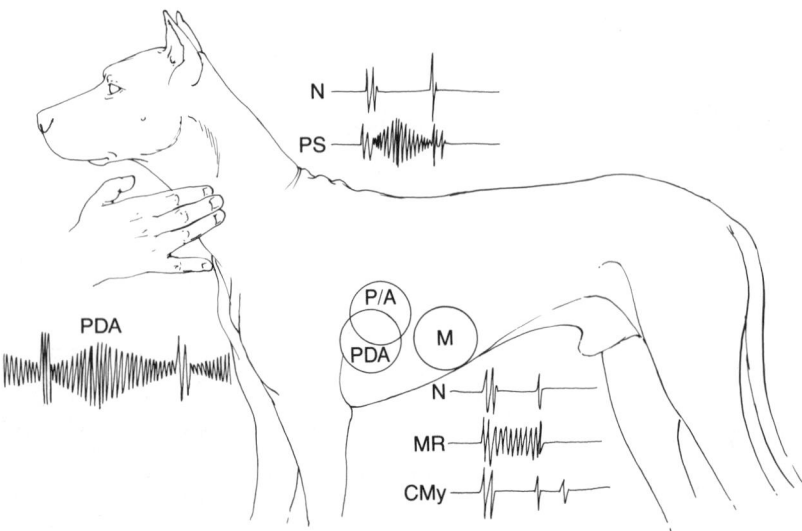

Figure 4. Regions where murmurs are heard best on the left hemithorax. Murmurs typical of specific defects are shown. Normal (N) heart sounds are indicated above the murmurs of pulmonic stenosis (PS) and mitral regurgitation (MR). The diastolic gallop heard with dilated cardiomyopathy (CMy) is shown below the murmur for mitral regurgitation. PDA is the continuous murmur of patent ductus arteriosus. P/A is the ejection murmur of pulmonic stenosis or aortic stenosis. (Note: Aortic stenosis may be heard equally on the right base as well.) M demonstrates systolic regurgitant murmur of mitral regurgitation.

Figure 5. Regions where murmurs are heard best on the right hemithorax. A is the systolic ejection murmur of aortic stenosis (AS) and may be equally loud at left and right hemithorax. Systolic regurgitant murmur of ventricular septal defect (VSD) is heard best at the right sternal border. A soft diastolic murmur may also be heard. T indicates where the systolic murmur of tricuspid regurgitation (TR) is heard best.

- Percussion note is dull because of fluid-filled parenchyma.
■ Pneumothorax (see sec. 6, ch. 24)
  - All breath sounds are softer than normal because the free air space between the stethoscope chest piece and the lung insulates against the transmission of sound.
  - Percussion note is hyper-resonant (i.e., sounds like thumping on a tympani drum) because the thoracic wall acts like a drumhead stretched over an air-filled chamber underneath.
■ Pleural effusion (see sec. 6, ch. 22)
  - All breath sounds are softer than normal because free liquid between pulmonary parenchyma and chest wall reflects sound away from its pathway to the stethoscope chest piece.
  - Percussion note is dull because water-filled cavity vibrates at high-frequency and low amplitude and is dampened rapidly.
  - Pulmonary retraction is an indention of the thoracic wall caused by fatigue of muscles of ventilation. Regions of the thoracic wall affected must generate greatest tension during ventilation and do not have assistance from thoracic limbs. Pulmonary retraction produces an "hourglass" configuration to the thorax in the dorsoventral radiograph.
■ Hepatic enlargement generates a dull note over a larger area than expected because the liver is an exceptionally dense structure.
■ Bloated (air-filled) stomach is distended and generates a hyper-resonant percussion note because skin serves as the head of the drum and the gas in the stomach serves as the air-filled kettle of the drum.
  Note: The abdomen bloated with gas produces an exceptional hourglass configuration with pulmonary retractions. It can be differentiated from organomegaly and/or ascites by the following:
  - It is tympanic (hyper-resonance).
  - It comes and goes quickly.
  - Air is often in the esophagus.
■ Cardiac auscultatory findings on the left hemithorax (see Fig. 4)

- Region at the left fifth intercostal space near approximately two to three fingerbreadths from the left sternal border
  S_1 is louder, longer in duration, and lower-pitched than S_2. S_1 is mimicked as a "lub"; S_2 is mimicked as a "dup."
  The murmur of mitral regurgitation extends from S_1 to, and often through, S_2.

KEY POINT ▶ The intensity of the murmurs of mitral and tricuspid regurgitation does *not* correlate with the severity of the regurgitation and is influenced profoundly by the force of contraction of the ventricle.

In dogs and cats with dilated cardiomyopathy, there is often an S_3 gallop producing a set of sounds like lub-dup-uh.

- Pulmonary artery region, where S_2 is heard the loudest
  Murmur of pulmonic stenosis (see sec. 6, ch. 12) is heard loudest.
    It is usually very loud and radiated dorsad; it is short in duration and very rough.
    There is often a pronounced splitting of S_2 caused by the pulmonic valve closing later than the aortic valve—this is particularly pronounced during inspiration.
  Murmur of aortic stenosis (see sec. 6, ch. 12) is heard equally loudly here and at the same position on the right hemithorax.

KEY POINT ▶ Intensity of murmurs of pulmonic and aortic stenoses correlate well with the severity of the stenosis.

- The continuous murmur of the patent ductus arteriosus (PDA) is heard the loudest in the PDA region. With this murmur, S_2 may not be heard because the murmur of blood rushing through the PDA is loudest during the time S_2 is generated. See sec. 6, chs. 12 & 13, for more on PDA.

- Cardiac auscultatory findings on the right hemithorax (see Fig. 5)
  - Region of the right fourth intercostal space at the sternal border
    S_1 louder than S_2.
    Systolic murmur of ventricular septal defect—louder during exhalation.
  - Region of right fifth intercostal space above the costochondral junction—systolic murmur of tricuspid regurgitation—louder during inspiration.
  - Region of the right base—systolic murmur of aortic stenosis is almost as loud as at the left base and is louder during exhalation than during inhalation.

2 Radiographic Evaluation

Wendy Myer
John D. Bonagura

Thoracic radiography is useful in the recognition and assessment of cardiovascular (CV) diseases. When combined with the results of the clinical examination, thoracic radiographs may contribute to the specific cardiac diagnosis, verify the presence of congestive heart failure (CHF), and assist in the differential diagnosis of respiratory signs such as coughing and dyspnea. Analysis of thoracic radiographs, including vascular patterns, is discussed in detail in sec. 6, ch. 17. This chapter describes specific aspects of radiography useful in cardiac diagnosis.

The importance of the technical quality of thoracic radiographs is often underestimated. A poor radiograph with inadequate penetration or poor patient positioning may be misleading and worse than no radiograph at all. This can be avoided by addressing the following technical aspects prior to radiographic evaluation for cardiac disease.

- Two views, a lateral projection (LAT) and either a dorsoventral (DV) or ventrodorsal (VD) projection, are needed for complete thoracic evaluation.
  - Cardiomegaly may be suspected on one view but may not be confirmed on the complementary projection.
  - The caudal lobar pulmonary arteries are best seen using DV projection.
- Radiographic technique:
  - Take films at the peak of inspiration.
  - Expiratory films are ineffective for evaluating the lung parenchyma for pulmonary edema.
  - A long-scale (high kV, low mAs) technique is most helpful for assessing thoracic disease. Underexposure mimics pulmonary disease by increasing apparent pulmonary density, whereas overexposure leads to an underestimation of the severity of pulmonary changes.
- Patient positioning:
  - Rotation often accentuates normal structures such as the main pulmonary artery on the VD projection or the left atrium or right ventricle on the lateral projection.
  - False apex shifting due to patient rotation on the VD projection may cause overestimation of ventricular size.

Once an adequately positioned and exposed radiograph has been obtained, attempt to answer the following general questions during the radiographic assessment of cardiac disease.

- Is cardiomegaly present or absent? If present, is this cardiac enlargement mild, moderate, or severe?
  - Species and conformational variations are important in this assessment (e.g., barrel-chested dogs normally have wider and more rounded hearts, and the cardiac size appears large relative to the thoracic volume).
- Which specific cardiac chambers are abnormal? Is more than one cardiac chamber affected? Is the abnormality restricted to one side of the heart or is it generalized?
  - Enlargement of one ventricle may cause the heart to rotate, leading to overestimation of the size of other cardiac chambers (e.g., right ventricular enlargement causes the apex to shift toward the left thoracic wall on the VD projection, mimicking left ventricular enlargement).
- Is the cardiac apex in its normal position? If not, is this shift due to poor patient positioning?
- Are the great vessels (aorta and main pulmonary artery) normal or abnormal in appearance?
- Are the pulmonary vessels normal, small, or enlarged (see sec. 6, ch. 17)? Are the changes restricted to the arteries (e.g., heartworm), veins (e.g., venous congestion), or are both altered in size (e.g., pulmonary under- or overcirculation)?
- Is the radiographic opacity of the lung normal, decreased, or increased? Are areas of increased opacity generalized or focal? If diffuse, what is the distribution of the pulmonary infiltrates (generalized, dorsal-caudal, or cranial-ventral)? See sec. 6, ch. 17 for more information on radiography of the respiratory tract.
- Is there evidence of pleural effusion?
  - This may be indicative of biventricular CHF or may be noncardiogenic in origin.
  - Thoracocentesis is necessary to determine the type of fluid present (see sec. 6, ch. 22).
  - The cardiac silhouette will be more obscured on a DV projection than on a VD projection in the presence of a mild to moderate amount of pleural fluid.
  - Patient stress may preclude a complete radiographic examination initially, but further films may be possible following thoracocentesis.
- Are the diaphragm and extrathoracic structures normal? If not, are the changes most likely congenital (e.g., peritoneopericardial hernia) or acquired (e.g., rib fractures indicating recent thoracic trauma)?

CARDIAC EVALUATION: NORMAL FINDINGS

Lateral View (Fig. 1)

Dogs

- Cardiac outline is roughly tear-shaped.
- Orientation—is at approximately 45° angle with the sternum (varies with breed).
- Location—extends from 3rd to 6th rib, and the heart and diaphragm usually touch or overlap.
- Size—ventricles occupy approximately three intercostal spaces.
- Cardiac borders represent:
  - Cranial—right ventricle and auricle (rounded border)
  - Caudal—left ventricle and atrium (straight border)
  - Dorsal—both atria, pulmonary arteries, both venae cavae, and aorta
- Quadrants:
  - Cranial three-fifths—right sided structures
  - Caudal two-fifths—left sided structures

Cats

- Cardiac outline is more elongated and elliptical than in the dog.
- Orientation is more variable than in the dog, with a more horizontal major cardiac axis.
- Location—heart and diaphragm are separated by one to two intercostal spaces.
- Size—the ventricles occupy approximately 2–2.5 intercostal spaces and the heart extends about two-thirds of ventrodorsal height of the thorax.
- Cardiac borders are similar to those in the dog.

Ventrodorsal (VD) or Dorsoventral (DV) Views (Fig. 2)

Dogs

- Cardiac outline has a curved right border and straight left border.

- Orientation—the apex is slightly to left of midline, approximately 30° angle with spine.
- Location—extends from 3rd to 8th vertebra; often touches the diaphragm.
- Size—cardiac-thoracic index (ratio) is about 60–65% of thorax as measured from right to left.
- Cardiac borders (using the clock-face analogy):
  - 11 to 1 o'clock—aortic arch
  - 1 to 2 o'clock—main pulmonary artery
  - 2 to 3 o'clock—left auricular appendage
  - 3 to 6 o'clock—left ventricle
  - 6 to 11 o'clock—right ventricle
  - 9 to 11 o'clock—right atrium

Cats

- Cardiac outline is slightly more elongated than in the dog.
- Orientation—the apex is at or slightly to the left of the midline.
- Location—heart and diaphragm are separated by one to two intercostal spaces.
- Cardiac borders are similar to those in the dog, except that the main pulmonary artery does not usually contribute to the 1 to 2 o'clock border.

Pulmonary Arteries and Veins

- Lateral view—artery (A) is dorsal to bronchus (B) and vein (V) (A-B-V from dorsal to ventral).
- VD or DV views:
  - Artery is lateral to bronchus and vein.
  - Arteries originate cranial to carina.
  - Veins terminate in left atrium caudal to the carina (veins are ventral and central).
- Size:
  - Artery and vein are approximately equal in size.
  - Normal vessel-to-rib ratio (compare to proximal one-third of 4th rib) is 0.75–0.8 (with a wide range of 0.5–1.25).

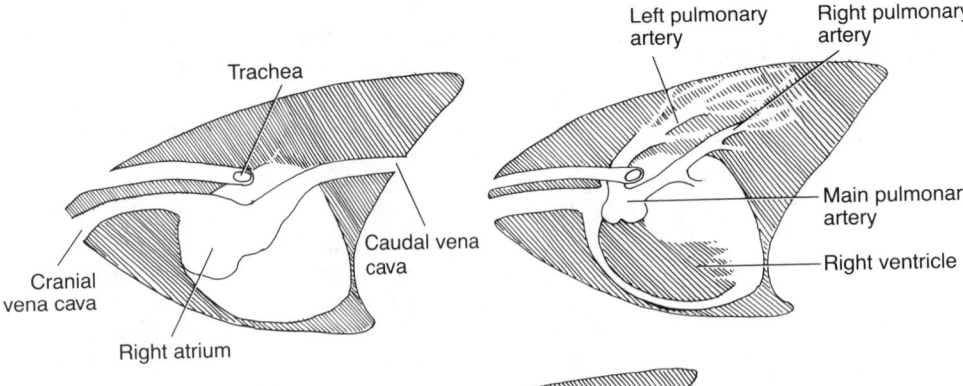

Figure 1. Three lateral views of the normal heart.

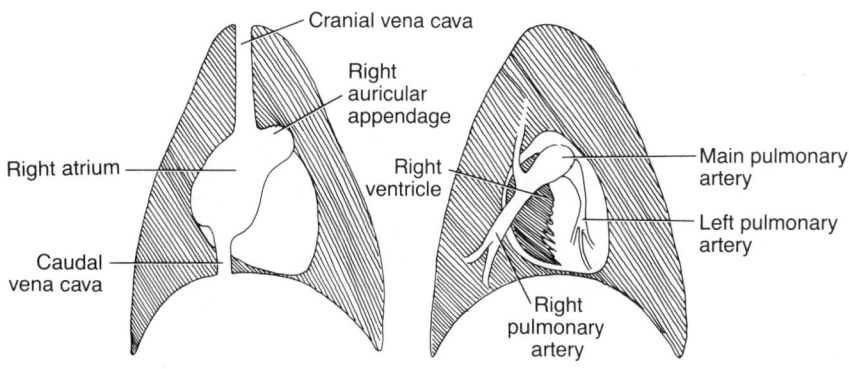

Figure 2. Four ventrodorsal views of the normal heart.

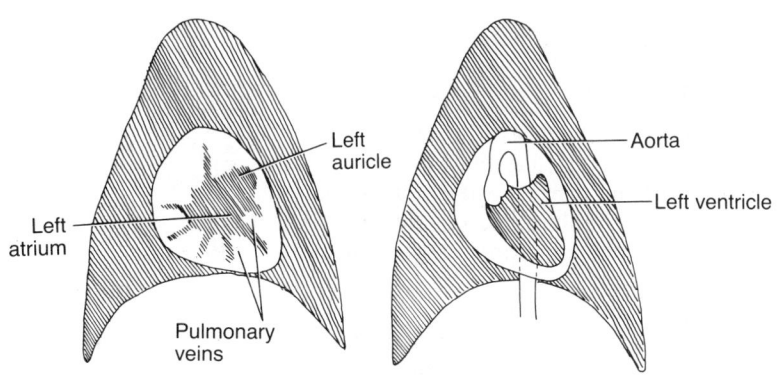

■ Margination:
  • Vessels are best seen on the lateral view as they extend into cranial lobes.
  • Vessels in lung farthest from cassette will be magnified.
■ Arteries are more dense than veins, slightly curved, and have dichotomous branching (branches of equal size).
■ Veins are less visible, are straighter and blunter than arteries, and have branches of unequal size.

RADIOGRAPHIC SIGNS OF CARDIOVASCULAR DISEASE

Right Atrial (RA) Enlargement

The right atrium is the most difficult chamber to detect radiographically (Fig. 3).

Lateral View

■ RA enlargement usually is not seen on this view.

■ Loss or filling in of the normal concave angle between the ventral edge of the cranial mediastinum and the cardiac silhouette (the cranial "waist") may be seen due to bulging of the right auricular appendage.

DV or VD Views

■ Bulging of the cranial right heart border (9 to 11 o'clock) is typical of RA dilation.
■ RA dilation is often masked by concurrent right ventricular enlargement.

Common Causes

■ Atrial septal defect (ASD)
■ Pulmonic stenosis
■ Tricuspid regurgitation
■ RA tumors
■ Atrial fibrillation
■ Advanced heartworm disease
■ Pulmonary hypertension (including cor pulmonale)

Figure 3. Radiographic signs of right atrial enlargement. The red areas denote the abnormal region.

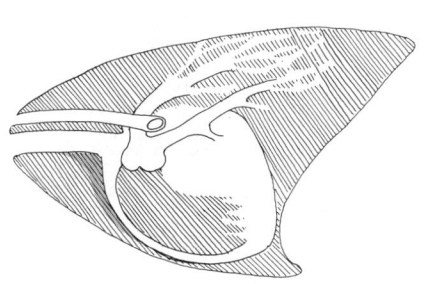
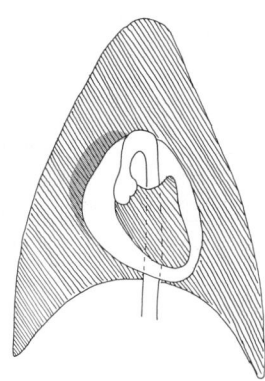

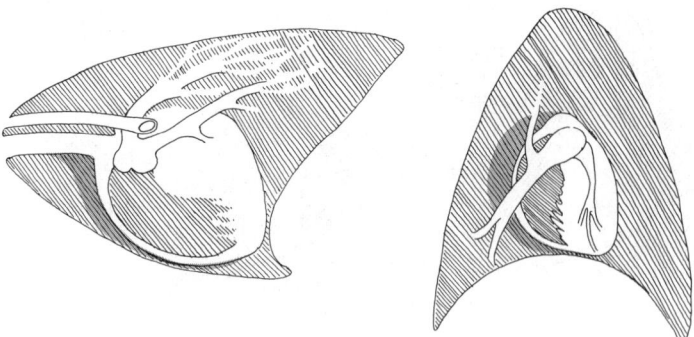

Figure 4. Radiographic signs of right ventricular enlargement. The red region denotes the abnormality.

Right Ventricular (RV) Enlargement (Fig. 4)

Lateral View

- Increased overall width of heart
- Rounding of the cranial heart border
- Elevation of the cardiac apex and caudal vena cava
- In severe RV enlargement, elevation of trachea cranial to carina and some degree of cardiac elongation

DV or VD View

- Rounding of the right heart border (6 to 11 o'clock)
- "Reversed D" appearance if the main pulmonary artery is also dilated
- Increased overall width of the heart
- Decreased distance between the right heart and thoracic wall or shifting of the apex to the left side

Common Causes

- Pulmonic stenosis
- Tricuspid regurgitation
- Pulmonary hypertension of any cause (heartworm disease, cor pulmonale, congenital disease with pulmonic stenosis
- Tetralogy of Fallot
- ASD
- Some ventricular septal defects

Left Atrial Enlargement (Fig. 5)

Lateral View

- Elevation of the distal end of the trachea with dorsal displacement and compression of the left main-stem bronchus between the left atrium and descending aorta
- Bulging of the caudal-dorsal heart border (dorsal to the caudal vena cava)
- Filling in and loss of the normal caudal indentation of the cardiac border (the caudal waist); or, with marked dilation, accentuation of the waist as the atrium projects caudodorsally

DV or VD View

- The left atrium, proper, is a midline structure and does not normally contribute to the heart border on this view.
- There is displacement and separation of the mainstem bronchi as they approach the cranial border of the left atrium and bifurcate around this chamber (producing a "bowlegged cowboy" appearance to the bronchial tree).
- On a well-exposed DV view, the enlarged atrium may be seen as a round, soft tissue mass summated on the caudal heart border.
- Left auricular dilation is seen in dogs as bulging of the left heart border at 2 to 3 o'clock, and in cats as a bulge from 1 to 3 o'clock.

Common Causes

- Mitral regurgitation (MR)
- Patent ductus arteriosus
- Ventricular septal defect
- Cardiomyopathy (all forms)
- Mitral dysplasia (causing MR ± mitral stenosis)
- Hyperthyroidism
- Hypertensive heart disease
- Left-sided CHF from any cause

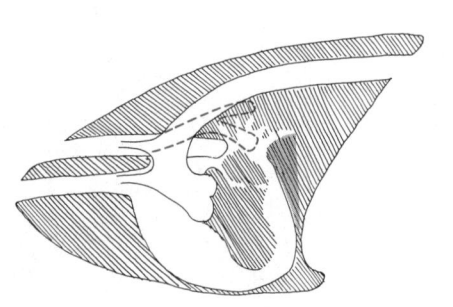
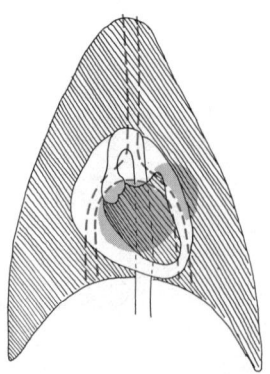

Figure 5. Radiographic signs of left atrial enlargement. The red region denotes the abnormality.

Left Ventricular (LV) Enlargement (Fig. 6)

Lateral View

- Elongation of the cardiac silhouette and possibly widening of the silhouette
- Rounding of the caudal heart border
- Elevation of the carina and distal end of the trachea (causing the trachea to more closely parallel the spine than the sternum; this finding depends on chest conformation and breed)

DV or VD View

- Elongation, rounding, and expansion of the left heart border
- Rounding of the cardiac apex
- Decreased distance between the left heart border and thoracic wall or shifting of the cardiac apex to the right (especially common in cats)

Common Causes

- Mitral regurgitation
- Patent ductus arteriosus
- Ventricular septal defect
- Aortic stenosis
- Aortic regurgitation (e.g., from bacterial endocarditis)
- Cardiomyopathy of any cause
- Hyperthyroidism
- Hypertensive heart disease

Generalized (Biventricular) Cardiac Enlargement

- This is a relatively common feature of many cardiac disorders.
- It usually is difficult to determine which ventricle is most enlarged on survey films alone; however, ancillary studies such as echocardiography may help to delineate exact chamber abnormalities.
- The heart appears generally rounded, and usually there is increased sternal contact on the lateral view.

Common Causes

- Chronic valvular heart disease (mitral and tricuspid regurgitation)
- Left-sided heart failure (any cause) with secondary pulmonary hypertension
- Ventricular septal defect

- Dilated cardiomyopathy
- Mild to moderate pericardial effusion (mimics cardiomegaly)

Microcardia

- A generalized decrease in cardiac size is most often associated with plasma volume contraction, shock, or trauma.
- Because the heart shifts off the thoracic midline, it appears elevated from the sternum on the lateral view.
- Pulmonary circulation often appears diminished.

Common Causes

- Hypovolemic shock
- Addison's disease
- Hemorrhage
- Protracted vomiting/diarrhea
- Obstructive hepatic circulation (cirrhosis, caudal vena cava obstruction)

Aortic Enlargement (Fig. 7)

- The direction of bulging depends on the underlying etiology.
  - Patent ductus arteriosus—some cranial bulging of aortic arch is seen, but the most pronounced bulging is toward the left side at the site of patent ductus ("ductus bump"). This is seen on the DV or VD view.
  - Aortic stenosis—there is dilation of the ascending aorta (cranioventrally) and aortic arch (cranially) caused by poststenotic turbulence; a similar feature is observed with tetralogy of Fallot and pulmonary atresia due to increased aortic blood flow (right → left shunt) and dextropositioned aorta.
- Persistent right fourth aortic arch—the aorta may descend to the right side (mirror-image arch) instead of left of the midline.
- Dilation and tortuosity of the ascending aorta, arch, or descending aorta may be observed in cats with hyperthyroidism or systemic hypertension or as an incidental senile change in aged cats.

Pulmonary Artery (PA) and Pulmonary Vascularity (Fig. 8)

Enlargement of the main PA leads to bulging of the left cranial cardiac border at 1 o'clock (DV or VD

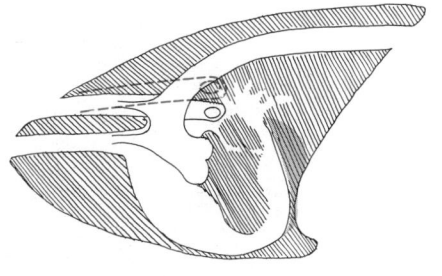
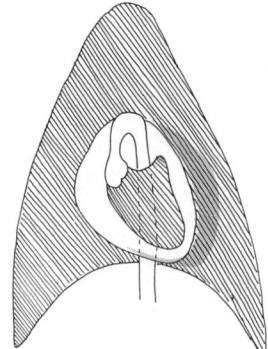

Figure 6. Radiographic signs of left ventricular enlargement. The red region denotes the abnormality.

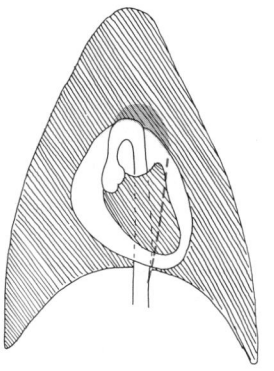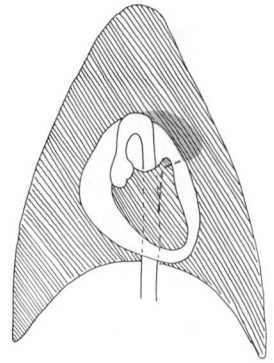

Figure 7. Radiographic signs of aortic enlargement. Left, aortic stenosis; right, patent ductus arteriosus.

view) in the dog (may not be evident in cats). There are three general causes of dilation of the main PA:

- Increased blood flow (PDA, VSD, ASD),
- Poststenotic dilation (pulmonic stenosis), and
- Pulmonary hypertension (heartworms or related to congenital disease).

Enlargement of the *lobar and peripheral pulmonary arteries and veins* has two general causes:

- Overcirculation (increased flow due to left to right shunts such as patent ductus arteriosus, ventricular and atrial septal defects, or hyperdynamic circulations as with severe anemia or thyrotoxicosis) leads to dilation of both pulmonary arteries and veins. Enhanced vascularity in the peripheral lung fields also may be evident.
- Pulmonary arterial and venous hypertension causes widening of the affected vessels. Left-sided CHF causes pulmonary venous hypertension. Pulmonary arterial hypertension is caused by heartworm disease, pulmonary embolism, and severe left-sided CHF. When arterial hypertension is caused by left-sided CHF, pulmonary venous distension also is prominent.

Assessment of pulmonary vascularity requires judgment and evaluation of other cardiac structures. General guidelines include:

- Lateral view: Evaluate vessels as they extend into the cranial lobes. The lobar artery is dorsal to the bronchus and vein. Peripheral vascular markings normally are prominent in deep-chested dogs and in many cats (following full inspiration).
- DV or VD view: Evaluate vessels as they extend beyond the heart border. The lobar artery is lateral to the bronchus and vein.
- The normal artery and vein should be equal in size and average 75% of the width of the proximal one-third of the rib at the same level (4th rib on lateral view).
- Decreased vascular markings are typical of undercirculation due to right-to-left cardiac shunts (e.g., tetralogy of Fallot), low cardiac output (e.g., tricuspid regurgitation, cardiac tamponade), or plasma volume contraction (e.g., shock).

Radiographic Signs of Congestive Heart Failure (CHF)

- Cardiomegaly is expected, particularly atrial enlargement (Fig. 9).
- Increased pulmonary venous size indicates elevated

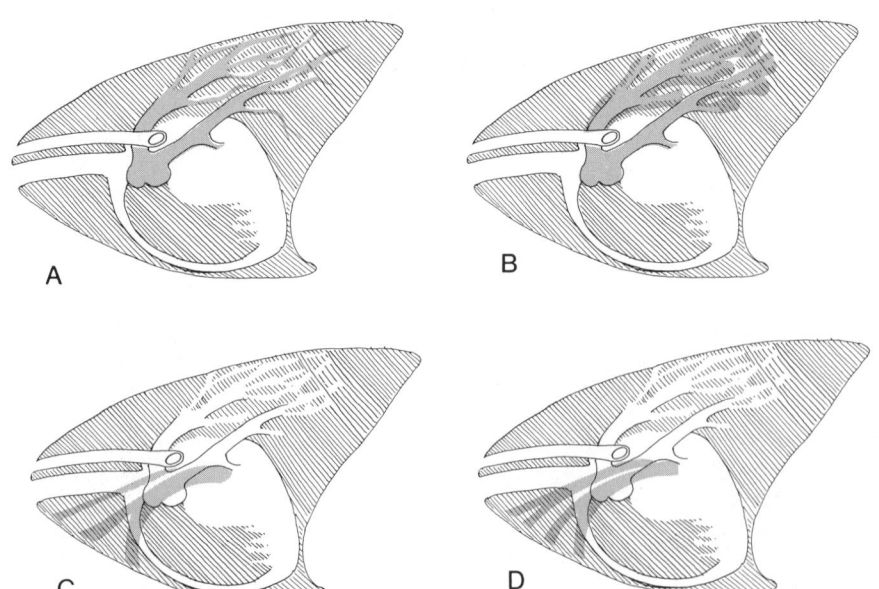

Figure 8. Radiographic signs of pulmonic circulatory disorders. *A,* Normal pulmonary circulation. *B,* Pulmonary arterial hypertension caused by heartworm disease. *C,* Effects of venous congestion due to mitral insufficiency. *D,* Signs of pulmonary overcirculation caused by left-to-right shunt.

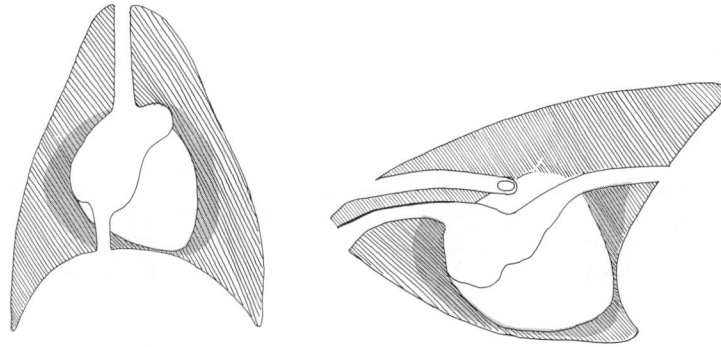

Figure 9. Radiographic signs of cardiomegaly. The red region denotes the abnormality.

pulmonary venous pressure ("congestion" or "venous hypertension"). Secondary pulmonary arterial hypertension may be observed as well.

Left Sided CHF

- Left-sided CHF is characterized by increased pulmonary density.
- Initially, perivascular interstitial densities that blur vascular margins are seen. These progress to a diffuse interstitial density and airway cuffing with ensuing alveolar flooding.
- Alveolar patterns are recognized by visualization of fluffy, coalescing densities with air bronchogram signs. Fluid density structures such as the heart and diaphragm may be obscured (silhouetted).
- Distribution of cardiac edema is usually perihilar, dorsal, and bilateral; however, right-sided prominence is common in severe edema due to different lymphatic drainage between sides. Diffuse or dependent infiltrates may be observed in fulminant cardiogenic edema.
- Expect mobilization of alveolar edema within 48–72 hours following aggressive therapy for CHF (see sec. 6, ch. 6). Radiographic changes often lag behind clinical improvement or deterioration by 12–18 hours. Failure to resolve increased pulmonary densities following appropriate treatment should prompt a reconsideration of the diagnosis of cardiogenic lung edema.
- Development of pleural fissure lines and pleural effusion is usually a sign of biventricular CHF. Severe pleural effusion usually indicates right ventricular decompensation associated with pulmonary hypertension secondary to left-sided disease. Cardiac tamponade is another cause of pleural effusion.

KEY POINT ▶ Chronic left-sided CHF is characterized by a fine interstitial lung density that may represent congestion-induced pulmonary fibrosis. Alveolar infiltrates are unlikely unless therapy is suspended or acute deterioration in heart function develops (e.g., ruptured mitral chorda tendinea or development of atrial fibrillation.

RADIOGRAPHIC FINDINGS IN SPECIFIC DISEASES

The radiographic features of many cardiac disorders are described in detail in other chapters in this section.

Table 1 summarizes typical features of common conditions. Some clinical pointers are offered below.

Valvular Heart Disease (see sec. 6, ch. 7)

- The severity of valvular regurgitation usually corresponds to the degree of atrial dilation observed radiographically.
- Chronic regurgitation allows the atrium to expand and increase its compliance; therefore, severe cardiomegaly can develop prior to onset of CHF.
- Compression of the left main-stem bronchus by the left atrium may persist following resolution of lung edema. This finding is often associated with recurrent coughing.

Cardiomyopathy (see sec. 6, ch. 8)

Hypertrophic Cardiomyopathy

Hypertrophic cardiomyopathy is now the most common cause of CHF in cats. The radiographic features are variable, and heart size can change dramatically following diuretic therapy. Advanced hyperthyroid heart disease can produce similar radiographic features.

- Dilation of the left atrium or auricle is the most consistent feature, and left auricular enlargement may produce a "valentine-shaped heart" on the VD projection.
- LV hypertrophy is concentric, but may lead to elongation of the heart.
- Pulmonary edema can be widespread or patchy, dependent, or dorsad.
- Pleural effusion develops in chronic cases secondary to pulmonary hypertension and biventricular CHF.

Dilated Cardiomyopathy

Dilated cardiomyopathy is characterized by biventricular dilation and often a rounded cardiac silhouette.

- A globoid appearance may mimic the changes seen with pericardial effusion; however, pulmonary venous congestion is usually evident with cardiomyopathy but absent in pericardial effusion.
- Left-sided or biventricular failure may develop.

KEY POINT ▶ The radiographic features of dilated cardiomyopathy cannot be reliably distinguished from those of chronic atrioventricular valve regurgitation.

TABLE 1. Common Radiographic Features of Heart Disease*

Disorder	LV	LA	Ao	RV	RA	MPA	Pulmonary Circulation	Additional Findings
Patent ductus arteriosus	+	+	+ Desc Ao	0 [a]	0		+ Artery + Vein	Left-sided CHF
Ventricular septal defect	+	+	0	+ [b]	0 [b]	+	+ Artery + Vein	Left-sided CHF
Atrial septal defect	0	0 [c]	0	+	+	+	+ Artery + Vein	Right-sided CHF
Mitral regurgitation	+	+	0	+ [b]	0	0	+ Vein 0/+ Artery [b]	Left-sided CHF
Tricuspid regurgitation	0	0	0	+	+	0	0	Dilated vena cava Right-sided CHF
Aortic stenosis	+	0/+	+ Asc Ao	0	0	0	0/+ Vein 0/+ Artery [b]	Left-sided CHF
Pulmonic stenosis	0	0	0	+	+	+	0/− Artery 0/− Vein	Right-sided CHF
Tetralogy of Fallot	0	0	+ [d]	+	+	[e]	− Artery − Vein	
Dilated cardiomyopathy	+	+	0	+	+	0	+ Vein 0/+ Artery	Biventricular CHF
Hypertrophic cardiomyopathy	+	+	0	0/+ [b]	0/+ [b]	0	+ Vein 0/+ Artery [b]	Left-sided or biventricular CHF
Restrictive cardiomyopathy	+	+	0	+	+	−	+ Vein 0/− Artery [b]	Variable findings
Pericardial effusion	+	+	0	+	+	0	0/− Artery 0/− Vein	Possible mass lesion
Hyperthyroidism	+	+	+	+	+	0	0/+ Artery 0/+ Vein	Dilated or tortuous aorta
Pulmonary hypertension	0/+ [f]	0/+ [f]	0	+	+	+	−/0+ Artery −/0/+ Vein [f, g]	Lungs may be abnormal or under-circulated
Heartworm disease	0	0	0	+	+	+	+ Artery 0 Vein	Pulmonary infiltrate

*LV = left ventricle; LA = left atrium; Ao = aorta; RV = right ventricle; RA = right atrium; MPA = main pulmonary artery; CHF = congestive heart failure; 0 = no change; + = enlarged or increased; − = decreased; desc = descending; asc = ascending.

[a] Although the RV may appear enlarged, echocardiograph demonstrates that left ventricular dilatation accounts for ventricular enlargement; in the rare case of reversed patent ductus arteriosus, the radiograph resembles that of pulmonary hypertension.

[b] Right-sided cardiomegaly will develop if there is pulmonary hypertension due to increased pulmonary flow, increased pulmonary vascular resistance, or both.

[c] In the typical ostium secundum (high) atrial septal defect (ASD), blood flows immediately into the RA and the LA doesn't enlarge. In cases of primum ASD with concurrent ventricular septal defect, or mitral dysplasia (endocardial cushion defect), LA dilation also develops.

[d] The aorta is dextropositioned and receives the most blood flow; this causes widening of the ventrocranial mediastinum on the lateral projection.

[e] The pulmonary artery is not dilated because blood preferentially shunts across the ventricular septal defect into the aorta.

[f] In cases of pulmonary hypertension secondary to left-sided CHF, left heart structures will be enlarged.

[g] In cases of pulmonary hypertension secondary to left-sided CHF, pulmonary venous distension will also be present; in pulmonary hypertension caused by pulmonary vascular disease (e.g., reversed patent ductus arteriosus, primary pulmonary hypertension), peripheral pulmonary vascularity will be decreased whereas central lobar vessels will be dilated from pressure.

Pericardial Disease

- One cannot differentiate the type of pericardial fluid radiographically.
- The radiographic appearance depends on the degree of hydropericardium. When there is only a small amount of fluid, the heart may appear normal or minimally enlarged.
- Progressive pericardial effusion causes the heart to appear globular in shape on both views ("pumpkin heart").
- Pleural effusion may be evident, as well as hepatomegaly and ascites.
- Pulmonary vascularity, when evident, is often diminished.
- Acute pericardial effusion in dogs with chronic mitral valve disease may indicate left atrial rupture.
- Heart base tumors are often associated with some degree of pericardial effusion. A bulge may be noted near the aortic arch (heart base).

- Peritoneopericardial hernia, very common in cats, leads to features of pericardial effusion. Other signs include:
  - The heart shadow cannot be separated from the diaphragm.
  - Gas-filled loops of bowel within the pericardial shadow may be seen (more common in dogs).
  - Fat density (omentum) may be noted in the caudal ventral pericardial space (especially in cats).
  - A persistent mesothelial remnant is evident ventral to and parallel to the caudal vena cava (which is displaced dorsally).
  - There may be an absence or malformation of the last sternebra or pectus excavatum.

Supplemental Readings

Suter PF: *Thoracic Radiography: A Text Atlas of Thoracic Diseases of the Dog and Cat.* Wettswil, Switzerland: Peter F. Suter, 1984, pp 351–516.

3 Electrocardiography

Francis W. K. Smith Jr.
Larry Patrick Tilley
Michael S. Miller

Electrocardiography is the graphic representation of the electrical activity of the heart. Electrocardiograms (ECGs) are easy to perform and readily available to practicing veterinarians. There are numerous indications for performing ECGs. This test provides a wealth of information that is useful in the diagnosis and management of cardiac and systemic disturbances.

GENERAL PRINCIPLES OF ELECTROCARDIOGRAPHY

Indications for Performing an ECG

- To diagnose an arrhythmia detected on physical examination (auscultation, arterial pulse deficits, palpable precordial heartbeat irregularities, or abnormal jugular venous pulsations)
  - The ECG is the most sensitive test for the diagnosis of arrhythmias and for monitoring the effect of antiarrhythmic therapy.

KEY POINT ▶ An ECG is performed on all animals with tachycardia or bradycardia and on all cats with any irregularity in rhythm. An ECG is also recommended in any dog with an irregularity in rhythm that is related to a pulse deficit or is not related to phases of respiration.

- To rule out arrhythmias or conduction disturbances in patients with a history of syncope, seizures, or exercise intolerance
- To monitor effectiveness of antiarrhythmic therapy
- To assess cardiac size in patients with known or suspected cardiac disease
  - The ECG is not a very sensitive indicator of heart size. The presence of a heart enlargement pattern on the ECG usually correlates with cardiac chamber enlargement or hypertrophy. The more criteria for heart enlargement that are present in a patient, the more likely the heart will be enlarged. Most dogs with normal hearts will not exhibit heart enlargement patterns on the ECGs.

KEY POINT ▶ A normal ECG does not rule out a diagnosis of heart enlargement. Thoracic radiographs and echocardiography are more sensitive tests for evaluating heart size.

- To help individualize and monitor therapy in patients with heart failure
  - The diagnosis of congestive heart failure (CHF) cannot be made based on an ECG alone.

KEY POINT ▶ The presence of an arrhythmia or a heart enlargement pattern supports the diagnosis of heart disease but does not confirm CHF. A thoracic radiograph is obtained along with the ECG in a patient suspected of having CHF. The ECG is useful in patients with heart failure for the diagnosis and treatment of associated arrhythmias.

- To evaluate patients with suspected digoxin or other cardiac drug toxicity
- To screen for electrolyte disturbances, especially hyperkalemia, hypercalcemia, and hypocalcemia
- To look for evidence to support a diagnosis of pericardial effusion, hypothyroidism, hyperthyroidism, or hypoadrenocorticism (Addison's disease).

Technique for Recording an ECG

1. For accurate measurements, place the patient in right lateral recumbency.

KEY POINT ▶ If the animal is dyspneic or if restraint would be dangerous to the patient, a rhythm strip can be obtained with the animal supported in any comfortable position.

2. Wet the skin with alcohol or ECG electrode gel and attach the electrodes just above the elbows and stifles.
3. Hold the upper limbs perpendicular to the long axis of the patient and parallel to the floor. If the thoracic limbs are not parallel, the mean electrical axis will be altered.
4. Record approximately 3 to 4 complexes in each of the six limb leads and then record a long lead II strip for rhythm evaluation. Push the standard calibration button at the beginning and end of each recording.
5. Chest leads can be obtained using the V lead electrode, while keeping the limb leads attached. See Table 1 for electrode placement.

Chest leads are not necessary for all patients. However, they may be quite useful when the ECG complexes in the limb leads are small and difficult to evaluate. Often, P waves that cannot be seen in the limb leads become apparent on a chest lead. Evaluation of chest leads may also be helpful in evaluating heart enlargement patterns. The chest leads most commonly used in veterinary patients are CV_5RL (rV_2), CV_6LL (V_2), CV_6LU (V_4), and V_{10}.

Normal Cardiac Conduction

The ECG records the electrical activity of the heart. Electrical impulses originate in specialized pacemaker tissue in the sinus node of the right atrium. The impulse rapidly traverses the atrium, causing atrial contraction and then slows, as it passes through the atrioventricular (AV) node located at the proximal portion of the interventricular septum. Electrical activity then rapidly passes through the bundle of His, the anterior and posterior branches of the left bundle branch, the right bundle branch, and the terminal Purkinje fibers. This causes activation of the interventricular septum and the left and right ventricular myocardium (Fig. 1).

Components of the Electrocardiographic Tracing (Fig. 2)

- P wave indicates atrial depolarization.
- P-R interval indicates time for conduction of the impulse from the sinoauricular (SA) node to the AV node and delay of the impulse in the AV node, His bundle, bundle branches, and Purkinje system.
- QRS complex indicates ventricular myocardium depolarization.
- Q wave (lead II) is associated with depolarization of the interventricular septum.
- R wave (lead II) is associated with depolarization of the left ventricle.
- S wave (lead II), when present, is associated with depolarization of the right ventricle.

TABLE 1. Electrode Placement

Chest Lead	Placement of the V Lead
CV_5RL (rV_2)	Fifth intercostal space on the right side near the sternum
CV_6LL (V_2)	Sixth intercostal space on the left side near the sternum
CV_6LU (V_4)	Sixth intercostal space on the left side at the costochondral junction
V_{10}	Over the dorsal spine of the seventh thoracic vertebra

- T wave indicates ventricular repolarization.
- Q-T interval indicates an approximate interval of ventricular systole.

How to Evaluate the ECG

- Always evaluate the ECG from left to right.
- Identify and label the ECG waveforms (P-QRS-T).
- Calculate the approximate heart rate (HR) by counting the number of R-R intervals in 3 seconds (2 sets of time markers at 50 mm/sec) and multiplying by 20.
- Determine the mean electrical axis.
  One of the easiest ways to approximate the axis is to identify the isoelectric lead (sum of the positive and negative deflections of the QRS complex closest to zero).
  • Determine the perpendicular lead, and evaluate that lead to see if the complexes are positive or negative.
  • Axis is in the direction of the main deflection of the perpendicular lead (see Figure 3 for an example).
  • If all leads are isoelectric, an axis cannot be determined in the frontal plane.

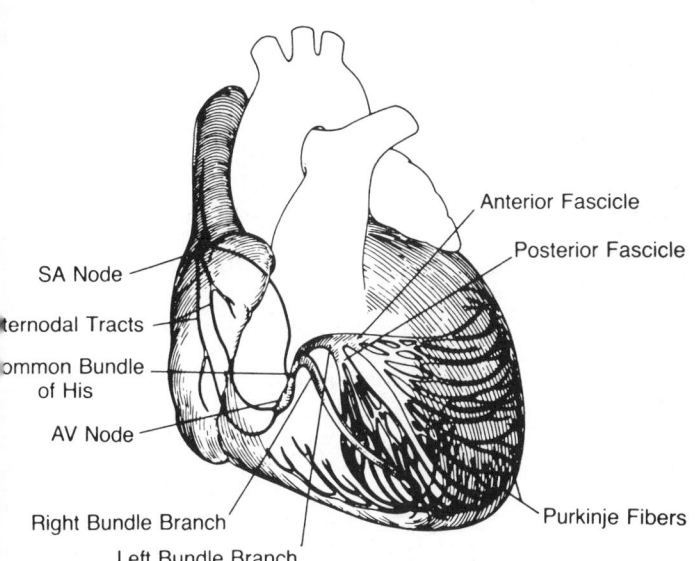

Figure 1. Normal conduction pathway in the heart. (From De Sanctis RW: Disturbances in cardiac rhythm and conduction. *In* Rubenstein R, ed.: *Scientific American Medicine,* section 1, subsection VI. © 1991 Scientific American, Inc. All rights reserved.)

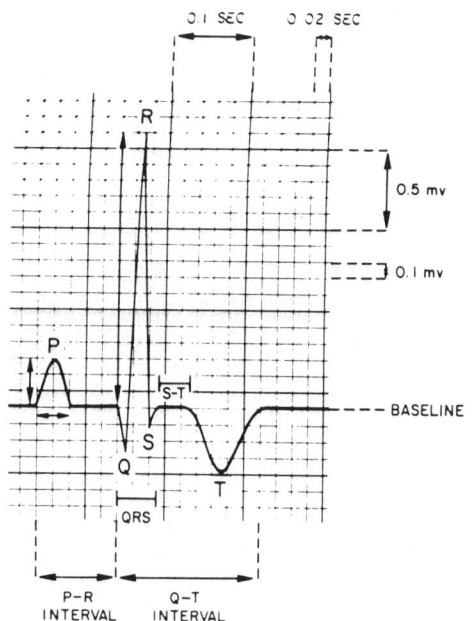

Figure 2. Normal electrocardiogram with components labeled. (From Tilley LP: *Essentials of Canine and Feline Electrocardiography,* 3rd ed. Philadelphia: Lea & Febiger, 1992.)

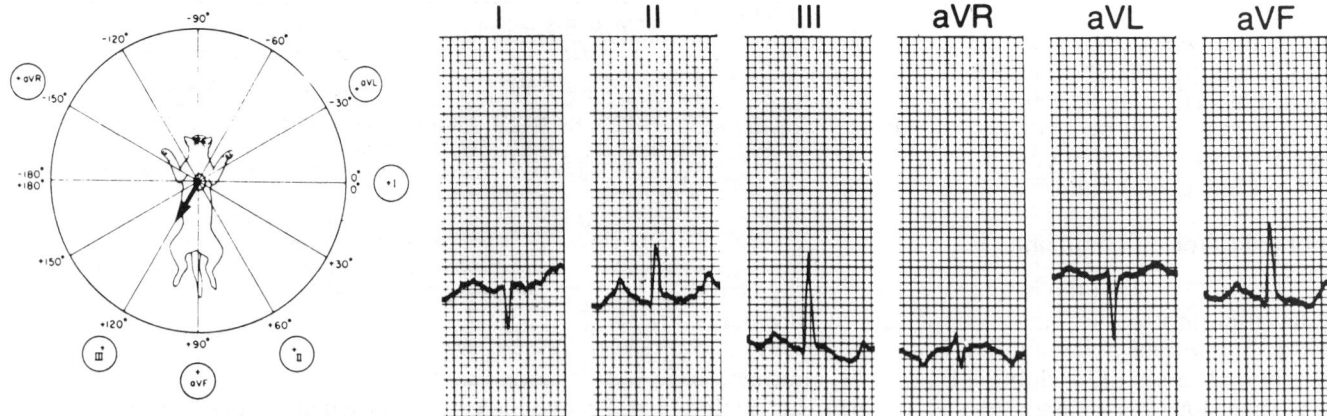

Figure 3. This electrocardiogram is from a cat. Lead aVR is isoelectric. Lead III is perpendicular to aVR. The QRS deflection in lead III is positive, making the axis +120. If lead III had been negative, the axis would have been −60. (From Tilley LP: *Essentials of Canine and Feline Electrocardiography,* 3rd ed. Philadelphia: Lea & Febiger, 1992.)

- Determine the rhythm.
  - A sinus rhythm has near constant P-R and R-R intervals.
  - A sinus arrhythmia has a near constant P-R interval, but the R-R interval varies, usually with the phase of respiration. For a more detailed discussion of arrhythmia evaluation, refer to sec. 6, ch. 4.
- Measure the height and width of the complexes.
- Determine the P-R and Q-T intervals and evaluate the S-T segment.

- Compare the heart rate, rhythm, and sizes of the complexes to the normal values (Table 2).

ECG ABNORMALITIES

Electrocardiographic abnormalities can be divided into those involving heart rate and rhythm and those involving the configuration of the complexes. This chapter discusses abnormalities involving the ECG complexes. Arrhythmias are discussed in sec. 6, ch. 4.

TABLE 2. Normal Canine and Feline Electrocardiogram Values*

	Canine	Feline
Heart rate (HR)	Puppy: up to 220 beats per minute Toy breeds: up to 180 beats per minute Standard: 70–160 beats per minute Giant breeds: 60–140 beats per minute	120–240 beats per minute
Rhythm	Sinus rhythm Sinus arrhythmia Wandering pacemaker	Sinus rhythm
P wave		
Height	Maximum: 0.4 mv	Maximum: 0.2 mv
Width	Maximum: 0.04 seconds (giant breeds 0.05 seconds)	Maximum: 0.04 seconds
PR interval	0.06–0.13 seconds (>0.13 seconds in giant breeds)	0.05–0.09 seconds
QRS		
Height	Small breeds: 2.5 mv maximum Large breeds: 3.0 mv maximum†	Maximum: 0.9 mv
Width	Small breeds: 0.05 seconds maximum Large breeds: 0.06 seconds maximum	Maximum: 0.04 seconds
S-T segment		
Depression	No more than 0.2 mv	None
Elevation	No more than 0.15 mv	None
Q-T interval	0.15–0.25 seconds at normal HR	0.12–0.18 seconds at normal HR
T waves	May be positive, negative, or biphasic Amplitude range +/− 0.05–1.0 mv in any lead	Usually positive
Electrical axis	+40° to +100°	0° to +/− 160°
Chest leads		
CV_5RL (rV_2)	T positive; R <3.0 mv	
CV_6LL (V_2)	S <0.8 mv; R <3.0 mv	R <1.0 mv
CV_6LU (V_4)	S <0.7 mv; R <3.0 mv	R <1.0 mv
V_{10}	QRS negative; T negative except in Chihuahua	T negative; R wave/Q wave <1

*Measurements are made in lead II unless otherwise stated.
†Not valid for thin, deep-chested dogs under 2 years of age.

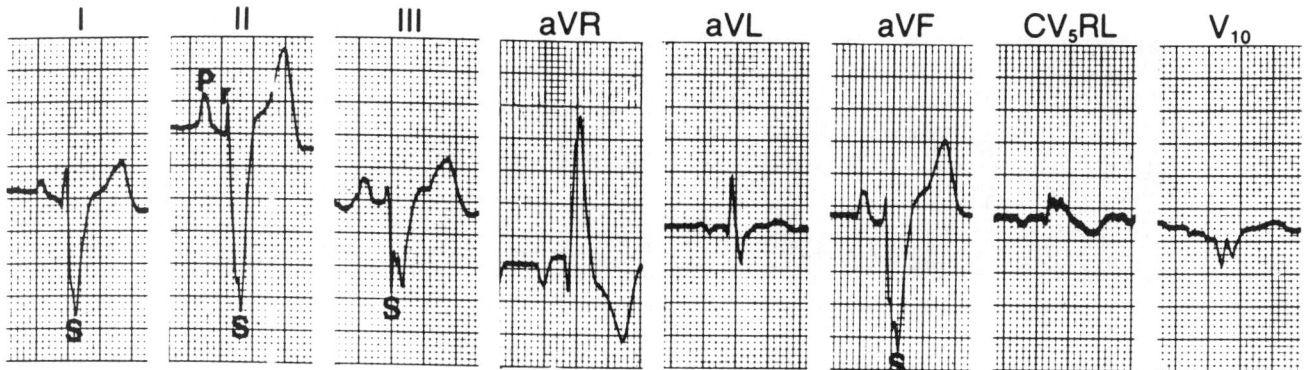

Figure 4. Example of right bundle branch block in the dog. Note the right axis (-110); the wide S wave in leads I, II, III, and aVF; and the M-shaped CV$_5$RL and W-shaped V$_{10}$. (From Tilley LP: *Essentials of Canine and Feline Electrocardiography*, 3rd ed. Philadelphia: Lea & Febiger, 1992.)

Interventricular Conduction Disturbances

- The right bundle branch is thinner and therefore more susceptible to injury than the left bundle branch.
- Injury to more than one bundle branch may result in first-, second-, or third-degree AV block.
- A bundle branch block does not cause hemodynamic changes and therefore does not warrant therapy.
- Rate-related bundle branch blocks can occur intermittently in association with either bradycardia or tachycardia. The right bundle branch cells have a longer refractory period than the left bundle branch cells. This makes the right bundle more sensitive to abrupt changes in the heart rate.

Right Bundle Branch Block (RBBB) (Fig. 4)

- ECG Characteristics
  - QRS width greater than 0.07 seconds (dog) or 0.06 seconds (cat)
  - Right axis deviation
  - Wide S waves in leads I, II, III, aVF, and lower left precordial leads, such as CV$_6$LL and CV$_6$LU
  - W-shaped pattern in V$_{10}$
  - Terminal QRS complex positive in aVR, aVL and M-shaped in CV$_5$RL
- Incomplete RBBB may be present if the aforementioned criteria are present but complexes are of normal width.
  - Must be differentiated from left posterior fascicular block.

- RBBB must be differentiated from right ventricular enlargement by radiographs or echocardiography. Right ventricular enlargement and RBBB can occur together.
- RBBB has been associated with the following conditions: congenital malformations, cardiac surgery, cardiac needle puncture or cardiac arrest, cardiac neoplasia, trauma, *Trypanosoma cruzi* infection (dog), cardiomyopathy, hyperkalemia (cat), acute ventricular dilation, balloon valvuloplasty, and doxorubicin cardiotoxicity. RBBB may be an incidental finding in patients without apparent cardiac disease (beagles).

Left Bundle Branch Block (LBBB) (Fig. 5)

- ECG Characteristics
  - QRS width greater than 0.07 seconds (dog) or 0.06 seconds (cat)
  - QRS positive in leads I, II, III, aVF, CV$_6$LL, and CV$_6$LU
  - QRS negative in leads aVR, aVL, and CV$_5$RL
  - Absent or small Q wave in leads I, CV$_6$LL, and CV$_6$LU (dog)
  - Q wave absent in leads I and CV$_6$LU (cat)
- LBBB indicates greater cardiac damage than RBBB—often cardiomyopathy
- LBBB must be differentiated from left ventricular enlargement by radiographs or echocardiography. Left ventricular enlargement and LBBB also can occur together.

Figure 5. Left bundle branch block in a dog. Note the wide QRS complexes (0.08 sec). This electrocardiogram could also be consistent with left ventricular enlargement. (From Tilley LP: *Essentials of Canine and Feline Electrocardiography*, 3rd ed. Philadelphia: Lea & Febiger, 1992.)

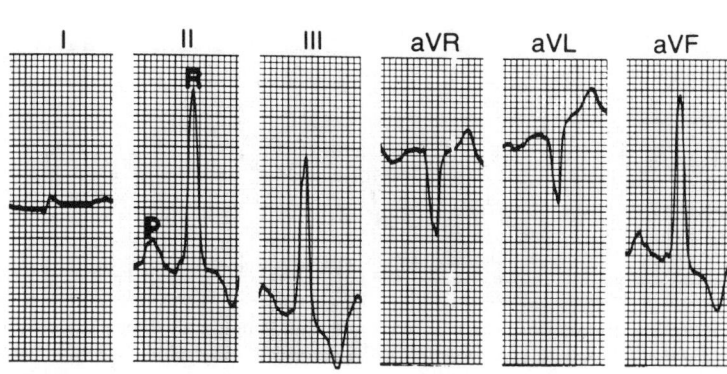

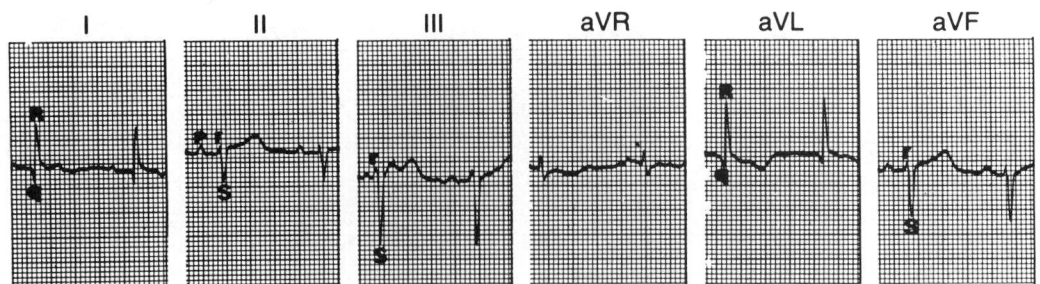

Figure 6. Left anterior fascicular block in a cat with hypertrophic cardiomyopathy. (Tilley LP: Feline electrocardiography. Vet Clin North Am 7:257, 1977.)

- LBBB is most often associated with the following conditions:
  - In dogs—cardiomyopathy, cardiac needle puncture, subaortic stenosis, and doxorubicin cardiotoxicity.
  - In cats—uncommon but associated with hypertrophic cardiomyopathy.

Left Anterior Fascicular Block (LAFB) (Fig. 6)

- ECG Characteristics
  - QRS width normal
  - Left axis deviation (dog< +40°, cat<0°)
  - Small Q and tall R in leads I and aVL (small Q not essential)
  - Deep S wave in leads II, III, and aVF (exceeding the R wave)
- Associated conditions include hypertrophic cardiomyopathy, causes of left ventricular hypertrophy, hyperkalemia, ischemic cardiomyopathy, and cardiac surgery.
- Must differentiate from left ventricular enlargement, altered position of the heart within the thorax, hyperkalemia, and ventricular pre-excitation.
- LAFB is considered a controversial entity in the cat.

Left Anterior Fascicular Block and Right Bundle Branch Block (Fig. 7)

- ECG Characteristics
  - QRS width greater than 0.07 seconds (dog) or 0.06 seconds (cat)
  - Left axis deviation
  - S waves deep and wide in leads I, II, III, aVF, and CV_6LU
  - Small Q and tall R in leads I and aVL
  - M-shaped QRS in lead CV_5RL
- Associated conditions: Same as for LAFB

Aberrant Conduction

- A premature beat is conducted through a bundle branch that is in an absolute or a relative refractory period.
- More common at slower heart rates or during sudden changes in R-R intervals. Aberrant complexes usually have an RBBB pattern, because of the longer refractory period of the right bundle branch cells.
- Aberrant beats are frequently confused with ventricular premature complexes (VPCs).
  - Look for P waves to differentiate the two.
  - An aberrantly conducted beat will have an associated P wave with a normal or slightly prolonged P-R interval.
  - VPCs do not have associated P waves with consistent P-R intervals. Refer to sec. 6, ch. 4 for further discussion.

Pre-excitation

- Anatomy. In some patients, accessory pathways exist that allow electrical impulses to bypass the AV node and go directly to the bundle of His or ventricular myocardium. Electrical impulses in these patients simultaneously go through the AV node. The bundles of Kent allow direct atrioventricular conduction. The James fibers bypass the AV node and connect to the bundle of His (Fig. 8).
- ECG characteristics. Electrical conduction through these accessory pathways is faster than through the AV node, resulting in a shortened P-R interval. If impulses are conducted over the bundles of Kent, the QRS complexes will be of longer duration and a delta wave will usually be present at the beginning of the complex (Fig. 9). The delta wave indicates the direct depolarization of the ventricular myocardium via the bypass tract. If the pre-excitation im-

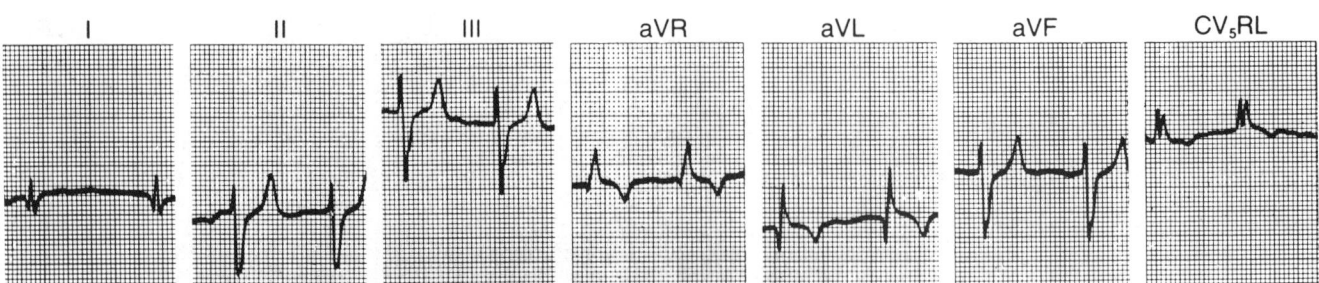

Figure 7. Left anterior fascicular block and right bundle branch block in a cat with hypertrophic cardiomyopathy. (From Tilley LP: *Essentials of Canine and Feline Electrocardiography,* 3rd ed. Philadelphia: Lea & Febiger, 1992.)

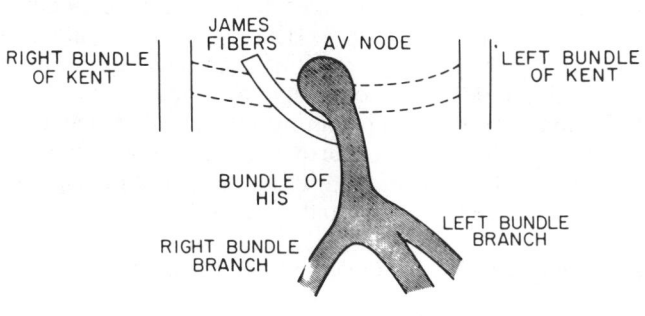

Figure 8. Anatomy of accessory pathways. (From Tilley LP: *Essentials of Canine and Feline Electrocardiography,* 3rd ed. Philadelphia: Lea & Febiger, 1992.)

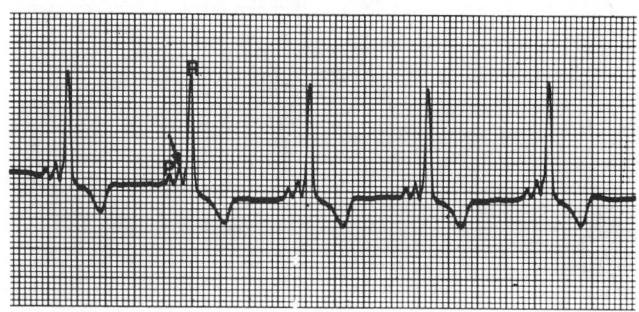

Figure 9. A dog with ventricular pre-excitation and a history of syncope. The arrow points out the delta wave. (From Tilley LP: *Essentials of Canine and Feline Electrocardiography,* 3rd ed. Philadelphia: Lea & Febiger, 1992.)

pulse is conducted by the James fibers, the P-R interval will be of short duration but the QRS complexes will be of normal duration with no delta waves. This finding is due to the impulses bypassing the AV node but still activating the ventricles through the bundle of His, the bundle branches, and the Purkinje system. P waves are normal, and a 1:1 relationship exists between P waves and QRS complexes. In most patients, no clinical symptomatology is associated with this conduction disturbance. However, re-entrant supraventricular tachycardia can develop in association with pre-excitation. These are discussed in sec. 6, ch. 4.

■ Associated conditions. Pre-excitation is often noted as a congenital finding without other evidence of organic heart disease. Pre-excitation may be seen in conjunction with other congenital cardiac diseases, such as atrial septal defect. In cats pre-excitation has been associated with hypertrophic cardiomyopathy.

Abnormalities of the QRS Complexes

■ Electrical alternans (Fig. 10)
  • Electrical alternans is a pattern of alternating configurations of the ECG complexes. The most common pattern is a variation in the height (taller:shorter) of the QRS complexes.
  • Electrical alternans is associated with a large pericardial effusion, a supraventricular tachycardia, and an alternating bundle branch block.

• Tachypnea (e.g., pleural effusion) can cause "pseudoalternans" when cardiac and respiratory rates are synchronized.
• Electrical alternans is not present in all cases of pericardial effusion.
■ Small complexes. Low amplitude complexes (R wave amplitude < 0.5 mv in lead II in dogs) may be a normal variant and may be associated with pericardial effusion, pleural effusion, pulmonary edema, hypothyroidism, obesity, pneumothorax, and hypoalbuminemia, and any cause of severe myocardial damage and loss of cardiac muscle mass.

Abnormalities of the S-T Segment

■ S-T elevation (dog > 0.15 mv in lead II, III, or aVF or those leads with dominant R waves) is seen with myocardial hypoxia, pericarditis, pericardial effusion, and digitalis toxicity.
■ Transmural myocardial infarction causes S-T segment elevation in leads overlying the infarcted myocardium.
■ S-T depression (dog > 0.2 mv in lead II, III, aVF, or those leads with dominant R waves) is seen with myocardial hypoxia, hyperkalemia or hypokalemia, and digitalis toxicity.
■ Subendocardial myocardial ischemia causes S-T segment depression in leads overlying the ischemic and infarcted myocardium.
■ Pseudodepression due to prominent T_a waves (atrial

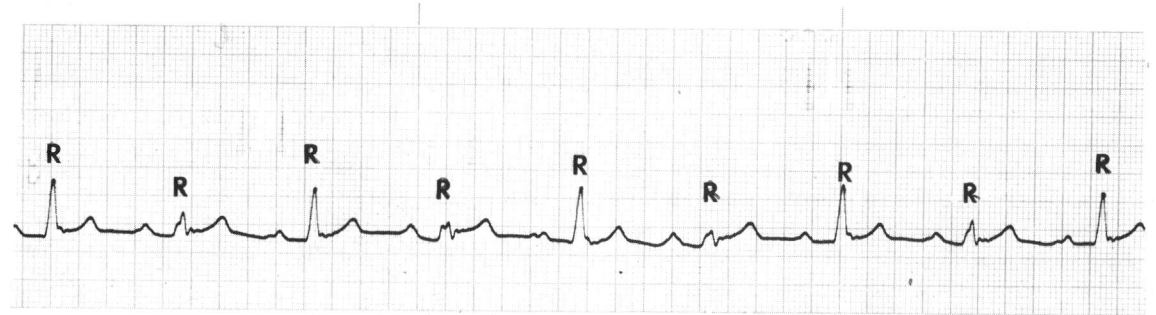

Figure 10. Electrical alternans in a dog with pericardial effusion.

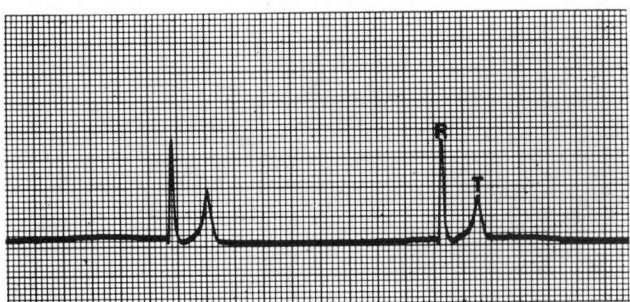

Figure 11. Atrial standstill and tall spiked T waves in a dog with severe hyperkalemia associated with Addison's disease.

repolarization) caused by atrial disease or tachycardia also causes S-T segment depression.

■ Miscellaneous S-T changes
  • S-T segment changes can occur secondary to bundle branch blocks, myocardial hypertrophy, and ventricular premature complexes. The changes in the S-T segment are in the opposite direction from the main QRS deflection. The S-T segment change in these conditions is often one of slurring or coving of the S wave into the T wave.
  • Artifact related to baseline motion
  • Normal variant

Abnormalities of the Q-T Interval

■ Q-T interval changes are relatively nonspecific. The Q-T interval is inversely related to the heart rate, being shorter with more rapid heart rates. As a general rule, the Q-T interval should be less than half the preceding R-R interval.
■ Q-T prolongation is associated with hypokalemia, hypocalcemia, hypothermia, quinidine administration, intraventricular conduction disturbance (associated with prolongation of the QRS complex), bradycardia, ethylene glycol toxicity, strenuous exercise, and central nervous system disturbance.
■ Q-T interval narrowing is associated with hypercalcemia, hyperkalemia, and digitalis administration.

Abnormalities Involving the T Waves

■ T wave changes are relatively nonspecific. In general, the T wave should not be more than one fourth the height of the associated R wave (Q or S wave, if either is larger than R), or more than 1.0 mv in any lead.
■ In most leads, normal T waves may be positive, negative, or biphasic.
■ Polarity should be consistent on serial electrocardiograms if HR is constant. T waves should be positive in CV$_5$RL in dogs over 2 months of age and negative in V$_{10}$, except in the Chihuahua.
■ Large T waves can be seen with myocardial hypoxia, intraventricular conduction disturbance, ventricular enlargement, hypothermia, and in animals with heart disease and bradycardia.
■ Large and sharply pointed (positive or negative) T waves are associated with hyperkalemia.

■ Small biphasic T waves can be seen with hypokalemia.
■ Nonspecific T wave changes can be seen secondary to metabolic disturbances (hypoglycemia, anemia, shock, fever), drug toxicities (digitalis, quinidine, procainamide), and neurologic disease.
■ T wave alternans (alternating positive and negative T waves) has been reported secondary to hypocalcemia, high levels of circulating catecholamines, and sudden increases in sympathetic tone.

Abnormalities of Electrolyte Derangements

The ECG is not very sensitive or specific in diagnosing systemic disturbances. However, it can be useful as a rapid screening test for certain electrolyte disturbances (predominantly moderate-to-severe hyperkalemia)

■ *Hyperkalemia.* ECG changes vary with the degree of hyperkalemia.
  • The earliest change is the development of sharply pointed (spiked) T waves (Fig. 11), followed by a reduction in the height of the P waves and prolongation of the P-R interval.
  • The QRS complexes then start to widen, and the P waves disappear (atrial standstill).
  • The QRS complexes become progressively wider and more bizarre in shape, and cardiac arrest or ventricular fibrillation follows.
  • AV block and escape beats may also be seen with hyperkalemia.
■ *Hypokalemia*
  • Q-T prolongation may develop along with prominent U waves. A U wave is a repolarization deflection of the Purkinje fibers that occurs after the T wave.
  • T waves may be small and notched.
  • The S-T segment becomes progressively depressed.
  • P-R prolongation and an increase in the height and width of the P and QRS complexes may be seen.
■ *Hypercalcemia*
  • Q-T interval may be shortened.
  • S-T segment shortening and depression have been reported.

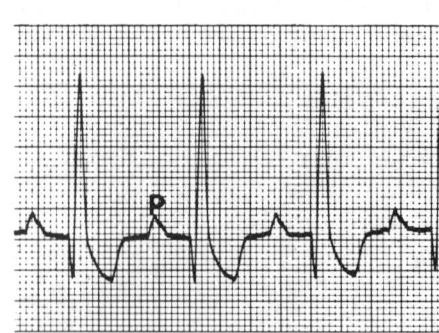

Figure 12. Wide and notched P waves in a dog with left atrial enlargement secondary to degenerative mitral valve disease. (From Tilley LP: *Essentials of Canine and Feline Electrocardiography,* 3rd ed. Philadelphia: Lea & Febiger, 1992.)

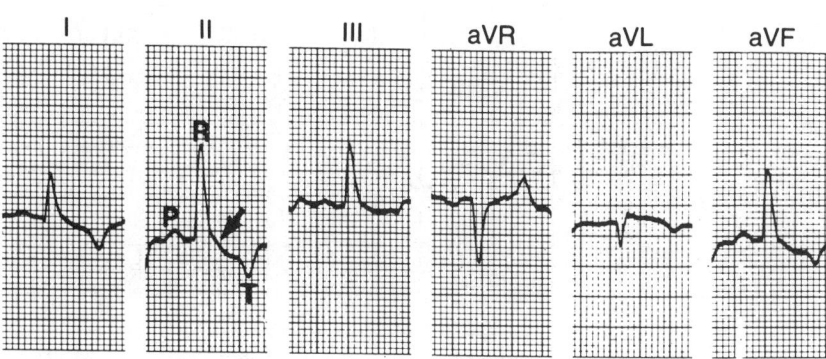

Figure 13. Tall and wide QRS complexes and S-T slurring indicate left ventricular enlargement in this cat with hypertrophic cardiomyopathy. (From Tilley LP: *Essentials of Canine and Feline Electrocardiography,* 3rd ed. Philadelphia: Lea & Febiger, 1992.)

■ *Hypocalcemia*
  • Q-T prolongation develops.
  • Duration of S-T segment correlates with the severity of hypocalcemia.
  • T wave alternans has been reported.
  • Deep wide T waves, tachycardia, and tall R waves may be present.

Heart Enlargement Patterns

■ Left atrial enlargement is characterized by wider than normal P waves in lead II (Fig. 12).
  • Dog and cat P > 0.04 seconds (> 0.05 seconds in giant breed dogs)
■ Left ventricular enlargement is characterized by one or more of the following (Fig. 13):
  • Left axis orientation (dog< +40°; cat<0°)
  • ST slurring or coving
  • QRS duration > 0.06 seconds (dog) or 0.04 seconds (cat)
  • Increased amplitude of the R waves
    Dog: R greater than 3.0 mv in leads II, aVF, V_6LU (V_4), CV_6LL (V_2), and CV_5RL (rV_2).
       R greater than 1.5 mv in lead I.
       Sum of R wave amplitude in leads I and aVF greater than 4.0 mv.
    Cat: CV_6LU (V_4): R > 1.0 mv
       Lead II or aVF: R > 0.9 mv
       V_{10}: R wave/Q wave > 1.0
■ Right atrial enlargement is characterized by taller than normal P waves in lead II (Fig. 14).
  • *Dog:* P > 0.4 mv (or prolonged P wave in some dogs)
  • *Cat:* P > 0.2 mv (may also indicate left atrial enlargement).

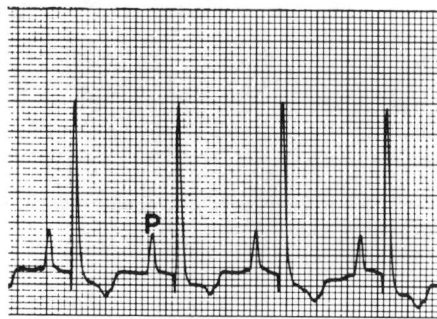

Figure 14. Tall P waves suggestive of right atrial enlargement. (From Tilley LP: *Essentials of Canine and Feline Electrocardiography,* 3rd ed. Philadelphia: Lea & Febiger, 1992.)

■ Right ventricular enlargement is characterized by one or more of the following (Fig. 15):
  • Right axis orientation (dog > + 100°; cat > +160°)
  • S wave in leads I, II, III, and aVF
  • S wave in lead I > 0.05 mv (dog)
  • Chest leads
    Dog: CV_6LL (V_2): S > 0.8 mv
       CV_6LU (V_4): S > 0.7 mv; R:S ratio < 0.87
       V_{10}: T positive (except Chihuahua) and W-shaped QRS complex
    Cat: Prominent S waves in CV_6LL (V_2) and CV_6LU (V_4)
       T positive in V_{10}

SPECIAL DIAGNOSTIC PROCEDURES
Post-Exercise ECG

Patients with suspected cardiac disease or arrhythmia, based on auscultation or history of syncope or exercise intolerance, may have normal resting ECGs. Sometimes, an arrhythmia can be documented by repeating an ECG after vigorous exercise. T wave changes or S-T segment abnormalities may become apparent following exercise, suggesting underlying myocardial disease.

Vagal Maneuvers

■ Indications
  • Vagal maneuvers are useful in evaluating supraventricular tachycardias and may terminate supraventricular tachycardia.
  • Vagal maneuvers may also help evaluate baroreceptor and sinus node functions.

Technique

1. While running a lead II rhythm strip, vigorously massage the carotid sinuses that are located under the mandible in the jugular furrow.
2. If this maneuver does not break the tachycardia, apply ocular pressure.
3. If still unsuccessful, apply ocular pressure along with carotid sinus massage.

■ Interpretation
  • If a supraventricular tachycardia breaks abruptly and the rhythm remains normal for at least a short time after stopping the vagal maneuver, the arrhythmia was probably re-entrant atrial (supraventricular) tachycardia.

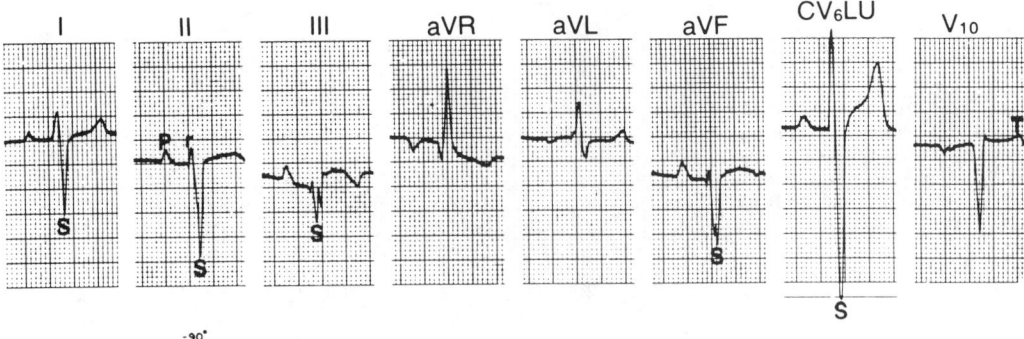

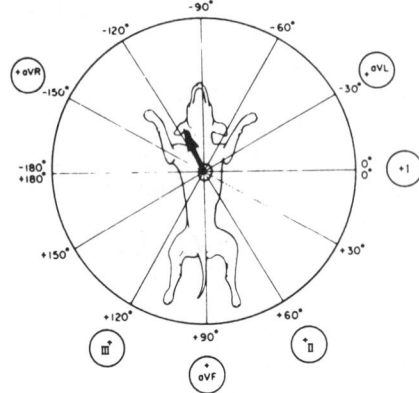

Figure 15. Marked right axis deviation in a dog with advanced heartworm disease and evidence of right sided heart failure. (From Tilley LP: *Essentials of Canine and Feline Electrocardiography*, 3rd ed. Philadelphia: Lea & Febiger, 1992.)

- If the rate gradually slows during the vagal maneuver and then speeds up again after the vagal maneuver, the rhythm is probably sinus tachycardia.
- If multiple P waves (> 300/minute) are observed, related to vagal-induced AV block, either atrial tachycardia or flutter is likely.
- If there is no change during the vagal maneuver, no conclusion can be made regarding the nature of the supraventricular tachycardia.
- Another area in which a vagal maneuver may be helpful is in trying to rule out a diagnosis of bradyarrhythmia as a cause of syncope.
- If the vagal maneuver results in prolonged periods of sinus arrest or produces AV block, this supports a diagnosis of sinus or AV nodal disease as a cause of syncope.

Holter Monitoring

In cases of syncope in which routine ECGs and laboratory evaluation do not confirm a diagnosis, a 24-hour Holter monitor recording can be useful in trying to rule out a diagnosis of intermittent arrhythmia. Holter monitoring is a specialized test that is offered through some veterinary cardiologists and sometimes can be arranged through a local medical cardiologist.

Lidocaine Response Test

Patients with sustained, wide complex tachycardia (ventricular tachycardia or atrial tachycardia with a bundle branch block) may be administered lidocaine (2 to 4 mg/kg IV) to help establish a diagnosis and to terminate the arrhythmia, if it is a lidocaine-responsive ventricular tachycardia. Occasionally, an atrial tachycardia will break following the administration of lidocaine.

Atropine Response Test

Patients with symptomatic bradyarrhythmia may be administered atropine (0.05 mg/kg IM or SC) and undergo an ECG 30 minutes later. This test is helpful in determining the role of vagal tone in the bradyarrhythmia and whether or not oral anticholinergic drugs (e.g., propantheline bromide and isopropamide iodide) might alleviate symptoms associated with the bradycardia, particularly if pacing is not an option.

Supplemental Readings

Bonagura JD: Cardiovascular diseases. *In* Sherding RG, ed.: *The Cat, Diseases and Clinical Management.* New York, Churchill Livingstone, 1989, p 649.

Edwards NJ: *Bolton's Handbook of Canine and Feline Electrocardiography,* 2nd ed. Philadelphia: W. B. Saunders, 1987.

Ettinger SJ, Suter PF: *Canine Cardiology.* Philadelphia: W. B. Saunders, 1970, p 102.

Harpster NK: The cardiovascular system. *In* Holzworth J, ed.: *Diseases of the Cat, Medicine and Surgery.* Philadelphia: W.B. Saunders, 1987, p 820.

Miller MS, Tilley LP: Electrocardiography. *In* Fox PR, ed.: *Canine and Feline Cardiology.* New York: Churchill Livingstone, 1988, p 43.

Tilley LP: *Essentials of Canine and Feline Electrocardiography.* 3rd ed. Philadelphia: Lea & Febiger, 1992.

Michael S. Miller
Larry Patrick Tilley
Francis W. K. Smith, Jr.

Cardiac arrhythmias include disorders of cardiac impulse formation, conduction, rate, and regularity. Terms such as dysrhythmia and ectopia also are used to identify arrhythmias. Cardiac arrhythmias can be benign and clinically insignificant, or they can cause clinical signs. They can even progress to malignant arrhythmias that lead to heart failure or sudden death.

Causes of cardiac arrhythmias include heart disease and disorders involving the autonomic nervous system, endocrine system, electrolytes, and other body systems. Cardiac arrhythmias are diagnosed and classified electrocardiographically; see sec. 6, ch. 3 for additional pertinent information.

ETIOLOGY

- Cardiac arrhythmias are classified in Table 1. They occur with congenital or acquired cardiac disease or systemic disorders (Table 2).
- Cardiac pathology does not necessarily correlate with the type and severity of arrhythmias.
- Arrhythmia variation in animals with cardiac or systemic disorders may be explained by the complex interactions among cardiac cell transmembrane potentials, the autonomic nervous system, and body fluids.

MECHANISM

- The normal cardiac impulse is generated automatically in the sinus node and is spread through the atria rapidly and sequentially via the His bundle, the bundle branches, and the intraventricular conduction system to the ventricular myocardium.
- The normal atrioventricular (AV) node serves as a bridge between the atria and the ventricles and slows the cardiac impulse prior to rapid impulse conduction through the ventricles.
- Reentry, a common arrhythmia mechanism, typically is caused by functional dissociation of cardiac tissue, unidirectional block in one pathway, and slowed conduction in the other pathway. The impulse then returns to the origination point by retrograde conduction through the unidirectionally blocked pathway.
- Triggered activity is caused by early or late afterdepolarizations.

DIAGNOSTIC APPROACH

Systematic Approach to the ECG Strip
(See Sec. 6, Ch. 3)

- Sinus rhythm or arrhythmia?
- Heart rate rapid, slow, or normal?
- Are P waves present?
  - Yes. Do the P (atria) waves occur at regular or irregular intervals? What is the height, width, direction?
  - No. What reason or abnormality explains the absence of the P wave? Is the P wave superimposed on a portion of the QRS complex, S-T segment, or T wave? Is the arrhythmia atrial standstill, atrial fibrillation, atrial flutter, AV junctional escape rhythm, or atrial tachycardia?
- Do the QRS (ventricular) complexes occur with regularity and uniformity? What is their morphology? If wide and bizarre, is this due to a ventricular arrhythmia or caused by a premature atrial impulse

TABLE 1. Classification of Cardiac Arrhythmias

Supraventricular Rhythms
Sinus rhythm
Sinus arrhythmia
Sinus bradycardia
Sinus tachycardia
Atrial premature complexes
Sinus block and/or arrest
Atrial tachycardia (reentrant)
Atrial flutter
Atrial fibrillation
Atrioventricular junctional rhythm

Ventricular Rhythms
Ventricular escape (rhythm)
Ventricular premature complexes
Idioventricular tachycardia
Ventricular tachycardia
Ventricular asystole
Ventricular fibrillation

Conduction Disorders
Atrial standstill
First-degree AV block
Second-degree AV block
Complete (third-degree) AV block

Arrhythmias and Conduction Disturbances
Sick sinus syndrome
Ventricular pre-excitation and the Wolff-Parkinson-White syndrome

TABLE 2. Causes of Cardiac Arrhythmias

Cardiac
Dogs
Heredity (genetics not documented in all cases)
   Doberman (His bundle degeneration)
   English springer spaniel (persistent atrial standstill)
   Miniature schnauzer, dachshund, cocker spaniel (sick sinus syndrome)
   Pug, Dalmatian (sinus node disease)
   Pug (stenosis and degeneration of the His bundle)
   Wolff-Parkinson-White syndrome
   Golden retriever (Duchenne muscular dystrophy)
   German shepherd (ventricular tachyarrhythmia)
Atrial and/or ventricular arrhythmias
   Atrial enlargement, secondary to congenital defects or acquired disease
   Cardiomyopathy
   Congenital heart disease
   Congestive heart failure
   Mitral valve disease (congenital and acquired)
   Myocarditis, endocarditis
   Myocardial ischemia
   Trauma
   Drugs
Conduction system disease
   Acquired sinus and AV node disease (sick sinus syndrome)
   Cardiomyopathy
   Neoplasia
   Surgical damage to conduction tissue
   Trauma
   Vascular (e.g., microscopic intramural myocardial infarction)
   Ventricular septal defect and other congenital defects
   Infection (Lyme disease)
   Drugs
   Degeneration
Cats
Heredity (rare)
   Wolff-Parkinson-White syndrome
Atrial and ventricular arrhythmias
   Cardiac enlargement secondary to congenital heart defects
   Cardiomyopathy
   Neoplasia
   Trauma
   Systemic diseases
Conduction system disease
   Cardiomyopathy
   Neoplasia
   Idiopathic fibrosis in older cats
Noncardiac
Dogs and Cats
Acidosis or alkalosis
Autonomic nervous system imbalance (parasympathetic or sympathetic); central nervous system (pain, excitement, fear); respiratory, gastrointestinal, organic brain disease
Drug toxicity (e.g., digitalis, preoperative sedatives, anesthetic agents, catecholamines, antiarrhythmic agents, bronchodilators)
Electrolyte disorders (hyperkalemia, hypercalcemia, hypokalemia, hypocalcemia, hypomagnesemia)
Endocrinopathies (hypothyroidism, hyperthyroidism, Addison's disease, pheochromocytoma)
Hypothermia
Hypovolemia
Hypoxia, anemia
Mechanical stimulation (cardiac catheterization, intravenous catheter)
Neoplasia
Shock
Toxemia, sepsis
Trauma

Adapted from Miller MS: Treatment of arrhythmias and conduction disturbances. *In* Tilley LP, Owens JM, eds.: *Manual of Small Animal Cardiology.* New York: Churchill Livingstone, 1985, with permission.

that is aberrantly conducted, or is bundle branch block evident?
■ What is the relationship between the P waves and the QRS complexes? Is the relationship consistent?
■ If AV dissociation is present, from where does the QRS complex evolve? Are AV junctional and/or Purkinje or idioventricular foci involved?

Questions to Be Answered in the Final Interpretation of Cardiac Arrhythmia

■ What is the possible mechanism for the arrhythmia?
■ Is it atrial, AV junctional, or ventricular in origin?
■ Is there a conduction abnormality?
■ What is the severity and frequency of the arrhythmia?

SUPRAVENTRICULAR RHYTHMS

Sinus Rhythm

Definition

■ Impulses originate in the sinus node.
■ The rhythm is regular with less than a 10% variation in the R-R interval.
■ There is a normal P wave for each QRS complex, with a constant P-R interval.
■ The heart rate is 60–180 beats per minute (bpm) in dogs and 120–240 bpm in cats.

Etiology and Clinical Significance

■ Sinus rhythm is a normal resting rhythm in dogs and cats and requires no therapy.
■ Animals with symptomatic cardiac disease or noncardiac disease may show a sinus rhythm.

Sinus Arrhythmia

Definition

■ Impulses originate in the sinus node.
■ The rhythm is irregular with more than a 10% variation in the R-R interval.
■ There is a normal P wave for each QRS complex, with a constant P-R interval.
■ A wandering pacemaker (change in morphology of the P wave due to a change in pacemaker location or conduction) is often present.
■ Heart rates are similar to sinus rhythm.

Etiology and Clinical Significance

■ Sinus arrhythmia is a normal rhythm variation in the resting dog, often correlated with varying levels of sinus node vagal tone, which changes with respiration (decreased vagal tone and increased heart rate during inspiration).
■ Sinus arrhythmia is unusual in cats.
■ Pronounced sinus arrhythmia occurs in the normal resting dog and in dogs and cats with respiratory disease.

Treatment

- No treatment is required unless there is symptomatic bradycardia, in which case anticholinergics may be helpful.

Sinus Bradycardia

Definition

- Impulses originate in the sinus node, but at a slower than normal frequency.
- The rhythm is regular.
- There is a normal P wave for each QRS complex, with a constant P-R interval.
- The heart rate is < 70 bpm in dogs (< 60 in giant breeds) and < 120 bpm in cats.

Etiology and Clinical Significance

- Sinus bradycardia may be a normal physiologic rhythm variation resulting from high levels of resting vagal tone.
- Hypothyroidism, sinus node disease (sick sinus syndrome), and hypothermia are pathologic causes of sinus bradycardia.
- Drugs that can cause a sinus bradycardia include acetylpromazine, xylazine, digoxin, propranolol, diltiazem, pilocarpine, and general anesthetics.
- Animals with sinus bradycardia are often asymptomatic.
- Clinical signs of weakness, lethargy, and syncope may accompany sinus bradycardia.

Treatment

- Asymptomatic dogs or cats require no specific therapy.
- When correlated with signs of weakness or syncope an atropine response test should be performed (0.04 mg/kg IM) followed by an ECG in 15 to 30 minutes.
  - If there is an increase in the cardiac rate following atropine administration, the animal may benefit from oral anticholinergic agents (Table 3).
  - A poor clinical response to atropine suggests the need for a temporary or permanent cardiac pacemaker.

- Congestive heart failure may also develop, in which case diuretics and vasodilators must be considered as adjunctive treatment. Digitalis may exacerbate the sinus arrest in these cases. Hypotension may develop from vasodilator therapy.

Sinus Block and/or Sinus Arrest (Fig. 1)

Definition

- A primary disorder of the sinus node resulting in lack of generation of the cardiac impulse or its poor propagation across surrounding tissue.
- It is not possible to distinguish between sinus block and arrest in dogs because of the normal variation in the R-R interval (sinus arrhythmia).
- The heart rate is variable and is often correlated with a bradycardia or slow sinus arrhythmia.
- The rhythm is regularly irregular or irregular with pauses.
- There is a normal P wave for each QRS complex with a pause equal to or greater than two times the normal R-R interval.
- The P wave may vary in shape if a concurrent wandering pacemaker is present.

Etiology and Clinical Significance

- Sinus arrest may be consistent with an increase in vagal tone (e.g., ocular pressure, irritation of the vagus nerve, brachycephalic breeds).
- Pathology of the atria including fibrosis, cardiomyopathy, neoplasia, and drug toxicity (e.g., digitalis, propranolol, quinidine, xylazine, and acetylpromazine) may result in sinus arrest.
- Sinus arrest is one of the arrhythmias in the sick sinus syndrome.

ECG Differentials

- Sinus block and/or sinus arrest can be confused with marked sinus arrhythmia and sinus bradycardia and nonconducted atrial premature complexes (APCs).

Treatment

- Treat the same as sinus bradycardia.

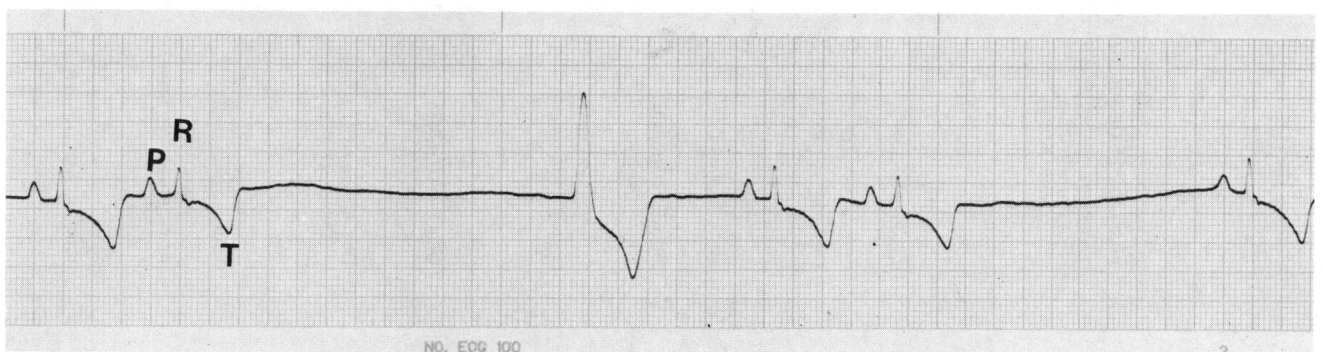

Figure 1. Sinus block and/or arrest with a ventricular escape beat, dog. (Selected arrhythmias; lead II rhythm strips; paper speed 50 mm/sec; 1 cm = 1 mV.)

TABLE 3. Common Antiarrhythmic Drugs

Generic Drug (Trade Name)	Formulation	Indications	Dosage for Dogs (D) and Cats (C)	Comments
Atenolol (Tenormin)	Tab: 25, 50, 100 mg	Atrial and ventricular arrhythmias, hypertrophic cardiomyopathy, hypertension	D: 0.25–1.0 mg/kg PO, q12h–q24h C: 6.25–12.5 mg q24h	Less bronchoconstriction, vasoconstriction, and interference with insulin therapy than with propranolol Taper dose when discontinuing therapy Decrease dose with renal disease
Atropine sulfate*	Inj: 0.1, 0.4, 0.5 mg/ml	Sinus bradycardia, AV block, SSS	D: 0.02 mg/kg IV; 0.045 mg/kg IM, SC q6h–q8h C: Same as D	May transiently worsen bradyarrhythmia More potent chronotropic effects than glycopyrrolate
Digitoxin* (Crystodigin)	Tab: 0.05, 0.1 mg	Supraventricular arrhythmias, myocardial failure	D: 0.033 mg/kg PO; small dogs q8h; large dogs q12h C: None	GI side effects less common than with digoxin Dose based on total body weight Toxicity potentiated by hypokalemia, hyponatremia, hypercalcemia, thyroid disorders, hypoxia Preferred to digoxin in renal failure
Digoxin* (Cardoxin, Lanoxin)	Tab: 0.125, 0.25, 0.5 mg Inj: 0.25 mg/ml Elixir: 0.05 mg/ml, 0.15 mg/ml Cap: 0.05, 0.1, 0.2 mg	Supraventricular arrhythmias, myocardial failure	D: 0.22 mg/M^2 q12h PO; 0.0055–0.01 mg/kg q12h PO; 0.01 mg/kg IV in divided dose 2 hours apart C: 0.01 mg/kg every other day (Tab preferred); 0.007 mg/kg every other day (with lasix and aspirin)	Toxicity potentiated by hypokalemia, hyponatremia, hypercalcemia, thyroid disorders, hypoxia Base dose on lean body weight; reduce dose 10–15% with elixirs Therapeutic range 1–2.4 ng/ml; 8 hours after dose Rapid digitalization not recommended except in emergency Reduce dose 50% with quinidine
Diltiazem (Cardizem)	Tab: 30, 60, 90, 120 mg	Supraventricular arrhythmias, hypertrophic cardiomyopathy, hypertension	D: 0.5–1.5 mg/kg q8h PO (titrate up to effect) C: 0.5–2.5 mg/kg q8h PO	Less myocardial depression than verapamil
Dobutamine HCl (Dobutrex)	Inj: 12.5 mg/ml	Short-term management of severe myocardial failure and brady-arrhythmias not responsive to atropine	D: 5–20 µg/kg/min (titrate up to effect); administer in D5W C: 2–5 µg/kg/min (titrate up to effect); administer in D5W	Monitor ECG, BP, and pulse quality Preferable to dopamine in CHF but more expensive Inotropic effect is dose dependent Less arrhythmigenic than most other catecholamines Intermittent use may result in sustained improvement
Epinephrine* (Adrenalin)	Inj: 1:1000 conc (1 mg/ml) 1:10000 conc (0.1 mg/ml)	Cardiac arrest	D: 0.2 mg/kg q3–5 min IV; double dose for IT administration C: Same as D	Monitor with ECG
Isoproterenol* (Isuprel)	Inj: 1:5000 (0.2 mg/ml)	Short-term management of sinus bradycardia, AV block, SSS	D: 0.04–0.09 µg/kg/min IV; 0.1–0.2 mg q4–6h IM SC C: Same as D	Expand volume with fluids to prevent hypotension

Drug	Preparations	Indications	Dosage	Comments
Lidocaine* (Xylocaine)	Inj: 5, 10, 15, 20 mg/ml (without epinephrine)	Ventricular arrhythmias	D: 2–8 mg/kg slowly IV in 2 mg/kg boluses followed by IV drip at 30–80 μg/kg/min CRI C: 0.25–1 mg/kg IV over 5 min	Drug of choice for initial control of ventricular tachycardia in dogs Use with caution in cats Effects increased by high potassium and decreased by low potassium Seizures controlled with diazepam Do not use formulations with epinephrine for arrhythmia control
Procainamide* (Procan SR, Pronestyl)	Cap: 250, 375, 500 mg Tab: 250, 375, 500 mg Tab SR: 250, 500, 750, 1000 mg Inj: 100, 500 mg/ml	Ventricular and supraventricular arrhythmias, WPW syndrome	D: 8–20 mg/kg IM q6h (SR q8h) 2 mg/kg IV over 3–5 min up to total dose of 20 mg/kg; 20–50 μg/kg/min CRI C: 3–8 mg/kg q8h IM or PO	Beware of hypotension with q6h dosage (switch to q8h) Effects increased by high potassium and decreased by low potassium Monitor ECG: 25% prolongation of QRS is sign of toxicity Fewer GI and CV side effects than quinidine Use with caution in cats Reduce dose with severe renal disease
Propanthelline bromide* (Pro-Banthine)	Tab: 7.5, 15 mg	Sinus bradycardia, AV block, SSS	D: small: 7.5 mg q8h PO; medium: 15 mg q8h PO; large: 30 mg q8h PO C: 7.5 mg SID-TID PO	
Propranolol* (Inderal)	Tab: 10, 20, 40, 60, 80, 90 mg Inj: 1 mg/ml	Atrial and ventricular arrhythmias, hypertrophic cardiomyopathy, hypertension, thyrotoxicosis	D: 0.2–1.0 mg/kg q8h PO; 0.02–0.06 mg/kg slowly IV C: <4.5 kg—2.5–5 mg q8h–q12h PO; >4.5 kg—5mg q8h–q12h PO; 0.02–0.06 mg/kg IV slowly	Nonselective blocker Start with low dose and titrate to effect Taper dose when discontinuing therapy
Quinidine gluconate* (Quinaglute Dura-tabs)	Tab: 324 mg Inj: 80 mg/ml	Ventricular and supraventricular arrhythmias, WPW syndrome, conversion of atrial fibrillation	D: 8–20 mg/kg q6h PO, IM; 8–20 mg/kg q8h PO with sustained release products; 5–10 mg/kg IV very slowly C: None	Decrease digoxin dose 50% with quinidine Effects increased by high potassium and decreased by low potassium Monitor ECG: 25% prolongation of QRS is sign of toxicity Has vagolytic, negative inotropic and vasodilating properties Hypotension is frequent with IV administration Reduce dose in CHF, hepatic disease, and hypoalbuminemia
Tocainide (Tonocard)	Tab: 400, 600 mg	Ventricular arrhythmias	D: 10–20 mg/kg q8h PO C: None	Oral analog of lidocaine Giving with food may decrease GI upset or neurologic side effects
Verapamil* (Calan, Isoptin)	Tab: 80, 120, 240 mg Inj: 2.5 mg/ml	Supraventricular arrhythmias, hypertrophic cardiomyopathy	D: 0.05–0.2 mg/kg IV slowly (5–10 min) in boluses of 0.05 mg/kg; 1–3 mg/kg q6h–q8h PO C: Same as D	Diltiazem is safer alternative in heart failure Potent vasodilator and negative inotrope

*Available in generic preparation.
Tab = tablets; Inj = injection; Cap = capsule; AV = atrioventricular; SSS = sick sinus syndrome; WPW = Wolff-Parkinson-White; GI = gastrointestinal; CV = cardiovascular; IT = intratracheal; CRI = constant rate infusion.

Sinus Tachycardia

Definition

- Impulses originate in the sinus node, but at a faster than normal frequency.
- The rhythm is regular.
- There are normal P waves for each QRS complex.
- The heart rate is > 140 bpm in the giant breeds, 180 bpm in toy breed dogs, and 240 bpm in cats.

Etiology and Clinical Significance

- Sinus tachycardia may be a normal physiologic rhythm variation resulting from high sympathetic tone occurring with exercise or excitement.
- Sinus tachycardia may also occur with conditions such as stress, anxiety, pain, shock, fever, anemia, congestive heart failure, hyperthyroidism, and pheochromocytoma.
- Drugs (atropine, sympathomimetic agents, ketamine, diazepam, and light anesthesia also can cause sinus tachycardia.

ECG Differentials

- Other supraventricular tachyarrhythmias confused with sinus tachycardia include paroxysmal (atrial or AV junctional) tachycardia, atrial flutter with 2:1 AV block, and ventricular tachycardia when sinus tachycardia is associated with wide QRS complexes.
- A vagal maneuver (e.g., carotid sinus or ocular stimulation for 5–10 seconds) may result in a transient, gradual slowing of the sinus tachycardia.

Treatment

- Identify and treat the underlying cause of the sinus tachycardia.
- Antiarrhythmic drugs are seldom required.
- Administer propranolol (2.5 mg q8–12h PO) to hyperthyroid cats with intractable tachycardia (i.e., unresponsive to antithyroid medication).
- Administer digitalis for sinus tachycardia in congestive heart failure. Digoxin will reestablish normal baroreceptor function and lessen sympathetic tone.

Atrial Premature Complexes (Fig. 2)

Definition

- Impulses originate from an atrial focus, often other than the sinus node.

- The rhythm is irregular and the heart rate varies with the sinus node rate.
- There is usually an abnormal P′ wave (premature P wave) followed by a normal QRS complex; the P′-R interval of the APC may vary from the sinus rhythm P-R interval. The P′ wave may have various morphologies and may be fused with the T wave of the preceding beat.
- The P′ wave may occur so early in the cardiac cycle that the AV conduction system will be refractory, and the impulse will not be conducted to the ventricles (e.g., APC with physiologic AV block).
- The pause following the APC is often less than fully compensatory, because of premature depolarization and resetting of the sinus node. Full compensatory pause occurs when the R wave–to–R wave interval surrounding the APC is equal to two normal R-R intervals.
- The QRS complex is usually normal, but the intraventricular conduction system may be, in a relative or absolute refractory period, causing a bizarre (abnormal shape or direction) QRS complex. This abnormality is termed an APC with aberrant ventricular conduction.

Etiology and Clinical Significance

- APCs often indicate underlying cardiac disease (e.g., chronic valvular fibrosis, cardiomyopathy, congenital defect, cor pulmonale).
- Other causes include electrolyte disturbances, thyrotoxicosis, hypoxia, anemia, drug toxicity (e.g., digitalis, dobutamine, dopamine), toxemia, and increased sympathetic tone.

ECG Differentials

- Sinus rhythm with APCs may be confused with marked sinus arrhythmia and VPCs during auscultation, and with VPCs on the ECG, when aberrant ventricular conduction follows an APC.
- A P′ wave preceding the abnormal QRS complex and a similarity of the initial deflection of the QRS complex compared with a preceding normal beat supports the diagnosis of aberrant conduction.

Treatment

- Infrequent APCs may be a normal variation and do not require treatment.

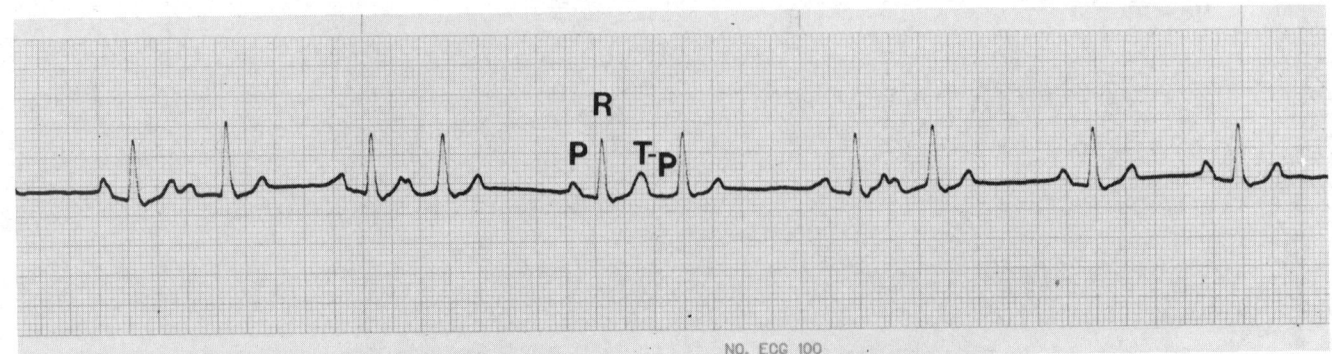

Figure 2. Atrial premature complexes, dog. (Selected arrhythmias; lead II rhythm strips; paper speed 50 mm/sec; 1 cm = 1 mV.)

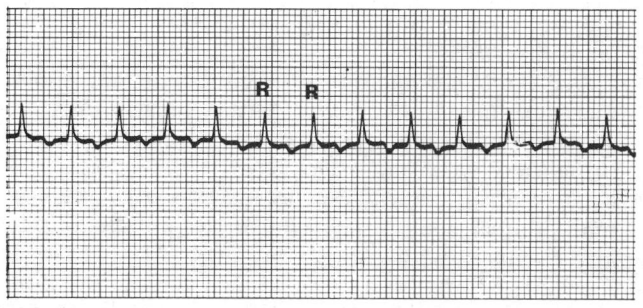 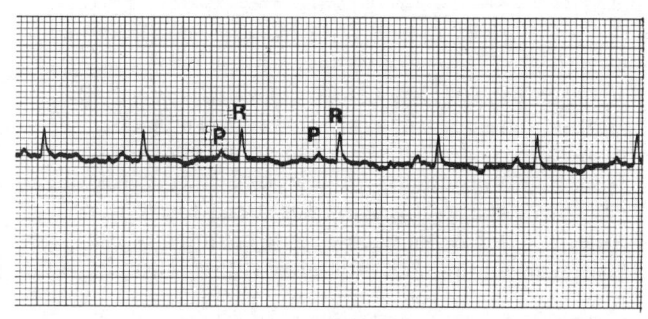

Figure 3. Paroxysmal atrial tachycardia (left) and after termination by a vagal maneuver (right), cat. (Selected arrhythmias; lead II rhythm strips; paper speed 50 mm/sec; 1 cm = 1 mV.)

- If this arrhythmia is correlated with congestive heart failure, treat the arrhythmia with digoxin.
- If the APCs are correlated with poor hemodynamic status without myocardial failure, prescribe digoxin, diltiazem, or propranolol (see Table 3).

Atrial Tachycardia (Figs. 3 and 4)

Definition

- Atrial tachycardia indicates rapid, abnormal impulses originating from an atrial site other than the sinus node.
- The atrium and/or AV junctional areas may be involved in a reentrant circuit that allows the impulse to restimulate the atrium as well as to pass to the ventricles. (A vagal maneuver may abolish this arrhythmia.)
- An abnormal automatic focus in the atrium may also be responsible for this arrhythmia (a vagal maneuver will cause AV block but not abolish the atrial tachycardia).
- The heart rate is > 140–180 bpm in dogs, > 240 bpm in cats and often approaches 300 bpm.
- The rhythm is usually regular but may be slightly irregular.
- There is a P' wave for each QRS complex, although the P' wave is usually of different morphology than the sinus P wave. The P-R interval is constant.
- The P' wave may not be evident because it may be fused with the preceding T wave or occur simultaneously with the preceding QRS complex.
- The QRS complex may also be of different morphology because of aberrant ventricular conduction.

- An irregular R-R interval may be caused by concurrent AV block or by multifocal atrial tachycardia (P' waves varying in shape; firing of two or more ectopic atrial foci).

Etiology and Clinical Significance

- Atrial tachycardia suggests severe myocardial or conduction system disease.
- This arrhythmia also may be secondary to digitalis toxicity or may occur under general anesthesia.
- Systemic disease that results in autonomic nervous systemic abnormalities also may be a cause.
- In cats, this arrhythmia is correlated with feline cardiomyopathy and hyperthyroidism.

Differential Diagnosis

- Atrial tachycardia can be confused with sinus tachycardia, AV junctional tachycardia, and atrial flutter.
- A vagal maneuver may abruptly terminate AV nodal reentry or cause transient AV block with atrial tachycardia or atrial flutter (P waves of flutter waves can then be identified on the baseline).

Treatment

- Sustained (nonparoxysmal) atrial tachycardia often is associated with weakness, hypotension, congestive heart failure, and syncope and requires immediate therapy.
- A vagal maneuver (ocular pressure or carotid sinus pressure; see sec. 6, ch. 3) may terminate a reentrant atrial tachycardia.

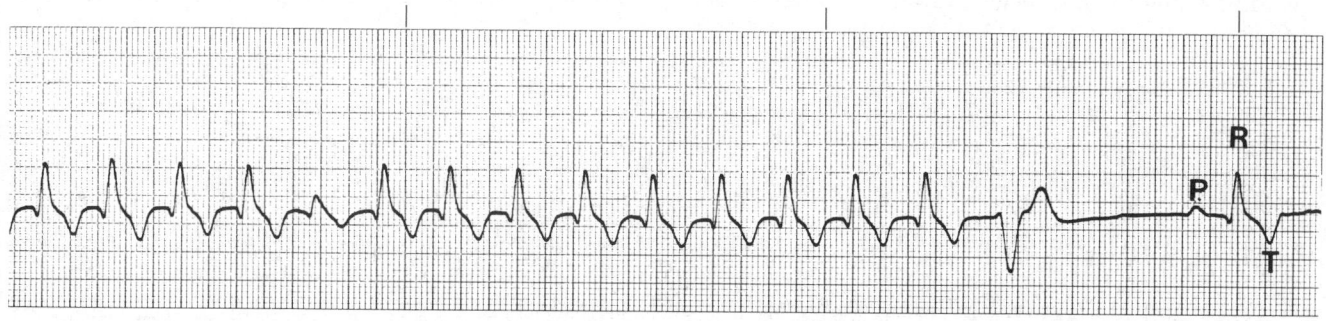

NO. ECG 100

Figure 4. Paroxysmal atrial tachycardia terminated after a ventricular premature complex, dog. (Selected arrhythmias; lead II rhythm strips; paper speed 50 mm/sec; 1 cm = 1 mV.)

- If congestive heart failure is present, administer digitalis for the arrhythmia. Intravenous digoxin, given cautiously, may slow the ventricular response and improve the clinical status (see Table 3).
- If digoxin is ineffective, intravenous adenosine, verapamil, diltiazem, or propranolol may convert supraventricular tachycardia (or atrial tachycardia) to sinus rhythm or slow the ventricular response rate. Use propranolol and verapamil with caution because they may decrease cardiac contractility and exacerbate congestive heart failure.
- For atrial tachycardia without congestive heart failure, initiate therapy with adenosine, verapamil, propranolol, or diltiazem.
- Intramuscular quinidine gluconate also has been used to convert atrial tachycardia to normal sinus rhythm in dogs with refractory atrial tachycardia.
- Reserve electrical cardioversion for refractory cases, to be administered only by an experienced veterinary cardiologist possessing the proper equipment.

Atrial Fibrillation (Fig. 5)

Definition

- A high number of disorganized atrial impulses, caused by a disorder of reentry within the atria, bombard the AV node, leading to an irregular rhythm.
- Many of these impulses approach the AV node in a refractory period and are not conducted to the ventricles, or they affect the conduction of subsequent impulses (concealed conduction).
- The heart rate is usually rapid (often > 180 bpm in dogs, and > 240 bpm in cats), and the rhythm is irregular.

KEY POINT ▶ The lack of P waves and an irregularly irregular rhythm on all ECG leads and an arterial pulse deficit are the hallmarks of atrial fibrillation.

- No P waves are seen, but there are normally shaped QRS complexes. Instead of P waves, small or large oscillations (f waves) are present.
- There may be some variation and widening of the QRS complexes due to aberrant ventricular conduction or bundle branch block.

Etiology and Clinical Significance

- Atrial fibrillation commonly occurs in patients with cardiomyopathy, advanced chronic valvular heart disease, pericarditis, and progressive congenital heart disease.
- Other etiologies include severe ischemia or shock (gastric dilatation/volvulus, after cardiac arrest), atrial tumor (hemangiosarcoma), and electrolyte disturbances (hyperkalemia).
- Loss of atrial contraction decreases the stroke volume and cardiac output. The rapid ventricular rate also results in poor cardiac output.
- Slow atrial fibrillation (< 100 bpm) may signify drug toxicity (e.g., digitalis), concurrent AV block, or low sympathetic tone (most often observed in giant breed dogs without CHF).

Differential Diagnosis

- Atrial fibrillation can be confused with frequent APCs, AV junctional tachycardia with AV block, atrial tachycardia with AV block, and atrial flutter with AV block.
- Atrial flutter usually shows a regular R-R interval, and the atrial oscillations (F waves) are larger than f waves.

Treatment

- Give digoxin (see Table 3) to slow the ventricular response. Rarely, a sinus rhythm will return.
- After approximately 3–7 days, if the ventricular rate is not controlled, add propranolol (begin with 0.2 mg/kg q8h) or diltiazem (begin with 0.5 mg/kg q8h) and increase the dose slowly until the resting ventricular rate is adequately controlled (< 140–160 bpm).
- Although it is unusual to convert atrial fibrillation to normal sinus rhythm in dogs, the antiarrhythmic drug quinidine or calcium channel blockers (verapamil, diltiazem) may be useful for this purpose. A normal-sized heart, recent onset of atrial fibrillation, and lack of congestive heart failure favor the use of quinidine. Use quinidine with caution because it may increase the ventricular response rate.
- Reserve electrical cardioversion for refractory cases without severe cardiomegaly. This requires experienced personnel and proper equipment.

Atrioventricular Junctional Rhythm

Definition

- Impulses are generated in the AV junctional tissue and spread backward (retrograde) through the atrium and forward (antegrade) to the ventricles.

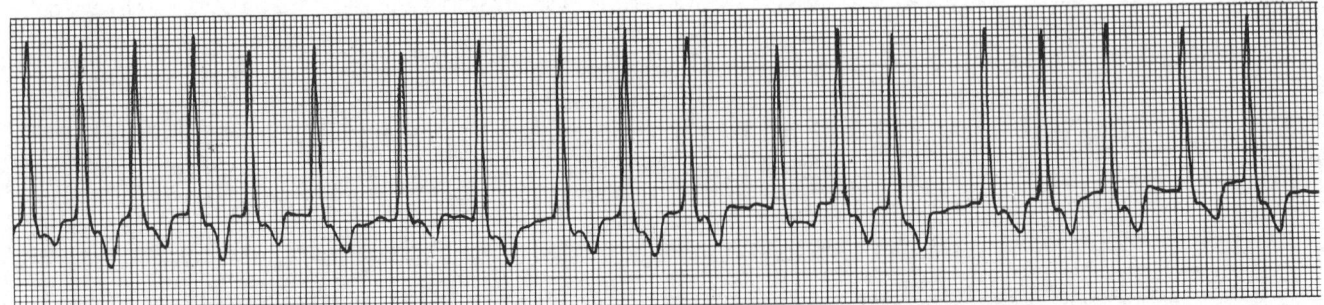

Figure 5. Atrial fibrillation, dog. (Selected arrhythmias; lead II rhythm strips; paper speed 50 mm/sec; 1 cm = 1 mV.)

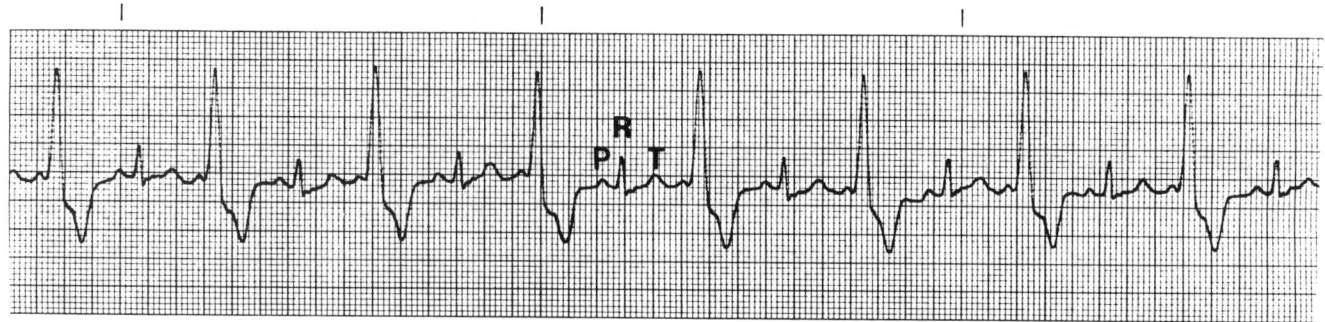

Figure 6. Ventricular premature complexes, cat. (Selected arrhythmias; lead II rhythm strips; paper speed 50 mm/sec; 1 cm = 1 mV.)

- The heart rate (usually > 60 bpm) varies with the mechanism; i.e., a passive escape rhythm (60 bpm) versus an enhanced AV junctional rhythm (> 60 bpm but < 100 bpm) versus a junctional tachycardia (> 100 bpm in the dog).
- The rhythm usually is regular.
- The negative P′ wave may occur before, during, or after the normal QRS complex. The P′-R or R-P′ interval is constant.
- The P′ wave location depends on the area of impulse generation and relative speed of retrograde conduction through the atrium compared with antegrade conduction through the AV node, His bundle, and ventricular conduction system.

Etiology and Clinical Significance

- Digitalis toxicity may cause an AV junctional rhythm. When abnormally rapid, this arrhythmia is difficult to distinguish from atrial tachycardia.
- An AV junctional escape rhythm may occur in patients with depressed sinus node function, as in the sick sinus syndrome.
- Myocarditis may be associated with an enhanced AV junctional rhythm or AV junctional tachycardia.

Differential Diagnosis

- AV junctional rhythm can be confused with atrial standstill and slow atrial fibrillation.

Treatment

- Usually no treatment is needed and the rhythm reverts spontaneously.

- If weakness or syncope is associated with a slow AV junctional rhythm, atropine, dobutamine, or isoproterenol may be used in an attempt to accelerate the sinus node in order to help regain function as the primary pacemaker.
- Oral anticholinergic agents also may be useful for chronic therapy.
- If congestive heart failure is present with an enhanced AV junctional rhythm, prescribe digitalis.

VENTRICULAR RHYTHMS

Ventricular Premature Complexes (VPCs)
(Figs. 6–8)

Definition

- Ectopic impulses originate from a focus below the AV node and AV junction.
- The heart rate is variable, depending on the frequency of VPCs; the rhythm is irregular.
- VPCs are usually related (coupled) to normal beats. If a VPC is not coupled to a normal beat, the origination site is referred to as a parasystolic focus.
- Usually there is a full compensatory pause following a VPC.
- Interpolated VPCs occur between normal beats and are not usually followed by a full compensatory pause.
- P waves that are seen are normal in shape, but are not associated with the QRS complex of the VPCs. The QRS complex often is wide and bizarre.
- If the major deflection of the QRS complex is negative in lead II, the ectopic focus likely is in the

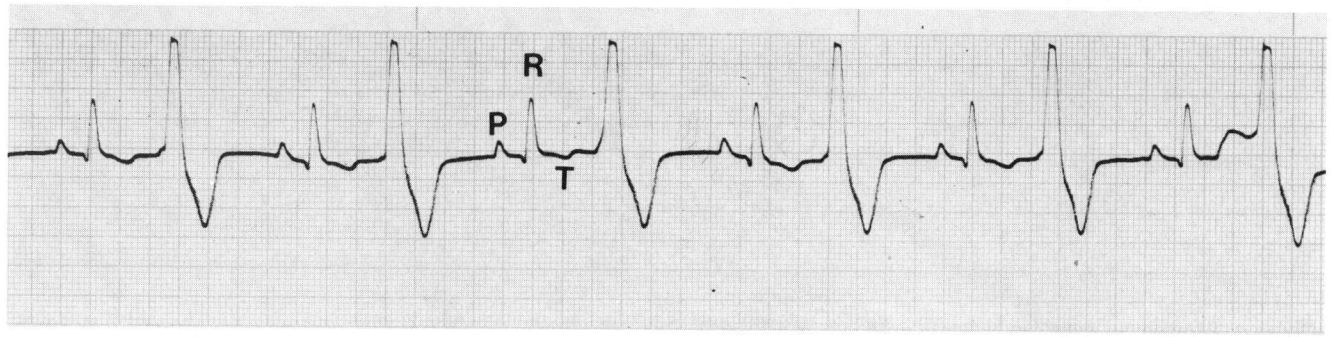

Figure 7. Ventricular premature complexes, dog. (Selected arrhythmias; lead II rhythm strips; paper speed 50 mm/sec; 1 cm = 1 mV.)

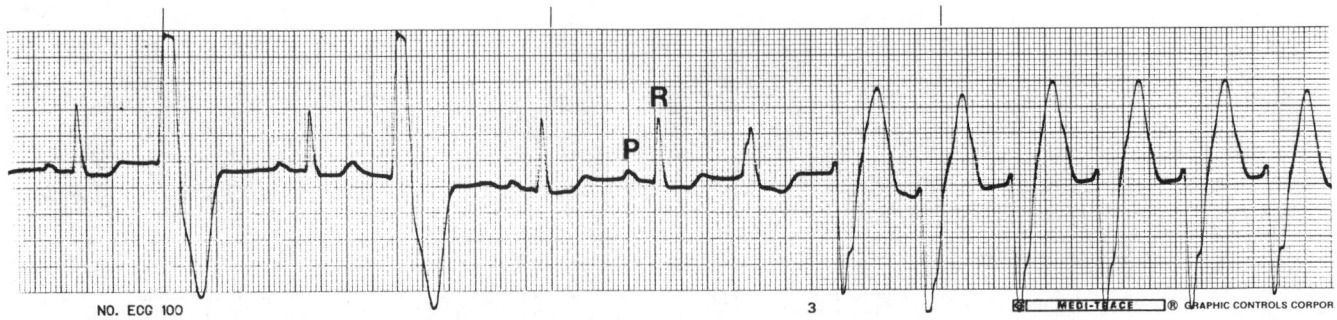

Figure 8. Sinus rhythm with ventricular premature complexes (right ventricular foci) and paroxysmal ventricular tachycardia (left ventricular foci), dog. (Selected arrhythmias; lead II rhythm strips; paper speed 50 mm/sec; 1 cm = 1 mV.)

left ventricle; if the major deflection is positive in lead II, the ectopic focus probably is in the right ventricle.

Etiology and Clinical Significance

- The ventricular arrhythmia may be due to cardiac disease (e.g., congestive heart failure, myocarditis, endocarditis).
- Secondary causes of VPCs include trauma, electrolyte disturbances, autonomic changes, hypoxia, systemic infections, ischemia, and drug toxicosis.
- Frequent VPCs may lead to hypotension, shock, or congestive heart failure.
- Frequent VPCs or VPCs occurring during the preceding Q-T interval may be electrically unstable (depending on underlying heart disease) and may progress to ventricular tachycardia and/or fibrillation and sudden death.
- A 24-hour tape-recorded (Holter) ECG may be necessary to assess a ventricular arrhythmia.

Differential Diagnosis

- VPCs can be confused with atrial premature complexes with aberrant ventricular conduction and right or left bundle branch block.

Treatment

- VPCs do not always require antiarrhythmic therapy.
- Antiarrhythmic therapy is recommended for:
  - Frequent symptomatic VPCs (greater than 20–30 per minute)

- Repetitive complexes or runs of VPCs
- Multifocal QRS configurations
- R on T phenomena (vulnerable period for development of ventricular fibrillation), in which the VPC occurs during the Q-T interval of the previous complex
- Associated clinical signs of poor cardiac output (e.g., weakness, dyspnea, syncope)
- Do not treat ventricular escape complexes (similar to VPC configuration but at the end of pauses) because they represent a safety mechanism for maintaining cardiac output.
- Antiarrhythmic drugs commonly used to control VPCs include intravenous lidocaine and parenteral or oral procainamide, quinidine, tocainide, propranolol, and phenytoin (for digitalis-induced VPCs).

Ventricular Tachycardia (Figs. 8, 9, and 10)

Definition

- Impulses are repetitively generated (greater than 3 VPCs in a row) from one or more ventricular foci.
- This arrhythmia may be paroxysmal or sustained.
- The rate usually is >100 bpm in dogs, and >150 bpm in cats.
- The rhythm is regular unless the arrhythmia is intermittent or variable exit block (Purkinje cells to ventricular myocardium) is present.
- The P waves that are seen are normal in shape but have no fixed relationship to wide and bizarre QRS complexes.
- A sustained ventricular rhythm slower than the above rates is termed an idioventricular rhythm.

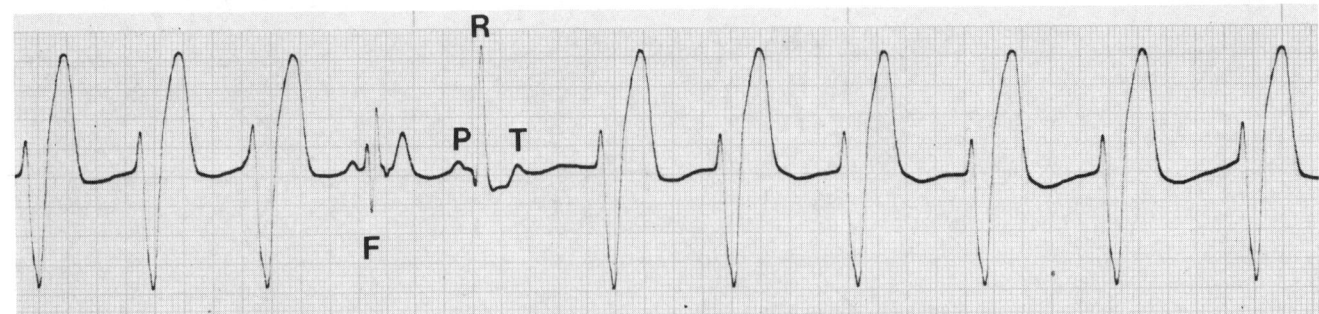

Figure 9. Paroxysmal ventricular tachycardia (fusion beat-F), dog. (Selected arrhythmias; lead II rhythm strips; paper speed 50 mm/sec; 1 cm = 1 mV.)

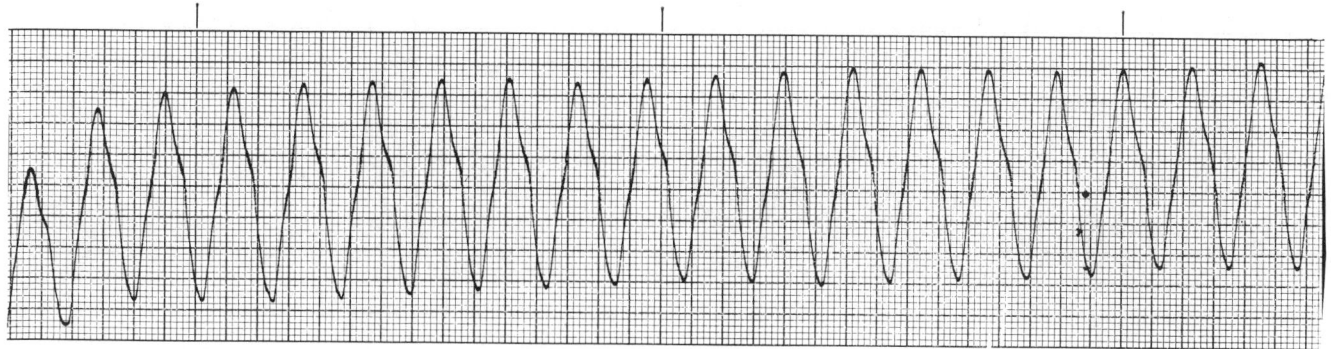

Figure 10. Ventricular tachycardia-flutter, dog. (Selected arrhythmias; lead II rhythm strips; paper speed 50 mm/sec; 1 cm = 1 mV.)

Etiology and Clinical Significance

KEY POINT ▶ Ventricular tachycardia is a life-threatening arrhythmia that, if sustained, may lead to hypotension, myocardial ischemia, syncope or seizures, shock, and sudden death.

- Some patients with ventricular tachycardia show no clinical signs, especially if there is no underlying primary cardiac disease.
- All etiologies of VPCs (e.g., primary and secondary cardiac disease) may lead to a ventricular tachycardia.

Differential Diagnosis

- Ventricular tachycardia can be confused with sinus tachycardia, atrial tachycardia, or atrial fibrillation with a conduction disturbance (e.g., left or right bundle branch block).

Treatment

- Antiarrhythmic therapy is required in most patients with sustained ventricular rhythms. Exceptions include patients with:
  - Complete heart block in which the ventricular rhythm may be an escape mechanism
  - "Slow" ventricular rhythms (also called idioventricular tachycardias in which the ectopic rate is <100 bpm and the rhythm alternates with the sinus rhythm)
- Severe acid-base or electrolyte disturbances, such as hypokalemia or hyperkalemia, which may respond to specific electrolyte or fluid therapy
- Lidocaine hydrochloride without epinephrine (2–3 mg/kg) via slow IV administration is the initial preferred treatment in the dog.
  - This drug may also be used in the cat (initial bolus of 0.25 mg/kg slow IV); beware of seizures.
  - Administer diazepam IV for seizures.
  - Hypotension also may occur if the bolus is administered too rapidly.
- If necessary, repeat the lidocaine bolus several times at 10 minute intervals, although the higher dosages will increase the incidence of toxicity.
- The maximum total dose for dogs is 8 mg/kg. Seizures and vomiting may occur in dogs at toxic doses.
- The therapeutic effect of lidocaine is short-term, and repeat boluses or constant-rate infusion may be required for a sustained antiarrhythmic effect. To calculate the amount of lidocaine to be added to fluids IV over 6 hours, use the following equation:

BW kg × 30–80 µg/kg/min × .36 = lidocaine in mg

- When the arrhythmia is controlled with lidocaine, initiate intramuscular or oral therapy with procainamide, quinidine, or tocainide (see Table 3), and slowly reduce the lidocaine infusion over a 24- to 48-hour period.
  - Treat hypokalemia and acidosis because they may cause therapeutic failure.
- When lidocaine therapy is not indicated or practical, give quinidine gluconate or procainamide IM to provide initial control of ventricular tachycardia.
- Prolonged therapy may be continued with oral quinidine or procainamide at appropriate doses. Other antiarrhythmic drugs that may be useful include propranolol, tocainide, and phenytoin (for digoxin toxicity).
- Reserve electrical cardioversion for refractory ventricular tachycardia. An experienced cardiologist and proper equipment are necessary.
- If the arrhythmia worsens, consider antiarrhythmic drug toxicity (proarrhythmia) as the cause rather than worsening disease.
  - Multiform ventricular tachycardia due to procainamide or quinidine toxicity may be a life-threatening complication of antiarrhythmic medication (torsades de pointes).
  - Treat this arrhythmic complication with drug withdrawal, bicarbonate, and isoproterenol or dopamine.
- If the arrhythmia is well controlled, consider discontinuing the antiarrhythmic agent after a 2- to 3-week period. This may avoid complications of long-term therapy and the expense of antiarrhythmic drugs. Evaluate the ECG before each decrease in dosage, or within 1 week after stopping the medication.
- In cases of refractory ventricular tachycardia, a cardiologist should be consulted.

Ventricular Fibrillation (Fig. 11)

Definition

- Cardiac impulses are generated and propagated in the ventricles in a chaotic, asynchronous manner.

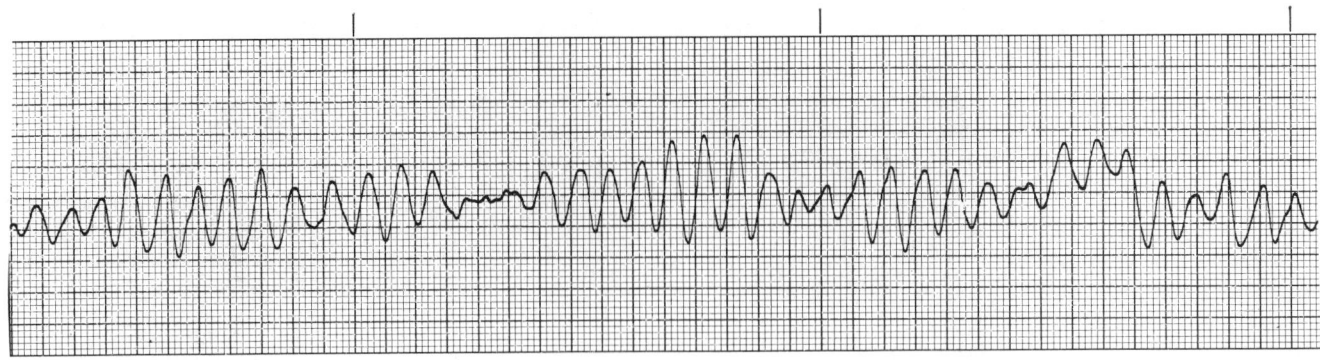

Figure 11. Ventricular fibrillation, dog. (Selected arrhythmias; lead II rhythm strips; paper speed 50 mm/sec; 1 cm = 1 mV.)

- The heart rate is rapid and disorganized.
- The rhythm is irregular.
- There are no P waves present and there are no recognizable QRS complexes. There are continuous positive and negative oscillations that are chaotic and bizarre. The oscillations may be large (coarse) or small (fine).

Etiology and Clinical Significance

KEY POINT ▶ The most common arrhythmia associated with cardiac arrest is ventricular fibrillation.

- There is no effective cardiac output.
- Conditions such as myocardial ischemia, electrolyte imbalance, autonomic nervous system imbalance, hypoxia, hypothermia, slow conduction, increased automaticity, drug toxicity, and unstable ventricular arrhythmias cause electrical instability and trigger ventricular fibrillation.
- Ventricular fibrillation carries a very grave prognosis.

Differential Diagnosis

- Differentiate ECG artifact (e.g., 60-cycle electrical interference, respiratory movement, use of electrocautery during surgery) from ventricular fibrillation. A palpable arterial pulse and rhythmic precordial heartbeat rule out ventricular fibrillation.

Treatment

- Perform cardiopulmonary resuscitation (CPR) immediately (see sec. 6, ch. 15).
- Electrical defibrillation is mandatory.
- Intracardiac lidocaine occasionally is successful in converting ventricular fibrillation to normal sinus rhythm.
- Open-chest cardiac massage may be effective in converting ventricular fibrillation to normal sinus rhythm if no defibrillation equipment is available (particularly in the cat). External blows to the chest (thump-version) are less effective.

Ventricular Asystole

Definition

- No impulses are generated from atrial, junctional, or ventricular pacemakers.

- There is no cardiac rate or ventricular rhythm.
- No QRS complexes are seen.

Etiology and Clinical Significance

- Ventricular asystole is associated with cardiac arrest and if left untreated is a lethal arrhythmia.

Differential Diagnosis

- Differentiate ECG artifact (e.g., electrocardiograph is not on a proper lead or is connected improperly) from ventricular asystole.

Treatment

- Perform CPR immediately (see sec. 6, ch. 15).
- Epinephrine, along with CPR, may be lifesaving.

CONDUCTION DISORDERS

Atrial Standstill

Definition

- Impulses are not generated in the sinus node and are poorly conducted or nonconducted through the atrial tissues.
- The heart rate is <60 bpm in dogs and <160 bpm in cats.
- No P waves are seen, and the QRS complexes are normal or bizarre depending on the intraventricular conduction. The S-T segment may be elevated or depressed. The T wave may be tall due to shortened repolarization.
- The rhythm may be regular or irregular.

Etiology and Clinical Significance

KEY POINT ▶ Atrial standstill is a life-threatening abnormality when associated with hyperkalemia (hypoadrenocorticism, acute renal failure, urinary obstruction, and diabetic ketoacidosis).

- Persistent atrial standstill occurs in English springer spaniels (may be correlated with a muscular dystrophy, as in humans) and other breeds and develops occasionally in cats with dilated cardiomyopathy in which there is degeneration and fibrosis of the atrial myocardial cells.

- There is cardiac enlargement, but electrolytes are normal, with persistent atrial standstill.

Differential Diagnosis

- Differentiate atrial standstill on multiple lead ECGs from AV junctional rhythm, idioventricular rhythm, and atrial fibrillation with complete heart block.

Treatment

- If hyperkalemia is suspected, perform emergency therapy, which is designed to dilute and transfer extracellular potassium into the cells, thereby restoring normokalemia.
- Administer 0.9% saline, 40–90 ml/kg/hr, until hyperkalemia and hypovolemia are corrected.
- In addition, administer 2 mEq/kg of sodium bicarbonate slowly IV. This may restore sinus rhythm within 15–30 minutes; beware of paradoxical cerebral acidosis.
- As an alternative therapy to sodium bicarbonate, administer 0.5 U/kg of regular insulin coupled with 2 g of dextrose per unit of insulin, slowly IV.
- For life-threatening conditions, give calcium gluconate (1 ml of 10% solution/10 kg BW, slowly IV) to counteract the cardiotoxic effects of hyperkalemia.
- If hyperadrenocorticism is the cause of hyperkalemia, mineralocorticoids and glucocorticoid replacement is necessary (see sec. 4, ch. 3).
- In the English springer spaniel with symptomatic atrial standstill, a permanent cardiac pacemaker is required.

Incomplete (First- and Second-Degree) AV Block

Definition

- The cardiac impulse is delayed or intermittently blocked in the region of the AV node or AV junction.
- The heart rate is variable, depending on the rate of the sinus node pacemaker and the AV conduction sequence.
- The rhythm usually is regular in first-degree AV block unless other arrhythmias are present.
- The rhythm usually is irregular in second-degree AV block.
- First-degree AV block shows a prolonged but constant P-R interval (AV conduction) with normal P wave and QRS complexes at a 1:1 ratio.
- Second-degree AV block has normal P wave and QRS complexes with a constant P-R interval and with intermittent P waves not followed by QRS complexes.
- In Mobitz type I (Wenckebach) AV block, the P-R interval is gradually prolonged before a dropped ventricular beat occurs. The rhythm is regularly irregular.
- In Mobitz type II AV block, a consistent P-R interval occurs prior to a dropped ventricular beat. The rhythm often is irregular.

Etiology and Clinical Significance

- First-degree and Mobitz type I second-degree AV blocks often are caused by an increase in vagal tone (e.g., in brachycephalic breeds and in patients with respiratory, gastrointestinal, or neurologic disease), digitalis, and sedatives (e.g., xylazine and acetylpromazine).
- Antiarrhythmic drugs (propranolol, quinidine, procainamide, and verapamil) and AV nodal disease are associated with these types of AV block.
- Physiologic AV block may occur following ectopic beats or atrial tachyarrhythmias that occur during the AV node's absolute or relative refractory periods (will slow down or block impulse).
- Mobitz type II AV block is a more advanced degree of block occurring in the AV junction, His bundle, or below. It may progress to complete heart block. Causes include:
  - Idiopathic fibrosis (older dogs and cats), hereditary stenosis of the His bundle in the Pug and Doberman pinscher, and hypertrophic cardiomyopathy in dogs and cats
  - Neoplastic infiltration secondary to metastatic neoplasia
  - Profound electrolyte disorders
  - Infection (e.g., Lyme disease)
- The development of clinical signs (e.g., weakness, syncope, congestive heart failure) depends on the degree of AV block, ventricular rate, and ventricular function.
- In cats there may be abrupt fluctuation between incomplete and complete AV block. Older cats (>12 years) may tolerate second- and third-degree AV block very well, and these bradyarrhythmias may be incidental findings.

Differential Diagnosis

- Differentiate complete AV block from advanced second-degree AV block on the ECG.

Treatment

- Treatment usually is not required for Mobitz type I AV block. If the block is related to drug toxicity, stop the drug or lower the dosage.
- Therapy for Mobitz type II AV block depends on the clinical signs. If the cardiac rate is slow and weakness or syncope is evident, begin therapy with atropine, dobutamine, isoproterenol, or a temporary or permanent cardiac pacemaker.

Complete (Third-Degree) AV Block (Fig. 12)
Definition

- The cardiac impulse is completely blocked in the region of the AV junction and/or the His bundle.
- The atrial rate (P-P interval) is within normal limits, and there is a slow idioventricular escape rhythm. The rhythm is usually regular. In dogs, an idioventricular escape rhythm has a rate of 40–60 bpm.
- An enhanced AV junctional or idioventricular

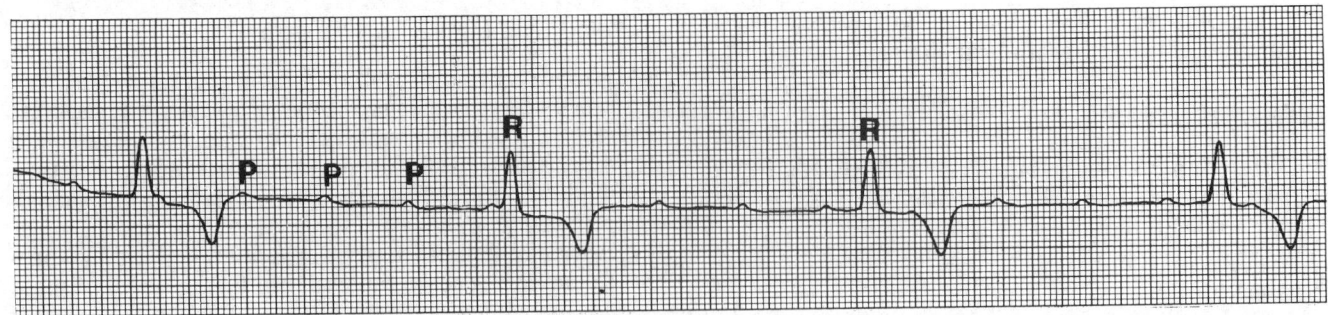

Figure 12. Complete (third degree) atrioventricular block, cat. (Selected arrhythmias; lead II rhythm strips; paper speed 50 mm/sec; 1 cm = 1 mV.)

rhythm (AV dissociation) has a more rapid rate, with the ventricular rate approaching the atrial rate.

- The P wave is completely dissociated from the QRS complex.
- The P-R interval is variable, and usually there are many P waves with few QRS complexes.
- The morphology of the QRS complexes varies depending on the location of the ventricular escape rhythm.

Etiology and Clinical Significance

- Complete AV block often is associated with the clinical signs of weakness, syncope, and congestive heart failure.

Differential Diagnosis

- Differentiate complete AV block on the ECG from advanced second-degree AV block, atrial standstill, and ventricular tachycardia (idioventricular rhythm).

Treatment

- A permanent cardiac pacemaker is the only consistently effective long-term treatment in symptomatic animals.
- Asymptomatic animals require no therapy.
- Drugs that may be useful for short-term stabilization and treatment include atropine, isoproterenol, dobutamine, and corticosteroids (anti-inflammatory). An IV dobutamine or isoproterenol infusion may be useful for increasing the rate of the ventricular escape rhythm during required surgical procedures.

OTHER ARRHYTHMIAS AND CONDUCTION DISTURBANCES

Sick Sinus Syndrome (SSS)

Definition

- Cardiac impulses are generated in the sinus node at a slower than normal rate or are blocked from exiting the sinus node.
- The atria and AV node may also be involved, resulting in an atrial tachyarrhythmia (e.g., atrial tachycardia, flutter, or fibrillation).
- A bradycardia-tachycardia syndrome may occur, with alternating periods of slow and rapid heart rates.

- There is a normal P wave for each QRS complex. The P-R interval is constant unless the bradyarrhythmia-tachyarrhythmia syndrome is present.

Differential Diagnosis

- Differentiate the multiple ECG abnormalities included in SSS from isolated sinus bradycardia, sinus block and/or arrest, and atrial tachycardia due to other causes. A poor (blunted) response to atropine (<50% increase in heart rate) supports the diagnosis of SSS.

Etiology and Clinical Significance

- SSS occurs predominantly in geriatric, small-breed females. Miniature schnauzers, cocker spaniels, and dachshunds are overrepresented.
- Clinical signs of SSS are variable but often include weakness and syncope.

Treatment

- If the animal is asymptomatic, no therapy is required.
- Anticholinergic drugs are rarely successful in symptomatic dogs.
- In animals with bradycardia-tachycardia syndrome, an artificial ventricular-demand pacemaker may be required for long-term control of bradyarrhythmias, and digoxin, propranolol, or diltiazem may control the tachyarrhythmia; do not use these drugs unless a pacemaker is implanted.

Ventricular Preexcitation and Wolff-Parkinson-White (WPW) Syndrome

Definition

- In ventricular preexcitation the cardiac impulses are generated in the sinus node but spread to the ventricle via an anomalous conduction pathway as well as the AV node.
- In WPW syndrome, a premature impulse finds the bypass pathway or AV node in its refractory period, allowing the development of a macro-reentry circuit that contributes to a tachycardia.
- During ventricular preexcitation, the cardiac rate and rhythm are normal. In the WPW syndrome, the rate may be very rapid (e.g., 300 bpm).
- The P waves are normal in ventricular preexcitation and are unrecognizable in WPW syndrome.

- The QRS complex is widened with notching of the R wave (delta wave) in ventricular preexcitation. In WPW syndrome, the QRS complex may be normal, wide, or bizarre, depending on the circuit of the atrial tachycardia.
- The P-R interval is short in ventricular preexcitation. In WPW syndrome, often there is a P wave for every QRS complex (1:1 conduction).
- A short P-R interval may be correlated with a normal QRS complex if the anomalous pathway bypasses the AV node to the area of the His bundle (Lown-Ganong-Levine syndrome in humans).

Etiology and Clinical Significance

- Ventricular preexcitation and WPW syndrome may be a congenital problem in the dog or cat that occurs with or without other congenital heart defects (e.g., atrial septal defect, valvular dysplasia, hypertrophic cardiomyopathy).

Differential Diagnosis

- Differentiate the tachycardia of WPW syndrome from AV junctional tachycardia, atrial tachycardia, and ventricular tachycardia.

Treatment

- Ventricular preexcitation without tachycardia requires no therapy.
- In animals with the WPW syndrome, control and/or convert the sustained tachycardia with a vagal maneuver (e.g., ocular or carotid sinus pressure), with drugs such as verapamil and adenosine, or with DC shock.

THERAPEUTIC PRINCIPLES

- Determine a precise diagnosis for the arrhythmia, if possible.
- Mechanisms for arrhythmias include isolated or concurrent disorders in impulse generation (automaticity), conduction (block or reentry), and triggered activity. These are often impossible to determine with certainty.
- Eliminate noncardiac causes (e.g., acid-base and electrolyte abnormalities, hypothermia, hypovolemia, hypoxemia, anemia, infections, and other sys-

temic problems) before using an antiarrhythmic drug.
- Stop other drug therapy if it may be the cause of the arrhythmia (e.g., digitalis, xylazine, acetylpromazine).
- Treat heart failure if present.
- Drug therapy for cardiac arrhythmias is intended to prevent clinical signs such as weakness, syncope, seizures, personality changes, and congestive heart failure. Also, drug therapy may decrease electrical instability and the likelihood of progression to a malignant arrhythmia (e.g., ventricular fibrillation).
- Select the antiarrhythmic drug best suited to the underlying cause of the arrhythmia (e.g., digoxin plus a beta blocker or calcium-channel blocker for atrial fibrillation, lidocaine to terminate ventricular arrhythmias). See sec. 6, ch. 5 for description of the various antiarrhythmic cardiac drugs.
- Be aware of synergistic effects of antiarrhythmic drugs (e.g., digoxin and propranolol may additively delay AV conduction) and antagonistic effects (e.g., quinidine may cause serum digoxin levels to rise, increasing the possibility of digoxin toxicity).
- Refractory arrhythmias may require a combination of antiarrhythmic agents, although these may increase the possibility of drug-related toxicity (e.g., digoxin and diltiazem or propranolol, procainamide and propranolol).
- Be aware that some arrhythmias may require antiarrhythmic drugs in addition to other therapeutic modalities (e.g., for SSS with bradyarrhythmia-tachyarrhythmias, a pacemaker for the bradyarrhythmia and an antiarrhythmic drug for the tachyarrhythmia).
- Be aware of the proarrhythmic potential of antiarrhythmic drugs. Digoxin can cause any arrhythmia and conduction disturbance. Monitor ECGs frequently.

Supplemental Readings

Miller MS: Treatment of arrhythmias and conduction disturbances. *In* Tilley LP, Owen JM, eds.: *Manual of Small Animal Cardiology.* New York: Churchill Livingstone, 1985, p 333.

Miller MS, Tilley LP: Electrocardiography. *In* Fox PR, ed.: *Canine and Feline Cardiology.* New York: Churchill Livingstone, 1988, p 43.

Tilley LP: *Essentials of Canine and Feline Electrocardiography,* 3rd ed. Philadelphia: Lea & Febiger, 1992.

Miller MS, Calvert CA: Special tests to diagnose arrhythmias. *In* Tilley LP, ed.: *Essentials of Canine and Feline Electrocardiography,* 3rd ed. Philadelphia: Lea & Febiger, 1992.

Miller MS: Quicksands of Electrocardiography. Annual Proceedings, A.C.V.I.M. 1991, p 707.

5 Drugs for Treatment of Cardiovascular Diseases

William W. Muir, III
John D. Bonagura

An understanding of cardiovascular pharmacology is best combined with a fundamental knowledge of the electrical and mechanical activity of the heart and vasculature. Therapy for heart failure may correct the underlying disorder or may merely palliate the clinical signs. Inotropic drugs, diuretics, vasodilators, antiarrhythmic drugs, and adjunctive therapy are described in this chapter. Specific drugs in each of these categories and recommended dosages are listed in Table 1.

DIGITALIS GLYCOSIDES

Digitalis glycosides, by poisoning the sodium-potassium pump and sensitizing baroreceptors, increase the force of cardiac contractions, slow the heart rate, and may affect cardiac rhythm. Because of variable patient response and untoward effects in normal patients individualization of digitalis dosages is indicated and the administration of digitalis as prophylactic therapy is at this time contraindicated.

Indications

- To increase cardiac contractile force—digitalis is potentially valuable in the therapy of heart failure caused by dilated and restrictive forms of cardiomyopathy (see sec. 6, ch. 8) and may improve congestive heart failure (CHF) resulting from chronic valvular disease, dirofilariasis, and congenital heart disease (see sec. 6, chs. 7, 10, and 12).
- To decrease heart rate—Digitalis glycosides may be effective against supraventricular tachyarrhythmias largely through a *parasympathetic* effect on atrial tissues and the atrioventricular (AV) node (see sec. 6, ch. 4). Specific effects include:
  - Decrease in sinus rate
  - Slowing of AV conduction
  - Reduction of ventricular rate response during atrial flutter or fibrillation
- As an antiarrhythmic (see sec. 6, ch. 4)—Antiarrhythmic activity is due to a decrease in heart size, parasympathetic action, and improved perfusion. Specific indications include:
  - Supraventricular arrhythmias
  - Atrial fibrillation

Contraindications

- Left ventricular outflow obstruction
- Constrictive pericarditis

- Cardiac tamponade
- Ventricular tachycardia and paroxysmal ventricular tachycardia
  - With caution in ventricular extrasystoles
- Cardiac disease without signs of heart failure
- Electrocardiographic evidence of AV nodal disease

Metabolism and Excretion

- Digoxin—This formulation of digitalis is primarily dependent on renal elimination.
- Digitoxin: This formulation is primarily (>85%) metabolized by the liver:
  - It is highly protein-bound.
  - Enterohepatic cycling is significant.
- Digitoxin and digoxin are well absorbed, although antacids, kaolin-pectin, food, and malabsorption states may interfere with gastrointestinal (GI) absorption:
  - Digitoxin is completely available when given orally.
  - The bioavailability of digoxin may be low in patients with congestive heart failure (CHF) at the beginning of therapy because of poor blood perfusion of the GI tract

Administration

- The route of administration and dosage of digitalis depend on the preparation (see Table 1).

KEY POINT ▶ An IV or oral loading dose of digitalis generally is not necessary in dogs, except for animals with atrial tachyarrhythmias associated with circulatory collapse, severe CHF, and high resting ventricular rates (i.e., >200/min).

- The daily dose of digitalis is *divided* q8–12h. This reduces the potential for drug toxicity and prevents low serum concentrations.
- Cats are more likely than dogs to become intoxicated during digitalis therapy. Therefore, use low doses of digoxin tablets in cats. The alcohol-based elixirs may be poorly tolerated due to an unacceptable taste.
- IV administration is very uncommon—Give one-fourth to one-half of the calculated total dose every 30 minutes to avoid toxicity.

436

TABLE 1. Drugs Commonly Used to Treat Cardiovascular Diseases in Dogs and Cats

Drug	Preparation(s)	Usual Dose
Inotropes		
Digoxin	Lanoxin, Cardioxin, Digoxin USP: 0.125, 0.25 and 0.5 mg tablets; 0.05 and 0.15 mg/ml elixirs; 0.25 mg/ml Lanoxin for injection	Digoxin loading dose: IV method, *dog*—0.0055–0.011 mg/kg IV q1h to effect (maximum total dose of 0.02 mg/kg, use ECG monitor); begin oral therapy 12h later; oral method, *dog*—twice the maintenance dose for 24–48 hrs. Maintenance dose: *dog*—0.0005–0.011 mg/kg q12h; *or* 0.22 mg/m² bsa q12h *Cat*—0.0035–0.0055 mg/kg once daily; or tablet (0.125 mg), ¼ tablet every other day
Digitoxin	Crystodigin: 0.1 mg tablet	Digitoxin: *dog*—0.02–.03 mg/kg q8h
Amrinone	Inocor: 5 mg/ml (20 ml vials)	1–3 mg/kg IV, followed by 30–100 µg/kg/min infusion
Dobutamine	Dobutrex, 250 mg vials, 20 ml per vial	*Dog and Cat*—2–10 µg/kg/min, constant rate infusion; higher doses to 20 µg/kg/min may be needed
Diuretics		
Furosemide	Lasix: 12.5 (VET) 20, 40, 50 (Vet), and 80 mg tablets; 1% syrup (10 mg/ml)	*Dog*—2–6 mg/kg repeated q8–12h as needed (IV, IM, SQ, PO) *Cat*—1–4 mg/kg repeated q12h as needed (IV, IM, SQ, PO)
Hydrochlorothiazide (HCT)/ spironolactone	Hydrodiuril USP: 25 and 50 mg tablets; Aldactazide: 25 mg HCT combined with 25 mg spironolactone	*Dog and cat*—2–4 mg/kg once or twice daily (either HCT or combined product)
Vasodilators		
Nitroglycerin (NTG) ointment (2%)	Nitrol, Nitro-bid, Nitrostat: 1 inch = 15 mg NTG; Minitran transderm patches 2.5, 5, 10, and 15 mg/24 hrs.	*Dog*—4–12 mg (up to 15 mg) topically q12h *Cat*—2–4 mg topically q12h (doses approximate)
Isosorbide dinitrate	Sorbitrate oral tabs, Isordil: 5 and 10 mg tablets	*Dog*—2.5–5 mg PO bid.
Hydralazine	Apresoline: 10, 25, and 50 mg tablets	*Dog*—1–3 mg/kg PO q12h (initial dose 0.5 mg/kg; titrate to effect or to at least 1 mg/kg q12h)
Captopril	Capoten: 12.5, 25, and 50 mg tablets	*Dog and cat*—0.5–2.0 (to 3.0) mg/kg PO q8h
Enalapril	Vasotec: 2.5, 5, 10, and 20 mg tablets	*Dog and cat*—0.25–0.5 mg/kg PO once or twice daily
Beta-Adrenergic Blockers		
Propranolol	Inderal, USP: 1 mg ampule for injection; 10, 20, 40, 60, and 80 mg tablets; 60, 80, 120, and 160 mg capsules (Inderal LA)	*Dog*—0.2–1.0 mg/kg PO q8h *Cat*—2.25–5.0 mg PO tid/IV dose: 20–60 µg/kg over 5–10 min
Atenolol	Tenormin: 50 and 100 mg tablets	*Dog*—6.25–25 mg q12h *Cat*—6.25–12.5 mg daily
Nadolol	Corgard: 20, 40, 80, and 120 mg tablets	*Dog and cat*—0.25–0.5 mg/kg q12h
Antiarrhythmics		
Quinidine	Quinidine gluconate: 80 mg/ml for injection; Quinidex (sulfate—SR) and Quinora (sulfate)/300 mg tablets (= 250 mg Q-base); Quinaglute (gluconate); 324 mg (= 202 mg Q-base)*	*Dog*—6–20 mg/kg IM q6h; 6–20 mg/kg PO q6–8h
Procainamide	Pronestyl, Pronestyl—SR, Procan SR: 250, 375, and 500 mg capsules and tablets	*Dog*—2 mg/kg IV up to a maximum total dose of 20 mg/kg over 30 min; 25–40 µg/kg/min IV infusion; 8–25 mg/kg IM q4–6h or PO q6–8h *Cat*—3–8 mg/kg IM or PO q6–8h
Lidocaine	Xylocaine, Lidocaine USP: 2% (20 mg/ml) for injection (without epinephrine)	*Dog*—2 mg/kg IV up to 8 mg/kg over 10 min; 25–75 µg (occasionally up to 100 µg) kg/min constant rate IV infusion *Cat*—0.25–0.75 mg/kg IV over 3–5 min.
Tocainide	Tonocard: 400, and 600 mg tablets	*Dog*—10–20 mg/kg q8h
Mexiletine	Mexitil: 150, 200, and 250 mg capsules	*Dog*—5–8 mg/kg PO q8–12h
Dilitiazem	Cardizem: 30, 60, 90, and 120 mg tablets	*Dog*—0.5–1.5 mg/kg PO q8h *Cat*—0.5–2.0 mg/kg q8–12h
Verapamil	Isoptin: 5 and 10 mg ampules for injection; Isoptin, Celan: 40, 80, and 120 tablets	*Dog*—0.05 mg/kg IV q10–30min to a maximum cumulative dose of 0.15 mg/kg; oral dose is uncertain *Cat*—as per dog

*The base-equivalent of quinidine (Q-base) varies with quinidine salt.
LA = long-acting; SR = sustained release, m² BSA = square meter of body surface area.

Digitalization

Effective digitalization is accompanied by diuresis, due to increased cardiac output and renal perfusion and inhibition of the renin-angiotensin system.

- Diuresis reduces clinical signs of CHF.
- Electrocardiographic changes are variable and include slowing of heart rate, ST-T segment change, reduction of ectopic depolarizations, and prolongation of the P-R interval.
- Serum digitalis levels should fall within the "therapeutic" range (1–2 ng/ml) in 8–12 h following dosing ("trough" levels for digoxin), with no signs of digitalis toxicosis.

Toxicity

Side effects include:

- Neurologic
  - Weakness
  - Lethargy
  - Depression
  - Restlessness
- Gastrointestinal
  - Anorexia
  - Nausea
  - Vomiting
  - Diarrhea
- Cardiac
  - Sinus bradycardia or ventricular bradycardia during atrial fibrillation
  - First- or second-degree AV block and ventricular conduction disturbances
  - Atrial and ventricular premature complexes, junctional tachycardia, and ventricular bigeminy

KEY POINT ▶ The most common signs of digitalis toxicity are lethargy, anorexia, vomiting, and arrhythmias. Renal failure and hypokalemia predispose to toxicity.

Drug Interactions

Digitalis serum concentrations are increased by:

- Hypokalemia
- Furosemide
- Quinidine
- Verapamil

DOBUTAMINE HCl

Dobutamine is a synthetic catecholamine with alpha- and beta-adrenergic agonist properties. Dobutamine is a potent, dose-dependent, positive inotropic drug helpful in the emergency management of life-threatening heart failure. Following infusion of dobutamine, the systemic vascular resistance decreases (low dose), increases (high dose), or remains unchanged.

Indications

- Severe, low-output, heart failure
- Cardiogenic shock characterized clinically by pulmonary edema with hypotension, hypothermia, pallor, and renal failure
- Cardiogenic shock caused by dilated cardiomyopathy

Contraindications

- Frequent, untreated ventricular extrasystole or ventricular tachycardia
- Systemic hypertension
- Subaortic stenosis
- Hypertrophic cardiomyopathy

Metabolism

- Dobutamine is an ultra-short–acting drug that is rapidly metabolized in the liver.

Administration

- Dobutamine is administered by slow, constant rate intravenous infusion following package-insert instructions for fluid compatibilities.
- The usual starting dose is less than 5 μg/kg/min. The dose can be increased to obtain the desired circulatory support or decreased if adverse effects develop. The duration of therapy is usually from 12 to 72 hours. Down regulation of beta receptors may necessitate an increasing dose during prolonged therapy.
- Therapeutic effects include increases in cardiac output, arterial blood pressure, tissue perfusion, urine production, and body temperature.
- Patients with atrial fibrillation are given digitalis to minimize the salutary effects of this drug on atrioventricular conduction.

Toxicity

- Adverse effects include tachycardia, excessive vasodilation (hypotension) or vasoconstriction (hypertension), induction of extrasystoles, and neurologic sympathomimetic effects.
- Adverse effects are treated by stopping the infusion and reestablishing therapy at a lower dosage.

BIPYRIDINE ANALOGS

The bipyridine analogs *amrinone* and *milrinone* work in part by inhibiting cardiac phosphodiesterase III. These drugs are mild to moderate arterial vasodilators. They usually do not slow the heart rate; thus, digoxin, a beta-blocker, or a calcium antagonist also may be needed if there is concurrent atrial fibrillation.

Indications

- To increase cardiac contractility
- To improve cardiac output
- To treat heart failure from dilated cardiomyopathy, valvular heart disease, and heartworm disease (see sec. 6, chs. 7, 8, and 10)

Contraindications

- Severe ventricular arrhythmias
- Constrictive pericarditis

- Cardiac tamponade
- Hypertrophic cardiomyopathy

Metabolism and Excretion

- Bipyridines are metabolized by the liver
- The mechanism of excretion is unknown.

Administration (see Table 1)

- Amrinone—Administer IV, following instructions for human use (considered extralabel use).

Toxicity

Signs of toxicity include:

- Vomiting and diarrhea
- Tachycardia and ventricular arrhythmias
- Hypotension (vasodilation)
- Blood dyscrasias (e.g., thrombocytopenia)

Drug Interactions

No drug interactions currently are recognized.

DIURETIC DRUGS

Diuretics are indicated for treatment of CHF, ascites, pleural effusion, and edema. Diuretic therapy reduces extracellular fluid (ECF) volume, relieving pulmonary congestion and improving pulmonary gas exchange. Diuretics may also reduce perivascular or vessel edema (vascular stiffness factors), thereby decreasing vascular resistance and facilitating the action of vasodilator drugs. The potent loop diuretics *furosemide* and *bumetanide* inhibit active chloride and sodium transport in the thick ascending portion of Henle's loop. This leads to diuresis, with loss of sodium, chloride, potassium, and water.

Indications

- Cardiovascular diseases that cause edema
  - Left ventricular failure—pulmonary edema
  - Right ventricular failure—ascites and edema
  - Biventricular CHF with pleural effusion
- Hypertension (see sec. 6, ch. 11)
- Oliguric renal failure and nephrotic syndrome (see sec. 8, ch. 1)
- Diabetes insipidus (thiazides; see sec. 4, ch. 6)
- Hypercalciuria (see sec. 4, ch. 2)
- Mobilization of ECF; changing composition of ECF

KEY POINT ▶ Diuretics are the most effective therapy for controlling fluid accumulation in CHF.

Contraindications

- Electrolyte disorders
  - Sodium depletion (hyponatremia), except in CHF
  - Potassium depletion (hypokalemia) (thiazides, loop diuretics)
- Acid-base disorders

- Extremely low cardiac output states
  - Shock
  - Hypoadrenocorticism (Addison's disease)
  - Hypovolemia
  - Prerenal azotemia

Administration

- CHF:
  - *Furosemide* is the diuretic of choice for treatment of moderate to severe CHF in dogs and cats.
  - In advanced CHF, administer furosemide IV and titrate to clinical effect (may be administered up to three times daily).
- Ascites—Parenteral administration may be required because of malabsorption (from intestinal congestion) in patients with ascites.
- Renal failure—may necessitate higher doses (4–10 mg/kg) to achieve sufficient concentration of drug in renal tubular fluid.
- Hypokalemia—Prevention
  - Salt substitutes (KCl salt) may be sprinkled on the food to increase dietary K+ intake and replace urinary K+ loss *or*
  - Potassium-sparing diuretics such as spironolactone and triamterene may be added to control serum potassium levels *or*
  - Angiotensin-converting enzyme (ACE) inhibitors to maintain serum potassium levels.

Metabolism and Excretion

Because the diuretic action of *bumetanide* and *furosemide* is a direct function of the concentration of unchanged drug within the renal tubule, prerenal metabolism of these agents, if it occurs, diminishes the pharmacologic effect.

Toxicity

- Volume depletion and metabolic abnormalities
- Volume depletion may result in:
  - Orthostatic hypotension
  - Prerenal azotemia
  - Decreased cardiac output
  - Tachycardia
- Metabolic abnormalities include:
  - Hypokalemia (thiazides, furosemide); hyperkalemia
  - Hyponatremia
  - Contraction alkalosis
  - Hypomagnesemia

Hypokalemia

Large losses of total body K+ may be reflected by relatively small changes in serum K+ concentration. Signs of hypokalemia include:

- Cardiovascular—tachycardia, arrhythmias, increased sensitivity to digitalis
- Skeletal muscle—weakness, hyporeflexia, flaccid paralysis
- Ileus

VASODILATOR AND ANTIHYPERTENSIVE DRUGS

Vasodilator and antihypertensive drug therapy falls into three main categories: vascular smooth muscle relaxants, sympatholytics, and angiotensin converting enzyme (ACE) inhibitors. Vasodilator drugs act by counteracting compensatory mechanisms evoked in an attempt to maintain blood pressure. More specifically, venodilation decreases preload by increasing venous capacitance, thereby decreasing symptoms caused by pulmonary congestion, including nervousness, tachycardia, hyperpnea, dyspnea, and crackles. Arteriolar dilation decreases afterload and reduces peripheral vascular resistance, thereby augmenting cardiac output, decreasing mitral regurgitation, and improving tissue perfusion. Myocardial O_2 demand also is decreased.

- Drugs producing direct-acting arteriolar vasodilator action (e.g., hydralazine) reduce arterial blood pressure and left ventricular afterload, which will increase stroke volume.
- Drugs with both venodilator and arteriolar dilator effects, such as prazosin (an alpha$_1$-adrenergic blocker), sodium nitroprusside (a direct smooth muscle vasodilator), and ACE inhibitors, also can be administered in cases of heart failure.
- ACE inhibitors such as captopril, enalapril, and lisinopril reduce the degradation of vasodilating kinins, resulting in vasodilation.
- Calcium channel blockers such as verapamil and diltiazem are arterial and venous vasodilators and are discussed in this chapter under Antiarrhythmic drugs.

Specific Vasodilators

Hydralazine

Hydralazine is a direct-acting arteriolar dilator that is effective orally and has a 12-hour duration of action in the dog.

- Hydralazine is metabolized by the liver, but elimination is influenced by renal excretion.
- This drug is used most often for controlling pulmonary edema in dogs with mitral regurgitation; it is used less often in patients with dilated cardiomyopathy.

Sodium Nitroprusside

Sodium nitroprusside and the nitrates nitroglycerin and isosorbide dinitrate are venodilators.

- Nitroglycerin is available as a transdermal ointment and patch, transmucosal spray, and IV injection.
- The IV preparations are balanced vasodilators that affect both the arteries and veins.
- Nitrate tolerance develops with repeated or constant administration; thus, intermittent use (q8–12h) is recommended.

Prazosin

This selective alpha$_1$-adrenergic blocker inhibits phosphodiesterase and stimulates alpha$_2$ adrenoreceptors, decreasing norepinephrine release.

- This drug is a "balanced" vasodilator that is effective orally and has a duration of action of 4–8 hours. It is metabolized by the liver.
- Prazosin is used infrequently for the management of chronic CHF but is effective as an antihypertensive drug.

ACE Inhibitors

This class of drugs includes *captopril, enalapril* (a prodrug that requires hepatic activation), and *lisinopril*.

- By blocking ACE, these drugs decrease angiotensin II levels. ACE inhibitors also retard the degradation of vasodilating kinins.
- ACE inhibitors are used in moderate to severe CHF caused by cardiomyopathy, and valvular heart disease, and in treatment of hypertension.
- Potential adverse effects include:
  - Hypotension
  - Acute renal failure
  - Neutropenia
  - Hyperkalemia (from decreased aldosterone levels; avoid KCl supplement and potassium-sparing diuretics)
  - Protracted anorexia that may require discontinuation of the drug

Indications

- Chronic CHF (see sec. 6, ch. 6)
- Valvular heart disease (see sec. 6, ch. 7):
  - Mitral regurgitation
  - Aortic regurgitation (use cautiously)
- Congenital heart disease (left-to-right shunt defects) (see sec. 6, ch. 12)
- Dilated cardiomyopathy (see sec. 6, ch. 8)
- Hypertrophic cardiomyopathy (use cautiously)
- Systemic hypertension (see sec. 6, ch. 11)

Contraindications

- Hypotension
- Shock
- Hyperkalemia

Toxicity

KEY POINT ▶ Arterial hypotension is the major adverse effect of vasodilator therapy.

Vascular smooth muscle relaxants may cause:

- Hypotension and fluid retention
- Depression
- Nausea and vomiting
- Reflex tachycardia (hydralazine)
- Bradycardia and AV block (verapamil)

ACE inhibitors may cause:

- Anorexia (with captopril)
- Hypotension
- Fainting, falling, and weakness
- Reversible agranulocytosis

KEY POINT ▶ ACE inhibitors may cause acute renal failure.

- Renal failure and proteinuria.
- Tachycardia

BETA-ADRENERGIC BLOCKING DRUGS

Most beta-adrenergic blocking drugs block both beta$_1$ and beta$_2$ receptors (i.e., they are nonselective beta-adrenergic blockers), although beta-adrenergic antagonists that demonstrate preferential beta$_1$ selectivity have been developed. The importance of the sympathetic nervous system in regulating the cardiovascular system and modulating various metabolic processes has resulted in the widespread use of beta-adrenergic blockers as therapy when increased beta-adrenergic receptor stimulation is likely to be harmful.

Propranolol and other beta-adrenergic blocking drugs are used to depress sinus node rate or AV nodal conduction and to decrease the ventricular rate in atrial fibrillation. These drugs occasionally are used with other antiarrhythmic agents when ventricular arrhythmias cannot be controlled.

KEY POINT ▶ Beta-adrenergic blockers with high lipophilicity (e.g., propranolol) interact with cimetidine and may prevent metabolism of other drugs (e.g., lidocaine).

Properties

Beta-adrenergic blockers are characterized by varying degrees of lipophilicity (dependent on liver metabolism), intrinsic sympathomimetic activity, membrane-stabilizing activity, and cardioselectivity.

Lipophilicity. Drugs with low lipophilicity are efficiently cleared by renal mechanisms because they are not reabsorbed to a significant extent by renal tubules.

Intrinsic Sympathomimetic Activity. Drugs possessing ISA produce less bronchoconstriction and peripheral vascular constriction and may help to support a failing myocardium.

Membrane Stabilizing Activity. Most beta-adrenergic blockers possess membrane-stabilizing, local anesthetic, or quinidine-like activity, but only at very high dosages.

Cardioselectivity (Beta$_1$). Beta$_1$-adrenergic blockers specifically block beta$_1$ receptors in the heart and exert minimal effects on beta$_2$-adrenergic receptors (e.g., bronchial smooth muscle).

Indications

- Cardiac arrhythmias (see sec. 6, ch. 4):
  - Sinus tachycardia (when harmful; e.g., in hypertrophic cardiomyopathy)
  - Supraventricular tachycardia (SVT)
  - Supraventricular ectopic activity
  - Paroxysmal SVT
  - Atrial flutter
  - Atrial fibrillation
  - Ventricular ectopic activity
  - Digitalis arrhythmias
  - Abnormal sympathetic activity (e.g., theobromine toxicity [chocolate poisoning])
- Heart disease:
  - Hypertrophic cardiomyopathy (see sec. 6, ch. 8)—to reduce heart rate and myocardial oxygen consumption
  - Obstructive cardiomyopathy—to decrease ventricular gradients
  - Dilated cardiomyopathy (see sec. 6, ch. 8)—to control heart rate after digitalization by blocking sympathetic activity
- Hypertension (see sec. 6, ch. 11)
- Thyrotoxicosis (see sec. 4, ch. 1)
- Pheochromocytoma in conjunction with an alpha-adrenergic blocker (see sec. 4, ch. 3)
- Glaucoma (intraocular)

Contraindications

- Bradycardia and heart block
- Impaired AV conduction

KEY POINT ▶ In cases of heart failure, *use cautiously* when heart function is dependent on sympathetic tone or when CHF is untreated.

- Untreated CHF
- Hypotension
- Severe bronchospastic disease
- Hypoglycemia

Metabolism and Excretion

- Highly lipophilic beta blockers are eliminated primarily by hepatic metabolism; there is extensive and variable first-pass extraction by the liver.
- Less lipophilic blockers are eliminated by hepatic metabolism and renal excretion (e.g., pindolol) or renal excretion (e.g., nadolol).

Administration

- Beta-adrenergic blockers usually are administered orally because of their negative inotropic effects; an exception is esmolol.
- Dosage is empirical and given to effect (e.g., predetermined heart rate, blood pressure)
  - Always start at a low dose and increase as needed

Toxicity

- Pulmonary signs of toxicity include *bronchoconstriction,* which can occur even with cardioselective antagonists when given in high doses.
- Cardiovascular adverse effects include:
  - Heart failure from bradycardia or myocardial depression
  - Acute hypotension

- Bradycardia
- Impaired AV conduction
- Central nervous system (CNS) depression may occur.
- Hypoglycemia is a possible side effect.

Drug Interactions

- Coadministration of cimetidine decreases extraction by the liver and may cause toxicosis.
- Calcium-entry blocking drugs (antagonists) and beta-adrenergic blockers administered concurrently can cause marked decreases in cardiac rate and contractility.

ANTIARRHYTHMIC DRUGS

A wide variety of drugs with diverse pharmacologic effects are capable of altering the heart rate and rhythm. Included in this category are the *digitalis glycosides* and *beta-adrenergic blocking drugs,* which have been described previously. See Table 1 for dosages of these and the other drugs discussed here.

Indications

The indications for cardiac antiarrhythmic drugs are based on a thorough assessment of the electrocardiogram and the ability to diagnose accurately the causes of the cardiac arrhythmias (see sec. 6, ch. 4).

Contraindications

- Bradyarrhythmias
- Atrioventricular block (first-, second-, and third-degree)
- Severe heart failure
- Hypotension

Metabolism and Excretion

The metabolism of most antiarrhythmic drugs is dependent on liver enzyme activity and liver blood flow.

Specific Antiarrhythmic Drugs

Quinidine and Procainamide

Indications

- Quinidine is a broad-spectrum antiarrhythmic drug that may convert atrial fibrillation to sinus rhythm, suppress atrial, junctional, and premature ventricular complexes (PVCs), and control ventricular tachycardia. It is used principally in dogs.
- Procainamide is similar to quinidine in its electrophysiologic actions; however, unlike quinidine, it does not block alpha-adrenergic receptors and has minimal anticholinergic effects. It is used primarily in the treatment of PVCs and ventricular tachycardia in dogs and cats.
- Quinidine and procainamide often are administered to control PVCs and to maintain sinus rhythm following conversion of sustained or paroxysmal ventricular tachycardia in dogs.

Metabolism. The route of excretion and elimination half-life of these drugs varies between species and accounts for differences in dosages.

Administration

- Quinidine—Administer IM or PO.
- Procainamide—Give IV or IM, and then PO to maintain sinus rhythm.

Toxicity

- Adverse effects include:
  - Hypotension
  - Decreased myocardial contractility
  - Anticholinergic effects (with quinidine)
  - Emesis and diarrhea
  - Atrioventricular block
  - Prolongation of QRS and QT intervals, with eventual development of ventricular fibrillation
  - Changes in skin or hair coat (with procainamide)
- As with any antiarrhythmic drug, exacerbation of ventricular arrhythmia (a *pro-arrhythmic* response) may occur.

Drug Interactions. Quinidine increases serum digoxin concentration.

Lidocaine, Phenytoin, Tocainide, and Mexiletine

These drugs decrease automaticity of cardiac tissues and are primarily given to treat ventricular arrhythmias and arrhythmias caused by digitalis toxicity (with lidocaine, phenytoin). Tocainide is a congener of lidocaine.

Metabolism and Administration

- *Lidocaine*—Administer IV. Lidocaine has a very rapid onset of action and is quickly metabolized by the liver (1–3 hours).
  - Repeat IV boluses every 10–20 minutes or supplement with constant-rate IV infusion.

KEY POINT ▶ The effectiveness of lidocaine therapy depends on the extracellular K^+ level, which must be maintained in the normal range. Most antiarrhythmic drugs are less effective during hypokalemia.

- *Phenytoin*—Administer PO or parenterally.
- *Tocainide and mexiletine*—These are available as oral preparations.

Toxicity

- CNS excitation with nervousness, vomiting, twitching, and generalized convulsions. These side effects can be controlled with diazepam (Valium).
- Depression of sinus or AV nodal function can occur, particularly in cats.
- Hypotension may develop with rapid injection.
- Loss of appetite.

Drug Interactions

- Propranolol and cimetidine reduce liver blood flow and delay excretion of lidocaine.

Calcium Channel Blockers

Verapamil and *diltiazem* block slow calcium channels and cause arterial and venous dilation.

Mechanism and Indications

- These drugs slow the ventricular response to atrial fibrillation and may cause conversion to normal sinus rhythm.
- The calcium-blocking effects cause peripheral vasodilation (verapamil also blocks alpha-adrenergic receptors) and reduce myocardial contractility.
- Verapamil is the drug of choice for acute, severe supraventricular tachycardias (HR > 280/min) because it can convert (reentrant tachycardia) or slow the ventricular response to atrial tachycardia, flutter, and fibrillation (see sec. 6, ch. 4).

Toxicity. Hypotension can be induced in seriously ill dogs, even at low IV doses of verapamil; accordingly, use calcium channel blockers cautiously in dogs with CHF.

Drug Interactions

- Diltiazem can be used with digoxin to slow the ventricular response to atrial fibrillation. Verapamil administration increases serum digoxin concentrations.
- Calcium chloride can be used to antagonize the hemodynamic depressant effects of verapamil and diltiazem.

6 Heart Failure

John D. Bonagura
John Rush

OVERVIEW

Heart failure is a state wherein the cardiac output is inadequate to meet the perfusion needs of the metabolizing tissues and exercise capacity is limited. In heart failure, venous filling pressures are normal to increased; the decrease in cardiac output is attributable to dysfunction of the active or passive tissues of the heart and circulation. The most common causes of heart failure are congenital or acquired defects that affect the following tissues (Table 1):

- Pericardium (pericardial effusion or constriction; see sec. 6, ch. 9)
- Myocardium (cardiomyopathy and myocarditis; see sec. 6, ch. 8)
- Endocardium and heart valves (valvular heart disease; see sec. 6, ch. 7)
- Cardiac impulse forming and conducting system (arrhythmia; see sec. 6, ch. 4)
- Development of the heart (congenital heart disease, in which shunts and valvular malformations are most common; see sec. 6, ch. 12)
- Blood vessels (vascular disease, including dirofilariasis; see sec. 6, chs. 10 and 11)

Clinical signs of heart failure can be subdivided into those related to low cardiac output and those stemming from pulmonary or systemic venous hypertension (congestive heart failure).

- Clinical signs of *low cardiac output* are secondary to reduced arterial blood pressure or decreased tissue perfusion.
- Clinical signs of *congestive heart failure* (CHF) are caused by inadequate cardiac pumping and compensatory mechanisms that lead to renal retention of sodium and water in the lung and body cavities.

Causes of Heart Failure

Causes of heart failure can be classified as etiologic (underlying cause), anatomic (tissues that are diseased), and physiologic (functional or hemodynamic abnormalities). Consider the history, physical examination, and results of diagnostic studies to determine the basis for heart failure in the individual patient. The following classification can be used to make a diagnosis of the pathophysiologic state of heart failure.

- *Etiologic diagnosis*—The cause can be a degenerative, anomalous, metabolic, nutritional, neoplastic, infectious, inflammatory, ischemic, immune, idiopathic, traumatic, or toxic condition (mnemonic = DAMNIT).
- *Anatomic diagnosis*—Area(s) of cardiovascular (CV) involvement include the endocardium and valves (both congenital and acquired valvar lesions); myocardium (including septal defects); pericardium; impulse-forming and conduction system; pulmonary, coronary, and systemic arteries (including patent ductus arteriosus); and veins.
- *Physiologic diagnosis*—This represents the consequence of an anatomic or functional lesion of the heart. Physiologic abnormalities include abnormal blood flow (e.g., valvular regurgitation or stenosis, shunting), abnormal blood pressure (e.g., hypotension, hypertension), cardiac arrhythmia, "low-output" and "congestive" heart failure, shock, syncope, and sudden death.

It is also useful, from a therapeutic perspective, to identify four pathophysiologic classes of cardiac failure:

- *Contractility failure* of the heart muscle (e.g., dilated cardiomyopathy)
- *Systolic hemodynamic (pressure or volume) overload* of the ventricle(s) (e.g., mitral regurgitation, pulmonic stenosis, heartworm disease)
- *Diastolic dysfunction or compliance failure* of the ventricle(s) (e.g., pericardial disease, hypertrophic cardiomyopathy)
- *Arrhythmia or conduction disturbance* of the heart

KEY POINT ▶ Identifying the cause and classifying the type of heart disease and pathophysiologic class of cardiac failure allows the clinician to direct appropriate therapy and render a more accurate prognosis.

In considering the development and therapy of cardiac failure, it is necessary to understand the following definitions and physiologic relationships:

- *Cardiac output* (CO) = stroke volume × heart rate/min (liters/min) = (ml blood ejected/beat) × (beats/min)/1000
- *Arterial blood pressure* (ABP) is related to CO × vascular resistance (mm Hg)
  - Thus, ABP is decreased by reduced CO or by vasodilation and can be increased by vasoconstriction.
- *Ventricular stroke volume* depends on ventricular systolic and diastolic functions; these include ven-

TABLE 1. Causes of Heart Failure in Dogs and Cats

Endocardial and Valvular Diseases
Bacterial endocarditis
Chronic valvular heart disease in dogs (endocardiosis)
Congenital endocardial fibroelastosis
Congenital valve malformation (pulmonic stenosis, subaortic
  stenosis, mitral and tricuspid valve dysplasia)
Rupture of mitral chorda tendinea
Myocardial Diseases
Cardiomyopathy
  Dilated cardiomyopathy
    Idiopathic dilated cardiomyopathy (dogs and cats)
    Taurine deficiency (cats, cocker spaniels?)
    Systemic or myocardial carnitine deficiency (dogs)
  Feline hypertrophic cardiomyopathy
    Idiopathic
    Secondary to growth hormone excess
  Feline intermediate or restrictive cardiomyopathy
Acute myocardial infarction
Secondary myocardial diseases
  Thyrotoxicosis (cats)
  Myocardial trauma
  Hypertensive heart disease (e.g., primary or secondary to
    chronic renal disease)
  Myocarditis (e.g., sepsis, parvovirus infection)
  Endotoxemia
  Chronic anemia
  Doxorubicin toxicity
Pericardial Diseases
Cardiac tamponade from pericardial effusion
  Idiopathic pericardial hemorrhage/pericarditis
  Infective pericarditis
Cardiac/pericardial neoplasia
  Causing pericardial effusion
  Causing intracardiac obstruction
Constrictive pericardial disease
  Constrictive-effusive disease
Congenital Heart Disease
Intracardiac and extracardiac shunts
  Patent ductus arteriosus
  Atrial septal and ventricular septal defects
  Endocardial cushion defect
Ventricular outflow obstruction
  Aortic and pulmonic stenosis
Tricuspid and mitral valve malformation leading to valvular
  regurgitation or stenosis
Cardiac Arrhythmias
Atrial arrhythmias (e.g., atrial tachycardia, flutter, and fibrillation)
Junctional (nodal) tachycardia
Ventricular tachycardia
Bradyarrhythmias
  Silent atrium (persistent atrial standstill)
  Third-degree AV block
Cor Pulmonale
Dirofilariasis
Pulmonary embolism
Miscellaneous Causes
Peripheral arteriovenous fistula
Drug toxicity

tricular filling and diastolic volume, myocardial contractility, and ventricular afterload (estimated by ABP in the absence of a stenotic semilunar valve).

PATHOPHYSIOLOGY: COMPENSATORY MECHANISMS: CLINICAL IMPLICATIONS

Principles

■ Blood pressure can be maintained through compensatory changes in the neuroendocrine system, kidney, and heart. The well-compensated cardiac patient can often maintain cardiac output and blood pressure that is within the normal range at rest (basal state) by activating the compensatory mechanisms enumerated below.
■ When the CV system is stressed (as with exertion, exercise, anesthesia, arrhythmia, anemia, or fever), cardiac output or blood pressure may not be commensurate with the physiologic state.
■ Patients with advanced heart failure generally have pronounced clinical signs at rest.
■ It is apparent that while compensatory mechanisms may be initially beneficial, these responses can injure the patient in the long term. Many of the clinical signs of CHF can be attributed to compensatory responses.

KEY POINT ▶ Excessive neurohumoral and renal compensatory responses contribute to the genesis of congestive heart failure. Therapy involves modulating these compensatory mechanisms.

Activation of the Sympathetic Nervous System

Heart failure is associated with increased activity of the sympathetic nervous system, increased circulating concentrations of norepinephrine and increased activity of the sympathetic modulating hormone angiotensin II. Some of the consequences of this enhanced sympathetic activity are:

■ Positive inotropic support
■ Tachycardia
■ Vasoconstriction
■ Activation of the renin-angiotensin system

Adverse Effects of Heightened Adrenergic Activity in CHF

■ Catecholamines can cause myocardial cell injury, increased oxygen demand, and cardiac arrhythmias.
■ Excessive heart rates may develop in patients with atrial fibrillation. Since atrial fibrillation also causes a chaotic ventricular response, cardiac filling time may be inadequate.
■ Decreased density of beta-receptors in the myocardium (the down-regulation in response to released catecholamines) may make the heart less responsive to sympathetic nervous system (SNS) traffic during exercise. There is some evidence that chronic beta-adrenergic blockade (e.g., via propranolol) may be beneficial to patients with heart failure, likely by counteracting some of these changes.

Vasoconstriction

Systemic arteriolar vasoconstriction develops to support arterial blood pressure.

■ Mechanisms involved are:
  • Enhanced SNS activity
  • Activation of the renin-angiotensin system
  • Release of arginine vasopressin (ADH)

Adverse Effects of Systemic Vasoconstriction in CHF

- There is a redistribution of flow away from "less vital" regional circulations such as exercising muscle, skin, kidney, and splanchnic circulation.
- Reduced perfusion can reduce tissue function with decreased ability to perform exercise in skeletal muscle.
- *Increased left ventricular afterload*—The failing ventricle is especially sensitive to peripheral vasoconstriction, and greater ventricular wall tension may be required to overcome systemic vascular resistance and aortic impedance; thus, the stroke volume may decrease.
- Potentiation of *mitral regurgitation* occurs by maintaining diastolic arterial pressure and prolonging the onset of aortic valve opening.

KEY POINT ▶ Modulating "excessive" arterial vasoconstriction with vasodilator drugs can be beneficial to the patient with heart failure. Inhibition of the renin-angiotensin system may be especially beneficial and may prolong survival.

Renal Retention of Sodium and Water

- The kidney behaves in cardiac failure as it does in hypovolemia and reabsorbs sodium and water in excess of "normal."
- Mechanisms that may contribute to sodium and water retention by the kidney include changes in renal blood flow and aldosterone and antidiuretic hormone levels, and insensitivity to atrial naturetic peptide.

Adverse Effects of Sodium and Water Retention in Heart Failure

- The most deleterious effect of fluid retention in heart failure is the excessive elevation of venous/capillary pressure and the formation of *edema* or *effusions*.
- Venous hypertension and elevated capillary hydrostatic pressure develop foremost in the vascular beds behind the failing ventricle.

KEY POINT ▶ The successful therapy of CHF almost always involves administration of diuretic drugs that counteract the renal reabsorption of sodium and water.

Body Cavity Effusions

- Serous body cavity effusions are manifestations of high capillary pressure with transudation of plasma into the body cavities.
- The effusions of CHF are classified cytologically as a transudate or modified transudate (or rarely chylous, from obstruction of lymphatic flow and dilation of lymphatics). Ascitic (peritoneal) fluid is relatively high in protein.
- Pleural effusion is usually a sign of biventricular CHF.
  - It seems likely that right ventricular (RV) failure

may lead to accumulation of pleural effusion fluid, but most experimental studies indicate that isolated RV failure often does not cause significant pleural effusion unless there is concurrent hypoalbuminemia.
- Pleural effusion is most commonly observed when there is a lesion or hemodynamic overload involving both ventricles or when left ventricular failure causes pulmonary hypertension and secondary right ventricular failure.
- Cardiac arrhythmias like atrial fibrillation also affect both sides of the heart and predispose to development of pleural effusion.

Cardiac Hypertrophy and Dilation

- Cardiac muscle hypertrophy develops in response to either volume or pressure work.
- Hypertrophy reduces wall stress (and hence afterload) during systole and may maintain stroke volume in the face of the increased work load.

Adverse Effects of Ventricular Hypertrophy and Dilation in Heart Failure

- The hypertrophied ventricle is less compliant, requiring higher venous and atrial pressures for filling. Active muscle relaxation may also be impaired. Oxygen demand is greater.
- The walls of the grossly dilated ventricle also may become stiffer during diastole, requiring higher venous pressure to maintain filling.
- The dilated heart is predisposed to arrhythmias.
- Atrioventricular valve regurgitation may develop.
- Myocardial failure can occur from chronic overload.

KEY POINT ▶ Diastolic dysfunction, often an unrecognized consequence of ventricular dilation or hypertrophy, predisposes the patient to venous congestion.

HEMODYNAMIC ABNORMALITIES

Hemodynamic variables include cardiac output, blood volume, blood pressure, and vascular resistances.

Cardiac Output

Basal CO is not a sensitive indicator of heart function because compensatory mechanisms can maintain the resting CO within the normal range for quite some time. CO in response to exercise is usually inadequate in heart failure, and in advanced heart failure the resting CO may be low.

Blood Volume

Circulating blood volume is increased in CHF.

Intravascular Pressures

Arterial Blood Pressure. The systemic ABP at rest generally is normal owing to compensatory mechanisms such as peripheral vasoconstriction and tachycardia.

Arterial hypotension can be observed in severe heart failure (e.g., dilated cardiomyopathy) or after administration of high doses of diuretics (reduced plasma volume) or vasodilator drugs.

Venous Blood Pressure. The systemic venous pressure, or central venous pressure (CVP), usually is increased as a result of decreased CO, venoconstriction, and increased blood volume. The CVP is higher in right ventricular failure than in left-sided CHF.

Pulmonary Blood Pressure. Pulmonary arterial blood pressure and pulmonary venous pressure (estimated by the pulmonary capillary occlusion or "wedge" pressure) are elevated in left-sided CHF.

CLINICAL SIGNS

Heart failure typically is described as left- or right-sided. This designation, while useful, neglects the fact that left and right ventricular outputs must be equal and that biventricular failure is common. Right-sided cardiac disorders like tricuspid regurgitation or pulmonary hypertension cause weakness and syncope by decreasing right ventricular, and consequently, left ventricular stroke volume. Similarly, left ventricular failure with pulmonary venous hypertension can cause the right ventricle to fail by increasing pulmonary venous pressure and elevating the right ventricular pressure required for pulmonary arterial perfusion.

Left Ventricular Failure

Clinical signs include:

- Exertional weakness, tiring, pallor, and syncope
- Oliguria and pre-renal azotemia
- Cardiac arrhythmias (possibly from myocardial ischemia)
- Pulmonary edema with tachypnea, "dyspnea," orthopnea, tiring, auscultable lung crackles, coughing, hemoptysis, and cyanosis (from mismatched ventilation and perfusion of the lung)
- Pleural effusion (more common in cats)

Right Ventricular Failure

Clinical signs are the result of reduced cardiac output and systemic venous hypertension and include:

- Exertional weakness, tiring, pallor, and syncope
- Systemic venous congestion with jugular venous distension and elevated central venous pressure
- Enlargement (congestion) of the liver and sometimes of the spleen
- Accumulation of fluid in extravascular spaces:
  - Small-volume pericardial effusion
  - Pleural effusion leading to atelectasis, tachypnea, respiratory distress, and cyanosis (more common with biventricular cardiac failure)
  - Peritoneal effusion (ascites)
  - Subcutaneous edema (uncommon in small animals)
  - Jugular venous distension and pulsations

KEY POINT ▶ The diagnosis of right-sided CHF is likely when the jugular venous pressure is elevated, cardiac auscultation is

abnormal, and hepatomegaly and abnormal fluid accumulation are present. Pulmonic stenosis, tricuspid regurgitation, heartworm disease, dilated cardiomyopathy, and pericardial effusion are the principal diagnostic considerations.

Other Findings

- Almost every case of heart failure is associated with some *abnormality of auscultation,* such as murmur, gallop, arrhythmia or muffled heart sounds.
- *Cardiac cachexia,* manifested as poor appetite and substantial loss of muscle mass is prominent in some patients, especially giant breed dogs with dilated cardiomyopathy. The proposed causes are multiple.
- Arterial *thromboembolism* may be detected in cats with any form of cardiomyopathy and in dogs and cats with bacterial endocarditis.
- A *thyroid tumor* may be palpable in cats with hyperthyroid heart disease.
- *Fever* or a history of fever is important in cases of bacterial endocarditis.

DIAGNOSIS

- The diagnosis of right-sided CHF is a physical diagnosis.
- Left-sided CHF usually requires ancillary tests to rule out other causes of respiratory disease.
- The exact cause of CHF requires a complete data base to detect radiographic, electrocardiographic, echocardiographic, and laboratory abnormalities.
- The exact abnormalities encountered depend on the cause of heart disease and the severity of the condition.
- Refer to other chapters within this section for specifics of diagnostic tests and of specific common disorders.

KEY POINT ▶ The usual data base includes the signalment and client history, results of cardiac auscultation and physical diagnosis, thoracic radiographs, electrocardiography, and routine blood tests. An echocardiogram can be very helpful for determining the cause of heart failure.

Radiography

In virtually all cases of CHF, the following radiographic features can be seen:

- Cardiomegaly (ventricular/atrial)
- Systemic or pulmonary venous dilation
- Abnormal fluid accumulation in the lung (pulmonary interstitial or alveolar edema) or pleural space (pleural effusion)

Electrocardiography

- The electrocardiogram (ECG) usually is abnormal in CHF and may contribute to the differential diag-

nosis (e.g., increased voltage or widened QRS complexes in dilated cardiomyopathy, attenuated QRS complexes in pericardial effusion).
■ Arrhythmias are common in heart failure but may also develop in noncardiac conditions such as systemic infections, metabolic diseases, and electrolyte imbalances.
■ Some arrhythmias, like atrial fibrillation, are characteristic of advanced heart disease and are likely to be associated with CHF.

KEY POINT ▶ A normal or equivocal ECG does not rule out CHF.

Echocardiography

This specialized imaging technique is very helpful in establishing the cause of CHF. Following are some characteristic echocardiographic features of common causes of heart failure:

■ Dilated cardiomyopathy—dilated cardiac chambers with a hypocontractile left ventricle
■ Hypertrophic cardiomyopathy (or hyperthyroidism)—thickened, normal or hypercontractile left ventricle with left atrial dilation
■ Pericardial effusion—an echo-free pericardial space with compression of the right heart chambers in cases of cardiac tamponade (cardiac masses may be evident as well)
■ Heartworm disease—right-sided dilation, dilated pulmonary arteries, and shifting of the septum into the left ventricle.

Routine Hematologic Tests

A complete blood count (CBC), biochemical profile, serum thyroxin, and urinalysis are indicated to evaluate metabolic function and may provide clues to the underlying disease.

■ Common abnormalities observed in CHF are prerenal azotemia, mild to moderate hypoproteinemia, and mild to moderate elevations in liver enzymes.
■ Hyponatremia is a feature of advanced CHF.
■ Hypokalemia is a common complication of diuretic therapy and anorexia.
■ Specialized tests such as plasma taurine concentration and blood cultures may be indicated for some patients.
■ Tests for heartworm microfilaria or immunologic tests for heartworm antigens are appropriate in cases of right-sided CHF.

Functional Classes of Heart Failure

It is common to speak in terms of "functional" classes of heart disease. These classes are extrapolated from the New York Heart Association criteria for humans and include:

■ Class I—objective signs of heart disease, but no clinical evidence of cardiac failure
■ Class II—objective signs of heart disease and clinical evidence of cardiac failure with exertion or vigorous activity

■ Class III—objective signs of cardiac failure with minimal activity or periodically while at rest (e.g., nocturnal orthopnea)
■ Class IV—objective signs of severe cardiac failure at rest

Most cases of CHF seen in animals have progressed to class III before the client seeks veterinary attention.

TREATMENT

Treatment of CHF can be divided into symptomatic and specific therapy.

■ Symptomatic therapy includes reducing activity and anxiety, improving blood and tissue oxygenation, decreasing edema, increasing cardiac output, and controlling cardiac arrhythmias.
■ Specific treatment includes measures that definitively correct the underlying disorder. Examples of specific therapy are shown in Table 2.
■ Many causes of heart failure such as chronic valvular disease and idiopathic cardiomyopathy cannot be definitively corrected; however, the hemodynamic abnormalities leading to CHF may be modulated by therapy, resulting in substantial improvement of quality and duration of life.

KEY POINT ▶ Delay diagnostic studies until pulmonary edema, pleural effusion, or cardiogenic shock have been controlled.

TABLE 2. Specific Therapies for Causes of Heart Failure

Congenital Heart Disease
Surgical repair of patent ductus arteriosus
Balloon valvulotomy or surgical repair of pulmonic stenosis
Palliative treatment for left-to-right shunts (e.g., large septal defects)
  Pulmonary artery banding
Open-heart surgery (usually experimental)
Endocardial and Valvular Disease
Congenital (see above)
Bactericidal antibiotics for endocarditis
Myocardial Disease
Taurine supplementation for taurine-deficiency dilated cardiomyopathy
Carnitine supplementation for carnitine-deficiency dilated cardiomyopathy
Antimicrobial therapy for infective myocarditis (e.g., Lyme carditis, trypanosomiasis)
Pericardial Disease
Pericardiocentesis for hemorrhagic pericardial effusion
Subtotal pericardiectomy for recurrent pericarditis/pericardial hemorrhage or for infective pericarditis or pericardial foreign body
Surgical removal of a constrictive pericardium
Surgery or chemotherapy for pericardial/cardiac tumors
Cor Pulmonale
Thiacetarsemide chemotherapy for dirofilariasis
Thrombolytic or surgical therapy for pulmonary embolism
Arterial Disease
Thrombolytic or surgical therapy for aortic or systemic thromboembolism
Cardiac Arrhythmias
Antiarrhythmic drugs
Cardiac pacing

When cardiogenic shock is present, begin emergency therapy (e.g., dobutamine infusion, pericardiocentesis).

Symptomatic Therapy

The initial steps in symptomatic therapy, which may be required at the time of admission, are summarized here. See sec. 6, ch. 5 for details of the drugs used to treat CHF. Specific treatment plans are covered in the chapters detailing myocardial, valvular, and pericardial diseases.

Oxygen Therapy

Place animals in severe congestive heart failure at rest in an oxygen-enriched environment (40–60% O_2). If an oxygen cage is unavailable, place the animal in a cool, well-ventilated area.

Sedation

Sedation may be indicated to reduce activity and anxiety and allow administration of further therapy with a minimum of stress.

- Give morphine sulfate 0.1 mg/kg IM or SC, to dogs.
  - Morphine decentralizes blood volume and may partially relieve pulmonary edema.
  - Morphine can release histamine, cause emesis, and depress respiration.
- Administer acepromazine maleate, 0.1 mg/kg SC, to cats. This drug and other promazine tranquilizers are peripheral vasodilators and negative inotropic agents.

Furosemide

For patients with severe pulmonary edema, give furosemide (Lasix), 2–6 mg/kg IV or IM, prior to performance of diagnostic studies.

Thoracocentesis

When there is a large pleural effusion leading to tachypnea or dyspnea, perform thoracocentesis with the patient in sternal recumbency (see sec. 1, ch. 3).

Nitroglycerin Ointment

A nitroglycerin (NTG) ointment or patch may be effective in reducing venous pressure by allowing translocation of pulmonary venous blood secondary to nitrate-induced pooling in systemic veins:

- NTG 2% ointment = 15 mg/inch
- Approximate dose: cats, 2–4 mg q12h; dogs, 4–15 mg q12h

Sodium Nitroprusside (Nipride)

This potent systemic arterial and venous dilator is used principally for life-threatening pulmonary edema caused by cardiomyopathy or mitral valvular disease.

- Use only when initial doses of furosemide and nitroglycerine fail to provide relief or when pulmonary edema is so fulminant that the patient is expectorating bloody froth.
- In patients with dilated cardiomyopathy, give infusions of dobutamine at the same time to prevent hypotension.
- Initial doses of 1–2 μg/kg/min generally are well tolerated. The infusion rate can be increased to 10 μg/kg/min; however, doses > 5 μg/kg/min are rarely required.

Dobutamine HCl (Dobutrex)

This synthetic catecholamine has beta- and alpha-adrenergic agonist properties.

- Administer infusions of 2–10 μg/kg/min when the patient shows signs of cardiogenic shock (hypothermia, severe weakness, mucous membrane pallor, low venous Po_2).

Amrinone (Inocor), a potent intravenous inotropic agent/vasodilator, also is available for intravenous infusion; however, dobutamine is more commonly used in patients with cardiogenic shock.

Hydralazine (Apresoline)

Hydrazaline is a direct-acting smooth muscle vasodilator that is useful in acute treatment of severe pulmonary edema associated with mitral regurgitation, particularly following rupture of a chorda tendinea.

Hydralazine is also used in dogs with severe mitral regurgitation when other treatments become ineffective (see subsequent discussion).

- By decreasing left ventricular afterload, hydralazine reduces mitral regurgitant fraction and increases cardiac output.
- Combination treatment with oxygen, furosemide, nitroglycerine, and hydralazine is effective for management of acute pulmonary edema due to mitral disease; the hydralazine-nitrate combination has benefits that are similar, although not as rapid-acting, to those of nitroprusside.
- Combine hydralazine with an angiotensin converting enzyme inhibitor; however, great care must be taken to avoid hypotension (see subsequent discussion).

Angiotensin-Converting Enzyme (ACE) Inhibitors

These agents, which have been demonstrated to prolong the life span in dogs with CHF, exert their therapeutic action through inhibition of the renin-angiotensin-aldosterone system.

- Onset of vasodilation is not as abrupt as with hydralazine or nitroprusside; however, ACE inhibitors are primary vasodilator therapy agents in long-term management of CHF.
- The most commonly used drugs are captopril (0.5–2 mg/kg, q8h PO) and enalapril maleate (0.25–0.5 mg/kg q12h PO).

Digitalis Glycosides

Digitalis glycosides play a minor role in the acute therapy of CHF; however, they are commonly used for chronic therapy of heart failure.

- In patients with atrial fibrillation, administer digoxin to slow the ventricular rate response (see sec. 6, ch. 4).
- The usual total daily dose is 0.01–0.02 mg/kg, divided q12h.
- Administer a loading dose (twice the calculated maintenance dose for two–four treatments) when the resting ventricular rate response exceeds 220/bpm.

Calcium Channel Blockers

- Drugs such as diltiazem (7.5 mg, q8h PO) may improve relaxation in cats with hypertrophic cardiomyopathy.
- Consider their use when furosemide, oxygen therapy, and nitrate therapy fail to mobilize pulmonary edema.

Pericardiocentesis

This is the treatment of choice for stabilization of the patient with cardiogenic shock and CHF caused by pericardial effusion (see sec. 6, ch. 9).

Chronic Therapy

A wide variety of drugs are available to treat diseases of the heart (Table 3). These agents, which include cardiotonics such as digoxin, diuretics, vasodilators, calcium channel blockes, beta blockers and antiarrhythmic drugs are used in various combinations for management of specific conditions. See chapters in this section for review of the clinical pharmacology of the most important agents and the specific use of these drugs for control of valvular, myocardial, pericardial, and electrical disturbances of the heart. Some typical treatment plans are discussed here.

Chronic Mitral Valve Regurgitation with Left-Sided CHF and Left Main-Stem Bronchial Compression

- Treatment includes dietary sodium restriction, furosemide, digoxin, and a vasodilator (typically enalapril).
- In advanced cases of left-sided CHF becoming refractory to increasing diuretic doses, give both enal-

TABLE 3. Drugs Commonly Used in the Treatment of Heart Failure

Type of Drug	Drugs	Principal Effects	Examples of Use
Cardiotonics	Digitalis glycosides (digoxin, digitoxin)	Positive inotropic; neurotropic (increases vagal tone); slows heart rate	CHF due to dilated cardiomyopathy; chronic valvular disease, atrial fibrillation, restrictive cardiomyopathy
	Dobutamine	Positive inotropic	Cardiogenic shock, severe CHF
	Amrinone	Positive inotropic/vasodilator	Cardiogenic shock, severe CHF
Diuretics	Furosemide	Diuretic	Pulmonary edema, ascites, pleural effusion
	Hydrochlorothiazide Spironolactone	Combination diuretic; antagonizes aldosterone; retains potassium	Refractory ascites or pleural effusion due to CHF
Vasodilators	Hydralazine	Systemic arteriolar vasodilator; decreases left ventricular afterload; reduces mitral regurgitation	Mitral regurgitation; pulmonary edema, concurrent systemic hypertension
	Nitroglycerin ointment	Systemic venodilator; pools blood in systemic veins	Pulmonary edema, left-sided CHF
	Enalapril Captopril	Angiotensin converting enzyme inhibitors; vasodilators; decrease aldosterone	Chronic CHF due to cardiomyopathy or valvular heart disease
	Sodium nitroprusside	Direct arteriolar vasodilator and venodilator	Emergency therapy for pulmonary edema
Calcium channel antagonists	Diltiazem	Decreases AV nodal conduction; improves ventricular relaxation; arterial vasodilator	Atrial fibrillation, hypertrophic cardiomyopathy
	Verapamil	Decreases AV nodal conduction	Acute therapy for supraventricular tachycardia
Beta Blockers	Propranolol Atenolol Nadolol Metroprolol	Decrease heart rate; slow AV nodal conduction; decrease outflow obstruction	Hypertrophic cardiomyopathy, atrial fibrillation, antiarrhythmic therapy
Antiarrhythmic drugs	Lidocaine Procainamide Quinidine Mexiletine Tocainide Amiodarone	Antiarrhythmic	Cardiac arrhythmias

See sec. 6, ch. 5 for pharmacology, adverse effects, and dosages of drugs listed.
CHF, congestive heart failure.

april (once daily) and hydralazine (twice daily) as well as maintenance doses of digoxin and furosemide.

■ If substantial mitral regurgitation causing left main stem bronchial compression is evident, decrease the dose of enalapril to once daily and add hydralazine (given q12h).

■ Cough suppressants (hydrocodone) may be beneficial for coughing secondary to bronchial compression; however, first ensure that effective diuretic and vasodilator treatment of pulmonary edema has occurred.

Chronic Tricuspid/Mitral Valve Regurgitation with Predominantly Right-Sided CHF

■ Treatment includes strict dietary sodium restriction (e.g., with prescription diet h/d; Hills) and digoxin, furosemide, and hydrochlorothiazide with spironolactone. Avoid vasodilator therapy in "pure" right-sided CHF.

■ In cases of refractory ascites, institute regular, SC furosemide therapy.

Dilated Cardiomyopathy with Left-Sided or Biventricular CHF

■ Give digoxin, furosemide, and enalapril, and restrict dietary sodium.

■ Antiarrhythmic drugs are often necessary for control of heart rate in atrial fibrillation (add diltiazem or a beta blocker) and for control of ventricular tachycardia (procainamide, tocainide, quinidine, or mexiletine).

Some patients respond to supplementation with taurine or carnitine (see sec. 6 ch. 8).

Feline Hypertrophic Cardiomyopathy

■ Restrict dietary sodium and give furosemide, and either a beta blocker (propranolol, atenolol), diltiazem, or both (see sec. 6, ch. 8).

■ If CHF worsens, add enalapril.

■ Give aspirin empirically as an antiplatelet drug to prevent systemic embolization.

Advanced Heartworm Disease Complicated by CHF

■ First stabilize the patient with strict cage rest, furosemide, and aspirin (3–5 mg/kg q12h) to reduce pulmonary vascular reaction, and restrict dietary sodium.

■ If these measures (including parenteral furosemide) fail to control ascites, add hydrochlorothiazide-spironolactone, given once daily, and a cautious maintenance dose of digoxin. After 2–4 weeks of stabilization, insititute heartworm adulticide therapy (see sec. 6, ch. 10).

Follow-up Examination of Patients with Chronic Heart Failure

■ Question the owner about current medication (exact dosage and frequency) and response to medication, including reactions that indicate the presence of drug toxicosis.

■ Ascertain the course of clinical events at home: activity level, exercise, diet and treats, fluid intake and availability, home environment, and resting heart rate (measured by owner).

■ Carefully examine the patient, with special emphasis on the heart rate and rhythm, arterial pulse, jugular venous pressure, mucous membranes, cardiac sounds, breath sounds and pattern of ventilation, liver size, abdominal girth and cavity, hydration, body weight, and assessment of the patient's overall sense of well-being.

■ Consider obtaining the following studies:
  • ECG (for arrhythmias, changes in rhythm, evidence of drug toxicosis)
  • Chest x-ray films (for assessment of heart and lungs)
  • Serum biochemistry (particularly blood urea nitrogen (BUN)/creatinine and electrolytes), packed cell volume (PCV), and total protein
  • Serum digoxin/digitoxin concentration (if currently receiving this medication)
  • Arterial blood pressure (if available)

■ Determine the patient's current functional class of heart failure and the trend of the heart disease.

■ Identify risk or complicating factors that might cause cardiac decompensation (see discussion of complications); correct these if possible.

Complications and Prognosis

■ CHF may worsen for a variety of reasons including:
  • Progression of valvular disease or myocardial dysfunction with enhanced neurohumoral compensation
  • Insufficient or inappropriate therapy for the stage of disease
  • Development of atrial fibrillation or other sustained arrhythmias
  • Ruptured mitral valve chorda tendineae
  • Ruptured left atrium with cardiac tamponade (in dogs with severe mitral regurgitation)
  • Excessive exercise
  • Hyperthyroidism (usually iatrogenic in dogs)
  • Anemia (increases cardiac workload)
  • Infections, fever (increase cardiac workload)
  • Excessive sodium intake
  • Compulsive drinking
  • Systemic hypertension (e.g., from chronic renal disease)
  • Environmental stress (heat, high humidity)

■ The patient may become depressed, anorectic, or weak due to:
  • Iatrogenic causes—excessive or inappropriate drug therapy causing hypotension, dehydration, or renal failure
  • Overt drug (e.g., digitalis) toxicosis
  • Multiorgan failure, especially renal failure or liver disease
  • Infections

- Arrhythmias
- Neoplasia
- Non-acceptance of dietary changes
- Change in owner's attitudes/behavior
- Progression of CHF with pleural effusion
■ The prognosis depends on the cause and severity of disease.
  - Once CHF has progressed to functional class IV, the outlook generally is guarded to poor and a prognosis of 3–12 months is typical.

- There are no critical studies examining prognostic criteria.

Supplemental Readings:

Keene BW, Rush JE: Therapy of heart failure. *In* Ettinger SJ, ed.: *Textbook of Veterinary Internal Medicine,* 3rd ed. Philadelphia: W. B. Saunders, 1989, pp 939–975.

Knight DH: Pathophysiology of heart failure. *In* Ettinger SJ, ed.: *Textbook of Veterinary Internal Medicine*, 3rd ed. Philadelphia: W. B. Saunders, 1989, pp 899–922.

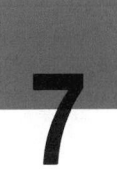

7 Valvular Heart Disease

John D. Bonagura
David Sisson

VALVE FUNCTION AND DYSFUNCTION

The Cardiac Valves

The heart contains four valves:

- The *mitral* or left atrioventricular (AV) valve
- The *tricuspid* or right AV valve
- The *aortic* or left semilunar valve
- The *pulmonic* or right semilunar valve

Structure

The semilunar valves consist of three individual leaflets that are closed during ventricular diastole and open during ventricular systole. The left and right AV valves consist of two major leaflets ("tricuspid" is a misnomer in dogs and cats), which are attached, via the chordae tendineae, to the papillary muscles (two for the mitral, three to five for the tricuspid). The base of each AV valve is supported by a valve annulus that is well defined for the mitral and poorly defined for the tricuspid valve.

Normal Function

The heart valves serve as one-way passages for blood and prevent retrograde (regurgitant) flow. The cardiac valves open and close in a cyclical pattern that is dictated by changes in pressure within the cardiac chambers and great vessels. Competent cardiac valves permit the development of high ventricular pressures during systole and facilitate the maintenance of low ventricular pressure during diastole. Vibrations attending closure of the AV and semilunar valves are manifested as the first and second heart sounds and herald the onset of ventricular systole and ventricular diastole, respectively.

Valve Dysfunction

Cardiac valves may be dysfunctional as a consequence of developmental or acquired heart disease. General patterns of disease include:

- Obstruction to flow, termed *valvular stenosis*
- Incompetent closure allowing *valvular regurgitation* (= insufficiency)

Valvular stenosis is almost always a congenital abnormality in animals. Valvular regurgitation may result from congenital malformation or acquired diseases. Common anatomic and functional causes of AV valvular regurgitation are listed in Table 1.

KEY POINT ▶ Because the AV valve consists of multiple anatomic components, disease of any portion of the apparatus, or geometric changes in the ventricle, can lead to AV valvular regurgitation.

Cardiac Murmurs

The hallmark clinical finding in valvular heart disease is a cardiac murmur. Murmurs are produced by high velocity and turbulent blood flow across the valve as the blood moves from a higher to a lower pressure

TABLE 1. Causes of Atrioventricular Valvular Regurgitation*

Mitral valve dysplasia (MR)
Tricuspid valve dysplasia (TR)
Myxomatous valvular disease (endocardiosis causing MR, TR)
Bacterial endocarditis (MR)
Ruptured chordae tendineae (MR)
Avulsion of the papillary muscle (MR, TR)
Transmural myocardial infarction (MR)
Causes of ventricular or atrial dilation
  Patent ductus arteriosus (MR)
  Ventricular septal defect/endocardial cushion defect (MR, TR)†
  Atrial septal defect (TR)
  Aortic regurgitation (MR)
  Pulmonary regurgitation (must be severe to cause TR)
  Myocarditis—for example, parvovirus, Chagas disease (MR, TR)
  Dilated cardiomyopathy (MR, TR)
  Intermediate/restrictive cardiomyopathy (MR, TR)
  Atrial muscular dystrophy—"silent atrium" (TR)
  Right ventricular cardiomyopathy—RV dysplasia (TR)
  Hyperdynamic circulation—AV fistula, hyperthyroidism (MR, TR)
  Chronic bradyarrhythmia—for example, complete AV block (MR, TR)
  Pulmonary hypertension including heartworm disease and chronic left-sided CHF (TR)
Causes of left ventricular hypertrophy (causing MR)
  Subaortic stenosis
  Hypertrophic cardiomyopathy
  Systemic hypertension—for example, chronic renal disease
  Hyperthyroidism
  Acromegaly
Causes of right ventricular hypertrophy (causing TR)
  Pulmonic stenosis
  Pulmonary hypertension
Cardiac arrhythmias preventing synchronous closure of AV valves—for example, ventricular premature beats

MR = mitral regurgitation; TR = tricuspid regurgitation.
*While this list is extensive, note that the most common causes of AV regurgitation are AV dysplasia, myxomatous degeneration, cardiomyopathy (any form), endocarditis, and hyperthyroidism (cats).
†May include mitral cleft or other AV valve malformation.

chamber or vessel. With few exceptions, the absence of a cardiac murmur virtually excludes the presence of clinically significant valvular disease (see sec. 6, ch. 1).

■ Semilunar valve stenosis or AV valve insufficiency can lead to systolic murmurs. Stenotic valves may also be incompetent, causing diastolic murmurs.
■ Cardiac murmurs may *not* be evident in the following situations:
  • Trivial valve regurgitation or stenosis (Note, however, that trivial stenosis may be relevant in breeding soundness examinations—for example, in dogs with subaortic stenosis.)
  • Massive, "wide-open" AV valve regurgitation in which the atrium and ventricle act as a common chamber and there is no pressure difference across the valve
  • Animals with very low cardiac outputs
  • Heart sounds muffled by lung sounds, pleural fluid, or pneumothorax

Valvular Diseases of Clinical Importance

Endocardiosis

Endocardiosis occurs primarily in dogs. It is also known as chronic "myxomatous" valvular heart disease or chronic mitral and tricuspid valvular fibrosis.

KEY POINT ▶ Endocardiosis, a degenerative disorder, is the most important cause of heart disease in veterinary medicine.

Congenital Aortic Stenosis

This lesion usually is a *subvalvular* fibrous obstruction that may extend to the valves proper (see sec. 6, ch. 12, for a discussion of congenital valvular disorders).

Congenital Pulmonic Valve Dysplasia Leading to Pulmonic Stenosis

A variety of anatomic lesions may contribute to narrowing of the right ventricular outflow tract.

Congenital Mitral and Tricuspid Valve Dysplasia

Anomalies of the chordae tendineae, papillary muscles, or valve cusps can lead to incompetency of the valves and in some cases stenosis as well.

Infective (Bacterial) Endocarditis

This condition almost always involves the left-sided heart valves in dogs and cats. Destruction of valve tissue commonly results in valvular insufficiency, and large vegetation(s) may obstruct the valve less often.

AV Valvular Regurgitation Due to Cardiomegaly

Valvular regurgitation may develop secondary to *ventricular dilation or hypertrophy*, which in turn results from a variety of causes (see Table 1).

KEY POINT ▶ When a cardiac murmur is a clinical sign, consider the possibility of valvular heart disease.

CHRONIC VALVULAR HEART DISEASE (ENDOCARDIOSIS) IN DOGS

Chronic valvular heart disease is a degenerative disorder of unknown cause affecting the subendocardial portions of the valve leaflets, primarily in middle-aged and older dogs. The AV valves are principally involved, with the mitral valve affected in nearly 100% of cases, the tricuspid in 34%, and the aortic valve in 3% of cases.

Pathology

■ The valve leaflets typically are thickened and distorted by nodular changes in the free edge and base of the valve. The valve surface glistens and the endocardium is intact, distinguishing this degenerative change from endocarditis.
■ The chordae are thickened near the valve attachment, and *chordal rupture* may be observed.
■ Focal subendocardial *myocardial fibrosis* may be evident, especially involving the papillary muscles.
■ Secondary *dilatation of the left atrium and ventricle* develops. Ventricular hypertrophy is of the eccentric type (with dilation of the ventricle), except when concurrent disorders (e.g., systemic hypertension from renal disease) stimulate the development of concentric hypertrophy (muscle wall thickening). The mitral valve annulus dilates as the ventricular dimensions increase.
■ Endocardial sclerosis develops in the left atrium secondary to mechanical irritation from regurgitant streams of blood. These "jet lesions" consist of fibrous and elastic tissue and smooth muscle. Fresh or healed linear left atrial tears are commonly found at necropsy, but rupture of the left atrium with pericardial tamponade is rarely encountered.
■ The right ventricle can be dilated due to concomitant tricuspid regurgitation or from pulmonary hypertension caused by chronic left ventricular failure.
■ In some dogs, *arteriosclerosis* (hyalinization) of the small intramural myocardial arterioles is present. Adjacent to these diseased vessels are focal areas of myocardial necrosis and fibrosis.

Pathophysiology

Endocardiosis represents a progressive process and does not cause detectable signs during the period of early structural changes. Progressive valvular distortion leads to detectable valvular insufficiency; yet not all animals develop heart failure. The entire process can take many years, although some breeds (e.g., Cavalier King Charles spaniel) are affected relatively early in life and may have a rapid progression to heart failure.

Mitral regurgitation (MR) causes left ventricular volume overload and left heart failure and predisposes to cardiac arrhythmias (Fig. 1).

KEY POINT ▶ Mitral valve disease is the most important cause of left-sided CHF in mature dogs.

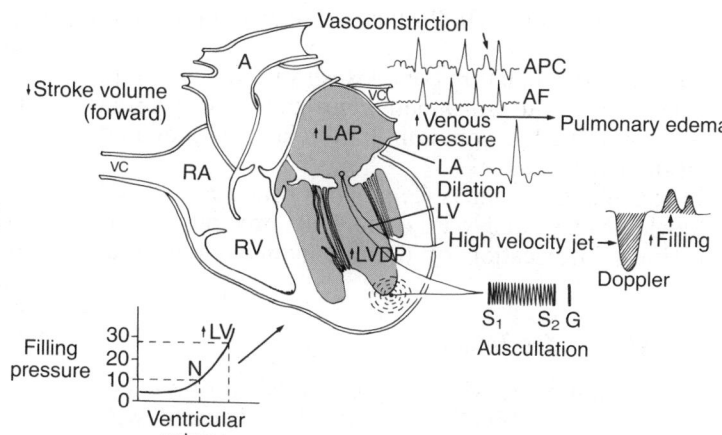

Figure 1. Diagrammatic representation of mitral regurgitation. Consult the text for an explanation of abbreviations and symbols.

Left-Sided Cardiomegaly

Chronic mitral insufficiency increases left atrial (LA) volume and pressure, causing LA dilatation. The increased atrial pressure increases left ventricular (LV) filling causing ventricular diastolic volume overload. Eccentric hypertrophy with dilatation of the left ventricular chamber ensues.

Mitral Regurgitant Volume

Total LV stroke volume is often greatly increased, but a large proportion of LV output is regurgitated into the left atrium. Therefore, the ability to eject blood in a forward direction is limited.

Pulmonary Venous Hypertension

LA and pulmonary venous (PV) pressures increase for a number of reasons:

■ Progressive MR increases LA pressure, initially during systole. If the regurgitant volume increases gradually, LA compliance increases, and the condition is well tolerated. This explains why many dogs have severe cardiomegaly but minimal clinical signs. If the regurgitant volume is very large, or if regurgitation develops suddenly (e.g., chordal rupture), the limits of atrial distensibility are exceeded and mean LA and PV pressures increase, leading to pulmonary edema.
■ The dilated left ventricle may become stiffer than normal, offering increased resistance to filling. This results in higher LV diastolic pressure, which is transmitted to the left atrium and pulmonary veins.
■ Reduced forward output may lead to retention of sodium and water by the kidneys (see sec. 6, ch. 6).

Pulmonary Edema

Substantial elevation of PV pressures leads to pulmonary capillary hypertension and pulmonary edema. Clinical consequences include tachypnea, hypoxemia, coughing, and exercise intolerance.

Bronchial Compression

The left main-stem bronchus is trapped between the pulsating aorta and the enlarging atrium. During sys-

tole, the bronchus is compressed by combined expansion of the aorta and the left atrium. As a result, exertional coughing and wheezing may occur even in the absence of lung edema.

Pulmonary Dysfunction

Chronic passive congestion of the lung causes ventilation perfusion inequalities (leading to hypoxemia) and, with chronicity, can also induce pulmonary fibrosis, which increases lung stiffness and the work of breathing.

Myocardial Failure

Chronic volume work by the left ventricle can cause biochemical and structural changes in the myocardium that lead to reduced LV contractility and cardiac muscle failure ("cardiomyopathy of overload"). However, CHF is often manifest prior to substantial myocardial failure.

Low Cardiac Output

If forward stroke volume is inadequate, signs of low output (weakness, exertional or cough-related syncope, and prerenal azotemia) may develop. Low output signs are often due to the concurrent development of tricuspid regurgitation and right-sided CHF.

Right Ventricular (RV) Failure

Left heart failure with secondary pulmonary hypertension combines with tricuspid regurgitation to cause RV dilation. RV failure may ensue, as evidenced by hepatomegaly and ascites. Low output signs often are exacerbated by the development of severe right-sided CHF; however, pulmonary edema may spontaneously resolve as blood flow to the left heart decreases.

Cardiac Arrhythmias

Arrhythmias are common and can further decrease cardiac output (see sec. 6, ch. 4).

■ Atrial arrhythmias are triggered by dilation of the atria. Atrial premature complexes (APC) frequently are recorded on the electrocardiogram (ECG). Atrial tachycardia and atrial fibrillation are evident in some cases.

■ Ventricular premature complexes (VPCs) develop in some dogs, but sustained ventricular tachycardia appears to be less common than in dogs with dilated cardiomyopathy.
■ Iatrogenic arrhythmias (e.g., sinus bradycardia, AV block, APCs, and VPCs) may be precipitated by digitalis intoxication or diuretic-induced hypokalemia.

Ruptured Chordae Tendineae

This condition is commonly observed during echocardiographic examination of dogs with advanced MR. Depending on the location of the chordal rupture, the added hemodynamic burden may be reasonably well tolerated, or severe CHF may supervene.

Left Atrial Rupture

Rupture of the left atrium, although uncommon, can cause acute cardiac tamponade, cardiogenic shock, and sudden death.

KEY POINT ▶ Rupture of the mitral valve chordae tendineae, the development of sustained atrial tachyarrhythmias, and LA rupture are important diagnostic considerations when rapid hemodynamic deterioration occurs in dogs with chronic MR. Appropriate therapeutic intervention can stabilize many of these patients, allowing sufficient time for further compensation.

Clinical Signs and Diagnosis

Signalment

Endocardiosis is most common in toy and small breeds of dogs (e.g., poodle, Yorkshire terrier, Cavalier King Charles spaniel, schnauzer, cocker spaniel). Some breeds, particularly the spaniels, German shepherds, and Afghan hounds, are prone to both valvular degeneration and dilated cardiomyopathy. Endocardiosis is an incidental finding in many aged dogs.

KEY POINT ▶ Occasionally, large-breed dogs develop CHF from primary valvular disease, but dilated cardiomyopathy is a more important cause of CHF in these dogs.

History

The presenting complaints typically are those attributable to pulmonary congestion or low cardiac output and include cough, tachypnea, tiring, and syncope. Weight loss is a frequent but subtle finding. Unless there are other metabolic problems such as hyperadrenocorticism, few dogs with CHF are obese. The opposite is true in dogs with chronic respiratory disease. In general, the clinical signs become gradually more severe, reflecting the progressive nature of the disease. Syncope may be related to one or more of the following problems:

■ Cough-syncope—fainting after vigorous coughing caused by decreased venous return or transient bradyarrhythmias.
■ Paroxysmal atrial or ventricular tachyarrhythmias that may be induced by exercise or excitement.
■ Orthostatic hypotension—sudden weakness following rising may be related to abnormal baroreceptor activity.
■ Insufficient forward flow from severe MR or from intercurrent RV failure, typically observed at the onset of exercise or with excitement.
■ Iatrogenic—hypotension secondary to diuretics, vasodilators, or angiotensin-converting enzyme inhibitors.

Physical Examination

Auscultation. As the disease progresses, the left apical systolic murmur of mitral insufficiency generally increases in intensity, and the duration increases from early systole (protosystolic) to midsystole (mesosystole) throughout systole (holosystolic). The murmur of MR radiates in the direction of the regurgitant jet, typically dorsal to the mitral valve on the left hemithorax, but often to the right hemithorax as well.

KEY POINT ▶ A systolic murmur heard best over the (palpable) left apex is almost always caused by MR. The murmur may radiate widely.

■ A short proto- or mesosystolic murmur usually indicates early disease but may also be heard in dogs with peracute CHF. The murmur of MR usually evolves from a soft decrescendo to a loud holosystolic murmur over a period of months to years.
■ Left apical midsystolic clicks often are detected in asymptomatic dogs and may be confused with a ventricular gallop.
■ A ventricular gallop (third heart sound) may be heard at the left apex in some dogs with untreated CHF. This sound resolves following successful therapy.
■ Cardiac arrhythmias and pulse deficits may be detected.

Precordial Palpation. The point of the left apical impulse shifts caudoventrally as the left ventricle enlarges. A precordial thrill reflecting valvular incompetency may be palpable over the left apex or tricuspid valve area.

Arterial Pulse. The arterial pulse is variable and depends on forward stroke volume, cardiac rhythm, and current therapy. Heart rate typically is increased when CHF is evident.

KEY POINT ▶ Pronounced sinus arrhythmia is atypical in dogs with untreated CHF caused by mitral valve disease but is common in patients with primary respiratory disease.

Pulmonary Auscultation. As lung congestion develops, ventilation and lung sounds become abnormal. Inspiratory/early expiratory crackles and cyanosis may be detectable. Wheezes, representing "cardiac asthma" from peribronchial edema (cuffing) or left main-stem bronchial compression, may be noted. Pleural effusion may cause muffling of heart sounds.

Right-Sided CHF. If the right heart fails, jugular venous pressure and liver size increase. Ascites is typical of advanced right-sided CHF. Occasionally, a dog is presented with predominant signs of RV failure due to severe tricuspid regurgitation (TR). Consider heartworm disease, pericardial effusion, dilated cardiomyopathy, and atrial muscular dystrophy/myocarditis in the differential diagnosis.

KEY POINT ▶ When there is pleural effusion in the absence of jugular venous distension, ascites, or atrial fibrillation, consider noncardiac causes for the effusion.

Imaging—Radiography and Echocardiography
(See also sec. 6, ch. 2)

- Progressive cardiomegaly is detected with left-sided heart enlargement predominating. LA enlargement typically is the first abnormality detected. As the disease progresses, LV enlargement, left main-stem bronchial compression, and pulmonary venous distension are observed.
- Left-sided CHF causes radiographic abnormalities that include increased lung density (interstitial and alveolar infiltrates) in the perihilar lung zones. These infiltrates characteristically are dorsal and bilaterally symmetric. However, owing to differences in pulmonary lymphatic drainage, edema may be worse in the right caudal lobe. Pleural effusion and ascites are present with right-sided or biventricular failure and commonly occur in association with atrial fibrillation.
- Echocardiographic findings include cardiomegaly, thickened AV valves, and variable changes in LV shortening fraction. In many cases, ventricular contractility appears normal to increased because the LV ejects a large portion of the total stroke volume backward into the low-resistance left atrium. The shortening fraction is rarely below the lower limits of normal reference values, helping to distinguish this condition from dilated cardiomyopathy. Ruptured chordae tendineae frequently are observed. Doppler studies can demonstrate mitral and tricuspid regurgitant flow. Often, aortic regurgitation (that is silent to auscultation) is evident as well.

Electrocardiography

- The ECG can be normal and does not rule out a diagnosis of CHF due to endocardiosis. Heart rate and rhythm usually are normal until significant cardiomegaly or CHF develops.
- Arrhythmias become common as the disease progresses. Sinus tachycardia, supraventricular premature beats, paroxysmal or sustained atrial or supraventricular tachycardia, atrial fibrillation, and VPCs may be recorded (see sec. 6, ch. 4).
- Cardiac enlargement often causes widening of the P wave (P mitrale) as well as increased amplitude. LV enlargement is suggested by increased voltages in leads II, III, and a V_F, widening of the QRS complex,

and slurring or coving of the ST segment (see sec. 6, ch. 3). Left axis deviation is uncommon.
- A tape-recorded, 24-hour ECG (Holter recording) is helpful for evaluating dogs with syncope, and for determining the need for and response to antiarrhythmic therapy.

Clinical Laboratory Tests

Laboratory changes that accompany advancing endocardiosis typically reflect the hemodynamic changes and renal responses that develop in dogs with CHF. Laboratory studies help to identify complications caused by extracardiac diseases (e.g., Cushing's disease, renal failure) and drug therapy (e.g., diuretics).

- Significant pulmonary edema or tissue hypoperfusion causes arterial hypoxemia (decreased PaO_2), and the associated increase in ventilatory effort can cause respiratory alkalosis.
- Mild to moderate increases in blood urea nitrogen (BUN), serum creatinine, and phosphorus are detected in many dogs with endocardiosis, as a result of chronic renal disease, decreased cardiac output, or hypotensive drug therapy. Diuretic therapy prevents use of urine specific gravity as a measure of interstitial-tubular function.
- Poor hepatic perfusion and hepatic congestion may cause mild to moderate elevations of serum alanine aminotransferase (ALT) and aspartate aminotransferase (AST). Persistently elevated liver enzymes usually indicate a noncardiac disorder of the liver, particularly when such changes are marked.
- Serum electrolyte abnormalities are uncommon. Hyponatremia is sometimes detected in dogs with severe biventricular heart failure, especially in those with marked ascites and polydipsia, and is a poor prognostic sign.
- Hypokalemia is usually iatrogenic as a result of diuretic therapy and anorexia.

Differential Diagnosis

The differential diagnosis of valvular heart disease includes the following:

Systolic Murmurs. For the systolic murmurs of MR or TR, consider the possibilities outlined in Table 1. The most important considerations in the diagnosis of MR and *left-sided CHF* are dilated cardiomyopathy and congenital AV valve malformations (especially in young to middle-aged, large-breed dogs) and bacterial endocarditis.

- The typical age, breeds, and clinical presentation make the diagnosis of endocardiosis straightforward in most cases.
- The echocardiogram is useful for distinguishing endocardiosis from congenital valve malformation or dilated cardiomyopathy.
- Endocarditis is associated with other clinical findings. Physical, radiographic, and echocardiographic features of healed mitral endocarditis may be difficult to distinguish from myxomatous changes.

Respiratory Disease. Because of similar signs, respiratory disease and CHF can be difficult to distinguish.

- When signs of tachypnea, cough, and dyspnea are present, consider tracheal collapse (especially in toy breeds), chronic bronchitis, pulmonary fibrosis, and other primary pulmonary disorders (e.g., pneumonia, neoplasia, allergic pulmonary disease, heartworm disease, and noncardiac causes of pleural effusions).
- CHF is commonly misdiagnosed in patients with chronic respiratory disease because these dogs often have cough, shortness of breath, and pulmonary crackles (which can be misinterpreted as "wet lungs," as opposed to small airway dysfunction).
  - The heart often appears enlarged in respiratory disease owing to inadequate expansion of the thorax, pericardial fat, or cor pulmonale (right heart enlargement secondary to chronic lung disease).
- Seek to identify positive findings of heart disease, such as murmur, arrhythmias, abnormal ECG, cardiomegaly with left atrial enlargement, and radiographic signs of pulmonary venous hypertension and edema. Do not consider endocardiosis in the diagnosis unless the definitive murmur of MR is evident.
- If CHF is a possibility, consider a trial course of furosemide (2 mg/kg, q12h) for 5 to 7 days. Anticipate a good response in cases of left-sided CHF. Some patients with chronic lung disease also respond partially to diuretics (mechanism uncertain).
- Pulmonary crackles without a murmur, a history of untreated, chronic (> 6 months) cough, right heart enlargement, and marked sinus arrhythmia are more typical of chronic respiratory disease than of chronic CHF. Thoracic radiography, airway cytology and culture, and bronchoscopy can usually establish the cause as respiratory.

Treatment

- Determine the functional class of heart disease (I, II, III, or IV; see sec. 6, ch. 6) and use appropriate cardiac drug therapy to control CHF (the pharmacology of cardiac drugs is discussed in sec. 6, ch. 5).
- Currently, treatment of asymptomatic dogs with a murmur (functional class I) is not recommended unless there is convincing evidence of impending heart failure (e.g., gross cardiomegaly with pulmonary venous distension).
- Traditional therapy with the "4 D's" (*d*iuretics, *d*ietary sodium restriction, *d*igoxin, and (vaso)*d*ilators) is appropriate for moderate to severe CHF (classes III–IV).
  - The order in which these drugs are used varies among clinicians; however, always administer a diuretic at the first indication of fluid accumulation. The current trend is for earlier use of combination therapy—diuretic, digoxin, and vasodilator—at the first objective sign of CHF.
  - In most cases, the vasodilator can be an angiotensin-converting enzyme (ACE) inhibitor; there are pros and cons for each agent, and judicious use of combination vasodilator (enalapril od and hydral-

azine bid) therapy has been effective in treatment of severe CHF.
  - Add antiarrhythmic therapy when appropriate (see also sec. 6, ch. 4)

Diuretics

Diuretics, a sodium-restricted diet, and some degree of exercise restriction are effective as initial therapy for many dogs with mild to moderate heart failure. Diuretic therapy is continued indefinitely, and the dose is titrated to effect.

- Furosemide (2–4 mg/kg, q12–24h PO) relieves pulmonary congestion in many cases. This drug is available in tablet and liquid forms for oral administration and in an injectable form.

KEY POINT ▶ Diuretics are a mainstay of therapy for dogs with CHF resulting from endocardiosis.

- Dogs with severe *right-sided* heart failure may not completely absorb furosemide, preventing sufficient drug concentration in the renal tubules. Substitution of the oral dose with an injectable form of furosemide often produces prompt diuresis and water-weight loss in such patients. Hospitalization and strict cage rest are often helpful in this circumstance. Other loop diuretics, such as bumetanide, may be better absorbed in such cases.
  - Other diuretic combinations, such as hydrochlorothiazide combined with spironolactone (Aldactazide; 2–4 mg/kg, q12–24h) or triamterene, may be useful in cases of refractory right-sided CHF or in dogs that develop hypokalemia. These diuretics usually are alternated with furosemide or another loop diuretic.
- Arterial vasodilators usually are more effective than combination diuretics for the relief of pulmonary edema that becomes refractory to furosemide.
- In cases of chronic *biventricular* CHF in which pleural effusion and ascites are marked and resist therapy, have the client weigh the dog daily as a guide to flexible diuretic dosing. Subcutaneous furosemide is substituted for the oral form and is given at home to control excessive fluid retention.

Digitalis Glycosides

The use of digitalis glycosides in dogs with MR has been controversial because echocardiographic studies indicate that LV myocardial function is relatively well preserved in dogs with endocardiosis. Some clinicians prefer to withhold digitalis glycosides, but most cardiologists now advocate its use in even mild cases of CHF. Data indicate that digitalis may exert favorable neurotropic effects and re-establish baroreceptor sensitivity even in dogs with normal sinus rhythm. Positive inotropic therapy may decrease the regurgitant fraction and slow the course of ventricular dilatation.

- Incontrovertible indications for digitalization in chronic valvular disease include:
  - Recurrent or sustained atrial arrhythmias including atrial fibrillation

- Biventricular or right-sided CHF
- Advanced (class IV) CHF
- Presence of a loud ventricular (S₃) gallop sound
- Echocardiographic evidence of impaired ventricular function

- The total daily maintenance dose of digoxin is 0.01–0.02 mg/kg, divided q12h (see sec. 6, ch. 5). After 5 to 10 days of therapy, measure serum digoxin concentrations 8 to 12 hours after the last dose and adjust the dosage accordingly.
- Highly potent positive inotropic drugs such as amrinone and dobutamine are used infrequently because cardiogenic shock is less common than in patients with dilated cardiomyopathy.

Vasodilators

Vasodilators are useful for increasing cardiac output, reducing the regurgitant fraction, and decreasing venous pressure. They usually cause detectable clinical improvement and may prolong life.

Hydralazine. Hydralazine effectively decreases mitral regurgitant fraction and increases forward flow; it can be used in the acute management of severe pulmonary edema and for chronic treatment of CHF caused by MR. Always give furosemide in conjunction with hydralazine. Use cautiously when combined with an ACE inhibitor.

- For severe *life-threatening pulmonary edema,* the combination of hydralazine, topical nitroglycerin, IV furosemide, morphine, and oxygen can be life-saving. The combination of nitroglycerin and hydralazine may be easier to administer and monitor than the more potent intravenously administered balanced vasodilator sodium nitroprusside (see sec. 6, ch. 6). Following resolution of pulmonary edema, an ACE inhibitor can be substituted for hydralazine.
- Hydralazine has a relatively rapid onset of action (near peak effect begins within 3 hours of administration) and also has a relatively long duration of action (about 12 hours). The effective dose can be titrated until there is clinical evidence of vasodilation (do this by starting with 0.5–1.0 mg/kg PO and repeat the dose q1–2h, up to a maximum cumulative dose of 3 mg/kg). Continue the effective dose q12h.
  - Signs of vasodilation include stronger pulse pressure, decreased capillary refill time, increased mixed venous PaO₂, and a lower mean arterial pressure following a cumulative dose of at least 1.0 mg/kg PO.
  - Adverse effects of hydralazine therapy include sinus tachycardia, anorexia, nausea, depression, weakness, and syncope. These signs often indicate that the dosage is too high. Combination vasodilator therapy plus diuretics causes significant hypotension in some dogs.
- As *long-term therapy* for CHF, hydralazine therapy may be initiated as MR worsens over time. This is most useful when there is severe bronchial compression indicating a large regurgitant fraction. When given to dogs receiving enalapril, the dose of enalapril is decreased by at least 50%.

ACE Inhibitors. ACE inhibitors such as enalapril and captopril are considered the initial vasodilators of choice for treatment of CHF in dogs. The afterload reducing effects of ACE inhibitors are less predictable than those of hydralazine in therapy for life-threatening pulmonary edema, but they have potential benefits for *long-term* use. Advantages include:

- They inhibit the renin-angiotensin-aldosterone axis, which theoretically decreases afterload and preload, relieving edema and augmenting forward blood flow. ACE inhibitors generally maintain serum potassium in the normal range.
- ACE inhibitors increase survival time in dogs (when enalapril is administered at 0.5 mg/kg, PO, once or twice daily).
- When ACE inhibitors are administered, the dose of furosemide may be decreased 25 to 50% (this practice also may be advantageous to prevent renal failure).

Adverse Effects
- Enalapril seems well tolerated. Captopril also is effective but often causes anorexia.
- Both drugs can cause hypotension. Initial doses should be low; increase the dose after 1 to 2 weeks of therapy.
- Decreased blood pressure, coupled with changes in intrarenal vascular resistance, may precipitate reversible acute renal failure (treat with fluids).

Nitroglycerin. Nitroglycerin 2% ointment (approximately 15 mg/inch) may be beneficial as a systemic venodilator, although efficacy and dosage studies are lacking. The major benefits are reduction of preload and venous pressures as a consequence of systemic venous pooling. Reduced preload also may decrease the mitral regurgitant orifice.

- Two principal uses are adjunct hospital treatment of severe pulmonary edema and home treatment of paroxysmal dyspnea due to chronic CHF (usual dose is 4–12 mg, q8–12h topically).
- Nitrate tolerance can develop; accordingly, do not give this drug more often than every 8 to 12 hours.
- Consider using a once-daily nitrate patch (2.5–10 mg) in home therapy of dogs that cannot readily be given pills. Patches may be placed on the inguinal skin or inside the pinna. Such treatment, however, is unlikely to be effective without concurrent administration of diuretics (e.g., furosemide).

Prazosin. Prazosin (1–2 mg, q8–12h PO) is an effective balanced vasodilator; however, long-term efficacy has not been evaluated and the capsule formulation makes dosing difficult. It is not commonly used for therapy of CHF but may be helpful in dogs with concomitant systemic hypertension as a result of chronic renal disease or hyperadrenocorticism.

Diltiazem. Diltiazem and other calcium channel blockers are effective arterial vasodilators; however, the principal use of diltiazem is for control of ventricular rate response in atrial fibrillation (see sec. 6, ch. 4).

Other Drugs

■ Other drugs such as *beta blockers* and *antiarrhythmic drugs* have specific uses for control of heart rate and rhythm (see sec. 6, ch. 4).
■ Prescribe a bronchodilator such as *aminophylline* when wheezes and crackles persist despite treatment with diuretics and vasodilators.
■ Bronchodilators, cough suppressants, and even low doses of prednisone can be helpful for controlling cough in dogs with left bronchial compression, concurrent chronic respiratory disease, or tracheal collapse (see sec. 6, ch. 20).

Follow-up and Complications

These are described in the chapter on heart failure (sec. 6, ch. 6).

Prognosis

The prognosis depends on the stage of the disease. No critical studies have examined prognostic criteria. Absence of cardiomegaly in asymptomatic dogs may allow a good prognosis for 2 to 4 years. In advanced cases, particularly when atrial fibrillation or biventricular failure is present, a prognosis of 3 to 12 months is appropriate.

INFECTIOUS (BACTERIAL) ENDOCARDITIS

Bacterial endocarditis (BE) is an infection of the valvular or mural endocardium. The mitral and aortic valves are the most common sites of cardiac infection in dogs and cats. Establishment of a cardiac infection requires a portal of bacterial entry into the circulation, subsequent bacteremia, and colonization of the endocardium. Because of the nature of the injury and the host's response to infection, a multisystemic disorder often develops. Acute and chronic forms of BE are recognized in dogs and cats.

Etiology

■ A diverse group of pathogenic bacteria have been identified in dogs and cats with endocarditis, including streptococci, staphylococci, corynebacteria, *Escherichia coli, Enterobacter aerogenes,* pseudomonas, pasteurella, and *Erysipelothrix*. Many of these bacteria are normal inhabitants of the skin, oral cavity, and respiratory and intestinal tracts.
■ Bacteria gain access to the circulation via external wounds, established infections, and a variety of surgical procedures and invasive medical interventions; however, in many cases there is no evidence of these sources. Endocarditis may also be a sequela to septic arthritis, osteomyelitis, infected catheters, and other infections.
■ Immunosuppressive drugs (e.g., corticosteroids, anticancer chemotherapy) also predispose to infection.
■ Injudicious use of antibiotics may predispose to infection by resistant or virulent organisms.

Pathogenesis

■ The pathogenesis of infective endocarditis involves entry of bacteria into the circulation and invasion of the valve endocardium by direct extension from the blood stream.
  • Virulent bacteria may attach themselves to the valve surface and aggressively ulcerate the endocardium and invade the valve stroma.
  • Previously diseased valves are believed to be more susceptible, particularly when the endocardium is disrupted. Dogs with subaortic stenosis are at increased risk for endocarditis, presumably because of jet lesions on the aortic valve. Dogs with endocardiosis, in which the endocardium is not usually eroded, rarely develop BE.
  • Some forms of endocarditis are associated with high titers of agglutinating antibodies that cause clumping of bacteria, thereby increasing the size of the infectious inoculum.
■ Collagen is exposed when microorganisms colonize and ulcerate the endocardium, causing platelet aggregation and the local accumulation of fibrin.
  • Vegetations resembling thrombi form on the valve surface. These vary in color from yellowish red to gray and are covered by a thin layer of clotted blood.
  • Lesions are usually localized to the valve but can extend to the mural endocardium, chordae tendineae (causing rupture), or sinuses of Valsalva (this may hasten the spread of septic foci via the coronary arteries to the myocardium).
■ Chronic valvular infections are established when layers of fibrin are repeatedly deposited at the site of infection, "protecting" the bacterial colonies from host responses and from many antibacterial agents.
■ Deformation of the valve usually results in *valvular insufficiency*. Exuberant vegetation may form in such a way as to produce valve stenosis, but this is uncommon.
■ Parts of the vegetation may break off, seeding the various tributaries of the systemic circulation, including the coronary arteries.
  • Intermittent bacteremia causes persistent or recurrent fever.
  • Thromboemboli, which can be septic or "bland" (aseptic), are shed.
■ Formation of immune complexes is an important host response; these may be filtered into the joints, kidneys, or other tissues, attract complement and leukocytes, and cause inflammation in these tissues.

Pathophysiology

The clinical signs of infective endocarditis result from cardiac injury, bacteremia and sepsis, thromboembolic complications, and immune-mediated processes (Fig. 2).

Cardiac Injury

A variety of cardiac manifestations are possible, including:

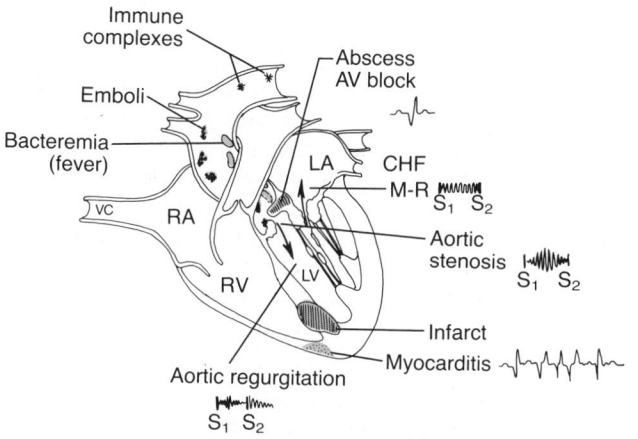

Figure 2. Diagrammatic representation of endocarditis. Consult the text for an explanation of abbreviations and symbols.

- Mitral and aortic valvular insufficiency
- Valvular stenosis (uncommon)
- Coronary occlusion with myocardial infarction
- Secondary myocardial invasion causing myocarditis or myocardial abscessation
- Pericarditis
- Left-sided CHF (from valvular injury)
- Arrhythmia
  - Arrhythmias may be related to endomyocarditis, "toxemia," or extension of aortic root abscesses into the conduction system causing AV block.

Bacteremia and Metastatic Infection

- Bacteremia causes fever, malaise, and anorexia.
- Other tissues may be seeded, resulting in brain abscesses, splenitis, osteomyelitis, arthritis, pyelonephritis, and other remote infections.
- In advanced cases it is difficult to distinguish a primary infection (portal of entry) from a metastatic infection.
- Bacteremia and sepsis may be associated with disseminated intravascular coagulopathy and lead to death from septic shock or organ failure.

Immune-Mediated Disease

Immune complexes may form and be trapped in many organs or tissues, with the following effects:

- The kidneys, leading to glomerulonephritis
- The brain and meninges, causing meningoencephalitis
- The joints, causing polyarthritis
- The skeletal muscles, causing myositis and myalgia
- The small blood vessels, leading to vasculitis, thrombosis, hemorrhages, or disseminated coagulopathy
- The eye, leading to chorioretinitis

KEY POINT ▶ Do not confuse the clinical findings seen in endocarditis of recurrent fever, multisystemic involvement, polyarthritis, and DIC with those of primary

immunologic or neoplastic diseases; such an assumption may prompt inappropriate therapy with corticosteroids.

Thromboembolic Complications

Septic or bland thrombi derived from the vegetation may be carried to distant tissues. Consequences include:

- Myocardial infarction and myocarditis
- Renal infarcts, abscess, pyelonephritis, and glomerulonephritis
- Stroke, meningitis, and encephalitis
- Bone infarcts and osteomyelitis
- Vascular obstruction including aortic-iliac occlusion
- Splenic infarcts
- Intestinal ischemia

Due to the low incidence of right-sided endocarditis in small animals, pulmonary embolism is uncommon.

Clinical Signs and Diagnosis

Signalment

Endocarditis is more common in certain large-breed male dogs (e.g., German shepherds) and dogs with congenital subaortic stenosis.

History

- The history may suggest previous or concurrent infection (especially of the skin, oral cavity, gut, bone, or urogenital tract).
- Certain diagnostic and therapeutic procedures predispose to BE by causing bacteremia (e.g., endoscopy, colonoscopy, dental extractions).
- Persistent use of corticosteroids or antineoplastic drugs or improper use of antibiotics may predispose to BE.

Physical Examination

Physical examination findings may include:

- Antibiotic-responsive fever, depression, anorexia, and shaking "chills."
- Polyarthritis (shifting lameness) with or without joint effusion and myalgia.
- Signs of vasculitis with hemorrhages (skin, eye, mucous membranes).
- Multifocal neurological deficits from meningitis or encephalitis.
- Physical signs of cardiac injury:
  - A cardiac murmur, particularly a "new" or changing murmur, is often detected.
  - BE destroys portions of the valve; therefore, regurgitant murmurs (MR, aortic regurgitation) usually are present in dogs and cats with BE. A systolic ejection murmur often accompanies the diastolic murmur of aortic insufficiency due to increased LV stroke volume. Large vegetation(s)

on the valves may also contribute to the genesis of murmurs in animals with BE.

- The pulse pressure increases with aortic insufficiency, which causes hyperkinetic femoral pulses with rapid run-off of diastolic pressure. Always consider BE when aortic regurgitation, which is uncommon in mature animals, is present.
- Signs of overt left-sided CHF or arrhythmias (especially ventricular premature complexes) may develop from cardiac injury.

Laboratory Studies

Complete Blood Count (CBC). Mild anemia and leukocytosis with neutrophilia and monocytosis may be present; red blood cell (RBC) fragments may suggest vasculitis (see sec. 6, ch. 11) or DIC.

Serum Biochemistries. These may reflect organ injury from infection, thrombosis, infarction, or poor perfusion from heart failure.

Autoimmunity Tests. Tests such as lupus erythematosus (LE) preparation and antinuclear antibody (ANA) assays can be positive in patients with BE.

Blood Cultures. Two or more positive blood cultures, obtained from a patient with compatible clinical signs, strongly suggest BE.

- Cultures are most rewarding if taken near febrile bouts when the animal is not receiving antibiotics. Cultures may be positive before, during, or after bouts of fever.
- Serial positive blood samples, taken 1 to 2 hours apart from different sites, help to rule out the possibility of skin contamination. (Surgically prepare the skin prior to obtaining the sample.)
- Transfer sufficient blood (5–10 ml) into special broth media tubes (usual blood:media ratio of 1:10). Aerobic and anaerobic culture and sensitivity are indicated. Special antibiotic adsorbing media are available for patients who have received antibiotic therapy.
- Consider culturing the catheter tip in patients suspected of being infected by an IV catheter.

Urinalysis. Hematuria, proteinuria, pyuria, or casts may be shown if pyelonephritis or glomerulitis is present. Culture the urine if there are any abnormalities, but do not automatically assume that organisms cultured from urine are responsible for the cardiac infection.

Cardiac Studies. Cardiac studies may substantiate the diagnosis and indicate the degree of cardiac injury. Serial studies following successful therapy are useful.

- Radiography may indicate cardiomegaly, valve calcification (from chronic BE), CHF, or (rarely) embolic pneumonia.
- Electrocardiography can be normal, but it may indicate chamber enlargement and detect arrhythmias (most often ventricular premature contractions).
  - ST-T changes, indicating ischemia or infarction, may be present (check precordial leads for these) (see sec. 6, ch. 3).
  - AV block likely indicates aortic valve involvement

with a perivalvular inflammation affecting the AV junction.

- Echocardiography is useful, especially for prognosis.
  - Routine 2-D or M-mode echocardiography may demonstrate a vegetation and signs of hemodynamic overload (cardiomegaly).
  - However, echocardiography cannot reliably differentiate mitral BE from mitral endocardiosis.
  - Doppler studies can document both abnormal valvular regurgitation and stenosis.
- Progressive cardiomegaly demonstrated by echocardiography or radiography indicates clinically significant valvular injury and regurgitation.

Other Studies. Other studies may be abnormal depending on the organ involved. *Cerebrospinal (CSF) fluid* and *joint fluid* cytology and culture may show evidence of septic or aseptic (immune complex) suppurative inflammation.

Treatment

Consider the following principles:

- Use bactericidal antibiotics. Because the bacteria are sequestered within the vegetation, normal defense and healing processes (e.g., granulation) are impeded.
- Because the drug must penetrate fibrin, exclude from consideration most sulfa drugs.
- Long-term (2–3 months) therapy is needed to ensure sterilization of the vegetation.
- Ideally, use IV therapy to obtain the highest possible plasma concentrations (this is sometimes impractical).
- Guide antibiotic therapy by monitoring blood cultures. It is appropriate to delay therapy for 2 to 4 hours while blood cultures are being obtained, unless the patient is demonstrating signs of septic shock.
- Empirical therapy for BE often includes the following drugs:
  - Penicillins (high doses) are safe and useful for streptococcal infections.
  - Aminoglycosides, combined with a synthetic penicillin or cephalosporin, provide wider antimicrobial coverage. Use of these drugs requires good patient hydration and careful monitoring for nephrotoxicity.
  - A patient with renal failure may be treated with a newer-generation cephalosporin (e.g., moxalactam) in lieu of an aminoglycoside.
- Treat for at least 4 weeks (at least 10–14 days when using an aminoglycoside, with continuation of the penicillin or cephalosporin for the full 4 weeks). Some cardiologists recommend treatment for 6–8 weeks. Repeat blood cultures following discontinuation of therapy or if fever should recur.
- If left-sided CHF develops, treat according to guidelines in sec. 6, ch. 6. Vasodilator therapy is not indicated for dogs with severe sepsis or septic shock.
- Use prophylactic antibiotics if the patient undergoes any procedure that may cause bacteremia. (The general subject of prophylactic therapy of BE is

unresolved and no firm recommendations can be made.)

Prognosis

The prognosis must be guarded.

■ Acute, ulcerative BE may cause dramatic clinical signs but, if promptly treated, may leave only mild cardiac dysfunction.

■ Chronic BE with severe valvular destruction is more difficult to treat because severe CHF may develop.
■ Echocardiographic evidence of diffuse, large vegetative lesions and documentation of volume overload imply a poor prognosis.

Supplemental Reading

Woodfield JA, Sisson D: Infective endocarditis. *In* Ettinger SJ, ed.: *Textbook of Veterinary Internal Medicine,* 3rd ed. Philadelphia: W.B. Saunders, 1989, pp 1151–1162.

8 Cardiomyopathy

John D. Bonagura
Linda B. Lehmkuhl

DEFINITIONS

- The ventricles react to increases in volume and pressure through the processes of myocardial dilatation and hypertrophy. These responses are commonly observed with valvular heart disease, cardiac shunts, thyrotoxicosis, chronic anemia, and arterial hypertension.
- Myocardial failure can develop secondary to increased workload, a process termed the *cardiomyopathy of overload*. Chronic tachyarrhythmias, especially ventricular tachycardia, can lead to a reversible loss of myocardial contractility. A model of congestive heart failure (CHF) in dogs is produced by rapidly pacing the ventricle for 1 to 2 weeks. The dog with spontaneous *sustained tachycardia* may develop a similar loss of contractility.
- The designation cardiomyopathy, however, usually pertains to a myocardial disease that cannot be explained by the presence of congenital or acquired cardiac or coronary artery lesions. When myocardial disease develops secondary to a systemic disorder, the designation "secondary" cardiomyopathy may be employed, although many clinicians and the World Health Organization usually restrict this designation to idiopathic myocardial disease.
- Cardiomyopathies are often classified by the postmortem anatomic appearance of the left ventricle (LV) and by the echocardiographic features of the ventricular anatomy and function. For the classification of myocardial disorders, see Table 1.
  - *Dilated (congestive) cardiomyopathy* (DCM) is characterized by dilatation of all cardiac chambers, markedly decreased myocardial contractility, and—when conventional methods, such as LV ejection fraction, are used to assess ventricular function—decreased systolic function. DCM is recognized in many species, particularly the dog and, to a lesser degree, the cat.

    DCM may be the end result of a diverse process that affects myocardial cell function, including deficiency of metabolic substrates (e.g., taurine, L-carnitine, selenium); myocarditis with necrosis of myocytes (e.g., parvovirus infection); severe global myocardial ischemia; or toxic injury to myocytes (e.g., doxorubicin, monensin) (see Table 1).

    Many cases of DCM in the dog are considered to be idiopathic or genetically predisposed.
  - *Hypertrophic cardiomyopathy* (HCM) is primarily

seen in cats and is characterized by *idiopathic* left ventricular posterior wall (LVPW) and interventricular septal (IVS) concentric hypertrophy. Ventricular hypertrophy decreases ventricular compliance and causes ventricular dysfunction primarily during diastole.

The LV ejection fraction (i.e., the volume of blood ejected divided by end diastolic volume) is usually high. The hypertrophy may be symmetric (LV wall = LV septal thickness); asymmetric (interventricular septum to LV > 1.3:1), or localized to areas of the LV free wall or IVS.

Obstructive cardiomyopathy describes the asymmetric septal myocardial hypertrophy associated with dynamic (i.e., not fixed) left ventricular outflow obstruction. Midsystolic pressure gradients develop in the left ventricular outflow tract (between the IVS and the anterior mitral leaflet), causing dynamic subaortic stenosis.

The clinical significance of this "obstruction" is controversial (see discussions of the Pathophysiology and Treatment of HCM).

Although LV anatomy may appear similar, established causes of LV hypertrophy (e.g., aortic stenosis, systemic hypertension, and hyperthyroidism), in our opinion, should not be designated as HCM.

- *Restrictive cardiomyopathy* (RCM, also called "intermediate" cardiomyopathy) is a poorly defined condition affecting the cat. The LV is characterized by (1) mild-to-moderate dilation and hypertrophy with mild-to-moderate depression of ejection fraction ("intermediate" between HCM and DCM) and (2) a variable degree of myocardial fibrosis (thought to restrict ventricular filling hence "restrictive"). There is almost always marked left atrial dilation because it must empty into a restricted, noncompliant LV.
- *Myocarditis* is inflammation of the myocardium. There are many potential causes of myocarditis (see Table 1).

  Idiopathic nonsuppurative myocarditis may also accompany the various forms of cardiomyopathy (CM) previously described.

  Potential sequelae of myocarditis include myocardial fibrosis, decreased myocyte contractility, and DCM.

KEY POINT ▶ Cardiomyopathies can cause CHF, cardiac arrhythmias, sudden death, and systemic arterial embolism (in cats).

TABLE 1. Spontaneous Cardiomyopathy (CM)

Disorder*	Feline	Canine
Myocarditis *Noninfective*	Idiopathic Thymoma [immune-mediated?]	Idiopathic Boxer dog† English bulldog Trauma
Infective	Toxoplasmosis FIP?	Bacterial Parvovirus Distemper virus Systemic mycoses Lyme carditis *(Borrelia)* Chagas disease *(Trypanosoma cruzi)*

Dilated CM (DCM) (also see infective and noninfective myocarditis because DCM can develop secondary to severe inflammatory disease)	Taurine deficiency
	Idiopathic
	Potassium iodide toxicity
	Hyperthyroidism
	Sustained ventricular or supraventricular tachycardia
	Chronic hypokalemia (causes taurine deficiency?)
		Idiopathic†
		Carnitine deficiency†
		Breed-"specific" DCM†
		  Doberman pinscher
		  Boxer dog
		  Cocker spaniel
		  "Giant" purebred dogs
		  Springer spaniel muscular dystrophy
		Doxorubicin toxicity†
		Global ischemia?

Hypertrophic CM	Idiopathic† (familial?, excess growth hormone?) Acromegaly Hypertension† Hyperthyroidism†	Idiopathic
Restrictive-intermediate CM	Idiopathic*	
Cardiotoxicity	Sodium iodide	Catecholamines Brain-heart syndrome Doxorubicin *Digitalis purpurea* (foxglove) and *Strophanthus* spp. Toad *(Bufo)* toxicity Chocolate toxicity

*Both primary (idiopathic) and secondary causes of cardiomyopathy are considered here. Some investigators prefer the designation "cardiomyopathy" to indicate only idiopathic conditions.
†Most important factors.

> Effective therapy of cardiomyopathy requires an accurate diagnosis.

See Table 2.

HYPERTROPHIC CARDIOMYOPATHY (HCM) IN THE CAT

Etiology

- The cause of HCM (Fig. 1) is unknown. Kittleson's group has reported an increased level of growth hormone in cats with HCM, but a causal relationship has not been proven. A genetic basis is suspected in some families of cats, which is similar to that in humans.

Pathology

- Left ventricular concentric hypertrophy includes the papillary muscles and the interventricular septum and results in a decreased LV chamber volume. Hypertrophy is either symmetric, asymmetric, or localized. Focal areas of LV myocardial fibrosis are common.
- Dilated and hypertrophied left atrium (LA)

- Dilated right ventricle (RV) with eccentric hypertrophy secondary to pulmonary hypertension
- Left atrial mural thrombus; systemic arterial thromboembolism—usually lodged in the terminal aorta.
- Pulmonary edema and pleural effusion due to CHF

Pathophysiology

- The hypertrophic LV is less distensible (decreased compliance) and the hypertrophied myocardium may not relax normally (decreased lusitropy). Papillary muscle hypertrophy further encroaches on the LV lumen. These abnormalities result in a decreased LV end-diastolic volume (EDV) and ventricular preload.
  - Cardiac output (CO) is maintained by increased sympathetic activity, vigorous ventricular contraction, high LV ejection fraction, and increased heart rate (HR); however, these responses can be deleterious (see subsequent discussion).
  - Anesthetics limit cardiac output and may precipitate LV failure.
- LV filling requires higher than normal venous and atrial pressures, causing the left atrium (LA) to dilate. This predisposes the cat to pulmonary venous hypertension and pulmonary edema.
  - Affected cats are poorly tolerant of infusions of crystalloid and of blood.

TABLE 2. Differential Diagnosis of Feline Cardiomyopathy and Heart Failure*

Other Causes of Dyspnea/Tachypnea
 Airway obstruction
  Nasopharyngeal polyp
  Laryngeal paresis
  Tracheal or esophageal foreign body, neoplasm, granuloma, abscess
  Mediastinal masses
   Lymphosarcoma or thymoma
 Primary bronchopulmonary disease
  Bronchial asthma
  Lungworms and lung flukes
  Pneumonia (viral, bacterial, fungal, toxoplasmic)
  Neoplasia
  Aspiration
 Pulmonary vascular disease/embolism
  Heartworms
 Noncardiogenic pulmonary edema
  Electrocution
  Trauma (shock lung)
  Anaphylaxis
 Trauma
  Diaphragmatic hernia
  Pulmonary hemorrhage/edema
  Pneumothorax
  Hemothorax
 Pleural effusion
  Pyothorax
  Hemothorax
  Feline infectious peritonitis (FIP)
  Lymphosarcoma-associated effusion
  Chylothorax
 Hyperthermia/fever
 Anemia
 Methemoglobinemia
  Acetaminophen toxicity
  Cetacaine
 Abnormal ventilatory pattern
  Metabolic acidosis
  CNS disease
Other Causes of Acute Lameness/Paresis/Gait Abnormality
 Musculoskeletal pain or injury
 Bite wounds
 Hypokalemia (weakness)
 Peripheral neuropathy
  Related to diabetes mellitus

 Spinal cord disease
  Injury
  Neoplasia
  FIP infection
  Extradural mass/granuloma
 Urinary obstruction
  Causing abdominal pain and reluctance to move

Other Causes of Cardiac Murmurs/Gallops/Arrhythmias/Cardiomegaly
 Congenital heart disease
  Especially septal defects and mitral valve dysplasia
 Congenital peritoneopericardial-diaphragmatic hernia
 Bacterial endocarditis
 Pericarditis
  FIP infection
  Idiopathic
  Bacterial
  Neoplastic
   Lymphosarcoma
   Mesothelioma
 Cardiac neoplasia
  Lymphosarcoma
 Cor pulmonale
  Heartworms
  Severe, chronic respiratory disease
 Chronic degenerative valvular disease (mitral, aortic)?
 Dilation of the aortic root with aortic regurgitation
 Cardiac arrhythmias (primary electrical disturbances)
  Chronic bradyarrhythmias
   AV block in aged cats
  Tachyarrhythmias and premature complexes
  Sedatives, tranquilizers, anesthetic drugs
 Chronic or severe anemia
 Hyperthyroidism
 Acromegaly
 Systemic hypertension
  Chronic renal disease
  Hyperthyroidism
  Idiopathic
 Electrolyte abnormalities
  Hyperkalemia
   Urinary obstruction
  Hypokalemia
   Renal disease

*The most common clinical presentations of feline cardiomyopathy are dyspnea from CHF, rear-limb paresis from aortic thromboembolism, and inactivity. The veterinarian often detects a murmur, gallop rhythm, arrhythmia, or cardiomegaly during examination.

- Diuretic drugs, such as furosemide, are highly effective in decreasing venous pressure and treating pulmonary edema, but excessive diuresis can decrease the ventricular preload and cardiac output.
- A vigorous atrial contraction (atrial "kick") from LA hypertrophy assists LV filling and helps maintain CO. Loss of LA contraction due to development of atrial fibrillation (AF)—a potential complication of atrial dilation—can be disastrous.
- Many cats develop mitral regurgitation (MR) because of the geometric changes in the ventricle, the altered papillary muscle support, or the abnormal anterior mitral leaflet movement during midsystole (see subsequent discussion). Large regurgitant volumes increase left atrial pressure (LAP) further.
- Tachycardia caused by stress (e.g., hospitalization), pain (e.g., due to aortic thrombus), arrhythmias (e.g., atrial fibrillation), or drugs (e.g., ketamine

HCl) is poorly tolerated. Even sinus tachycardia will do the following:
- Shorten ventricular filling and coronary artery perfusion time while increasing the myocardial oxygen consumption.
- Promote myocardial ischemia, which further impairs myocardial relaxation and LV compliance.
- In cases of "obstructive" cardiomyopathy, intraventricular pressure gradients develop during systole. This finding is associated with the movement of the anterior mitral leaflet towards the ventricular septum (systolic anterior motion of the mitral valve).
- Mitral regurgitation develops.
- Increased LV pressure contributes to further subendocardial ischemia.
- The overall significance of the ejection gradient is debated; however, drugs that reduce the contractility and the dynamic outflow gradient (beta blockers and calcium channel blockers) are often effec-

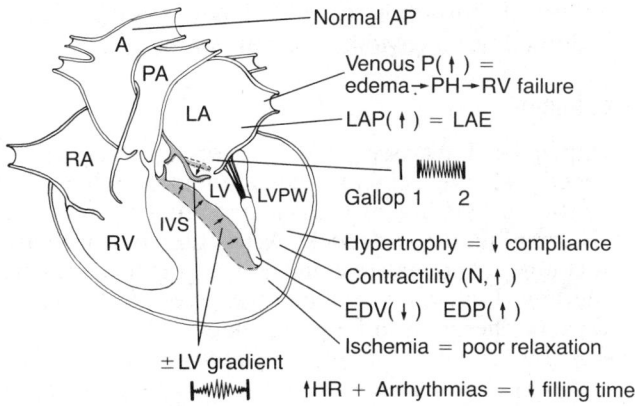

Figure 1. Diagrammatic representation of hypertrophic cardiomyopathy. Explanation of the abbreviations can be found in the text.

tive in management of HCM (see the discussion of therapy for HCM).

■ Chronic LA and pulmonary venous hypertension lead to pulmonary arterial hypertension, right ventricular overload, and biventricular CHF. The usual result is development of pleural effusion.

■ Hemodynamic abnormalities include high LV end-diastolic pressures and a prominent left atrial "a" wave. Pulmonary venous and arterial hypertension are present in cats with CHF. Intraventricular systolic gradients can be measured in hypertrophic "obstructive" CM.

Clinical Signs

■ Signalment. Mean age is 6 to 9 years, with a wide range of 6 months to 13 years. Male cats are affected more commonly. Persian cats may be predisposed. HCM may be more common in urban areas.

■ History. The cat may or may not be symptomatic.
  • Nonspecific signs of disease include anorexia, depression, inactivity, and reluctance to move.
  • Dyspnea or tachypnea is commonly observed and is related to pulmonary edema or pleural effusion. Cough is very unusual in cats with CM. Some cats vomit or retch, but the mechanism is unknown.
  • Thromboemboli can cause paralysis, especially of the rear limbs. The cat may present to the veterinarian because of relentless crying secondary to pain from an aortic embolism.
  • Most owners do not notice significant premonitory signs of CHF owing to the fastidious nature of the cat. Some cats are reportedly normal until they undergo some stressful event.
  • Asymptomatic cats may be identified during the course of a routine physical examination and auscultation.

■ Physical examination
  • Arterial pulse (AP) is normal unless there is an aortic embolus or a cardiac arrhythmia.
  • Jugular venous pressure/pulses may be elevated if there is pulmonary hypertension (PH) or biventricular CHF.
  • Cardiac auscultation is usually abnormal.
    Mitral regurgitation is evident in most cats as a holosystolic murmur heard best over the left apex/

left sternal border. The left apical impulse is typically strong.
    A murmur due to ventricular outflow obstruction is uncommon, even in cases of obstructive HCM.
    An atrial gallop (S$_4$), due to reduced ventricular compliance, is common.
    Sinus tachycardia is typical, owing to high adrenergic tone. Premature atrial or ventricular complexes or AF may be detected.
  • Respiratory distress, sternal recumbency, open-mouth breathing, and cyanosis are signs of CHF. Auscultation of pulmonary crackles and wheezes indicates pulmonary edema due to left-sided CHF. Pleural effusion, subsequent to biventricular failure, is indicated by muffled heart and breath sounds and dull thoracic percussion ventrally.
  • Clinical signs of aortic embolism may be detected (see subsequent discussion).
  • Abdominal palpation. Hepatomegaly is likely if there is biventricular CHF; however, ascites from CHF is much less common in the cat than in the dog. The kidneys may be painful or "pitted" on palpation if current or prior renal embolization has occurred.

Diagnosis

■ A presumptive diagnosis of HCM is made by recognizing signs of heart disease from history and physical examination, by identifying left-sided cardiomegaly from radiography and ECG, and by ruling out other known causes of LV hypertrophy, such as the following disorders:
  • *Hyperthyroidism* is detected by an elevated serum thyroxin (T$_4$) in cats older than 7 years (see subsequent discussion of hyperthyroid heart disease).
  • *Systemic hypertension* is particularly common in cats with chronic renal disease, but may also be idiopathic. Evaluate creatinine, urinalysis, and if necessary renal size by radiography or ultrasonography. This is a highly unlikely diagnosis in a cat with CHF or a thrombus, because hypertensive heart disease does not seem to progress to heart failure or to be associated with thromboembolic complications.
  • *Acromegaly* must be excluded from the diagnosis in cats with diabetes mellitus or facial deformity (see sec. 4, ch. 6). If available, measure plasma growth hormone activity.
  • *Congenital aortic stenosis* or *mitral dysplasia* is considered in young cats or in cats with a long history of cardiac murmur.

Radiography

■ Concentric LV hypertrophy and secondary left auricular dilation with shifting of the apex to the midline cause a typical "valentine"-shaped cardiac silhouette on the ventrodorsal view in many cases (see sec. 6, ch. 2). Elongation of the heart shadow is also typical.

■ Radiographic signs of left-sided heart failure include pulmonary venous dilation, pulmonary edema, and pulmonary arterial (PA) enlargement, with or without pleural effusion. Although classic cardiogenic perihilar infiltrates may be present, diffuse or dependent pulmonary edema is not uncommon.

KEY POINT ▶ Overlap exists between the radiographic features of the different forms of feline cardiomyopathy; thus, a definitive anatomic diagnosis of HCM is not possible from survey x-ray films.

■ Nonselective angiography, through a short cephalic vein catheter using 1 to 2 ml/kg of 80% iothalamate sodium, Angioconray (Mallinckrodt), or equivalent contrast agent, helps distinguish the various anatomic forms of feline CM. Therefore, this method can be used to make a definitive diagnosis.
  • With HCM, the LV lumen is small, the LV wall thick, the papillary muscles prominent, the outflow tract possibly narrowed, the LA dilated, and the aorta (A) normal or widened.
  • Filling defects in the LA indicate thrombus formation.

Echocardiography

■ The test of choice for the noninvasive diagnosis of HCM and other forms of cardiomyopathy. Anatomic abnormalities can be identified. Ventricular shortening fraction and ejection fraction are usually greater than normal.
■ Doppler studies can document valvular regurgitation and outflow obstruction.

Electrocardiography

■ Rhythm. Sinus tachycardia is typical, but premature complexes and atrial arrhythmias, including AF, are not uncommon. Ventricular pre-excitation occurs occasionally.
■ P waves. Increased P-wave amplitude (>0.25 mV) or duration (>0.035 sec) suggests LA enlargement (LAE).
■ QRS complexes. Left axis deviation secondary to LV hypertrophy or left anterior fascicular block is characteristic of HCM and perhaps related to lesions in the left bundle branch. A normal axis with increased voltage of R waves in leads II and aV_F (>0.7 mV) is common.

Laboratory Abnormalities

■ Laboratory abnormalities encountered in cats with HCM are quite variable but may include the following:
  • Azotemia secondary to CHF, aortic thrombosis, renal embolization, or dehydration.
  • Serum skeletal muscle enzyme levels, such as creatine kinase and aspartate aminotransferase (AST), are elevated in cats with aortic thrombosis. Elevated levels of alanine aminotransferase (ALT) are also common with thrombosis, and these may reflect a liver cell injury or a skeletal muscle isoenzyme.
  • Disseminated intravascular coagulation (DIC) is common in cats with thrombosis.

• Pleural effusion is typically a modified transudate. Sometimes a chylous effusion is present.

Treatment

■ Principles. First assess and categorize the degree of functional impairment: asymptomatic, CHF (left ventricular or biventricular), arrhythmia, thrombosis, renal failure, or shock. Acute pulmonary edema is common and may respond completely to aggressive therapy. Following treatment of severe CHF, maintenance therapy can be prescribed.
■ For the acutely symptomatic patient with CHF:
  • Avoid stress, sedate the cat if necessary using low doses (0.05 to 0.2 mg/kg) of SC acepromazine (Acepromazine; Ayerst). Acepromazine (an alpha-adrenergic blocker) is potentially hypotensive; thus, use cautiously in cats with marked hypothermia.
  • Treat hypoxemia with oxygen administration (40 to 60%).
  • For pulmonary edema administer furosemide (Lasix; Hoerst) initially at 2 mg/kg, IM or IV, then at 0.5 to 1.0 mg/kg, q8–12h, over the first 24 to 48 hours of therapy. In addition, apply 2% topical nitroglycerine ointment (Nitrol; Nitrobid) cutaneously. The usual dose is 1/4 inch, q8–12h.
  • Aminophylline (4 to 6 mg/kg, slowly IV) may improve ventilation but has disadvantageous sympathomimetic and inotropic effects and is rarely used.
  • If there is significant pleural effusion, aseptically drain each hemithorax with a 21- to 23-gauge butterfly needle, while the cat is resting in sternal recumbency.
  • Prevent heat loss if necessary by placing the cat in a warm environment.
  • Administer parenteral fluids only after lung edema is controlled or any pleural effusion has been aspirated. Fluid therapy is particularly important in dehydrated cats and in those with complicating metabolic disorders, such as azotemia. The usual fluid choice is 0.45% NaCl in 2.5% dextrose with 8 mEq KCl added per 250 ml fluid, if the cat is not oliguric or hyperkalemic.
■ Therapy of thromboembolism (see the subsequent discussion of the complications of cardiomyopathy)
■ Long-term therapy of feline HCM
  • Aspirin is often prescribed to prevent thrombosis (25 mg/kg, usually one children's aspirin given every 3 days or 3 times weekly). Efficacy is unproven and disputed.
  • Furosemide is continued with the dosage titrated to prevent recurrent pulmonary edema and pleural effusion.
    For cats with HCM that completely respond to treatment for an acute episode of pulmonary edema, the dosage of furosemide (Lasix; 12.5 mg tablets or 10 mg/ml syrup) can be tapered over 2 to 3 weeks to 1.0 mg/kg given two to three times weekly. Cats with progressive CHF may require furosemide daily at dosages up to 1 to 2 mg/kg q8h in addition to other treatments.

Clients can monitor diuretic efficacy by observing respiratory rate and activity. Periodic veterinary examinations and serum biochemical profiles are needed to insure efficacy and circumvent development of edema, hypokalemia, and prerenal azotemia.

- Prescribe a low sodium diet, e.g., Prescription Diet Feline h/d (Hill's) or its equivalent.
- Administer enalapril (Vasotec; Merck), an angiotensin converting enzyme inhibitor, for cats with progressive fluid accumulation, especially when pleural effusion occurs. Initial dosage is 0.25 mg/kg, PO, once daily. This can be increased to twice daily dosing.
- Diltiazem (Cardizem; Marian), a calcium channel blocker, may be beneficial in cats with HCM by the following mechanisms: improved LV relaxation (decreases LV end-diastolic pressure), coronary vasodilation (decreases ischemia), negative inotropism (decreases outflow obstruction), and negative chronotropism (decreases myocardial oxygen consumption). One feline study suggests that diltiazem may decrease LV hypertrophy.

  The initial dose is one fourth of a 30 mg tablet, PO, q8h.

  Diltiazem can be given as initial therapy in asymptomatic cats or added to the therapy in cats with poorly responding CHF currently receiving furosemide or enalapril.

  HR does not appear to be as well controlled by diltiazem as by beta blockade. The effects of calcium channel blockers on outflow gradients have not been evaluated in cats.

- Beta-adrenergic blockade with propranolol HCl (Inderal; Ayerst; 10-mg tablet) or atenolol (Tenormin; Stuart; 50-mg tablet) has been advocated in HCM for the following purposes: to slow heart rate (which decreases myocardial oxygen consumption and increases time for coronary and ventricular filling), to decrease LV outflow obstruction, and to exert antiarrhythmic actions.

  Beta blockers like propranolol also block bronchial and vascular beta-$_2$ receptors and, therefore, are contraindicated in arterial thrombosis, untreated CHF, and asthma.

  Propranolol (2.5 to 5 mg, q8h) or atenolol (one fourth of a 50-mg tablet, once or twice daily) may be prescribed as initial therapy in asymptomatic cats with documented HCM or added to a diuretic regimen following successful therapy of CHF.

  Heart rate is well controlled with beta blockers and can be used to monitor therapy. A target resting rate of 130 to 150 beats per minute (bpm) is appropriate. LV outflow obstruction is usually minimized by beta blockers; however, it is doubtful that these drugs improve relaxation.

- The treatment of choice between a beta blocker and a calcium channel blocker is unresolved. Both drugs could be used together, but this is not the usual approach. When LV outflow obstruction is documented by Doppler, choose a beta blocker first. Otherwise, diltiazem (plus a diuretic) is our initial choice for maintenance therapy of HCM.

KEY POINT ▶ When progressive CHF develops in a cat with HCM that is currently receiving both furosemide and beta blocker, substitute diltiazem for the beta blocker and add enalapril to the therapeutic regimen.

- The 2% nitroglycerin ointment (1/4-inch, cutaneously, q12h) may be applied for treatment or prevention of pulmonary edema; however, we prefer enalapril if vasodilator therapy is necessary.

  Nitroglycerin treatment may be useful for clients who cannot administer tablets.

  When lung edema develops suddenly at home, improvement may be obtained by administering the nitroglycerin ointment in combination with an extra dose of furosemide.

- Minimize stress because reflex tachycardia might worsen ventricular dynamics.
- Perform periodic thoracocentesis in cats with refractory pleural effusion.

Prognosis

- The natural history and prognosis of HCM are often quite favorable provided acute bouts of CHF can be controlled and complications such as aortic thrombosis do not develop. Many cats live for more than 2 years following a documented bout of pulmonary edema or a successful resolution of a thromboembolic event. With progressive heart disease, CHF episodes become worse. Development of pleural effusion and atrial fibrillation in cats with long-standing HCM are poor prognostic indicators (see subsequent discussion of the complications of cardiomyopathy).

DILATED CARDIOMYOPATHY (DCM) IN THE CAT

Etiology

- Most cases of DCM (Fig. 2) in the cat have developed secondary to a dietary deficiency in taurine. This form of feline DCM is reversible. Metabolic differences may also occur in cats in their ability to use taurine. Exclusive feeding of single diets may help to explain the predominance of DCM observed in some breeds (Burmese, Abyssinian). Some cats with DCM have normal plasma and whole blood taurine levels, and the condition may represent a different process such as postmyocarditis DCM.

Pathology

- Lesions that are often observed in advanced cases include dilatation of all cardiac chambers, particularly the LV and LA, a subjectively "flabby" myocardium, atrophied papillary muscles, increased heart weight compatible with eccentric hypertrophy, and left atrial and systemic arterial thrombi.
- Histologic lesions are nonspecific and include focal endocardial fibrosis, muscle cell degeneration and necrosis, and separation of cells by edematous extracellular ground substance or connective tissue.

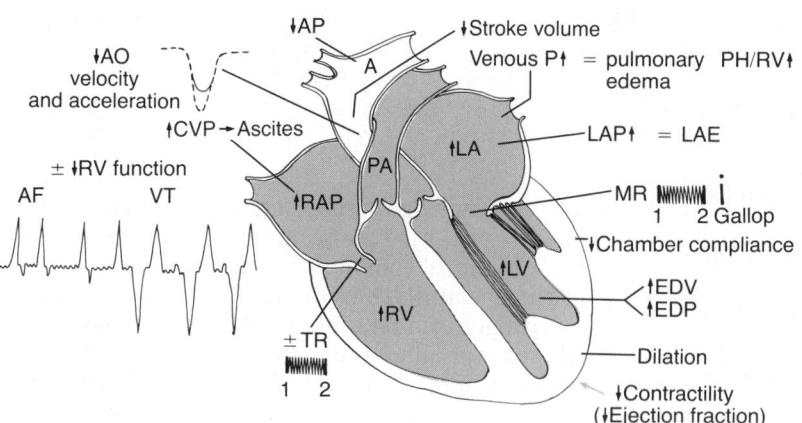

Figure 2. Diagrammatic representation of dilated cardiomyopathy. Explanation of the abbreviations can be found in the text.

Pathophysiology

- Myocardial inotropism is markedly depressed, leading to regional and eventually global ventricular myocardial failure.
- LV ejection fraction is depressed and stroke volume and cardiac output are limited.
- Neurohumoral compensations lead to sympathetic activation and to renal retention of sodium and water (see discussion of heart failure, sec. 6, ch. 6).
- The ventricles progressively dilate in most cases.
- Diastolic function is also compromised, owing to ventricular dilatation and fibrosis. Ventricular diastolic pressures increase.
- Atrioventricular (AV) valve annulus dilatation and altered papillary muscle function cause mitral regurgitation (MR) and tricuspid regurgitation (TR).
- Ventricular dilation and failure, valvular regurgitation, and renal sodium and water retention combine to increase atrial and venous pressures.
- CHF ensues and is usually characterized by biventricular failure.

Clinical Signs

- Signalment. Cats of any age can be affected, with both males and females affected in approximately equal numbers. Burmese, Abyssinian, and Siamese cats are over-represented in some reports.
- History. Historical abnormalities are identical to those described for feline HCM. Dietary history is important. Some cats eat only a single commercial diet. In particular, "off-brand" diets are often suspected as potentially deficient in taurine. Most, but not all, feline diets seem to have been sufficiently supplemented with taurine.
- Physical examination
  - Arterial pulse (AP) is usually hypokinetic, and it may be absent if there is aortic embolus or irregular if cardiac arrhythmia is present.
  - Jugular venous distension is usually present if there is CHF.
  - Cardiac auscultation/palpation is usually abnormal.
    Mitral regurgitation or tricuspid regurgitation murmurs are common. Often heart sounds are soft, even in the absence of pleural effusion, suggesting decreased contractility. The left apical impulse is typically weak.

A ventricular gallop (S_3) or summation gallop (S_3 and S_4) is typically present as a result of ventricular dilation and reduced ventricular compliance.

Sinus tachycardia, sinus bradycardia, or arrhythmias may be detected.

- Hypothermia, severe depression, weakness, pallor, and slow capillary refill time (from vasoconstriction) are evidence of cardiogenic shock.
- Examination of the ocular fundus may reveal abnormal hyper-reflective areas of retinal degeneration adjacent to the optic disc, which are typical of taurine deficiency.
- Other respiratory, abdominal, and physical findings—including those of aortic thrombosis—are similar to those of feline HCM.

Diagnosis

- Presumptive diagnosis of feline DCM is made by considering the breed and dietary history, recognizing the signs of heart disease from history and physical examination, identifying the cardiomegaly from radiography and ECG, detecting the retinal lesions of taurine deficiency, and ruling out the diagnosis of hyperthyroidism.
- Definitive diagnosis of feline DCM requires echocardiography or angiography. Taurine deficiency as the cause of DCM can be verified by measuring the plasma or whole blood taurine concentration and monitoring the response to supplementation.

Radiography

- Generalized cardiomegaly is evident with rounding of the cardiac apex. The valentine-shaped heart (ventrodorsal view) is far less common than in HCM.
  - The heart may not appear substantially enlarged following volume contraction with diuretic drugs.
  - Pleural effusion is typical; however, some cats manifest signs of pulmonary edema only.
  - Nonselective angiography delineates dilated RV and LV lumina; thin ventricular walls; LA dilation; and poorly contrasted aorta (A), indicative of low cardiac output. Angiography can cause cardiac arrest in cats with DCM. Stabilization with treatment is, therefore, advised.

Echocardiography

- Echocardiography is the diagnostic procedure of choice for DCM. Anatomic abnormalities can be identified. End-systolic dimension is increased owing to low LV shortening fraction, which is usually between 5 and 20%. Normal shortening fraction is more than 30%. Doppler studies can document valvular regurgitation and low aortic outflow velocity.

Electrocardiography

- A variety of arrhythmias are possible. Sinus bradycardia is not uncommon. Sinus arrest and junctional (nodal) rhythms may be observed.
- P waves that are increased in amplitude (>0.25 mV) or duration (>0.035 sec) suggest LA enlargement.
- A normal axis with increased voltage R waves in leads II and aV_F (>0.7 mV) is common and indicates LV dilation. Right axis deviation secondary to RV dilation or right bundle branch block may be present.

Laboratory Abnormalities

- Laboratory abnormalities in cats with DCM are similar to those in cats with HCM, with the following exceptions:
  - Plasma taurine concentration is usually below the reference range for the laboratory and, typically, ≤ 20 nmol/ml before clinical DCM develops. Both plasma and whole blood levels are helpful; however, some evidence suggests that taurine concentration in whole blood is a better diagnostic index of taurine status. Whole blood taurine of >250 nmol/ml appears to indicate an adequate level. The clinician is encouraged to contact the laboratory regarding handling and interpretation.
  - Cats with persistent hypokalemia may be predisposed to taurine depletion.
  - Occasionally, cats with hyperthyroidism develop DCM; therefore, serum thyroxin (T_4) is measured in cats older than 7 years of age. Hyperthyroidism also can complicate DCM and precipitate CHF.
  - Moderate-to-severe anemia (packed cell volume $<18\%$) in cats with underlying DCM may rarely develop into CHF owing to increased cardiac output demands.

Treatment

- Principles. Assess the degree of functional impairment: asymptomatic, CHF (left ventricular or biventricular), arrhythmia, thrombosis, renal failure, shock. Recognize that cardiogenic shock requires aggressive therapy to prevent death from hypoxia and hypotension. Following the initial therapy for severe CHF, maintenance therapy can be prescribed.
- For the acutely symptomatic patient with CHF:
  - Minimize stress but use sedatives cautiously, because even low doses of SC acepromazine (Acepromazine; Ayerst), 0.05 to 0.1 mg/kg, may potentiate hypotension and hypothermia.
  - Administer oxygen (40 to 60%).
  - For pulmonary edema or pleural effusion administer furosemide (Lasix; Hoerst) initially at 2 mg/kg IM or IV, and then 0.5 to 1.0 mg/kg q8–12h over the first 24 hours of therapy. In addition, apply 2% topical nitroglycerin ointment (Nitrol; Nitrobid) cutaneously. The usual dose is 1/4-inch, q8–12h.
  - Using a 21- or 23-gauge butterfly needle, aseptically drain each hemithorax as required to relieve pleural effusion.

KEY POINT ▶ Thoracocentesis is essential for the management of large pleural effusions in cats with DCM.

  - Aminophylline (4 mg/kg, slowly IV) can be administered to improve ventilation.
  - Prevent heat loss if necessary by placing the cat in a warm environment.
  - Place an IV catheter, and administer warmed IV or SC fluids only after lung edema is controlled or pleural effusion is aspirated. Usually one can provide 0.45% NaCl in 2.5% dextrose solution IV or lactated Ringer's solution SC, with 8 mEq KCl per 250 ml fluid, if the cat is not oliguric or hyperkalemic. The usual rate of infusion is 30 to 60 ml/kg over 24 hours provided the effusion has been drained and diuresis has been attained.
  - Cardiogenic shock is treated by infusion of dobutamine (Dobutrex; Lilly, 2 to 5 µgm/kg/min) or dopamine (Intropin; Armour, 2 to 5 µgm/kg/min) for up to 36 hours. Alternatively, the inotropic-dilator amrinone (Inocor; Winthrop) can be administered at the labeled human dose.
- For therapy of thromboembolism see the subsequent discussion of the complications of cardiomyopathy.
- For long-term therapy of feline DCM
  - Prescribe aspirin as described for HCM.
  - Titrate furosemide to prevent recurrent pulmonary edema and pleural effusion as described for HCM. Daily furosemide is required unless the cat has taurine-responsive CHF (see subsequent discussion).
  - Feed a low sodium diet, e.g., Prescription Diet Feline h/d (Hill's) or its equivalent. A diet supplemented with taurine is always recommended.
  - Prescribe enalapril (Vasotec; Merck) for cats with an initial dosage of 0.25 mg/kg, PO, once daily. If necessary, increase to twice daily.
  - Prescribe digoxin (Lanoxin; Burroughs-Wellcome; or Cardoxin; Evsco) at a dosage of 0.01 mg/kg, q48h for elixirs; or one fourth of a 0.125 mg digoxin tablet, q48h. Avoid digoxin if the serum creatinine level remains higher than 2.5 mg/dl.
  - Beta-adrenergic blockers and calcium channel blockers are not typically prescribed, owing to the negative inotropic effects of these drugs.
  - DCM secondary to taurine deficiency (i.e., low plasma levels) still occurs sporadically. Some cats with DCM have normal plasma levels. Nonetheless, after a plasma or whole blood sample for taurine concentration has been obtained, it is prudent to treat *all* cats with echocardiographic or angiocardiographic evidence of DCM with taurine (250 mg, PO, q8–12h) for at least 12 weeks.

DCM is reversible after 4 to 6 weeks of taurine supplementation in cats with taurine-induced DCM.

In cats with taurine-deficiency DCM, therapy for CHF may be gradually withdrawn after 4 to 6 weeks if there is radiographic and echocardiographic documentation of improved myocardial function.

Periodically evaluate plasma and whole blood taurine concentrations.

RESTRICTIVE (INTERMEDIATE) CARDIOMYOPATHY (RCM) IN THE CAT

Etiology

- RCM (Fig. 3) is a poorly defined condition of unknown cause.
- Cats with RCM have clinical and functional disorders that are similar to those in cats with both HCM and DCM.
- Most cats with RCM have normal plasma taurine levels. Previous myocarditis is a plausible (but unproven) etiology, because inflammation can lead to myocyte degeneration and fibrosis.

Pathology

- Lesions that are often observed in advanced cases are as follows:

  - Dilatation of all cardiac chambers may be evident. The left ventricular cavity is dilated near the basilar portion. The LV wall thickness may be increased, especially apically and in the area of the papillary muscles.
  - Prominent areas of diffuse or focal (involving papillary muscles) myocardial fibrosis are seen in the LV.
  - Often prominent moderator bands (trabeculae septomarginalis) are evident spanning the LV wall or septum to the papillary muscles.
  - The LA is dilated to a greater degree than that typical for DCM. A large spherical thrombus ("ball thrombus") may be evident in the auricle or atrium proper.
  - Although myocardial fibrosis is prominent, detailed histologic studies have not been reported.

Pathophysiology

- Pathophysiology is presumptive. Myocardial inotropism is mildly to moderately depressed, as indicated by echocardiographic indices of systolic function. LV ejection fraction is depressed, and stroke volume and cardiac output are limited.
- LV is probably stiffened from myocardial fibrosis, and this may contribute to LA dilation.
- Neurohumoral compensations lead to sympathetic activation and to renal retention of sodium and water (see sec. 6, ch. 6).
- RV dysfunction probably develops from pulmonary hypertension secondary to left-sided heart failure.
- AV valve annulus dilatation and altered papillary muscle function cause mitral and tricuspid regurgitation that ranges from mild to severe. (Note: Severe cases may resemble those in cats with AV valve dysplasia).
- Ventricular dilation and failure, valvular regurgitation, and renal sodium and water retention combine to increase atrial and venous pressures.
- CHF ensues and is usually characterized by biventricular failure.
- Atrial arrhythmias, including atrial fibrillation, are not uncommon.

Clinical Signs

- Signalment. Cats of any age or sex can be affected; most are mature.
- History is typical of feline heart disease. The signs of CHF or arterial thromboembolism (TE) are reported.
- Physical examination findings are characterized by the signs of heart disease (murmur, gallop, arrhythmia), CHF, or TE. These have been described previously for HCM and DCM.
  - Arterial pulse is normal to hypokinetic.
  - Jugular venous distension occurs if there is CHF.
  - Pulmonary edema is evident in cases of early CHF.
  - In severe CHF, both pleural effusion and ascites may be observed, especially if atrial fibrillation has developed.

Diagnosis

- Presumptive diagnosis of feline RCM is made by obtaining the history, recognizing the signs of heart disease during the physical examination, identifying cardiomegaly by radiography and ECG, and ruling out the possibility of hyperthyroidism. Definitive diagnosis of feline RCM requires echocardiography or angiography. One of these studies is undertaken, once the initial signs of CHF have been controlled.

Radiography

- Generalized cardiomegaly is evident. The apex may be pointed or rounded. A valentine-shaped heart may be observed on the ventrodorsal radiograph, or the atria may be markedly enlarged and dominate the cardiac shadow.
  - Nonselective angiography delineates dilated RV and RA lumina. The LV cavity is usually very

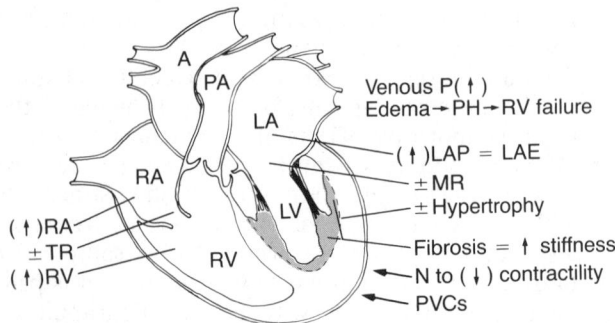

Figure 3. Diagrammatic representation of restrictive cardiomyopathy. Explanation of the abbreviations can be found in the text.

irregular with filling defects caused by fibrosis or abnormal papillary muscle hypertrophy.
- The LA is often enormous and filling defects (thrombi) may be evident.

Echocardiography

- Dilation of the atria and RV can be identified. The LV is often dilated near the mitral valve. Regional areas of hypertrophy may be observed. The papillary muscles project prominently into the LV lumen and often appear "rigid."
- LV shortening fraction is mildly to moderately decreased (usually <25% but >15%) and regional LV wall motion abnormalities may be observed.
- Prominent moderator bands are commonly observed. Focal areas of heightened echogenicity in the LV suggest myocardial fibrosis.
- Doppler studies can document valvular regurgitation when present.

Electrocardiography

- Rhythm. A variety of arrhythmias are possible, especially atrial premature complexes and atrial fibrillation.
- Increased amplitude of P waves (>0.25 mV) or duration (>0.035 sec) suggests LA enlargement.
- Axis deviations and intraventricular conduction disturbances (e.g., bundle branch blocks) are common. Increased voltage R waves or widened QRS complexes suggest LV dilation.

Laboratory Abnormalities

Laboratory abnormalities in cats with RCM are similar to those in cats with HCM. In some cats, plasma taurine levels may be decreased; however, unlike cats with DCM, supplementation with taurine does not reverse the anatomic and functional disorders of the heart.

Treatment

- Therapy most resembles that given to cats with DCM, using the same agents and dosages given in the HCM and DCM discussions of this chapter.
- Myocardial contractility is somewhat diminished; therefore, digoxin, enalapril (an angiotensin-converting enzyme inhibitor), dietary sodium restriction, and taurine supplementation are prescribed as for DCM.
- Furosemide is administered, and the dose titrated as for HCM and DCM.
- Thoracocentesis is often required for initial management.
- When CHF persists despite this therapy, diltiazem can be considered to possibly improve diastolic function of the heart.
- If atrial fibrillation develops, diltiazem is added to therapy to control the ventricular rate response.
- Fluid therapy may be required during initial stabilization to prevent dehydration and progressive renal failure.
- Aspirin is prescribed to alter platelet aggregation.

COMPLICATIONS OF FELINE CARDIOMYOPATHY

Systemic Thromboembolism

- *Systemic thromboembolism* (TE) is common, especially involving the terminal aortic trifurcation. Signs are often acute in onset and associated with substantial anxiety and pain. The stress and associated tachycardia may precipitate CHF. Less common thromboembolic sites cause acute foreleg paresis, acute renal failure due to suprarenal or renal thrombus, or colic related to gut ischemia. Cats with renal thrombosis or mesenteric ischemia may display *severe* abdominal pain.

Clinical Signs

- *Signs* of aortic embolism include vascular, neurologic, and skeletal muscle dysfunction.
  - Vascular. Loss of femoral pulse and coccygeal pulse (via rectal examination); cool, pale limbs; and absence of bleeding from cut nail beds.
  - Neurologic. Lower motor neuron paresis is usually present, and the cat may be paralyzed. Involvement may be unilateral or bilateral. The tail may or may not be involved. Severe ischemic neuropathy is characterized by paralysis, areflexia, and loss of deep pain.
  - Musculoskeletal. Muscle contracture (gastrocnemius, semitendinosus, quadriceps), muscle pain, and eventual muscle necrosis characterized by persistent blue discoloration and progressive softness with edema.
    Skeletal muscle enzymes (creatine kinase or CK, AST) leak into the serum, and levels are severely elevated.
    Serum ALT levels may also be elevated. The source of this enzyme (from the liver or from a massive skeletal muscle necrosis) is uncertain.
    Although enzyme concentrations are increased within hours of the insult and ischemic myopathy develops almost immediately, it may take 3 to 10 days for severe skeletal muscle injury to be evident clinically.

Laboratory Abnormalities

- Laboratory abnormalities depend on the site of obstruction and severity of tissue injury.
  - Elevated serum CK, AST, and sometimes ALT
  - Hyperkalemia often develops from reperfusion of injured and necrotic tissues following spontaneous, drug-induced, or surgical revascularization.
  - Metabolic acidosis is common (lactic acidosis?).
  - Disseminated intravascular coagulopathy is common and may contribute to bleeding in other organs.
  - Renal infarction or suprarenal thrombosis is associated with elevated BUN and serum creatinine concentrations.
  - Leucocytosis with a left shift usually occurs after 2 to 5 days.

Diagnosis

■ In most cats, the diagnosis of TE is made from the history and physical examination. Markedly elevated skeletal muscle enzyme concentrations support the diagnosis. Angiography is almost never required for diagnosis and may be a dangerous added stress in the clinical setting of acute embolism with uncontrolled CHF.

- Differential diagnosis includes bacterial endocarditis of the aortic or mitral valve; tumor infiltration of the pelvic canal or iliac trifurcation; missile-like foreign body (pellet), which is very rare; and trauma to the caudal abdomen.

- The client is advised that arterial TE in the cat is almost always associated with underlying heart disease. This concern may limit the use of anesthesia and surgery for treatment of this condition.

Treatment

■ A number of therapeutic options are available.
- General therapy applicable for all cats includes the following:

Management of CHF.

Analgesics are prescribed for this painful condition, such as butorphanol (Torbugesic; Fort Dodge), 0.1 to 0.4 mg/kg, IV, SC, IM but not in rear limbs. Alternatively, use buprenorphine (Buprenex; Norwich Eaton) 0.01 to 0.02 mg/kg, IM. If combined with a tranquilizer expect substantial sedation, which may be beneficial.

Prevent hypothermia, but do not subject the limbs to external temperatures exceeding normal body temperature.

Administer sodium bicarbonate for presumed metabolic acidosis (1 mEq/kg, slowly IV over 5 minutes, and repeat thereafter based on ECG monitoring and measurement of blood gas and serum potassium values).

Administer maintenance fluid therapy (as for feline DCM) to prevent acute renal failure and hyperkalemia. This treatment is delayed until CHF is controlled.

Determine the baseline clotting times for monitoring anticoagulant therapy (e.g., partial thromboplastin time, prothrombin time, and activated clotting time) (see sec. 3, ch. 2).

- Conservative—but empirical—medical therapy has been associated with a favorable outcome. The goals are to increase collateral circulation and to prevent further thrombosis.

Sodium heparin is provided at 200 IU/kg IV followed by 200 IU/kg SC, q8h, to prolong the clotting times 2 to 3 times those over baseline. Continue therapy for at least 72 hours.

Aspirin is given at 20 to 25 mg/kg, PO, every 3 days or three times weekly, indefinitely.

Acepromazine is administered initially at 0.1 mg/kg IM in an unaffected muscle; thereafter, repeat SC, q8h until the cat is tranquilized and the nictitating membranes are prolapsed. The goals are alpha-adrenergic blockade and collateral vasodilation. The initial dosage can be subsequently increased by 0.1 mg/kg increments as necessary to achieve these goals. Acepromazine tablets of 1 to 2 mg/kg, q8–12h, can be substituted after 2 or 3 days. Continue therapy up to 4 weeks.

Ampicillin (10 to 20 mg/kg, q8–12h, SC or PO) is administered prophylactically.

- Thrombolytic therapy with either streptokinase or tissue plasminogen activator (t-PA) is highly effective in dissolving clots in some cats.

Strongly consider such treatment in cats with symptoms that have been present for less than 12 hours.

The cost of t-PA is probably too great to be practical. Streptokinase, which activates plasminogen, can be obtained at reasonable cost from most human hospitals.

The greatest dangers of therapy are uncontrolled bleeding and reperfusion hyperkalemia.

KEY POINT ▶ Thrombolytic therapy, when selected, proceeds without delay to prevent further tissue injury and to obtain the best thrombolytic effect. Such therapy is likely to decrease the clot size; however, there are substantial risks, such as hyperkalemia.

Doses extrapolated from Killingsworth's study are streptokinase at 90,000 IU by constant rate infusion over 30 minutes, followed by constant rate infusion of 45,000 IU/hour. We recommend treatment for up to 6 hours or until arterial pulses return.

Serum potassium concentration is monitored three to four times daily, and the ECG monitored almost continuously. If serum potassium level exceeds 8 mEq/L, or if atrial standstill develops, temporarily discontinue the infusion and treat the cat with sodium bicarbonate (1 to 2 mEq/kg, IV); IV fluids; and, if needed, calcium gluconate (0.1 ml of the 10% solution per kg, very slowly, IV), until the ECG rhythm returns to normal.

- Surgical removal of the thrombus via a ventral midline incision is considered in cats with clinical and laboratory signs of suprarenal or mesenteric thrombus.

Surgery in most cats is not advocated owing to a high perioperative mortality rate. However, cats without CHF may benefit from surgery. This option, therefore, can be considered in selected cases.

Fogarty embolectomy catheters may be used to remove clots, but this procedure is technically difficult in a cat with a femoral artery obstruction.

Natural History and Prognosis

■ Provided the cat does not die of CHF, arrhythmia, or reperfusion hyperkalemia, a significant percentage (40 to 50%) may develop spontaneous revascularization of the limbs and progressive improvement in motor function over the next 2 to 4 weeks.

- It is not always possible to predict the outcome based on initial evaluation. Some cats with severe embolism improve dramatically.

- Unfortunately, some cats develop such severe skeletal muscle necrosis and ischemic neuropathy that the limb atrophies and becomes a fibrotic and useless appendage.

- Gangrene also may develop and is considered in any cat with a soft, edematous limb and progressive, antibiotic-resistant fever. Sepsis is another potential complication.
- Amputation of such severely affected limbs may be required 1 to 4 weeks after the initial insult (see sec. 9, ch. 22). Some cats do well following amputation.

■ Recurrent arterial TE can occur in some cats. In some cases, a rapid return to limb function ensues, perhaps related to development of collateral vessels. Other cats die or are euthanatized because of severe tissue injury or client-related concerns.

Atrial Fibrillation

■ *Atrial fibrillation* is more common with hypertrophic and restrictive forms of feline CM. This condition is disastrous in cats with stiff ventricles because the atrial contribution to filling is lost.

- Some cats develop paroxysmal AF. This may convert to sinus rhythm spontaneously or following therapy with a calcium channel blocker.
- Initial management for cats with acute onset AF or a ventricular rate response more than 320/minute is verapamil at 0.05 mg/kg, IV, q30 minutes to a maximum cumulative dose of 0.2 mg/kg (see sec. 6, ch. 4).
- For persistent or chronic AF, digoxin (see discussion of feline DCM) is administered along with diltiazem (see discussion of feline HCM). The goal is control of ventricular rate response to less than 200/minute. Diltiazem dose is titrated to the desired heart rate.
- Pleural effusion often develops in cats with AF, and thoracocentesis may be required.

Pleural Effusion

■ *Pleural effusion* is a consequence of biventricular CHF and may develop as an end-stage feature of CHF in cats with chronic left-sided heart failure.

■ *Chylothorax* secondary to CHF is not uncommon and can be controlled only when the underlying cardiac condition can be managed. The following are considered in treatment:

- Optimize furosemide therapy (1 to 3 mg/kg, q8–12h), insuring that serum creatinine concentration does not increase and serum potassium concentration does not decrease. Consider intermittent SC dosing by the client to insure maximum effect.
- Digitalize the cat and measure the serum digoxin concentration after 10 days of therapy. Obtain a blood sample 8 hours post dose.
- Prescribe enalapril (Vasotec; Merck) up to a maximum dosage of 0.25 mg/kg, PO, q12h. Monitor serum creatinine levels periodically.
- For cats with HCM or RCM, prescribe diltiazem to improve diastolic function (see discussion of feline HCM).
- When atrial fibrillation supervenes, control the

ventricular rate response (see preceding discussion of atrial fibrillation).

- Instruct the client to feed the patient a sodium-restricted diet.
- Perform thoracocentesis for moderate to severe effusions.

MYOCARDITIS

Etiology

■ Inflammation of the myocardium may develop secondary to infectious agents (see Table 1) or in association with cardiomyopathy (e.g., feline cardiomyopathy and boxer dog cardiomyopathy), trauma, ischemic injury, or toxicity. It can also be idiopathic in origin. Myocarditis may eventually cause dilated cardiomyopathy and may be the underlying cause of "idiopathic" DCM in some animals.

Pathology

■ Myocarditis is classified histologically based on the predominant cellular infiltrate. The cellular infiltrate varies, depending on the cause and duration. The heart can respond to injury in a limited number of ways, so that most inflammations are nonsuppurative (consisting of mononuclear cells, predominantly lymphocytic-plasmacytic), granulomatous, suppurative, or, rarely, eosinophilic. Infective agents may or may not be present.

- A predominantly nonsuppurative endomyocarditis has been observed in most forms of feline CM. Inflammation often involves the conduction system and may explain the conduction disturbances that occur in some cats with CM.
- CHF due to acute necrotizing myocarditis can be fatal in litters of pups infected neonatally by parvovirus (see sec. 2, ch. 7).
- Boxer dogs with "boxer myocarditis" may have nonsuppurative myocarditis that is associated with development of malignant ventricular arrhythmias (see subsequent discussion of canine dilated cardiomyopathy).
- Dogs, in the southwestern United States, with Chagas disease develop granulomatous myocarditis that can cause heart failure, arrhythmias, or AV conduction block.

■ Myocardial degeneration and necrosis are noted in association with myocarditis. Advanced stages have significant subendocardial infiltrate, with macrophages and histiocytes accompanying the predominant inflammatory cells. The myocardium is replaced by granulation tissue consisting of histiocytes, Anitschkow's cells, hemorrhage, and inflammatory cells. In chronic myocarditis, fibrosis may be the principal lesion and may be evidenced grossly at necropsy as a white, unraised discoloration of the myocardium.

Clinical Signs

■ When myocarditis causes decreased myocardial contractility, either exercise intolerance or overt CHF may develop (e.g., necrotizing myocarditis caused by parvovirus in pups leads to death from pulmonary edema). Clinical features in this situation are virtually identical to those in DCM of the cat or dog.

■ Most often, myocarditis becomes evident because cardiac arrhythmias develop.
  • Clinical signs can include weakness and syncope, CHF, abnormal heart sounds and pulses, and sudden death.
  • Ventricular premature complexes and ventricular tachycardia are most commonly associated with myocarditis; however, atrial arrhythmias and AV block also can occur.
  • Myocarditis associated with trauma or with infectious agents (e.g., *Trypanosoma, Borrelia*) may be unrecognized if other clinical signs dominate.

Diagnosis

■ Clinical recognition of myocarditis may not be easy because no test specifically confirms a diagnosis of myocardial inflammation other than biopsy. Transvenous endomyocardial biopsy can be done with little risk; however, it requires special equipment and training and is rarely done.
■ Laboratory diagnosis of myocarditis—elevated myocardial fractions of the serum muscle enzymes (creatine kinase, lactic dehydrogenase (LDH), and AST)—is suggestive of myocarditis, but these isoenzyme fractions must be measured in a laboratory using human standards. There is little laboratory experience interpreting these test results in animals.

Treatment

■ Management of myocarditis or secondary myocardial injury has the following objectives:
  • Treatment of the primary cause, if it can be identified.
  • Treatment of cardiac arrhythmias (see discussion of the management of cardiac arrhythmias).
  • Treatment of CHF when present (see discussion of DCM).
  • Possible role of corticosteroids in the treatment of certain types of myocarditis remains uncertain.

DILATED CARDIOMYOPATHY IN DOGS

Etiology

■ DCM is common in dogs. The causes are unknown; however, a number of explanations have been proposed (see Table 1).
  • DCM occurs following a presumed change in the myocardial environment induced by inflammation, toxins, lack of essential cellular nutrients, inborn errors of myocardial metabolism, and so forth.

    The underlying cause of DCM is unknown in the majority of cases. Because it is most common in certain large and "giant" breeds and in a number of spaniel breeds, a genetic or familial link is proposed. *Giant breed cardiomyopathy* is considered synonymous with DCM.

Keene's group has demonstrated a deficiency of L-carnitine (used for fatty acid energy metabolism in the mitochondria) in a substantial number of dogs with DCM. Partial reversal of DCM is observed in some, but not all, dogs given L-carnitine supplementation.

Kittleson's group has found plasma taurine levels to be low in some American cocker spaniels; however, when all breeds are considered, taurine deficiency is *not* likely to be important in the pathogenesis of DCM in the dog.

Toxic injury to the myocardium can lead to DCM. This may occur with long-term administration of doxorubicin (Adriamycin), an anticancer chemotherapeutic.

  • Although myocytes cannot undergo hyperplasia, myocardial cell proteins and myosin enzymes frequently turn over in the heart. A change in their structure or function leads to a loss of myocardial cell contractility. Thus, DCM can develop slowly or somewhat rapidly.
  • Progressive global myocardial failure and chamber dilatation lead to dilated cardiomyopathy.

Pathology

■ Dilatation of all the cardiac chambers is accompanied by mild-to-moderate (eccentric) hypertrophy. The papillary muscles may appear flattened and atrophic.
■ Dilatation of the LV and RV also causes dilatation of the mitral and tricuspid valve rings, predisposing the dog to mitral and tricuspid regurgitation.
■ Mild-to-moderate myxomatous valvular changes also can be present (AV valve endocardiosis), but these are not the primary lesions of this condition.
■ Lesions of CHF include serous cavity effusions, hepatomegaly, and pulmonary edema.
■ Histologic lesions are minimal in most cases and may include the following: congestion, mononuclear and occasional neutrophilic infiltration, hemorrhage, necrosis, fibrosis (possibly resolved inflammation or the result of myocyte degeneration), and fatty change. Histologic lesions do *not* satisfactorily provide the explanation for the development of DCM.

Pathophysiology

■ Similar to feline DCM, this condition in the dog represents principally a "systolic dysfunction" syndrome due to myocardial failure. The left ventricular ejection fraction is decreased.
■ The AV valve annulus dilatation or the geometric changes in the papillary muscles often result in mitral and tricuspid valvular insufficiency.
■ Lord has also demonstrated decreases in ventricular diastolic compliance probably secondary to the presence of fibrosis and marked dilation of the ventricle.
■ Arrhythmias are common. *Atrial fibrillation* and *ventricular tachycardia* are the most important, because these tachyarrhythmias further depress ventricular function in the following ways:
  • Tachycardia decreases coronary perfusion time while myocardial oxygen consumption increases.
  • Ventricular filling time is erratic and shortened.

- With atrial fibrillation, the normal atrial "kick" is lost, which further decreases ventricular preload, especially at rapid ventricular heart rates.
- Ventricular tachycardia activates the ventricle abnormally, causing a less forceful beat. Moreover, the heart is made less electrically stable, and ventricular premature beats may progress suddenly to a fatal rhythm, i.e., ventricular fibrillation or cardiac arrest.
- Decreased cardiac output and renal and hormonal compensatory mechanisms lead to venous congestion with left ventricular or biventricular CHF.
- Acute and severe ventricular arrhythmias may cause sudden death prior to or following the onset of CHF.

Clinical Signs

- Signalment. "Giant" breeds and other large dogs (>15 kg) are predisposed. The spaniel breeds, particularly springer and cocker spaniels, are also predisposed. A male predominance is reported in most surveys. The affected dogs are often relatively young, with most between 2 and 5 years of age.
- Client complaints and history. Animals are usually presented for signs referable to progressive heart disease, CHF, or cardiac arrhythmia, including the following:
  - Exercise intolerance, lethargy, and tiring
  - Respiratory problems, such as tachypnea, dyspnea, orthopnea, or coughing
  - Fulminant pulmonary edema may cause hemoptysis, which is particularly common in the Doberman pinscher breed.
  - Weight loss is often dramatic and may occur within a short period of time (e.g., 2 to 4 weeks). This sign probably represents cardiac cachexia or a generalized disorder of striated muscle metabolism.
  - Abdominal distension (from ascites)
  - Sudden weakness or syncope (probably from an arrhythmia)

KEY POINT ▶ The two major clinical syndromes of DCM in the dog are CHF and paroxysmal or sustained cardiac arrhythmias. Often, these two problems occur together.

- Physical examination findings
  - Weight loss, poor body condition, and depression
  - Slow capillary refill time due to peripheral vasoconstriction and reduced cardiac output
  - Cyanosis due to pulmonary dysfunction from CHF or severe vasoconstriction
  - Typical pulse abnormalities include (1) hypokinetic pulses due to decreased stroke volume or cardiac arrhythmias; (2) rapid, erratic pulse with pulse deficits suggesting atrial fibrillation or ventricular arrhythmias; and (3) alternating intensity pulse (pulsus alternans) indicating severe myocardial failure or bigeminal arrhythmia.
  - Prominent jugular pulses and increased jugular venous pressures usually indicate right-sided CHF.

- Abnormalities of cardiac auscultation may include the following: (1) soft first sound, which signifies myocardial failure; (2) ventricular (S_3) or summation ($S_3 + S_4$) gallop, which is common (the gallop is easiest to detect when the dog is in sinus rhythm and may diminish following successful therapy of CHF); (3) left or right apical systolic murmurs, which are common and due to mitral or tricuspid regurgitation (when compared with the murmurs commonly detected with canine endocardiosis, the murmurs of DCM are typically less intense—usually grade 2 to 4 of 6); and (4) auscultatory evidence of cardiac arrhythmia, which is typical.

  Rapid, irregular, chaotic, variable intensity heart sounds typify atrial fibrillation, which is the *most common arrhythmia.*

  Isolated premature beats may be heard in the dog with a rhythm that is otherwise sinus, suggesting atrial or ventricular premature beats.

  Periods of rapid, regular rhythm with variable intensity (or split) sounds that start and stop abruptly typify paroxysmal ventricular tachycardia.
- Respiratory examination in symptomatic dogs usually demonstrates signs of left-sided or biventricular CHF: (1) tachypnea and dyspnea are common because of pulmonary edema or pleural effusion; (2) inspiratory/early expiratory pulmonary crackles suggest pulmonary edema; and (3) inspiratory dyspnea with muffled heart and breath sounds (and dull percussion) ventrally suggest pleural effusion.
- Hepatomegaly with or without ascites indicates right-sided CHF.
- Signs of cardiogenic shock may include severe weakness, depression, hypothermia, and mucous membrane pallor.

Diagnosis

Radiography

- Advanced DCM is characterized by generalized cardiomegaly and radiographic signs of CHF. Dilation of the LV and LA are most evident in some dogs.
  - Of note is the Doberman pinscher breed in which marked dilation of the left atrium with pulmonary edema is often the principal finding.
  - Pulmonary venous congestion is a feature of DCM prior to the onset of lung edema.
  - Pulmonary edema can be severe and diffuse, particularly in Doberman pinschers and in dogs that suddenly develop atrial fibrillation.
  - Pleural effusion is common.

Echocardiography

Echocardiography is the current clinical "gold standard" for diagnosis of DCM. The cardinal findings are ventricular and atrial dilatation with depressed myocardial systolic function (fractional shortening is low, <25% and usually <15% in symptomatic dogs). Doppler studies can document mitral or tricuspid regurgitation and decreased aortic ejection velocity typical of myocardial failure.

Electrocardiography

- Electrocardiography. The ECG is abnormal in most dogs with DCM. Common abnormalities include the following:
  - Tachycardia is often due to sinus or atrial tachycardia, atrial fibrillation, or ventricular tachycardia.
  - Isolated atrial or ventricular premature complexes (PVCs) may be observed. They can be the earliest detectable sign of DCM in some asymptomatic dogs.
  - Ventricular tachycardia is very common in Doberman pinschers and in Boxer dogs with DCM.

    Harpster's classification of "boxer cardiomyopathy" is based on ECG and clinical criteria:

    I—asymptomatic with isolated PVCs

    II—symptomatic (weakness, syncope) due to periods of sustained ventricular tachycardia

    III—symptomatic for CHF with concurrent atrial or ventricular arrhythmias. This last group is virtually indistinguishable from giant breed DCM and is treated in the same manner in our hospital.

    The best method by which to evaluate the severity and therapy of ventricular arrhythmias in DCM is 24-hour Holter monitoring.

KEY POINT ▶ Atrial fibrillation is the most common arrhythmia associated with CHF in giant breeds.

- P waves are often prolonged (>0.04 seconds), indicating atrial dilation.
- QRS prolongation (>0.06 seconds) or increased QRS voltages suggests ventricular LV dilatation.

  A widened QRS with a slurred R wave descent (leads II and aVF), associated with *ST-T slurring,* strongly suggests myocardial disease.

  Left (more common) or right bundle branch block may occur (see sec. 6, ch. 3).
- The ST-T segment may be depressed secondary to myocardial ischemia.
- Low QRS voltages suggest pleural effusion or concurrent hypothyroidism.

Laboratory Abnormalities

- Routine hematologic and urinalysis findings are usually normal unless altered by severe heart failure, therapy for heart failure, or concurrent disease.
  - Prerenal azotemia, generally mild, occurs in about 25% of cases.
  - Mild hypoproteinemia is observed in about 25% of cases.
  - Hypokalemia, hypochloremia, and metabolic alkalosis can be observed following vigorous diuretic therapy.
  - Hyponatremia is usually a sign of severe heart failure and an indication for aggressive medical therapy.
  - Hypothyroidism may be present in some dogs as a complicating disease.
  - Low plasma taurine concentration is found in some American cocker spaniels.
  - Low plasma or myocardial L-carnitine concentration can be measured in some dogs with DCM. If these tests become more available, they should become part of the routine data base in canine DCM.
  - Pleural effusions and ascitic fluid are typically found to be transudates or modified transudates and, rarely, chylous.
- A presumptive diagnosis of DCM is not difficult to make, because most large and giant breeds seldom develop severe endocardiosis. Conversely, DCM is rare in most toy and miniature breeds. Many dogs with DCM are relatively young.
  - Congenital heart disease can usually be eliminated from the differential diagnosis by noting the lack of prior clinical signs or indicators of congenital heart disease (no murmur).
  - DCM must be distinguished from heartworm disease, bacterial endocarditis, cardiac tumors, and pericardial disease. (See other sections in the text for typical features of these conditions.)
  - Some breeds—spaniels, standard Schnauzers, Afghan hounds, German shepherds—are at risk for both DCM and endocardiosis. Echocardiography may be required to determine if one or both conditions are present.

KEY POINT ▶ Definitive diagnosis is made by echocardiography. The low LV shortening fraction is uncharacteristic of any other condition. Even a dog with a chronic workload (e.g., mitral regurgitation from endocardiosis) rarely develops marked reduction in LV shortening fraction.

- Dogs with primary tachyarrhythmias (e.g., atrial tachycardia, ventricular tachycardia) may appear to have DCM; however, following successful resolution of the arrhythmia, LV function returns to normal. This is not the case with DCM.

Treatment

- Principles. Treatment of acute CHF and cardiogenic shock are described more fully in sec. 6, ch. 6. General principles of therapy include administration of positive inotropic drugs, diuretics, and vasodilators. Cardiac arrhythmias must be controlled. Exercise restriction and sodium restriction are also appropriate.
- Digoxin. Administer digoxin (Lanoxin; Burroughs Wellcome or Cardoxin; Evsco) at an initial dosage of 0.005 to 0.007 mg/kg, PO, q12h.
  - Digoxin increases myocardial contractility and improves baroreceptor activity to slow heart rate.
  - For atrial fibrillation, initiate therapy with digitalis to help slow ventricular rate response. An oral loading dose (twice the daily maintenance dose) can be used for the first 24 to 48 hours (see sec. 6, ch. 4).
  - Digoxin therapy, alone or in combination with a beta blocker or calcium channel blocker, does not typically lead to conversion to normal sinus rhythm. However, combination therapy does slow the ventricular rate response (see the following discussion).

- Doberman pinschers are very sensitive to digoxin. Usual *total daily dosage* in this breed is 0.25 to 0.375 mg.
■ Furosemide is administered parenterally (2 to 4 mg/kg, q8h) to mobilize edema and ascites. An oral dosage is then initiated, which is titrated to the patient's response (see sec. 6, ch. 6).
■ Initial vasodilator therapy for pulmonary edema can include nitroglycerin ointment (see sec. 6, ch. 6), which can be discontinued in 24 to 48 hours. Then prescribe enalapril (Vasotec; Merck) at an initial dosage of 0.25 mg/kg, PO, q12h, and gradually increase (over 1 to 2 weeks), if necessary, to 0.5 mg/kg, q12h. We prefer enalapril to hydralazine in chronic canine DCM. If a dog with DCM also has severe mitral regurgitation, a combination of hydralazine (Apresoline; CIBA), 1 mg/kg, PO, q12h, and enalapril (0.25 mg/kg, q12h) may be most effective.
■ Oral supplementation with taurine (500 mg, q8h) is considered in cocker spaniels with DCM, particularly if a low plasma taurine level has been documented. Oral administration of L-carnitine (50 to 100 mg/kg, q8h) may be helpful in dogs with deficiency of L-carnitine; however, no readily available method exists for assessing myocardial carnitine and L-carnitine is very expensive. Consequently, we do not routinely prescribe this drug unless we document low plasma or myocardial L-carnitine concentration and the client understands the empirical and costly nature of the treatment. (Note: Do not use D-carnitine.)
■ Drugs to slow heart rate. Successful therapy of CHF, combined with digitalization, should slow the resting heart rate in a dog with DCM and underlying sinus mechanism. Persistent sinus tachycardia may indicate arterial hypotension, excessive drug dosages (e.g., diuretic, vasodilator), or presence of an ectopic atrial (not sinus) tachycardia.
  - The tachycardia associated with *atrial fibrillation,* in contrast, does not generally respond to simple therapy with digoxin. In order to decrease the resting heart rate, either a calcium channel or a beta blocker is added to therapy after digoxin has been administered for at least 24 to 36 hours.
  - Judicious use of diltiazem (Cardizem; Marion), beginning at 0.5 mg/kg, PO, q8h, and increasing the dosage over 48 to 72 hours to 1.0 to 1.5 mg/kg, q8h, will usually reduce the ventricular rate response.
  - Alternatively, a beta blocker, such as propranolol (Inderal; Wyeth-Ayerst) or atenolol (Tenormin; Stuart), can be administered to slow rate response. Begin propranolol at 0.2 mg/kg, PO, q8h, and increase over 48 to 72 hours up to 1.0 mg/kg, q8h. The initial dosage of atenolol for a giant breed dog is 6.25 to 12.5 mg, PO, q12h.
  - Diltiazem and beta blockers are negative inotropic drugs and must be used with caution and only after initial stabilization of CHF. The doses are titrated to obtain a resting ventricular rate of 120 to 160 beats/minute.
  - The aforementioned therapy merely controls the ventricular rate by depressing AV nodal conduction. It generally does not convert the rhythm from atrial fibrillation to sinus rhythm.
  - Cardioversion and quinidine are not consistent in achieving a permanent conversion in dogs with DCM and CHF. These methods are therefore not recommended.
■ Ventricular arrhythmias. When sustained or recurrent ventricular tachycardia or frequent (>30 beats/minute) or multiform PVCs are present, prescribe either procainamide or tocainide (see sec. 6, ch. 4).
  - Antiarrhythmic drug therapy is best monitored by 24-hour ECG analysis (Holter monitor), because antiarrhythmic drugs can promote arrhythmias (leading to ventricular fibrillation), suppress escape rhythms during cardiac arrest (ventricular standstill), and depress myocardial inotropism.
  - Abrupt symptoms of low output and cardiac syncope in dogs with documented ventricular arrhythmias are indications for antiarrhythmic therapy provided drug-induced hypotension is excluded as the cause.
■ Concurrent medications
  - L-thyroxine. Dogs with documented hypothyroidism are given L-thyroxine at the lowest possible dose needed to prevent signs of hypothyroidism. Higher doses commonly used for dermatologic manifestations (e.g., 20 to 25 μgm/kg, daily) are avoided to circumvent taxing the circulatory system or inducing tachycardia or atrial arrhythmias. When initiating therapy with thyroid hormone, gradually increase the dose every 2 to 3 weeks until the target dosage is attained.
  - Anti-inflammatory drugs. Dogs with musculoskeletal disorders that require either aspirin or corticosteroids can receive these medications; however, the potential for gastrointestinal ulceration may be higher than usual. Aspirin inhibits vasodilatory prostaglandins, which may be a problem in severe CHF. Glucocorticoids are unlikely to cause sodium retention in dogs and can be prescribed along with cardiac medications.

Prognosis

■ The prognosis of symptomatic DCM with CHF, atrial fibrillation, or recurrent ventricular tachycardia is guarded. With excellent home care and regular veterinary attention, most dogs live for 6 to 12 months following the initial onset of CHF or syncope. Experience with Doberman pinschers is most unfavorable, and those presented in cardiogenic shock, even when stabilized, often die within 3 to 6 months. Some breeds—Irish wolfhound, Saint Bernard, Great Dane, cocker spaniels—seem to stabilize after 1 to 2 months of therapy and may have a good quality of life for extended periods, often more than 1 year.
  - The echocardiogram findings have minimal prognostic value.
  - Clients must be made aware of the possibility of sudden death in these dogs. Recurrent ventricular arrhythmias increase the possibility of sudden arrhythmic death, even when CHF is controlled.

- Intractable CHF, unresponsive to the most aggressive therapy, is an indication for euthanasia.

HYPERTHYROID HEART DISEASE

Cause

- Hyperthyroid heart disease develops most often in older (>8 years) cats with spontaneous hyperthyroidism due to thyroid adenoma (see sec. 4, ch. 1). Rarely, iatrogenic hyperthyroidism (from oversupplementation) or spontaneous hyperthyroidism (from a functional tumor) is diagnosed in the dog.

Pathology

- Spontaneous hyperthyroidism in the cat leads to myocardial hypertrophy and dilatation. Marked increases in ventricular mass can develop over a matter of weeks.

Pathophysiology

- The noncardiac effects of thyrotoxicosis are described in sec. 4, ch. 1. Most cats with hyperthyroid heart disease manifest increased cardiac demand from the hypermetabolic state, peripheral vasodilation, systemic hypertension, and the direct effects of thyroid hormone on the heart.
  - The majority of cats have a hypertrophied hyperdynamic LV. A minority develop myocardial failure that resembles DCM.
  - The cardiac lesions—both functional and anatomical—are largely reversible with appropriate therapy.

Clinical Signs

History and Physical Examination

- The clinical signs of hyperthyroidism are described elsewhere (see sec. 4, ch. 1). Cardiac manifestations include tachycardia, arrhythmias, and systolic murmurs and/or gallop rhythm. Biventricular CHF may develop.
- Most commonly, a systolic murmur of mitral regurgitation or a systolic flow murmur along the cranial sternal border is detected. Less often, a murmur compatible with tricuspid regurgitation is heard.
- The heart rate may be very high, often more than 250 beats/minute.
- CHF is not common but when present is generally characterized by development of pleural effusion.
- Systemic hypertension may be present.

Diagnosis

Radiography

- Cardiac elongation, typical of LV enlargement, and left auricular enlargement are typical; right-sided heart enlargement is variable. The aorta may be dilated, especially the ascending aorta and aortic arch (possibly an age-related change or caused by increased cardiac output or systemic hypertension).
- Pulmonary edema and pleural effusion are uncommon.

Electrocardiography

- Increased voltages typical of ventricular enlargement are common.
- Axis deviations and conduction blocks—left anterior fascicular block and right bundle branch block—may be detected.
- AV block, when present, is typically an incidental finding of senile degeneration of the conduction system, which is a common problem in aged cats.
- Sinus tachycardia and atrial and ventricular premature beats are common.

Echocardiography

- The LV is dilated and hyperkinetic; the LV wall and interventricular septum are hypertrophied; the LA and RA are dilated; and the aorta is increased in diameter.
- In cats with CHF, the right-sided chambers are markedly dilated.
- Doppler studies show AV valve regurgitation and turbulence in the ascending aorta.

Laboratory Abnormalities

- Laboratory studies are typical of hyperthyroidism (increased thyroxin, elevated liver enzyme levels) and make the diagnosis of hyperthyroid heart disease a straightforward one in most cases. Failure of cardiac disease to regress (or stop progressing) following appropriate therapy prompts the reconsideration of the diagnosis (e.g., could there also be idiopathic cardiomyopathy?). Blood taurine levels are measured in cats with CHF.

Treatment

- Hyperthyroid heart disease usually responds to control of hyperthyroidism with antithyroid medication (e.g., methimazole, Tapazol, 2.5 to 5 mg, PO, q8–12h), surgery, or radioactive iodine treatment, as described in sec. 4, ch. 1.
  - Prognosis is good unless CHF has developed. In this case, prognosis is guarded but therapy can be successful and ventricular function may improve over time.
  - Cats with severe depression of shortening fraction may not respond and die of CHF.
  - When CHF develops, administer furosemide (Lasix; 1 to 2 mg/kg, q12h) and enalapril (Vasotec; 0.25 mg/kg, PO, q12h), and recommend rest.
  - Thoracocentesis is performed for initial stabilization.
  - Methimazole is prescribed, and the cat is treated medically for 2 to 4 weeks until CHF is stabilized.
  - At that time, radioactive iodine therapy or surgery can be considered (see sec. 4, ch. 4).

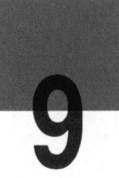

9 Pericardial Disease and Cardiac Neoplasia

John R. Reed
Steven E. Crow

The parietal pericardium is a strong, flasked-shaped sac that surrounds and attaches via the visceral pericardium to the heart and its major arteries. Under normal conditions, the pericardium serves to protect the heart and major vessels. When diseased, however, it can cause life-threatening restriction of ventricular function. If pericardial disease remains unrecognized, signs of heart failure and potentially death will ensue.

KEY POINT ▶ Pericardial diseases is a very important cause of right-sided heart failure in the dog.

Clinically significant pericardial disease is uncommon in cats. The most common causes of pericardial dysfunction are the acquired disorders (Table 1).

ETIOLOGY
Congenital Disorders

- *Pericardial defects* are rare and clinically insignificant.
- *Diaphragmatic peritoneopericardial hernia* (DPPH) may be recognized in patients ranging from 4 weeks to 15 years of age. The majority of cases are diagnosed within the first year of life. Of reported cases, 58% occur in males. Evidence suggests that the Weimaraner breed may be predisposed. This condition is common in cats.
- *Pericardial cysts* are uncommon but clinically significant. The origin of the cysts may be incarcerated omentum. This defect is manifested clinically in relatively young patients. Affected patients may develop pericardial effusion.

Acquired Disorders

KEY POINT ▶ *Pericardial effusion* is the most common type of pericardial disease (PD).

Insignificant amounts of pericardial effusion develop in patients with many forms of heart disease and with certain metabolic disorders. Clinically significant effusion is either exudative or hemorrhagic. It may be idiopathic or caused by hemangiosarcoma, heart base tumor, mesothelioma, ruptured left atrium due to chronic mitral regurgitation, or infections. Hemorrhagic effusion is more commonly diagnosed in large breed dogs over 6 years of age. The German shepherd and golden retriever appear to be predisposed. Small breeds (e.g., dachshund) are predisposed to ruptured left atria. Pericardial effusion in a large breed dog has approximately a 50% chance of being caused by idiopathic or neoplastic conditions. Clinically significant pericardial effusion in cats are usually due to infectious or neoplastic causes.

- *Constrictive pericarditis* is not as common as pericardial effusion. It primarily occurs in large breed dogs and causes compression and/or restriction to myocardial diastolic filling. The causes are listed in Table 1.

CLINICAL SIGNS
Cardiac Displacement

- In DPPH the degree of herniation can be variable. Clinical signs often occur acutely. Clinical signs may

TABLE 1. Causes of Pericardial Disease in the Dog and Cat

Congenital Disorders
Diaphragmatic peritoneopericardial hernia (DPPH)
Pericardial cyst

Acquired Disorders
Pericardial effusions
  Transudates*
    Congestive heart failure
    DPPH
    Hypoalbuminemia
  Exudate
    Infection (bacterial, fungal)
    Sterile uremic
    Feline infectious peritonitis
  Hemorrhagic
    Neoplasia (hemangiosarcoma, heart base tumor, mesothelioma, carcinoma, lymphosarcoma)
    Trauma
    Cardiac rupture (left atrial tear)
    Idiopathic
Constrictive pericardial disease
  Infection (fungal, bacterial)
  Neoplasia
  Pericardial foreign body
  Idiopathic
Pericardial mass lesions
  Pericardial abscess
  Pericardial cyst

*Conditions that rarely cause significant cardiac compression

481

be absent, and the hernia diagnosed as an incidental finding. A large hernia tends to displace the heart dorsally and forward. The clinician may hear heart sounds in unlikely locations. Common clinical signs are as follows:

- Gastrointestinal signs (vomiting, diarrhea, colic, anorexia, weight loss) are most common.
- Respiratory signs (dyspnea, cough, wheeze) are the second most common.

■ Pericardial effusion (no matter what the cause) does not cause cardiac displacement.
■ Some forms of constrictive pericarditis (e.g., infection) and pericardial mass lesions commonly impinge upon the right side of the heart.

Cardiac Compression

■ The principal hemodynamic effect of pericardial disease is a decrease in ventricular diastolic compliance. As a result, end diastolic pressure increases and end diastolic volume decreases (Fig. 1). Decreased cardiac output and increased venous pressure cause right-sided heart failure (pleural effusion, ascites). As the diastolic pressures of all chambers rise, signs of cardiac tamponade occur and cardiogenic shock may develop. Obvious signs of left-sided heart failure are absent. Systolic function including contractility in these patients is usually normal.
■ DPPH infrequently causes diastolic impairment.

Cardiac Dysfunction

■ Patients with a left atrial tear due to chronic mitral regurgitation have both diastolic and systolic dysfunction. The systolic dysfunction is a result of chronic mitral regurgitation.
■ Systolic cardiac dysfunction rarely occurs in pericardial diseases.
- Hemangiosarcoma can impair cardiac function via metastasis throughout the myocardium. Systolic function is reduced via destruction of muscle and arrhythmias. In some cases, this tumor may grow into the chambers of the right side of the heart, impairing inflow and outflow.

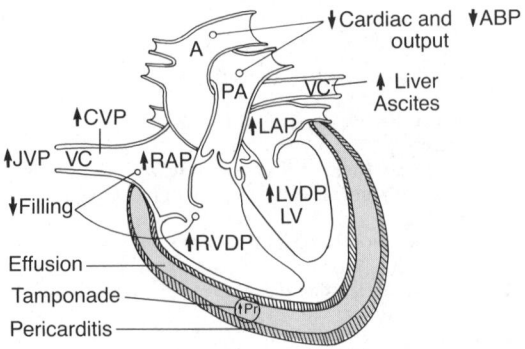

Figure 1. Diagrammatic representation of pericardial effusion. See text for explanation (A = aorta; PA = pulmonary artery; VC = vena cava; LAP = left atrial pressure; LVDP = left ventricular diastolic pressure; LV = left ventricle; RVDP = right ventricular diastolic pressure; Pr = pressure; RAP = right atrial pressure; JVP = jugular venous pressure; CVP = central venous pressure).

- Some heart-based tumors reduce cardiac function because of both infiltration of myocardium and induction of severe arrhythmias.
- Pericardial mass lesions may impinge upon the right ventricle to the point of significantly reducing inflow and outflow.

DIAGNOSIS

Physical Examination

■ Abnormal respiratory efforts may be seen in all cases of pericardial disease.
■ In effusive and constrictive pericardial diseases, the femoral arterial pulse may be weak and/or pulsus paradoxus (an exaggerated increase and decrease in arterial pulse pressure during expiration and inspiration) may occur.
■ Jugular vein distension results from systemic venous hypertension and is frequently seen in pericardial disease.

KEY POINT ▶ Ascites is a very common finding in pericardial disease. Systemic venous hypertension causes right-sided heart failure.

■ Auscultation
- In DPPH, heart sounds can be displaced cranially and/or dorsally.
- With pericardial effusion, heart sounds are often muffled; however, in small dogs and cats heart sounds may be normal. Arrhythmias sometimes are present.
- In constrictive pericarditis, heart sounds are usually diminished. A pericardial friction rub is very rare.
- Pericardial masses may cause displaced heart sounds.
■ Increases in body temperature are commonly seen in diseases of infectious origin.

Electrocardiogram (ECG)

■ The ECG may be normal or have an axis deviation in DPPH.
■ Pericardial effusion
- In dogs, the QRS amplitudes are diminished to less than 1.0 mV in all leads. ECGs in cats are normal.
- Nonspecific ST segment changes are uncommon.
- Electrical alternans occurs in approximately 50% of dogs with high-volume effusion. This finding has not been reported in cats.
- Myocardial infiltration will sometimes produce supraventricular and ventricular arrhythmias.
■ Constrictive pericardial disease
- Diminished QRS voltages
- Increased P wave duration (>0.45 sec)
- Sinus rhythm is usually normal. Supraventricular arrhythmias are sometimes noted.

Thoracic Radiographs

■ In DPPH, radiographic findings are dependent upon the volume of the hernia. Some common features are as follows:
- "Silhouetting" of the diaphragm and heart
- A very enlarged elongated or spherical cardiac silhouette
- Gas patterns within the cardiac silhouette
- A double density cardiac shadow due to omental fat and/or liver and spleen (Fig. 2)
- Deformities of the sternum (e.g., pectus excavatum)
- When barium is given, it may outline stomach or intestines that are displaced into the pericardial sac.

■ With pericardial effusion, a rounded cardiac silhouette in both views is a common feature. Small effusions may cause only mild changes in the size and shape of the cardiac silhouette, whereas large effusions may cause marked enlargement of the cardiac silhouette.
- Pleural effusion and/or enlarged caudal vena cava is a frequent finding. In animals with pleural effusions, adequate pleural fluid drainage is necessary before the cardiac silhouette can be seen.
- A cardiac silhouette that is enlarged and has the same shape as that prior to enlargement is typical of a left atrial tear. The left atrium is usually prominent.
- Tracheal elevation or deviation can indicate the presence of a heart base tumor.
- Pulmonary metastatic lesions are suggestive of a right atrial hemangiosarcoma.
- Pneumopericardiography is useful when echocardiography is unavailable. Mass lesions may be outlined at the heart base, over the right atrium, or within the pericardial space itself.
- In affected cats, the cardiac silhouette varies in shape. Sometimes the silhouette appears rounded and is suggestive of pericardial effusion. Frequently the cardiac silhouette has a normal morphology, yet it is enlarged. In these situations, it is difficult to differentiate pericardial effusion from other forms of cardiac disease.

■ Radiographic findings of constrictive pericardial disease are subtle and may include mild-to-moderate

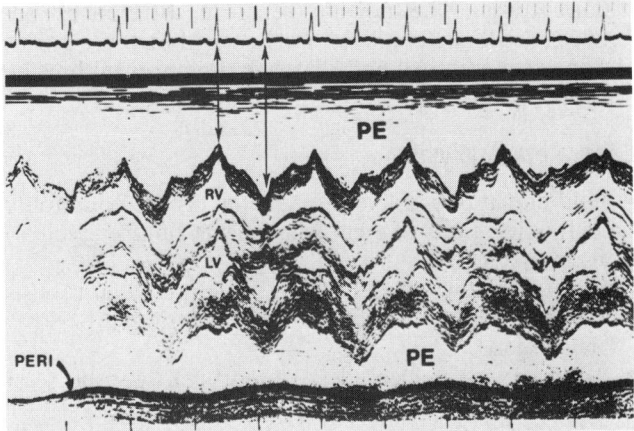

Figure 3. Echocardiogram revealing the echo-free space caused by pericardial effusion (PE) (RV = right ventricle; PERI = pericardium).

cardiac enlargement, rounding of the right side of the heart in one or both views, enlarged caudal vena cava, and pleural effusion.

Echocardiography

■ DPPH can be detected routinely when the liver and omentum are displaced forward into the pericardial sac. When the intestines are displaced forward, a poorer quality image may result because of the presence of air.

KEY POINT ▶ Echocardiography is the most sensitive procedure for documenting pericardial effusion and for detecting pericardial and cardiac masses.

- Effusion causes an echo-free space (fluid) surrounding all four chambers of the heart (Fig. 3).
- Compression of all cardiac chambers is indicative of cardiac tamponade.
- Congenital pericardial cysts are seen near the apex. These cysts are attached to the pericardium and not the heart.
- Hemangiosarcoma lesions are seen at the junction between the right atrium and ventricle. Sometimes this tumor grows inward, causing partial obstruction to inflow into the right ventricle.
- Heart base tumors are observed.
- Pericardial abscesses impinge on the right ventricle. Right ventricular collapse can be observed.
■ Echocardiography is less reliable in determining constrictive pericardial disease. Sometimes pericardial thickening or loculated effusion can be observed.

Magnetic Resonance Imaging (MRI)

This noninvasive imaging technique (see sec. 1, ch. 4) is useful for identifying cardiac tumors associated with pericardial effusion and for determining whether tumors are operable.

Hemodynamic Studies

■ Cardiac catheterization may be necessary in the diagnosis of constrictive and effusive-constrictive

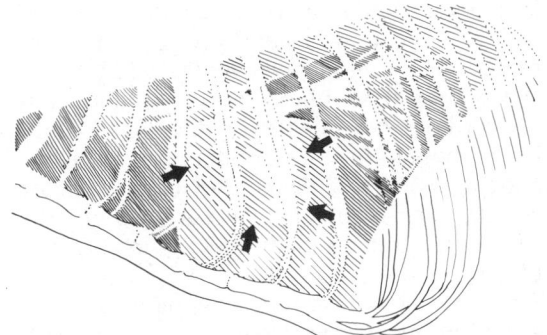

Figure 2. Representation of the enlarged cardiac silhouette and double density cardiac shadow (*arrows*) caused by omental fat in a patient with diaphragmatic peritoneopericardial hernia (DPPH).

pericarditis. The normal pressure differences between cardiac chambers are lost within these forms of pericarditis. All end-diastolic pressures within the heart equilibrate.

Laboratory Analysis

- Mild elevations of liver enzyme levels are commonly seen when signs of right-sided heart failure (ascites) are present.
- Normal-to-low normal serum protein concentrations may be present in effusive and constrictive pericardial disease.
- Anemia with nucleated red blood cells can be seen with hemangiosarcoma (see sec. 3, ch. 7).
- Cases of infectious pericarditis or pericardial abscesses can demonstrate leukocytosis with a left shift.
- Pericardial fluid analysis yields variable diagnostic results.
  - Identifying a purulent, serosanguineous, chylous, and transudative effusion is not difficult.
  - It is very difficult to differentiate between idiopathic and neoplastic effusion, because both are serosanguineous. It is also difficult to differentiate cytologically between neoplastic cells and reactive mesothelial cells (Table 2).

TREATMENT

KEY POINT ▶ To relieve cardiac compression due to pericardial effusion, pericardiocentesis is the treatment of choice.

- A needle, or over-the-needle catheter, is directed through the right side of the chest between the fourth and fifth intercostal space at the level of the costal chondral junction and into the pericardial space.
- Aspirate as much of the pericardial fluid as possible.
- In idiopathic pericardial effusion, pericardial taps can be repeated as needed. Approximately 50% of idiopathic cases will have return of the effusion. Corticosteroid therapy has not been shown to be of benefit in preventing this recurrence.
- In neoplastic effusions, repeated taps or surgery are necessary.
- For hemangiosarcoma the prognosis is poor; however, options are repeated pericardial taps and surgery/chemotherapy (see sec. 3, ch. 7). Euthanasia

must be considered because of the aggressive nature of this form of cancer.
- Infectious pericarditis can sometimes be treated by placing an indwelling catheter for infusion of selected antibiotics directly into the pericardial space.

Surgery

- Patients, especially dogs, with DPPH require surgical correction (see sec. 6, ch. 24).
  - Even if the hernia is small and contains only fat, there is a potential risk for a hernia of abdominal viscera in the future.
- Pericardial cysts and abscesses require thoracotomy or sternotomy (see sec. 6, ch. 25). The incision site depends upon the location of the abnormal structure. These structures generally are found on the right side of the heart.
- Recurrent idiopathic and infectious pericardial effusions require pericardiectomy.
  - Either a right-sided or left-sided thoracotomy or a sternotomy is performed (see sec. 6, ch. 25). A subtotal pericardiectomy is performed ventral to the phrenic nerve.

Technique for Pericardectomy
1. Identify the phrenic nerves on the dorsal right and left side of the pericardial sac.
2. After placing pericardial stay sutures make a stab incision 1 cm ventral to the nerve.
3. Remove pericardial fluid via suction.
4. Incise the pericardium circumferentially using scissors.
   Avoid trauma to the myocardium.
5. Control hemorrhage via electrocautery.
6. Place a chest tube.
   Close the thoracotomy or sternotomy routinely.

  - Histopathology is always performed on the pericardium to rule out neoplasia (e.g., mesothelioma).
- When heart base tumors have been determined by echocardiography or by MRI to be small and not invading major vessels, the tumors can be surgically removed.
  - A sternotomy approach is made to give the surgeon better access to the tumor.
  - Several hours of very delicate and intense surgery is necessary to remove these tumors.
  - A pericardiectomy is performed as well.
  - In the rare situation in which the tumor is completely resectable, a good prognosis may be warranted. The tumor rarely metastasizes.
  - When heart base tumors are inoperable, continued pericardiocentesis or pericardiectomy is necessary. Even though the tumor increases in size, many patients live 1 to 2 years after pericardiectomy.
- A small, suspected hemangiosarcoma requires immediate attention. A right-sided thoracotomy is performed.
  - The lungs are viewed for possible metastasis.
  - The right atrial lesion is removed if it is both small and easily isolated. The tissue is then submitted for histopathologic study.

TABLE 2. Classification of Hemorrhagic Pericardial Effusions

	Idiopathic	Hemangio-sarcoma	Heart Base Tumor
Protein	0.9–5.7 gm/dL	3.0–6.0 gm/dL	1.3–3.0 gm/dL
Red blood cell count (RBC)	0.01–8.75 × 10⁶/mcL	0.13–12.5 × 10⁶/mcL	0.89–4.1 × 10⁶/mcL
Nucleated RBC	1.1–18.0 × 10³/mcL	1.8–30.9 × 10³/mcL	0.9–4.6 × 10³/mcL
Mesothelial cells*	Reactive	Reactive	Less reactive

*Reactive mesothelial cells are easily misinterpreted as neoplastic cells.

Technique for Removal of Atrial Appendage Tumors

1. Double clamp the atrial appendage with Satinsky clamps proximal to the tumor.
2. Incise the tissue between the clamps, and remove the tumor.
3. Oversew the appendage over the clamp using 4-0 polypropylene (Prolene; Ethicon) with simple continuous sutures. Carefully remove the clamps, and place a second simple continuous suture layer. Place additional sutures at areas of bleeding.
4. Alternatively, use surgical staples (TA; US Surgical) to close the atrial tissue prior to tumor removal.
5. Place an indwelling chest tube, and close the incision routinely.
   - Once healing has occurred, chemotherapy follows (see sec. 3, ch. 7). In the majority of cases, by the time a suspected hemangiosarcoma lesion is seen, it has already metastasized; thus, the prognosis is very poor.

■ Constrictive pericarditis requires surgery.
   - Pericardiectomy is curative when the parietal pericardium only is affected. A favorable prognosis exists under these circumstances.
   - When epicardial fibrosis is present, epicardial stripping is required. This is a very difficult, high-risk procedure.
   - Patients with both have high rates of postoperative complications (pulmonary embolization).

Chemotherapy

Experience in the chemical treatment of cardiac and pericardial neoplasms is limited, with only a few cases reported. Consequently, recommendations are based on theoretic considerations and reports from cases in human medicine.

■ Hemangiosarcoma is a rapidly metastasizing malignant neoplasm. Presumption of dissemination at the time of diagnosis is appropriate, even if no gross evidence of distant disease exists.
   - Chemotherapy is instituted aggressively following diagnosis, especially when surgery appears to have rendered the patient free of gross tumor.
   - Combination chemotherapy regimens, such as vincristine/Adriamycin/cyclophosphamide (VAC) or Adriamycin/dacarbazine (ADIC) (Table 3), have been advocated.

     Objective responses have been reported using several of these agents singly or in combination.

     The therapy regimens are generally well tolerated by dogs if cardiac and renal function are not severely compromised. The major toxicity of both combinations is myelosuppression. Monitor blood counts every 7–14 days to detect neutropenia. Occasionally, thrombocytopenia may require the temporary discontinuation of chemotherapy.

     Radiographs and/or ultrasound examinations are repeated regularly (every 3 weeks) to monitor the response to chemotherapy.
■ Heart base tumors tend to be slow growing, invasive neoplasms with minimal metastatic potential.

TABLE 3. Chemotherapy for Cardiac and Pericardial Neoplasms

Single Agents		
Cyclophosphamide (Cytoxan)	50 mg/m²	PO every other day
	250 mg/m²	IV every 14 days
Melphalan (Alkeran)	2 mg/m²	PO daily
Thiotepa	7.5–15 mg	IC every 7–14 days
Cisplatin	50–70 mg/m²	IV every 21–28 days
Combination Protocols		
VAC (21-day cycle)		
Vincristine (Oncovin)	0.6 mg/m²	IV on day 8 and day 15
Doxorubicin (Adriamycin)	30 mg/m²	IV on day 1
Cyclophosphamide	100–200 mg/m²	IV on day 1
ADIC		
Doxorubicin	30 mg/m²	IV every 21 days
DTIC	1000 mg/m²	IV as an 8-hour drip every 21 days

IC = intracavitary; IV = intravenously; PO = orally; VAC = vincristine/adriamycin/cyclophosphamide; ADIC = Adriamycin/dacarbazine; DTIC = imidazole carboxanide.

   - Aggressive chemotherapy is rarely indicated because of the relatively small growth fraction (percentage of dividing cells) characteristic of these well-differentiated neoplasms.
   - Chemotherapy may be advisable when surgical resection is impossible.
   - Cyclophosphamide and melphalan are good therapy choices because they can be administered orally. Observe the animal carefully for sterile hemorrhagic cystitis when providing cyclophosphamide, especially with prolonged therapy. Other drugs to be considered include vincristine and dactinomycin.
■ Mesothelioma is typically a rapidly progressive neoplastic disorder that spreads to adjacent tissues, primarily by transcoelomic implantation. It is one of the most treatment-resistant malignancies in human beings. Anecdotal reports in the veterinary literature suggest a similar behavior for this neoplasm in dogs.
   - Systemic chemotherapy is largely ineffective.
   - Intrathoracic instillation of triethylenethiophosphoramide (thioTEPA) or cisplatin has been advocated following pericardiectomy for the management of malignant effusion caused by mesothelioma.
   - Treatment with radioactive phosphorus (³²P) has occasionally controlled the severity of effusions caused by mesothelioma.

PROGNOSIS

Although a complete cure cannot be expected using chemotherapy for any of these neoplasms, some prolongation of life is possible for animals with hemangiosarcomas but less so for those with mesotheliomas. Cardiac drugs do not cure mitral insufficiency, but they can prolong life by relieving the signs of congestive heart failure. Similarly, chemotherapy may "stem the tide" in pericardial neoplasia, temporarily improving the quality of the animal's life, with dramatic results in the occasional case.

Supplemental Readings

Bonagura JD, Pipers FS: Echocardiographic features of pericardial effusion in dogs. J Am Vet Med Assoc 179:49, 1981.

Evans SM, Biery DN: Congenital peritoneopericardial diaphragmatic hernia in the dog and cat: A literature review and 17 additional case histories. Vet Radiol 21:108, 1980.

Reed JR: Pericardial diseases. *In* Fox PR, ed.: *Canine and Feline Cardiology.* New York: Churchill Livingstone, 1988.

Sutter PF: Thoracic radiography. *In* Sutter PF, ed.: *A Text Atlas of Thoracic Diseases of the Dog and Cat.* Switzerland: Wettswill, 1984.

Thomas WP: Pericardial disorders. *In* Ettinger SJ, ed.: *Textbook of Veterinary Internal Medicine,* 3rd ed. Philadelphia: W.B. Saunders, 1989.

Thomas WP, Sisson D, Bauer TG, Reed, JR: Detection of cardiac masses in dogs by two-dimensional echocardiography. Vet Radiol 25:65, 1984.

Wagner SD, Breznock EM: Surgical management of pericardial and intramyocardial diseases including Chemodectomas. *In* Bojrab MJ, ed.: *Current Techniques in Small Animal Surgery,* 2nd ed. Philadelphia: Lea & Febiger, 1983.

10 Heartworm Disease

Clay A. Calvert

Heartworm disease is a common problem in many areas of the world, particularly in tropical and subtropical regions. The disease has been endemic along the southeast Atlantic and Gulf coasts of the United States as far as Texas for over fifty years. Heartworm infection has spread north and west to most areas of the United States, but the prevalence is still low at high elevations and in most areas of the northern tier of states.

ETIOLOGY

Heartworm infection is the result of *Dirofilaria immitis* infection and is transmitted to dogs during the feeding of many species of mosquitos.

Life Cycle

- Female mosquitos are the intermediate hosts and acquire the first-stage larvae (microfilariae) during feeding on infected dogs.
  - Larvae develop within the mosquito to the third stage in 2–2.5 weeks.
  - Third-stage larvae (L_3) infect the dog via the bite wound created during the feeding of the mosquito. Transmission is unlikely to occur during the dry cold months of the year.
- Larvae migrate through the subcutaneous tissues and vascular adventitial tissues for approximately 100 days.
  - During this time two molts occur.
  - Young adults (fifth-stage, or L_5, larvae) enter the vascular system at 3–3.5 months postinfection.
  - Young adult *Dirofilaria immitis* worms arrive in the small pulmonary arteries 5–6 months postinfection.

KEY POINT ▶ Patent infection, as evidenced by microfilaremia, occurs approximately 6 months following transmission from the mosquito.

- Microfilarial concentrations increase for the next 6 months and then decrease if superinfection does not occur.
- Immune-mediated (microfilaria-specific antibody–mediated) occult infections occur in the presence of persistent host antibody excess. Antibody-dependent leukocyte adhesion results in entrapment of microfilariae in the pulmonary microcirculation.
- Microfilaria-leukocyte (neutrophils and eosinophils) complexes are engulfed by phagocytic cells of the mononuclear phagocyte system, resulting in granulomatous inflammation.

- Progressive granulomatous inflammation occasionally leads to pulmonary eosinophilic granulomatosis.
- Predominately eosinophilic inflammation results in allergic pneumonitis.
- Other causes of occult infections are unisex infections, drug-induced microfilaremia associated with monthly heartworm prophylaxis, and high-dose ivermectin administration.

Epizootiology

Prevalence

Heartworm infection is most common in tropical and subtropical climates.

- Infection rates approach 50% along the Atlantic and Gulf coasts as far inland as 150 miles.
- Virtually all unprotected dogs in highly endemic regions will become infected.

Signalment

- Male dogs are more often infected, probably related to increased outdoor exposure.

KEY POINT ▶ Dogs housed outdoors have a four- to fivefold increased risk of infection with heartworms.

- Large and medium-sized dogs are more often infected, probably because of increased outdoors exposure compared to toy and miniature breeds.
- Infection is diagnosed most often in dogs 4–7 years of age. In highly endemic regions it is common in younger dogs.
- Cats are relatively resistant but can be affected, especially in highly endemic areas.

Pathogenesis

Disease onset and severity largely reflects the number of adult heartworms, which can vary from one to more than 250 per dog. In infected cats, the average number of adult worms is three. Acute dyspnea and even sudden death are more common in cats and are not always associated with high worm burden.

Worm Location

- Until the adult worm burden exceeds 50 in a 25-kg dog, nearly all worms are located in the pulmonary arteries.
- Worm burdens of approximately 75 are associated with worms located in the right atrium.

■ The vena cava syndrome typically is associated with worm burdens of about 100.

Response to Live Worms

■ Pulmonary arterial endothelial damage and subsequent myointimal proliferation most often affects the caudal and intermediate lung lobes.
■ Pulmonary lobar arterial enlargement, tortuosity, and obstruction of smaller branches begin within a few weeks of worm arrival.
■ Intrapulmonary blood flow is obstructed as the disease progresses and blood is diverted to less severely affected lobes.
■ Small downstream arterioles become damaged and leak plasma and inflammatory cells into the surrounding lung parenchyma. This causes interstitial and alveolar lung disease with signs of fever, coughing, leukocytosis, and dyspnea.

Response to Dead Worms

The most severe disease is seen in response to dead worm fragments that are swept into small arterioles.

■ Pulmonary vascular compliance and blood flow become severely impaired, resulting in pulmonary hypertension and increased right ventricular afterload.
■ Parenchymal lung disease (infarction and consolidation) occurs secondary to pulmonary arterial thromboembolism and increased vascular permeability.

CLINICAL SIGNS

The clinical signs associated with heartworm infection reflect the adult worm burden, duration of infection, and host-parasite interaction.

Common Pulmonary Signs

■ Exercise intolerance, coughing, dyspnea, and respiratory crackles occur in dogs with moderate and advanced heartworm disease. Coughing is common in cats with chronic disease.
■ Hemoptysis occurs in severe disease associated with pulmonary thromboembolism. It can be seen prior to but more often following treatment.
■ Acute dyspnea and increased pulmonary alveolar densities may develop secondary to spontaneous worm death. This is most common in cats.

Syncope

Syncope is associated with severe pulmonary arterial disease and hypertension.

Elevated Central Venous Pressure

Signs of elevated central venous pressure are associated with severe pulmonary hypertension with right-sided congestive heart failure (CHF) (e.g., jugular pulse, distended jugular veins, ascites).

Hemoglobinuria

Hemoglobinuria commonly occurs in association with the vena cava syndrome (i.e., acute hemolytic crisis caused by obstruction of the vena cava by adult worms) and occasionally when severe pulmonary arterial disease results in thrombocytopenia and hemolysis due to disseminated intravascular coagulation (DIC).

Nephrotic Syndrome

This syndrome occasionally occurs as the result of severe glomerular disease in the form of amyloidosis or immune complex glomerulonephritis (see sec. 8, ch. 1). Manifestations include hypoalbuminemia, ascites, peripheral edema, hypercholesterolemia, and variable azotemia.

Intermittent Vomiting

Intermittent vomiting is a frequent sign of heartworm disease in cats.

DIAGNOSIS

The diagnosis of heartworm infection is based on the presence of microfilariae in the peripheral blood and/or a positive immunodiagnostic test in dogs with clinical or radiographic findings consistent with the disease. Cats are usually negative for microfilariae but may have characteristic radiographs and a positive enzyme-linked immunosorbent assay (ELISA) test for heartworm antigen.

History

The history in dogs with heartworm infection varies considerably.

■ Some dogs are totally without signs; others have an unexplained tachypnea, exercise intolerance, or cough.
■ Signs consistent with pulmonary hypertension with or without overt right-sided CHF are associated with severe heartworm disease (Table 1).
■ Most heartworm-infected dogs have not received prophylactic therapy.
■ Coughing, emesis, and sudden dyspnea are typical in cats.

Physical Examination

■ Findings vary from clinically normal to signs of right-sided CHF (see sec. 6, ch. 6).

TABLE 1. Historical and Clinical Signs of Heartworm Disease

Severity of Disease	Historical Findings and Clinical Signs
Asymptomatic	None
Mild	Cough
Moderate	Cough, exercise intolerance, abnormal lung sounds
Severe	Cough, exercise intolerance, dyspnea, abnormal lung sounds, hepatomegaly, syncope, ascites, tricuspid regurgitation, loud or split S_2 heart sounds

■ Pulmonary crackles, rhonchi, and loud bronchial sounds may be auscultated.
■ Signs of pulmonary hypertension and cardiac decompensation may be evident (see Table 1).

Laboratory Studies

Standard laboratory studies vary, depending on the patient's age, clinical signs, and preference of individual clinicians.

■ As the minimum pretreatment data base for all dogs suspected of having heartworm infection, include packed cell volume (PCV), blood urea nitrogen (BUN), urine specific gravity, direct blood smear, and microfilariae concentration test.
■ Middle-aged and older dogs and dogs with moderate to severe signs, occult infections, infection of unknown duration, and concomitant problems should have an extended data base (Table 2).
■ Cats always require thoracic radiographs. Fecal studies for lungworms, cardiac ultrasound, and/or a nonselective angiogram are often indicated for diagnosis. A tracheal or bronchial wash can rule out other lung disease.

Microfilaria Detection

■ Perform a direct blood smear immediately following procurement of a diagnostic blood sample. If the direct smear is negative, a concentration test is indicated.
■ The Knott test (a centrifugal, concentration test) or a millipore filter test (e.g., Difil Test, Evsco) is acceptable for the detection of microfilariae. Each methodology has advantages and disadvantages, but efficacy is similar.
■ If results are negative, an immunodiagnostic test is indicated in order to ensure that infection is absent.

Immunodiagnostic Tests

■ Immunodiagnostic tests are indicated when heartworm infection is suspected but microfilaremia is absent; in cats, microfilaria tests usually are negative.
■ Serodiagnosis of adult heartworm antigens in dogs is readily accomplished by ELISA and latex agglutination tests. A number of very specific and sensitive tests are available.
  • Some clinicians routinely perform serodiagnostic screens because the general incidence of occult infections is 15–20%. If results are positive, a microfilaria concentration test is indicated.
  • In some highly endemic regions, such as Hawaii,

as many as 50% of infected dogs lack circulating microfilariae.
■ The Cite SemiQuant test (Idexx) is useful not only to diagnose heartworm disease but also to estimate low versus high worm burdens.
■ Immunodiagnostic tests are the tests of choice in dogs receiving chronic preventive therapy with ivermectin, mibemycin, or moxidectin.
■ Immunodiagnostic tests are specific but less sensitive in the detection of heartworms in cats.

KEY POINT ▶ Thoracic radiography is the most important diagnostic test for determining the severity of heartworm disease.

Radiography

Pulmonary Arterial Disease

■ The degree of arterial disease is best assessed by the dorsoventral projection.
■ The caudal lobar arteries, especially the right, are the first to enlarge and typically are the most severely diseased. The diameters of the caudal lobar arteries should not exceed that of the ninth rib.
■ Tortuosity and pruning of the arteries (the latter due to thromboembolism) are best seen on the dorsoventral projection; the caudal lobar vessels are most severely affected.
■ The cranial lobar arteries are best evaluated on the lateral projection; their diameters should not exceed that of the proximal portions of the third rib. In cats, angiograms can delineate these vessels more clearly.
■ Nonselective angiography may be diagnostic in cats with heartworm disease and is useful in suspected cases when the ELISA is negative.

Parenchymal Lung Disease

■ Parenchymal lung disease results from the pulmonary arteriolar thromboembolism with leakage of plasma and inflammatory cells into the adjacent tissues.
■ Severity varies; disease is most prevalent in the caudal and intermediate lung lobes and is most concentrated surrounding the lobar arteries.

Allergic Pneumonitis

■ This mixed diffuse interstitial-alveolar lung disease is best visualized in the caudal lobes.
■ It often occurs with minimal pulmonary arterial enlargement.
■ It is associated with occult infections, eosinophilia, coughing, and dyspnea.

Clinical Pathology

No abnormalities are pathognomonic for heartworm infection.

■ Eosinophilia and basophilia are the most common abnormalities in dogs.
  • Eosinophilia is more common; the highest eosinophil and basophil counts tend to occur in occult infections.
  • *Dipetalonema reconditum* infections produce eo-

TABLE 2. Data Bases for Dogs with Heartworm Infection

Criteria	Data Base
Asymptomatic; young dogs	PCV, BUN, urine specific gravity
Middle-aged or old; symptomatic; occult infection; unknown duration	CBC, serum biochemical profile, urinalysis, thoracic radiographs

sinophilia equal to or greater than that associated with heartworm disease.
- Neutrophilic leukocytosis, often with a left shift, occurs with pulmonary thromboembolism.
- Azotemia may occur in dogs with complicated infections.
  - Prerenal azotemia can be due to dehydration or right-sided CHF.
  - Primary azotemia can result from glomerulopathies, including immune complex disease and amyloidosis.
- Increased serum hepatic enzyme levels may occur; however, increases up to ten-fold do not affect treatment, complications, or survival.
- Hepatic insufficiency, evidenced by increased serum bile acid levels, can occur, but mild to moderate increases do not affect treatment.
- Proteinuria is common and is most pronounced in patients with severe infections or renal amyloidosis.
  - Nephrotic syndrome is a contraindication to treatment.
  - In the absence of hypoalbuminemia, most cases of proteinuria resolve following effective heartworm treatment.
- Hypoalbuminemia occurs in some dogs with severe infections; hyperglobulinemia is common in dogs and cats with chronic heartworm disease.
  - Loss of albumin into the third space occurs with right-sided CHF and is complicated by hepatic insufficiency and intestinal congestion.
  - Proteinuria, when severe, will produce hypoalbuminemia.
- Thrombocytopenia is commonly associated with severe pulmonary arterial and parenchymal lung disease.
  - Activated clotting time is marginally increased in many cases.
  - DIC develops in some animals with severe thromboembolic disease.
- Hemoglobinuria, usually accompanied by thrombocytopenia, is seen with the vena cava syndrome and with severe pulmonary thromboembolic disease.
  - Heparin, 100–200 U/kg tid SC, usually reduces hemoglobinuria due to severe lung disease.
  - Do not administer in the presence of frank hemorrhage or when the coagulogram is markedly abnormal.

Electrocardiography

Electrocardiography (ECG) is sometimes helpful in animals with severe heartworm disease, especially for evaluation of arrhythmias.

- A right ventricular hypertrophy pattern is common in dogs with severe pulmonary hypertension and is found in 90% of dogs with overt right-sided CHF (ascites). However, significant pulmonary hypertension may exist in the absence of ECG abnormalities.
- Occasionally, cardiac rhythm disturbances occur in dogs with severe infections. Atrial fibrillation is the most common arrhythmia, especially in larger breeds.

Ultrasonography

- Evidence of right ventricular enlargement can be detected by M-mode and two-dimensional (2-D) ultrasonography in patients with moderate to severe pulmonary hypertension.
- Worms may be detected in the right ventricle and the main pulmonary artery during 2-D ultrasonography.
- Ultrasonography is particularly useful in cats in which the diagnosis is often difficult.

TREATMENT

The goal of treatment is to kill all adult heartworms with an adulticide and all microfilariae with a microfilaricide and to accomplish this with minimal drug toxicity and a tolerable degree of pulmonary thromboembolism due to the dying worms.

Patient Selection

Although the majority of heartworm-infected dogs can be treated successfully, there are exceptions. Most clinicians consider the mortality associated with thiacetarsamide therapy in cats to be unacceptably high; consequently adulticide therapy is not recommended for cats.

- Experience is limited in the treatment of older dogs. Heartworm disease may be nonprogressive in old dogs that have chronic infections with low worm burdens. Aspirin therapy alone is a reasonable alternative.
- Treat pulmonary signs in cats with prednisolone (1.0–2.0 mg/kg, daily for 10 days; then taper the dose to prevent signs of disease). Do not use aspirin or thiacetarsamide.

Adulticide Therapy

The only approved adulticidal agent is thiacetarsamide sodium (Caparsolate; Sanofi). The following regimen has proved effective in dogs. (See *Aspirin*, this chapter.)

Pretreatment Measures

- Feed the patient approximately one-half hour prior to injection to evaluate for anorexia.
- Examine for bilirubinuria, jaundice, fever, depression, and dyspnea.
- Correct concurrent problems such as dehydration, prerenal azotemia, and primary azotemia (BUN 40–120 mg/dl).

Drug Administration

- Give thiacetarsamide sodium, 2.2 mg/kg (0.22 ml/kg), q8–15h IV, for a total of four injections.
- Give each injection in a peripheral vein at a different site as distal as possible.
- Eliminate the possibility of extravasation in each instance by a test injection of saline (facilitated by the use of a butterfly, or scalp infusion needle).

KEY POINT ▶ Do not use indwelling catheters (except jugular catheters) because they contribute to phlebitis and vein rupture and tend to produce a false sense of security. Do not give multiple injections at one site.

Drug Storage

- Store thiacetarsamide in the refrigerator.
- Discard if yellow discoloration and precipitates occur.

Contraindications

- Hepatic failure
- Nephrotic syndrome
- Advanced renal failure
- Combination of right-sided CHF and severe azotemia
- Concomitant life-threatening disorders such as metastatic cancer

Investigational Therapy

RM 340 is a very effective adulticide therapy that offers a number of advantages over thiacetarsamide sodium.

- IM route of injection (2.5 mg/kg), two doses at 24-hour intervals and repeat in 4 months.
- Better therapeutic index
- More efficacious against various aged worms of both sexes

Microfilaricide Therapy

Always complete adulticide treatment before initiating microfilaricide therapy.

KEY POINT ▶ Ivermectin is the most effective microfilaricide drug; it is associated with fewest complications and is the easiest to use.

Ivermectin (Ivomec; MSD Agvet)

- Administer 50 μ/kg as a 1:9 dilution (1 ml Ivomec added to 9 ml propylene glycol or water, respectively) at a dosage of 1 ml/20 kg PO.
- Give at 4 weeks post-adulticidal treatment.
- Administer the drug in the morning and observe the patient throughout the day for signs of toxicity such as vomiting, depression, diarrhea, and hemodynamic embarrassment. If cardiovascular instability is suspected give IV lactated Ringer's solution (20 ml/kg), with a soluble corticosteroid (dexamethasone SP, 2 mg/kg, IV).
- Perform microfilarial concentration test in 3 weeks.
  - If positive—repeat the ivermectin protocol; then repeat microfilarial concentration test in 3 weeks. Positive results in this test indicate that persistent adult worms are likely present, requiring repetition of the adulticide phase of therapy.
  - If negative—begin prophylactic therapy (see discussion on heartworm prevention).
- Safe for use in collies as prescribed.

Mibemycin Oxide

(Interceptor; Ciba-Geigy) is also a microfilaricideal agent but should not be used for this purpose.

Therapy Variations

Occult Infections

Microfilaricide therapy is not indicated in the absence of microfilaremia.

Persistence of Young Adult Female Worms

- After adulticidal therapy, young, female worms may be refractory to thiacetarsamide sodium. This should be suspected when:
  - Microfilariae are not eliminated by microfilaricidal therapy (e.g., after two treatments with ivermectin, 50 μg/kg).
  - Repeated adulticide treatment is ineffective.
  - Management: place on Heartgard (see discussion on prevention) repeat adulticide therapy in 1 year.

Adjuncts in Adulticide Therapy

- Aspirin
  - Reduces pulmonary arterial lesions and improves intrapulmonary blood flow.
  - For dogs with severe disease, give 5 mg/kg, q24h, PO, beginning 14–21 days before adulticide therapy and continuing for 30 days after.
- Corticosteroids
  - Reduce parenchymal disease in the lung but exacerbate pulmonary arterial disease.
  - Do not use routinely but only as needed to control sequelae (see the following discussion).

Treatment of Sequelae

Occult Heartworm Allergic Pneumonitis

This complication occurs in 10–15% of patients with occult infections.

- Clinical signs include dyspnea, coughing, respiratory crackles, and exercise intolerance.
- Thoracic radiographs reveal diffuse interstitial-alveolar infiltrates.
- Eosinophilia is common, and in tracheal lavage cytology eosinophils usually predominate.
- The syndrome responds well to oral prednisone (1–2 mg/kg, q24h for several days). Stop prednisone therapy after 3–7 days and begin adulticide therapy.

Pulmonary Eosinophilic Granulomatosis

This uncommon complication of occult heartworm disease probably results from the granulomatous inflammation known to be associated with occult infections. The reaction in some cases is progressive and assumes a neoplastic-like behavior.

- Clinical signs are coughing and dyspnea.
- Eosinophilia and basophilia are common findings, and hyperglobulinemia may occur.
- Pleural effusion (eosinophilic) occurs occasionally.

- Intrathoracic lymphadenopathy is always present.
- Multiple pulmonary nodules develop simultaneously and sequentially, grow at variable rates, and are 1–10 cm in diameter or larger.
- The trachea, liver, spleen, kidneys, abdominal lymph nodes, and intestines are sometimes infiltrated with eosinophils and eosinophilic granulomas.
- Combination chemotherapy is recommended (see sec. 3, ch. 5 for details of chemotherapy):
  - Prednisone (50 mg/m² q24h) plus azathioprine (Imuran) (50 mg/m², q24h PO for 7–10 days; then alternate days).
- Therapy usually results initially in partial or complete remission, but relapse is common even with continued aggressive therapy or when drug dosages are reduced.
- The duration of therapy is indefinite and the prognosis is poor.
- Consider lung lobectomy for isolated lesions.

Thromboembolic Lung Disease

This common sequela of moderate to severe pulmonary arterial disease can occur prior to adulticide therapy (especially in cats) but is most common 7–21 days following adulticide therapy.

- Clinical signs include coughing, dyspnea, fever, and occasionally hemoptysis.
- A regenerative leukocytosis with thrombocytopenia usually is present.
- Thoracic radiographs reveal severe pulmonary arterial disease with periarterial parenchymal disease of variable severity.
- The following therapy usually is successful:
  - Initiate cage confinement for 5–10 days.
  - Administer prednisone (1.0 mg/kg, q24h for 3–10 days).
  - Use intranasal oxygen for severely affected patients.
  - Administer broad-spectrum antibiotics (e.g., trimethoprim-sulfa, cephalosporins, enrofloxacin) empirically to control bacterial pneumonia.

Pulmonary Arterial Disease

Severe pulmonary arterial disease occurs in 10% of infected dogs in highly endemic regions.
Option 1. Forceps extraction of adult worms from the pulmonary arteries.

- Requires fluoroscopy and a long, flexible, alligator forceps which is introduced into the jugular vein via a surgical approach and manipulated through the heart into the pulmonary arteries. Numerous attempts to grasp worms are required.
- This procedure is highly effective in experienced hands.
- Follow with microfilaricide therapy when appropriate.

Option 2. Cage confinement and aspirin in conjunction with adulticide therapy.

- Place patient in cage confinement for 2–3 weeks prior to, during, and for 3–4 weeks following adulticide therapy.

- Begin adulticide therapy after 2–3 weeks of cage confinement.
- Give aspirin (5 mg/kg daily) throughout the treatment period, beginning at least 2 weeks before adulticide therapy and continuing at least 4 weeks after treatment.
- Prescribe a diuretic and low-salt diet for patients with concomitant, overt right-sided CHF.
- Survival rate is 70–80%, compared with 40–50% in patients given standard treatment.

Investigational Therapy

A modified adulticide protocol utilizing RM 340 has been successful for the treatment of severe heartworm disease.

- One IM injection (2.5 mg/kg) is given initially.
- Two doses (2.5 mg/kg) are given 24 hours apart, 1 month later.
- Exercise restriction is maintained during and for 1 month after completion of drug therapy.

Postcaval Syndrome

The postcaval syndrome develops when massive retrograde worm migration leads to severe tricuspid regurgitation, acute hepatic congestion, cardiogenic shock, and DIC. Therapy includes local anesthesia, jugular venotomy, and removal of worms using long forceps or sterile endoscopic basket-retrieval devices.

Prevention

Diethylcarbamazine

Diethylcarbamazine (2.5–3.0 mg/kg, PO) given daily is an effective prophylactic drug (Table 3). If the owner skips more than 2 days of treatment, do not reinstitute preventive treatment before performing a microfilarial concentration test.

- Duration of efficacy is short because the drug affects the L_3-L_4 (larval) molt 9–12 days postinfection.
- Begin therapy prior to the mosquito season and continue for 1 month following the first frost (or year-round in regions that have mosquitos all year).
- All diethylcarbamazine products are equally effective.
- Combination diethylcarbamazine and oxybendazole (Filarbits Plus; Smith-Kline) is a popular product in regions where intestinal helminths are prevalent. An occasional side effect of oxybendazole is characterized by increased liver enzyme activity, icterus, and hepatic insufficiency.

TABLE 3. Dosage Recommendations for Ivermectin (Heartgard-30) Prophylaxis in Dogs (6 µg/kg, PO monthly)

Weight (lb)	Total Dosage/Tablet
1–25	68 µg (1 tablet; blue box)
26–50	136 µg (1 tablet; green box)
51–100	272 µg (1 tablet; brown box)
>100	Combination of above

TABLE 4. Dosage Recommendations for Mibemycin Oxide (Interceptor) Prophylaxis in Dogs (0.5–0.99 mg/kg, PO monthly)

Weight (lb)	Total Dosage/Tablet
1–10	2.3 mg (brown tablet)
11–25	5.75 mg (green tablet)
26–50	11.5 mg (yellow tablet)
51–100	23 mg (white tablet)
>100	Combination of above

KEY POINT ▶ Never initiate diethylcarbamazine treatment in microfilaremic dogs because an anaphylactoid reaction may develop.

Ivermectin

Ivermectin (Heartgard; MSD Ag Vet), 5–6 mg/kg given monthly, is an effective preventive drug (see Table 3). If a monthly dosage is missed reinstitute preventive treatment and perform a heartworm antigen test in 7–8 months. A chewable formulation of Ivermectin plus pyrantel pamoate is an effective heartworm preventative that also clears ascarid and hookworm infections.

- Infection with larvae (L_3) as long as 2 months prior to initiation of ivermectin prophylaxis will be blocked.
- Drug reactions are rare at the recommended dosage.
- Chronic administration of ivermectin suppresses microfilariae in heartworm-positive dogs; however, adult worms are not killed.
- Safe for collies when used as prescribed.

- A dose of 24 μg/kg is an effective prophylaxis in cats.

Mibemycin Oxide

Mibemycin (Interceptor; Ciba-Geigy), 0.5–0.99 mg/kg, is an effective once-a-month preventive agent for heartworm disease in dogs and cats (see Table 4).
- Also controls hookworm, roundworm, and whipworm infestations.

Moxidectin

Moxidectin (American Cyanamid), 1–3 μg/kg, is an effective once-a-month heartworm preventative.

KEY POINT ▶ All preventive drugs may kill microfilariae; for this reason chronic dosing with ivermectin or mibemycin can lead to "occult" nonmicrofilaremic infections.

Supplemental Readings

Calvert CA: Feline heartworm disease. *In* Sherding RG ed.: *The Cat: Diseases and Clinical Management*. New York: Churchill Livingstone, 1989, p 495.

Calvert CA, Rawlings CA: Canine heartworm disease. *In* Fox PR, ed.: *Canine and Feline Cardiology*. New York: Churchill Livingstone, 1988, p 519.

Hribernik TN: Canine and feline heartworm disease. *In* Kirk RW, ed. *Current Veterinary Therapy, X*. Philadelphia: W.B. Saunders, 1989, p 263.

Rawlings CA, Calvert CA: Heartworm disease. *In* Ettinger SJ, ed.: *Textbook of Veterinary Internal Medicine*. Philadelphia: W.B. Saunders, 1990, p 1163.

11 Vascular Diseases

John Bonagura
Rebecca L. Stepien

THROMBOSIS AND EMBOLISM

Thrombosis refers to the presence of a clot in a blood vessel that may obstruct blood flow. *Arterial embolism* is the sudden occlusion of an artery that occurs when a thrombus (or other substance) is introduced into one part of the body and is carried to another tissue via the vascular system.

- In typical cases, the embolus is carried from the left side of the heart to a systemic artery or from a systemic vein through the right side of the heart and then into a pulmonary artery.
- A thrombus or embolus that originates in the left side of the heart or in a systemic artery may obstruct systemic blood flow, causing *ischemia* and necrosis of tissues nourished by that vessel.
- Thrombus formation in a systemic vein or in the right side of the heart may obstruct systemic venous flow or be carried to the lungs and cause a *pulmonary embolism*.
- Thrombi usually form by slightly different mechanisms:
  - A venous thrombus (red thrombus) is related to stasis of blood and activation of clotting factors. Deficiency of plasma antithrombin III predisposes to thrombosis.
  - An arterial thrombus (white thrombus) follows activation and aggregation of platelets and is frequently related to injury of vascular endothelium or endocardium, as well as stasis of blood.

Etiology

The following conditions may be associated with development of thrombosis:

- Inflammation of the vessel wall (arteritis)
- Physical (e.g., trauma, IV catheter) or chemical (e.g., chemotherapy, thiacetarsemide) injury to a vessel
- Feline cardiomyopathy (all forms)
- Bacterial endocarditis
- Verminous arteritis (e.g., heartworm disease)
- Degenerative arterial disease (e.g., atherosclerosis)
- Hypercoagulable states including those related to deficiency of antithrombin III, such as renal amyloidosis, disseminated intravascular coagulation (DIC), polycythemia, immune-mediated hemolytic anemia, and Cushing's disease
- Air emboli (from radiographic procedures such as cystography or from cryosurgery)
- Fat emboli (from long bone fractures)
- Missiles such as shotgun pellets that directly penetrate the vascular system
- Torsion of a vascular pedicle (e.g., splenic torsion)
- Fibrocartilaginous embolism of the spinal cord vessels
- Aberrant filarial parasites in systemic arteries (e.g., *Dirofilaria immitis*)
- Venous stasis or obstruction

Pathophysiology

The pathophysiology and pathogenesis of clinical signs in thrombosis depend on the acuteness of injury, location of obstruction, degree of thrombosis, and presence or absence of collateral circulation.

Pathologic consequences include:

- *Myocardium*—myocardial ischemia causing infarction, arrhythmias, hypokinetic ventricular wall motion, and myocardial failure
- *Limbs*—muscle ischemia, rhabdomyocytolysis, peripheral neuropathy
- *Spinal cord*—neuronal degeneration, ischemic or hemorrhagic necrosis
- *Brain*—hemorrhage, necrosis, and ischemia-induced neuronal damage
- *Lung*—pulmonary embolism
  - A massive embolus can obstruct the left or right pulmonary artery leading to severe obstruction of right ventricular output, low cardiac output, systemic hypotension, myocardial ischemia, and cardiac arrest.
  - Embolization of smaller vessels can initiate the release of vasoactive chemicals and cause pulmonary edema, inflammation, and vascular narrowing with increased pulmonary vascular resistance.
  - Heartworm death following adulticidal therapy is a common example of pulmonary embolization that leads to pulmonary injury and may precipitate heart failure (see sec. 6, ch. 10).
- *Kidneys, adrenal glands, liver, spleen, and skin*—infarcts, hemorrhages, and parenchymal necrosis.
- *Systemic veins*—obstruction to venous return and subsequent elevation of venous pressure

Diagnosis

The clinical diagnosis of thrombosis or embolism requires a high level of suspicion. Sudden onset of clinical signs is typical. Certain conditions (listed previously) predispose to thrombosis or embolism (refer to appropriate chapter for further information).

Physical Examination and Laboratory Studies

Physical examination and laboratory signs of embolism depend on the vessels involved and may be obvious or subtle.

- *Myocardium*—ischemia that causes discomfort and anxiety, electrocardiographic (ECG) abnormalities (ST-T segment deviation, infarction patterns, ventricular arrhythmias), elevation of cardiac muscle enzymes (myocardial-MB-band of creatine kinase), and echocardiographic abnormalities such as regional hypokinetic wall motion.
- *Limbs*—limb weakness and pallor, loss of pulse, ischemic myopathy (pain, contracture, elevated serum muscle enzymes), and lower motor neuron sensory and motor neuropathy
- *Spinal cord*—segmental spinal cord disease (upper or lower motor neuron)
- *Brain*—ischemic neuropathy or "stroke" with attendant seizures or neurologic deficits
- *Lungs*—numerous clinical abnormalities including:
  - Shock, hypotension, sudden death with a massive thrombus or embolus of air, heartworms, or fat
  - Tachypnea, dyspnea, tachycardia, increased interstitial/alveolar infiltrates, dilated pulmonary arteries with peripheral hypoperfusion, pleural effusion, right-sided congestive heart failure (CHF), and hypoxemia when the embolism is not lethal
- *Kidneys, adrenal glands, liver, spleen, and skin*—renal or abdominal pain or colic, cutaneous hemorrhages, serum biochemical abnormalities reflecting end-organ injury (e.g., azotemia, hypoadrenocortical crisis of hyperkalemia with hyponatremia)
- *Systemic venous obstruction*—swelling of cutaneous vessels that do not collapse and may be warm and painful (thrombophlebitis); edema distal to the obstruction likely (deep venous thrombosis may lead to bilateral limb edema or thrombosis in the liver or spleen.)

Special Laboratory Studies

Certain laboratory studies can be useful in confirming the diagnosis of thrombosis or embolism, depending on the suspected cause and regions of injury. Consult specialists regarding radiographic, ultrasonic, angiographic, radionuclide (perfusion studies), and clinical laboratory tests. These studies may demonstrate changes attributable to decreased blood flow, organ ischemia, or tissue necrosis.

Treatment

KEY POINT ▶ Principles of therapy for thrombosis or embolism include removal or disintegration of the clot, control of the underlying disorder, and supportive care to damaged tissues.

Thrombolysis

- Consult a specialist (hematologist, internist, cardiologist) prior to the use of IV thrombolytic therapy

because this treatment is aggressive and can be associated with high morbidity and mortality.
- Tissue plasminogen activator (t-PA) and streptokinase are effective in dissolving arterial clots and restoring tissue perfusion, particularly if used during the first 12 hours following thromboembolism formation.
  - Uncontrolled bleeding and metabolic complications (e.g., hyperkalemia from reperfusion of ischemic muscle) can be lethal complications.

Surgery

- Surgical intervention is rarely employed in cats with cardiomyopathy owing to the risk of anesthesia and development of DIC.
- Surgical removal of the thrombus (or thrombolytic therapy) is recommended in cases of suprarenal aortic thrombosis, splenic thrombosis, and thrombosis with associated mechanical compression (e.g., spinal injury).
- The inaccessibility of some blood vessels makes surgery an ineffective option in some cases.

Embolectomy Catheters (Fogarty)

Embolectomy catheters have not been satisfactorily evaluated in animals.

Anticoagulants

Anticoagulants such as heparin and drugs such as aspirin that interfere with platelet function will not dissolve clots but are commonly administered to prevent further arterial and venous embolism.

- The dosages of aspirin are empirical, and there are doubts regarding its efficacy. Commonly used doses are:
  - In dogs with heartworm disease, 5–10 mg/kg daily.
  - In cats with cardiomyopathy, one child's aspirin tablet every other day.
- Sodium heparin (100–200 I.U./kg, SC, q8h) can be used in cases of pulmonary embolism, aortic embolism, or deep venous thrombosis.
  - Monitor clotting profiles to maintain the activated partial thromboplastin time (APTT) or one-stage prothrombin time (OSPT) at two to three times normal.
- Mini- or low-dose heparin (regimens vary between 10 and 75 I.U./kg, given q8h SC) may be used prophylactically or, in cases of DIC, to prevent further thrombosis (e.g., immune-mediated hemolytic anemia, DIC, jugular venous thrombosis).

Thrombophlebitis

- Treatment includes removal and culture of any catheters from the affected limb, hotpacks of the affected limb, and antibiotic therapy.
- Treat chemical phlebitis (e.g., thiacetarsemide) with topical DMSO and corticosteroid ointment (q8–12h) with concurrent administration of prednisolone (0.5 mg/kg, q12h).
- Gently wrap the limb to prevent self-trauma.

- Consider a mini- or low-dose heparin regimen (10–75 I.U./kg, q8h SC for 5–14 days) in cases of severe thrombophlebitis.

ARTERIAL HYPERTENSION

An increase in systemic or pulmonary arterial blood pressures is termed *hypertension*. Hypertension can be systolic, diastolic, or both. Identification of systemic hypertension is impeded by technical aspects of blood pressure determination in animals and by the wide variation in normal values. Detection of pulmonary hypertension requires cardiac catheterization.

Etiology

Systemic hypertension can be secondary to:

- Renal disease (particularly glomerular disease)
- Cushing's disease
- Pheochromocytoma
- Hyperthyroidism
- Drugs (e.g., alpha-adrenergic agonists)
- Central nervous system (CNS) disease

Causes of *pulmonary hypertension* include:

- Dirofilariasis
- Pulmonary embolism
- Congenital heart disease—large left-to-right shunts (increased flow) or left-to-right shunts that lead to pulmonary vascular injury and subsequent pulmonary hypertension as in reversed patent ductus arteriosus (PDA)
- Severe pulmonary disease (e.g., chronic pulmonary fibrosis, chronic bronchial disease)
- Pulmonary parenchymal disease/alveolar hypoxemia (reactive pulmonary vasoconstriction)
- Idiopathic (primary pulmonary hypertension)
- Severe or chronic left-sided heart failure

Pathophysiology

The pathogenesis of *systemic hypertension* in animals is unresolved and, as in human patients, is probably multifactorial. Potential causes include:

- Inability to regulate plasma volume, which occurs in renal disease (see sec. 8, ch. 1)
- Hyperadrenocorticism (see sec. 4, ch. 3)
- Excessive adrenergic activity (e.g., pheochromocytoma; see sec. 4, ch. 3)
- Renin-angiotensin system abnormalities

The pathogenesis of *pulmonary hypertension* varies with the underlying etiology:

- Left-sided heart failure leading to pulmonary venous and subsequently pulmonary arterial hypertension
- Pulmonary vascular injury or vasoconstriction with reduced vascular cross-sectional area (e.g., heartworm disease, [see sec. 6, ch. 10] pulmonary disease, alveolar hypoxia)
- Increased pulmonary blood flow (e.g., large left-to-right shunt, as with a septal defect or PDA)

Clinical Signs

Systemic hypertension most often affects the brain, heart, and kidneys. Associated clinical features include:

- CNS deficits from cerebral or brainstem vascular rupture and hemorrhage
- Blindness from retinal edema, hemorrhage, and detachments
- Epistaxis
- Abnormal renal contour or size (related to underlying morphologic lesion) with proteinuria and azotemia
- A systolic murmur (from mitral regurgitation) and atrial (S_4) gallop sound (from increased ventricular stiffness)
- Left ventricular hypertrophy and cardiomegaly; changes that may be demonstrated by radiography, ECG, or echocardiography

Clinical findings of *pulmonary hypertension* usually are dominated by the associated pulmonary or cardiac disease. Possible clinical signs include:

- Exercise intolerance
- Tachypnea and dyspnea, abnormal lung sounds (e.g., crackles), cyanosis, hemoptysis (coughing up blood)
- Abnormal heart sounds (loud or split second heart sound, tricuspid regurgitation, other associated heart lesions)
- Hypoxemia (low arterial PaO_2), and possibly polycythemia if the hypoxia is chronic
- Radiographic evidence of right-sided heart enlargement, dilation of the pulmonary arteries, and increased parenchymal densities (depending on the underlying cause)
- Right ventricular hypertrophy or dilation demonstrated by ECG, radiography, or echocardiography

Diagnosis

A presumptive diagnosis may be made based upon the clinical findings previously listed.

KEY POINT ▶ Systolic pressures >160 mm Hg and diastolic pressures >95 mm Hg are generally considered abnormal in the resting dog and cat with a normal heart rate.

- A definitive diagnosis of *systemic hypertension* requires an arterial puncture or an indirect pressure determination that is repeatable and uses a reliable technology.
  - Oscillometric and Doppler flow methods have been used successfully in dogs.
  - Cats are difficult to evaluate noninvasively, but systolic pressure can be determined with a Doppler flow crystal and occlusion cuff.
- Diagnose *pulmonary hypertension* using catheterization or Doppler echocardiographic methods that detect the velocity of associated tricuspid or pulmonary regurgitation across the right-sided heart valves.
  - Systolic pulmonary artery pressures of >30 mm Hg generally are considered abnormal.

Treatment

Systemic Hypertension

Detailed studies of therapy for systemic arterial hypertension in animals are unavailable. Treatment usually involves a stepwise method, beginning with diuretic therapy and dietary sodium restriction and proceeding to vasodilator therapy or treatment with a beta blocker. Consider the possibility of drug interactions when prescribing multiple drug regimens. Listed are some commonly used procedures and therapies:

- Treatment of the underlying problem (e.g., hyperthyroidism)
- Dietary sodium restriction (e.g., Prescription Diet h/d or k/d; Hill's Pet Foods)
- Diuretics (furosemide, 1–3 mg/kg, q12h; or hydrochlorothiazide-spironolactone, 2–4 mg/kg of combined product, q12h)
- Alpha-adrenergic blocker such as prazosin (Minipress; Squibb), 1–2 mg capsule q8–12h
- Angiotensin-converting enzyme (ACE) inhibitor (enalapril, 0.25–0.5 mg/kg, q12h; or captopril, 0.5–2.0 mg/kg, q8h)
- Beta-adrenergic blocker (propranolol 0.5–1.0 mg/kg, q8h or equivalent)
- Direct-acting arterial vasodilator drug (hydralazine, 1–2 mg/kg, q12h).
- Calcium channel blocker (diltiazem, 0.5–1.5 mg/kg, q8h)
- For emergency treatment, give an IV infusion of sodium nitroprusside, 1–5 mg/kg/minute at a constant rate.
- Check blood pressure regularly to ensure efficacy and prevent further organ injury.
- Anticipate signs of hypotension (weakness, depression, syncope, acute renal failure) and treat by reducing medication dosages.
- Initial therapy with vasodilator drugs such as prazosin may cause immediate hypotension; reducing the dose for the first 1–2 days may prevent complications.

Drug Selection. Choice of antihypertensive drug therapy varies.

- When retinal detachments are present, the authors recommend aggressive treatment with either nitroprusside or a combination of furosemide, prazosin or hydralazine, and propranolol (such treatment has been associated with reattachment of the retina).
- Consider the combination of furosemide, dietary sodium restriction, and either prazosin in the dog or enalapril in the cat in initial treatment of chronic moderate to severe hypertension.
- A beta blocker can be added if blood pressure remains elevated, or hydralazine (in the dog or cat) can be substituted for the vasodilator.

KEY POINT ▶ Monotherapy (e.g., furosemide) is rarely successful in the treatment of moderate to severe hypertension. A diuretic plus a vasodilator or ACE inhibitor is more likely to be effective.

Pulmonary Hypertension

- Therapy of pulmonary hypertension always involves treatment of the underlying condition.
- Oxygen therapy may decrease pulmonary arterial pressure if there is associated reactive pulmonary arterial vasoconstriction.
- Vasodilator drugs are contraindicated in patients with pulmonary hypertension because severe systemic hypotension may develop.

VASCULITIS

Arteritis

Arteritis (i.e., inflammation involving arterioles or arteries) can be caused by infection with various microorganisms and is often a component of *multisystemic infections*, including infectious canine hepatitis, (see sec. 2, ch. 9), infectious feline peritonitis (FIP) (see sec. 2, ch. 3), and Rocky Mountain spotted fever (see sec. 2, ch. 10). Immune-mediated arteritis is believed to be important in FIP, systemic lupus erythematosus, idiopathic vasculitis in Akita, spitz, and Doberman pinscher dogs, and some drug reactions. Cutaneous manifestations of vasculitis are discussed in other chapters in this text.

Clinical Signs

Clinical signs are related to inflammatory mediators, increased vascular permeability, and interruption of the vascular endothelial lining and include:

- Fever
- Subcutaneous edema
- Cutaneous hemorrhages
- Coagulation disorders including thrombocytopenia and disseminated intravascular coagulopathy that develop secondary to vasculitis
- Thrombosis and ischemic injury (see previous discussion of thrombosis)

Vasculitis Syndromes

Specific clinical vasculitis syndromes commonly seen in cats and dogs include:

- FIP (see sec. 2, ch. 3)
- Verminous arteritis associated with dirofilariasis and angiostrongyliasis (damage occurring primarily within the pulmonary arteries; angiostrongyliasis is uncommon in the United States).
- *Rocky Mountain spotted fever*, which is a tick-borne infection caused by *Rickettsia rickettsii* that affects dogs and human beings (see sec.2, ch.10). Invasion of vascular endothelial cells causes vasculitis with mononuclear inflammation, microscopic thrombosis, and microinfarction. Thrombocytopenia is common.
  - Multiple organs are affected, including the heart (myocarditis and arrhythmias), brain (stupor, coma), blood (thrombocytopenia, neutropenia), and skin (edema, rash).
  - Fever is common and death may occur.

- Blood from affected dogs has public health significance (contagion).
- Diagnosis is made by clinical and laboratory signs and serology.
■ *Uremic vasculitis*, which causes myoarteritis of small arteries, particularly in the stomach. This leads to hemorrhage and necrosis, predisposing to uremic gastritis and gastrointestinal ulceration and melena.

Treatment

■ Treatment depends on the underlying cause.
■ Management of FIP (sec. 2, ch. 3), systemic lupus erythematosus and immune-mediated vasculitis (sec. 3, ch. 3), and spotted fever (sec. 2, ch. 10) are discussed elsewhere in this text.
■ Immunosuppressive doses of glucocorticoids are indicated for management of some vasculitides.
■ Thrombotic complications may require prophylactic heparin (10–100 I.U./kg, q8h SC)

ARTERIOSCLEROSIS

Arteriosclerosis is a chronic arterial metamorphosis characterized by loss of elasticity, luminal narrowing, and proliferative and degenerative lesions of the intima and media. *Atherosclerosis* pertains to the arteriosclerotic state that also includes fatty degenerative changes in the arterial wall. This is the typical underlying lesion of coronary artery disease in human patients.

■ Coronary arteriosclerosis, prominent in older dogs with endocardiosis, has been related to small and microscopic areas of myocardial fibrosis. Presumably this is due to ischemic necrosis and infarction of myocytes secondary to reduced perfusion.
■ Similar lesions also have been observed in dogs with congenital subaortic stenosis, in dogs with diabetes mellitus, and in cats with hypertrophic cardiomyopathy.
■ Naturally occurring atherosclerosis occurs in severe canine hypothyroidism (see sec. 4, ch. 1) when serum cholesterol concentrations are extraordinarily high (generally >750 mg/dl).
■ In canine and feline patients, clinically important hyaline arteriosclerosis is primarily related to the coronary vasculature. The overall clinical significance of arterial degenerative changes in animals is relatively small compared with that in human beings.

Diagnosis

The diagnosis of arteriosclerosis is difficult. Suspect this condition in patients with severe hypercholesterolemia and in association with the aforementioned cardiac disorders.

■ Small-vessel (intramural) arteriosclerosis may contribute to the morbidity of other cardiac disorders by causing ischemia-induced arrhythmias (e.g., premature ventricular contractions) or increased myocardial stiffness (e.g., hypertrophic cardiomyopathy, subaortic stenosis).
■ Suspect acute myocardial infarction due to extra-

mural coronary thrombosis in dogs with respiratory distress, ventricular arrhythmias, and severe ST-T segment changes on the ECG (particularly ST-T segment elevation). Diagnosis is presumptive because coronary angiography and myocardial enzyme analysis are rarely done in animals.
■ In the differential diagnosis of extramural coronary artery obstruction or thrombosis, rule out embolic complications of bacterial endocarditis.

Treatment

Management includes treatment of the underlying disease and the complications of ischemia (e.g., ventricular antiarrhythmic therapy).

■ In cases of presumed myocardial infarction, administer oxygen and nitroglycerin ointment (see discussion of cardiac drugs) empirically.
■ Beta blockers (e.g., propranolol, 0.4–1.0 mg/kg, q8h PO), by decreasing myocardial oxygen consumption, may be cardioprotective in animals with multifocal small vessel coronary arteriosclerosis.
■ Calcium channel blockers (e.g., diltiazem, 0.5–2.0 mg/kg, q8h PO) may act as a coronary vasodilator and prevent coronary vascular spasms (see discussion of feline hypertrophic cardiomyopathy).

VASCULAR NEOPLASIA

Etiology

Vascular tumors can be primary or metastatic. The endocardium and vascular elements of the heart also may become neoplastic.

■ *Primary* arterial and venous tumors are uncommon:
  - Aortic and carotid body tumors (chemodectomas) can act as space-occupying lesions in the thorax or about the ascending aorta.
  - Aortic body tumors are an important cause of hemorrhagic pericardial effusion in older brachycephalic dogs. These tumors also may be an incidental finding at necropsy (see discussion of pericardial diseases, sec. 6, ch. 9).
■ *Tumors from vascular elements* (e.g., hemangiosarcoma) and malignancies metastatic to blood vessels are described in detail in sec. 3, ch. 7. Hemangiosarcoma is the most common intracardiac tumor. Multicentric involvement (e.g., liver, spleen, heart) is common. Pulmonary metastasis is frequent.
■ *Extravascular neoplasms* may invade blood vessels; for example, obstruction of the caudal vena cava can develop secondary to ingrowth of a pheochromocytoma from the adrenal medulla (see sec. 4, ch. 3).

Pathophysiology

■ Tumor-related hemorrhage into the pericardial space can cause cardiac tamponade.
■ Intraluminal obstruction to venous return (usually of the caudal vena cava) causes ascites. This is most common with hemangiosarcoma; however, other primary intracardiac tumors, such as myxoma and fibrosarcoma, can cause similar problems.

Clinical Signs

- Clinical signs of cardiac or vena caval neoplasia are usually those of right-sided CHF (hepatomegaly, ascites, pleural effusion).
- Compression of the cranial vena cava (e.g., from mediastinal lymphosarcoma) can cause intermandibular and ventrocervical subcutaneous edema.

Differential Diagnosis

- Differential diagnosis of caudal vena cava obstruction includes idiopathic sclerosis, neoplasia, kinking, or trauma of the caudal vena cava.

Imaging Studies

- Radiographic studies may demonstrate mass lesions; however, the cardiac silhouette may be radiographically normal when the obstruction is intraluminal. Nonselective angiography (peripheral venous injection) may demonstrate vascular obstruction or interruption.
- Ultrasound studies may demonstrate dilated hepatic veins typical of obstructed hepatic venous drainage or solid tissue mass lesions.
- Echocardiography can reveal intracardiac mass lesions.

Treatment

Therapy for vascular neoplasia is complicated and requires surgery, and possibly chemotherapy (see sec. 3, ch. 5). Most patients should be transferred to a referral hospital.

ARTERIOVENOUS FISTULA

An arteriovenous (AV) fistula is a congenital or acquired communication between artery and vein.

- Congenital lesions tend to be multiple and involve the limbs, whereas a post-traumatic fistula is usually a single direct connection associated with abnormal healing of the injured blood vessels.
- Declawing operations and tumors have been rarely associated with AV fistula formation in the feline paw.
- Thyroid carcinoma may lead to a cervical AV communication in dogs. AV fistulas have been reported secondary to other tumors.
- A hepatic AV fistula is a special type of congenital vascular malformation. This condition usually is associated with portal hypertension and ascites (sec. 7, ch. 8).

Clinical Signs

Clinical signs include local vascular changes (due to venous hypertension) and cardiac manifestations (due to increased cardiac output required to perfuse the shunt). Any combination of the following signs may be observed:

- Edema, pain, inability to use the limb, a warm or cool extremity, and abnormal tissue growth
- A continuous murmur (bruit) detectable over the affected area as blood shunts continuously through the fistula

KEY POINT ▶ A positive Branham sign may be present in large AV shunts; slowing of the heart rate follows digital occlusion of the artery—the result of a sudden increase in arterial resistance and pressure.

- An overall increase in cardiac output (equal to the shunt flow), which may be manifested by tachycardia, cardiomegaly, and increased pulmonary vascularity
  - Increased cardiac work, cardiac dilation, renal retention of sodium and water, elevation of venous filling pressures, and eventually congestive heart failure can develop; this is particularly true of large shunts.

Diagnosis

The diagnosis is made by clinical signs, ultrasonography (including Doppler studies), and angiography. These studies generally require transfer of the patient to a referral hospital.

Treatment

- Ligation or removal of the shunt is the treatment of choice.
- The surgical approach usually is guided by imaging and vascular contrast studies.
- Other methods of vessel occlusion (e.g., catheter-delivered "umbrellas") have not been used routinely in veterinary practice.

Complications and Prognosis

- The prognosis is good for an acquired AV fistula that is not associated with malignancy.
- Congenital AV fistulas may be problematic and difficult surgical procedures.
- Limb amputation may be necessary if the exact location of the shunt cannot be isolated and ligated or if the limb becomes devitalized.
- Management of hepatic AV fistulas may require partial hepatectomy of the involved lobe.

Supplemental Readings

Suter PF: Peripheral vascular disease. *In* Ettinger SJ, ed.: *Textbook of Veterinary Internal Medicine*, 3rd ed. Philadelphia: W. B. Saunders, 1989, p 1185.
Olivier NB: Pathophysiology of arteriovenous fistulae. *In* Slatter DH, ed.: *Textbook of Small Animal Surgery*. Philadelphia: W. B. Saunders, 1985, p 1051.

12 Congenital Heart Disease

Matthew W. Miller
John D. Bonagura

ETIOLOGY

KEY POINT ▶ Congenital heart disease (CHD) is the most common cause of cardiovascular disease in animals less than 1 year of age.

- Common defects include patient ductus arteriosus (PDA); subvalvular aortic stenosis (SAS); pulmonic stenosis (PS); mitral and tricuspid dysplasia, causing insufficiency or stenosis of the valve; atrial and ventricular septal defects (ASD, VSD); and the tetralogy of Fallot. Congenital peritoneopericardial diaphragmatic hernia is a common defect of the diaphragm and pericardium (see sec. 6, ch. 9).
- Signalment, physical examination, thoracic radiography, and electrocardiography often provide an accurate diagnosis. Definitive diagnosis of the type and severity of CHD requires more sophisticated tests, including echocardiography and selective angiocardiography. Although the management of CHD is often interesting and challenging to the practicing veterinarian, one must consider the following points:
  - Some dogs with seemingly simple defects, such as PDA, may have complicating conditions, such as myocardial failure, tricuspid dysplasia, VSD, or subaortic stenosis. These complications are particularly common in larger breeds of dogs.
  - Most congenital heart defects have a genetic basis, but the mode of inheritance is rarely a simple mendelian pattern.
  - Mildly affected dogs, such as those with trivial subaortic stenosis, may be clinically normal; however, owners are usually advised not to breed these animals. Doppler or catheterization studies may be required to diagnose such conditions.
  - Young animals may appear to tolerate even severe congenital defects for quite some time. Heart failure may develop suddenly and unexpectedly. When the veterinarian suspects CHD and clients are interested in optimal care, especially if cardiac surgery is a possibility, referral is not delayed.

KEY POINT ▶ Following a tentative diagnosis of CHD, the best course of action for the patient is generally referral to a cardiologist or a specialist with training with experience in the management of CHD.

- The balance of this chapter discusses the approach to a recognition of cardiac malformations and an overview of the options available in the management of CHD.

CLINICAL SIGNS

- Most animals with CHD are asymptomatic.
- Stunted growth
  - Most commonly associated with right-to-left shunts (cyanotic heart disease) or CHF.
  - Respiratory distress, exercise intolerance, and tachypnea are typical in cases of CHF or cyanotic heart disease (e.g., tetralogy of Fallot).
- Fainting and exertional collapse are signs of severe CHD and may be related to:
  - Right-to-left shunts (hypoxemia)
  - Paroxysmal arrhythmias
  - Ventricular outflow tract obstruction (e.g., aortic and pulmonic stenosis)
  - CHF.
- Exercise intolerance is usually a sign of moderate-to-severe CHD.

DIAGNOSIS (Fig. 1)

Signalment

- Breed, age, and sex predilection are used in conjunction with physical examination findings to formulate an initial list of differential diagnoses, (Table 1).

Physical Examination

- Besides complete physical examination, cardiac auscultation is the key to recognition of CHD.
  - Cardiac murmurs
    May be absent in right-to-left shunting defects with polycythemia, with pulmonary or aortic atresia and large (unrestrictive) VSD, or with severe pulmonary hypertension.
    May be characteristic of a particular cardiac defect (see Fig. 1). See the discussion of a cardiovascular examination in section 6, chapter 1.
    May be soft and possible for the veterinarian to confuse with an innocent murmur (e.g., mild subaortic stenosis).
    The intensity of the murmur does not correlate with the severity of the cardiac lesion except in ventricular outlet obstruction in which louder

TABLE 1. Breed and Sex Predilections for Certain Congenital Cardiac Defects

Defect	Predilection
Patent ductus arteriosus (PDA)	Poodle, collie, Pomeranian, German shepherd, Shetland sheepdog (female:male, 2.2:1)
Pulmonic stenosis (PS)	Beagle, bulldog, fox terrier, miniature schnauzer, Chihuahua, Samoyed, Labrador retriever
Subaortic stenosis (SAS)	Newfoundland, boxer, German shepherd, German shorthaired pointer, golden retriever, rottweiler, bull terrier
Ventricular septal defect (VSD)	English bulldog
Atrial septal defect (ASD)	Samoyed, boxer, Doberman pinscher
Mitral dysplasia	Great Dane, German shepherd (male>female), bull terrier
Tricuspid dysplasia	Great Dane, German shepherd, Weimaraner, Labrador retriever (male>female)
Tetralogy of Fallot	Keeshond, English bulldog

Note: PDA, PS, and SAS are the most common defects in dogs. ASD/VSD and atrioventricular valve dysplasias are the most common defects in cats.

and later peaking murmurs usually indicate a progressively tighter obstruction.
■ Precordial palpation (palpation of the thorax over the heart)
  • Apical impulse identifies the relative areas of the mitral and tricuspid valve sounds and murmurs and is thereby useful in localizing cardiac murmurs.
  • Strong left apical impulse suggests ventricular hypertrophy (e.g., AS).
  • Right-sided impulse equal to or greater than that on the left suggests right ventricular hypertrophy (e.g., PS).
  • Precordial thrill is a vibration that identifies the point of maximum intensity (PMI) of a loud murmur.
■ Arterial pulse
  • Often normal. Weak (hypokinetic) pulses suggest left ventricular outflow obstruction or cardiac failure.
  • Bounding (hyperkinetic) pulses are most commonly associated with PDA or congenital aortic insufficiency.
  • Severe right-sided lesions or CHF may be associated with weak arterial pulses.
■ Venous pulses
  • Distended or pulsating jugular vein suggests a right-sided heart lesion (e.g., PS, tricuspid dysplasia) or pulmonary hypertension.
■ Mucous membranes
  • Pink membranes are typical.
  • Pallor with prolonged capillary refill time suggests cardiac failure or concurrent anemia.
  • Cyanotic membranes may indicate pulmonary dys-

function, from left-sided CHF or pneumonia, or may suggest right-to-left shunting.
  Tetralogy of Fallot
  Reversed ASD, VSD, PDA
  Differential cyanosis—oral membranes pink, caudal membranes (vulva, prepuce) cyanotic—suggests a reversed PDA (i.e., blood flow from the pulmonary artery to the aorta).

Electrocardiography

See section 6, chapter 3.

■ Especially valuable in CHD for diagnosis of cardiac chamber enlargement when there is moderate-to-severe cardiomegaly. The electrocardiogram is of little value in mild CHD (e.g., mild AS).
■ Chamber enlargement patterns
  • Atrial enlargement patterns (P wave > 0.04 sec; > 0.4 mV) are relatively insensitive for predicting right vs. left atrial dilation.
  • Left ventricular enlargement (R wave > 2.5–3.0 mV in lead II or left-axis deviation)—PDA, VSD, mitral dysplasia, subaortic stenosis.
  • Right ventricular hypertrophy (right-axis deviation with prominent S waves in leads I, II, III, AVF, and V_2 to V_6); ± widened QRS (right bundle branch block)—PS, ASD, VSD (some cases); tricuspid dysplasia; tetralogy of Fallot; pulmonary hypertension associated with right-to-left shunts.

Thoracic Radiography

■ Normal pups have relatively dominant right ventricular shadow until approximately 8–12 weeks of age. Right-sided dilation often causes apical shifts leading to overestimation of the left side of the heart. Radiographic interpretation focuses on the following (see Fig. 1 and the discussion of cardiac radiography in sec. 6, ch. 2).
  • Cardiac size and shape; specific chamber enlargement
  • Great vessels (aorta, pulmonary artery)
  • Pulmonary vascularity (overcirculation and undercirculation; left-sided CHF).

Echocardiography (Table 2)

■ In certain defects the anatomic abnormality may be visualized, for example, in ASD, VSD, and subaortic narrowing. A normal, two-dimensional echocardiographic study does not rule out the diagnosis of mild congenital heart disease. Doppler or cardiac catheterization studies may be needed to identify minor lesions in potential breeding animals.
■ Determination of the degree of cardiac enlargement/hypertrophy is useful in assessing the overall significance of the lesion, because mild lesions do not lead to substantial cardiomegaly.
■ Saline injections (contrast echocardiography) into a peripheral vein readily demonstrate right-to-left shunting lesions.
■ Doppler echocardiography is highly effective for noninvasive quantitation of the severity of the lesion and is supplanting cardiac catheterization for routine

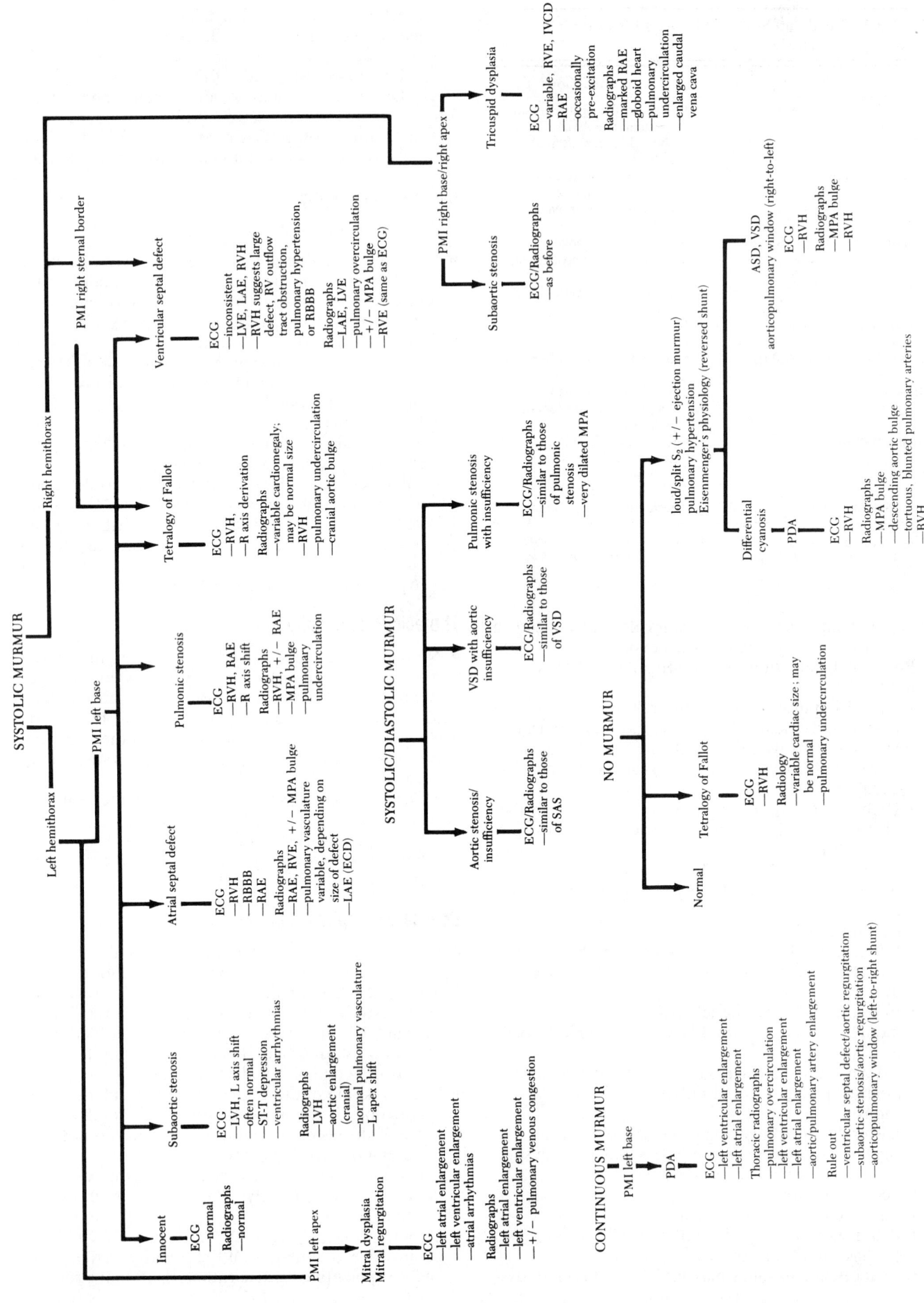

TABLE 2. Echocardiographic (Doppler) Features of Select Congenital Heart Defects

Defects	Echocardiographic (Doppler) Features
Patent ductus arteriosus (PDA)	Dilated left atrium, left ventricle, and pulmonary trunk; possible identification of PDA; turbulent flow in main pulmonary artery, with retrograde diastolic flow and increased transmitral and aortic flow velocities
Pulmonic stenosis (PS)	Right ventricular hypertrophy, right atrial and pulmonary artery enlargement, outflow tract obstruction, thickened valve leaflets, septal flattening and/or paradoxical septal motion, high-velocity flow (>1.5 m/sec) across the pulmonic valve
Subaortic stenosis (SAS)	Left ventricular hypertrophy, dilated aorta, subvalvular narrowing, high velocity flow (>2.0 m/sec) across the aortic valve
Ventricular septal defect (VSD)	Variable chamber enlargement, most commonly left atrial and ventricular, possible identification of defect, right ventricular hypertrophy if pulmonary hypertension (PH) or very large defect, visualization of flow across defect, may be bidirectional; increased transmitral and PA flow velocity, right to left in the case of PH
Atrial septal defect (ASD)	Right atrial and ventricular enlargement, possible identification of defect, main pulmonary artery enlargement, flow across defect, increased velocity flow across tricuspid (diastole) and pulmonic (systole) valves
Mitral valve dysplasia	Left atrial and left ventricular enlargement, abnormal mitral valve anatomy, increased transmitral diastolic flow velocity, turbulent retrograde systolic transmitral flow
Tricuspid valve dysplasia	Right atrial and ventricular enlargement, abnormal tricuspid valve anatomy, increased transtricuspid diastolic flow velocity, turbulent retrograde systolic transtricuspid flow
Tetralogy of Fallot	Right ventricular hypertrophy, right ventricular outflow tract obstruction, identification of VSD, over-riding aorta, small left heart, contrast study indicating right-to-left shunting, septal flattening and/or paradoxical septal motion, right-to-left flow across VSD, decreased diastolic transmitral flow, possibly increased transaortic systolic flow, increased flow velocity across the pulmonic valve
Pulmonary hypertension (PH)	Right ventricular hypertrophy, right atrial enlargement, dilated main pulmonary artery, visualization of associated shunt, right-to-left shunt by Doppler or bubble study, increased flow acceleration across pulmonary valve

diagnosis. A complete Doppler study (with color flow imaging) can provide anatomic detail; blood flow information, including abnormally high velocity of flow; and intracardiac pressure estimates.

Cardiac Catheterization

- Useful when echocardiographic-Doppler study findings are equivocal or when therapeutic intervention is necessary. Of possible assistance when outlining the surgical anatomy.
- Usually necessitates referral to a cardiologist or a specialist with training and experience in the diagnosis and management of CHD.
- Can involve therapeutic manipulations in some cases (e.g., balloon valvulotomy for PS; ± subaortic stenosis).

THERAPY

Definitive treatment of CHD usually requires cardiac surgery. In addition, complications such as CHF and arrhythmias may necessitate medical management.

Congestive Heart Failure (CHF)

- Similar to the therapy of left-sided CHF that is associated with acquired diseases (see sec. 6, ch. 6).
  - Digoxin (0.005–0.01 mg/kg, q12h, PO)

- Diuretics (furosemide [Lasix], 0.5–2.0 mg/kg, q12h, q8h)
- Vasodilators may control CHF and reduce left-to-right shunting (e.g., VSD). Enalapril (Vasotec, 0.25–0.5 mg/kg, q12h) is given for CHF unless there is a left-to-right shunt. In this case, the lower dose of enalapril is provided, and hydralazine (0.5–2 mg/kg, q12h) is titrated to decrease shunting.
- Exercise limitation and dietary sodium restriction are prescribed.
- Use vasodilators with caution—if at all—in patients with subaortic stenosis (SAS).

Arrhythmias

See section 6, chapter 4.

- Supraventricular (atrial tachycardia, flutter, fibrillation)
  - Digoxin (0.005–0.01 mg/kg, q12h, PO)
  - Propranolol or equivalent beta blocker (0.5–1.0 mg/kg q8h, PO)
  - Diltiazem (1.0–1.5 mg/kg, q8h, PO)
  - Combinations of the aforementioned when necessary
- Ventricular tachycardia
  - Procainamide (2–20 mg/kg, IV or IM; 25–40 mcg/kg/min constant rate infusion; 12–20 mg/kg, q8h to q6h, PO)
  - Tocainide (Tonocard, 10–20 mg/kg, q8h, PO)

Figure 1. ASD, atrial septal defect; ECD, endocardial cushion defect; IVCD, intraventricular conduction defect; LAE, left atrial enlargement; LVE, left ventricular enlargement; LVH, left ventricular hypertrophy; MPA, main pulmonary artery; PDA, patent ductus arteriosus; PMI, point of maximal intensity; RAE, right atrial enlargement; RBBB, right bundle branch block; RV, right ventricle; RVE, right ventricular enlargement; RVH, right ventricular hypertrophy; SAS, subaortic stenosis; VSD, ventricular septal defect.

- Lidocaine (50–75 mcg/kg/min constant rate infusion for intraoperative, perioperative control)
- Propranolol (0.5–1.0 mg/kg, q8h, PO) or equivalent beta blocker has been used for empirical prophylactic therapy in dogs with subaortic stenosis to prevent arrhythmias and sudden death.

Surgical Correction

- Surgical management of cardiac defects must not be undertaken without proper training and experience in thoracic surgery (see sec. 6, ch. 25).
- For PDA, surgical ligation is the therapy of choice and is associated with an intraoperative mortality of < 5% at most institutions (see sec. 6, ch. 13).
- VSD, ASD
  - Definitive repair has been reported with varying degrees of success. Requires cardiopulmonary bypass.
  - Pulmonary artery banding may reduce the left-to-right shunt and is useful for patients with CHF or for those developing pulmonary hypertension.
- Pulmonic stenosis
  - Patch graft, pulmonary valvulectomy, surgical or balloon valvuloplasty, or their combination has been utilized.
- Minimal success has been obtained thus far for subaortic stenosis.
- Palliative therapy for tetralogy of Fallot involves the creation of an extracardiac shunt between a systemic artery (aorta or subclavian) and the pulmonary artery to increase pulmonary circulation and left-sided venous return. This therapy may produce significant clinical improvement.
  - For polycythemia, phlebotomy with replacement of blood with isotonic saline may provide symptomatic improvement (see sec. 3, ch. 1).

NATURAL HISTORY AND PROGNOSIS

Cardiac Shunts

- PDA has an excellent prognosis with surgery. Approximately 60% of pups die within 1 year without surgery. Prognosis with reversed PDA is grave, and surgery is contraindicated.
- Prognosis for small and restrictive VSD is good; however, large, unrestrictive VSD leads to CHF or pulmonary hypertension.
- ASD is similar to VSD.
- In endocardial cushion defect (ASD, VSD, AV valvular malformation), CHF is common.

Valvular Malformations

- In pulmonic stenosis, the prognosis is good unless the obstruction is severe and the transvalve catheterization gradient exceeds 75 mm Hg, in which case CHF or sudden death may occur.
- Subaortic stenosis has a guarded to good prognosis unless the obstruction causes >100 mm Hg catheterization gradient, in which case CHF or sudden death is likely.
- Mitral and tricuspid valve dysplasia lesions are well-tolerated if mild; however, severe stenosis or severe regurgitation often leads to CHF or atrial fibrillation.

Tetralogy of Fallot

- Progressive hypoxemia, polycythemia, tachypnea, and exercise intolerance are typical, usually leading to sudden death.

Pulmonary Hypertension

- Pulmonary hypertension due to high vascular resistance may develop secondary to a left-to-right shunt. This condition usually occurs before 6 months of age. Prognosis is poor, and surgery is contraindicated. Polycythemia is controlled by intermittent phlebotomy. Medical therapy is ineffective.

Supplemental Readings

Bonagura JD: Congenital heart disease. *In* Ettinger SJ, ed.: *Textbook of Veterinary Internal Medicine,* 3rd ed. Philadelphia: W.B. Saunders, 1989.

Miller MW, Bonagura JD.: Congenital heart disease. *In* Kirk RW, ed.: *Current Veterinary Therapy X.* Philadelphia: W.B. Saunders, 1989.

13 Surgical Correction of Patent Ductus Arteriosus

Eric R. Schertel

Ligation of the patent ductus arteriosus (PDA) in dogs and cats is a rewarding surgical procedure. When performed by an experienced surgeon, the combined operative/postoperative mortality rate is relatively low (8–10%) compared with surgery of other forms of congenital heart disease. The long-term prognosis after correction is excellent. However, like any thoracic or cardiovascular procedure, special attention to the details of anesthetic and surgical techniques is necessary for success. An accurate diagnosis is important, as is a thorough knowledge of the anatomy and physiology of the cardiovascular system.

ANATOMY AND PHYSIOLOGY

- The ductus arteriosus is a remnant of the left sixth aortic arch and connects the pulmonary artery and the descending aorta in the fetus and newborn. Its continued patency post partum results in left-to-right shunting of blood causing volume overload of the left atrium and ventricle. In severe cases, left ventricular failure may be present.
- The relationship of the descending aorta, main pulmonary artery, and right and left pulmonary arteries with the PDA must be appreciated (Fig. 1).
- The PDA may vary in size and shape but generally is approximately one-fifth to one-fourth the diameter of the aorta, or slightly smaller than the left main pulmonary artery. The PDA is usually short (0.5–

1.0 cm), bridging the small distance between the aorta and pulmonary artery.
- The left vagus nerve lies over the ductus and is immediately underneath the visceral pleura. The recurrent laryngeal nerve arises from the vagus and courses caudal and medial to the PDA.
- Rarely, a persistent left cranial vena cava may be found coursing over the pulmonary artery. This does not pose a surgical problem in PDA ligation.

PREOPERATIVE AND PERIOPERATIVE CONSIDERATIONS

- Consult the chapter on congenital heart disease (sec. 6, ch. 12) for details of diagnosis and medical management.
- Institute conservative medical management prior to surgery when there is evidence of heart failure. More aggressive medical management may not benefit the patient as much as surgery.
- Mortality with surgery is higher when congestive heart failure (CHF) or atrial fibrillation is present; however, the mortality of nonsurgically managed PDA patients also is high. Thus, if conservative therapy for heart failure is not effective in 24–48 hours, surgery combined with intensive medical management is the appropriate course of action.
- Administer IV fluids carefully during anesthesia and surgery, especially in animals with heart failure.

Figure 1. Retraction of the left cranial lobe of the lung allows exposure of the region of the ductus.

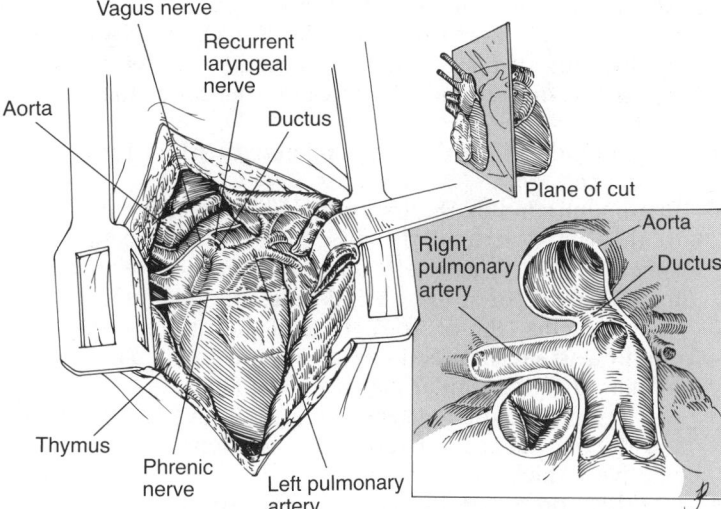

505

- Perioperative mortality is 8–10% according to recently published reports.
- Perioperative complications occur in 10–15% of cases.

Ligation of the Patent Ductus Arteriosus

Objectives

- Careful exposure and definition of the ductus arteriosus through a left fourth intercostal space thoracotomy. (The left fifth space may be indicated in cats.)
- Double ligation of the ductus without trauma to the vessels.

Equipment

- General surgery pack and standard suture, plus instruments required for thoracic surgery (see sec. 6, ch. 25)
- Assorted sizes of right-angle forceps
- Vascular clamps, preferably pediatric/infant ductus clamps (3 pairs)
- Multipurpose peripheral vascular clamps (2 pairs)
- Suture; nonabsorbable, 5-0 or 6-0, on a cardiovascular needle

Technique

1. Utilize an appropriate anesthetic regimen based on the preoperative assessment of cardiac function (see sec. 1, ch. 2 for discussion of anesthesia techniques). Positive pressure ventilation is required during the majority of the procedure.
2. Place the patient in right lateral recumbency. The left thorax is clipped and aseptically prepared from cranial border of the scapula to rib 13, and from the dorsal to the ventral midline. In preparation, include the left shoulder and extend past the elbow.
3. Perform a standard left fourth intercostal space thoracotomy (see sec. 6, ch. 25).
4. Identify the region of the ductus following caudal retraction of the left cranial lung lobe (see Fig. 1). Pack the lobe with a moist sponge or laparotomy pad.
5. Elevate the vagus nerve and encircle with umbilical tape for retraction to expose the PDA. Identify the location of the recurrent laryngeal nerve as it courses from the vagus to the caudal aspect of the ductus.
6. Palpate the thrill in the main pulmonary artery for reference.
7. Begin blunt and sharp dissection cranial and caudal to the PDA. Extend the dissection caudally between the aorta and left main pulmonary artery for a distance of at least 1.5–2 times the diameter of the ductus (Fig. 2, top). Extend the dissection cranioventrally between the aorta and main pulmonary artery a similar distance. The depth of the dissection should be at least equal to the width of the ductus. Dissection should be adjacent to the relatively thick-walled aorta.
8. Consider preparing the craniodorsal aspect of the

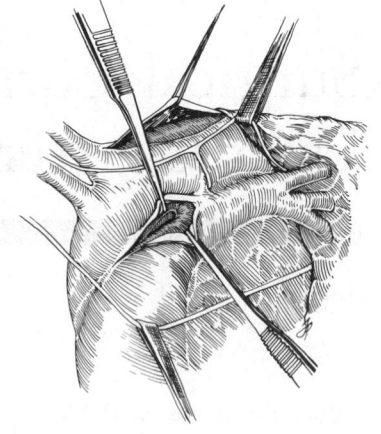

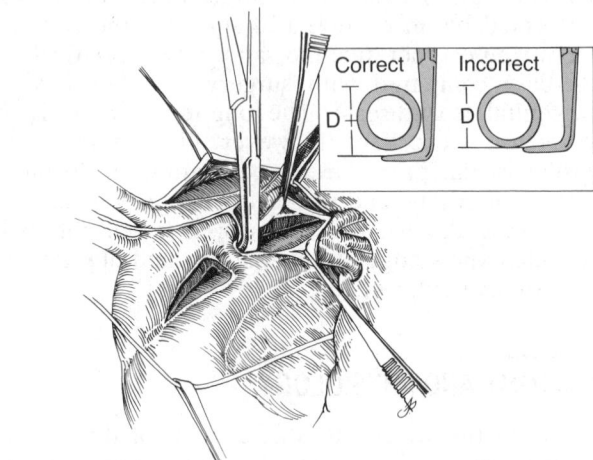

Figure 2. Exposure of the ductus. Top, initial areas of the section. Bottom, use closed right-angle forceps to dissect the region behind the patent ductus arteriosus. See text for further instructions.

aorta just distal to the left subclavian artery by reflecting the pleura and adjacent mediastinal tissues. This requires a small amount of time and ensures a clear path for clamp placement if hemorrhage control is necessary (see below).

9. The pericardium has a variable insertion at the level of the ductus. It may insert on the aortic side or on the main pulmonary artery side of the ductus. Thus, the ductus occasionally is within the pericardium. In these circumstances, open and incise the pericardium at its insertion on the ductus or aorta.
10. Once the cranial and caudal aspects of the ductus are exposed, initiate blunt dissection behind the PDA using right-angle forceps (Fig. 2, bottom). Take care to visualize the depth of the ductus. Accomplish dissection behind the ductus by inserting closed forceps, spreading gently, and removing the forceps. Carry out dissection *adjacent* and *parallel* to the surface of the aorta.
11. The author prefers caudal to cranial dissection to avoid repeated work in the cranial aspect of the ductus. The vascular structures of the cranial region are under greater tension and are most prone to hemorrhage. However, minor medial dissection in this area often is necessary.
12. When the majority of the medial dissection is complete, gently separate the aorta and main pul-

monary artery cranial to the ductus to allow visualization of the tips of the right-angle forceps as they are passed from caudal to cranial. When the tips are visible, carefully incise the remaining *fascia* over the tips of the forceps with a No. 15 blade. This is preferable to repeated efforts at pressing through this fascia.

KEY POINT ▶ Do not cut any tissue unless it is certain that it is fascia and not vessel wall.

13. Individually pass two strands of 1-0 to 2-0 silk suture, depending on the size of the dog and the ductus (Fig. 3, top).
14. Attenuate the ductus prior to ligation to observe the hemodynamic effects. If bradycardia is observed, atropine may be given. Double-ligate the ductus, aortic side first. Palpate the pulmonary artery again for ductal-related thrill or turbulence.
15. If hemorrhage is encountered from perivascular structures, pressure, ligation, or cautery may be used for control. If the ductus ruptures and aggressive hemorrhage is encountered, first place vascular clamps on the aorta in the previously prepared region just caudal to the left subclavian artery and cranial to the ductus (Fig. 3, bottom).

Also place clamps caudal to the ductus on the aorta and across the base of the ductal origin from the pulmonary artery. Identify the region of hemorrhage and suture with 5-0 or 6-0 nonabsorbable suture on a cardiovascular needle.

16. Subcutaneously tunnel a No. 5 Or 8 Fr. red rubber tube from a small wound made caudal to the skin incision. Place the tube in the chest through the thoracotomy. Close the chest in a routine manner, incorporating the temporary chest tube.
17. After evacuating the chest of air and fluid, remove the temporary chest tube. If hemorrhage or inadvertent lung injury occurs, place a standard indwelling chest tube (see sec. 1, ch. 3).

POSTOPERATIVE CARE AND COMPLICATIONS
Short-Term

KEY POINT ▶ Close monitoring in an intensive care setting is of the utmost importance.

■ Monitor the following parameters/signs:
  • Mucous membrane color, capillary refill time, respiratory rate
  • Dyspnea, urine output
  • Recovery of body temperature, pulse, chest auscultation
■ Analgesic therapy is indicated in animals with pain (see sec. 6, ch. 25, for discussion of post-thoracotomy analgesics).
■ Some surgeons treat routinely with furosemide (1–2 mg/kg) during the preoperative and immediate postoperative periods. This may be guided by the preoperative status, course of surgery, patient size, and operative fluid balance. If preoperative medical management was instituted, continue it postoperatively until clinical signs resolve.
■ Perform frequent intermittent evacuation of the chest (e.g., q2h) if a tube was left in place. Remove the chest tube when negative pressure is achieved or danger of hemorrhage has subsided.
■ Limit fluid therapy but maintain a sterile intravenous catheter for 24 hours.
■ Auscultate the heart postoperatively for persistent murmur. A systolic murmur of mitral insufficiency, caused by left ventricular dilation, may be present. There should be no diastolic murmur if ligation is successful.

Long-Term

■ Reevaluate heart sounds at 2 weeks when sutures are removed, at 6 months, and then yearly thereafter to detect the uncommon occurrence of recanalization. The murmur of mitral regurgitation may disappear in days or weeks following ligation.
■ PDA ligation has excellent long-term results if ligation is complete.
■ Recanalization of the PDA occurs rarely (1–2% of cases) and is treated by religation.

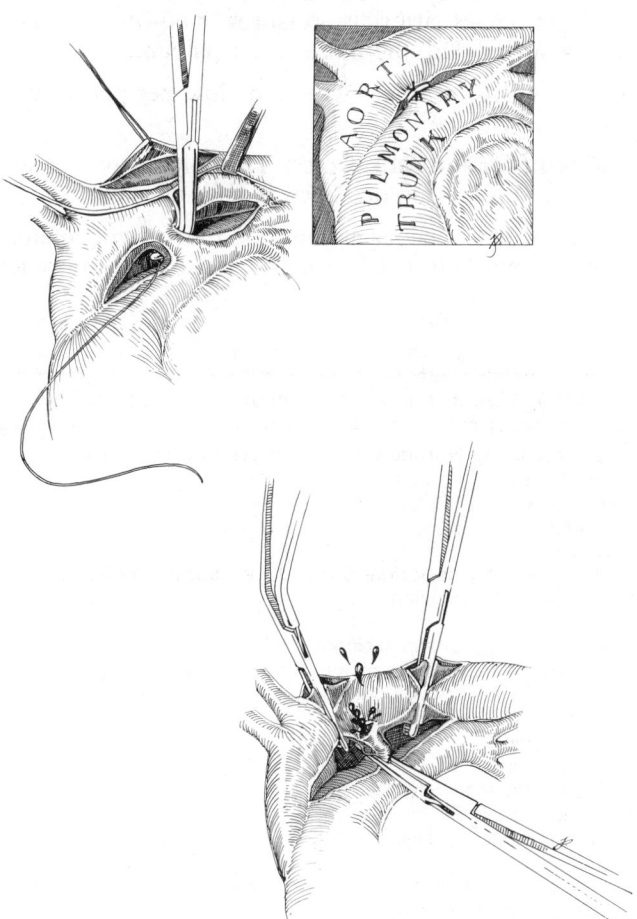

Figure 3. Top initial suture placement for double ligation of the ductus. Bottom, procedure for alleviating ductus rupture.

14 Shock

Eric R. Schertel

KEY POINT ▶ Shock is the clinical state resulting from an inadequate supply of oxygen to the tissue or an inability of the tissues to utilize oxygen properly.

Shock involves numerous physiologic disturbances and pathologic changes that affect multiple organ systems in different ways. Veterinarians often are alerted to the presence of shock in their patients by the physical findings of depressed mentation, pale mucous membranes, tachycardia, and weak pulse pressure. These clinical signs are the manifestations of a complex process and do not represent the full extent of the problem. The objective of this chapter is to provide a simplified approach to the diagnosis, monitoring and treatment of shock. Information on the various manifestations, mechanisms, and temporal patterns of shock is not provided, but is considered important to appropriate and successful therapy. Therapy for shock caused by acute heart failure is discussed in sec. 6, ch. 6. See appropriate chapters for discussion of specific diseases that can cause shock.

ETIOLOGY AND CLASSIFICATION

Shock generally is classified by etiology because each cause of shock may produce distinct primary and secondary pathophysiologic changes and temporal patterns. Shock etiologies can be organized into those forms that result from:

- An abnormality or inadequacy of the vehicle of oxygen transport (blood)
- An abnormality of the transport system (cardiovascular system)

Hypovolemia and hypoxemia (anemic, hypoxic) are examples of the first category (Table 1). Diseases that disrupt the cardiovascular system and its control mechanisms (circulatory control mechanisms) also cause shock.

- The three important circulatory control mechanisms regulate:
- Blood pressure and blood flow distribution
- Blood volume distribution
- Cardiac function

Shock may develop from a disruption of one or more of these systems.

- Sepsis is an example of a condition in which shock is caused by a loss of control of blood flow distribution.

- Endotoxemia and gastric dilation-volvulus also cause shock by interfering with the distribution of blood volume, but via different mechanisms.
- Heart failure creates shock due to inadequate cardiac function.

CLINICAL SIGNS

Mental Attitude. Depressed mentation often is the most apparent physical finding. This parameter is subjective and may be complicated by head injury.

- *Causes:* Decreased cerebral blood flow and oxygen delivery, circulating toxins, or head injury.

Arterial Pulse Pressure. A weak pulse is common but not necessary for shock to exist. The pulse feels weak at mean arterial pressures <60–70 mm Hg. Below 40 mm Hg, the pulse is not palpable.

- *Causes:* Low cardiac output or low peripheral vascular resistance.

Mucous Membrane Color. The color may be pale, gray (muddy), cyanotic, brick-red, or normal.

- *Causes:* Pale mucous membranes reflect hypovolemia or anemia. Gray or cyanotic mucous membranes

---

TABLE 1. Classification and Common Etiologies of Shock

Shock Involving Normal Circulatory Control Mechanisms
Hypovolemia
Hypoxemia
  Anemia
  Hypoxia
Shock Involving Abnormal Circulatory Control Mechanisms
Blood flow maldistribution
  Sepsis
  Trauma—surgical and accidental
Blood volume maldistribution
  Endotoxemia
  Anesthesia
  Neurogenic
  Anaphylactic
  Gastric dilatation-volvulus
Impaired Cardiac Function
  Systolic functional failure
    Cardiomyopathy
    Valvular heart disease
    Myocardial ischemia
    Myocardial contusion
    Arrhythmias
  Diastolic functional failure
    Pericardial disease—tamponade
    Myocardial disease—decreased diastolic compliance

generally indicate severe cardiovascular compromise or arterial hypoxemia. Brick-red mucous membranes are common in septic shock. Mucous membrane color may be normal.

Body/Extremity Temperature. Hypothermia (<99°C) and cold extremities are common. Patients that are septic may be hyperthermic (<130°C) with warm extremities.

■ *Causes:* Decreased cardiac output, oxygen delivery, and ambient temperature. Cold extremities result from severe vasoconstriction. Hyperthermia results from the increased metabolic rate that commonly accompanies sepsis. Warm extremities reflect peripheral vasodilatation.

Capillary Refill Time. Capillary refill time typically is prolonged (>2 seconds), but may be normal.

■ *Causes:* Prolonged capillary refill time reflects hypovolemia and poor peripheral blood flow.

Heart Rate. Heart rate is commonly elevated; >140 beats per minute (bpm) in large-breed dogs, >160 bpm in small-breed dogs, and >180 bpm in cats. Begin monitoring with electrocardiography (ECG) if an irregular rhythm is detected.

■ *Causes:* Hypotension, hypovolemia, pain, stress, and fever may cause tachycardia. Irregular rapid heart rhythms result from ventricular tachycardia and atrial tachyarrhythmias, including atrial fibrillation (see sec. 6, ch. 4).

Respiratory Rate. Increased respiratory rate (tachypnea) is common, but may be due to excitement or fever.

■ *Causes:* Hypoxemia, metabolic acidosis, pain, fever, and excitement.

Urine Output. Urine output is decreased (normal = 1.2 ml/kg/h).

■ *Causes:* Urine formation virtually ceases when mean arterial pressure falls <60 mm Hg. Blood pressure may be normal in mild to moderate hypovolemia.

MONITORING AND TREATMENT
Goals

The goals of management of the shock patient are to optimize the physical and functional characteristics of the cardiovascular system. These characteristics are blood volume, cardiac output, arterial blood pressure, and oxygen delivery. Employ monitoring techniques that provide accurate information about these characteristics.

Cardiac output, arterial blood pressure, and oxygen delivery are dependent on blood volume. When blood volume is expanded these other parameters commonly return to normal.

KEY POINT ▶ Blood volume is the most important parameter to optimize and monitor in shock patients.

Monitoring
Blood Volume

■ Physical signs and findings do not accurately reflect blood volume.
■ Central venous pressure (CVP) is the simplest measurement that reflects blood volume. It may be obtained via a jugular catheter positioned so that its tip is within the thorax (see sec. 1, ch. 3). CVP is equivalent to right atrial pressure and reflects the function of the systemic circulation and the right heart (Fig. 1).
■ CVP is easily measured by a water manometer attached to the jugular catheter (see sec. 1, ch. 3).
■ Normal CVP ranges from 0 to 5 cm H_2O. In shock, CVP usually is −3 to 2 cm H_2O but may be as low as −5 cm H_2O. The goal of fluid therapy in shock is to optimize blood volume by administering fluid in an amount that increases CVP to 5–12 cm H_2O.
■ Plasma proteins, particularly albumin, maintain plasma volume. Assess total plasma proteins prior to fluid therapy and frequently during treatment to ensure that values remain above 4.0 gm/dl (albumin >1.5 gm/dl).

Arterial Pressure

■ Digital palpation may be used to assess mean arterial pressure (MAP). Strong pulse pressure usually reflects an MAP of >70 mm Hg. A weak pulse is detected when MAP is <70 mm Hg. When MAP is <40 mm Hg, the pulse is difficult or impossible to palpate.
■ Arterial pressure also may be assessed using Doppler and oscillometric methods. These techniques are noninvasive and accurate, except when arterial pressure is low.

Cardiac Output

■ Capillary refill time, body temperature, and mentation are the physical findings that best reflect cardiac output. However, these are not always accurate.
■ Urine output is a good indicator of cardiac output. When cardiac output is reduced, sympathetic nervous system activity may maintain blood pressure within normal limits but may decrease renal blood flow. Consequently, urine output will be decreased

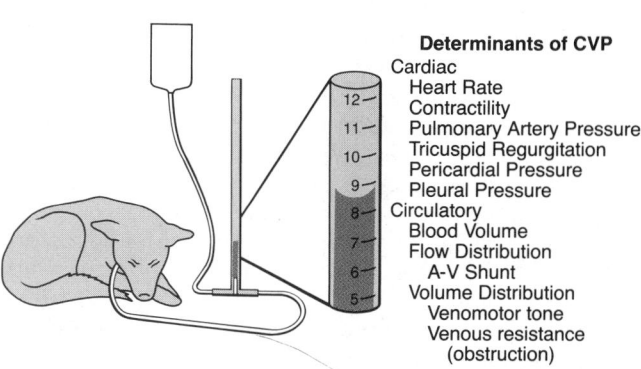

Figure 1. Determinants of central venous pressure (CVP).

(<1 ml/kg/h). However, other causes of reduced urine formation must be considered.

■ Cardiac rhythm influences cardiac output and can be monitored by ECG.

Oxygen Delivery

■ Oxygen delivery is determined by cardiac output as assessed above; pulmonary function, assessed by arterial oxygen pressure (PaO_2); and hemoglobin, assessed by hematocrit.

■ Mucous membrane color, mentation, body temperature, and respiratory rate are the physical findings that best reflect oxygen delivery.

■ Obtain blood samples for hematocrit measurement prior to treatment for shock. Repeat measurements frequently during aggressive fluid therapy (e.g., q1–2h). Maintain hematocrit >20%; in severe shock, it should be >30%.

Treatment

Preliminary Measures

■ Establish an airway and ventilate if necessary. Supplement with 100% oxygen via an endotracheal tube, mask, nasal tube, or tracheal catheter.

■ To evaluate the patient for the cause of shock, perform a physical examination and obtain a history. The time allotted for these efforts depends on the condition of the patient.

■ Place and secure a large-gauge IV catheter, preferably jugular. The catheter should be long enough to reach the thoracic cavity.
  • Jugular catheterization has the advantages of allowing the use of a large-gauge catheter even in small patients, ease of placement, access for blood sampling, rapid fluid administration, CVP measurement, and catheter security. The major disadvantage is that jugular catheters are slightly more expensive.

■ Obtain blood for storage in EDTA and clot tubes. Measure hematocrit and total protein, serum electrolytes, serum creatinine, and blood glucose. Obtain a CBC.

Optimize Blood Volume

■ Initially, administer sodium-rich isotonic crystalloid fluids (e.g., 0.9% NaCl, lactated Ringer's solution) at a rate of 60–90 ml/kg/h (Table 2). To ensure effective plasma volume expansion, maintain the sodium concentration of the isotonic fluid at >130 mEq/liter.

■ Administration of 7% NaCl (hypertonic saline) is an alternative resuscitation regimen. Deliver the initial dosage of 4–6 ml/kg over 5–10 minutes (Table 3). The hypertonic saline may be combined with 6% dextran 70 and given at the same dosage.

■ The goal of the initial rapid rate of fluid administration is to establish a normal arterial pressure and optimize blood volume. An adequate arterial pressure is easily determined by palpation of pulse pressure. Physical signs, including pulse pressure, may

be normal despite continuing tissue hypoxia and less than optimal or unstable blood volume.

■ Blood volume is optimized when CVP is 5–12 cm H_2O.

■ To treat hypoproteinemia, fresh or frozen plasma may be administered at a dosage of 10–20 ml/kg/day.

■ Alternatively, synthetic colloids may be used to treat hypoproteinemia. Those useful in small animal patients include 6% dextran 70 and 6% hetastarch. The dosages are similar to those for plasma (10–20 ml/kg/day) and commonly are divided into 5–10 ml/kg slow IV infusions (10–20 min).

■ Fresh or stored blood may be given to optimize blood volume if the hematocrit and total protein are decreased below acceptable levels. Blood collected from the abdominal or thoracic cavity may be autotransfused if other, more acceptable sources are unavailable. This blood must be free of bacterial and neoplastic contamination and should be administered via a blood administration set (including filter). Autotransfused blood will have decreased platelets, clotting factors, and fibrinogen concentration.

Optimize Blood Flow

■ Cardiac output increases and is often optimized as a result of aggressive volume expansion.

■ If volume expansion has increased the CVP to 5–12 cm H_2O but urine output and other physical signs reflecting cardiac output are not normalized, evaluate cardiac function with ECG.

■ If the ECG is normal, administer a positive inotropic agent. Dobutamine (Dobutrex, Lilly) and dopamine (Intropin, DuPont) are inotropic drugs (see sec. 6, ch. 5) that are commonly used to enhance cardiac function in shock.
  • Dobutamine produces dose-dependent increases in contractility when administered at a dosage of 2–15 μg/kg/min (Fig. 2).
  • Dopamine administered at dosages of 1–3 μg/kg/min improves renal and mesenteric blood flow. At dosages of 3–5 μg/kg/min, dopamine improves contractility and increases cardiac output and peripheral vascular resistance, causing renal and mesenteric arterial vasoconstriction.

■ Cardiac arrhythmias may contribute to low cardiac output. Consider causes of arrhythmias (myocardial hypoxia, myocardial contusion, and electrolyte disturbances) and correct them if possible (see sec. 6, ch. 4). Ventricular arrhythmias are the most common and may be treated with lidocaine administered IV at 1–2 mg/kg or as a continuous infusion of 25–75 μg/kg/min (see sec. 6, ch. 5).

Optimize Blood Pressure

■ Arterial blood pressure often is returned to normal by fluid therapy.

KEY POINT ▶ When arterial blood pressure is <40 mm Hg (pulse weak or not palpable), increase blood pressure immediately.

TABLE 2. Treatment of Shock

Therapeutic Goal	Therapy	Specific Objectives	Dosage Recommendations

Optimize blood volume	Crystalloids
	  Isotonic
	  Hypertonic
	Colloids
	Whole blood
		CVP 5–12 cm H_2O
		Wedge pressure 7–20 mm Hg
		Total protein >4.0 gm/dl
		Albumin >1.5 gm/dl
		Normal skin turgor
			Isotonic fluids: 0.9% NaCl, LRS:
			  60–90 ml/kg/h to effect
			Hypertonic saline/dextran: 7% NaCl or
			  7% NaCl in 6% dextran 70, 4–6 ml/
			  kg slowly IV
			Whole blood: 20–30 ml/kg
			Plasma: 10–20 ml/kg
			6% Dextran 70: 10–20 ml/kg/day
			6% Hetastarch: 10–20 ml/kg/day

Optimize blood flow	Fluids Inotropic agents	Urine output >1 ml/kg/h CRT < 2 sec Pv_{O_2} > 35 torr Cardiac index 150–200 ml/min/kg	See Optimize Blood Volume Dopamine: 2–10 μg/kg/min Dobutamine: 2–15 μg/kg/min
Optimize oxygen delivery and consumption	Fluids Whole blood Packed red cells O_2 supplementation Mechanical ventilation Respiratory care	Pa_{O_2} > 70 torr Pv_{O_2} > 35 torr Hct > 25 Pink mucous membranes Patient bright, alert, responsive	See Optimize Blood Volume Packed red cells: 10–20 ml/kg FIO_2: 40–100%

Optimize blood pressure	Fluids
	Vasopressors
		Arterial pressure:
		  Systolic, 100–160 mm Hg
		  Mean, 70–120 mm Hg
		  Diastolic, 50–100 mm Hg
		Strong pulse
			See Optimize Blood Volume in text
			Dopamine: 5–10 μg/kg/min IV
			Epinephrine: 0.1–0.3 μg/kg/min IV
			Phenylephrine: 0.01–0.1 μg/kg/min IV
			Methoxamine: 0.2 μg/kg IV

Optimize heart rate/rhythm	Fluids Antiarrhythmics	70–160 bpm Sinus rhythm	See Optimize Blood Volume in text Lidocaine: 1–2 mg/kg bolus, 25–75 μg/kg/min IV Procainamide: 15–20 mg/kg IM
Correct acid-base imbalance	$NaHCO_3$	pH >7.3 and < 7.5	Sodium bicarbonate: 0.5–5.0 mEq/kg IV or mEq = 0.3 × base deficit × kg
Optimize urine output	Fluids	1–2 ml/kg/h urine production	Furosemide: 2–4 mg/kg Mannitol (20%): 1–2 g/kg IV
Control sepsis	Antibiotics Surgery Culture and sensitivity	Negative culture Wound/infection management	Cephalothin: 20 mg/kg IV q6h Ampicillin: 20 mg/kg IV q6h Gentamicin: 2 mg/kg IV q8h
Optimize blood glucose	Glucose Insulin	Blood glucose 60–120 mg/dl	Dextrose 5% in maintenance fluids Dextrose 50%: 0.5–2.0 g/kg/h Insulin (regular): 0.5–2 units/kg q2–6h IV (if hyperglycemic)

Immune/inflammatory
modulation
	Corticosteroids	Same as Therapeutic Goal	Dexamethasone sodium phosphate:
			  1–2 ml/kg IV
			Prednisolone sodium succinate:
			  10–20 mg/kg IV

CVP = central venous pressure; LRS = lactated Ringer's solution; CRT = capillary refill time; Hct = hematocrit; Pv_{O_2} = venous oxygen partial pressure; Pa_{O_2} = arterial oxygen partial pressure; FIO_2 = inspired oxygen fraction.

TABLE 3. Hypertonic Saline and Synthetic Colloid Therapy*

	Sodium Chloride Solutions			Synthetic Colloids	
	3% NaCl	5% NaCl	7% NaCl	6% Dextran 70	6% Hetastarch
Approximate osmolality (mOsm/kg)	1000	1800	2400	N/A	N/A
Maximum dosage range (ml/kg)	20	6–10	4–8	10–20	10–20
Maximum infusion rate (ml/kg/min)	2	1	1	1	1
Available products Manufacturers	3% NaCl Baxter, Kendall McGaw	5% NaCl Baxter, Abbott, Kendall McGaw	7% NaCl Butler	Gentran 70 Baxter	Hespan DuPont

*Indications: hypovolemia, traumatic shock, endotoxemia, septicemia, gastric dilatation-volvulus. Contraindications: dehydration, hypernatremia, hyperosmolality, heart/renal failure.

- Administer epinephrine to increase peripheral vascular resistance and cardiac output until fluid therapy can be initiated and blood volume expanded.
  - The intravenous dosage of epinephrine for cardiac arrest is 0.02–0.2 mg/kg (0.02–0.2 ml/kg of 1:1000 dilution).
  - When the primary problem is severe hypotension, not cardiac arrest, administer epinephrine continuously at a dosage of 0.1–0.3 µg/kg/min (see Fig. 2).
  - Once blood volume is expanded and cardiac output and mean arterial pressure are restored, discontinue epinephrine.
- Use of an abdominal wrap or "belly band" to augment arterial blood pressure and to tamponade abdominal bleeding may be dangerous and is not recommended. Any increase in arterial resistance (arterial pressure) created by an abdominal wrap may be counteracted by obstruction of the vena cava and portal vein and by decreased venous return. Furthermore, the abdominal wrap may compromise respiratory function, exacerbate diaphragmatic hernia, and lead to hypotension when it is removed.
  - Manage uncontrolled intra-abdominal hemorrhage by aggressive fluid replacement, and perform surgical exploration if the condition fails to stabilize.

Optimize Oxygen Delivery

- Optimal oxygen delivery is often attained by aggressive volume replacement.
- Hemodilution or preexisting anemia may limit oxygen delivery. Red blood cell (RBC) replacement (whole blood, packed red cells) is necessary when hematocrit decreases <20%. Whole blood may be administered at a dosage of 20–30 ml/kg and packed RBCs at 10–20 ml/kg (see sec. 3, ch. 1).
- Administration of corticosteroids (e.g., prednisolone sodium succinate, 10–20 mg/kg) prior to transfusion will minimize the risk of severe transfusion reaction and improve the RBC function of stored blood.
- Oxygen supplementation will improve arterial blood oxygen content and may be administered via mask, nasal catheter (see sec. 1, ch. 3), oxygen cage, or transtracheal catheter and is particularly crucial when the patient is anemic.
- In cases of severe lung injury, ventilatory assistance must be provided. This requires anesthetizing the patient and placement of an endotracheal tube. Alternatively, a tracheostomy may be performed.

Correction of Acid-Base and Electrolyte Disturbances

- The metabolic acidosis that results from shock that is mild or of short duration often can be managed effectively by fluid replacement therapy.
- The degree of metabolic acidosis that develops in shock depends on the severity and duration of the oxygen delivery deficit. If blood gas analysis can be performed, the milliequivalent (mEq) dosage of $NaHCO_3$ required to correct the acidosis may be calculated by the following formula:

$$NaHCO_3 \text{ (mEq)} = 0.3 \times \text{body weight (kg)} \times \text{base deficit}$$

- If blood gas analysis is not available, an estimate of the base deficit may be made based on the severity of the shock state and its duration. Mild, moderate, and severe shock may be treated with $NaHCO_3$ dosages of 1.0, 3.0 and 5.0 mEq/kg of body weight, respectively (see sec. 1, ch. 5 for more information on treatment of acidosis).
- Hyperkalemia is the most common serum electrolyte concentration abnormality observed in shock. Hyperkalemia generally responds to aggressive volume replacement, increased urine output, and improvement of metabolic status. Glucose and $NaHCO_3$ infusions facilitate reduction of serum potassium concentration (see sec. 1, ch. 5).
- Hypokalemia often occurs after aggressive volume replacement. Once maintenance fluids are started, they should contain 15–20 mEq/liter of KCl (see sec. 1, ch. 5).

Corticosteroid Therapy

- Corticosteroids may be of benefit in most forms of shock. Administer early in the course of therapy to derive maximum benefits.
- Use water-soluble drugs, including dexamethasone sodium phosphate (Azium-SP, Schering) (1–2 mg/kg) and prednisolone sodium succinate (Solu-Delta-Cortef, Upjohn) (10–20 mg/kg).

Miscellaneous Treatments

- Broad-spectrum antibiotics are indicated in most forms of severe shock, particularly septic shock.
- Surgical management of a septic focus should be performed as soon as cardiorespiratory stability is established.
- Intravenous glucose can provide some of the caloric requirements of the shock patient. Maintenance fluids should contain 5% dextrose. This treatment is helpful over the short term, but supplies only a fraction of the caloric requirements. More complete caloric supplementation may be achieved by administration of 50% dextrose at an hourly dosage of 0.5–2.0 g/kg.

Supplemental Readings

Schertel ER, Tobias TA: Hypertonic fluid therapy. *In* DiBartola SP, ed.: *Fluid Therapy in Small Animal Practice*. Philadelphia: W. B. Saunders, 1992, p 471.

Tobias TA, Schertel ER: Shock: Concepts and management. *In* DiBartola SP, ed.: *Fluid Therapy in Small Animal Practice*. Philadelphia: W. B. Saunders, 1992, p 436.

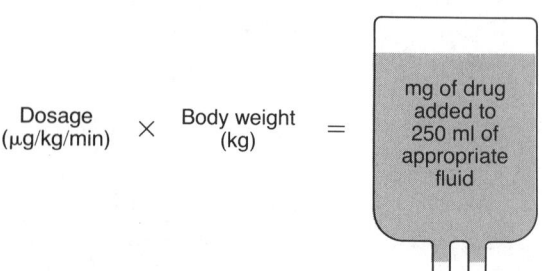

Figure 2. Simplified method of dosage formulation for continuous-infusion drugs. Once formulated, administer at 15 ml/h or 1 drop/4 sec from a 60-drop/ml administration set to achieve desired dosage.

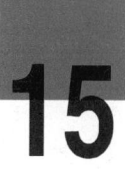15 Cardiopulmonary Cerebral Resuscitation

William W. Muir, III

Resuscitation is the restoration of life after apparent death. Cardiopulmonary resuscitation (CPR) includes therapy specifically oriented toward restoring heart and lung function to normal. Most resuscitative techniques incorporate methods to maximize and maintain cerebral blood flow and have redefined CPR as cardiopulmonary cerebral resuscitation (CPCR). Preparedness and early recognition of the signs of sudden death are the major factors that determine long-term outcome (Tables 1 and 2).

CPCR is divided into three phases:

- Phase 1, basic life support (BLS), consists of establishing an airway (A), breathing (B), and circulatory support (C).
- Phase 2, advanced life support (ALS), incorporates the use of drugs (D), electrocardiography (E), and methods to convert ventricular fibrillation (F) to sinus rhythm.
- Phase 3, prolonged life support (PLS), includes measures that focus on treating the causes of cardiac arrest and deciding whether to continue resuscitative efforts. Gauging (G) (monitoring of patient trends), hypnogenesis (H) (use of sedation, anesthesia, and pain control), utilization of methods to restore cerebral function, and intensive care (I) oriented toward preventing multiorgan failure are also elements of PLS.

BASIC LIFE SUPPORT: AIRWAY, BREATHING, AND CIRCULATION

Airway

KEY POINT ▶ Establishing a patent functional airway is the first and most important step when performing CPCR.

Establishing an Airway

Mouth to Muzzle. Tightly cup hands around the muzzle of small dogs and cats, or place mouth directly over the patient's muzzle. Blow exhaled air into the animal's lungs.

Mouth to Mask. A variety of masks have been developed for use in dogs and cats for the delivery of oxygen or inhaled anesthetics.

Mouth to Endotracheal Tube. The insertion of a cuffed endotracheal tube of appropriate size is facilitated by placing the patient on the sternum, opening the mouth widely, and maximally extending the head and neck. The larynx is visualized and intubation accomplished. A laryngoscope can facilitate intubation.

Tracheotomy. A tracheotomy may be necessary in animals with upper airway obstruction, brachycephalic animals, or in dogs and cats that are successfully resuscitated, regain consciousness and object to oral-tracheal intubation (This procedure is described in sec. 1, ch. 3.)

TABLE 1. Signs and Symptoms of Cardiopulmonary Arrest

Evaluations	Clinical Signs and Observations
Effort, rate, and rhythm of breathing	Dyspnea (abdominal breathing) Gasps (gurgling sounds) Tachypnea Bradypnea Altered patterns of breathing: Cheyne-Stokes Biot's (periodic breathing) Agonal
Heart rate and rhythm	Tachycardia Bradycardia Irregular rhythm
Pulse	Peripheral arterial pulse is difficult or impossible to palpate at ABPs <50–60 mm Hg
Heart sounds	Heart sounds are inaudible at ABPs <50 mm Hg
Bleeding	Absence of bleeding Change in color of blood from red to blue during surgical procedure
Peripheral perfusion	Change in mucous membrane color: Pale or white Blue or cyanotic—5 g/dl of reduced Hb imparts bluish discoloration to mucous membranes regardless of Hb concentration; anemic animals <5 dl Hb) do not demonstrate cyanosis
Pupils	Pupils dilate within 1–2 min after cardiac arrest
Mental state	Altered consciousness Coma

ABPs = arterial blood pressures; Hb = hemoglobin.

TABLE 2. Essential Equipment to Perform CPCR*

1. Assortment of cuffed endotracheal tubes with inside diameter of 2–15 mm
2. Oxygen supply source
   a. Small animal anesthetic machine
   b. Demand valve
   c. Oxygen hose for the delivery of nasal oxygen
   d. Respirator (pressure or volume cycled)
   e. Oxygen chamber
3. Fluid and drug administration equipment
   a. Assortment of intravenous needles and catheters
      (1) Needles—18–25 gauge
      (2) Over-the-needle or through-the-needle catheters—17–22 gauge
   b. Assortment of syringes—1, 3, 6, 12, and 60 ml
   c. Solution administration sets
      (1) Standard solution administration sets (10 drops/ml) for animals over 5 kg
      (2) Mini-drop solution administration sets (60 drops/ml) for animals < 5 kg and to deliver drugs that must be administered by infusion
   d. Venous extension tubing to prolong the time until drug effect, by increasing distance between fluids and patient
   e. Three-way stopcocks and catheter plugs
4. Fluids
   a. Balanced electrolyte solutions to be administered IV in most emergency situations; rate of fluid administration is determined by circumstances (see text for dosages):
      (1) 20 ml/kg/h during hypotension
      (2) 40 ml/kg/h following acute cardiac arrest
      (3) 80 to 90 ml/kg/h following circulatory failure due to hemorrhage
   b. Other solutions
      (1) 5% dextrose in water to supply volume and additional calories and dilute plasma potassium concentration
      (2) Normal saline (0.9% NaCl) to supply volume and dilute plasma potassium concentration
      (3) Colloid solutions (6% dextran 70) to supply volume and oncotic value
      (4) Mannitol (20% Osmotrol) to be used as an osmotic diuretic and as an oxygen free radical scavenger
   c. Special solutions
      (1) Hypertonic saline solutions (usually 3% or 7%) to restore vascular volume; the appropriate quantity of NaCl may be mixed in 6% dextran 70; 7% NaCl in 6% dextran 70 can be administered IV, 4 ml/kg, over 1–2 min.
5. Drugs (see text for dosages)
   a. Anticholinergics (atropine or glycopyrrolate)
   b. Epinephrine (1:1000 and 1:10,000)
   c. Dopamine or dobutamine
   d. Calcium chloride
   e. Lidocaine (2%)
   f. Injectable procainamide
   g. Glucocorticosteroids (dexamethasone, prednisolone sodium succinate)
   h. Furosemide
   i. Mannitol
   j. Diazepam, thiobarbiturates (thiamylal, thiopental), phenytoin
   k. Oxymorphone, other opioids
   l. Doxapram
6. Surgical instruments
   a. Scalpel and several #10 blades
   b. Mosquito and Kelly hemostats
   c. Rib retractors
   d. Thumb forceps
   e. Suture and tissue (Metzenbaum) scissors, needle holders
7. Bandage material (1, 2, and 4 inch)
   a. Sterile 4 × 4 gauze sponges
   b. Cotton bandage
   c. Elastic bandage
   d. Tape
8. Other equipment
   a. Clippers
   b. Leg splints (tongue depressors can be used in animals under 10 kg)
   c. Water circulating heating pad
   d. Electrocardiographic machine
   e. Electrical defibrillator
   f. Aspiration or suction device and tubing
   g. Assortment of suture material

*This material should be kept in one place, preferably on an emergency cart or in a large tool chest.

Proper Endotracheal Tube Placement

Correct placement of the endotracheal tube can be verified by:

- Direct observation of the tube positioned through the larynx (most reliable technique)
- Palpation of the endotracheal tube in the trachea
- The appearance of water vapor on clear endotracheal tubes
- The inability of the animal to vocalize
- Gas exiting the endotracheal tube during exhalation. This sign, which frequently is used clinically, should not be the only method used to ensure proper endotracheal tube placement.

Air or Oxygen Delivery Systems (Fig. 1, *top*)

- *Self-refilling bags* connected to oxygen (Ambu bag) can be used to provide an air or oxygen source during controlled breathing.
- *Demand valves,* which are oxygen-powered manually triggered ventilatory devices, permit both the initiation and termination of ventilation.
- Anesthetic machines are the most readily available source of oxygen in most hospitals.

- Automatic pressure- or volume-cycled ventilators can be used to assist (control volume) or control (control rate and volume) breathing.
- In *translaryngeal or tracheal insufflation* (Fig. 1, *bottom*), an over-the-needle catheter (Surflo, Terumo Medical Corp.) (17–14 gauge) is positioned in the trachea and attached to a three-way stopcock and venous extension tubing and oxygen supply.

Breathing

Use of a ventilator, delivering 50–100% oxygen, to assist or control breathing, must not be delayed. In the meantime, the resuscitator's exhaled air, which contains 16–18% oxygen, is adequate for maintaining PaO_2 values if large tidal volumes are used.

Maximal oxygenation of arterial blood with minimal hemodynamic impairment can be obtained by:

- Providing a source of 100% oxygen
- Proper placement of an endotracheal tube
- Slow (1–2 sec) inflation of the lungs
- Providing adequate (14–20 ml/kg) tidal volume
- Providing adequate (25–30 cm H_2O) but not excessive inspiratory pressure
  - Rapid inflation of the lung (mouth to muzzle) with

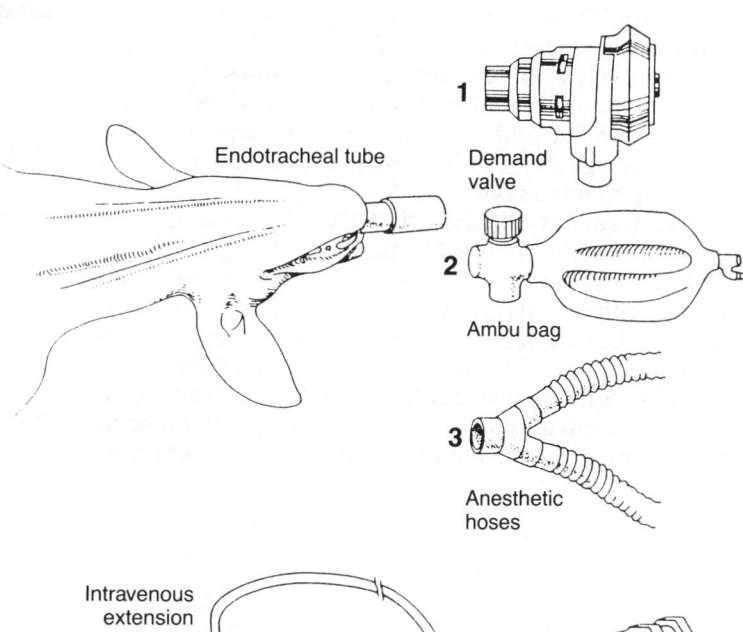

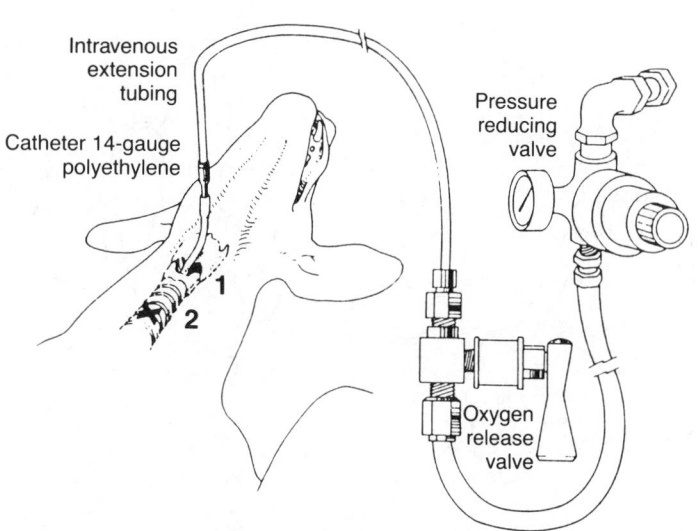

Figure 1. Methods of oxygen administration *(top);* transtracheal oxygen administration *(bottom).* (Modified from Sherding RG: *Medical Emergencies.* New York: Churchill Livingstone, 1985.)

large volumes of gas predisposes to inflation of the stomach with gas, which interferes with lung inflation and may provoke regurgitation and aspiration.

■ Using any of the following drugs for sedation and anesthesia, which frequently are necessary in order to control ventilation in the conscious or semiconscious patient (see sec. 1, ch. 2 for details concerning pharmacologic actions):
  • Diazepam, 0.2–0.5 mg/kg IV
  • Thiamylal or thiopental, 4–8 mg/kg IV
  • Pentobarbital, 2–6 mg/kg IV
  • Isoflurane, 1–2%
■ Providing minimal (1–5 cm H_2O) positive end expiratory pressure (PEEP)

Circulation

The early reestablishment of normal or near-normal hemodynamics, particularly cerebral blood flow, is vital to long-term survival.

KEY POINT ▶ External chest compression is effective in restoring blood flow to the systemic circulation and brain if proper techniques are utilized.

One-Rescuer CPCR with Intermittent Positive Pressure Ventilation (IPPV). One-rescuer chest compression (80–100 compressions/min) can be accomplished by placing the animal in lateral recumbency and manually compressing the thorax from side to side, using the thumb and first two index fingers in animals less than 5 kg and the palm of the hand in larger animals (Fig. 2). Ventilate the lungs following every 15 chest compressions.

Two-Rescuer CPCR with IPPV. The technique for compressing the chest is identical to that in one-rescuer CPCR (see above). Ventilation may be provided intermittently without slowing the rate of chest compression (1 breath for each 15 chest compressions) or simultaneously with chest compression (SVC or simultaneous compression ventilation–CPCR). Take care not to overinflate the lungs (<60 cm H_2O), in order to prevent or minimize pulmonary barotrauma and pneumothorax.

Three-Rescuer CPCR with IPPV and Abdominal Pressure. Applying steady or intermittent abdominal pressure during CPCR or SVC-CPCR may augment carotid arterial pressures, cerebral and myocardial blood flow, and cardiac output.

■ The palm of the hand (third rescuer) may be used to compress the abdomen against the backbone for periods of 5–10 seconds. Repeat this procedure 4 times per minute.
■ Synchronize abdominal compression with chest compression. Apply abdominal compression to the midabdomen during the relaxation phase of chest compression.

ADVANCED LIFE SUPPORT

The primary purpose of advanced life support techniques is to restore adequate spontaneous circulation. Open-chest CPCR is considered an advanced life support technique. Antiarrhythmic, inotropic, and antishock drugs (glucocorticosteroids, free radical scavengers) are frequently used in conjunction with fluid therapy in order to restore normal hemodynamics.

Drug Therapy

Drugs and fluids are preferably administered intravenously (see Table 3 for dosages and side effects; also see sec. 6, ch. 5 for additional details regarding the pharmacologic actions of cardiovascular and antiarrhythmic drugs). Place a large-bore catheter (18–14 gauge) in the cephalic or jugular veins, depending on the size of the patient. Placement of an IV catheter may require a "cutdown" because the veins usually collapse shortly after cardiac arrest (see sec. 1, ch. 3).

Epinephrine

KEY POINT ▶ Epinephrine is the initial drug of choice for the treatment of cardiac arrest regardless of cause (Table 4).

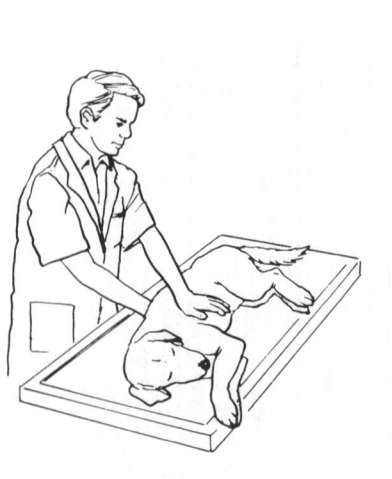 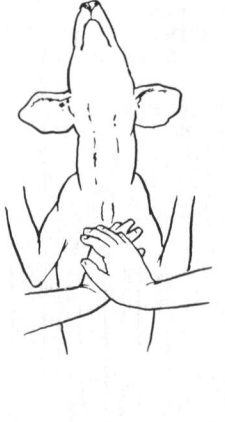 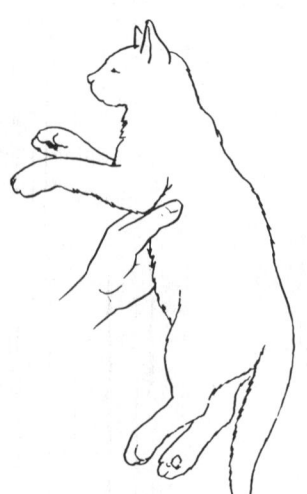

Figure 2. Chest compression in the dog *(left, middle);* chest compression in the cat *(right).*

- Large doses of epinephrine (0.2 mg/kg IV) produce dramatic increases in cerebral blood flow in dogs and cats suffering from cardiac arrest but may induce ventricular arrhythmias and ventricular fibrillation in animals that are in sinus or idioventricular rhythms.
- Initial doses of 0.01 mg/kg IV are adequate in most patients with hypotension or bradycardia and may be adjusted upward according to the patient's response.

Lidocaine

Lidocaine is an appropriate first choice antiarrhythmic for the treatment of ventricular arrhythmias in dogs and cats.

- It is the drug of choice for the treatment of cardiac arrhythmias induced by catecholamines and digitalis glycosides, and cardiac sensitization produced by inhalation anesthetics (halothane) and thiobarbiturates.
- Initial bolus dosages should not exceed 4 mg/kg in dogs and 1.0 mg/kg in cats. A lidocaine infusion of 40–60 μg/kg/min, used to produce a sustained antiarrhythmic effect, is made by mixing 25 ml of 2% lidocaine in 500 ml of lactated Ringer's solution (infuse 0.5 ml/10 kg/min).

Sodium Bicarbonate

Sodium bicarbonate administration helps to combat the development of metabolic acidosis and, more specifically, lactic acidosis produced by anaerobic metabolism secondary to arrested circulation.

- The initial dose of sodium bicarbonate is 1 mEq/kg followed by 0.5 mEq/kg IV every 10 minutes until resuscitative efforts are successful or terminated.

Anticholinergics

Atropine or glycopyrrolate is effective for the treatment of heart block produced by increases in parasympathetic nerve activity.

- The recommended dosage for atropine is 0.01–0.02 mg/kg IV; the dosage for glycopyrrolate is 0.005–0.01 mg/kg IV.

Calcium Chloride

Calcium chloride and calcium gluconate have the potential to increase the force of myocardial contraction and thereby increase cardiac output and peripheral blood flow.

- IV administration of calcium chloride (1 ml/10kg of a 10% solution) is indicated for the treatment of hyperkalemia, hypocalcemia, and inhalation anesthetic or calcium antagonist overdose. Calcium chloride administration is also recommended for electromechanical dissociation.
- The routine use of calcium during the initial phases of CPR cannot be recommended because calcium-mediated cardiac injury (calcium overload) may occur.

Isoproterenol

Isoproterenol is a mixed (β_1, β_2) beta-adrenoceptor agonist that produces marked increases in heart rate and the force of cardiac contraction. Concurrent vasodilation makes it a poor drug for CPCR.

- Isoproterenol is effective (5 μg/kg IV; 0.05–1 μg/kg/min) in some cases of bradycardia (e.g., third-degree atrioventricular block).

Procainamide

Procainamide is a membrane-stabilizing antiarrhythmic drug used for acute therapy of both supraventricular and ventricular arrhythmias (see Table 4).

- Dosages range from 6–20 mg/kg IV slowly, followed by an infusion of 40–60 μg/kg/min if necessary. Procainamide can also be administered IM, at a dose of 10–20 mg/kg.

Parenteral Fluids

The administration of fluids is mandatory following cardiac arrest from any cause in order to treat the associated vasodilation (relative hypovolemia) and hypotension and to establish a diuresis. The basic principles of IV administration of drugs described previously also apply to parenteral fluid administration.

Crystalloids

- Approximately 10–15 ml/kg of crystalloids (e.g., lactated Ringer's solution) are needed to reverse the relative blood loss due to venous pooling and vasodilation caused by cardiac arrest.
- Blood loss should be replaced by at least three times as much crystalloid and guided by changes in the packed cell volume (PCV), total protein concentration, and central venous pressure when appropriate.

Colloids

Colloids (e.g., 6% dextran 70 [Gentran], Travenol) provide colloid osmotic pressure benefits and produce marked improvement in cardiac output and arterial blood pressure while helping to prevent blood sludging and capillary microembolization.

- Colloids are relatively confined to the intravascular volume and are used to replace blood loss in a ratio of 1:1 (thereby producing less hemodilution than crystalloids). Otherwise, colloids can be administered up to 10ml/kg IV to a total of 20 ml/kg.

Hypertonic Saline

- Hypertonic sodium chloride solutions (3% and 7%) are extremely effective as an adjunctive and temporary replacement fluid for increasing cardiac output and arterial blood pressure and restoring peripheral perfusion in hemorrhaging dogs and cats.
- The effects of hypertonic saline solutions can be prolonged by mixing them with 6% dextran 70

TABLE 3. Therapeutic Management of Problems Associated with Cardiac Arrest

Problem	Treatment	Trade Name or Device (Manufacturer)	Dosage	Side Effects or Contraindications
Hypovolemia Fluid loss	Crystalloid Hypertonic saline (7%)	Lactated Ringer's solution	50–90 ml/kg/hr IV 4 ml/kg IV	Hypervolemia, pulmonary edema, hypoproteinemia Hypokalemia, hypernatremia, acidosis, arrhythmias
Plasma loss	Colloid expander	Gentran 40 (Travenol)	20–40 ml/kg IV	Hypervolemia, pulmonary edema, allergic reactions
Blood loss	Whole blood		10–40 ml/kg IV	Hypervolemia, allergic reactions
Hypotension	See Hypovolemia Phenylephrine	Neo-Synephrine (Winthrop)	10–50 μg/kg IV	Hypertension, tachycardia, arrhythmias
	Epinephrine	Adrenalin (Parke-Davis)	3–5 μg/kg IV	
	Dopamine Dobutamine	Intropin (Arnar Stone) Dobutrex (Lilly)	3–10 μg/kg/min IV 3–10 μg/kg/min IV	
Cardiac arrhythmias Bradycardia	Atropine Glycopyrrolate	Atropine (Elkins-Sinn) Robinul (Robins)	0.01–0.02 mg/kg IV 0.005–0.01 mg/kg IV	Tachycardia Tachycardia
Tachycardia Atrial arrhythmias	Propranolol Quinidine	Inderal (Ayerst) Quinidine gluconate (Lilly)	0.05–0.01 mg/kg IV 4–8 mg/kg/10 min IV	Bradycardia, cardiac failure Hypotension
	Diltiazem	Cardiazem	1–3 mg/kg PO q8h; 5–10 μg/kg/min	Hypotension, AV block
Ventricular arrhythmias	Lidocaine	Xylocaine (Astra)	2–4 mg/kg IV dogs; 1 mg/ kg IV cats 40–60 μg/kg/min IV	CNS excitement
	Procainamide	Pronestyl (Squibb)	6–20 mg/kg/10 min IV	Hypotension
Acute heart failure	Calcium chloride Epinephrine Dopamine Dobutamine	Adrenalin (Parke-Davis) Intropin (Arnar Stone) Dobutrex (Lilly)	1 ml 10% /10 kg IV 3–5 μg/kg IV 3–10 μg/kg/min IV 3–10 μg/kg/min IV	Hypertension, tachycardia, cardiac arrhythmias
Respiratory failure Hypoxia	O₂, nasal catheter; oxygen cage Ventilation		2–4 liters/min Tidal volume = 14 ml/kg	Decreased venous return, respiratory alkalosis
Hypercarbia	Doxapram Ventilation	Dopram V (Robins)	1.0–2.0 mg/kg Tidal volume = 14 ml/kg	CNS excitement Decreased venous return, respiratory alkalosis
Dyspnea	Tracheostomy Chest tubes Ventilation	Heimlich valve	Tidal volume = 14 ml/kg	Decreased venous return, respiratory alkalosis

Sepsis	Surgery		
	Gentamicin	Gentocin (Schering)	1–3 mg/kg q6–8h IM, IV	Muscle weakness, renal toxicity
	Kanamycin	Kantrim (Bristol)	10 mg/kg q6h IM	Muscle weakness, renal toxicity
	Ampicillin	Omnipen (Wyeth)	10 mg/kg q6h IV	Phlebitis, myositis
	Cephalothin	Keflin	20–30 mg/kg IV q6h	
Metabolic acidosis	Sodium lactate*		Bicarbonate dose = base deficit × 0.3 × wt (kg) or 0.5 mEq/kg/10 min IV to effect	Metabolic alkalosis, hyperosmolarity, CSF acidosis
	Sodium acetate*			hyperkalemia, hypocalcemia
	Sodium bicarbonate			
Hyperkalemia	Sodium bicarbonate		0.5–2.0 mg/kg IV	As above
	NaCl 0.9% solution		10–40 ml/kg/h IV	Hypervolemia, hypoproteinemia
	Calcium gluconate		0.5 ml/kg of 10% solution IV	Tachycardia
	Hyperventilation			Decreased venous return, respiratory alkalosis
Hypoglycemia	Dextrose 50%		1–2 ml/kg IV 0.5–1.0 g/kg/h, 10% glucose	Hyperosmolarity
Renal ischemia	Fluids	Lactated Ringer's solution	10–40 ml/kg/h IV	Hypervolemia, hypoproteinemia, pulmonary edema
	Mannitol 20%	Osmitrol (Travenol)	0.5–2.0 g/kg IV	Hyperosmolality
	Furosemide	Lasix (Hoechst)	1.0–2.0 mg/kg IM, IV	Decreased cardiac output
Hypothermia (<36°C)	Fluids	Lactated Ringer's solution	10–40 ml/kg/h, warmed to 37°C	Hypervolemia, hypoproteinemia, pulmonary edema
	H₂O-filled heating pad		Warmed slowly to 38°C	
Disseminated intravascular coagulation	Correct hypotension	Lactated Ringer's solution	10–40 ml/kg/h IV	Hypervolemia, hypoproteinemia, pulmonary edema
	Correct hypoxemia	Nasal catheter Ventilation	2–4 liters/min Tidal volume = 14 ml/kg	Decreased venous return, respiratory alkalosis
	Correct acidosis	Sodium bicarbonate (Lipomed)	0.5–1.0 mg/kg IV	
	Heparin		Dog: 500 units/kg SC q8h for 24h Cat: 250–400 units/kg SC q8h for 24h	Bleeding
Cellular ischemia	Fluids	Lactated Ringer's solution	10–40 ml/kg/h IV	Hypervolemia, hypoproteinemia, pulmonary edema
	Mannitol	Osmitrol	0.5–2.0 g/kg IV	
	Oxygen	Nasal catheter	2–4 liters/min	
	Dexamethasone sodium phosphate	Azium (Schering)	4–6 mg/kg IV	
	Prednisolone sodium succinate	Solu-Delta-Cortef (Upjohn)	>10 mg/kg IV	

Hypothermia (<36°C) — Tidal volume = 14 ml/kg

Modified from: Muir WW, Bonagura JD: Cardiovascular emergencies. *In* Sherding RG, ed.: *Medical Emergencies*. New York: Churchill-Livingstone, 1985, p. 52.
*Questionable efficacy during severe low-flow states.

TABLE 4. Emergency Doses of Epinephrine

Route	Dose	Comments
Intravenous		
Arrest/		
fibrillation	0.2 mg/kg	Dose determined by heart
Bradycardia	0.01–0.1 mg/kg	rate. Begin at low dose
Intracardiac	0.05–0.1 mg/kg	Potentially arrhythmogenic
Intratracheal	0.05 mg/kg	Ineffective during cardiac arrest/fibrillation

(Gentran, Travenol). A 3% or 7% solution of hypertonic saline in 6% dextran 70 is produced by adding 30 mg or 70 mg of sodium chloride to each ml of 6% dextran 70, respectively. The doses of 3% or 7% sodium chloride are 8 and 4 ml/kg IV, respectively.

Blood

- Blood replacement therapy is indicated whenever hemorrhage is severe (> 25–30 ml/kg), the PCV is < 20% or the total protein is < 2.5 g/dl.
- Like colloids, blood replacement therapy is administered in a ratio of 1:1 with blood loss.

Electrocardiography

Electrocardiography (ECG) can be used to distinguish between asystole, ventricular fibrillation, and electromechanical dissociation, which helps to determine initial therapy (Fig. 3; Table 5).

Treatment of Ventricular Fibrillation

KEY POINT ▶ The only good method for treating ventricular fibrillation is by electrical defibrillation.

- Both external and internal techniques for converting ventricular fibrillation to sinus rhythm are highly successful in an otherwise healthy patient (Table 6).
- The prior administration of epinephrine and lidocaine help to reduce the energy required for defibrillation and the possibility of post-defibrillation ventricular arrhythmias, respectively.
- Use extreme care to avoid electrical injury to personnel.

Open-Chest Cardiac Massage

Open chest cardiac massage may be the only way to provide adequate systemic blood flow in some patients (barrel-chested dogs, and animals with penetrating chest trauma, broken ribs, pneumothorax, hemotho-

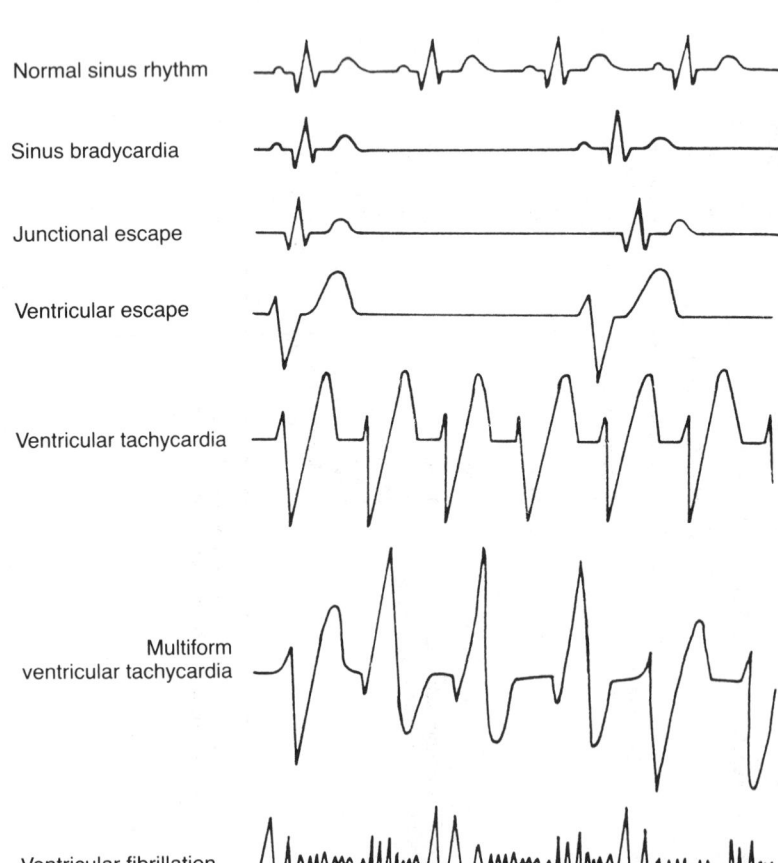

Normal sinus rhythm

Sinus bradycardia

Junctional escape

Ventricular escape

Ventricular tachycardia

Multiform ventricular tachycardia

Ventricular fibrillation

Ventricular arrest

Figure 3. Significant cardiac rhythm patterns during cardiopulmonary cerebral resuscitation. (From Muir WW, and Bonagura J: Cardiac emergencies. *In* Sherding R, ed.: *Medical Emergencies.* New York: Churchill Livingstone, 1985, pp 37–93.)

TABLE 5. Distinguishing Characteristics of Several Types of Cardiac Failure and Arrest

Cause	Peripheral Pulse	Auscultation of Heart Sounds	ECG	Visual Observation
Ventricular tachycardia	Weak, rapid pulse deficit	Muffled; may be variable intensity	Wide QRS-T complexes; absence of P-QRS relationship (see Fig. 3)	Disorganized, rapidly beating heart
Ventricular fibrillation	None	None	Absence of QRS-T complexes; fibrillation waves (see Fig. 3)	Fine to coarse ripping of ventricular myocardium
Bradycardia	Slow; may be irregular	Normal or muffled; infrequent	Infrequent, or irregular P-QRS-T complexes; junctional or ventricular escape complexes (see Fig. 3)	Infrequent coordinated ventricular contractions
Ventricular asystole	None	None	Absence of QRS-T complexes; straight-line ECG	No cardiac improvement
Electromechanical dissociation	None	None	Normal P-QRS-T complexes	Feeble or absent cardiac contractions

Modified from Muir WW, Bonagura JD: Cardiovascular emergencies. *In* Sherding RG, ed.: *Medical Emergencies.* New York: Churchill-Livingstone, 1985, p 80.

rax, pericardial effusion, or thoracic masses) and should be considered early (within the first 3–5 minutes) if chest compressions are ineffective.

Technique

1. After minimal skin preparation, make a skin incision at the fourth or fifth intercostal space on the left side.
2. Make a small hole in the pericardium near the apex of the heart and reflect the pericardium dorsally.

TABLE 6. Defibrillation Techniques

Ventricular Tachycardia with Severe Hypotension or Ventricular Fibrillation
Direct-current fibrillators: 0.5–2.0 ws/kg internal; 5–10 ws/kg external
  Small patient (<7 kg):
    5–15 ws internal
    50–100 ws external
  Large patient (>10 kg):
    20–80 ws internal
    100–400 ws external
Alternating-current defibrillators
  Small patient:
    30–50 V internal
    50–100 V external
  Large patient:
    50–100 V internal
    150–250 V external

Unresponsive Ventricular Fibrillation
Evaluate ventilation
Evaluate chest or cardiac compression
Repeat epinephrine (calcium chloride administration if electromechanical dissociation)
Repeat sodium bicarbonate administration
Administer lidocaine
Repeat electrical defibrillation (direct current; see above)

Modified from Muir WW, Bonagura JD: Cardiovascular emergencies. *In* Sherding RG, ed.: *Medical Emergencies.* New York: Churchill Livingstone, 1985, p. 90.
WS = watt seconds; V = volts.

3. Compress the heart between the thumb and forefingers or in the palm of the hand, concentrating effort on the left ventricle. The usual compression rate is 80–100/minute.

PROLONGED LIFE SUPPORT

Prolonged life support incorporates all the medical and surgical methods necessary to prevent central nervous system and multiple organ failure following cardiac arrest (Table 7).

Drug Therapy
Catecholamines

Dopamine and dobutamine produce dose-dependent increases in cardiac output and peripheral perfusion.

■ Initial dosages for continuous IV infusion are 1–5 μg/kg/min but may be increased to 15–20 μg/kg/min, depending on the patient's response.

Diuretics

Furosemide and Bumetanide. These highly potent loop diuretics are used to treat edema (e.g., pulmonary edema), promote diuresis, and "mobilize fluids."

■ The IV dose of furosemide is 1–2 mg/kg.
■ The dose for bumetanide is 0.005–0.01 mg/kg IV, depending on the desired effect.

Mannitol. Mannitol (osmotherapy) produces an osmotic gradient that moves water from the extravascular fluid compartment and the brain into the intravascular space. It can be used routinely or if the period of cardiac arrest exceeds 3 minutes.

■ The recommended dose for mannitol is 0.5–1.0 mg/kg IV. This dose can be repeated at approximately 2–4 hours.

TABLE 7. Brain-Oriented Resuscitation

Problem	Therapy/Drug	Dose
Hypotension	Lactated Ringer's solution	35–70 ml/kg IV
	6% Dextran 70	10 ml/kg IV
	7% NaCl	5 ml/kg IV
	7% NaCl in 6% Dextran 70	5 ml/kg IV
	Dopamine	2–5 μg/kg/min IV
	Dobutamine	1–3 μg/kg/min IV
Seizures	Pentobarbital	1–3 mg/kg IV
	Thiamylal, thiopental	1–3 mg/kg IV
	Phenytoin	10–20 mg/kg IV
	Diazepam	0.1–0.2 mg/kg IV
Cerebral edema or increased ICP	Hyperventilation	$Paco_2$ 25–35 mm Hg
	Oxygenation	Pao_2 60 mm Hg
	Furosemide	1 mg/kg IV
	Mannitol	0.5–1.0 g/kg IV
	Methylprednisolone sodium succinate	5–10 mg/kg IV
Cerebral vasospasm	Nimodipine	10 μg/kg IV
		10 μg/kg/min
	Diltiazem	2–3 mg/kg q8h PO
Toxic cellular products*	Desferoxamine	25–50 mg/kg IV slowly
	Superoxide dismutase	5–50 mg SC
	Dimethyl sulfoxide	250–500 mg/kg IV
	Allopurinol	10 mg/kg PO

Modified from Muir WW: Brain hypoperfusion post-resuscitation. Vet Clin North Am [Small Anim Prac] 19:1151, 1989.
*These therapies await clinical verification of efficacy.

Glucocorticosteroids

Therapy with dexamethasone or prednisolone sodium succinate has multiple benefits. These drugs can:

- Stabilize lysosomal membranes
- Reduce and prevent histamine release
- Protect against increases in capillary membrane permeability
- Cause vasodilation and inhibit phospholipase A_2 breakdown of arachidonic acid to prostaglandins and leukotrienes.
- Dosages are 3–5 mg/kg of dexamethasone (Azium, Schering) and 10–20 mg/kg for prednisolone sodium succinate (Solu-Delta-Cortef, Upjohn).

Calcium Entry Blockers

Calcium entry blockers, or calcium antagonists, are potentially beneficial in preventing reperfusion and reoxygenation injury, thereby limiting the detrimental effects of platelet aggregation, and the vasoactive and membrane damaging effects of prostaglandins and leukotrienes and other post-insult necrotizing cascades.

- Experimentally, nimodipine has been administered at a dose of 10 μg/kg IV, followed by an infusion of 1 μg/kg/min.
- Diltiazem is available only for oral use and is administered in doses of 1–3 mg/kg/q8h PO or 5–10 μg/kg/min for 10 minutes.
- Calcium solutions (chloride, gluconate) can be used to antagonize the negative inotropic actions of any of the calcium entry blockers.

Iron Chelators

Deferoxamine, a selective chelator of ferric iron, is potentially useful in preventing the deleterious effects of increases in intracellular free iron concentration.

- Doses of 5–15 mg/kg IV, IM, or SQ have been used in experimental studies.

Free Radical Scavengers

Dimethyl sulfoxide (DMSO) (250–500 mg/kg, IV) allopurinol (10 mg/kg, PO), and tromethamine (0.5–1.0 mg/kg, IV) are experimental drugs potentially useful as oxygen-free radical scavengers. Mannitol (see previous discussion) is also an oxygen free radial scavenger.

Heparinization

The administration of 100 IU/kg of heparin is of questionable value in the post-arrest period (once hemorrhage has been controlled); it may limit the clotting cascade and microcirculatory plugging.

Sedation

- Dosages of pentobarbital of 1–3 mg/kg IV are adequate to reduce cerebral oxygen requirements and prevent seizures in most dogs and cats.
- Phenytoin, 15 mg/kg IV, may be used for the same purpose.
- Diazepam, 0.1–0.3 mg/kg IV, is an excellent alternative to pentobarbital and produces less CNS depression.

Antibiotics

The choice of antibiotics is based on the potential for efficacy (see Table 4).

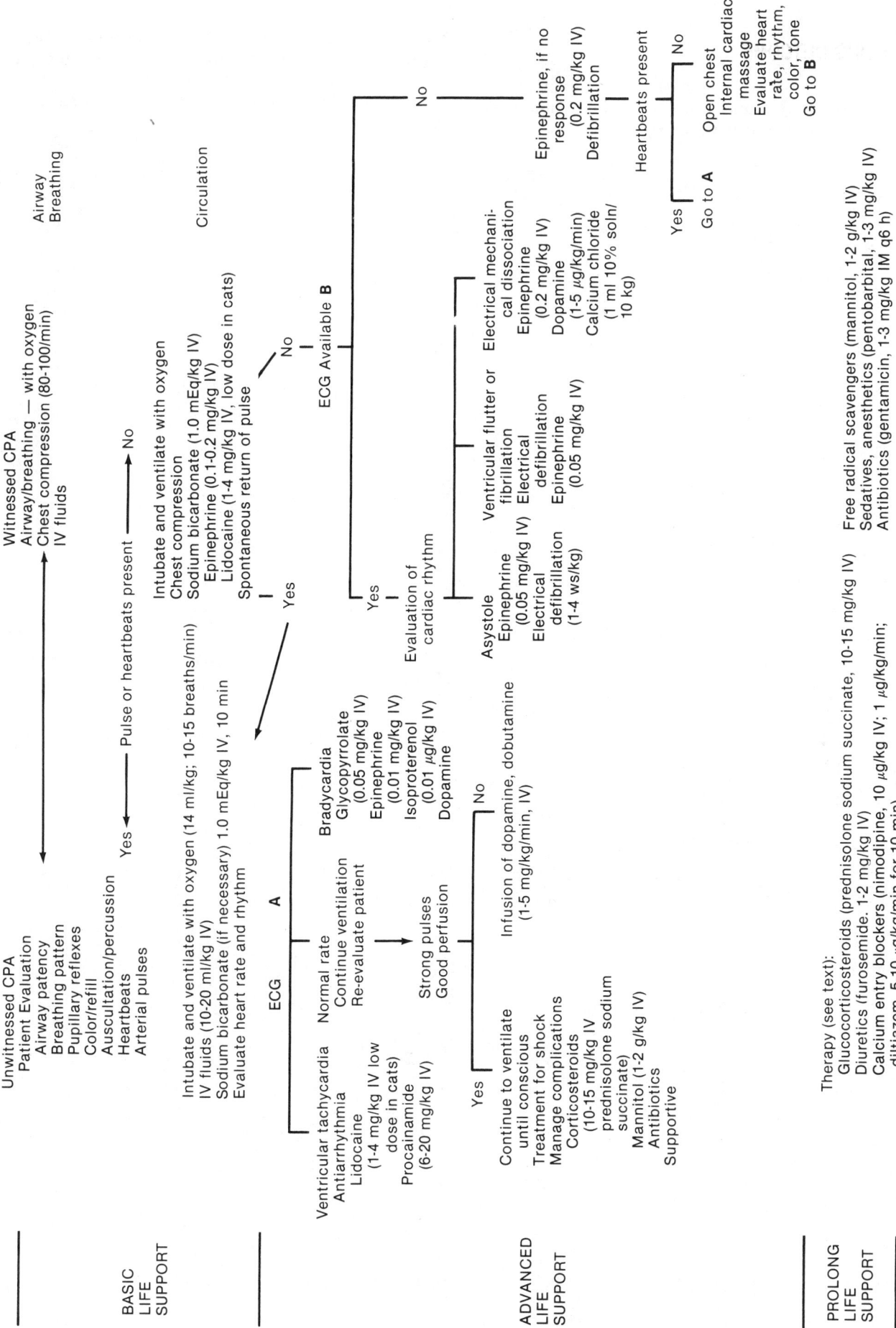

Figure 4. Flow chart for decision-making during cardiopulmonary resuscitation.

523

PREDICTING OUTCOME

■ Rapid recovery of eye (corneal), upper airway (swallowing, sneezing), and chest wall (lung inflation) reflexes are a good prognostic sign.

■ Continued unconsciousness, nonresponsive pupils, and progressive deterioration of reflexes after initial partial recovery are poor prognostic signs.

A simple algorithm for CPCR is illustrated in Figure 4.

16 Diagnostic Methods for Respiratory Disorders

Larry Berkwitt
James Prueter

UPPER RESPIRATORY TRACT DISORDERS

Nasal Cavity Disorders

Sneezing and nasal discharge are the principal clinical problems associated with nasal cavity and sinus diseases.

History

When taking the history, include:

- The chronology, progression, and duration of clinical signs, such as sneezing
- Type of nasal discharge
- Site of involvement (unilateral or bilateral)

Sneezing
- Acute paroxysmal sneezing typically is associated with viral rhinitis, nasal foreign body, allergic rhinitis, and trauma.
- Chronic sneezing suggests neoplasia, parasites, prolonged infection or inflammation (e.g., fungal rhinitis), long-term foreign body, and trauma with secondary infection or osteomyelitis.

Nasal Discharge
- Serous discharge typically is associated with foreign body, allergy, and viral infection.
- Mucopurulent and/or serosanguineous discharge typically is associated with viral infections (complicated by), bacterial; mycotic, and parasitic infections; long-term foreign body; neoplasia; and lymphocytic-plasmocytic inflammation.
- Hemorrhagic discharges suggest trauma, neoplasia, coagulopathy, and prolonged infection.
- Foodstuffs in the discharge suggest a communicating congenital defect (cleft palate) and acquired oral nasal fistula.

Duration of Clinical Signs
- Recent onset of acute signs suggests foreign body, viral infection, trauma, and coagulopathy.
- Chronic signs are associated with neoplasia, infection, foreign body, small parasite infection, chronic inflammation, or congenital defect.

Site of Involvement
- Unilateral discharge suggests early neoplasia, foreign body, early infection, dental disease, or trauma.
- Bilateral discharge suggests chronic infection or inflammation, prolonged foreign body with resulting infection/osteomyelitis, prolonged neoplasia, coagulopathy, pneumonia, parasite, allergy, or trauma.

Physical Examination

A complete physical examination includes a thorough evaluation of the oral cavity, mucous membranes, tonsils, hard and soft palate, retropharyngeal area, regional lymph nodes, and teeth. Sedation and/or anesthesia may be required. The use of dental mirrors and a spay hook or an endoscope (in the retroflexed position) for visualization above the soft palate also is often necessary.

- Look for swelling and asymmetry of the face, palate, or eyes (exophthalmos) that might suggest neoplasia, fungal infection, and trauma.
- Identify areas of pain that may identify the primary area of the disorder.
- Evaluate for loss of patency of one or both nasal passages.
- Note ocular discharge that may be associated with nasal lacrimal duct inflammation and/or obstruction secondary to inflammation or neoplasia.
- Identify cracked, loose, and infected teeth.

Complete Blood Count (CBC), Serum Chemical Profile, and Coagulation Screen

These studies are important when systemic diseases may be an underlying cause of signs. Although clotting disorders can cause epistaxis, it is usually associated with platelet disorders such as immune-mediated thrombocytopenia, von Willebrand's disease, thrombocytopathia, and ehrlichiosis.

Serology

- Serologic tests such as immunodiffusion and enzyme-linked immunosorbent assay (ELISA) for aspergillosis and penicilliosis antibodies and for cryptococcal capsular antigen can be used for diagnosis of mycotic rhinitis. However, false–negative results are common, limiting the usefulness of serology.
- Cytology, culture, and biopsy are more reliable for identifying nasal fungi.

525

Radiography

- General anesthesia is essential for proper positioning and for prevention of motion artifacts.
- Include the following radiographic views:
  - Open-mouth ventrodorsal
  - Intraoral (occlusal)
  - Rostral-caudal frontal skyline
  - Lateral
  - Oblique skull views, particularly if dental arcade problems are suspected.

See section 1, chapter 4.

Nasal Flushing or Cytology

Nasal cytologic evaluation is often of little to no value unless it is performed with aggressive nasal flushing or by rhinoscopic visualization with the animal under anesthesia.

- Perform aggressive nasal flushing with a polypropylene (rigid) male urinary catheter. Measure the length (nares to medial canthus) prior to insertion to avoid penetrating past the cribriform plate.
- Perform intermittent flushing and suctioning via syringe to obtain as much nasal fluid and/or tissue fragments as possible.
- Place gauze sponges in the nasal pharynx to catch any tissue that may be extracted during the flushing procedure.
- Submit samples for culture, cytology, and histopathology.

Rhinoscopy

Rhinoscopic examination under anesthesia allows visualization, biopsy, and procurement of specimens for cytology and culture and sensitivity. Instrumentation can include any of the following:

- Otoscope with bright light source
- Arthroscope or otoscope with outer diameter of 1.9–5 mm
- Bronchoscope with outer diameter of 2.9–5 mm
- Flexible pediatric bronchoscope

Surgery

- Exploratory rhinotomy with removal of a bone flap (see sec. 6, ch. 18) provides complete exposure of the nasal cavity for biopsy, foreign body retrieval, culture, and debridement of diseased tissue.
- Placement of drains can be performed at the time of surgery for treatment of bacterial and/or fungal infections.

Laryngeal Disorders

History

Clinical signs of laryngeal disease often are slowly progressive, and the owner may have noted them for an extended period of time.

- The owner may report hoarseness, progressive changes in voice, or complete loss of voice.
- Noisy respirations characterized by high-pitched inspiratory stridor or by mild, raspy, or fluid-sounding noise are common.
- Choking, gagging, and coughing may be observed, particularly while the animal is eating and/or drinking. This often worsens as the disease progresses.
- Exertional dyspnea, cyanosis, and syncope may be observed in patients with laryngeal obstructions (e.g., laryngeal collapse, paralysis, foreign body, or neoplasia).

Physical Findings

- The most frequent physical findings in laryngeal disease are inspiratory dyspnea and stridor. Auscultation can detect upper respiratory inspiratory stridor ("wheeze") centered over the larynx.
- Palpation of the laryngeal area may detect site of pain, fractures, and subcutaneous emphysema in cases of trauma and asymmetry due to neoplasia, granulomas, laryngitis, or unilateral muscle atrophy.

Laryngoscopy/Bronchoscopy

- Perform direct visualization under *light* planes of anesthesia for evaluation of pharyngeal structures, soft palate, and laryngeal motor function.
- Observe laryngeal (arytenoid) movement during both phases of respiration. Often asymmetry is observed between the left and right arytenoids and vocal folds.
- A bronchoscope allows the best evaluation of the pharynx and the subglottic area for masses, infiltrates (areas of discoloration), granulomas, and polyps.
- Aspiration or brush cytology and endoscopic biopsy may be performed at the time of examination, if appropriate.

Radiography

- A lateral radiograph of the larynx is rarely diagnostic but may demonstrate:
  - Dilated lateral sacculus in cases of paralysis
  - Soft tissue swelling and/or asymmetry in cases of neoplasia and trauma
  - Fractures, dislocations, and subcutaneous air in cases of trauma
  - Elongated soft palate
  - Collapsed or ruptured trachea
- Thoracic radiographs may reveal chronic pulmonary or cardiac disease associated with upper respiratory diseases.

Electromyography

Abnormal electromyographic studies of the laryngeal muscles may be associated with neuromuscular, immune-mediated, and hypothyroid-related laryngeal disorders.

Thyroid Function Testing

Patients with acquired laryngeal paralysis may have subnormal levels of triiodothyronine (T_3) and thyroxine (T_4), as well as abnormal results of TSH stimulation tests (see sec. 4, ch. 1).

Histopathology

Histopathology of any abnormal growth or mass is important in order to differentiate chronic granulomatous disease and neoplasia and may also be useful in a generalized case of polyneuropathy.

Tracheal Disorders (see also sec. 6, ch. 19)

History

- Usually there is a chronic, unproductive, dry "honking" cough with intermittent attacks of dyspnea, particularly elicited on excitement, exercise, drinking, or eating, and with tracheal pressure (e.g., digital pressure or collar).
- Dyspnea and occasionally cyanosis may be demonstrated.
  - Inspiratory dyspnea and stridor develop if the trachea collapses in the cervical area (extrathoracic).
  - Expiratory dyspnea is evident with intrathoracic collapse.
- Both phases of ventilation (although worse on expiration) are abnormal if the entire trachea is involved.

Physical Examination

- Tracheal palpation may demonstrate "sharp" edges or angles of the collapsible margins of the trachea.
- Cardiac examination is important to differentiate tracheal disease from primary heart disease and for evaluation of coexisting chronic heart disease.
- Auscultate the entire respiratory tract to localize primary abnormalities and to differentiate primary parenchymal disease and coexisting bronchopulmonary disease (chronic bronchitis) (see sec. 6, ch. 20).

Radiography

Radiographic examination (ventrodorsal and lateral views) is mandatory for routine evaluation of the cervical and thoracic trachea.

- Be careful in positioning to avoid artifactual deviations of the trachea.
- Attempt to obtain both inspiratory and expiratory films in order to identify an intermittently collapsing trachea or bronchus (this may be difficult or impossible in small-breed dogs).
- Survey radiography has limited sensitivity and specificity for diagnosis.
- Fluoroscopy or tracheoscopy is necessary to evaluate dynamic tracheal functions and intermittent tracheal collapse.

Transtracheal Wash

Perform the tracheal wash (via a sterile endotracheal tube) for cytology, fluid analysis, and microbiologic evaluations to identify initiating or complicating factors that may be important in the treatment regimens. See Bronchopulmonary and Pleural Space Disorders in this chapter for a description of this procedure.

Tracheoscopy

Tracheoscopy can be used to visualize the area of collapse. Extreme care must be taken because of the potential of worsening the collapse by trauma and iatrogenic irritation. Tracheoscopy is best utilized in those cases where there is concern for neoplasia, mass lesion, congenital defects, or concurrent mainstem bronchial collapse. See Bronchoscopy in the Bronchopulmonary section for further discussion of this procedure.

BRONCHOPULMONARY AND PLEURAL SPACE DISORDERS

The diagnosis of diseases of the respiratory tract and pleural space depends on information obtained from a thorough history, a physical examination, and a series of ancillary tests that are well conceived and organized so as to limit the patient's discomfort and stress.

When evaluating the dyspneic patient, use sound clinical judgment in selecting tests that will aid in the diagnosis but will not place the patient in further respiratory distress. Often these patients must be stabilized, based on the physical examination, history, and a dorsoventral thoracic radiograph prior to performing other tests.

History

Coughing, tachypnea, dyspnea, and exercise intolerance are the principal signs associated with bronchopulmonary and pleural disease.

- Determine the patient's signalment, because certain breeds or age groups are more susceptible to particular diseases. For example, small-breed dogs such as the Yorkshire terrier are more susceptible than large-breed dogs to lower respiratory disease secondary to a collapsing trachea.
- Note the client's complaint. Determine if the patient's problem is acute or chronic and if it is improving, stagnant, or progressive.
- When evaluating a cough, determine the time of day of the cough. Cardiac coughs are usually nocturnal, whereas an infectious cough will occur throughout the day.
  - Determine the quality of the cough, such as dry hacking (nonproductive) or moist (productive).
- Note prior medical and travel history.
  - It is imperative to know what medications have been given previously and what medical response was obtained.
  - Consider geographically distributed diseases (e.g., systemic mycoses) in pets that travel or have lived in various locations.
  - Determine the patient's past exposure to other pets (e.g., in a kennel or grooming situation).
- Note the patient's current medical history. Do not overlook routine history questions about water consumption, change in appetite, or elimination, because this information can give insight into the diagnosis of systemic diseases.

Physical Examination

A complete physical examination is imperative.

■ It is important to evaluate each body system, because key diagnostic physical findings may be present and pulmonary complications of heart disease may be evident. If we evaluate only the respiratory system, we may miss important pieces of the puzzle:
  • A remote lesion such as a rectal carcinoma may be the source of metastases that cause dyspnea and abnormal lung sounds.
  • Skin lesions and lymphadenopathy suggest a diagnosis of blastomycosis in a coughing patient.
■ Physical examination of the lower respiratory system and pleural space includes observation, auscultation, and percussion (see also sec. 6, ch. 1).

Observation. Observe the patient's rate and pattern of breathing. Certain diseases cause inspiratory vs. expiratory dyspnea.

■ Note whether the patient is barrel-chested or overweight.
  • Barrel chest may indicate chronic obstructive pulmonary disease. Pickwickian syndrome in overweight animals may account for possible breathing problems.
■ Slow, deep breathing with inspiratory difficulty can be due to obstructive disease.
■ Short, shallow breathing may be associated with restrictive disease.

Pulmonary Auscultation. Pulmonary sounds usually are classified as normal or vesicular, bronchial, or bronchovesicular. Adventitious sounds include crackles (rales), wheezes, stridor, rhonchi, and rubs.

■ As air travels through the lung, it produces vesicular or bronchovesicular sounds. Depending on the medium through which the air travels (e.g., fluid or mucus) or if there are changes in diameter of diseased airways, the sound is modified (e.g., crackles, rhonchi, wheezes).
■ Identification of crackles (small airway/parenchymal disease), rhonchi (airway disease or exudate), and wheezes (airway obstruction) indicates a need for additional diagnostic studies.

Percussion. The lungs and thoracic cavity emit a specific resonance when percussed by striking the second phalanx (p) of the middle finger positioned on the chest with the knuckle joint (p1–p2) fully extended.

■ Dull resonance is associated with increased density (fluid or mass lesion) within the underlying pleural space or lung.
■ Increased resonance (bass drum) is associated with increased air within the pleural space or lung.

As an example of incorporating all parts of the physical examination, consider the patient that has a mammary mass with louder or adventitious lung sounds on auscultation and dull percussion on the left side of the thoracic wall. This patient may have pleural effusion associated with metastatic disease. If dull percussion is present without lung sounds, suspect a consolidating mass lesion.

Thoracic Radiography (See also sec. 6, ch. 17)

Standard radiographic views include inspiratory lateral and ventrodorsal views.

■ To evaluate for metastatic lung disease use a right and left lateral projection with the ventrodorsal view.
■ In a dyspneic animal, a single dorsoventral view is recommended to avoid unnecessary stress and to enable the clinician to initiate stabilizing therapy prior to further evaluation.

Evaluation. Good-quality radiographs are important because excess motion or underexposure may result in false information regarding the pulmonary interstitium. Expiratory films may cause the pulmonary interstitium to have an increased density that can be mistaken as abnormal.

To evaluate thoracic radiographs:

■ Determine the type of radiographic infiltrative pattern present, such as interstitial, alveolar, bronchial, and vascular, or combinations of these.
■ Characterize the location of the infiltrate as localized or diffuse; cranial or caudal; and ventral, dorsal, or hilar.
■ Pleural effusion appears as blunting of the costophrenic angles, pleural fissure lines, and ventral scalloping of the lungs on the lateral projection.

CBC and Serum Chemistry Profile

The CBC may be helpful in evaluation of respiratory disease. For example:

■ Leukocytosis can indicate infection or inflammation.
■ Polycythemia is associated with chronic hypoxemia.
■ Eosinophilia may suggest a parasitic or allergic disease.

No single segment of the standard automated serum chemistry profile is pathognomonic for respiratory system disease; however this study is useful as a baseline to evaluate other organ systems. For example:

■ If a patient has a localized anterior ventral alveolar infiltrate, calcification of the airways, neutrophilic leukocytosis, lymphopenia, and eosinopenia with elevated alkaline phosphatase and cholesterol levels, a tentative diagnosis of bacterial pneumonia secondary to hyperadrenocorticism might be made pending confirmatory tests.

Arterial Blood Gas (ABG) Analysis

The ABG specimen usually is drawn from the femoral artery or dorsal pedal artery or via an indwelling arterial catheter. ABG arterial analysis evaluates the patient's ability to oxygenate arterial blood.

■ In the normal patient breathing room air, the partial pressure of oxygen is >95 mm Hg.
■ When the level is <60 mm Hg, a severe degree of respiratory failure is present.

Serology

Specific serologic evaluations aid in the diagnosis of fungal, rickettsial, and immune-mediated disease as a possible cause of intrathoracic disorders.

Fecal Examination

To establish the diagnosis of parasitic lung disease, evaluate fecal specimens by direct smear, flotation, and sedimentation (available from commercial laboratories) techniques. Fecal sedimentation is important for detection of lungworm larvae (e.g., *filaroides, Aelurostrongylus*) that can be overlooked if flotation is used.

Tracheal Washing

Tracheal washing is a simple inexpensive procedure in which warm sterile saline is placed in the lower respiratory tract and then retrieved. Use this technique to obtain specimens for cytologic and microbiologic evaluation of the lower respiratory tract to aid in the diagnosis of bronchopulmonary disease.

Technique

1. In *dogs,* insert a long through-the-needle catheter (12 or 18 inches) percutaneously through the tracheal rings and then advance it into the lower airway.
   a. In *cats,* use an open-end urinary catheter placed through a sterile endotracheal tube.
2. The catheter may be passed through the cricothyroid membrane; however, it is preferable to place the catheter between the tracheal rings of the proximal trachea.
3. Inject warm sterile saline (6 ml in cats and small dogs; up to 20 ml in large dogs) through the catheter.
4. Retrieve the fluid from the airway by aspiration.
5. Prepare samples of the lavage fluid for cytology, culture, and sensitivity testing.
6. Any fluid remaining in the airways is harmless because it is rapidly absorbed by the pulmonary lymphatics.

Bronchoalveolar Lavage and Bronchoscopy

Bronchoalveolar Lavage. This is an effective method for retrieving diagnostic material from the lung and is particularly useful in alveolar-interstitial lung diseases and in tachypnea/dyspnea when prominent cough is absent.

Technique

1. Advance a flexible fiberoptic bronchoscope into the bronchial tree.
2. Visually locate the diseased area and wedge the bronchoscope within the bronchus.
3. Instill 20–30 ml of warm saline (for a 30 lb dog) through the bronchoscope channel and then retrieve it.

4. Prepare samples for cytology or quantitative cell counts, culture, and sensitivity testing.

Bronchoscopy. Bronchoscopy allows direct visualization of the lower airway to the level of bronchial divisions 3–5, depending on the size of the patient and the length and diameter of the bronchoscope.

- Bronchoscopy is a valuable alternative when no diagnostic material is obtained using the tracheal wash procedure. (This can occur because there is not enough cellular material present within the airway or because the catheter is too short to retrieve any material)
- Diseased areas can be directly visualized, and the exudate or tissue can be removed for cytology or histopathology.
- If there is no visible material present, bronchial brushing or bronchoalveolar lavage can retrieve cells that may aid in a diagnosis.
- Direct biopsy of visible lesions can be performed through the bronchoscope as well as transbronchial lung biopsy described as follows.

Lung Biopsy

When the cause of diffuse lung disease cannot be determined using one of the methods described previously, consider a lung biopsy. Three types of lung biopsy procedures are performed in small animals:

- Fine-needle aspiration
- Bronchoscopy
- Mini-thoracotomy

Fine-Needle Aspiration. The simplest, most cost-effective procedure is fine-needle aspiration. This is usually performed on diffuse or large superficial lesions within the parenchyma or pleural space.

Technique for Fine-Needle Aspiration
1. Clip and surgically prepare the thoracic wall and instill a local anesthetic at the site.
2. Insert a 22-gauge biopsy needle through the chest wall, staying on the cranial aspect of the rib in order to avoid the intercostal vessels.
3. Apply suction to obtain samples for cytologic evaluation and biopsy.

Bronchoscopy. A lung biopsy can be obtained utilizing the bronchoscope. This method is used with deeper, more central lesions and ideally should be performed under fluoroscopy. The biopsy forceps are passed through the bronchial wall into the pulmonary parenchyma.

Mini-Thoracotomy. The third type of biopsy is performed via a mini-thoracotomy.

Technique for Open Lung Biopsy via Mini-Thoracotomy
1. Make an incision 2–4 cm long between the ninth and tenth ribs.
2. Bring the lung tissue into the incision, place a ligature around the lung, and remove the sample.

Potential Risks. Because of the risk of hemorrhage and pneumothorax with all these procedures, post-biopsy monitoring is essential.

- Open lung biopsy decreases the risk of pneumothorax because the biopsy site is visualized and all leakage can be controlled.
- In fine-needle aspiration, withdrawal of infectious material can contaminate the pleural space and cause pyothorax.

Thoracocentesis

The diagnosis of pleural effusion generally depends upon analysis of pleural fluid obtained by thoracocentesis (see sec. 1, ch. 3). Thoracocentesis can also be therapeutically beneficial. Perform the procedure with minimal stress to the patient.

Electrocardiography and Ultrasonography

Often, it is difficult to determine whether a patient's problem is respiratory or cardiovascular.

- With pulmonary hypertension secondary to thoracic disease, the electrocardiogram may show pulmonale evidenced by p waves >0.4 mV and deep s waves in leads I, II, III, and aVF.
- Ultrasonography can identify specific cardiac abnormalities and masses within the mediastinum, pleural space, and pulmonary parenchyma (see sec. 1, ch. 4).

Other Specialized Diagnostic Tests

Other useful tests include bronchography, lymphangiographic studies for evaluation of chylothorax, computed tomography, magnetic resonance imaging, and vascular and radioisotopic studies to identify pulmonary thromboembolism. These procedures, if necessary, are performed at referral diagnostic centers.

Supplemental Readings

Ettinger SJ: *Textbook of Veterinary Internal Medicine,* 3rd Ed. Philadelphia: W. B. Saunders, 1989.

Fenner W: *Quick Reference to Veterinary Medicine,* 2nd Ed. Philadelphia: J. B. Lippincott, 1991.

Morgan RV: *Handbook of Small Animal Practice.* New York: Churchill-Livingstone, 1988.

17 Diagnostic Imaging of the Respiratory System

Wendy Myer

INDICATIONS FOR RADIOGRAPHIC EVALUATION

Radiography is a widely available, rapidly performed, and noninvasive method for evaluating respiratory disease in small animals. It also has the advantage of allowing repeated evaluations of an animal. Although radiography is a sensitive method for detecting respiratory disease, changes are nonspecific, and similar radiographic patterns are seen in many different disease processes. Therefore, radiographic findings should be considered morphologic, rather than etiologic, in nature.

RADIOGRAPHIC ANATOMY

- Radiographic evaluation of the *upper airways* is best accomplished with the animal in lateral recumbency. The soft palate and epiglottis are well outlined by air within the oral and nasal pharynx. Mineralization of the laryngeal cartilages, including the epiglottis, is a common finding in dogs. The normal *larynx* is slightly wider than the *trachea*; the remainder of the trachea is uniform in diameter throughout its length.

KEY POINT ▶ The trachea normally should be no smaller than three times the diameter of the proximal end of the third rib.

- The following structures should be visible on a normal thoracic radiograph (Fig. 1): the cardiac silhouette, pulmonary arteries and veins, caudal vena cava, descending aorta, trachea, diaphragm, and (in young animals) the thymus.
- The following structures usually are *not* visible on a normal thoracic radiograph: the cranial vena cava, aortic arch, great vessels, esophagus, interlobar pleural fissures, bronchial walls (except in the hilar area), and the mediastinal, hilar, and sternal lymph nodes.
- Radiographically the *pulmonary vessels* account for the majority of the pulmonary pattern. The pulmonary arteries and veins are approximately equal in size.
  - On the lateral view the arteries are dorsal to the bronchi and veins; on the ventrodorsal (VD) view, the arteries are lateral to the veins (i.e., "veins are ventral, veins are central").
  - On the lateral view the ratio of the cranial lobar vessels to the proximal one-third of the fourth rib should be approximately 0.75. Measure the vessels at the point where they cross the cardiac silhouette.
- The bronchi normally are thin-walled and seen clearly only in the hilar area. They may appear as pairs of faint, soft tissue density lines running between and parallel to the vessels, and in cross section are seen as small thin-walled doughnuts.

TECHNICAL CONSIDERATIONS

For a general discussion of radiographic equipment and techniques, see sec. 1, ch. 4.

Inspiration Versus Expiration

KEY POINT ▶ All thoracic radiographs should be taken at the height of inspiration. This allows the best evaluation of the lung and gives a more accurate assessment of cardiac size.

A poorly aerated lung will appear diffusely increased in density and may lead to an erroneous impression of pulmonary disease. Inspiratory and expiratory films taken during the same examination may be used to demonstrate dynamic problems such as expiratory airway collapse and paralysis of the diaphragm.

Respiratory Motion

Failure to control respiratory motion is one of the major causes of nondiagnostic thoracic radiographs in small animals. Use of a low Mas technique helps to decrease necessary exposure time and to minimize respiratory motion. In tachypneic animals, temporarily holding off or blowing into the animal's nose may briefly arrest respiratory motion.

Effect of Gravity on the Dependent Lung

When an animal is placed in lateral recumbency, the lung closest to the cassette becomes partially atelectatic and receives more blood and less air than normal. This decreases the air available to contrast normal or abnormal soft tissue density structures or areas of consolidation within the dependent lung. Therefore, masses that are seen on other thoracic views may seem to disappear when they are in the dependent portion of the lung. This is especially evident in the part of the lung adjacent to the heart or diaphragm. Thus, soft

531

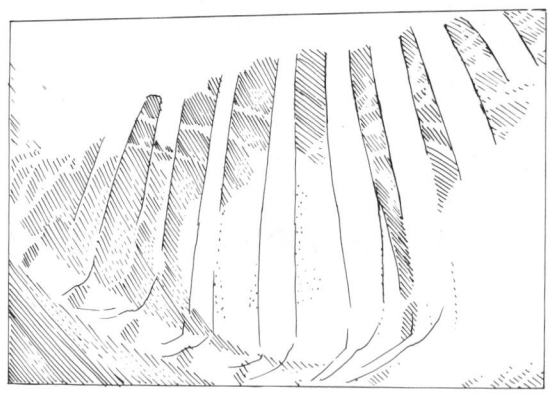 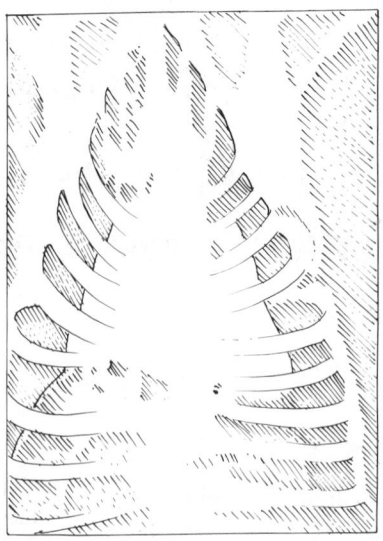

Figure 1. Radiographic appearance of the normal chest. Left, lateral view; right, ventrodorsal view.

tissue density pulmonary structures are best seen radiographically when they are in the better aerated, *nondependent* portion of the lung. For this reason, both right and left lateral views are sometimes useful (e.g., for detecting early pulmonary metastases).

Follow-up Studies

KEY POINT ▶ When repeating examinations for the purpose of following disease progression, utilize the same radiographic technique and the same radiographic positioning as in the initial examination to provide the most accurate comparison with the animal's previous state.

This is especially critical in animals with pneumonia, because pathologic changes in the dependent lung may not be well appreciated on the lateral view. Accurate assessment of pleural fluid volume is also difficult when comparing dorsoventral (DV) and VD projections even when the two radiographs are taken during the same examination.

RADIOGRAPHIC ABNORMALITIES OF THE NASAL CAVITY AND LARYNX

- Upper airway disease such as brachycephalic upper airway obstruction syndrome, laryngeal paralysis, and laryngospasm are best evaluated using visual examination externally or endoscopically. Laryngeal masses or foreign bodies may appear radiographically as soft tissue densities within the airway.
- The nasal passages are best evaluated using occlusal DV or open-mouth VD views of the maxilla. On these views the turbinates should appear as thin, lacy mineralized structures surrounded by air.
  - Rhinitis, foreign bodies, and nasal neoplasms may cause focal or diffuse increases in radiographic density of the nasal passages. Turbinate destruction is often present in animals with neoplasia or erosive rhinitis. Most cases of bacterial or foreign

body rhinitis tend to involve primarily the middle and rostral portions of one or both nasal passages.
  - Neoplastic processes often appear more destructive and primarily involve the caudal portion of the nasal passages. Despite these characteristics, a definitive diagnosis of nasal disease usually is not possible by radiography alone.

RADIOGRAPHIC ABNORMALITIES OF THE TRACHEA (Fig. 2)

- *Tracheal hypoplasia* is manifested as a uniform decrease in tracheal diameter owing to decreased size of the dorsal tracheal muscle. In severely affected animals, the tracheal diameter may be reduced to 50% of the laryngeal diameter. This condition is congenital and is most commonly seen in brachycephalic breeds, especially English bulldogs.
- *Tracheal edema* and *pseudomembranous tracheal inflammation* can also result in a diffuse decrease in tracheal diameter and must be considered in animals with an apparent decrease in tracheal diameter.
- *Focal tracheal stenosis* is manifested as a focal area of narrowed tracheal lumen and is usually the result of trauma or stricture following tracheal perforation from a dog fight or prolonged intubation with an endotracheal tube with an overinflated cuff. Tracheal perforation also usually results in air density in the peritracheal cervical region and pneumomediastinum or pneumothorax.
- *Tracheal collapse* is manifested as a focal or diffuse decrease in the dorsoventral diameter of the trachea. The collapse can be persistent or it can be intermittent, occurring during periods of excitement or coughing (see also sec. 6, ch. 19).
- To assess tracheal dynamics adequately, obtain lateral thoracic radiographs at the peaks of inspiration and of expiration. The extrathoracic (cervical and thoracic inlet) portion of the trachea will collapse during inspiration, whereas the intrathoracic portion of the trachea will collapse during expiration. In some dogs, the degenerative cartilaginous changes

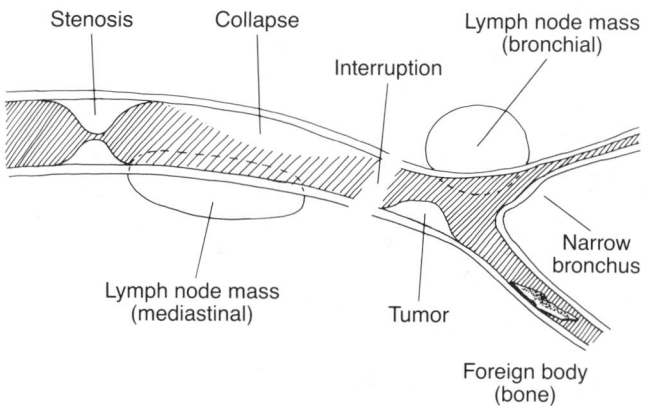

Figure 2. Schematic representation of various causes of tracheal disease.

may extend into the main stem bronchi, causing them to collapse severely during expiration.

KEY POINT ▶ Superimposition of the esophagus over the dorsal aspect of the trachea is a common finding that may lead to the misdiagnosis of tracheal collapse in a normal dog. This appearance will not change during respiration; however, the tracheal diameter in an animal with true tracheal collapse will vary during the various phases of the respiratory cycle.

■ *Tracheal masses or foreign bodies* appear as soft tissue or mineral-dense objects within the tracheal lumen. Small foreign bodies often pass into the bronchi, causing obstruction or pulmonary abscessation. Exudate within the trachea usually is not evident, because of the recumbent positioning used in small animals; however, it may be evident if horizontal beam films are obtained.

RADIOGRAPHIC ABNORMALITIES OF THE EXTRAPLEURAL SPACE

■ The extrapleural space communicates with many of the fascial planes of the body via the thoracic inlet. It can be divided into two areas:
  • The potential space between the parietal pleura and the body wall
  • The potential space within the mediastinum
■ Conditions affecting the extrapleural space include abscesses, hematomas, granulomas, and neoplasms.
■ Radiographically, most extrapleural diseases appear as relatively spherical, smoothly marginated masses that have a convex surface facing the lung and tapered or concave cranial and caudal borders, and that do not involve the pleural space until late in the disease process.
■ Mediastinal lymphadenopathy and rib tumors with secondary rib destruction are common extrapleural lesions.

The Thoracic Lymph Nodes (Fig. 3)

KEY POINT ▶ Thoracic lymph nodes are not seen radiographically in normal animals.

■ The thoracic lymph nodes are located in three areas within the mediastinum:
  • Dorsal to the second sternebra (sternal lymph nodes)
  • In the dorsal portion of the cranial mediastinum (mediastinal lymph nodes)
  • At the hilar area of the lung surrounding the bifurcation of the trachea (tracheobronchial lymph nodes)
■ When any of these nodes are substantially enlarged, they will appear as soft tissue density masses in these locations, causing the mediastinum to appear widened on the VD view and often displacing the trachea.

Thymic or Cranial Mediastinal Lymphosarcoma

■ In the cat, this disorder frequently causes a large cranial thoracic mass (see sec. 3, ch. 6).
■ Radiographic signs include dorsal tracheal deviation, a variable amount of pleural fluid, and caudal displacement of the heart, cranial lung borders, and tracheal bifurcation. It is not uncommon for the tracheal bifurcation to be displaced to the level of the seventh or eighth ribs from its normal position at the fifth to sixth ribs.

Pneumomediastinum

■ Pneumomediastinum (i.e., air within the mediastinum) may result from perforating injury of the esophagus, trachea, or bronchus near the hilus, usually in association with penetrating wounds of the cervical soft tissues or thoracic inlet.
■ This condition allows radiographic visualization of the normally invisible mediastinal structures such as the esophagus, cranial vena cava, and other mediastinal vessels.

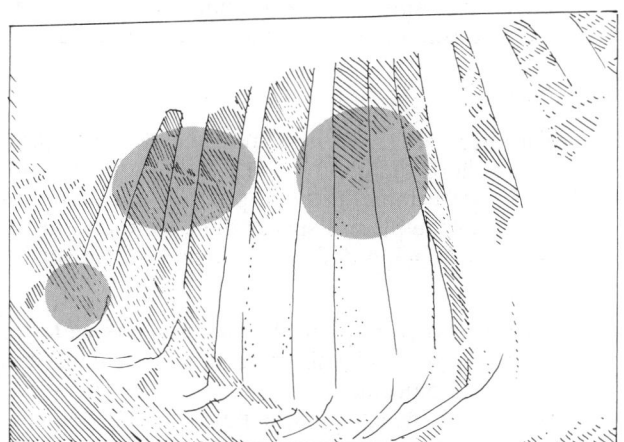

Figure 3. Location of thoracic lymph nodes.

■ Because of its communication with the fascial planes of the body, extensive subcutaneous emphysema is a common complication of this condition.

RADIOGRAPHIC ABNORMALITIES OF THE PLEURAL SPACE

The normal pleural space is not visible radiographically. Filling of this space with air (pneumothorax), fluid (hydrothorax), or viscera (diaphragmatic hernia) will cause the space to enlarge and become apparent radiographically.

Pneumothorax

In animals with pneumothorax, the pleural space appears widened and radiolucent, the lung appears smaller than normal and relatively radiopaque, and the heart appears elevated off of the sternum on the recumbent lateral view, due to shifting of the heart off the midline. Pneumothorax may be classified as:

■ *Open pneumothorax*, in which there is a defect in the body wall
■ *Closed pneumothorax*, in which the pleural air comes from the lung (see sec. 6, ch. 24).
Closed pneumothorax can be further subdivided into simple and tension forms.

■ *Simple closed pneumothorax* is caused by a puncture wound or laceration of the lung that allows free movement of air through the defect during both inspiration and expiration. There is rapid equilibration between the lung and pleural cavity, and the severity of the condition depends upon the size of the injured area.
■ *Tension pneumothorax* is due to a flaplike lesion that allows air to enter the pleural space during inspiration but closes and does not allow air to leave during expiration. Thus, pressure within the pleural space may continue to increase, and progressive pulmonary atelectasis and cardiovascular compromise may develop. This condition is a medical emergency.
■ Radiographically, tension pneumothorax is characterized by flattening of the diaphragm, severe and progressive pulmonary atelectasis, and microcardia.

Hydrothorax

Hydrothorax (Fig. 4) is a nonspecific term that indicates filling of the pleural space with fluid. It is not possible to determine radiographically the type of effusion within the pleural space; thus, thoracocentesis is necessary to reach a definitive diagnosis (see sec. 1, ch. 3).

■ Radiographically the pleural space appears widened and radiopaque and the lung appears small and relatively radiolucent.
■ The ease with which pleural fluid can be detected depends on the amount and distribution of the pleural fluid. Small amounts of fluid gravitate to the dependent portions of the thorax.

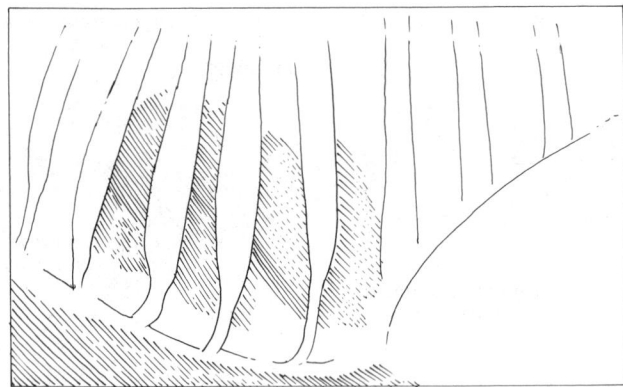

Figure 4. Radiographic appearance of hydrothorax.

● Thus, on the DV view the fluid may result in a diffuse haziness of the thorax and decreased visualization of the cardiac apex.
● On the lateral and VD views, the fluid is seen surrounding retracted lung borders, and the heart and diaphragm will be obscured in areas where they contact fluid.

KEY POINT ▶ If fluid accumulation is limited to one side of the thorax or if the caudal lobar edges are persistently rounded, consider the possibility of restrictive pleuritis due to chronic pyothorax or chylothorax.

Diaphragmatic Hernias

Most diaphragmatic hernias are traumatic in origin, although hiatal, peritoneal-pericardial, and mediastinal hernias also occur.

■ The radiographic appearance of a diaphragmatic hernia varies, depending on the size and location of the defect and the amount of herniated viscera. The most obvious radiographic signs are discontinuity of the diaphragm and herniation of abdominal viscera into the thorax. The lungs, heart, and mediastinum often will be shifted cranially or laterally. The heart and part of the diaphragm adjacent to the hernia may be obscured owing to their contact with herniated viscera or with pleural fluid, which also may be present.
■ Herniation of the liver through a small diaphragmatic rent may result in strangulation of a portion of liver with secondary pleural effusion. Cranial gastric displacement may be a helpful radiographic sign in these cases.
■ Although gas is often present within herniated small bowel or stomach, administration of a small amount of barium (1.0 ml/kg) may be helpful to verify herniation of a portion of the gastrointestinal tract.
■ Herniation of the stomach may result in acute gastric dilation and is a potential source of life-threatening cardiovascular compromise.

Positive-Contrast Peritonography. If the diagnosis of a diaphragmatic hernia is uncertain, abdominal ultrasound or positive-contrast peritonography may be helpful to assess diaphragmatic integrity. Prior to peritonography, remove pleural and abdominal fluid.

The procedure is as follows:

- Administer 1–2 ml/kg of sterile aqueous tri-iodidinated contrast agent such as that used for intravenous urography (see sec. 1, ch. 4). Warm the contrast agent to body temperature and mix with 0.1 ml/kg of lidocaine prior to intraperitoneal administration.

- Shave, surgically prepare, and locally anesthetize a small area just to the right of the umbilicus. Pass a needle/catheter combination, such as an Intrafusor (Abbott Labs.) into the abdomen, avoiding trauma to the spleen, bladder, or bowel. Perform aspiration to verify that there has been no perforation of a hollow viscus or laceration of a blood vessel.

- Slowly introduce the warmed contrast agent/lidocaine mixture into the peritoneal cavity, remove the needle, and gently roll the animal to facilitate distribution of the contrast agent.

- Obtain radiographs immediately; if findings are inconclusive, repeat in 15–20 minutes.

- Optimally, obtain all four views of the abdomen (right and left laterals, DV and VD). However, if the clinical state of the animal is compromised and only limited views can be taken, place the area of the suspected rent dependently (i.e., left lateral and DV views for a suspected ventral left-sided tear).

- In a normal animal the contrast material will coat the abdominal surface of the diaphragm. Discontinuity of this silhouette or extension of the contrast material into the thorax indicates the presence of a diaphragmatic tear.

RADIOGRAPHIC ABNORMALITIES IN PULMONARY DISEASE

Principles of Interpretation

A number of different methods have been used to describe the radiographic findings associated with pulmonary disease. One common technique uses a pattern approach that is based on the microscopic pathologic changes involved in the disease process.

KEY POINT ▶ The radiographic patterns of pulmonary disease are alveolar, interstitial, bronchial, vascular, and mixed.

Evaluate the extent of a lesion (diffuse or focal), the location of the lesion within the lung, and any associated abnormalities of other thoracic structures (such as the heart, large blood vessels, and thoracic wall) when making a radiographic differential diagnosis. Two radiographic signs important in the evaluation of pulmonary disease are the *silhouette sign* and the principle of *summation*.

Silhouette Sign. The silhouette sign occurs when two objects of the same radiographic density contact one another and are oriented in such a way that there is a gradual rather than an abrupt change in thickness at their borders (Fig. 5, left).

- Radiographically these objects appear to blend together and the borders between them are obscured. Therefore, it is not possible to perceive where one object ends and the other begins.

- This sign is most commonly seen in the thorax when

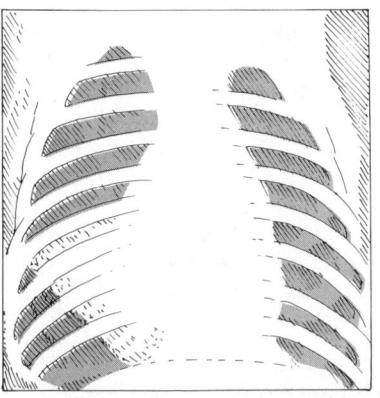
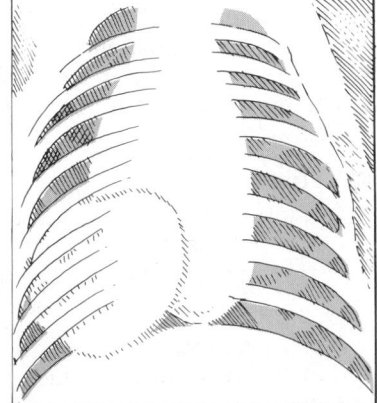
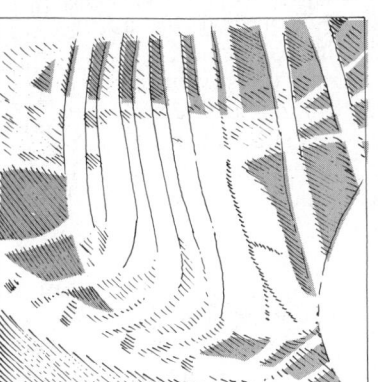
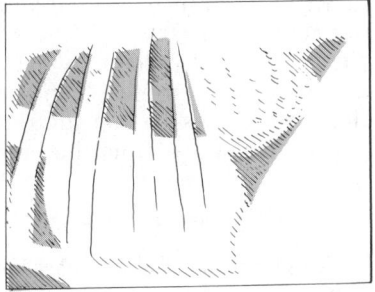

Figure 5. Representation of silhouette sign (left) and summation (right).

abnormal fluid density within the lung or pleural space contacts the heart or diaphragm, and the borders of these structures become indistinct.

Summation. The opposite effect occurs with "summation" (Fig. 5, right). Summation occurs when two objects are superimposed in such a way that there is an abrupt change in thickness at the border where these structures overlap or when they are separated by material of a different radiographic density.

- This occurs when a soft tissue density mass is within a well-aerated portion of lung and is superimposed over the heart or diaphragm. In this case the heart and mass are separated by air and the densities of the mass and the heart will be additive.
- Thus, the margin where the two objects overlap will be enhanced and the mass will appear denser than it actually is.

Alveolar Pattern

The alveolar pattern of pulmonary disease indicates decreased air within the lung as the result of alveolar collapse or filling of the alveolar air spaces with fluid or cellular debris. It is not possible to determine radiographically what type of fluid (especially if present only 1–2 days) is within the alveoli. Often there is a lag period, both at the beginning and at the end of a disease process, in which radiographic signs may not correlate with the severity of clinical signs; thus, the history, signalment, and other clinical information are extremely important in arriving at a definitive diagnosis.

Characteristics of alveolar disease include:

- Patchy, ill-defined areas of infiltration that fade into adjacent normal lung ("cotton candy" effect)
- The tendency for these lesions to coalesce, leading to lobar consolidation
- Rapid progression or regression of the infiltrates
- The presence of "air bronchograms" and the silhouette sign

KEY POINT ▶ The *air bronchogram* sign is one of the most reliable characteristics of alveolar disease. Air bronchograms are due to the presence of an air-filled bronchus within an area of fluid-filled alveoli.

Air Bronchogram. In an air bronchogram, the air within the bronchus provides excellent contrast with the fluid-filled lung, and the bronchus appears as a faint, gray, branching tube within the abnormally radiopaque lung (Fig. 6). The soft tissue density bronchial walls and pulmonary vessels within the affected portion of lung are not seen because of silhouetting of these structures by the infiltrated lung (these distinguish the alveolar from the bronchial pattern).

Associated Disease Processes

Common disease processes that cause an alveolar pattern include bronchopneumonia, pulmonary edema, and pulmonary contusions. The distribution of the

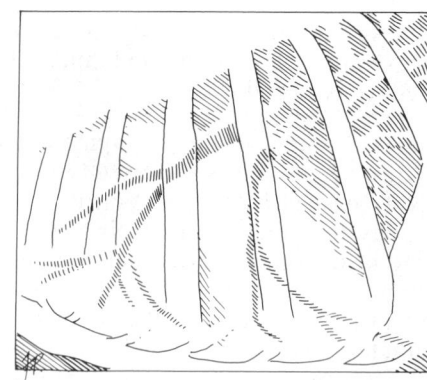

Figure 6. Alveolar lung consolidation with air bronchograms.

alveolar pattern in the lung may be helpful in the differential diagnosis of these conditions.

Bronchopneumonia

- Inhalation pneumonia, or bronchopneumonia, usually leads to focal or diffuse alveolar infiltration of the cranioventral portion of the lung. The right middle lobe is one of the most commonly affected lobes. Air bronchograms and lobar consolidation are common findings in patients with bronchopneumonia.
- In contrast, pneumonia due to hematogenous spread of bacteria, fungi, or other infectious agents often has a diffuse or dorsocaudal distribution. For further discussion of diagnosis and treatment of bronchopneumonia, see sec. 6, ch. 21.

Pulmonary Edema

- Pulmonary edema, whether cardiogenic or noncardiogenic, usually has a dorsal or dorsocaudal distribution.
- Edema of allergic origin or caused by congestive left-sided heart failure or electrocution usually is most dense in the hilar area of the lung.
- Air bronchograms may not be a prominent feature of cardiogenic edema secondary to mitral insufficiency, possibly because of the slow onset and chronic nature of this type of heart failure. Animals with acute onset of pulmonary edema from any cause are more likely to have air bronchograms because of the rapid accumulation of pulmonary fluid.
- Edema secondary to seizures or head trauma ("neurogenic") tends to affect the more peripheral portions of the caudal lobes.
- Acute upper airway obstruction is a relatively uncommon cause of pulmonary edema. When it occurs, it is often similar in distribution to cardiogenic edema.

Interstitial Patterns

The interstitium surrounds and supports the pulmonary vessels, lymphatics, bronchi, and alveoli; therefore, diseases of these structures may be reflected in the interstitium. The interstitial pattern can be subdivided into structured (nodular) and unstructured patterns.

Nodular Interstitial Pattern

■ The nodular interstitial pattern is one of the most common pulmonary patterns. The ease of detection of pulmonary nodules depends on a number of factors including the size and number of nodules, their distribution within the lung, and their margination and density. Soft tissue nodules less than 0.5 cm in diameter are extremely difficult to detect unless they are numerous, mineralized, or superimposed over soft tissues structures such as the heart or diaphragm.

■ Nodules with smooth, well-defined borders suggest a slowly progressive process with minimal involvement of the surrounding alveoli. Examples include primary and metastatic neoplasia and chronic (inactive) pulmonary granulomas and abscesses.

  • An indistinct nodular margin suggests a more active process that extends into the adjacent alveoli or is causing associated edema.

  • Highly aggressive neoplasms, active granulomas, and pulmonary abscesses often appear irregular or indistinct in margination.

■ Metastatic neoplasia generally appears as multiple, variably sized nodules randomly distributed throughout the lung. When small, these nodules are occasionally confused with cross-sectional views of pulmonary vessels.

■ On-end pulmonary vessels can be identified because they are:

  • More numerous in the hilar area

  • Consistently more dense than the adjacent vasculature

  • Associated with a longitudinal vessel of which they are a branch

  • Progressively less numerous and smaller in the periphery of the lung

■ In contrast, tumor nodules are:

  • Randomly distributed throughout the lung (i.e., small nodules may be seen centrally and large nodules peripherally)

  • Often less dense or have the same density as the pulmonary vascular pattern

  • Frequently cannot be associated with a vessel of similar or greater size.

■ Parasitic granulomas such as those secondary to *Paragonimus kellicotti* (see sec. 6, ch. 21) may be solitary or multiple and may occur anywhere in the lung.

  • Radiographic appearance varies from lesions that are almost entirely cystic to those that are primarily granulomatous with only a small cystic cavity.

  • Spontaneous pneumothorax may occur secondary to this condition.

■ Primary lung tumors are relatively uncommon and are usually carcinomas.

  • Bronchogenic carcinoma is usually hilar in location and occurs most commonly as a large, irregularly marginated soft tissue mass in the caudal lobes, especially on the right side.

  • Cavitation is uncommon but may develop in large necrotic tumors. Intrapulmonary metastasis also may be seen.

  • Although pulmonary carcinomas commonly metastasize to hilar lymph nodes, these metastases generally are not large enough to be evident radiographically. (For further discussion of lung neoplasia, see sec. 6, ch. 23).

Unstructured Interstitial Pattern

■ This pattern is one of the most difficult to diagnose because it is commonly mimicked by poor radiographic technique. The lung generally appears denser than normal, with blurring of the vascular shadows (Fig. 7). Diseases causing diffuse unstructured interstitial infiltration usually have a widespread or dorsocaudal distribution.

KEY POINT ▶ The unstructured interstitial pattern must be differentiated from respiratory motion, poor inflation of the lung such as might occur in a recumbent or obese animal, and radiographic underexposure.

■ Pulmonary edema, both cardiogenic and noncardiogenic, usually appears initially as an interstitial pattern. As the disease progresses, fluid extends further into the alveoli resulting in an alveolar pattern.

■ Interstitial pneumonia of fungal, parasitic, and especially viral etiology typically causes a diffuse increase in interstitial density of the dorsal and hilar lung areas. Secondary bacterial bronchopneumonia can simultaneously produce a mixed or alveolar infiltrate of the cranioventral portions of the lung.

■ Lung fibrosis is a very common cause of diffuse interstitial density especially in older dogs.

■ Most neoplastic processes of the lung tend to be nodular; however, in some neoplasms there is a less structured and more diffuse increase in interstitial pulmonary density. These neoplastic cells may reach the lung lymphogenously (e.g., pulmonary lymphosarcoma) or hematogenously (e.g., the scirrhous form of mammary adenocarcinoma). Differentiation of this type of neoplastic infiltration from other causes of diffuse interstitial density is difficult.

  • Clinically affected animals may present with a degree of respiratory distress disproportionate to the degree of pulmonary infiltration.

  • Fine needle aspiration of the lung, bronchoalveolar lavage, or lung biopsy may be needed for diagnosis.

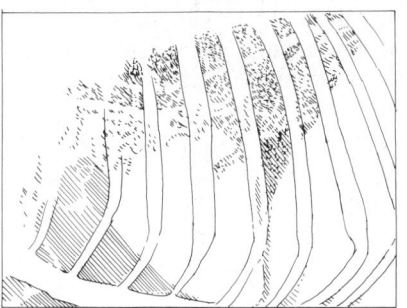

Figure 7. Diffuse interstitial pattern.

Vascular Pattern

- The vascular pattern of pulmonary disease is primarily determined by the size of the pulmonary arteries and veins.
- As mentioned previously, the vessels are best appreciated on the lateral thoracic radiograph as they extend from the hilar area into the cranial lobes.
- On the DV and VD views they are seen just lateral to the spine.
- The arteries extend into the caudal lobes from their origin at the left cranial heart border, and the veins enter the left atrium at the caudal aspect of the heart.

Hypovascularity. This appears as a decrease in the size of both the arteries and veins and is associated with relative pulmonary underperfusion, which may be due to:

- Congenital shunting of blood in a right-to-left direction, as in tetralogy of Fallot
- Acquired circulatory problems, such as acute blood loss, shock, and cardiac tamponade

Hypervascularity. Hypervascularity can refer to enlargement of both the arteries and veins, the arteries alone (arterial pulmonary hypertension), or the veins alone (venous congestion).

- Enlargement of both the pulmonary arteries and veins usually is associated with overhydration with intravenous fluids or with some type of congenital cardiac left-to-right shunt, resulting in pulmonary overcirculation. Examples include patent ductus arteriosus and ventricular septal defects (see sec. 6, ch. 12).
- High-output states such as hyperthyroidism also may produce prominent pulmonary vascularity.
- Severe left-sided heart failure due to hypertrophic cardiomyopathy or chronic mitral insufficiency with longstanding venous congestion and secondary pulmonary hypertension also may lead to enlarged arteries and veins.

Acquired Arterial Hypertension

- In the dog, this condition most commonly is the result of heartworm disease (see sec. 6, ch. 10).
  - In early heartworm disease, there is right heart enlargement and a mild to moderate increase in interstitial pulmonary density in the dorsal lung fields.
  - As the condition progresses, the right ventricle becomes more rounded, giving a "reversed D" shape to the cardiac silhouette on the VD view, and the main pulmonary artery segment and peripheral pulmonary arteries become enlarged and tortuous (Fig. 8).

KEY POINT ▶ Truncation or abrupt termination of the peripheral vessels, also called the "pruned tree" effect, is commonly seen in the caudal lobar vessels in advanced cases of heartworm disease.

  - Focal areas of pulmonary infarction appear as patchy alveolar densities, primarily around the caudal lobar vessels.

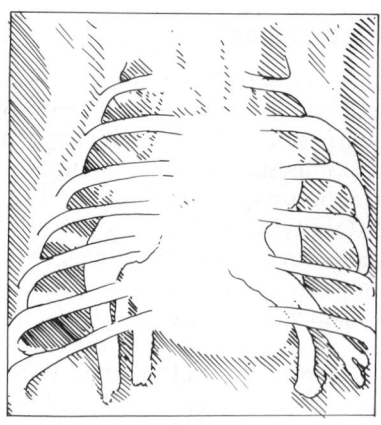

Figure 8. Radiographic appearance of heartworm disease.

- Arterial hypertension also occurs in the cat and may be due to heartworm disease or aleurostrongylosis.

Venous Congestion. Venous congestion, characterized by increased pulmonary venous size, usually is associated with left heart failure (see sec. 6, ch. 6) from congenital or acquired cardiac disease.

- Early interstitial edema, which in the dog is usually restricted to the hilar area, causes a symmetric increase in interstitial density of the hilar area of the lung, with blurring and decreased visualization of the veins.
- As the pulmonary edema progresses, alveolar infiltrates become evident in the caudal lobes.
- In the cat, pulmonary edema is somewhat less predictable in its distribution and may appear more focal and asymmetric than that in the dog.

Bronchial Pattern

- Increased bronchial prominence in the dog may occur as a normal aging change or may be secondary to chronic bronchial inflammation.
- Radiographic changes in animals with acute bronchitis may be restricted to pulmonary overinflation or air trapping.
- As the disease progresses, the bronchial walls tend to appear thickened. This often results in a relative decrease in luminal diameter and is best appreciated on cross-sectional views in which the bronchi appear as "thick-walled doughnuts" (Fig. 9).
- When viewed longitudinally, the bronchial walls appear as paired nearly parallel linear densities or "tram lines" extending into the lung periphery.
- Bronchial mineralization is a common sequel of chronic bronchitis, especially in cases with an allergic or immune-mediated etiology.

Bronchial Prominence in Cats. This pattern in cats is most commonly associated with *bronchitis* or *feline asthma*, although infection with *Aleurostrongylus abstrus* may occasionally cause this appearance.

- Cats presenting with acute respiratory distress generally show evidence of thoracic overexpansion with a flattened diaphragm and a barrel-shaped thorax in addition to bronchial prominence.
- Asymptomatic animals may appear radiographically

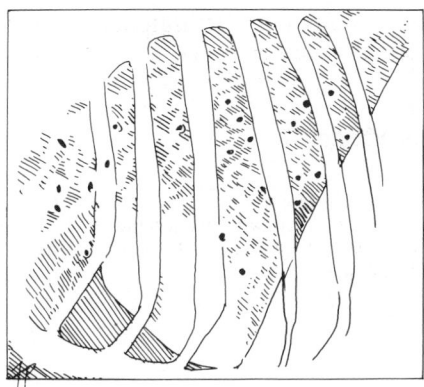

Figure 9. Bronchial pattern.

normal unless the disease is chronic and the animal has had several acute episodes of dyspnea.

- Some cats with chronic bronchitis have chronic consolidation or atelectasis of the right middle lung lobe, the result of chronic fibrosis and volume loss in this lobe.

Bronchiectasis. Bronchiectasis, or irreversible bronchial dilatation, generally occurs secondary to chronic bronchial disease.

- It may be cylindrical or saccular, and on cross-sectional views the affected bronchi have prominent walls that appear relatively thin compared with the enlarged bronchial lumen.
- Animals with bronchiectasis are prone to secondary bronchopneumonia because of poor mucociliary pulmonary clearance.

Mixed Patterns

Although the pattern approach to pulmonary evaluation is helpful in arriving at a differential diagnosis, many disease processes result in a mixture of the aforementioned patterns. These patterns often vary depending on the stage of the disease process during which the animal is evaluated. Diseases commonly causing a mixed pattern include heartworm disease, heart failure, and pneumonia.

Increased Pulmonary Radiolucency

- Abnormal pulmonary radiolucency is probably easiest to recognize when it is focal.
- Thin-walled bullae or blebs often occur secondary to pulmonary trauma. They are generally subpleural in location and resolve spontaneously.
- Thicker-walled cavitary lesions may be the result of parasitic cysts (e.g., *Paragonimus kellicotti*), congenital bronchial cysts, and cavitated abscesses, neoplasms, and granulomas. These may be single or multiple, and their location within the lung is variable.
- Horizontal beam radiographs may be helpful in determining if fluid or cellular debris is present in the "cystic" areas.

Emphysema. Emphysema may occur as a compensatory change following surgical removal of a lung lobe or volume loss in one of the lung lobes; it also can be the result of aging or of true histologic breakdown of the alveolar septa. True emphysema, as seen in humans, is relatively uncommon in dog and cats.

- Radiographically, hyperinflation is recognized by:
  - Relative pulmonary hyperlucency
  - Flattening of the diaphragm
  - Increased separation of the heart and diaphragm
  - Apparent decreased size of the pulmonary vessels
  - A barrel-shaped chest
  - Decreased differences in diaphragmatic excursion between inspiratory and expiratory films
- Radiographic overexposure and severe hypovolemia (e.g., hypoadrenocorticism) are other causes of apparent pulmonary hyperlucency but usually are not accompanied by the other radiographic signs seen in generalized emphysema.

ALTERNATE IMAGING MODALITIES

Ultrasonographic Evaluation of the Lung and Mediastinum

- It is not possible to evaluate the normally aerated lung utilizing ultrasonography, because of the large acoustic mismatch between air and soft tissue and the reflection of most of the ultrasound beam at the pleural/lung interface.
- Focal areas of pulmonary infiltration may be evaluated as long as they extend to the pulmonary periphery. Fine-needle aspiration of these areas also can be done for microscopic evaluation and culture (see sec. 1, ch. 4).
- In animals with pleural effusion, the lung is displaced away from the body wall, allowing assessment of the character of the pleural fluid to determine if it is cellular or noncellular or contains fibrin.
- Large mediastinal masses also displace the lung, allowing assessment of whether these masses are single or multiple, solid or cystic, and mineralized or nonmineralized and whether the heart or great vessels are affected. These masses are usually imaged through the intercostal spaces or through the thoracic inlet.
- Thymomas, ectopic thyroid neoplasia, and lymphosarcoma are among the mediastinal masses that can be evaluated and aspirated using ultrasonographic guidance.

Nuclear Medicine

- Nuclear medicine in pulmonary evaluation of animals is mostly limited to referral centers associated with veterinary colleges.
- Perfusion/ventilation studies are commonly done in humans and were first used in dogs to evaluate the effects of heartworm disease.
- Special aerosol masks and trapping mechanisms are used to deliver the radioactivity for the ventilation portion of the study.

■ The perfusion part of the study involves IV administration of technetium 99m macroaggregated albumin (MAA). Because this agent is trapped in the capillary network of the lung on the first pass following an IV injection, it can be used to detect areas of decreased pulmonary perfusion.

These studies are done relatively infrequently in animals, because of various technical problems. Further improvements in the technical and radiation safety aspects of this study may facilitate its more widespread use in veterinary medicine.

Supplemental Readings

Suter PF: *Thoracic Radiography: A Text Atlas of Thoracic Diseases of the Dog and Cat.* Wettswil, Switzerland: P. F. Suter, 1984.
Thrall DE: *Textbook of Veterinary Diagnostic Radiology.* Philadelphia: W. B. Saunders, 1986.

18 Surgical Management of Chronic Nasal Cavity and Paranasal Sinus Disease

Cheryl S. Hedlund

Signs in dogs and cats with chronic nasal and paranasal sinus disease may include nasal discharge, epistaxis, sneezing, gagging, stertorous breathing, nasal discomfort, and nasal deformity. Causes of nasal cavity and paranasal sinus diseases can be difficult to identify, but most cases are traumatic, infectious, inflammatory, or neoplastic in origin. Rhinotomy may be necessary to arrive at a definitive diagnosis and may facilitate treatment of the disease. Hemostatic abnormalities may lead to epistaxis.

ANATOMY

Nasal Cavity

- The nasal cavity is divided into two chambers by the nasal septum. The rostral portion of the nasal septum is cartilaginous and difficult to evaluate radiographically.
- The rostral nasal chambers are occupied by the dorsal and ventral nasal turbinates (endoturbinates) (Fig. 1).
- The caudal nasal chamber is filled with ethmoturbinates (ectoturbinates). The ethmoturbinates extend into the frontal sinus, forming narrow communicating ostia between the frontal sinus and nasal cavity (see Fig. 1).
- In the cat, the nasal cavity is shorter, the ethmoturbinates are larger, and the nasal turbinates are smaller than in the dog.
- The cribriform plate is a sievelike partition between the nasal and cranial cavities (see Fig. 1). It articulates with the frontal bones dorsally and the presphenoid bones ventrally and laterally.
- The blood supply to the nasal cavity originates from the external carotid arteries via branches of the maxillary artery, including the sphenopalatine, ethmoid, greater palatine, dorsal nasal, lateral nasal, and maxillary labial arteries.

Paranasal Sinuses

- The paranasal sinuses enlarge with age and vary in size depending on the breed of the animal.
- The frontal sinus extends roughly from the medial canthus of the eyes to the temporal line. In dogs (but not in cats), it is divided into rostral, lateral, and medial compartments (see Fig. 1). The frontal sinus varies more in size than other cavities in the skull. The lateral compartment is particularly large in dolichocephalic breeds. Brachycephalic breeds have small lateral compartments, and the medial compartment may be absent.
- The maxillary sinus or recess is found dorsal to the roots of the third and fourth premolars and medial to the infraorbital canal. The maxillary recess in the cat is very narrow.
- Cats have a small sphenoid sinus. Dogs do not have a sphenoid sinus.

PREOPERATIVE CONSIDERATIONS

Disease Conditions

- Signs of chronic nasal disease include unilateral or bilateral nasal discharge, sneezing, nasal discomfort, gagging, stertorous breathing, and facial or nasopharyngeal distortion.
- The most frequent causes of chronic nasal and paranasal sinus disease are neoplasms and infections.
- Other causes include parasites *(Pneumonyssus caninum, Linguatula serrata),* dental disease, trauma, lymphocytic-plasmocytic inflammation, and congenital anomalies. Nasal polyps, which are benign lesions, occur rarely.

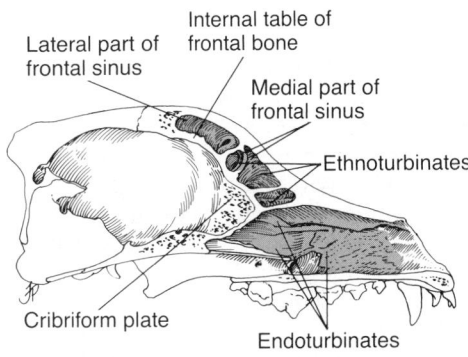

Figure 1. Sagittal section of the skull illustrating the anatomy of the nasal cavity and paranasal sinuses in relationship to the cranium. (Redrawn with permission from Evans HE, ed.: *Miller's Anatomy of the Dog,* 3rd ed. Philadelphia: W.B. Saunders, 1992.)

Tumors

- Tumors of the nasal cavity and paranasal sinuses account for approximately 1% of all neoplasms in cats and dogs.
- Most intranasal tumors are diagnosed in older dogs and cats (>8–10 years) and in large-breed dogs.
- Tumors in the nasal cavity are usually found in the caudal third of the nasal passages.
- Most intranasal tumors are malignant (80%). Adenocarcinomas are most common, but squamous cell carcinoma, fibrosarcoma, chondrosarcoma, osteosarcoma, lymphosarcoma, hemangiosarcoma, undifferentiated sarcomas or carcinomas, and transmissible venereal tumors also occur.
- The prognosis for malignant nasal neoplasms is guarded because of rapid local invasion and recurrence after therapy. Typically, these tumors do not metastasize until late in the course of the disease.
- Therapies that may help control some tumors include radiotherapy, immunotherapy, cryotherapy, and chemotherapy. These modalities are sometimes combined with surgically debulking the lesion.

Infections

- Infections, especially those caused by fungal organisms, are the frequent cause of infectious nasal and paranasal cavity disease.
- Systemic diseases such as distemper, feline upper respiratory viral infections, and Rocky Mountain spotted fever can also cause acute or chronic rhinitis.
- Primary bacterial rhinitis is uncommon and usually is associated with foreign bodies, immunosuppression (feline leukemia virus [FeLV], feline immunodeficiency virus [FIV]), or dental disease.

Fungal Rhinitis. The most commonly reported pathogenic fungi are *Aspergillus* and *Penicillium* species in dogs and *Cryptococcus neoformans* in cats. Other reported pathogens are *Rhinosporidium* and *Alternaria alternata*.

- Dogs with fungal rhinitis due to *Aspergillus* or *Penicillium* are usually young (1–7 years).
- Patients with fungal rhinitis generally do not have facial distortion but may exhibit ulceration of the nares and more nasal discomfort than dogs with nasal neoplasia.
- Treatment of fungal rhinitis is primarily medical, although surgery may be necessary for definitive diagnosis or creating ports for medical therapy.
- Medical therapy may be systemic (ketoconazole, thiabendazole, itraconazole, enilconazole), topical (same as systemic or iodine administered directly into the nasal cavity), or both.
  - Topical therapy is accomplished by implanting fenestrated tubes or creating a nasal stoma for nasal irrigation or swabbing.
- Nasal rhinosporidiosis is treated by surgical excision of the lesion.

Diagnosis

Follow a standard protocol of evaluation, including a thorough history and physical examination, for all dogs and cats presenting with chronic nasal disease. Besides a complete blood count (CBC), serum chemistry profile, and urinalysis, consider a coagulation profile, radiography, enzyme-linked immunosorbent assay (ELISA) for FELV and FIV, computed tomography (CT), fungal serology, rhinoscopy, and nasal biopsy.

Clinical History

The clinical history can provide important diagnostic clues.

- Suspect a destructive process if the discharge changes from unilateral to bilateral.
- Sneezing suggests involvement of the mid and rostral nasal chambers.
- Gagging suggests nasopharyngeal involvement or postnasal drainage.
- A history of trauma or dental disease suggests an oronasal fistula.

Physical Examination Findings

- Facial or palatal deformity suggests neoplasia.
- Mouth breathing indicates nasopharyngeal obstruction.
- An ocular discharge may indicate nasolacrimal duct erosion.

Laboratory Studies

- A CBC, serum chemistry profile, and urinalysis can assess the patient's overall status.
- A coagulation profile is indicated if exploratory rhinotomy is planned or if epistaxis is a major clinical sign.

Imaging Studies

Radiography. Radiographs of the thorax are taken in the conscious patient, whereas those of the nasal cavity and paranasal sinuses are taken with the patient under general anesthesia.

- Include lateral, ventrodorsal, rostrocaudal, and rostroventral-caudodorsal open mouth or occlusal radiographic views.
- The two most useful radiographic views are the ventrodorsal view of the maxilla using intraoral radiographic film and the rostrocaudal projection highlighting the frontal sinuses.
- To avoid iatrogenic fluid densities within the cavities, schedule radiography before performing any rhinoscopic, flush, or biopsy procedures.

CT. Although not widely available, CT should be performed when possible to localize lesions more accurately than is possible with radiography.

Rhinoscopy

Rhinoscopy is performed in the anesthetized patient following skull radiography. The nasal mucosa is very sensitive to manipulation, and visualization can be obliterated by hemorrhage. Therefore, the gentlest techniques and suction are used.

- The rostral aspect of the nasal cavity may be visualized with an otoscope or a cystoscope. A flexible pediatric bronchoscope facilitates visualization of the remainder of the cavity and allows retropharyngeal examination of the choanae.
- It may be impossible to perform a rhinoscopic examination on very small dogs and cats because of the size discrepancies between the scope and nasal passages. However, examine the pharynx and choanae in these animals.

Biopsy

- During the rhinoscopic procedure, lesions can be biopsied using endoscopic biopsy instruments.

Other Diagnostic Procedures

- *Nasal flushing* or coring procedures are performed with the patient still under anesthesia if endoscopic biopsy was not possible or successful.
  - In this procedure, a stiff plastic tube (e.g., the plastic cover of a Sovereign indwelling catheter) is moved vigorously in and out of the nasal passages (inserted through the nares and not extending beyond the medial canthus) while flushing and aspirating saline.
  - Pre-measure the catheter to avoid trauma to or beyond the cribriform plate.
  - Collect the lavage fluid and debris and examine for tissue fragments.
- *Nasal swabs* for culture or cytologic evaluation are of limited value. Positive fungal cultures can be obtained in about 40% of normal dogs. Occasionally, cryptococcosis organisms are identified by examining a stained, direct smear.
- *Serologic evaluation* for *Aspergillus* and *Penicillium* species is useful, but false-positive results are possible.
- *Rhinotomy* is performed as a diagnostic procedure if a diagnosis is not achieved by other means.

Anesthesia

- Induce and maintain routine general anesthesia for diagnostic and surgical procedures (see sec. 1, ch. 2).
- Prior to extubation it is advisable to examine and suction the nasopharyngeal area. Leave the endotracheal tube cuff partially inflated to prevent tracheal aspiration of blood clots, fluid, and debris.

SURGICAL PROCEDURES

Objectives

- Obtain sufficient tissue samples to achieve a definitive diagnosis for the patient's chronic rhinitis/sinusitis.
- Completely remove or debulk the lesion.
- Facilitate administration of or effectiveness of adjuvant therapy.
- Minimize blood loss.
- Maintain a cosmetically acceptable appearance.

Equipment

- Standard general surgical pack and suture
- Umbilical tape, vascular tape (Vas-Tie; Sil-Med Corp., Taunton, MA), or bulldog vascular clamps for temporary carotid ligation
- Periosteal elevator
- Oscillating saw, air drill, pins and pin chuck, and/or osteotome and mallet to create bone flap
- Gelpi retractor
- Bone curet, rasp, bur, rongeur, and trephine
- Fenestrated, indwelling tubes (e.g., Sovereign indwelling catheter cover) to facilitate application of topical medications.
- Synthetic mesh to span the bony defect (usually not needed).

Temporary Bilateral Carotid Artery Occlusion

This procedure is performed prior to entry into the nasal cavity or paranasal sinuses if major surgery such as rhinotomy and turbinectomy is to be performed. Carotid artery occlusion decreases blood loss and improves visualization during rhinotomy. *Not all surgeons choose to use this technique.*

Technique

1. Place the dog in dorsal recumbency with the front legs secured caudally and a rolled towel placed under the neck.
2. Clip and aseptically prepare the ventral neck from the caudal aspect of the mandibles to the manubrium.
3. Incise the skin and subcutis on the ventral cervical midline from the larynx to the mid trachea.
4. Separate the paired sternohyoideus muscles to expose the ventral trachea.
5. Bluntly dissect lateral to the trachea and palpate the carotid pulse.
6. Exteriorize the carotid sheath and separate the external carotid artery from the vagosympathetic trunk and internal jugular vein (Fig. 2).
7. Occlude the carotid artery with a vascular tie, umbilical tape, or vascular clamp (see Fig. 2).
8. Repeat the procedure on the opposite carotid.

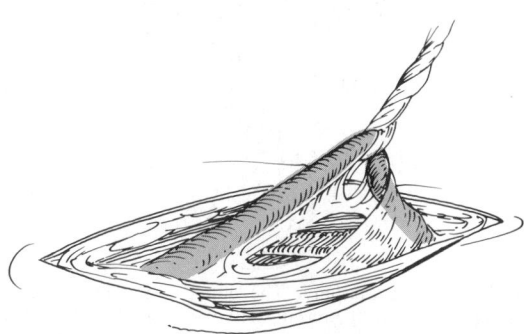

Figure 2. The carotid sheath is located lateral to the trachea, exteriorized, and incised. The common carotid artery (top) is separated from the vagosympathetic trunk and internal jugular vein (bottom) and occluded.

9. Appose the separated sternohyoid muscles and skin in two layers with simple continuous suture patterns.
10. Cover the surgical site with sterile draping material and, if necessary, reposition the patient for rhinotomy.
11. Following rhinotomy, re-expose the carotids and release occlusion. Lavage the area and routinely close in three layers (muscle, subcutis, and skin).

Dorsal Rhinotomy

Following carotid occlusion, the nasal cavity and frontal sinuses are exposed for exploration and biopsy.

Technique

1. Position the patient in ventral recumbency.
2. Prepare the nasal and frontal sinus areas for aseptic surgery.
3. Incise the skin and subcutis along the dorsal midline (Fig. 3).
4. Elevate the dense fascia and periosteum with a periosteal elevator and retract these tissues laterally with Gelpi retractors.
5. Create a unilateral or bilateral bone flap with an oscillating saw or drill.
   a. Alternatively, make holes (drill or pin chuck) at the edges of the proposed flap and connect them with an osteotome and mallet.
   b. Another method is to make a hole into the nasal cavity with a trephine or pin and chuck; the adjacent bone is rongeured and discarded.
   Expose the nasal cavity and the rostral portion of the frontal sinus for complete exploration (see Fig. 3).
6. Remove or debulk the lesion and involved turbinates, using forceps, Metzenbaum scissors, and/or

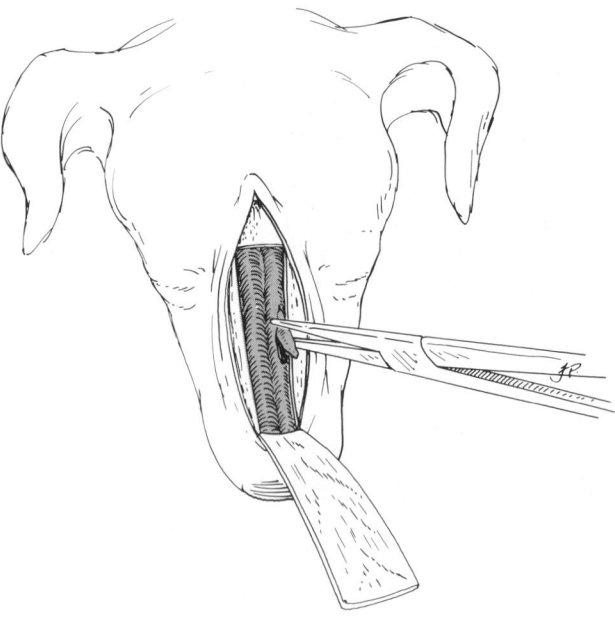

Figure 4. The bone flap is reflected rostrally or removed. Turbinectomy is performed using forceps, scissors, and curets. (Redrawn with permission from Bojrab MJ, ed.: *Current Techniques in Small Animal Surgery,* 3rd ed. Philadelphia: Lea & Febiger, 1990.)

a bone curet (Fig. 4). Save all tissues for culture and histologic evaluation.
7. Remove exudate from the frontal sinus, curet the lining to remove all diseased tissue, and enlarge the ostia to facilitate drainage.
8. Lavage and suction the nasal cavity and sinuses thoroughly with copious amounts of saline to dislodge debris and blood clots.
9. If required for adjuvant therapy or to minimize subcutaneous emphysema, place a fenestrated, indwelling tube into the frontal sinus and extending into the nasal cavity. Create the opening in the frontal sinus with a trephine, drill, or pin chuck.
10. To replace the nondiseased bone flap, drill holes in the bone flap and rhinotomy margins and place nonmetallic sutures through adjacent holes to secure the flap (Fig. 5).
11. Close, using continuous suture patterns in the fascial and periosteal layer, subcutaneous tissues, and the skin.
    a. Alternatively, close the soft tissues in an identical manner after discarding the bone flap.
    b. When the defect is large and cosmetic appearance is critical, a synthetic mesh (e.g., Marlex mesh) can be stretched across the bony defect and secured.
13. The skin edges may be secured directly to the margins of the bony defect, creating a stoma into the nasal cavity to facilitate topical therapy or to prevent subcutaneous emphysema (Fig. 6).
14. If the stoma is small it may heal by second intention; otherwise, following conclusion of medical therapy, debride, undermine, and appose the skin edges.
15. Dogs tolerate rhinotomy very well. Aggressive rhinotomy in cats can be associated with higher rates of morbidity and mortality.

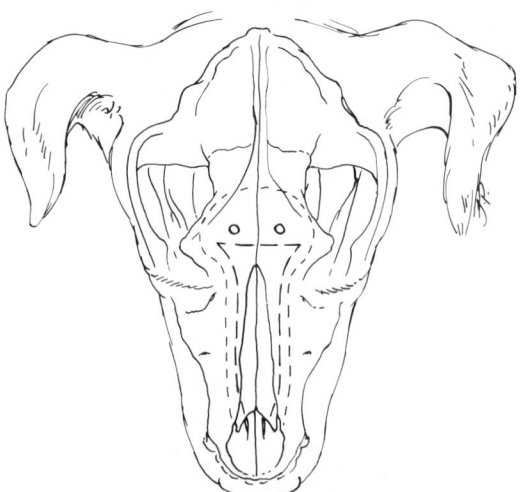

Figure 3. Dorsal rhinotomy. The outer dotted line describes the approximate extent of the nasal cavity and frontal sinuses. The inner dashed lines demonstrate the bone flap for a unilateral or bilateral approach. The holes over the frontal sinuses indicate the site for insertion of drains. (Redrawn with permission from Bojrab MJ, ed. *Current Techniques in Small Animal Surgery,* 3rd ed. Philadelphia: Lea & Febiger, 1990.)

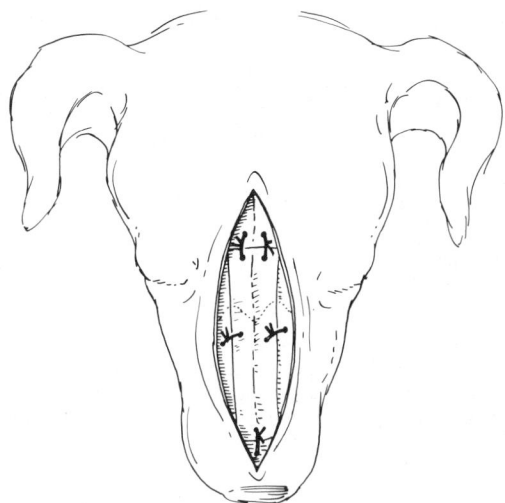

Figure 5. The bone flap is replaced by placing sutures through holes drilled in the flap and margins of the defect. (Redrawn with permission from Bojrab MJ, ed.: *Current Techniques in Small Animal Surgery,* 3rd ed. Philadelphia: Lea & Febiger, 1990.)

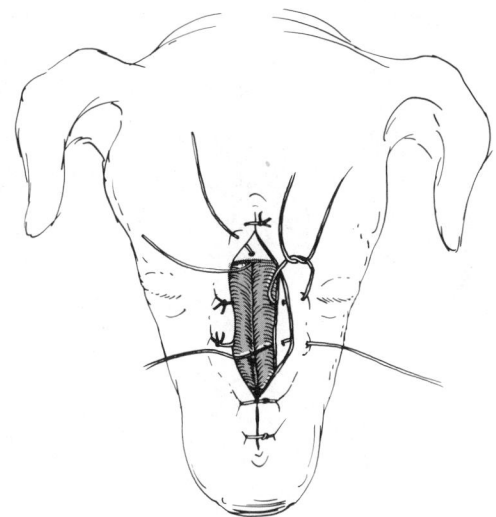

Figure 6. Creation of a stoma following rhinotomy is accomplished by drilling holes in the margins of the defect and passing sutures through these holes and the skin.

Ventral Rhinotomy

The nasal cavity and nasopharynx can be explored using a ventral approach. With this technique, evaluation of the frontal sinuses is limited to the rostral half.

Technique

1. Position the patient in dorsal recumbency with the oral cavity exposed by hanging and securing the mandible in a wide, open-mouth position (Fig. 7).
2. Cleanse the oral cavity, dental arcade, and nasopharyngeal area with a mild antiseptic solution (dilute chlorhexidine or povidone-iodine).
3. Incise the mucoperiosteum of the hard palate on the midline from the level of the canine teeth caudally to the fourth premolar or continue through the mucosa of the soft palate if the lesion extends into the nasopharyngeal area (Fig. 8).
   a. Alternatively, a U-shaped mucoperiosteal incision parallel to the dental arcade can be used (Fig. 8).
4. Bilaterally reflect and retract the mucoperiosteum laterally.
5. Identify and preserve the major palatine arteries. They penetrate the hard palate near the caudal aspect of the fourth premolar and parallel the course of the dental arcade about midway between it and the midline of the hard palate (see Fig. 8).
6. Create a window into the nasal cavity by removing

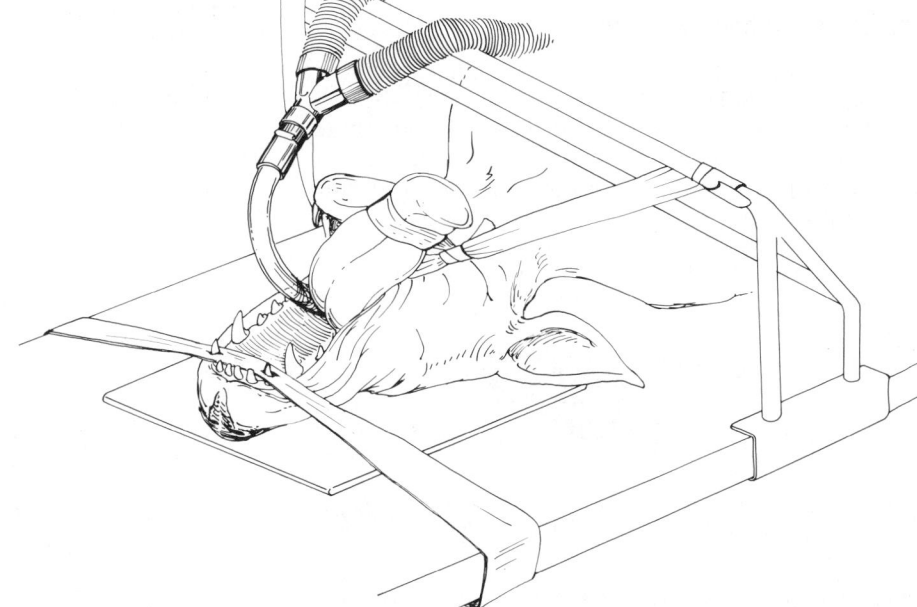

Figure 7. Positioning for ventral rhinotomy. (Redrawn with permission from Slatter DH, ed.: *Textbook of Small Animal Surgery.* Philadelphia: W.B. Saunders, 1985.)

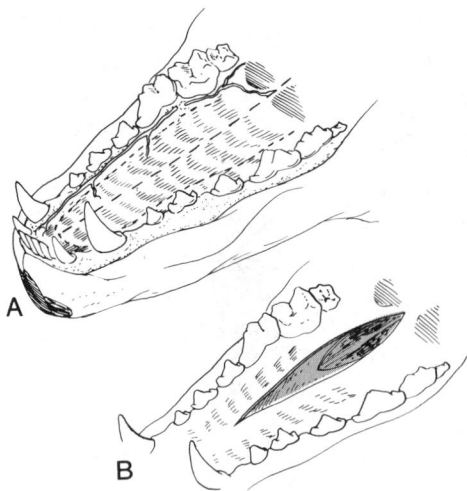

Figure 8. Ventral rhinotomy. Incise the mucoperiosteum on the midline or in the shape of a U, which parallels the dental arcade *(A)*. The incision may extend into the soft palate to expose lesions extending into the nasopharynx *(B)*.

a flap of hard palate with an oscillating saw, air drill, or osteotome and mallet (Fig. 9). Enlarge the window with rongeurs, if necessary.

7. Remove the lesion and involved turbinates with forceps and curettage.
8. Lavage and suction blood clots and debris from the area with copious amounts of saline.
9. Replace or discard the bone flap as for dorsal rhinotomy.
10. Close the mucoperiosteum with simple interrupted sutures. If possible, close the soft palate incision in two or three layers (nasal mucosa, muscle and connective tissue, pharyngeal mucosa) (Fig. 10).

Frontal Sinus Procedures

Chronic rhinitis/sinusitis (especially in cats) generally recurs in a variable period of time with either of the following procedures.

Technique for Sinus Flushing

1. Insert tubes for frontal sinus flushing by first trephining a hole into the sinus.
2. Make an incision in the soft tissues and trephine a hole in the bone just lateral to the midline, on a line connecting the rostral margins of the supraorbital processes.

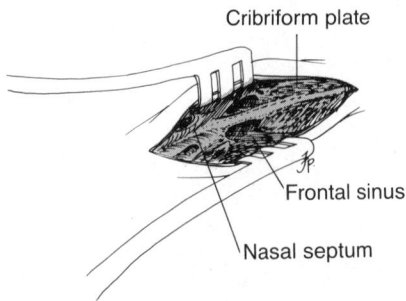

Figure 9. Exposure using ventral rhinotomy: cribriform plate, frontal sinuses, remnant of nasal septum.

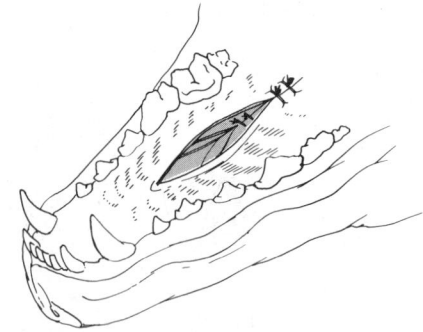

Figure 10. Following ventral rhinotomy the mucoperiosteum is apposed with simple interrupted sutures. The soft palate is apposed using two or three layers of simple interrupted or simple continuous sutures.

3. Collect biopsy and culture specimens.
4. Insert the fenestrated tube into the sinus and secure it to the skin (Fig. 11).
5. Following tube removal, allow the hole to heal by second intention.

Technique for Sinus Obliteration

1. Create a bone flap to expose the frontal sinuses and caudal nasal cavity.
2. Remove the compartment divisions and mucosal lining of the frontal sinus and aperture with a pneumatic bone bur.
3. Cover the aperture of the frontal sinus into the nasal cavity with a free fascial or muscle patch.
4. Lavage the area and fill the sinus with fat harvested from a secondary site (e.g., falciform ligament).
5. Close the periosteum, subcutaneous tissue, and skin.

POSTOPERATIVE CARE AND COMPLICATIONS

Recovery and Expectations

- Following rhinotomy, place the patient in a slightly head-down position and remove the endotracheal tube with the cuff slightly inflated to help remove fluid and debris.

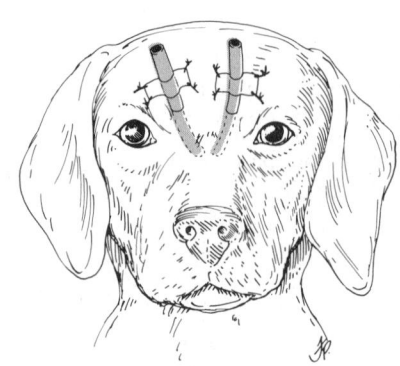

Figure 11. Position of tubes inserted into the frontal sinus and nasal cavity for topical treatment of chronic rhinitis and sinusitis. (Redrawn with permission from Slatter DH, ed.: *Textbook of Small Animal Surgery.* Philadelphia: W.B. Saunders, 1985.)

- Give postoperative analgesics such as buprenorphine (Buprenex; Norwich Eaton), 0.02 mg/kg IM or IV, for the first 24 hours as needed.
- Expect sneezing and mild epistaxis for several days.
- Breathing sounds are harsh and resonant, often sounding "hollow."
- Appetite may be depressed for several days.
- A serous to serosanguineous discharge occurs for several days to weeks, depending on the primary disease condition and the effectiveness of adjuvant therapy.
- Inward and outward movement of the skin flap may occur if the bone flap is discarded, but is usually temporary.
- Chewing on hard objects is forbidden if the bone flap from the hard palate is discarded.
- Prior to creating a nasal stoma, graphically describe to the client the postoperative appearance of the patient (optimally by viewing pictures of other patients). Many clients are initially reluctant to accept their pets' appearance following rhinostomy.
- Following rhinotomy, patients are discharged from the hospital within 2–3 days unless complications or adjuvant therapy dictates longer hospitalization.
- Survival following various combinations of therapy for nasal neoplasms ranges from 4 months to longer than 24 months.
- Fungal rhinitis is refractory to antifungal agents currently available in about 50% of the cases. Antifungal agents are usually given for 6–8 weeks.

Complications

- Chronic rhinitis/sinusitis and its causative agents will persist or recur if rhinotomy and turbinectomy are performed without appropriate medical therapy (see sec. 6, ch. 21). Exceptions may include nasal disease caused by foreign bodies or *Rhinosporidium* organisms.
- If carotid artery occlusion is not employed, blood loss during surgery may be excessive, requiring transfusions and vigorous fluid therapy.
- Indwelling catheters can be dislodged by the patient; therefore, some surgeons advocate the creation of temporary rhinostomies to facilitate topical therapy.
- Subcutaneous emphysema may occur. It is usually localized to the head and resorbs without treatment. If emphysema is excessive, place a tube in the frontal sinus to vent the air.
- Nasocutaneous or oronasal fistulas may form if healing is interrupted.
- Replaced bone flaps may sequestrate secondary to infection or radiation therapy.
- The chronic nasal discharge may persist because it is not possible to remove all diseased tissue during turbinectomy, and the epithelium may have undergone squamous metaplasia.

Supplemental Readings

Birchard SJ: A simplified method for rhinotomy and temporary rhinostomy in dogs and cats. J Am Anim Hosp Assoc 24:69, 1988.

Hedlund CS, Tangner CH, Elkins AD, Hobson HP: Temporary bilateral carotid artery occlusion during surgical exploration of the nasal cavity in the dog. Vet Surg 12:83, 1983.

Holmberg DL, Fries C, Cockshutt J, Van Pelt D: Ventral rhinotomy in the dog and cat. Vet Surg 18:446, 1989.

Pavletic MM, Clark GN: Open nasal cavity and frontal sinus treatment of chronic canine aspergillosis. Vet Surg 20:43, 1991.

Sharp NJH, McEntee M, Gilson S, Thrall D: Nasal cavity and frontal sinuses. Problems in Veterinary Medicine: Head and Neck Surgery 3:170, 1991.

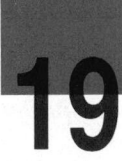# 19 Diagnosis and Surgical Management of Obstructive Upper Airway Diseases

Roger B. Fingland

Obstructive upper airway diseases typically are insidious in onset and result in progressively worsening respiratory stridor and dyspnea. The dimensions of the upper airway play a fundamental role in the efficiency of breathing and progression of disease. In narrowed regions of the upper airway, air velocity is higher and pressure is correspondingly lower than elsewhere (Bernoulli effect) which tends to narrow susceptible regions of the upper airway still more.

ETIOLOGY

Congenital obstructive upper airway diseases are diagnosed so commonly in brachycephalic dogs that they are referred to collectively as the brachycephalic syndrome. Most other obstructive upper airway diseases are acquired and are diagnosed in middle-aged and older dogs. Obstructive upper airway diseases are diagnosed less frequently in cats.

Brachycephalic Syndrome. The brachycephalic syndrome consists of stenotic nares, elongated soft palate, and everted laryngeal saccules.

Tracheal hypoplasia is a generalized narrowing of the tracheal lumen diameter diagnosed commonly in English bulldogs and, less commonly, in other brachycephalic breeds.

Stenotic nares and elongated soft palate are congenital conditions diagnosed quite frequently in brachycephalic dogs.

Laryngeal saccule eversion is a consequence of chronic upper airway obstruction.

Laryngeal Collapse. Laryngeal collapse is recognized most commonly in brachycephalic dogs with chronic obstructive upper respiratory disease (brachycephalic syndrome). Loss of the supporting function of the laryngeal cartilages results from pressure changes within the larynx induced by obstruction rostral to the rima glottidis. Laryngeal collapse is a progressive, end-stage disease.

Laryngeal Paralysis. This condition is seen primarily in old, large and giant-breed dogs. Interruption of the innervation to the intrinsic muscles of the larynx, particularly the cricoarytenoideus dorsalis muscle, results in failure of the arytenoid cartilages and vocal folds to abduct during inspiration. The condition is congenital in the Bouvier des Flandres breed and is related to an inherited degenerative process in the nucleus ambiguus. Laryngeal paralysis also has been associated with hypothyroidism (see sec. 4, ch. 1) and diffuse polyneuropathies in dogs (see sec. 10, ch. 6). In many cases laryngeal paralysis is idiopathic.

Nasopharyngeal Polyps. These inflammatory masses arise from the epithelium of the nasopharynx, auditory canal, or tympanic cavity (see sec. 5, ch. 24).

- Polyps commonly occur in cats and may be congenital in young cats.
- Masses that arise from or involve the nasopharynx result in upper airway obstruction. Although nasopharyngeal polyps are rare in dogs, upper airway obstruction related to soft-tissue proliferation can develop in dogs with hyperprogesteronism secondary to drug administration or excessive hormone production in the bitch.

Tracheal Collapse. This condition is seen primarily in old, toy-breed dogs. Occasionally it is diagnosed in young dogs and may be congenital.

- The etiology of tracheal collapse is not known, but most likely is multifactorial, and related to changes in airflow dynamics due to primary small airway or upper airway disease. Potential etiologic factors include:
- Predisposition in small-breed dogs
  - Obesity
  - Degeneration of tracheal cartilages
  - Chronic bronchitis.

Tracheal Stenosis. Tracheal stenosis is usually a sequela of traumatic tracheal disruption.

- Animal bite wounds, traumatic intubation or extubation, and cervical gunshot wounds are common causes of tracheal disruption.
- Intraluminal foreign bodies and tracheal neoplasia can cause tracheal stenosis.
- Tracheal foreign bodies rarely cause complete obstruction; large items usually are retained at the carina while small ones often pass into the bronchi, leading to bronchial obstruction and pneumonia.

Primary Tracheal Neoplasia. These tumors are uncommon in dogs and rare in cats.

- Primary tracheal tumors reported in dogs include osteosarcoma, osteochondroma, chondrosarcoma, leiomyoma, mast cell tumor, adenocarcinoma, and squamous cell carcinoma.

■ Primary tracheal lymphosarcoma and adenocarcinoma have been reported in cats.

Extraluminal Compression of the Trachea. Segmental tracheal stenosis can be caused by compression from extraluminal masses such as parasitic granulomas *(Filaroides osleri)*, thyroid carcinoma (see sec. 4, ch. 1), hilar lymphadenopathy (see sec. 6, ch. 23), left atrial enlargement (see sec. 6, ch. 2), mediastinal lymphosarcoma (see sec. 3, ch. 6), and mediastinal lipoma.

CLINICAL SIGNS

Stertor and Stridor. These signs of obstructive upper respiratory disease are so common in brachycephalic dogs that owners frequently do not recognize noisy breathing as abnormal.

■ Stridor is a high-pitched inspiratory sound generated from obstruction of laryngeal air flow.

■ Dogs with an elongated soft palate often have characteristic stertorous "gurgling" respiratory sounds that result from occlusion of the rima glottidis by the excessively long soft palate.

■ Stridor and voice change are common in cats with nasopharyngeal polyps and in dogs with laryngeal paralysis.

Dyspnea. Dyspnea is observed in most animals with obstructive upper respiratory disease.

■ Inspiratory dyspnea, expiratory dyspnea, or a combination may be present, depending on the location and severity of obstruction.

■ Collapse of the cervical segment of the trachea results in primarily inspiratory dyspnea, whereas collapse of the thoracic segment of the trachea often is associated with expiratory dyspnea.

■ Animals with fixed upper respiratory obstruction such as tracheal stenosis and laryngeal collapse usually are continually dyspneic. Dyspnea may be intermittent and exacerbated by exercise, stress, or high ambient temperature in dogs with tracheal collapse or laryngeal paralysis.

Cough. Coughing is common in dogs with tracheal collapse and, with less frequency, in dogs with tracheal stenosis or laryngeal paralysis.

■ Approximately 50% of dogs with tracheal collapse have a characteristic "goose honk" cough associated with vibration in the collapsing segment. Many dogs with tracheal collapse do not have a characteristic cough, and some do not cough.

■ Dogs with tracheal collapse rarely cough continuously. The cough may be intermittent, and paroxysms usually are exacerbated by stress, excitement, and mechanical stimulation of the trachea.

Decreased Exercise Tolerance. Occasionally, decreased exercise tolerance is observed in dogs with laryngeal paralysis, tracheal stenosis, or brachycephalic syndrome.

Voice change. This may be an early clinical sign in dogs with laryngeal paralysis. It is also common in cats with nasopharyngeal polyps.

Hyperthermia. Symptoms of laryngeal paralysis frequently are not apparent until the animal is exposed to high ambient temperature; some dogs with laryngeal paralysis are presented with profound hyperthermia.

KEY POINT ▶ Evaluate laryngeal function in large-breed dogs requiring treatment for hyperthermia.

Gagging. Occasionally, gagging is observed early in the course of obstructive upper airway diseases such as laryngeal paralysis and elongated soft palate.

Dysphagia. Dysphagia may occur in cats with nasopharyngeal polyps and, rarely, in dogs with laryngeal paralysis.

Syncope. Fainting associated with exercise (overexertion), excitement, or coughing spells is common in dogs with tracheal collapse.

DIAGNOSIS

History

■ Animals in the early stages of obstructive upper airway disease typically are asymptomatic at rest.

■ Excitement or stress leads to varying degrees of coughing, dyspnea, and stridor.

■ Clinical signs may progress to constant, severe coughing and dyspnea.

■ Some animals with severe obstructive upper respiratory disease are presented with a history of cyanosis or syncope.

General Physical Examination

The physical examination often is unremarkable in dogs with obstructive upper respiratory diseases.

■ Distinct lateral tracheal borders may be identified on cervical palpation in dogs with tracheal collapse. Gentle tracheal palpation may cause paroxysms of coughing.

■ An ear discharge occasionally is identified in cats with nasopharyngeal polyps. Otoscopic examination may reveal polypoid masses within the external ear canal.

■ Stenosis of the external nares may be evident in brachycephalic dogs.

Oral Examination

A thorough oral examination under light general anesthesia is diagnostic for most obstructive upper airway diseases.

Brachycephalic Syndrome

■ The soft palate overlaps the tip of the epiglottis.

■ Everted laryngeal saccules are identified as oval mucosal masses projecting into the ventral rima glottidis, lateral to the vocal folds.

■ Enlarged tonsils and edematous pharyngeal mucosa are common.

Laryngeal Paralysis

■ Animals with laryngeal paralysis are unable to abduct the arytenoid cartilages and vocal folds during inspiration.

KEY POINT ▶ Use *light* anesthesia for evaluation of laryngeal function. A surgical plane of anesthesia will obliterate normal laryngeal reflexes.

■ Slight, asynchronous abduction of the arytenoids may be observed.
■ The majority of dogs with laryngeal paralysis have bilateral dysfunction of the cricoarytenoideus dorsalis muscle. Unilateral laryngeal paralysis (hemiplegia) is identified infrequently, perhaps because animals with unilateral involvement remain asymptomatic.
■ Laryngeal edema and inflammation also may be seen.

Laryngeal Collapse

■ The corniculate and cuneiform processes of the arytenoid cartilages are apposed or overlap, causing collapse of the airway.
■ Abduction of the arytenoids is not observed.

Nasopharyngeal Polyp

■ Expose the polyp by gently retracting the soft palate ventrally and rostrally.

Radiography

Radiographs of the pharyngeal, cervical, and thoracic regions are beneficial.

■ A soft tissue density cranial to the pharynx or increased radiodensity of one of the osseous bullae may be identified on skull radiographs of cats with nasopharyngeal polyps.
■ The soft palate may appear thickened and lengthened in dogs with elongated soft palate. Normally, the soft palate does not extend beyond the tip of the epiglottis.
■ Narrowing of the tracheal diameter may be evident on lateral cervical and thoracic radiographs in dogs with tracheal collapse. Collapse occurs most commonly at the thoracic inlet. Tracheal collapse is a dynamic disease, especially in the early stages. Obtain full inspiratory and expiratory views because the trachea may not be collapsed during all phases of respiration. A normal or near-normal tracheal diameter on plain film radiographs does not rule out tracheal collapse.
■ Tracheal stenosis is identified on a lateral cervical or thoracic radiograph as a focal reduction of the tracheal lumen diameter. Radiographs usually are adequate to establish a diagnosis of tracheal stenosis, owing to the static nature of the condition.
■ Aspiration pneumonia is an infrequent sequela of obstructive upper respiratory disease. Aspiration pneumonia typically is characterized by a mixed alveolar-interstitial density in the dependent portions of the cranial and middle lung lobes (see sec. 6, ch. 21).

Fluoroscopy

This modality allows continual assessment of the tracheal lumen diameter during all phases of the respiratory cycle. In dogs suspected of having tracheal collapse, evaluate the entire trachea and both mainstream bronchi during quiet respiration and induced coughing.

Tracheoscopy

Tracheoscopy is beneficial in assessing the location and severity of stenotic tracheal lesions. This procedure requires general anesthesia and close attention to patient oxygenation.

TREATMENT

Brachycephalic Syndrome

Nasal Wedge Resection

Surgical Anatomy. In the dog, the nasal vestibule is occupied by the end of the ventral nasal concha called the alar fold.

Preoperative Considerations

■ Administration of oxygen through a face mask for 3 to 5 minutes prior to induction (preoxygenation) is beneficial if it can be accomplished with little stress to the patient.
■ Tracheostomy may be desirable in brachycephalic dogs undergoing upper respiratory tract surgery.
■ Rapid induction of anesthesia and control of the airway is essential. Mask induction is discouraged.
■ A thorough evaluation of the upper airway is essential in animals with stenotic nares. Staphylectomy (soft palate excision) and laryngeal sacculectomy probably will be necessary.

Surgical Procedure
Objective. To increase the cross-sectional area of the nasal vestibule.
Equipment

■ #15 or #11 blade
■ 4-0 or 5-0 monofilament nylon or polypropylene suture material
■ Standard minor surgery pack

Technique

1. Excise a vertical triangular or elliptical wedge of tissue extending from the wing of the nostril caudally to include part of the alar cartilage. The base of the wedge should include one-third to one-half of the free edge of the nostril (Fig. 1).
2. Close the incision with 4-0 or 5-0 nylon suture material in a simple interrupted pattern.
3. If the cross-sectional area of the nasal vestibule has not been increased adequately, remove the sutures and excise more tissue.

Postoperative Care and Complications

■ Carefully monitor the dog during recovery and for several hours after surgery.

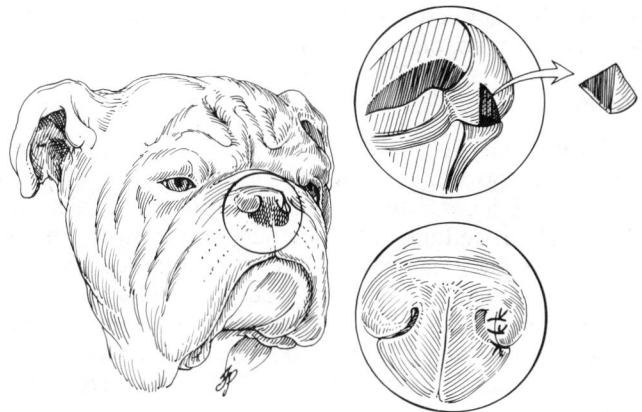

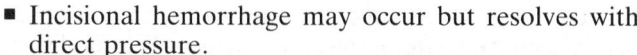

Figure 1. Wedge resection for stenotic nares.

■ Incisional hemorrhage may occur but resolves with direct pressure.
■ Signs of respiratory obstruction will persist following nasal wedge resection if concurrent obstructive upper respiratory diseases have not been managed properly.

Staphylectomy

Surgical Anatomy

■ The soft palate is a valve-like partition composed of mucosal and muscular layers.
■ The free edge of the soft palate should appose or slightly overlap the epiglottis.

Preoperative Considerations. See preceding discussion of nasal wedge resection.

Surgical Procedure
Objectives

■ To shorten the soft palate so that the free edge apposes or barely overlaps the epiglottis
■ To minimize pharyngeal and laryngeal edema by using an atraumatic technique

Equipment

■ Standard instrument pack and suture
■ Babcock forceps

Technique (Fig. 2)

1. Position the dog in ventral recumbency with the mouth held open with an oral speculum or adhesive tape sling.
2. Determine the portion of the soft palate that is excessive by placing it adjacent to the epiglottis.
3. Place traction sutures of 4-0 absorbable suture material in the lateral aspect of the soft palate adjacent to the point at which the epiglottis touches the soft palate.
4. Grasp the free border of the soft palate with Babcock forceps and retract it rostrally.
5. Incise approximately one third the width of the soft palate with Metzenbaum scissors. Suture the incised mucosal edges with 4-0 absorbable suture material in a simple continuous pattern. The nasal mucosa tends to retract caudally.

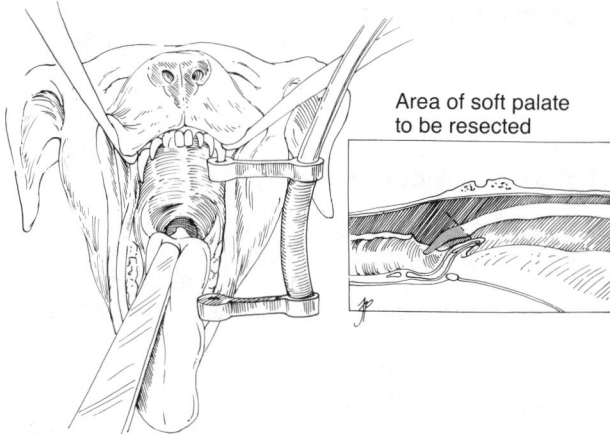

Area of soft palate to be resected

Figure 2. Staphylectomy. The area of soft palate to be resected is in red.

6. Continue the "cut-and-sew" technique (Fig. 3) until the palate is resected and closure is complete.
7. Avoid use of crushing clamps and electrocautery.

Postoperative Care and Complications

■ Laryngeal edema is a common postoperative complication in brachycephalic dogs that have had surgery on the upper respiratory tract.
  • At the conclusion of the surgical procedure administer a combination of prednisolone sodium succinate (2.5–5.0 mg/kg IV) and dexamethasone (0.5 mg/kg IV) or dexamethasone sodium phosphate alone (0.5 mg/kg IV), to reduce laryngeal edema.

KEY POINT ▶ Excessive resection of the soft palate may allow aspiration of food postoperatively because the shortened palate is unable to close off the nasopharynx during swallowing.

■ Clinical signs may persist if resection of the palate was inadequate.

Laryngeal Sacculectomy

Surgical Anatomy. Laryngeal saccules are small, mucosa-lined outpouchings that lie lateral to the vestibular folds.
Preoperative Considerations. See discussion of nasal wedge resection.

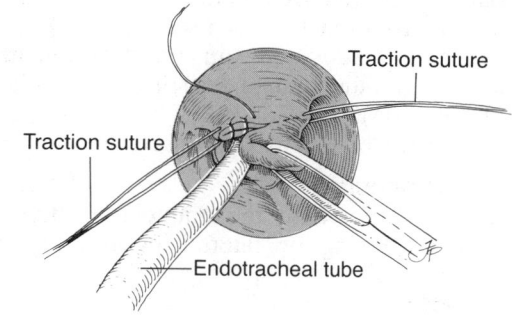

Traction suture
Traction suture
Endotracheal tube

Figure 3. "Cut-and-sew" procedure for palate resection.

Surgical Procedure

Objective. To remove the everted laryngeal saccules.

Equipment

- Metzenbaum scissors
- Babcock or Allis tissue forceps

Technique

1. Position the dog in ventral recumbency with the mouth held open with an oral speculum or adhesive tape sling.
2. Grasp the saccule with Babcock or Allis tissue forceps and retract it rostrally.
3. Amputate the saccule at its base with Metzenbaum scissors.
4. Use direct pressure to control hemorrhage. The cuff of the endotracheal tube can be used to apply pressure.

Postoperative Care and Complications. See discussion of soft palate resection.

Laryngeal Paralysis

Surgical Anatomy

- The larynx is supported by the cricoid and thyroid cartilages.
- Left and right arytenoid cartilages covered with mucous membrane are positioned at the rostral end of the larynx and form the dorsal part of the glottal cleft. The corniculate and cuneiform processes of the arytenoid cartilages project into the glottal cleft.
- The vocal folds form the ventral part of the glottal cleft.
- The cricoarytenoideus dorsalis muscles are innervated by the recurrent laryngeal nerves and are the only abductors of the arytenoid cartilages and vocal folds.

Preoperative Considerations

- Medical therapy for hyperthermic dogs in acute cyanotic crisis includes oxygen administration, alcohol or ice water baths, intravenous fluid therapy, and corticosteroids (prednisolone sodium succinate, 2.5–5.0 mg/kg IV, and dexamethasone, 0.5 mg/kg IV).
  - Sedation may be necessary (e.g., acepromazine) to calm hyperthermic animals.
  - Temporary tracheostomy (see sec. 1, ch. 3) may be necessary for animals that do not respond to initial conservative treatment.
- Evaluate thyroid function (see sec. 4, ch. 1).
- Preoxygenate the dog and gain control of the airway rapidly during induction of anesthesia (i.e. via tracheal intubation).
- Prepare for tracheostomy tube insertion.

Surgical Procedure

Objective. To increase the diameter of the rima glottidis by removing or lateralizing the arytenoid cartilages

Equipment

- Standard surgical pack and suture

- Long Metzenbaum scissors or laryngeal cup forceps
- Narrow malleable retractors

Technique

Several laryngoplasty techniques have been described. Reported success rates for the different procedures are inconsistent, making it difficult to identify the ideal procedure. The simplest procedure, per os partial arytenoidectomy and ventriculocordectomy, is used commonly as an initial procedure. More complicated procedures such as castellated laryngofissure and arytenoid lateralization may be performed initially or as a follow-up procedure to failed partial arytenoidectomy.

Partial Arytenoidectomy and Ventriculocordectomy

The objective of this procedure is to resect enough tissue to provide a functional airway without significantly compromising laryngeal function. Bilateral ventriculocordectomy combined with unilateral arytenoidectomy (Fig. 4) usually provides an adequate airway while minimizing webbing across the glottis and maintaining laryngeal function. The contralateral arytenoid may be removed at a later date if unilateral resection proves inadequate; however, excessive scar formation and resultant laryngeal stenosis is more common if this is done.

1. Perform a temporary tracheostomy and place the endotracheal tube through this approach.
2. Place the dog in ventral recumbency with the mouth held open with an oral speculum or adhesive tape sling.
3. Elevate the soft palate dorsally and depress the tongue with malleable retractors.
4. Remove the laryngeal saccules if they are everted.
5. Remove both vocal folds (ventriculocordectomy) and a portion of the cuneiform, corniculate, and vocal processes of the most affected arytenoid cartilage, using long Metzenbaum scissors or laryngeal cup forceps.
6. Avoid the dorsal commissure, where the arytenoid cartilages join dorsally, and the ventral commissure, where the vocal folds meet ventrally.
7. Control bleeding by direct pressure with gauze sponges.

Arytenoid Lateralization

Arytenoid lateralization involves freeing the arytenoid cartilage from its cartilaginous attachments and placing a nonabsorbable suture to permanently abduct

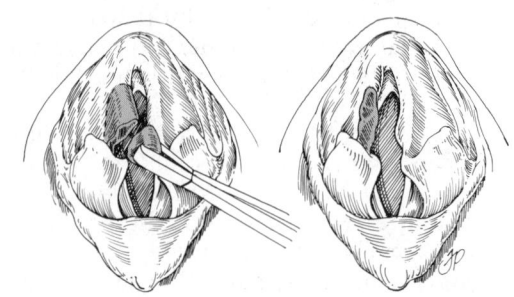

Figure 4. Partial arytenoidectomy.

the cartilage, thus increasing the diameter of the rima glottidis. The procedure can be performed unilaterally or bilaterally. Unilateral lateralization can be successful in alleviating clinical signs; however, results are not consistent.

Advantages of arytenoid lateralization are:

- The incidence of intraoperative hemorrhage and postoperative edema is less compared with intraoral procedures.
- Postoperative laryngeal scar formation is uncommon.
- Voice change is minimal because a ventriculo-cordectomy is not performed.
- Temporary tracheostomy seldom is needed.

1. Prepare the ventral cervical region for aseptic surgery.
2. Position the dog in dorsal recumbency with the neck extended over a small rolled towel.
3. Make a paramedian incision adjacent to the larynx, approximately in the jugular furrow. If bilateral arytenoid lateralization is planned, make a ventral midline incision from 2 cm rostral to 2 cm caudal to the larynx.
4. Continue the incision through the superficial muscle and subcutaneous fat and identify the sterno-thyroideus, thyrohyoideus, cricopharyngeus, and thyropharyngeus muscles (Fig. 5).
5. Grasp the dorsal edge of the thyroid cartilage through the thyropharyngeus muscle. Rotate the thyroid cartilage ventrally.
6. Transect the thyropharyngeus muscle along the dorsal edge of the thyroid cartilage (Fig. 6).
7. Elevate the exposed dorsal edge of the thyroid cartilage and incise the articulation of the thyroid

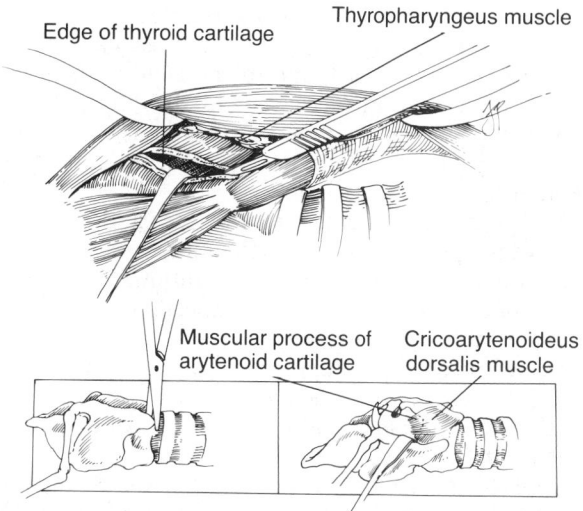

Figure 6. Arytenoid lateralization. Transect the thyropharyngeus muscle and expose the arytenoid cartilage. Below left, transect the cricothyroid articulation; below right, expose the arytenoid cartilage, accomplished by retracting thyroid cartilage.

and cricoid cartilages. The intrinsic muscles of the larynx are exposed. Identify the cricoarytenoideus dorsalis muscle.

8. Transect the cricoarytenoideus dorsalis muscle near its insertion on the muscular process of the arytenoid cartilage (Fig. 7). Preserve a section of the muscle for histologic analysis.
9. Retract the remainder of the cricoarytenoideus dorsalis muscle rostrally and visualize the cricoarytenoid articulation.
10. Separate the cricoarytenoid articulation with Mayo scissors.
11. Retract the arytenoid cartilage laterally.
12. Pass Mayo scissors between the arytenoid and cricoid cartilages and transect the arytenoid-arytenoid articulation on the dorsal midline of the larynx. Avoid incising the laryngeal mucosa.

KEY POINT ▶ Wound infection and postoperative stricture formation are more likely if the laryngeal mucosa is incised during this procedure.

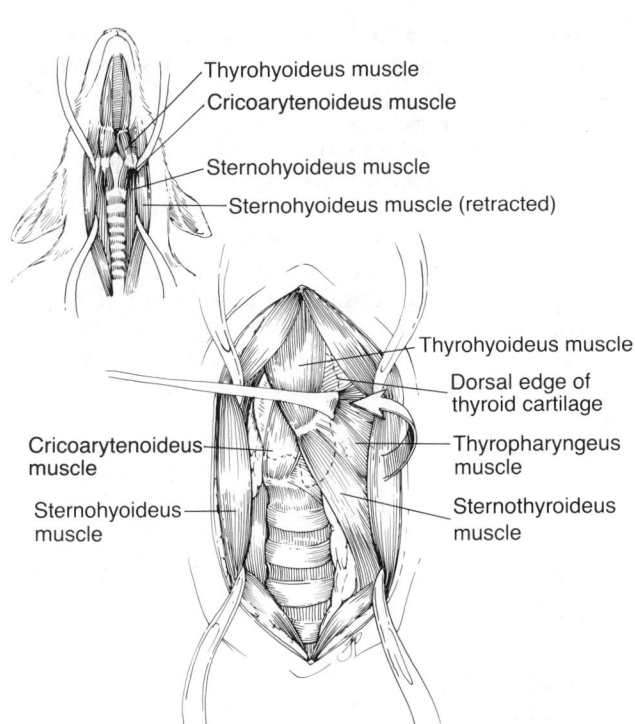

Figure 5. Arytenoid lateralization. Expose the surgical area and rotate the thyroid cartilage.

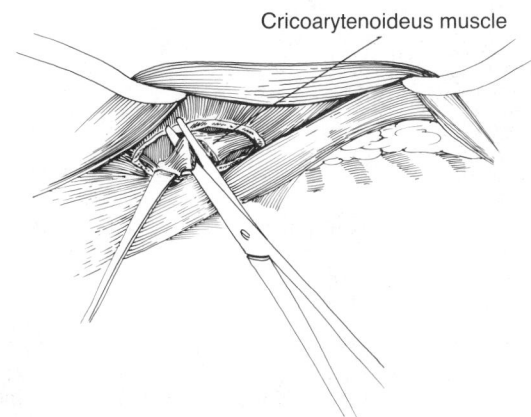

Figure 7. Arytenoid lateralization. Transect cricoarytenoideus dorsalis muscle.

13. Pass a monofilament nonabsorbable suture (0 nylon or polypropylene) from the muscular process of the arytenoid cartilage to the caudodorsal portion of the thyroid cartilage (Fig. 8). Alternatively, pass the suture from the muscular process of the arytenoid cartilage to the caudodorsal aspect of the cricoid cartilage (see Fig. 8).

14. Temporarily extubate the patient and have an assistant perform an oral examination to evaluate the degree of arytenoid lateralization. Temporary extubation is not necessary if anesthetic gasses are being delivered through an endotracheal tube passed through a temporary tracheostomy.

15. Tighten the suture as an assistant evaluates the position of the arytenoid cartilage. Knot the suture at the point of maximal abduction.

16. Replace the endotracheal tube if it was removed.

17. Close the thyropharyngeus muscle with 3-0 absorbable suture in a simple continuous pattern.

18. If indicated, perform the procedure on the contralateral side.

KEY POINT ▶ If the diameter of the rima glottidis is not adequate following unilateral lateralization, perform the procedure on the contralateral side.

19. Close the subcutaneous and skin layers routinely.

Postoperative Care and Complications

■ Laryngeal edema is a common sequelae of laryngoplasty. Carefully monitor postoperative laryngoplasty patients that do not have a tracheostomy tube for signs of upper respiratory obstruction. Administer corticosteroids and supplemental oxygen if laryngeal edema develops. Be prepared for emergency tracheostomy.

■ Manage tracheostomy tubes meticulously. Clean the tube as needed (at least every 2 hours). Double-cannula tracheostomy tubes are ideal (see sec. 1, ch. 3)

■ Laryngeal web formation resulting in cranial glottic stenosis is a potential complication of laryngoplasty, especially when excision of the vocal folds or arytenoid cartilages extends into the dorsal or ventral commisures. Laryngeal webbing can be managed surgically in some patients.

■ Failure to open the rima glottidis adequately may result in recurrence or persistence of clinical signs after surgery.
  • Consider contralateral arytenoidectomy, castellated laryngofissure, or arytenoid lateralization if signs recur after partial arytenoidectomy.
  • Consider lateralization of the contralateral arytenoid cartilage if signs recur or persist after unilateral arytenoid lateralization.

■ Bilateral arytenoidectomy or excision of excessive arytenoid tissue during partial arytenoidectomy may result in laryngeal dysfunction characterized by episodes of aspiration pneumonia and gagging. Surgical amelioration of this condition is unlikely. Permanent tracheostomy can be performed as a salvage procedure.

Laryngeal Collapse

Treat the predisposing factors, such as stenotic nares, everted laryngeal saccules, and elongated soft palate. If clinical signs persist, reevaluate the respiratory tract. Persistence of clinical signs after appropriate surgical management of predisposing factors may necessitate a permanent tracheostomy.

Permanent Tracheostomy

Preoperative Considerations

■ Permanent tracheostomy is a salvage procedure that usually is indicated for treatment of end-stage laryngeal disease. Permanent tracheostomy is performed following laryngectomy for laryngeal neoplasia.

■ Detailed client communication is vital prior to performing permanent tracheostomy. Explain the procedure, potential postoperative complications, and activity restrictions (see below).

■ Make certain the segment of the trachea distal to the proposed tracheostomy site is normal. Tracheoscopy or fluoroscopy is preferable; however, inspiratory and expiratory cervical and thoracic radiographs may be adequate to evaluate the integrity of the distal trachea.

■ Use an endotracheal tube with a high-volume, low-pressure cuff that has been checked for leaks. Position the cuff distal to the proposed tracheostomy site.

Surgical Procedure
Objective. To create a permanent stoma in the cervical segment of the trachea.

Equipment
■ Standard surgical pack and suture
■ Tracheostomy tube with a high-volume, low-pressure cuff (tube must be long enough to allow positioning of the cuff in the caudal cervical trachea).

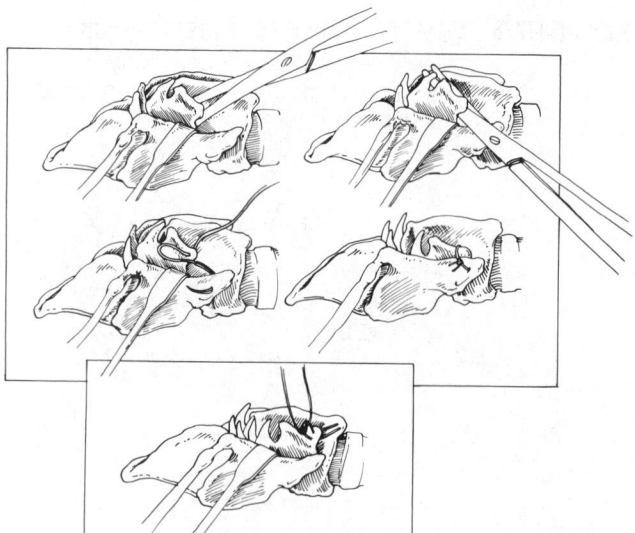

Figure 8. Arytenoid lateralization. Suture adduction. Top, transect the arytenoid-arytenoid articulation carefully, avoiding incising the laryngeal mucosa; suture the muscular process of the arytenoid cartilage to the caudodorsal portion of the thyroid cartilage. Inset, the alternate Lattue approach.

Technique

1. Position the dog in dorsal recumbency with the neck extended over a rolled towel. Prepare the ventral cervical region for aseptic surgery.
2. Make a ventral cervical midline incision through the skin and subcutaneous tissues, beginning at the larynx and extending caudally approximately 10 cm. Center the incision over the proposed tracheostomy site.
3. Separate the paired sternohyoideus muscles, exposing the trachea.
4. Bluntly dissect the cervical fascia from the entire circumference of the trachea between the second and sixth tracheal cartilages.

KEY POINT ▶ Identify and avoid the recurrent laryngeal nerves when dissecting the cervical fascia from the trachea.

5. Preplace two horizontal mattress sutures (2-0 polyglycolic) between the sternohyoideus muscles, passing *dorsal* to the trachea where the cervical fascia was dissected.
6. Tie the horizontal mattress sutures. This apposes the sternohyoideus muscles dorsal to the trachea, decreasing tension on the mucocutaneous anastomosis by deviating the trachea ventrally to the level of the skin.
7. Make a partial-thickness rectangular incision in the tracheal wall. Make the segment to be excised three tracheal cartilages long (include the third, fourth, and fifth cartilages) and approximately one-third the width of the the tracheal circumference (Fig. 9).

KEY POINT ▶ Do not make a full-thickness incision in the tracheal wall. Incise the tracheal wall to the level of the mucosa.

8. Bluntly elevate the tracheal cartilages and annular ligaments from the tracheal mucosa inside the boundaries of the rectangular incision. Remove the cartilages and annular ligaments, leaving the mucosa intact.
9. Excise a rectangular section of skin adjacent to the stoma bilaterally. Make each section equal to the

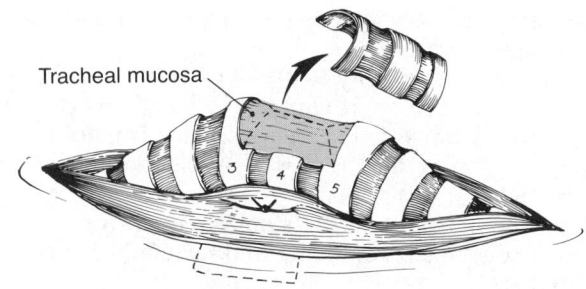

Figure 9. Permanent tracheostomy. Remove the segment of ventral trachea with remaining mucosa intact (red). The dotted line indicates the area of mucosa and skin to be incised to complete the stoma.

length and approximately one-half the width of the tracheal stoma (Fig. 10).

10. Secure the skin to the trachea by placing simple interrupted sutures (2-0 polyglycolic) between the dermis (not the skin edge) and the fascia on the lateral aspect of the trachea.
11. Check the endotracheal tube position and make certain that the cuff is inflated. The cuff should be positioned approximately 2 cm distal to the stoma.
12. Incise the tracheal mucosa, as shown in Figure 10.
13. Place simple interrupted sutures (4-0 monofilament nylon) 2 mm apart between the skin and tracheal mucosa. Precise apposition is important.

KEY POINT ▶ Make certain that there is no tension on the mucocutaneous sutures. Tension predisposes to dehiscence and stenosis.

14. Close the skin incision cranial and caudal to the stoma.
15. Gently suction the tracheal lumen proximal to the cuff to remove clotted blood.

Postoperative Care and Complications

▪ Clean the stoma every 4–6 hours for 48 hours after surgery. Cleaning is needed less frequently after 48 hours. Instruct the owner to clean the stoma once a day.

▪ Protect the stoma from self-trauma. Elizabethan collars are not recommended. Rarely, rear-limb hob-

Figure 10. Permanent tracheostomy. After the mucosa is incised and removed, suture the skin directly to the peritracheal fascia and the annular ligament. Complete the stoma by closing the mucosa and skin with simple interrupted sutures.

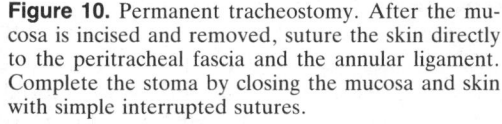
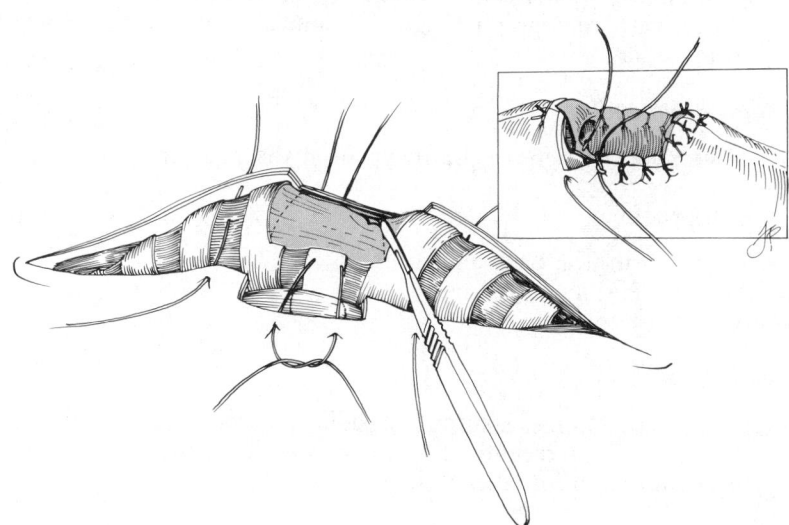

bles are necessary to keep the animal from scratching the surgery site.

- Apply petroleum jelly to the skin around the stoma once a day for approximately 2 weeks to prevent irritation from dried secretions. This usually is not necessary after hair regrows. Avoid putting petroleum jelly in the stoma.
- Trim the hair around the stoma frequently.
- Dirty, dusty environments and swimming must be avoided.
- Skin-fold occlusion of the stoma resulting in episodes of respiratory distress is the most common postoperative complication. Excision of redundant skin may be necessary, especially in brachycephalic breeds.
- Approximately 60% of dogs and cats are unable to bark or purr after permanent tracheostomy.
- All tracheostomies stenose approximately 20 to 40%. The degree of stenosis is variable and can be minimized by meticulous surgical technique.
- Closure of the stoma rarely is indicated. Closure is accomplished by resection of the stomal segment and primary anastomosis (see discussion of tracheal resection and anastomosis).

Nasopharyngeal Polyp

Surgical Anatomy

- The auditory (Eustachian) tube extends from the nasal pharynx to the rostral portion of the tympanic cavity. The pharyngeal opening of the auditory tube is an oblique, slit-like opening that lies on the lateral wall of the nasal pharynx above the middle of the soft palate.
- The tympanic bulla is a smooth bulbous enlargement of the temporal bone, located between the retroarticular and jugular processes.

Preoperative Considerations

- Obtain skull radiographs preoperatively. Evaluate the tympanic bulla and petrous-temporal bones for evidence of middle-ear infection, including osseous bulla thickening, increased density within the tympanic cavity, and sclerosis of the petrous-temporal bone.
- Be prepared to perform a ventral bulla osteotomy in cats with radiographic signs or clinical signs of otitis media.

Surgical Procedure

Objective. To remove the polyp from the pharynx and bulla.

Equipment

- Standard surgical pack and suture
- Atraumatic spay hook
- Allis tissue forceps

Technique

1. If a ventral bulla osteotomy is indicated, position the cat in dorsal recumbency and prepare the ventral cervical region for aseptic surgery.

2. Perform a ventral bulla osteotomy (see sec. 5, chap. 24) on the side with radiographic evidence of otitis media. If the cat is affected bilaterally, perform the osteotomy on the side of origin of the polyp. If the side of origin can not be determined, perform the osteotomy on the side with the most pronounced radiographic changes.
3. Expose both the dorsomedial and ventrolateral compartments of the tympanic cavity and carefully remove all inflammatory tissue. Submit tissues for histologic analysis. Avoid curettage of the dorsomedial aspect of the tympanic cavity.
4. Submit material from the bulla for bacterial culture and sensitivity testing.
5. Place a small rubber drain in the bulla that exits from an opening in the skin adjacent to the primary incision.
6. Position the cat in sternal recumbency with the mouth held open by a mouth speculum or adhesive tape sling.
7. Retract the soft palate cranially and ventrally with an atraumatic spay hook.
8. Grasp the nasopharyngeal polyp with an Allis tissue forceps and apply slow steady traction until the mass is removed. A long stalk should be attached at the base.
9. Submit the excised tissue for histologic evaluation.

Postoperative Care and Complications

- Observe for laryngeal edema postoperatively.
- Horner's syndrome is a common complication of bulla osteotomy in cats. Symptoms typically resolve within 4 weeks.
- Leave the drain in the bulla osteotomy site for 3 to 5 days.
- Administer antibiotics based on results of culture and sensitivity testing.
- Nasopharyngeal polyps may recur as a result of incomplete excision of inflammatory tissue. Failure to perform a bulla osteotomy in cats with middle ear involvement is a common cause of recurrence.

Tracheal Collapse

Application of Extraluminal Prostheses

Surgical Anatomy

- Individual C-shaped cartilage rings provide structural rigidity for the trachea.
- The space left by failure of the cartilage rings to meet dorsally is spanned by the transversely oriented trachealis muscle and connective tissue, collectively referred to as the dorsal tracheal membrane.
- The left recurrent laryngeal nerve lies on the left lateral or dorsolateral aspect of the trachea.
- The trachea is supplied by the cranial thyroid, caudal thyroid, and bronchoesophageal arteries. These arteries are enmeshed in delicate sheets of connective tissue on the lateral aspects of the trachea called lateral pedicles. Small, transversely oriented branches penetrate between tracheal rings and arborize in the tracheal submucosa.

Preoperative Considerations

- Consider surgical management on initial presentation only in dogs that are experiencing life-threatening dyspnea or syncope. Treat other dogs medically (Table 1) for approximately 4 weeks before considering surgical management. Dogs with mild to moderate tracheal collapse that respond well to medical management may not require surgery.
- Perform a transtracheal wash and submit samples for bacterial culture and sensitivity testing.
- Be certain that the location of collapse has been identified.
- Anesthesia (see sec. 1, ch. 2 for details on drug dosages):

TABLE 1. Medical Treatment of Tracheal Collapse

Avoid airborne irritants or allergens
  If any can be identified.

Identify and then minimize exacerbating factors
  Such as excitement, stress, extremes of air temperature and humidity, etc.

Control daily activity
  At limits that minimize fatigue, episodes of exercise-induced cough, or dyspnea.

Nutritional counseling
  To correct overweight body condition.

Routine preventive dental care
  To reduce bacterial contamination of the pharynx and upper airway.

Prevent dehydration
  To maintain low viscosity of airway secretions and thereby promote clearance.

Promote clearance of airway secretions
  By first liquefying them, using humidifier/vaporizer treatments (probably more effective than expectorant drugs), and then facilitating their removal, using physiotherapy (light exercise, coupage, or percussion).

Prevent infectious tracheobronchitis (kennel cough complex)
  Through vaccination for parainfluenza, adenovirus, and *Bordetella*.

Antibiotics
  If complicating bacterial airway infections are suspected use cephalosporins, trimethoprim-sulfa, or others as guided by tracheobronchial cultures; aerosol administration (gentamycin, 50 mg q12h for 5–7 days) may be more effective for eliminating *Bordetella* from the airways.

Reduce airway inflammation
  Use an oral glucocorticosteroid (prednisone, 1–2 mg/kg/day for 1–2 weeks; if improvement is noted, then continue with alternate-day maintenance.

Bronchodilator therapy (see sec. 6, ch. 20 for table of drug dosages)
  Administer drugs such as aminophylline, theophylline, oxtriphylline, or terbutaline, although the reversibility of lower airway obstruction in canine bronchitis and tracheobronchitis may be limited.

Antitussive therapy (see sec. 6, ch. 20 for table of drug dosages)
  Administer drugs such as hydrocodone to control cough that is distressful to the owner or that causes exhaustion or episodic collapse in the animal; use cautiously and only intermittently if possible, because suppression of the cough reflex may be detrimental to clearance of airway secretions in chronic bronchitis.

- Choose an endotracheal tube that is long enough to reach the thoracic inlet. Test the cuff.
- Premedicate with diazepam.
- Administer a *light* dose of thiobarbiturate. Evaluate laryngeal function.
- Induce anesthesia and rapidly gain control of the airway.
- Prepare for mechanical ventilation.

- Administer cefazolin (25 mg/kg IV) at induction of anesthesia and 2 hours after the first dose.

Surgical Procedure
Objective. To provide rigid support for the collapsed tracheal segment and maintain function of the mucociliary system.

Equipment

- Spiral- or ring-shaped prostheses made from the case and barrel of a 3-ml polypropylene syringe case (Fig. 11).
- 4-0 polypropylene suture material with a tapercut needle.
- Standard instrument pack and suture
- Small Gelpi retractors

Technique

1. Position the dog in dorsal recumbency with the neck extended over a small rolled towel.
2. Prepare the ventral cervical region for aseptic surgery.
3. Incise the skin on the ventral cervical midline from the larynx to the manubrium.
4. Separate the paired sternohyoideus and sternothyroideus muscles on the midline and retract the muscles laterally with Gelpi retractors. Partially myotomize the sternocephalicus muscles at the manubrial attachment.
5. Identify the left recurrent laryngeal nerve.
6. Beginning approximately 2 cm caudal to the larynx and preserving the caudal thyroid artery, dissect the lateral pedicle from the left side of the trachea to the level of the thoracic inlet.
7. Make a 5-mm window in the right lateral pedicle 2 cm caudal to the larynx, preserving the caudal thyroid artery.
8. Position a right-angle forceps dorsal to the trachea through the window in the right lateral pedicle; grasp the spiral prosthesis and direct the prosthesis around the trachea.

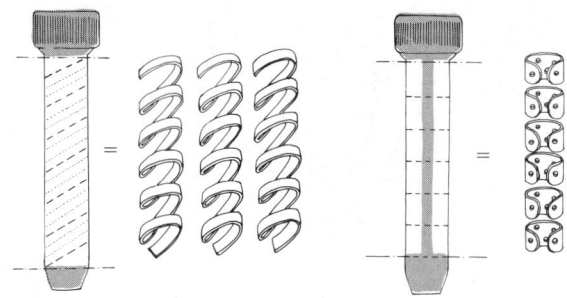

Figure 11. Extraluminal prosthesis. The barrel of a 3-cc polypropylene syringe case can be used to make spiral or ring-shaped tracheal prostheses.

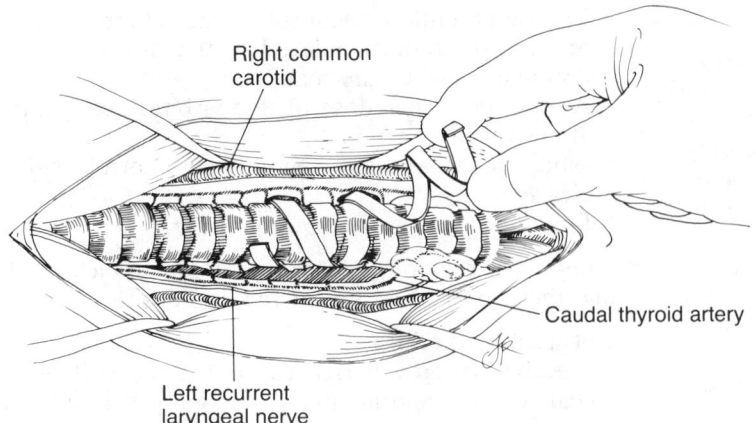

Right common
carotid

Caudal thyroid artery

Left recurrent
laryngeal nerve

Figure 12. Extraluminal prosthesis. Rotate the prosthesis onto the trachea.

9. Rotate the prosthesis onto the trachea, making a small window in the right lateral pedicle where the prosthesis passes around the right lateral aspect of the trachea. Position the prosthesis over the collapsed segment of the trachea (Fig. 12).
10. When applying total ring prostheses, segmentally dissect both the right and left lateral pedicles.
11. Deflate the endotracheal tube cuff and reposition the tube either cranial or caudal to the prosthesis. Reinflate the endotracheal tube cuff.
12. Suture the prosthesis to the trachea with 4-0 polypropylene suture material placed in simple interrupted fashion. Place a row of sutures laterally, ventrally, and dorsally, including the dorsal tracheal membrane. All sutures enter the tracheal lumen (Fig. 13).
13. Apply additional protheses caudally as needed. Gentle cranial traction on the cervical trachea affords limited exposure to the segment of the trachea in the thoracic inlet.
14. Deflate the endotracheal tube cuff and gently move the tube in the trachea to ensure that sutures have not been placed through the endotracheal tube cuff. Reinflate the cuff.
15. Appose the sternocephalicus, sternohyoideus, and

sternothyroideus muscles. Close the subcutaneous tissue and skin in a routine manner.
16. The intrathoracic segment of the trachea can be supported by performing a right third intercostal thoracotomy (see sec. 6, ch. 25) and applying prostheses as described above.

Postoperative Care and Complications

- Leave the endotracheal tube in place with the cuff inflated until the dog has a strong swallowing reflex. Deflate the cuff prior to removing the tube.
- Administer supplemental oxygen postoperatively as needed.
- Administer corticosteroids immediately postoperatively and at 6 hours postoperatively to minimize tracheal mucosal swelling (see discussion of soft palate resection for drugs and dosages).
- Continue antibiotic therapy for 14 days after surgery.
- Continue antitussive and bronchodilator therapy as needed to control coughing (see Table 1).
- Observe the dog for subcutaneous emphysema and signs of tracheal obstruction for 5 days after surgery.
- Ischemic necrosis of the trachea resulting from dissection of the lateral pedicles occurs in a limited number of cases. Gentle tissue handling and mini-

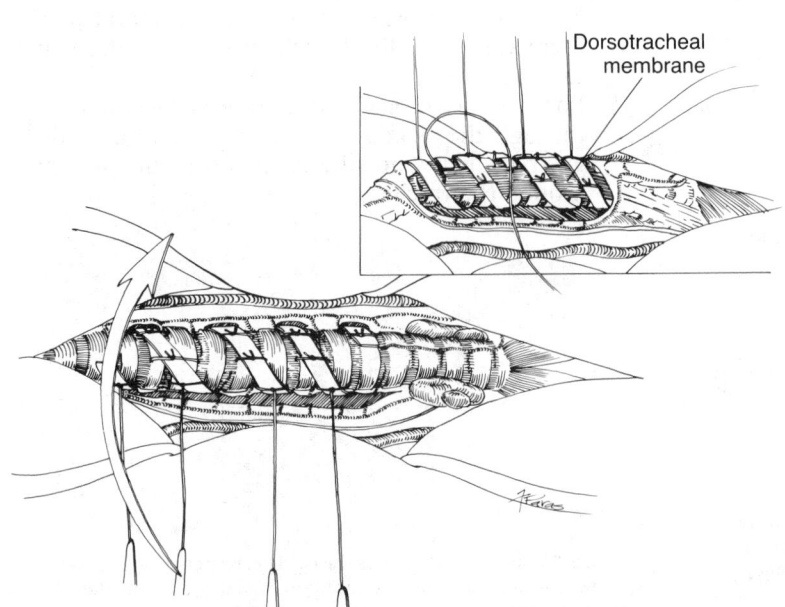

Dorsotracheal
membrane

Figure 13. Extraluminal prosthesis. Suture the prosthesis to the trachea laterally, ventrally, and dorsally. All sutures enter the tracheal lumen.

mizing dissection of the lateral pedicles reduces the incidence of this complication.

Segmental Stenosis

Tracheoscopy

Tracheal foreign bodies often can be removed with a fiberoptic endoscope. Various transendoscopic retrieval devices are available for flexible and rigid endoscopes.

Technique

General anesthesia is required for this procedure:

1. Attach a Y-shaped swivel adapter that has a self-sealing port for passage of the endoscope (Fiberoptic Scope/Suction Catheter Adapter with Swivel, Portex, Inc., Wilmington, ME) to the endotracheal tube. This allows simultaneous tracheoscopy and inhalation anesthesia in dogs intubated with a tube with an inner diameter > 7.5 mm.
2. Anesthetize small dogs and cats with an intravenous anesthetic and pass the endoscope directly into the trachea.
3. Position the animal in sternal recumbency with the head elevated.
4. Insert an oral speculum to prevent the animal from biting and damaging the endoscope.
5. Carefully insert the endoscope into the trachea. Examine the trachea and bronchi and locate the foreign body.
6. Critically evaluate the type and position of the foreign body before attempting to remove it. Foreign bodies embedded in the tracheal mucosa or that have sharp edges may not be amenable to transendoscopic removal.
7. Pass the retrieval instrument through the operative port of the endoscope. Position the retrieval instrument either proximal (forceps) or distal (basket device) to the foreign body.
8. Grasp the foreign body and *gently* retract the endoscope and foreign body together. Tracheotomy or tracheal resection and anastomosis may be necessary if the foreign body is firmly lodged in the trachea.

KEY POINT ▶ Excessive traction on a foreign body firmly lodged in the trachea may cause severe tracheal trauma.

9. After the foreign body has been removed, replace the endoscope and perform a thorough, systematic inspection of all accessible parts of the trachea and bronchial tree.

Postoperative Care and Complications

- Complications are rare after transendoscopic removal of a tracheal foreign body.
- Moderate coughing from tracheal irritation is common but transient.
- If the foreign body was firmly lodged in the trachea and removal was difficult, closely monitor the animal for signs of tracheal trauma (e.g. subcutaneous emphysema) for 48–72 hours.

Tracheal Resection and Anastomosis

Tracheal resection and anastomosis is indicated for treatment of tracheal stricture, tracheal neoplasia, and, rarely, for removal of a tracheal foreign body. Meticulous surgical technique is imperative to minimize postanastomotic stenosis.

Surgical Anatomy
- Review surgical anatomy in the tracheal collapse section.
- The tracheal cartilages are joined ventrally and laterally by 1-mm wide fibroelastic bands called annular ligaments.

Preoperative Considerations
- Identify the extent of the stenotic lesion radiographically and/or endoscopically.
- Anesthesia:
  - Endotracheal intubation may be difficult or impossible when the cranial cervical segment of the trachea is stenotic. Be prepared to perform a tracheostomy for delivery of anesthetic gases.
  - Gain control of the airway rapidly. Mask induction is not advisable.
- Administer cefazolin (25 mg/kg IV) at induction of anesthesia and 2 hours after the first dose.

Surgical Procedure
Objective. To remove the stenotic segment of the trachea and create an airtight anastomosis under minimal tension.

Equipment
- Standard surgical pack and suture
- Gelpi retractors
- 2-0 and 3-0 polypropylene suture material with a tapercut needle

Technique

Many techniques for tracheal resection and anastomosis have been described. The split-cartilage technique is ideal because the technique is easy to perform and results in more precise anatomic alignment with less luminal stenosis compared with other anastomotic techniques.

1. Patient positioning and surgical approach are the same as for application of tracheal prostheses.
2. Dissect the right and left lateral pedicles from the stenotic segment of the trachea.
3. Place stay sutures one cartilage cranial and one cartilage caudal to the stenotic segment to prevent retraction and facilitate manipulation of the incised ends.
4. Reposition the endotracheal tube so that the cuff is distal to the stenotic segment. Perform the resection and anastomosis over the endotracheal tube if possible. Do not manipulate the distal segment with the endotracheal tube cuff inflated.
5. Using a #10 blade, circumferentially split in half one tracheal cartilage at each end of the stenotic segment. Incise the stenotic segment longitudinally and remove it. Submit the diseased segment for histologic evaluation.

6. Preplace four to six simple interrupted tension-relieving sutures with 2-0 polypropylene suture material between the cranial and caudal tracheal segments. Pass each suture around the second or third tracheal cartilage cranial and caudal to the anastomotic site.

7. Bring the cranial and caudal segments into apposition by tying the tension sutures.

8. Place eight to 12 simple interrupted sutures, encompassing the split tracheal cartilage at the end of the cranial and caudal segment. Penetrate the tracheal lumen and tie knots on the outside of the trachea. Make certain that the edges of the dorsal tracheal membrane are apposed.

Postoperative Care and Complications

- Leave the endotracheal tube in place with the cuff inflated until the dog has a strong swallowing reflex. Deflate the cuff and then carefully remove the tube.
- Observe for signs of tracheal obstruction. Mucosal swelling rarely is a problem after resection and anastomosis.
- Discourage extension of the neck if the resected segment was large (i.e., more than five tracheal cartilages).
- Obtain cervical radiographs 1, 2, and 3 months after surgery. Follow-up tracheoscopy to assess healing is ideal.
- Postanastomotic stenosis is the most common complication. Excessive anastomotic tension usually is the cause. Complications such as air leakage, infection, mucostasis, and dehiscence occur rarely.

Supplemental Readings

Evans HE, Christensen GC: *Miller's Anatomy of the Dog*, Philadelphia: W. B. Saunders, 1979.

Fingland RB, DeHoff WD, Birchard SJ: Surgical management of cervical and thoracic tracheal collapse in dogs using extraluminal spiral prostheses. J Am Anim Hosp Assoc 23:501, 1987.

Hedlund CS: Surgical diseases of the trachea. Vet Clin North Am: [Small Anim Pract] 17:301, 1987.

Rosin E, Greenwood K: Bilateral arytenoid cartilage lateralization for laryngeal paralysis in the dog. J Am Vet Med Assoc 180:515, 1982.

20 Bronchopulmonary Disorders

John D. Bonagura

OVERVIEW

Causes in Dogs

Dogs frequently are afflicted with diseases of the trachea, bronchial tree, alveoli, and pulmonary interstitium.

- Chronic bronchitis and pulmonary fibrosis are probably the most frequent causes of chronic coughing and shortness of breath.
- Noninfectious inflammatory conditions (e.g., pulmonary granulomatosis, pulmonary infiltrates with eosinophils) and pulmonary neoplasia (see sec. 6, ch. 23) are important causes of acute and chronic respiratory signs.
- Infectious causes of chronic respiratory disease include bacterial bronchitis (see sec. 6, ch. 21), paragonimiasis and other lungworm infections, heartworm disease (see sec. 6, ch. 10), and systemic mycotic infections (see sec. 2, ch. 12).
- Infectious tracheobronchitis can be caused by agents of canine kennel cough complex (i.e., adenoviruses, parainfluenza virus, and *Bordetella bronchiseptica*) (see sec. 2, ch. 5).
- Canine distemper virus can cause bronchopulmonary signs (see sec. 2, ch. 6).
- Pulmonary edema (both cardiogenic and noncardiogenic) (see sec. 6, ch. 6), sepsis, thoracic trauma (see sec. 6, ch. 23), pulmonary embolism (including heartworm disease), and diffuse metastatic neoplasia (see sec. 6, ch. 22) can cause acute pulmonary injury and respiratory distress in dogs.

Causes in Cats

Cats often are presented for acute or chronic respiratory signs caused by bronchopulmonary disorders.

- Chronic bronchitis, including bronchial "asthma," is a frequent cause of coughing, gagging, and dyspnea.
- Pulmonary neoplasia, although less common in cats than in dogs, is an important consideration when acute or chronic respiratory signs are present.
- Lungworm and heartworm infections may cause acute or chronic respiratory problems.
- In cats with chronic infectious bronchitis or middle lung lobe pneumonia, consider an underlying immunosuppressive disease such as feline leukemia virus (FeLV) (see sec. 2, ch. 1) and feline immunodeficiency virus (FIV) (see sec. 2, ch. 2).
- Infectious agents that can attack the respiratory tract include herpesvirus, calcivirus, and chlamydia, which are the agents of the feline infectious respiratory disease complex (see sec. 2, ch. 5).
- Thoracic trauma is a common cause of respiratory distress in cats.

Clinical Signs

The clinical manifestations of chronic bronchopulmonary disorders often are characterized by a long history of respiratory dysfunction. Because initial signs of pulmonary disease may be subtle or intermittent, clients may not present their pets for evaluation until considerable disability has developed.

- The most frequent clinical signs include tachypnea, dyspnea, and cough.
- Distinguish signs associated with bronchopulmonary disease from upper airway disorders such as tracheal collapse (see sec. 6, ch. 17), tracheobronchial tumors or foreign bodies, nasopharyngeal tumors or polyps, and congestive heart failure (CHF) caused by mitral regurgitation (see sec. 6, ch. 7) or cardiomyopathy. (see sec. 6, ch. 8).

CHRONIC BRONCHITIS IN THE DOG

Etiology

The etiology of chronic bronchitis in the dog in most cases is unknown.

- Some cases of chronic or recurrent viral or bacterial infection clearly suggest an abnormality of local immunity (e.g., IgA) or in mechanical airway defense mechanisms.
- Always consider chronic infection with *Bordetella bronchiseptica* in younger dogs with lingering "kennel-cough" (see sec. 2, ch. 5).
- Rarely, bronchitis can be associated with ciliary dyskinesia, a congenital abnormality of respiratory cilia. These dogs typically have recurrent bacterial sinusitis, bronchitis, and pneumonia.
- Environmental pollutants, including passive exposure to cigarette smoke, and hypersensitivity reactions are speculated to be causes of chronic airway irritation and injury, but it is difficult to document this.
- A relationship of chronic respiratory diseases to poor oral health is suggested but unproved.
- Migrating intestinal larvae may provoke bronchopulmonary hypersensitivity.

Pathophysiology

Chronic bronchitis is a persistent inflammatory change in the bronchial tree that may involve lobar bronchi or the smaller airways.

- Chronic bronchial inflammation or irritation, regardless of cause, seems to promote the predictable responses of increased tracheobronchial secretions (mucus and "sputum"), cough, and progressive architectural changes in the bronchial tree that alter air flow.
- Morphologic changes associated with chronic bronchitis can include proliferation of goblet cells, narrowing of bronchial lumina, ectasia (or bronchiectasis) of larger airways, and alteration in the normal respiratory epithelium predisposing the airways to secondary infection.
- Visual examination of the bronchial tree (e.g., by fiberoptic bronchoscopy) demonstrates hyperemia and granularity of the mucosa, mucus hypersecretion, and exudate that may occlude smaller bronchi. Bronchiectasis (irreversible saccular dilation of bronchi), pneumonia, pulmonary fibrosis, and large airway disease (tracheal, main-stem bronchi) also are evident in some dogs.
- Histologic lesions in chronic bronchitis include mucosal hyperemia, mucosal proliferation with focal ulceration and squamous metaplasia, infiltration of the lamina propria by mononuclear cells and neutrophils, and edema and fibrosis of the bronchial walls.
  - Bronchial mucus glands and goblet cells increase in size and number. The bronchial luminal dimensions are reduced from weakened walls and edema, contributing to decreased air flow.
  - Mild emphysematous changes due to loss of interalveolar septa produce increased air spaces distal to terminal bronchioles. These areas of emphysema are noted at the periphery of the lung. Uncommonly, severe gas trapping develops and the lungs appear histologically and grossly overinflated.
- Although mild changes have little functional significance, severe alterations obstruct air flow and also cause ventilation:perfusion (V/Q) inequalities in the lung.
  - Small airway obstruction leads to increased work of breathing, which can be compounded by dynamic, expiratory collapse of the large airways. Lobar bronchi and the intrathoracic trachea may totally collapse during forced expiration or with coughing.
  - Mucus and bronchial secretions stimulate coughing. Mucus plugs may further obstruct gas flow and lead to reabsorption atelectasis. Bronchiectasis predisposes to recurrent respiratory infection.

Clinical Signs

Signalment

The typical signalment of dogs with chronic noninfective bronchitis is an adult dog of a small or medium-sized breed. Chronic infective tracheobronchitis is more common in dogs less than 1 year of age.

History

Regardless of etiology, coughing is the hallmark of chronic bronchitis and is usually progressive in frequency and severity.

- Clinical findings in dogs with chronic noninfective bronchitis include "dry" or productive cough (depending on whether the sputum is swallowed or coughed up), tachypnea, shortness of breath with exercise, and intermittent expectoration or gagging (misinterpreted as vomiting by many owners). Wheezing may be evident following exertion.
- Frequently, the pet has coughed for years prior to the owner's seeking veterinary help. The cough is worsened by exercise and may be exacerbated at variable times of the day.
- Severely affected dogs become cyanotic with exertion and may faint after coughing (cough-syncope).
- Appetite generally is unaffected and weight loss is uncommon, which helps to distinguish bronchitis from chronic CHF, which often is characterized by weight loss. Anorexia, marked depression, or fever in the dog with chronic bronchitis suggests complicating respiratory infection or pneumonia.

Physical Examination

The dog usually is well-fleshed, except in advanced cases.

- Coughing can be elicited upon palpation of the trachea or during excitement. Tracheal sensitivity is a nonspecific finding, however, and does not necessarily indicate tracheitis.
- The respiratory rate may be increased, and shortness of breath may be severe, particularly in dogs with concurrent pulmonary fibrosis.
- The dog may appear to be "barrel-chested," and some dogs exhibit cyanosis with dyspnea during both inspiration and expiration.
- Auscultation of the lungs is abnormal.
  - Auscultate while the dog is breathing deeply, because abnormal lung sounds (especially crackles) may be overlooked if the lung is not adequately expanded. Close the mouth to prevent referral of tracheal sounds to the thorax. If necessary, occlude the nostrils for 10–15 seconds to force the dog to inspire deeply.
  - Some dogs have wheezing due to mucus plugging and dynamic expiratory collapse of intrathoracic airways. In advanced cases, bilateral crackles will be evident during inspiration and possibly expiration. These crackles frequently are louder than those heard with cardiogenic pulmonary edema.
  - A snapping sound heard over the trachea or the carina suggests concurrent tracheal collapse or collapsing of the main-stem bronchus.
  - In most cases, the heart sounds are normal, permitting the clinician to virtually eliminate valvular heart disease from the differential diagnosis.

Diagnosis

The diagnosis of chronic bronchitis is based on the history, physical examination, thoracic radiographs, and tracheobronchial examination and cytology. Several conditions can lead to similar clinical signs and must be considered and ruled out (Table 1).

Many dogs with chronic bronchitis and/or pulmonary fibrosis are overweight, whereas chronic CHF, pulmonary neoplasia, and inflammatory lung diseases usually cause considerable weight loss.

The absence of a cardiac murmur in a small-breed dog virtually excludes the diagnosis of chronic left-sided CHF resulting from mitral valve disease.

TABLE 1. Causes of Coughing, Dyspnea, or Tachypnea

Respiratory infection
 Viral
 Bacterial
 Toxoplasmosis
 Systemic or localized fungal infection
 Parasitic

Pharyngeal disease
 Redundant soft palate (brachycephalic-breed dogs)
 Nasopharyngeal polyp (cats)

Laryngeal paralysis, collapse, or eversion of the saccules
Chronic food aspiration (esophageal disease)
Tracheal or main-stem bronchial collapse
Tracheal or bronchial compression
 Mediastinal mass (lymphosarcoma, thymoma)
 Hilar lymphadenopathy (neoplasia, systemic mycosis,
  granulomatous disease)
 Mediastinal granuloma
 Mediastinal abscess
 Left atrial enlargement

Intraluminal mass lesion or obstruction
 Congenital hypoplasia
 Tumor
 Foreign body
  Esophageal foreign body
 Hematoma

Tracheal-esophageal fistula
Lungworms
 Filaroides osleri tracheal granuloma (dogs)
 Paragonimiasis
 Capillariasis
 Aleurostrongylosis (cats)

Heartworm disease
Bronchitis
Pulmonary edema
 Cardiac
 Noncardiac

Pneumonia
 Infectious
 Granulomatous
 Pulmonary infiltrates of eosinophils (dogs)

Pulmonary fibrosis (dogs)
Pulmonary contusion, hemorrhage
Pulmonary neoplasia
 Primary lung tumors
 Metastatic/multicentric pulmonary neoplasia

Pulmonary microlithiasis
Pulmonary embolism
Primary pulmonary hypertension
Pleural effusion
 Pleural fibrosis

Pneumothorax
Diaphragmatic hernia
Obesity
Abdominal masses
Neuromuscular disease
Diaphragmatic paralysis
Altered ventilatory pattern
 Central nervous system and metabolic diseases
 Fever
 Acidosis
 Anemia, methemoglobinemia, toxicity
 Benzyl alcohol toxicity (cats)

Radiography

The thoracic radiograph is abnormal in most cases.

- Typical findings include increased interstitial density with prominent peribronchial infiltrates. It may be difficult to distinguish these findings from normal aging changes of the canine thorax.
- Variable degrees of bronchiectasis may be evident.
- Cranial and middle lung lobe consolidation or alveolar infiltrates indicate complicating bacterial pneumonia.
- In some dogs, the right middle lung lobe is atelectatic from bronchial occlusion by mucus plugs, with subsequent resorption of air.
- The overall volume of the lung is usually normal for the breed and size of the patient; however, in some dogs gas trapping with pulmonary overinflation (emphysema) causes a barrel-chested appearance. In other cases, retraction of the lung borders, typical of diffuse pulmonary fibrosis, is observed.
- Dynamic expiratory collapse of a lobar bronchus or the intrathoracic trachea is not uncommon.
- Do not be surprised to find apparent cardiomegaly or cor pulmonale in dogs with chronic respiratory disease.
  - A common error is to overinterpret the heart size on thoracic radiographs in dogs with chronic bronchitis or interstitial lung disease.
  - Possible reasons for cardiomegaly in these cases include cor pulmonale (right heart enlargement from lung disease), increased intrapericardial fat, concurrent valvular disease, and inadequate pulmonary expansion that artificially increases the cardiac:thoracic ratio.

Tracheobronchial Examination, Cytology, and Culture

Sputum samples may be obtained by a transtracheal wash, via a sterile endotracheal tube, or during bronchoscopic examination.

Transtracheal Wash

- Use a large-bore intravenous through-the-needle catheter (Delmed-Icath or Sovereign, 14 or 17 gauge, 8–14 inches long) or a 14-gauge intravascular cannula through which a 3.5 Fr., polyethylene urinary catheter is passed into the tracheal lumen.
- It is helpful to lightly sedate some patients to prevent struggling (acepromazine: 0.05–0.1 mg/kg SC, 30 minutes prior to the procedure; or acepromazine, 0.03 mg/kg, plus diazepam, 0.1–0.2 mg/kg IV, 10 minutes prior to the procedure). Restrain the dog in either a standing or sitting position.
- Following tranquilization and local anesthesia, most mature dogs tolerate the procedure well, and tracheobronchial secretions ("sputum") are reliably obtained in this manner unless the cough is nonproductive.

Luminal Tracheal or Bronchial Wash. A tracheal or bronchial wash through a sterile endotracheal tube is another option, suitable for intractable dogs, puppies with chronic infective tracheobronchitis, and older dogs who will undergo subsequent dental procedures.

■ The animal is tranquilized and then lightly anesthetized with a thiobarbiturate or with IV ketamine-diazepam (or midazolam) combination (for dosages, see sec. 1, ch. 2), intubated carefully with a sterile endotracheal tube, and allowed to breathe room air.
■ The tracheobronchial tree is lavaged, using a sterile male urinary catheter that has been advanced through the endotracheal tube.
■ Disadvantages of this technique are inadequate cough due to anesthesia and pooling of lavaged secretions in the endotracheal tube. Also, it is difficult to avoid contamination of culture specimens with oral flora.
■ Greater yield of sputum can be obtained using constant suction and a sterile mucus trap while gently moving the catheter in the airways.

Bronchoscopy. Bronchoscopy can be used to obtain a sample of the tracheobronchial sputum. A sterilized bronchoscopic port is required to obtain samples for culture.

■ An advantage of bronchoscopy is that it permits direct visualization of the airways for:
  • Identification of intraluminal mass lesions, inflamed mucosal surfaces, and exudates
  • Evaluation of airway dynamics and collapse under light planes of anesthesia
  • Performance of lavage and sampling of multiple bronchi
  • Diagnosis of focal lung disease, bronchial foreign bodies, lung parasites, endobronchial tumors, hemoptysis, and tracheal or bronchial collapse
■ Typical bronchoscopic features of chronic bronchitis include:

  • Hyperemia, granularity, and friability of the bronchial mucosa
  • Increased intraluminal mucus, mucoid plaques, and roughening of the surface
  • Occlusion of airways with exudate and mucus, and variable degrees of airway collapse.
■ Mucosal redundancy and polypoid structures also may be found.

Evaluation of Collected Sputum Specimens. The sputum sample is cultured aerobically for bacteria, sensitivity testing is done, and a cytofuge preparation is evaluated cytologically. The sputum obtained via tracheal or bronchial washings from affected lobes can provide insight about the type of inflammatory process.

■ Normal findings include a small number of neutrophils, alveolar macrophages, epithelial and goblet cells (more likely with bronchial brushings), and, rarely, lymphocytes and eosinophils.
  • Cytologic findings in most dogs with chronic bronchitis are nonspecific and characterized by a mixed inflammatory cell population dominated by neutro-

phils, and accompanied by some reactive epithelial cells, eosinophils (<15%), and macrophages.
■ Intracellular bacteria are present in some cases, but the majority of specimens are sterile.
  • Frequently, nonresistant organisms such as *Pasteurella multocida* are cultured, but it is difficult to assess the overall significance of this type of isolate to the bronchial disorder.
  • Bacteria cultured from young dogs with chronic tracheobronchitis or from mature dogs with concurrent bronchiectasis or pneumonia are more likely to be significant.
■ Mucopurulent or suppurative inflammation with intracellular bacteria is sometimes found, particularly in younger dogs with chronic infective tracheobronchitis.
■ Chronic bronchitis that becomes complicated by secondary bacterial infection can lead to an acute exacerbation of the disease. While awaiting culture results, Gram stain results can be used to guide the choice of antibiotics.
■ In some dogs, the tracheobronchial sputum is sterile but is characterized by an increased number of cells, predominated by eosinophils and reactive epithelial cells. These findings are suggestive of an allergic etiology (hypersensitivity) or parasitic infection.

Other Laboratory Tests. Electrocardiography (ECG), a complete blood count (CBC), packed cell volume (PCV), and arterial blood gas analysis may be helpful in assessing the heart and lungs and in refining the differential diagnosis.

■ ECG in dogs with chronic bronchitis generally reveals pronounced sinus arrhythmia (with faster heart rate during inspiration), a wandering atrial pacemaker, and peaked P waves (P-pulmonale). Rarely, right axis deviation is present. Some dogs have increased QRS voltages (R wave > 3.0 mV in leads II and aVF) for unexplained reasons.

KEY POINT ▶ The CBC is frequently normal; thus, a normal white blood cell count does not rule out bronchitis.

■ Neutrophilia or monocytosis may indicate bacterial pneumonia. Peripheral eosinophilia is seen in only a small percentage of dogs found to have sputum compatible with "allergic bronchitis." Eosinophilia is also observed in dogs with respiratory parasites or heartworm disease. Mild polycythemia (possibly caused by chronic hypoxia) may be encountered in some dogs; however, the elevation of the PCV can also be explained in some dogs by hemoconcentration secondary to inappropriate diuretic therapy and dehydration.
■ Arterial blood gas analysis is variable but most commonly demonstrates arterial hypoxemia that partially improves after oxygenation; hypocarbia; and a mixed metabolic acidosis and respiratory alkalosis. If respiratory failure ($Pa_{O_2} < 60$ torr, increased Pa_{CO_2}) ensues, artificial ventilation and vigorous medical therapy may be necessary.

Treatment

Therapy of chronic bronchitis is guided by the cytology and culture of the tracheobronchial secretions ("sputum"), by the extent of radiographic changes (e.g., pneumonia), and by response to therapy. Chronic, intermittent antibiotic or corticosteroid therapy, combined with the use of bronchodilators, antitussives, and supportive care of the respiratory system form the basis of chronic therapy.

- Rarely is a cure obtained; however, with diligent home care, significant improvement of clinical signs does occur in many dogs.
- Patients with advanced changes including bronchiectasis or lobar atelectasis generally respond poorly to medical therapy.

General Supportive Measures

The following general recommendations may be helpful in dogs with chronic bronchitis, regardless of cause.

- Obesity can accentuate respiratory problems because diaphragmatic function is impaired, small airways close earlier than normal, and ventilation may be impeded. Therefore, recommend weight reduction over a 2–3 month period, using dietary restriction or a special diet such as Prescription Diet r/d (Hill's Pet Foods).
- If a restraint collar is worn, replace it with a harness to decrease airway irritation.
- Avoid environmental stresses, including house dust, vapors, chemical fumes, and tobacco smoke.
- Inhalation of humidified air, via a vaporizer or nebulizer may liquefy secretions, hydrate the airways, and reduce coughing. Instruct the owner to exercise the pet lightly following these procedures to encourage cough.
- Treatment of dental disease and oral cavity infections is prudent in dogs with chronic bronchitis (see sec. 7, ch. 1). At the time of the dentistry, a tracheal wash can be obtained during induction of anesthesia, thereby permitting examination of tracheobronchial secretions. Intravenous antibiotics (e.g., cephalothin) can then be given and the dental procedures completed.
- In dogs with eosinophilic inflammations, be sure to eliminate heartworm disease and treat empirically

for nematode and fluke infections with fenbendazole, 25–50 mg/kg PO for 10 days.

Antitussive Therapy

The use of cough suppressants varies on a case-by-case basis. In dogs with nonbacterial bronchitis, breaking the cough cycle is an essential part of treatment. For central-acting antitussive products and dosages, see Table 2.

KEY POINT ▶ Cough suppressants are contraindicated in cases complicated by lobar pneumonia.

- Initial treatment with codeine-derivative cough suppressants such as hydrocodone (Tussionex; Fisons; or Hycodan; Dupont) at a total dose of 2.5–5 mg PO, q8–12h, often is effective. The dosage can be reduced gradually to the lowest effective dose. Sedation is a common side effect, but this actually may be beneficial if coughing is triggered by excitement or stress.
- Butorphenol (Torbutrol; Bristol), 0.5–1.0 mg/kg PO, q8–12h, can also be prescribed but is less potent for reducing cough.

Bronchodilator Therapy

Bronchodilator drugs include xanthine derivatives and beta$_2$ adrenergic (sympathomimetic) agonists. Bronchodilators also may increase the vigor of contraction of the respiratory muscles which may be useful in dogs with chronic dyspnea. Theophylline and its various salts are most commonly chosen. For bronchodilator drugs and their dosages, refer to Table 3.

- The author prefers long-acting theophylline, (Theo-Dur; Key Pharmaceuticals), 20–25 mg/kg PO, q12h, or oxtriphylline (Choledyl or Brondecon [plus guaifenesin], Parke-Davis), 6–11 mg/kg PO, q8–12h. Adjust the dose to individual patient response.
- Serum concentrations of theophylline, obtained after 1 week of therapy, can be used to guide dosage (10–20 μg/ml) or follow therapeutic levels for human hospital laboratories).
- Some dogs cannot tolerate the adverse effects of the methylxanthines, which include anxiety, restlessness, tachycardia, polyuria, and emesis.
- The beta$_2$ agonist terbutaline (Brethine, Geigy; Bricanyl, Marion Merrell Dow), 2.5 mg PO, q8–12h,

---

TABLE 2. Central-Acting Antitussives

Drug	Trade Name	Manufacturer	Preparation	Suggested Dosage
Butorphanol	Torbutrol	Fort Dodge	Injectable: 0.5 mg/ml Tablet: 1, 5, 10 mg	Injectable: 0.05–0.1 mg/kg SC, q6–12h Tablet: 0.5–1 mg/kg PO, q6–12h
Hydrocodone*	Hycodan	DuPont	Tablet: 5 mg Liquids: 1 mg/ml	0.25 mg/kg PO, q6–12h
Codeine	Many generic brands	Many	Tablet and liquid	1–2 mg/kg PO, q6–12h
Dextromethorphan	Many generic brands	Many	Syrup and liquid	1–2 mg/kg PO, q6–8h

*Hydrocodone also available in the following combinations: hydrocodone plus antihistamine (chlorpheniramine), (Tussionex, Fisons); hydrocodone plus expectorant (guaifenesin) (Entuss, Hauck); hydrocodone plus expectorant (guaifenesin) and decongestant (pseudoephedrine) (Entuss-D, Hauck).

TABLE 3. Bronchodilators

Drug	Trade Name	Manufacturer	Preparation	Suggested Dosage†
Theophylline	Many generic brands	Many	Liquid: 3, 5, 20 mg/ml	4–8 mg/kg PO, q6–8h
Theophylline (long-acting)	Theo-Dur	Key	Tablet: 200, 300, 450 mg Sprinkle*: 50, 75, 125, 200 mg	10–25 mg/kg PO, q12h
	Slo-Phyllin	Rhone-Poulenc Rorer	Tablet: 100, 200 mg	
	Slo-bid Gyrocaps	Rhone-Poulenc Rorer	Sprinkle*: 50, 75, 125, 200 mg	
Theophylline and guaifenesin	Quibron	Bristol	Capsule, Elixir (15 ml); 150 mg theophylline, 90 mg guafenesin	1 cap/20–30 kg PO, q6–8h 0.2–0.6 ml/kg PO, q6–8h
Aminophylline	Many generic brands Somophyllin	Many Fisons	Tablet: 100, 200 mg Liquid: 21 mg/ml	6–10 mg/kg PO, IM, or IV, q6–8h
Oxtriphylline	Choledyl	Parke-Davis	Tablet: 100, 200 mg Liquid: 20 mg/ml	6–10 mg/kg PO, q6–8h
Oxtriphylline (long-acting)	Choledyl SA	Parke-Davis	Tablet: 400 mg, 600 mg	10–20 mg/kg PO, q12h
Terbutaline	Brethine Bricanyl	Geigy Marion Merrell Dow	Tablet: 2.5, 5 mg	1.25–5 mg PO, q8–12h
Ephedrine	Many generic brands	Many	Many	2 mg/kg PO, q8–12h

†These doses may not be tolerated by some dogs and may require medication adjustments.
*Theophylline sprinkle preparations (Theo-Dur Sprinkle, Slo-bid Gyrocaps) are capsules that contain sustained-action microencapsuled beads of theophylline. The capsule can be given whole, or it can be opened and its bead contents sprinkled on the animal's food.

can be given as an alternative agent to dogs without heart disease. Adverse effects are similar to those caused by the methylxanthines.

■ Lowering the dose of terbutaline by 50% and combining this with a low dose of theophylline (6–10 mg/kg q12h) may be tried in some dogs who cannot tolerate full doses of either drug.

Antibacterial Therapy

Dogs with chronic bronchitis often have shown no improvement after receiving previous courses of antibiotics. In the patients with primary bacterial tracheobronchitis with complicating bacterial infection, a good response may be obtained if the organism is susceptible to the chosen drug. In many dogs, however, antibiotic treatment causes little improvement, presumably because of a nonbacterial cause or lack of suitable culture and sensitivity testing.

Signs of Bacterial Infection. Suspect bacterial infection in any of the following situations:

■ Acute exacerbation of cough in a dog with previously stable chronic bronchitis
■ Cough associated with anorexia, mucopurulent nasal discharge, or fever
■ Radiographic evidence of bronchiectasis or lobar consolidation/atelectasis
■ Recurrent signs of bronchitis in a previously documented case of bacterial tracheobronchitis
■ Severe periodontal or dental disease.

Antibiotic Therapy. Use sputum culture and sensitivity as a guide to antibiotic treatment in the following situations:

■ Pending culture results, evaluate cytology and Gram stain and administer a broad-spectrum antibiotic, such as amoxicillin-clavulinic acid, trimethoprim-sulfonamide, cephalothin or cefalexin, quinolone (enrofloxacin), or tetracycline. Continue treatment for a minimum of 3 weeks.

■ Some dogs develop a recurrent bacterial bronchitis that responds well to antibiotic treatment until a relapse occurs. Especially in younger dogs this may indicate an unusual or resistant microorganism (e.g., mycoplasma, bronchopulmonary aspergillosis), an anatomic lesion in a bronchus, an endobronchial foreign body, lack of local immunity, or abnormal cilia (ciliary dyskinesis). Such animals may benefit from cultures and bronchoscopy, particularly if a single lung lobe remains infiltrated or pneumonic.

■ To mobilize secretion in dogs with bacterial bronchitis or pneumonia, combine breathing of humidified air or nebulization with coupage of the chest. Administer bronchodilators to prevent reflex bronchospasm from nebulized fluid: avoid cough suppressants.

■ When *Bordetella bronchiseptica* is cultured, consider the use of gentamicin nebulization using an anesthetic face mask interfaced with a glass nebulizer (Devilbiss model #40) and the oxygen output line of a gas anesthetic machine.
  ● Combine gentamicin (4–6mg/kg) with 0.5 ml of saline in the nebulization pot, and use 1–3 liter/min of oxygen flow to transport the solution into the face mask. Administer therapy twice daily for 5 days.
  ● Current data indicate that gentamicin is not absorbed systemically from the lung.

Anti-Inflammatory Therapy

Prednisolone or prednisone can be effective for control of nonbacterial bronchitis and is the most efficacious treatment for eosinophilic bronchitis. Presumably, bronchitis associated with eosinophilia or eosinophil-laden sputum represents a hypersensitivity reaction (also see pulmonary infiltrates of eosinophils). Such dogs with "allergic" bronchitis respond very well to decreasing doses of prednisone.

- Give prednisone initially at 0.5–1.0 mg/kg PO, q12h, for 10–14 days. Then taper the daily dose over the next month to the lowest effective maintenance dose given once q24–48h.
- Some dogs require pulsed monthly therapy (1 week per month) or treatment every other day to maintain remission.
- Explain the adverse effects of long-term prednisone to the owner.
- Bronchodilators, cough suppressants, and antibiotics when indicated may reduce the need for continuous or high dosages of corticosteroids. Some dogs develop secondary infection, and prednisone therapy may need to be discontinued.
- The response to treatment varies, some pets make near-recoveries, and others require relatively high doses and varying combinations of medication throughout their lives.

FELINE CHRONIC BRONCHITIS AND BRONCHIAL ASTHMA

Etiology

Feline chronic bronchial diseases include reactive bronchoconstriction ("asthma"), bronchial inflammation, and recurrent bronchopulmonary infections. The causes of chronic bronchial diseases in the cat are unknown, although hypersensitivity, environmental pollutants, genetic predisposition (Siamese cats?), and infectious agents (e.g., mycoplasma, viruses) are likely.

- Most cases of bronchitis are attributed to asthma, but not all cats exhibit the classic signs of hypersensitivity airway disease and mixed patterns of bronchial disease are recognized.
- Parasitic infections such as *Aleurostrongylus abstrusus*, *Paragonimus kellicotti*, and *Capillaria aerophilia* can cause chronic bronchial problems in cats.

Pathophysiology

Typical features of chronic bronchitis include bronchial luminal narrowing, mucosal edema, excessive mucus, proliferation of goblet cells, and inflammation. Smooth muscle hypertrophy further predisposes to reactive bronchoconstriction in cats with signs typical of asthma.

- The pathologic changes seen in chronic bronchitis lead to airway obstruction and gas trapping (emphysema).
- Acute reversible bronchoconstriction with sudden onset of cough and dyspnea is typical of asthma.
- Progressive dyspnea, coughing, gagging, and exercise intolerance develop with chronic bronchitis.
- Pulmonary parenchymal involvement with lobar pneumonia is suggestive of recurrent or complicating bacterial infection.

- Collapse or lobar infiltration of the right middle lung lobe is not uncommon and suggests bacterial infection (possibly attributable to immunosuppression) or mucus plugging of the bronchus with reabsorption atelectasis.

Clinical Signs

Chronic bronchial disease is characterized by coughing, wheezing, dyspnea, gagging or vomiting (probably expectoration of tracheobronchial secretions), and sometimes sneezing.

- Episodic and seasonal occurrences of respiratory signs are not uncommon, but often the condition becomes persistent and nonseasonal.
- Exposure to environmental pollutants may exacerbate clinical signs.
- A previous beneficial response to corticosteroid therapy is typical of asthma.
- Body condition tends to be normal except in advanced cases and in cats suffering from bacterial infection or immunosuppression.

Diagnosis

The diagnosis is based on history, physical examination, and thoracic radiographs. Definitive diagnosis is made following examination of tracheobronchial secretions and elimination of other causes of respiratory disease (see Table 1). Important considerations are heartworm disease, acute viral respiratory infections, and pulmonary parasites.

Physical Examination Findings

These vary, depending on the stage and severity of disease.

- Severe dyspnea or tachypnea and orthopnea are evident in some cats. A cough may be evident or elicited.
- Fever suggests bacterial infection, although hyperthermia may develop from anxiety and increased work of breathing.
- Abnormal lung sounds detected by auscultation include loud bronchial sounds, wheezes (typically expiratory), rhonchi, and crackles. Percussion may indicate a hyperresonant thorax.
- Cyanosis is evident in some cats.
- Cardiac auscultation is usually normal; however, a systolic murmur of uncertain origin is detectable in some cats. Sinus arrhythmia, otherwise uncommon in cats, has been observed in cats with bronchitis.

KEY POINT ▶ Coughing, a hallmark of bronchial disease and parasitic infections, is uncommon in cats with heart failure.

Radiography

Radiographs of the thorax may be normal or may show evidence of pulmonary hyperinflation, with a flattened diaphragm, peribronchial infiltration, and mild diffuse or patchy interstitial infiltrates. Aerophagia is common.

■ Cardiac size is normal or slightly enlarged.
■ Pulmonary consolidation or atelectasis may be evident, most often in the right middle lung lobe. Radiographic abnormalities may, but do not invariably improve following successful therapy.

Laboratory Studies

Laboratory abnormalities are inconsistent.

■ Eosinophilia is present in less than one-third of the cases of bronchitis. Neutrophilia is less common.
■ Hyperglobulinemia is observed in some cats with chronic bronchitis.
■ Serum biochemistries are unremarkable.
■ Arterial hypoxemia develops during acute asthma and in cats with chronic bronchopulmonary disease.
■ In some cats, enzyme-linked immunosorbent assay tests for FeLV (see sec. 2, ch. 1) or FIV (see sec. 2, ch. 2) may be positive, especially in cats with bacterial bronchitis, recurrent middle lung lobe pneumonia, or chronic sinusitis.
■ Perform heartworm (ELISA), fecal flotation, and fecal sedimentation technique to rule out parasitic infection.

Cardiopulmonary Evaluations

■ The ECG, although typically normal, may demonstrate right ventricular hypertrophy (cor pulmonale) or right bundle branch block.
■ An echocardiogram can be used to exclude heart failure as a cause of similar signs.
■ Pulmonary function tests such as tidal breathing flow-volume loop analysis can be used to detect airway hyperreactivity; however, these tests are not yet routinely available.

Tracheobronchial Washes

Culture and cytologic examination of bronchial secretions are important.

■ Technique:
  • Wash the airways by intubating the cat with a sterile endotracheal tube.
  • Use a sterile syringe adaptor or sterile urinary catheter to obtain samples for culture (bacterial, including culture for mycoplasma) and cytology.
■ Bacterial growth may indicate primary bacterial bronchitis or a secondary infection. *Pasteurella multocida* is the most frequently isolated organism.
■ Cytologic examination is variable. Cats with bronchitis have increased mucus and increased numbers of inflammatory cells.
  • The presence of eosinophils in bronchial cytologic specimens is *not* diagnostic of asthma. Inasmuch as the normal cats may have 25% eosinophils in bronchoalveolar lavage fluid (normal route of extrusion for these cells), the cell count must be interpreted in conjunction with other findings. When the majority of cells are eosinophils and are accompanied by mast cells, neutrophils, and mucus, "allergic" pulmonary disease or parasitic infection is likely.

• Many cats with bronchitis and clinical signs of asthma exhibit a predominately neutrophilic response.
• Examine cytologic specimens carefully for parasitic larvae and ova, especially when the majority of cells are eosinophils.

Bronchoscopy

■ Bronchoscopy is indicated when the cat does not respond to appropriate therapy for asthma and bronchitis, or when other diagnoses must be excluded, such as nasopharyngeal polyp, laryngeal disease, major airway obstruction, intraluminal foreign body, or mucosal tumor (adenocarcinoma).
■ Mucosal edema and increased mucus are typical findings in bronchitis.

Treatment

Treatment of bronchitis includes both symptomatic and specific aspects of therapy. The modulation of autonomic activity and inflammatory mediators such as leukotrienes will undoubtedly play an increasing role in the treatment of bronchial disease in cats.

Emergency Treatment

Acute asthmatic attacks may require emergency treatment.

■ Handle the cat gently, and place it in an oxygen cage. Delay additional diagnostic studies until respiratory distress is stabilized.
■ Administer aminophylline (not a sustained release preparation) either orally (5 mg/kg, q8h for 24 h) or parenterally (5 mg/kg, slowly IV over 10 minutes, followed by oral therapy). Oral absorption is rapid and avoids the stress of restraint necessary for IV administration.
■ Administer corticosteroids, either prednisolone (1 mg/kg IM, q12h) or prednisolone sodium succinate (Solu Delta Cortef; Upjohn), 10 mg/kg IV) followed by oral prednisolone therapy as described below.
■ Inadequate response within 2 hours indicates the need for additional treatment. Choose *one* of the following drugs with beta$_2$ agonist activity:
  • Subcutaneous isoproterenol (Isuprel; Winthrop), 1:5000 solution, 0.1–0.2 ml
  • Epinephrine, 1:10,000 solution, 1–2 ml SC
  • Terbutaline HCl (Brethine; Geigy), 2.5 mg tablet, ¼ tablet orally
■ For non-responders, consider atropine (to decrease cholinergic tone), 0.04 mg/kg IM.

Intermediate and Long-Term Therapy

The underlying cause and results of tracheal washings determine intermediate and long-term therapy. Some cats with true asthma may require only intermittent treatment during exacerbations of their disease. Other cats need recurrent or chronic treatment to control clinical signs.

General Measures. Try to eliminate dusts (kitty litter), smoke (including tobacco), powders (flea products, carpet cleaners), sprays, and other potentially inciting substances from the cat's environment. Dust-free and plastic reusable cat litter are available from different manufacturers. Decrease body weight in obese cats to reduce the restrictive effect of fat on ventilation. Consider a 10-day course of fenbendazole in cats with a marked eosinophilic bronchial reaction.

Bronchodilators. Prescribe bronchodilators for periods of symptomatic bronchial disease (see Table 3).

- Administer sustained release theophylline (Theo-Dur tablets, Key; Slo-bid Gyrocaps, Rhone-Poulenc Rorer), of 25 mg/kg PO q24h.
  - Monitor for clinical signs of toxicosis such as anxiety, emesis, and tremors.
  - After 7–14 days of therapy, measure plasma theophylline trough blood level (10–12 hours post pill administration); therapeutic levels according to Dye are probably 5–20 µg/ml.
  - Chronic therapy with theophylline is indicated in cats with progressive, nonseasonal disease.
- Alternative therapy to theophylline is terbutaline (Brethine; Geigy), ⅛–¼ of a 2.5 mg tablet daily, gradually titrated up to a maximum of ¼ tablet q12h. Caution: Side effects include anxiety, tachycardia, hypotension.
- Consider combination therapy with theophylline and low-dose terbutaline for refractory cases.

Antibiotics. Antibiotic therapy, ideally guided by culture and sensitivity testing of tracheobronchial secretions, is indicated for cats with evidence of respiratory infection. If empirical therapy is needed, choose drugs effective against *Pasteurella* species (ampicillin, cephalosporins). Consider quinolones for cats with diffuse pulmonary infiltration that might indicate mycoplasma infection.

Suspect bacterial infection in the following situations:

- Fever
- Positive airway culture
- Suppurative airway inflammation with degenerative neutrophils
- Mixed inflammatory processes with a predominance of well-preserved neutrophils (empiric antibiotic therapy can be initiated in mixed inflammatory responses, or antibiotic treatment can be withheld pending tracheobronchial fluid culture)
- Lobar consolidation or alveolar pulmonary pattern
- Mucopurulent sinusitis
- Clinical signs of respiratory disease in FeLV- or FIV-positive cats.

Prednisolone. Administer prednisolone, 0.5–1.0 mg/kg PO, q12h, in cats with asthma or with eosinophilic (or mixed) bronchial inflammations when the likelihood of concurrent infection is remote. Because most cats do not have a positive airway culture, the backbone of treatment consists of chronic corticosteroid therapy along with theophylline.

- Continue the initial dose of prednisolone for 10–14 days. If symptoms regress, switch the dose to alternate days and taper over 2–4 weeks to the lowest effective maintenance dose.

- When the owner cannot administer pills, administer a reposital corticosteroid preparation, methylprednisolone acetate (Depo-Medrol; Upjohn), 10–20 mg/kg, IM, once every 3 weeks. Lower doses may suffice for some cats.
- Discontinue prednisolone if all signs of disease are eliminated. Be judicious when making this decision because many cats do not require chronic treatment but may need intermittent therapy when a relapse occurs.
- Advise the client about adverse effects of glucocorticoid therapy in cats, including development of diabetes mellitus.

Prognosis

The prognosis for bronchial disease in cats is always guarded. Initial bouts of bronchitis may be easily controlled, but many cats experience recurrent or progressive clinical signs.

- This disease requires diligence on the part of the client to administer medications and observe for exacerbations of disease.
- The veterinarian is obligated to perform a thorough initial diagnostic evaluation and to maintain suspicion of complications of bronchial disease, especially bacterial infection and pneumonia.

PULMONARY ALVEOLITIS AND INTERSTITIAL FIBROSIS IN THE DOG

Etiology

The etiopathogenesis of spontaneous pulmonary fibrosis in the dog has not been identified.

- Fibrosis is the end-result of tissue injury caused by underlying progressive interstitial inflammatory disease.
- It is likely that severe, diffuse lung fibrosis in middle-aged and older dogs is preceded by multifocal alveolitis similar to that associated with chronic pulmonary fibrosis in humans and reproduced in experimental canine models.
- Hundreds of inhaled, ingested, and administered chemicals, dusts, gases, pollutants, and drugs are capable of inducing pulmonary alveolitis and fibrosis in humans. Presumably, dogs may react in a similar manner to such inciting agents. Inorganic and organic dusts, gases and vapors, drugs, and infectious agents, as well as chronic passive lung congestion (e.g., from chronic mitral disease) and chronic uremia can cause lung fibrosis. In canine models of pulmonary interstitial disease, alveolitis precedes development of fibrosis.

Pathophysiology

The pathophysiology is believed to involve an injury stimulus or allergen that causes lung alveolitis, recruitment of effector cells into the alveolar interstitium, release of inflammatory mediators, and eventual destruction and derangement of alveolar tissues.

■ These changes lead to a loss of functional alveolar capillary units. Resolution leaves end stage interstitial fibrosis.

■ Effector cells, including neutrophils and activated mononuclear cells, are found in increased numbers in the affected tissue and in bronchoalveolar washes.

■ Noncardiogenic pulmonary edema of the alveolar septa occurs in acute cases. Fibrosis is diffuse but piecemeal and may not be adequately assessed by small transbronchoscopic biopsies.

Clinical Signs

■ Typically there is a long and progressive history of shortness of breath and exercise intolerance. Small terrier breeds, especially West Highland white terriers are predisposed.

■ Coughing is slight or remarkably absent except when fibrosis is associated concurrently with bronchitis.

Diagnosis

Physical Examination

The most significant physical examination finding is bilateral, ventral, end-inspiratory and early-expiratory crackles that are most evident on full inspiration. The dog seldom sighs or takes deep inspirations.

■ In advanced cases, crackles are audible without a stethoscope.

■ Forced exercise usually results in tachypnea or gasping and often provokes cyanosis. If there is concurrent bronchitis, physical findings may be similar to those previously described for chronic bronchitis.

KEY POINT ▶ Because physical examination findings in dogs with pulmonary fibrosis can be quite subtle, careful auscultation and observation are essential.

Radiography

■ Optimal radiographic exposure is necessary because several technical factors can affect the amount of interstitial infiltrates that will be perceived. Expiratory radiographs and obesity increase overall lung density. The amount of lung density compatible with normal aging is unresolved.

■ Usually a mild, diffuse increase in interstitial lung densities is evident throughout the lung.

■ Retraction of the peripheral lung edges from the ribs may be evident, and the diaphragm may be flat with poor lung expansion in some cases.

■ A moderate degree of cardiomegaly is commonly seen as the result of cor pulmonale or incomplete thoracic expansion.

■ Radiograph features of concurrent bronchial disease may be seen (see discussion of bronchitis).

Laboratory Studies

■ The CBC is almost always normal.

■ Arterial blood gas analysis is a sensitive and often overlooked method for verifying the presence of significant lung disease. Arterial hypocarbia (hyperventilation) and hypoxemia (generally in the range of 65–85 mm Hg) are present; improvement occurs when the dog is given 100% oxygen by face mask, indicating a ventilation perfusion inequality.

■ Tracheal washes are unlikely to be useful if the dog is only short of breath and does not have a productive cough.

■ Although an open lung biopsy can definitively diagnose alveolitis and lung fibrosis, it is invasive and not required in most cases. A fine-needle lung aspirate, useful for identifying diffuse increases in pulmonary density caused by neoplasia or infection (e.g., systemic mycosis), is not helpful for diagnosis of pulmonary fibrosis.

■ Bronchoalveolar lavage: In dogs with typical historical, auscultatory, radiographic, and blood gas findings, bronchoscopy can establish the diagnosis. Provided there is no significant bronchitis (absence of productive cough and lack of bronchial erythema and mucous hypersecretion at endoscopy), bronchoalveolar lavage can be used to obtain samples from the alveoli and to diagnose lower airway inflammation.

• Under direct visualization of the airways, wedge the bronchoscope in a bronchus. Rapidly lavage the airway and its lobe with 0.9% saline. Repeat in at least 3 different lobes.

• The lavage fluid obtained from the different lobes is pooled (or can be examined separately), centrifuged, and the sediment is examined by a pathologist for cellularity and for percentage distribution of cells.

• Normal dogs have a predominance of alveolar macrophages and a low neutrophil count (typically < 12%) and variable numbers of eosinophils. Dogs with alveolitis/fibrosis typically have neutrophil counts >25% with reactive macrophages.

• Bronchoalveolar lavage is not as valuable for documenting alveolitis when the dog has concurrent bronchitis and upper airway exudates that contaminate the aspirated fluid.

Treatment

Treatment of idiopathic pulmonary fibrosis is frustrating because the underlying cause of alveolitis is rarely determined or controlled and because therapy does not reverse preexistent fibrosis.

■ If the animal is exposed to smoke, dusts, or fumes, eliminate the source.

■ Control obesity.

■ Because many drugs are associated with pulmonary fibrosis in humans, scrutinize current medications being given to the dog and read the drug insert carefully relative to adverse pulmonary effects.

■ Consider a trial course of bronchodilators using sustained-release theophylline, aminophylline, or oxtriphylline (see discussion of chronic bronchitis section and Table 3) because small airway function may be compromised and these drugs also may increase diaphragmatic contractility.

■ Treat initially with immunosuppressive doses of prednisone, 1 mg/kg PO, q12h, for 2 weeks, and then taper the dose over the next month. This will not reverse the existing fibrosis but may decrease ongoing alveolitis. Chronic treatment is empirical, but one approach is to prescribe pulsed prednisone (for example, 1 mg/kg q12h for 1 week per month).

■ The benefits, if any, of cyclophosphamide have not been evaluated in the dog; however, this is commonly used in humans with pulmonary fibrosis.

■ Serial blood gas determinations and bronchoalveolar lavage cytologies can be used to monitor therapy and the clinical course of the disease; however, most clients refuse this type of follow-up.

■ If coughing is a prominent clinical sign, bronchitis is probably present (see discussion of chronic bronchitis).

Prognosis

The prognosis is unfavorable, and gradual clinical deterioration is expected. Severe hypoxemia or progressive right-sided cardiac dysfunction may be observed in advanced cases.

PULMONARY INFILTRATES OF EOSINOPHILS

Etiology

Pulmonary infiltrates of eosinophils (PIE) is an uncommon, poorly-defined condition that most often affects the dog. This idiopathic condition resembles a pulmonary hypersensitivity reaction observed in human patients, from which the term PIE is derived. Eosinophilic pneumonitis is a synonym.

Clinical Signs

Clinical signs include weight loss, cough, tachypnea, and fever.

Diagnosis

The history, physical examination, and radiographic, and laboratory findings indicate alveolar pulmonary infiltration and secondary lung dysfunction.

Diagnostic criteria include the following:

■ Diffuse pulmonary alveolar-interstitial density with minimal, if any, thoracic lymphadenopathy

■ Peripheral eosinophilia (often > 10,000 eosinophils/μl)

■ Eosinophil-laden tracheobronchial secretions (e.g., seen in tracheal washes and bronchoalveolar lavage)

■ Response to corticosteroids

■ In some cases, lung biopsy can be used to confirm the lesion of diffuse infiltration of eosinophils into the pulmonary interstitium.

Differential Diagnosis

Before a diagnosis can be made, all other known causes of pulmonary eosinophilia should be ruled out, including:

■ Parasites, such as heartworms, lungworms, lung flukes, migrating intestinal parasites

■ Fungal infections, including histoplasmosis and endobronchial aspergillosis (more likely with chronic steroid therapy)

■ Lymphosarcoma (eosinophilic chemotaxis; "hypereosinophilic syndrome")

■ Pulmonary eosinophilic granulomas, characterized by radiographic evidence of mass lesions and hilar lymphadenopathy

Treatment

■ Administer immunosuppressive doses of prednisolone (2 mg/kg PO, q12h) for 10–14 days, followed by a gradual tapering of glucocorticoid dose over several weeks.

■ Relapses may occur, but many dogs seem to recover fully.

■ This condition is relatively uncommon if known causes of pulmonary eosinophilic infiltration are first excluded.

GRANULOMATOUS PULMONARY DISORDERS

Etiology

A variety of pulmonary disorders are characterized by granulomatous inflammation, hilar lymphadenopathy, and increased lung density. Important conditions include:

■ Systemic mycoses (sec. 2, ch. 12)

■ Eosinophilic pulmonary granulomatosis (usually heartworm-positive)

■ Lymphomatoid granulomatosis (especially common in Bernese Mountain dogs)

■ Pulmonary tuberculosis (rare in most countries)

■ Idiopathic (immune-mediated?) pulmonary granulomatosis

Clinical Signs

These conditions share the following clinical features.

■ Systemic signs of illness, such as inappetence, weight loss, lethargy, and fever

■ Objective signs of pulmonary disease, especially tachypnea and cough

■ A natural history of progression and death or spontaneous arrest/resolution of the disease

Diagnosis

The characteristics of the granulomas depend on the underlying cause, location of the lesions, and the involved inflammatory cells (e.g., eosinophilic, lymphomatoid). The diagnosis of pulmonary granulomatous disease usually requires a lung biopsy unless the diagnosis can be made by other means (e.g. cytology, culture, and serology for systemic mycoses). A thoracotomy for pulmonary and lymph node biopsy usually is required. The biopsy usually reveals:

■ Hilar (and sometimes generalized) lymphadenopathy

■ Pulmonary infiltration and pulmonary parenchymal lesions.

Treatment

Therapy of eosinophilic and lymphomatoid granulomatosis requires immunosuppressive doses of prednisolone and administration of cyclophosphamide (Cytoxan, Mead Johnson) at doses employed for severe immune system disorders or for lymphoma (sec. 3, ch. 6 for details).

Prognosis

The prognosis for eosinophilic, lymphomatoid and idiopathic pulmonary granulomatosis disorders is guarded; however, good response is obtained in some animals with aggressive therapy.

NONCARDIOGENIC PULMONARY EDEMA

Etiology

■ Pulmonary edema is characterized by an increase in lung water and solute.
■ Most cases of lung edema develop secondary to high pulmonary capillary pressure caused by left-sided heart failure (see chapter VI-6) or overinfusion of crystalloid fluids.
■ Noncardiogenic pulmonary edema (NCPE) can develop following injury to the pulmonary capillaries, with a resultant increase in vascular permeability. The mechanisms by which NCPE edema develops in some conditions are controversial.
■ Often-used synonyms for NCPE are *adult* or *acute* respiratory distress syndrome and *shock lung*, terms extrapolated from the human medical literature.
■ There are numerous causes of NCPE; some of the more important are listed in Table 4.

Pathophysiology

Pulmonary edema interferes with gas exchange, alters pulmonary compliance, and causes ventilation perfusion mismatching and hypoxemia. Depending on the underlying cause of NCPE (e.g., aspiration of gastric contents), intrapulmonary shunting also may occur.

Clinical Signs

The principal clinical signs of pulmonary edema are tachypnea and respiratory distress. Coughing may not be evident unless there is fulminant alveolar edema or cardiomegaly with bronchial compression.

■ Cats assume sternal recumbency with abducted elbows; dogs are reluctant to lie down and often sit up with neck extended.
■ Auscultable pulmonary crackles become evident during inspiration and early expiration.
■ Mucous membranes may be dusky or cyanotic, corresponding to the decrease in arterial PaO_2.

TABLE 4. Causes of Pulmonary Edema

High-Capillary Pressure Pulmonary Edema
Left-sided heart failure*
Overinfusion of crystalloid fluids

Increased Pulmonary Capillary Permeability
Sepsis
Shock
Pulmonary thromboembolism
Disseminated intravascular coagulopathy
Inhalation of smoke or other noxious gases
Aspiration of gastric contents
Uremia
Near-drowning
Pancreatitis
Immunologic reactions
 Transfusion reactions
Snake bite (envenomation)
Pulmonary infection
Ingested toxins

Lymphatic Insufficiency
Pulmonary neoplasia

Pulmonary Edema of Undetermined or Multiple Origin
Neurogenic
 Seizure
 Head trauma
Electrocution
Upper airway obstruction
 Brachycephalic dogs
Reexpansion lung edema (rapid removal of pleural fluid or air)
Drug-induced
 Ketamine
 Narcotic overdosage

---

*Hypoalbuminemia potentiates high-pressure pulmonary edema.

Diagnosis

■ Radiographs of the thorax demonstrate increased lung density of an interstitial and alveolar nature; however, the location of the infiltrate varies depending on the cause.
 • With heart failure, edema is typically perihilar, although severe untreated cardiogenic edema can be diffuse.
 • NCPE may be diffuse but is often dorsal and peripheral (especially neurogenic edema).
 • Lung densities may not be bilaterally symmetric owing to differences in lymphatic drainage (in such instances, the right side is generally more fluid-dense).
 • A lag of 12–24 hours may occur between onset of clinical signs and obvious radiographic change.
 • Depending on the underlying condition, other radiographic abnormalities may be seen (e.g., cardiomegaly, dilated pulmonary artery, trauma, mass lesions).
■ When pulmonary edema is identified radiographically, evaluate for historical, physical, laboratory, and radiographic findings that may indicate a noncardiogenic cause (see Table 4).
■ In some cases, cardiac evaluations (ECG, echocardiography, angiography) may be required to diagnosis cardiogenic pulmonary edema of left-sided congestive heart failure (see 6, ch. 6).

KEY POINT ▶ Maintain a high index of suspicion when diagnosing noncardiogenic pulmonary edema. Consider this diagnosis, as well as the diagnosis of acute pulmonary embolism, whenever unexplained tachypnea develops.

Treatment

Treatment of cardiogenic lung edema is described in sec. 6, ch. 6. Noncardiogenic edema is more difficult to treat because simply lowering pulmonary capillary pressure is insufficient. General goals of therapy are:

- Treat the underlying condition.
- Increase inspiratory oxygen concentration by placing the animal in oxygen cage or administering nasal oxygen (see sec. 1, ch. 3) or mechanical ventilation.
- Maintain airway patency.
- Stop or minimize IV fluids and lower pulmonary capillary pressure with furosemide (initially 4 mg/kg IV; thereafter, 2 mg/kg IV q8h). The use of vasodilators to lower capillary pressure is controversial.
  - If hypotension develops, infuse dopamine, 2–5 kg/min, do not infuse large volumes of crystalloid or blood.
  - Provide minimal fluids (20–30 ml/kg/day): err towards the side of dehydration until life-threatening edema has resolved.
- If sedation is required, use morphine in dogs (0.1 mg/kg IM) or acepromazine in cats (0.1–0.2 mg/kg SC).
- Consider one shock dose of glucocorticoid (10–20 mg/kg of prednisolone sodium succinate IV).
- Administer aminophylline or theophylline to increase respiratory muscle strength and to produce bronchodilation (see discussion of bronchitis and Table 3).
- Correct metabolic acidosis.

- Consider prophylactic IV administration of broad-spectrum antibiotics.
- Monitor respiratory rate and effort, and arterial blood gases if possible.
- Consider mechanical ventilation if supplemental oxygen fails to relieve hypoxemia, respiratory distress, or cyanosis.
  - Indications for artificial ventilation include persistent hypoxemia with $Pao_2 < 60$ torr; hypercarbia with $Paco_2 > 50$ torr (first, be certain that airways are patent), and obvious respiratory distress and fatigue (such patients invariably develop apnea and cardiopulmonary arrest).
  - Unfortunately, artificial ventilation is usually delayed excessively because of the technical problems associated with this treatment in animals.
  - Always culture tracheal secretions after 24–48 hours of ventilation to anticipate the presence of a respiratory infection.

Prognosis

The prognosis is always guarded and depends on the underlying disorder and the ability to provide intensive therapy, including artificial ventilation. Clinical and radiographic improvement often require days; nevertheless, steadfastness when the underlying disorder is potentially reversible can yield gratifying results.

Supplemental Readings

Brown NO, Noone KE, Kurzman ID: Alveolar lavage in dogs. Am J Vet Research 44:335, 1983.

Dungworth DL: Interstitial pulmonary diseases. Adv Vet Sci Comp Med 26:173, 1982.

Bonagura JD, Hamlin RL, Gaber CE: Chronic respiratory disease in the dog. *In* Kirk RW, ed.: *Current Veterinary Therapy X.* Philadelphia: W. B. Saunders, 1989, p 361.

Wheeldon EB, Pirie HM, Fisher EW, et al.: Chronic respiratory disease in the dog. J Small Animal Pract 18:229, 1977.

21 Respiratory Infection

John D. Bonagura
Robert G. Sherding

The respiratory system is a common portal of entry for infectious agents of all types. A large number of infectious agents have been identified as respiratory pathogens (Table 1). The purpose of this chapter is to emphasize important causes of respiratory infections in dogs and cats. For details concerning specific infectious diseases, the reader is referred to sec. 2, ch. 4 for respiratory virus and chlamydia infections of the cat; sec. 2, ch. 5 for *Bordetella* and viral tracheobronchitis of the dog; sec. 2, ch. 6 for canine distemper; sec. 2, ch. 12 for the systemic mycoses; and sec. 2, ch. 13 for toxoplasmosis. Diagnostic procedures for respiratory infections are described in sec. 6, ch. 16 and for radiography in sec. 6, ch. 17. Management of noninfective bronchopulmonary diseases and chronic bronchitis in the dog and cat is described in sec. 6, ch. 20. Management of pyothorax and pleural infections is described in sec. 6, ch. 22.

The subject of infectious disease is extensive; for more detailed information on specific infections, consult textbooks dedicated to this subject, such as *Greene's Infectious Diseases of the Dog and Cat.*

TYPES OF INFECTION

Primary

Many infectious agents are primary pathogens of the respiratory epithelium, pulmonary interstitium, or pleural space. This is particularly true of upper respiratory infections caused by viral agents or bacteria such as *Bordetella bronchiseptica.*

Secondary

The nasal cavity, nasopharynx, larynx, and the trachea normally are inhabited by a variety of microorganisms. The tracheobronchial tree is intermittently populated by aspirated bacteria from the upper respiratory tract. Thus, the potential for secondary opportunistic infection is high when underlying pulmonary injury is present or when the host is immunologically compromised.

Multisystemic

The respiratory system also may be involved in multisystemic infections. This is common with the systemic mycoses, *Blastomyces dermatidis* and *Histoplasma capsulatum.*

CLASSIFICATION

It is helpful to determine the principal anatomic sites of infection, because many infectious agents produce a characteristic pattern of respiratory disease that focuses the clinician on specific diagnostic considerations. The viral upper respiratory infections of cats and canine infectious tracheobronchitis are good examples of localized respiratory disease. Rhinitis, sinusitis, tracheitis, bronchitis, pneumonia, and pleuritis-respiratory infections are discussed using anatomic classification (Table 2) because clinicians generally speak in terms of the anatomic diagnosis.

KEY POINT ▶ Because many respiratory infections are secondary to another condition, consider the possibility of underlying respiratory disease or the possibility of host immunosuppression.

RHINITIS AND SINUSITIS

Etiology

Infections of the nasal cavity and nasal sinuses are not uncommon, especially those associated with acute, contagious viral infections in dogs and cats (see Table 2).

- Acute viral rhinitis is usually self-limiting within 1–2 weeks.
- Viral or bacterial rhinitis or sinusitis can persist in immunocompromised cats infected with feline leukemia virus (FeLV) or feline immunodeficiency virus (FIV). In addition, feline herpesvirus persists in a latent subclinical carrier form in recovered cats, and this occasionally recrudesces to result in episodic or persistent rhinitis.
- Primary bacterial rhinitis and sinusitis are uncommon; however, secondary bacterial infection can develop as a sequela to mucosal injury or obstructed nasal passages caused by: upper respiratory viral infection, foreign body, periodontal disease and tooth root abscesses, oro-nasal fistula or cleft palate, trauma (sequestrum), allergic rhinitis, lymphocytic-plasmacytic rhinitis, congenital ciliary dyskinesia (Kartagener's syndrome), neoplasia, and fungal infection.
- Chronic sinusitis may occur in dogs or cats with recurrent bronchitis or lobar pneumonia. It is likely that sinobronchial route of migration reinforces each

574

TABLE 1. Etiologic Classification of Respiratory System Infections

Viruses
Feline calicivirus, herpesviruses (canine, feline rhinotracheitis virus), canine parainfluenza virus, canine distemper virus, canine adenovirus-2, reoviruses, feline infectious peritonitis coronavirus

Rickettsia
Rocky Mountain spotted fever, *Erhlichia canis,* salmon poisoning disease

Bacteria
Gram-positive and gram-negative bacteria, anaerobes, *Bordetella bronchiseptica, Actinomyces* spp, *Nocardia asteroides,* mycobacteria

***Mycoplasma* spp**

Chlamydia psittaci

Fungi
Cryptococcus neoformans, Histoplasma capsulatum, Blastomyces dermatidides, Coccidioides immitis, Aspergillus spp, *Penicillium* spp, *Rhinosporidium seeberi*

Protozoa
Toxoplasma gondii, Leishmania donovani

Nematodes/Trematodes
Aelurostrongylus abstrusus, Capillaria aerophilia, Filaroides (F. osleri, F. milksi, F. hirthi), Paragonimus kellicotti

infection. *Bordetella bronchiseptica* infection in dogs, especially pups, leads to significant rhinitis as well as tracheobronchitis.

■ Bacterial isolates in rhinitis/sinusitis are variable and typify bacteria normally encountered in the nasopharynx, including gram-positive, gram-negative, and anaerobic organisms.

■ Fungal infection of the nasal cavity or sinuses (see Table 2) can be associated with immunosuppression; however, this may be difficult to demonstrate in dogs. *Aspergillus flavus* is a normal inhabitant but may invade respiratory epithelium in dogs with altered immunity or preexistent inflammation (e.g., lymphocytic-plasmacytic rhinitis, foreign body, trauma).

■ Nasal parasites, such as the nasal mite *Pneumonyssus caninum,* are rare.

Clinical Signs

■ Sneezing, nasal discharge, and gagging or retching from postnasal drip are the cardinal signs of rhinitis and sinusitis. Cough may indicate involvement of the tracheobronchial tree. Some dogs retch and expectorate secretions that have accumulated in the pharynx.

■ A serous discharge is typical of acute viral or allergic disease, whereas mucopurulent nasal exudate suggests a bacterial or fungal component.

■ Other clinical findings such as fever, bony swelling, regional lymphadenopathy, oral ulceration, and ocular or neurologic involvement depend on the underlying cause of the disease.

Diagnosis

■ In most cases, the age and vaccination status of the animal, along with other aspects of the history and physical examination, focus the diagnostic considerations. The diagnostic studies chosen depend on the presumptive diagnosis and response to initial therapy (Table 3).

● Primary infectious diseases and foreign bodies with secondary infection are the most important causes of rhinitis and sinusitis in younger dogs and cats.

● Older pets (> 8 years) tend to be afflicted with

TABLE 2. Anatomic Classification of Common Respiratory Infections*

Rhinitis and Sinusitis
Herpesvirus (rhinotracheitis) [F]†
Calicivirus [F]†‡
Chlamydia psittaci†
Parainfluenza virus [C]†
Canine distemper virus [C]†‡
Adenovirus-2 [C]†‡
Bordetella bronchiseptica [C]†‡
Secondary bacterial infection (find predisposing cause)
Aspergillus flavum [C]
Penicillium spp. [C]
Rhinosporidium seeberi [C]
Cryptococcus neoformans [F]
Pneumonyssus caninum [C]
Salmon poisoning rickettsial agent [C]

Tracheitis
Upper respiratory viruses (see above)
Bordetella bronchiseptica [C]‡
Filaroides osleri [C]

Pulmonary Infections§
Some upper respiratory viruses (see above)
Bacteria bronchopneumonia (both gram-positive and gram-negative)
  Bordetella bronchiseptica
  Gram-negative bacteria: *Escherichia coli* and *Klebsiella, Pseudomonas,* and *Pasteurella* spp
  Gram-positive bacteria: *Streptococcus, Staphylococcus,* and *Mycoplasma* spp
Parasitic Infections: *Aelurostrongylus abstrusus* [F], *Paragonimus kellicotti* [C, F], *Capillaria aerophilia* [C, F], *Filaroides (F. milksi, F. hirthi)* [C]
Aspergillosis (endobronchial infection)
Viral infections: feline calicivirus; canine distemper virus
Chlamydia psittaci
Rickettsial infections: *Ehrlichia canis,* Rocky Mountain spotted fever
Toxoplasma gondii [F > C]
Nocardia spp, *Actinomyces,* anaerobes‖
Leishmania donovani
Systemic mycoses: *Histoplasma capsulatum, Blastomyces dermatidides, Coccidioides immitis, Cryptococcus neoformans*
Response to parasitic infection: migrating nematodes, *Dirofilaria immitis,* lungworms and flukes

Pleuritis and Pleuropneumonia
Feline infectious peritonitis
Anaerobic bacteria
Aerobic bacteria (*Pasteurella* spp, *E. coli,* etc.)
Nocardia asteroides
Actinomyces spp
Blastomyces dermatididis
Toxoplasma gondii

*This list is not comprehensive; important clinical conditions are indicated, and the most commonly affected species are designated as [C] = canine and [F] = feline.
†Infection commonly extends to the larynx and trachea.
‡Infection commonly extends to the bronchi and may cause pneumonia.
§Alveolar involvement may develop in some cases of interstitial pneumonia.
‖Pulmonary abscess, pleuropneumonia, and pyothorax may develop.

TABLE 3. Diagnosis of Respiratory Infections

Rhinitis and Sinusitis

Signalment (age, breed, sex), vaccination status, history

Physical examination (emphasis: head, eyes, nose, oral cavity, regional lymph nodes)

Serologic tests for aspergillosis, FeLV, FIV, and *Cryptococcus neoformans*

Skull and nasal radiographs

Rhinoscopy and dental and oral cavity examinations under anesthesia

Nasal culture (bacterial, fungal)

Aspiration biopsy/cytology (traumatic nasal flush) or forceps mucosal biopsy of nasal cavities

Fine-needle aspiration biopsy/cytology of regional lymph nodes or masses

Surgical exploration of nasal cavity and paranasal sinuses for culture, biopsy, and debridement.

Virology: Immunocytologic identification of viruses (e.g., immunofluorescence for canine distemper, feline herpesvirus) and virus isolation (e.g., feline calicivirus)

Bronchopulmonary Infections

History and physical examination (observation, auscultation, percussion of thorax)

Thoracic radiography

Hemogram (to characterize inflammatory responses)

Heartworm tests

Transtracheal or endotracheal wash (aspiration cytology; culture and sensitivity testing)

Bronchoscopy (visual examination and bronchoalveolar lavage cytology)

Fecal examinations: (flotation and Baermann sedimentation to detect lung parasites)

Serologic testing when appropriate (e.g., immunodiffusion for systemic mycoses, IgM ELISA for toxoplasmosis)

Pleuritis/Pyothorax

History and physical examination (observation, auscultation, percussion of thorax)

Thoracic radiography (pre- and post-thoracocentesis)

Thoracocentesis

Cytology, culture and sensitivity testing of pleural effusate

Serological testing when appropriate (FIV, feline infectious peritonitis)

---

nasal tumors (see sec. 6, ch. 23) or dental disease complicated by secondary nasal infection.
- Radiographs demonstrate increased fluid density in the nasal cavity or sinuses; various degrees of bony destruction may be evident with chronic infection or with neoplasia.
- Idiopathic lymphocytic-plasmacytic inflammation in dogs, which may be allergic, may facilitate secondary mucosal invasion by bacteria or fungi. Biopsy is required for diagnosis.
- Some infections caused by *Aspergillus* and *Penicillium* species require histologic examination of nasal tissue with special stains (e.g., silver) to detect hyphae.
- High-quality rhinoscopy and radiography, and possible surgical exploration, may be required to identify *Rhinosporidium* infection, foreign bodies, and mass lesions. A retroflexed bronchoscope or a dental mirror may be needed to identify lesions at the caudal choanae.
- Because bacteria and fungi normally can be cultured from the nasal cavities, it is essential to exclude any underlying conditions and to avoid overinterpretations of positive cultures.

Treatment

Treatment depends on the underlying condition.

Viral and Bacterial Infections

- Management of acute upper respiratory infection involves: supportive nursing care, maintenance of hydration, and prevention of secondary bacterial infections by administration of a broad-spectrum antibiotic (do not use tetracycline in young animals or chloramphenicol in cats) (see sec. 2, ch. 4 for further details regarding feline viral rhinitis).
- Dogs > 8 months of age with bordetellosis may be treated with tetracycline; however, this brush-border inhabitant is difficult to eradicate with systemic antibiotics. When *B. bronchiseptica* has been definitively diagnosed, consider empirical therapy with nebulized gentamicin (3–5 mg/kg q12h for 5 days:
  - Use a DeVilbiss #40 nebulizer, remove the bulb and attach the unit to an oxygen source to vaporize a 1:1 gentamicin:saline mixture through an attached anesthetic mask that is lightly placed over the muzzle.
  - Gentamicin is not absorbed systemically by this route.
- Treat immunosuppressed patients with secondary bacterial rhinitis with broad-spectrum antibiotics when clinical signs worsen or if lower respiratory infection develops.

Fungal Infections

A variety of treatments have been suggested for fungal rhinitis/sinusitis, and treatment can be complicated and, in many cases, unsuccessful. The use of surgical curettage and drainage tubes combined with medical therapy is one method (see sec. 6, ch. 18). An alternative is medical therapy alone, which is preferred by the authors unless enilconazole is to be used. Drug selection depends on the infective agents.

- In cases of rhinosporidiosis, surgical extraction of the "puff-balls" is recommended.
- *Aspergillus flavus* and *Penicillium* species have been treated with a variety of medications:
  - Enilconazole (10 mg/kg, q12h, infused topically for 6–8 weeks) is effective but not yet available. To instill enilconazole, nasal tubes (rhinostomy) are placed in the frontal sinus.
  - Itraconazole (Janssen), another azole derivative not yet available, is effective when given for 6–8 weeks at a dosage of 5 mg/kg PO, q12h.
  - Thiabendazole (Mintezol; Merck), (10–20 mg/kg PO, q12h [start at lower dose] for 6–8 weeks), is less effective (40–50% positive response) and is hepatotoxic.
  - Ketoconazole (Nizoral, Janssen) (5–10 mg/kg PO, q12h for 6–8 weeks), is as effective as thiabendazole.
- Treat *Cryptococcus neoformans* infection of the upper airways with ketoconazole, amphotericin B (alone or in combination with ketoconazole or flucytosine), or itraconazole (see sec. 2, ch. 12 for description of antifungal drugs and their dosages).

BRONCHOPNEUMONIA

Etiology

Bronchopneumonia in dogs and cats is almost always related to bacterial infection. Common microorganisms responsible for bacterial pneumonia are indicated in Table 2. Bacterial pneumonia is an important cause of morbidity and mortality in dogs and cats, especially in hospitalized animals. The route of infection is typically inhalation. Hematogenous spread to the lungs is less common and can be very difficult to treat. Prompt recognition and treatment of bronchopneumonia is important; moreover, it is essential that the clinician also consider the underlying risk factors and predispositions for pneumonia, including:

- Contagious upper respiratory infection (e.g., infective tracheobronchitis after boarding)
- Preexistent bronchopulmonary disease (lungworms, systemic mycoses, lung contusion, heartworm disease, smoke inhalation, thromboembolic disease)
- Pulmonary atelectasis
- Inhalation or aspiration of pharyngeal or gastric fluid or contents as the result of anesthesia, swallowing disorders, megaesophagus, neuromuscular disease, laryngeal paralysis, posterior fossa brain-stem disorder, stupor, vomiting, prolonged recumbency
- Oronasal sources of infection (sinusitis, dental disease) with oro- or sinobronchial route of infection
- Immunosuppression caused by another virus (FeLV, FIV, canine distemper, parvovirus) or disease (hyperadrenocorticism, diabetes mellitus, generalized demodecosis)
- Immunosuppressive drug therapy (glucocorticoids, anticancer chemotherapy)
- Abnormal respiratory defense mechanisms (Cushing's disease, chronic bronchitis, ciliary dyskinesia, neutrophil dysfunction syndromes)
- Bronchial foreign body
- Foreign body (food; mineral oil in cats) aspiration pneumonia
- Debilitation, hospitalization, nosocomial infection
- Indwelling intravenous catheter sepsis (hematogenous spread)
- Contaminated endotracheal tube, tracheostomy tube, or bronchoscope
- Aspiration or inhalation of liquid foreign material during diagnostic or therapeutic procedures (barium sulfate, medications, mineral oil, nutritional supplements)
- Following thoracic surgery

Clinical Signs

- The history often indicates a predisposing factor for bronchopneumonia.
- Tachypnea, respiratory distress, productive cough, and fever are typical features.
- Constitutional signs such as depression, anorexia, and listlessness may be observed as the only features of disease.
- Mucopurulent nasal exudate may be present.
- Pulmonary adventitious sounds, especially rhonchi and crackles, may be auscultated; however, loud or asymmetric bronchial sounds may be the only auscultatory finding.

Diagnosis

Clinical signs, radiography, and a hemogram are usually sufficient to make a presumptive diagnosis of bacteria pneumonia. Airway cytology and culture can confirm the diagnosis.

- Thoracic radiography indicates increased lung density that most commonly is alveolar in nature (manifested as air bronchograms) and cranioventral in distribution. Lung consolidation may occur, leading to an eventual loss of air bronchograms except for the most proximal portion of the lobe.
  - Hilar or sternal lymphadenopathy is uncommon in animals with bacterial infection.
  - Pleural effusion (pyothorax) is uncommon and, when present with pneumonia, suggests an atypical infectious agent such as *Nocardia* or *Actinomyces* species, a pleural foreign body, associated malignancy, or pulmonary embolus.
  - Hematogenous pneumonia (e.g., from catheter sepsis) may be diffuse, beginning as an interstitial pattern and progressing to alveolar.
  - Viral, protozoal (e.g., toxoplasmosis), and fungal pneumonia typically are interstitial in distribution. Fungal and *Toxoplasma* infections produce granulomatous lesions in the lung, and, with systemic mycoses, hilar lymphadenopathy can be pronounced.

KEY POINT ▶ The right middle lung lobe is most prone to bacterial infection; the cranial lobes frequently also are involved. A *cranioventral* distribution of bacterial bronchopneumonia is typical.

- Leukocytosis, left shift, and monocytosis are typical; however, the magnitude of change is not consistently related to the extent of infection. Overwhelming fulminant bacterial pneumonia may cause a neutropenia with degenerative left shift.
- Infected cats also may be FIV- or FeLV-positive (see sec. 2, chs. 1 and 2).
- Transtracheal or endotracheal aspiration cytology demonstrates neutrophilic inflammation, often with degenerative polymorphonuclear neutrophils (PMNs) and intracellular bacteria. Cocci are usually streptococci, and rods are usually gram-negative bacteria. The culture typically is positive for bacterial growth (see Tables 1 and 2).
  - Avoid percutaneous needle aspiration of the lung in order to prevent inoculation of the pleural space.
- The condition that predisposed the animal to bronchopneumonia may be evident from the history, physical, and neurologic examinations or may require additional studies such as:
  - Barium swallow to identify swallowing disorders
  - Bronchoscopy to identify a bronchial foreign body

Treatment

General Measures

- Keep the patient well hydrated and warm. Fluid therapy is often required to prevent dehydration, which can cause inspissation of respiratory secretions.
- Perform thoracic coupage 4–6 times daily. When the patient has recovered sufficiently, brief walks followed by coupage help to mobilize tracheobronchial secretions.
- Airway humidification may assist in expectoration of secretions.
- Expectorants such as guaifenesin are of uncertain merit and usually are not prescribed.
- Bronchodilator therapy is not of proven efficacy but may reverse irritative bronchoconstriction and strengthen respiratory muscle effort in dyspneic animals (see Table 3 in sec. 6, ch. 20 for specific drugs and dosages).
- Cough suppressants are contraindicated.
- Administer humidified oxygen to dyspneic, cyanotic, or hypoxemic animals.

Antibiotics

Give antibiotics at least 3 weeks; duration of therapy may be longer, depending on clinical results and radiographs.

- Base antibiotic choice on culture and sensitivity testing (obtained by transtracheal washes) and on current or prior antibiotic therapy.
- Consider initial treatment while awaiting culture results) with an extended-spectrum antibiotic such as cephalosporin, sulfadiazine-trimethoprim, quinolone (enrofloxacin), amoxicillin-clavulanic acid, tetracycline (mature dogs), and chloramphenicol (not in cats).
  - In life-threatening sepsis, consider the combination of intravenous cephalothin (20 mg/kg, q8h) or ampicillin (20 mg/kg, q8h) plus amikacin (5 mg/kg q8h).
  - Newer-generation cephalosporins (e.g., moxalactam) are very expensive and usually reserved for resistant infections.
- Diffuse pulmonary infiltration in cats may be associated with mycoplasma or hematogenous bacterial infections. The quinolones, tetracyclines, and erythromycin have demonstrated activity against mycoplasma organisms.

Follow-up Radiography

Obtain radiographs to ensure resolution of infection.

- It may take 2–6 weeks for areas of lobar consolidation to become totally clear. If there is a lack of steady clinical and radiographic improvement, reevaluate the patient and consider a tracheal wash or bronchoscopy with bronchial fluid aspiration.
- Recurrent pneumonia is common, particularly in animals with persistence of predisposing factors such as swallowing disorders, anticancer therapy, ciliary dyskinesis, and acquired or congenital immune deficiencies.
- Infrequently, an unresponsive or refractory single lobe infection requires surgical lobectomy for resolution of the problem (see sec. 6, ch. 25).

Bacterial Pyothorax

Management of bacterial pyothorax requires thoracostomy tube drainage and antibiotics (see sec. 6, ch. 22). Because anaerobic organisms commonly are involved in pyothorax, one of the following treatment regimens is recommended:

- Penicillin (20,000–40,000 units/kg PO or IV, q6–8h) alone or in combination with either sulfadiazine-trimethoprim (Tribrissen, 15 mg/kg PO, q12h) or clindamycin (Antirobe; Upjohn) (5–10 mg/kg, PO, q12h)

RESPIRATORY PARASITES

Etiology

A number of respiratory parasites have been identified in dogs and cats. The life cycle of some of these is complex and involves intermediate and transport hosts. Clinically, the most important infections are:

- *Aelurostrongylus abstrusus:* This nematode is a feline parasite; the intermediate host is a snail or slug; transport hosts include birds, small mammals, and reptiles.
- *Paragonimus kellicotti:* A fluke of the dog and cat. Infection follows ingestion of an intermediate host (crayfish, aquatic snail) or transport host (e.g., raccoon).
- *Capillaria aerophilia:* A nematode parasite of the dog and cat that has a direct life cycle.
- *Filaroides* spp.: These nematodes parasitize the respiratory tract of the dog and exhibit a direct life cycle. Three species have been associated with respiratory disease: *F. osleri* (lives in granulomas near the tracheal bifurcation), *F. milksi* (bronchopulmonary parasite), and *F. hirthi* (lung parasite).
- *Toxoplasma gondii:* A multisystemic protozoal infection that usually is subclinical but occasionally can cause pneumonia (see sec. 2, ch. 13 for further details of this infection).

Clinical Signs

- Signs depend on the specific parasite, the severity of infection, and the magnitude of the host reaction.
- Mild cases are asymptomatic and detected only if ova or larvae are identified during routine fecal examination.
- Clinically apparent infections occur most often in younger animals (< 2 years) that are heavily infested.
- Coughing is the most common sign of lungworm infections. Exercise intolerance and weight loss also may occur.
- Fever and tachypnea are typical of toxoplasmosis but not of other respiratory parasitic infections.
- Multisystemic disease may be present in animals with

toxoplasmosis, including neurologic signs, anterior uveitis, chorioretinitis, and hepatitis.

Diagnosis

Diagnosis of lungworms is based on the clinical examination, radiography, and identification of ova or larvae in fecal samples or respiratory secretions.

- Transtracheal washes or aspirations of tracheobronchial secretions may demonstrate parasitic ova or larvae. In some cases, ova are scarce. An eosinophilic pulmonary infiltrate with accompanying neutrophilia is typical. Peripheral eosinophilia is not uncommon in lungworm or fluke infections.
- Radiographs are helpful in the recognition of advanced lungworm infections.
  - Aelurostrongylosis: An indistinct interstitial-nodular pattern may be detected. Distribution of infiltrates varies but caudal lung lobes are typically involved.
  - Paragonimiasis: Granulomas with interstitial reaction are typical, and the appearance of air-filled cystic structures (especially in the dog) is characteristic of this parasitic infection.
  - *Filaroides* infection: The more common parasite *F. osleri* causes no obvious radiographic changes unless soft tissue granulomas are observed in the air-filled distal trachea and carina. *F. milksi* can cause a diffuse and severe interstitial infiltrate. *F. hirthi* generally is present in research kennels and seldom leads to clinical disease.
  - Toxoplasmosis: The pulmonary form of toxoplasmosis leads to a mixed interstitial-alveolar infiltrate seen radiographically
- Use fecal flotation to identify ova (double-operculated *Capillaria* ova, single-operculated *Paragonimus* ova) and larvae of *Aelurostrongylus* or *Filaroides* organisms. Special fecal sedimentation techniques may be required to identify larvae.
- Diagnosis of *F. osleri* usually requires bronchoscopy,

identification of nodules (containing small, filamentous worms), or biopsy of a granuloma.
- Diagnosis of pulmonary toxoplasmosis depends on clinical signs and serologic evaluation (see sec. 2, ch. 13).

Treatment

Treatment of respiratory parasites involves destroying the infective organism, reducing parenchymal reaction, and instructing the owner about the prevention of further infection.

A number of drugs have demonstrated efficacy against respiratory parasites. Fenbendazole (Panacur) generally is the safest. In cases of severe eosinophilic pulmonary reaction, adjunctive therapy with prednisolone (0.25 mg/kg PO, once or twice daily for 7–14 days) may be helpful.

- Aelurostrongylosis: Fenbendazole (Panacur), 50 mg/kg PO, q24h for 10 days
- Paragonimiasis (give one):
  - Fenbendazole (as for aelurostrongylosis)
  - Praziquantel (Droncit), 25 mg/kg PO, q8h for 2 days)
  - Albendazole (25–50 mg/kg PO, q12h for 10–20 days)
- *Filaroides* infection: Administer fenbendazole or albendazole (as preceding infections) or oral ivermectin, 200 μg/kg/week for 3 doses or 400 μg/kg once; do not give to collies.
- *Capillaria* infection often is asymptomatic but can be treated as for *Filaroides* infection.

Prognosis for recovery and elimination of signs is good unless severe granulomatous disease has developed, in which case, residual cough may occur.

Supplemental Readings

Greene CE: *Infectious Diseases of the Dog and Cat*, 2nd ed. Philadelphia: W.B. Saunders, 1990, pp 114, 259, 669, 909.

22 Pleural Effusion

Theresa W. Fossum

Pleural effusion, the abnormal accumulation of fluid in the pleural space, is a common diagnostic problem encountered by veterinarians. Regardless of cause, fluid in the pleural space requires investigation because it may signify serious and frequently life-threatening disease.

ETIOLOGY

- The amount of fluid in the thoracic cavity is governed by factors that affect the production and resorption of fluid. Normally a small amount of fluid is present in the thorax and serves to lubricate the pleural surfaces.
- Changes in hydrostatic and oncotic pressures and vascular or lymphatic permeability may increase pleural fluid production and/or decrease its resorption, resulting in pleural effusion. Etiologies of pleural effusion are classified according to these mechanisms in Table 1.

CLINICAL SIGNS

Clinical signs associated with pleural effusion vary, depending on the underlying etiology, rapidity of fluid accumulation, and volume of fluid. Accumulation of fluid within the pleural space restricts lung expansion and ventilation. Most animals do not exhibit clinical signs until there is significant impairment of ventilation; hence, pleural effusion may first be noted by the veterinarian on careful physical examination, prior to the presence of obvious clinical signs.

Common clinical signs include:

- Tachypnea and inspiratory dyspnea that may worsen with exercise or exertion
- Open-mouth breathing, cyanosis, and preference for sternal recumbency, often seen in advanced pleural effusion
- Muffled heart and lung sounds on auscultation
- Coughing, that may be the result of tracheobronchial compression from a mediastinal mass, simultaneous lung involvement, or severe pleuritis (as in some animals with chylothorax and pyothorax)
- Cardiogenic pleural effusion, which can be accompanied by ascites, pericardial effusion, jugular venous distension/pulsation, arrhythmias, or murmurs

Additional nonspecific findings include

- Fever (e.g., pyothorax, feline infectious peritonitis [FIP]).
- Depression
- Anorexia, weight loss, and pale mucous membranes.

DIAGNOSIS

The cause of pleural effusion may be obvious, as when it is associated with underlying cardiac disease. In most cases, the combination of physical examination, radiography, and fluid analysis is required for accurate diagnosis. Occasionally, despite these evaluations, because the etiology of the fluid remains obscure and undefined, further diagnostic procedures are required.

Radiography

- Radiographic signs associated with pleural effusion are listed in Table 2.
- Preferred views
  - If small amount of fluid: ventrodorsal and lateral; expiratory.
  - If large amount of fluid and animal is severely dyspneic: standing lateral and dorsoventral.
- Evaluate radiographs for underlying cardiomegaly, intrapulmonary lesions (masses, infiltrates, vascular changes), diaphragmatic hernia, lung lobe torsion, and thoracic trauma. These abnormalities may be more easily identified on post-thoracentesis radiographs.
- Other radiographic findings of diagnostic significance include:
  - Unilateral pleural effusion (fluid encapsulation), which occurs most often in pyothorax and chylothorax but also occasionally in hemothorax, lung neoplasia, diaphragmatic hernia, and lung lobe torsion.
  - Rounded lung lobe edges (fibrosing pleuritis) that most often are the result of fibrosing visceral pleural reaction in chylothorax and pyothorax (occasionally FIP).
  - Concurrent ascites, seen in congestive heart failure (CHF) (dogs > cats), FIP, severe hypoproteinemia, diaphragmatic hernia, and disseminated neoplasia
  - Mediastinal mass, such as lymphoma
  - Fluid-dense lung lobe, which occurs in lung lobe torsion and primary lung tumors
  - Displaced abdominal organs, which may occur in diaphragmatic hernia
- In selected cases (see sec.1, ch. 4), contrast radiography may be indicated to evaluate:

TABLE 1. Etiologies of Pleural Effusion

Pathogenetic Mechanisms	Etiologies
Increased hydrostatic pressure	Congestive heart failure (e.g., cardiomyopathy, valvular diseases, pericardial effusion; see sec. 6, ch. 9)
	Overinfusion of fluids
	Intrathoracic neoplasia (see sec. 6, ch. 22)
Decreased oncotic pressure (due to hypoalbuminemia)	Protein-losing enteropathy (see sec. 7, ch. 6)
	Liver disease (see sec. 7, ch. 9)
	Protein-losing nephropathy (nephrotic syndrome; see sec. 8, ch. 1)
Vascular/lymphatic permeability or obstruction	Infectious pleuritis
	Bacterial (pyothorax; see Table 4)
	Viral (FIP: see sec. 2, ch. 3)
	Fungal (blastomycosis; see sec. 2, ch. 12)
	Noninfectious pleuritis
	Uremia (see sec. 8, ch. 1)
	Pancreatitis (see sec. 7, ch. 10)
	Foreign body penetration of the pleural space
	Hemorrhage (trauma, coagulopathy, neoplasia)
	Diaphragmatic hernia (see sec. 6, chs. 23 and 24)
	Lung lobe torsion
	Pulmonary thromboembolism
	Neoplasia (see sec. 6, ch. 22)
	Mediastinal lymphosarcoma
	Metastatic neoplasia (e.g., mammary)
	Primary lung tumors
	Mesothelioma
	Chylothorax
	Idiopathic (etiology undetermined)
	Secondary to primary disease
	Congestive heart failure, pericardial disease
	Obstruction of cranial vena cava (thrombosis)
	Blastomycosis
	Occult heartworm disease in cats
	Neoplasia (e.g., lymphosarcoma)
	Immune-mediated

- The thoracic duct in chylothorax by contrast lymphangiography
- Esophageal compression by mediastinal masses-barium by contrast esophography
- For diaphragmatic hernia (positive contrast [iodide] peritoneography)
- Cardiac disease, especially congenital types (contrast angiocardiography)

KEY POINT ▶ Avoid radiography if the patient is extremely dyspneic. Perform thoracocentesis first to stabilize the animal.

Ultrasonography

Perform ultrasonography to evaluate:
- Cardiac function (cardiogenic versus noncardiogenic effusion)

TABLE 2. Radiographic Signs of Pleural Effusion

Blurring of cardiac silhouette
Fluid-filled interlobar fissures
Rounding or blunting of lung margins at costophrenic angles (ventrodorsal view)
Scalloping of lung margins at sternal border (lateral view)
Widening of mediastinum
Separation of lung borders from thoracic wall by fluid density

- Valvular lesions
- Congenital cardiac abnormalities
- Pericardial effusion
- Mediastinal and cardiac masses

KEY POINT ▶ Perform ultrasonography prior to removal of pleural fluid.

Thoracocentesis

The technique for thoracocentesis is described in sec. 1, ch. 3. Collect fluid for analysis as follows:

- For nucleated cell count: 5 ml in EDTA tube.
- For cytology: 6–8 direct smears or 5 ml EDTA tube for cytocentrifuge preparation
- For biochemical parameters (e.g., triglyceride): 5 ml in clot tube
- For culture: inoculation of aerobic and anaerobic media

Fluid Analysis

The characteristics of various pleural effusion patterns and their clinical associations are described in Table 3.

Color, Clarity, and Viscosity

- Clear and colorless: transudate
- Clear, amber to red-tinged: transudate or modified transudate

TABLE 3. Guidelines for Categorization of Feline Pleural Effusions

	Transudate	Modified Transudate	Nonseptic Exudate	Septic Exudate	Chylous Effusion	Hemorrhage
Color	Colorless to pale yellow	Yellow or pink	Yellow or pink	Yellow to red-brown	Milky white	Red
Turbidity	Clear	Clear to cloudy	Clear to cloudy	Cloudy to opaque; flocculent	Opaque	Opaque
Protein (g/dl)	<1.5	1.5–3.0	2.5–6.0 (FIP: 3.5–8.5)	3.0–7.0	2.5–6.0*	>3.0
Fibrin†	Absent	Absent	Present	Present	Variable	Present
Triglyceride‡	Absent	Absent	Absent	Absent	Present	Absent
Bacteria§	Absent	Absent	Absent	Present	Absent	Absent
Nucleated cells/µl	<1000	1000–5000 (LSA: 1000–100,000)	1000–20,000 (LSA: 1000–100,000)	5000–300,000	500–20,000	Similar to that of peripheral blood
Cytologic features	Mostly mesothelial cells	Mostly macrophages and mesothelial cells; few nondegenerate PMNs; neoplastic cells (LSA, carcinoma) in some cases	Mostly nondegenerate PMN and macrophages; neoplastic cells (LSA, carcinoma) in some cases	Mostly degenerate PMN; also macrophages	Lymphocytes, PMN, and macrophages in variable proportions	Mostly erythrocytes; some leukocytes
Disease associations	Hypoproteinemia Early CHF (rare)	Chronic CHF Neoplasia (LSA, carcinoma) Diaphragmatic hernia	FIP Neoplasia Diaphragmatic hernia Lung lobe torsion	septic pleuritis (pyothorax)	Chylothorax; Obstructed thoracic duct Ruptured thoracic duct CHF Neoplasia (LSA)	Hemothorax: Trauma Hemostatic disorders Neoplasia

*Protein concentration is artifactually increased by the lipid content of the fluid.
†Fibrin is evidenced by the presence of flecks, strands, or clots.
‡Triglyceride concentration exceeds that of serum; cholesterol/triglyceride ratio is <1; chylomicrons are seen microscopically; milky opalescence clears when either is added.
§Bacteria demonstrated cytologically or by culture.
FIP = feline infectious peritonitis; LSA = lymphosarcoma; CHF = congestive heart failure; PMNs = polymorphonuclear leukocytes or neutrophils.
Adapted from Sherding RG: Diseases of the pleura and pleural space. *In* Sherding RG, ed.: *The Cat: Diseases and Clinical Management.* New York: Churchill Livingstone, 1989.

- Mildly turbid, amber to red-tinged: usually modified transudate
- Moderately to markedly turbid, amber to red-tinged: exudate
- Yellow, tan, or white and opaque: exudate (e.g., chylothorax, pyothorax)
- Red, opaque: exudate (e.g., hemothorax)
- Viscous fluid: associated with FIP or highly cellular fluids with large numbers of ruptured cells.

Specific Gravity, Total Protein, and Nucleated Cell Count

See Table 3.

Cytology (Determine Predominant Cell Type)

- Mesothelial cells and macrophages: transudate, modified transudate
- Neutrophils and macrophages: modified transudate or exudate (e.g., pyothorax, chylothorax, mycoses, immune-mediated disease, neoplasia)
- Lymphocytes
  - If mature: consider chylothorax or heart failure
  - If lymphoblasts: consider lymphoma
- Eosinophils (> 10%): consider pneumothorax, neoplasia, parasites, immune-mediated infections
- Neoplastic cells: search for primary tumor

KEY POINT ▶ Be sure to differentiate reactive mesothelial cells from neoplastic cells. Many primary and metastatic neoplasms do not exfoliate into pleural fluid.

- Peripheral blood: intrapleural hemorrhage due to coagulopathy, neoplasia, lung-lobe torsion, traumatic vascular injury
- Chylomicrons: very suggestive of chylous effusion
- Degenerative neutrophils
  - Culture
  - See Table 1 and discussion of pyothorax for common etiologic agents in septic pleuritis.

Miscellaneous Evaluations

Ether Clearance Test. This can be used as a rapid screening test for chyle. An advantage is its practicality: however, it is not as accurate as cholesterol and triglyceride analysis.

Technique

1. Divide 6 ml of pleural fluid equally into two test tubes.
2. Alkalinize both samples by adding 3 drops of 10% KOH to each tube.
3. Add 3 ml of ether to one tube and 3 ml of water to the other.
4. Shake the tubes several times and compare. If the fluid is chyle, the ether mixture will appear clearer than the control.

Cholesterol and Triglyceride Concentration in Fluid Versus Serum

- Chylothorax
  - Pleural fluid cholesterol ≤ serum cholesterol

- Pleural fluid triglyceride > serum triglyceride.
- Pseudochylous effusion (extremely rare in animals)
  - Pleural fluid cholesterol > serum cholesterol.
  - Pleural fluid triglyceride ≤ serum triglyceride.
- Protein electrophoresis
  - Consider as aid to diagnosis of effusive FIP in cats
  - Values predictive of FIP: albumin < 48% of total protein, gamma globulin > 32% of total protein, A/G ratio < 0.82

Miscellaneous. Common tests whose usefulness in animals has not been established include pH measurement, glucose concentration, and amylase/lipase concentrations.

Laboratory Evaluations

Depending on suspected etiologies for pleural effusion, the following laboratory evaluations may be indicated.

- Complete blood count (CBC) to evaluate leukocyte responses (e.g., pyothorax, FIP, neoplasia)
- Serum chemistry profile
  - To screen for concurrent systemic diseases or complications
  - To evaluate serum proteins for hypoalbuminemia as a cause of transudative effusion and for hyperglobulinemia as a marker of chronic immune stimulation (e.g., FIP)
- Tests for feline infectious diseases
  - Coronaviral serologic test (for FIP; see sec. 2, ch. 3)
  - Feline leukemia virus antigen test (in mediastinal lymphoma; see sec. 2, ch. 1)
  - Feline immunodeficiency virus serologic test (in pyothorax; see sec. 2, ch. 2)
- Tests for underlying causes of feline cardiomyopathic pleural effusion
  - Serum thyroxin (T4) determination (for hyperthyroidism; see sec. 4, ch. 1)
  - Plasma taurine concentration (for taurine deficiency; see sec. 6, ch. 8)
  - Heartworm ELISA (for heartworm-induced chylothorax; see sec. 6, ch. 10)

Exploratory Thoracotomy

Indications

- To identify and remove migrating pleural foreign bodies
- For biopsy of lung or mediastinal lesions
- For treatment of pyothorax or chylothorax
- For lung lobectomy (e.g., lung lobe torsion, neoplasia)

Technique

See sec. 6, ch. 25.

TREATMENT

The treatment of pleural effusion varies depending on the underlying etiology. Only the specific treatment of chylothorax and pyothorax are described here. For the various other underlying causes of pleural effusion, the reader is referred to the respective chapters on those diseases.

Chylothorax

- When possible, identify and treat the underlying disorder including:
  - Cardiovascular disease (e.g., congestive heart failure, thrombosis, heartworms)
  - Mediastinal lymphoma (by chemotherapy)

Idiopathic Chylothorax

Medical Management

- Thoracocentesis as needed (see sec. 1, ch. 3 for technique)
- Feed a low-fat diet (e.g., r/d Prescription Diet; Hill's) or a homemade diet consisting of 1 cup of boiled rice or potato, oatmeal, or pasta and 1 cup low-fat (2%) cottage cheese, supplemented with 1 vitamin/mineral tablet, ½ tsp calcium carbonate (e.g., Tums), and 15 ml of MCT oil. This meets the daily needs of a 6 to 7-kg dog.
  - Skinned, boiled chicken breast or water-packed tuna may be substituted for cottage cheese.
  - Supplement with MCT oil (Mead Johnson), 1–2 ml/kg/day PO, because short- and medium-chain triglycerides are absorbed directly into the portal system, bypassing the thoracic duct.

Surgery. Surgical options include mesenteric lymphangiography and thoracic duct ligation, passive pleuroperitoneal shunting, active pleuroperitoneal or pleurovenous shunting, and pleurodesis.

Mesenteric Lymphangiography and Thoracic Duct Ligation. Thoracic duct ligation causes the formation of abdominal lymphatic anastomoses for transport of chyle to the venous system, thereby bypassing the thoracic duct. Preoperative lymphangiography helps to identify the thoracic duct and its branches.

- Procedure:
  - To aid in visualization of a mesenteric lymphatic for cannulation, feed animal corn oil or cream 3 hours prior to surgery; alternatively, inject methylene blue (American Quinine, Shirley, NY) into a mesenteric lymph node at surgery.
  - Via a right (dogs) or left (cats) paracostal incision or a ventral midline abdominal approach, cannulate a mesenteric lymphatic.
  - Take thoracic radiographs following injection of a contrast agent (e.g., Conray or Renovist, 0.5 ml/kg diluted in an equal volume of saline). The lymphangiogram helps to identify the location and number of branches of the thoracic duct to be ligated.
  - Perform ligation of the thoracic duct and its branches through a ninth or tenth space intercostal thoracotomy (right-sided approach in dogs; left-sided in cats), or transdiaphragmatically, using 2-0 or 3-0 silk suture and hemoclips.

- Verify complete ligation by repeating the lymphangiogram following ligation.
- Thoracic duct ligation results in complete resolution of pleural effusion approximately 50% of the time in dogs and <30% of the time in cats.
- Advantage: If successful, thoracic duct ligation results in complete resolution of pleural fluid, in contrast to the palliative procedures described later.
- Disadvantages:
  - Prolonged surgery time
  - High incidence of continued or recurrent chylous or nonchylous (from pulmonary lymphatics) effusion.
  - Difficulty in performing mesenteric lymphangiography (particularly in cats).
  - Ligation of all branches of the thoracic duct may not be assured, even though dye does not enter the thoracic duct after ligation.

Passive Pleuroperitoneal Shunting (PPS). This procedure allows palliative treatment of animals with chylothorax by shunting chyle into the abdominal cavity, where it is absorbed owing to the increased surface area. PPS may be performed in conjunction with thoracic duct ligation or alone.

- Procedure:
  - Cut medical-grade silastic sheeting (Dow Corning, Midland, MI) to fit defects created in the diaphragm. Make perforations in the sheeting with a 3- or 6-mm biopsy punch.
  - Suture sheeting to the edges of the diaphragmatic defect using nonabsorbable suture material (Prolene; Ethicon, Somerville, NJ).
- Success rates have not been reported in a large number of animals; however, spontaneous resolution of pleural fluid has occurred in some animals following placement.
- *Advantage:* PPS is inexpensive and easy to perform, shortening the duration of surgery, which is especially beneficial in debilitated animals.
- *Disadvantage:* Patients are at risk for developing fibrosing pleuritis if chylothorax continues. Also, inadequate drainage frequently occurs if the holes become plugged with fibrin or abdominal organs.

KEY POINT ▶ Do not use PPS in animals with cardiac disease or portal hypertension because the effusion may not be reabsorbed from the abdominal cavity.

Active Pleuroperitoneal or Pleurovenous Shunting

- Procedure:
  - Place one arm of a commercially made shunt catheter (Denver Double-Valve Peritoneous Shunt; Denver Biomaterials Inc., Evergreen, CO) into the thorax, place the other arm into the abdomen or venous system (jugular or azygous vein or caudal vena cava).
  - Position the pump chamber over the rib cage so that it can be effectively compressed.
  - Manually pump pleural fluid into the abdomen or

TABLE 4. Morphologic and Culture Characteristics of Bacteria Commonly Associated with Pyothorax in Small Animals

Bacterial Genus	Oxygen Requirements	Gram Stain	Morphology	Antibiotic Sensitivity*
Actinomyces	Facultative to strict anaerobe	Gram-positive	Small bacilli; may form filaments; often beaded and difficult to discern in clinical specimens; may form sulfur granules	**Penicillin** (penicillin G, ampicillin and amoxicillin), cephalosporin, clindamycin, chloramphenicol, erythromycin
Bacteroides	Obligate anaerobe	Gram-negative	Bacilli; pleomorphic and may be beaded or cocci; often stain poorly and are difficult to see	Most *Bacteroides* spp—**Penicillin**, cephalosporin, clindamycin, chloramphenicol, metronidazole
				B. fragilis—amoxicillin plus clavulanic acid, clindamycin, chloramphenicol, metronidazole
Clostridium	Obligate anaerobe	Gram-positive	Bacilli; large, frequently encapsulated, motile; spores uncommon from clinical specimens	Most Clostridia spp—penicillin, chloramphenicol, metronidazole
				C. perfringens—**penicillin**, cefoxitin, clindamycin, chloramphenicol, metronidazole, erythromycin
Fusobacterium	Obligate anaerobe	Gram-negative	Bacilli; often have a cigar-shaped appearance; may be filamentous	**Penicillin**, clindamycin, chloramphenicol, metronidazole
Klebsiella	Facultative anaerobe	Gram-negative	Bacilli; encapsulated	**Cephalosporin**, gentamicin, tobramycin, ticarcillin
Nocardia	Aerobe	Gram-positive (partially acid-fast)	Small bacilli; may form filaments; often beaded and difficult to discern in clinical specimens; may form sulfur granules	**Trimethoprim-sulfa**, tetracycline, gentamicin, amikacin
Pasteurella	Facultative anaerobe	Gram-negative	Coccobacilli; pleomorphic; biopolar staining from tissues	Penicillin, ampicillin
Pseudomonas	Aerobe	Gram-negative	Bacilli; slender, motile	**Carbenicillin**, gentamicin, tobramycin, amikacin, ticarcillin, cefotaxime, moxalactam

*Bold type indicates drug of choice.
Reprinted with permission of author and publisher. Fossum TW: Pleural cavity diseases. *In* Morgan R, ed.: *Handbook of Small Animal Practice.* New York: Churchill Livingstone, 1992.

venous system by compressing the pump chamber (may require 200–300 times 3 to 4 times a day).

■ *Advantages:* Drainage of the thorax may be more complete than with PPP. Pleurovenous shunting overcomes problems with inadequate peritoneal absorption that may occur with pleuroperitoneal shunting.

■ *Disadvantages:*
  • The shunts are expensive, may easily occlude with fibrin, and require a high degree of owner compliance and dedication.
  • Some animals will not tolerate compression of the pump chamber.
  • Thrombosis, venous occlusion, sepsis, and electrolyte abnormalities may occur.

Pleurodesis. Pleurodesis is the formation of generalized adhesions between the visceral and parietal pleura.

■ Adhesions may occur spontaneously in association with pleural effusion. In some species they can be induced following instillation of an irritating substance into the pleural cavity

■ Advantage: Inexpensive and easily performed (does not require a thoracotomy or general anesthetic, except for chest tube placement).

■ Disadvantages:
  • Seldom causes generalized adhesions to form.
  • Appropriate dosages, concentrations, and dwell times of the pleurodesis agent have not been determined for dogs or cats, and little experimental data are available in animals.
  • In order for pleurodesis to occur the lungs must be able to contact the body wall; however, many animals with chronic chylothorax have some thickening of their visceral pleura that prohibits normal lung expansion.

Pyothorax

Management of pyothorax includes the following measures:

■ Diagnosis and treatment of underlying etiology if possible (foreign body, bite wound, etc.)
■ Placement of indwelling thoracic tube for pleural drainage (see sec. 1, ch. 3)
■ Thoracic lavage (see Technique)
■ Systemic antibiotic therapy
■ Surgery

Technique for Thoracic Lavage

1. Following pleural evacuation, infuse warmed lactated Ringer's solution (10 ml/kg) through tube by slow injection.

a. Heparin may be added (1500 units/100 ml of lavage solution).
b. Antibiotics may be added at half the systemic dose (unproven benefit and may cause toxicity).
2. Evacuate lavage solution after 30 minutes by syringe aspiration or by constant drainage/suction (see sec. 1, ch. 3).
3. Perform drainage and lavage 2–4 times per day.
4. Continue drainage and lavage until effusion clears and no bacteria are seen on smears.

Systemic Antibiotic Therapy

Choice of antibiotics is based on culture and sensitivity testing results.

■ See Table 4 for choice of antibiotic while waiting for culture results.
■ Continue therapy for a minimum of 3–4 weeks.

KEY POINT ▶ For treatment of pyothorax, choose an antibiotic regimen with efficacy against anaerobic bacteria because these are often involved.

Surgery

Perform thoracotomy in refractory cases (see sec. 6, ch. 25). The objectives of this procedure are to:

■ Explore for intrapleural foreign bodies
■ Break down intrapleural adhesions
■ Drain abscesses or pockets of exudate
■ Lobectomize severely diseased lung lobes
■ Allow optimal indwelling drainage tube placement

Supplemental Readings

Forrester SD, Troy GC, Fossum TW: Pleural effusions: Pathophysiology and diagnostic considerations. Comp Contin Educ Pract Vet 10:121, 1988.

Fossum TW, Birchard SJ, Jacobs RM: Chylothorax in thirty-four dogs. J Am Vet Med Assoc 188:1315, 1986.

Fossum TW, Forrester SD, Swenson CL, et al: Feline chylothorax: 37 cases (1969–1989) J Am Vet Med Assoc. 198:672–678, 1991.

Fossum TW, Evering WN, Forrester SD, et al.: Severe bilateral fibrosing pleuritis associated with chronic chylothorax in five cats and two dogs. J Am Vet Med Assoc 201:317–324, 1992.

Orton EC: Pleura and pleural space. *In* Slatter DH, ed.: *Textbook of Small Animal Surgery*. Philadelphia: W. B. Saunders, 1985, p 547.

Shelly SM, Scarlet-Kranz J, Blue J: Protein electrophoresis on effusions from cats as a diagnostic test for feline infectious peritonitis. J Am Anim Hosp Assoc 24:495, 1988.

Stewart A, Padrid P, Lobinger R. Diagnostic utility of differential cell counts and measurement of LDH, total protein, glucose and pH in the analysis of feline pleural fluid. *Proceedings,* Eighth Annu Vet Med Forum, Washington, D.C., 1990, p 1121.

23 Respiratory Neoplasia

Marcia Carothers

Neoplasms of the respiratory tract are relatively rare in small animals, representing 4–5% of all neoplasms in the dog and cat. More than 80% of respiratory tract tumors are malignant. In addition to primary tumors affecting the respiratory tract, the lungs are common sites of metastatic neoplasia.

NEOPLASMS OF THE NASAL PASSAGES AND PARANASAL SINUSES

Neoplasms of the nasal cavity are more common in dogs than in cats and constitute approximately 75% of all respiratory tract tumors in dogs. Approximately 80% of primary nasal tumors are malignant. Nasal tumors are more likely to originate in the caudal two-thirds of the nasal passages and often invade the sinuses. Local invasion of the surrounding tissues is typical of these tumors. Paraneoplastic syndromes are rare and include hypercalcemia (associated with an adenocarcinoma) and polycythemia (associated with fibrosarcoma).

Tumor Types

Histologically, epithelial tumors are more common than mesenchymal tumors. Benign tumors are rare. Table 1 lists tumors of the nasal passages and paranasal sinus occurring in dogs and cats.

KEY POINT ▶ Malignant nasal tumors usually are locally invasive, with metastasis occurring late in the course of the disease.

Signalment

- Nasal tumors are more common in older animals.
- There is no sex predilection in the dog; male cats appear to be at higher risk than female cats.
- Dolichocephalic and medium- to large-breed dogs are predisposed to developing nasal neoplasms. Canine breeds reported to be at high risk for the development of nasal neoplasms include the Airedale terrier, bassett hound, Old English sheepdog, Scottish terrier, collie, German shepherd, Keeshond, and German short-haired pointer.

History

- The average duration of clinical signs prior to diagnosis is approximately 3 months.
- Sneezing, nasal discharge, and epistaxis are the most common complaints.

- A partial response to antibiotic therapy can be observed initially; however, intermittent and progressive signs continue.

Clinical Signs

- *Unilateral or bilateral nasal discharge* (hemorrhagic, serohemorrhagic or mucopurulent) and/or ocular discharge are the most common signs noted.
- Sneezing, snoring, or reverse sneezing may also be reported by the owner.
- Facial deformity (i.e., exophthalmos and nasal swelling) may occur late in the course of the disease.
- Seizures, blindness, and behavioral changes may result from invasion of the central nervous system (CNS) by direct extension.

KEY POINT ▶ Chronic nasal discharge unresponsive to antibiotic therapy is most likely caused by neoplasia.

Diagnosis

Imaging Studies

- Plain radiographs (occlusal dorsoventral, open-mouth ventrodorsal, lateral, frontal sinuses, and ventrodorsal views) may demonstrate loss of trabecular pattern, increase in soft tissue density, septal destruction, facial bone destruction, frontal sinus opacification, and/or periosteal bone formation.
- Computed tomography (CT) may be useful in evaluating the extent of the tumor.

TABLE 1. Types of Neoplasms of Nasal Passages and Paranasal Sinuses Occurring in Dogs and Cats*

Malignant Tumors in Dogs
Adenocarcinoma
Chondrosarcoma
Squamous cell carcinoma
Fibrosarcoma
Mast cell tumor
Osteosarcoma
Transmissible venereal tumor

Malignant Tumors in Cats
Squamous cell carcinoma
Adenocarcinoma
Lymphoma—usually feline leukemia virus (FeLV) negative

Benign Tumors in Dogs and Cats
Polyps (more common in cats)
Adenoma
Fibroma

*Listed in decreasing order of frequency.

587

Cytologic and Histopathologic Studies

Cytologic and/or histologic confirmation is diagnostic. Procedures (and their specific uses) include:

- Rhinoscopy (performed with cystoscope or arthroscope)—for viewing tumor and acquiring tissue for cytology, histopathology, and culture
- Nasal flushes—for cytologic identification
- Blind biopsy procedures using biopsy needle, catheter, or polypropylene tube (covering of IV catheter)—to obtain diagnostic specimen for cytology/ histopathology

KEY POINT ▶ Pre-measure nasal biopsy devices to avoid penetration of cribriform plate.

- Rhinotomy and nasal exploratory surgery—for direct visualization of tumor and to obtain larger biopsy specimens
- Transnasal curettage (through nostril)—to obtain tissues for cytology and histopathology

Treatment

Surgical Cytoreduction

Surgical cytoreduction alone or followed by radiation therapy has been reported.

- Rhinotomy (nasal flap) with curettage or turbinectomy is the most common procedure (see sec. 6, ch. 18).
- Transnasal curettage using a uterine curette and suction may be less invasive.
- Survival times for animals treated with surgical cytoreduction alone are similar to that for untreated animals.
- Survival times are improved with combination surgical cytoreduction and radiation therapy.

Radiation Therapy

In radiation therapy (Orthovoltage, cesium, cobalt, and linear accelerator), the dose and fractionation of treatment is determined by tumor type and source of radiation (for specific recommendations, consult a radiologist or oncologist).

The following post-treatment complications have been reported:

- Rhinitis may be severe but usually subsides within 2 months.
- A slight nasal discharge and sneezing may persist.
- Ulcerative dermatitis usually occurs at the irradiated site but generally responds to topical therapy.
- Ocular complications of nasal radiation may include keratoconjunctivitis sicca, corneal ulcers, uveitis, and cataract formation.

Chemotherapy

Chemotherapy may be effective in certain tumor types (see sec. 3, ch. 5 for discussion of chemotherapy).

- Combination drugs (doxorubicin, cyclophosphamide, vincristine, 5-fluorouracil) have been used in therapy for adenocarcinoma, lymphoma, and transmissible venereal tumor.
- Single-agent therapy with dactinomycin, doxorubicin, cisplatin, and mitoxantrone has had variable results.
- Myelosuppression, anorexia, vomiting, diarrhea, and lethargy may occur secondary to chemotherapy.

KEY POINT ▶ To maximize survival times, follow tumor cytoreduction with radiation therapy.

Prognosis

Prognostic factors include histologic type and tumor size.

- Prognosis for nasal polyps is good, but recurrence is possible.
- Dogs with adenocarcinoma or sarcoma have longer median survival times than dogs with undifferentiated or squamous cell carcinoma.
- Larger and more extensive tumors have a poorer prognosis.
- In cats with nasal lymphoma, radiation therapy has had good results.

NEOPLASMS OF THE LARYNX

Table 2 lists the types of laryngeal neoplasms seen in dogs and cats. These tumors are uncommon and usually are locally invasive; however, distant metastasis has been reported.

Malignant neoplasms are more common than benign tumors. However, oncocytomas, which are usually benign, are the second most common laryngeal tumor in dogs. Most common are malignant (i.e., squamous cell carcinoma). (Oncocytes are epithelial cells sporadically present within the seromucinous glands of the upper airway.)

TABLE 2. Types of Neoplasms of the Larynx Occurring in Dogs and Cats

Primary Malignant Tumors in Dogs
Squamous cell carcinoma
Lymphoma
Osteosarcoma
Melanoma
Mast cell tumor
Adenocarcinoma

Metastatic Tumors in Dogs
Thyroid carcinoma
Lymphoma
Pharyngeal rhabdomyosarcoma

Primary Malignant Tumors in Cats
Lymphoma
Squamous cell carcinoma
Adenocarcinoma

Benign Tumors in Dogs and Cats (Uncommon)
Unilateral polyps, generally inflammatory in origin
Oncocytoma*

*The second most common laryngeal tumor in dogs. See text for description.

Signalment

- Laryngeal tumors occur in middle-aged to older animals (5–15 years) with the exception of oncocytomas, which occur in young to middle-aged dogs (2–8 years).
- Males appear to be at increased risk.

History

- *Noisy breathing and respiratory distress* are the most common complaints reported.
- *Exercise intolerance, change in voice, and loss of bark or purr* may be noted by the owner.

Clinical Signs

- *Inspiratory dyspnea and cyanosis* usually occur when the animal is stressed.
- Coughing due to *aspiration pneumonia* may occur secondary to laryngeal dysfunction.
- Palpable laryngeal masses are uncommon.

KEY POINT ▶ Inspiratory dyspnea is the most common sign of laryngeal obstructive disease. Neoplasia must be differentiated from laryngeal paralysis or foreign body via laryngoscopy.

Diagnosis

- The history and physical findings may suggest laryngeal disease.
- Radiography may demonstrate laryngeal distortion, increased soft tissue density of the larynx, and decreased laryngeal space.
- Laryngoscopic evaluation (using a laryngoscope or endoscope) may reveal a laryngeal swelling or mass.
- Biopsy and histopathology provide a definitive diagnosis. Biopsy via direct visualization with alligator biopsy forceps, needle biopsy instruments, or bronchoscopic biopsy forceps is usually successful in obtaining a diagnosis.

Treatment

Surgery

Surgical excision may be curative if the tumor is benign, but it only provides palliation for malignant disease. Complete laryngectomy with a permanent tracheostomy (see sec. 6, ch. 19) has been done rarely in veterinary medicine.

Radiation Therapy

Radiation may be beneficial in the treatment of some laryngeal tumors (e.g., squamous cell carcinomas, mast cell tumors, lymphomas); however, little information is available.

Chemotherapy

Chemotherapy for laryngeal tumors has been reported rarely.

- Lymphomas usually respond to combination chemotherapy (see sec. 3, ch. 6), but little information is available concerning laryngeal tumors.
- Mast cell tumors, adenocarcinomas, and sarcomas may respond to chemotherapy (See sec. 3, chs. 5 and 7).

Prognosis

The prognosis for most laryngeal tumors is guarded because advanced disease usually is present at the time of diagnosis. However, if tumors are benign (e.g., polyps, oncocytomas), the prognosis is good with surgical excision.

NEOPLASMS OF THE TRACHEA

Tracheal tumors are rare in dogs and cats. See Table 3 for common types of tumors.

Signalment

Young animals are at higher risk for osteochondroma.

KEY POINT ▶ Tracheal tumors are rare; consider them malignant in older animals.

History

Exercise intolerance, panting, and cough may be present for weeks prior to presentation.

Clinical Signs

- *Cough,* usually nonproductive, is the most common sign.
- *Stridor,* usually inspiratory, may be noted during exercise or panting.
- Tumors located at the carina cause both inspiratory and expiratory respiratory distress.
- *Cyanosis, dyspnea, and collapse* may occur with severe obstruction.

TABLE 3. Types of Neoplasms of the Trachea Occurring in Dogs and Cats

Malignant Tumors in Dogs
Osteosarcoma
Chondrosarcoma
Lymphoma
Mast cell tumor
Adenocarcinoma
Malignant Tumors in Cats
Adenocarcinoma
Lymphoma
Squamous cell carcinoma
Benign Tumors in Dogs and Cats
Osteochondroma (dogs)
Leiomyoma
Polyps
Eosinophilic granuloma (cats)
Nodular amyloidosis (dogs)

Diagnosis

- *Radiography* may demonstrate a soft tissue density within the tracheal lumen or decrease in lumen size.
- *Bronchoscopy* may be needed to reveal a tracheal mass.
- *Biopsy and histopathology* are diagnostic.

Treatment

Surgical Excision

Surgery is the primary treatment for tracheal masses (see sec. 6, ch. 19).

- Benign lesions may be cured with surgical resection.
- Tracheal reconstruction with wedge resection and side-to-side, telescoping, and end-to-end anastomosis have been used (see sec. 6, ch. 19).

Chemotherapy

Cyclophosphamide, vincristine, and prednisone can prolong survival in animals with lymphoma (see sec. 3, ch. 6).

Prognosis

Benign tumors respond well to surgical excision. Little information regarding treatment and prognosis is available about most tracheal tumors.

NEOPLASMS OF THE LUNG

Primary pulmonary neoplasms represent approximately 1.2% and 0.5% of all tumors in the dog and cat, respectively. Primary lung tumors may metastasize to bronchial lymph nodes, lung, brain, bone, and pleura via lymphatics, airways, blood vessels, and transpleural routes.

Paraneoplastic syndromes may be associated with primary pulmonary neoplasms.

- Hypertrophic osteopathy is the most common paraneoplastic syndrome associated with large lung masses and has been reported in 3–15% of animals with pulmonary neoplasia.
- Other paraneoplastic syndromes include paraplegia and subclinical neuromyopathy, hypercalcemia, neutrophilic leukocytosis associated with metastatic fibrosarcoma, and secretion of adrenocorticotropic hormone resulting in clinical signs of hyperadrenocorticism.

KEY POINT ▶ Pulmonary neoplasia is the most likely diagnosis in dogs with hypertrophic osteopathy.

Tumor Types (see Table 4)

Primary Pulmonary Neoplasms. Carcinomas are the most common primary lung tumors in dogs. In primary pulmonary adenocarcinomas and epidermoid carcinomas, 50% and 80%, respectively, have metastasized at the time of diagnosis.

Metastatic Pulmonary Neoplasms. These tumors

TABLE 4. Types of Pulmonary Neoplasms Occurring in Dogs and Cats

Primary Tumors in Dogs
Carcinoma
  Bronchoalveolar adenocarcinoma (>70%)
  Epidermoid (squamous cell)
  Bronchogenic or bronchial gland
  Anaplastic or alveolar (small cell, large cell, adenomatous)
Sarcoma (uncommon)
  Lymphoma
  Fibrosarcoma
  Hemangiosarcoma
  Osteosarcoma
Other
  Lymphomatoid granulomatosis
  Malignant histiocytosis (in Bernese mountain dogs)

Primary Tumors in Cats
Carcinoma
  Adenocarcinoma (papillary, bronchoalveolar)
  Epidermoid (squamous cell)
  Bronchial gland
Sarcoma (rare)
  Hemangiosarcoma
  Spindle cell
  Reticulum cell
Benign (rare)
  Bronchial adenoma
  Hemangioma

Metastatic Tumors in Dogs and Cats
Mammary carcinoma
Osteosarcoma
Thyroid carcinoma
Transitional cell carcinoma
Melanoma
Hemangiosarcoma
Squamous cell carcinoma

---

are more common than primary pulmonary neoplasms. Metastasis occurs by spread of tumor emboli via lymphatic or blood vessels. Because of the capillary network in the lungs, these tumor emboli are trapped and may proliferate and form nodules. See Table 4 for a list of common metastatic tumors.

Signalment

- Pulmonary neoplasms occur in older animals (>10 years), except lymphomatoid granulomatosis, which occurs in young dogs (1–6 years).
- Most studies do not recognize a breed or sex predilection; however, boxers and Bernese mountain dogs have been reported to be at increased risk for primary lung tumors.

History

History may vary depending on the tumor type, size, and doubling time. Many dogs are asymptomatic, and pulmonary nodules are discovered during a medical work-up.

Clinical Signs

- *Cough* (harsh, nonproductive) is one of the most common presenting signs. The duration is usually chronic, and occasionally hemoptysis is also present.

- *Dyspnea, tachypnea, and cyanosis* may be present and associated with pleural effusion and/or diffuse disease.
- *Decreased exercise tolerance* is usually related to respiratory compromise.
- Less common signs include anorexia, fever, weight loss, dysphagia, vomiting, and regurgitation.
- *Lameness* may be associated with hypertrophic osteopathy or with skeletal muscle and/or bone metastasis.

Diagnosis

Radiography

Plain thoracic radiography usually establishes the diagnosis. However, approximately 11% of pulmonary neoplasms are missed on survey radiographs because of:

- Small size of the lesions (<5–10 mm).
- Lack of tumor contrast with pulmonary parenchyma, tumor site in a hidden location (e.g., the subpleural space or paraspinal recesses).
- Presence of pleural fluid.
- Atelectasis of one or more lung lobes.

KEY POINT ▶ Evaluate three radiographic views (ventrodorsal, right, and left lateral) of the thorax when primary or metastatic pulmonary neoplasia is suspected.

Radiographic Pattern. The most common radiographic pattern seen in dogs and cats with metastatic neoplasms is that of circumscribed nodules. Patterns include:

- Solitary circumscribed nodule
- Multiple circumscribed nodules
- Interstitial disseminated reticulonodular pattern
- Mixed disseminated alveolar pattern
- Homogeneous lobar consolidation

Other Diagnostic Signs

- Radiographic changes associated with pulmonary tumors include pleural effusions, pleural thickening, and thoracic lymphadenopathy.
- Calcification and cavitation of masses have been associated with adenocarcinomas.
- The right side and caudal lung lobes are the most common locations of primary pulmonary neoplasms in dogs. The left lung lobes are affected more often than the right side in cats.

Other Studies

- *Percutaneous transthoracic fine-needle aspiration or biopsy* for cytologic or histologic evaluation may provide a diagnosis in 50% of cases.
- *Cytologic evaluation* of tracheal wash fluid, bronchoalveolar lavage fluid, and pleural fluid may detect neoplastic cells in some cases.
- *Bronchoscopy* may be valuable in perihilar masses.
- *Exploratory thoracotomy* (see sec. 6, ch. 25) and biopsy will provide a definitive diagnosis and aid in staging the tumor.

Treatment

Surgical Excision

Surgical excision and/or lobectomy is the treatment of choice for solitary lung tumors (see sec. 6, ch. 25).

- Obtain biopsy samples from regional lymph nodes when possible.
- Adjunctive chemotherapy may improve survival in some cases in which metastasis or local invasion is present.

KEY POINT ▶ Always submit lung tumors for biopsy to establish diagnosis and prognosis.

Chemotherapy

Chemotherapy may be beneficial in some tumors.

- Lymphomatoid granulomatosis may respond to combination chemotherapy with prednisone, vincristine, and cyclophosphamide (see sec. 3, ch. 5 for dosages).
- Malignant histiocytosis in Bernese mountain dogs may respond to doxorubicin, cyclophosphamide, and vincristine (see sec. 3, ch. 5 for dosages).
- Complete and partial responses have been reported in the treatment of metastatic neoplasms (hemangiosarcoma, thyroid carcinomas, squamous cell carcinoma, mammary adenocarcinomas) with doxorubicin, cyclophosphamide, and vincristine (see sec. 3, ch. 5 for dosages).

Prognosis

- Factors that decrease survival time include large tumor burden, thoracic lymph node involvement, and other metastases.
- Small (<5 cm), solitary primary lung tumors without metastasis or malignant effusion are associated with prolonged survival (>1 year). Even large lobar masses can be removed successfully with a reasonable (>6 months) survival time, provided metastases have not yet developed.
- In cats, the prognosis is poor because >75% of primary lung tumors are inoperable at the time of diagnosis.
- Following treatment, monitor with routine thoracic radiographs every 1–3 months.

Supplemental Readings

Adams WM, Withrow SJ, Walshaw R, et al: Radiotherapy of malignant nasal tumors in 67 dogs. J Am Vet Med Assoc 191:311, 1987.

Bell FW: Neoplastic diseases of the thorax. Vet Clin North Am 17:387, 1987.

Carothers MA, Couto GC: Respiratory neoplasia. *In* Kirk RW, ed.: *Current Veterinary Therapy X.* Philadelphia: W. B. Saunders, 1989, p 399.

Carpenter JL, Andrews LK, Holzworth J: Tumors and tumor-like lesions. *In* Holzworth J, ed.: *Diseases of the Cat.* Philadelphia, W. B. Saunders, 1987, p 468.

Lang J, Wortman FA, Glickman LT, et al.: Sensitivity of radiographic detection of lung metastases in the dog. Vet Radiol 27:74, 1986.

MacEwen EG, Withrow SJ, Patnaik AK: Nasal tumors in the dog:

Retrospective evaluation of diagnosis, prognosis, and treatment. J Am Vet Med Assoc 170:45, 1977.

Madewell BR, Priester WA, Gillette EL, Snyder SP: Neoplasms of the nasal passages and paranasal sinuses in domesticated animals as reported by 13 veterinary colleges. Am J Vet Res 37:851, 1976.

Madewell BR, Theilen GH: Tumors of the respiratory tract and thorax. *In* Theilen GH, Madewell BR, ed.: *Veterinary Cancer Medicine*. Philadelphia: Lea & Febiger, 1987, p 535.

Mehlhaff CJ, Mooney BA: Primary pulmonary neoplasia in the dog and cat. Vet Clin North Am 15:1061, 1985.

Ogilvie GK, Haschek WM, Withrow SJ, et al.: Classification of primary lung tumors in dogs: 210 cases (1975–1985). J Am Vet Med Assoc 195:106, 1989.

Ogilvie GK, Weigel RM, Haschek WM, et al.: Prognostic factors for tumor remission and survival in dogs after surgery for primary lung tumor: 76 cases (1975–1985). J Am Vet Med Assoc 195:106, 1989.

Saik JE, Toll SL, Diters RW, Goldschmidt MH: Canine and feline laryngeal neoplasia: A 10-year survey. J Am Anim Hosp Assoc 22:359, 1986.

Suter PF, Carrig CB, O'Brien TR, Koller D: Radiographic recognition of primary and metastatic pulmonary neoplasms of dogs and cats. J Am Vet Radiol Soc 15:3, 1974.

Thrall DE, Harvery CE: Radiotherapy of malignant nasal tumors in 21 dogs. J Am Vet Med Assoc 183:663, 1983.

Wheeldon EB, Suter PF, Jenkins T: Neoplasia of the larynx in the dog. J Am Vet Med Assoc 180:642, 1982.

Withrow SJ: Tumors of the respiratory system. *In* Withrow SJ, MacEwen EG, ed.: *Clinical Veterinary Oncology*. Philadelphia: J. B. Lippincott 1989, p 215.

24 Management of Thoracic Trauma

Dale E. Bjorling

Thoracic trauma in dogs and cats most often is the result of automobile accidents. The lack of apparent external injuries often is misleading; the diaphragm, thoracic wall, heart, or lungs may be severely damaged with little apparent damage to the overlying skin. Evaluate animals presented for treatment of thoracic trauma thoroughly but rapidly; if necessary, institute treatment prior to completing a full patient assessment. Animals with thoracic trauma may suffer concurrent abdominal injuries.

Surgical correction of injuries associated with thoracic trauma may be required on an emergency basis; however, in general veterinary practice it is preferable to avoid emergency surgery of animals suffering thoracic trauma unless this is absolutely necessary.

This chapter discusses the major disorders caused by thoracic trauma: pulmonary and myocardial contusions, pneumothorax, rib fractures and flail chest, hemothorax, and diaphragmatic hernia; see sec. 6, ch. 22 for discussion of chylothorax.

Injuries to abdominal viscera are discussed in respective chapters.

ETIOLOGY

Blunt Trauma

- Blunt trauma to the thoracic cavity usually is the result of automobile accidents. It may also be the result of a kick by a human or farm animal (horse, cow), being struck by a heavy object, or falling from heights (e.g., a cat falling from a window of high-rise buildings).
- The severity of injury depends upon the mass of the object delivering the blow, the velocity of the object, and the area to which the blow is delivered. It has been shown experimentally that when a blow equivalent to that delivered by a car is administered to the thorax of anesthetized dogs, the thoracic viscera may be compressed until the opposing parietal pleural surfaces underlying the ribs may almost be brought into contact.
- Blunt trauma can cause pneumothorax, hemothorax, pulmonary contusions, fractured ribs, and any combination of these.

Penetrating Trauma

- Penetrating trauma usually is the result of a gunshot. It may also result from a sharp instrument (e.g., a knife, screwdriver, stick, arrow) and from deep bite wounds inflicted by a big dog on a smaller dog or cat.

- Consider the type of projectile, point of entry, and path of the penetrating object when attempting to determine the presence of thoracic trauma, even if wound entry is distant to the thoracic cavity. The path of a projectile may be altered if it strikes bony structures.
- It is often unclear whether thoracic injuries have resulted from penetrating wounds. Depending on the extent of injury, signs of cardiovascular collapse or respiratory distress may develop more slowly in patients suffering penetrating injuries of the thorax.

CLINICAL SIGNS

- Dogs and cats that suffer thoracic trauma usually are presented for evaluation of tachypnea or dyspnea (difficulty breathing). The animal may have an anxious or distressed appearance. The owner may or may not have observed occurrence of the injury. Clinical signs of thoracic trauma may be delayed in onset, especially those associated with diaphragmatic hernia.
- Hypovolemic shock may result from internal or external hemorrhage or accumulation of fluid within tissue spaces. An animal suffering from hypovolemic shock has increased heart rate, weak peripheral arterial pulses, cold extremities, and pale mucous membranes, and often appears depressed or stuporous (see sec. 6, ch. 14 for a complete discussion of shock).
- Gastrointestinal signs (diarrhea or vomiting due to obstruction) may be observed if a portion of the gastrointestinal tract has been displaced across the diaphragm into the thoracic cavity through a diaphragmatic hernia. These signs are not commonly present immediately after the injury has occurred.

DIAGNOSIS

KEY POINT ▶ Treatment of hypovolemic shock or other life-threatening disorders takes precedence over patient evaluation.

History

- Attempt to identify recent or past traumatic episodes.
- Question the owner regarding the onset and progression of the current clinical signs.
- Take the history while initial evaluation of vital signs is in progress so that life-threatening injuries (e.g.,

593

tension pneumothorax) can be detected and treated immediately.

Physical Examination

After initially determining the animal's vital signs (e.g., heart rate, respiratory rate, mucous membrane color and refill, temperature, level of consciousness), examine the respiratory system by:

- Observation (of breathing)
- Palpation
- Auscultation
- Percussion
- Radiography

Observation

Observe the rate, depth, and effort of respirations.

- Rapidly developing dyspnea usually is the result of pneumothorax or pulmonary contusion.
- Rapid, shallow, choppy breathing can result from restriction of the thoracic wall because of painful rib fracture.
- Paradoxical motion of the chest wall is caused by collapse of a portion of the rib cage on inspiration when multiple rib fractures create an unstable flail chest wall.
- Decreased hemithorax movement (fixation) can be seen on the side into which abdominal viscera have herniated through a ruptured diaphragm.
- Herniation of the lung into the intercostal space countercurrent with each respiration indicates torn intercostal muscles.

Palpation

- Palpate the thoracic wall for rib fractures, unstable (flail) segments, hematomas (usually adjacent to rib fractures), subcutaneous emphysea (crepitus), intercostal muscle tears (usually under intact skin), and abnormal location of the cardiac apex beat (displaced by herniation of abdominal viscera).
- Also palpate the abdominal cavity for concurrent intrabdominal injuries. The absence of viscera suggests their displacement into the thoracic cavity.

Auscultation

- Carefully auscultate the entire thoracic cavity to determine whether functional lung tissue can be identified throughout the thoracic cavity. The absence of respiratory sounds strongly suggests displacement of the lungs by air, fluid (e.g., blood), or abdominal viscera.
- Auscultate the heart as well. A change in the location or pitch of heart sounds suggests displacement of the heart by air, fluid, or viscera. Ventricular arrhythmias frequently occur as the result of traumatic myocarditis or myocardial ischemia; however, their onset is more frequently observed 24–48 hours after the traumatic episode.

Percussion

- Perform percussion of the thoracic wall to determine increased or decreased resonance. By placing one hand flat on the thoracic wall and tapping the knuckle of the middle finger with the tips of the fingers of the opposite hand, a sound of consistent frequency is produced in normal animals.
- In animals with air or air-filled viscera underlying the thoracic wall, the pitch will be deeper and more resonant, whereas the sound produced in animals with fluid or solid viscera immediately under the thoracic wall will be dull and less resonant.
- Percussion aids detection of pneumothorax, pleural effusion (e.g., hemothorax, chylothorax), diaphragmatic hernia, and consolidation of lung lobes.
- Skilled use of this technique requires frequent practice on normal animals to allow a distinction between normal and abnormal sounds.

Fractures

- Examine the animal for the presence of fractures; do not be distracted by the obvious presence of broken bones but continue searching for evidence of more serious internal injuries.
- If spinal fractures are suspected, handle the animal with great care until these have been stabilized or it is determined radiographically that the spine is intact (see sec. 1, ch. 4).
- The presence of fractures suggests that trauma of sufficient force to inflict injury to the thorax and its contents has occurred. A survey of dogs injured in motor vehicle accidents found that over 50% of animals with intrathoracic injuries also had fractured bones.

Surface Wounds and Abrasions

Clip hair from the thoracic wall area as necessary to identify abrasions, bruises, or wounds that may point to likely sites of intrathoracic injury.

- Open wounds that freely communicate with the pleural space can cause progressive pneumothorax; seal them immediately.

Thoracic Radiography

Take radiographs to evaluate the heart, lungs, pleural space, and thoracic wall (see sec. 6, chs. 2 and 17 for discussion of thoracic radiography).

- It is sometimes advisable to delay thoracic radiography of the injured animal until after higher-priority conditions such as shock have been stabilized by emergency treatment. Pulmonary contusion, characterized by hemorrhage and fluid accumulation within the lungs, may not reach its greatest extent for 6–12 hours and then often may not appear radiographically to be improved for 7–10 days after injury.

KEY POINT ▶ The full severity of pulmonary contusions may not be apparent on thoracic radiographs made within 1–2 hours of injury.

- A narrowed cardiac silhouette may suggest hypovolemia.

- Evaluate the pleural space carefully for the presence of fluid, air or abdominal viscera, and evaluate the integrity of the diaphragmatic outline.
- Look for radiographic evidence of fracture or dislocation of skeletal structures and the presence of subcutaneous emphysema, which indicates leakage of air into the subcutaneous space from the environment, the thoracic cavity, or a major airway.
- Pneumomediastinum is seen as air outlining the mediastinal contents and is indicative of tracheobronchial rupture.
- If the animal's condition does not preclude this, two radiographic projections are desirable.
- Often it is difficult to identify the presence of a diaphragmatic hernia on thoracic radiographs, particularly if obscured by accumulation of fluid within the pleural space. If a large quantity of pleural fluid is present, remove it and repeat the radiographs (see sec. 6, ch. 17).
  - Observations suggesting the presence of diaphragmatic hernia include cranial displacement of the stomach, loss of the caudal outline of the liver, and the presence of gas-filled viscous organs within the thoracic cavity.
  - If a diaphragmatic hernia is suspected but unconfirmed by plain radiographs, consider positive contrast coelography or abdominal ultrasonography.

Thoracocentesis

If indicated, perform thoracocentesis to obtain a sample of pleural fluid or to drain air from the pleural space (see sec. 1, ch. 3 for technique).

- Analyze the fluid for the presence and concentration of red blood cells (RBCs) and plasma protein. It may be apparent that the fluid is whole blood, or the fluid may be a combination of transudate, exudate, chyle, or blood, depending on the severity and duration of injury and the organs affected.
- Centrifuge an aliquot of the fluid and examine the cellular portion of the fluid microscopically for the presence of degenerative neutrophils, bacteria, and organic matter (see sec. 6, ch. 22). These findings may suggest a severe inflammatory process and possibly perforation of the esophagus or gastrointestinal tract.
- On rare occasions, the biliary tract may be ruptured in the presence of diaphragmatic hernia, and this can be identified by determining the concentration of bilirubin within pleural fluid.

Blood Samples

- Draw blood samples and store in an anticoagulant and serum tube (preferably prior to initiating treatment).
- Although these samples may not be needed, often it is helpful to determine the biochemical status of the animal at the time of hospital admission when attempting to distinguish between preexistent disease and that which has developed acutely after injury. These same considerations apply to the collection and storage of urine samples.

Packed Cell Volume (PCV) and Plasma Protein Concentration (PPC)

- Determine the PCV and PPC as soon as possible after the initial examination.
- It is critical to record these values because the diagnosis of continuing hemorrhage often relies on the comparison of serial determinations of PCV and PPC.
- If hemorrhage is ongoing, these two values will continue to decline at a similar rate. If, however, hemorrhage has ceased, it is not uncommon for the PPC to stabilize while the PCV continues to decline.
- The administration of IV fluids may further decrease these values; consider this fact when evaluating these parameters.

Arterial pH and Blood Gas Tensions

- These values give an indication of ventilatory function.
- Satisfactory oxygenation of the blood by the lungs requires adequate cardiac output, and decreased cardiac output caused by hypovolemic shock or depressed cardiac function may profoundly effect blood gas values.

Electrocardiography (ECG)

- If available, perform serial ECGs to check for arrhythmias associated with myocardial injury.
- If ECG is not available, closely monitor the animal's heart rate and rhythm and the occurrence of pulse deficits.

TREATMENT

Modify treatment to suit the individual needs of each animal. It is advisable to place and maintain at least one IV catheter for administration of fluid and drugs early in the course of treatment. In severely traumatized animals, it is advisable to place two IV catheters (one may be a central venous line) to allow more rapid infusion of IV fluids.

When confronted with a seriously injured animal, often it is difficult to develop a logical, disciplined treatment plan. The ABC approach is a consistent, comprehensive plan for initial treatment of animals with thoracic trauma.

ABC Approach

Airway

Be sure that the animal has a patent airway.

- Remove debris from the trachea and bronchi by forceps or suction or by passing an endotracheal tube.
- If the pharynx, larynx or cranial portion of the trachea is severely damaged, consider performing a tracheostomy (see sec. 1, ch. 3).

Breathing (Spontaneous or Assisted) and Oxygen Therapy

Restore thoracic wall integrity by sealing open ("sucking") chest wounds with an occlusive dressing and stabilizing flail segments so the animal can ventilate effectively. If the animal is not able to ventilate satisfactorily, institute assisted breathing.

- This requires the presence of an endotracheal or tracheostomy tube and may necessitate anesthetizing the animal or giving neuromuscular blocking drugs to paralyze the animal (see sec. 1, ch. 2).
- Supplemental oxygen may be provided by an incubator or oxygen cage, face mask, nasal catheter (see sec. 1, ch. 3), transtracheal cannula or catheter, or endotracheal or tracheostomy tube.
  - When supplemental oxygen is administered to the animal in such a manner that it does not pass through the nasal passages, prewarm and humidify the air.
- A transtracheal catheter may be placed using a large-gauge (12–18) jugular catheter passed between the rings of the trachea.
  - Secure the catheter to the skin and attach to the oxygen source. Deliver oxygen via the transtracheal catheter at an initial rate of 10–20 ml/kg/min.

Circulation

If myocardial function is satisfactory, administer IV fluids as needed to increase the circulating blood volume and cardiac output.

- In most cases of hypovolemic shock, administer a blood volume (90 ml/kg in dogs and 65 ml/kg in cats) as rapidly as gravity flow will allow.
- In the presence of significant ongoing hemorrhage, fluid bags may be pressurized to increase the rate of administration.
- After the rapid infusion of a bolus of IV fluids equivalent to 1 blood volume, reassess the status of the patient and determine the need for ongoing fluid administration.
  - If signs of hypovolemic shock have abated and hemorrhage has ceased, continue to administer fluids at a rate of 30–50 ml/kg/24 h (see sec. 6, ch. 14).
  - If the animal's condition does not stabilize, continue rapid fluid administration.
- Auscultate the lungs for evidence of pulmonary edema and carefully monitor for other signs of edema (e.g., chemosis, tearing, tissue swelling, decreasing PCV and PPC).
- If necessary, monitor the central venous pressure (CVP) to determine the ability of the right side of the heart to eject the volume of blood presented to it (see sec. 1, ch. 3 for CVP techniques). The relative change in CVP is more significant than the absolute value, and an increase of 7–10 cm H_2O indicates that the rate of fluid administration should be slowed.
- Because of the low oncotic pressure of the crystalloid fluid that may contribute to fluid loss into the tissue space, a general rule for replacement of blood loss by crystalloid fluids is:
  - For every 1 ml of blood lost, administer 3 ml of crystalloid fluid.

Pleural Space Drainage

- The pleural space may be drained intermittently by thoracocentesis using a hypodermic needle.
- If continuous or prolonged pleural drainage for removal of fluid or air is required, place a thoracostomy tube (see sec. 1, ch. 3 for thoracic drainage techniques).
  - Attach thoracostomy tubes to a three-way stopcock to allow intermittent aspiration of the tube (e.g., q2–4h) or to a continuous suction device.
  - If continuous suction is used, carefully control the negative pressure; it should not be less than −5 to −10 cm H_2O.
- Alternatively, attach the thoracostomy tube to a Heimlich one-way flutter valve.
  - If using this valve, carefully monitor the animal for complications.
  - Be aware that if the valve becomes cracked or the valve's diaphragm becomes wet, the one-way function of the valve may be lost and severe pneumothorax may develop.
  - Animals weighing < 20 lb frequently are incapable of activating the valve, resulting in continued accumulation of air within the thoracic cavity.
- If fluid or air cannot be aspirated from the thoracostomy tube, the pleural space may be completely evacuated or the tube may be obstructed by a fibrin clot or by the tube's bending upon itself. Obtain thoracic radiographs and flush the tube with sterile saline to confirm patency.

Tube Removal. Remove the tube when it is no longer needed.

- The presence of the thoracostomy tube will result in continued production of a small volume (at least 30–60 ml of fluid/24 h in a dog weighing 25 kg).
- It also is possible that a small volume of air may continue to accumulate within the pleural space due to air migration along the external surface of the chest tube or through leaks in the tubing.

Therefore, often it is not possible to wait until there is no air or fluid accumulation within the thorax to remove the thoracostomy tube, and the tube usually is removed when the volume of air and fluid has reached insignificant levels.

Treatment of Pneumothorax

Pneumothorax can be closed or open; in *closed* pneumothorax, the most common type, air escapes from the injured lung or airway into the pleural space; in *open* pneumothorax, air enters the pleural space through an open wound in the chest wall (e.g., bites, sharp objects, projectiles).

Simple Pneumothorax. Accumulation of air in the pleural space that is not progressive is termed simple pneumothorax and is a common complication of thoracic trauma.

- Conservative treatment with chest drainage and cage rest usually is adequate. The air leak will usually seal itself within hours, and residual intrapleural air will be reabsorbed within a few days.
- Occasionally, oxygen therapy may be needed as initial treatment in animals that are severely dyspneic on presentation until the chest can be evacuated.
- Simple pneumothorax frequently is accompanied by other thoracic problems, such as pulmonary contusions and rib fractures, that can combine to cause serious ventilatory problems.

Tension Pneumothorax. Laceration of the lung, bronchus, or trachea may result in tension pneumothorax, which is the progressive accumulation of air in the pleural space that results in positive intrapleural pressure.

- Animals with tension pneumothorax need immediate life-saving chest drainage via a thoracostomy tube to prevent lung collapse, decreased systemic venous return to the heart, and rapid death. This reestablishes negative intrapleural pressure and allows lung reexpansion.
- Intermittent chest drainage may not be adequate to allow proper ventilation, and continuous suction drainage frequently is necessary. In this case, connect the chest tube to a suction drainage unit such as Pleurevac (Deknatel, Inc.).
- Consider exploratory thoracotomy (see later discussion in this chapter; also see sec. 6, ch. 25) if the patient's condition fails to stabilize.

Treatment of Pulmonary Contusions

A pulmonary contusion is analogous to a bruise, with disruption of the tissues and capillaries resulting in extravasation of blood and accumulation of fluid within the pulmonary parenchyma. As previously mentioned in the discussion of IV fluid administration, aggressive fluid therapy may result in fluid accumulation within the lungs. This most likely is the result of decreased plasma oncotic pressure. IV infusion of the equivalent of 1 blood volume of crystalloid fluids over the course of 1 hour does not increase the extent of experimentally created pulmonary contusions in dogs. It is unlikely that IV fluid administration will increase fluid accumulation within pulmonary contusions unless the plasma protein concentration is < 3.0 gm/dl or the plasma albumin concentration is < 1.5 gm/dl.

- Transfusions of plasma or whole blood help to maintain plasma oncotic pressure.
- The administration of corticosteroids (2–4 mg/kg dexamethasone phosphate or 30 mg/kg methylprednisolone sodium succinate) may be useful in limiting the size of pulmonary contusions if administered soon after injury.
- Diuretics have been recommended to remove excess water and limit the size of contusions; however, diuretics may act to reduce total body fluid at a time when volume expansion is critical to resuscitate the animal.
- Administer antibiotics to animals with pulmonary contusions to minimize the potential for development of bacterial pneumonia (antibiotic therapy for animals with thoracic trauma is discussed at the end of this chapter).
- In animals that are recumbent, frequent repositioning may help to prevent hypostatic congestion, atelectasis, and pneumonia.
- Administer oxygen to treat or prevent hypoxemia.
- Bronchodilators (e.g., aminophylline, 6–10 mg/kg, q8h, PO or IV) may improve ventilation by keeping airways open.
- Closely monitor animals with moderate to severe contusions. If deterioration of respiratory function continues despite the above-mentioned measures, positive-pressure assisted ventilation may be necessary.

Treatment of Myocardial Contusions

Administration of corticosteroids as described for treatment of pulmonary contusions may be beneficial in the treatment of myocardial contusions, but the efficacy of any form of treatment is uncertain.

- Monitor ventricular arrhythmias (see sec. 6, ch. 4) that develop as a result of traumatic myocarditis by continuous ECG and treat initially with IV administration of lidocaine (2 mg/kg boluses to a maximum of 8 mg/kg/h).
  - If lidocaine therapy is effective but a constant infusion is required, administer lidocaine at a rate of 50–80 µg/kg/min. Adjust the rate to achieve the desired effect.
- Procainamide may also be given (8–20mg/kg q4–6h, PO or IM).

Treatment of Hemothorax

Hemothorax (blood accumulation in the pleural space) occurs secondary to any form of trauma that causes laceration of blood vessels, heart, lung, or thoracic wall. (Diseases other than trauma can cause hemothorax and are discussed in sec. 6, ch. 22.) Hemothorax causes two major problems: hypovolemic shock and impairment of ventilation. Massive hemorrhage from rupture of the heart or one of the great vessels usually causes rapid death.

- Treatment of traumatically induced hemothorax involves aggressive and rapid supportive care consisting of IV fluids and/or blood transfusions and pleural drainage (see sec. 6, ch. 14 for details of treatment of hypovolemic shock).
- Consider autotransfusions for animals with significant hemothorax not complicated by an infectious or neoplastic process in the chest.
  - Aseptically collect the blood via a chest tube and return to the patient using a blood administration set.
  - Closely monitor the patient's vital signs, PCV, and PPC.
- Consider exploratory thoracotomy for animals that fail to stabilize (see subsequent discussion in this chapter). However, surgical treatment of hemothorax may be unsuccessful because the source of hemorrhage is rarely identifiable.

Stabilization of Rib Fractures and Flail Chest

KEY POINT ▶ Stabilization of rib fractures is required when a gross deformity has occurred; displacement of the fragments results in ongoing damage to the underlying viscera or displacement or instability of the fragments interferes with ventilation (e.g., flail chest).

Potential complications of rib fractures include:

- Pneumothorax (from lung laceration by the sharp end of a fragment)
- Pulmonary contusions
- Hemothorax (bleeding from torn intercostal vessels, lacerated lung, or exposed rib marrow cavity)
- Unstable chest wall (flail chest).

Flail chest occurs when two or more adjacent ribs are fractured or dislocated both dorsally and ventrally, resulting in the paradoxical movement of a segment of the thoracic wall during respiration. This may diminish lung volume and damage the underlying viscera as the flail segment is displaced during respiration.

- Rib fractures may be stabilized by open fixation using pins and wires.
- Alternatively, the ribs may be secured to an external frame by percutaneous placement of sutures around the ribs (this procedure has been used successfully to stabilize flail chest).
  - A frame made of malleable rodding used to construct splints is contoured to the normal curvature of the thoracic wall. Bars pass over the dorsal and ventral aspects of the flail segment. At least two sutures are placed around the ribs of the flail segment, dorsally and ventrally, and are tied to the frame to displace the flail segment in a lateral or outward direction (Fig. 1).
  - Damage to the underlying lung tissue usually does not occur during passage of the suture needle around the rib because of the presence of pneumothorax. The potential for injury of the underlying lungs also can be minimized by grasping a rib with a towel forceps and retracting the flail segment laterally.
  - Keep the frame in place for at least 3 weeks.
- Do not apply tight bandages for stabilization of rib fractures, because this displaces the ribs medially, resulting in continued damage to the underlying viscera and healing of the ribs in such a position that lung volume is permanently decreased.
- Adjunctive therapy for rib fracture includes analgesia and intercostal nerve blocks to control pain, thereby promoting uninhibited cough and deeper, less restrictive breathing that helps to prevent hypoventilation, atelectasis, retained secretions, and pneumonia.

Treatment of Open Chest Wounds

- Immediate treatment of open chest wounds consists of minor cleansing of the wound and application of a bandage to restore continuity of the chest wall.
- Treat the resultant pneumothorax with thoracentesis or chest tube.

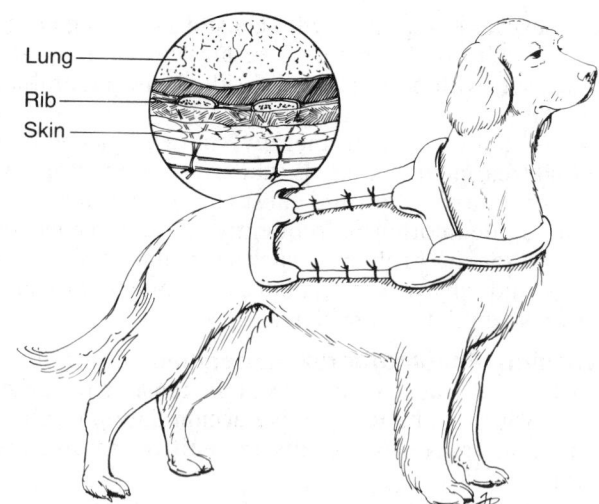

Figure 1. Fractured ribs can be secured to an external frame contoured to the body wall. Sutures are passed around the ribs dorsally and ventrally and tied around the bars of the frame. (Redrawn from Bjorling DE, et al.: Flail chest: Review, clinical experience, and new method of stabilization. J Am Anim Hosp Assoc 18:269–276, 1982.)

- Allow small penetrating wounds to heal in an open manner (if air is not leaking into the pleural space), or they may be explored, debrided, and sutured. Surgically explore, debride, and close large open wounds of the thoracic wall.
- It may be necessary to remove ribs that are devoid of musculature and vascular supply.
  - Up to four adjacent ribs can be removed and the thoracic wall closed by apposing the remaining ribs.
  - Larger defects require the use of synthetic mesh (e.g., polyprophylene) to compensate for the tissue lost.

Diaphragmatic Hernia Repair

Some hernias remain undetected for months or years before signs of pleural effusion, weight loss, gastrointestinal dysfunction, or jaundice occur (see sec. 6, ch. 17 for radiographic diagnosis of diaphragmatic hernia).

- Minor perforations of the diaphragm usually seal without treatment.
- Surgically repair diaphragmatic defects (most can be closed by suture) that result in displacement of viscera into the thoracic cavity (see Technique). The liver, spleen, omentum, and gastrointestinal tract commonly are herniated.
- Timing of diaphragmatic hernia repair depends on the patient's condition.
  - It is preferable to delay diaphragmatic hernia repair until the condition is stabilized; however, if respiratory function cannot be stabilized despite aggressive supportive care, it may be necessary to repair the diaphragmatic hernia on an emergency basis.
  - Acute dilatation of herniated stomach or strangulation of herniated bowel requires emergency surgery.

Technique

1. Keep the animal on mechanical ventilation throughout the repair.
2. Approach the diaphragm through a ventral midline abdominal incision.
3. Initially it may be necessary to enlarge the diaphragmatic rent in order to reduce the herniated viscera. If so, make the incision ventrally to simplify repair.
4. In cases of chronic hernia, adhesions between viscera and diaphragm or lungs may be present. Break these down carefully.
5. Following reduction of displaced organs and examination of the lungs and pleural space, close the rent with synthetic absorbable or monofilament nonabsorbable suture (simple continuous or horizontal mattress pattern).
6. Begin with the most dorsal aspect of the hernia and work ventrally to close the repair.
7. Grasp large "bites" of the abdominal wall musculature or ribs when suturing diaphragm that has avulsed from the ventrolateral body wall.
8. If large portions of diaphragm have been destroyed, repair the defect with synthetic mesh or transposition of a transversus abdominis muscle flap.
9. Place a thoracostomy tube to remove air and fluid after surgery.

Postoperative Care and Complications

■ Remove the chest tube when no longer needed.
■ Advise the owner to limit the patient's activity for 2–4 weeks.
■ Complications are rare and the prognosis usually is good.

Exploratory Thoracotomy

Thoracotomy for treatment of ongoing hemorrhage or air leakage on an emergency basis is difficult and may be unrewarding. The animal is at significant risk due to the effects of anesthesia, and often it is difficult to identify and effectively treat the site of hemorrhage or air leakage.

■ Before undertaking an exploratory thoracotomy, be sure that adequate equipment and personnel are available to successfully complete the procedure.

■ Perform exploratory thoracotomy for treatment of traumatic injuries of the thoracic cavity only after aggressive medical therapy and tube drainage have failed to stabilize the animal's condition.
  • If the site of injury can be identified, a lateral thoracotomy approach may be used (see sec. 6, ch. 25). Unfortunately, this rarely is possible.
  • A midsternal approach (splitting the sternum) allows exploration of both sides of the thorax (see sec. 6, ch. 25).

Antibiotic Therapy

■ Administer antibiotics to prevent:
  • Development of bacterial pneumonia resulting from traumatic injuries of the lungs
  • Wound infection as a result of disruption of the thoracic wall.
■ Initially give antibiotics intravenously to establish satisfactory tissue concentrations. This can be followed by oral administration of antibiotics.
■ Prophylactic antibiotic treatment for pulmonary injuries should provide broad-spectrum antibacterial activity. A satisfactory combination is cephazolin (20 mg/kg q8h, IM or IV) and gentamicin (2–4 mg/kg q12h or 4–8 mg/kg q24h, SC, IM, or IV).
■ Wound infections due to contamination of tissues with dirt most often are caused by gram-positive bacteria. Cephazolin or other cephalosporin antibiotics have good activity against the most common organisms involved.

Supplemental Readings

Bjorling DE, DeNovo RC, Kolata RJ: Flail chest: Review and clinical experience. J Am Anim Hosp Assoc 18:269, 1982.

Craven KD, Oppenheimer L, Wood LDH: Effects of contusion and flail chest on pulmonary profusion and oxygen exchange. J Appl Physiol 47:729, 1979.

Fitzpatrick RK, Crowe DT Jr: Nasal oxygen administration in dogs and cats: Experimental and clinical investigations. J Am Anim Hosp Assoc 22:293, 1986.

Kolata RJ: Surgical emergencies. In Gourley IM, Vasseur PB, Eds.: General Small Animal Surgery. Philadelphia: J. B. Lippincott, 1985, p 65.

Trinkle JK, Furman RW, Hinshaw MA, et al.: Pulmonary contusion. Ann Thorac Surg 16:568, 1973.

25 Principles of Thoracic Surgery

Stephen J. Birchard
Eric R. Schertel

Thoracic surgery frequently is performed in small animals, especially in referral centers. Thoracotomy is commonly performed to correct routine cardiovascular defects such as patent ductus arteriosus and to evaluate and correct respiratory diseases such as pulmonary neoplasia. Exploratory thoracotomy may be recommended to determine the extent of diseases such as neoplasia and diffuse infection and to obtain biopsies to help establish a definitive diagnosis. It is important to be well versed in the anatomy and physiology of the thoracic cavity and its major structures and to be familiar with the principles of anesthetic management of the thoracic surgery patient.

This chapter discusses the surgical anatomy and physiology of the thorax, thoracic surgical technique, and patient care before, during, and after thoracic surgery.

SURGICAL ANATOMY

Bony Structures

- The bony structures of the thorax usually consist of 13 pairs of ribs and costal cartilages, 13 vertebrae, and eight sternebrae.
- The first nine ribs, called the sternal ribs, articulate with the sternum. The last four ribs are called the asternal ribs. The costal cartilages of ribs 10–12 make up the costal arch. The thirteenth pair of ribs are also called the floating ribs.
- The manubrium is the most cranial aspect of the sternum, and the xyphoid is located caudally. The xyphoid cartilage is the caudal extension of the xyphoid. Intersternebral cartilages are located between each sternebra. The sternebrae are very narrow structures, making midline division somewhat difficult. The sternebral midline is characterized by a slight bony ridge.

Soft Tissues

Muscles

- The external and internal intercostal muscles are located between each rib and are important for inspiration.
- Other surgically important muscles of the lateral thoracic wall are the serratus ventralis and serratus cranialis dorsalis, scalenus, and external abdominal oblique. The latissimus dorsi, a large fan-shaped muscle extending from the ribs to the forelimb, is the first major muscle encountered during lateral thoracotomy.

Vessels and Nerves

- The intercostal arteries, veins, and nerves are located on the caudal aspect of each rib. The internal thoracic artery and veins run horizontally just lateral to the sternum, within the thorax.
- The cutaneous and muscular branches of the thoracodorsal artery are frequently encountered during lateral thoracotomy.

PREOPERATIVE CONSIDERATIONS

History, Physical Examination, and Diagnostic Tests

- Review the animal's history and perform a thorough physical examination.
  - Give special consideration to the patient's cardiopulmonary status (mucous membrane color and refill time, heart rate and rhythm, pulse rate and character, heart and lung sounds, ventilation, thoracic palpation and percussion).
- Review diagnostic tests already performed and repeat if necessary.
  - Evaluate thoracic radiographs to become familiar with the animal's disease and to plan the surgical approach.
  - Evaluate blood tests, such as complete blood count (CBC) and serum chemistry profile, to establish the patient's baseline before surgery. If the condition is severe, blood gas analysis may be helpful to further evaluate the patient's respiratory status.

Preoperative Treatment and Stabilization

General Supportive Care

- Administer appropriate medical therapy that will stabilize the animal and reduce the level of anesthetic and surgical risk.
  - For example, if a dog with patent ductus arteriosus is in congestive heart failure, treat with the appropriate drugs to improve cardiopulmonary function before anesthesia and surgery.
- Correct fluid and electrolyte deficiencies.
- Maintain the animal's nutritional status. Consider placing a nasogastric or pharyngostomy tube if the animal will not eat and is becoming debilitated (see sec. 1, ch. 3).

■ Closely observe the patient's condition. Animals with thoracic disease may rapidly show changes in their clinical status.

Chest Drainage

■ If pleural fluid or air is present, tap the chest before anesthesia to allow better ventilation.
■ Place an indwelling thoracic drainage tube if fluid or air accumulation is recurrent (see sec. 1, ch. 3).
  • Use intermittent or continuous suction drainage.
  • Quantify amount of fluid or air recovered to establish a baseline before surgery.

Oxygen

■ Administer oxygen to severely dyspneic or cyanotic animals.
  • Place the animal in an oxygen cage at 40–50% concentration or place a nasal oxygen tube to raise the concentration of inspired oxygen (see sec. 1, ch. 3).
■ If possible, analyze blood gases before and after oxygen administration to establish its effectiveness.

Prophylactic Antibiotics

■ Use prophylactic antibiotics if the planned operation will be a clean-contaminated, contaminated, or "dirty" procedure.
■ Thoracotomy to open and/or resect a portion of the respiratory tract is considered a clean-contaminated procedure. However, the author uses prophylactic antibiotics only if there is a strong suspicion that significant contamination of the surgical field will occur (e.g., foreign bodies, abscess, necrotic tumor, bacterial pneumonia). Thoracotomy for drainage and resection of the pericardium for pericarditis is a good example of the need for preoperative use of antibiotics.
■ Administer the prophylactic antibiotic immediately before surgery to ensure sufficient blood concentrations of the drug at the time of surgery. Discontinue antibiotic administration 24–48 hours postoperatively unless evidence of infection is present.
■ Choose an antibiotic that is effective against the suspected contaminant and that reaches therapeutic concentrations in the target tissues.

Blood

■ Cardiac surgery or removal of large, vascular neoplasms may be associated with acute blood loss.
■ Have a blood donor or packed cells available if significant blood loss is anticipated.
■ Cross-match or type the donor's blood if multiple transfusions are anticipated.

Client Communication

Risks

■ Major cardiac and respiratory surgery is associated with a high incidence of morbidity and mortality.
■ Review the incidence of complications and death associated with the planned procedure and discuss this information with the client.

Cost

Thoracic surgery and patient care may be quite expensive.

■ Discuss the cost of preoperative diagnosis and therapy, anesthesia and surgery, and postoperative intensive care with the client.

ANESTHETIC CONSIDERATIONS

The general principles of anesthesia described in sec. 1, ch. 2 apply to thoracic surgery patients. Special considerations for thoracic surgery patients are outlined in this section.

Premedication

■ Avoid phenothiazines such as acepromazine because of possible side effects of hypotension and myocardial depression. However, at low doses (0.1 mg/kg, SC or IM), they may be beneficial for calming animals with respiratory compromise but no cardiac involvement.
■ Diazepam (Valium) is a safe drug that can be used as a premedicant (0.2 mg/kg, IV); it has minimal effects on the cardiovascular and respiratory systems.
■ Xylazine (Rompun) is a commonly used drug but has significant drawbacks such as cardiac and respiratory depression, making it a poor choice for thoracic surgery.
■ Anticholinergics (e.g., atropine) are not used routinely because they increase viscosity of respiratory secretions, can increase anatomic dead space, and may induce cardiac arrhythmias.

Induction

■ Diazepam (0.2mg/kg IV) followed by administration of a thiobarbiturate (e.g., Thiopental) (6–10 mg/kg, IV) provides relatively safe and rapid induction. Rapid, smooth induction which allows immediate intubation and control of ventilation is preferable.
■ The combination of ketamine and diazepam (1:1 mixture; 1 ml of mixture/10 kg) also can be used for thoracic surgery patients. Hemodynamics are minimally compromised by this combination. However, ventilatory support may be necessary.

Maintenance

■ Any of the commonly used inhalation anesthetics can be used successfully for thoracic procedures. Isoflurane is preferred because of less myocardial depression and better maintenance of blood pressure, although hypotension commonly occurs.
■ Avoid nitrous oxide in patients with respiratory disease, pneumothorax, anemia, or hypoxia.
■ Provide positive pressure ventilation by manual compression of the bag or with a mechanical ventilator (see Table 1 for ventilation guidelines).

KEY POINT ▶ Adequate positive pressure ventilation in the thoracic surgery patient is critical to prevent hypoxia, respiratory acidosis, and atelectasis.

TABLE 1. General Guidelines for Controlled Ventilation

Physiologic Parameter	Value
Respiratory	8–12 breaths/min
Tidal volume	15–20 ml/kg ideal body weight
Peak airway pressure	15–20 cm H_2O–closed
	20–30 cm H_2O—open
Inspiratory time	1–1.5 sec
Expiratory time	2–3 sec
Inspiratory:expiratory ratio	1:2–1:4

Modified from Faggella AM, Raffe MR: Anesthetic management of thoracotomy. Vet Clin North Am 17:480, 1987.

Fluids

- Thoracotomy diminishes the functional reserve of the heart by decreasing effective filling pressures. This may be compensated for, in part, by fluid therapy.
- Place one or two intravenous catheters for fluid administration.
- Administer balanced electrolyte solutions at a surgical maintenance rate of 10–20 ml/kg/h.

Monitoring

Cardiovascular

- The standard methods of cardiovascular monitoring (e.g., heart rate, color, pulse quality, capillary refill) are very important, because alterations due to the disease or surgical manipulations are common.
- Monitoring with electrocardiography (ECG) is helpful to determine when and why cardiac problems arise.
- Blood pressure recording is being used with increasing frequency. Direct measurements are obtained with an arterial catheter or a Doppler unit with a pneumatic cuff placed over an accessible artery (e.g., metatarsal artery). Blood pressure measurements help determine circulatory status during the anesthetic period.

Respiratory

- Carefully monitor the respiratory rate and depth. In the patient with respiratory compromise, be especially aware of respirations before thoracotomy and immediately after chest closure.
- Monitor blood gas analysis to determine respiratory status; make necessary adjustments.

Other

- Use standard techniques for monitoring anesthetic depth (see sec. 1, ch. 2).
- Ensure good communication between anesthesiologist and surgeon, which is essential for a smooth and successful procedure. Indicate to the anesthesiologist when major manipulations of the heart and lungs are imminent, and point out when problems arise such as atelectasis due to inadequate ventilation. The anesthetist should keep the surgeon informed of the patient's overall status.

SURGICAL PROCEDURES

Instruments. A standard general pack is needed. In addition, see Table 2 for instruments that are particularly useful in thoracic surgery.

Lateral Thoracotomy

Indications

- This is the standard approach to most intrathoracic structures. See Table 3 for location of structures exposed through intercostal thoracotomy.

Objective

- To gain access for the right or left hemithorax and expose heart, lungs, or other structures

Equipment

- See Table 2 for specific instruments useful in thoracic surgery.

Technique

1. Place the animal in lateral recumbency and prepare the lateral thorax for aseptic surgery.
2. Count the intercostal spaces to approximate the location of the incision.
3. Incise the skin, subcutaneous tissues, and cutaneous trunci muscle, from dorsal to ventral, from the costovertebral junction to the sternum.
4. Incise the latissimus dorsi muscle from ventral to dorsal (Fig. 1).
5. Recount the intercostal spaces from cranial to caudal unless the incision is located in the caudal thorax.

TABLE 2. Special Instruments Recommended for Thoracic Surgery

Scissors
Long-handled Metzenbaum
Potts

Needle Holders
Mayo-Hegar (long-handled)
DeBakey
French eye

Tissue Forceps
DeBakey general thoracic
DeBakey vascular

Other Forceps
Satinsky clamps
Angled or curved forceps
   Gallbladder
   Rumel thoracic and dissecting
   Mixter hemostatic, thoracic
   Lahey gall duct thoracic
Bronchus clamps
Vascular clamps

Retractors
Finnochietto rib
Burford rib

Other
Rib approximator

TABLE 3. Location of Thoracic Structures via Intercostal Thoracotomy

Thoracic Structure	Intercostal Space	
	Left	Right
Heart and pericardium	4, 5	4, 5
PDA, PRAA	4 (5)	
Pulmonic valve	4	
Trachea		3
Lungs	4–6	4–6
Cranial lobe	(4) 5	(4) 5
Intermediate lobe		5
Caudal lobe	5 (6)	5 (6)
Esophagus		
Cranial		3, 4
Caudal	7–10	7–10
Caudal vena cava	(6–7)	7–10
Diaphragm	7–10	7–10
Thoracic duct (caudal)		
Dog		8–10
Cat	8–10	

Modified from Orton C: Thoracic wall. *In* Slatter DH, ed.: *Textbook of Small Animal Surgery.* Philadelphia: W. B. Saunders, 1985, p 539.
PDA = patent ductus arteriosus; PRAA = persistent right aortic arch

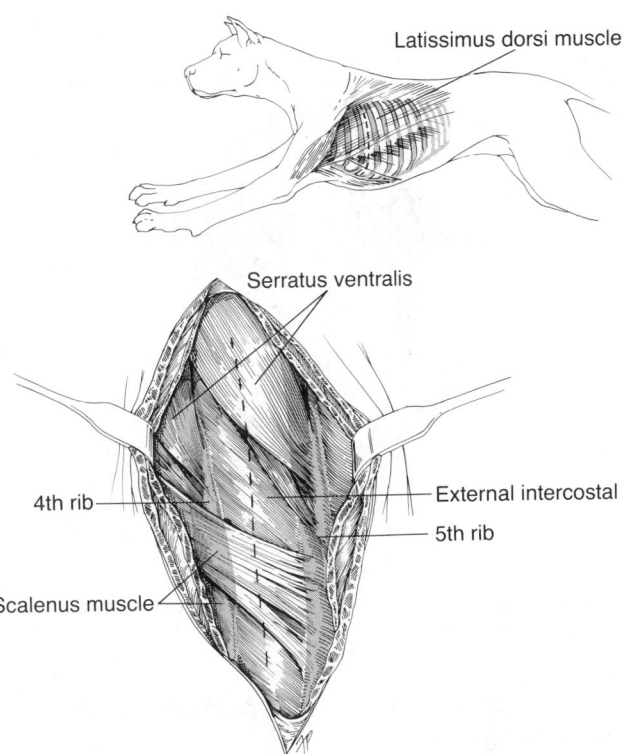

Figure 1. Thoracotomy technique. Top, incise the skin at the intercostal space between ribs 4 and 5 (dotted line). Below, cut the latissimus dorsi muscle and retract to expose the serratus ventralis, dorsalis, scalenus, and external intercostal muscles.

6. Incise through the remainder of muscles: serratus ventralis (can be bluntly separated rather than incised), scalenus, external abdominal oblique, and external and internal intercostal (Fig. 2). Penetrate the pleura (instruct the anesthetist to stop positive pressure ventilation before introducing sharp instruments into the thorax), and incise the pleura dorsally and ventrally with scissors. Avoid trauma to
7. the internal thoracic artery when incising ventrally. Protect the ribs and muscle tissue with moistened sponges and insert a self-retaining rib retractor to
8. expose the thoracic viscera (Fig. 3).
   Closure
   a. Preplace a temporary or permanent thoracic drain tube.
   b. Preplace several large (2–0, 0, or 1) absorbable sutures around the ribs. Hug the caudal rib during suture passage to avoid damage to the intercostal vessels and nerve.
   c. While the assistant approximates the ribs with one of the sutures, tie the rib sutures using a surgeon's knot (Fig. 4).
   d. Close the deep muscles in one layer (serratus, scalenus, external abdominal oblique, and intercostal muscles) in a simple continuous pattern.
   e. Close the latissimus dorsi muscle in a simple continuous pattern (Fig. 5).
   f. Close the cutaneous trunci muscle and subcutaneous tissues in the next layer in a simple continuous pattern; then close skin in pattern of your choice.
   g. Perform thoracocentesis using the chest tube to evacuate air or fluid.
   h. Place a light, loosely fitting bandage over the incision and chest tube.

Median Sternotomy

Median sternotomy is indicated when bilateral exposure of the thorax is necessary.
Examples are:

■ Multiple lung lesions
■ Pericardectomy
■ Mediastinal tumors (e.g., thymoma)

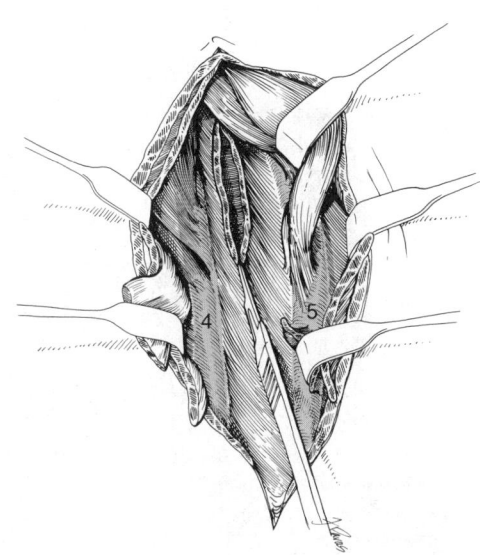

Figure 2. Cut or separate the serratus and scalenus muscles between ribs 4 and 5 so that an incision can be made in the intercostal muscles and the pleura.

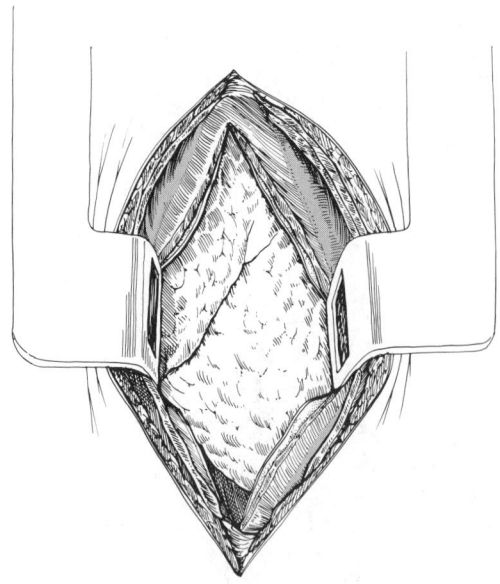

Figure 3. After the intercostal muscles and pleura are cut, retract the ribs to expose the lung.

- Alternate approach to pulmonic valve or other cardiac procedures
- Hepatic surgery
- Complicated diaphragmatic hernia or other diaphragmatic surgery

Objective

- Bilateral exposure of the thorax

Equipment

- See Table 2 for special equipment needed for thoracic surgery
- Oscillating bone saw for medium to large dogs
- Osteotome and mallet
- Orthopedic wire (0.028–0.035 gauge) for medium to large dogs; wire cutters; wire twisting instrument
- Electrocautery

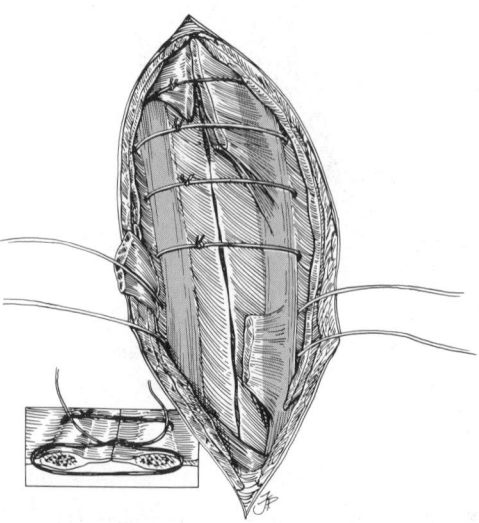

Figure 4. Place sutures around ribs 4 and 5 and secure each with a surgeon's knot.

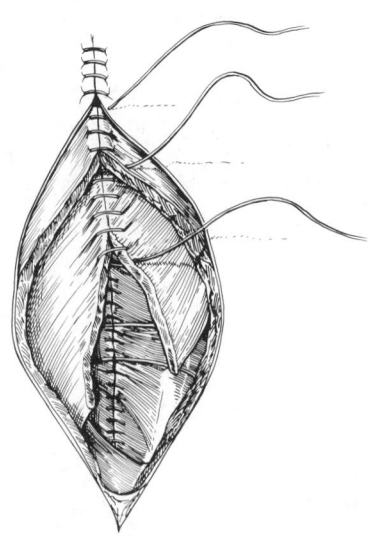

Figure 5. Close the latissimus dorsi muscle (simple continuous), the subcutaneous tissue (simple continuous), and the skin (simple continuous or interrupted).

Technique

1. Place the dog in dorsal recumbency.
2. Prepare the sternum and ventral half of the thorax for aseptic surgery.
3. Incise the skin and subcutaneous tissues from manubrium to xyphoid.
4. Divide the muscular attachments to the sternum along the thin, white fascial raphe to expose the sternum. This is best performed using electrocautery (Fig. 6).
5. Score the sternebrae on the ventral midline with a scalpel or electrocautery (see Fig. 6).
6. Cut two-thirds of the thickness of the sternebrae with the bone saw. Finish the cut with an osteotome and mallet, being careful not to injure the heart or internal thoracic vessels.

KEY POINT ▶ When performing sternotomy, make the sternal cut exactly on the midline to facilitate secure closure with full cerclage wire.

7. Protect the sternum with moistened sponges and retract with a rib retractor.
8. Closure
   a. Place a temporary or permanent thoracic drain tube.
   b. Preplace cerclage wire or heavy suture (e.g., 0 or 1 polypropylene) around each sternebra, using hemostatic forceps (Fig. 7). Stay close to the bone to avoid the internal thoracic vessels. Tighten the wire, using wire holding forceps.
   c. Close the muscle tissue, using an absorbable suture in a simple continuous pattern.
   d. Close the subcutaneous tissue and skin in a routine fashion.
   e. Perform thoracocentesis, using the chest tube to evacuate air and fluid.
   f. Loosely place a lightly padded bandage over the incision and chest tube.

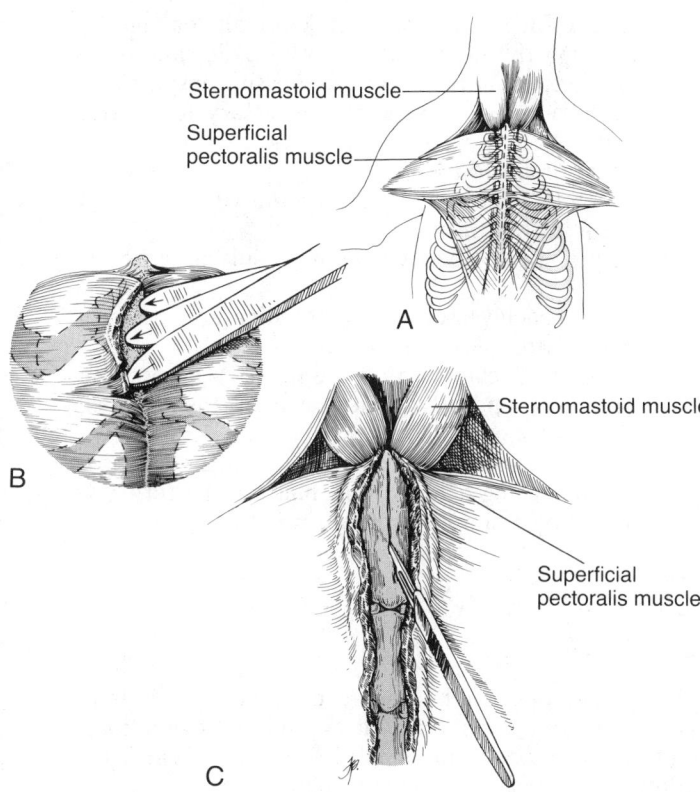

Figure 6. Technique for median sternotomy. *A*, Determine the middle of the sternum and associated muscle attachments; *B*, bluntly dissect muscle off the sternum; *C*, score the exposed periosteum on the midline.

Lung Lobectomy

Indications for lung lobectomy include:

- Neoplasia
- Abscesses or granuloma of the lung
- Lung lobe torsion
- Irreversible atelectasis
- Bronchoesophageal fistula

Objectives

- Remove part or all of a lung lobe.
- Maintain good hemostasis, especially of the major pulmonary blood vessels.
- Establish an air-tight seal of the bronchus.
- Leave adequate pulmonary tissue to avoid compromise of the patient's cardiopulmonary status.

Equipment

- The same equipment used for lateral thoracotomy or median sternotomy

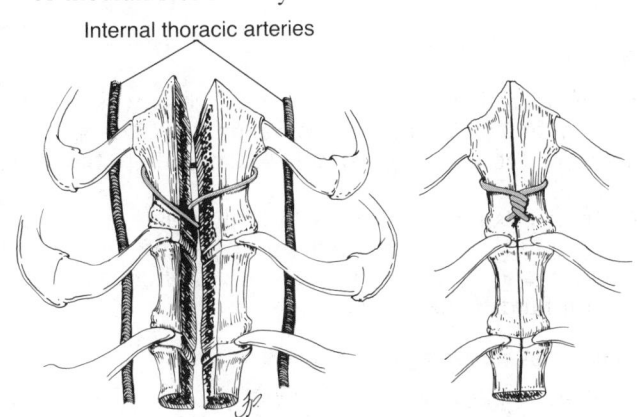

Figure 7. Close each sternebra with full cerclage wire twisted with a needle holder or wire twister.

- Babcock tissue-holding forceps
- Small suture with swaged needle (e.g., 4-0 silk, nylon, or polypropylene)
- Tissue stapling device (TA 55 or 90 U.S. Surgical Thoracoabdominal Autosuture stapler) (optional)

Technique

1. See preceding surgical techniques for description of approaches to the lung lobes.
2. Explore the thorax and determine the extent of disease and which lobes are involved.
3. Determine which bronchus or bronchi supply the affected lobe(s).
4. Mobilize the lobe.
   a. Caudal lung lobe—incise the pulmonary ligament that attaches the caudal aspect of the lobe to parietal pleura.
   b. Incise the pleural attachments between the affected lobe and adjacent lobes.
   c. Gently incise or dissect adhesions between the lobe and surrounding tissues (especially a problem in pulmonary neoplasia).
5. Partial lobectomy
   a. Place a noncrushing clamp (e.g., Satinsky) between the lesion and the hilus and incise distally to the clamp with scalpel or scissors.
   b. Close the remaining lobe with 4-0 or 5-0 silk, nylon, or polypropylene in a continuous horizontal mattress pattern. Oversew the incised tissue with a simple continuous pattern, if necessary, to prevent air leakage.
   c. Alternatively, place the Autosuture stapler between the lesion and the hilus. Staple the lung, incise above the stapler, and remove the diseased tissue.

   d. Check for hemostasis; check for air leakage by flooding the lung incision with sterile saline and giving the animal a positive pressure inspiration. Place additional sutures if necessary to control leaks.

6. Complete lobectomy
   a. Dissect the pulmonary artery and vein free from the adjacent bronchus.
   b. Triple ligate each vessel with silk or chromic catgut.
   c. Divide each vessel between the ligatures, leaving two ligatures with the animal.
   d. Place two clamps (e.g., Satinsky) across the bronchus and divide it between the clamps. Remove the lung lobe.
   e. Close the bronchus with silk, nylon, or polypropylene, using a horizontal mattress pattern followed by a simple continuous pattern.

POSTOPERATIVE CARE AND COMPLICATIONS

Chest Tubes

- If a chest tube has been placed, leave it in as long as necessary, depending on the animal's condition and production of air or fluid (see sec. 1, ch. 3 for details on chest tube management).
- In routine procedures in patients without recurrent pneumothorax or effusion, pull the tube as soon as negative pressure has been reestablished after completion of surgical closure.
- After major pulmonary resection, consider leaving a chest tube in place for a minimum of 24 hours even if no air or fluid is recovered. Otherwise, leave the tube in until insignificant amounts of air or fluids are being recovered (< 2 ml/kg/day).
- Obtain thoracic radiographs prior to removal of the chest tube to ensure that there is no significant pleural air or fluid.
- See sec. 1, ch. 3 for more details on chest tube management.

Pain

- Thoracic surgery is associated with postoperative pain that causes discomfort and can inhibit ventilation by making the animal reluctant to expand the thorax.
- Be careful when handling the animal, especially around the thoracotomy site. Unilateral forelimb lameness is common after lateral thoracotomy but should resolve within several days.
- Local analgesia can be used as a method of decreasing postoperative discomfort. Inject 0.5 ml of bupivacaine (0.5%; Marcaine) locally (using a 25-gauge 1-inch needle) at the dorsal aspect of the intercostal nerves before thoracotomy closure; two or three intercostal nerves adjacent to the thoracotomy incision are anesthetized.
- Systemic analgesia can also be used for those animals exhibiting significant pain.
  - Administer morphine (0.2–0.4 mg/kg, IM or SC), for 2–5 hours of analgesia. Respiratory depression or nausea may occur.

  - Other opioids that can be used are butorphanol (Torbutrol) (0.4 mg/kg, IM), for 2–3 hours of analgesia, and buprenorphine (Buprenex) (.01–.03 mg/kg, IM), for 4–8 hours of analgesia.

Pneumothorax

- Residual air in the pleural space is common after thoracic surgery and rarely causes a clinical problem.
- Persistent postoperative pneumothorax can be a serious problem after surgery of the lung or airways if leakage occurs at the site of incision or excision.
- If pneumothorax causes respiratory compromise and a chest tube is not already present, tap the animal's chest with a butterfly needle, syringe, and stopcock. Place a chest tube and consider performing thoracic radiography if improvement in the animal's condition does not occur or if the pneumothorax is recurrent. Evaluate the heart, lungs, pleural space, and location of the chest tube.

Hemothorax

- Postoperative hemothorax can occur after any thoracic surgery but is more common after major cardiac or vascular surgery, or after removal of large, highly vascular tumors. This can be a difficult complication to manage because re-operation does not usually reveal the source of bleeding.
- If large quantities of bloody fluid are aspirated from the thorax, obtain a PCV assay of the fluid. If the fluid is consistent with whole blood and the animal is losing considerable volume (i.e., clinical evidence of shock or PCV <20), use supportive care to replace volume (isotonic or hypertonic fluids).
- Perform autotransfusion if the blood is not contaminated. Give whole blood from a donor dog if autotransfusion is not possible.
- Monitor peripheral PCV and total protein until the animal's condition is stabilized.
- As a general rule, some surgeons recommend re-exploration of the thorax if blood loss is > 2ml/kg/h for 3–4 hours and unresponsive to conservative therapy.

Ventricular Arrhythmias

- Cardiac arrhythmias are not uncommon and may develop 24–48 hours postoperatively (see sec. 6, ch. 4).

Infection

- Postoperative infection after thoracotomy is uncommon but may occur if contamination was present during the surgery or occurs secondarily to the chest tube.
- Treat pleural infection with appropriate antibiotics (based upon culture and sensitivity of the pleural fluid) and chest drainage. Rarely, thoracic lavage with fluids is necessary.

Supplemental Readings

Evans HE, Christensen GC, eds.: *Miller's Anatomy of the Dog,* 2nd ed. Philadelphia: W. B. Saunders, 1979, p 317.
Orton C: Thoracic Wall. *In* Slatter DH, ed.: *Textbook of Small Animal Surgery.* Philadelphia: W. B. Saunders, 1985, p 536.

Gastrointestinal Disorders

Susan E. Johnson

1 Oropharynx

Sandra Manfra Marretta

Diseases of the oropharynx are common in dogs and cats. These diseases can be divided into categories including oral surgical disease, periodontal disease, endodontic disease, orthodontic disease, stomatitis/gingivitis, neoplastic disease, and salivary gland disease. Neoplastic disease of the maxilla and mandible is discussed in sec. 9, ch. 4.

ORAL SURGICAL DISEASE

The two major categories of oral surgical (non-neoplastic) disease are:

- Diseases requiring dental extraction
- Oronasal fistulas and palatal defects that can be surgically corrected

Diseases Requiring Dental Extraction

Etiology

Dental diseases in which extraction is a treatment option include retained deciduous and supernumerary teeth, maloccluded teeth, advanced periodontal disease, fractured teeth, gross decay/erosions, diseased teeth in the fracture site of the mandible or maxilla, periapical abscess, and impacted and deformed teeth.

Clinical Signs

Common historical findings and signs of dental disease include changes in eating habits, halitosis, pawing at the mouth, abnormal salivation, oral hypersensitivity, facial swelling, oral hemorrhage, sneezing, nasal discharge, and abnormal behavior.

Diagnosis and Indications for Extraction

The decision to perform dental extraction depends not only on the dental disease present but also on the client's ability and desire to pursue alternatives to extraction, such as periodontal, endodontic, and orthodontic therapy.

KEY POINT ▶ If a client is unwilling to pursue alternatives for treatment of a painful tooth, then the tooth should be extracted.

Retained Deciduous and Supernumerary Teeth. Deciduous teeth are considered overly retained if they are firmly attached following the initial stage of eruption of the permanent tooth. Failure to extract deciduous teeth during this initial stage frequently results in malocclusion of the permanent tooth. Retained deciduous teeth and supernumerary teeth can be diagnosed as extra teeth present in the dental arcade. Deciduous teeth may be differentiated from supernumerary permanent teeth by their smaller crown size grossly and smaller root structure radiographically.

Maloccluded Teeth. Extraction may be required for maloccluded teeth that cause traumatic soft tissue occlusion or interfere with proper closing of the mouth. Orthodontic therapy is a viable alternative in these cases.

Advanced Periodontal Disease. Extremely mobile teeth caused by severe periodontal disease should be extracted. Other indications for extraction of teeth affected by periodontal disease include periodontal pockets extending to the apex of the tooth, pockets that reach the nasal cavity or maxillary sinus, and periapical abscess (discussed later).

Fractured Teeth. Extract fractured teeth with exposed pulp tissue if endodontic therapy is not an option. To diagnose pulpal exposure, place a dental explorer over the suspected exposure site. If the explorer penetrates into the tooth, the pulp is exposed.

Gross Decay/Dental Erosion. This condition, characterized by soft areas of demineralized enamel or cementum, is rare in dogs and cats.

- In dogs, gross decay, which usually occurs on the occlusal or biting surface of the maxillary first molar, can be identified with a dental explorer placed into the soft carious lesion. Penetration of the explorer into the soft demineralized enamel confirms gross decay. Radiographs of the affected tooth will show the extent of the lesion.
- Subgingival and cervical erosive lesions are very common in cats. These defects are called external root resorptions (ERRs) or neck lesions.
- ERRs often are extensive and painful and usually are covered by granulation tissue. Removal of the granulation tissue reveals the underlying erosion.
  - Determine the extent of the erosion in the neck and crown of the tooth with a dental explorer.
  - Radiographs are imperative to determine the severity of root resorption, because minor erosions in the crown may be associated with major root resorption.
- Treat dental caries and external root resorptive lesions that extend into the pulp with extraction. Minor lesions can be restored with various dental restorative materials.

Diseased Teeth in a Mandible or Maxilla Fracture Site. Extract teeth in a fracture site that are severely affected with periodontal disease or that have fractured roots. If the fracture line in the jaw is located along the periodontal ligament and communicates with the apex of the tooth, the tooth is extracted. Careful gross assessment and radiographic examination of the fracture site can determine if an extraction is necessary.

Periapical Abscess. In small animals, a periapical abscess (infection around the apex of a tooth) usually is secondary to periodontal or endodontic disease and is characterized by acute, severe painful swelling in the area of the affected tooth.

- Carefully examine teeth in the area of acute facial swelling for deep periodontal pockets with a periodontal probe and for pulpal exposure with a dental explorer.
- Periapical lysis will be present around the apex of the affected root. Radiographs can confirm the diagnosis.
- Extraction of the affected tooth is recommended.

Impacted Teeth. Impacted (unerupted) teeth may cause nasal discharge, orthodontic problems, and pain.

- Dentigerous cysts may occur and can cause expansion of bone with subsequent facial asymmetry, extreme displacement of teeth, severe root resorption of adjacent teeth, and pain.
  - Dentigerous cysts may give rise to ameloblastomas.
- Radiography can diagnose impacted teeth. Extraction is recommended if they are causing problems.

TABLE 1. Deciduous and Permanent Dental Formulas for Dogs and Cats

Deciduous Dentition
Dog: 2(I3/3 C1/1 P3/3) = 28
Cat: 2(I3/3 C1/1 P3/2) = 26
Permanent Dentition
Dog: 2(I3/3 C1/1 P4/4 M2/3) = 42
Cat: 2(I3/3 C1/1 P3/2 M1/1) = 30

I = incisor; C = canine; P = premolar; M = molar.

Deformed Teeth. Diagnose deformed teeth based on gross and radiographic appearance. Usually they result from trauma or fever that occurred during tooth development.

- Diagnose minor dental deformities such as enamel hypoplasia based on the observation of symmetric defects and staining of enamel combined with a history of illness during tooth development. No treatment is required in these cases.
- Extract severely deformed teeth, secondary to dental trauma, that are causing pain.

Surgical Anatomy

Proper performance of dental extractions requires a thorough knowledge of dental formulas, dental root structure, and dental anatomy.

KEY POINT ▶ Determine the number of roots in any tooth to be extracted to ensure that all roots are removed during extraction.

- Deciduous and permanent dental formulas for dogs and cats are listed in Table 1.
- In both dogs and cats, all incisors and canines have only a single root. The dentition, including root structure, of dogs and cats is illustrated in Figures 1 and 2, respectively. Tooth roots for both species are listed in Table 2.
- Basic anatomic structures of the teeth and related areas are illustrated in Figure 3 and defined in Table 3.

Preoperative Considerations

- Prior to performing dental extractions, perform a thorough physical examination, standard laboratory tests including a complete blood count (CBC), serum biochemistry, and urinalysis.

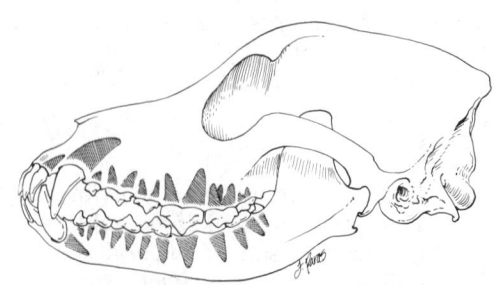

Figure 1. Dental root structure in the dog.

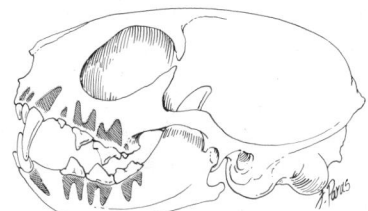

Figure 2. Dental root structure in the cat.

- Perform appropriate radiographic procedures, based on the animal's clinical signs, physical examination findings, and age.
- Correct any underlying metabolic abnormalities such as dehydration, azotemia, electrolyte imbalances, hyperglycemia, and hypoglycemia.

Surgical Procedure

There are three basic types of extractions: simple, multirooted, and complicated surgical. See Tables 4–6 for equipment and materials recommended for all types of dental procedures.

Simple Extraction. Simple extraction refers to the extraction of a small single-rooted tooth such as an incisor.

Technique

1. Place an appropriate-size dental elevator in the gingival sulcus to sever the attachments of the gingiva around the tooth.

TABLE 2. Tooth Roots in Dogs and Cats

Type of Tooth	No. of Roots
In Dogs	
Incisor	1
Canine	1
Maxillary (upper) cheek:	
1st (1st P)	1
2nd and 3rd (2nd and 3rd P)	2
4th–6th (4th P; 1st and 2nd M)	3
Mandibular (lower) cheek:	
1st and last (1st P; 3rd M)	1
2nd–6th (2nd–4th P; 1st and 2nd M)	2
In Cats	
Incisor	1
Canine	1
Maxillary (upper) cheek:	
1st (2nd P)	1
3rd (4th P)	3
All others	2
Mandibular (lower) cheek:	
All	2

P = premolar; M = molar.

2. Advance the elevator apically (toward the apex or tip of the root) between the alveolar bone and root.
3. Rotate the elevator 90° and hold for 15-second intervals to tear the periodontal ligament (Fig. 4A).
4. Advance the elevator again apically, rotate it 90°, and hold for 15 seconds.
5. When the tooth is loose, place an appropriate-size dental extraction forcep on the crown near the gingival margin and rotate and remove the tooth from the alveolus (Fig. 4B).

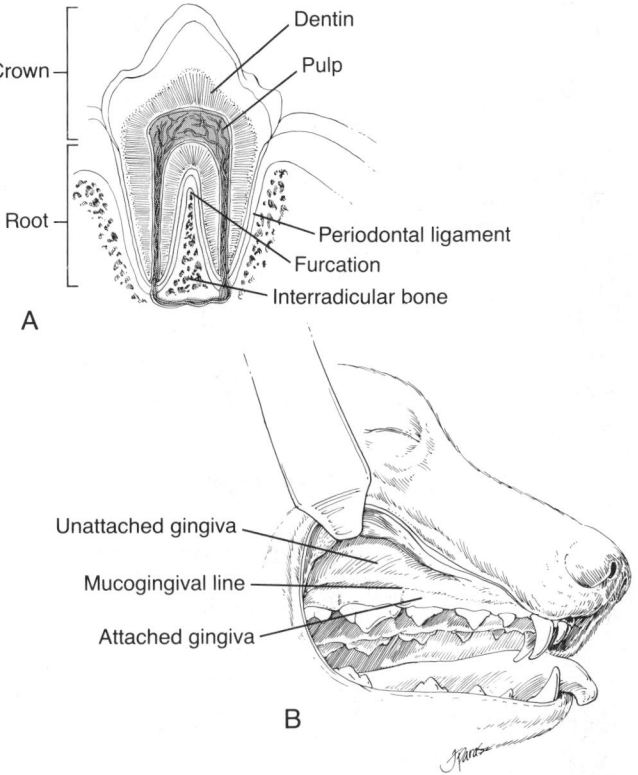

Figure 3. *A,* Anatomy of the tooth. *B,* Gingival anatomy.

TABLE 3. Basic Anatomic Structures of the Dentition

Crown:	Portion of the tooth located in the oral cavity. It is covered by enamel.
Root:	Portion of the tooth that lies within the alveolar bone. It is covered by cementum.
Furcation:	The space between the roots of a multirooted tooth.
Periodontal ligament:	Ligament that attaches the root of the tooth to the alveolar bone.
Interradicular bone:	Bone located between the roots.
Buccal bone:	Bone located on the buccal or cheek side of the tooth root.
Attached gingiva:	Keratinized gingiva firmly attached to the underlying alveolar bone.
Alveolar mucosa:	Mucosa that is loosely attached to the underlying bone.
Mucogingival line:	Anatomic landmark that separates the attached gingiva from the alveolar mucosa.

6. Examine the tooth to confirm that the root has been removed completely.

Multirooted Extraction. Multirooted teeth such as premolars and molars are more difficult to extract than incisors. Often only one root is affected and the other root(s) are firmly attached to the alveolar bone. Furthermore, most roots are embedded in the alveolar bone at divergent angles, making removal of the intact tooth difficult.

KEY POINT ▶ Sectioning of a multirooted tooth into two or three sections converts the procedure into multiple simple extractions. A high-speed handpiece or a low-speed electric handpiece with adequate irrigation can be used for sectioning teeth.

Technique

1. Locate the furcation with a dental elevator.
2. Place a tapered fissure bur (#701 in small animals and #702 in larger animals) at the furcation and direct it through the crown (Fig. 5A).
3. Advance the elevator apically between two roots.

TABLE 4. Dental Equipment

Equipment	Applications
Portable electric dental drill with low-speed handpiece and prophy angle (VC-30; Schein)	Sectioning teeth, removal of alveolar bone, polishing teeth
Mobile delivery system with high-speed handpiece, low-speed handpiece, water and air syringe (Vet-Base; Schein)	Sectioning teeth, removal of alveolar bone, polishing teeth, cavity and crown preparations
Ultrasonic scaler (Micro-son; Butler)	Permits rapid, easy removal of dental calculus
Dental radiography unit (MinXray; Butler)	Permits rapid, easy exposure of dental radiographs

4. Rotate the elevator 90° and hold for 15 seconds to gently force the roots apart (Fig. 5B).
5. Advance the elevator further apically, rotate it 90°, and hold for 15 seconds.
6. Place a dental extraction forceps on each crown segment and rotate to extract each root independently (Fig. 5C).

Complicated Surgical Extraction. This procedure involves the removal of teeth with large roots, such as the canine teeth in dogs, or large multirooted teeth, such as the mandibular first molars.

Technique

1. Reflect a mucoperiosteal flap to expose buccal alveolar bone overlying the root (Fig. 6A).
2. Remove the buccal alveolar bone overlying the root with a large round bur (Fig. 6B).
3. If the tooth is multirooted, section it with a #702 bur.
4. Elevate and extract the tooth.
5. Perform an alveoloplasty to remove the rough edges of the alveolus, using a large, round bur.

TABLE 5. Dental Instrumentation

Instrumentation*	Applications
Oral Surgery	
Dental elevator (ST8/ST9)	Tears periodontal ligament during extraction
Extraction forceps (ST5/ST6)	Completes breakdown of periodontal ligament and removal of tooth from alveolus during extraction
Root tip pick (ST11)	Removal of small-breed deciduous teeth or broken root tips
Bone curette (ST10)	Debridement of alveolus following extraction
Periosteal elevator (ST7)	Elevation of mucoperiosteum during oronasal fistula repair and palatal surgery
Periodontic	
Periodontal probe/explorer (ST4)	Measurement of depth of periodontal pocket (probe); detection of pulpal exposures and carious lesions (explorer)
Hand scalers (ST2)	Subgingival scaling
Curette (Columbia #13/14)	Removal of accretions on the root surface and of granulation tissue from the pocket wall
Prophylaxis paste (Zircon F)	Polishing teeth following scaling
Endodontic	
Endodontic files (Hedstrom/K-Files)	Debridement of necrotic pulpal tissue from canal
Lentulo spiral filler	Placement of zinc oxide and eugenol in canal
10:1 Reduction gear (Contra Angle)	Attachment of lentulo spiral filler to low-speed handpiece
Root canal plugger	Compression of gutta percha into the apex

*Available from H. Schein, Port Washington, N.Y.

TABLE 6. Dental Materials

Material	Applications
Amalgam (Strat-O-Caps, Schein; Contour, Kerr)	Restorations following endodontic therapy or cavity preparation
Composite resins (Concise, 3M; Adaptic, Johnson & Johnson)	Esthetic restorations following endodontic therapy or cavity preparation
Glass ionomers (Ketac-Bond, Espe-Premier)	Restoration of feline external root resorptive lesions
Eugenol–zinc oxide pastes (Schein)	Endodontic filling
Calcium hydroxide paste (Dycal, Caulk)	Stimulates closure of an apex and reparative dentin formation following pulpotomies
Gutta percha	Fills the pulp canal following debridement during root canal therapy
Zinc phosphate cement	Used as base following the placement of endodontic filling material and prior to placement of final restorative material

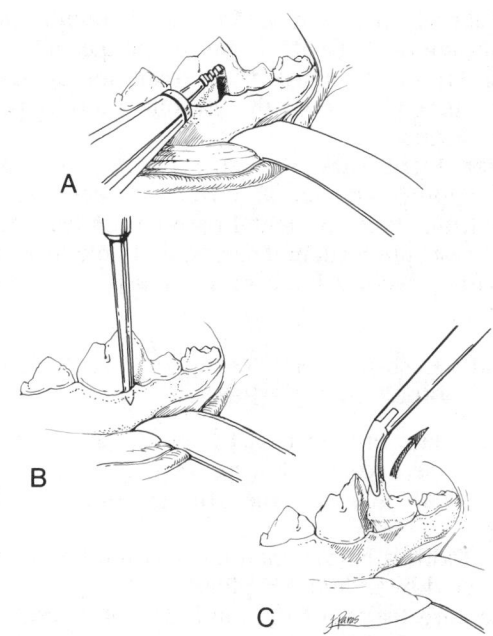

Figure 5. *A,* Tooth is sectioned with a tapered fissure bur. *B,* Elevator is rotated 90°. *C,* Extraction forceps is used to extract each root separately.

6. Curettage and flush the alveolus.
7. Replace and suture the mucoperiosteal flap to the adjacent gingiva with 2–0 chromic catgut suture in a simple interrupted pattern (Fig. 6*C*).

Postoperative Care and Complications

- Offer a soft diet for 3–10 days, depending on the number and complexity of dental extractions.
- Administer antibiotics (e.g., amoxicillin, 10–20 mg/kg q12h, PO) for 3–7 days when infection is present.

Hemorrhage. Hemorrhage is a common complica-

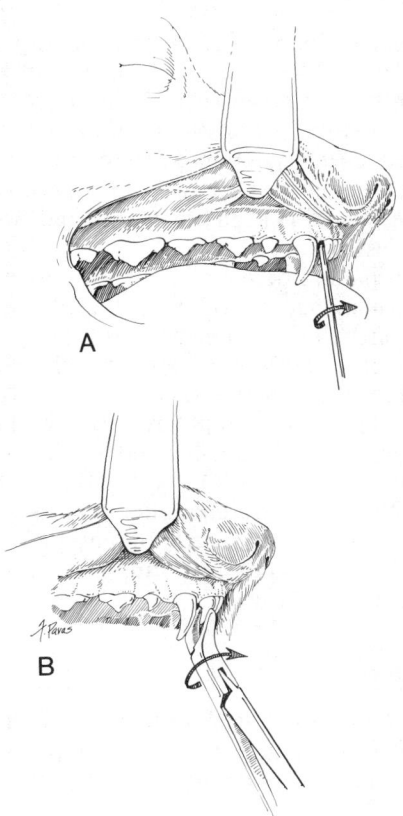

Figure 4. *A,* Dental elevator in gingival sulcus is rotated 90°. *B,* Tooth is rotated with extraction forceps.

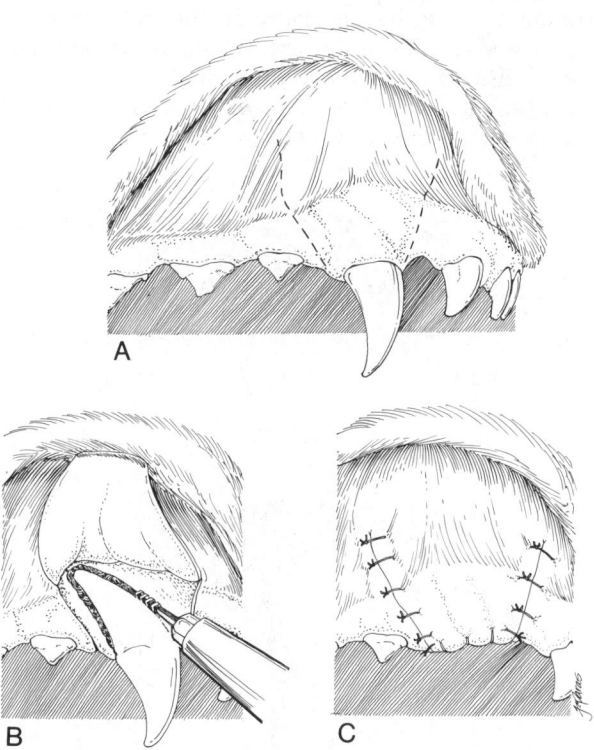

Figure 6. *A,* Proposed mucoperiosteal flap incision site for extraction of a maxillary canine tooth. *B,* Buccal alveolar bone is removed. *C,* Mucoperiosteal flap is replaced and sutured.

tion of dental extractions and usually is minor and can be easily controlled with a gauze sponge and digital pressure. Control persistent alveolar hemorrhage by suturing the gingiva over the alveolus thereby permitting clot formation.

Broken Root Tips. Broken root tips are common when inappropriate dental extraction techniques are used. Various types of dental pathology such as external root resorption, dental caries, and ankylosis of the root to the alveolar bone may predispose to broken root tips.

KEY POINT ▶ Always remove any tooth roots that break during extraction.

■ Differentiate broken root tips from surrounding alveolar bone by the following features:
  • The tooth is whiter than the surrounding yellow bone.
  • The tooth is harder than the surrounding bone, as detected by a dental explorer.
  • The hard tissues of the tooth do not bleed.
■ Remove root tips with a root tip pick or obliterate with an appropriate-size round bur (Fig. 7).

KEY POINT ▶ Permanent teeth may be damaged during the extraction of deciduous teeth.

Damage to Permanent Teeth. Careful extraction of deciduous teeth can help minimize this complication. However, extraction of deciduous teeth prior to complete formation of the permanent crowns (especially at 8–12 weeks of age) can result in enamel hypocalcification, enamel hypoplasia, crown deformity, and eruption failure.

Misplaced Tooth or Root Tip. A tooth or root tip infrequently may be misplaced in the nasal cavity or maxillary sinus during an extraction. Advanced periodontal disease in combination with aggressive extraction techniques can force a tooth or root tip into the nasal cavity or maxillary sinus.

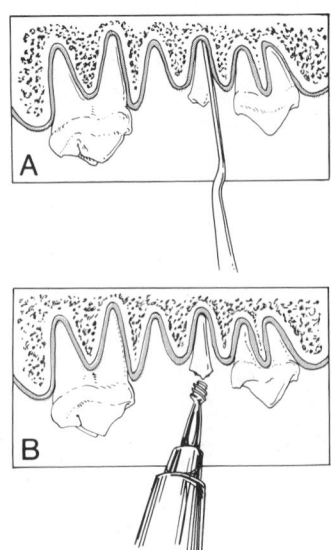

Figure 7. *A,* Elevation of root tip with root tip pick. *B,* Obliteration of root tip with round bur.

■ Enlarge the defect in the floor of the extraction site to remove a misplaced tooth or root tip.

Iatrogenic Fractures. Severe periodontal disease, inappropriate extraction techniques, and metabolic bone disease in geriatric animals may be predisposing factors in iatrogenic mandibular fractures.

■ Careful elevation of the tooth, digital support of the mandible during extraction, and a rotational movement with the dental extractor can help prevent iatrogenic mandibular fractures.

Osteomyelitis and Bony Sequestra. Osteomyelitis following extraction of teeth may be caused by retained tooth roots, exposed alveolar bone, and osseous necrosis. A bone sequestrum may develop when a segment of alveolar bone is fractured off during a dental extraction and left in the extraction site.

■ Treat osteomyelitis and bony sequestra by removing retained tooth roots and bony sequestra and by curettage of necrotic bone to the level of healthy, bleeding bone.

Oronasal Fistulas and Palatal Defects

Oronasal fistulas are abnormal communications between the oral and nasal cavity. Palatal defects may occur anywhere in the palate and result in a communication between the oral and nasal cavity or the oral cavity and the maxillary sinus.

Etiology

Palatal defects may be congenital or acquired. Congenital palatal defects occur primarily in brachiocephalic breeds, miniature schnauzers, cocker spaniels, beagles, and cats. Congenital abnormalities of the primary palate (incisive bone) are referred to as a hare lip. These defects may occur concomitantly or independent of secondary palate (hard and soft palate) abnormalities.

Acquired palatal defects are most frequently caused by a deep maxillary periodontal pocket that has progressed to the apex of the tooth, resulting in lysis of the thin layer of bone that separates the apex of the maxillary tooth and the nasal cavity or maxillary sinus. Acquired palatal defects that have etiologies other than dental disease usually are located in the hard palate and may be caused by various types of trauma including dog bites, blunt head trauma, electrical shock, gunshot wounds, foreign body penetration and pressure necrosis. They also may occur as a complication of maxillectomy for oral neoplasia.

Clinical Signs

■ Clinical signs associated with oronasal fistulas and palatal defects include unilateral or bilateral mucopurulent and occasionally hemorrhagic nasal discharge.
■ Animals often are presented because of recurrent episodes of sneezing, especially after eating.

Diagnosis

- Defects located in the hard palate usually are confirmed by an oral examination.
- Perform thorough periodontal examination to identify oronasal and oroantral fistulas secondary to periodontal disease. This requires tranquilization or general anesthesia.
  - Insert a probe into the suspected periodontal pocket, which often is located on the palatal aspect of the maxillary canine tooth but may be located anywhere along the periodontal ligament of the maxillary cheek teeth.
  - If the probe penetrates easily into the nasal cavity or maxillary sinus, when the nose is tipped ventrally, immediate ipsilateral nasal hemorrhage confirms the presence of an oronasal or oroantral fistula.

Surgical Anatomy

KEY POINT ▶ Oronasal fistulas are associated most frequently with defects in the area of the maxillary canine tooth.

The surgical anatomy varies with the location of the defect. The mucoperiosteal flap used in the repair of oronasal fistulas extends from the margins of the defect across the mucogingival line (the anatomic landmark separating the attached gingiva from the unattached gingiva). Surgical techniques used to repair defects in the hard palate often require preservation of the palatine arteries, which arise approximately 1 cm palatal to the maxillary 4th premolar and course nostrally along the hard palate (Fig. 8).

Preoperative Considerations

KEY POINT ▶ Tube- or bottle-feed animals with congenital hard palatal defects until they are 3 months of age to decrease the incidence of inhalation pneumonia.

- Perform surgery when the animal is 3 months of age following thoracic radiography to check for pneumonia.

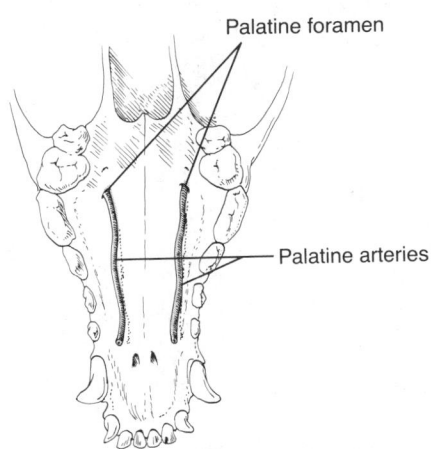

Figure 8. Palatine arteries.

- Give animals with severe, purulent rhinitis or pneumonia antibiotics prior to surgery.

Surgical Procedure

Two techniques used frequently for the repair of oronasal fistulas include the single-layer and the double-layer mucoperiosteal flap. The overlapping flap technique is used frequently for the repair of hard palatal defects.

Single-Layer Mucoperiosteal Flap

Technique

1. Place the animal in lateral recumbency.
2. Debride the epithelial margin of the fistula with a #15 scalpel blade.
3. Make two divergent incisions in the mucosa, beginning at the mesial and distal aspects of the fistula and extending across the mucogingival line (Fig. 9A).
4. Using a periosteal elevator, gently raise the flap (Fig. 9B).
5. Reflect the flap apically and incise the deepest layer of the flap (the periosteal layer) the entire width of the flap at its most dorsal aspect (Fig. 9C).
6. If necessary, remove excess buccal bony plate with a rongeur or dental bur to permit tensionless apposition of tissues (Fig. 9D).
7. Prior to closure, remove all infected bone and soft tissue, and irrigate the surgical site with sterile saline.
8. Suture the flap to the palatal and gingival mucosa with 2–0 or 3–0 chromic catgut suture or PDS (polydioxanone; Ethicon) in a simple interrupted pattern (Fig. 9E).

Double-Layer Mucoperiosteal Flap. Use to repair large chronic or recurrent oronasal fistulas.

Technique

1. Debride the mesial, distal, and buccal epithelial margins of the fistula with a #15 blade. The palatal epithelial margin does not need to be debrided.
2. Elevate an elliptical palatal mucoperiosteal flap with a periosteal elevator, preserving the lateral attachment of the base of the flap (Fig. 10A).
3. Fold over and suture the flap to the edges of the defect with 2–0 or 3–0 chromic catgut suture or PDS in a simple interrupted pattern (Fig. 10B).
4. Elevate a buccal mucoperiosteal flap dorsal to the oronasal fistula (see Figs. 9A–C).
5. Advance the buccal mucoperiosteal flap palatally to cover the inverted flap and the denuded palatine bone (Fig. 10C).
6. Suture the flap to the palatal and gingival mucosa with 2–0 or 3–0 chromic catgut suture or PDS in a simple interrupted pattern (Fig. 10D).

Overlapping Flap Technique. Use for repair of hard palatal defects, especially on the midline.

Technique

1. Make an incision the length of the palatal defect in the palatal mucosa just palatal to the maxillary

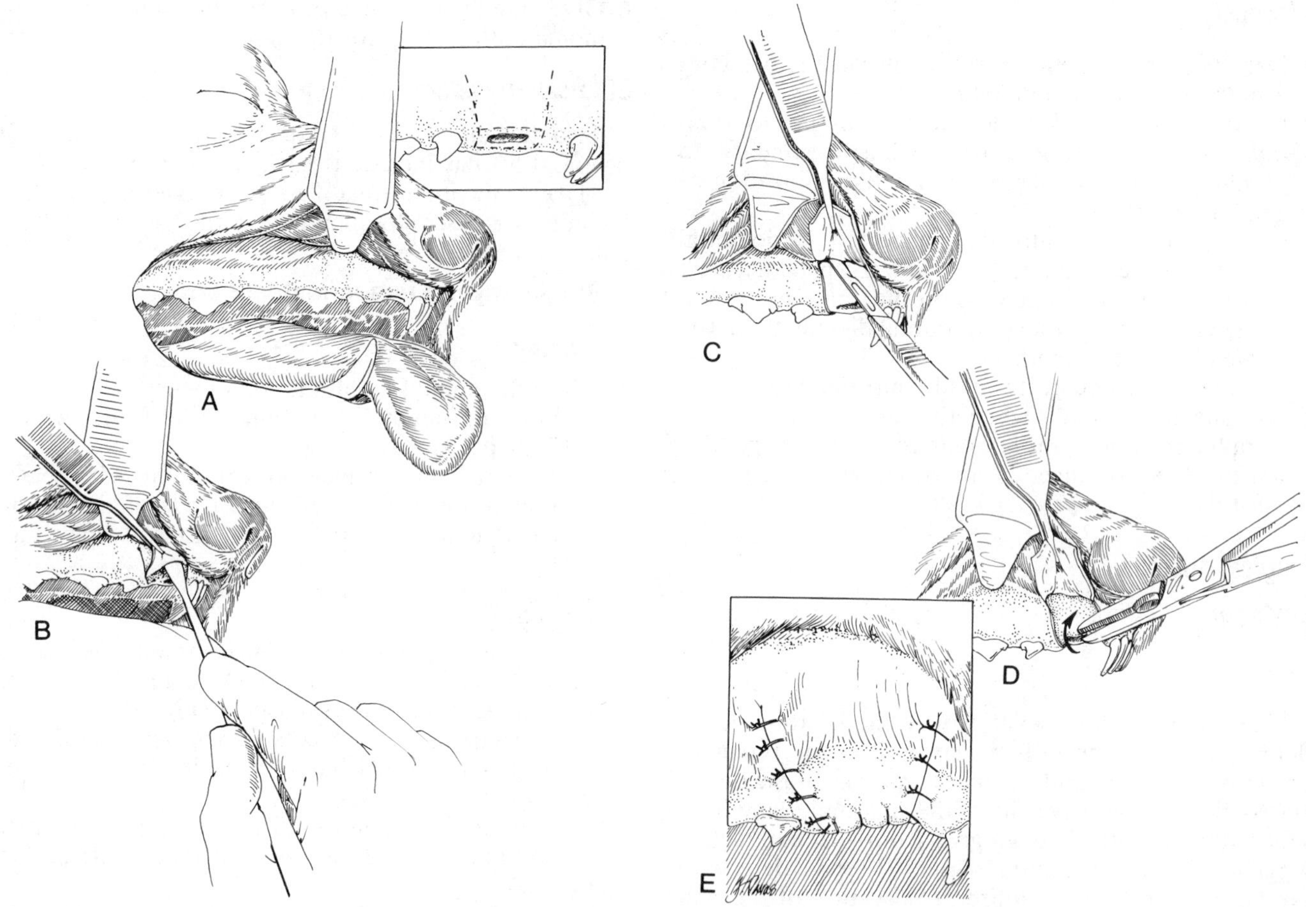

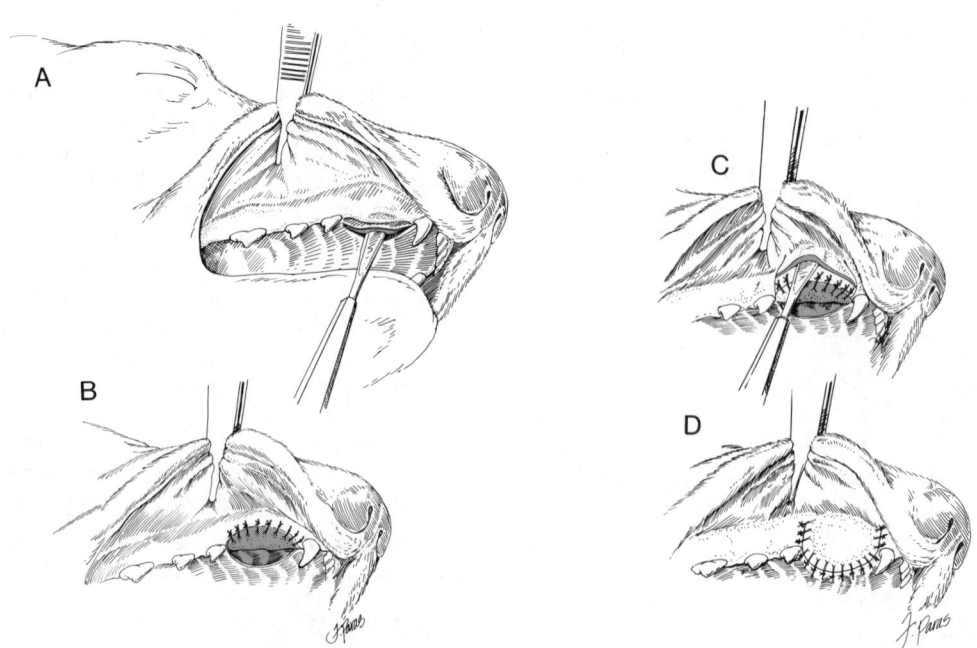

Figure 9. *A,* Proposed incision sites in mucosa for oronasal fistula repair. *B,* Elevation of mucoperiosteal flap. *C,* Incision of periosteal layer flap. *D,* Removal of rough edges of buccal alveolar bone with rongeurs. *E,* Mucoperiosteal flap is replaced and sutured.

Figure 10. *A,* Periosteal elevation of palatal flap. *B,* Palatal flap is sutured to debrided edges of defect. *C,* Buccal mucoperiosteal flap elevated and advanced palatally. *D,* Flap sutured to palatal and gingival mucosa.

dental arcade. The rostral and caudal aspects of these incisions are connected to the rostral and caudal aspects of the palatal defect (Fig. 11*A*).

2. Incise the opposite side of the palatal defect along the entire length of the defect and gently elevate with a periosteal elevator to create a recipient site for the mucoperiosteal flap. Carefully elevate the mucoperiosteal flap with a periosteal elevator, preserving the palatine artery that arises approximately 1 cm palatal to the upper 4th premolar (Fig. 11*B*).

3. Hinge the mucoperiosteal flap at the end of the palatal defect and place beneath the mucosa on the other side of the defect.

4. Preplace 3–0 polyglactin 910 sutures in an interrupted horizontal mattress pattern through the recipient site and the flap.

5. Tie the sutures from caudal to rostral to complete the procedure (Fig. 11*C*).

Postoperative Care and Complications

■ Feed a soft diet (gruel or liquid) for 2–3 weeks. For animals requiring complicated repair, consider using pharyngostomy or gastrotomy tube feeding (see sec. 1, ch. 3). Place Elizabethan collars on patients that paw at the oral cavity.

■ In 3 weeks, reexamine the patient to assess the integrity of the repair.
  • If the repair is intact, gradually return to a normal diet over the next 1–2 weeks.
  • If the repair was unsuccessful, schedule a second operation in approximately 4 weeks.

PERIODONTAL DISEASE

KEY POINT ▶ Periodontal disease is the most common cause of oral infection and tooth loss in dogs.

Periodontal disease occurs in two forms: gingivitis and periodontitis. Gingivitis is a reversible inflammation of the gingiva. Periodontitis involves deeper inflammation with loss of tooth support and permanent damage.

The purpose of periodontal therapy is to prevent gingivitis from progressing to periodontitis and to delay the progression of periodontitis once it is established.

Etiology

■ Periodontal disease is initiated by an accumulation of large amounts of bacteria at the junction of the tooth and the gingiva. Prolonged retention of these bacteria results in a change of the predominant flora from gram-positive aerobic coccoid bacteria to more motile gram-negative anaerobic rod-shaped bacteria.
  • *Bacteroides asaccharolyticus, Fusobacterium nucleatum, Actinomyces viscosus,* and *A. odontolyticus* are important pathogens in causing periodontal disease in dogs.

■ Tissue destruction occurs secondary to inflammation, resulting in a loss of periodontal support. Over a period of time (usually years), the presence of plaque, calculus, and gingivitis results in loss of periodontal support.

Clinical Signs

■ Common signs include mobile teeth, periodontal and periapical abscesses, facial swelling, gingival pockets, nasal discharge, and oronasal and oroantral fistulas.

■ Severe gingival sulcus hemorrhage, pathologic mandibular fractures, intranasal tooth migration, and osteomyelitis with or without bone sequestra develop uncommonly.

Diagnosis

The diagnosis of periodontal disease is based on a thorough oral and periodontal examination and dental radiography.

Gingivitis

■ Animals with gingivitis have swollen gingival margins that bleed after the application of light pressure. Serous or purulent exudate may be produced from the gingival sulcus. Halitosis commonly is present.

■ Examination with a periodontal probe is normal and

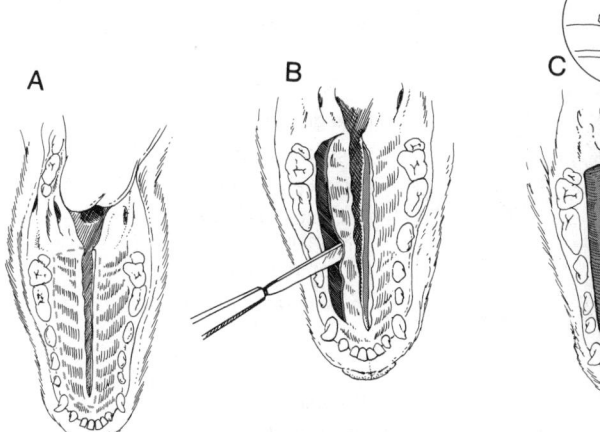

Figure 11. *A,* Palatal incisions to create flaps for overlapping flap technique. *B,* Periosteal elevation of flap. *C,* The larger flap is placed beneath the smaller flap and the flaps are sutured together.

there is no radiographic evidence of bone loss around the teeth.

Periodontitis

- Hyperplasia and gingival recession are seen, as well as severe gingival inflammation with various amounts of calculus and debris.
- Periodontal probing will reveal the presence of periodontal pockets that can progress to tooth loss if untreated.
- Dental radiographs can identify bone loss, which most frequently is horizontal or parallel to the cemento-enamel (CE) junction, separating the crown from the root. Less frequently the bone loss is vertical or parallel to the long axis of the root.

Surgical Anatomy

The periodontal tissues are composed of the gingiva, cementum, periodontal ligament, and alveolar bone. An accurate estimate of the amount of support that has been lost around a tooth depends on the appropriate use of a periodontal probe and the recognition of a few anatomic landmarks.

- Locate the cemento-enamel junction that separates the anatomic crown from the anatomic root, 1–2 mm below the normal gingival margin (Fig. 12).
- The free gingival margin, an important anatomic landmark when assessing periodontal disease, is the highest point of gingival tissue that lies on the tooth. In normal tissues, the free gingival margin is just above the CE junction (see Fig. 12).
  - When gingival recession is present, the free gingival margin is below the CE junction.
  - In cases of gingival hyperplasia, it is >2 mm above the CE junction.
- Measure and record the depth of the pocket in millimeters. Also note the relationship of the free gingival margin to the CE junction. These values will adequately assess the level of attachment and thereby dictate the appropriate therapy.

Preoperative Considerations

- Prior to treatment, a thorough physical examination and clinical laboratory testing are recommended to rule out the presence of concurrent disease.
- In severe cases, administer antibiotics (amoxicillin) prior to the dental procedure so that adequate blood levels are present during dentistry.

Surgical Procedures

Several procedures are used in the treatment of periodontal disease. These include scaling, root planing, polishing, gingivectomy, and open-flap curettage.

Dental Scaling

Dental scaling can be divided into two main categories; supragingival and subgingival.

Supragingival Scaling. This involves the removal of calculus located above the gingival margin. It is most easily performed with an ultrasonic scaler.

Technique

1. A universal tip is most appropriate for use in small animals.
2. Place the side of the tip below the edge of the calculus and gently lift to remove calculus.
3. Move the tip gently across the surface of the tooth with a paint brush–type movement.
4. Continuously move the tip across the dentition during scaling; never hold it on one tooth continuously for more than 10–15 seconds.
5. Spray copiously with water to prevent overheating of the tooth and to wash away dislodged calculus.

Subgingival Scaling. Following supragingival scaling, perform subgingival scaling, root planing, and curettage with an ultrasonic scaler and hand scaler.

Technique

1. Use an ultrasonic scaler with a universal tip subgingivally with a light touch, copious water spraying, and constant motion to remove the major portion of subgingival calculus.
2. With a hand instrument such as the Columbia 13/14 curette, complete the root cleaning. Place the curette at the bottom of the pocket; engage the root with the edge of the curette and pull the curette coronally along the surface of the root (Fig. 13).

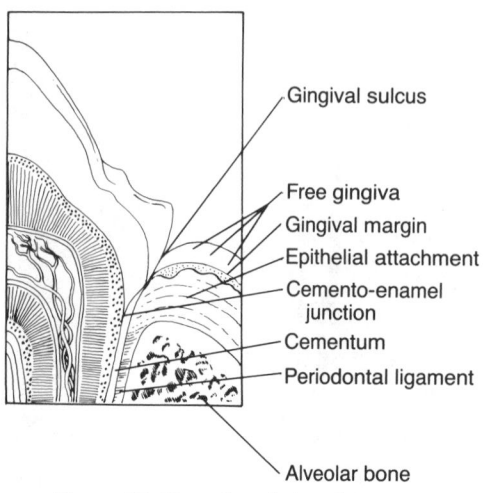

Figure 12. Normal periodontal anatomy.

Gingival sulcus

Free gingiva
Gingival margin
Epithelial attachment
Cemento-enamel junction
Cementum
Periodontal ligament

Alveolar bone

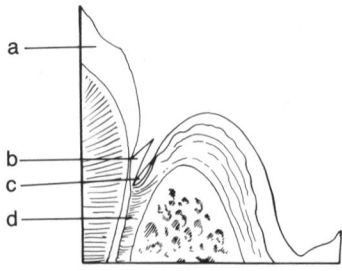

Figure 13. Cross-section of curette placed beneath calculus for subgingival scaling: (a) enamel, (b) calculus, (c) curette in cross-section, (d) gingiva.

3. Continue subgingival scaling and root planing (scaling of the root) until the root is smooth and clean.
4. Following removal of subgingival calculus, record areas of pathologic deepening (>3mm) on a dental chart.
5. Perform subgingival curettage by gently scraping the soft tissue lining of the pocket with a sharp curette until all epithelial and granulation tissue is removed.

Polishing Technique

1. Place a prophylaxis angle on a slow-speed handpiece. Fill the cup with medium-grit prophylaxis paste.
2. Rotate the cup over the entire exposed surface of the teeth, smoothing the surface of the enamel.
3. Rinse the teeth with forced air and water spray to remove any residual debris.

Gingivectomy

Gingivectomy is the resection of unsupported gingival tissue. This technique is used to eliminate periodontal pockets >5mm deep that are caused by horizontal bone loss. Gingivectomy is also used to remove hyperplastic gingival tissue.

KEY POINT ▶ Do not perform gingivectomy unless sufficient attached gingiva (>3mm) can be retained following the procedure, because removal of tissue below this point may result in dehiscence of the gingiva.

Technique

1. With a periodontal probe, mark the depth of the periodontal pocket on the gingiva opposite the affected tooth (Fig. 14A).
2. Make a beveled incision in the gingiva, slightly apical to the pocket mark, to create a natural gingival contour to the gingiva following the gingivectomy (Fig. 14B). The incision can be made with a gingivectomy knife, scalpel blade, or electrosurgery tip. If electrosurgery is used, surgical cutting modes are recommended.
3. Following the removal of excessive hyperplastic tissue and pocket elimination, scale and polish the exposed tooth surface.

Open-Flap Curettage

This technique is used to treat periodontal pockets that extend beneath the level of the alveolar crest. Open-flap curettage permits access to intrabony defects without loss of attached gingiva.

Technique

1. Make an incision with a #11 or #15 scalpel blade 1–2 mm from the tooth and directed toward the alveolar crest (Fig. 15A).
2. Make a scalloped incision on the buccal and lingual or palatal surfaces of the affected tooth, dipping interproximally (between the teeth) to preserve most of the gingival tissue.
3. Elevate the mucoperiosteal flaps 3–5 mm from the

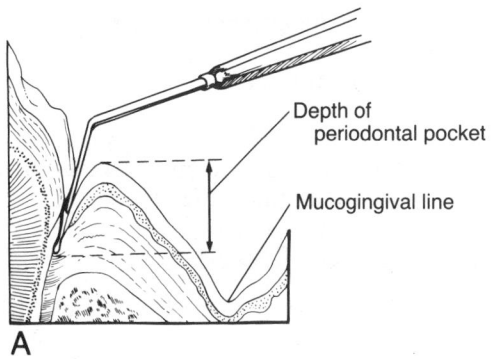

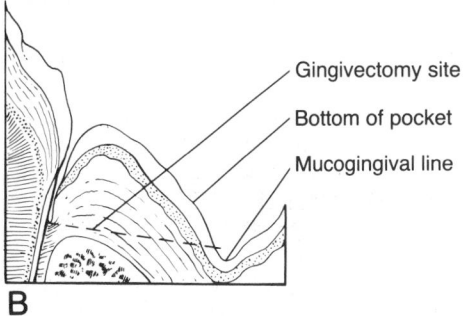

Figure 14. *A,* Periodontal probe measures pocket depth. *B,* Proposed gingivectomy site.

edge of the incision, using a sharp periosteal elevator (Fig. 15B).
4. Remove the collar of gingival tissue around the tooth with curettes.

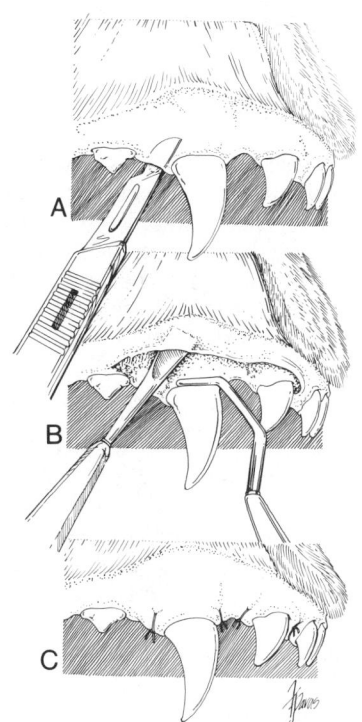

Figure 15. *A,* Open-flap curettage is initiated with an incision directed toward the alveolar crest. *B,* Mucoperiosteal flaps are elevated 3–5 mm to permit open curettage. *C,* The flaps are repositioned with 4–0 chromic sutures.

5. Perform scaling and root planing on the exposed tooth surface.
6. Polish the tooth and liberally irrigate the area with sterile saline.
7. Reposition the flaps and hold in place with 4–0 chromic catgut sutures in a simple interrupted pattern, placed interdentally (Fig. 15C).

Postoperative Care and Complications

- To retard the recurrence of plaque and calculus accumulation, instruct the owner to irrigate the animal's mouth with a 0.2% chlorhexidine (Nolvasan, Ft. Dodge) solution for 2 weeks. Additionally, recommend daily toothbrushing with warm water, C.E.J. toothpaste (VRx Products), or Nolvadent (Ft. Dodge).
- If significant stomatitis (discussed later in this chapter) or abscess secondary to periodontal disease occurs, give broad-spectrum antibiotics such as amoxicillin (10–20 mg/kg q12h, PO) and metronidazole (25 mg/kg q12h, PO) or Clavamox (14 mg/kg q12h, PO).
- Reevaluate the animal in 2 weeks. Annual or semiannual scaling is recommended.
- Complications are minimal when procedures are properly performed.

KEY POINT ▶ Prolonged application of an ultrasonic tip to a tooth without adequate water spraying can result in pulpal necrosis.

- Failure to remove subgingival calculus adequately can result in progressive periodontal disease.
- Inadequate irrigation of the gingival sulcus following therapy can result in entrapment of debris subgingivally and subsequent periodontal abscess.

ENDODONTIC DISEASE

Endodontic disease refers to disease of the pulp (the inner aspect of the tooth). It occurs frequently in small animals and may cause significant pain. Pulp cap, pulpotomy, apexogenesis, apexification, and nonsurgical and surgical endodontic therapy can result in the resolution of endodontic disease and retention of a functional, painless tooth.

Etiology

- The most common cause of endodontic disease in small animals is a fractured tooth with pulpal exposure.
- Less common causes include rapid dental attrition (tooth wear), deep external root resorptive lesions, deep caries, severe periodontal disease with secondary endodontic disease, and dental trauma with secondary pulpal hemorrhage or damage to the apical vessels.

Clinical Signs

Pulpal exposure can result in the progressive development of the following conditions:

- Bacterial pulpitis
- Pulp necrosis
- Apical granuloma
- Periapical abscess
- Acute alveolar periodontitis
- Osteomyelitis
- Sepsis

The time required for this progression varies from months to years. When a tooth is fractured and the pulp is exposed, the pulp will bleed.

KEY POINT ▶ Pulpal exposure is extremely painful, and animals with a fractured tooth with pulpal exposure hypersalivate, are reluctant to eat, and exhibit other abnormal behaviors.

Over a period of several months, the pulp becomes necrotic and the animal no longer has signs of pain until an inflammatory reaction occurs around the apex of the tooth, at which time the pain recurs.

Diagnosis

The diagnosis is based on a thorough oral examination and dental radiography.

Physical Examination

- Differentiate teeth suspected of being diseased secondary to fractures from worn teeth. Worn teeth, or dental attrition, rarely result in pulpal exposure.
  - A dental explorer will penetrate into the pulp canal when the pulp is exposed.
  - When dental attrition is the cause of a shortened crown, the explorer will not penetrate the tooth but will be stopped by the reparative dentin, or "brown spot," that fills in the area of receded pulp.
- Evaluate the color of the tooth. A discolored tooth (red, purple, or gray) may be diseased.
- Percussion of a tooth with endodontic disease may be painful because of the presence of periapical inflammation.
- Soft-tissue fistulas may occur secondary to endodontic disease. Usually they are located apical to the mucogingival line. When probed, they will be found to originate from the apex of an endodontically diseased tooth.
- Severe maxillary or mandibular swelling may be present with endodontic disease when the disease process has progressed to a periapical abscess or osteomyelitis.

Radiography

Perform dental radiography to delineate the endodontic system and confirm endodontic disease. Radiography reveals the stage of apical development.

- Chronic endodontically diseased teeth have an area of periapical lysis around one or more roots.
- When soft-tissue fistulas are present, radiopaque material such as a gutta percha point may be placed into the fistula prior to radiography to confirm that the fistula arises from the apex of the affected tooth.

Surgical Anatomy

Surgical anatomy varies with each tooth. The endodontic system is divided into two parts: the pulp chamber and the pulp canal.

■ The endodontic system generally follows the external anatomic contours of the tooth, including its root structure.
■ The size of the endodontic system also varies with the age of the patient. Young animals have immature teeth with open apices. As the tooth develops, the apex is formed and, as the tooth matures, the dentinal layer thickens, resulting in a thinner endodontic system.

Preoperative Considerations

■ Examine the teeth for concurrent periodontal disease with a periodontal probe.

KEY POINT ▶ Teeth with combined periodontal and endodontic lesions have a poorer prognosis than teeth with only endodontic lesions.

Surgical Procedures

Numerous endodontic procedures are available (Table 7). The type selected depends on the status of the endodontic system and the following factors:

■ Vital pulp versus nonvital pulp
■ Mature versus immature tooth
■ Closed versus opened apex
■ Exposure time

Pulp Cap

This procedure is used when the pulp of a vital tooth is inadvertently exposed during a dental procedure.

Technique

1. Flush exposed pulp with sterile saline.
2. Control pulpal hemorrhage with a cotton pellet or paper point.

TABLE 7. Endodontic Procedures Recommended for Common Endodontic Problems

Procedure	Problem
Pulp cap	Vital tooth with iatrogenic pulpal exposure
Pulpotomy and apexogenesis	Vital immature tooth with open apex and traumatic pulpal exposure <5 days
Apexification	Immature nonvital tooth with open apex
Nonsurgical root canal	Nonvital mature tooth with closed apex
Vital mature tooth with prolonged pulpal exposure
Surgical root canal	Nonvital mature tooth with apical lysis
Immature nonvital tooth with open apex

3. Apply calcium hydroxide powder (Schein) to the exposed pulp with a sterile amalgam carrier.
4. Apply a layer of hard-setting calcium hydroxide paste (Schein). In larger teeth, apply a cement base (Schein).
5. Apply a restoration material such as composite or amalgam.

Pulpotomy

This is similar to a pulp capping procedure, except that the coronal portion of the pulp is removed. Removal of this pulp is indicated in immature vital teeth that have extended pulpal exposure of up to 5 days, which results in coronal pulp contamination.

Technique

1. Remove the contaminated pulp with a sterile #2 or #3 round bur.
2. Place a sterile, moist cotton pellet over the pulp for 3–5 minutes to control hemorrhage.
3. Persistent hemorrhage for >5 minutes may indicate an irreversibly affected pulp. Perform a more apical amputation to reach healthier tissue.
4. Apply calcium hydroxide powder to the pulp with a sterile amalgam carrier, and condense lightly with a sterile amalgam plugger to a thickness of 2–4 mm.
5. Apply a layer of firm-setting zinc-oxide eugenol.
6. Place a permanent restorative material.

Apexogenesis

This endodontic procedure allows the root to continue to grow. Apexogenesis is useful in cases in which apical development and closure are not complete and the pulp is not irreversibly compromised. Maintenance of vitality of an immature tooth is desirable so that the tooth will continue to develop, resulting in a thicker dentinal layer and a formed apex.

Technique

Remove the involved or injured portion of the pulp as described for pulpotomy.

Apexification

This procedure is used in the treatment of immature teeth in which there is an absence of vital tissue. Teeth in which early pulp death has occurred have large open apices, making root canal filling by nonsurgical techniques difficult. Apexification permits closure of the apex by cementum formation, which is stimulated by the application of calcium hydroxide.

Technique

1. Remove the necrotic contents of the immature root canal just short of the radiographic apex. *Note:* During debridement, do not disrupt the root-forming tissues beyond the apex.
2. Irrigate the canal with 2.5% sodium hypochlorite.
3. Carefully dry the canal with premeasured paper points to prevent penetration into the apical tissue, which can result in additional hemorrhage.
4. Mix calcium hydroxide powder and sterile saline to a thick consistency and place in the root canal with a sterile amalgam carrier, and condense with a sterile amalgam plugger.

5. Place a layer of quick-setting calcium hydroxide paste.
6. Restore the access hole with composite or amalgam.
7. Replace the calcium hydroxide every 3–6 months until apexification is complete.
8. Following formation of the apex, perform nonsurgical root canal procedure.

Nonsurgical (Conventional) Root Canal

This procedure is used to treat nonvital mature teeth with closed apices and vital mature teeth with pulpal exposure of >8 hours.

KEY POINT ▶ Nonsurgical root canal therapy is preferable to surgical treatment in most cases of endodontic disease because of its relative ease and speed of completion, noninvasive nature, and relative decreased cost.

Technique

1. Using an appropriate size round bur, obtain access to the pulp at a point that will permit straight delivery of the files to the apex of the tooth (Fig. 16).
2. Begin debridement of the canal with a #15 file inserted to the apex of the tooth. Use a rubber stop to mark the length of the file, and insert all subsequent files to that depth.
3. Introduce progressively larger files into the canal. Flush the canal with 2.5% sodium hypochlorite solution before changing files.
4. Debridement is complete when white dentinal shavings are present on the file and there is no further bleeding from the canal.
5. Dry the canal with paper points.
6. Transfer a mixture of zinc oxide and eugenol to the root canal with a slowly rotating spiral paste filler.
7. Cut a gutta percha point the same size as the largest file that reaches the apex to the appropriate length, and use a plugger to compress the gutta percha to the apex.
8. Remove any excess zinc oxide and eugenol from the access site.
9. Place an intermediate cement layer.
10. The access site is undercut with an inverted cone bur.
11. Apply restorative material (silver amalgam or composite) to the access site to complete the procedure.

Surgical Nonconventional Endodontic Therapy

This is the treatment of endodontic problems with an approach through oral soft tissue and bone rather than through the crown of the tooth. (In a nonsurgical root canal procedure, the pulp canal is accessed by the crown only.)

Indications for surgical endodontic therapy include:

- Apical root resorption
- Incomplete root development
- Complications during conventional root canal therapy (broken files)
- Recurrent apical abscessation following nonsurgical root canal therapy (recurrent swelling over the apex of the tooth root or periapical draining fistulous tracts)
- Size, length, or curvature of the canal that makes instrumentation impossible

Technique

1. Perform a conventional root canal procedure prior to surgical endodontic therapy.
2. An apical approach for most teeth is through a mucoperiosteal incision just apical to the mucogingival line. However, access to the apex of the mandibular canine is most easily gained through a cutaneous incision overlying the ventral border of the mandible.
3. Access to the apex is achieved by removing the buccal alveolar bone overlying the apex with a #4 or #6 round bur.
4. Perform apical curettage to remove necrotic and fibrotic granulation tissue surrounding the periapical region.
5. Perform an apicoectomy (amputation of the apex of the tooth) using a #701 bur. The exposed face of the cut root tip is beveled at a 45° angle to increase exposure of the canal access site.
6. Flush the periapical region with sterile saline solution.
7. Pack the periapical region with #0 cotton pellets or a hemostatic agent to control hemorrhage.
8. Create an undercut in the root canal of the apex with an inverted #33 cone bur.
9. Place a 2–4 mm layer of zinc-free amalgam in the apical end of the canal, using a retrograde amalgam carrier, and condense the amalgam with a small amalgam plugger.
10. Prior to closure, remove all cotton pellets and flush the periapical region with sterile saline solution.
11. Reposition the mucoperiosteal flap and suture with 3–0 chromic catgut in a simple interrupted pattern. Procedures involving the mandibular canine teeth are closed with nonabsorbable suture material in the skin.

Postoperative Care and Complications

- Immediately following endodontic therapy, take a radiograph to document and assess the procedure.

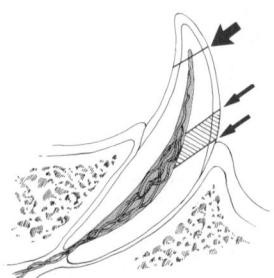

Figure 16. *Large arrow,* fracture site; *small arrows,* straight access site to apex.

- Administer a broad-spectrum antibiotic, such as amoxicillin (10–20 mg/kg q12h, PO), for 1 week.
- Reexamine and radiograph the treated tooth 6 months postoperatively, and then annually, to evaluate the success of the endodontic therapy.

Intraoperative Complications

Intraoperative complications usually are associated with improper use of instrumentation or inappropriate technique. Examples are:

- Broken endodontic files lodged in the root canal
- Perforation of the root canal or pulpal floor

Postoperative Complications

Postoperative complications usually are associated with improper technique, inadequate apical seal, or inadequate follow-up.

- Vital endodontic procedures such as pulp cap, pulpotomy and apexogenesis require oral and radiographic reevaluations 3–6 months postoperatively and then annually. If there are persistent signs such as periapical swelling, periapical fistulas, painful tooth percussion, and progressive radiographic periapical lysis in teeth previously treated with vital endodontic techniques, schedule retreatment with nonvital techniques.
- Nonvital techniques include apexification and non-surgical and surgical root canal therapy.
  - Perform surgical root canal therapy on teeth unsuccessfully treated with apexification and nonsurgical root canal techniques.
  - Where there is persistent endodontic pathology following surgical root canal therapy, retreatment or extraction is recommended.

ORTHODONTIC DISEASE

Orthodontic disease refers to malocclusions. Veterinary orthodontics involves the movement and repositioning of teeth to a more normal position.

KEY POINT ▶ Veterinary orthodontic therapy is indicated to alleviate traumatic malocclusions that result in pain or in inability to function or eat; it should not be used to correct cosmetic or genetic dental alignment defects.

Etiology

The majority of malocclusions are genetic in origin. Previous trauma or an eruption pattern discrepancy resulting from retained deciduous teeth may also result in a malocclusion of the permanent dentition.

Clinical Signs

Clinical signs depend on the severity of the malocclusion.

- Animals with pronounced prognathic occlusion (mandibular teeth are rostral to their normal position in relation to the maxillary dentition) may be presented because of difficulty in prehending food. This condition is not severe enough to cause nutritional problems.
- Animals with brachygnathic occlusion (maxillary teeth are rostral to their normal position in relation to the mandibular dentition), may be presented because of drooling, but this is usually not severe.
- The majority of dental malocclusions are cosmetic and cause no clinically significant problems. However, animals with lingually displaced mandibular canines may have painful palatal defects caused by traumatic occlusion.
- A dental malocclusion in which one tooth traumatically occludes against another tooth can result in dental attrition of the affected teeth.

Diagnosis

The diagnosis is based on a thorough oral examination. Assess the following factors:

- *Incisor relationship:* The maxillary incisors should overlap the facial surface of the mandibular incisors.
- *Canine tooth relationship:* The lower canines should be centered between and not touching either the upper canine or the upper lateral incisor.
- *Lower fourth premolar:* The large cusp of the lower fourth premolar should be centered between the upper third and fourth premolar.
- *Interdigitation of other premolars:* The cusp tips of the upper premolars should interdigitate with the cusp tips of the lower premolars.
- *Premolar horizontal alignment:* The space between the upper and lower premolars should have good horizontal alignment.
- *Head symmetry:* The midlines of the maxillary and mandibular dental arches are centered over each other, and these must also be in alignment with the midplane of the head.

Deviations from these criteria for normal occlusion results in malocclusions of varying severities.

Surgical Anatomy and Orthodontic Principles

Tipping is the most common type of corrective movement used in veterinary orthodontics. A single force is applied to the crown of a tooth, resulting in a tipping action. During orthodontic movement, alveolar bone is *resorbed* (osteoclastic activity) on the side of the tooth with less tension on the periodontal ligament. Conversely, alveolar bone is *deposited* (osteoblastic activity) on the side of the tooth with more tension on the periodontal ligament.

Preoperative Considerations

Prior to correction of orthodontic defects, attempt to determine the etiology of the problem. Correction of genetically induced, cosmetic orthodontic defects is contraindicated. Attempt to correct orthodontic defects resulting in a traumatic occlusion. The timing of orthodontic movement is important.

KEY POINT ▶ Delay orthodontic movement until the animal is 1–2 years of age unless simple, quick interceptive movements of the tooth can be achieved.

Surgical Procedures

KEY POINT ▶ Extraction of overly retained deciduous teeth can prevent malocclusions of the permanent dentition.

Extraction of retained deciduous teeth is referred to as *interceptive orthodontics*. Extract a deciduous tooth that is still firmly attached when the permanent tooth starts to erupt to allow the permanent tooth to erupt in its normal position. Perform extraction carefully to avoid disruption of the permanent tooth.

Correction of Lingually Displaced Mandibular Canines. A technique that can be easily applied in one visit is the intraorally fabricated acrylic inclined plane.

Technique

1. Clean and polish the teeth.
2. Create a retaining wall around the proposed site of the inclined plane with modeling clay.
3. Fabricate an acrylic splint in layers by the addition of the powder and liquid components of the acrylic material until the splint is approximately 1-cm thick.
4. When the splint is hard, remove the retaining wall and create the appropriate inclined plane with an acrylic bur, so that when the lingually displaced mandibular canine hits the side of the acrylic splint it will be deflected labially into a normal position.
5. Add additional acrylic to create a band around the canine teeth to provide retention for the splint.

Postoperative Care and Complications

- Instruct the client to:
  - Restrict the animal's chewing activities and to feed a soft diet.
  - Observe the orthodontic device daily, making sure that it is not displaced or causing excessive soft tissue trauma.
  - Gently clean the acrylic splints daily with a stream of water from a water pick or a syringe with a catheter attached.
- Leave the orthodontic appliance in place until the appropriate movement has been achieved. This usually takes about 6 weeks.
- Complications usually are caused by application of inappropriate techniques or inadequate postoperative care.
  - Misapplication of orthodontic forces can result in resorbed roots, devitalized teeth (necrotic pulp), avulsed teeth, periodontal pockets, gingivitis, and failure to achieve the desired orthodontic movement.

STOMATITIS/GINGIVITIS

Stomatitis/gingivitis is a common clinical problem. Always attempt to identify a specific underlying cause, because this can determine therapeutic approach and prognosis. When a specific cause cannot be identified or specific therapy is not available, treatment is symptomatic and supportive. Chronic relapsing stomatitis can be particularly frustrating to manage.

Etiology

Causes of stomatitis/gingivitis are listed in Table 8. Many systemic diseases that cause stomatitis/gingivitis are discussed in detail elsewhere in this book, including viral upper respiratory infections of cats (sec. 2, ch. 4), feline leukemia virus (FeLV) (sec. 2, ch. 1), feline immunodeficiency virus (FIV) (sec. 2, ch. 2), renal failure (sec. 8, ch. 1), autoimmune diseases such as systemic lupus erythematosus (LE) (sec. 3, ch. 3) and pemphigus (sec. 3, ch. 3), and eosinophilic granuloma complex (sec. 5, ch. 14).

Periodontal Disease

Periodontal disease is a common predisposing cause of stomatitis/gingivitis in dogs and cats (see previous discussion).

KEY POINT ▶ In any animal with stomatitis/gingivitis, perform a complete periodontal examination and dental prophylaxis, including tooth extractions if necessary, to eliminate periodontal disease as a contributing factor.

Physical Injury

Foreign bodies (plant awns, sticks, bones, oral trauma, and thermal, electrical, and radiation burns can cause stomatitis/gingivitis. A history of exposure combined with the oral examination may be diagnostic.

- Plant awn stomatitis (bur tongue, vegetative stomatitis) occurs in outdoor dogs who groom burs from their coat or eat horse feces containing burs. The awns become embedded in the tongue and gingiva, causing glossitis, gingivitis, and gingival hyperplasia.
  - On oral examination, close inspection will reveal tiny plant spicules embedded in tissue, and plant material may be seen on biopsy.

Chemical Injury

Strong alkalis (lye solutions) and acids, petroleum distillates, and phenols can damage the oral cavity. In many cases, the specific agent is not identified and the diagnosis is based on circumstantial evidence. Concurrent esophageal and gastrointestinal mucosal involvement supports the diagnosis of ingestion of a caustic substance.

Infection Nocardia

Nocardia spp have been associated with severe halitosis, gingivitis, and oral ulcerations in dogs. In severe cases, necrosis and pseudomembranes are present. Lesions are most severe in periodontal areas. Rarely, mandibular lymph nodes and adjacent skin may be involved.

TABLE 8. Diagnosis and Treatment of Stomatitis

Disorders	Diagnosis	Treatment*
Periodontal Disease	Oral exam, dental radiography	Dental prophylaxis, antibiotics
Physical Injury		
Foreign bodies (e.g., plant awns, sticks, bones, fiberglass); trauma; thermal, electrical, radiation burns	Exposure history, oral exam, tissue biopsy for microscopic agents	Remove foreign bodies; for plant awns, scrape with dry 4″ × 4″ sponge or scalpel blade Debride necrotic tissue
Chemical Injury		
Strong alkalis (lye solutions); acids; petroleum distillates; phenol	Exposure history, oral exam (lesions may extend into esophagus and GI tract)	Immediate therapy; rinse mouth with water Alkaline chemicals: flush with vinegar solution or citrus juice Acid chemicals: flush with bicarbonate solution
Drug- or Toxin-Induced		
Drug reaction; toxic epidermal necrolysis; heavy metal poisoning (thallium); *Dieffenbachia* (house plant) ingestion	Exposure history	Symptomatic therapy only
Infection		
Feline herpesvirus/calicivirus	History, physical exam (naso-ocular discharges, fever)	Symptomatic therapy only
Ulcerative necrotizing stomatitis	Oral exam, bacterial culture, impression smears for spirochetes	Treat with antibiotics for at least 3 weeks
Candidiasis	Oral exam, fungal culture	Ketoconazole (Nizoral) 5–10 mg/kg, q12h, PO, or Nystatin 2% in Orabase applied topically
Nocardiosis	Oral exam, bacterial culture	Sulfadiazine, 80 mg/kg q8h, PO
Immunodeficiency or Immunosuppression		
Feline leukemia virus (FeLV)	FeLV antigen test	Symptomatic therapy only
Feline immunodeficiency virus (FIV)	FIV antibody test	Same as above
Metabolic Disorders		
Renal failure	Creatinine, BUN, urinalysis	Correct or control underlying disorder
Diabetes mellitus	Blood and urine glucose	Same as above
Hypothyroidism	T_4, TSH stimulation tests	Same as above
Autoimmune Disorders		
Systemic LE; pemphigus complex; bullous pemphigoid	Physical exam (other mucocutaneous areas affected); biopsy (including IFA test); ANA and LE tests	Immunosuppressant therapy (e.g., glucocorticoids, azathioprine, cyclophosphamide, gold salts)
Neutropenia		
Cyclic neutropenia; agranulocytosis; leukemia	CBC, bone marrow aspiration	Symptomatic therapy only
Nutritional Deficiencies†		
Niacin deficiency (black tongue)	Diet history	Vitamin supplementation
Idiopathic		
Feline plasma cell stomatitis	Biopsy, total serum protein; protein electrophoresis; dental radiography	Symptomatic therapy including antibiotics and dental prophylaxis initially; other therapies include prednisolone, megestrol acetate, gold therapy and low-dose azathioprine; results are inconsistent Dental extractions in refractory cases
Eosinophilic granuloma complex	Physical exam (may have other dermatologic involvement); biopsy	Cats: Depo-medrol, 20 mg/cat, SC, every 2 weeks for at least 30 days; alternate therapy for refractory cases includes megestrol acetate, surgery, cryosurgery, CO_2 laser, radiation therapy, levamisole, gold salts; correct underlying problem (flea control, hypoallergenic diet, hyposensitization) Dogs: Prednisolone, 0.5–1.0 mg/kg q12h, PO for 7 days; then taper dose over 2–3 weeks
Underlying Oral Neoplasia	Physical exam (enlarged regional lymph node with metastases); biopsy and needle aspirate of lesion and lymph nodes; thoracic and skull radiography	Treat underlying neoplasia (see text)

*Symptomatic therapy appropriate for all causes of stomatitis may include systemic, oral antibiotics, especially for severe gingivitis or necrotic oral ulcerations, such as amoxicillin (20 mg/kg q12h), metronidazole (25 mg/kg q12h), clindamycin (10 mg/kg q12h), and tetracycline (20 mg/kg q8h); oral rinses with 0.1–0.2% chlorhexidine or 1% hydrogen peroxide, 3–4× daily; dental prophylaxis as needed; and soft food (canned or gruel).
†Rare in clinical practice.
BUN = blood urea nitrogen; T_4 = thyroxine; TSH = thyroid-stimulating hormone; IFA = indirect fluorescent antibody; LE = lupus erythematosus; CBC = complete blood count.

Oral Candidiasis

This uncommon cause of stomatitis is characterized by white plaques or pseudomembranes on the oral mucosa. Conditions that may predispose to candidal stomatitis include immunosuppression (including che-motherapy), systemic diseases, and long-term antibiotic therapy.

Necrotizing Ulcerative Stomatitis

This form of stomatitis is characterized by gingivitis, oral ulcerations, tissue necrosis, severe halitosis, and pain on eating. Numerous bacteria have been incriminated as contributing to this disorder, including spirochetes and fusiform bacilli.

Immunosuppression

Immunosuppression secondary to FeLV and FIV infection is an important predisposing cause of chronic stomatitis/gingivitis in cats.

KEY POINT ▶ Always test for FeLV and FIV in cats with chronic gingivitis.

Uremia

Uremia is a common cause of stomatitis and oral ulcerations. Urease-containing bacteria metabolize urea to ammonia, which is irritating to the oral mucosa. Dehydration and drying of the oral mucous membranes may contribute to the problem. In uremic animals, the rostral portion of the tongue may slough, possibly owing to uremic vasculitis and thrombosis.

Plasma Cell Stomatitis

Plasma cell stomatitis in cats is a disease of unknown etiology characterized by proliferative, often symmetric, hyperemic friable lesions at the glossopalatine arches.

- Concurrent pharyngitis is common.
- Ulcerative gingivitis may occur. This condition is extremely painful and can cause difficulty on eating. Some cats have concurrent plasma cell pododermatitis.
- An association with chronic calicivirus infection has been noted in some cases.
- On biopsy, lesions are characterized by plasma cells infiltrated with lesser numbers of lymphocytes, neutrophils, and histiocytes.
- Hyperglobulinemia, characterized as a polyclonal gammopathy, is often present and probably indicates chronic immune stimulation. An immune-mediated basis for the disease is suspected.

KEY POINT ▶ Underlying dental disease, especially external root resorptive lesions, may be an important contributing factor in plasma cell stomatitis of cats.

- Perform dental radiography to identify resorptive lesions, broken teeth, and retained roots. Some cases respond to extraction of adjacent teeth.
- FeLV and FIV infection does not appear to be a predisposing factor.
- The disease is often refractory to medical treatment, and relapse is common after treatment is discontinued.

Feline Eosinophilic Granuloma Complex

This disorder is an important cause of oral lesions in cats.

- Any of three forms (indolent ulcer, collagenolytic [linear] granuloma, and eosinophilic plaque) may occur in the oral cavity. The indolent ulcer involving the upper lips is most common.
- Differentiate lesions from squamous cell carcinoma.
- Oral lesions may coexist with dermatologic involvement. The disorder may be a hypersensitivity reaction associated with underlying atopy, food allergy, or flea bite hypersensitivity. Diagnosis and treatment are discussed in sec. 5, ch. 14.

Canine Oral Eosinophilic Granuloma

This disorder occurs in all breeds of dogs, but especially in young Siberian huskies.

- The cause is unknown but a hypersensitivity reaction to an as yet unidentified antigen is suspected, based on the dramatic response that occurs with corticosteroid therapy. Spontaneous regression also may occur. Hereditary factors may play a role.
- Lesions are characterized by proliferative tissue with superficial ulcerations that occur primarily on the lateral and ventral surfaces of the tongue. Soft palate involvement may also occur.
- Peripheral eosinophilia is common. Histologically, the lesion appears identical to collagenolytic (linear) granuloma in cats. Degenerating collagen is surrounded by granulomatous inflammation with an eosinophilic component.
- Differentiate lesions from neoplasia (especially mast cell tumor), mycotic infections, and foreign body reaction.

Clinical Signs

Clinical signs include hypersalivation, drooling, halitosis, oral bleeding, reluctance to eat dry food, dysphagia, anorexia, and weight loss.

KEY POINT ▶ Chronic stomatitis/gingivitis can be extremely painful and can cause behavioral changes such as reclusive behavior, dropping food while eating, and running away from the food dish because of pain on eating.

Diagnosis

Base the overall strategy for diagnosis of stomatitis/gingivitis without an obvious underlying cause (e.g., foreign body) on the following measures:

- Rule out underlying systemic disorders with appropriate laboratory testing.
- Pursue specific diagnostics such as dental evaluation and oral biopsies and cultures.
- Perform dental prophylaxis (as needed) and initiate symptomatic therapy while awaiting test results (see Table 8).

History

- Obtain a complete history, with special emphasis on potential exposure to foreign bodies, chemicals, drugs, and toxins.
- Look for signs suggesting underlying systemic disease (see Table 8).

Physical and Oral Examinations

- Perform a general physical examination. In particular, evaluate for concurrent dermatologic lesions, especially at mucocutaneous junctions (e.g., nail beds, anus, vulva, prepuce) that suggest an underlying autoimmune disorder.
- Oculonasal discharges and fever in a cat supports the diagnosis of an underlying viral upper respiratory infection (see sec. 2, ch. 4).
- Perform a complete oral examination, including periodontal evaluation, to identify and characterize the nature and extent of the lesions. This usually requires sedation or general anesthesia. A specific diagnosis can sometimes be made on oral examination (e.g., foreign body, periodontal disease).

Laboratory Evaluation

- Perform routine laboratory tests including a CBC, biochemical profile, and urinalysis to identify underlying systemic diseases such as renal failure (see sec. 8, ch. 1) and diabetes mellitus (see sec. 4, ch. 4).
- If general anesthesia is required for complete oral examination, obtain results of laboratory tests prior to anesthesia.
- Perform ancillary tests as suggested by specific historical and physical examination findings, such as FeLV and FIV tests in cats with chronic stomatitis/gingivitis, fine-needle aspiration of enlarged mandibular lymph nodes for suspected neoplasia, and antinuclear antibody (ANA) and LE tests for suspected systemic LE.
- Bacterial and fungal cultures of the oral cavity can be performed on scrapings, swabs, or pieces of tissue. Unfortunately, cultures are not usually helpful, owing to the large number of potentially pathogenic organisms present as normal flora. Exceptions include isolation of *Candida* and *Nocardia* organisms.
- If bacterial cultures yield a large growth of a single organism, antibiotic therapy based on sensitivity patterns may be warranted.

Radiography

- In animals with periodontal disease, radiograph involved areas to identify periodontal defects, retained root tips, and external root resorptive lesions, as discussed elsewhere in this chapter.
- Skull radiographs may show lysis of bone secondary to neoplastic disease.

Biopsy and Histopathologic Evaluation

Tissue biopsy is essential when evaluating chronic stomatitis, especially when proliferative lesions are present. Histopathology is useful to characterize the cellular response, identify specific causes, and differentiate neoplastic from non-neoplastic lesions.

- If autoimmune disease is suspected, place some tissue in Michel's solution and submit for direct immunofluorescence if warranted by histopathologic results.
- Cytology can be performed on impression smears of

exudates or biopsied tissue and may be useful to diagnose underlying neoplasia (e.g., melanoma) and infection (e.g., *Nocardia* and *Candida* spp).

Treatment

Treatment is based on the initiating cause. Whenever possible, institute specific therapy, such as removal of foreign bodies, immunosuppressive therapy for autoimmune diseases, corticosteroids for eosinophilic granuloma complex, sulfadiazine for nocardiosis, and ketoconazole for candidiasis (see Table 8). Symptomatic treatment of stomatitis usually is warranted, regardless of whether specific therapy is available.

- Because periodontal disease may be the underlying cause of stomatitis or, at the very least, an important contributing factor, perform thorough dental prophylaxis in all animals.
  - Apply a 0.1 to 0.2% chlorhexidine solution topically at the gingival margin once a day to retard plaque formation and provide local antibacterial activity.
  - Cleanse the oral cavity in animals with stomatitis with cotton-wrapped applicators soaked in saline or an oral rinse such as 0.1–0.2% chlorhexidine solution 3–4 × daily.
- Administer systemic antibiotics such as amoxicillin, metronidazole, clindamycin, Clavamox, and tetracycline to control secondary bacterial infections, particularly in cases of severe gingivitis or oral ulcerations (see Table 8).
- Initiate fluid therapy (see sec. 1, ch. 5) and tube feeding (nasogastric or gastrostomy tube) as needed in animals with severe stomatitis/gingivitis that refuse food and water.
- Consider extraction of the teeth (at least of the premolars and molars) in animals with severe stomatitis/gingivitis that is refractory to medical management and for which extensive diagnostic tests do not reveal an underlying cause.
  - Cats with plasma cell stomatitis/gingivitis/pharyngitis, in particular, may have an excellent response when adjacent molars and premolars are removed. Inflammation of the gingiva and buccal mucosa may significantly improve, but persistent pharyngeal inflammation may warrant continued medical management with antibiotics and corticosteroids.

KEY POINT ▶ Advise owners of animals with chronic nonresponsive stomatitis/gingivitis that long-term therapy often is necessary to control the problem.

- Re-examine animals with chronic stomatitis/gingivitis 2 weeks after initial therapy, and then every 1–3 months to assess and re-evaluate response to treatment.
- In animals with chronic nonresponsive stomatitis/gingivitis treated with tooth extraction, thoroughly examine the oral cavity 1 month postoperatively to assess proper gingivial healing. Take radiographs of regional areas of gingival hyperemia to reveal retained roots. Extraction of these roots will permit normal gingival healing.

TONSILLITIS

Tonsillitis is seen occasionally in dogs, and less frequently in cats.

KEY POINT ▶ Tonsillitis usually occurs secondary to other diseases associated with chronic irritation or contamination of the pharynx.

Etiology

Disorders that predispose to tonsillitis (and pharyngitis) include chronic vomiting or regurgitation, chronic productive cough, and chronic contamination of the nasopharynx (e.g., severe periodontal disease, cleft palate, nasal disease with discharge). Primary tonsillitis is rare but may occur in young, small-breed dogs.

The spectrum of bacteria cultured from dogs with pharyngitis/tonsillitis is similar to that cultured from the pharynx of healthy dogs, including *Escherichia coli,* and *Streptococcus, Staphylococcus, Pasteurella, Proteus, Pseudomonas,* and *Diplococcus* organisms.

Group A *Streptococcus pyogenes,* the cause of "strep throat" in humans, does not cause signs of pharyngitis/tonsillitis in dogs and cats, and the prevalence of infection appears to be low. Dogs and cats can acquire a transient infection from close contact with infected humans; thus, they may serve as a reservoir for human reinfection. When recurrent group A *S. pyogenes* infection in humans in the household is a problem, treatment of pets as well as humans is warranted to prevent reinfection. In dogs and cats, effective antibiotics include penicillin, erythromycin, and chloramphenicol.

Clinical Signs

- Signs of tonsillitis include retching, cough, fever, anorexia, and lethargy.
- When tonsillitis is secondary to other disorders, signs of the primary disease overshadow those of the tonsillitis.

Diagnosis

- The diagnosis of tonsillitis is based on the gross appearance of the tonsils, which may be swollen and bright red with small hemorrhages or punctate white foci (abscesses). Concurrent pharyngitis is common.
- Attempt to identify important predisposing disorders (see Etiology) with a complete history, physical examination, and appropriate laboratory tests.
- Perform bacterial cultures in cases of primary tonsillitis refractory to routine antibiotic therapy.
- Differentiate for chronic enlargement of the tonsils from underlying neoplasia (e.g., lymphosarcoma, squamous cell carcinoma), which can be diagnosed by tonsillar biopsy.

Treatment

Secondary tonsillitis is usually resolved with identification and treatment of the predisposing disorder. When a predisposing disorder cannot be identified, administer a course of broad-spectrum antibiotics such as ampicillin or amoxicillin (20 mg/kg q8h, PO) for 2 weeks. Tonsillectomy rarely is necessary.

TONSILLAR NEOPLASIA

Etiology

Squamous cell carcinoma and lymphosarcoma are the most common tumors of the tonsil.

Clinical Signs

- Retching and coughing may occur owing to pharyngeal irritation by the mass.
- A cervical mass may be present as a result of metastasis to regional lymph nodes.

KEY POINT ▶ Carefully examine the tonsils in all dogs with a cranial cervical mass.

Diagnosis

- Diagnosis is based on oral examination and biopsy (tonsillectomy) findings. The tonsils appear enlarged and inflamed, and may have an obvious irregular mass.
- Perform partial or complete tonsillectomy to obtain tissue for histopathology.
- The most common tonsillar neoplasms in dogs and cats are lymphosarcoma and squamous cell carcinoma.

Technique

Tonsillectomy (Biopsy)

1. Place the animal in ventral recumbency. Place an oral speculum.
2. Grasp the tonsil with an Allis tissue forceps.
3. Cut the base of the tonsil with scissors or a tonsillectomy snare and remove the tissue.
4. Control hemorrhage with electrocautery or with direct pressure, using a surgical sponge.
5. If a large defect remains, close the tissue using a continuous pattern with 3-0 chromic catgut.
6. Submit the tissue for histopathology.

Treatment

- For the management of tonsillar lymphosarcoma, see sec. 3, ch. 6.
- In animals with tonsillar squamous cell carcinoma, combination chemotherapy (doxorubicin and cisplatin) and radiation therapy have been reported to give the best results.

Prognosis

The prognosis is poor.

SALIVARY GLAND DISEASES

Diseases of the salivary glands that may be encountered include:

- Mucoceles

- Fistulae
- Sialoadenitis
- Neoplasia

Etiology

Mucoceles. Salivary mucoceles, or sialoceles, result from damage to the duct or gland, with subsequent leakage of saliva into the tissues. Salivary mucoceles are lined with granulation tissue rather than epithelium. The sublingual and mandibular salivary glands are most commonly involved. The sites for mucoceles include the cervical mucoceles, sublingual mucoceles (ranula), and, less commonly, the pharyngeal and orbital region.

Fistulae. Salivary gland fistulae occur infrequently in small animals and they are usually the result of trauma to the parotid salivary gland or duct.

Sialoadenitis. Sialoadenitis (an inflammatory reaction in the salivary glands) occurs infrequently in small animals. The zygomatic salivary gland is most commonly involved.

Neoplasia. Tumors of the salivary glands (e.g., adenocarcinoma) are rare. The parotid and submandibular salivary glands are most susceptible to tumor formation.

Clinical Signs

Clinical signs depend on the salivary gland affected and the type of disease present.

Mucoceles. Clinical signs depend on the location of the mucocele.

- Animals with cervical mucoceles usually are presented because of a soft, fluctuant nonpainful mass in the cervical area.
- Animals with a ranula often are presented because of abnormal tongue movements, reluctance to eat, dysphagia, and blood-tinged saliva.
- Animals with a pharyngeal mucocele usually are presented because of difficulty breathing or swallowing.
- Animals with zygomatic mucoceles usually have exophthalmos, divergent strabismus, and a fluctuant nonpainful swelling in the orbital area.

Fistulae

- Clinical signs include a small skin opening in an area overlying a salivary gland that drains serous fluid. The amount of drainage increases when the animal is eating.

Sialoadenitis

- *Zygomatic sialoadenitis*—exophthalmos, tearing, divergent strabismus, reluctance to eat, extreme pain on opening the mouth, inflammation of the oral mucosa near the papilla, and mucopurulent discharge from the duct
- *Parotid sialoadenitis*—a painful, warm, firm parotid salivary gland with mucopurulent discharge from the duct

Neoplasia

- Most dogs and cats with salivary gland tumors are presented because of an asymptomatic palpable mass in the region of a salivary gland.

- Associated clinical signs from enlargement, impingement on adjacent structures, and local infiltration can occur.

Diagnosis

The diagnosis of salivary gland disease is based on history, clinical signs, clinical pathologic findings, radiography, and histopathology.

- The diagnosis of mucoceles usually is based on palpation and aspiration of a clear or blood-tinged, ropey fluid that is consistent with saliva.

KEY POINT ▶ Perform aspiration of mucoceles under aseptic conditions to prevent infection of a mucocele.

Sialography also can be used; however, it is somewhat difficult to perform and is usually not necessary.

- Base the diagnosis of sialoadenitis on clinical signs, an elevated white blood cell count, and histopathology.
- Histopathology is necessary to diagnose salivary gland neoplasia. Thoracic radiography can evaluate for metastatic disease.

Surgical Anatomy

There are four pairs of major salivary glands in the dog and cat: parotid, mandibular, sublingual, and zygomatic (Fig. 17).

The *parotid salivary gland* is located at the base of the auricular cartilage. The parotid duct is formed by two or three short radicles and passes lateral to the masseter muscle. It enters the oral cavity opposite the maxillary fourth premolar.

The *mandibular salivary gland* is located at the junction of the maxillary and linguofacial veins. It is covered by a dense capsule. The mandibular duct leaves the medial surface of the gland and courses between the masseter muscle and mandible laterally and the digastricus muscle medially and then passes over the digastricus muscle and between the styloglossus muscle medially and the mylohyoides muscle laterally. The mandibular duct enters the mouth on a papilla lateral to the rostral end of the frenulum.

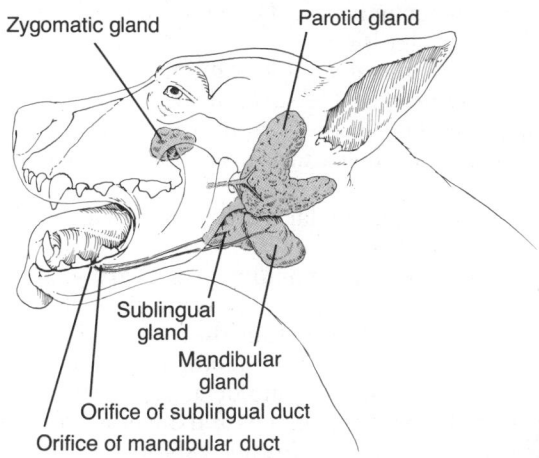

Zygomatic gland

Parotid gland

Sublingual gland

Mandibular gland

Orifice of sublingual duct

Orifice of mandibular duct

Figure 17. Salivary glands in the dog.

The *sublingual salivary glands* consist of a caudal portion (monostomatic) located at the rostral pole of the mandibular gland and a rostral portion (polystomatic) that lies directly below the oral mucosa lateral to the tongue. The sublingual salivary duct originates at the caudal portion of the gland and accompanies the mandibular duct to a common or separate opening on the papilla at the rostral end of the frenulum.

The *zygomatic salivary glands* are located ventral to the zygomatic arch. The major zygomatic duct opens about 1 cm caudal to the parotid papilla on a ridge of mucosa.

Preoperative Considerations

- Prior to salivary gland surgery, perform a thorough physical examination and appropriate laboratory tests and radiographic procedures, based on the animal's clinical signs, physical examination findings, and age.
- Diagnosis of the type of salivary disease is necessary prior to surgical intervention.

KEY POINT ▶ Surgery is not recommended for animals with sialoadenitis. Treat with systemic antibiotics, drainage of the abscess, and application of warm compresses.

Surgical Procedure

Several surgical procedures have been described in the treatment of salivary gland diseases, including:

- Excision of the mandibular and sublingual salivary glands
- Marsupialization of ranulas
- Drainage and excision of the zygomatic salivary gland
- Management of pharyngeal mucoceles

Excision

The technique for surgical excision of the mandibular and sublingual salivary glands (Fig. 18) follows.

Technique

1. Determine the affected side by placing the animal in dorsal recumbency. The mucocele will gravitate to the affected side.
2. Place the animal in dorsolateral recumbency and routinely prepare the surgical site.
3. Make a skin incision from the junction of the maxillary and linguofacial veins to the angle of the mandible.
4. Locate the mandibular salivary gland and make an incision in the capsule.
5. Bluntly dissect the mandibular salivary gland from the capsule, ligating and severing the arteries and veins that enter the dorsomedial aspect of the gland.
6. Continue dissecting the sublingual gland rostrally between the masseter and digastricus muscles.
7. Clamp and ligate the glands and ducts as far rostrally as possible with 2–0 chromic catgut.
8. Using a simple interrupted pattern, close the dead

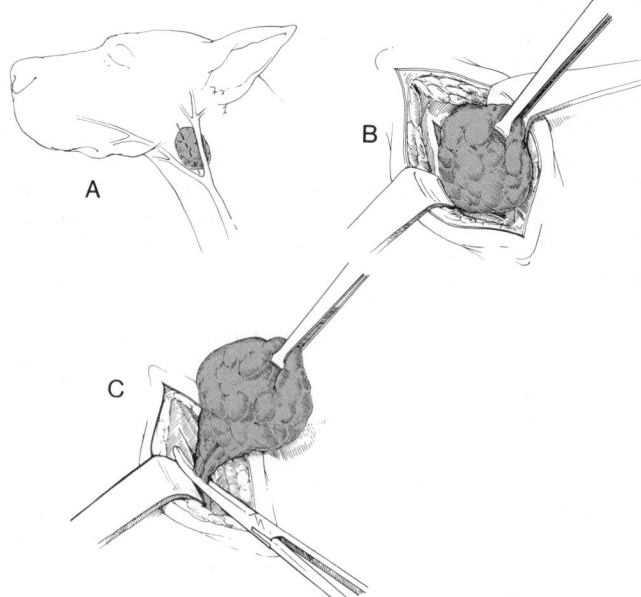

Figure 18. *A–D,* Surgical excision of the mandibular and sublingual salivary glands. See text for details.

space with a few sutures in the capsule and deep tissue.

KEY POINT ▶ To prevent the formation of seromas, place a Penrose drain from the site of the excised gland to the most ventral aspect of the mucocele.

9. Close the skin routinely.

Technique

Marsupialization (Surgical Management of Ranula)

1. Place the animal in lateral recumbency and routinely prepare the surgical site.
2. Incise the ranula longitudinally and remove the redundant portion of the mucosa.
3. Join the mucosal edges of the ranula to the adjacent oral mucosa with a few 4–0 chromic catgut sutures.

If the ranula recurs, removal of the mandibular-sublingual salivary gland complex is recommended.

Technique

Drainage of Zygomatic Salivary Gland (Treatment of Sialoadenitis)

1. Place the animal in lateral recumbency and routinely prepare the surgical site.
2. Advance a mosquito forceps through a small stab incision in the inflamed oral mucosa caudal to the last maxillary molar.
3. Use caution to prevent damage to the maxillary artery and nerve that course ventromedial to the orbit.

Technique

Surgical Excision of Zygomatic Salivary Gland (Treatment of Mucocele)

1. Place the animal in lateral recumbency and routinely prepare the surgical site.

2. Protect the animal's eyes from irritants with ophthalmic ointment.
3. Make an incision along the dorsal aspect of the zygomatic arch.
4. Reflect the periosteum of the zygomatic arch ventrally and retract the palpebral fascia dorsally.
5. Remove the dorsal aspect of the zygomatic arch, using rongeurs.
6. Retract the globe dorsally to expose the zygomatic salivary gland beneath the periorbital fat.
7. Retract the gland dorsally, ligate the vessels supplying the gland, and remove the gland.
8. Suture the palpebral fascia to the periosteum of the zygomatic arch, using absorbable sutures.
9. Close the subcutaneous tissues and skin routinely.

Management of Pharyngeal Mucoceles

■ Treat by marsupialization or by excision of the entire mucocele.
■ If the mucocele recurs, remove the mandibular and sublingual salivary glands.

Postoperative Care and Complications

■ Administer broad-spectrum antibiotics immediately before and following surgery.
■ Feed a soft diet for 1 week postoperatively.

Complications

Complications vary according to the initial problem.

■ If salivary mucoceles recur, re-explore for residual salivary tissue. Removal of residual tissue is curative.
■ Sialoadenitis—clinical response is good if drainage is adequate and appropriate antibiotics, based on bacterial culture and sensitivity testing, are given.
■ Neoplasia—recurrence is possible. Postoperative orthovoltage radiation therapy may be beneficial in animals with salivary gland adenocarcinomas.

SUPPLEMENTAL READINGS

Bojrab MJ, Tholen M: *Small Animal Oral Medicine and Surgery*. Philadelphia: Lea & Febiger, 1990.

Brooks MB, Matus RE, Leifer CE, et al.: Chemotherapy versus chemotherapy plus radiotherapy in the treatment of tonsillar squamous cell carcinoma in the dog. J Vet Intern Med 2:206, 1988.

Harvey CE: *Veterinary Dentistry*. Philadelphia: W.B. Saunders, 1985.

Knecht CD: Salivary glands. *In* Bojrab MJ, ed.: *Current Techniques in Small Animal Surgery*. Philadelphia: Lea & Febiger, 1990, p 197.

Manfra Marretta S: *Problems in Veterinary Medicine "Dentistry."* Philadelphia: JB Lippincott, 1990.

2 Diseases of the Esophagus and Disorders of Swallowing

Susan E. Johnson
Robert G. Sherding

OVERVIEW

Etiology

Esophageal disease in dogs and cats can be classified as structural disorders (e.g., foreign body, stricture, vascular ring anomaly) and motility disorders (e.g., oropharyngeal dysphagia, megaesophagus). Motility disorders may be caused by primary neuromuscular disease of the esophagus or may be secondary to systemic neuromuscular disorders.

Clinical Signs

Clinical signs of esophageal disease include regurgitation, dysphagia, odynophagia (pain on swallowing), ptyalism, and exaggerated swallowing. Weight loss, polyphagia, anorexia, cough, dyspnea, and fever also may be seen.

Regurgitation. Regurgitation is the passive expulsion of food or fluid from the esophagus and is influenced by mechanical events in the esophagus. The timing of regurgitation in relation to eating is determined by the location of esophageal dysfunction, degree of obstruction, and presence or absence of esophageal dilation.

- Regurgitation immediately after eating is most likely to occur with proximal esophageal lesions or esophageal obstruction.
- Regurgitation may be unassociated with eating when the esophagus is dilated, because this provides a reservoir for food and fluid.
- Selective retention of fluids over solid food is more likely with partial obstruction.

KEY POINT ▶ Differentiate regurgitation, which is the passive expulsion of esophageal contents, from vomiting, which is the centrally mediated reflex expulsion of contents from the stomach and duodenum.

- In contrast to regurgitation, vomiting is preceded by hypersalivation, retching, and abdominal contractions.

Dysphagia, Odynophagia, Ptyalism, and Exaggerated Swallowing. These signs are most likely to occur with oropharyngeal and proximal esophageal disorders.

Weight Loss. Weight loss occurs secondary to inadequate food intake and is related to the severity of esophageal dysfunction.

Polyphagia. Polyphagia occurs when an animal is otherwise healthy but unable to retain ingested food owing to partial or complete esophageal obstruction (e.g., esophageal stricture).

Anorexia, Cough, Dyspnea, and Fever. These signs may be seen with secondary aspiration pneumonia, esophageal perforation, or bronchoesophageal fistula.

Diagnosis

The diagnosis of esophageal disease requires an accurate history, radiographic evaluation of the esophagus, and, in many cases, esophagoscopy.

KEY POINT ▶ Aspiration pneumonia is a frequent and serious complication of esophageal disease that must be detected and treated appropriately (see sec. 6, ch. 21).

Signalment

The signalment may suggest certain breed predispositions for esophageal disease (Table 1). The age of onset is also important because regurgitation caused by a vascular ring anomaly or congenital idiopathic megaesophagus usually begins at the time of weaning.

History

- Obtain a complete history with emphasis on exposure to foreign bodies or chemicals, recent anesthesia (reflux esophagitis, esophageal stricture), and systemic signs such as neurologic dysfunction or muscle weakness, atrophy, or pain (central nervous system [CNS] disease, generalized peripheral neuromuscular disorders).
- The onset and duration of clinical signs may provide important clues to the underlying disorder. For example:
  - When the onset of regurgitation is acute, consider an esophageal foreign body or caustic esophagitis.
  - A long-standing history of regurgitation is consistent with disorders such as idiopathic megaesophagus, vascular ring anomaly, and esophageal neoplasia.

630

TABLE 1. Profiles for Esophageal Disease Based on Signalment

Parameter	Clinical Association
Age	
Young	Vascular ring anomaly; idiopathic megaesophagus; foreign body
Mature	Esophageal neoplasia
Breed	
Boston terrier	Vascular ring anomaly (PRAA)
Bouvier	Dysphagia due to hereditary muscular dystrophy (oropharyngeal dysphagia and megaesophagus)
Cocker spaniel	Cricopharyngeal achalasia
Collie	Familial canine dermatomyositis (oropharyngeal dysphagia and megaesophagus)
English bulldog	Vascular ring anomaly (esophageal compression by left subclavian artery and brachiocephalic artery) Esophageal deviation cranial to the heart (normal variant)
German shepherd	Idiopathic megaesophagus Vascular ring anomaly (PRAA) Acquired myasthenia gravis Giant axonal neuropathy
Golden retriever	Idiopathic megaesophagus Acquired myasthenia gravis
Great Dane	Idiopathic megaesophagus Vascular ring anomaly (PRAA)
Greyhound	Idiopathic megaesophagus
Irish setter	Idiopathic megaesophagus Vascular ring anomaly (PRAA)
Jack Russell terrier	Congenital myasthenia gravis
Labrador retriever	Idiopathic megaesophagus Hereditary myopathy (megaesophagus)
Miniature schnauzer	Idiopathic megaesophagus
Newfoundland	Idiopathic megaesophagus
Rottweiler	Spinal muscular atrophy (megaesophagus)
Shar pei	Idiopathic megaesophagus Hiatal hernia Esophageal deviation cranial to the heart (mild regurgitation)
Smooth fox terrier	Congenital myasthenia gravis
Springer spaniel	Cricopharyngeal achalasia Polymyopathy (megaesophagus) Congenital myasthenia gravis
Wire-haired fox terrier	Idiopathic megaesophagus
Siamese cat	Idiopathic megaesophagus

PRAA = persistent right aortic arch.

- Intermittent signs often are seen with hiatal hernia and secondary reflux esophagitis.
- If both regurgitation and vomiting occur, give special consideration to a hiatal hernia/intussusception or reflux esophagitis secondary to disorders causing chronic vomiting.
- In the southern United States, consider *Spirocerca lupi*–associated granuloma and neoplasia of the esophagus.

Physical Examination

Perform a complete physical examination.

- Palpate the cervical esophagus to detect masses and foreign bodies.
- Distension of the cervical esophagus may occur with mechanical obstruction or diffuse motility disorders and frequently can be induced in animals with megaesophagus by compressing the thorax while the nostrils are occluded.
- A mucopurulent nasal discharge, pulmonary crackles, and fever suggest secondary aspiration pneumonia.
- A rigid stance, in conjunction with fever and depression, may be seen with mediastinitis secondary to esophageal perforation.
- Weight loss and emaciation can be seen with severe, long-standing esophageal disease.
- Other physical findings depend on the underlying cause of esophageal disease and include:
  - Horner's syndrome and noncompressible cranial thorax secondary to a mediastinal mass
  - Muscle weakness, atrophy, or pain with generalized muscle disorders
  - Neurologic deficits with primary CNS disease and esophageal denervation
- Observe how the animal eats (using both dry and canned food) to detect abnormalities of prehension and swallowing (suggesting oropharyngeal dysphagia) and to confirm that regurgitation rather than vomiting is occurring.

Radiography

Radiography is the most important tool available for diagnosis of esophageal disease. Survey and contrast radiography provide adequate information to diagnose structural disorders. Esophageal motility disorders are best characterized with fluoroscopy.

- Perform survey thoracic and cervical films to evaluate the entire esophagus. The esophagus is not normally visible unless it contains air, fluid, food, or foreign material. Evaluate thoracic radiographs for complications of esophageal disease such as aspiration pneumonia and esophageal perforation.
- Perform a contrast esophagram using barium sulfate paste or an aqueous organic iodine (see sec. 1, ch. 4).

KEY POINT ▶ If esophageal perforation is suspected, use an aqueous organic iodine rather than barium when performing contrast esophagography, because it is less irritating to periesophageal tissues.

- Esophageal motility disorders, especially those causing oropharyngeal dysphagia, are best evaluated with image-intensified fluoroscopy and rapid-sequence filming. Use of fluoroscopy is limited to universities and large referral centers because of the cost of equipment.

Endoscopy

Endoscopic evaluation of the esophagus is a unique, noninvasive method for diagnosis of esophageal disorders. The gross appearance of the mucosa can be assessed and tissue obtained for biopsy, cytology, and culture. In addition, esophageal foreign body removal or dilation of esophageal strictures with endoscopy can be therapeutic. Either rigid or flexible endoscopes can be used for esophagoscopy.

Esophageal Manometry

This modality evaluates intraluminal esophageal pressures and is useful for evaluation of esophageal motility disorders. Unfortunately, this procedure is infrequently performed in veterinary patients because of lack of availability of equipment and lack of patient cooperation.

Treatment

Treatment of esophageal disease is discussed under the specific disorder. General management of esophageal disease involves fluid therapy as needed (see sec. 1, ch. 5), management of complications such as secondary aspiration pneumonia (see sec. 6, ch. 21), and in severe cases, nutritional support by tube gastrostomy (see sec. 1, ch. 3).

OROPHARYNGEAL DYSPHAGIA

Oropharyngeal dysphagia is defined as difficulty in moving a bolus of food or water from the oral cavity to the cervical esophagus. This disorder can be subclassified as oral dysphagia or pharyngeal dysphagia, based on the clinical findings (Table 2).

- *Oral dysphagia* involves difficulty with prehension or aboral transport of ingesta to the hypopharynx during bolus formation.
- *Pharyngeal dysphagia* is defined as interrupted transport of a bolus from the oropharynx through the cranial esophageal sphincter into the cervical esophagus. It includes disorders of the cranial esophageal sphincter (cricopharyngeus muscle) such as failure of the sphincter to open (cricopharyngeal achalasia), failure to close (cricopharyngeal chalasia), or lack of coordination between cranial esophageal sphincter relaxation and pharyngeal contraction during swallowing.

Etiology

Oropharyngeal dysphagia usually is caused by morphologic disease that interferes with normal prehension and swallowing (see Table 2). Functional oropharyngeal dysphagia is associated with neuromuscular disorders that affect the tongue, muscles of mastication, or the cranial nerves involved in voluntary and involuntary swallowing.

Clinical Signs

- Oral dysphagia is characterized by abnormalities of prehension and mastication. Weight loss is not a

problem because animals compensate for their deficits and maintain food intake. Secondary aspiration pneumonia is uncommon because pharyngeal function is unaffected.
- Pharyngeal dysphagia is characterized by repeated unsuccessful attempts to swallow, with gagging, retching, and spitting out of saliva-covered food. Aspiration pneumonia is a common and serious complication.
- Regurgitation may be a prominent clinical sign since many of the systemic neuromuscular disorders causing oropharyngeal dysfunction can also cause esophageal hypomotility (megaesophagus).
- When a neuromuscular disorder is the underlying cause of oropharyngeal dysphagia, generalized signs of muscle weakness, atrophy, and neurologic deficits often are present.

Diagnosis

The strategy for diagnosis of oropharyngeal dysphagia includes the following:

- Identify underlying morphologic disorders with a complete oropharyngeal and radiographic evaluation.
- Characterize functional dysphagia as to the affected stage of swallowing.
- Pursue ancillary testing to identify underlying neuromuscular disorders that may be associated with functional dysphagia (see Table 2).

Signalment

The signalment may suggest certain breed predispositions for congenital neuromuscular disorders associated with oropharyngeal dysphagia (see Table 1).

History

Obtain a complete history, including a description of eating and drinking. Evaluate for signs suggestive of aspiration pneumonia (cough, dyspnea, anorexia, depression), or a systemic neuromuscular disorder (weakness, muscle pain, gait abnormalities).

Physical Examination

Many of the morphologic diseases that cause dysphagia are detected initially by oropharyngeal examination. Tranquilization or general anesthesia may be required for a thorough oropharyngeal evaluation. A general physical and neurologic examination (see sec. 10, ch. 1) is particularly important to identify focal and generalized neuromuscular abnormalities that may be associated with functional oropharyngeal dysphagia.

KEY POINT ▶ Observation of the animal eating and drinking is an important extension of the physical examination to confirm that dysphagia is present and to characterize it as an oral or pharyngeal problem (see Table 2).

Radiography

- Perform survey radiographs of the skull and pharyngeal area to identify morphologic disorders such as

TABLE 2. Diagnosis of Oropharyngeal Dysphagia*

	Anatomic Association	Clinical Findings	Etiology	Diagnosis	Treatment
Oral Dysphagia: (Abnormalities of prehension and mastication)	Teeth, tongue, hard palate, bony structures, and TMJ	Difficulty prehending food or lapping water	***Morphologic Disorders:*** Dental disease	Oral exam, radiography	See sec. 7, ch. 1
		Excessive chewing and chomping	Oral foreign body	Oral exam, radiography	See sec. 7, ch. 1
		Exaggerated head movements when eating	Oral neoplasia	Oral exam, radiography, biopsy	See sec. 7, ch. 1
			Severe stomatitis	Oral exam, biopsy	See sec. 7, ch. 1
		Submerging muzzle to drink	Cleft palate	Oral exam	See sec. 7, ch. 1
		Dropping food from mouth	Persistent frenulum	Oral exam	See sec. 7, ch. 1
		Pawing at face	Skeletal disorders (e.g., TMJ, craniomandibular osteopathy)	Oral exam, skull radiography	See sec. 7, ch. 1
		Excess salivation			
		No weight loss or aspiration pneumonia			
			Functional Disorders: CNS disease or peripheral neuropathy (cranial nerves V, VII, XII)	Oral exam (atrophy or deviation of tongue secondary to denervation), neurologic exam, EMG, nerve biopsy, CSF tap, CT scan (see sec. 10, Ch. 1)	See sec. 10, chs. 2 and 5
			Neuromuscular disease (e.g., myasthenia gravis, botulism)	Neurologic exam, EMG with repetitive nerve stimulation, tensilon test, ACA titer (see sec. 10, ch. 6)	See sec. 10, ch. 6
			Myopathy or myositis (e.g., masticatory myositis, immune polymyositis, hypothyroidism)	EMG, muscle biopsy, CK, AST, ANA, LE, TSH stimulation tests (see sec. 10, ch. 6)	See sec. 10, ch. 6
Pharyngeal Dysphagia: (Abnormalities of bolus transport from the oropharynx through the cranial esophageal sphincter)	Pharyngeal constrictor muscles, soft palate, cranial esophageal sphincter	Normal food and water uptake but repeated unsuccessful attempts to swallow	***Morphologic Disorders:*** Inflammatory or neoplastic diseases of the pharynx, tonsils, or retropharyngeal lymph nodes	Oral exam, skull and pharyngeal radiography, biopsy of inflammatory or mass lesions, fine-needle aspiration of lymph nodes, endoscopy	See sec. 7, ch. 1
		Spitting out saliva-covered food	Retropharyngeal foreign body or abscess	Oral exam, pharyngeal radiography, fine-needle aspiration, endoscopy	See sec. 7, ch. 1
		Eating with head and neck tucked ventrally	Soft palate disorders (e.g., cleft soft palate or iatrogenic shortening)	Oral exam	See sec. 7, ch. 1
		Pharyngeal food retention and secondary pharyngitis	***Functional Disorders:*** CNS disease or peripheral neuropathy (cranial nerves V, VII, IX, X)	Neurologic exam, EMG, nerve biopsy, CSF tap, CT scan (see sec. 10, ch. 1)	See sec. 10, chs. 2 and 5
		Gagging, retching Regurgitation Nasal discharge	Myopathy or myositis (e.g., immune polymyositis, hypothyroidism)	EMG, muscle biopsy, CK, AST, ANA, LE, TSH stimulation tests (see sec. 10, ch. 6)	
		Cough, fever (pneumonia)	Neuromuscular disease (e.g., myasthenia gravis, botulism)	Neurologic exam, EMG with repetitive nerve stimulation, tensilon test, ACA titer (see sec. 10, ch. 6)	See sec. 10, ch. 6
		Weight loss	Congenital cricopharyngeal achalasia	Barium swallow with fluoroscopy, response to myotomy	Cricopharyngeal myotomy; see sec. 7, ch. 3
			Cricopharyngeal dysphagia†	Barium swallow with fluoroscopy	Cricopharyngeal myotomy is contraindicated

*The type of dysphagia is first characterized as oral dysphagia versus pharyngeal dysphagia based on observing animal eat (e.g., prehension of food and water, swallowing). Barium swallow with fluoroscopy is useful to characterize functional oropharyngeal dysphagia but is not indicated for evaluation of morphologic disorders.

†Includes failure of the cranial esophageal sphincter to close or lack of coordination between cranial esophageal sphincter opening and pharyngeal contraction.

TMJ = temporomandibular joints; CNS = central nervous system; EMG = electromyography; CSF = cerebrospinal fluid; CT = computed tomography; ACA = acetylcholine antibody; CK = creatine kinase; AST = aspartate aminotransferase; ANA = antinuclear antibody; LE = lupus erythematosus; TSH = thyroid-stimulating hormone.

a pharyngeal foreign body or retropharyngeal abscess that can cause oropharyngeal dysphagia.

■ Perform thoracic radiographs to detect aspiration pneumonia and associated megaesophagus.

■ A barium swallow with fluoroscopic examination is required for definitive characterization of functional swallowing abnormalities, and it is essential for the diagnosis of cricopharyngeal achalasia. Unfortunately, fluoroscopy is available only at large referral centers.

Ancillary Testing

Ancillary tests frequently indicated for further diagnosis of causes of functional oropharyngeal dysphagia include:

■ Tensilon test, acetylcholine antibody titer, and electromyography (EMG) for myasthenia gravis (see sec. 10, ch. 6)

■ EMG and muscle biopsy for polymyositis and polymyopathy (see sec. 10, ch. 6)

■ Cerebrospinal fluid (CSF) tap and computed tomography (CT) scan for primary CNS diseases (see sec. 10, ch. 1).

Treatment

■ The treatment and prognosis of oropharyngeal dysphagia depends on the underlying disorder (see Table 2).

■ Supportive care is especially important with pharyngeal dysphagia. Detect and treat aspiration pneumonia (see sec. 6, ch. 21) and provide appropriate nutritional support, including a gastrostomy tube in severely emaciated animals (see sec. 1, ch. 3).

ESOPHAGEAL HYPOMOTILITY (MEGAESOPHAGUS)

Esophageal hypomotility refers to a decrease in esophageal tone or peristalsis that may be segmental or diffuse. The term megaesophagus commonly is used when a diffuse severe motility disorder results in a large, flaccid esophagus. In most cases, the primary disturbance is an abnormality of the body of the esophagus rather than failure of the gastroesophageal sphincter to relax (achalasia), as occurs in humans. Clinical findings associated with megaesophagus reflect impaired esophageal transport with secondary complications such as weight loss and aspiration pneumonia.

Etiology

■ Esophageal hypomotility disorders may be congenital or acquired. A familial predisposition for congenital idiopathic megaesophagus has been suggested for many breeds of dogs and Siamese cats (see Table 1). Breeding of affected animals is not recommended.

■ Acquired megaesophagus may occur secondary to many disorders, especially diseases causing diffuse neuromuscular dysfunction (Table 3). However, in

TABLE 3. Causes of Esophageal Hypomotility (Megaesophagus)

Idiopathic
Congenital
Acquired

Central and Peripheral Neuropathies
CNS (caudal brain stem) disorders (e.g., distemper, trauma, neoplasia)
Immune polyneuritis
Polyradiculoneuritis (coonhound paralysis)
Bilateral vagal nerve damage (e.g., surgery, trauma, neoplasia)
Giant axonal neuropathy
Hereditary spinal muscular atrophy
Dysautonomia
Ganglioradiculitis

Neuromuscular Junctionopathies
Myasthenia gravis (congenital or acquired)
Botulism
Tick paralysis

Myopathy or Myositis
Polymyositis (e.g., SLE, idiopathic, infectious)
Muscular dystrophy
Hereditary myopathy
Familial canine dermatomyositis
Glycogen storage disease type II

Miscellaneous
Hypothyroidism
Hypoadrenocorticism
Lead toxicity
Thallium toxicity
Cholinesterase inhibitor administration (prolonged)
Thymoma
Pituitary dwarfism
Esophagitis
Esophageal fistula
Tetanus

CNS = central nervous system; SLE = systemic lupus erythematosus.

most cases, a cause is not identified and the diagnosis is idiopathic megaesophagus.

■ The underlying pathophysiologic mechanism for idiopathic megaesophagus is unknown. Efferent neuromuscular pathways appear to be intact and a defective afferent component of the neural reflex is suspected. Mechanisms may be similar for both congenital and acquired idiopathic megaesophagus.

Clinical Signs

■ The primary clinical sign is regurgitation, which may or may not be related to eating. In most cases, the more liquid the food, the less likely it is to be regurgitated. Weight loss and emaciation occur secondary to inadequate food intake.

■ Dyspnea, cough, and fever are indicative of secondary aspiration pneumonia, a common complication of megaesophagus.

■ In cases in which megaesophagus is associated with an underlying disorder (see Table 3), additional clinical signs may be detected, including:
  • Generalized muscle weakness with myasthenia gravis, polymyositis, polymyopathy, or hypoadrenocorticism
  • Neurologic deficits with CNS disease or polyneuropathy

- Generalized muscle atrophy or pain with polymyositis
- Obesity and alopecia with hypothyroidism
- Oropharyngeal dysphagia with generalized neuromuscular dysfunction.

Diagnosis

Idiopathic megaesophagus is a diagnosis of exclusion. Strategies for diagnosis of megaesophagus should include:

- Confirmation of a persistently dilated esophagus
- Evaluation for underlying obstructive esophageal disease
- Evaluation for underlying causes of megaesophagus (see Table 3)

Signalment

The signalment is important since idiopathic megaesophagus is a common disorder in young animals with regurgitation and certain breeds are predisposed (see Table 1).

History

Obtain a complete history. In young animals with congenital idiopathic megaesophagus, regurgitation is often noted at weaning when solid food is first introduced. Multiple animals in a litter may be affected. Historical findings that indicate the need for a more complete evaluation for predisposing causes include systemic lethargy or weakness, concurrent oropharyngeal dysphagia, and neurologic abnormalities.

Physical Examination

The physical examination may be unremarkable except for weight loss.

- Distension of the cervical esophagus can be accentuated by compressing the thorax while the nostrils are occluded.
- A mucopurulent nasal discharge, pulmonary crackles, and fever suggest secondary aspiration pneumonia.
- Perform a complete neurologic examination with emphasis on cranial nerves IX (glossopharyngeal) and X (vagus).
- Evaluate all skeletal muscles (especially temporal and limb muscles) for weakness, atrophy, or pain.
- Additional physical examination findings are determined by the underlying cause (see Table 3).

Radiography

- Survey thoracic radiographs usually show distension of the entire intrathoracic esophagus with gas, fluid, or food. If hypomotility is mild, radiographs may be unremarkable. Evaluate for evidence of aspiration pneumonia.
- A barium esophagram can be useful to confirm persistent dilation of the esophagus and to evaluate for possible mechanical obstruction at the gastroesophageal junction.

- Esophageal motility disorders are best evaluated with fluoroscopy, which provides a means of subjectively assessing the intensity and coordination of esophageal peristalsis and is the only modality that can detect subtle esophageal motility disorders.

Routine Laboratory Tests

Perform a minimum data base of tests, including:

- *Biochemical profile* to screen for changes associated with underlying systemic disorders causing megaesophagus (e.g., hyponatremia and hyperkalemia with hypoadrenocorticism; hypercholesterolemia with hypothyroidism; increased creatine kinase (CK) and aspartate aminotransferase (AST) levels with polymyositis)
- *Complete blood count* (CBC) to detect a neutrophilia and left shift consistent with aspiration pneumonia
- *Acetylcholine antibody titer* to evaluate for acquired myasthenia gravis (MG), even in the absence of generalized muscle weakness, because acquired focal MG may mimic idiopathic megaesophagus (see sec. 10, ch. 6).

Other Tests

- Perform other tests as indicated by clinical and laboratory findings to detect underlying causes of megaesophagus, such as:
  - Adrenocorticotropic hormone (ACTH) stimulation test for hypoadrenocorticism
  - Thyroid-stimulating hormone (TSH) test for hypothyroidism
  - Antinuclear antibody (ANA) and lupus erythematosus (LE) tests for systemic LE
  - Blood lead assay for lead poisoning
  - Tensilon test for MG
  - EMG for polymyopathy, polymyositis, polyneuropathy, and MG
  - Muscle biopsy for polymyopathy and polymyositis
  - CSF tap for CNS disease (see sec. 10, ch. 1)
- Transtracheal wash for cytology, and culture and sensitivity testing if aspiration pneumonia is suspected (see sec. 6, ch. 21).

Esophagoscopy

Esophagoscopy is not routinely indicated for evaluation of megaesophagus unless obstructive disease of the gastroesophageal sphincter is suspected. With idiopathic megaesophagus, the esophagus appears dilated and contains variable amounts of froth, fluid, or food. The esophageal mucosa is usually normal.

Esophageal Manometry

This is an extremely useful diagnostic tool to detect and characterize esophageal motility disorders in humans, but it is not widely used in veterinary medicine because of the expense and the lack of patient cooperation.

Treatment

KEY POINT ▶ Treatment of megaesophagus is primarily supportive and symptomatic, unless a reversible underlying disorder can be identified.

- Offer frequent small meals with the animal in an upright position. Maintain the upright position for 10–15 minutes after eating, so that gravity can assist entry of food into the stomach. In most cases, the more liquid the diet, the easier it is to reach the stomach. However, different types of food should be given on a trial basis to identify that which is best tolerated.
- Place a gastrostomy tube for temporary nutritional support of animals with severe malnutrition (see sec. 1, ch. 3).
- Give antibiotics for treatment of aspiration pneumonia, based on results of culture and sensitivity testing (see sec. 6, ch. 21). Caution the owner that recurrent pneumonia is a common problem and that early detection and treatment are essential for long-term success.
- Treat the underlying disorder whenever possible (see Table 3).
- Surgical myotomy of the gastroesophageal sphincter is not recommended because "achalasia" of the sphincter is not usually present.

Prognosis

- Some animals with congenital idiopathic megaesophagus may improve in time with diligent supportive care.
- Idiopathic acquired megaesophagus is usually irreversible. The animal may do well for months to years if the owner is dedicated to performing appropriate feeding procedures and if pneumonia is detected and treated early.
- Aspiration pneumonia and euthanasia are the most common causes of death in animals with megaesophagus.

ESOPHAGEAL FOREIGN BODY

Esophageal foreign bodies are common. They usually lodge at narrowed areas of the esophagus including the thoracic inlet, at the base of the heart, or at the hiatus of the diaphragm. The extent of secondary esophageal damage depends on the type of object, its size and shape, and the duration of time in contact with the mucosa. Complications of esophageal foreign body include esophagitis, esophageal perforation and mediastinitis, esophageal stricture, and, rarely, bronchoesophageal fistula.

Etiology

The most commonly encountered esophageal foreign bodies are bones. Other objects include needles, fish hooks, string, toys, and, in cats, hairballs.

Clinical Signs

- Most dogs and cats with esophageal foreign bodies are presented for evaluation of acute onset of gagging, salivation, dysphagia, and regurgitation.

- If esophageal foreign bodies go undiagnosed initially, they may cause chronic regurgitation and dysphagia.

Diagnosis

History

Foreign body ingestion may be reported by the owner.

Physical Examination

- The physical examination often is normal except for dysphagia, excess salivation, or gagging and retching.
- Cervical esophageal foreign bodies may be palpable.
- Findings of depression, anorexia, fever, cough, and dyspnea may suggest secondary aspiration pneumonia or esophageal perforation. Cervical swelling may be palpated with foreign body–induced perforation of the cervical esophagus.

Radiography

- Thoracic and cervical radiographs usually are diagnostic for metal or bone foreign bodies. Evaluate thoracic radiographs for aspiration pneumonia. Findings of pneumomediastinum, pneumothorax, and mediastinal or pleural effusion suggest esophageal perforation.
- Contrast radiography may be necessary to identify radiolucent objects. Use an organic iodine (Gastrografin; Squibb, New Brunswick, NJ) rather than barium sulfate if perforation is a possibility (see sec. 1, ch. 4).

Routine Laboratory Tests

A CBC, serum biochemical profile, and urinalysis, may be indicated.

- Perform routine blood work prior to general anesthesia for foreign body removal, especially in older animals with possible concurrent systemic diseases (e.g., renal failure), that might warrant special anesthetic considerations.
- With secondary aspiration pneumonia or esophageal perforation, the CBC may indicate a neutrophilia and left shift.

Esophagoscopy

Esophagoscopy is indicated to confirm the diagnosis, remove the object, and assess secondary mucosal damage.

Treatment

Esophageal foreign bodies should be considered an emergency situation. Do not delay foreign body removal, as the likelihood of complications increases with time. Institute fluid therapy as needed to correct secondary fluid and electrolyte imbalances prior to general anesthesia.

KEY POINT ▶ Endoscopic removal of esophageal foreign bodies usually is successful and should be attempted prior to surgery.

Technique for Foreign Body Removal

1. Perform esophagoscopy with the animal under general anesthesia.
2. Use a rigid or flexible endoscope with foreign body retrieval (grasping) instruments.
3. Grasp the object and attempt to dislodge it by gentle rotation. Perform all manipulations cautiously to prevent further mucosal damage or perforation.
4. If the object cannot be extracted orally without trauma, advance it into the stomach and remove it by gastrotomy. Gastrotomy is not required for bone foreign bodies, as they dissolve rapidly once reaching the stomach. In this situation, perform serial abdominal radiographs to confirm that the bone has dissolved and does not cause obstruction.
5. Once the object is removed, assess the mucosa for hemorrhage, erosions, lacerations, and perforations.
6. Following an uncomplicated foreign body retrieval, withhold oral food and water for 24 to 48 hours and give parenteral fluids and parenteral broad spectrum antibiotics such as ampicillin (22 mg/kg q8h, SC, IM, or IV) if mild esophagitis is detected. (See elsewhere in this chapter for diagnosis and management of complications of esophageal foreign bodies such as esophagitis, esophageal perforation, and esophageal stricture.)
7. If the foreign body cannot be removed endoscopically and cannot be advanced into the stomach, an esophagotomy is indicated (see sec. 7, ch. 3).

Prognosis

The prognosis for recovery after endoscopic foreign body removal is excellent unless secondary complications occur. With perforation and mediastinitis, the prognosis is guarded.

ESOPHAGEAL PERFORATION

Perforation of the intrathoracic esophagus is more likely to be associated with significant morbidity than is perforation of the cervical esophagus.

Etiology

- *Esophageal foreign bodies* are the most common cause of esophageal perforation, especially objects with irregular or sharp edges, such as bones, and chronically lodged foreign bodies that cause secondary pressure necrosis.
- *Iatrogenic perforation* may occur during esophagoscopy for foreign body removal and during therapeutic dilation of an esophageal stricture.
- *Penetrating injuries* of the cervical esophagus can be caused by bite wounds and gunshot injuries.

Clinical Signs

- Anorexia, depression, odynophagia, and a rigid stance are seen with esophageal perforation.
- Cough and dyspnea may occur with perforation of the thoracic esophagus that leads to mediastinitis and pleuritis.

Diagnosis

History

Exposure to potential foreign bodies or trauma to the cervical esophagus may be elicited in the history.

Physical Examination

Findings suggesting perforation include depression, fever, and pain. With cervical perforations, there may be cervical swelling, cellulitis, and drainage.

Routine Laboratory Tests

A CBC usually reveals neutrophilia and a left shift.

Radiography

- With esophageal perforation, thoracic radiography shows pneumomediastinum, pneumothorax, and mediastinal or pleural effusion.
- Perform a contrast esophagram using an organic iodine (Gastrografin) to confirm perforation (see sec. 1, ch. 4).

Esophagoscopy

Esophageal perforation may be detected by esophagoscopy.

KEY POINT ▶ If perforation is present or occurs during endoscopy, life-threatening tension pneumothorax may require immediate thoracentesis and chest tube placement (see sec. 1, ch. 3).

Treatment

- If a small tear occurs secondary to a sharp foreign body or during endoscopic manipulations, conservative medical management may be sufficient.
- Give broad-spectrum antibiotics such as gentamicin (2.2 mg/kg q8h, IV, SC, or IM) combined with cephalothin (20 mg/kg q8h, IV), fluid therapy, and nothing per os for 5 to 7 days; monitor closely for clinical deterioration.
- Consider nutritional support by tube gastrostomy or parenteral alimentation (see sec. 1, ch. 3).
- Perform repeated thoracic radiographs (for thoracic perforations) on a daily basis to monitor response to therapy and to detect evidence of mediastinitis and pleuritis.
- If perforation is accompanied by fever, and mediastinitis or pleuritis, surgical exploration for primary repair is indicated (see sec. 7, ch. 3).

ESOPHAGITIS

Etiology

- *Foreign bodies* are a common cause of esophagitis.
- *Chemical irritants or caustic substances* may cause

esophagitis. Concurrent stomatitis (see sec. 7, ch. 1) and gastritis (see sec. 7, ch. 4) may occur.

- *Thermal injury* may occur with overheating of food (e.g., in a microwave).
- *Gastroesophageal reflux* is a common cause of esophagitis. Predisposing factors that may contribute to reflux esophagitis include general anesthesia, use of a head-down tilt table for surgery, indwelling nasogastric tube or pharyngostomy tube, hiatal hernia, chronic vomiting, and delayed gastric emptying.

Clinical Signs

- Signs of esophagitis are nonspecific for esophageal disease in general and include dysphagia, regurgitation, repeated swallowing, and excess salivation.
- Anorexia, depression, and fever suggest secondary aspiration pneumonia or perforation.
- Weight loss and dehydration may occur with chronic or severe esophagitis.
- With mild esophagitis, signs may be absent.

Diagnosis

History

Look for potential predisposing factors such as exposure to foreign bodies or caustic materials and recent general anesthesia.

Physical Examination

Oral ulcerations or stomatitis may be present if caustic injury occurred. Weight loss and dehydration may be detected with severe esophagitis.

Radiography

- Survey radiographs usually are unremarkable. Occasionally, small amounts of gas may be seen in the esophagus and mild focal esophageal dilation may occur secondary to delayed motility.
- Contrast studies often are normal. When esophagitis is severe, the mucosa may appear irregular. Segmental luminal narrowing can occur with involvement of the submucosa and tunica muscularis. This radiographic appearance can be difficult to distinguish from a fibrous stricture.

Endoscopy

Endoscopic evaluation of the esophageal mucosa is the most sensitive method for detecting esophagitis.

- Findings include mucosal erythema, hemorrhage, increased friability, erosions or ulcers, and in severe cases, pseudomembranes.
- If gastroesophageal reflux is the cause of esophagitis, lesions are most severe in the distal esophagus and the gastroesophageal junction may appear dilated.
- Reflux of gastric contents into the esophagus may be noted during endoscopy.

Treatment

Mild esophagitis frequently resolves without treatment and may not require additional therapy, especially when the cause (e.g., foreign body) can be easily resolved.

General Therapy

- Administer antibiotics (e.g., as ampicillin, amoxicillin, cephalosporins) routinely to prevent or control infection of the altered mucosa by oral bacteria.
- Maintain adequate nutrition in mild cases with frequent oral feeding of small portions of a nonabrasive, soft food. Place a gastrostomy tube in animals with severe esophagitis, prolonged anorexia, or inability to retain food.

Reflux Esophagitis

- Give metoclopramide (Reglan) to decrease gastroesophageal reflux (by increasing gastroesophageal sphincter pressure), promote gastric emptying, and possibly improve esophageal clearance (see sec. 7, ch. 4, Table 3, for drug dosage).
- Decrease acidity of refluxed gastric juice by giving an H_2 receptor blocker such as cimetidine (Tagamet), ranitidine, (Zantac), and famotidine (Pepcid) (see sec. 7, ch. 4, Table 3, for drug dosages). H_2 receptor blockers are preferable to antacids for control of acid secretion because of their potency and ease of administration.
- Sucralfate suspension is beneficial in the treatment of reflux esophagitis. Sucralfate (Carafate) is an aluminum salt that binds selectively to injured gastroesophageal mucosa, and acts as an effective barrier against the damaging actions of acid, pepsin, and bile acids associated with reflux esophagitis (see sec. 7, ch. 4, Table 3, for drug dosage). Unfortunately, sucralfate suspension is not commercially available, although it can be specially prepared by a pharmacist. It is not known whether the tablet form is as effective as the liquid for treatment of reflux esophagitis.
- Consider omeprazole (Prilosec) therapy for treatment of severe reflux esophagitis in dogs that is unresponsive to the previously described treatments (see sec. 7, ch. 4, Table 3, for drug dosage).
- Give prednisolone (0.5 mg/kg q12h) in animals with severe esophagitis to prevent healing by stricture formation. Be sure to control any infection (e.g., aspiration pneumonia) prior to starting corticosteroid therapy.

Prognosis

The prognosis is good for mild to moderate esophagitis and guarded or poor for severe esophagitis, especially when accompanied by perforation. Strictures may occur secondary to severe esophagitis (see below).

ESOPHAGEAL STRICTURE

An intramural esophageal stricture results when severe esophagitis involving the submucosa and tunica muscularis heals by fibrosis. Multiple strictures may occur secondary to diffuse esophagitis.

Etiology

- Esophageal stricture may occur secondary to severe esophagitis of any etiology.
- *Reflux esophagitis* associated with gastroesophageal reflux of gastric acid and enzymes during general anesthesia and *esophageal foreign bodies* are the most commonly recognized causes.
- Esophageal surgery may be complicated by healing with stricture formation.

Clinical Signs

- Regurgitation usually occurs immediately after eating. If the stricture is chronic, regurgitation may not be related to eating because esophageal distension cranial to the stricture acts as a food reservoir.
- A ravenous appetite is common because of inability to get food past the strictured area.

Diagnosis

History

Progressive dysphagia for solid foods with preferential retention of liquids is common. Clinical signs from a stricture usually occur 5–14 days after onset of esophageal injury and esophagitis.

Physical Examination

The physical examination is often unremarkable unless the stricture has been present for a long time, resulting in weight loss. Animals are often otherwise bright and alert.

Radiography

- Survey radiographs usually are normal unless the esophagus is distended with food or fluid proximal to the stricture. Evaluate for aspiration pneumonia.
- A contrast study of the esophagus using barium paste or barium mixed with food will demonstrate the stricture (see sec. 1, ch. 4). A contrast study is useful to assess the number and length of strictures.

Endoscopy

Endoscopy can diagnose an esophageal stricture and, at the same time, allow visualization of the stricture during treatment by bougienage or balloon dilation.

At endoscopy, a stricture appears as a ring of white fibrous tissue which narrows the esophageal lumen and fails to distend with insufflation. Multiple strictures are sometimes present. Esophagitis, erosions, and ulcers may also be detected.

Procedure

- If possible, pass the endoscope through the stricture to assess its length and to evaluate the esophagus distal to the strictured area.
- Perform a complete endoscopic examination of the esophagus and stomach to evaluate for severity of esophagitis and to identify potential underlying causes of esophagitis and stricture formation (e.g., foreign bodies, hiatal hernia/intussusception).

- If the endoscope cannot be passed through the stricture, contrast studies may be necessary (if not previously performed) for complete evaluation of number and length of strictures. Balloon dilation of the stricture may allow subsequent passage of the endoscope.
- Mucosal biopsies of the strictured area may be warranted in some cases to rule out underlying neoplasia, especially when the stricture is associated with a mass effect or mucosal irregularities, or fails to respond to therapy.

Complications. Gastric overdistension can be a significant complication of endoscopy in animals with esophageal stricture; thus, use insufflation sparingly. If the stricture precludes passage of the endoscope into the stomach, air introduced during insufflation will pass through the stricture and accumulate in the stomach, and it cannot be suctioned off through the endoscope.

Treatment

Esophageal strictures can be managed surgically or endoscopically. Surgery may be indicated if the stricture is too small to pass a dilator or if inadequate dilation is achieved after multiple attempts (see sec. 7, ch. 3). Mechanical dilation of the stricture is performed under general anesthesia with endoscopic visualization.

KEY POINT ▶ Conservative management of esophageal strictures with endoscopically guided balloon catheter dilation or bougienage is preferable to surgery.

Bougienage

- A well-lubricated dilator, such as a bougie or tapered probe (or the endoscope itself), is passed through the stricture. Avoid excessive force because esophageal perforation is a life-threatening complication.
- Passage of progressively larger bougies results in stretching and dilation of the stricture.
- The procedure is repeated at intervals of 5–7 days as needed to maintain clinical improvement.
- The total number of dilations (3–10) is determined by the severity of the stricture and the clinical response.

Balloon Catheter Dilation

This technique, which is the preferred method for dilation of esophageal strictures, appears to be superior to bougienage because there is less likelihood of perforation, fewer repeated dilations are required, and there is a longer response time between dilations.

Balloon catheters (Rigiflex Dilator; Microvasive Inc., Milford, MA) are available in 10-mm, 15-mm, and 20-mm diameters. These catheters can be passed down a 2.8-mm endoscopic biopsy channel, or they can be carefully passed adjacent to the endoscope using endoscopic or fluoroscopic guidance.

- Procedure—Distend the balloon with water (or contrast material for fluoroscopy) to the pressure recommended by the manufacturer (usually 45–50 psi).

Use a pressure gauge to avoid overdistension and inadvertent balloon rupture. Distend the balloon for 1–2 minutes, and then deflate it to evaluate the size of the stricture and the extent of secondary mucosal hemorrhage. The procedure can be repeated immediately using the next larger balloon.
  • Balloon dilations are usually performed 2–5 times at intervals of 5–7 days.
■ Give prednisolone (0.5 mg/kg q12h) for 10–14 days to prevent further healing by stricture formation; taper dosage over the remaining period of time that the stricture requires dilation.
■ If concurrent esophagitis is detected, institute therapy as described in the discussion of esophagitis.
■ An esophageal diameter of 1 cm is usually adequate for a cat or small dog to be maintained on canned food. Larger dogs may require an opening 1.5–2 cm in diameter.

ESOPHAGEAL DIVERTICULA

Etiology

■ Esophageal diverticula are pouch-like dilations of the esophageal wall that may be congenital or acquired. They are rare in veterinary medicine. Diverticula most commonly affect the distal esophagus.
■ Acquired diverticula are classified as *pulsion* or *traction* diverticula. Pulsion diverticula are believed to occur because of increased intraluminal pressure secondary to obstruction or altered motility. They have been associated with foreign bodies, stricture, vascular ring anomalies, esophagitis, hypomotility, and hiatal hernia.
■ Traction diverticula occur secondary to periesophageal inflammation that results in fibrosis and contraction, which pulls out the wall of the esophagus into a pouch.

Clinical Signs

■ Large diverticula cause clinical signs because they predispose to impaction with foreign bodies or food, which may lead to esophagitis and even perforation.
  • Signs include regurgitation, distress after eating, anorexia, weight loss, intermittent thoracic or abdominal pain, and respiratory signs.
■ Clinical signs may not occur with small diverticula.

Diagnosis

Radiography

■ Thoracic radiography frequently reveals a gas or food-filled mass in the area of the esophagus.
■ A barium esophagram will confirm that a pouch communicates with the esophageal lumen.

Treatment

■ Large diverticula require surgical resection (see sec. 7, ch. 3).
■ Small diverticula can be managed medically with upright feeding of frequent small meals of a soft food diet.

■ Identify predisposing causes and treat when possible.

ESOPHAGEAL FISTULA

Esophagotracheal, esophagobronchial, and *esophagopulmonary fistulas* are patent communications between the esophagus and the respective airways. They occur rarely in dogs and cats. Of these, esophagobronchial (bronchoesophageal) fistulas are most commonly described. Clinical signs are related to contamination of the airways with esophageal secretions and food.

Etiology

Esophageal fistulas may be congenital or acquired. Acquired fistulas are most likely and are usually associated with esophageal foreign bodies, especially bones. Other causes include trauma, malignancy, and severe infection.

In most cases, a lodged esophageal foreign body is suspected to cause esophageal wall necrosis with subsequent development of a fistula.

■ Most esophagobronchial fistulas occur in the caudal esophagus, probably due to the close anatomic proximity of caudal esophagus and bronchi in this region.
■ Esophagobronchial fistulas commonly are accompanied by an esophageal diverticulum.
  • A traction diverticulum may develop secondary to periesophageal inflammation and fibrosis in the region of the fistula.
  • A pulsion diverticulum may develop secondary to lodging of a foreign body.
  • The diverticulum may occur first, and predispose to foreign body lodging and subsequent fistula formation.

Clinical Signs

■ Clinical signs are primarily associated with the respiratory tract. Coughing, especially after drinking liquids, is a common presenting sign. Anorexia, fever, dyspnea, and weight loss are attributed to aspiration pneumonia.
■ Signs of esophageal disease such as regurgitation, gagging, and retching may be seen but are not consistently described.
■ Contamination of the airways can lead to recurrent localized bacterial pneumonia, pulmonary abscesses, and pleuritis.

Diagnosis

History

Suspect an esophageal fistula when there is a history of chronic cough, recurrent localized pneumonia and signs of esophageal disease.

Physical Examination

Findings reflect the secondary pulmonary involvement and may include fever, pulmonary crackles, muffled heart sounds (pleural effusion), and weight loss.

Radiography

- Thoracic radiographic abnormalities are primarily indicative of pulmonary complications and include localized alveolar, bronchial, or interstitial patterns, pulmonary consolidation, and pleural effusion. Radiopaque esophageal foreign bodies may be identified. The caudal lung lobes are most commonly affected.
- A barium esophagram is required for definitive diagnosis. Contrast material will outline the communicating airway. Use a thin mixture of barium sulfate (20–30% weight/volume) to enhance filling of small fistulas.

KEY POINT ▶ Do not use oral iodinated contrast material because it is hypertonic and may cause pulmonary edema.

- Esophagoscopy and bronchoscopy can be performed, but a contrast study is more reliable in detecting fistulas.

Treatment

- Treatment of esophageal fistulas requires surgery for esophagotomy, foreign body removal, fistula resection, and lobectomy.
- Perform culture and sensitivity testing of involved tissues for appropriate antibiotic therapy.

Prognosis

If severe complications such as pneumonia, pulmonary abscesses, and pleuritis are present, the prognosis is poor.

VASCULAR RING ANOMALIES

Etiology

Vascular ring anomalies are congenital malformations of the great vessels and their branches that entrap the intrathoracic esophagus and cause clinical signs of esophageal obstruction.

Persistent Right Aortic Arch (PRAA)

This malformation accounts for 95% of vascular ring anomalies in dogs and cats. PRAA occurs when the embryonic right rather than the left fourth aortic arch becomes the functional adult aorta. The ductus arteriosus continues to develop from the left side, forming a band that crosses over the esophagus to connect the main pulmonary artery and the anomalous aorta (Fig. 1). Esophageal compression occurs by the aorta on the right, the ligamentum arteriosum (remnant of the ductus arteriosus) dorsolaterally on the left, the pulmonary trunk on the left, and the base of the heart ventrally.

Persistent right aortic arch appears to have a familial tendency, because certain breeds, especially German shepherds and Irish setters (see Table 1), appear to be predisposed and multiple animals in a litter may be affected. The mechanism of inheritance may involve single or multiple recessive genes. Breeding of affected animals is not recommended.

Other Anomalies

Other anomalies that have been described include double aortic arch, persistent right ductus arteriosus (with normal left aortic arch), aberrant left or right subclavian arteries, and (in English bulldogs) esophageal compression by the left subclavian and brachiocephalic arteries.

Clinical Signs

- Affected animals are usually presented for regurgitation of solid food that began at the time of weaning. Regurgitation of undigested food commonly occurs immediately after eating but is sometimes delayed, as a large esophageal pouch develops cranial to the obstruction. Liquids and semi-solid food are preferentially retained because they can pass through the constricted area.
- Weight loss or failure to gain weight despite a good appetite is common.
- Cough and dyspnea suggest aspiration pneumonia.

Diagnosis

Differentiate vascular ring anomalies from other causes of regurgitation in young animals such as congenital megaesophagus and, less frequently, esophageal foreign bodies. Diffuse esophageal hypomotility (megaesophagus) occasionally complicates vascular ring anomalies in dogs.

History

Regurgitation since weaning is very suggestive of a vascular ring anomaly. Most animals are presented by 6 months of age, although occasionally signs are mild and a diagnosis is not made until later in life.

Physical Examination

The cervical esophagus may be distended secondary to partial obstruction and development of a pouch. Cough, dyspnea, pulmonary crackles, and fever indicate aspiration pneumonia.

Radiography

- Survey thoracic radiographs often suggest a vascular ring anomaly. The dilated esophagus appears as a food- or fluid-filled density cranial to the heart, which tapers to normal at the base of the heart. With PRAA, the normal bulge of the aortic arch to the left is absent.
- Perform a barium esophagram (see sec. 1, ch. 4) to confirm the location of esophageal obstruction and severity of esophageal distension. Differential diagnoses for this radiographic appearance include an intramural stricture, segmental motility disorder, or congenital diverticulum.
- Fluoroscopy is useful to evaluate generalized esophageal hypomotility.

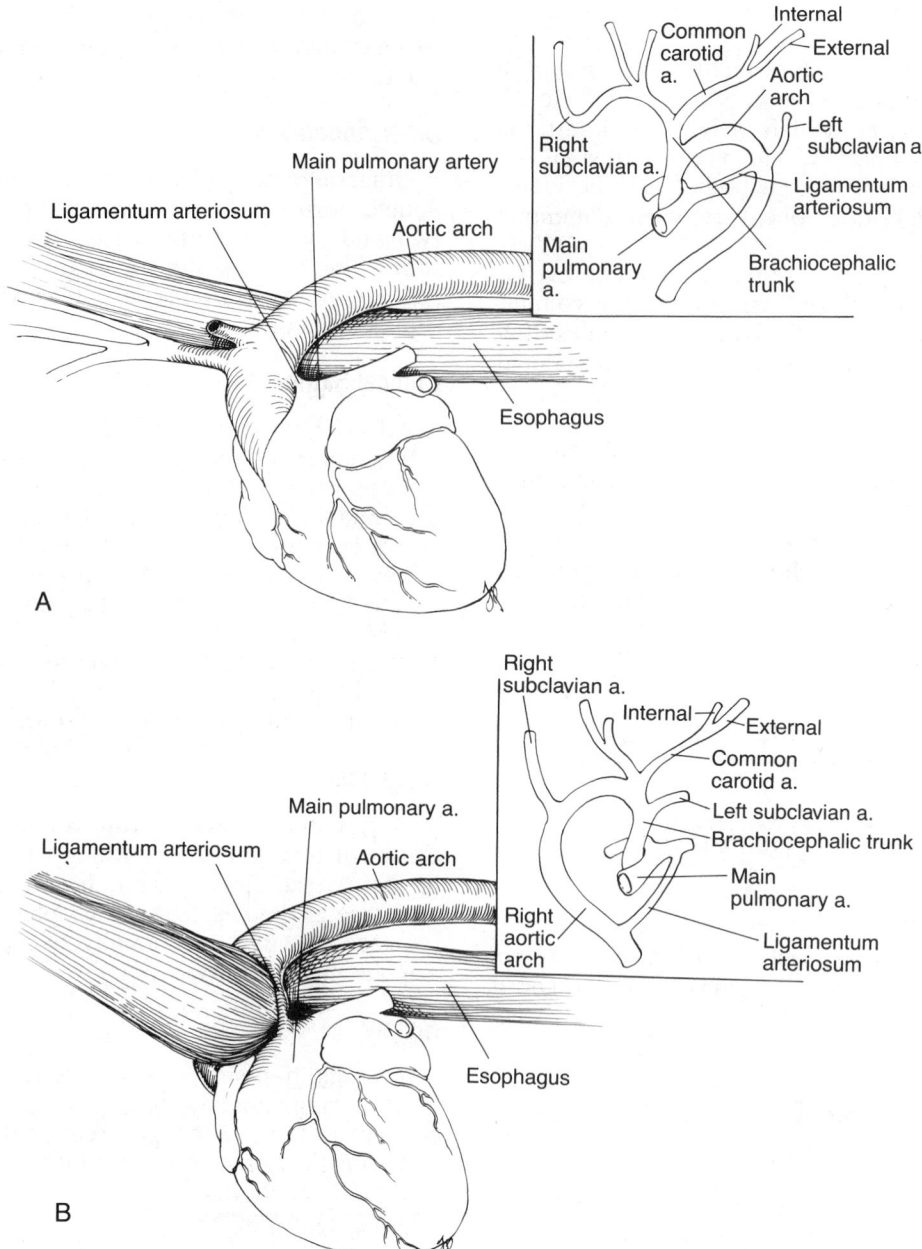

Figure 1. Persistent right aortic arch. *A,* Normal development of the aortic arch viewed from the animal's left side. Inset shows normal embryonic development of the great vessels from a dorsoventral view. *B,* When the embryonic right fourth aortic arch becomes the adult aorta, esophageal constriction occurs. Inset shows dorsoventral view of the vascular malformation.

- Angiography is seldom necessary, but in selected cases can be used for definitive confirmation of the type and location of vascular ring anomaly prior to surgery.

Endoscopy

Endoscopy can distinguish a mural lesion from extraluminal compression. In animals with PRAA, the indentation in the esophagus caused by external compression by the ligamentum arteriosum may be visible.

Treatment

- Definitive therapy for vascular ring anomaly is surgical ligation and transection of the ligamentum

arteriosum in animals with PRAA (see sec. 7, ch. 3).
- If the animal is debilitated and malnourished, improve nutritional status prior to surgery. Give frequent elevated feedings of small amounts of a semimoist or liquid diet. If this diet is poorly tolerated, consider feeding through a gastrostomy tube (see sec. 1, ch. 3).
- Control aspiration pneumonia with antibiotics prior to surgery (see sec. 6, ch. 21).
- Clinical improvement is usually noted after surgery, although mild esophageal distension often persists, especially if a large cranial pouch was present.
- Management as described for megaesophagus is indicated if regurgitation persists.

■ Recovery of normal esophageal function is more likely if surgery is performed at an early age and esophageal dilation is not severe.

HIATAL DISORDERS

Anatomic abnormalities of the hiatus include hiatal hernia and gastroesophageal intussusception (GEI).

■ A *sliding* hiatal hernia is a protrusion of any structure (usually the distal esophagus and stomach) through the esophageal hiatus of the diaphragm into the thorax.
■ A *paraesophageal* hiatal hernia involves displacement of a portion of the stomach through a diaphragmatic defect adjacent to the esophageal hiatus, and is rare in veterinary medicine.

Differentiate hiatal hernia from GEI, in which the stomach (and occasionally other structures such as the spleen, proximal duodenum, pancreas, and omentum) invaginates or prolapses into the distal lumen of the esophagus. Hiatal hernias and GEI may be intermittent or persistent.

Etiology

Congenital or acquired enlargement of the esophageal hiatus or laxity of the surrounding ligaments may predispose to hiatal hernias and GEI. Most hiatal hernias are probably congenital and Shar pei dogs appear to have an increased incidence.

■ Acquired hiatal hernias may occur secondary to blunt abdominal trauma.
■ Reversible hiatal hernia and megaesophagus may be seen as a complication of tetanus in dogs.
■ Young male dogs appear to be predisposed to GEI.
■ Congenital idiopathic megaesophagus predisposes to GEI, presumably due to decreased esophageal motility and decreased gastroesophageal sphincter pressure.

Clinical Signs

■ Small hiatal hernias or intussusceptions may not be associated with clinical signs. If the hernia or intussusception occurs intermittently, clinical signs also may be intermittent. Common signs include vomiting, regurgitation, hypersalivation, and weight loss. Dyspnea also is common and may be due to aspiration pneumonia or compression of the lungs secondary to large hernias.
■ *Hiatal hernias*—signs are due primarily to impaired gastroesophageal sphincter function, which predisposes to gastroesophageal reflux and reflux esophagitis. If large portions of the stomach are displaced through the diaphragm, signs occur because of esophageal and gastric obstruction.
■ *GEI*—GEI can cause both esophagitis and esophageal obstruction. When a large portion of the stomach is intussuscepted, rapid clinical deterioration is evidenced by signs of dyspnea, hematemesis, profound depression, collapse, and sudden death.

Diagnosis

History

Regurgitation prior to the onset of GEI suggests that megaesophagus may be a predisposing factor. When GEI causes esophageal obstruction, the acuteness of onset and rapid progression to death often precludes an antemortem diagnosis.

Physical Examination

Findings often are unremarkable unless a large hernia or intussusception is causing esophageal obstruction. In this situation, dyspnea, collapse, and shock predominate.

Radiography

■ Survey thoracic radiography may confirm both hiatal hernia and GEI if they are large and persistently present. A soft tissue and gas density mass (the stomach) can be seen in the caudal dorsal mediastinum. The normal gastric gas bubble usually seen in the cranial abdomen may be diminished in size.
■ Perform a barium esophagram to confirm a hernia or GEI and to distinguish masses arising from other mediastinal structures or the esophagus. With a hiatal hernia, the gastroesophageal junction and gastric rugae are visible cranial to the diaphragm but the linear relationship between the esophagus and the stomach is preserved. Gastroesophageal reflux also may be demonstrated. With GEI, gastric rugae are seen within the esophageal lumen and esophageal obstruction is present.
■ Hiatal hernias and GEI that are small and reduce spontaneously are a diagnostic challenge. Because of their intermittent nature, they may not be identified routinely on either survey or contrast radiographs. Application of pressure to the abdomen during radiography, especially fluoroscopy, may be useful for detection of small hernias and gastroesophageal reflux.

Endoscopy

Endoscopy can assess secondary reflux esophagitis and may confirm a GEI (gastric rugal folds are seen bulging within the lumen of the distal esophagus).

Treatment

■ Surgery is indicated for treatment of large hiatal hernias and intussusceptions (see sec. 7, ch. 3). Emergency surgery is required for reduction of a large GEI, along with intensive fluid therapy for treatment of shock (see sec. 6, ch. 14).
■ Small intermittent hiatal hernias or intussusceptions do not usually require surgery. Medical management of reflux esophagitis (see earlier in this chapter) usually will control clinical signs. In refractory cases, consider other causes of regurgitation and vomiting prior to surgical intervention.

PERIESOPHAGEAL OBSTRUCTION

Etiology

- Mass lesions arising from the periesophageal tissues may cause signs of esophageal disease because of esophageal compression with partial or complete obstruction.
- Examples include thyroid tumors (cervical esophagus) or tumors arising from mediastinal structures (e.g., lymph node, thymus, heart base), lung tumors, and intrathoracic abscesses.

Clinical Signs

- Clinical signs associated with external compression of the esophagus by mass lesions (especially neoplasia) include chronic progressive regurgitation, dysphagia, and hypersalivation.
- Signs of esophageal disease may be overshadowed by signs reflecting involvement of other systems (e.g., pulmonary metastases, pleural and pericardial effusion), such as dyspnea, cough, and exercise intolerance.

Diagnosis

Radiography

- Survey thoracic radiographs will usually identify an intrathoracic mass.
- If survey films are unremarkable, a barium esophagram is indicated to identify the location and severity of obstruction.

Endoscopy

Endoscopy is helpful to characterize whether mucosal or mural involvement of the esophagus is present, or whether obstruction is predominantly extramural.

Biopsy

The diagnosis depends on identifying the cause of the offending mass lesion with fine-needle aspiration or biopsy via thoracotomy (see sec. 6, ch. 25).

Treatment

Treatment and prognosis are determined by the underlying cause of esophageal compression.

ESOPHAGEAL NEOPLASIA

Etiology

Primary esophageal neoplasms are rare. Malignant tumors of the esophagus include squamous cell carcinoma, osteosarcoma, fibrosarcoma, and undifferentiated carcinoma. Metastatic tumors occasionally involve the esophagus but unless the tumor is large, clinical signs of esophageal disease are absent.

- Esophageal fibrosarcoma and osteosarcoma in dogs can develop after malignant transformation of esophageal granulomas associated with infection by the helminth parasite *Spirocerca lupi*. Infection with this parasite occurs in the southeastern United States. The life cycle involves a coprophagous beetle that is eaten by the dog or a transport host (mouse, chicken, bird, reptiles) that is subsequently eaten by the dog.
- Squamous cell carcinoma is the most commonly reported esophageal tumor in cats.
- The most common benign esophageal tumor is leiomyoma.

Clinical Signs

- Animals with esophageal neoplasia have signs of chronic regurgitation, dysphagia, and ptyalism that are slowly but relentlessly progressive.
- Anorexia, weight loss, and cachexia result from inability to retain food or are secondary to metastatic disease and the systemic effects of cancer.
- Signs associated with *S. lupi* infection are often subclinical until late in the disease, and include anorexia, lethargy, regurgitation, and dyspnea (with large masses).

Diagnosis

History

Chronic progressive signs of obstructive esophageal disease in an older animal suggest esophageal neoplasia.

Physical Examination

- Findings may include weight loss and emaciation consistent with the secondary effects of chronic malnutrition.
- Cervical esophageal tumors may be palpable.
- Dyspnea may occur with a large intrathoracic mass or pulmonary metastatic disease.

Radiography

- Survey thoracic radiographs may be normal or may reveal a mass in the region of the esophagus. With partial to complete esophageal obstruction, the esophagus may be dilated proximal to the mass and contain air, fluid, or food.
- Evaluate the lungs for metastases.
- Spondylitis of the caudal thoracic vertebrae or hypertrophic osteopathy may be associated with *S. lupi* esophageal granulomas.
- A barium esophagram can confirm the presence of a mass or obstruction, characterize the mass as esophageal or periesophageal in origin, and evaluate the extent of esophageal wall involvement.

Endoscopy/Biopsy

Endoscopy and biopsy are required for definitive diagnosis of esophageal neoplasia. If esophageal sarcoma is caused by *S. lupi* infection, adult worms may be seen protruding into the lumen of the esophagus from the affected tissue. *S. lupi* eggs may be detected on fecal sedimentation.

Treatment

- Successful treatment of esophageal neoplasia requires surgical resection of the tumor (see sec. 7, ch. 3).
  - For best results, it is important to make an early diagnosis before metastasis or extensive esophageal involvement has occurred.
  - In many cases, the tumor is too extensive for complete surgical resection, and thus the prognosis is poor.
- Results of anthelmintic therapy for *S. lupi* infection are inconsistent.
  - The standard recommendations for treatment of adult *S. lupi* include disophenol as a single dose (10 mg/kg SC) that is repeated in 7 days if no improvement is noted, or diethylcarbamazine (20–500 mg/kg PO) daily until no more ova are found in the feces. The efficacy of diethylcarbamazine has been questioned, however.
  - Although unproven, fenbendazole (50 mg/kg) or ivermectin (200 µg/kg, single oral dose) may be effective against larvae.
  - Levamisole is not recommended because it sterilizes but does not kill adult *S. lupi* organisms.

Supplemental Readings

Johnson SE: Diseases of the esophagus. *In* Sherding RG, ed.: *The Cat: Diseases and Clinical Management, Vol 2*. New York: Churchill Livingstone, 1989, p 907.

Jones BD, Jergens AE, Guilford WG: Diseases of the esophagus. *In* Ettinger SJ, ed.: *Textbook of Veterinary Internal Medicine, Vol 2*, 3rd ed. Philadelphia: W. B. Saunders, 1989, p 1255.

Surgery of the Esophagus

Ronald M. Bright

In general, the signs of esophageal disease are related to loss of function, to obstruction, or to inflammation of the esophagus and the surrounding structures. Surgery on the esophagus probably requires more skill and precision than any other portion of the alimentary tract. The esophagus is constantly moving, lacks a serosal layer, and does not have omentum to help seal small leaks. If suture line reinforcement is necessary, adjacent muscle, diaphragmatic tissue, or pericardium may be used.

ANATOMY

Upper Esophageal Sphincter

The upper esophageal sphincter is located at the proximal end of the esophagus. There is no obvious thickening of the esophageal tissue.

- The sphincter function is performed primarily by the cricopharyngeal muscle.
- Innervation of the cricopharyngeal muscle is from branches of the glossopharyngeal and vagus nerves.
- The blood supply is derived primarily from branches of the cranial thyroid artery.

Lower Esophageal Sphincter

The distal two centimeters of the esophagus is located intra-abdominally below the diaphragm and is thought to have a slightly thickened inner circular muscle that acts as a sphincter.

- Sling fibers from the lesser curvature of the stomach may reinforce the sphincteric function.
- The pinch-cock effect of the diaphragmatic hiatus is thought to assist in preventing gastroesophageal reflux.
- Innervation is primarily from the vagus.
- The major portion of the blood supply is derived from the esophageal branch of the left gastric artery.

Body of the Esophagus

- The esophagus has a cervical and thoracic portion.
- The esophagus has four layers—adventitia, muscularis (striated in the dog, smooth muscle in the caudal one-third of the cat), a thin submucosal layer, and mucosa composed of stratified squamous epithelium.
- The blood supply is from the thyroid and esophageal branches of the carotid artery proximally; the bronchoesophageal artery supplies the thoracic and distal portion of the esophagus. A few branches from the

left gastric artery are located just above and below the lower esophageal sphincter.

CRICOPHARYNGEAL ACHALASIA

This rare form of dysphagia is characterized by inadequate relaxation of the cricopharyngeal muscle and affects primarily young animals.

Preoperative Considerations

As described in sec. 1, ch. 4, barium swallow fluoroscopy ideally is performed preoperatively to distinguish cricopharyngeal achalasia from other forms of oropharyngeal dysphagia and to evaluate motility of the body of the esophagus.

Surgical Procedure (Cricopharyngeal Myectomy)

Objectives

- Surgically relieve the constriction by removing fibers of the cricopharyngeal muscle.
- Allow unobstructed movement of food from the pharynx to the esophagus while decreasing the incidence of aspiration pneumonia.

Equipment

- Standard surgical pack
- Gelpi or Weitlaner retractors
- Surgical suction and cautery

Technique

1. Place the animal in dorsal recumbency with the legs tied caudally.
2. Aseptically prepare the ventral portion of the neck, from the angle of the mandible to the manubrium.
3. Make a ventral midline cervical incision, starting just cranial to the larynx and extending caudally 15–20 cm.
4. Separate the sternohyoideus muscles to expose the trachea and cricothyroideus muscles.
5. Expose the dorsum of the trachea by rotating the larynx and trachea 180 degrees in either direction. If working on the dog's right side, pull the trachea to the right.
6. Remove a thin layer of connective tissue, exposing the cricopharyngeal musculature.
7. Incise the cricopharyngeal musculature on its midline. Gently elevate the muscle from the underlying esophagus with meticulous and careful blunt dis-

section. Consider placing a Foley catheter or endotracheal tube in the esophagus to help delineate the structures.

8. Elevate the cricopharyngeal muscle laterally and then cranially to the thyropharyngeal muscles.
9. Cut the halves of the muscle belly along their lateral attachments and remove the muscle (Fig. 1).
10. Allow the larynx and trachea to return to the normal position, and appose the sternohyoideus muscle with a continuous suture, using 4–0 synthetic absorbable suture.

Postoperative Care and Complications

Short-Term

■ Give blenderized food for 48 hours.
■ Slowly return to normal diet over the next 48–72 hours.
■ If *oral phase dysphagia* is present (see sec. 7, ch. 2), there may not be any improvement seen following surgery.
■ If *pharyngeal phase dysphagia* is present (see sec. 7, ch. 2) concurrently, a cricopharyngeal myectomy may worsen the animal's signs and the aspiration pneumonia.
■ Esophageal hypomotility, especially if proximal in location, may interfere with a successful outcome. Food and liquids will pass more easily through the cricopharyngeal sphincter, but decreased clearance by the esophagus enhances the likelihood of stasis and retrograde movement of material into the trachea. Aspiration pneumonia will continue to be a problem.

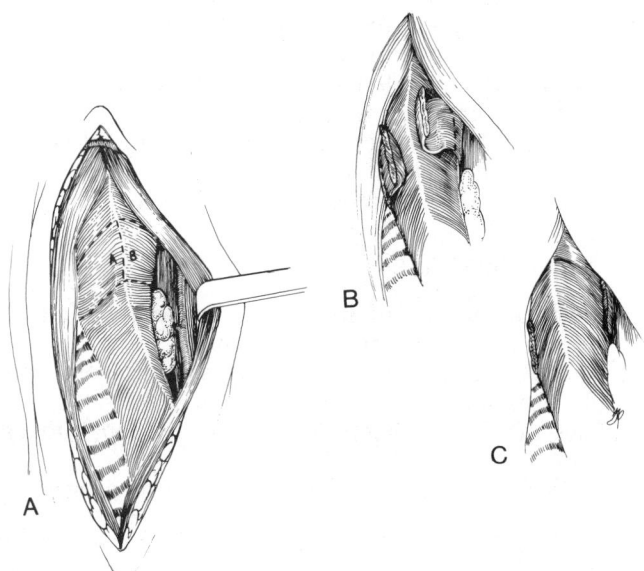

Figure 1. Myotomy of the cricopharyngeus muscle for cricopharyngeal achalasia. The cranial esophagus has been exposed via a ventral midline cervical approach. *A*, The esophagus is rotated so that the dorsal aspect is exposed and the cricopharyngeal muscles are seen. *B*, Initially incise on the midline (raphe) to separate the paired muscles. Use care not to perforate the esophagus. *C*, Make two longitudinal incisions laterally, one in each muscle belly, in the cricopharyngeal muscles. Remove each section of muscle.

Long-Term

■ If concurrent disease is present, as described above, feeding a gruel with the animal in a standing position may be necessary to prevent aspiration pneumonia while allowing passage of nutrients into the stomach.

Prognosis

■ If there is no concurrent oropharyngeal or esophageal neuromuscular disorder, the prognosis is fair to good.

VASCULAR RING ANOMALY

Preoperative Considerations

■ Any young dog or cat with regurgitation should be suspected of having a vascular ring anomaly.
■ Most animals with a vascular ring anomaly are presented to the veterinarian at the age of 4–10 weeks. Rarely, an animal may reach adulthood before a vascular ring anomaly is diagnosed.
■ Persistent right aortic arch (PRAA) accounts for 95% of vascular ring anomalies in dogs.
■ Rule out other causes of megaesophagus.
■ Confirm the diagnosis by contrast esophagography and endoscopy of the esophagus.
■ Fluoroscopy can evaluate motility of the esophagus above and below the site of constriction.
■ Evaluate the lungs radiographically for aspiration pneumonia. If necessary, treat with antibiotics for several days preoperatively.
■ Debilitated animals may benefit from hyperalimentation via a gastrostomy tube (see sec. 1, ch. 3) for 7–10 days prior to surgery.

Surgical Procedure

Objectives

■ Relieve the constricted portion of the esophagus caused by the vascular ring.
■ Allow unobstructed passage of food to the stomach.
■ Avoid perforation of the esophagus.

Equipment

■ Finochietto rib retractors
■ Suction and cautery
■ Right-angle forceps
■ DeBakey thumb forceps
■ Foley catheter or balloon dilator

Technique

1. Place the animal in right lateral recumbency.
2. Aseptically prepare the left lateral thoracic wall from three intercostal spaces above to five spaces below the fourth intercostal space.
3. To approach the vascular ring, perform a thoracotomy through the fourth intercostal space (see sec. 6, ch. 25 for thoracotomy technique).
4. Identify the ligamentum arteriosus, which is a constricting band encircling the esophagus. In a PRAA,

the aorta is on the animal's right side and cannot be seen through a left thoracotomy (see Fig. 1 in sec. 7, ch. 2).

5. If a PRAA is not the problem, consider vascular anomaly variations, including a left subclavian artery originating from the brachiocephalic trunk and, less commonly, a double aortic arch.

6. Double-ligate (e.g., with 3–0 or 4–0 silk) and divide the constricting vessel.

7. Gently dissect the mediastinum and adventitia away from the esophagus 1–2 cm above and below the constricted portion.

KEY POINT ▶ The esophageal wall usually is very thin; use great care to avoid perforation during dissection.

8. Pass a large Foley catheter or balloon dilator into the esophagus per os to further expand the esophagus at the site of constriction.

Closure

1. Administer a long-acting local anesthetic agent (e.g., mepivacaine) caudal to the head of the rib above and below the thoracotomy incision.

2. Place a chest tube prior to closure.

3. Close the thoracotomy incision routinely (see sec. 6, ch. 25).

Postoperative Care and Complications

Short-Term

- The chest tube usually can be removed within 24 hours.

- Regurgitation may continue to be a problem early in the postoperative period. Feeding blenderized food with the animal in a standing position may be necessary because of concurrent esophageal hypomotility.

Long-Term

- Amelioration of signs followed by a return of regurgitation several weeks after surgery may signal extraluminal scar formation acting as a constricting band.

- Repeated endoscopic balloon dilation (see sec. 7, ch. 2) of these strictures will sometimes ameliorate signs.

- An esophagoplasty or resection of the stenotic segment may be necessary.

Prognosis

- The prognosis is guarded to poor in most animals.

- Although not well documented, it is believed that the younger the patient at the time of surgical correction, the better the prognosis.

- The prognosis is thought to be better in animals in which preoperative fluoroscopy shows:
  - Normal or near-normal motility of the esophagus above and below the constriction
  - Absence of severe esophageal dilation cranial to the obstruction

ESOPHAGOTOMY

The most common indication for an esophagotomy is to remove a foreign body that could not be removed by intraluminal retrieval methods.

Preoperative Considerations

- Place a large-bore tube in the esophagus just prior to an esophagotomy to aspirate esophageal contents, act as a support while incising into the lumen of the esophagus, and help immobilize the esophagus.

- Treat aspiration pneumonia, a condition often accompanying esophageal diseases, aggressively before and after esophagotomy.

- Although surgery of the esophagus carries a low risk of postoperative infection, some contamination will occur. Perioperative antibiotics are recommended (given 30 minutes before surgery and repeated once or twice). The antibiotic chosen should be effective against gram-positive pathogens (e.g., a cephalosporin).

- Make the incision over healthy esophageal tissue.

Surgical Procedure

Objectives

- Gain access to the lumen of the esophagus to assist in the removal of a foreign body.

- Handle esophageal tissues gently to preserve blood supply and optimize healing.

- Establish a water-tight seal with closure.

Equipment

- Standard general surgery pack and suction unit

- Laparotomy pads to pack off the esophagus and prevent contamination of the surrounding tissues

- Fine-tipped needle holders to assist in delicate placement of sutures during closure

- Long-handled Metzenbaum scissors for thoracic esophagus dissection

- DeBakey thumb forceps

Technique (Cervical)

1. Make a ventral midline cervical incision extending from the manubrium to the larynx.

2. Retract the trachea and carotid sheaths gently to the right side.

3. Pack off the esophagus with moistened laparotomy pads.

4. Following the insertion of a large-bore orogastric tube, make an incision into the esophagus.

Closure

1. A two-layer closure is preferred:
   a. The first layer incorporates the submucosa and mucosa; use 3–0 or 4–0 monofilament nonabsorbable sutures with the knots tied in the lumen.
   b. The second layer incorporates the muscle and adventitia. Use an absorbable synthetic suture for this layer.

2. Close both layers with a single interrupted appositional suture pattern. Place sutures 2–3 mm deep and at intervals of 2–3 mm.
3. Irrigate the surgical field with a copious amount of sterile saline.
4. If infection is present or tissue trauma excessive, use a closed drainage system, using silicone tubing, for 3–5 days.

Technique (Cranial Thoracic)

1. To approach the cranial esophagus (T2–T6), perform a right-sided third or fourth intercostal space thoracotomy.
2. Pack off the cranial and middle lung lobes caudally with moistened sponges.
3. If necessary, dissect the azygous vein free and ligate.
4. Dissect the mediastinal pleura overlapping the esophagus to just above and below the proposed site of esophagotomy.

KEY POINT ▶ Avoid trauma to the vagal trunks located laterally along the esophagus.

Technique (Caudal Thoracic)

1. Perform right seventh or eighth intercostal space thoracotomy to gain exposure to the caudal one-half of the esophagus.

Closure

1. Closure of an esophagotomy incision is similar to that described under cervical technique.
2. Place a chest tube prior to thoracotomy closure.

Postoperative Care and Complications

■ Remove the chest tube 24–48 hours postoperatively unless esophageal perforation and mediastinitis were present.
■ Withhold all food and water (NPO) and give IV fluid therapy for at least 48 hours.
  • If esophageal tissue was devitalized or compromised at the time of esophagotomy, it may be necessary to maintain the NPO period for several weeks.
  • Ideally, use a gastrostomy tube for nutritional support during the NPO period (see sec. 1, ch. 3).
■ For the next 5–7 days, feed a blenderized diet. Gradually return to a normal diet by postoperative day 10.
■ If infection was present at the time of esophagotomy, submit a tissue sample for culture and sensitivity testing and initiate appropriate antimicrobial therapy.

Prognosis

■ The prognosis is good if the tissue was viable at the time of esophagotomy.
■ If perforation has already occurred and infection is present, the prognosis is poor.

ESOPHAGEAL RESECTION AND ANASTOMOSIS

Indications for resection and anastomosis include foreign bodies, esophageal strictures, neoplasia, and granulomas.

Preoperative Considerations

KEY POINT ▶ Some type of nutritional support (e.g., via gastrostomy tube) for patients undergoing an esophageal resection and anastomosis should always be part of preoperative treatment strategy.

■ If the site of anastomosis is unhealthy or compromised, a reinforcement or grafting technique may be necessary.
■ Many patients requiring esophageal resection are dehydrated and malnourished and may have aspiration pneumonia. Ideally, correct these conditions prior to resection and anastomosis.

Surgical Procedure

Approaches to the various parts of the esophagus are described under Esophagotomy. Closure following anastomosis and resection is described here.

Objectives

■ Resect the lesion and reappose the esophagus under minimal tension.
■ Restore esophageal continuity while minimizing the risk of early postoperative leakage and stricture at a later date.

Equipment

■ Similar to that for esophagotomy plus intestinal non-crushing forceps

Technique—Closure

1. A two-layer closure, using a simple interrupted appositional suture pattern, is preferred (Fig. 2).
   a. Use non-crushing forceps (or fingers) to occlude esophageal ends during closure.
   b. Use multiple stay sutures to maintain alignment of the tissues.

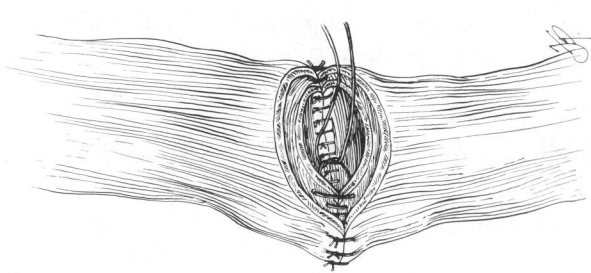

Figure 2. Esophageal resection and anastomosis. Close the esophageal layers in the following order: far wall, seromuscular layer; far wall, mucosal layer (knots in the lumen); near wall, mucosal layer (knots in the lumen); near wall, seromuscular layer.

2. Close the contralateral adventitial and muscular layers, using 3–0 or 4–0 synthetic nonabsorbable sutures.
3. Appose the contralateral mucosal-submucosal layers with 3–0 or 4–0 monofilament nonabsorbable sutures with the knot tied in the lumen; follow with closure of the ipsilateral mucosa-submucosa.
4. Close the ipsilateral superficial layers as in Step 2.
5. To relieve excessive tension across the suture line, a circular myotomy (including only the outer muscular layer) adjacent to the anastomosis can be performed. Injecting saline between the muscle layers helps to identify the outer layer.
   a. Mobilizing the stomach cranially through an enlarged hiatal opening can also help to reduce tension across the suture line.
6. If necessary, reinforce the sutures by bringing omentum on a pedicle through a small rent in the diaphragm or by using pericardial tissue or intercostal musculature.
7. Place a chest tube prior to thoracotomy closure.

Postoperative Care and Complications

Short-Term

KEY POINT ▶ By-pass the esophageal anastomotic site and provide nutrition via gastrostomy tube for a minimum of 7 days.

- Monitor closely for fever, which will often signal an infection secondary to leakage.
- Allow water consumption and return to oral feeding beginning on day 7. Retain the gastrostomy tube until normal food and water intake can be restored.

Long-Term

- Dysphagia or regurgitation occurring 3–6 weeks postoperatively probably indicates a stricture.
- Bougienage or balloon dilation may be necessary to relieve the postoperative stricture (see sec. 7, ch. 2 for discussion of esophageal stricture).

Prognosis

- Esophageal surgery of any kind carries a poorer prognosis than surgery on any other portion of the alimentary tract.
- If the anastomosis is done with precision and the tension across the suture line is minimal, fair to good results can be expected.
- Any compromise of the tissue at the anastomotic site carries a guarded to poor prognosis.

ESOPHAGOTRACHEAL/ESOPHAGOBRONCHIAL FISTULAE

Preoperative Considerations

- These fistulae usually are sequelae to the chronic presence of a foreign body.
- Most affected animals are high-risk patients because of the presence of severe bronchopneumonia.

- It may be necessary to sacrifice a lung lobe to achieve a cure.
- The use of gas anesthesia may cause the stomach to become overinflated if the endotracheal tube is located cranial to the fistula.

Surgical Procedure

Objectives

- Isolate the esophagus and the trachea or bronchus associated with the fistula.
- Close the abnormal communication between the alimentary and respiratory tracts.

Equipment

- General surgical pack
- Laparotomy pads
- Finochietto retractors
- TA stapler (U.S. Surgical) (optional for lung lobectomy)
- Chest tube

Technique

1. If a lobectomy is contemplated, the approach is through the sixth or seventh intercostal space.
2. Isolate the esophagus and trachea or affected bronchus and dissect free around the fistula. Take samples for culture and sensitivity testing.
3. Sever the fistula near its respiratory attachment; debride the opening and close using 3–0 or 4–0 nonabsorbable sutures.
4. If necessary, enlarge the opening to the esophagus to remove the foreign body if it is still present. The wound is then debrided and the esophageal defect closed in two layers as described previously under Esophagotomy.
5. Remove the affected lung if it is irreversibly damaged.
6. Place a chest tube prior to the thoracotomy closure.

Postoperative Care and Complications

Short-Term

- Treat concurrent pneumonia, emphysema or septicemia aggressively, and administer a broad-spectrum antibiotic pending culture and sensitivity testing results.
- If empyema is present, the chest tube may be retained for an extended period of time (see sec. 1, ch. 3).
- Maintain enteral feeding for an extended period of time via a tube gastrostomy to allow esophageal healing and decrease the likelihood of leakage from the esophageal wound.

Long-Term

- Stricture is always a potential sequela to esophageal surgery.

Prognosis

- In most cases, pulmonary involvement is significant, and the mortality rate is high.

■ If the degree of pulmonary involvement and esophageal trauma are minimal, the prognosis is better.

ESOPHAGEAL DIVERTICULECTOMY
Preoperative Considerations

■ Perioperative antibiotics are necessary to decrease the potentially deleterious effects of bacterial leakage.
■ If regurgitation is severe, dehydration may occur; correct this condition prior to surgery.

Surgical Procedure
Objectives

■ Resect the large diverticula and reconstruct the esophageal wall.
■ Remove the primary cause of the diverticulum, including strictures or periesophageal adhesions.

Equipment

■ General surgical pack
■ Finochietto rib retractors
■ Chest tube
■ Non-crushing intestinal or vascular clamp

Technique

1. A left eighth intercostal space thoracotomy is used to approach most diverticulae because of their epiphrenic location (just cranial to the diaphragm).
2. Isolate the diverticulum by blunt dissection down to its base.
3. Place a non-crushing clamp across the base of the diverticulum.
4. Excise the diverticulum below the clamp and close the esophagus in an open two-layer technique as described previously under Esophagotomy.
5. Place a chest tube prior to thoracotomy closure.

Postoperative Care and Complications
Short-Term

■ Dietary restrictions are the same as those used following esophagotomy. A gastrostomy tube usually is not necessary.
■ Monitor elevated temperature and neutrophilia closely, because these suggest esophageal dehiscence and mediastinitis.
■ Prior to discharge, perform contrast esophagography to evaluate esophageal motility.

Long-Term

■ Stricture formation may be a sequela to extensive excision of the esophagus.
■ Special dietary management may be necessary for the life of the animal if motility dysfunction remains.

Prognosis

■ The prognosis is good if the underlying cause can be corrected.

ESOPHAGEAL STRICTURE REPAIR
Preoperative Considerations

KEY POINT ▶ Attempt surgical correction of esophageal stricture only after bougienage or balloon dilation (as described in sec. 7, ch. 2) is unsuccessful.

■ Cervical strictures carry less risk with surgical correction than do those involving the thoracic esophagus.
■ Correction of fluid and electrolyte imbalances is imperative prior to any surgical procedure.

Surgical Procedure
Objectives

■ Increase the size of the esophageal lumen by reconstructive procedures or resection.
■ Resection of a lesion > 3 cm in length may require an esophageal lengthening procedure or a suture line reinforcement technique.

Equipment

■ Standard general surgery pack
■ Cervical location—Gelpi retractors; thoracic location—Finochietto retractors
■ Chest tube (thoracic repair)
■ Intestinal non-crushing clamps

Technique

Esophagoplasty
If the stricture is not too wide, a longitudinal full-thickness incision followed by a transverse closure (two-layer) may be adequate to increase lumen size. This is similar to Heineke-Mikulicz pyloroplasty (see sec. 7, ch. 5).

Patch-Grafting Technique in Cervical Region
1. Resect a partial circumference stricture, leaving a defect.
2. Separate a belly of one of the paired sternohyoideus or sternocephalicus muscles from its attachment to the other belly and reflect it laterally.
3. Transpose the muscle to lie deeply against the esophageal defect. Suture the muscle to the edges of the defect. Be sure that the muscle fills the entire defect.
4. The muscle graft must be mobile enough and of sufficient width to prevent postoperative stricture.

Resection and Anastomosis
This is described previously under Esophageal Resection and Anastomosis.

Postoperative Care and Complications
Short-Term

■ Monitor signs of infection that may suggest leakage from the surgical site; the more extensive the resection, the more likely that signs of early leakage will occur.

■ Placement of a gastrostomy tube is probably necessary in most cases to enhance esophageal healing and prevent leakage.

Long-Term

■ Stricture is likely to recur.
■ Life-long tube gastrostomy to by-pass the stricture may be necessary if surgery fails and if the owner is willing to maintain nutrition by this method.

Prognosis

■ The more extensive the surgery, the poorer the prognosis.
■ Less aggressive procedures (e.g., esophagoplasty) carry a better prognosis.

HIATAL HERNIA

Preoperative Considerations

KEY POINT ▶ The radiographic presence of a hiatal hernia does not by itself indicate the need for surgical repair.

■ Most cases of reflux esophagitis can be managed successfully with medical therapy alone (see sec. 7, ch. 2).
■ Sphincter reinforcement procedures (e.g., fundoplication) probably are not indicated in most cases of hiatal hernia, because incompetence of the lower esophageal sphincter usually is not a factor in dogs and cats (in contrast to humans).
■ Treat gastroesophageal intussusception with using similar surgical techniques as described below.

Surgical Procedure

Objectives

■ Restore the anatomic relationship of the stomach, diaphragm, and distal esophagus.
■ Decrease the size of the enlarged hiatus.
■ "Fix" the distal esophagus and stomach to structures below the diaphragm.

Equipment

■ General surgery pack
■ Abdominal self-retaining retractors
■ 28 French orogastric tube
■ Malleable (ribbon) retractors

Technique

1. Place the animal in dorsal recumbency with the forelimbs gently drawn forward.
2. Aseptically prepare the ventral midline from the mid-sternum to 2–3 cm cranial to the pubis.
3. Pass a 28 Fr. orogastric tube into the stomach per os.
4. Incise the skin and underlying tissues from just below the xiphoid to several centimeters caudal to the umbilicus.
5. Cover the left side of the liver with a saline-soaked laparotomy pad and retract the liver to the right and caudally with a wide malleable retractor.
6. Evaluate the esophageal hiatus for size. Gently dissect the surrounding tissue to expose the margins of the hiatus. Identify and protect the vagus nerves.
7. While an assistant places caudal traction on the stomach, plicate the hiatus with 1–0 or 2–0 nonabsorbable sutures (Fig. 3).
8. When plication is completed, it should be possible to insert two fingers through the hiatus.
9. Perform esophagopexy by placing 2–0 nonabsorbable sutures between the diaphragm and the lateral aspect of the distal esophagus as it passes through the hiatus; incorporate the muscle layers of the esophagus (see Fig. 3).
10. Fix the fundus of the stomach to the left abdominal wall by performing an incisional or tube gastropexy.
11. Make an incision 3–4 cm long through the serosa and muscular layers of the stomach. Make a similar incision in the peritoneum and transversalis musculature.
12. Appose the margins of the two surgical wounds, using six–eight 1–0 nonabsorbable sutures.

Postoperative Care and Complications

Short-Term

■ Feed a gruel diet for 3–5 days. A return to a normal ration usually is possible.

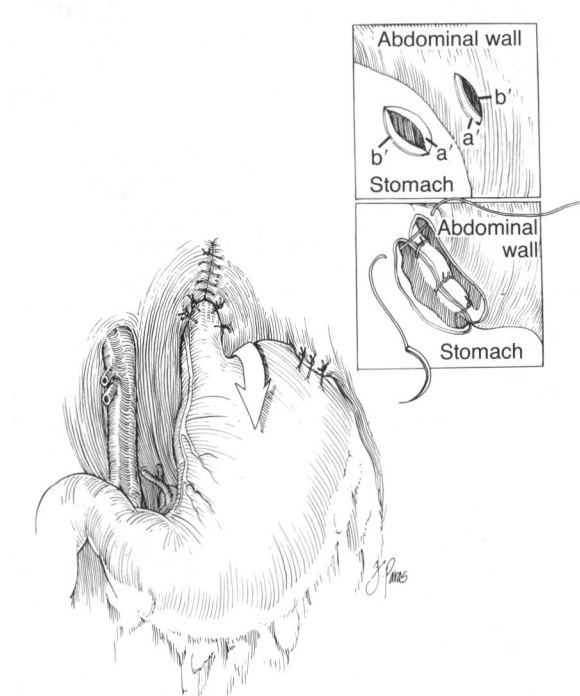

Figure 3. Hiatal plication for hiatal hernia. Place the stomach in its normal position and put slight caudal traction on the stomach to expose the distal esophagus and esophageal hiatus. Plicate the esophageal hiatus with nonabsorbable sutures, then perform an esophagopexy by placing sutures from the diaphragm to the esophageal wall being careful not to penetrate the lumen and not to injure the vagus nerves. Perform a pexy of the fundus to the interior body wall (insets). Incise the seromuscular layer of the fundus and then incise the peritoneum and underlying muscle adjacent to the fundic incision. Suture the stomach wall to the body wall as shown.

■ Some animals may need to be fed from an elevated position for an indefinite period of time.
■ If severe esophagitis was present prior to surgery, continue medical therapy for reflux esophagitis (see sec. 7, ch. 2) with a systemic antacid postoperatively.
  • Omeprazole (0.7 mg/kg per os, once daily) is the preferred antacid. Ranitidine (2–4 mg/kg q8h per os) or cimetidine (5 mg/kg q8h) can be substituted.
  • Administer metoclopramide (0.2–0.4 mg/kg q8h) to most patients for 2–3 weeks postoperatively.
■ Some dysphagia is common for several days following surgery. However, unrelenting dysphagia suggests that the hiatus has been narrowed too much. Reoperation is necessary in those cases that do not respond to medical therapy and when there are signs of dysphagia beyond 1 week.

Long-Term

■ Perform esophagography if signs of regurgitation continue in spite of surgery and follow-up medical therapy.
■ If failure of the "pexy" procedure or if incompetence of the lower esophageal sphincter is suspected, surgical intervention is necessary.
  • If a sphincter-reinforcement procedure is indicated, a Nissen fundoplication procedure is recommended (Fig. 4).

Prognosis

■ The prognosis is good if aspiration pneumonia is controlled.
■ Chronic reflux esophagitis associated with a hiatal hernia may cause various degrees of esophageal stricture. If the pathology is advanced to this degree, the prognosis is poor.

Supplemental Readings

CRICOPHARYNGEAL

Rosin E: Cricopharyngeal achalasia. *In* Bojrab MJ, ed.: *Current Techniques in Small Animal Surgery I.* Philadelphia: Lea & Febiger, 1975, p 190.

Shelton GD: Swallowing disorders in the dog. Comp Contin Educ Pract Vet 4:607, 1982.
Suter PF, Watrous BJ: Oropharyngeal dysphagias in the dog: A cineradiographic analysis of experimentally induced and spontaneously occurring swallowing disorders. Oral stage and pharyngeal stage dysphagia. Vet Radiol 21:24, 1980.

VASCULAR RING ANOMALY

DeHoff WD: Persistent right aortic arch. *In* Bojrab MJ, ed.: *Current Techniques in Small Animal Surgery I.* Philadelphia: Lea & Febiger, 1975, p 301.
Lawson DD, Purie HM: Conditions of the canine esophagus II: Vascular rings, achalasia, tumors, and perioesophageal lesions. J Small Anim Pract 7:117, 1966.
Shires PK, Liu W: Persistent right aortic arch in dogs: A long-term follow-up after surgical correction. J Am Anim Hosp Assoc 17:773, 1981.

ESOPHAGOTOMY

Flanders JA: Problems and complications associated with esophageal surgery. *In* Matthesen DT, ed.: *Problems in Veterinary Medicine: Gastrointestinal Surgical Problems*, Vol. 1. Philadelphia: J B Lippincott, 1989.
Parker N, Caywood D: Surgical diseases of the esophagus. Vet Clin North Am 17:333, 1987.

ESOPHAGEAL RESECTION AND ANASTOMOSIS

Bright RM: Esophagus and stomach. *In* Harvey C, Newton C, and Schwartz A, eds.: *Small Animal Surgery.* Philadelphia: J B Lippincott, 1990, p 323.
Flanders JA: Problems and complications associated with esophageal surgery. *In* Matthesen DT, ed.: *Problems in Veterinary Medicine, Gastrointestinal Surgical Problems*, Vol. 1. Philadelphia: J B Lippincott, 1989.

ESOPHAGOTRACHEAL/BRONCHIAL FISTULAE

Park RD: Bronchoesophageal fistula in the dog: Literature survey, case presentations, and radiographic manifestations. Comp Contin Educ Pract Vet 6:669, 1984.
vanEe R, Dodd VM, Pope E: Bronchoesophageal fistula and transient megaesophagus in a dog. J Am Vet Med Assoc 188:874, 1986.

ESOPHAGEAL DIVERTICULECTOMY

Lantz GC, Bojrab MJ, Jones BD: Epiphrenic esophageal diverticulectomy. J Am Anim Hosp Assoc 12:629, 1976.

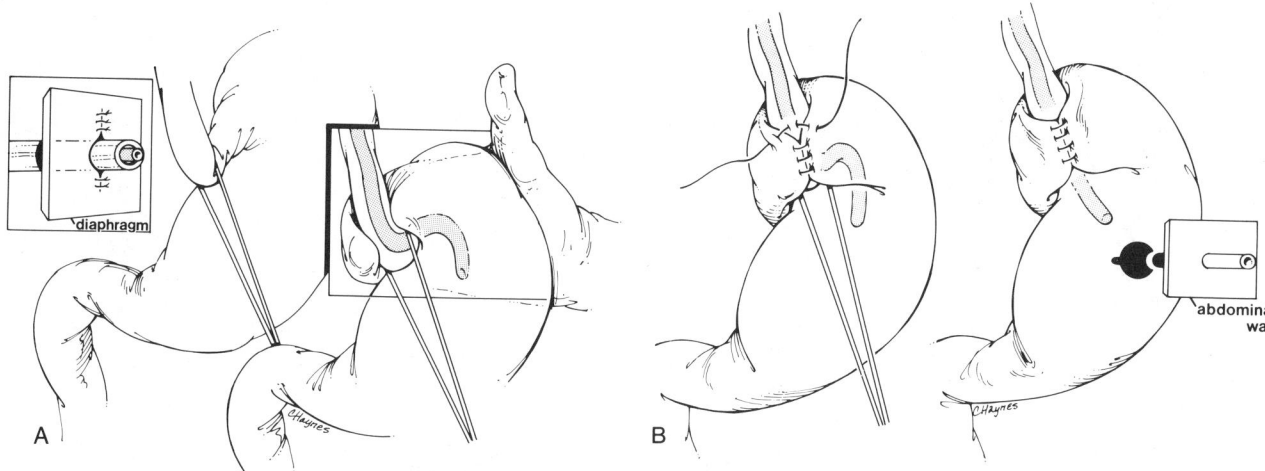

Figure 4. Surgical treatment of hiatal hernia. *A*, Place traction on the distal esophagus and wrap the fundus around the esophagus. *B*, Plicate the fundus around the distal esophagus and place a tube gastrostomy.

ESOPHAGEAL STRICTURE

Craig D, Todhunter R: Surgical repair of an esophageal stricture in a horse. Vet Surg 16:251, 1987.

Pearson H, Darke PG, Gibbs C, et al.: Reflux oesophagitis and stricture formation after anesthesia: A review of seven cases in dogs and cats. J Small Anim Pract 19:507, 1978.

Sooy TE, Adams W, Pitts RP, et al.: Balloon catheter dilatation of alimentary tract strictures in the dog and cat. Vet Radiol 28:131, 1987.

HIATAL HERNIA

Bright RM, Sackman JE, DeNovo RC, et al.: Hiatal hernia in the dog and cat: A retrospective study of 16 cases. J Small Anim Pract 31:244, 1990.

Ellison GW, Lewis DD, Phillips L, et al.: Esophageal hiatal hernia in small animals: literature review and a modified surgical technique. J Am Anim Hosp Assoc 23:391, 1987.

Prymak, Saunders HM, Washabau RJ: Hiatal hernia repair by restoration and stabilization of normal anatomy. An evaluation in four dogs and one cat. Vet Surg 18:386, 1989.

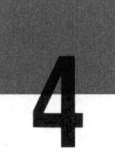

4 Diseases of the Stomach

Susan E. Johnson
Robert G. Sherding
Ronald M. Bright

VOMITING

Vomiting is a common clinical sign associated with many gastrointestinal (GI) and nongastrointestinal (non-GI) disorders of dogs and cats. Vomiting is a central nervous system reflex that is integrated in the vomiting center of the brain stem. Afferent stimuli can originate from the cerebral cortex, chemoreceptor trigger zone, pharynx, peritoneum, or abdominal viscera. Vomiting must be differentiated from regurgitation, which is the passive expulsion of undigested food indicating a pharyngeal (swallowing) or esophageal disorder (see sec. 7, ch. 2).

The metabolic consequences of vomiting vary, depending on the volume and composition of the expulsed fluid. Mild vomiting of short duration usually is not accompanied by overt fluid, electrolyte, or acid-base imbalances. Frequent or profuse vomiting can cause metabolic complications such as dehydration, electrolyte imbalances including hypokalemia, hyponatremia, and hypochloremia, and acid-base imbalances such as metabolic acidosis or metabolic alkalosis. Metabolic alkalosis is most likely to occur in dogs and cats with vomiting secondary to pyloric obstruction. Other potential complications of vomiting include aspiration pneumonia and reflux esophagitis.

Etiology

Vomiting is a clinical sign, rather than a diagnosis, and can be associated with numerous GI and non-GI disorders (Table 1).

KEY POINT ▶ Remember that non-GI disorders commonly cause vomiting; do not overlook these prior to evaluating for primary GI causes of vomiting.

Clinical Signs

- Vomiting frequently is preceded by nausea (evidenced by hypersalivation, licking of the lips, repeated swallowing), retching, and abdominal contractions.
- Vomitus consists of stomach and duodenal contents such as food, mucus, and foamy or bile-stained fluid with a neutral or acidic pH.
- The term *hematemesis* is used when vomitus contains blood flecks, blood clots, or brown coffee grounds–like material (digested blood).
- Vomitus may contain hair, plant material, or other ingested foreign material that can irritate the stomach.
- Vomiting of undigested or partially digested food more than 12–16 hours after eating suggests delayed gastric emptying (functional or mechanical).
- Projectile vomiting (the forceful ejection of vomitus from the mouth that may be expelled a considerable distance) usually indicates gastric or upper small bowel obstruction.
- Other clinical signs may be present depending on the underlying cause of vomiting and the presence of complications such as dehydration or electrolyte and acid-base imbalances.

Diagnosis

The diagnostic approach to vomiting is directed toward identifying the underlying disorder (see Table 1) and is influenced by whether vomiting is acute or chronic and the associated historical and physical abnormalities.

Acute Vomiting. Acute vomiting is a common problem in dogs and cats and may be caused by benign, self-limiting disorders such as acute gastritis or serious life-threatening diseases such as acute pancreatitis, intestinal obstruction, or acute renal or hepatic failure (see Table 1).

- Extensive diagnostic testing is not necessarily warranted in every dog or cat with acute vomiting, because nonspecific, self-limiting acute gastritis is a common cause of acute vomiting.
- Base the decision to perform further testing in an acutely vomiting dog or cat on historical and physical findings.
  - Further evaluation is usually warranted at initial presentation if abnormal physical findings such as fever, lethargy, depression, weakness, dehydration, or palpable abdominal abnormalities are detected.
  - A history of possible GI foreign body exposure may warrant abdominal radiographs even if the physical examination is normal.
- If the history and physical examination are unremarkable, further diagnostic evaluation may be postponed and symptomatic therapy given on an outpatient basis.
- If vomiting does not resolve in 2–3 days or if addi-

TABLE 1. Causes of Vomiting in Dogs and Cats

Acute Vomiting (<1 wk)	Chronic Vomiting (>1–2 wk)
Gastrointestinal Disorders	***Gastrointestinal Disorders***
Diet-related	Diet-related
Sudden diet change	Food intolerance
Food intolerance or allergy	Food allergy
Dietary indiscretion (e.g., garbage)	Chronic gastritis
Acute gastritis or enteritis	Lymphocytic plasmacytic
Ingested bacterial enterotoxins	Eosinophilic
Foreign bodies (e.g., bones, plants, plastic, rocks, hairballs)	Granulomatous (e.g., Zygomycetes)
Ingested chemical irritants or toxins	Foreign bodies (including hairballs)
Drug-induced (e.g., aspirin and other NSAIDs, glucocorticoids, antineoplastics, erythromycin)	Parasites (*Ollulanus, Physaloptera*)
	Reflux gastritis
Viral enteritis (e.g., canine parvovirus, feline panleukopenia, canine distemper)	Hypertrophic gastropathy
	Gastrointestinal ulceration
	Gastric neoplasia
Bacterial infection (e.g., *Gastrospirillum*-like organisms)	Gastric outflow obstruction
	Foreign bodies
Parasites	Gastric neoplasia
Gastric or intestinal obstruction	Gastric polyps
Foreign bodies	Hypertrophic gastropathy
Intestinal volvulus	Pyloric stenosis
Intestinal intussusception	Chronic gastritis
Gastric dilatation-volvulus	Granuloma (Zygomycetes)
	External compression
	Partial gastric dilatation-volvulus
Nongastrointestinal Disorders	Gastric motility disorder
Acute pancreatitis	Hiatal hernia
Acute renal failure	Diaphragmatic hernia
Acute hepatic failure	Chronic colitis
Ketoacidotic diabetes mellitus	Obstipation
Pyometra	Partial distal intestinal obstruction
Prostatitis	
Peritonitis	***Nongastrointestinal Disorders***
Drug-induced (e.g., cardiac glycosides, narcotics, antineoplastics)	Renal failure
	Hepatic disease
	Hypoadrenocorticism
Sepsis	Hyperthyroidism (feline)
CNS disorders (inflammation, edema)	Chronic pancreatitis (feline)
	Heartworm (feline)
Motion sickness	CNS disorders (e.g., inflammatory, neoplastic, visceral epilepsy)
Vestibular disease	
	Lead toxicity

NSAIDs = nonsteroidal anti-inflammatory drugs; CNS = central nervous system.

tional clinical signs develop, further evaluation is indicated.

Chronic Vomiting. Chronic or persistent vomiting is always an indication for further work-up.

History

- Perform a complete history.
- Characterize vomiting as to duration, frequency, progression, relationship to eating, and other specific features (e.g., presence of hematemesis, foreign material, partially digested food).
- Determine if there are other associated clinical signs.
  - Is the appetite decreased or increased?
  - Has there been weight loss?
  - Has there been a change in attitude (depression)?
  - Has there been any diarrhea?
  - Is polyuria or polydipsia present?
  - Is there a history of cough or dyspnea?
- Determine the past medical and worming history.
- Determine the vaccination status.
- Determine the diet.
- Determine if there has been any recent exposure to medications, toxins, plants, string or other foreign bodies, garbage, or other sick animals.

Physical Examination

- The physical examination is often unremarkable in animals with gastric disorders.
- Perform a complete oropharyngeal examination to detect a sublingual string foreign body (especially in cats).
- Palpate the GI tract for masses, foreign bodies, trichobezoars, thickenings, distension, plication, or pain.
- Evaluate for evidence of non-GI causes of vomiting (e.g., lumpy, enlarged, or small kidneys with renal failure; cranial abdominal pain and fever with pancreatitis; icterus or hepatomegaly with liver failure; palpable thyroid nodule with feline hyperthyroidism).
- Perform a digital rectal examination to evaluate the character of the feces (e.g., presence of melena, foreign material, blood, and mucus) and to obtain a sample for fecal evaluation.
- Evaluate for systemic effects or complications of vomiting (e.g., dehydration, weakness, cachexia).
- Findings that suggest potentially serious underlying disease include hematemesis, weakness, severe depression, anorexia, abdominal mass, fever, abdominal pain, abdominal distension, dehydration, and shock.

Laboratory Evaluation

- When further diagnostic testing is indicated, a stepwise strategy is recommended.
- Perform routine hematology, biochemistries (including serum amylase and lipase), urinalysis, survey abdominal radiographs, and miscellaneous ancillary tests, such as serum T_4 in cats > 6 years of age, feline leukemia virus (FeLV) antigen test, feline immunodeficiency virus (FIV) antibody test, as indicated by the history and physical examination. These evaluations are necessary to rule out non-GI disorders that cause vomiting prior to evaluating for primary GI disorders with contrast radiology, endoscopy, or exploratory laparotomy.
- Routine blood tests are also helpful to detect and characterize metabolic complications of vomiting such as dehydration and electrolyte imbalances.
- Perform a fecal flotation test to diagnose GI parasitism, especially if vomiting is accompanied by diarrhea.
- Perform a fecal occult blood test to detect occult GI bleeding when blood loss is suspected but overt melena is absent.

Radiography

- Perform routine ventrodorsal and lateral abdominal radiographs to identify radiopaque foreign bodies, gastric or intestinal obstruction, and abdominal masses or abnormalities of the kidneys, liver, and pancreas.
- Perform contrast radiography to evaluate for GI causes of vomiting such as radiolucent foreign bodies, obstruction, and mural thickening or irregularity. Barium administered by stomach tube is usually recommended (see sec. 1, ch. 4). Barium mixed with food may be better than liquid barium to detect a gastric retention disorder. Double air-barium contrast gastrography can also be performed.
  - Use aqueous iodide contrast (Gastrografin, Squibb Diagnostics) rather than barium if perforation is suspected.
- Perform abdominal ultrasonography to evaluate for non-GI disorders associated with vomiting that are suspected based on initial blood work (e.g., pancreatitis, hepatic or renal disease). Ultrasonography may also be helpful to evaluate primary GI disorders such as intussusception and gastric outflow obstruction.

Endoscopy

Endoscopy of the stomach and proximal duodenum is a noninvasive technique for evaluation of primary upper GI disorders associated with vomiting. Endoscopy is used to obtain biopsies, remove foreign bodies, and collect intraluminal juices.

- Endoscopy requires general anesthesia and a flexible fiberoptic endoscope. The most versatile endoscope for use in evaluating the GI tract of dogs and cats is one at least 100 cm long with a 7.9-mm diameter shaft, 2.0- to 2.8-mm biopsy channel, four-way angulation of the tip, and flush and suction capabilities.
- Routinely evaluate the esophagus, stomach, pylorus, and proximal duodenum. Perform mucosal biopsies in all cases because abnormal histologic findings may be present despite a normal gross appearance.

Laparotomy

- Exploratory laparotomy is sometimes indicated for diagnosis or treatment of primary GI disorders, especially when endoscopy is not available.
- Obtain full-thickness gastric and intestinal biopsies (see sec. 7, chs. 5 and 7).

Treatment

Treatment strategies in the vomiting animal are directed toward:

- Correction of the underlying cause of vomiting, whenever possible
- Symptomatic and supportive therapy of vomiting and its metabolic complications.
- Surgery is indicated to remove large gastric foreign bodies, excise localized tumors and deep ulcers, and correct gastric outflow obstruction.

Fluid Therapy

- Give fluids parenterally because vomiting usually precludes adequate oral intake of fluid. Treat mild dehydration, in the absence of other systemic signs, with subcutaneous fluid administration. Intravenous fluid therapy is preferred for animals with moderate to severe dehydration. Daily fluid therapy requirements in the vomiting dog or cat depend on the degree of dehydration, ongoing fluid losses, and maintenance needs (see sec. 1, ch. 5).
- Ideally, base the choice of replacement fluid on serum electrolyte concentrations and blood gas analysis, because the electrolyte and acid-base changes that occur secondary to vomiting may vary considerably. In the absence of such information, use a balanced electrolyte solution such as Ringer's or 0.9% saline. Additional potassium supplementation (see sec. 1, ch. 5) usually will be necessary because hypokalemia is a common complication of vomiting.
- If metabolic acidosis is present, use an alkalinizing solution such as lactated Ringer's. Sodium bicarbonate administration is necessary only in treatment of severe metabolic acidosis (pH < 7.1–7.2)(see sec. 1, ch. 5).
- Hypochloremic metabolic alkalosis is most likely to occur with pyloric obstruction. Give 0.9% saline supplemented with potassium chloride.

Dietary Management of Acute Vomiting

- Restrict oral intake of food to minimize vomiting and further fluid loss. Withhold food for at least 12 to 24 hours.
- If vomiting resolves, offer a bland, digestible, moderately fat-restricted diet such as Prescription Diet i/d (Hill's Pet), chicken and rice, or low-fat cottage cheese and rice.
- After 2 to 3 days on the bland diet, gradually reintroduce the animal's routine diet over a period of 2–3 days.

Antiemetics

Antiemetics are used for symptomatic control of acute vomiting on a short-term basis or to control profuse vomiting that results in fluid, electrolyte, or acid-base imbalances.

Phenothiazines. Phenothiazine derivatives are broad-spectrum, central-acting antiemetics that inhibit the chemoreceptor trigger zone (CRTZ) at low doses and depress the vomiting center at higher doses. Phenothiazines, especially chlorpromazine (0.5 mg/kg q6–8h, SC or IM; 0.05 mg/kg IV) and prochlorperazine (0.5 mg/kg q6–8h, IV, SC, or IM) are the most widely used antiemetics.

- Hypotension, a potentially serious side effect, is caused by alpha-adrenergic receptor blockade. Consequently, use phenothiazines cautiously in patients with pre-existing dehydration.
- Sedation may occur because of concurrent tranquilizing properties; however, the dose required for antiemetic activity is lower than the sedative dose.

Metoclopramide. Metoclopramide (Reglan, A. H. Robins) (0.2–0.4 mg/kg q8h, PO, IM, or SC; or 1–2 mg/kg/24h as a constant-rate IV infusion) possesses both central and peripheral antiemetic properties. Central effects are attributed to antidopaminergic activity at the CRTZ; the peripheral antiemetic effect is due to its stimulant effect on GI motility. Metoclopramide promotes gastric emptying by increasing the tone and amplitude of gastric contractions and relaxation of the pylorus (Fig. 1). Because gastric relaxation and retroperistalsis are key events preceding vomiting, their inhibition may account in part for the drug's peripheral antiemetic effect.

- Metoclopramide is particularly effective in preventing chemotherapy-induced nausea and vomiting.
- It is indicated for control of vomiting associated with parvoviral gastroenteritis because this disorder may be complicated by delayed gastric emptying.

Anticholinergic Drugs. Avoid the use of anticholinergic drugs such as isopropamide, atropine, and aminopentamide hydrogen sulfate (Centrine, Fort Dodge) for routine symptomatic control of vomiting.

- Although anticholinergics may decrease peripheral afferent stimulation of the vomiting center by relieving GI smooth muscle spasms or inhibiting intestinal secretions, their side effects include xerostomia, mydriasis, tachycardia, urinary retention, ileus, and gastric retention.
- Because delayed gastric emptying caused by anticholinergics can in itself cause vomiting, these drugs should not be used any longer than three days in a vomiting patient.

ACUTE GASTRITIS

Acute gastritis is a common disease in dogs and cats. It is usually a mild, self-limiting condition that rarely warrants biopsy confirmation. Clinical diagnosis of acute gastritis often is made when acute vomiting occurs without apparent cause and resolves on its own in 24–48 hours.

Etiology

There are numerous potential etiologies of acute gastritis (see Table 1), but the cause often is not determined. Possible causes include the following:

- *Dietary indiscretion* is frequently associated with acute gastritis and vomiting. Gastritis is most likely due to ingestion of rancid or spoiled foods that contain fermentation by-products, bacterial enterotoxins, or mycotoxins.
- *Foreign-body ingestion* (e.g., rocks, aluminum foil, small toys, food wrappings, or plastic) can cause mechanical irritation of the gastric mucosa.
- *Ingested plant material* including grass and house plants is a common cause of acute gastritis.
- *Chemical irritants or toxins* (e.g., fertilizers, herbicides, cleaning agents, heavy metals such as lead) can cause gastric irritation.
- *Drugs* (e.g., aspirin, phenylbutazone, glucocorticoids) can cause acute gastritis which is frequently accompanied by erosions and ulceration.
- *Viral infections* such as canine parvovirus, feline panleukopenia, or canine distemper can cause lesions of gastritis in addition to more diffuse intestinal and systemic involvement.
- *Bacterial infections* causing gastritis are uncommon. Gastric spirillum-like organisms may play a role in gastritis in some dogs and cats but can also be present in asymptomatic animals.
- *Parasitic infections* of the stomach are uncommon. *Physaloptera* spp infect dogs and cats but the infection is not consistently associated with clinical signs. *Ollulanus tricuspis* is a cause of chronic gastritis in cats.
- *Systemic disorders* such as uremia, liver disease, neurologic disease, shock, stress, and sepsis may be associated with acute gastritis by altering the gastric mucosal barrier, mucosal blood flow, or gastric acidity.

Clinical Signs

- Acute onset of vomiting
- Acute anorexia, lethargy, and diarrhea

Diagnosis

Because acute gastritis is usually self-limiting, diagnostic evaluations are not usually warranted unless specific historical or physical findings suggest a more serious problem. Response to supportive therapy in 1–3 days indirectly supports the diagnosis of uncomplicated acute gastritis as the cause of vomiting.

History

- Acute vomiting in an otherwise healthy animal suggests the possibility of acute gastritis.
- Perform a detailed historical evaluation including

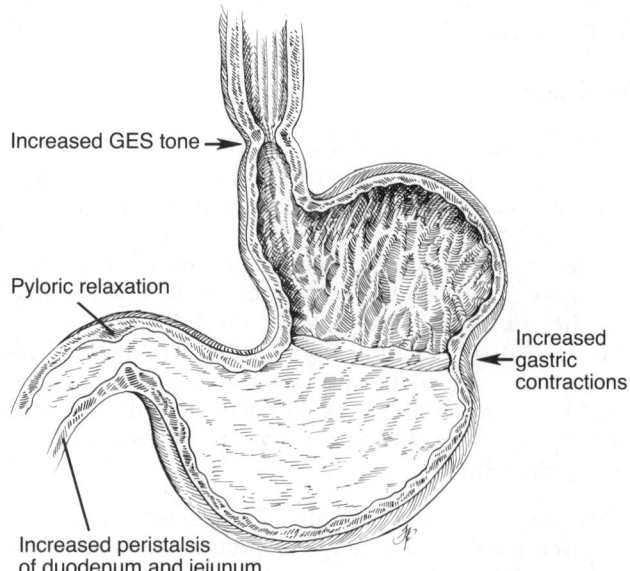

Increased GES tone →

Pyloric relaxation

Increased gastric contractions ←

Increased peristalsis of duodenum and jejunum

Figure 1. Effects of the promotility agent metoclopramide on the gastrointestinal tract. Metoclopramide increases gastroesophageal sphincter tone and promotes gastric emptying by coordinating increased gastric contractions with pyloric relaxation and increased intestinal peristalsis.

recent exposure to drugs or other sick animals and the potential for dietary indiscretion.

Physical Examination

- The physical examination is usually unremarkable unless acute gastritis is complicated by dehydration.

Treatment

Identify and treat underlying causes when possible.

Dietary Restriction

- Withhold food for 12–24 hours.
- Reintroduce food when vomiting has ceased for > 24 hours. Offer a bland, digestible, moderately fat-restricted diet such as Prescription Diet i/d (Hill's Pet), chicken and rice, or low-fat cottage cheese and rice.
- After 2–3 days on the bland diet, gradually reintroduce the animal's routine diet over a period of 2–3 days.

Maintenance of Hydration

- For oral hydration, offer ice cubes, small amounts of water, or oral electrolyte solutions such as Pedialyte (Ross Labs.) and Entrolyte (Beecham Labs.). Give at frequent intervals to provide daily maintenance requirements.
- Parenteral fluid therapy is indicated to treat dehydration (see previous discussion of fluid therapy in the vomiting patient and refer to sec. 1, ch. 5).
- Consider using antiemetics for short term symptomatic control of vomiting (see previous discussion).
- If vomiting does not resolve in 1–3 days, pursue further diagnostic evaluation (see previous discussion).

GASTRIC FOREIGN BODIES

Gastric foreign bodies are most common in dogs owing to their dietary habits and indiscriminant chewing behavior.

Etiology

- Gastric foreign bodies frequently seen in dogs include needles, coins, stones, sticks, peach pits, plastic, aluminum foil, Super Balls, and small toys.
- String and other linear foreign bodies are more likely in cats.
- Gastric foreign bodies cause clinical signs because of mechanical irritation (e.g., acute or chronic gastritis) or gastric outflow obstruction.

Clinical Signs

- Most dogs and cats with a gastric foreign body are presented for acute onset of vomiting. However, if the foreign body goes undiagnosed initially, chronic vomiting may be the primary complaint.
- Additional clinical signs may be seen if systemic absorption of a toxic component occurs. For example:

- Zinc-induced hemolytic anemia has been described secondary to ingestion of zinc-containing nuts and bolts or pennies minted after 1983.
- Lead-containing foreign bodies may be associated with significant lead absorption and toxicity.
- Neurologic signs due to absorption of aluminum also have been described.

Diagnosis

Consider gastric foreign bodies in all animals with acute vomiting and a history of chewing on foreign objects.

Physical Examination

- This is often unremarkable except when gastric foreign bodies are very large and palpable.

Radiography

- Abdominal radiographs can identify radiopaque objects (e.g., coins, needles, other metal objects), radiodense objects, and gastric outflow obstruction (gas-, fluid-, or food-distended stomach).
- A contrast gastrogram may be necessary to detect radiolucent gastric foreign bodies.

Endoscopy

- Endoscopy can confirm a suspected gastric foreign body and, more important, can remove most objects noninvasively. For this reason, endoscopy often is preferable to a barium-contrast study, unless general anesthesia is contraindicated.

Treatment

When a gastric foreign body is identified radiographically, consider whether immediate removal is necessary.

- Remove the object promptly if it is large, sharp, or potentially toxic (e.g., pennies, nuts and bolts, lead objects) or if the animal is persistently vomiting, anorexic, or dehydrated.
- Small, nontoxic foreign bodies may pass through the GI tract uneventfully and thus can be managed conservatively if the animal is not symptomatic. Allow a period of 7–10 days while periodically repeating radiographs to monitor progress. If clinical signs develop, immediate removal is recommended.

Endoscopic Removal

Attempt endoscopic removal of gastric foreign bodies prior to gastrotomy, because most foreign bodies can be removed in this manner.

- Fast the animal 8–12 hours prior to anesthesia to be sure that the stomach is empty, because food can obscure the endoscopic view. Correct fluid, electrolyte, and acid-base imbalances prior to general anesthesia.
- Repeat abdominal radiographs immediately prior to induction of anesthesia to confirm that the object is

still in the stomach. This will avoid an unnecessary procedure if the object has already entered the intestinal tract and is beyond the reach of the endoscope.

- The key to removing foreign bodies endoscopically is to get a firm grip on the object, using a grasping forceps or a basket retrieval instrument.
  - Use forceps for retrieval of needles, coins, and small soft objects. To remove the foreign body, grasp the object, pull it up near the end of the endoscope, and remove the endoscope, instrument, and foreign body as one unit.
  - Use the basket for retrieval of small round objects such as marbles or stones that cannot be grasped with the forceps. Large smooth objects are also removed with a basket, but they can be especially difficult to maneuver back through the gastroesophageal sphincter (or upper esophageal sphincter).
  - Use an overtube (a plastic tube that fits over the shaft of the endoscope and can be advanced off the end of the endoscope) to protect the esophageal mucosa when sharp or pointed objects are withdrawn. An overtube is also useful to assist removal of objects through the gastroesophageal sphincter by maintaining sphincter dilation.
- After removing the foreign body, perform a thorough examination of the stomach to look for other objects or mucosal lesions. This should be done even if only one object is seen radiographically, because radiolucent objects may not have been detected or multiple objects may have previously adhered to each other. If food obscures the endoscopic view, reposition the animal in the alternate lateral position or a ventral dorsal position.

Gastrotomy

If endoscopic equipment is unavailable or the object cannot be retrieved endoscopically, gastrotomy is indicated (see sec. 7, ch. 5).

Postoperative Care and Complications

- Food and water can be given orally 12–24 hours after removal.
- If mucosal injury is severe, treat as for gastric ulcer (see below).

GASTRODUODENAL ULCERATION

For the purposes of this discussion, gastroduodenal ulceration is defined as mucosal defects associated with bleeding, which includes petechiations, erosions, and ulcers. Clinical recognition of gastroduodenal ulceration as a complicating factor in many disorders is becoming more common, most likely due to the increased use of endoscopy.

Etiology

Many disorders have been associated with gastroduodenal ulceration (Table 2). Ulceration is more likely when two or more risk factors are present. General mechanisms of gastroduodenal ulceration include direct damage to the gastric mucosal barrier, increased gastric acid secretion, delayed gastric epithelial renewal, and decreased gastric mucosal blood flow.

Non-Steroidal Anti-Inflammatory Drugs (NSAIDs). NSAIDs (Table 2) are frequent causes of gastric ulceration. These drugs inhibit prostaglandin synthesis, which decreases mucosal blood flow and alters gastric mucus production, thus predisposing to ulceration.

- Both gastric hemorrhage and large perforating ulcers may occur. A predilection for ulceration of the pyloroantral region has been recognized.
- Ulceration is most likely to occur when NSAIDs are given to animals with other risk factors (see Table 2).
- Dogs are more susceptible to the ulcerogenic effects of NSAIDs than are humans.

Glucocorticoids

- Glucocorticoid therapy has been associated with gastric erosions and bleeding but usually only when combined with other risk factors for ulceration such as NSAIDs (see Table 2).
- Dexamethasone, especially at high doses, is more likely to cause gastrointestinal bleeding than is prednisolone.

Hepatic Disease. Hepatic diseases of all types are commonly associated with ulceration. Potential mechanisms include decreased mucosal blood flow secondary to portal hypertension, decreased gastric epithelial cell turnover associated with negative nitrogen balance and hypoalbuminemia, increased gastric acid secretion

---

TABLE 2. Risk Factors for Gastroduodenal Ulceration

Drug-induced gastrointestinal damage
  Aspirin
  Flunixin
  Ibuprofen
  Indomethacin
  Meclofenamic acid
  Naproxen
  Phenylbutazone
  Piroxicam
  Glucocorticoids
Infiltrative disease
  Gastric neoplasia
  Eosinophilic gastroenteritis
  Lymphocytic plasmacytic gastroenteritis
  Gastric Zygomycetes
Liver disease
Renal failure
Mast cell tumor
Spinal cord disease
Stress conditions
  Severe illness
  Major surgery
  Hypotension
  Trauma
  Shock
Hypoadrenocorticism
Lead poisoning
Cyclic hematopoiesis (gray collies)
Enterogastric reflux
Gastrinoma (Zollinger-Ellison syndrome)

due to impaired degradation of a secretagogue (possibly histamine), or stimulation of gastrin release by increased serum bile acids.

■ Coexisting coagulopathies will magnify GI blood loss.
■ Duodenal ulceration is more common than gastric ulceration.

Renal Failure. Renal failure may be associated with GI hemorrhage and ulceration. Multiple factors probably contribute, including damage of the gastric mucosal barrier by urea, uremic vasculitis, and increased concentrations of gastrin with hypersecretion of gastric acid.

Gastritis. Eosinophilic gastritis, lymphocytic-plasmacytic gastritis, and granulomatous gastritis may be complicated by mucosal ulcerations.

Neoplasia. Gastric neoplasia, especially adenocarcinoma, frequently is associated with mucosal hemorrhage and erosions.

Mast Cell Tumors. These tumors can cause GI ulceration due to histamine-induced gastric acid hypersecretion.

■ Perform a thorough search for cutaneous masses in all animals with GI bleeding and ulceration to identify a predisposing mast cell tumor.

Gastrinoma. This rare gastrin-producing tumor, arising from the APUD cells of the pancreas, causes gastric acid hypersecretion and gastroduodenal ulceration.

■ Suspect gastrinoma when ulceration is associated with gastric mucosal hypertrophy or when ulcers respond to medical management but relapse when therapy is discontinued and no underlying cause can be identified.
■ Diagnosis is made by documenting hypergastrinemia and finding the tumor on surgical exploration.
■ Most pancreatic gastrinomas are small (<2 cm) and have metastasized to regional lymph nodes and liver at the time of diagnosis.
■ Tumor cytoreduction may be a useful palliative procedure to temporarily control clinical signs along with medical therapy to control ulceration (see under Treatment).

Neurologic Disease. Neurologic disease can predispose to GI ulceration, especially in dogs with spinal cord disease that are receiving corticosteroids. Colonic perforation, septic peritonitis, and sudden death have been described.

Stress Conditions. Severe illness, major surgery, trauma, shock, and hypotension can all predispose to gastroduodenal bleeding and ulceration.

■ Acutely ill, intensive-care patients are most at risk.
■ Consider a presumptive diagnosis of gastroduodenal ulceration when vomiting or hematemesis occurs in this clinical setting.

Clinical Signs

■ Signs include anorexia, vomiting, melena, abdominal pain, and weight loss. The vomitus may contain digested blood (coffee-grounds appearance) or fresh blood with clots. Overt hematemesis and melena may not be consistently observed by the owner. Weakness associated with blood loss anemia may occur.
■ Ulcer perforation and septic peritonitis are suggested by acute onset of abdominal pain, depression, collapse, and shock.

Diagnosis

History

Perform a detailed history. Determine if any ulcerogenic drugs have been administered recently (see Table 2).

Physical Examination

■ Palpate the abdomen for abdominal pain.
■ Evaluate the mucous membranes for evidence of anemia.
■ Perform a rectal examination to evaluate for melena.
■ If hematemesis and melena are present, evaluate the skin and mucous membranes for hemorrhages, which may suggest that GI bleeding is secondary to a systemic coagulopathy.
■ Perform a thorough examination for cutaneous masses that may be mast cell tumors.

Laboratory Evaluation

Complete Blood Count (CBC). Perform a CBC to assess for anemia.

■ Acute GI bleeding is associated with a normocytic normochromic regenerative anemia, whereas chronic blood loss is characterized by iron deficiency and microcytic hypochromic anemia (see sec. 3, ch. 1).
■ With peracute GI bleeding, nonregenerative anemia may be detected initially until the bone marrow has adequate time to respond (3–5 days).
■ Iron deficiency is further characterized by decreased serum iron concentration and decreased per cent saturation.
■ With active bleeding, anemia is accompanied by hypoproteinemia.
■ A neutrophilia and left shift may be seen with severe inflammation and ulcer perforation.

Other Laboratory Tests
■ A biochemistry profile is indicated to identify underlying liver disease (see sec. 7, ch. 8), renal failure (see sec. 8, ch. 1), and hypoadrenocorticism (see sec. 4, ch. 3). Decreased total protein and albumin levels are common with blood loss, but liver disease, renal disease, and malnutrition also may contribute to these changes.
■ Evaluate for dehydration and electrolyte imbalances secondary to vomiting.
■ Perform blood gas analysis to assess acid-base imbalances.
■ Perform a urinalysis to screen for underlying systemic disorders.
■ If GI blood loss is suspected and the stool is grossly normal, perform a fecal occult blood test. Perform

- a fecal flotation to diagnose hookworm infection as a cause of GI blood loss.
- Screen for underlying bleeding disorders with evaluations such as one-stage prothrombin time, activated partial thromboplastin time, platelet count, fibrinogen, and fibrin degradation products (FDPs).
- Perform fine-needle aspiration (or biopsy) of any cutaneous masses to diagnose mast cell tumor.
- If gastrinoma is suspected, evaluate a fasting serum gastrin concentration and measure gastrin after a provocative secretin injection.

Radiography

- Survey abdominal radiographs usually are unremarkable unless ulcer perforation results in pneumoperitoneum or peritoneal effusion (peritonitis).
- A GI contrast study will usually outline large ulcers but is an insensitive method for detecting small ulcers and erosions. If perforation is suspected, use an iodide contrast agent rather than barium.

Abdominocentesis

Perform abdominocentesis to detect septic peritonitis secondary to ulcer perforation. Submit a sample for bacterial culture and antibiotic sensitivity testing.

Endoscopy

Endoscopy is indicated to characterize the location and severity of upper GI bleeding.

KEY POINT ▶ Endoscopy is more reliable for detection of mucosal ulcers and erosions and is preferred over contrast radiography, unless general anesthesia is contraindicated.

- Concurrent gastric mucosal thickening or mass lesions suggest an underlying neoplastic or inflammatory disorder.
- Perform mucosal biopsies regardless of the gross appearance, to identify predisposing causes such as gastritis or gastric neoplasia.
- If perforation is suspected, perform exploratory laparotomy.

Laparotomy

Laparotomy can be used to diagnose and resect gastroduodenal ulcers.

- Evaluate other abdominal organs, including the kidneys and liver.
- Carefully palpate the pancreas to identify gastrinoma nodules.

Treatment

The goals of management of gastroduodenal ulceration include the following:

- Eliminate or control predisposing factors (see Table 2). Correct fluid, electrolyte, and acid-base imbalances.

- Control any GI bleeding and correct resulting anemia. If the packed cell volume (PCV) is <15%, give a blood transfusion (see sec. 3, ch. 1).
- Control gastric acid secretion (Fig. 2).
- Promote mucosal cytoprotection.

Agents that Control Gastric Acid Secretion

Antacids. Antacids can effectively neutralize gastric acid secretion; however, H$_2$ blockers are preferred because of their ease of administration and potency (Table 3).

H$_2$ Blockers. These drugs are most commonly used to control acid secretion. They inhibit basal, nocturnal, and meal-stimulated acid secretion by blocking the H$_2$ receptors on gastric parietal cells (see Fig. 2). H$_2$ blockers inhibit acid secretion stimulated by histamine but have less of an inhibitory effect against other secretagogues such as gastrin and acetylcholine. Several H$_2$ blockers (e.g., cimetidine, ranitidine, famotidine) are available that are equally effective but differ in potency, frequency of administration, and potential to inhibit hepatic p-450 enzymes (see Table 3).

Omeprazole. Omeprazole (Prilosec, Merck Sharp & Dohme) is a potent inhibitor of gastric acid secretion that acts by inhibiting hydrogen potassium ATPase (the proton pump) of the gastric parietal cell (see Fig. 2). This drug has broad-spectrum antisecretory activity because the proton pump is the final common pathway for hydrochloric acid production, regardless of initiating stimulus. Because of its long duration of action, omeprazole can be given on a once-daily basis (see Table 3). It is more expensive than the H$_2$ blockers but is indicated when ulcers do not respond to treatment with H$_2$ blockers and sucralfate.

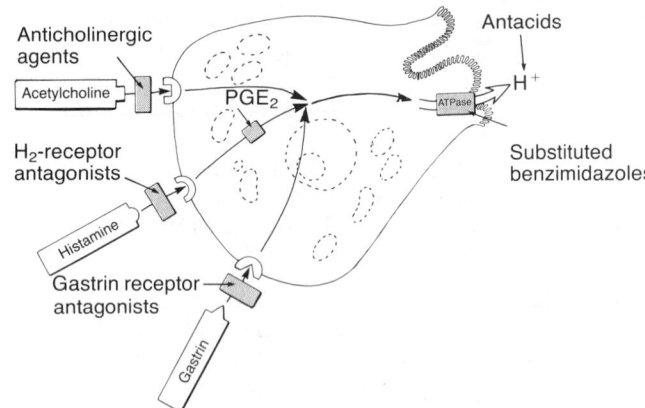

Figure 2. Representation of a gastric parietal cell showing the site of action of various therapeutic agents used to decrease gastric acidity. Acid secretion may occur via acetylcholine, histamine, or gastrin stimulation of their respective receptors. H$_2$-receptor antagonists (blockers) primarily inhibit histamine-induced acid secretion. Prostaglandin (PGE$_2$) analogs, such as misoprostol, inhibit acid secretion by blocking histamine-induced cAMP production. Use of anticholinergic drugs to inhibit acid secretion is limited by systemic side effects. The gastrin receptor antagonist proglumide is given for experimental purposes only. Substituted benzimidazoles, such as omeprazole, have broad-spectrum antisecretory activity because they interrupt the final common pathway of acid secretion by inhibiting hydrogen potassium ATPase. Antacids neutralize luminal gastric acid.

Agents that Promote Mucosal Cytoprotection

Sucralfate. Sucralfate (Carafate, Marion Merrell Dow) is an aluminum salt that selectively binds to injured gastroesophageal mucosa, forming a protective "bandage." Sucralfate neutralizes acid, inactivates pepsin, adsorbs bile acids and pancreatic enzymes, and stimulates local prostaglandins which are cytoprotective. It is a safe drug with minimal systemic absorption.

KEY POINT ▶ For initial treatment of gastric ulcers and erosions, combine an H_2 blocker for acid control with sucralfate for mucosal cytoprotection.

Misoprostol. Misoprostol (Cytotec, Searle) is a synthetic prostaglandin analog that at low doses (3–5 μg/kg) is cytoprotective and at high doses (10 μg/kg) has antisecretory activity (see Fig. 2). The primary indication for use of misoprostol in humans is to prevent NSAID-induced gastric injury. Preliminary evaluation in dogs suggests a similar indication. Side effects (especially at the higher dose) include diarrhea and abortion (see Table 3).

Antibiotic Therapy

- Give systemic antibiotics when ulcer perforation is suspected or confirmed.
- Select the antibiotic based on results of culture and sensitivity testing of abdominal fluid or affected tissue.
- Give an aminoglycoside (e.g., amikacin, gentamicin) combined with a cephalosporin (e.g., cephalothin) while awaiting culture results. Avoid aminoglycosides in the presence of renal insufficiency.

Laparotomy

Emergency exploratory laparotomy is indicated when perforation of a gastroduodenal ulcer is suspected or confirmed (see sec. 7, ch. 13 for detailed description of treatment for peritonitis).

- Correct fluid, electrolyte, and acid-base imbalances as rapidly as possible prior to surgery.
- Treat shock as described in sec. 6, ch. 14.

Prevention

- Avoid giving NSAIDs other than aspirin to dogs and cats. Use recommended doses of aspirin and monitor for occult bleeding, melena, or vomiting to detect early GI bleeding. Do not give glucocorticoids concurrently.
  - Misoprostol is probably the drug of choice to prevent NSAID-induced injury; however, this drug is relatively new and its clinical use in dogs is only preliminary. In humans, misoprostol is preferred to sucralfate for this purpose.
  - Omeprazole provides some protection against the development of aspirin-induced GI damage in dogs, but cimetidine appears to be ineffective.
- The use of an H_2 blocker or sucralfate to prevent ulceration in animals being given glucocorticoids is probably not warranted on a routine basis.

- Consider use of these drugs if multiple risk factors are present or if any degree of GI bleeding would be poorly tolerated by the patient.

CHRONIC GASTRITIS

Chronic gastritis is a common cause of chronic and episodic vomiting in dogs and cats. Chronic gastritis is classified based on histologic features such as type of inflammatory infiltrate and the presence of fibrosis, atrophy, or mucosal hypertrophy. The most common histologic category is lymphocytic-plasmacytic gastritis, which is a nonspecific tissue reaction to many insults.

Etiology

Regardless of the initial insult, damage to the gastric mucosa allows back-diffusion of gastric acid, which, in turn, promotes further mucosal injury. Immune-mediated mechanisms may occur secondary to mucosal damage that further promote inflammation.

- The underlying etiology of chronic gastritis is seldom determined. Possible causes include all factors capable of causing acute gastritis (see Table 1) where repeated or persistent exposure occurs.
- In cats, lymphocytic-plasmacytic gastritis is often accompanied by diffuse inflammatory bowel disease.
- Gastroduodenal ulcerations may be associated with secondary lymphocytic-plasmacytic gastritis that resolves after ulcer therapy. Conversely, lymphocytic-plasmacytic gastritis may be complicated by gastric erosions and ulcerations.
- *Ollulanus tricuspis* is associated with chronic fibrosing gastritis in cats.
- Granulomatous gastritis occurs rarely and has been described in association with fungal infection caused by Zygomycetes.
- Reflux gastritis (or bilious vomiting syndrome) refers to gastric mucosal damage caused by persistent enterogastric reflux of potentially damaging constituents such as bile and pancreatic enzymes. Inappropriate pyloric relaxation predisposes to excess reflux, and impaired gastric motility contributes to delay in clearing previously refluxed material from the stomach. Reflux gastritis is a poorly documented clinical entity in dogs.
- Gastric *Spirillum*-like bacteria may play a role in chronic gastritis in some dogs and cats but can also be present in asymptomatic animals.
- Eosinophilic gastritis is discussed in this chapter.

Clinical Signs

- Animals with *chronic gastritis* have intermittent vomiting, usually over a period of weeks to months. Vomiting is not consistently associated with eating. Hematemesis and melena may occur if gastritis is associated with mucosal erosions or ulcers.
- Other signs such as depression, anorexia, weight loss, and abdominal pain are present less frequently.
- Signs of *reflux gastritis* include nausea, vomiting of bile-stained fluid or foam early in the morning when the stomach is empty, and abdominal pain. Most

TABLE 3. Drugs Used for Treatment of Gastric Disease

	Product (Manufacturer)	Preparations	Dosage	Special Indications	Comments*
H₂ Blockers					
Cimetidine	Tagamet (Smith Kline Beecham)	Liquid: 60 mg/ml Tabs: 200 mg, 300 mg, 400 mg, 800 mg Injectable: 150 mg/ml	5–10 mg/kg PO or IV q6–8h	First choice to decrease gastric acid secretion.	Inhibits hepatic P-450 drug metabolizing enzymes. Decrease the dose of the following drugs if used concurrently: lidocaine, propranolol, theophylline, diazepam, phenytoin, warfarin. Does not decrease hepatic blood flow. Simultaneous oral administration of cimetidine and sucralfate or cimetidine and metoclopramide is acceptable if using the higher dose range for cimetidine. Separate oral administration from antacids by ≥ 1 hour. Decrease dosage in renal failure.
Ranitidine	Zantac (Glaxo)	Liquid: 15 mg/ml Tabs: 150 mg, 300 mg Injectable: 25 mg/ml	2.0 mg/kg PO or IV q8–12h (dog); 2.5 mg/kg IV q12h or 3.5 mg/kg PO q12h (cat)	Decrease gastric acid secretion. Preferred over cimetidine when concurrently administering drugs dependent on hepatic metabolism.† Less frequent administration than cimetidine.	4–10 × as potent as cimetidine. Minimal inhibition of hepatic P-450 enzymes. No effect on hepatic blood flow. Separate oral administration from antacids by ≥1 hour. Decrease dose in renal failure.
Famotidine	Pepcid (Merck Sharp & Dohme)	Liquid: 8 mg/ml Tabs: 20 mg, 40 mg Injectable: 10 mg/ml	0.5–1.0 mg/kg PO or IV q12–24h	Decrease gastric acid secretion. Preferred over cimetidine when concurrently administering drugs dependent on hepatic metabolism.† Once-a-day dosing convenience.	20–50 × as potent as cimetidine. No inhibition of hepatic drug metabolizing enzymes and no effect on hepatic blood flow. Decrease dose in renal failure.
Mucosal Protectants					
Sucralfate	Carafate (Marion)	Tabs: 1 gm	1 gm–large dogs, 0.5 gm–small dogs, 0.25 gm–cats; PO q8–12h	GI erosions and ulcers; NSAID-induced gastritis; reflux esophagitis (suspension).	Safe local-acting drug. Potential for nonspecific binding with impaired absorption of simultaneously administered oral drugs. No effect (in dogs) on absorption of the following drugs: digoxin, quinidine, propranolol, aminophylline, diazepam, imipramine, chlorpromazine. Minor effect on cimetidine absorption; not clinically significant at higher doses of cimetidine (and other H₂ blockers?). Separate phenytoin, tetracycline, and fluoroquinolone antibiotics from sucralfate by ≥ 2 hours. Antacids interfere with sucralfate binding—give antacids ≥ 30 min after sucralfate. Contains aluminum—use cautiously in renal failure. Side effect: constipation.
Proton Pump Inhibitors					
Omeprazole‡	Prilosec (Merck Sharp & Dohme)	Caps: 20 mg (delayed release)	0.75–1.0 mg/kg PO q24h§ *or* 20 mg/day (1 cap) for animals > 20 kg 10 mg/day (½ cap) for animals > 5 kg < 20 kg 5 mg/day (1/4 cap) for animals < 5 kg	Severe GI ulceration, unresponsive to H₂ blockers. Severe reflux esophagitis, unresponsive to metoclopramide and H₂ blockers. Gastrinoma (Zollinger-Ellison syndrome).	Inhibits subset of hepatic P-450 drug metabolizing enzymes. Decrease the dose of concurrently administered diazepam and phenytoin but not theophylline or propranolol. 2–7 × as potent as cimetidine. No dose adjustment necessary in hepatic or renal failure. Sustained-release capsule (20 mg) limits dosing option.§

Drug	Product (Manufacturer)	Formulation	Dosage	Indication	Comments
Prostaglandin Analogs					
Misoprostol‡	Cytotec (Searle)	Tabs: 100 μg, 200 μg	3–5 μg/kg PO q6h	Prevention of NSAID-induced GI injury.	Gastric mucosal cytoprotection at low doses; inhibits gastric acid secretion at higher doses. Side effects: diarrhea, abortion.
Promotility Agents					
Metoclopramide	Reglan (A. H. Robins)	Syrup: 1 mg/ml Tabs: 5 mg, 10mg Injectable: 5 mg/ml	0.2–0.4 mg/kg PO, IM, or SC 30 min before eating, q8h *or* 1–2 mg/kg/24h given in fluids as constant-rate infusion	Central antiemetic chemoreceptor trigger zone (CRTZ): drug-induced vomiting, parvoviral enteritis, uremic gastritis. Reflux esophagitis, functional gastric emptying disorder, recurrent gastric hairballs, reflux gastritis, gastric stasis 2° to gastric surgery, ileus.	Side effects: anxiety, agitation, constipation. Contraindicated in patients with mechanical gastric outflow obstruction or epilepsy. Should not be used in combination with phenothiazines, butyrophenones, or narcotics. Atropine or other anticholinergic drugs antagonize effects of metoclopramide. When oral metoclopramide is given simultaneously with oral cimetidine, decreased cimetidine absorption occurs; probably not clinically significant if cimetidine is given at higher dosage range. Decrease dose in renal failure. Metoclopramide is physically incompatible when mixed with cephalothin sodium, sodium bicarbonate, chloramphenicol sodium succinate, or tetracycline. Light sensitivity of metoclopramide occurs in dextrose solutions after 24 hours.
Cisapride‡	Prepulsid (Jansen Pharm.) (not currently available in U.S.A.)	Tabs: 10 mg	0.5 mg/kg PO	Same indications as metoclopramide except: no antiemetic effect, has effects on motility of distal small bowel and colon, possible effect on esophageal motility of smooth muscle.	Decrease dose in hepatic but not renal failure.
Antacids					
Many available	Maalox (Al + Mg) Mylanta II (Al + Mg) + simethicone) Amphogel (AlOH) Tums tabs (CaCO₃)	Tabs and liquid	5–10 ml PO q4–6h	Safe and inexpensive treatment of GI ulceration.	Potency varies between products. Crush tablets for maximum effectiveness. Difficult to administer in animals. Potential side effects: constipation (AlOH, CaCO₃), diarrhea (Mg salts), hypernatremia and alkalosis (NaHCO₃), hypercalcemia and acid rebound (CaCO₃), phosphate depletion (AlOH); impaired excretion of aluminum and magnesium in renal failure; nonspecific binding of concurrently administered drugs (e.g., cimetidine, ranitidine); interference with binding of sucralfate to GI ulcers.

*All drugs that decrease gastric acidity will decrease absorption of orally administered drugs that are weak bases (e.g., ketoconazole) and increase absorption of drugs that are weak acids (e.g., diazepam, aspirin, furosemide).
†E.g., lidocaine, propranolol, theophylline, diazepam, phenytoin, warfarin.
‡Limited experience with use in cats.
§When dosages < 20 mg are used, repackage the enteric-coated granules in a gelatin capsule to avoid gastric acid degradation.

animals are otherwise healthy and do not usually vomit any other time of day.

Diagnosis

Confirmation of chronic gastritis requires a gastric mucosal biopsy, obtained by endoscopy or laparotomy.

History

Obtain a complete history, emphasizing potential exposure to ingested drugs, foreign bodies, chemicals, irritants, and unusual diets (see Table 1).

■ Response to previous therapy (e.g., a change in diet) may indirectly suggest a dietary intolerance or allergy.

Physical Examination

The physical examination often is unremarkable.

Laboratory Evaluation

■ A CBC, biochemical profile, and urinalysis are indicated to exclude non-GI causes of vomiting and to characterize any fluid, electrolyte, or acid-base imbalances secondary to vomiting.
■ Test results usually are normal in animals with chronic gastritis unless vomiting is profuse, mucosal erosions or ulcers cause blood loss anemia, or inflammation of the antral and pyloric region results in gastric outflow obstruction.

Radiography

■ Survey abdominal radiographs usually are unremarkable.
■ Upper GI contrast studies may be normal or show thickening of gastric rugal folds, mucosal irregularity, mass lesions, or delayed gastric emptying. These findings are nonspecific, and gastric biopsy is required to distinguish chronic gastritis from other disorders such as gastric neoplasia.

Endoscopy

This is the diagnostic method of choice to obtain mucosal biopsies to confirm chronic gastritis.

■ Endoscopically, the gastric mucosa may appear grossly normal or show thickened rugae, mucosal irregularity or friability, hemorrhage and ulceration, or firm areas of fibrosis.
■ Severe chronic gastritis may have a diffuse nodular appearance that must be differentiated from gastric lymphosarcoma.

KEY POINT ▶ Always obtain biopsies because histologic changes in chronic gastritis may be present despite a normal gross appearance.

■ If *O. tricuspis* is suspected, aspirate gastric juice for microscopic examination for adult and larval forms.
■ Gastric foreign bodies can be detected and removed.
■ In patients with reflux gastritis, large amounts of bile-stained fluid may be present in the stomach and the pylorus may appear wide open.

Laparotomy

■ Perform laparotomy to obtain full-thickness gastric biopsies and to correct associated gastric outflow obstruction.
■ Full-thickness biopsy may be necessary to differentiate severe lymphocytic gastritis diagnosed by endoscopic biopsy from gastric lymphosarcoma.

Treatment

Eliminate underlying causes of gastritis whenever possible. For example:

■ Discontinue suspected drugs (e.g., aspirin)
■ Remove gastric foreign bodies
■ Treat *O. tricuspis* infections
■ Avoid further exposure to plants, chemicals, and other irritants

In most cases, a specific cause cannot be identified, and therefore specific therapy is unavailable.

Dietary Trials

■ Perform dietary trials in all animals with chronic gastritis because dietary factors or antigens could be the inciting cause. Feed a bland, predominantly carbohydrate diet in frequent small meals.
  • Commercial diets such as Prescription Diet i/d (Hill's Pet) or homemade diets of boiled rice and cottage cheese can be used in dogs.
  • Consider using Prescription Diet c/d (Hill's Pet), Feline Science Diet (Hill's Pet), or Feline Diet (Iams) for cats.
  • Homemade turkey-, lamb-, or chicken-based diets without additives or preservatives can also be tried for both dogs and cats. Commercial or homemade hypoallergenic diets can also be offered.
■ Avoid high-fiber diets or feeding only one large meal per day.
■ Perform dietary trials for at least 2–4 weeks before assessing response to therapy.
■ If gastritis is mild, dietary modification may be all that is required to control clinical signs.
■ Reflux gastritis often responds to frequent feedings or feeding a late bedtime meal. Food may be effective because it buffers refluxed duodenal contents or stimulates gastric motility. Metoclopramide (Reglan, A. H. Robins), discussed below, also may be effective.

H₂ Blockers

Reduction of acid secretion with H_2 blockers (discussed previously) may be useful in animals with chronic gastritis even if gross mucosal erosions or ulcerations are absent (see Table 3). A 2-week trial is recommended, but long-term therapy may be required, depending on clinical response.

Anti-Inflammatory/Immunosuppressant Drugs

Prednisolone

- If no response is obtained with dietary control and H₂ blocker therapy, give prednisolone (1 mg/kg/day in divided doses) for a 2-week trial period.
- If remission occurs, taper this dose over a period of 6–8 weeks, and maintain alternate-day therapy using the lowest effective dose.

Azathioprine

- Azathioprine (Imuran, Burroughs Wellcome), an immunosuppressive drug, may be useful for treatment of chronic gastritis in dogs and cats that have not responded to prednisolone or when glucocorticoid side effects are a problem.
- The initial dose for dogs is 2.0 mg/kg, q24h, PO. The dose can be tapered after a clinical response is obtained, usually by giving the same dose on an alternate-day basis.
- Administer a lower dose (0.3 mg/kg q24–48h PO) in cats.
- Because of azathioprine's ability to suppress the bone marrow, periodically monitor the CBC to detect neutropenia and thrombocytopenia.

Metoclopramide

- Secondary motility disorders may accompany chronic gastritis. If postprandial vomiting occurs, add metoclopramide to the above therapy (see Table 3).
- This central-acting antiemetic also improves gastric emptying (see Fig. 1).

Antibacterial Drugs

Gastric *Spirillum* infection is treated as in humans with combinations of bismuth, amoxicillin, and metronidazole, although the clinical significance of these bacteria in animals is not yet determined.

Prognosis

The prognosis for chronic gastritis is variable.

- If the underlying cause can be identified and corrected, the prognosis for recovery is good.
- In animals with idiopathic chronic gastritis, long-term dietary and medical management may be required.

EOSINOPHILIC GASTRITIS AND GRANULOMA

Eosinophilic gastritis is characterized by diffuse or focal infiltration of mature eosinophils into the mucosa, submucosa, or muscularis. Variable increases in lymphocytes, plasma cells, and neutrophils may also occur.

- Eosinophilic inflammation of the stomach in dogs occurs as two distinct pathologic entities:
  - Diffuse eosinophilic infiltration of the gastric mucosa and submucosa is most common and is usually associated with generalized eosinophilic gastroenterocolitis.
  - Single or multiple eosinophilic granulomatous lesions (scirrhous eosinophilic gastritis) with transmural eosinophilic inflammation, severe arteritis, and fibrosis occur less frequently.

- In cats, eosinophilic gastritis is usually a manifestation of hypereosinophilic syndrome (see sec. 7, ch. 6).

Etiology

- The cause of eosinophilic gastritis or granuloma in dogs is unknown. The presence of increased numbers of circulating and tissue eosinophils suggests an allergic or immunologic hypersensitivity, possibly in response to dietary components or parasites.
- Food allergy or hypersensitivity has been proposed but not proven as a cause of eosinophilic gastritis in dogs.
- Microfilaria have been observed on histologic sections in a dog with diffuse eosinophilic gastritis.
- Eosinophilic gastroenteritis with multiple focal eosinophilic granulomas has been described in German shepherds with visceral larva migrans but is not an important clinical cause of eosinophilic gastroenteritis.

Clinical Signs

- Dogs with eosinophilic gastritis usually have signs of chronic vomiting, anorexia, and weight loss. Eosinophilic gastritis is more likely to be associated with mucosal ulceration and bleeding (suggested by hematemesis and melena) than are other types of chronic gastritis.
- Additional clinical signs may be present if gastritis is a component of diffuse eosinophilic gastroenterocolitis. Small intestinal involvement is characterized by malabsorption and voluminous watery diarrhea, whereas colonic or rectal involvement is characterized by bloody-mucoid diarrhea with tenesmus (see sec. 7, ch. 6).

Diagnosis

History

- Determine previous diets and clinical response to dietary changes.
- A dramatic response to previous corticosteroid therapy is consistent with but not specific for eosinophilic gastritis.

Physical Examination

- Weight loss is common.
- Less common findings include pain on palpation of the stomach, or the stomach may feel diffusely rigid and firm. With large focal granulomas, a mass in the stomach wall may be palpated.
- Additional findings that indicate more extensive intestinal involvement include focal or diffuse thickening of the small intestine or colon or mesenteric lymphadenopathy.

Laboratory Evaluation

- A hemogram often reveals eosinophilia, but not in all cases.
- Gastric erosions and ulcerations can cause anemia and hypoproteinemia.

■ Heartworm and fecal flotation tests are indicated to identify underlying parasitism.

Radiography

■ Abdominal radiography is usually normal unless gastric outflow obstruction occurs secondary to transmural involvement or granuloma formation at the antral or pyloric region.
■ Contrast radiography may demonstrate irregularity of the gastric mucosa or diffuse or focal thickening of the gastric wall.
■ With concurrent intestinal involvement, associated radiographic changes may be identified.
■ Abdominal ultrasonography may identify gastric wall thickness or enlarged mesenteric lymph nodes.

Endoscopy

■ Abnormalities of the gastric mucosa usually can be detected endoscopically, although the gross appearance may be normal.
■ Visual endoscopic findings are nonspecific and may mimic other inflammatory and neoplastic diseases.
■ Involved areas of the stomach may appear diffusely thickened, with hemorrhages, erosions, or ulcers. Granulomas appear as focal mass lesions.
■ Endoscopy is the preferred method for biopsy rather than laparotomy, unless mechanical obstruction requiring surgical decompression is present.
  • Obtain multiple biopsies from the stomach and duodenum.
  • Cytologic examination of mucosal biopsies reveals increased numbers of eosinophils.
■ A disadvantage of endoscopically obtained biopsies is that the depth of the biopsy generally is limited to the mucosa, and deeper layers may be predominantly involved in eosinophilic gastritis.

Laparotomy

■ Exploratory laparotomy may show diffuse or focal thickening in affected regions of the stomach and GI tract.
■ Diffuse involvement of the stomach wall or large focal granulomas may grossly resemble neoplasia.
■ Regional lymphadenopathy is common.

Treatment

The treatment of choice for eosinophilic gastritis in dogs is glucocorticoid therapy combined with dietary management.

■ If a broad-spectrum anthelmintic has not been administered recently, prior to initiating glucocorticoids, treat with fenbendazole (Panacur, Hoechst-Roussel Agri-Vet) (50 mg/kg daily for 3 days) to eliminate undetected GI parasites as a potential cause of the clinical signs.
■ Treatment of eosinophilic gastritis in cats that is a manifestation of hypereosinophilic syndrome is discussed in sec. 7, ch. 6. Rarely, eosinophilic gastritis or gastroenteritis in cats is associated with focal GI involvement that resembles canine eosinophilic gas-

troenterocolitis and can be managed as outlined below for dogs.

Anti-inflammatory/Immunosuppressant Drug Therapy

■ Administer prednisolone, 1 mg/kg q12h, PO. Response is prompt and dramatic, usually occurring within 24–48 hours.
■ Gradually taper dosage over the following 6–8 weeks, decreasing to once daily (given in the morning) and then to alternate days. If the initial treatment period is too short, relapse may occur. If relapse does not occur while tapering the dosage, discontinue therapy at the end of the 6–8 week period. Continue to monitor for relapse.
■ If side effects are a problem or if higher dosage or continued daily therapy is required, give azathioprine concurrently, as described previously for chronic gastritis.

Dietary Recommendations

■ Because food hypersensitivity is a potential cause of eosinophilic gastritis, consider a trial with a hypoallergenic diet. Some dogs with eosinophilic gastritis may respond to a hypoallergenic diet alone. Institute a dietary trial if corticosteroids are being given, because it may decrease the dose of corticosteroids required to control clinical signs.
■ Suggested hypoallergenic diets include home-cooked (boiled) lamb and rice in a 1:1 mixture, or one part low-fat cottage cheese or tofu to three parts rice. Commercial hypoallergenic diets consisting of lamb and rice, egg and rice, or venison and rice are available.
  • Feed the diet exclusively for at least 3–4 weeks before determining effectiveness.
■ If a hypoallergenic diet is ineffective, try a controlled diet such as Prescription Diet i/d (Hill's Pet) or Eukanuba (Iams).

Surgery

Perform surgical resection of obstructing granulomas at the antral and pyloric region and followup with glucocorticoid therapy.

Prognosis

The prognosis for eosinophilic gastritis in dogs is good. Most dogs respond to therapy and many have complete resolution of clinical signs on a long-term basis. In others, relapses occur, and a hypoallergenic diet or corticosteroid therapy is required on a long-term basis.

GASTRIC OUTFLOW OBSTRUCTION

Etiology

Gastric outflow obstruction most commonly is caused by mural, mucosal, and luminal abnormalities involving the antral and pyloric regions of the stomach (see

Table 1). External compression of the gastric outflow tract is identified less frequently. Common causes of outflow obstruction include the following.

- Foreign bodies commonly lodge in the pylorus and cause partial or complete outflow obstruction.
- Chronic hypertrophic pyloric gastropathy (CHPG) is a benign disorder of middle- to older-aged small-breed dogs that frequently results in outflow obstruction. (See discussion later in this chapter under Hypertrophic Gastropathy.)
- Pyloric stenosis is hypertrophy of the circular muscle fibers of the pylorus. Congenital pyloric stenosis occurs in young dogs and cats. Acquired muscular pyloric stenosis is sometimes a component of CHPG in older animals.
- Chronic gastritis, especially eosinophilic gastritis and granuloma, that involves the antral and pyloric region can result in outflow obstruction. Obstructing granulomas may be a manifestation of fungal gastritis caused by Zygomycetes or histoplasmosis.
- Gastric ulcers at the pylorus may cause outflow obstruction.
- Gastric neoplasia, especially adenocarcinoma, has been associated with obstruction (see under Gastric Neoplasia).
- Gastric dilatation-volvulus is a well-recognized cause of acute outflow obstruction and is discussed later in this chapter.
- Extrinsic outflow compression may be caused by hepatic or pancreatic inflammation, abscesses, and neoplasia; marked regional lymphadenopathy; and diaphragmatic hernia with gastric displacement.

Clinical Signs

- Vomiting is a consistent sign of gastric outflow obstruction. Typically, undigested food is present in the vomitus >12–16 hours after eating (the stomach normally empties by 8–10 hours after eating).
  - Bile-staining of vomitus is usually absent.
  - Projectile vomiting suggests outflow obstruction.
  - Complete obstruction results in severe, profuse vomiting.
- Abdominal distension caused by an enlarged fluid- or food-filled stomach may occur, especially after eating.
- Anorexia may occur because of a sense of fullness characteristic of gastric overdistension.
- Belching may indicate an attempt to release gas from the stomach.
- Weight loss and dehydration may result from chronic vomiting.

Diagnosis

History and Signalment

The history and signalment often can suggest a possible underlying cause.

- In young animals, persistent vomiting since weaning suggests a congenital pyloric stenosis.
- Acute onset of vomiting in young animals may indicate a foreign body.

- Chronic vomiting with hematemesis is seen with gastric neoplasia, chronic gastritis, and gastric ulcer.
- Chronic intermittent vomiting over weeks to months in middle-aged and older small-breed dogs is consistent with CHPG.
- Acute onset of nonproductive retching and gagging accompanied by abdominal distension in large-breed dogs suggests gastric dilatation-volvulus.

Physical Examination

- The examination may be unremarkable.
- Potential findings include abdominal distension and signs associated with metabolic abnormalities secondary to profuse vomiting such as weakness and dehydration.

Laboratory Evaluation

- Laboratory findings usually are unremarkable unless profuse vomiting results in fluid, electrolyte, or acid-base imbalances such as dehydration, hypokalemia, hyponatremia, hypochloremia, or metabolic alkalosis.
  - Gastric outflow obstruction is an important cause of hypochloremic metabolic alkalosis.
- Other laboratory findings are variable and depend on the underlying cause of obstruction.

Radiography

Survey Abdominal Radiography
This is helpful to confirm gastric outflow obstruction.

- The finding of a distended fluid-filled stomach or food present in the stomach >12–16 hours after eating suggests delayed gastric emptying. The stomach normally empties by 8–10 hours after eating; however, emptying times up to 16 hours are normal in some dogs, especially when fed dry food.
  - Identification of the underlying cause of delayed gastric emptying requires further evaluation with contrast radiography, endoscopy, or exploratory laparotomy.

Contrast Gastrography
- A contrast gastrogram is useful to further evaluate gastric emptying. Liquid barium normally begins to leave the stomach in 5–15 minutes and the stomach is usually empty in 30–60 minutes in cats and 1–2 hours in dogs.
  - The presence of barium in the stomach after 12–24 hours confirms delayed gastric emptying.
  - If the lesion affects the emptying of food more than that of liquids, emptying studies using contrast material mixed with canned food may be helpful (see sec. 1, ch. 4).
- Contrast studies can provide important information about the cause of delayed gastric emptying. Potential findings include foreign bodies, thickening or mass lesions of the antral and pyloric region, and narrowing of the pyloric canal (the "beak" sign).

Fluoroscopy/Ultrasonography
- Fluoroscopy and ultrasonography may provide information about the outflow tract including intrinsic

thickening of the wall of the pyloric antrum or extrinsic compression of the antrum and pylorus by hepatic and pancreatic lesions.

Endoscopy

Endoscopy is useful to identify and remove foreign bodies and to evaluate the antral and pyloric region for outflow obstruction.

- Fast the patient with suspected delayed gastric emptying for at least 24 hours prior to endoscopy to assure that the stomach is empty. If large volumes of fluid are still present, aspirate the fluid through the endoscope to improve visualization.
- Foreign bodies, masses, mucosal proliferations (e.g., CHPG) or thickenings, and ulcers can readily be identified at endoscopy.
- Endoscopic biopsies of affected tissues can be obtained; however, if mechanical outflow obstruction is detected, immediate surgical relief of obstruction and full-thickness biopsies are preferred.
- If the outflow area looks normal and the endoscope is readily passed through the pylorus into the duodenum, mechanical outflow obstruction is much less likely. However, extrinisic compression of the outflow region cannot be fully appreciated with endoscopy and may require an exploratory laparotomy.
- An alternative consideration when the pylorus appears normal is that delayed gastric emptying is caused by a motility disturbance (see under Gastric Motility Disorders) of the stomach rather than by mechanical outflow obstruction.

Treatment

- Give appropriate fluid therapy to correct fluid, electrolyte, and acid-base disturbances prior to general anesthesia for surgery or endoscopy. Because metabolic imbalances are variable, base the choice of fluid composition on results of electrolyte and blood gas analysis (see previous discussion of fluid therapy for vomiting).
- Metabolic alkalosis may occur secondary to outflow obstruction; manage with non-alkalinizing solutions such as 0.9% saline and Ringer's solution, supplemented with potassium chloride, as described in sec. 1, ch. 5.
- Surgery is indicated for definitive treatment of gastric outflow obstruction (see sec. 7, ch. 5).
- If gastric stasis persists after surgical relief of outflow obstruction, give metoclopramide to improve gastric emptying (see Fig. 1). Metoclopramide is contraindicated in the presence of mechanical outflow obstruction.

GASTRIC MOTILITY DISORDERS

Gastric motility disorders that result in weak or ineffective gastric contractions can cause delayed gastric emptying in dogs and cats. These disorders are not well documented in veterinary medicine. Currently, the diagnosis of a gastric motility disorder is presumptive and is based on clinical findings consistent with delayed gastric emptying in the absence of an obstructive lesion.

Etiology

The causes and pathophysiologic mechanisms of gastric motility disorders are poorly understood. Gastric motility is dependent on normal electrical and mechanical activity of the stomach. Control of gastric motility and emptying is influenced by the composition of the food. Emptying is prolonged when the fat and protein content, acidity, osmolality, and viscosity of the gastric contents increase. Hormonal and autonomic nervous input also are important factors.

The following factors may be associated with functional delays in gastric emptying.

- Drug therapy with anticholinergic drugs or narcotic analgesics can delay gastric emptying.
- Inflammatory lesions such as gastritis, gastric ulcers, and parvoviral gastroenteritis are associated with gastric motility disorders.
- Nervous inhibition associated with stress, trauma, pain, or psychogenic input may cause a transient delay in gastric emptying due to increased sympathetic stimulation.
- Metabolic disturbances such as hypokalemia, uremia, hepatic encephalopathy, and hypothyroidism may delay gastric emptying.
- Prolonged gastric obstruction may be complicated by secondary motility dysfunction.
- In many cases, functional gastric emptying disorders are idiopathic. These disorders may be associated with abnormal gastric electrical conduction disturbances such as tachyarrhythmias.
- Chronic trichobezoar formation in cats may be related to abnormal migrating motor complexes that impair gastric emptying of indigestible material during fasting.

Clinical Signs

The clinical signs of a gastric motility disorder causing delayed gastric emptying are similar to those of gastric outflow obstruction. These include:

- Vomiting with undigested food present in the vomitus >12–16 hours after eating
- Abdominal distension after eating
- Anorexia and belching.

Diagnosis

History

Perform a complete history to determine if anticholinergics or narcotics are currently being administered.

Laboratory Evaluation

Perform routine screening tests including a CBC, biochemical profile, and urinalysis to detect predisposing metabolic abnormalities.

- The finding of neutropenia in a young dog with acute onset of vomiting and bloody diarrhea suggests parvoviral gastroenteritis as a cause of gastric retention.

Radiography

- Perform abdominal radiographs. Delayed gastric emptying is suggested by the finding of a distended fluid-filled stomach or food present in the stomach >12–16 hours after eating.
- Perform a contrast gastrogram to assess gastric emptying, as described previously for gastric outflow obstruction. Normal gastric emptying of barium does not exclude a gastric motility disorder because it evaluates only the ability of the stomach to empty liquids and not solids. In functional gastric motility disorders, the gastric outflow region appears normal, but barium may not leave the stomach in a timely fashion.

Endoscopy

- Electrogastrograms have been used on a research basis to document abnormal gastric electrical rhythms and may have clinical applications in the future.
- Endoscopy is a useful noninvasive method to exclude mechanical outflow obstruction as a cause of delayed gastric emptying.
- Fast the patient for at least 24 hours prior to endoscopy to assure that the stomach is empty. Large volumes of fluid are often present and should be aspirated through the endoscope to improve visualization.
- In idiopathic gastric motility disorders, the gastric mucosa and pyloric outflow area appear normal. If gastritis is a predisposing cause, gross and microscopic changes will be detected.

Treatment

Whenever possible, identify and correct the underlying cause of a gastric motility disorder. For example, discontinue any anticholinergic drug therapy.

Fluid Therapy

Institute fluid therapy as needed. (See previous discussion of fluid therapy for vomiting.)

Dietary Management

This is an important aspect of treatment of gastric motility disorders.

- The diet should be low in fat, high in carbohydrate, and fed in small amounts at frequent intervals.
- The consistency of the diet can be altered. In many instances, the more liquid the diet, the better it empties from the stomach.

Drug Therapy

The treatment of choice for idiopathic gastric motility disorders is the motility modifier metoclopramide (see Table 3). The effects of metoclopramide on the stomach are shown in Figure 1. Cisapride, another motility modifier, has similar actions on the stomach but is not commercially available at this time.

- Administer metoclopramide one-half hour before a meal, 0.2–0.4 mg/kg, q8h, PO.
- If effective, oral metoclopramide can be given on a long-term basis to improve gastric emptying.

HYPERTROPHIC GASTROPATHY

The term hypertrophic gastropathy is used to describe a heterogeneous group of poorly understood disorders associated with focal, multifocal, or diffuse hypertrophic changes of the gastric mucosa of dogs. Hypertrophic gastropathy appears to be quite rare in cats. Various other names have been used, including chronic hypertrophic pyloric gastropathy, hypertrophic gastritis, gastric polyps, and acquired pyloric stenosis or hypertrophy. These disorders may be variations of the same disease process. Microscopic changes are variable and include hyperplasia of mucosal epithelial cells, glandular hypertrophy, variable inflammatory infiltrates, and mucosal ulceration. The most commonly recognized form of hypertrophic gastropathy in dogs is a benign disorder associated with mucosal hypertrophy of the antral and pyloric region, resulting in gastric outflow obstruction. Some affected dogs have a component of pyloric muscular hypertrophy. This disorder has been termed chronic hypertrophic pyloric gastropathy (CHPG).

Etiology

Little is known about the underlying etiology and pathophysiologic mechanisms of hypertrophic gastropathy. Environmental, hormonal, genetic, and immune-mediated mechanisms may play a role.

- Chronic irritation associated with aspirin therapy can result in focal gastric hypertrophy.
- Hormones such as gastrin, cholecystokinin, acetylcholine, and histamine can be trophic to the gastric mucosa. Causes of hypergastrinemia such as chronic renal failure, chronic gastric distension, gastrin-secreting tumors, and idiopathic hypertrophy of the antral G-cells (gastrin-secreting cells) may be important considerations in some cases.
- Basenji dogs have hypertrophic gastritis in association with immunoproliferative enteropathy; genetic, immune-mediated, and hormonal (gastrin) factors may play a role.
- CHPG is most common in highly excitable, nervous small-breed dogs; underlying neuroendocrine or stress-related mechanisms have been proposed.

Clinical Signs

- Chronic vomiting is the most consistent clinical sign in dogs. Vomiting occurs at variable intervals after eating.
  - If hypertrophic changes cause outflow obstruction, undigested food may be present in the vomitus >12–16 hours after eating.
  - Hematemesis and melena may be detected in association with mucosal ulceration.
  - Dogs with CHPG often are otherwise healthy and are presented because of chronic intermittent vom-

iting for a duration of weeks to months (sometimes years).

■ Anorexia, weight loss, abdominal distension, and belching are less frequent signs.

■ Basenji dogs with immunoproliferative enteropathy and hypertrophic gastritis usually have concurrent chronic diarrhea, anorexia, and weight loss.

Diagnosis

History and Signalment

■ CHPG is most common in middle-aged or older small-breed dogs such as Lhasa Apsos, Shih Tzus, and miniature poodles.

■ Males are affected more commonly than females.

■ A history of chronic intermittent vomiting is typical.

Physical Examination

■ Potential findings include weight loss and abdominal distension due to a fluid- or food-filled stomach.

■ If significant gastrointestinal blood loss occurs, pale mucous membranes due to anemia may be detected.

Laboratory Evaluation

Laboratory evaluation often is unremarkable.

■ If profuse vomiting has occurred, laboratory findings may reflect dehydration or electrolyte imbalances.

■ Metabolic alkalosis may occur secondary to gastric outflow obstruction.

■ If hypertrophic gastropathy is associated with gastric ulceration, evaluate serum gastrin concentration to detect underlying hypergastrinemia (e.g., gastrinoma).

■ Iron deficiency anemia may result from chronic GI blood loss.

Radiography

■ Perform survey abdominal radiographs to detect a fluid-filled distended stomach or food remaining in the stomach >12–16 hours after eating. These findings are consistent with a gastric retention disorder.

■ Perform a contrast gastrogram.
  • Findings consistent with CHPG include delayed gastric emptying, filling defects in the antral and pyloric region due to hypertrophied mucosa, and narrowing of the pyloric canal.
  • With other types of hypertrophic gastropathy, potential findings include focal, multifocal, or diffusely thickened gastric rugae.
  • Radiographic features of hypertrophic gastropathy are not specific and mimic other inflammatory and infiltrative disorders.

■ Ultrasonography can demonstrate thickening of the gastric wall at the antral and pyloric region.

Endoscopy

■ Endoscopy can confirm focal, multifocal, or diffusely thickened mucosal folds. Moderate gastric distension with air is required so that normal-sized gastric rugal folds do not appear falsely thickened.

■ With CHPG, the lesion predominantly involves the antrum and pyloric region, causing partial or complete pyloric obstruction. Mucosal ulceration or hemorrhage is not typical.

■ Endoscopically obtained biopsies are inadequate to diagnose hypertrophic gastropathy because they are too superficial to demonstrate the lesion.

Surgery

■ Definitive diagnosis of hypertrophic gastritis requires full-thickness biopsies obtained surgically.

■ Excisional biopsies are indicated when possible to help relieve the obstruction.

Treatment

■ Surgical excision of abnormal tissue and relief of outflow obstruction is the treatment of choice for CHPG (see sec. 7, ch. 5). Response to surgery is usually good to excellent and most dogs are clinically normal after relief of obstruction. If gastric atony persists after surgery, a trial of metoclopramide may be warranted.

■ If hypertrophic gastropathy is associated with gastric erosions or ulcerations, institute anti-ulcer therapy with H_2 blockers and sucralfate as described under Gastroduodenal Ulceration.

■ When hypertrophic gastropathy is accompanied by a significant inflammatory infiltrate, consider treatment with prednisolone as described under Chronic Gastritis.

■ For treatment of Basenji dogs with hypertrophic gastritis and immunoproliferative enteropathy, see sec. 7, ch. 6.

GASTRIC NEOPLASIA

The clinical presentation of gastric neoplasia in dogs and cats is influenced by the size and location of the tumor, whether it is benign or malignant, and whether it is associated with outflow obstruction, altered gastric motility, or mucosal ulceration.

Etiology

Malignant Neoplasia

KEY POINT ▶ Gastric adenocarcinoma is the most common gastric neoplasm in dogs.

■ In dogs, gastric adenocarcinoma occurs most commonly in the antral and pyloric region and may appear as a raised plaque or mass with a central ulcerated area or as diffuse infiltration of the gastric wall. Metastases to the regional lymph nodes, liver, adrenals, and lungs are common. Gastric adenocarcinoma is rare in cats.

KEY POINT ▶ Lymphosarcoma is the most common malignant gastric neoplasm in cats.

■ Cats with gastric lymphosarcoma usually are FeLV-negative. Lymphosarcoma may appear as multiple, raised white masses or as diffuse infiltration of the gastric wall. Mucosal ulceration is common.

- Other, less common primary malignant neoplasms include leiomyosarcoma and fibrosarcoma.

Benign Neoplasia

- Benign adenomatous polyps occur infrequently in dogs and cats. Polyps probably develop in response to chronic gastric mucosal damage or irritation. They appear as single or multiple, pedunculated or polypoid nodules that vary in size from millimeters to centimeters. Clinical signs usually are absent unless pyloric obstruction occurs. Polyps usually are an incidental finding at endoscopy or necropsy.
- Leiomyomas are the second-most common gastric tumor in dogs. These tumors arise from the muscle layers of the gastric wall; clinical signs may be absent unless the mechanical effects of the mass alter motility or cause outflow obstruction. Mucosal ulceration occasionally occurs.

Clinical Signs

Malignant Neoplasia

- Dogs and cats with malignant gastric neoplasia are usually presented because of chronic progressive vomiting.
- If outflow obstruction occurs, clinical signs reflect delayed gastric emptying.
- Hematemesis and melena are common with adenocarcinoma because of mucosal ulceration. Other signs include anorexia, weight loss, and chronic debilitation.

Benign Neoplasia

- Clinical signs may be absent with benign neoplasms or polyps unless pyloric obstruction occurs.

Diagnosis

Gastric neoplasia is an important consideration in older dogs and cats with a history of chronic progressive vomiting and hematemesis.

Physical Examination

- Findings often include weight loss and cachexia.
- Palpable abnormalities of the stomach usually are absent, although, rarely, a gastric mass may be palpable.
- Pale mucous membranes and melena are consistent with mucosal ulceration and blood loss anemia.
- Gastric perforation and peritonitis are associated with abdominal distension, pain, collapse, and shock.
- Additional findings such as ascites, jaundice, and dyspnea reflect metastatic disease.

Laboratory Evaluation

Laboratory evaluation is variable and depends on secondary complications such as blood loss, perforation, metastatic disease, and metabolic complications of vomiting.

Radiography

- Survey films may be unremarkable or suggest outflow obstruction, a thickened gastric wall, or mass lesions.
- Contrast radiography is helpful to confirm mass lesions and diffuse thickening of the gastric wall.
- Rigidity of the gastric wall when compared on multiple films suggests an infiltrative lesion.
- Other potential findings include filling defects, ulcers, and delayed gastric emptying.
- Perform thoracic films to screen for pulmonary metastases.

Endoscopy

Endoscopy is useful to confirm lesions suggested on radiography and to obtain biopsies of affected tissues. Gastric neoplasia that does not involve the mucosa or result in a mass effect can be difficult to detect endoscopically, and a full-thickness biopsy obtained surgically is necessary.

- Adenocarcinoma may appear as raised plaques, polypoid lesions, or a diffuse infiltrating lesion. Mucosal ulceration is common.
- Gastric lymphosarcoma appears as multiple white nodules or diffuse infiltration of the mucosa with irregularity and thickening of the mucosal folds. With diffuse infiltration of the gastric wall, the stomach may lack distensibility.
- Leiomyomas are smooth mass lesions with a normal overlying mucosa unless complicated by ulceration.
- Polyps appear as small, smooth or raspberry-like masses on a stalk.

Surgery

Surgical exploration is an important method to evaluate gastric neoplasia.

- Palpate all areas of the stomach to identify affected areas.
- Obtain full-thickness biopsies.
- Evaluate regional lymph nodes and the liver for metastases.

Treatment

- The treatment of choice for gastric neoplasia is surgical resection of the tumor by partial gastrectomy (see sec. 7, ch. 5). Because the antral and pyloric region are often involved, a gastroduodenostomy or gastrojejunostomy may be necessary (see sec. 7, ch. 5).
- For treatment of lymphosarcoma, surgical removal of large solitary masses can be followed by chemotherapy with cyclophosphamide, vincristine, and prednisone, as described in sec. 3, ch. 5.

Prognosis

- The prognosis for benign neoplasms after surgical removal is good.
- The prognosis for adenocarcinoma is poor.
- Diffuse infiltration of wall with lymphosarcoma is not responsive to treatment and has a poor prog-

nosis. However, some cats with lymphosarcoma localized to the stomach may have a good to excellent response to chemotherapy.

GASTRIC DILATATION-VOLVULUS

Gastric dilatation-volvulus (GDV) is an acute, life-threatening disorder that is a medical and surgical emergency. Early recognition and treatment are essential for a successful outcome. Gastric dilatation refers to distension of the stomach, usually with swallowed air. Gastric dilatation may or may not be complicated by volvulus. GDV occurs when the stomach rotates on its long axis, resulting in complete gastric outflow obstruction. Concurrent obstruction of the gastroesophageal junction precludes relief of fluid and gas accumulation by vomiting or belching. Massive gastric distension impairs venous return through the portal vein and caudal vena cava, causing hypovolemic and endotoxic shock. Passive congestion of the abdominal viscera predisposes to local acidosis and disseminated intravascular coagulation (DIC). The spleen often is displaced concurrently, causing splenic vascular occlusion, congestion, and splenomegaly. Strangulation necrosis of the gastric wall occurs secondary to twisting of the stomach.

Etiology

The cause of GDV is unknown.

- An anatomic predisposition may play a role; large-breed, deep-chested dogs are most commonly affected, and the disorder is rare in small dogs and cats.
- Gastric dilatation due to excessive swallowed air is generally believed to precede volvulus; thus, causes of aerophagia such as gulping of food may be important.
- Delayed gastric emptying has also been suspected in some dogs with GDV.
- Overeating, postprandial exercise, and dry, cereal-based diets have been suggested to predispose to GDV but have not been substantiated clinically or experimentally.

Clinical Signs

Signs include:

- Acute onset of abdominal distension with tympany
- Nonproductive retching
- Salivating, restlessness, and respiratory distress.

Diagnosis

History and Signalment

- Consider GDV in the differential diagnosis of any large-breed, deep-chested dog with acute onset of abdominal distension.

Physical Examination

- Examination usually reveals abdominal distension and findings indicative of hypovolemia and/or shock,

including increased heart rate, weak femoral pulses, decreased capillary refill time, and pale oral mucous membranes.

Laboratory Evaluation

- After initial stabilization (see below) submit blood for a CBC and biochemical evaluation to characterize secondary metabolic imbalances and to identify any other co-existent abnormalities.
- Hypokalemia is the most common electrolyte abnormality in dogs with GDV. Although serum potassium concentration may be normal initially, hypokalemia frequently develops after aggressive fluid therapy and, if surgery is necessary, postoperatively. Prevention of hypokalemia may decrease the frequency of postoperative cardiac arrhythmias and muscle weakness.
- Because a variety of acid-base imbalances may occur secondary to GDV, repeated laboratory assessment and frequent monitoring of blood gases and electrolyte concentrations are recommended.
  - Metabolic acidosis is most common and occurs because of decreased effective circulating blood volume, arterial hypoxemia, and lactic acid accumulation.
  - Metabolic alkalosis, respiratory alkalosis, respiratory acidosis, and mixed acid-base disorders may also develop.

Radiography

- Perform abdominal radiography only after the patient is stabilized medically (see below). Minimize stress to the patient during the procedure.
- Right lateral and ventral-dorsal abdominal radiographs are most useful to evaluate for GDV.
- Radiographic findings suggestive of GDV include:
  - Pyloric displacement dorsally and to the left, with gastric fundic displacement caudally and to the right
  - Compartmentalization of the stomach on the lateral view
  - Splenomegaly
- Pneumoperitoneum suggests gastric perforation and requires immediate surgery.
- Thoracic radiography is not essential but may demonstrate microcardia due to hypovolemia, megaesophagus, or aspiration pneumonia.
- In cases of intermittent bloating or failure of surgical correction following tube decompression, perform a contrast gastrogram (see sec. 1, ch. 4) to identify malposition of the stomach.

Initial Medical Management

Decompress the Stomach by Orogastric Intubation

- Sedation may be necessary to pass an orogastric tube. Give diazepam (0.1 mg/kg IV slowly) alone or in combination with butorphanol (0.5 mg/kg IV). An alternative is the combination of fentanyl-droperidol (1 ml/10–35 kg IV).
- Perform gastric decompression by passing a well-

lubricated large-bore orogastric tube. Remove all air and fluid from the stomach and lavage the stomach with 4–5 liters of warm saline or water. Repeat orogastric decompression as needed during the stabilization period.

■ If orogastric decompression is not possible with a tube, use several 18-gauge needles to trocarize the distended stomach. Following decompression with needle trocarization, a subsequent attempt to pass the orogastric tube often is successful.

■ If decompression cannot be accomplished, perform a temporary gastrostomy via a right paracostal approach. The gastrostomy is subsequently repaired at the time of definitive surgery.

Place an Intravenous Catheter and Administer Fluids

■ While decompression is being performed, place a large-bore catheter in each cephalic vein.

■ Give isotonic crystalloid fluids such as lactated Ringer's solution at an initial rapid rate of 90 ml/kg for the first hour. Add potassium chloride to the fluid (30–40 mEq KCl/liter of fluid) after the initial shock dose of fluids has been given. When blood gas analysis is not available, routine addition of $NaHCO_3$ to fluids is not recommended, because many dogs with GDV have relatively normal blood pH at presentation. Correction of volume depletion and mild metabolic acidosis by lactated Ringer's solution is sufficient unless severe metabolic acidosis is present.

■ Alternatively, administer small-volume fluid therapy using 7% NaCl (5 ml/kg) in 6% Dextran 70 (HS/D70). Give over 5–10 minutes and follow with 20 ml/kg/hour 0.9% NaCl.

■ Place a Foley catheter in the bladder to monitor urine output.

Control Infection and Endotoxemia

■ To treat endotoxemia, give prednisolone sodium succinate (10 ml/kg) IV. Give a single dose of flunixin meglumine (Banamine, Schering) intravenously (1 mg/kg) during the initial phase of therapy.

■ Give a broad-spectrum antibiotic (cefmetazole, 15 mg/kg IV) or combination drug therapy (cefazolin, 20 mg/kg IV, and gentamicin, 2 mg/kg IV).

Monitor and Treat Cardiac Arrhythmias

See section 6, chapter 4.

■ Ventricular arrhythmias are the most common.

■ To treat ventricular arrhythmias, give a bolus of lidocaine (1–2 mg/kg) IV while monitoring the ECG. If no conversion is noted within 3–5 minutes, repeat this dose.

■ If only temporary conversion occurs, start a lidocaine drip. A maintenance effect is achieved with a constant rate infusion of lidocaine at a rate of 40–60 μg/kg/minute added to the intravenous fluids. Lidocaine's effectiveness may be impaired in the presence of hypokalemia.

■ If lidocaine boluses are ineffective for controlling ventricular arrhythmias, consider giving procainamide (10–15 mg/kg, q6h, IM) or quinidine sulfate (6–15 mg/kg q6h, IM). If arrhythmias are controlled with parenteral administration of procainamide or quinidine, an oral antiarrhythmic can later be substituted, as described in sec. 6, ch. 4.

Surgical Management

The goals of surgical intervention for acute GDV include:

■ Repositioning of the stomach and spleen

■ Resecting devitalized gastric and splenic tissue

■ Permanently fixing the stomach to the abdominal wall to prevent future occurrences of volvulus (see sec. 7, ch. 5).

Prevention

If medical therapy alone is successful and no evidence of gastric volvulus is detected subsequently on a contrast gastrogram, there is still a 70–75% likelihood that the dog will have another episode of GDV. Owner education can help to lessen the probability of recurrence.

Instruct the owner to:

■ Feed the dog frequent, small portions of food 3–5 times per day.

■ Limit water intake and do not allow access to water for 1 hour after eating.

■ Restrict exercise after eating, because this may predispose to GDV.

■ Be aware of the early warning signs of GDV (e.g., depression, restlessness, belching, excessive flatulence, abdominal enlargement), especially when there is a change in the dog's environment—for example, when the dog is boarded or hospitalized, or when a new adult, child, or pet is introduced into the household.

Supplemental Readings

Allen DA, Schertel ER, Muir WW, et al.: Hypertonic saline/dextran resuscitation of dogs with experimentally induced gastric-dilatation-volvulus shock. Am J Vet Res 52:92, 1991.

Johnson SE: Medical emergencies of the digestive tract and abdomen. In Sherding RG, ed.: Contemporary Issues in Small Animal Practice: Medical Emergencies. New York: Churchill Livingstone, 1985, p 213.

Orton EC: Gastric dilatation-volvulus. In Kirk RW, ed.: Current Veterinary Therapy IX. Philadelphia: W. B. Saunders, 1985, p 856.

Strombeck DR, Guilford WG, eds.: Small Animal Gastroenterology, 2nd Ed. Stonegate: Davis, CA, 1990, p 167.

Twedt DC, Magne ML: Diseases of the stomach. In Ettinger SJ, ed.: Textbook of Veterinary Internal Medicine, Vol 2., 3rd Ed. Philadelphia: W. B. Saunders, 1989, p 1289.

Twedt DC, Tams TR: Diseases of the stomach. In Sherding RG, ed.: The Cat: Diseases and Clinical Management, Vol. 2. New York: Churchill Livingstone, 1989, p 929.

Whitney WO: Complications associated with the medical and surgical management of gastric-dilatation-volvulus in the dog. Problems in Veterinary Medicine, Vol. 1, No. 2, Philadelphia: W. B. Saunders, 1989, p 268.

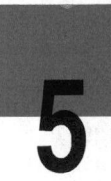

5 Surgery of the Stomach

Ronald M. Bright

Retrieval of foreign bodies is the most common reason for surgery on the stomach. Surgery of the pylorus is most often indicated for some forms of gastric outflow obstruction. The most common sign related to surgical disease of the stomach is emesis. The stomach has an excellent blood supply and heals rapidly (10–14 days).

ANATOMY

Stomach

- The stomach is a musculoglandular organ capable of undergoing a great amount of distension.
- The stomach is C-shaped and a partially coiled, bulging tube.
- The stomach lies in a transverse plane. The larger part of the stomach (fundus) lies to the left of the midline.
- The esophageal entrance and duodenal exit are dorsal—the former lying to the left of the midline, the latter to the right.
- In the fasting dog, the stomach does not extend caudally beyond the costal arch and is rarely palpable.
- The stomach is divided into four regions: cardia, fundus, body (corpus), and pylorus.
- The stomach has four tunics: mucosa, submucosa, muscularis, and serosa. The submucosa and mucosa layers are easily separated from the overlying seromuscular layers.
- The blood supply to the distal stomach is from a branch of the hepatic artery giving rise to the right gastric and gastroepiploic arteries.
  - The splenic artery gives rise to the left gastroepiploic artery, which supplies the greater curvature.
  - The left gastric supplies blood to the lesser curvature of the stomach and the distal esophagus.
- Veins are satellites to the arterial branches. Most blood drains from the left side of the stomach via the gastrosplenic vein and from the right side via the gastroduodenal vein. These veins ultimately drain into the portal vein.
- The major innervation is parasympathetic from the vagi and sympathetic from the celiac plexus.

Omentum

- The greater omentum extends caudally from the greater curvature to the urinary bladder forming a double-layered cover of the small intestine.
- A splenic portion of the omentum attaches the greater curvature to the spleen and a smaller portion attaches to the pancreas.
- The lesser omentum extends from the lesser curvature of the stomach and attaches to the diaphragm, liver, and duodenum.
- The hepatoduodenal and hepatogastric ligaments are loose attachments between the respective components.

Pylorus

- The pylorus is comprised of two segments, the antrum and the canal. The antrum is a narrow funnel-shaped chamber leading to the narrowed pyloric canal.
- The inner circular muscle layer is thickened in the pyloric region and functions as a powerful sphincter. An outer longitudinal muscle layer is also present.
- The pylorus has two major functions—to control the emptying of solid food once it becomes reduced to an appropriate size and to prevent excessive amounts of duodenogastric reflux.

GASTROTOMY

Preoperative Considerations

KEY POINT ▶ Serious water and electrolyte abnormalities often accompany conditions that affect the stomach and require gastrotomy. Fluid and electrolyte resuscitation precedes gastrotomy.

- The most common indication for gastrotomy is to retrieve foreign bodies.
- Endoscopic retrieval of gastric foreign bodies is preferred. When this approach fails, a gastrotomy is indicated.

Surgical Procedure

Objectives

- Access and visualization of intraluminal contents
- Collection of biopsy specimens
- Avoidance of contamination of the peritoneal cavity

Equipment

- General surgical pack
- Babcock forceps (optional)
- Abdominal self-retaining Balfour retractors
- Laparotomy pads

Technique

1. A cranial ventral midline abdominal approach is made with the skin incision extending from the xiphoid to the umbilicus.
2. The stomach is exteriorized and well packed with moistened laparotomy pads.
3. Two Babcock forceps or two stay sutures are placed 10–15 cm apart on a hypovascular area of the stomach, halfway between the lesser and greater curvature.
4. A stab incision into the lumen is made with a # 11 blade.
5. The stomach is suctioned free of liquid contents.
6. An extension of the stab incision is made with scissors.
7. A visual and tactile exploration of the entire stomach is done.

Closure

1. The first layer is a continuous inverting horizontal mattress (Connell) suture pattern involving only the submucosal and mucosal layers. A simple continuous suture pattern can be substituted. Synthetic 3–0 absorbable suture material is preferred. Use of chromic gut suture material is discouraged, because it breaks down too rapidly when placed in the stomach's lumen.
2. The second layer is closed utilizing similar sutures in a vertical (Lembert) or horizontal (Cushing) continuous inverting pattern.
3. If the gastrotomy closure incorporates diseased or devitalized tissue, a section of vascularized omentum or a serosal patch employing a loop of jejunum is sutured over the wound for additional reinforcement.

Postoperative Care and Complications

Short-term

- No food for 24 hours; water ad libitum.
- Monitor the patient for leakage, especially if the gastrotomy closure involves diseased tissue (neoplasia).
- Emesis may be noted once or twice following gastric surgery and treatment is usually not required.
- Systemic antacids are indicated if ulcers or severe gastritis is observed during surgery.

Prognosis

- Good to excellent if the reason for surgery is related to a foreign body.

PARTIAL GASTRECTOMY RELATED TO GASTRIC DILATATION-VOLVULUS

Preoperative Considerations

- Gastrectomy in the dilatation-volvulus case is a high risk procedure.
- Initially, attempt to stabilize metabolic abnormalities—but, rapidly proceed with surgery because gastric rupture may occur.

Surgical Procedure

Objectives

- Resect nonviable gastric tissue and restore gastric continuity.
- Use a stapling technique, if possible, to expedite this high risk procedure.

Equipment

- General pack
- LDS stapler (U.S. Surgical) (optional)
- TA stapler (U.S. Surgical) (optional)
- Abdominal self-retaining retractor
- Laparotomy pads
- Noncrushing straight Doyen intestinal clamps

Technique

1. The approach to the stomach is similar to that for a gastrotomy.
2. Nonviable tissue is recognized by its lack of bleeding on cut surfaces, bluish-black or greenish discoloration, and severe thinning of the stomach wall on palpation.

KEY POINT ▶ Do not rely on the appearance of the mucosa alone to determine if full-thickness stomach wall necrosis has occurred.

3. The appropriate short gastric vessels are ligated and divided. LDS stapler apparatus is optimal. This procedure may not be necessary because these vessels are frequently torn.
4. After placement of stay sutures, intestinal forceps are applied 2 cm lateral to the junction of viable and nonviable tissue. The tips of the forceps meet at an approximate 45° angle.
5. Use a # 10 scalpel blade to cut along the intestinal clamps, leaving a 1-cm margin of healthy tissue outside the intestinal clamps.

Alternate method of resection

1. A TA stapler is placed parallel to the junction of viable and nonviable tissue, leaving a 1-cm width of normal tissue.
2. After the stapler is engaged and the staples are placed in the tissue, the stomach wall is cut next to the blade of the stapler and the necrotic tissue is removed.

Closure

1. Without a stapler, the closure is similar to that for a gastrotomy incision.
2. With a stapler, the closure is done before cutting the nonviable tissue away from the TA stapler's blade.
3. The abdomen is closed routinely. If gastric rupture has occurred, the abdomen may remain partially open (see sec. 7, ch. 13).

Postoperative Care and Complications

Short-term

- Refer to the discussion of gastric dilatation-volvulus surgery for postoperative management of metabolic problems.

- Feeding is delayed for 24 hours.
- Monitor very closely for signs of gastric leakage (fever, vomiting, pneumoperitoneum, peritonitis), especially during the first 96 hours postoperatively.

KEY POINT ▶ When a partial gastrectomy is performed during surgical therapy for gastric dilatation-volvulus complex, the mortality rate doubles to approximately 60%.

PARTIAL GASTRECTOMY (DISTAL STOMACH)

Preoperative Considerations

KEY POINT ▶ Attempts to define the extent and nature of the disease (benign polyp, malignancy, fungal infiltrative, chronic gastric ulcer) by radiography and endoscopic biopsy are extremely important when planning surgical therapy.

Many animals with gastric neoplasia are old and debilitated and are at greater risk during surgery than others.

Surgical Procedure—Partial Gastrectomy and Gastroduodenostomy (Billroth 1)

Objectives
- To remove diseased tissue that is benign or, if malignant, is limited to the antrum and/or body of the stomach.
- To correct failed pyloroplasty procedures
- To maintain an adequate outflow lumen

Equipment
- Same as that for partial gastrectomy associated with the gastric dilatation-volvulus complex.
- If a stapler technique is used, a GIA stapler is recommended.
- Large straight intestinal clamps

Technique

1. The dog is placed in dorsal recumbency with surgical preparation similar to that for gastrotomy.
2. Stapling devices (e.g., the GIA stapler) can be substituted for more traditional suturing techniques.
3. If the pathology is limited to the pylorus, a modification of a Billroth I (von Haberer) technique can be done (Fig. 1).
4. If a partial gastrectomy is performed to control ulcer disease, the entire antrum should be resected.
5. More extensive resection of the pylorus or distal stomach can be done and reconstructed with the original Billroth I (Shoemaker) procedure (see Fig. 1).
6. After the line of resection is determined, the blood vessels supplying the lesser and greater curvature and attached omentum are ligated and divided.
7. The pylorus is mobilized after incising the gastro-hepatic ligament. Avoid cutting the common bile duct and hepatic arteries.

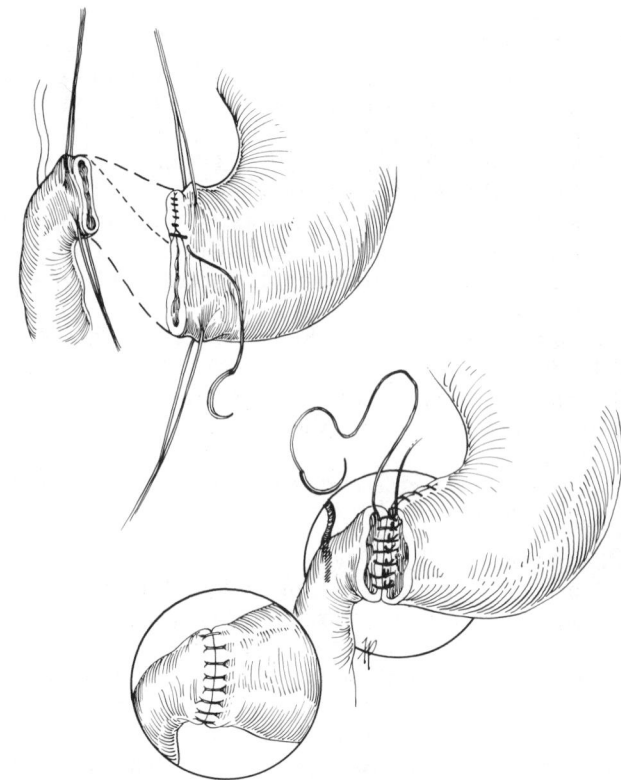

Figure 1. Partial gastrectomy with a Billroth I (gastroduodenostomy) repair. *Above,* Close lesser curvature of the stomach until lumen disparity is corrected. *Below,* Close with single interrupted sutures.

8. The area to be resected is isolated from the abdominal cavity with moistened laparotomy sponges.
9. Large, straight noncrushing intestinal forceps are placed above and below the proposed lines of incision.

Closure
1. A single layer interrupted appositional suture pattern is used to appose the stomach and duodenum. With unequal lumen sizes, the lesser curvature side of the stomach is closed first until the lumen disparity is corrected (Fig. 1, *top*).
2. The back (far) wall is apposed first, placing the knots into the lumen. Synthetic 3-0 absorbable suture (e.g., polydioxanone (PDS), Ethicon) is recommended.
3. The near wall is then apposed.

Surgical Procedure—Partial Gastrectomy and Gastrojejunostomy (Billroth II)

Objectives
- Resect a significant portion of the diseased stomach and all or part of the duodenum.
- Remove duodenum distal to the common bile duct opening.
- Re-establish continuity of the stomach to small bowel with a gastrojejunostomy.
- Restore a biliary connection to the duodenal or jejunal stump via a cholecystenterostomy.

Equipment
Same as that for the Billroth I.

Technique

1. Ligate and divide the appropriate vessels and the common bile duct.
2. The duodenal or jejunal stump is closed with a simple interrupted appositional suture pattern using 3-0 synthetic absorbable suture material or staples (TA, U.S. Surgical).
3. The original Billroth II reconstruction is done by closing the gastric stoma followed by a side-to-side anastomosis of the jejunum to an incision made in the ventral aspect of the stomach (Fig. 2).
4. A simple interrupted appositional suture pattern is used to appose the gastric and jejunal segments.
5. For more extensive resections, the entire width of the gastric stump is apposed to a longitudinal incision made in the jejunum (Fig. 3).
6. A suture pattern as described in step 4 is employed for closure.
7. A cholecystenterostomy is then performed to complete the procedure (see sec. 7, ch. 9).
8. Placement of a jejunostomy tube is done to provide nutrition in the debilitated patient.

Postoperative Care and Complications

Short-term

- Monitor temperature and abdominal pain for early signs of leakage peritonitis.
- Nothing by mouth (NPO) for 24 hours

- Initiate small amounts of food by mouth (per os) 24 hours after surgery.
- Dumping syndrome (passage of undigested food directly into the jejunum) may initially be a problem.

Long-term

- Dumping syndrome, due to disruption of the normal storage function of the stomach and excessive dumping of ingested food into the small intestine, may cause chronic postprandial discomfort, vomiting, and diarrhea.
- Alkaline reflux gastritis may result from loss of pyloric function.
- After extensive gastrectomy, multiple small feedings are necessary.

Prognosis

- Good—if the underlying disease is benign or inflammatory.
- Poor—if malignancy is the indication for surgery.

PYLOROMYOTOMY

Preoperative Considerations

- A pyloromyotomy is delayed until hypochloremic hypokalemic metabolic alkalosis, which often accom-

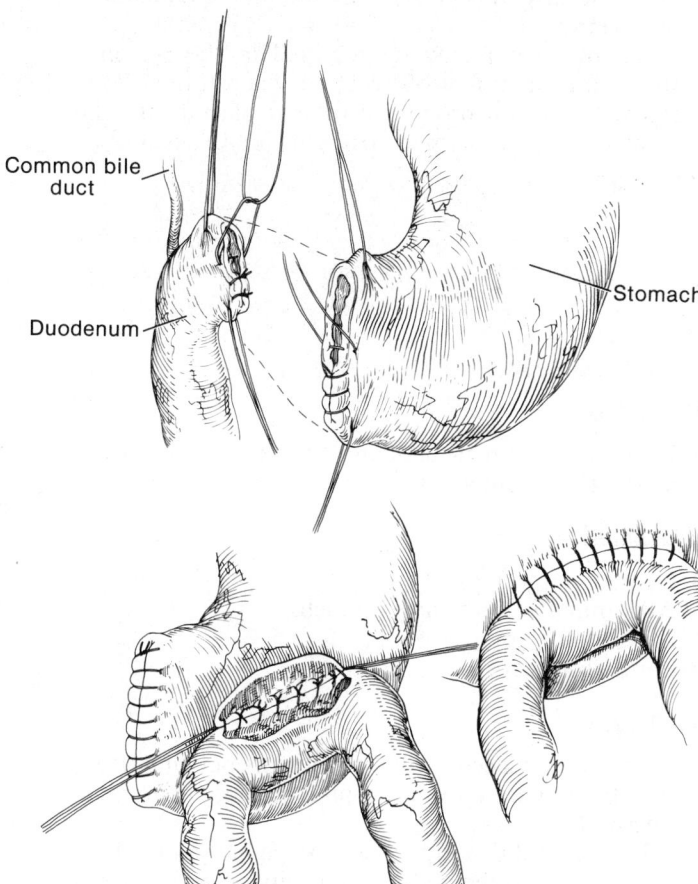

Figure 2. Billroth II procedure with side-to-side gastrojejunostomy.

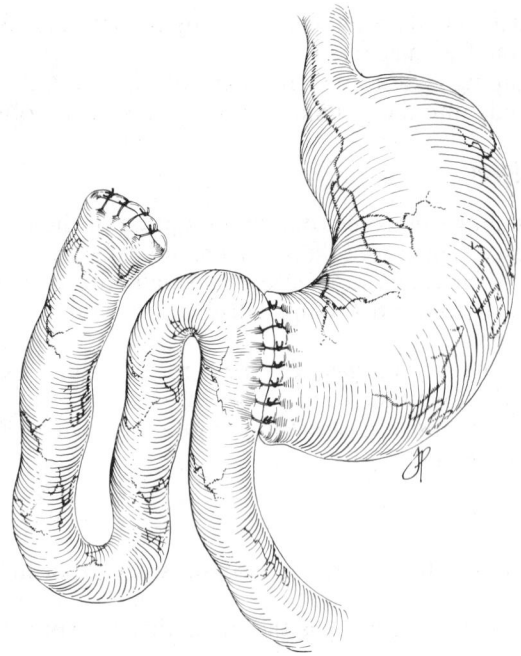

Figure 3. Billroth II with anastomosis of the entire gastric stump to a longitudinal incision of the jejunum.

panies the conditions requiring pyloromyotomy, is corrected.

■ Fluid therapy is directed toward restoring electrolyte *and* water abnormalities.

■ In the younger dog or cat, dextrose is added to the fluid therapy regimen in an attempt to maintain euglycemia.

■ Food and water may be retained in the patient's stomach with outflow obstruction. Therefore, following sedation, an orogastric tube is placed into the stomach and the stomach contents are evacuated.

KEY POINT ▶ Pyloromyotomy will *not* effectively relieve outflow obstruction caused by mucosal hypertrophy. Pyloromyotomy is primarily indicated for dogs with muscular hypertrophy only (see sec. 7, ch. 4).

Surgical Procedure

Objectives

■ Increase the lumen diameter of the pylorus to enhance gastric emptying.

Equipment

■ General surgery pack
■ Abdominal self-retaining retractor
■ Laparotomy sponges
■ Babcock forceps

Technique

1. The dog is placed in dorsal recumbency and aseptically prepared for a cranial midline abdominal incision.
2. The skin and underlying tissues are incised to allow an opening to the abdominal cavity extending from the xiphoid to 4–5 cm below the umbilicus.

3. The gastrohepatic ligament is partially incised to allow the pylorus to be mobilized.
4. The stomach is isolated and packed with laparotomy sponges.
5. A stay suture or a Babcock forceps is placed 3–5 cm proximal and distal to the pyloric ring.
6. An incision 4–5 cm long is made into a hypovascular area of the serosa overlying the pyloric antrum and canal and extended distally into the proximal duodenum. The pylorus is at the midpoint of the incision (Fig. 4, *top*).
7. All muscle fibers are gently incised or dissected away, using a curved hemostat, to allow the submucosa and mucosa to bulge (Fig. 4, *middle* and *bottom*).
8. The stomach is gently replaced into the abdomen.
9. Routine ventral abdominal closure is performed.

Postoperative Care and Complications

Short-term

■ Emesis extending beyond 6–8 hours postoperatively is treated with metoclopramide SC q6h at a dose of 0.2–0.4 mg/kg, as needed. Constant-rate IV infusion of metoclopramide 1–2 mg/kg/day is most effective.

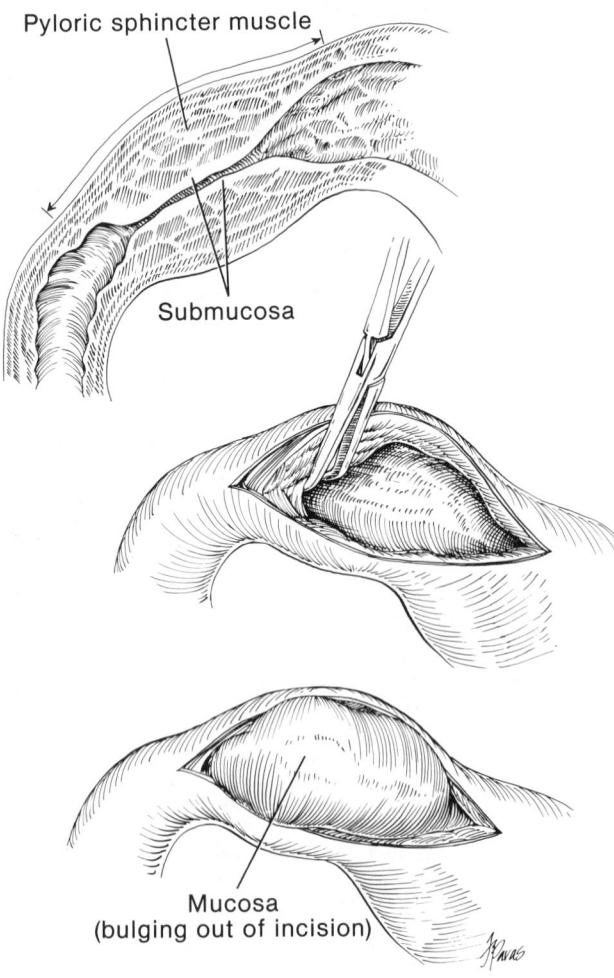

Figure 4. Technique for pyloromyotomy.

- Fluid therapy is maintained for 36–48 hours post-operatively.
- Frequent monitoring of the packed cell volume, albumin, and blood glucose values is done, especially in the very young animal.
- Electrolyte values are monitored closely in all animals the first 24 hours.
- Soft food is begun 24 hours after surgery unless vomiting continues.

Long-term

- Emesis may continue with little to no improvement noted. This sign may suggest a need to reoperate and perform a more extensive procedure (e.g., pyloroplasty).
- Signs of vomiting may recur several days or weeks following surgery. If other causes of vomiting are not identified, reoperation may be necessary.

Prognosis

Because the underlying disease in most cases is benign, the prognosis is good to excellent.

PYLOROPLASTY

Preoperative Considerations

- See pyloromyotomy.
- Pyloroplasty is indicated for pyloric hypertrophy involving muscle and mucosa or mucosa alone (see sec. 7, ch. 4). Dogs with severe pyloric hypertrophy may require the Billroth I procedure (see previous discussion).
- Manual and visual inspection of the lumen of the distal stomach, pylorus, and proximal duodenum is possible with a pyloroplasty.

Surgical Procedure

Objectives

- Inspect the distal stomach and pylorus for pathology.
- Increase the diameter of the gastric outflow tract.

Equipment

See pyloromyotomy.

Technique

Heineke-Mikulicz Pyloroplasty

1. Temporary stay sutures or Babcock forceps are placed on the antrum and proximal duodenum proximal and distal to the pyloric ring.
2. A full-thickness stab incision is made into the pylorus using a # 11 Bard-Parker scalpel blade. A suction tip is placed into the stomach to evacuate contents and bile.
3. The incision is extended with scissors to 1–2 cm above and below the pylorus (Fig. 5).
4. The stay sutures or Babcock forceps are removed.
5. The longitudinal incision is closed transversely with 3-0 synthetic absorbable sutures in a simple interrupted appositional pattern. Stay sutures can be

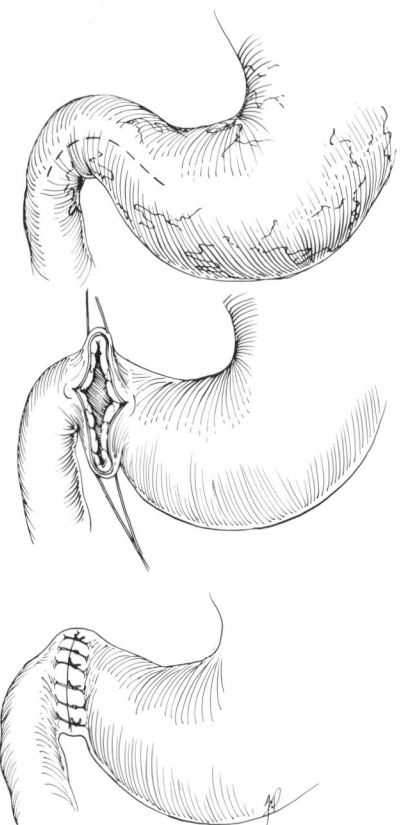

Figure 5. Technique for Heineke-Mikulicz pyloroplasty.

placed on both sides of the incision to help orient the tissues for closure.
6. Routine abdominal closure follows warm saline lavage of the surgical site.

Technique

Y-U Pyloroplasty (Antral Flap Advancement)

1. The pylorus is mobilized as described for pyloromyotomy.
2. Temporary stay sutures are placed 4–5 cm above and below the pylorus.
3. A Y-shaped incision is made through the seromuscular tissue overlying the pylorus and distal stomach (Fig. 6).
4. Each limb of the Y is approximately 3–4 cm in length depending on the size of the animal.
5. The base of the Y extends a small distance (3–4 mm) into the antrum proximal to the pylorus.
6. The V-shaped antral flap is trimmed to a U-shape. The resected tissue is employed as a biopsy specimen and placed in formalin.
7. Extensive palpation and visualization of the stomach and proximal duodenum are done.
8. Hypertrophied tissue is excised via a submucosal resection. Adjacent mucosa/submucosa is closed in a continuous pattern with 3-0 or 4-0 synthetic absorbable suture.
9. Pyloroplasty closure is begun by suturing the base of the U-shaped flap distally to the proximal duodenum with 3-0 or 4-0 synthetic absorbable suture (see Fig. 6).

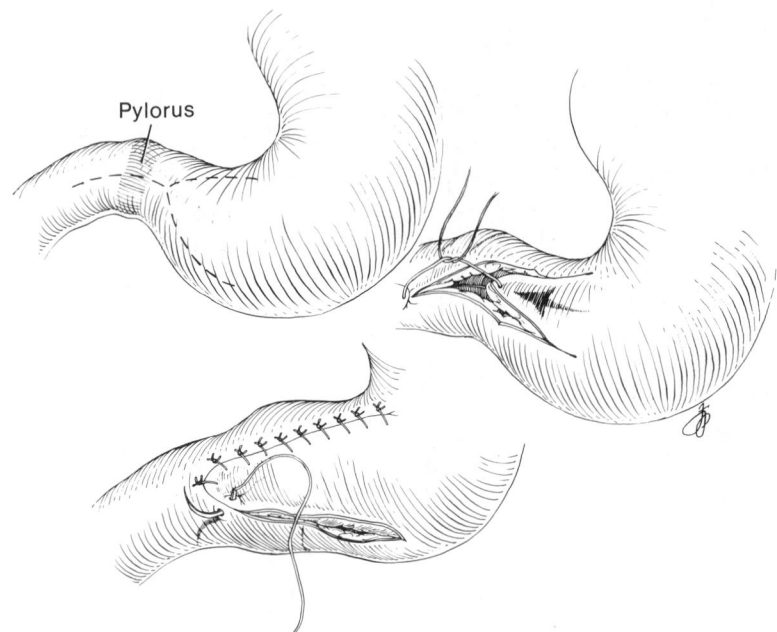

Pylorus

Figure 6. Technique for Y-U pyloroplasty.

10. A simple interrupted appositional pattern is recommended. If necessary, preplace the sutures to ensure accuracy.
11. The lesser curvature limb of the Y is closed, followed by the greater curvature limb (see Fig. 6).

Postoperative Care and Complications

Short-term

■ Same as that for pyloromyotomy.

Long-term

■ Emesis containing a significant amount of bile several weeks after surgery may suggest duodenogastric reflux. Consider treatment with metoclopramide.
■ Alkaline reflux gastritis resulting from duodenogastric reflux may require long-term therapy.

Prognosis

■ Good—if the disease being treated is benign.

ACUTE GASTRIC-DILATATION VOLVULUS

Preoperative Considerations

■ Aggressive fluid therapy, cardiac arrhythmia therapy, and orogastric decompression are necessary prior to any surgical intervention (see Ch. 7 sec. 4).
■ Stabilization of most patients can be accomplished in 2–3 hours.
■ Gastric perforation is considered a surgical emergency.

Surgical Procedure

Objectives

■ Reposition stomach and spleen to their normal anatomic relationship.

■ Fix ("pexy") the stomach to the abdominal wall to prevent future episodes of volvulus.
■ Resect devitalized tissue (spleen, stomach).

Equipment

■ General surgical pack
■ Self-retaining abdominal retractor (Balfour)
■ Foley catheter (22–26 Fr.)
■ Orogastric tube

Technique

1. The dog is placed in dorsal recumbency and surgically prepared from the midsternum to 6–8 cm below the umbilicus. If a tube gastropexy is utilized, the right side of the abdominal wall is prepared aseptically, halfway up the side of the thoracic and abdominal wall that corresponds with the length of the midline incision.
2. An orogastric tube is gently placed into the esophagus and advanced until there is resistance.
3. Derotation of the stomach is accomplished by grasping the pylorus and duodenum, usually located near the gastroesophageal junction, and elevating them to the right side of the body.
4. The fundus, usually on the right side, is depressed and rotated to the left side while the pylorus is being repositioned.
5. The orogastric tube is now placed within the stomach, and the stomach is decompressed.
6. The viability of the stomach is assessed, and resection of necrotic tissue done if necessary (see discussion of partial gastrectomy).
7. Splenectomy is usually not done unless there is evidence of splenic torsion or necrosis.
8. A gastropexy procedure is performed on the right side of the dog regardless of the technique employed. All of the gastropexy techniques described subsequently are effective. The technique chosen depends on the surgeon's preference.

Technique

Tube Gastropexy (22–26 Fr. Foley Catheter)

1. A full-thickness pursestring suture is placed in the midantrum area using 2-0 or 3-0 nonabsorbable suture. This suture is left untied (Fig. 7).
2. The tip of a Foley catheter is pulled through a small right paracostal incision using Carmalt forceps, approximately 4 cm caudal to the costal arch and 4 cm lateral to the incision.
3. A stab incision is made into the middle of the pursestring suture area and the tip of the Foley catheter advanced through this and into the stomach (Fig. 7).
4. The balloon portion of the catheter is inflated.
5. The pursestring suture is drawn tightly and tied.
6. The stomach is now moved to the abdominal wall with traction on the Foley catheter.
7. Six to eight interrupted sutures are now preplaced between the stomach, being sure to penetrate to the submucosa, and abdominal wall. Nonabsorbable # 1 or 1-0 suture material is used (see Fig. 7).
8. The sutures are now tied starting dorsally and ending ventrally.
9. The catheter is affixed to the skin with a traction suture.

Technique

Circumcostal Gastropexy

1. Two retention sutures utilizing 1-0 or 2-0 nonabsorbable suture material are placed in the antrum approximately 6 cm apart and midway between the lesser and greater curvature.
2. A 3 × 3–cm incision is made through the seromuscular layer forming an I-shaped configuration (Fig. 8, *inset*).
3. The seromuscular flaps are formed by careful dissection between the muscular and submucosa tunics. Two stay sutures are placed on each flap.
4. The 11th or 12th rib below the costochondral junction is isolated and rotated laterally with two towel clamps placed 6 cm apart.

5. A 4–5 cm length of the rib is exposed by incising through the peritoneum and muscle.
6. Blunt dissection removes all tissue attached to the rib.
7. One arm of each stay suture is passed under the rib.
8. Another stay suture is placed midway down the seromuscular flap found on the greater curvature side. This placement helps pull this flap around the exposed rib.
9. Once the flap is pulled around the rib, the two retention sutures are tied.
10. The seromuscular flap is sutured to the opposite flap using 2-0 synthetic absorbable or nonabsorbable suture (see Fig. 8). A simple interrupted full-thickness suture pattern is employed.
11. The peritoneum and musculature on the lateral aspect of the completed flap repair are now sutured to the seromuscular layer of the stomach with six to eight sutures. This bridges and supports the seromuscular flap suture line.

Technique

Belt Loop Gastropexy

1. A belt loop of muscle is produced by making two parallel transverse incisions 2–3 cm apart and 2–3 cm in length through the peritoneum and fascia of the transversus abdominis muscle.
2. The muscle fibers are bluntly separated with scissors (Fig. 9A).
3. A 2 × 4–cm tongue-shaped seromuscular flap is made with the base of the flap along the greater curvature of the antrum (Fig. 9B).
4. A branch of the gastroepiploic artery is centered at the base of the flap.
5. When creating the flap, the base is a little wider than the tip of the tongue-shaped flap.
6. The stomach flap is now passed through the belt loop in a cranial to caudal direction (Fig. 9C).
7. The flap is now repositioned over its original anatomic location and reattached to adjacent seromuscular tissue with 1-0 monofilament synthetic absorbable or nonabsorbable suture (Fig. 9D).

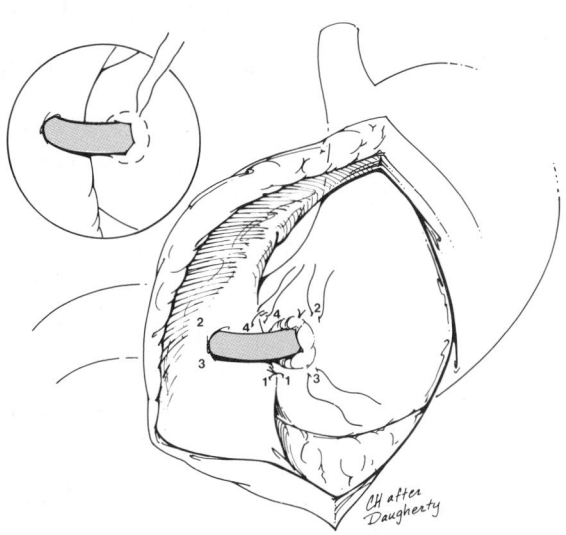

Figure 7. Technique for tube gastrotomy, for treatment of gastric dilatation volvulus. *Inset,* Place an untied pursestring suture in the mid-antrum area. Connect the stomach and abdominal wall with interrupted sutures. In the figure, points 1 are connected, as are points 2 to each other, and so forth. (Drawing by Carol Haynes, after Dougherty.)

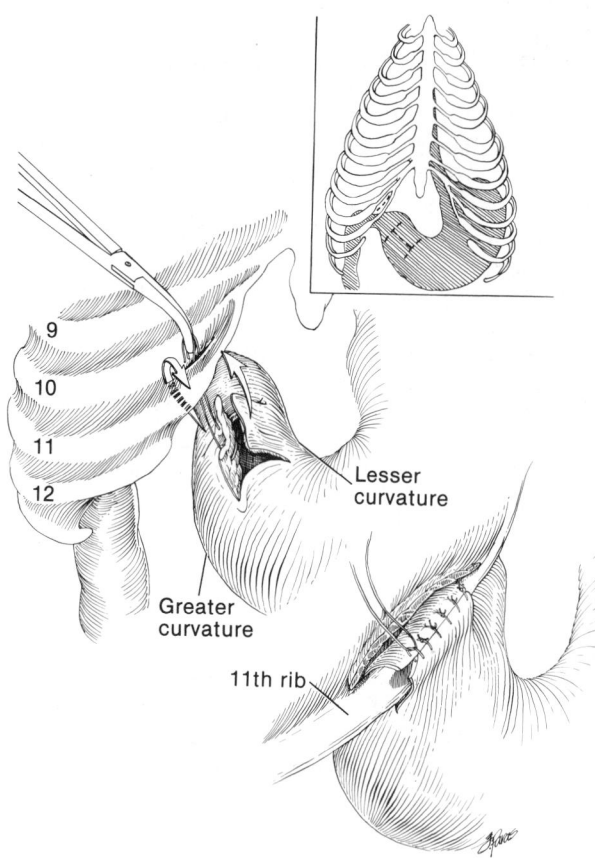

9
10
11
12

Lesser
curvature

Greater
curvature

11th rib

Figure 8. Technique for circumcostal gastrostomy (for gastric dilatation volvulus).

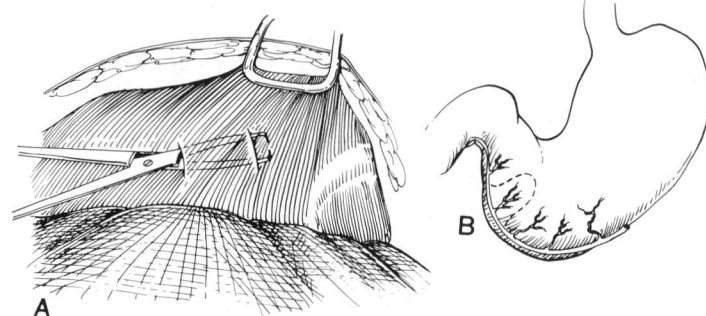

A

B

Figure 9. Technique for belt loop gastropexy (for gastric dilatation volvulus).

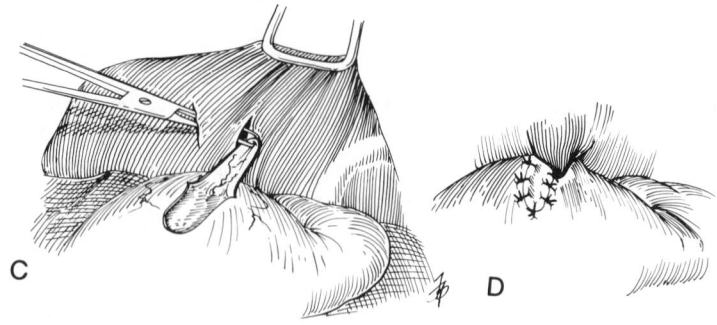

C

D

Technique

Muscle Flap Gastropexy

1. A U-shaped incision is made through the peritoneum and transversus abdominis muscle caudal to the 13th rib on the right lateral side.
2. The muscle flap is undermined and reflected ventrally.
3. Two horizontal mattress sutures using 1-0 nonabsorbable material are preplaced from the base of the U through the seromuscular layer of the antrum that is drawn laterally to the right abdominal wall (Fig. 10*A*).
4. The sutures are tied and secured against the body wall (Fig. 10*B*).
5. The remaining base of the U is secured to the stomach wall employing a simple continuous suture pattern (Fig. 10*C*).
6. The muscle flap is brought to the gastric surface advancing it a few millimeters beyond the previous suture line.
7. The flap is then sutured with the same material to the stomach wall to close the myotomy (Fig. 10*C*).

Postoperative Care and Complications

Short-term

■ Monitor closely for a minimum of 4 days for cardiac arrhythmias, especially ventricular arrhythmias, (see sec. 6, ch. 4, for details of treatment); hemodynamic abnormalities or circulatory collapse; recurrent gastric retention; and gastric perforation with subsequent peritonitis.

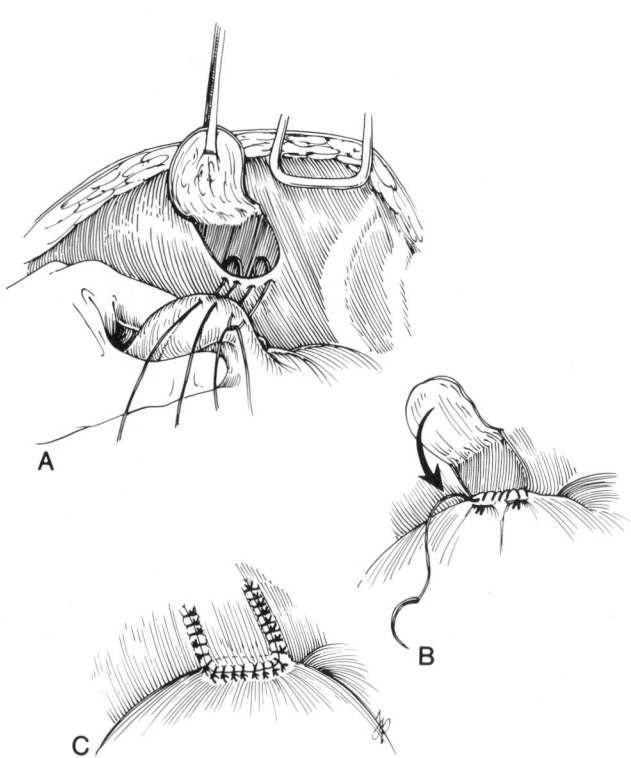

Figure 10. Technique for muscle flap gastropexy (for gastric dilatation volvulus).

■ Maintain fluid therapy and supplement with potassium for a minimum of 48 hours.
■ Monitor serum electrolyte, blood gas, hematocrit, total protein, urinary output, and central venous pressure values as necessary.
■ Promote gastrointestinal motility with metoclopramide 0.2–0.4 mg/kg SC or PO q6–8h. Treat with systemic antacids and sucralfate (see sec. 7, ch. 4) if ulcers or necrosis was present at surgery, or if vomiting of bloody fluid is present postoperatively.
■ Tube gastropexy is maintained under a soft padded bandage so that chewing or dislodgement of tube is prevented.
■ The tube can be used for decompression and administration of fluids, gruel, and medication.
■ Feeding can resume 24 to 48 hours after surgery.

Long-term

■ Remove the tube (tube gastropexy) 5–7 days after placement. Allow the fistula to heal by second intention (contraction and epithelialization).
■ Wean the animal slowly off antiarrhythmic drugs if cardiac arrhythmia was a problem and so treated.
■ Encourage three to four feedings per day at home.

Prognosis

■ Fair to good if partial gastrectomy is not indicated.
■ Grave to poor when partial gastrectomy is done—approximately 60% mortality.

Supplemental Readings

GASTROTOMY

Arnockzy SP, Ryan WW: Gastrotomy and pyloroplasty. Vet Clin North Am 5:343, 1975.
Dulisch ML: Gastrotomy. *Current Techniques in Small Animal Surgery II.* Philadelphia: Lea & Febiger, 1983, p 157.

PARTIAL GASTRECTOMY RELATED TO GASTRIC DILATATION-VOLVULUS

Clark GN, Pavletic MM: Partial gastrectomy with an automatic stapling instrument for treatment of gastric necrosis secondary to gastric dilatation-volvulus. Vet Surg 20:61, 1991.
Matthiesen DT: Partial gastrectomy as a treatment of gastric volvulus: results of 30 dogs. Vet Surg 14:185, 1985.

PARTIAL GASTRECTOMY (DISTAL STOMACH)

Ahmadu-Suka F, Withrow SJ, Nelson AW, et al.: Billroth II gastrojejunostomy in dogs. Stapling techniques and postoperative complications. Vet Surg 17:211, 1988.
Bright RM: Esophagus and stomach. Harvey CE, Newton CD, Schwartz A, eds.: *Small Animal Surgery.* Philadelphia: J.B. Lippincott, 1990, p 323.

PYLOROMYOTOMY

Dulisch ML: Pyloromyotomy and pyloroplasty. *Current Techniques in Small Animal Surgery II.* Philadelphia: Lea & Febiger, 1983, p 158.
Fox SM, Burns J: The effect of pyloric surgery on gastric emptying in the dog: comparison of three techniques. J Am Anim Hosp Assoc 22:783, 1986.

PYLOROPLASTY

Bright RM, Richardson DC, Stanton ME: Y-U antral flap advancement pyloroplasty in dogs. Comp Cont Educ Pract Vet 10:139, 1988.

Stanton ME, Bright RM, Toal R, et al.: Chronic hypertrophic pyloric gastropathy as a cause of pyloric obstruction in the dog. J Am Vet Med Assoc 186:157, 1985.

Walters MC, Goldschmidt MH, Stone EA, et al.: Chronic hypertrophic pyloric gastropathy as a cause of pyloric obstruction in the dog. J Am Vet Med Assoc 186:157, 1985.

GASTRIC DILATATION-VOLVULUS (SURGERY)

Fallah AM, Lumb WV, Nelson AW, et al.: Circumcostal gastropexy in the dog, a preliminary study. Vet Surg 11:9, 1982.

MacCoy DM, Sykes GP, Hoffer RE, et al.: A gastropexy technique for permanent fixation of the pyloric antrum. J Am Anim Hosp 18:763, 1982.

Schulman AJ, Lusk R, Lippincott CL, et al.: Muscular flap gastropexy: A new surgical technique to prevent recurrences of gastric dilatation-volvulus syndrome. J Am Anim Hosp Assoc 22:339, 1986.

Whitney WO, Scavelli TD, Matthiesen DT: Belt-loop gastropexy: Technique and surgical results in 20 dogs. J Am Anim Hosp 25:75, 1989.

6 Diseases of the Intestines

Robert G. Sherding
Susan E. Johnson

DIARRHEA AS A CLINICAL SIGN OF INTESTINAL DISEASE

Diarrhea results from excessive fecal water content and is the most important clinical sign of intestinal disease in the dog and cat. It is characterized by an abnormal increase in the frequency, fluidity, and volume of feces. The pathogenesis involves derangement of transmucosal water and solute fluxes caused by abnormal digestion, absorption, secretion, permeability, or motility or a combination of these.

Acute Versus Chronic Diarrhea

For initial management of diarrhea, determine if diarrhea is acute or chronic (based on history).

Acute Diarrhea

Acute diarrhea is a common clinical sign. It is characterized by sudden onset and short duration (3 weeks or less) of watery or watery-mucoid diarrhea that may be overtly bloody in severe cases. Inappetence, lethargy, and vomiting are frequent associated signs; fever, abdominal pain, and significant dehydration suggest more serious intestinal disease.

- Acute diarrhea in dogs and cats may be caused by dietary indiscretion or intolerance, drugs and toxins, intestinal parasites, infectious agents (viral, bacterial, rickettsial), and systemic or metabolic disturbances.
- Although there are exceptions, acute diarrhea associated with diet, parasites, and medications generally tends to be mild and self-limiting, whereas acute diarrhea that is severe and life-threatening occurs most frequently in young animals with infectious enteritis (e.g., parvoviral enteritis).
- Diagnostic evaluations in acute diarrhea need not be extensive. Because treatment is mainly supportive and nonspecific, many animals can be managed without determination of a definitive diagnosis. Nevertheless, it is important to identify parasites and enteropathogens that require specific treatments and to identify surgical diseases (e.g., foreign bodies, intussusception).
- Treatment of acute diarrhea is based on rehydration therapy and dietary restriction. Symptomatic therapy with antidiarrheal agents may be considered. Nonspecific or mild acute diarrhea often is self-limiting in a day or two without treatment or with restriction of food intake.

Chronic Diarrhea

- Diarrhea is categorized as chronic if it has been persistent (3–4 weeks or longer) or has a pattern of episodic recurrence. Chronicity generally excludes simple dietary indiscretion, intoxication, and viral enteritis as causes.

KEY POINT ▶ Base management of chronic diarrhea on diagnosis rather than symptomatic treatment. Specific intervention or treatment usually is necessary, requiring a specific diagnosis or histopathologic characterization.

- The first step in management is to classify the diarrhea as large or small bowel in origin, based on the history and physical examination. Diagnostic tests and procedures include routine hematologic and serum chemistry evaluations, tests of enteropancreatic function, fecal examinations, radiographic procedures, and endoscopic procedures. Biopsy of the small or large intestine often is necessary.

Small Bowel Versus Large Bowel Diarrhea

The anatomic localization of the disease process to the small or large bowel is based on the fecal characteristics (frequency, volume, consistency, color, odor, composition) and defecation patterns (Table 1). This distinction is important because it determines the direction of subsequent diagnostic evaluations. Diffuse diseases of the gastrointestinal tract may produce concurrent small and large bowel signs, and sometimes gastric signs such as vomiting.

Small Bowel Diarrhea

- Chronic small bowel diarrhea can be associated with maldigestion and malabsorption and is characterized by a high volume without urgency, tenesmus, or increased frequency. Weight loss and decline in body condition (malnutrition) may occur.
- Because of unabsorbed nutrients that are degraded and fermented by intestinal bacteria, the feces are rancid and foul-smelling. Increased production of luminal gas by bacteria results in excessive flatulence and borborygmus.
- Steatorrhea (feces containing an excess of unabsorbed fat) can be a prominent manifestation of small bowel diarrhea. In extreme cases, the feces may appear oily, greasy, and light in color. Hair

TABLE 1. Differentiation of Small Bowel Diarrhea from Large Bowel Diarrhea

Observation	Small Intestine	Large Intestine
Frequency of defecation	Normal to slightly increased	Very frequent
Fecal output	Large volumes	Small volumes frequently
Urgency or tenesmus	Absent	Present
Dyschezia	Absent	Present with rectal disease
Mucus in feces	Absent	Present
Hematochezia (red blood)	Absent (except in acute hemorrhagic diarrhea)	Present sometimes
Melena (digested blood)	Present sometimes	Absent
Steatorrhea	Present in maldigestive or malabsorptive disease	Absent
Flatulence & borborygmus	Present in maldigestive or malabsorptive disease	Absent
Weight loss	Present in maldigestive or malabsorptive disease	Rare
Vomiting	Present sometimes in inflammatory bowel disease	Rare

around the perineum may also have an oily texture from contact with fatty feces.

■ Small bowel diarrhea is generally free of grossly visible mucus or blood. When there is bleeding from a lesion in the proximal gastrointestinal (GI) tract, the luminal blood pigment produces dark black discoloration of the feces (melena) during transit. In the absence of gastric bleeding, melena generally indicates intestinal parasitism (hookworms), infection (viral, bacterial, fungal), ulceration (e.g., drug-induced), severe inflammation, or neoplasia.

Large Bowel Diarrhea

■ Large bowel diarrhea is characterized by frequent urges to defecate (usually greater than three times normal frequency), each defecation producing small quantities of feces that contain excessive mucus and sometimes fresh red blood.

■ Urgency resulting from irritability or inflammation of the distal colon causes frequent premature expulsions of small quantities of feces that would otherwise be insufficient to trigger the defecation reflex. Lapses in house-training ("accidents") may be caused by urgency and inability to control urges to defecate.

■ Straining (tenesmus) may be noted as the animal remains in a squatting posture for an extended period of time after defecation or makes repeated attempts to defecate within a few minutes. These attempts may produce little or no feces, or sometimes a small amount of feces composed almost entirely of mucus, exudate, and blood.

■ Because colonic diseases often are associated with mucosal injury, inflammation, or ulceration, abnormal fecal constituents frequently are present, including fresh red blood (hematochezia) that originates from sites of erosion or ulceration, mucus that originates from the abundant goblet cells in the colon that respond to mucosal injury by an outpouring of mucus, exudate (leukocytes) that originates from the site of inflammation.
  • Blood may coat the feces, streaks of blood may be mixed within the feces, or drops of blood may be passed at the end of defecation.
  • Excessive mucus may give the feces a glistening or jelly-like appearance.
  • Exudates are detected by the positive identification of fecal leukocytes, using cytology stains.

KEY POINT ▶ Abnormal fecal constituents such as fresh red blood, mucus, and leukocytes are localizing signs indicative of colonic disease.

■ Because the principal function of the colon is absorption of water and electrolytes rather than digestion and absorption of nutrients, nutrient malabsorption and steatorrhea are absent in large bowel diarrhea. Thus, dramatic weight loss and wasting are unlikely if the animal is eating, and the daily fecal output (volume or weight of feces) usually is only minimally increased.

Protein-Losing Enteropathy

Gastrointestinal loss accounts for approximately 40% of the normal daily turnover of plasma proteins. The term *protein-losing enteropathy* refers to a variety of intestinal diseases that are associated with hypoproteinemia caused by an accelerated loss of plasma proteins into the gut.

■ Mechanisms of excessive enteric loss of protein include:
  • Impaired intestinal lymphatic drainage (e.g., lymphangiectasia) that results in extravasation of protein-rich lymph into the lumen.
  • Disruption of the mucosal barrier (e.g., inflammation) that results in protein leakage from sites of exudation, bleeding, or increased permeability.
■ Protein-losing enteropathy occurs most frequently in association with chronic enteropathies such as:
  • Idiopathic canine intestinal lymphangiectasia
  • Chronic inflammatory small bowel diseases (lymphocytic-plasmacytic enteritis, granulomatous enteritis, eosinophilic enteritis, immunoproliferative enteropathy of basenjis)
  • Intestinal histoplasmosis
  • Intestinal lymphosarcoma

DIAGNOSTIC APPROACH TO DIARRHEA

History

The history is especially helpful for localizing the disease process to the small or large bowel. It also may indicate underlying extraintestinal causes of diarrhea

TABLE 2. Clinical Significance of Abnormal Physical Findings Associated with Intestinal Disease

Physical Finding	Potential Clinical Associations
General Physical Examination	
Dehydration	Diarrheal fluid loss
Depression/weakness	Electrolyte imbalance, severe debilitation
Emaciation/malnutrition	Chronic malabsorption, protein-losing enteropathy
Dull unthrifty haircoat	Malabsorption of fatty acids, protein, and vitamins
Fever	Infection, transmural inflammation, neoplasia
Edema, ascites, pleural effusion	Protein-losing enteropathy
Pallor (anemia)	Gastrointestinal blood loss, anemia of chronic illness or inflammation
Intestinal Palpation	
Masses	Foreign body, neoplasia, granuloma
Thickened loops	Infiltration (inflammatory, neoplastic)
"Sausage loop"	Intussusception
Aggregated loops	Linear intestinal foreign body, peritoneal adhesions
Pain	Inflammation, obstruction, ischemia
Gas or fluid distension	Obstruction, ileus
Mesenteric lymphadenopathy	Inflammation, infection, neoplasia
Rectal Palpation	
Masses	Polyp, granuloma, neoplasia
Circumferential narrowing	Stricture, spasm, neoplasia
Coarse mucosal texture	Colitis, neoplasia

(e.g., renal failure, hypoadrenocorticism, or hyperthyroidism) and identify important predisposing factors such as breed, diet, environmental factors, current medications, and exposure to parasites, infectious agents, and toxins. The following historical aspects of the diarrhea may be diagnostically useful:

- Mode of onset (abrupt versus gradual)
- Duration (acute versus chronic)
- Clinical course (intermittent, continuous, or progressive)
- Fecal characteristics (small bowel versus large bowel; see previous discussion)
- Correlation with diet (food intolerances, dietary indiscretions)
- Correlation with medication usage (drug side effects)
- Correlation with stressful events (psychogenic, anxiety or "irritability" factors)
- Response to previous treatments (prescribed diets, antibiotics, corticosteroids, anthelmintics)
- Association with other signs (weight loss, vomiting, dyschezia)

Physical Examination

A complete physical examination may reveal important clues about the severity, nature, and cause of diarrhea (Table 2), although in many patients the findings are nonspecific.

- Identify physical findings that may indicate underlying systemic disease that could be a cause or consequence of diarrhea.

- Identify abnormalities on abdominal palpation of the intestinal loops and digital palpation of the rectum.
- Inspect the fecal material obtained on the palpation glove for abrasive particles (such as bone chips), blood, and mucus. If indicated, examine the material microscopically for parasites and inflammatory cells or submit for culture.

Routine Laboratory Tests

- Evaluate the complete blood count (CBC) for leukocyte responses and anemia that may be associated with intestinal disease (Table 3).
- Perform a serum biochemical profile and urinalysis to identify metabolic or systemic disorders that could cause or result from diarrhea (see Table 3).
- Measure serum thyroxin levels in older cats with diarrhea and weight loss to exclude hyperthyroidism as a cause (see sec. 4, ch. 1).

TABLE 3. Implications of Various Laboratory Findings in Intestinal Disease

Abnormal Laboratory Findings	Clinical Associations
Hematologic Findings	
Eosinophilia	Parasitism, eosinophilic enteritis, hypoadrenocorticism
Neutrophilia	Bowel inflammation, necrosis, or neoplasia
Neutropenia	Parvovirus, endotoxemia, or overwhelming sepsis (e.g., leakage peritonitis from bowel perforation)
Monocytosis	Chronic or granulomatous inflammation (e.g., mycosis)
Lymphopenia	Loss of lymphocytes from intestinal lymphangiectasia
Anemia	Enteric blood loss, depressed erythropoiesis from chronic inflammation or malnutrition
Elevated hematocrit	Hemoconcentration from GI fluid loss
RBC microcytosis	Iron deficiency from chronic GI blood loss
RBC macrocytosis	RBC regeneration, feline hyperthyroidism, feline leukemia virus, nutritional deficiencies (rare)
Serum Biochemical Findings	
Panhypoproteinemia	Protein-losing enteropathy
Hyperglobulinemia	Chronic immune stimulation, basenji enteropathy
Azotemia	Dehydration, primary renal failure
Hypokalemia	GI loss of fluid and electrolytes, anorexia
Hyperkalemia/ hyponatremia	Hypoadrenocorticism, trichuriasis (rare)
Hypocalcemia	Hypoalbuminemia, lymphangiectasia, pancreatitis
Hypocholesterolemia	Lymphangiectasia, liver disease
Elevated liver enzymes/ bile acids	Liver disease
Elevated amylase/lipase	Pancreatitis, mild elevations in enteritis or azotemia
Elevated thyroxine (T4)	Feline hyperthyroidism

GI = gastrointestinal; RBC = red blood cell.

Fecal Examinations

Fecal examinations are an important aspect of the diagnostic approach to diarrhea and may involve gross inspection (as previously described), parasite and microscopic examinations, quantitative fecal collection and analysis, chemical determinations, and cultures.

■ Examination of feces for parasites should be part of the minimum data base for all animals with diarrhea.
■ In cases of chronic unresponsive diarrhea, expand the data base to include microscopic examination of stained fecal smears for fat, starch, and leukocytes.
■ If circumstances suggest infection, perform fecal culture for specific enteropathogenic bacteria (Salmonella, Campylobacter).
■ Diagnostic methods for intestinal parasites and infectious agents are listed in Table 4.

Fecal Examinations for Parasites

■ Perform conventional fecal flotations to identify metazoan ova.
■ In warm, humid regions (e.g., Southern United States) endemic for Strongyloides spp., perform a direct smear, sedimentation, or Baermann technique to identify larvae in feces.
■ Giardia, the most important protozoan parasite, is best diagnosed by identification of cysts using a zinc sulfate centrifugation-flotation method. Motile trophozoites of protozoan parasites, including Giardia spp., Trichomonas spp., Entamoeba histolytica, and Balantidium coli, can be identified microscopically in a drop of fresh feces suspended in a few drops of isotonic saline. The distinguishing characteristics of each of these protozoa are discussed in the section Protozoan Infections of the Intestines in this chapter.

TABLE 4. Diagnosis of Intestinal Pathogens of Dogs and Cats

Pathogen	Method of Diagnosis
Helminths	
Ascarids (Toxocara, Toxascaris leonina)	Routine fecal flotation for ova
Hookworms (Ancylostoma)	Routine fecal flotation for ova
Whipworms (Trichuris vulpis)	Routine fecal flotation for ova; Rx trial
Tapeworms (Taenia, Dipylidium caninum)	Fecal proglottids or flotation for ova
Strongyloides	Fecal sediment or Baermann test for larvae
Others (flukes)	Zinc sulfate fecal flotation for ova
Protozoa	
Coccidia (Isospora, Cryptosporidium)	Sheather's fecal flotation for oocysts
Giardia	Zinc sulfate fecal flotation for cysts; fecal smear for trophozoites; fecal ELISA; Rx trial
Pentatrichomonas hominas	Saline fecal smear for trophozoites
Entamoeba histolytica	Saline fecal smear for trophozoites
Balantidium coli	Saline fecal smear for trophozoites
Viruses	
Parvovirus:	
Canine parvovirus	Fecal ELISA for viral antigen; EM
Feline panleukopenia virus	Signs, leukopenia
Coronavirus:	
Canine coronavirus	Fecal EM
Feline enteric coronavirus, FIP	Signs, serology, fecal EM, biopsies
Rotaviruses	Fecal EM
Astrovirus	Fecal EM
Others:	
Canine distemper virus	Signs
Retroviruses (FeLV, FIV)	Signs, serology
Rickettsia	
Salmon poisoning disease (Neorickettsiae helminthoeca)	Operculated trematode eggs in feces; rickettsia in lymph node cytology (Giemsa stain)
Bacteria	
Salmonella	Fecal culture
Campylobacter jejuni	Fecal microscopy and culture
Yersinia enterocolitica, Y. pseudotuberculosis	Fecal culture
Bacillus piliformis (Tyzzer's)	Biopsy (gut, liver) for filamentous bacteria; mouse inoculation
Mycobacteria	Biopsy for acid-fast bacteria
Clostridium perfringens, C. dificile (?)	Fecal microscopy, culture and toxin assays
Enteropathogenic E. coli (?)	Fecal culture and toxin assays
Fungi	
Histoplasma capsulatum	Fungi in biopsies/cytologies; serology
Pythium, Zygomycetes	Poorly septate hyphae in biopsies
Others (Candida albicans, Aspergillus)	Yeast or hyphae in biopsies
Algae (Prototheca)	Unicellular algae in cytologies or biopsies; fecal culture (Sabouraud's)

Rx = therapeutic response trial; ELISA = enzyme-linked immunosorbent assay; EM = electron microscopy; FIP = feline infectious peritonitis; FeLV = feline leukemia virus; FIV = feline immunodeficiency virus.

- Use Sheather's sugar flotation method to identify small coccidia such as *Cryptosporidia* spp.
- Diagnosis of occult parasite infections (e.g., *Giardia*, whipworms) can be based on response to a therapeutic trial.

KEY POINT ▶ Intestinal parasitism can mimic virtually any of the more complex small and large bowel disorders, and in many areas parasites are the most frequent cause of diarrhea. The most important enteropathogens are hookworms, whipworms, and *Giardia*.

Fecal Examinations for Infectious Agents

The diagnosis of infectious diarrhea often depends on the detection of the offending viral, bacterial, or fungal organisms in the feces. Details of diagnosis of these various enteric infections are found in the respective sections of this chapter.

Viruses. Viral diarrhea generally is acute and is confirmed by identification of virus in the feces serologically or by electron microscopy (see sec. 2, ch. 7).

Bacteria
- Specific enteropathogenic bacteria such as *Salmonella*, *Campylobacter*, *Clostridium*, and *Yersinia* can be isolated from fresh feces using specialized culture media. Such cultures are indicated when:
  - Examination of fecal cytology preparations reveals the presence of numerous fecal leukocytes, *Campylobacter*-like bacteria, or a predominance of *Clostridium* spp. (large, gram-positive endospore-forming rods).
  - There is an outbreak of diarrhea in groups of animals.
- Feces may be assayed for the diarrheogenic enterotoxins of *Clostridium perfringens* and *C. difficile*.

Fungi. The diagnosis of fungal *(Histoplasma, Aspergillus, Pythium, Candida)* and protothecal infection usually is based on identification of the organisms in fecal cytologies or intestinal biopsies.

- Sabouraud's media can be used to culture feces for *Histoplasma*, other fungi, and *Prototheca* (a rare cause of colitis), but culture growth is slow (up to 2 weeks) and the isolation rate is low.
- Serodiagnostic tests for histoplasmosis also are available (see sec. 2, ch. 12).

Fecal Examination Using Special Stains

Feces can be examined microscopically for abnormal constituents using stains such as direct and indirect Sudan, Lugol's iodine, Gram, and various other cytologic stains. In each test, 1–2 drops of feces and 1–2 drops of stain are mixed well on a microscope slide, coverslipped, and examined. In general, these procedures are only appropriate as initial screening tests because they are relatively insensitive and nonspecific and are dependent on the diet.

Sudan Stain
- *Direct Sudan Staining* (Sudan III stain) identifies excessive undigested (unsplit) fat in the feces as numerous, large, refractile orange droplets, indicating steatorrhea due to pancreatic maldigestion.
- *Indirect Sudan Staining* (Sudan stain with 36% acetic acid and heating) identifies unabsorbed fatty acids (split fat) as well as undigested fat. Thus, numerous large orange lipid droplets on an indirect Sudan stain in an animal with a negative direct Sudan stain suggest steatorrhea due to intestinal malabsorption of fatty acids.

Lugol's Iodine Stain (2%). This method identifies excessive undigested starch in the feces (amylorrhea) as dark blue-black granules or identifies light brown, undigested striated muscle fibers in meat-fed animals; either of these findings suggest maldigestion due to pancreatic maldigestion. *Giardia* trophozoites and cysts also stain light brown with iodine.

Cytology Stain. Cytology staining (e.g., new methylene blue, Wright's, Diff-Quik) identifies fecal leukocytes, which appear in exudative inflammatory bowel diseases when there is disruption of distal intestinal or colonic mucosa. Cytology may occasionally identify neoplastic cells or *Histoplasma* or *Prototheca* organisms. It is advisable to follow up patients that are positive for fecal leukocytes with colonoscopy and fecal cultures for invasive bacteria such as *Campylobacter* and *Salmonella*.

Gram Stain. Gram staining identifies an overabundance of large, gram-positive endosporulating rods *(Clostridia)* or *Campylobacter*-like organisms.

Tests for Fecal Occult Blood

These include a simple, in-office qualitative screening test (Hemoccult Test) and a more accurate, semi-quantitative send-out test (HemoQuant; SmithKline). These tests are sensitive for detecting even very small amounts of gastrointestinal hemorrhage. Because of this sensitivity, it is recommended to exclude meat from the animal's diet for at least 3 days prior to testing to avoid false positive results.

- The presence of fecal occult blood signifies a bleeding lesion of the GI tract, which suggests an ulcerative, inflammatory, or neoplastic condition.
- The fecal occult blood test is also indicated to document GI bleeding as a cause of blood loss anemia.

Quantitative Fecal Fat Analysis

This can be used as an intestinal function test to confirm steatorrhea, but it is extremely cumbersome and impractical to perform and does not differentiate pancreatic maldigestion from intestinal malabsorption. Feces must be collected for a 24- to 72-hour period while the animal is confined and fed a standard diet. The feces are weighed and sent to a commercial laboratory for analysis. Normally, less than 10% of ingested fat is excreted in the feces, or less than 0.3 g/kg/day in dogs and less than 0.4 g/kg/day in cats.

Tests for Fecal Proteolytic Activity

This can be assayed as an indicator of pancreatic secretion of proteases (trypsin) for the diagnosis of exocrine pancreatic insufficiency (EPI), especially in cats. The serum trypsin-like immunoreactivity (TLI) assay is more accurate and is preferred for diagnosis of EPI in dogs (see sec. 7, ch. 10).

Tests to Document GI Protein Loss

For the documentation of protein-losing enteropathy, GI loss of plasma proteins can be measured using the fecal excretion of intravenously administered radiolabeled proteins and macromolecules, such as ^{51}chromium-labeled albumin. However, these radiolabeled substrates are difficult to obtain and the procedures are impractical for use in the clinical setting.

Tests of Digestive and Absorptive Function

Exocrine Pancreatic Function Tests

Tests for exocrine pancreatic insufficiency (pancreatic maldigestion), such as serum trypsin-like immunoreactivity (TLI), oral bentiromide (BT-PABA) digestion, and fecal assays for proteolytic activity are described in sec. 7, ch. 10.

Quantitative Fecal Fat Analysis

See preceding discussion.

Xylose Absorption Test

The xylose absorption test is the standard test for evaluating canine intestinal absorptive function; however, it is relatively insensitive and does not help to differentiate the numerous small intestinal diseases capable of causing malabsorption.

- In normal dogs, following a 12-hour fast and oral administration of xylose (0.5 g/kg as a 5–10% solution), plasma xylose concentration peaks at 60 mg/dL in 60–120 minutes. Intestinal malabsorption is indicated by an abnormally low plasma xylose level.
- In cats, the xylose absorption test provides inconsistent results; thus, the test is difficult to interpret and not recommended.

Serum Folate and Cobalamin Assays

Serum levels of folate and cobalamin (vitamin B_{12}) reflect intestinal absorptive function and the status of the intestinal flora. Serum folate levels (normal, 3.5–11.0 μg/liter) depend on the absorptive function of the jejunum, whereas serum levels of cobalamin (normal, 300–700 ng/liter) depend on secretion of pancreatic intrinsic factor and absorption in the ileum.

- Serum folate may be decreased in enteropathies that impair absorption in the proximal small intestine.
- Serum cobalamin may be decreased in exocrine pancreatic insufficiency and enteropathies that impair absorption in the distal small intestine.
- The levels of both vitamins may be decreased in diseases that cause diffuse intestinal malabsorption.
- In small intestinal bacterial overgrowth, serum folate levels may actually be increased due to synthesis of folate by the overgrown bacteria, whereas cobalamin may be decreased because bacteria can utilize or

bind the vitamin, making it unavailable for absorption.

Radiography and Ultrasonography

Plain Abdominal Radiography

Plain radiography is indicated for detection of intestinal masses or abnormal gas-fluid patterns when mechanical or obstructive disorders are suspected (intestinal mass, foreign body, intussusception).

Upper GI Barium Contrast Radiography

This is indicated when other tests fail to determine the cause of small bowel diarrhea or when intestinal obstruction is suspected (see sec. 1, ch. 4). The study may help to detect obstructive lesions, stagnant loops, and neoplastic or inflammatory lesions that cause an irregular mucosal pattern or distortion of the bowel wall. In most cases, however, diarrhea involves microscopic or functional changes in the bowel that are not detected by barium radiography.

Barium Enema Contrast Radiography

This may be useful in selected cases of large bowel diarrhea for evaluating the colon and cecum for intussusceptions, neoplasms, polyps, strictures, inflammatory lesions, and colonic displacement or shortening. Colonoscopy is generally preferred over barium enema for evaluating the colon because it yields more definitive diagnostic information.

Abdominal Ultrasonography

Ultrasonography can define intestinal and other abdominal masses and evaluate the mesenteric lymph nodes, pancreas, liver, biliary tract, and prostate (see sec. 1, ch. 4).

Endoscopy

KEY POINT ▶ Endoscopic examination with mucosal biopsy is required for definitive diagnosis or accurate characterization of the disease in most cases of chronic intractable diarrhea in which extraintestinal, dietary, parasitic, and infectious causes have been excluded.

Upper GI Endoscopy

- Duodenoscopy with a flexible fiberoptic endoscope can be performed in the anesthetized animal for visual examination of the duodenum, for duodenal aspiration (for quantitative bacterial culture or detection of *Giardia*), and for directed forceps biopsy of the intestinal mucosa (see sec. 7, ch. 4 for a description of endoscopic equipment and discussion of gastroscopy).
- The normal duodenal mucosa appears pale pink with a uniformly granular villus pattern. Biliary and pancreatic duct papillae and Peyer's lymphoid patches are normally seen. The mucosa is nonfriable and free of excessive granularity, ulcers, thickened folds, masses, or strictures.

Colonoscopy

- Colonoscopy allows direct visualization of the lumen of the colon, sampling of luminal content for culture and exfoliative cytology, and directed forceps biopsy of the ileocolonic mucosa.
- Suitable rigid colonoscopes are relatively inexpensive and easy to use. Because colonic diseases are often diffuse, examination of the descending colon with a rigid instrument is sufficient for diagnosis in many patients.
- When lesions are located predominantly in the ascending or transverse colon, areas inaccessible with a rigid colonoscope, use a flexible fiberoptic colonoscope. A flexible colonoscope often can be navigated through the ileocolic sphincter for examination and biopsy of the ileum.
- The normal colonic mucosa appears pale pink through the colonoscope and reflects light uniformly. It is nonfriable, thin enough that the submucosal vessels are visible, and free of ulcers, thickened folds, masses, or strictures.

Intestinal Biopsy

The least invasive and, in many cases, preferred method for procurement of intestinal biopsies is endoscopy; if this is unavailable or if endoscopic biopsies are inconclusive, consider full-thickness intestinal biopsy by laparotomy (see sec. 7, ch. 7).

- Obtain multiple biopsies along the length of the gut even if no lesions are visible by gross inspection, which is often the case.
- Biopsy mesenteric lymph nodes and evaluate other abdominal organs, especially the pancreas, liver, and colon.
- Duodenal aspirates or duodenal mucosal impression smears may be examined for *Giardia* or cultured quantitatively for aerobic and anaerobic bacterial overgrowth.

NONSPECIFIC SYMPTOMATIC TREATMENT OF DIARRHEA

Dietary, supportive, and symptomatic therapy often is beneficial in diarrhea, especially acute diarrhea. In severe acute diarrhea, rehydration therapy can be life-saving.

Diet

Acute Diarrhea

The initial goal is to put the GI tract to rest by restricting food intake for at least 24 hrs.

- When resuming feeding give bland low-fat foods in small amounts at frequent intervals. Examples of appropriate foods include boiled rice, potatoes, and pasta as carbohydrate sources combined with boiled skinless chicken, yogurt, or low-fat cottage cheese as protein sources. Ready-made prescription diets (e.g., Prescription Canine Diet i/d; Hill's Pet) can also be used.
- When the diarrhea has been resolved for 48 hrs, gradually reintroduce the animal's regular diet.

Chronic Diarrhea

Divide daily food intake into 3 to 4 feedings; use low-fat diets with high digestibility for small bowel diarrhea, hypoallergenic diets for idiopathic inflammatory bowel diseases, and high-fiber diets for large bowel diarrhea (refer to respective disease sections of this chapter).

Fluid Therapy

- In severe acute diarrhea, such as occurs with parvoviral enteritis, fluid and electrolyte replacement is essential for management of intestinal fluid loss which may lead to serious dehydration, shock, and death (see sec. 1, ch. 5).
- Parenteral methods of fluid therapy are preferred in most cases; however, oral glucose-electrolyte solutions (e.g., Entrolyte, SmithKline) are available for counterbalancing intestinal fluid losses in cases of mild diarrhea.

Antidiarrheal Drugs

Symptomatic treatment is based on drugs that modify motility and fluid secretion/absorption or that act locally within the lumen as protectants/adsorbents. In most cases, these drugs are reserved for short-term use, usually for periods of 5 days or less. Some commonly used antidiarrheal drugs and their dosages are listed in Table 5.

Opiate and Opioid Narcotic Analgesics

These are probably the most effective all-purpose antidiarrheal agents.

- Mechanism:
  - They inhibit intestinal fluid loss through modification of mucosal fluid and electrolyte transport.
  - They impede bowel transit by stimulating nonpropulsive contractions (segmentation) and decreasing propulsive motility (peristalsis), thereby allowing more contact time for absorption.
- Examples include paregoric, diphenoxylate (Lomotil), and loperamide (Imodium).

Anticholinergic/Antispasmodic Drugs

- Mechanism:
  - They inhibit intestinal fluid loss, presumably through an antisecretory effect.
  - They cause a generalized suppression of gut motility that may potentiate ileus; however, their "atropine-like" antispasmodic action may be beneficial for controlling the urgency and discomfort of colitis.
- Examples include dicyclomine (Bentyl), isopropamide (Darbazine), aminopentamide (Centrine), and propantheline (Pro-Banthine).

Prostaglandin-Inhibitors

- These drugs have an anti-inflammatory/antisecretory action.

TABLE 5. Drugs Used for Symptomatic Treatment of Diarrhea

Drug	Product (Manufacturer)	Preparation	Dosage	Frequency
Narcotic Analgesics*				
Diphenoxylate	Lotomil (Searle)	Tab—2.5 mg; Liq—0.5 mg/ml	0.1–0.2 mg/kg	q6–8h
Loperamide	Imodium A-D (McNeil)	Cap—2 mg; Liq—0.2 mg/ml	0.1–0.2 mg/kg	q6–8h
Codeine	Many	Tab; Cap; Liq	0.25–0.5 mg/kg	q6–8h
Anticholinergics/Antispasmodics				
Aminopentamide	Centrine (Fort Dodge)	Tab—0.2 mg, Inj–0.5 mg/ml	0.1–0.5 mg total	q8–12h
Dicyclomine	Bentyl (Marion Merrell-Dow)	Tab—20 mg, Cap—10 mg, Liq—2 mg/ml, Inj—10 mg/ml	0.2 mg/kg	q8–12h
Propantheline	Pro-Banthine (Schiapparelli Searle)	Tab—7.5–15 mg	0.25 mg/kg	q8–12h
Methscopolamine	Pamine (Upjohn)	Tab—2.5 mg	0.3–1.5 mg/kg	q8–12h
Hyoscyamine	Levsin (Schwarz)	Tab—0.125 mg; Liq—0.025 mg/ml, 0.125 mg/ml	0.003–0.006 mg/kg	q8–12h
Clidinium	Quarzan (Roche)	Cap—2.5 mg, 5 mg	0.1–0.25 mg/kg	q8–12h
Anticholinergics plus CNS Depressant				
Isopropamide plus prochlorperazine	Darbazine (SmithKline)	Cap	Refer to product label	q8–12h
Clidinium plus chlordiazepoxide	Librax (Roche)	Cap—2.5 mg (clidinium)	0.1–0.25 mg/kg (clidinium)	q8–12h
Hyoscyamine plus phenobarbital	Donnatal (Robins)	Tab; Cap; Liq	0.003–0.006 mg/kg (hyoscyamine)	q8–12h
Antisecretory/Protectant				
Bismuth subsalicylate†	Pepto-Bismol (Procter & Gamble)	Liq—9 and 16 mg salicylate/ml	0.5–1.0 ml/kg	q6–8h

*Narcotic analgesics are not recommended for cats or for cases of bacterial enteritis or liver disease.
†Avoid long-term (>3 days) use in cats because of low tolerance for salicylates.
Tab = tablets; Cap = capsules; Liq = elixir, suspension, or drops; Inj = injectable; CNS = central nervous system.

- They can be used for intraluminal delivery of antiprostaglandin to the proximal GI tract (bismuth subsalicylate [Pepto-Bismol]) and to the lower GI tract or colon (sulfasalazine [Azulfidine], olsalazine, [Dipentum], mesalamine [Asacol]) for treatment of chronic colitis (see Chronic Inflammatory Bowel Disease later in this chapter).
- Avoid use of systemic prostaglandin inhibitors (nonsteroidal anti-inflammatory drugs) because they tend to cause gastric ulceration.

Protectant/Adsorbent Drugs

- These oral agents work in the lumen to adsorb injurious bacteria and toxins and to provide a protective coating on inflamed mucosal surfaces.
- The efficacy of these drugs remains unproven; large doses are often required, and they may be difficult to administer.
- Examples include kaolin-pectin, bismuth, activated charcoal, and barium.

Antibiotic Therapy

- Do not use antibiotics routinely as empirical therapy in cases of uncomplicated diarrhea of undetermined cause because of their adverse effects on the normal intestinal flora and their tendency to promote resistant strains of bacteria.
- Antibiotics are indicated when specific bacterial or rickettsial enteropathogens, such as *Salmonella*, *Clostridium*, or *Campylobacter*, are suspected causes.
- Antibiotics are appropriate in conditions associated

with severe mucosal damage and a high risk of secondary sepsis or endotoxemia (e.g., parvoviral enteritis and hemorrhagic gastroenteritis). Thus, indications for antibacterial therapy in the animal with acute GI disease include bloody diarrhea, fever, leukocytosis, leukopenia, fecal leukocytes, and shock.

DIETARY DIARRHEA

Etiology

- Diarrhea as a result of indiscriminant eating and chewing behavior is particularly common in dogs. Dietary indiscretions include overeating, ingestion of spoiled garbage or decomposing carrion, and ingestion of abrasive or indigestible foreign material (e.g., bones, stones, hair, plants, wood, cloth, carpeting, foil, plastic) that can traumatize the GI mucosa.
- Diarrhea may result from an abrupt change in diet. Any change in the composition of the diet should be made in gradual increments over a period of several days to allow for adaptation.
- Animals may be intolerant of certain foods, such as lactose ingested as milk, fatty foods, spicy foods, and food additives found in certain commercial diets. Food hypersensitivity to specific protein sources is implicated as a cause of inflammatory bowel disease in dogs and cats.

Diagnosis

Dietary causes of diarrhea usually are identified by careful history-taking and the response to a restricted diet.

- Carefully question the owner about all aspects of diet and environment, including recent changes in type and brand of food, all supplemental feeding practices using "people foods," patterns of chewing behavior involving nonfood items (including toys, plants, haircoat), likelihood of garbage ingestion, and potential for unobserved indiscretions in free-roaming animals.
- Examine the feces for abrasive particles.

Treatment

Dietary diarrhea is self-limiting with feeding of a restricted diet, elimination of identifiable offending substances from the diet, and prevention of indiscriminant eating or chewing behavior. Management of dietary hypersensitivity is discussed under Chronic Inflammatory Bowel Disease later in this chapter.

DRUG AND TOXIN-INDUCED DIARRHEA

Etiology

- Diarrhea is a frequent adverse side effect of many medications, including nonsteroidal anti-inflammatory agents (NSAIDs) (e.g., aspirin, ibuprofen, indomethacin, phenylbutazone, flunixin meglumine), digitalis and other cardiac drugs, dithiazanine (Dizan), magnesium-containing compounds, lactulose (for hepatic encephalopathy), some anthelmintics, most anticancer drugs, and many antibacterial drugs (partly from adverse effects on the flora).
- Dexamethasone has been associated with hemorrhagic gastroenterocolitis characterized by erosion, ulceration, necrosis, and sometimes fatal colonic perforation, especially in dogs treated for intervertebral disc disease.
- Many exogenous toxins cause diarrhea, including biologic toxins such as the enterotoxin that causes staphylococcal food poisoning and various diarrheogenic chemical poisons such as heavy metals (lead, arsenic, thallium), insecticides (organophosphate dips, flea treatments), lawn and garden products (insecticides, herbicides, fungicides), and some house plants.
- Free-roaming animals may drink from stagnant or run-off water polluted or potentially contaminated with toxic industrial, petroleum, or agricultural chemicals.

Clinical Signs

- Many medications and most toxins that cause diarrhea also cause vomiting.
- Some toxicities are associated with various extraintestinal signs (e.g., neurologic manifestations of lead and organophosphate toxicity).

Diagnosis

Suspect drug and toxin-induced diarrhea on the basis of history of exposure (or opportunity for exposure), clinical signs, and exclusion of other causes of diarrhea.

Treatment

- Drug-induced diarrhea usually resolves after discontinuation of the offending medication or a reduction in its dosage.
- Toxin-induced diarrhea resolves with symptomatic antidiarrheal therapy, prevention of further exposure to the toxin, and gradual elimination of the substance from the body. However, if the exact toxin is known, consult other sources of information for additional specific treatments and antidotes.

METAZOAN PARASITES OF THE INTESTINES

The majority of intestinal parasite infections are asymptomatic: when clinical signs do occur, diarrhea and weight loss are most common. Young growing animals generally are more frequently and severely parasitized, but never overlook endoparasitism as a possible cause of acute or chronic diarrhea of either the small or large bowel type in dogs and cats of all ages. Other intestinal diseases, such as viral or bacterial enteritis, often are complicated by intestinal parasite infection.

The diagnosis of parasitism depends on the identification of eggs, cysts, larvae, trophozoites, or proglottids in the feces (see Table 4). Parasites that are notorious for evading detection include *Giardia* in dogs and cats with small bowel diarrhea, and whipworms in dogs with large bowel diarrhea. In such cases, response to a therapeutic trial is an indirect method of diagnosis. Anthelmintics used to treat the common parasites are listed in Table 6.

Ascarids

Etiology

Ascarid nematodes are the most prevalent parasites of dogs and cats worldwide. The ascarids of the dog are *Toxocara canis* and the less common *Toxascaris leonina*; those in the cat are *Toxocara cati* and *T. leonina*.

Life Cycle

- Ascarid infection occurs by four routes:
  - Prenatal infection as a result of transplacental migration, which occurs only with *T. canis*
  - Milk-borne infection as a result of transmammary migration, which occurs with both *T. canis* and *T. cati*
  - Infection by ingestion of infective eggs, which occurs with all three ascarids (*T. canis, T. cati, and T. leonina*)
  - Infection by ingestion of a paratenic (transport) host (*T. canis, T. cati*) or intermediate host (*T. leonina*)

TABLE 6. Anthelmintics for Dogs and Cats

Drug	Product (Manufacturer)	Dosage	Ascarids	Hook-worms	Whip-worms	Tapeworms
					Efficacy	
Butamisole*	Styquin (Haver/ Diamond)	Dog—2.4 mg/kg, SC	−	+ +	+ + +	−
Dichlorophene/toluene	Many products	Dog—capsule size as directed	+ +	+ +	−	+
Dichlorvos*	Task (Fermenta)	Dog—27–33 mg/kg; cat & pups—11 mg/kg, PO	+ +	+ +	+ +	−
Diethylcarbamazine (DEC)† plus oxibendazole (OXI)†	Many products	Dog—6.6 mg/kg daily or 110 mg/kg once, PO	+ +	−	−	−
	Filarabits Plus (SmithKline Beecham)	Dog—6.6 mg/kg DEC & 5 mg/kg OXI daily, PO	+ +	+ +	+	−
Disophenol*	DNP (Haver/Diamond)	Dog—10 mg/kg, SC	−	+ + +	−	−
Epsiprantel	Cestex (SmithKline Beecham)	Dog—5.5 mg/kg, PO; Cat—2.75 mg/kg, PO	−	−	−	+ + +
Febantel (FEB) plus praziquantel (PRA)	Rintal (Haver/Diamond)	Dog/Cat— 15 mg/kg, PO, for 3 days	+ + +	+ + +	+ + +	
	Vercom (Haver/ Diamond)	Dog/Cat—15 mg/kg FEB & 1.5 mg/kg PRA, PO, for 3 days	+ + +	+ + +	+ + +	+ + +
Fenbendazole	Panacur (Hoescht-Roussel)	Dog/Cat—50 mg/kg, PO, for 3–5 days	+ + +	+ + +	+ + +	+ +¶
Ivermectin*†§	Heartgard (MSD Agvet)	Dog—200 mcg/kg, PO or SC, once	+ +	+ +	+ +	−
Mebendazole*	Telmintic (Pitman-Moore)	Dog—22 mg/kg, PO, for 3 days	+ + +	+ + +	+ + +	+ +¶
Milbemycin oxime†	Interceptor (Ciba-Geigy)	Dog—0.5 mg/kg, PO, monthly	+ +	+ +	+ +	−
Piperazine	Many products	Dog/Cat—110 mg/kg, PO	+ +	−	−	−
Praziquantel	Droncit (Haver/ Diamond)	Dog/Cat—See label; PO, SC, IM	−	−	−	+ + +
Pyrantel pamoate	Nemex (Pfizer)	Dog/Cat—10 mg/kg, PO, if < 2.5 kg; 5 mg/kg, PO, if > 2.5 kg	+ + +	+ + +	−	−
Thenium closylate* plus piperazine	Canopar (Coopers)	Dog—see label; PO	−	+ +	−	−
	Thenatol (Coopers)	Dog—see label; PO	+ +	+ +	−	−

*Consult package insert because of special safety precautions or potential for serious side effects.
†Drugs used concomitantly as heartworm preventatives (see sec. 6, ch. 10).
¶Efficacious for *Taenia* spp. of tapeworms only; not effective against *Dipylidium caninum*.
§Not approved for treatment of intestinal parasites or for use at this dosage.

- Nearly all puppies are born infected with ascarids because of transplacental migration of the bitch's somatic *T. canis* larvae into the fetus (prenatal infection).
- Milk-borne infection during nursing is the major source of ascariasis in kittens.
- Three types of migration patterns occur when an animal is infected:
  - Liver-lung migration (*T. canis, T. cati*)
  - Migration within the wall of the GI tract (all three ascarids)
  - Somatic tissue migration (*T. canis, T. cati*)

Clinical Signs

- Signs of ascariasis occur most often in young puppies and kittens, in which the adult worms in the small intestine may cause abdominal discomfort, whimpering and groaning, potbellied appearance, dull haircoat, unthriftiness, stunted growth, and diarrhea. Worms frequently are passed in vomitus or diarrhea.
- Rarely, large tangled masses of worms occlude the lumen in young pups and cause death from intestinal obstruction, intussusception, or intestinal perforation.
- In the neonatal pup, the migration of large numbers of *T. canis* larvae through the lungs can cause severe damage and fatal pneumonia.
- In young animals with light infections and in adults, infection is most commonly asymptomatic, or evidenced merely by a loss of body condition.

Diagnosis

- The diagnosis of ascariasis is readily established by the identification of ascarid eggs in routine fecal flotation.
- Most pups begin passing large numbers of eggs in their feces at about 3 weeks of age and continue to shed eggs for most of early puppyhood (4 to 6 months) until treated.

Treatment

- Numerous effective anthelmintics for ascarids are available (see Table 6). Pyrantel pamoate is well tolerated in puppies and kittens and also is effective in controlling hookworms.
- Because most pups are born infected with *T. canis*, treatment is recommended at 2 weeks of age, before eggs are first passed in the feces, and repeated at 4, 6, and 8 weeks to kill all worms derived from prenatal, milk-borne, and ingestion routes of infection.
- Toxocaral visceral larva migrans (VLM) is a serious disease of humans (especially children) produced by the invasion of visceral tissues by migrating *T. canis*; thus, infected pups are considered public health hazards.

Hookworms

Etiology

- *Ancylostoma caninum*, the most common hookworm in the dog, is a voracious bloodsucker.
- *A. tubaeforme*, the common hookworm in the cat, is more of a tissue feeder than a bloodsucker and is far less pathogenic than *A. caninum* in dogs.
- *A. braziliense* (southern United States) and *Uncinaria stenocephala* (Canada) affect both dogs and cats but are less common than *A. caninum* and *A. tubaeforme* and are only mildly pathogenic.

Life Cycle

Hookworm infection can occur by five routes: prenatal, milk-borne, ingestion of infective larvae (L3), skin penetration by infective larvae, and ingestion of paratenic hosts. Ingestion and cutaneous migration probably are the most common routes of infection. With all routes of infection, eggs are passed in feces after 2–3 weeks.

Clinical Signs

Pathogenicity is directly related to the hookworm's bloodsucking activity and capacity for causing intestinal blood loss. Hookworms embed their mouthparts in the mucosa to suck blood and tissue fluid, leaving bleeding, punctiform ulcers as they "graze." Hence, an important consequence of severe hookworm infection is blood loss anemia.

- The clinical signs of ancylostomiasis include tarry (melena) or bloody diarrhea accompanied by pallor, weakness, emaciation, and dehydration.
- Rapidly progressive blood loss anemia may result in acute death of neonates. In other animals, chronic blood loss may cause iron deficiency anemia characterized by erythrocytes that show hypochromasia and microcytosis.
- Acute, pruritic dermatitis occasionally is associated with the active penetration of skin by hookworm larvae.
- Hookworm infections in mature animals often are asymptomatic.

Diagnosis

Young dogs are most often affected, and the diagnosis usually is readily established by identification of the characteristic strongyloid hookworm ova by routine fecal flotation. Ancylostomiasis often is associated with eosinophilia on the CBC.

Treatment

Anthelmintics effective for eradicating hookworms include pyrantel pamoate (safest for young animals), fenbendazole, febantel, butamisole HCl, mebendazole, and dichlorvos (see Table 6 for product names and dosages).

- In areas in which *A. caninum* is a frequent problem, routinely treat bitches and pups. Because of prenatal and milk-borne infection, initiate treatment of pups at 2 weeks of age, along with treatment for *T. canis*.

KEY POINT ▶ Pyrantel pamoate suspension is an excellent anthelmintic for nursing pups because it is safe and active against both hookworms and ascarids.

- Severely anemic animals should receive whole blood transfusions, iron supplementation, and supportive therapy.

Prevention

- Parasite control is aided by good sanitation and impervious flooring in kennels and dog runs.
- Various commercial products have combined effect as preventive agents against both heartworms and hookworms (e.g., oxibendazole and milbemycin; see Table 6).

Whipworms

Etiology

The canine whipworm, *Trichuris vulpis*, is a common cause of large bowel diarrhea in dogs in many areas. The adult nematode has a predilection for the proximal colon and cecum, where its distinctive threadlike head end, or "whip," firmly embeds deep within the mucosa to feed on blood and tissue fluids, thereby causing colitis and typhlitis.

The feline whipworms, *T. campanula* and *T. serrata*, are rare and usually are not associated with clinical signs.

Life Cycle

- Whipworm infections occur by ingestion of infective ova, and the life cycle is direct.
- The prepatent period is approximately 3 months. Ova may survive and remain infectious in the environment for 4 to 5 years; hence, contaminated ground is probably the major reservoir of infection.

Clinical Signs

- Whipworms infect dogs of all ages. Although there may be minimal clinical signs in light infestations, trichuriasis frequently causes acute, chronic, or intermittent signs of mucoid large bowel-type diarrhea with urgency and sometimes hematochezia.
- Pseudohypoadrenocorticism, characterized by hyperkalemia and hyponatremia in the presence of normal adrenal function, has been associated with severe whipworm diarrhea in several dogs.

Diagnosis

- Definitive diagnosis of whipworm infection requires identification of the characteristic brown, bipolar-operculated football-shaped ova by routine fecal flotation.
- Repeated fecal examinations may be necessary to identify ova because of the unusually long prepatent period and because it is not uncommon for active

infection to be characterized by prolonged periods when ova are not shed in the feces.
- Alternative means of diagnosis of ova-negative, or so-called occult, infections, include:
  - Colonoscopic observation of adult whipworms in the bowel lumen
  - Resolution of signs in response to a therapeutic trial of an effective anthelmintic

Treatment

- Give fenbendazole (Panacur) or febantel (Rintal or Vercom) for 3 days (see Table 6). In refractory cases, a 5-day course is recommended. Routinely repeat treatment at 3 weeks and 3 months, because whipworms are difficult to eradicate.
- Other whipcidal anthelmintics include mebendazole (Telmintic), butamisole (Styquin), and dichlorvos (Task), but these drugs have less efficacy and greater toxicity (see Table 6).
- Rarely, trichuriasis has been associated with severe transmural granulomatous typhlitis that may be palpable as a tender right-midabdominal mass. This lesion may be refractory to anthelmintics and require typhlectomy.

Prevention

- Because it is virtually impossible to eradicate the parasite from infected ground, frequent reinfection is a common problem. For this reason, collect and properly dispose of feces whenever possible.
- In dogs with frequent access to ground that has been heavily contaminated with whipworm ova (a common situation in many public parks and backyards), reinfection is so frequent that retreatment every 2 to 3 months may be necessary.
- Disinfect concrete runs with dilute sodium hypochlorite bleach.

Strongyloides spp.

Etiology

Strongyloides spp. are tiny (2 mm) rhabdoid nematodes found in warm, humid tropical regions such as the southern Gulf states of the United States.

- In dogs, strongyloidiasis is caused by *S. stercoralis*, a parasite that burrows in the mucosa of the proximal small bowel.
- In cats, strongyloidiasis is caused by *S. tumefaciens*, a parasite that burrows within the mucosa of the large intestine.

Life Cycle

- Infection with third-stage larvae is by the oral or cutaneous route, and adult worms develop in the small intestine following migration in the circulation and lung.
- Parthenogenetic female adults produce eggs that hatch within the gut lumen, so that first-stage (rhabdoid) larvae are passed in the feces. These larvae may develop into infectious third-stage (filariform) larvae or free-living adults.

Clinical Signs

- *S. stercoralis* is mainly a problem in pups, in which it causes acute hemorrhagic enteritis that is often fatal.
- *S. tumefaciens* infection in cats is usually asymptomatic, but in some cats the parasite causes peculiar tumor-like white nodular (2–3 mm) proliferations in the colonic mucosa and submucosa that are associated with chronic diarrhea and debilitation.

Diagnosis

- Ova containing first-stage *Strongyloides* larvae can be identified in feces by flotation techniques. Free larvae (0.8–1.6 mm long × 30–80 μ) may be identified by direct microscopic examination of fresh feces or by the Baermann technique.
- In cats, the diagnosis of *S. tumefaciens* also can be established by colonoscopic observation and biopsy of mucosal nodules filled with adult worms.

Treatment

Treat with fenbendazole (50 mg/kg/day, PO, for 5 days), diethylcarbamazine (100 mg/kg, PO, once), or pyrantel pamoate (20 mg/kg/day, PO, for 5 days).

Tapeworms

Etiology

- The most common tapeworm (cestode) of dogs and cats in *Dipylidium caninum*. Fleas and lice are intermediate hosts.
- Several species of *Taenia* can be acquired by dogs and cats (most commonly *T. pisiformis* in the dog, *T. taeniaeformis* in the cat) from ingestion of cysticercus-infected tissues from intermediate hosts (e.g., rabbits, rodents, sheep, and ungulates).
- Other cestodes that rarely cause infection include *Echinococcus, Multiceps, Mesocestoides,* and *Spirometra*.

Clinical Signs

- Tapeworms that parasitize the small bowel of dogs and cats are relatively harmless, rarely causing more than a subtle decline in body condition.
- The proglottids of *D. caninum* are highly motile and may cause anal pruritus as they crawl on the perineum; crawling proglottids are often detected by observant owners in the animal's stool or on the perineum.

Diagnosis

- Tapeworms are diagnosed by the identification of proglottids or ova in feces.
- *D. caninum* proglottids are distinguished from *Taenia* spp. by their barrel shape and double genital pore. Also, a proglottid can be squashed in a drop of water between a slide and coverslip to identify the characteristic *D. caninum* egg capsules that contain up to 20 eggs.

Treatment

- Praziquantel and epsiquantel are the most effective all-around drugs for treatment of cestodiasis (see Table 6).
- Mebendazole and fenbendazole are effective against *Taenia* spp. but not *Dipylidium caninum*.
- Flea and lice control is important for preventing *D. caninum* reinfection; control of predation and scavenging helps prevent infection with other cestodes.

PROTOZOAN PARASITES OF THE INTESTINES

Coccidia

Etiology

Canine and feline intestinal coccidia are protozoan parasites that belong to the genera *Isospora*, *Besnoitia*, *Hammondia*, *Sarcocystis*, *Neosporum*, *Toxoplasma*, and *Cryptosporidium*. Most enteric coccidial infections of dogs and cats are commensal and nonpathogenic.

- Primary enteric disease in small animals has been described only with *Isospora* (discussed later) and *Cryptosporidium* (which is uncommon and is not discussed here).
- *T. gondii* and *N. canis* cause multisystemic infection and are discussed in sec. 2, ch. 13.
- *Isospora* spp. that infect dogs include *I. canis*, *I. ohioensis*, *I. burrowsi*, and *I. neorivolta*; *I. felis* and *I. rivolta* infect cats.

Life Cycle

- Infection occurs most commonly by ingestion of infective (sporulated) oocysts from a feces-contaminated environment.
- Infection occurs occasionally from ingestion of infective cyst-containing tissues of paratenic (transport) hosts such as rodents and other prey and ingestion of uncooked meat of herbivores.

Clinical Signs

- Coccidiosis in most animals is an asymptomatic, incidental infection.
- *Coccidia* are opportunists and clinical disease is usually related to massive oocyst ingestion in newborn animals and is associated with overcrowded, unsanitary, high-stress conditions in settings such as pet shops, kennels, pounds, catteries, and laboratory colonies. Concurrent disease, malnutrition, or immunosuppression are predisposing factors.
- Clinical disease usually is characterized by diarrhea that varies from soft to fluid and is occasionally mucoid or bloody. Other signs can include vomiting, lethargy, weight loss, and dehydration. *Isospora* spp. occasionally have been associated with chronic malabsorption.

Diagnosis

- Coccidiosis is diagnosed by the identification of oocysts in fresh feces.

- Because many normal dogs and cats harbor intestinal coccidia and these protozoa are generally regarded as minimally pathogenic, the clinical significance of finding coccidial oocysts often is questionable. Even in animals with diarrhea, oocysts are usually incidental findings and other causes for the diarrhea should be sought.

Treatment

Identification of oocysts in a healthy animal with normal feces indicates a self-limiting commensal infection and does not necessarily warrant treatment, although treatment may help to reduce environmental contamination with oocysts.

If clinical signs are attributed to coccidiosis, as in young puppies and kittens with diarrhea, treat with one of the following coccidiostats:

- sulfadimethoxine—50–60 mg/kg/day, PO, for 1 to 3 weeks
- trimethoprim-sulfa—15–30 mg/kg q12–24h, PO, for 1 week
- furazolidone—8–20 mg/kg/day, PO, for 1 week
- amprolium (unapproved for use in dogs but often recommended for treating animals in kennels or other groups of dogs)—20% powder in gelatin capsules, 100 mg q24h for small-breed pups or 200 mg q24h for larger-breed pups, PO, for 7–12 days; alternatively, ¼ tsp 20% powder per 4 pups mixed with puppy ration, or 1 ounce (30 ml) of 9.6%, solution per gallon of free-choice water

Giardia spp.

Giardia spp. are pear-shaped, binucleated, flagellated protozoa that infect the small intestine, interfere with mucosal absorption, and sometimes produce diarrhea. There are two forms: motile trophozoites and nonmotile infective cysts.

Giardia has a worldwide distribution, with a prevalence of at least 5% in most populations. The incidence is highest in young animals and animals confined together in groups.

Life Cycle

The life cycle of *Giardia* is direct, and the usual source of infection is the ingestion of food or water contaminated with cysts. Wild animals are potential reservoirs.

Clinical Signs

- The majority of *Giardia* infections are subclinical, especially in mature animals.
- Clinically apparent giardiasis occurs most frequently in young dogs and cats and is characterized by intestinal malabsorption with large volumes of foul-smelling, light-colored, watery or "cow paddy–like" diarrhea, steatorrhea, and weight loss. Diarrhea may be acute or chronic, intermittent or continuous and self-limiting or persistent.
- The severity of giardiasis is enhanced by concomitant viral, bacterial, or helminth infections.

Diagnosis

- Definitive diagnosis of giardiasis depends on identification of cysts (oval; 8–12 μm × 7–10 μm) by zinc sulfate centrifugation-flotation of feces or of motile flagellated trophozoites (pear-shaped; 9–21 μm × 5–15 μm × 2–4 μm) in fresh diarrheic feces suspended in saline or in duodenal specimens (aspirates, brushings, or impression smears of mucosal biopsies).
- Negative fecal examinations do not exclude a diagnosis of giardiasis. When fecal examinations are negative, "occult" giardiasis may be diagnosed indirectly by the response to a therapeutic trial of an antigiardial drug such as metronidazole.
- New methods of detecting *Giardia* by enzyme-linked immunosorbent assay (ELISA) and immunofluorescent antibody (IFA) techniques are becoming more available.

Treatment

Three drugs currently available in the United States are effective in the treatment of giardiasis: metronidazole, quinicrine, and furazolidone.

- Metronidazole (Flagyl; Searle) (25–30 mg/kg q12h, PO, for 5–10 days) usually is effective with minimal side effects, although up to one-third of infections may be metronidazole-resistant.
- Quinicrine (Atabrine; Winthrop) (6.6 mg/kg q12h, PO, for 5 days) is effective in the treatment of canine giardiasis but is associated with a high incidence of side effects (anorexia, lethargy, vomiting, fever).
- Furazolidone (Furoxone; SmithKline) (4 mg/kg q12h, PO, for 5 days) is effective and convenient for cats, as it is available in a suspension form.

Trichomonads

Pentatrichomonas hominas organisms are motile, pear-shaped, flagellated protozoa that inhabit the colon of dogs and cats. Trichomonads have been found in both normal and diarrheic feces, but pathogenicity is unproven.

Diagnosis

The diagnosis of trichomoniasis is based on identification in saline fecal smears of motile, pear-shaped, flagellated trophozoites with the characteristic wavelike motion of an undulating membrane and a constant erratic turning and rolling motion.

Treatment

Metronidazole (25–30 mg/kg q12h, PO, for 5 days) is an effective treatment.

Entamoeba spp.

E. histolytica, primarily a human pathogen, rarely may cause amebic colitis (bloody-mucoid diarrhea) in dogs and cats that drink polluted water.

Diagnosis

Diagnosis is based on identification of ameboid trophozoites with pseudopodial movement in saline smears of fresh diarrheic feces; amebic cysts in zinc sulfate flotation of formed feces; or trophozoites in colon biopsies.

Treatment

Amebic colitis responds to metronidazole (25–30 mg/kg q12h, PO, for 5–10 days) or furazolidone (2.2 mg/kg q8h, PO, for 7 days).

Balantidium spp.

B. coli, a ciliated protozoan that primarily infects swine, is a rare cause of chronic ulcerative colitis in dogs.

Diagnosis

Diagnosis is based on identification of large (40–80 μm × 25–45 μm), oval, brown, rapidly swimming ciliated trophozoites with prominent macronuclei in saline suspensions of fresh feces or identification of protozoal cysts in zinc sulfate or sedimentation preparations of feces.

Treatment

Metronidazole (25–30 mg/kg q12h, PO, for 5–10 days) is effective.

VIRAL INFECTIONS OF THE INTESTINES

Canine Intestinal Viruses

- Canine parvovirus, canine coronavirus, and rotavirus cause viral enteritis and diarrhea in dogs. Canine parvovirus is an acute, severe, highly contagious enteritis that is prevalent worldwide. Coronavirus and rotavirus are less prevalent and cause relatively mild clinical signs except in neonates. For details concerning intestinal viruses, see sec. 2, ch. 7.
- Because of its epitheliotropism, canine distemper virus also causes diarrhea (sec. 2, ch. 6).

Feline Intestinal Viruses

- The most clinically important primary enteric virus is feline panleukopenia virus (FPV), a parvovirus. Other feline intestinal viruses include enteric coronavirus, rotavirus, and astrovirus (see sec. 2, ch. 7).
- The intestine may be involved as part of generalized viral infections such as feline leukemia virus (FeLV; see sec. 2, ch. 1), feline immunodeficiency virus (FIV; see sec. 2, ch. 2) and feline infectious peritonitis (FIP), a coronavirus (see sec. 2, ch. 3).

BACTERIAL INFECTIONS OF THE INTESTINES

Most enteropathogenic bacteria produce intestinal disease by invading the epithelium (invasive bacteria) or by remaining attached to the mucosal surface without penetrating it and liberating a diarrheogenic enterotoxin (noninvasive or enterotoxigenic bacteria).

Enteropathogenic bacteria of clinical importance include *Salmonella* spp., *Campylobacter jejuni*, and *Clostridium* spp. (*Yersinia* spp. and *Bacillus piliformis* are rare and are not discussed here.) These bacteria primarily invade the colon and distal small bowel, causing mucosal damage that leads to inflammation, exudation, mucus secretion, and bleeding. Thus, typical signs of large bowel diarrhea and hematochezia are characteristic of these infections. Bacterial enterotoxins may also play a role in the pathogenesis of diarrhea.

KEY POINT ▶ Because *Salmonella, Campylobacter,* and *Yersinia* also are human pathogens, pets occasionally are reservoirs for human infection.

Salmonella

Etiology

- Salmonellosis is caused by gram-negative bacilli belonging to the genus *Salmonella* of the family Enterobacteriaceae. *Salmonella* spp. frequently are isolated from the feces of normal dogs and cats, but clinical signs of salmonellosis are uncommon, indicating a prevalent asymptomatic carrier state.
- Salmonella infection is transmitted by the feco-oral route, mainly through ingestion of contaminated food or water. The organisms can survive in the environment for long periods outside the host, thus, fomite transmission also can occur.
- Infection risk depends on infectivity of the strain, size of the inoculum, competition from the established flora, age of the host, and host defense factors. Infection rates are greatest in young animals and in group confinement situations with overcrowding and poor sanitation.

Clinical Signs

Manifestations of *Salmonella* infection may be categorized into three syndromes: the subclinical carrier state, enterocolitis, and enterocolitis with bacteremia.

- Clinical salmonellosis is relatively uncommon compared with the prevalence of the subclinical carrier state.
- *Salmonella* enterocolitis is characterized by acute watery or mucoid diarrhea (containing blood in severe cases), vomiting, tenesmus, fever, anorexia, lethargy, abdominal pain, and dehydration. Most animals recover in 3–4 weeks, although shedding of organisms often persists for up to 6 weeks, and sometimes longer.
- *Salmonella* can cause chronic or intermittent diarrhea in some animals.
- Rarely, *Salmonella* enterocolitis progresses to a potentially fatal bacteremia or endotoxemia with signs of endotoxic shock and disseminated intravascular coagulation (DIC).

Diagnosis

- Suspect the salmonellosis in animals that develop acute diarrhea and have identifiable risk factors, such as known or probable exposure, young age, immune deficiency, debilitating illness, or housing in overcrowded or unsanitary conditions.
- Nosocomial outbreaks with high morbidity and mortality have been recorded in hospitalized animals, the greatest risk occurring in animals:
  - With severe illness
  - Undergoing major surgery
  - Hospitalized for 5 or more days
  - Receiving glucocorticosteroids, anticancer chemotherapy, or oral antibiotics (especially ampicillin) that upset the normal flora
- Routine diagnostic tests usually are noncontributory, except that a degenerative neutropenia may be found in severe cases with bacteremia and endotoxemia.
- Confirmation of the diagnosis depends on isolation of *Salmonella* spp. from properly cultured fecal specimens or from blood cultures in bacteremic animals.

Treatment

The use of antibiotics in the treatment of salmonellosis is controversial. *Salmonella* invasion that is confined locally to the mucosa produces enterocolitis that is self-limiting and is not likely to be affected by antibiotics.

KEY POINT ▶ Antibacterial therapy, especially oral nonabsorbable antibiotics which alter the flora, may actually prolong shedding of *Salmonella* organisms and encourage development of a prolonged convalescent carrier state.

Antibiotics are indicated when *Salmonella* invasion becomes severe or complicated by bacteremia and endotoxemia, as indicated by signs such as shock, dehydration, high fever or hypothermia, and extreme depression; or by laboratory findings such as azotemia, electrolyte imbalances, neutropenia, hypoglycemia, hypoproteinemia, or coagulopathy. Peracute onset and severe hematochezia may also be an indication of impending systemic invasion and should prompt antibiotic therapy.

- Base antibiotic selection on culture and sensitivity testing. Most isolates are susceptible to enrofloxacin (Baytril; Haver/Diamond) (5 mg/kg q12h, PO) or trimethoprim-sulfa (15 mg/kg q12h, PO). Administer antibiotics for 7–10 days and reculture feces 1 and 4 weeks after treatment.
- In addition to antibiotics, fluid and electrolyte replacement and identification and correction of underlying predisposing conditions are important aspects of therapy.
- Proper hygiene in handling of infected animals is necessary to prevent feco-oral or fomite transmission of infection to other animals or to humans.

Prognosis

The prognosis for most animals with salmonellosis is good, although the mortality rate can be high in outbreaks in extremely susceptible populations (e.g., hospital patients, neonates).

Campylobacter spp.

Campylobacter jejuni organisms are fastidious, microaerophilic, gram-negative, motile, slender curved bacteria that are important pathogens of animals and humans worldwide.

Etiology

Many clinically normal dogs and cats shed *Campylobacter* in their feces. Isolation rates vary widely, from less than 1% in confined pet populations to 50% or more in some animal pounds and shelters. Thus, conditions of close confinement and poor sanitation apparently provide the greatest opportunity for exposure.

Clinical Signs

Because it is difficult to produce enteritis with *Campylobacter* experimentally in dogs and cats and because many of the animals that harbor these organisms are asymptomatic, it has been debated whether *Campylobacter* by itself causes diarrhea in dogs and cats unless superimposed on other enteropathogenic infections with viruses, other bacteria, *Giardia*, or helminths.

- Clinical signs associated with *Campylobacter* infection in dogs and cats have been attributed to superficial erosive enterocolitis or enterotoxin-mediated secretory diarrhea and are characterized by watery-mucoid diarrhea lasting 5–15 days that occasionally contains blood and may be accompanied by vomiting or tenesmus.
- Fever is usually mild or absent.
- In some animals the diarrhea appears to be chronic or intermittent.

Diagnosis

- *Presumptive* diagnosis of campylobacteriosis can be made by fecal microscopy; however, this requires an experienced examiner, because spirochetes and other motile bacteria that are part of the normal flora may be mistaken as *Campylobacter*. The presence of fecal leukocytes may also be noted.

KEY POINT ▶ *Campylobacter* are identified as slender curved gram-negative rods that are characteristically W-shaped in stained fecal smears and as highly motile, darting, spiral, or S-shaped bacteria in fresh saline fecal smears examined by dark-field or phase-contrast microscopy.

- *Definitive* diagnosis requires isolation of *Campylobacter* from fresh feces using special selective media. Since *Campylobacter* organisms are microaerophilic and difficult to isolate, obtain fecal specimens directly from the rectum and culture or place in transport media immediately after collection.

Treatment

- The antibiotic of choice is erythromycin (10–15 mg/kg q8h, PO, for 7 days). Anorexia and vomiting are frequent side effects.
- Other effective oral antibiotics include neomycin (10 mg/kg, q8h, PO), enrofloxacin (Baytril,Haver/Diamond) (5 mg/kg q8h, PO), chloramphenicol, furazolidone, and doxycycline.
- Antibiotics are rapidly effective for eliminating fecal shedding of the organisms. Repeat fecal cultures 1 and 4 weeks after treatment.
- Because contact with feces from infected animals is a potential source of infection for humans as well as other animals, advise owners of infected pets to take standard precautions such as proper disposal of potentially infectious feces, hand washing after handling infected animals, and separating infected animals from infants and small children until post-treatment cultures confirm that infection has been eliminated.

Prognosis

The prognosis is considered good, although rare fatalities in dogs and cats have been reported.

Clostridia

Etiology

- *Clostridium perfringens* is part of the normal anaerobic intestinal microflora in dogs and cats. These toxin-producing bacteria may be involved in acute and chronic diarrhea.
- *C. difficile* causes severe pseudomembranous colitis in humans, usually subsequent to antimicrobial suppression of the normal flora. Toxigenic *C. difficile* and its toxin have been isolated from normal dogs and cats and from a few dogs with chronic diarrhea, but the significance of this organism as a pathogen in dogs and cats remains to be established.

Clinical Signs

Clostridia have been associated with canine hemorrhagic gastroenteritis (see subsequent section), acute necrotizing hemorrhagic enterocolitis, acute nosocomial diarrhea, and chronic diarrhea, but the evidence implicating these bacteria as primary pathogens is only circumstantial.

- Clostridial diarrhea is watery or soft, with or without mucus, blood, and tenesmus.
- Onset is usually acute, although chronic and recurrent diarrhea have been attributed to *Clostridium perfringens* in some animals.

Diagnosis

- Presumptive diagnosis of *C. perfringens* infection is based on identification of fecal leukocytes and predominance of large gram-positive rods with endospores by fecal cytology. Greater than 2–3 spores (identified on Diff-Quik or Wright's staining by their "safety-pin" appearance) per high power oil immersion field is considered abnormal.

- Definitive diagnosis is based on detection of enterotoxin by fecal assay.
- Diagnosis of *C. difficile* infection is based on a positive fecal assay for *C. difficile* toxin.

Treatment

Standard dosages of amoxicillin, ampicillin, metronidazole, tylosin, tetracycline, or chloramphenicol for 5–7 days are effective for treating *C. perfringens* infection. Most cases are self-limiting or responsive to antibiotics in 2–3 days; however, fatalities have been reported. Chronic *C. perfringens* diarrhea may require long-term treatment with antibiotics to prevent recurrences. *C. difficile* is susceptible to metronidazole, tetracycline, or vancomycin.

FUNGAL INFECTIONS OF THE INTESTINES

Mycotic infections of the bowel are uncommon; however, fungi are opportunists that capitalize on predisposing factors such as lowered host resistance, malnutrition, antecedent debilitating illness, and prolonged therapy with antimicrobials or corticosteroids. Fungi may cause acute, dysentery-like diarrhea, or chronic diarrhea accompanied by emaciation.

Causes of mycotic intestinal disease include *Histoplasma capsulatum*, *Pythium* spp., *Aspergillus* spp., *Candida albicans*, and other saprophytes. Histoplasmosis is a multisystemic mycotic infection and is discussed in sec. 2, ch. 12. Intestinal aspergillosis and candidiasis are rare and will not be discussed further.

Intestinal Pythiosis and Zygomycosis

Various poorly septate saprophytic molds and fungi that include *Pythium* spp. (pythiosis) and several genera of Zygomycetes (zygomycosis) can deeply invade the tissues of the gastrointestinal tract. These infections were formerly misnamed phycomycosis.

Pythiosis is most common in young, large-breed dogs that live in the southern Gulf states of the United States. Rare feline cases are characterized by ulcerative gastroenteritis.

Clinical Signs

Pythium and Zygomycetes can infect any part of the digestive tract, but lesions most commonly involve the stomach, small intestine, mesentery, and mesenteric lymph nodes, resulting in an extensive granulomatous tissue reaction.

- Signs include chronic intractable diarrhea and vomiting, anorexia, depression, and progressive weight loss.
- Bowel necrosis and ulceration may cause bloody diarrhea in some cases.
- Regions of extensive granulomatous inflammation may produce palpable enteromesenteric masses.
- The infection may disseminate beyond the GI tract to other abdominal viscera.

Diagnosis

- Physical examination may reveal an abdominal mass or marked regional thickening of the bowel.
- The CBC may reveal mild to moderate nonregenerative anemia and mild neutrophilia, with or without a left shift.
- Routine abdominal radiography frequently demonstrates an abdominal mass; barium contrast GI radiography often delineates a thickened, stenosed segment of bowel.
- Confirmation depends on histologic identification of broad, nonseptate or sparsely septate hyphae in biopsies of the stomach, intestine, or abdominal lymph nodes. The organisms stain with Gridley's or methenamine silver stains and are found mostly within the necrotic regions of granulomas in the submucosa and muscularis mucosa.
- Differentiate intestinal pythiosis from other granulomatous and neoplastic proliferations of the GI tract, including histoplasmosis, lymphosarcoma, and regional (granulomatous) enteritis.
- The extensive tissue reaction can easily be mistaken for neoplasia at laparotomy (or necropsy); thus, careful histologic evaluation including use of fungal stains is essential for accurate diagnosis.

Treatment

Because these fungi are not affected by standard antifungal drugs, treatment requires radical surgical excision of the severely involved segments of bowel (for surgical technique, see sec. 7, ch. 7).

Prognosis

The prognosis is guarded.

INTESTINAL PROTOTHECOSIS

Etiology

Prototheca spp. are ubiquitous unicellular algae that may rarely colonize the lamina propria and submucosa of the intestinal tract of dogs and cause severe necrotizing or ulcerating enterocolitis.

Clinical Signs

- The algae appear to have a predilection for initially invading the colon, resulting in signs of chronic large bowel diarrhea with hematochezia.
- The organisms typically disseminate widely throughout the body and most frequently involve other visceral organs, the eyes, and the central nervous system (CNS).
- Only a cutaneous form has been described in cats.

Diagnosis

- Colonoscopy reveals thickened, corrugated mucosal folds that may be friable or ulcerated.
- Organisms can be identified in feces, cytology preparations (Wright's or Gram stain), and biopsies (Go-

mori's or periodic acid–Schiff stain) as clusters of endosporulated ovoid structures (5–16 μ in length).
- *Prototheca* can also be cultured on Sabouraud's cyclohexamide-free dextrose media.

Treatment

Successful treatment of prototheca in animals has not been reported.

CANINE HEMORRHAGIC GASTROENTERITIS

Etiology

Hemorrhagic gastroenteritis (HGE) is a syndrome of unknown etiology characterized by sudden onset of vomiting, profuse bloody diarrhea, and marked hemoconcentration. Despite its name, HGE does not appear to be primarily an inflammatory disease but rather is a condition of altered intestinal mucosal permeability and perhaps mucosal hypersecretion.

Cultures of intestinal contents from dogs with HGE have yielded large numbers of *C. perfringens*, leading to speculation that this organism or its toxins are the cause.

Signalment

HGE has a predilection for toy and miniature breeds, particularly schnauzers and toy poodles, but any breed can be affected. Dogs of any age can be affected, but especially young adults 2–4 years of age.

Clinical Signs

The first signs are usually sudden onset of vomiting and severe depression, followed within hours by a profuse, bloody, fluid diarrhea with a fetid odor. Progressive prolongation of capillary refill time and other indicators of circulatory failure are noted as shock develops.

Diagnosis

- The diagnosis of HGE is suggested by evidence of extreme hemoconcentration (packed cell volume [PCV] > 60%, reaching 70–80% in some dogs) along with fetid, bloody diarrhea.
- Radiography and other laboratory findings are generally unremarkable, but they are useful for excluding other causes of bloody diarrhea.
- The high PCV and lack of fever or leukopenia help distinguish HGE from parvoviral enteritis; however, for greater certainty, a fecal test for parvovirus may be necessary.
- Evaluate dogs with HGE for *Clostridium perfringens* (see previous discussion).

Treatment

The mortality from HGE is low if treated promptly by vigorous fluid volume replacement.

- Rapidly infuse a balanced multiple electrolyte solution, preferably by indwelling IV catheter, at a rate of 90 ml/kg/h until capillary refill time and PCV are normal; then continue IV fluids at a maintenance rate for the next 24 hours.

KEY POINT ▶ Without volume expansion using IV fluid therapy, HGE can cause circulatory failure and death in < 24 hours.

- Occasionally, if shock appears to be refractory to IV fluid therapy, a dose of corticosteroids may be needed during the initial hours.
- Use antibiotics effective against *C. perfringens*, such as ampicillin or amoxicillin, empirically.
- Restrict food and water initially until vomiting and bloody or fluid diarrhea have ceased; then feed small amounts of bland food. Nonspecific antidiarrheal and antiemetic therapy may be helpful.

Most animals show marked improvement within hours, although the diarrhea may not subside for 24–48 hours. Failure of the animal to improve dramatically in 24–48 hours should prompt a search for other diseases that may mimic HGE (e.g., parvovirus, GI foreign body, intussusception, volvulus).

CHRONIC INFLAMMATORY BOWEL DISEASE

The term inflammatory bowel disease (IBD) refers to a diverse group of chronic enteropathies characterized by idiopathic infiltration of the GI tract mucosa and (sometimes) submucosa with inflammatory cells. The infiltration may involve the stomach, small intestine, colon, or a combination of these, and is classified on the basis of the predominant cell type as lymphocytic-plasmacytic, eosinophilic, neutrophilic, granulomatous, or histiocytic. A mixture of inflammatory cells in some lesions makes classification difficult.

Lymphocytic-Plasmacytic IBD

Etiology

- Lymphocytic-plasmacytic IBD is by far the most common form of IBD in both dogs and cats. The etiology is not determined in most cases; however, genetic, dietary, bacterial, immunologic, and mucosal permeability factors have been suggested to play a role.
- The pathogenesis of lymphocytic-plasmacytic IBD may involve a hypersensitivity reaction to antigens (bacterial, food, or self-antigens) in the bowel lumen or mucosa. This may result from a primary disorder of the intestinal immune system or its regulation, or from immune events that occur secondary to mucosal injury and permeability. Chronic inflammation of the bowel may become self-perpetuating when loss of mucosal integrity allows bacterial or dietary proteins to enter the lamina propria, where they incite further immune reaction and inflammation.
- Genetic factors appear to be involved in predisposing certain breeds to lymphocytic-plasmacytic IBD (e.g., basenji, soft-coated Wheaton terrier, and Shar pei). Basenjis develop a severe form of IBD (also called immunoproliferative enteropathy) that is thought to

be related to a genetic disorder of immune regulation and that is progressive in nature and exacerbated by stress.

Clinical Signs

■ *Lymphocytic-plasmacytic gastroduodenitis* causes intermittent vomiting and occurs most frequently in cats with IBD.
■ *Diffuse lymphocytic-plasmacytic enteritis* causes chronic unresponsive small bowel diarrhea and progressive weight loss. Signs may be intermittent or persistent. In severely affected dogs, protein-losing enteropathy (ascites, hydrothorax, edema) can occur.
  • Some animals with a biopsy diagnosis of lymphocytic-plasmacytic enteritis that fail to respond to treatment or that later relapse and deteriorate rapidly are found to have diffuse intestinal lymphosarcoma.
■ *Lymphocytic-plasmacytic colitis* causes chronic large bowel diarrhea characterized by increased frequency of defecation, urgency, tenesmus, increased fecal mucus, and hematochezia. Intermittent hematochezia may be the only sign of IBD in some cats.

Diagnosis

■ In the diagnostic evaluation, exclude parasitic (*Giardia*, canine whipworms) and infectious (*Campylobacter, Salmonella, Histoplasma*) causes of IBD.
■ The differential diagnosis of lymphocytic-plasmacytic IBD includes dietary hypersensitivity, bacterial overgrowth syndrome, intestinal lymphosarcoma, intestinal lymphangiectasia, and the other types of chronic inflammatory bowel disease.
  • To exclude dietary hypersensitivity as a cause of IBD, use a feeding trial with a controlled "hypoallergenic" diet as described under Treatment.
■ Routine hematologic and biochemical parameters typically are unremarkable except for occasional nonspecific findings such as a stress leukogram, hypoproteinemia, hypokalemia, and mildly elevated serum liver enzymes. Basenji enteropathy is associated with hypoalbuminemia and hyperglobulinemia, whereas affected soft-coated Wheaton terriers may have hypoalbuminemia with concurrent glomerulonephropathy.
■ Radiography (including barium contrast) usually is unremarkable.
■ Serum vitamin levels (cobalamin, folate, vitamin K) can be decreased from malabsorption. Bleeding and abnormal hemostasis have been associated with vitamin K deficiency in some cats with IBD. Markedly decreased serum cobalamin is common in affected Shar peis.
■ Intestinal biopsy (usually via endoscopy) is required for definitive diagnosis.
  • Endoscopically, the mucosa in IBD often appears thickened, friable, and abnormally granular. In the colon there is decreased visibility of the submucosal vessels and replacement of the glistening appearance of the mucosa with a dry granular surface covered with strands of mucus. Ulceration

is uncommon. Mild cases of IBD may appear endoscopically normal, such that lesions can only be detected histopathologically.
  • Histopathologically, the lesion of lymphocytic-plasmacytic IBD is characterized by diffuse infiltration of the mucosa with mature lymphocytes and plasma cells.
  • Additional findings can include atrophic or fused villi, fibrosis, epithelial abnormalities (hyperplasia, degeneration, erosion, ulceration, glandular dilatation, loss of goblet cells), and mixed infiltration of other types of inflammatory cells (neutrophils, eosinophils, macrophages).

Treatment

The initial treatment strategy is directed toward dietary manipulation; if this is unsuccessful, medical therapy is usually required using anti-inflammatory-immunosuppressive drugs as single agents or in combination, such as 5-aminosalicylates (e.g., sulfasalazine, olsalazine, mesalamine), corticosteroids (prednisone), metronidazole (Flagyl), and azathioprine (Imuran). Motility-modifying antidiarrheal drugs may help to alleviate some of the clinical signs. Various drugs used to treat IBD and their suggested dosages are indicated in Table 7.

Dietary Therapy

In some dogs and cats with lymphocytic-plasmacytic IBD, dietary modification produces complete or partial resolution of the signs and sometimes even regression of the lesions. This suggests that dietary hypersensitivity may be involved in the pathogenesis of the disease in some animals. Other potential explanations for a beneficial response to dietary modification include the effects of the diet on bowel motility, composition of the flora, mucosal morphology and function, and exclusion of food-borne antigens or irritating additives.

The dietary approach to treatment of IBD is based on the controlled feeding of a well-defined, additive-free diet that contains a single highly digestible or novel source of protein combined with an easily assimilated carbohydrate such as white rice. Both homemade and commercial lamb and rice diets are reported to maintain remission of lymphocytic-plasmacytic IBD in many dogs and cats, especially in those with colitis.

■ Several specialized commercial diets are marketed for dietary hypersensitivity, but many of these are relatively new products that have not yet received enough clinical evaluation in the treatment of IBD to determine efficacy. Products include:
  • Egg-based diets (e.g., dry Canine Prescription Diet d/d, Hill's Pet).
  • Lamb-based diets (e.g., canned Canine Prescription Diet d/d and Feline Prescription Diet d/d, Hill's Pet; Natural Pack, Eagle; Lamaderm, Natural Life; Natural Choice, Nutro; Wayne Sensible Choice, Royal Canin; Anergen I, Wysong; and Nature's Recipe Lamb & Rice).
  • Rabbit-based diets (e.g., Nature's Recipe Rabbit & Rice; Protocol).
  • Venison-based diets (e.g., Nature's Recipe Venison & Rice).

TABLE 7. Drugs Used for Treatment of Idiopathic Chronic Inflammatory Bowel Disease

Drug	Product (Manufacturer)	Preparations	Dosage
Anti-inflammatory/immunosuppressives			
Prednisone**	Many	Tab—5, 10, 20, 50 mg	Dog—1–2 mg/kg, PO, q24h
			Cat—2–3 mg/kg, PO, q24h
Methylprednisolone acetate	Depo-Medrol (Upjohn)	Inj—40 mg/ml	Cat—20 mg, IM, q2–4wk
Azathioprine†	Imuran (Burroughs Wellcome)	Tab—50 mg	Dog—1–2 mg/kg, PO, q24–48h
			Cat—0.3–0.5 mg/kg, PO, q24–48h
Colonic Anti-inflammatory Drugs			
Sulfasalazine*	Azulfidine (Kabi Pharmacia)	Tab—500 mg	Dog—10–30 mg/kg, PO, q8–12h
			Cat—10–20 mg/kg, PO, q12–24h
Olsalazine	Dipentum (Kabi Pharmacia)	Cap—250 mg	Dog—10–20 mg/kg, PO, q12
Mesalamine	Asacol (Procter & Gamble)	Tab—400 mg	Dog—10–20 mg/kg, PO q8–12h
Anti-inflammatory Retention Enemas‡			
5-Aminosalicylate	Rowasa (Reid-Rowell)	Enema—4 g/60 ml	Needs to be determined
Hydrocortisone	Cortenema (Reid-Rowell)	Enema—100 mg/60 ml	20–60 ml, rectally, q24h
Antibiotics			
Metronidazole	Flagyl (Searle)	Tab—250 mg, 500 mg	10–15 mg/kg, PO, q8–12h
Tylosin§	Tylan-Plus (Elanco)	Powder—470 mg/tsp	Dog—20–40 mg/kg, PO, q12h
			Cat—10–20 mg/kg, PO, q12h

Tab = tablets; Liq = elixir, suspension or drops; Cap = capsules; Inj = injectable.

*Dosage may need to be increased to 25–50 mg/kg q8h to achieve effect in some dogs; may cause keratoconjunctivitis sicca in dogs and salicylate toxicosis in cats.

**In some cats with severe colitis, prednisone dosage may need to be increased to 5 mg/kg/day, divided bid. In dogs, if steroidal side effects become a problem, decrease dosage and combine with azathioprine or metronidazole or both.

†May cause myelotoxicity, so monitor CBC; tablet can be crushed and added to VAL Syrup (Fort Dodge) for accurate dosing of cats.

‡Retention enemas for topical therapy of the distal colon may relieve signs of tenesmus and urgency in some animals with proctitis.

§Tylosin powder is bitter-tasting and thus best tolerated when mixed with food.

- Homemade diets for a feeding trial can be made from one part low-fat cottage cheese, tofu, or lamb (cooked or baby food) combined with 3 parts rice.
- A cooperative and patient owner is needed for success; allow a minimum of 3–4 weeks for the trial feeding period; in some cases 6 weeks or more may be required before improvement is complete.
- Eliminate intake of all other foods or sources of antigen throughout the feeding trial, including table scraps, treats, dog biscuits, rawhide chew toys, and flavored medications such as vitamins and heartworm preventatives.
- If there is a substantial response to the dietary trial, the animal can be re-challenged with its original diet.
  - Recurrence of signs confirms dietary intolerance or hypersensitivity.
  - Once remission is restored with the controlled diet, the animal can then be challenged sequentially with individual dietary components to identify the specific offenders. To do this, individual components of the original diet are added one at a time to the controlled diet while the animal is in remission. With each challenge the animal is monitored for recurrence of signs for 7–10 days. If signs recur, that substance is implicated as an offender.
- After several weeks of remission on the controlled diet, some animals can be returned to their original diet and remain asymptomatic; however, most animals will need specially formulated or hypoallergenic diets indefinitely to prevent relapse.
- If there is no response to dietary management within 4–6 weeks, institute medical therapy.

Other Dietary Adjustments. In cases in which hypoallergenic diets are not effective, other dietary adjustments may be beneficial.

- Various special-formulation diets can be helpful in IBD, such as Eukanuba (Iams) for dogs and Prescription Diet c/d (Hill's Pet) for cats.
- In animals with colitis, fiber supplementation of the diet (see sec. 7, ch. 11) or feeding of a commercial high-fiber diet (e.g., Canine or Feline Prescription Diet w/d, Hill's Pet) may improve colonic function and control diarrhea.
- Animals with small intestinal disease may improve on a highly digestible low-fiber diet (e.g., Prescription Diet i/d, Hill's Pet).

5-Aminosalicylic Acid (5-ASA, Mesalamine Drugs)

These drugs exert an anti-inflammatory effect in colitis through local inhibition of mucosal leukotrienes and prostaglandins. In dogs with IBD, 5-ASA drugs are the initial drugs of choice when the colon alone is involved. Cats generally tolerate corticosteroids better than salicylates; thus, prednisone is the first choice for feline IBD, and 5-ASA drugs generally are reserved for steroid-resistant feline colitis. For 5-ASA drugs to be effective in treating colitis they must reach the lumen of the colon; thus, each orally administered 5-ASA drug has a delivery vehicle mechanism that prevents significant absorption during passage through the small intestine.

Sulfasalazine (Azulfidine; Kabi Pharmacia). In this drug, 5-ASA is combined with sulfapyridine by an azo bond that prevents significant absorption of the drug, so that 75% of it reaches the colon where the bacteria split the bond and release the 5-ASA for its local effect in the colon (see Table 7 for dosages).

- The most common adverse side effect of sulfasalazine is keratoconjunctivitis sicca. When it occurs, the decline in tear production is often irreversible. For this reason, it is recommended that a baseline Schirmer tear test be performed at the start of therapy and monitored subsequently at monthly intervals if treatment is long-term.

- Less common side effects include allergic dermatitis, nausea and vomiting, and cholestatic jaundice. Rarely, cats may develop anemia.
- Because up to 30% of the salicylate is absorbed and cats metabolize salicylates very slowly, use caution when treating cats with this drug in order to avoid salicylate toxicity.

Olsalazine (Dipentum; Kabi Pharmacia). This newer derivative, consisting of two molecules of azo-bonded 5-ASA, is poorly absorbed, so that 98% reaches the colon where the two 5-ASA molecules are then released by the action of colonic bacteria on the azo bond (see Table 7 for dosages).

- The advantages of olsalazine over sulfasalazine are that olsalazine contains only 5-ASA (without sulfa) and that a greater percentage of the drug reaches the colon.
- Unfortunately, olsalazine is currently available only in 250-mg capsules, an inconvenient size for dosing most animals.

Polymer-Coated Mesalamine (Asacol; Procter & Gamble). A pH-sensitive coating prevents release of 5-ASA until the drug reaches the site of inflammation in the colon.

Mesalamine Suspension Enema (RowASA; Reid-Rowell). This form of 5-ASA is available for direct instillation into the rectum. In animals, enema administration of 5-ASA is probably not as effective as the oral route except when proctitis is the principal manifestation.

Corticosteroids

Oral prednisone is the preferred initial therapy for dogs with concurrent IBD of the small intestine and for all cats with IBD. In addition, dogs with severe colitis or colitis that is refractory to 5-ASA drugs alone may respond best to prednisone used as a single agent or in combination with a 5-ASA drug (e.g., sulfasalazine, olasalazine) or metronidazole.

- Clinical response, using the dosage in Table 7, should be noted within 1–2 weeks. After 2 weeks of remission, taper the dosage over an additional 4-week period to the lowest effective alternate-day dosage (usually about 0.25–0.5 mg/kg in dogs and 0.5–1.0 mg/kg in cats).
- In cats that are too difficult to medicate orally, periodic injections of methylprednisolone acetate may be used instead (see Table 7).
- Corticosteroid therapy may be discontinued on a trial basis after 8–12 weeks of remission; however, continuous therapy is required in many cases to prevent relapse.
- Hydrocortisone retention enemas (Cortenema) may be useful for controlling severe urgency or tenesmus associated with proctitis. One dose in the evening is usually adequate, but in cases of severe proctitis, treatment can be given q8h (see Table 7).

Antibiotics

- Antibiotics such as metronidazole (Flagyl) and tylosin (Tylan-Plus) are sometimes beneficial in animals with colitis (see Table 7). These can be used alone as single agents, but they are most effective in combination with the previously mentioned treatment measures.
- The beneficial effects of metronidazole, as shown in human patients and experimental animals with colitis, may be attributed to the drug's intraluminal antibacterial action (reduction of bacterial-derived antigens) or to its suppressive effect on cell-mediated immune responses in the colon.

Azathioprine

- In IBD patients refractory to 5-ASA drugs, prednisone, and metronidazole, the combination of azathioprine (Imuran) with prednisone may be a more effective immunosuppressive regimen for producing remission of the disease (see Table 7). In addition to treating refractory IBD, the addition of azathioprine enables use of a lower dose of corticosteroid to control the disease and thereby minimizes steroidal side effects.
- Azathioprine usually is given as a daily treatment until remission occurs and then decreased to an alternate-day treatment (alternating with every-other-day prednisone) for maintenance. Because of its myelosuppressive toxicity (leukopenia), periodically monitor the CBC of azathioprine-treated animals.

Motility-Modifying Antidiarrheal Drugs

Adjunctive use of colonic motility-modifying drugs may provide some symptomatic relief for animals with colitis (see Table 5 for dosages).

- Opioid drugs such as loperamide (Imodium) and diphenoxylate (Lomotil) may aid control of diarrhea by acting on colonic smooth muscle to inhibit propulsive movements and by inhibiting mucosal efflux of water and electrolytes.
- Anticholinergic antispasmodics such as dicyclomine (Bentyl) may be beneficial in colitis patients with severe tenesmus and urgency associated with rectocolonic spasm.

Prognosis

- Inform the owner that persistence or recurrence of IBD is likely despite therapy; thus, a realistic expectation is maintenance of remission or control of relapses rather than a permanent cure.
- The clinical course in basenjis, soft-coated Wheaton terriers, and Shar peis is often progressive despite treatment.

Eosinophilic Gastroenteritis

Eosinophilic gastroenteritis (EGE) is a relatively uncommon form of IBD that is characterized by diffuse or segmental infiltration of some portion of the GI tract with mature eosinophils, often accompanied by a peripheral eosinophilia.

Etiology

Allergy and parasitism have been proposed as causes, but in most patients evidence for these is lacking, and the disease must be considered idiopathic.

Clinical Signs

- One or more layers of the stomach, small intestine, or colon may be affected, resulting in clinical syndromes of chronic vomiting (eosinophilic gastritis, see sec. 7, ch. 4), chronic small bowel–type diarrhea (eosinophilic enteritis), chronic large bowel–type diarrhea (eosinophilic colitis), or any combination of these.
- Diffuse infiltration of the intestinal tract with eosinophils may result in malabsorption (watery diarrhea and weight loss) or protein-losing enteropathy.
- Diarrhea or vomitus may contain blood from mucosal erosions or ulcers.
- Eosinophilic granuloma of the deeper layers of the bowel wall occasionally produces segmental tumor-like thickening that can cause partial intestinal obstruction.

Diagnosis

- The history may indicate dramatic responsiveness to prior glucocorticoid therapy.
- Palpation may reveal diffusely thickened intestinal loops or a tumor-like intestinal mass (eosinophilic granuloma).
- Laboratory evaluation may reveal peripheral eosinophilia (although not present in all cases), hypoproteinemia, or impaired absorptive function tests.
- Routine fecal flotation is indicated because parasitism can also cause eosinophilic inflammation; it is important to exclude occult whipworm or hookworm infection in dogs by response to a therapeutic trial of an anthelmintic such as fenbendazole (see Table 6).
- Barium radiography may be normal, or may indicate thickening and irregularity (mucosal filling defects) of bowel loops, or may delineate sites of partial luminal obstruction caused by eosinophilic granulomas.
- The diagnosis is based on demonstration of eosinophilic inflammation in intestinal biopsies. The endoscopic appearance is similar to that described for lymphocytic-plasmacytic IBD except that mucosal ulceration is more common in EGE. Occasionally lesions are deep in the submucosa and found only by full-thickness biopsy.

Treatment

- Because food allergy is a potential cause of EGE in some animals, a feeding trial using an elimination or hypoallergenic diet (as described for lymphocytic-plasmacytic IBD) can be considered initially; however, dietary therapy alone is seldom effective.
- Oral prednisone usually is the most effective treatment for EGE, at an initial dosage of 1–2 mg/kg/day for dogs and 2–3 mg/kg/day for cats. Clinical signs typically improve rapidly, especially when infiltration is limited to the mucosa. When remission has been maintained for 2 weeks, gradually taper the dosage over an additional 2–4 weeks to the lowest effective maintenance dose.
  - In some animals the treatment can eventually be discontinued, but in others alternate-day maintenance therapy is required.
- In some patients it may be necessary to add azathioprine to the corticosteroid regimen (as described for lymphocytic-plasmacytic IBD) to facilitate reduction of corticosteroid dosage and side effects or to provide more effective control of the disease.
- Obstructing transmural eosinophilic granulomas involving a localized segment of bowel wall occasionally require surgical excision followed by corticosteroid therapy.

Feline Hypereosinophilic Syndrome

Feline hypereosinophilic syndrome (FHS), a rare disease of cats, is characterized by severe eosinophilic gastrointestinal infiltration accompanied by widespread infiltration of various other organs (liver, spleen, lymph nodes, bone marrow, lung, pancreas, adrenals, skin).

Etiology

The etiopathogenesis is not known. The aggressive course and high mortality associated with this syndrome indicate that it should be considered distinct from the more benign eosinophilic gastroenteritis that is confined to the GI tract; in fact, FHS in many ways resembles neoplasia more than an inflammatory bowel disease.

Clinical Signs

- Vomiting, diarrhea (sometimes bloody), anorexia, and weight loss are the most consistent clinical signs.
- Clinical deterioration is rapidly progressive and fatalities are common.

Diagnosis

- Abdominal palpation may reveal intestinal thickening, hepatosplenomegaly, or mesenteric lymphadenopathy because of the disseminated visceral infiltration of eosinophils.
- Persistent, severe eosinophilia is a consistent finding in affected cats.
- The diagnosis depends on histopathologic confirmation of tissue infiltration and effacement by eosinophils in biopsies of affected organs.

Treatment

- Use high-dose prednisolone (4–6 mg/kg/day for 2–4 weeks) to induce remission, followed by half this dose for 2–4 weeks, and then by 1–2 mg/kg daily or on alternate days for maintenance. Add azathioprine or alkylating cancer chemotherapeutics in refractory patients.

Prognosis

Unlike EGE confined to the GI tract, FHS has a poor prognosis despite treatment.

Regional Granulomatous Enterocolitis

Regional granulomatous enterocolitis (RGE) is an uncommon form of IBD characterized by transmural granulomatous inflammation that results in a stenosing, masslike thickening of a region of the bowel wall. The ileocolic junction is most often involved, and the mass may incorporate adjacent lymph nodes and mesentery. In some dogs the granulomatous lesion also contains numerous eosinophils (eosinophilic granuloma).

Clinical Signs

The principal clinical sign of RGE is chronic large bowel diarrhea containing mucus and fresh blood, sometimes accompanied by tenesmus and abdominal pain. Additional signs may include weight loss, anorexia, and depression.

Diagnosis

- The diseased segment of bowel may be palpable as a firm mass in the midabdomen. The adjacent intestinal loops and mesentery may also be thickened and regional lymph nodes may be enlarged.
- A routine CBC may reveal eosinophilia, neutrophilia, or monocytosis. Panhypoproteinemia due to excessive enteric loss of protein may be found in some animals.
- Barium contrast radiography of the ileum and colon may delineate a thickened or stenosed segment of bowel.
- Definitive diagnosis of RGE requires biopsy by colonoscopy or laparotomy. The key feature is transmural granulomatous inflammation. Fibrosis and aggregates of epithelioid cells, giant cells, and eosinophils often are found deep in the lesion. Deep ulceration is common.
- Differentiate RGE from intestinal neoplasia and infectious causes of granulomatous bowel lesions, such as histoplasmosis, pythiosis, and mycobacteriosis. Examine granulomatous lesions by special stains to detect fungi and acid-fast organisms. In cats, feline immunodeficiency virus (sec. 2, ch. 2) and FIP coronavirus (sec. 2, ch. 3) occasionally are associated with pyogranulomatous IBD.

Treatment

- Medical treatment of regional granulomatous colitis is based on the use of anti-inflammatory and immunosuppressive agents such as olsalazine or sulfasalazine, prednisone, azathioprine, and metronidazole, as described for treatment of lymphocytic-plasmacytic IBD.
- If the degree of thickening and cicatrization of the affected segment of bowel produces severe stenosis and obliteration of the lumen, surgical excision of the lesion may be necessary, followed by medical therapy for 6–8 weeks or longer to prevent recurrence of the lesion at the surgical site.

Histiocytic Ulcerative Colitis

- Histiocytic ulcerative colitis is a chronic idiopathic IBD of young boxer dogs characterized by infiltration of the lamina propria and submucosa of the colon by distinctive histiocytes engorged with deposits that stain positive with periodic acid–Schiff (PAS) stain.
- In addition to boxers, there have been isolated case reports of histiocytic colitis in a cat and a French bulldog, but it is not known if this is the same disease that occurs in boxers.

Clinical Signs

- Affected boxers generally develop severe, unresponsive, bloody-mucoid large bowel diarrhea before 2 years of age.
- Severe weight loss and debilitation occurs in dogs with long-standing disease.

Diagnosis

The diagnosis is based on the known breed predisposition and the presence of numerous PAS-positive histiocytes in a colonoscopic biopsy. A mixture of other types of inflammatory cells are also found in the lesion, and usually there is severe mucosal ulceration.

Treatment

- Give olsalazine or sulfasalazine, prednisone, azathioprine, and metronidazole in single-agent or combination regimens as described for lymphocytic-plasmacytic colitis (see Table 7); however, lifetime therapy is needed, and the probability of effective control of the disease is poor.
- In general, these dogs seem to have less diarrhea on a highly digestible diet than on a high-fiber diet.

Neutrophilic (Suppurative) Enterocolitis

Etiology

- Bacterial enterocolitis (see under Bacterial Infections of the Intestines)
- Idiopathic (i.e., neutrophilic IBD in the absence of an identifiable infectious cause)

Clinical Signs

- Large bowel diarrhea that can be either acute or chronic.

Diagnosis

- Colonoscopic biopsy shows infiltration of predominantly neutrophils, with variable mucosal ulceration, necrosis, or crypt abscesses.
- Diagnosis is based on tests to exclude bacterial enteropathogens (see under Bacterial Infections of the Intestines).

Treatment

Give antibiotics (e.g., trimethoprim-sulfa, enrofloxacin, chloramphenicol) or regimens consisting of sulfasalazine, metronidazole, or anti-inflammatory/immunosuppressive drugs, as described for lymphocytic-plasmacytic IBD (see Table 7).

IRRITABLE BOWEL SYNDROME

Etiology

Irritable bowel syndrome (IBS) is characterized by noninflammatory mucoid large bowel diarrhea associated with episodic disturbances of colonic myoelectrical function (spastic colon). Psychological and emotional factors are implicated in humans afflicted with IBS.

Clinical Signs

- Signs associated with myoelectrical dysfunction in humans with IBS are alternating patterns of diarrhea, constipation, and abdominal cramping.
- Evidence for the existence of IBS in animals is circumstantial; but psychomotor diarrhea due to colonic motility dysfunction or IBS may be a consideration in animals that have intermittent mucoid diarrhea but lack evidence of organic disease.
- Large breeds, especially those used as working dogs (e.g., police dogs, Seeing Eye dogs), and temperamental or excitable dogs seem to be predisposed to IBS.

Diagnosis

- By definition, irritable bowel syndrome is a functional disorder lacking in any identifiable lesions; therefore, the diagnosis can be established only by normal colonoscopic biopsy and diligent exclusion of the other known causes of colonic disease such as dietary, parasitic, infectious, and idiopathic colitis (IBD).
- At colonoscopy, the colon may appear to be hypermotile or spastic. The mucosa appears normal except for increased intraluminal mucus.

Treatment

Dietary modification. Supplementing dietary fiber in the form of unprocessed wheat bran (1–5 tbsp per meal) or a commercial high-fiber diet (Prescription Diet w/d; Hills Pet) can normalize colonic myoelectrical activity and decrease functional diarrhea in some dogs.

Motility modification. If dietary fiber supplementation is unsuccessful, consider medication to alter motility; anticholinergics (antispasmodics) such as propantheline, clidinium, or dicyclomine or opioid drugs such as diphenoxylate or loperamide can be used (see Table 5 for dosages).

Mood modification. Light sedation during stressful times with acetylpromazine, chlorpromazine, or phenobarbital may be helpful in excessively nervous or excitable animals. Anticholinergic CNS depressant drug combinations such as clidinium-chlordiazepoxide (Librax) also can be effective.

INTESTINAL LYMPHANGIECTASIA

Etiology

Lymphangiectasia is a chronic protein-losing enteropathy in dogs, characterized by marked dilatation and dysfunction of the intestinal lymphatic network. Impaired intestinal lymph drainage is presumably caused by obstruction to the normal lymphaticovenous flow. It leads to stasis of chyle within dilated lacteals and lymphatics of the bowel wall and mesentery. Overdistended lacteals release intestinal lymph into the gut lumen by rupture or extravasation, causing loss of the constituents of chyle—plasma proteins, lymphocytes, and lipid (chylomicrons).

Clinical Signs

- The presenting signs of lymphangiectasia usually are attributable to protein-losing enteropathy and include dependent pitting edema of subcutis and limbs, fluid distension of the abdomen (ascites), and respiratory distress (hydrothorax). These manifestations of fluid transudation are the result of hypoalbuminemia and reduced plasma colloidal osmotic pressure.
- Chronic intermittent or persistent diarrhea with a watery or semisolid consistency often is observed, but not all patients have diarrhea.
- Progressive weight loss is common. Clinical signs often develop insidiously.

Diagnosis

KEY POINT ▶ Typical laboratory findings in intestinal lymphangiectasia include hypoalbuminemia, hypoglobulinemia, lymphocytopenia, hypocholesterolemia, and hypocalcemia.

- Differentiate protein-losing enteropathy from nonenteric causes of hypoproteinemia, such as liver failure (impaired hepatic synthesis of albumin) and renal disease (protein-losing glomerulonephropathies), through liver function testing (sec. 7, ch. 8) and urine protein determinations (sec. 8, ch. 1).
- Ancillary diagnostic procedures may be helpful:
  - Radiography can detect or confirm ascites and pleural effusion
  - Fluid analysis of body cavity effusions may be helpful. The effusion associated with lymphangiectasia is usually a transudate. Chylous ascites and chylothorax are found occasionally.
  - Cardiac evaluations can exclude right-sided congestive heart failure (see various chs. in sec. 6), which is a rare cause of lymphangiectasia.
- Definitive diagnosis of lymphangiectasia is based on identification of the characteristic lymphatic lesions in biopsies obtained via laparotomy, or less invasively by endoscopy or suction biopsy capsule. Laparotomy may reveal the mesentery and serosa to have a prominent, weblike network of distended, milky-white lymphatics along with small yellow-white nodules and foamy granular deposits (lipogranulomas) adjacent to lymphatics.

Treatment

The major goal in treating intestinal lymphangiectasia is to decrease the enteric loss of plasma proteins so that normal plasma protein levels can be restored and edema and effusions controlled. This is accomplished with dietary manipulation and anti-inflammatory therapy.

Dietary Therapy

Because absorption of dietary long-chain triglycerides (LCTs) is a major stimulus of intestinal lymph flow, restriction of dietary intake of LCTs may reduce lymph flow, lymphatic distension, and protein loss in lymphangiectasia.

- The ideal diet contains minimal fat (LCT) and provides an ample quantity of high-biologic quality protein; for example, Prescription Diet r/d (Hill's Pet) or a homemade diet consisting of one part low-fat cottage cheese or yogurt as the protein source and three parts rice or potatoes as the carbohydrate source. Supplement diets with fat-soluble vitamins.
- Low-fat diets are inherently low in calories, but another goal of therapy is to promote regain of lost weight. Medium-chain triglycerides (MCT Oil; Mead Johnson) 1 to 2 ml/kg, can be added to the diet to replace the calories lost by restriction of conventional fat (LCT). MCTs are hydrolyzed more rapidly and efficiently than LCTs and are absorbed directly into the portal venous system, bypassing the dysfunctional lymphatics.
- The plasma protein loss and diarrhea of lymphangiectasia often benefit from anti-inflammatory doses of corticosteroids (prednisone, 2–3 mg/kg/day, PO). When remission has been achieved, adjust the dosage to the lowest effective maintenance level.

Prognosis

The prognosis and response to therapy is unpredictable. Many patients achieve a remission of months to years in duration with combined dietary and anti-inflammatory therapy. However, some animals fail to respond and many eventually relapse to finally succumb to severe protein-calorie depletion, incapacitating effusions, or intractable diarrhea.

VILLOUS ATROPHY

Etiology

Villous atrophy is a lesion of the small intestine characterized by short, blunted mucosal villi and is associated with intestinal malabsorption and chronic diarrhea. The forms of villous atrophy may be categorized as primary or secondary.

Primary Forms

- Wheat-sensitive enteropathy of Irish setters resembles gluten enteropathy of humans (celiac disease, nontropical sprue). This is apparently hereditary in Irish setters in Great Britain and is characterized by partial villous atrophy, deficiency or delayed development of specific microvillus enzymes, and dietary sensitivity to wheat.
- Idiopathic canine villous atrophy is recognized most often in German shepherds.

Secondary Forms

- Sequelae of diffuse infiltrative diseases of the intestines, such as chronic inflammatory bowel disease and lymphoma
- Sequelae of enteric infections, such as viruses (coronavirus, rotavirus), bacteria (small intestinal bacterial overgrowth syndrome), and parasites (Giardia)

Clinical Signs

Villous atrophy generally causes chronic small bowel–type diarrhea and weight loss. The severity of signs depends on the degree of disruption of the villous absorptive surface area.

Diagnosis

Histologic examination usually is adequate for documentation of villous atrophy. However, because this can be a nonspecific secondary lesion found in various enteropathies, the diagnosis is mainly based on:

- Breed predilection (German shepherd dogs, Irish setters in Great Britain)
- Response to withdrawal of wheat from the diet
- Tests or procedures to identify enteric infections (e.g., Giardia) or bacterial overgrowth
- Characterization of morphologic and biochemical abnormalities in jejunal biopsies

In some cases, infiltration of lymphocytes and plasma cells and fibrosis make it difficult to determine if the lesion should be categorized as a primary idiopathic villous atrophy or as a chronic inflammatory disease (lymphocytic-plasmacytic enteritis) with secondary villous atrophy (see under Lymphocytic-Plasmacytic Enteritis).

Treatment

Wheat-Sensitive Enteropathy

In wheat-sensitive Irish setters, the signs and lesions of villous atrophy promptly resolve with complete elimination of wheat and possibly other gluten-containing cereal grains from the diet. Most commercial dog foods contain gluten; however, diets that are based on rice or corn rather than wheat or gluten-containing grains are available (e.g., Hill's Pet Food products such as Prescription Diets d/d and i/d and Science Canine Growth Diet; and Iams Pet Food products such as Chunks, Plus, and Eukanuba). Wheat restriction must continue for life, and breeding of affected animals is discouraged.

Idiopathic Villous Atrophy

- Dietary management with a gluten-restricted hypoallergenic diet (e.g., Prescription Diet d/d; Hill's Pet) is sometimes beneficial.
- Vitamin therapy with folate (5 mg daily, PO) and cobalamin (500 μg monthly, IM for 6 months) is indicated if serum levels of these are low.
- Antibiotic therapy is sometimes beneficial, using antibiotics such as oxytetracycline, tylosin, or metro-

nidazole to empirically treat bacterial overgrowth (see under Small Intestinal Bacterial Overgrowth).

■ Prednisone as used for treatment of inflammatory bowel disease (1–3 mg/kg/day, PO, for 4 weeks, followed by tapering to lowest effective alternate-day dosage) may produce clinical improvement in dogs with idiopathic villous atrophy that fail to respond to dietary modification, vitamins, or antibiotics.

Prognosis

The prognosis is guarded, as diarrhea and weight loss often persist despite treatment.

SMALL INTESTINAL BACTERIAL OVERGROWTH

Bacterial overgrowth syndrome is an overproliferation of microflora within the proximal small intestine that results in malabsorption and diarrhea. In the dog, bacterial overgrowth is defined as a fasting bacterial count in duodenal juice of greater than 10^5 organisms per milliliter of intestinal contents.

Etiology

The normal small intestinal microflora is a sparse but stable population of aerobic and facultative anaerobic bacteria whose growth is regulated and influenced by a combination of host factors, bacterial interactions, and dietary composition. Mechanical self-cleansing action of normal intestinal motility and continuous downstream flow of ingesta are especially important for preventing bacterial overgrowth.

Because documentation of bacterial overgrowth is difficult, the syndrome may occur more frequently in dogs and cats than is generally recognized. Development of an abnormal small bowel flora should be considered a potential secondary complication in the following situations:

■ Intestinal surgery
■ Stasis-producing mechanical obstructions such as chronic intestinal foreign bodies and stenosing neoplastic or inflammatory lesions of the gut
■ Destructive lesions of the ileocecocolonic junction that allow colonoenteric reflux
■ Motility disorders such as idiopathic intestinal pseudo-obstruction
■ Immune deficiency states (proposed as the explanation for an apparent breed predilection for overgrowth in German shepherds, basenjis, and Shar peis)
■ Conditions associated with hyposecretion of gastric acid
■ Exocrine pancreatic insufficiency

Clinical Signs

■ Bacterial overgrowth typically causes chronic, foul-smelling watery diarrhea, steatorrhea, and weight loss; however, additional presenting clinical signs can depend somewhat on the underlying cause of the abnormal proliferation of flora.

■ Diarrhea caused by overgrowth usually does not contain blood or mucus.
■ Bacterial overgrowth may be responsible for failure of some dogs with exocrine pancreatic insufficiency to respond adequately to enzyme supplementation.

Diagnosis

Definitive diagnosis of small intestinal bacterial overgrowth requires quantitative aerobic and anaerobic cultures that yield greater than 10^5 organisms/ml of duodenal juice. Duodenal culture specimens are taken by endoscopy, intestinal intubation, or laparotomy after an 18-hour fast. This is impractical for routine clinical application.

Indirect evidence of bacterial overgrowth in animals with unexplained small bowel diarrhea and malabsorption include the following observations:

■ Responsiveness to antibiotics (e.g., tetracyclines, tylosin, or metronidazole)
■ Delayed intestinal transit of barium on radiographs (obstruction or poor motility)
■ Idiopathic pseudo-obstruction manifested by a dilated, hypomotile segment of gut
■ Elevated serum folate and decreased serum cobalamin (because bacteria may synthesize folate and bind or compete for cobalamin)
■ Minimal morphologic abnormalities in intestinal biopsies
  • Unlike many other enteropathies, mucosal morphology in bacterial overgrowth may be normal or characterized by mild atrophy of villi and minimal increase in mononuclear cells in the lamina propria.
■ Failure to obtain the expected treatment response in other intestinal disorders known to be conducive to bacterial overgrowth (such as exocrine pancreatic insufficiency)

Treatment

■ Identify and treat underlying disorders or predisposing factors. In animals with stasis caused by anatomic abnormalities, this may include surgery.
■ Antibiotic therapy:
  • Oral broad-spectrum antimicrobials and those with activity against anaerobes are recommended, such as tetracycline, oxytetracycline, doxycycline, metronidazole, ampicillin, chloramphenicol, tylosin, and erythromycin.
  • Continue treatment for at least 10–14 days and repeat as necessary. Some animals need treatment at frequent intervals or even continuously, others may remain in remission for months after one course of antibiotics.
  • Clinical signs and abnormal function tests usually resolve within the first week of therapy, which in itself is good indirect evidence in support of the diagnosis.
■ Treatment with *Lactobacillus* or live yogurt culture usually is not effective for altering the enteric microflora.

INTESTINAL NEOPLASIA

Benign tumors of the intestinal tract include adenomatous polyps, adenomas, and leiomyomas. In dogs, these occur most commonly in the rectum and terminal colon. The most common malignant neoplasms of the intestinal tract are adenocarcinoma and lymphosarcoma. Less common malignancies include carcinoid tumors, leiomyosarcoma, fibrosarcoma, mastocytoma, hemangiosarcoma, and anaplastic sarcoma.

Adenocarcinoma

- Adenocarcinomas are locally invasive and slow-growing and are usually seen in older animals. The most common sites in dogs are the duodenum and colon; in cats, the ileum and distal jejunum.
- Morphologically there are three forms of adenocarcinoma:
  - Infiltrative—thickened stenotic region of bowel that obstructs the lumen
  - Ulcerative—deep indurated mucosal ulcer with raised edges
  - Proliferative—lobulated expanding intestinal mass
- Mucosal ulceration is frequent, sometimes resulting in melena and blood loss anemia.
- Local invasion of the mesentery, omentum, and regional lymph nodes is common. More widespread metastasis also may occur.

Lymphoma

- GI lymphoma arises from B lymphocytes of the gut-associated lymphoid tissue (GALT) and is the most common extranodal lymphoma in dogs and cats (see sec. 3, ch. 6).
- In cats, intestinal lymphoma occurs mostly over 8 years of age and is caused by feline leukemia virus (see sec. 2, ch. 1), although as few as 30% are viremic.
- Morphologically there are two types of intestinal lymphoma:
  - Diffuse lymphoma—diffuse infiltration of the lamina propria and submucosa with neoplastic lymphocytes causes malabsorption and occasionally deep ulceration
  - Nodular lymphoma—expanding intestinal mass, most often in the ileocecocolic region, causing progressive luminal obstruction
- Metastasis to regional lymph nodes and other organs is common.

Clinical Signs

- Small intestinal neoplasia typically develops insidiously with initial vague signs of anorexia and lethargy, progressing to diarrhea and intermittent vomiting. Weight loss develops and progresses in severity in parallel with tumor growth. Melena, hematemesis, anemia, fever, icterus, and abdominal effusion may also occur.
- Colonic polyps and tumors cause hematochezia, dyschezia, and tenesmus, sometimes with mucoid diarrhea; thus, they are easily confused with inflammatory diseases of the colon.
- Multifocal GI lymphoma may invade the stomach, small intestine, or colon, in any combination, thereby varying the clinical presentation. Furthermore, signs of extraintestinal involvement of organs such as the liver, spleen, or kidney may add to the clinical signs and physical findings.

Diagnosis

- Abdominal palpation often detects intestinal neoplasia as a firm mid-abdominal mass, thickened intestinal loops, or mesenteric lymphadenopathy.
- Rectal palpation detects stenosing or polypoid rectal masses. Most adenomatous rectal polyps can be exposed at the anus by everting the rectal mucosa with gentle traction. Polyps usually appear dark red and lobulated, are extremely friable, and bleed easily.
- Laboratory evaluation may reveal blood loss anemia, neutrophilic leukocytosis with left shift, hypoproteinemia, or elevated serum hepatic enzyme concentrations.
- Radiography, particularly barium-contrast, can be helpful for delineating regions of mucosal irregularity, luminal narrowing, and intramural infiltration, thickening, or nodularity. Thoracic radiography is indicated for detection of metastasis.
- Abdominal ultrasonography may be used to better define abdominal mass lesions.
- Surgical excision or biopsy of the affected segment of bowel provides a definitive diagnosis:
  - Gastric, duodenal, or colonic lesions are accessible to endoscopic biopsy.
  - Percutaneous fine-needle aspiration can be used to make a cytologic diagnosis in selected cases in which the neoplastic intestinal mass or loop can be well delineated and stabilized by palpation.

Treatment

- Surgical resection is the treatment of choice for benign tumors such as polyps and, when feasible, for adenocarcinomas and other nonlymphomatous tumors. Unfortunately, many malignant tumors of the intestinal tract are too advanced for successful resection by the time they are recognized clinically. Always submit excised tissue for thorough histopathologic examination, including evaluation of surgical margins.
- Intestinal lymphoma can be treated with anticancer chemotherapy (see sec. 3, chs. 5 and 6).
- Treatment strategy and prognosis may be affected by complications such as malabsorption, protein-losing enteropathy, intestinal blood loss anemia, intestinal obstruction, intussusception, intestinal perforation and peritonitis, and metastasis to the liver or kidneys.

INTESTINAL OBSTRUCTION
Etiology

Intestinal obstruction in dogs and cats may be caused by intraluminal objects, intramural thickening or stenosis, and extramural compression. Specific causes include:

- Foreign bodies (e.g., bones, toys, cloth, metallic objects, stones, peach pits, acorns, rubber nipples, rubber balls, and linear objects such as string and thread)
- Intussusception
- Volvulus
- Intestinal torsion
- Incarceration of bowel in a hernia (includes abdominal hernias of all types, diaphragmatic hernia, and internal herniation of gut loops through a tear in the mesentery)
- Adhesions or stricture (post-trauma or postsurgery)
- Intramural abscess, granuloma, or hematoma
- Congenital malformation (stenosis or atresia)
- Intestinal neoplasia

Pathophysiology

Proximal Versus Distal Obstruction

The more proximal and complete the obstruction, the more acute and severe the signs and the greater the likelihood of dehydration, electrolye imbalance, and shock.

- *Proximal obstructions* cause gastric outlet occlusion, leading to persistent vomiting, loss of gastric secretions (hydrochloric acid), and metabolic alkalosis.
- *Distal obstructions* cause varying degrees of metabolic acidosis. Distal and incomplete obstructions can be insidious, with vague, intermittent signs of chronic anorexia and occasional vomiting that span several days or even weeks, leading to progressive starvation.

Simple Versus Strangulated Obstruction

Vascular compromise of obstructed bowel worsens the severity of the condition.

- *Simple obstructions* occlude the lumen without compromising vascular integrity.
- *Strangulated obstructions* cause vascular compromise of the obstructed bowel segment. This occurs most often with intussusception, volvulus, and incarcerated hernia. The sequence of events following strangulation are edema and engorgement of the affected loop, tissue hypoxia and infarction of the bowel wall, accumulation of gut bacteria and toxins in the peritoneal fluid, and rapidly progressive toxemia and shock, culminating in death.

Clinical Signs

The clinical manifestations and consequences of obstruction depend on its location, completeness, and duration, as well as the vascular integrity of the affected bowel segment.

- Acute onset of vomiting, anorexia, and depression are the most consistent clinical signs.
- Other signs may include abdominal distension, diarrhea (watery, hemorrhagic, or melenic), abdominal pain (restlessness, panting, or abnormal body posture), and shock (acute collapse).

Diagnosis

- Abdominal palpation may identify intestinal foreign bodies, intussusceptions ("sausage loop"), or gas- and fluid-distended loops of bowel proximal to the obstruction.
- Radiography often confirms the presence of obstruction and delineates the cause, especially when contrast studies are used.
  - Radiographic findings suggesting obstruction include gas or fluid distension (mechanical ileus) of the bowel, delayed transit of contrast material, fixation or displacement of gut loops, luminal filling defects, and foreign objects within the lumen.
- Cats commonly ingest radiolucent linear intestinal foreign bodies (e.g., thread, string, cloth, fishing line, dental floss, and decorative tinsel) that cause aggregation and plication of the bowel and have a distinctive radiographic pattern.
- Laboratory findings often reflect fluid, electrolyte, and acid-base derangements; these vary with location, completeness, and duration of obstruction.
- Leukocytosis with a left shift or degenerative leukopenia accompanied by septic abdominal effusion indicates intestinal ischemia or perforation with peritonitis (see sec. 7, ch. 13).

Treatment

- Intestinal obstructions are treated surgically. Give close attention to supportive care, especially maintenance of fluid, electrolyte, and acid-base homeostasis before, during, and after surgery (for further information on intestinal surgery, see sec. 7, ch. 7).
- Treatment includes management of complications such as necrosis or perforation of the bowel, peritonitis (see sec. 7, ch. 13), and endotoxic shock (see sec. 6, ch. 13).

Supplemental Readings

Burrows CF: Medical diseases of the colon. *In* Jones BD, ed.: *Canine and Feline Gastroenterology*. Philadelphia: W. B. Saunders, 1986, p 221.
Leib MS, Hay WH, Roth L: Plasmacytic-lymphocytic colitis in dogs. *In* Kirk RW, ed.: *Current Veterinary Therapy X*. Philadelphia: W. B. Saunders, 1989, p 939.
Nelson RW, Stookey LJ, Kazacos E: Nutritional management of idiopathic chronic colitis in the dog. J Vet Intern Med 2:133, 1988.
Richter KP: Diseases of the large bowel. *In* Ettinger SJ, ed.: *Textbook of Veterinary Internal Medicine*, 3rd Ed. Philadelphia: W. B. Saunders, 1989, p 1397.
Sherding RG: Chronic diarrhea. *In* Ford RB, ed.: *Clinical Signs and Diagnosis in Small Animal Practice*. New York: Churchill Livingstone, 1988, p 473.
Sherding RG: Diseases of the intestines. *In* Sherding RG, ed.: *The Cat—Diseases and Clinical Management*. New York: Churchill Livingstone, 1989, p 955.
Sherding RG: Diseases of the small bowel. *In* Ettinger SJ, ed.: *Textbook of Veterinary Internal Medicine*, 3rd Ed. Philadelphia: W. B. Saunders, 1989, p 1323.
Strombeck DR, Guilford WG: Idiopathic inflammatory bowel diseases. *In Small Animal Gastroenterology*, 2nd Ed. Davis, CA: Stonegate Publishing, 1990, p 357.

7

Surgery of the Intestines

Ronald M. Bright

Surgical therapy is indicated for structural disease of the bowel. Most animals that require surgery of the small bowel are physiologically compromised. When obstruction of the small bowel is proximal in location, serious electrolyte and water abnormalities can place these patients at high risk.

Prophylactic antibiotics administered perioperatively are indicated in small bowel surgery.

- Prior to surgery of the upper and middle small bowel, give a first-generation cephalosporin such as cefazolin (20 mg/kg) IV and IM initially; repeat IV 1½–2 hours later.
- Prior to surgery of the distal small bowel and large intestine, give a second-generation cephalosporin such as cefmetazole (15 mg/kg) IV or cefoxitin (30 mg/kg) IV and IM; repeat IV 1½ hours later.

ANATOMY

- The small intestine extends from the pylorus to the cecum.
- The duodenocolic ligament restricts the movement of the distal duodenum.
- The jejunum is the major portion of the small bowel and is a very mobile structure.
- The major blood supply is from the cranial mesenteric artery.
- A portion of the proximal duodenum is supplied by the celiac artery and shares a source of blood with the right lobe of the pancreas via the pancreatico-duodenal artery.
- The tunica of the small intestine includes the mucosa, submucosa, muscularis, and serosa.
- The submucosal layer provides blood vessels, lymphatics, and nerves. It is also the support or "holding" layer for sutures.

ENTEROTOMY

Preoperative Considerations

- Give perioperative antibiotics, as previously described.
- Attempt to correct electrolyte and water abnormalities prior to surgery.
- Low albumin levels affect the choice of suture materials (nonabsorbable) and the need for suture-line reinforcement technique such as serosal patch techniques.

Surgical Procedure

Objectives

- Gain access to the lumen of small bowel to remove a foreign body.
- Help define a disease by acquiring a full-thickness biopsy.
- Avoid contamination of the peritoneal cavity.

Equipment

- General surgical pack
- Babcock forceps
- Laparotomy sponges
- Doyen non-crushing intestinal clamps
- #11 Bard-Parker blade

Technique

1. Make a midline abdominal incision to allow access to the small bowel.
2. Pack off the segment of bowel to be entered with moistened laparotomy sponges.
3. Place a 3–0 silk stay suture at both ends of the proposed enterotomy incision (Babcock forceps may be substituted).
4. Milk bowel contents away from the proposed enterotomy site; place non-crushing intestinal forceps (or an assistant's fingers) across the bowel to minimize spillage.
5. Make a full-thickness stab incision into the lumen, using a #11 Bard-Parker scalpel blade. Place a suction tip in the bowel lumen and remove its contents. Enlarge the incision as needed with Metzenbaum scissors.
6. If removing a foreign body, perform the enterotomy over healthy bowel distal to the foreign body.
7. If a biopsy is needed, excise a 2–3 mm strip of bowel parallel to the enterotomy incision.
8. Trim any everted mucosa with scissors.
9. Close the enterotomy incision with 3–0 or 4–0 synthetic absorbable or monofilament nonabsorbable suture material on a swaged-on taper-point needle. A simple interrupted or continuous appositional suture pattern is preferred.
10. Rinse the enterotomy site thoroughly with warm saline.
11. Use omentum or a jejunal onlay patch to reinforce the suture line. The author prefers to use omentum, even in relatively healthy tissue.
12. Some severely debilitated animals may benefit from a jejunostomy tube placement for postoper-

ative enteral nutritional support (See sec. 1, ch. 3 for nutritional support of critical patients.)

13. Perform routine closure of the abdomen.

Postoperative Care and Complications

Short-Term

■ Monitor for signs of leakage peritonitis by abdominal palpation, body temperature measurements, and a complete blood count (CBC).
■ Give food and water the day after surgery.
■ Gradually taper off fluid and electrolyte therapy as the animal returns to normal eating and drinking.

Long-Term

■ Strictures are rare unless an excessive amount of tissue was removed for biopsy and the lumen diameter was compromised.
■ Slow leakage from an enterotomy site may become walled off and later be manifested as an abscess.

Prognosis

■ The prognosis is good if the enterotomy was done for a foreign body.
■ If biopsy indicates neoplasia, the prognosis is poor.
■ If biopsy reveals a protein-losing enteropathy due to benign infiltrative disease, the prognosis is poor to guarded (see sec. 7, ch. 6).

INTESTINAL RESECTION AND ANASTOMOSIS

Indications for intestinal resection and anastomosis include:

■ Diseases causing bowel necrosis (e.g., foreign body, volvulus, trauma)
■ Neoplasia
■ Intussusception
■ Severe, focal infiltrative bowel disease (e.g., phycomycosis)

Preoperative Considerations

■ Administer perioperative antibiotics starting 20–40 minutes before surgery, as described previously.
■ Although controversy surrounds the choice of suture pattern for intestinal anastomosis, any of several techniques probably is acceptable in the hands of a competent surgeon who follows sound intestinal surgery principles.
  • The author prefers the simple interrupted appositional (SIA) suture pattern for intestinal (large or small) anastomoses. This non-crushing technique causes little compromise of the blood supply of the intestinal segments. (Disruption of vascularity is the most common biological cause of failure of an anastomosis.)

KEY POINT ▶ Accurate and atraumatic placement of sutures and gentle handling of the bowel gives the best results. Failure of an anastomosis usually is due to poor surgical technique.

■ Assess bowel viability before determining the amount of bowel to be resected. Standard clinical criteria include color, peristalsis, and arterial pulsations.
■ In the rare case in which standard criteria are not adequate to determine bowel viability, an intravenous fluorescein dye technique can be used.
  • Inject 2 ml of 5% fluorescein dye IV; in a darkened surgery room, evaluate the pattern of fluorescence using #3600 ultraviolet illumination (Wood's lamp).
  • A smooth, uniform green-gold color or a finely mottled pattern with no areas of nonfluorescence > 3 mm denotes acceptable bowel viability.

Surgical Procedure

Objectives

■ Remove diseased or nonviable segment of bowel and restore bowel continuity with an end-to-end anastomosis.
■ Preserve lumen diameter and tissue blood supply.
■ Avoid spillage of bowel contents.

Equipment

■ General surgical pack
■ Doyen non-crushing clamps
■ Laparotomy pads
■ Abdominal retractors

Technique

1. Make a midline abdominal incision long enough to accommodate a thorough abdominal exploratory procedure.
2. Isolate the affected bowel segment and pack off with saline-moistened laparotomy sponges.
3. Isolate and ligate the mesenteric vessels to the affected area. Ligate the arcadial vessels within the mesenteric fat similarly.
4. Place crushing clamps across the bowel at a 60-degree angle to the long axis of the bowel and just inside the arcadial vessels.
5. Milk the ingesta away from the crushing clamps. Place a non-crushing clamp across the viable segments of bowel to be anastomosed, or have an assistant gently hold the bowel segments during the anastomosis.
6. Excise the diseased bowel by incising between the crushing clamp and the arcadial vessel ligation.
7. The mucosal collar may evert around the ends of the transected bowel. This can be trimmed with scissors.
8. Correct any lumen disparity by cutting the small lumen at a more acute angle, longitudinally incising the antimesenteric edge of the small end, or oversewing the larger end.
9. Use a 3–0 or 4–0 suture on a small taper-point needle to place the sutures. All knots are extraluminal.
10. Carefully place the first suture at the mesenteric border. The second suture apposes the antimesenteric border. Place sutures approximately 2–3 mm

apart along the "near" side of the anastomosis. Include the entire thickness of the bowel. Pull down the sutures slowly so as to gently appose the edges of the bowel (SIA pattern).

11. Appose the "far" side or back wall similarly.
12. Gently flush warm sterile saline over the anastomotic site and adjacent lengths of bowel.

KEY POINT ▶ Do not flush the entire abdominal cavity unless there is gross contamination from the surgery or pre-existing peritonitis.

13. Wrap a piece of omentum around the line of anastomosis and gently tack it to the bowel above and below the anastomosis.
14. Close the defect in the mesentery with a continuous suture.
15. Use fresh gloves and a sterile set of instruments for abdominal wall closure.
16. If nutritional support is necessary, place a jejunostomy tube prior to closure of the abdomen.

Postoperative Care and Complications

- Maintain intravenous fluid and electrolyte supplementation until the animal is drinking water.
- Withhold food and fluids for 12–24 hours, after which the regular diet can be fed.
- Discontinue antibiotics 2–4 hours postoperatively, unless peritonitis was present. In this case, continue therapy, basing choice of antibiotic on bacterial culture taken at time of surgery.
- Monitor for signs of depression, high fever, excessive abdominal tenderness, vomiting, and ileus, which may indicate leakage peritonitis. If warranted, initiate appropriate diagnostic (e.g., abdominocentesis) and therapeutic measures (see sec. 7, ch. 13).

ENTEROENTEROPEXY/ENTEROPEXY (COLOPEXY)

- Enteroenteropexy, or plication of loops of bowel, is done to prevent recurrence of intussusception and is usually performed at the time of definitive surgical repair of the intussusception.
- Enteropexy, or fixation of bowel to the abdominal wall, is done as part of a tube jejunostomy placement procedure, as a colopexy for treatment of rectal prolapse, or as an adjunctive procedure for correcting rectal sacculation related to a perineal hernia (see sec. 7, ch. 12).
- These procedures have limited use in dogs and cats.

Surgical Procedures

Objectives

- Prevent telescoping of bowel following surgical repair of intussusception.
- Diminish likelihood of leakage around a jejunostomy tube as it exits the bowel and enters the abdominal wall.
- Prevent caudal movement of the colon and rectum (colopexy).

Equipment

General surgical pack
Balfour abdominal retractor

Technique

Enteroenteropexy

1. Place loops of small bowel side-by-side to form a series of gentle loops. Suture loops to each other by engaging the seromuscular layers with monofilament nonabsorbable suture (Fig. 1). Place sutures approximately 6–10 cm apart.
2. The amount of bowel to include in the "pexy" procedure is controversial. Some surgeons include the entire small bowel, starting at the descending duodenum and finishing at the ileocecocolic junction. Others include only two or three loops of bowel above and below the point of intussusception. Another option is to include only the distal jejunum and ileum, because most of the intussusceptions involve the distal small bowel.

Colopexy

1. Scarify an 8–10 cm portion of the descending colon with a surgical blade along the antimesenteric border.
2. Alternately, make a longitudinal seromuscular incision along the antimesenteric border. This may result in a more consistent colopexy. Avoid entering the lumen.
3. Make an incision into the peritoneum and underlying musculature in the abdominal wall opposite the segment of prepared colon.
4. Preplace four to six horizontal mattress sutures between the colon and the exposed surface of the abdominal wall (Fig. 2). Monofilament nonabsorbable suture is preferred.
5. Tie the sutures to securely appose the fresh bleeding surfaces of the colon and abdominal wall (see Fig. 2).

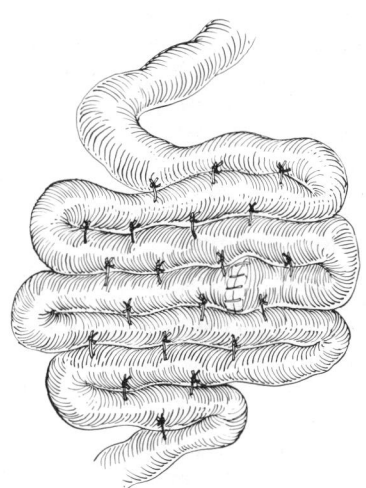

Figure 1. Jejunal enteroenteropexy to prevent intussusception via a ventral midline abdominal approach.

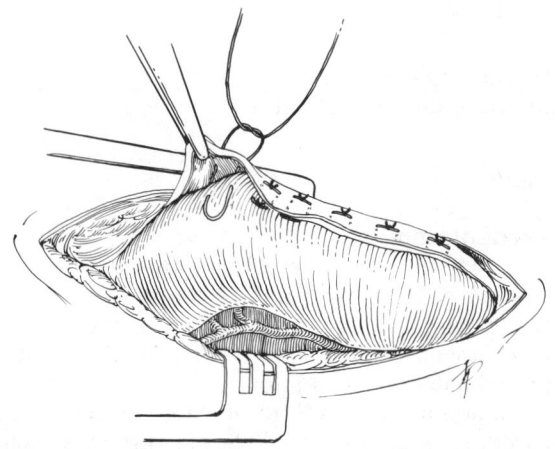

Figure 2. Technique for colopexy to prevent recurrence of rectal prolapse.

Postoperative Care and Complications

- No special feeding limitations are necessary.
- Recurrence of intussusception (following enteroenteropexy) or rectal prolapse (following colopexy) suggests that the pexy site has broken down.

COLOTOMY

The most common indication for a colotomy is a full-thickness biopsy when diagnosis has eluded other diagnostic procedures. Whenever possible, colonoscopic methods of biopsy are preferred (see sec. 7, ch. 6). Rarely, a colotomy is done to remove a foreign body.

Preoperative Considerations

- Surgical procedures involving the colon are more likely to be associated with dehiscence than those involving other portions of the gastrointestinal tract.

KEY POINT ▶ Gentle handling of the colon and the prevention of excessive tension across the suture line will help preserve a good blood supply and promote ideal wound healing.

- The risk of a serious abdominal infection is considerable with colonic surgery.
- To reduce the risk of postoperative sepsis, administer perioperative antibiotics for gram-negative aerobes and anaerobes. Give cefmetazole (15 mg/kg) IV q1½h for two or three doses, starting 20–30 minutes before surgery. Cefoxitin (30 mg/kg) may be substituted.
- Preoperative mechanical cleansing of the colon via multiple enemas may be indicated. This can be especially helpful to improve exposure of colonic polyps or neoplasms during resection.

Surgical Procedure

Objectives

- Collect tissue for biopsy.
- Remove foreign body in cases of low bowel obstruction.
- Prevent spillage of colonic contents.

Equipment

- General surgery pack
- Babcock forceps
- Laparotomy sponges
- Doyen non-crushing intestinal clamps
- #11 Bard-Parker blade

Technique

1. Make a caudal midline abdominal incision for access to the colon.
2. Pack off the colon with laparotomy sponges at the proposed incision site.
3. Place stay sutures at either end of the proposed colotomy incision (Babcock forceps can be substituted).
4. Milk the colonic contents away from the incision site and cross-clamp the bowel segment with Doyen clamps.
5. Using a #11 Bard-Parker surgical blade, stab into the lumen of the colon. Remove a full-thickness elliptical piece of tissue with Metzenbaum scissors.
6. Close the colotomy incision side-to-side with 3–0 or 4–0 synthetic absorbable suture (e.g., polydioxanone, PDS) in a simple interrupted appositional pattern. A nonabsorbable suture (e.g., polypropylene) may be substituted.
7. Gently irrigate the bowel immediately adjacent to the colotomy incision with warm saline before removing the laparotomy pad. Do not allow irrigation fluid to enter the peritoneal cavity.
8. Cover the colotomy incision line with a piece of omentum.
9. Perform routine closure of the abdomen.

Postoperative Care and Complications

Short-Term

- Monitor closely for signs of leakage peritonitis for 48 hours.
- Abdominal pain, an unusually high fever, and a neutrophilia with a left shift suggest a need for further diagnostic tests such as radiography and diagnostic peritoneal lavage.

Long-Term

- Strictures occur rarely.
- Slow-leakage peritonitis may be masked by antibiotics, or the infected area may be walled off, only to be manifested later as an abscess.

Prognosis

- The prognosis is good if the colotomy is done to remove a foreign body.

- If the biopsy suggests a non-neoplastic process, the prognosis depends on the underlying disease (see sec. 7, ch. 6).

SUBTOTAL COLECTOMY

The primary indication for subtotal (90–95%) removal of the colon is for palliation of constipation (obstipation related to megacolon). Idiopathic megacolon in the cat (see sec. 7, ch. 6) is the most common disease for which surgery is indicated.

KEY POINT ▶ Meticulous handling and careful apposition of tissue and a tension-free anastomosis are critical for the success of subtotal colectomy.

Preoperative Considerations

- In cats, the ileocolic valve can be resected with few postoperative problems. Reestablishing bowel continuity with an ileocolostomy versus a colocolostomy (when the ileocolic valve is preserved) is technically easier. However, it is preferable to preserve the ileocolic valve. The postoperative convalescent period is shorter and the likelihood of intractable diarrhea secondary to small bowel bacterial overgrowth is diminished.
- Administer prophylactic antibiotics, as described previously.
- Preoperative enemas are not necessary.

Surgical Procedure

Objectives

- Palliate signs of constipation or obstipation that are associated with megacolon.
- Remove most of the colon with restoration of continuity by ileocolostomy or colocolostomy.
- Allow interrupted movement of ingesta from the small bowel to the rectum.
- Prevent spillage of colonic contents.

Equipment

- General surgery pack
- Balfour abdominal retractors
- Laparotomy sponges
- Doyen non-crushing straight intestinal clamps
- Carmalt crushing forceps

Technique

1. Make a ventral midline abdominal incision, starting from midway between the xiphoid and umbilicus and coursing caudally to the brim of the pelvis.
2. Exteriorize and carefully pack off the colon and distal small bowel from the rest of the abdominal viscera outside the abdominal cavity.
3. Isolate the appropriate colic vessels approximately 1–2 cm from the mesenteric side of the colon. Ligate and divide these (Fig. 3).
4. If the ileocolic valve is being removed, ligate an additional set of vessels (ileocecocolic artery and vein) (see Fig. 3).

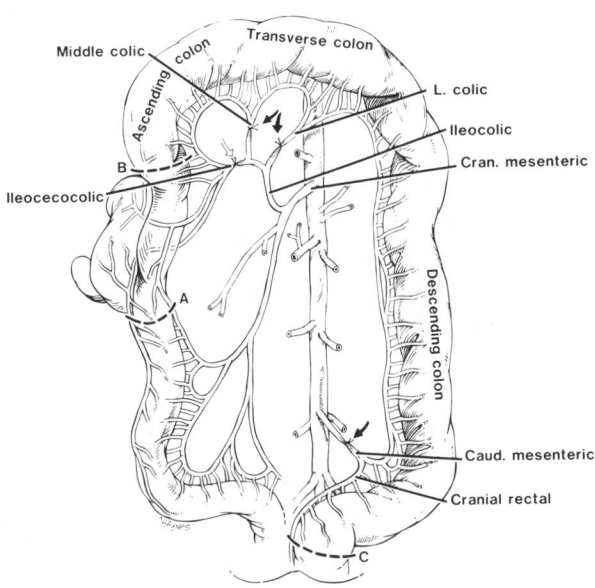

Figure 3. Subtotal colectomy. Sites of ligation of colic blood vessels prior to resection and anastomosis.

5. Caudally, ligate the caudal mesenteric artery and vein.
6. Milk the fecal contents toward the center of the segment of colon to be removed.
7. Place a non-crushing intestinal clamp across the distal colon approximately 1 cm cranial to the brim of the pelvis; if the ileocolic valve is being preserved, place another clamp across the short 1-cm segment of proximal colon remaining below the ileocolic valve.
8. If the ileocolic valve is being resected, place a non-crushing clamp across the ileum just proximal to the ileocolic valve.
9. Use crushing forceps to clamp the colon approximately 1 cm to the inside of the previously placed non-crushing clamps. Transect the colon next to the crushing forceps and the segment of bowel being removed.
10. Perform an end-to-end anastomosis using 4/0 polypropylene or a monofilament synthetic absorbable suture in a simple interrupted appositional suture pattern.
11. Correct any lumen disparity by longitudinally incising the antimesenteric side of the bowel with the smaller lumen. Lumen disparity can also be corrected by partial closure of the larger colonic segment, using the same suture and pattern (Fig. 4).
12. Be careful to incorporate the serosa and to ensure accurate and gentle placement of all sutures. Place the sutures at 2–3 mm intervals.
13. Gently irrigate the anastomotic site and adjacent 4–5 cm of bowel with warm saline. Do not allow fluid to enter the peritoneal cavity.
14. Place an omental patch over the site of anastomosis and gently tack it with 1 or 2 sutures below the line of anastomosis.
15. Remove the laparotomy sponges and replace the bowel in the abdominal cavity.

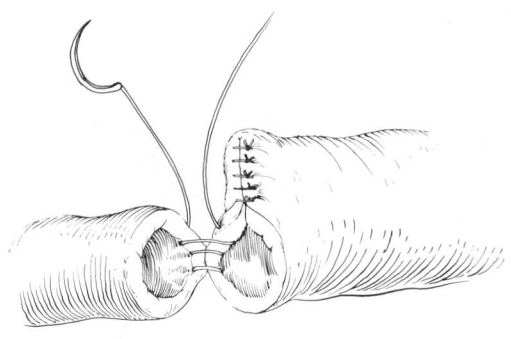

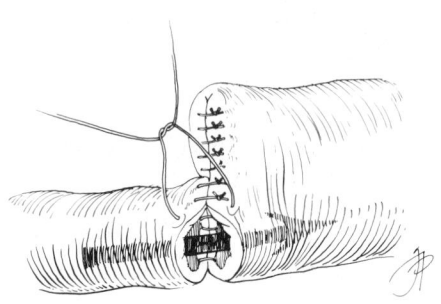

Figure 4. Subtotal colectomy. Correction of lumenal disparity of the bowel by partial closure of larger segment prior to anastomosis.

16. Use fresh gloves and a sterile set of instruments for closure of the midline incision.

Postoperative Care and Complications

Short-Term

- Withhold food and liquids for 24 hours.
- Monitor closely for signs of leakage from the anastomosis for 48–72 hours.
- Some animals continue to have some tenesmus for 7–10 days after surgery.
- Loose stools and increased frequency of defecation occur but usually improve somewhat over a period of weeks to months.
- Continue intravenous fluids for 36–48 hours.

Long-Term

- The frequency of defecation generally increases by 30–50%.
- The stools remain soft indefinitely but often become less fluid and more semiformed within a few weeks.
- Cats do not need a special diet.
- It may be necessary to keep animals on a diet low in volume and high in caloric density for 10–14 days. Thereafter, feed a diet that minimizes diarrhea and results in solidly formed stools.

TYPHLECTOMY

Indications for typhlectomy, or surgical removal of the cecum, include:

- Typhlitis (cecal inflammation) caused by chronic whipworm infection
- Cecal inversion
- Cecal neoplasia

Preoperative Considerations

- If possible, evert the inverted cecum prior to its amputation.
- If manual reduction of cecal inversion is not possible because of adhesions, reduction may need to be done through a colotomy incision.
- The cecum is attached to the terminal ileum by the ileocecal fold, which consists of fascia and peritoneum.

Surgical Procedure

Objective

- Remove the cecum without interfering with ileocolic anatomy and function.

Equipment

- General surgery pack
- Doyen non-crushing straight intestinal forceps
- Abdominal retractor

Technique

1. Bluntly dissect the ileocecal fold to free the cecum from its attachments to the ileum.
2. Preserve the ileocecal vessels while ligating and dividing the cecal branches.
3. Carefully incise the remaining attachments of the cecum to the proximal colon.
4. When the cecum is isolated from its attachments and blood supply, double-clamp the base of the cecum with straight intestinal forceps.
5. Amputate the cecum between the two forceps.
6. Oversew the forceps remaining on the base of the cecum with 2–0 or 3–0 synthetic absorbable suture using a Parker-Kerr suture pattern.
7. Place a second layer of a continuous Lembert inverting suture.

Postoperative Care and Complications

Short-Term

Give food and liquids the day after surgery.

Long-Term

Complications are rare.

Prognosis

- The prognosis is good.

Supplemental Readings

ENTEROTOMY

Oates JA, Wood AJJ: Antimicrobial prophylaxis in surgery. N Engl J Med 315:1129, 1986.

Richardson DC: Intestinal surgery—a review. Comp Contin Educ Pract Vet 3:259, 1981.

Rosen E: Principles of intestinal surgery. *In* Slatter DH, ed.: *Textbook of Small Animal Surgery*. Philadelphia: W. B. Saunders, 1985, p 720.

RESECTION AND ANASTOMOSIS

Bauer MS, Matthiesen DT: Complications and decision making associated with small intestinal surgery. *Problems in Veterinary Medicine—Gastrointestinal Surgical Complications* 1:316, 1989.

Ellison GW, Jokinen MP, Park RD: End-to-end approximating intestinal anastomosis in the dog: A comparison fluorescein dye, angiographic and histopathologic evaluation. J Am Anim Hosp Assoc 18:729, 1982.

Richardson DC: Intestinal surgery—a review. Comp Cont Educ Pract Vet 3:259, 1981.

Sullins KE, Stashak TS, Mero KN: Evaluation of fluorescein dye as an indication of small intestinal viability in the horse. J Am Vet Med Assoc 186:257, 1985.

Wheaton LG, Strandberg JD, Hamilton SR, et al.: A comparison of three techniques for intraoperative prediction of small intestinal injury. J Am Anim Hosp 19:897, 1983.

ENTEROPEXY, ENTEROENTEROPEXY, AND COLOPEXY

Bauer MS, Matthiesen DT: Complications and decision making associated with small intestinal surgery. *Problems in Veterinary Medicine—Gastrointestinal Surgical Complications* 1:316, 1989.

Enger MH: Management of rectal prolapse. *In* Bojrab MJ, ed.: *Current Techniques in Small Animal Surgery II*. Philadelphia: Lea & Febiger, 1983, p 184.

Lewis DD: Intussusception in dogs and cats. Comp Cont Educ Pract Vet 9:523, 1987.

Orton EC: Enteral hyperalimentation administered via needle catheter—jejunostoma as an adjunct to cranial abdominal surgery in dogs and cats. J Am Vet Med Assoc 188:1406, 1986.

COLOTOMY

Orsher RJ: Problems and complications associated with colorectal surgery. *Problems in Veterinary Medicine—Gastrointestinal Surgical Complications* 1:243, 1989.

Richardson DC, Krahwinkel DJ: Surgery of the colon. *In* Bojrab MJ, ed.: *Current Techniques in Small Animal Surgery II*. Philadelphia: Lea & Febiger, 1983, p 162.

SUBTOTAL COLECTOMY

Bright RM, Burrows CF, Goring R, et al.: Subtotal colectomy for the treatment of acquired megacolon in the dog and cat. J Am Vet Med Assoc 188:1412, 1986.

Richardson DC, Duckett KE, Krahwinkel DJ, et al.: Colonic anastomosis: evaluation of an end to end crushing and inverting technique. Am J Vet Res 43:436, 1982.

Rosin E, Walshaw R, Mehlhoff C, et al.: Subtotal colectomy for treatment of chronic constipation associated with idiopathic megacolon in cats: 38 cases (1979–1985). J Am Vet Med Assoc 193:850, 1988.

TYPHLECTOMY

Greiner T, Christie T: The cecum, colon, rectum, and anus. *In* Bojrab MJ, ed.: *Current Techniques in Small Animal Surgery I*. Philadelphia: Lea & Febiger, 1975, p 126.

8 Diseases of the Liver and Biliary Tract

Susan E. Johnson
Robert G. Sherding

General Comments

The liver has many diverse functions related to hepatic blood flow; protein, carbohydrate, and fat metabolism; detoxification and excretion of drugs and toxins; and formation and elimination of bile. Consequently, the clinical and laboratory abnormalities associated with liver failure are diverse.

The diagnostic strategy includes:

- Clinical, laboratory, and radiographic studies to identify liver disease is the problem
- Characterization of the functional aspects of the hepatic disease
- Determination of an etiologic or histologic diagnosis, which usually requires a liver biopsy

The clinical approach and management of patients with hepatic disease is dictated largely by the acute versus chronic nature of the hepatic disorder. Historical, physical, laboratory, and radiographic findings may suggest whether the hepatic disease is acute or chronic but hepatic biopsy often is required for definitive evaluation. Classifying a disorder as acute or chronic has both diagnostic, therapeutic, and prognostic implications.

- In acute hepatic failure, toxic or infectious causes are common, and intensive supportive care is warranted to allow time for hepatic regeneration. The long-term prognosis for recovery is favorable if the animal survives the initial stages.
- Chronic hepatic disorders are more likely to be accompanied by irreversible changes (cirrhosis); thus, the long term prognosis may not be favorable.

Clinical Signs

Clinical signs of liver disease include those typically associated with hepatic dysfunction, such as jaundice, hepatic encephalopathy, ascites, and excessive bleeding, and nonspecific signs such as vomiting, anorexia, lethargy, and weight loss, which overlap with signs of other body system disorders.

- Vomiting is a common sign of liver disease. Hematemesis suggests gastroduodenal ulceration, a recognized complication of hepatobiliary disease.
- Diarrhea occurs less frequently than vomiting and is characteristically small-bowel diarrhea (see sec. 7, ch. 6).
- Anorexia is a common but nonspecific sign of hepatobiliary disease.
- Weight loss and stunted growth are nonspecific signs that suggest chronic rather than acute hepatic disease.
- Polyuria and polydipsia (PU/PD) may be important presenting clinical signs in dogs with liver disease. The mechanism is multifactorial and includes psychogenic polydipsia and renal concentrating defects.
- Pigmented urine (bilirubinuria) and jaundice (icterus) of the sclera, oral mucous membranes, and skin are classic signs of cholestatic liver disease. However, these findings are not specific for hepatobiliary disease and can also be caused by hemolytic disorders.
- Acholic (gray-colored) feces occur secondary to severe cholestasis (usually from common bile duct obstruction), which prevents bilirubin in the bile from entering the intestinal tract and imparting the normal brown color to the feces.
- Excessive bleeding (i.e., hemorrhages of the skin and mucous membranes, melena, hematuria) occasionally is associated with liver disease, especially if hepatic damage is severe or is associated with common bile duct obstruction. Subclinical clotting abnormalities may become clinically apparent after liver biopsy, surgery, and development of gastroduodenal ulcers. Potential mechanisms for bleeding include disseminated intravascular coagulation (DIC) (see sec. 3, ch. 2), primary failure of the hepatocytes to synthesize clotting factors, and vitamin K malabsorption caused by biliary obstruction.
- Hepatic encephalopathy is a metabolic encephalopathy that occurs secondary to severe liver disease and portosystemic shunting of blood. Clinical signs include depression, hypersalivation, behavioral changes, altered consciousness, motor disturbances, seizures, and coma. As with other metabolic encephalopathies, signs typically wax and wane and are interspersed with normal periods.
  - Ammonia, mercaptans, short-chain fatty acids, and gamma-aminobutyric acid (GABA) are potential encephalopathic toxins that are produced in the colon by bacterial action on various substrates. Because the liver normally detoxifies these substances, systemic concentrations are low. With severe liver disease or portosystemic shunting, these potential toxins reach high concentrations in

the systemic circulation and the central nervous system (CNS), resulting in clinical signs.
- Exacerbation of encephalopathy occurs after eating a meal high in protein because protein is a substrate for toxins such as ammonia and mercaptans.
- It is important to differentiate hepatic encephalopathy from other metabolic encephalopathies and from primary CNS disorders.
■ Ascites is a common feature of severe chronic liver disease. Mechanisms of ascites and edema formation in liver disease include hypoalbuminemia, portal hypertension, and renal retention of sodium and water. Rupture of the biliary tract causing bile peritonitis also is associated with abdominal fluid accumulation.

Signalment and History

■ The signalment often provides important clinical information, because breed predilections for specific liver diseases have been recognized, and young animals are more likely to be presented for congenital hepatic disorders such as portosystemic shunt.
■ The history is helpful to characterize the clinical course of liver disease as acute or chronic. Recent onset of signs in an animal that was previously healthy suggests acute hepatic failure. However, because of the large functional reserve capacity of the liver, in occult chronic liver disease the clinical signs may be vague and may not be recognized by the owner until the final phase of hepatic decompensation.
- Chronic hepatic disease can be associated with recent onset of clinical signs and can initially seem to be an acute disease.
- Persisting signs of weight loss and ascites and findings of hypoalbuminemia and microhepatica on subsequent diagnostic evaluation are more likely with chronic hepatic disease.
■ The history may provide important information regarding the potential for exposure to known causes of hepatic injury such as drug therapy, surgical and anesthetic procedures, and toxins or infectious agents.
■ Determine if the animal has a history of intolerance to drugs normally metabolized by the liver, such as sedatives, tranquilizers, anticonvulsants, and anesthetics.
■ Determine the current vaccination status and exposure potential for infectious agents known to affect the liver, such as leptospirosis, infectious canine hepatitis, and feline infectious peritonitis (FIP).

Physical Examination

■ Evaluate the sclera, oral mucous membranes, and skin for jaundice. Jaundice is not clinically detectable until serum bilirubin concentrations are >2.5–3.0 gm/dl. In cats, subtle jaundice often is best detected on the palatine mucosa.
■ Palpate the abdomen carefully. The normal liver can be difficult to palpate in dogs and cats, and the edges are normally sharp, not rounded.
- Hepatomegaly is caused by passive venous congestion, diffuse inflammation, nodular hyperplasia, bile engorgement, and infiltration by fat, glycogen, and neoplastic cells.
- Pain on palpation of the liver (hepatodynia) usually indicates acute liver disease. The pain is caused by stretching of the liver capsule and must be differentiated from pain arising in the pancreas, stomach, or spleen.
- Moderate to severe abdominal effusion may be detected.
■ Perform a neurologic examination in animals with a history of neurologic signs. With hepatic encephalopathy, the neurologic examination may be normal or suggestive of diffuse cerebral disease (e.g., depression and dementia, disorientation, pacing, circling, head-pressing, hypersalivation, seizures, or coma).
■ Perform a rectal examination and obtain a fecal sample to evaluate for melena (indicative of gastrointestinal bleeding) and acholic feces.
■ Evaluate the skin and mucous membranes for evidence of bleeding. Pallor may be detected with blood loss anemia.

Laboratory Evaluation

Because clinical findings in hepatobiliary disease often are vague and nonspecific, hepatic disease may not be suspected until biochemical tests identify elevated liver enzyme activity or other evidence of hepatic dysfunction (e.g., hyperbilirubinemia, hypoalbuminemia). Liver function studies such as serum bile acid (SBA) concentrations are used to:

■ Identify occult liver disease
■ Assess liver function when there is increased liver enzyme activity
■ Determine whether significant hepatic dysfunction is present to warrant performing a liver biopsy
■ Monitor response to therapy

Findings consistent with liver disease on routine laboratory tests are described below.

Complete Blood Count (CBC)

■ Mild to moderate anemia may occur secondary to liver disease because of blood loss (e.g., gastroduodenal ulceration, coagulopathy) or may be associated with normocytic-normochromic anemia of chronic disease.
■ Erythrocytic microcytosis without hypochromia or anemia is a common finding in dogs and cats with portosystemic shunts. The mechanism for microcytosis is unknown; however, iron deficiency is not typically present.
■ Target cells and acanthocytes may occur in dogs and cats with various types of hepatic disease, due to altered red blood cell (RBC) membranes.

Urinalysis

■ The urine specific gravity may be isosthenuric or hyposthenuric if liver disease is associated with PU/PD.

- Bilirubinuria is a sensitive indicator of abnormal bilirubin metabolism, and this finding precedes hyperbilirubinemia and jaundice. Bilirubinuria imparts a yellow-orange color to the urine. Bilirubin crystals may form in the presence of bilirubinuria.
  - Trace amounts of bilirubin may be found in concentrated urine of normal dogs (especially males).
  - Bilirubinuria is always abnormal in cats and suggests underlying hemolytic or hepatobiliary disease.
- Urine urobilinogen is a colorless product of enteric bacterial degradation of bilirubin that is absorbed from the gut. A small portion of urobilinogen escapes the enterohepatic circulation and is excreted in the urine. The finding of urobilinogenuria supports an intact enterohepatic circulation of bilirubin pigments. The absence of urobilinogenuria in a jaundiced animal suggests common bile duct obstruction.
  - However, this test is not reliable in a clinical setting because many nonhepatic factors affect urine urobilinogen concentration, including altered intestinal flora, gastrointestinal bleeding, intestinal absorption, renal excretion, urine pH, urine volume, and urine storage.
- Ammonium biurate crystals are commonly detected in animals with portosystemic shunts but occasionally may be a finding in normal animals.

Liver Enzymes

Evaluation of liver enzyme activity in the serum is used as a screening test to detect liver disease. Increases in liver enzyme activity are not specific for the underlying hepatic disorder. However, liver enzymes can be used to categorize the underlying pathophysiologic mechanism. Increases in liver enzyme activity may occur secondary to hepatocellular injury and leakage (Fig. 1) or due to accelerated production stimulated by bile retention (cholestasis) or drug induction (Fig. 2).

Many systemic diseases can secondarily affect the liver, causing increased liver enzyme activity, but these are not necessarily associated with clinical liver disease. An important example is feline hyperthyroidism, which is commonly associated with increased liver enzyme activity without significant hepatic dysfunction.

KEY POINT ▶ Liver enzymes do not evaluate liver function. Thus, severe hepatic dysfunction may coexist with normal liver enzyme activity; conversely, increased liver enzyme activity may be detected in animals without significant hepatic dysfunction.

Alanine Aminotransferase (ALT)*

- Increased ALT activity indicates hepatocyte injury with leakage of enzyme from the cytoplasm of the hepatocyte (see Fig. 1).

KEY POINT ▶ ALT is considered liver-specific in dogs and cats; the magnitude of ALT increase

---

*Formerly called serum glutamic pyruvic transaminase (SGPT).

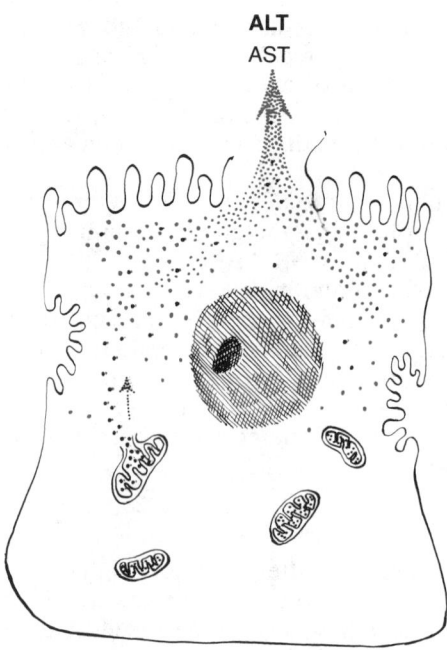

Figure 1. With hepatocyte injury, leakage of alanine aminotransferase (ALT) from the cytoplasm results in increased serum activity. Aspartate aminotransferase (AST) is primarily associated with mitochondria but is also present in the cytoplasm. Release of AST from the mitochondria requires a severe insult. Thus, with hepatocyte injury, ALT is more readily released and its activity level will usually be higher than that of serum AST.

generally correlates with the number of injured hepatocytes.

- The largest increases in ALT activity occur with hepatocellular necrosis and inflammation (up to 100 × normal). Increases also occur with increased hepatocyte membrane permeability, such as that caused by hypoxia. Severe cholestasis can also cause secondary hepatocyte injury, with increases in ALT up to 20–40 × normal. Increased production of ALT by regenerating hepatocytes may account for persisting increases in enzyme activity after resolution of the initial injury.
- Anticonvulsant drug therapy in dogs can be associated with mild increases in ALT activity (4 × normal) in the absence of obvious hepatocellular injury. Corticosteroid therapy or hyperadrenocorticism also is associated with mild to moderate (2–10 × normal) increases in ALT activity.
- Small amounts of ALT are present in canine skeletal muscle; recently it has been shown that severe skeletal muscle injury may be associated with increases in ALT activity of 5–25 × normal.

Aspartate Aminotransferase (AST)*

- Hepatocyte injury is associated with increased AST activity secondary to leakage from mitochondria and cytoplasm of hepatocytes (see Fig. 1).
- AST is not liver-specific in dogs and cats; it is present in significant quantities in hepatocytes and skeletal muscle tissue.

---

*Formerly called serum glutamic oxaloacetic transaminase (SGOT).

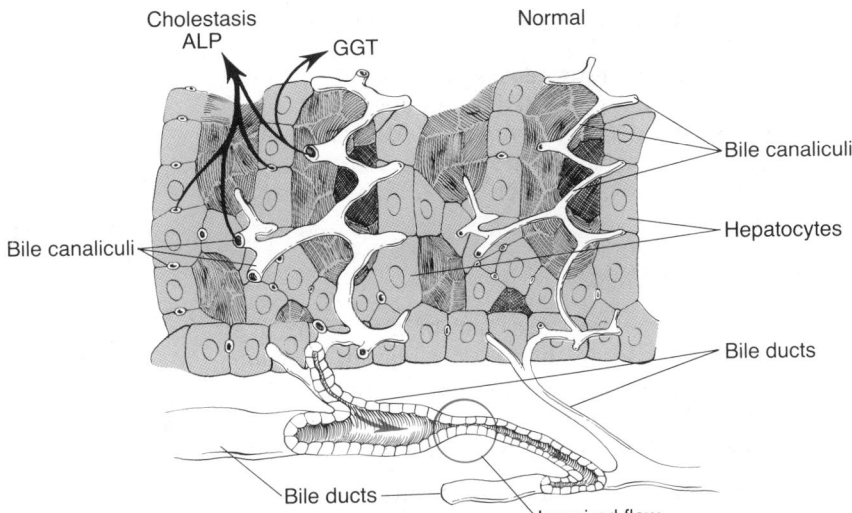

Figure 2. Impaired bile flow (cholestasis) causes increased synthesis of alkaline phosphatase (ALP) and gamma-glutamyltransferase (GGT). Alkaline phosphatase is a sensitive indicator of cholestasis in dogs but is less sensitive in cats (see text). With cholestatic disorders, increased ALP activity precedes hyperbilirubinemia. ALP and GGT lack specificity in differentiating between intrahepatic and extrahepatic cholestasis.

■ Comparison of activities of ALT, AST, and creatine kinase (CK), a muscle enzyme, can indicate whether AST activity is increased due to hepatic or muscle injury.

KEY POINT ▶ Increased AST activity associated with hepatic injury generally parallels but is less than the increase in ALT activity, and CK is normal. Increased AST activity due to skeletal muscle injury is associated with increased CK activity and normal or mildly increased ALT activity.

■ In some cats with liver disease, AST may be more sensitive than ALT in detecting hepatic disease.

Alkaline Phosphatase (ALP)

Increases in serum ALP activity are due to accelerated production of this enzyme, stimulated by cholestasis or drug induction (see Fig. 2). ALP is a membrane-associated enzyme present in many tissues; however, only liver, bone, and corticosteroid-induced isoenzymes contribute to serum ALP activity. Serum ALP activity in normal dogs and cats is usually due to the liver isoenzyme. An increase in this type of ALP activity indicates intrahepatic or extrahepatic cholestasis.

■ Young growing animals or animals with severe bone disease may have mild increases in ALP activity due to the bone isoenzyme.
■ Cats generally have smaller increases in serum ALP activity with hepatobiliary disease than do dogs, owing to a limited capacity for ALP production and a short serum half-life. Therefore, even small increases in serum ALP activity in cats suggest significant cholestasis.
■ Exogenous or endogenous glucocorticoids are associated with hepatic production of a novel isoenzyme of ALP, corticosteroid-induced ALP (CIALP), in dogs, but not in cats. The isoenzyme of CIALP can be distinguished electrophoretically from bone and liver isoenzymes. In cases with excess glucocorticoid levels, CIALP activity usually accounts for at least 70% of total serum ALP activity.

KEY POINT ▶ Hypercortisolism caused by glucocorticoid therapy or hyperadrenocorticism (Cushing's) is the most common cause of increased serum ALP activity in dogs; it is usually attributed to an increase in CIALP.

■ Increase in ALP activity associated with corticosteroid therapy varies considerably with the individual animal and the drug, dose, and duration of therapy. Oral, systemic, and topical preparations (including ear and eye medications) are capable of inducing ALP activity. This increase does not necessarily imply the presence of iatrogenic hyperadrenocorticism, a suppressed pituitary-adrenal axis, corticosteroid-induced hepatopathy, or indicate that corticosteroid therapy must be discontinued.
■ Increased CIALP activity is a sensitive but not specific test for exposure to excess glucocorticoids (iatrogenic or endogenous). Increases in CIALP activity may be detected with diabetes mellitus, anticonvulsant drug therapy, primary hepatic disorders including neoplasia, hypothyroidism, and chronic illnesses. In this setting, CIALP usually accounts for less than 50% of total ALP activity.
■ Increased CIALP activity may be accompanied by mild to moderate (2–10 × normal) increases in ALT activity that typically are of lesser magnitude than increases in ALP activity.
■ Anticonvulsant drug therapy is associated with enzyme induction of the liver isoenzyme of ALP in dogs (but not in cats) in the absence of obvious hepatocellular injury. CIALP activity also may be increased in some dogs. Reported maximal increases for induced serum ALP activity include those caused by phenobarbital (30 × normal), primidone (5 × normal), and diphenylhydantoin (3 × normal).

Gamma Glutamyltransferase (GGT). This membrane-associated enzyme is present in many tissues. Increased serum GGT activity usually reflects cholestasis and increased production by hepatocytes (see Fig. 2).

■ Increased GGT activity parallels increased ALP activity in dogs, including increases associated with excess corticosteroids.

- Anticonvulsant therapy causes mild (2–3 × normal) increases in serum GGT activity in dogs.
- In cats, serum GGT activity exceeds serum ALP activity in most hepatobiliary diseases; an exception is hepatic lipidosis, in which GGT activity may be normal.

Other Biochemical Tests

Numerous biochemical tests can be altered by liver disease, including serum bilirubin, albumin, globulin, urea nitrogen, glucose, and cholesterol. Many of these parameters reflect some aspect of liver function; however, they lack sensitivity or specificity for liver disease.

- Increased serum bilirubin concentration occurs secondary to hemolysis or cholestasis. Evaluate for underlying hemolytic disorders by performing a CBC to detect anemia.
  - Fractionation of the total serum bilirubin into conjugated and unconjugated components (van den Bergh's test) to distinguish the mechanism of hyperbilirubinemia is of little diagnostic value because there is considerable overlap in hemolytic, hepatocellular, and extrahepatic biliary disorders.
  - Lipemia falsely elevates serum bilirubin concentration; the absence of concurrent bilirubinuria suggests pseudohyperbilirubinemia.
- Albumin is synthesized exclusively by the liver. Because of a large reserve capacity for albumin production, hypoalbuminemia does not occur until the functional hepatic mass is reduced 70–80%. Hypoalbuminemia associated with hepatic disease implies chronicity because of the long half-life of albumin. With chronic liver disease, fluid retention and dilution of existing serum albumin may also contribute to hypoalbuminemia. When the serum albumin is <1.5 gm/dl, hypoalbuminemia contributes to the development of ascites and edema.
  - Hypoalbuminemia is not specific for liver disease, and other causes of hypoalbuminemia such as urinary and gastrointestinal (GI) loss must be excluded.
- Hyperglobulinemia due to increased gamma globulins occurs in some dogs and cats with chronic liver disease. The most likely mechanism is a systemic response to antigens that escape from the GI tract because of impaired hepatic mononuclear phagocyte system function or portosystemic shunting. Significant hypoglobulinemia does not usually occur with liver disease despite the liver's role in the synthesis of alpha and beta globulins.
- Blood urea nitrogen (BUN) concentration may be decreased secondary to liver disease because the liver is responsible for converting ammonia to urea. However, many nonhepatic factors (e.g., PU/PD, fluid diuresis, low-protein diet) can also decrease BUN levels.
- Hypoglycemia may occur secondary to hepatic dysfunction because of impaired hepatic gluconeogenesis, decreased hepatic glycogen stores, and decreased hepatic insulin degradation. However, because <30%

of liver function is sufficient to maintain euglycemia, hypoglycemia is an insensitive indicator of hepatic function.

- Because it indicates severe liver dysfunction, liver-associated hypoglycemia is a poor prognostic factor, except in dogs and cats with congenital portosystemic shunts.
- Some hepatic neoplasms such as hepatocellular carcinoma and adenoma, leiomyosarcoma, and hemangiosarcoma have been associated with profound hypoglycemia.
- Also consider nonhepatic causes of hypoglycemia such as sepsis, hypoadrenocorticism, and insulinoma (see sec. 4, ch. 5).
- Hypercholesterolemia occurs with acute cholestatic disorders because of increased synthesis of cholesterol and decreased incorportion of cholesterol into bile acids; however, there are many nonhepatic causes of hypercholesterolemia. Although cholesterol is synthesized in the liver, hypocholesterolemia secondary to liver disease is rare; it has been noted with congenital portosystemic shunts and anticonvulsant-induced hepatic disease.
- Serum electrolyte changes secondary to liver disease are variable. In acute liver failure, serum electrolyte concentrations are usually normal. With chronic liver disease, total body potassium depletion and sodium retention are common, and the serum sodium concentration is usually normal or decreased.

Liver Function Tests

Liver function tests can document clinically significant hepatic dysfunction when liver disease is suspected, based on historical, clinical, laboratory, and radiographic findings. SBA determinations have largely replaced the use of organic anion dyes such as sulfobromophthalein (Bromsulphalein; BSP) and indocyanine green (ICG). Blood ammonia concentration and ammonia tolerance tests can specifically evaluate the portal circulation (for portosystemic shunts) and detect hepatic encephalopathy.

KEY POINT ▶ The test of choice for clinical evaluation of liver function is a combined fasting and 2–hour postprandial SBA concentration.

Serum Bile Acid (SBA) Concentrations. The normal physiology of bile acid metabolism is shown in Figure 3A. In health, bile acids are confined to the enterohepatic circulation, and systemic concentrations are low. SBA concentrations increase in the systemic circulation with all types of liver disease (Fig. 3B). Because the liver has a large reserve capacity for synthesis of bile acids, even severe hepatic dysfunction does not cause decreased SBA concentrations.

Fasting Serum Bile Acid (FSBA) Concentration. An FSBA concentration obtained after a 12-hour fast is a sensitive, specific measure of hepatobiliary function in dogs and cats.

- Increased concentrations occur with hepatocellular and cholestatic disorders that interfere with hepatic uptake or secretion of bile acids and with portosys-

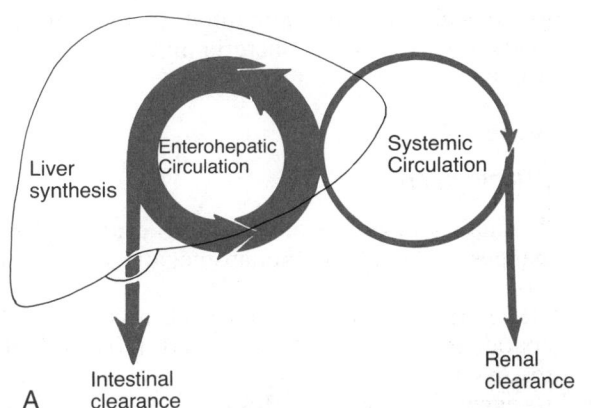
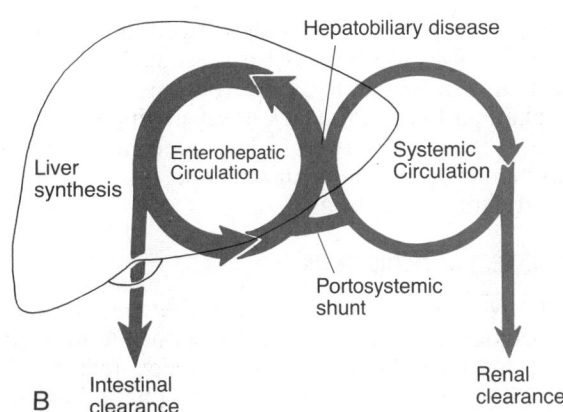

Figure 3. *A*, Bile acids are synthesized in the liver, secreted into the biliary system, and stored in the gallbladder during fasting. With ingestion of a meal, cholecystokinin release stimulates gallbladder contraction and entry of bile acids into the intestinal tract. Bile acids are efficiently reabsorbed in the distal ileum and carried in the portal blood back to the liver, thus completing the enterohepatic circulation. In the healthy animal, the liver removes 90 to 95% of bile acids from the portal circulation during the first pass of the enterohepatic circulation. This allows only small amounts of bile acids to escape to the systemic circulation. Normal serum concentrations are therefore low. (Fasting < 10 μmole/L; postprandial < 15 μmole/L).

B, Hepatocellular dysfunction or cholestasis interferes with hepatic uptake, storage, and secretion of bile acids. Thus, impaired extraction of bile acids from the portal blood results in increased serum bile acid concentrations. With portosystemic shunting, bile acids in the portal blood are diverted directly into the systemic circulation.

temic shunting, in which bile acids are diverted directly into the systemic circulation (see Fig. 3*B*).
■ Normal FSBA values in dogs and cats are <10 μmol/liter. When concentrations exceed 30 μmol/liter, a liver biopsy may be warranted to evaluate the underlying liver disease.

Postprandial Serum Bile Acid (PPSBA) Concentration.
PPSBA concentration is an endogenous challenge test of liver function. Evaluation of PPSBA concentration, compared with FSBA concentration, increases the sensitivity for detection of liver dysfunction, especially in cases of portosystemic shunting, in which FSBA concentrations may be normal after a prolonged fast but PPSBA concentrations are consistently increased.

■ To perform the PPSBA concentration test:
  • Obtain a serum sample for FSBA concentration, and then feed at least 2 tablespoons of food to dogs and at least 1 tablespoon to cats (the more the better).
  • To ensure gallbladder contraction, feed a diet high in fat (e.g., Prescription Diet p/d [Hill's Pet]; Prescription Diet c/d [Hill's Pet] for cats). For encephalopathic animals in which a high-protein diet is contraindicated, substitute a protein-restricted diet and add a few milliliters of corn oil per feeding.
  • Obtain a second serum sample 2 hours after feeding.
■ *Results*: In normal dogs and cats, PPSBA concentrations are <25 μmol/liter and peak 2 hours after a meal. A liver biopsy may be indicated when concentrations are >30 μmol/liter.

Blood Ammonia (BA) Concentration.
Ammonia is metabolized by the liver, and normal plasma concentrations are low.

■ Measurement of BA concentration primarily is in-

dicated to document hepatic encephalopathy. However, normal values do not exclude this diagnosis, because other toxins can contribute to the encephalopathy.
■ Portosystemic shunting is the most common mechanism of hyperammonemia, but severe, diffuse hepatic disease (especially acute hepatic necrosis) also increases BA concentrations.
■ Congenital urea cycle enzyme deficiency is a rare cause of hyperammonemia.

Ammonia Tolerance Test (ATT).
This is a more sensitive test than BA concentration measurement for documenting portosystemic shunting. However, the ATT is contraindicated if resting ammonia levels are already increased, because no further diagnostic information will be obtained and performing an ATT can cause signs of hepatic encephalopathy. *Note*: The ATT is not recommended for use in cats.

■ To perform the ATT:
  • Fast the dog for 12 hours, and then give 100 mg/kg of ammonium chloride (do not exceed a total dose of 3 g), either as a solution by stomach tube or as a powder in a gelatin capsule.
  • Take a heparinized blood sample before and 30 minutes (stomach tube) or 45 minutes (capsule method) after administering the ammonium chloride. Vomiting may occur but does not invalidate the test.
■ *Results*: In normal dogs, there is no increase in BA concentration or a mild increase (<2 × greater than baseline). In dogs with portosystemic shunting, results are consistently abnormal (up to 10 × baseline values); however, results may be normal in the presence of other hepatic disorders, especially those unaccompanied by portosystemic shunting.
■ *Contraindications*: Measurement of ammonia is technically difficult, and appropriate sample handling requires heparinized blood samples to be stored

immediately on ice, cold-centrifuged, and assayed as soon as possible. Because of these technical difficulties, the potential for exacerbation of hepatic encephalopathy, and the lack of sensitivity for detecting many hepatic disorders, SBA concentration measurement is preferable for assessing liver function in most clinical situations.

Parameters of Hemostasis

The liver plays a central role in the coagulation and fibrinolytic systems. The liver is responsible for synthesis of all coagulation factors (except factor VIII), plasminogen, antithrombin III, and alpha$_2$ antiplasmin. Activated coagulation factors and fibrinolytic enzymes are also cleared by the liver.

- Mechanisms of excessive bleeding associated with liver failure include primary failure of hepatocytes to synthesize clotting factors, DIC, and malabsorption of vitamin K caused by complete biliary obstruction. Clinical evidence of bleeding secondary to liver disease is uncommon, and the frequency of abnormal coagulation tests is much higher.
- Measure prothrombin time (PT) to evaluate the extrinsic coagulation system and activated partial thromboplastin time (APTT) to evaluate the intrinsic coagulation system. These tests can be abnormal in the presence of liver disease. Activated coagulation time (ACT) also can be used as a rapid screening test for abnormalities of the intrinsic coagulation system. For further discussion of these tests, see sec. 3, ch. 2.
- Thrombocytopenia may occur secondary to splenic sequestration of platelets associated with portal hypertension or consumption of platelets from DIC. Platelet function defects also have been documented in dogs with liver disease, which may account for clinical bleeding tendencies in the presence of normal coagulation tests and platelet numbers.
- The combination of prolonged PT and APTT, low plasma fibrinogen, increased fibrin degradation products, fragmented RBCs, and thrombocytopenia suggests DIC (see sec. 3, ch. 2).

Blood Gas Analysis

Various acid-base imbalances may occur secondary to liver disease, including respiratory alkalosis, metabolic alkalosis, metabolic acidosis, and mixed acid-base disturbances.

Abdominal Fluid Analysis

- Ascitic fluid that accumulates secondary to liver disease and hypoalbuminemia is usually a transudate. With hepatic venous congestion from vena caval obstruction or cardiac causes, the fluid typically is a modified transudate with protein concentration >2.5 gm/dl.
- Rupture of the biliary tract is associated with bile peritonitis. Grossly, the abdominal fluid appears yellow or green. Chemical tests for bilirubin are positive, and concentrations of bilirubin are higher in abdominal fluid than in serum. Cytologic examination reveals a mixed inflammatory infiltrate and bile-laden macrophages. Bacteria may be seen if bile peritonitis is complicated by sepsis.

Radiographic Evaluation

Survey Radiography

- Abdominal radiographs are useful to evaluate for:
  - Changes in liver size (hepatomegaly, microhepatica)
  - Altered tissue characteristics such as mineralized hepatic densities (choleliths) and radiolucencies (abscesses)
  - Presence of abdominal effusion
- If hepatic neoplasia is suspected, take thoracic films to evaluate for pulmonary metastases.

Ultrasonography

Ultrasonography can be used to image the liver noninvasively, especially when abdominal effusion precludes survey radiographic evaluation. A normal ultrasonographic appearance of the liver does not eliminate the possibility of significant hepatic pathology; however, ultrasonography is diagnostically useful to:

- Detect focal parenchymal abnormalities such as masses, abscesses, cysts, and regenerative nodules. The ultrasonographic appearance of these focal lesions often is similar, and biopsy is required for differentiation.
- Document that a palpable mass is associated with the liver.
- Investigate disorders of the biliary tract, such as biliary obstruction and biliary calculi.
- Detect vascular lesions such as portosystemic shunts, hepatic arteriovenous fistulae, and hepatic venous congestion.
- Obtain percutaneous liver biopsies (see below).

Angiography

Angiography is useful to diagnose vascular disorders involving the liver such as congenital and acquired portosystemic shunts, hepatic arteriovenous fistulae, and vena caval obstruction causing hepatic venous obstruction (see under Congenital Portosystemic Shunts in this chapter).

Liver Biopsy

Liver biopsy often is required to definitively characterize the nature and severity of hepatic disease, to differentiate acute from chronic disorders, and to assess response to therapy. Selection of the best procedure for obtaining a liver biopsy depends on numerous factors including liver size, presence of coagulopathy, diffuse versus focal hepatic lesions, presence of biliary tract obstruction, presence of other intra-abdominal abnormalities, likelihood of surgical resection of a mass, tolerance of general anesthesia, available equipment, and expertise of the clinician.

KEY POINT ▶ Perform a hemostasis screen prior to liver biopsy to detect coagulopathy. After the biopsy is performed, monitor for bleeding from the biopsy site.

Biopsy Methods

Fine-Needle Aspiration. Fine-needle aspiration for cytologic evaluation of the liver is most useful if the pathologic process is diffuse and architectural relationships (that can be obtained only by histopathology) are not essential to the diagnosis. Examples include feline hepatic lipidosis, hepatic neoplasia, and liver disease associated with infectious agents such as histoplasmosis.

Blind Percutaneous Needle Biopsy. Transabdominal and transthoracic needle biopsies are most likely to be successful when the liver is enlarged and pathologic changes are diffuse. The transabdominal approach is preferred, using a Tru-Cut (Travenol Labs.) or Menghini (V. Mueller Co.) biopsy needle.

- The advantage of percutaneous techniques is that they require minimal sedation and take little time.
- Potential disadvantages are that trauma to adjacent organs may occur undetected, and an adequate tissue sample may not be obtained. Recognition of complications such as excessive bleeding or rupture of the biliary tract often is delayed.
- Feed a high-fat meal to cause gallbladder contraction prior to blind percutaneous needle biopsy to minimize the likelihood of inadvertently puncturing the gallbladder.
- Blind biopsy procedures are contraindicated with suspected hepatic abscess or cyst, vascular tumors, bile duct obstruction, peritonitis, abdominal adhesions, and extreme obesity.

Ultrasound-Guided Needle Biopsy. This technique is the percutaneous procedure of choice, depending on the availability of equipment and clinician expertise.

- In addition to the advantages of blind percutaneous techniques, it is possible to obtain tissue from focal lesions, avoid structures adjacent to the liver, and monitor post-biopsy bleeding.
- Ultrasound-guided biopsy may be difficult if the liver is small.

Keyhole Needle Biopsy. Keyhole needle biopsy is performed under general anesthesia similarly to the percutaneous techniques. However, with this technique, a small incision is made, and a sterile, gloved finger localizes the liver lobe to be biopsied and helps guide the needle into the appropriate area.

Laparoscopy. Laparoscopy provides direct visualization of the liver and adjacent structures such as the pancreas and extrahepatic biliary tract. Biopsies also are obtained under direct visualization.

- When the liver is small, laparoscopy is a useful alternative method to ultrasound-guided needle biopsy.
- It is preferable to percutaneous techniques when excess bleeding is anticipated and to laparotomy when delayed wound healing (hypoalbuminemia) is anticipated.
- This technique requires heavy sedation or anesthesia

and is subject to equipment availability and clinician expertise.

Laparotomy. Laparotomy is indicated for liver biopsy when a surgically correctable disease is suspected, such as extrahepatic biliary tract obstruction or a single, large hepatic mass (see sec. 7, ch. 9 for description of the procedure for surgical biopsy).

- This technique makes it possible to:
  - Obtain large samples of liver tissue
  - Monitor for postbiopsy bleeding
- Disadvantages include:
  - The requirement for general anesthesia
  - A relatively high risk of complications
  - Delayed wound healing in hypoalbuminemic patients

Biopsy Analysis

- To prepare biopsy tissue for histopathology, place samples in 10% buffered formalin and allow to fix for 24 hours. The volume of fixative should be 20 times the volume of biopsy tissue.
- To prepare needle biopsy samples, gently remove liver tissue from the biopsy needle and place on tissue paper; fold paper and place in formalin jar.
- Perform routine light microscopy on liver tissue stained with hematoxylin and eosin (H&E).
- Additional stains may be requested, including trichrome for fibrous connective tissue; periodic acid–Schiff (PAS) for glycogen; rhodanine or rubeanic acid for copper; Prussian blue for iron; Congo red for amyloid; oil red O for fat; and silver or acid-fast stains for infectious organisms.
- Submit fresh liver tissue for bacterial and fungal culture.
- Perform quantitative copper analysis on fresh or formalin-fixed hepatic tissue.
- Place samples for electron microscopy in chilled, buffered 2.5% glutaraldehyde.

PRINCIPLES OF TREATMENT FOR LIVER DISEASE

General Considerations

Objectives

- Whenever possible, identify and eliminate the inciting or predisposing causes of liver disease.
- Prevent or manage complications of liver failure, including hepatic encephalopathy, ascites, GI ulceration, coagulopathy, infection, and endotoxemia.

Identification of the underlying cause of hepatobiliary disease can provide insight into specific therapy, the likelihood and nature of potential complications, and the prognosis for recovery. (Therapy for individual hepatobiliary disorders is discussed later under specific diseases.)

In patients in which hepatic regeneration and recovery are possible, supportive care allows time for this to occur. In other cases, clinical manifestations of hepatic failure may be minimized for variable periods.

TABLE 1. General Therapy for Hepatic Failure

Therapeutic Goals	Therapeutic Regimen
Fluid Therapy	
Maintain hydration	Use 0.9% NaCl or Ringer's solution IV.* Use 0.45% NaCl in chronic disease.
Prevent hypokalemia	Add 20–30 mEq KCl to each liter of maintenance fluid. Monitor serum potassium daily and adjust as necessary.
Maintain acid-base balance	Avoid alkalosis in HE. Give NaHCO$_3$ rather than lactated fluids for treatment of severe metabolic acidosis.
Prevent or control hypoglycemia	To treat hypoglycemia, give 50% dextrose (0.5–1 ml/kg) IV to effect. To maintain normoglycemia, add dextrose to fluids to achieve 2.5–5.0% solution.
Nutritional Support	
Maintain caloric intake	Provide 60–100 kcal/kg/per day of good-quality diet.
Provide adequate vitamins and minerals	Add B vitamins to fluids of anorexic cats. For long-term therapy, give oral vitamin-mineral supplement. Give parenteral vitamin K$_1$ (1–3 mg/kg q24h, IM or SC) in biliary obstruction.
Modify diet to control complications	See specific complications (e.g., HE, ascites).
Control of HE	
Modify diet and prevent formation and absorption of enteric toxins	Give NPO in initial stages of HE. For long-term management, provide low-protein, low-fat, high-carbohydrate diet (Prescription Diet k/d or u/d,† cottage cheese, avoid meats). In hepatic coma, use retention enemas q6h containing neomycin (15 mg/kg) and lactulose (diluted 1:2 with water; 50–200 ml total) or povidone iodine solution (diluted 1:10 with water; 50–200 ml total). For maintenance therapy, give neomycin (10–20 mg/kg q6–8h, PO) or metronidazole (7.5 mg/kg q8h, PO) and lactulose (0.5 ml/kg q6–8h, PO).
Control gastrointestinal hemorrhage	Correct coagulopathy; treat GI parasites; treat gastric ulcer (cimetidine or ranitidine); avoid drugs that exacerbate GI hemorrhage (e.g., aspirin, glucocorticoids).
Correct metabolic imbalances (e.g., dehydration, azotemia, hypokalemia, alkalosis, hypoglycemia)	See Fluid Therapy above.
Avoid drugs or therapies that exacerbate HE	Do not administer sedatives, tranquilizers, analgesics, anesthetics, methionine-containing products, diuretics, stored blood, or commercial protein hydrolysates.
Control seizures	Use intravenous phenobarbital at reduced doses for refractory seizures. Oral phenobarbital can be used for long-term therapy; reduce dosage; monitor serum concentrations to adjust dose. Potassium bromide is an alternative to phenobarbital for long-term control of seizures.
Control infection	Give systemic antibiotics (see below).
Control Ascites and Edema	Give low-sodium diet (Prescription Diet k/d or h/d† or homemade diet); spironolactone (1–2 mg/kg q12h, PO)‡; furosemide (1–2 mg/kg q12h, PO)‡; paracentesis for relief of dyspnea only; plasma transfusion or colloids such as hetastarch or dextrans.
Control Coagulopathy and Anemia	Give vitamin K$_1$ (1–3 mg/kg q12h, IM or SC); fresh plasma or blood transfusion. For DIC, give heparin (5–10 IU/kg q8–12h, SC).
Control Gastrointestinal Ulceration	Give cimetidine (5–10 mg/kg q8h, PO or IV); ranitidine§ (2 mg/kg q8–12h, PO or IV); sucralfate (1-g tablet/25 kg q8h, PO).
Control Infection and Endotoxemia	Give systemic antibiotics (e.g., penicillin, ampicillin, cephalosporins, aminoglycosides); intestinal antibiotics (e.g., neomycin); toxin binders (e.g., cholestyramine).

*May be given SC if animal is mildly dehydrated and is not vomiting.
†Hill's Pet Products, Topeka, KS.
‡Dose may be doubled if there is no effect in 4–7 days.
§May be preferable to cimetidine because there is no inhibition of hepatic microsomal enzymes.
HE = hepatic encephalopathy; NPO = nothing per os; GI = gastrointestinal; DIC = disseminated intravascular coagulation.
Adapted from Johnson SE: Liver and Biliary Tract. *In* Anderson NV, ed.: *Veterinary Gastroenterology*, 2nd Ed. Philadelphia: Lea & Febiger, 1992, p 504.

KEY POINT ▶ Prior to administering any drug to a patient with hepatic disease, consider whether the drug is metabolized or excreted by the liver, is potentially hepatotoxic, or may exacerbate signs of liver failure.

Drug Metabolism

The liver is a major site of drug metabolism, and liver disease may alter drug metabolism. In many cases, hepatic disease is associated with decreased hepatic clearance of a drug with subsequent potential toxicity. Avoid drugs that:

- Are known to depend primarily on the liver for inactivation or excretion
- Are potential hepatotoxins such as thiacetarsamide
- May worsen signs of hepatic failure, such as methionine-containing products, tranquilizers, sedatives, analgesics, and diuretics (may exacerbate hepatic encephalopathy); and aspirin and corticosteroids (may cause GI bleeding and exacerbate hepatic encephalopathy).

Supportive Therapy for Liver Disease (Table 1)
Restore Fluid, Electrolyte, and Acid-base Balance

- Maintain normal fluid balance to support hepatic blood flow and microcirculation and prevent complications such as hepatic encephalopathy, DIC, shock, and renal failure. The composition of the fluid to be given is influenced by the patient's electrolyte and acid-base status and the presence or potential for hypoglycemia (see Table 1 for guidelines).

■ Avoid alkalinizing agents (e.g., lactate in lactated Ringer's solution; sodium bicarbonate) when hepatic encephalopathy is present or impending, because alkalosis augments the entry of ammonia into the CNS and can exacerbate signs of hepatic encephalopathy.

Give Nutritional Support

Nutritional support is important for promoting hepatic regeneration and maintenance of body weight.

■ Modify the diet as needed to control complications of hepatic disease, such as hepatic encephalopathy, hypoproteinemia, and ascites (see Table 1).
■ Supply the bulk of the calories by carbohydrates, which provide an easily assimilated source of non-protein calories.
■ Avoid high-protein or high-fat diets that may exacerbate signs of hepatic encephalopathy. Indiscriminate protein restriction is discouraged, however, because adequate protein intake is important for normal hepatic regeneration and to counteract hypoproteinemia.
■ When voluntary food intake is lacking, provide other methods of nutritional support, such as feeding through a gastrostomy tube (see sec. 1, ch. 3).

Control Complications

Hepatic Encephalopathy

Goals for treatment of hepatic encephalopathy are summarized in Table 1.

■ Restrict dietary protein intake.
■ Prevent formation and absorption of enteric toxins.
  • Give antibiotics (e.g., neomycin, metronidazole) to alter the urease-producing bacterial population in the colon, thus decreasing conversion of urea to ammonia (see Table 1).
  • Lactulose, a synthetic disaccharide, often is effective in controlling signs of hepatic encephalopathy and decreasing arterial blood ammonia concentrations through its actions as a cathartic and colonic acidifier (see Table 1). It usually is given in combination with antibiotics.

KEY POINT ▶ Detect and control GI hemorrhage, which could provide enteric bacteria with a source of protein for toxin production. Give fresh rather than stored blood if a transfusion is required, because stored blood contains substantial amounts of ammonia.

Ascites and Edema

Ascites in liver disease usually is associated with hypoalbuminemia, portal hypertension, and renal retention of sodium and water.

■ Direct treatment of ascites primarily at dietary sodium restriction and use of diuretics to promote urinary sodium and water excretion (see Table 1).
■ For temporarily supporting plasma colloid osmotic pressure in hypoproteinemic animals, consider plasma transfusion to supply albumin or volume expanders such as hetastarch or dextran.

Coagulopathy and Anemia

Hemostatic defects associated with hepatobiliary disease can be attributed to DIC, primary failure of hepatocytes to synthesize clotting factors, or vitamin K deficiency caused by biliary obstruction.

■ Parenteral administration of vitamin K_1 corrects coagulopathy caused by vitamin K malabsorption within 24–48 hours, but no response is seen when bleeding is caused by hepatocyte failure or DIC (see Table 1).
■ For treatment of DIC and other coagulopathies, see sec. 3, ch. 2.

Gastrointestinal Ulceration

Dogs with hepatobiliary disease are at increased risk to develop GI ulceration. Possible mechanisms include gastric acid hypersecretion, impaired gastric mucosal blood flow secondary to portal hypertension, and decreased gastric epithelial cell turnover.

■ GI bleeding is deleterious in patients with hepatic encephalopathy because blood is a substrate for ammonia production.
■ Manage GI ulceration with an H_2 blocker for control of acid secretion and with sucralfate for mucosal cytoprotection, as described in sec. 7, ch. 4. Ranitidine may be preferable to cimetidine as an H_2 blocker in animals with liver disease, because it does not inhibit hepatic microsomal enzymes.

Infection and Endotoxemia

An increased incidence of infection may be seen in animals with hepatic disease as enteric bacteria and endotoxins gain access to the systemic circulation as a result of impaired hepatic mononuclear phagocyte system function or portosystemic shunting. Septicemia and endotoxemia may, in turn, perpetuate liver injury.

■ Give systemic antibiotics to control extrahepatic infections or sepsis. Penicillins, cephalosporins, or aminoglycosides are good choices because they are eliminated primarily by renal mechanisms.

Renal Failure

Renal dysfunction and azotemia may complicate liver disease, especially chronic liver dysfunction, and can be prerenal, primary renal, or both.

■ Prerenal mechanisms that decrease effective circulating volume and renal perfusion include dehydration (including that induced by diuretics), hypoalbuminemia, ascites, and overzealous abdominal paracentesis. Appropriate fluid therapy is essential to avoid prerenal azotemia.

TABLE 2. Causes of Acute Hepatic Failure

Hepatotoxins	Infectious and Parasitic Agents	Systemic Conditions
Chemicals	**Viruses**	Acute pancreatitis
Arsenic	Infectious canine hepatitis	Hemolytic anemia
Carbon tetrachloride	(adenovirus I)	Heat stroke
Chlordane	Canine herpesvirus	Surgical hypotension/hypoxia
Chlorinated biphenyls, hydrocarbons,	Feline infectious peritonitis	Shock
naphthalenes	(coronavirus)	Inflammatory bowel disease/colitis
Chloroform	**Bacteria**	Sepsis and extrahepatic infections
Dieldrin	Cholangiohepatitis	
Dimethylnitrosamine	Hepatic abscess	
Heavy metals (copper, iron, lead, mercury)	*Leptospira* spp	
Phosphorus	*Bacillus piliformis*	
Selenium	(Tyzzer's disease)	
Tannic acid	**Fungi**	
Drugs	*Histoplasma*	
Analgesics (salicylates, acetaminophen,	*Coccidioides*	
phenylbutazone)	*Blastomyces*	
Anticonvulsants (phenytoin, phenobarbital,	Others	
primidone, valproic acid)	**Protozoa**	
Antineoplastics (methotrexate)	*Toxoplasma*	
Aprindine	*Babesia*	
Azathioprine	**Dirofilaria (Postcaval Syndrome)**	
Glipizide (in cats)		
Griseofulvin (in cats)		
Isoniazid		
Itraconazole		
Ketoconazole		
Mebendazole		
Megestrol acetate (in cats)		
Methimazole (in cats)		
Mibolerone		
Oxibendazole plus diethylcarbamazine		
Phenazopyridine (in cats)		
Sulfonamides (sulfadiazine/trimethoprim)		
Tetracycline		
Thiacetarsamide		
Tolbutamide		
Anesthetics		
Halothane		
Methoxyflurane		
Biologic Toxins		
Aflatoxin		
Blue-green algae endotoxin		
Amanita mushroom toxin		
Cycads (cycasin toxin)		
Pyrrolizidine alkaloids		
Pennyroyal oil		

■ Primary renal failure may occur with pre-existing renal disease or may result from infectious or toxic agents (e.g., leptospirosis) that affect the liver and kidneys concurrently or secondary to advanced liver disease.

ACUTE HEPATIC FAILURE

Acute hepatic failure occurs when a sudden severe insult to the liver compromises at least 70–80% of functional hepatic tissue. The clinical manifestations and laboratory findings associated with acute hepatic failure reflect general liver failure and are not specific for the underlying cause of injury.

Etiology

Causes of acute hepatic failure in dogs and cats include hepatotoxins, infectious and parasitic agents,

and miscellaneous disorders (Table 2). In many cases, a specific cause cannot be identified.

Toxin-Induced Injury

Hepatic injury may occur after exposure to a wide variety of industrial chemicals, organic solvents, pesticides, heavy metals, and biologic toxins (see Table 2). Exposure can be unobserved in a free-roaming animal that drinks from a contaminated water source. When hepatic necrosis is severe and widespread, rapid deterioration and death in 3–4 days often occur. With less extensive damage, complete recovery is possible.

Drug-Induced Injury

Drug-induced injury is a recognized cause of acute hepatic failure in dogs and cats. The incidence of drug-induced hepatic disease is unknown but is probably underestimated, based on the fact that 25% of human cases of fulminant hepatic failure and 5% of all human cases of jaundice are attributed to adverse drug reactions. Hepatic drug reactions are categorized as *intrinsic* or *idiosyncratic*.

Intrinsic Hepatotoxins. These hepatotoxins predictably damage the liver in an exposed population. The effect is dose-related and reproducible experimentally. An example is thiacetarsamide, the arsenic compound used to treat adult heartworms.

Idiosyncratic Hepatotoxins. These hepatotoxins cause hepatic injury in only a small number of individuals that are unusually susceptible. The mechanism may be an allergy-like response or a unique metabolic pathway whereby the drug is metabolized to a toxic intermediate. The hepatotoxic effect is not time- or dose-dependent. Because of the unpredictability of an idiosyncratic reaction, a cause-and-effect relationship is difficult to establish. Examples include halothane and methoxyflurane, anticonvulsants, mebendazole, oxibendazole, trimethoprim-sulfadiazine, and methimazole.

Drugs that have been incriminated as potential hepatotoxins include analgesics, anthelmintics, anticonvulsants, and antimicrobials (see Table 2). Specific clinical details regarding known drug reactions in dogs and cats are summarized in Table 3.

Infectious Agents

Infectious causes of acute hepatic failure (see Table 2) include leptospirosis (see sec. 2, ch. 11), toxoplasmosis (see sec. 2, ch. 13), histoplasmosis (see sec. 2, ch. 12), FIP virus (see sec. 2, ch. 3), and infectious canine hepatitis virus (see sec. 2, ch. 9).

Miscellaneous Systemic Diseases

Hepatic injury can occur secondary to various systemic conditions, including those discussed below.

Hemolytic Anemia. Hemolysis, especially immune-mediated hemolytic anemia in dogs, can be complicated by centrilobular necrosis attributed to acute hepatocellular hypoxia or DIC-induced sinusoidal thrombosis. The hepatic injury generally resolves with resolution of the anemia crisis.

Anesthesia, Surgical Hypotension, Hypoxia, and Shock. Conditions that decrease liver blood flow can lead to hypoxia and hepatic damage. In the postoperative period it is difficult to differentiate hepatic damage or jaundice caused by the hypoxic effects of anesthesia and surgery from other potential causes, such as toxic injury induced by anesthetic agents (e.g., halothane, methoxyflurane) and other drugs, postoperative infections, and endotoxemia, or a combination of these factors.

Acute Pancreatitis. Pancreatitis in dogs often is characterized by increased serum concentrations of liver enzymes resulting from secondary hepatic injury from released toxins, enzymes, and vasoactive substances (see sec. 7, ch. 10). Hepatic lesions usually resolve with resolution of the pancreatitis and require no special treatment. Less commonly, jaundice results from partial to complete obstruction of the common

bile duct associated with peripancreatic inflammation, pancreatic abscess, or pancreatic healing by fibrosis. Surgical intervention to relieve biliary obstruction is indicated in animals with pancreatic abscess or if jaundice persists after resolution of acute pancreatitis, which usually indicates pancreatic fibrosis as a cause of biliary obstruction (see sec. 7, ch. 10).

Extrahepatic Bacterial Infections. Septic conditions such as pneumonia, pyometra, peritonitis, and abscesses can be associated with jaundice, mild to moderate increases in liver enzyme activity (especially ALP), and increased SBA concentration. Liver biopsy reveals intrahepatic cholestasis without significant necrosis or inflammation. The hepatic injury resolves when the infection is controlled.

Clinical Signs

Clinical signs of acute hepatic failure often are nonspecific and overlap signs of disorders of other body systems. Clinical signs reflect general hepatic dysfunction rather than the specific underlying cause. Signs of extrahepatic or multisystemic disease often provide important diagnostic clues when hepatic injury occurs secondary to acute pancreatitis, hemolytic disease, septicemia/endotoxemia, and many infectious diseases.

- Acute onset of anorexia, lethargy, vomiting, and diarrhea are the most common presenting signs of acute hepatic failure.
- Other potential findings include PU/PD, jaundice, excessive bleeding, and hepatic encephalopathy.

Diagnosis

- When acute hepatic failure is diagnosed, attempt to identify the underlying cause with a complete history, ancillary diagnostic testing, and, if indicated, a liver biopsy. In many instances, a specific cause cannot be identified.
- When acute hepatic failure is accompanied by jaundice, consider diseases of the extrahepatic biliary tract such as biliary obstruction and rupture; surgical intervention may provide both diagnostic and therapeutic benefit.

History

Attempt to document recent or potential exposure to any drug, toxin, or infectious disease, especially those listed in Table 2.

- Suspect a drug- or toxin-induced cause of acute hepatic failure when clinical and biochemical evidence of acute hepatic dysfunction is associated with recent exposure to a potential hepatotoxin.
- Consider toxin-induced injury in the absence of known exposure to toxins, because potential hepatotoxins can be present in contaminated dog food (aflatoxins), pond water (blue-green algae), and many other unobserved sources.
- Although numerous drugs have been incriminated (see Tables 2 and 3), remember that an idiosyncratic reaction can occur with *any* drug. With most drug-

TABLE 3. Selected Hepatotoxic Drug Reactions in Dogs and Cats

Drug(s)	Species	Onset of Signs and Key Features	Hepatic Lesions	Suggested Mechanism	Comments
Analgesics					
Acetaminophen (Tylenol, McNeil)	Canine and feline	Initial toxicity is cyanosis and methemoglobinemia, especially in cats	Centrilobular necrosis and congestion; vacuolar hepatopathy and bile stasis	Intrinsic	Dose-related injury (dosages exceeding 200 mg/kg in dogs and 120 mg/kg in cats); Phenazopyridine causes toxicity by similar mechanism in cats. Treatment: *N*-acetylcysteine (140 mg/kg PO initially; then 70 mg/kg q6h for 36 h total) and ascorbic acid (30 mg/kg q6h for 36 h).
Anesthetics					
Halothane (Fluothane, Ayerst) Methoxyflurane (Metofane, Pitman-Moore)	Canine	Acute hepatic failure* within 1 week of most recent exposure	Centrilobular necrosis	Idiosyncratic	Rare reaction in clinical veterinary medicine; difficult to separate from other potential causes of injury (e.g., other drugs, surgical trauma, hypoxia, concurrent infection); multiple exposures may predispose; potential for concurrent renal damage.
Anthelmintics					
Mebendazole (Telminic, Pitman-Moore)	Canine	Acute hepatic failure* 1–14 days following administration	Centrilobular necrosis	Idiosyncratic	High mortality.
Oxibendazole plus diethylcarbamazine (Filaribits Plus, SmithKline Beecham)	Canine	Acute hepatic failure* 2–4 weeks after starting drug; possible chronic hepatic failure	Periportal hepatitis and vacuolar hepatopathy	Idiosyncratic	Clinical signs improve within days of stopping drug. Biochemical abnormalities may persist >6 months.
Thiacetarsamide (Caparsolate, Ceva Labs.)	Canine	Acute hepatic failure* after 1–2 injections	Centrilobular or massive necrosis; intrahepatic cholestasis	Intrinsic	Dogs more susceptible to hepatic injury than cats. Can readminister uneventfully in 2–4 weeks.
Anticonvulsants					
Primidone, phenytoin, phenobarbital or combinations	Canine	Chronic liver disease and cirrhosis; anorexia, lethargy, weight loss, PU/PD, icterus, ascites, encephalopathy; ↑ ALP, ↑ ALT, ↑ GGT, ↑ total bilirubin, ↑ SBA and BSP; coagulopathy.	Hepatocellular hypertrophy; intrahepatic cholestasis, lobular hepatitis, bridging necrosis, cirrhosis	Idiosyncratic or Intrinsic†	Liver disease is most likely with chronic administration of primidone or combination of primidone and phenytoin at higher doses. Phenobarbital alone may cause chronic liver disease and cirrhosis, especially at higher doses. Dogs with phenobarbital hepatotoxicity may improve when dosage is decreased to therapeutic range as determined by serum phenobarbital levels. Incidence of chronic hepatic disease from long-term anticonvulsant therapy is approximately 6–14%.

734

Drug	Species	Clinical/Laboratory Features	Histopathology	Type	Comments
Antimicrobials					
Ketoconazole (Nizoral, Janssen Pharmaceutica)	Canine and feline	Asymptomatic with ↑ ALT, ↑ ALP or acute hepatic failure†	Not characterized	Idiosyncratic‡	May be dose-related phenomenon: >40 mg/kg/day in dogs. In humans, asymptomatic serum enzyme elevations are considered harmless, and enzymes usually return to normal despite continued therapy. Discontinue therapy if clinical signs or jaundice occur. Recovery usually is uneventful.
Tetracycline	Canine	Not characterized	Vacuolar hepatopathy	Intrinsic	Experimental hepatic injury is induced by high doses given IV. Avoid in animals with PSS; unlikely to be a clinically important hepatotoxin.
Trimethoprim-sulfadiazine	Canine	Acute hepatic failure* 2–4 weeks after starting therapy	Massive necrosis or periportal hepatitis and intrahepatic cholestasis	Idiosyncratic	Multiple exposures may predispose to reaction; recovery is rapid after drug withdrawal.
Steroids					
Glucocorticoids (various types)	Canine	Chronic hepatopathy but hepatic failure rare; signs indicative of hypercortisolism (e.g., PU/PD, polyphagia, hepatomegaly, lethargy); ↑↑ ALP, usually with induction of steroid isoenzyme of ALP. Mildly ↑ ALT; normal total bilirubin; SBA within normal limits or mildly ↑ (<60 μmol/liter)	Centrilobular vacuolization due to glycogen accumulation	Intrinsic but considerable individual variation	Lesions are reversible after treatment is discontinued; does not occur in cats.
Megesterol acetate (Ovaban, Schering)	Feline	Chronic liver disease, jaundice	Not characterized	Idiosyncratic	Rare
Mibolerone (Cheque, Upjohn)	Canine	Chronic liver disease, jaundice	Not characterized	Idiosyncratic	Rare
Miscellaneous					
Methimazole (Tapazole, Lilly)	Feline	Acute hepatic failure* within 2 months of starting therapy	Necrosis and cholestasis	Idiosyncratic	Clinical signs resolve within 7 days of stopping therapy; biochemical resolution by 45 days.

*Typical manifestations of acute hepatic failure include anorexia, depression, vomiting, and jaundice accompanied by ↑ ALT, ↑ ALP, and ↑ serum bilirubin.
†For drug reaction accompanied by clinical signs and hyperbilirubinemia.
‡See text for further information.
PU/PD = polyuria/polydipsia; ALP = alkaline phosphatase; ALT = alanine aminotransferase; GGT = gamma glutamyltransferase; SBA = serum bile acids; BSP = Bromsulphalein (sulfobromophthalein); PSS = portosystemic shunt.

and toxin-induced disorders, the diagnosis is presumptive and cannot be proved.

■ To confirm the diagnosis:
  • Discontinue the drug and observe for clinical improvement, which usually occurs within several weeks, even after chronic drug administration.
  • Recurrence of hepatic damage after a challenge dose of the same drug (or inadvertent re-exposure) supports the diagnosis of drug-induced hepatotoxicity. *Note*: This is not recommended as a diagnostic procedure because it is potentially dangerous, especially with a drug that causes hepatic necrosis.
■ Determine if there is a history of recent surgical or anesthetic procedures that may be associated with drug- or hypoxia-related hepatic damage.
■ Evaluate the animal's vaccination status for infectious diseases that can involve the liver, such as leptospirosis and infectious canine hepatitis.
■ Determine if there are any subtle chronic signs of illness that suggest that the underlying liver disease may be chronic rather than acute and that the current illness may be exacerbation or decompensation of chronic liver disease.

Physical Examination

Physical findings often reflect general hepatic dysfunction rather than the specific etiology (see previous discussion of physical examination findings under Diagnostic Strategy for Liver Disease).

■ Hepatodynia may occur with any cause of acute hepatic injury that results in swelling and stretching of the liver capsule.
■ Findings of weight loss and ascites are indicative of a chronic rather than an acute process.
■ Signs of extrahepatic or multisystemic disease may be important clues when liver injury occurs secondary to systemic disorders.
  • For example, fever may be present with infectious causes of hepatic injury such as leptospirosis, infectious canine hepatitis, bacterial cholangiohepatitis, liver abscess, systemic mycoses, and extrahepatic infections that secondarily involve the liver.
  • Fever and acute abdominal pain are presenting signs of acute pancreatitis but can also occur with cholangiohepatitis and hepatic abscess.
  • When jaundice is accompanied by pallor, consider immune hemolytic anemia.

Laboratory Evaluation

Acute hepatotoxicity frequently is associated with abnormal serum biochemistry analysis, liver function tests, and urinalysis.

■ Because diffuse hepatic necrosis is the most common lesion associated with acute hepatic failure, increased ALT activity is the most consistent finding, and values are often markedly increased. Increased ALP activity may also occur.
■ Other potential findings include hyperbilirubinemia, increased serum bile acid concentrations, hypogly-

cemia, hyperammonemia, and coagulopathy. Hypoalbuminemia usually suggests chronic rather than acute liver disease.

■ Some hepatotoxins (e.g., thiacetarsamide, inhalation anesthetics) and infectious agents (e.g., leptospirosis) may concurrently damage the kidneys; thus, biochemical evidence of concomitant renal failure may be present.
■ An inflammatory CBC suggests possible acute pancreatitis or underlying infectious disease. Evaluate serum amylase and lipase to diagnose acute pancreatitis.

Radiography

■ Liver size usually is normal to increased unless massive hepatic necrosis causes parenchymal collapse and microhepatica.
■ A small liver suggests chronic rather than acute hepatic disease.
■ Additional radiographic findings may be noted, depending on the underlying disorder (Table 4).

Liver Biopsy

Perform a liver biopsy when the cause of acute hepatic failure is not suggested by preliminary laboratory evaluation.

TABLE 4. Ancillary Diagnostic Evaluations for Acute Hepatic Failure

Diagnostic Evaluation	Intended Diagnosis (Rule Out)
Bacterial cultures: Liver and bile	Bacterial invasion of the liver
Blood, urine, infected tissues	Sepsis, endotoxemia
Serologic tests (antibody titers)	Mycoses (histoplasmosis, coccidioidomycosis, blastomycosis) Toxoplasmosis Feline infectious peritonitis
Urine darkfield examination (for spirocheturia)	Leptospirosis
Lymph node aspiration cytology	Mycoses Lymphoid neoplasia
Hepatic fine-needle aspiration cytology	Infectious agents (mycoses) Neoplasia Lipidosis
Microfilaria examination	Heartworm disease
Serum amylase and lipase	Acute pancreatitis
Coombs test	Immune hemolytic anemia
Thoracic radiography	Mycoses Toxoplasmosis Heartworm disease Metastases
Abdominal radiography	Hepatic abscesses Emphysematous cholecystitis Cholelithiasis Pancreatitis
Abdominal ultrasonography	Pancreatic disease Hepatic abscesses Biliary or gallbladder disease

Modified from Sherding, RG: Acute hepatic failure. Vet Clin North Am 15:119, 1985.

- Histopathologic examination of hepatic tissue can help to establish the cause and to distinguish between acute and chronic liver disease. Diffuse hepatic necrosis is the histologic lesion most consistently associated with acute hepatic failure.
- If overt bleeding is present, liver biopsy may be contraindicated.

Ancillary Diagnostic Procedures

Perform ancillary diagnostic procedures (see Table 4) to diagnose underlying causes of acute hepatic failure.

Treatment

Management of the patient with acute hepatic failure is first directed toward supportive therapy (see Table 1).

- Maintenance of fluid, electrolyte, and acid-base balance is the cornerstone of supportive therapy.
- Prevent or control complications such as hypoglycemia, hepatic encephalopathy, coagulopathy, and endotoxemia.

Whenever possible, institute specific treatment for the underlying cause; for example, administer injectable penicillin for treatment of leptospirosis. Although specific antidotal therapy usually is not available for drug-induced liver damage, discontinuing use of the suspect drug will prevent further hepatic injury and may be associated with clinical improvement.

In many cases, even though the cause remains unidentified or specific therapy is unavailable, supportive care alone may allow adequate time for hepatic regeneration to occur.

INFECTIOUS AND PARASITIC HEPATIC DISEASE

The liver can be involved in many systemic infections (Table 5). In some disorders, such as leptospirosis and infectious canine hepatitis, the liver is a target organ, and evidence of liver failure dominates the clinical presentation. In other infections, such as many of the systemic protozoal infections, the liver is involved as a result of widespread invasion of organs with a large mononuclear phagocyte population, such as the spleen, lymph nodes, and bone marrow (see Table 5). Signs of hepatic dysfunction may or may not be present, and may be overshadowed by more obvious extrahepatic involvement. Liver cytology and biopsy can be diagnostically useful for identification of these organisms.

Systemic infections are covered in detail elsewhere in this book (sec. 2). Infections localized to the hepatobiliary tract are covered in greater detail here.

Hepatic Abscess

Hepatic abscesses from bacterial infection of the liver occur rarely in dogs and cats. Multifocal microabscesses or discrete unifocal abscesses may develop.

Etiology

- Potential sources of bacteria include hematogeneous spread, ascension via bile ducts, penetrating abdominal and caudal thoracic wounds, and direct extension from local suppurative diseases. Umbilical infections are the most common cause of hepatic abscesses in puppies (*Staphylococcus*) and kittens (*Streptococcus*).
- Hypoxia of hepatic tissue caused by hepatic neoplasia or trauma may predispose to abscess formation, because small numbers of anaerobes (e.g., *Clostridium* spp) normally are present in the liver and can proliferate under these conditions.
- Systemic diseases that are associated with immunosuppression (e.g., feline leukemia virus [FeLV], feline immunodeficiency virus [FIV]) or that predispose to infection (e.g., diabetes mellitus) may predispose to hepatic abscesses.

Clinical Signs

- Signs are attributed to sepsis, inflammation, and hepatic dysfunction and include anorexia, fever, and vomiting.
- Rupture of a hepatic abscess leads rapidly to peritonitis, septic shock, and death.

Diagnosis

- Physical examination findings are often vague but may include depression, fever, hepatomegaly, abdominal tenderness, and abdominal effusion.
- Potential laboratory findings include neutrophilia with a left shift (or neutropenia and degenerative left shift if rupture occurs), markedly increased ALT activity (although it may be in the normal range), hyperglobulinemia, mild hyperbilirubinemia, hypoglycemia, and septic suppurative abdominal effusion.
- Radiolucent areas may be seen on abdominal radiographs when gas-producing organisms are involved. Ultrasonography may reveal a parenchymal abscess cavity. Ultrasound-guided fine-needle aspiration for cytology and culture may be diagnostic.
- Diagnosis often is established at exploratory laparotomy to determine the cause of septic peritonitis.
- Perform aerobic and anaerobic cultures of abdominal effusion, blood, and hepatic tissue.

Treatment

- Treatment of large, unifocal hepatic abscesses requires surgical excision of affected liver lobes (see sec. 7, ch. 9).
- Initiate broad-spectrum antibiotics such as intravenous penicillin combined with an aminoglycoside (e.g., gentamicin, amikacin) while awaiting culture results. Monitor renal function during aminoglycoside therapy, and base further therapy on results of sensitivity testing. Give long-term antibiotic therapy (but not aminoglycosides) for at least 6–8 weeks.

Cholangiohepatitis and Cholangitis

Cholangiohepatitis is an inflammatory disorder of the bile ducts and adjacent hepatocytes. The term *cholangitis* is used when inflammation is confined to the bile ducts; the term *cholangiohepatitis* implies secondary hepatocyte involvement. Cholangitis and

TABLE 5. Infectious Diseases with Potential Hepatobiliary Involvement*

Disease	Agent	Refer to
Viral		
Infectious canine hepatitis (ICH)	Canine adenovirus I	Sec. 2, ch. 9
Systemic neonatal herpesvirus	Canine herpesvirus	Sec. 2, ch. 9
Canine acidophil cell hepatitis	Unknown	Sec. 2, ch. 9
Feline infectious peritonitis	Feline coronavirus	Sec. 2, ch. 3
Bacterial		
Leptospirosis:	*Leptospira interrogans:*	Sec. 2, ch. 11
Acute hepatic failure	Serovars *L. icterohemorrhagiae* and *L. canicola*	
Chronic hepatitis	Serovar *L. grippotyphosa*	
Tyzzer's disease	*Bacillus piliformis*	Sec. 7, ch. 6
Nocardiosis	*Nocardia* spp.	Sec. 2, ch. 11
Actinomycosis	*Actinomyces* spp.	Sec. 2, ch. 11
Tuberculosis	*Mycobacterium tuberculosis, M. bovis, M. avium*	Sec. 2, ch. 11
Salmonellosis	*Salmonella typhimurium*	Sec. 7, ch. 6
Brucellosis	*Brucella canis*	Sec. 2, ch. 11
Hepatic abscess	*Staphylococcus* spp (dogs) *Streptococcus* spp (cats) *Escherichia coli,* anaerobes	
Cholangitis/cholangiohepatitis	Gram-negative bacteria (esp. *E. coli*), anaerobes	
Cholecystitis	Gram-negative bacteria (esp. *E. coli*), *Clostridium* spp	
Yersiniosis	*Yersinia pestis*	Sec. 2, ch. 11
Tularemia	*Francisella tularensis*	Sec. 2, ch. 11
Fungal		
Histoplasmosis	*Histoplasma capsulatum*	Sec. 2, ch. 12
Blastomycosis	*Blastomyces dermatitidis*	Sec. 2, ch. 12
Coccidioidomycosis	*Coccidioides immitis*	Sec. 2, ch. 12
Aspergillosis	*Aspergillus terreus*	Sec. 2, ch. 12
Protozoal		
Toxoplasmosis	*Toxoplasma gondii*	Sec. 2, ch. 13
Babesiosis	*Babesia canis, B. gibsoni*	Sec. 3, ch. 1
Cytauxzoonosis	*Cytauxzoon felis*	Sec. 2, ch. 13
Hepatozoonosis	*Hepatozoon canis*	Sec. 2, ch. 13
Leishmaniasis	*Leishmania* spp	Sec. 2, ch. 13
Encephalitozoonosis	*Encephalitozoon cuniculi*	Sec. 2, ch. 13
Rickettsial		
Ehrlichiosis	*Ehrlichia* spp	Sec. 2, ch. 10
Algal		
Prototothecosis	*Prototheca* spp	Sec. 7, ch. 6

*But not necessarily associated with clinical hepatobiliary disease.

cholangiohepatitis are characterized by inflammatory infiltrates (suppurative versus nonsuppurative or lymphocytic) within and around the bile ducts. Cholangiohepatitis is one of the most common hepatobiliary disorders of cats but is recognized much less frequently in dogs. The following discussion focuses on cholangiohepatitis in cats; however, similar principles of diagnosis and therapy apply to cholangiohepatitis in dogs.

Etiology and Clinical Associations

■ Bacterial infection is a possible cause when there is histologic evidence of suppurative inflammation. Gram-negative bacteria (especially *Escherichia coli*) are most commonly cultured from the bile of affected cats. Their role has yet to be defined; it is unknown whether they initiate cholangiohepatitis or are a secondary complication. Factors that predispose to bacterial infection include biliary obstruction and bile stasis, cholelithiasis, and anatomic malformations of the biliary tract.

■ Infectious agents infrequently associated with lesions of cholangiohepatitis in cats include liver flukes (see the following discussion), *Toxoplasma*-like organisms, and *Hepatozoon canis*.

■ The cause of nonsuppurative cholangitis/cholangiohepatitis is unknown. Bacterial infection is documented infrequently with this form. It is possible that nonsuppurative cholangiohepatitis is preceded by the suppurative form. Self-perpetuating immunologic mechanisms may perpetuate further inflammation.

■ In cats, lesions of cholangiohepatitis commonly are associated with chronic pancreatitis, cholecystitis, and duodenitis. Associated cholelithiasis and sludging of bile may cause partial or complete biliary obstruction. Chronic cholangiohepatitis can progress to biliary cirrhosis.

Clinical Signs

- Common signs include anorexia, depression, weight loss, fever, vomiting, jaundice, and dehydration. Hepatic encephalopathy, ascites, and excessive bleeding are uncommon unless cholangiohepatitis has progressed to biliary cirrhosis.
- Signs may be acute or chronic, intermittent or persistent.

Diagnosis

Suspect cholangiohepatitis in any cat with fever and jaundice (although not all cases are febrile). Definitive diagnosis requires liver biopsy to distinguish this disease from other hepatic disorders such as hepatic lipidosis, hepatic FIP, and neoplasia.

History and Physical Examination

- Persian cats may have a genetic predisposition for lymphocytic cholangitis.
- Cats with bacterial cholangiohepatitis may have a history of previous episodes responsive to antibiotic therapy.
- Physical examination findings include fever, jaundice, and hepatomegaly. If chronic cholangiohepatitis has progressed to cirrhosis, ascites may occur.

Laboratory Evaluation

- Findings include an inflammatory CBC with mild nonregenerative anemia; hyperbilirubinemia and bilirubinuria; increased ALP, ALT, and GGT activity; and increased FSBA and PPSBA concentrations. Hyperglobulinemia is an inconsistent finding.
- A coagulopathy may occur secondary to vitamin K malabsorption or hepatocyte failure.
- Hypoalbuminemia, decreased BUN, and hyperammonemia suggest advanced disease.

Radiography

- Radiographic features of cholangiohepatitis include hepatomegaly and, in some cases, cholelithiasis.
- Ultrasonography is useful to evaluate concurrent abnormalities of the extrahepatic biliary system, such as cholecystitis, cholelithiasis, sludging of bile, common bile duct obstruction, and pancreatic abnormalities.
  - *Note*: a small amount of sludged bile may be detected ultrasonographically in anorectic, sick animals that do not have biliary tract disease.

Liver Biopsy and Histopathologic Evaluation

- If concurrent biliary obstruction occurs, obtain a liver biopsy specimen and aerobic and anaerobic bile cultures at laparotomy during surgical relief of the obstruction.
- At laparotomy, the gallbladder and common bile duct frequently are thickened, firm, and distended. Inspissated bile and choleliths may be present.
- In the absence of obstruction, percutaneous liver biopsy is adequate for diagnosis.
- In suppurative cholangitis and cholangiohepatitis, biopsy findings include neutrophils within and around intrahepatic bile ducts, intrahepatic cholestasis, and, in chronic cases, portal fibrosis. In the nonsuppurative form, lymphocytic portal infiltrates are seen, and lymphoid aggregates may be quite marked.
- Other features include bile duct hyperplasia, biliary fibrosis, and, eventually, cirrhosis. Marked segmental periductal fibrosis (sclerosing cholangitis) is seen in some cases.

Treatment

Drug Therapy

Systemic Antibiotics. Systemic antibiotic therapy is indicated if a bacterial bile culture is positive or if suppurative cholangitis or cholangiohepatitis is diagnosed. (In the initial treatment, administer antibiotics before starting glucocorticoid therapy in order to eliminate any bacterial component.) If possible, base the choice of drug on culture and sensitivity testing results; otherwise, consider the following recommendations.

- Antibiotics effective against aerobic gram-negative organisms include ampicillin, amoxicillin, cephalosporins, chloramphenicol, and aminoglycosides such as kanamycin and gentamicin; those effective against anaerobic organisms include metronidazole, clindamycin, chloramphenicol, ampicillin, and amoxicillin.
- Consider ampicillin or amoxicillin (11–22 mg/kg q8h, PO, IV, or SC) as first-choice therapy or combine these drugs with kanamycin (5 mg/kg q8–12h, IM or SC) or gentamicin (2.2 mg/kg q8h, IV, IM, or SC) if systemic signs of infection are severe. Do not start aminoglycoside therapy until dehydration is corrected; then monitor closely for nephrotoxicity.
- Metronidazole (10–15 mg/kg q8–12h, IV or PO) is probably the drug of choice for anaerobic infections because of its broad spectrum and high concentrations in the bile.
- Tetracycline and chloramphenicol have been recommended because of their spectrum of activity and high biliary concentrations; however, they are considered poor first-choice drugs for animals with hepatic dysfunction because tetracycline is potentially hepatotoxic and chloramphenicol depends on hepatic metabolism and causes anorexia in cats.

Prednisolone. Prednisolone is used empirically in the treatment of lymphocytic cholangitis because of its anti-inflammatory and immunosuppressive properties.

- Give 1–2 mg/kg daily, PO, and taper after the first 1–2 weeks if clinical improvement occurs. Continuous or intermittent therapy may be required on a long-term basis, using the lowest dose possible that will control signs.

Dehydrocholic Acid. Because of its hydrocholeretic properties, dehydrocholic acid (Decholin, Miles Lab.) (10–15 mg/kg q8h, PO) has been recommended on an empirical basis to prevent bile sludging.

Surgery

- Surgical relief of obstruction is necessary if extrahepatic biliary obstruction due to sludged bile or cholelithiasis occurs (see sec. 7, ch. 9).

General Supportive Care

- Fluid therapy, maintenance of nutritional intake, and vitamin supplementation are especially important in debilitated cats with hepatic disease.

- Control complications such as ascites, hepatic encephalopathy, and excessive bleeding as previously discussed (see Table 1).

Cholecystitis

Cholecystitis, or inflammation of the gallbladder, is a clinical problem that occurs uncommonly in both dogs and cats. Cholecystitis may be associated with cholangitis, cholangiohepatitis, cholelithiasis, and choledocholithiasis. Acute necrotic cholecystitis in dogs frequently is complicated by rupture of the gallbladder and septic bile peritonitis.

Etiology

- Bacteria appear to play an important role in cholecystitis. An enteric origin of bacteria seems most likely, because isolates are usually aerobic gram-negative bacteria (especially *E. coli*, but also *Klebsiella, Pseudomonas,* and *Salmonella* spp) or anaerobes (*Clostridium* spp). Intestinal bacteria may be refluxed into the gallbladder or they may be bloodborne from the hepatic circulation.
- Gas-producing organisms, such as *E. coli* and *Clostridium*, can cause emphysema of the gallbladder wall. Emphysematous cholecystitis is recognized most frequently in diabetic dogs.
- Cholelithiasis can predispose to cholecystitis by obstructing the cystic duct, causing gallbladder overdistension and stasis, which enables proliferation of anaerobic organisms.
- Anatomic malformations of the gallbladder, biliary obstruction from any cause, and biliary surgery also predispose to biliary infections.

Clinical Signs

- Signs include anorexia, lethargy, fever, abdominal pain, hepatomegaly, vomiting, diarrhea, and jaundice. In addition, acute rupture of the gallbladder with septic bile peritonitis causes abdominal distension, collapse, and septic shock.
- Signs may be acute or chronic, persistent or episodic.

Diagnosis

Differentiate cholecystitis from other cholestatic hepatobiliary disorders that are characterized by fever, inflammation, and similar clinical findings, such as acute pancreatitis or pancreatic abscess, cholangiohepatitis, cholelithiasis, hepatic abscess, and septicemia/endotoxemia.

- Physical examination findings include fever, cranial abdominal pain, jaundice, and shock (bile or septic peritonitis).
- Laboratory findings are characteristic of severe cholestatic hepatobiliary disease, including hyperbilirubinemia, markedly increased ALP and GGT activity, increased ALT activity, increased serum bile acid concentrations, and hypercholesterolemia. Other findings suggestive of inflammation or sepsis are neutrophilia with a left shift and hypoglycemia.
  - Increased amylase and lipase levels have been reported in dogs with cholecystitis in the absence of clinical pancreatitis.
  - Prolonged PT and APTT occur if chronic biliary obstruction causes vitamin K malabsorption.
  - Other laboratory findings reflect dehydration and electrolyte and acid-base imbalances secondary to vomiting, dehydration, and sepsis.
- If cholecystitis is complicated by rupture of the gallbladder or biliary tract, abdominal fluid analysis is consistent with septic bile peritonitis. For a general discussion of peritonitis, see sec. 7, ch. 13.
- Potential radiographic findings include cholecystolithiasis, emphysema of the gallbladder wall, and, if perforation occurs, abdominal effusion.
- Ultrasonographic findings include distension of the gallbladder and cystic duct, thickening of the gallbladder wall, cholecystoliths, and inspissated bile. Small amounts of abdominal effusion not evident on survey radiographs may also be identified.
- Findings at exploratory surgery include thickening, necrosis, and rupture of the gallbladder, localized or generalized peritonitis, and calculi or inspissated bile in the gallbladder, cystic duct, or bile duct. Previous gallbladder rupture may be associated with omental or hepatic adhesions.
  - Obtain aerobic and anaerobic cultures of the gallbladder mucosa and bile.
- Histologic examination of the gallbladder reveals varying degrees of necrosis, inflammation, and fibrosis.

Treatment

- Give parenteral vitamin K_1 prior to surgery to correct coagulopathy (see Table 1).
- Administer antibiotic therapy effective against aerobic gram-negative and anaerobic bacteria, as described previously for bacterial cholangitis and cholangiohepatitis. Long-term treatment (4–6 weeks) is indicated.
- Cholecystectomy is required in most cases (see sec. 7, ch. 9). Surgically manage complications such as biliary obstruction, cholelithiasis, inspissated bile, and abdominal drainage for septic bile peritonitis (see sec. 7, ch. 13).

Postoperative Care and Complications

- Correct any fluid, electrolyte, and acid-base imbalances.
- Common postoperative complications include vomiting, diarrhea, anorexia, hypoproteinemia, and hypokalemia.

Prognosis

- Death usually is attributed to sepsis and peritonitis.
- If the animal survives the immediate postoperative period, the long-term prognosis is good, and recurrence of biliary or hepatic disease is unlikely.

Liver Fluke Infection

Liver fluke infection is uncommon in cats and rare in dogs. Infection usually is asymptomatic but may cause clinical biliary tract disease when associated with marked biliary fibrosis, cholangitis, cholangiohepatitis, or extrahepatic bile duct obstruction.

Etiology

- *Platynosomum concinnum (P. fastosum)* is the most important liver fluke in cats and is found in tropical and subtropical geographic areas, including Hawaii, Florida, and the Caribbean. In endemic areas, the prevalence of infection is high.
- Other liver flukes that have been identified in cats include *Amphimerus pseudofelineus (Opistorchis pseudofelineus)*, *O. tenuicollis*, *O. sinensis*, and *Metorchis conjunctus (M. complexus)*.
- Liver flukes require two intermediate hosts for their life cycle. Adult flukes reside in the gallbladder and bile ducts. Embryonated eggs are shed in the feces and ingested by a snail, the first intermediate host for all liver flukes. The house gecko, skink, lizard, and Bufo toad are second intermediate hosts for *P. concinnum*; fish are second intermediate hosts for the other species of flukes.

Clinical Signs

- Most infected cats are asymptomatic for liver fluke infection.
- Liver fluke infection occasionally is associated with anorexia, weight loss, diarrhea, vomiting, jaundice, hepatomegaly, abdominal distension, and death.

Diagnosis

- Operculated fluke eggs can be identified in feces by a formalin-ether technique (a sedimentation procedure). Routine methods for flotation do not consistently identify eggs.
- Other laboratory findings are inconsistent and often unremarkable. Eosinophilia, hyperbilirubinemia, and increased serum ALP and ALT activity is sometimes detected.
- At laparotomy or necropsy, the bile ducts and gallbladder may be distended and thick-walled and contain inspissated bile and small (<12 mm long) adult flukes. The liver frequently is enlarged. In many cases, no visible abnormalities are present.

Treatment

Little information is available about treatment of liver flukes.

- Praziquantel (Droncit, Haver), 40 mg/kg, given orally or parenterally once a day for 3 consecutive days, has been suggested. Drugs used unsuccessfully include mebendazole, levamisole, thiabendazole, diamphenethide, and rafoxanide.
- Manage complications such as biliary obstruction and secondary bacterial cholangitis/cholangiohepatitis as described elsewhere in this chapter.

ANTICONVULSANT-ASSOCIATED HEPATIC DISEASE

Long-term anticonvulsant therapy for control of seizures has been associated with hepatic injury in dogs (see Table 3). Severe hepatic dysfunction is estimated to develop in 6–14% of dogs treated with anticonvulsants for more than 6 months. Two types of hepatotoxic injury have been identified: hepatic cirrhosis and cholestatic hepatopathy.

Etiology

- Long-term therapy with primidone, alone or in combination with other anticonvulsants, and with phenobarbital have been associated with cirrhosis and liver failure. Phenobarbital hepatotoxicity appears more likely when high oral dosages are used and serum concentrations are maintained at ≥40 μg/ml. Idiosyncratic hepatotoxicity is suspected.
- High-dose phenytoin therapy, in combination with primidone or phenobarbital, has been associated with a cholestatic hepatopathy and hepatic failure. Hepatic damage is reproducible experimentally in dogs, suggesting intrinsic hepatotoxicity.

Clinical Signs

- Clinical signs are those of chronic hepatic disease and include anorexia, lethargy, weight loss, weakness, polydipsia, polyuria, and jaundice. Ascites and hepatic encephalopathy are most likely with advanced hepatic disease.
- When impaired hepatic inactivation of phenobarbital causes increased blood levels, seizure frequency may decrease or dogs may show signs of overdosage such as ataxia, weakness, and depression.
- Increased frequency of seizures may be related to the development of hepatic encephalopathy or to failure of the liver to convert primidone to its active anticonvulsant metabolites (phenobarbital and phenylethylmalonic acid).

Diagnosis

Suspect anticonvulsant-associated hepatopathy in any dog with a history of chronic anticonvulsant therapy and clinical and biochemical evidence of hepatic injury.

Laboratory Evaluation

- Phenobarbital, phenytoin, and primidone are potent inducers of serum ALP activity. Increased ALP activity occurs in the absence of morphologic evidence of hepatic injury. Increases usually are due to induction of the liver isoenzyme of ALP but sometimes the result of increased corticosteroid-induced isoenzyme. Increases in ALT activity (up to 4 × normal) with anticonvulsant therapy are less consistent. Greater increases in ALT activity suggest hepatocellular injury.
- Findings of hyperbilirubinemia, hypoalbuminemia, and hypocholesterolemia suggest hepatic failure and should be further pursued with a liver function test such as FSBA and PPSBA. Increased SBA concentrations are a consistent finding in anticonvulsant-induced hepatic disease.

Radiography

- Radiographic findings may suggest microhepatica with cirrhosis, or hepatomegaly with phenytoin-induced cholestatic hepatopathy.
- Ultrasonography is useful to further characterize liver changes and to evaluate for other hepatic disorders.

Liver Biopsy and Histopathologic Evaluation

Perform liver biopsy when SBA concentrations are increased, liver enzyme activities are greatly increased, or clinical signs of hepatic dysfunction are present.

- The most consistent histologic finding in dogs on anticonvulsant therapy is hepatocellular hypertrophy with a ground-glass appearance of the cytoplasm. Hypertrophy is due to hyperplasia of smooth endoplasmic reticulum. This finding is commonly identified in dogs without clinical or biochemical evidence of hepatic dysfunction and does not warrant a change in drug therapy.
- Cirrhosis is characterized by bridging necrosis, lobular hepatitis, nodular hyperplasia, and fibrosis. Micro- or macronodular cirrhosis may occur.
- Features of cholestatic hepatopathy include intrahepatic cholestasis, biliary hyperplasia, cytoplasmic vacuolization, disorganization of hepatocellular plates, and small, multifocal areas of necrosis.

Treatment

- Discontinue or modify, if possible, the anticonvulsant therapy in dogs with biochemical and histologic evidence of hepatic disease (see sec. 10, ch. 3). In general, the earlier hepatic damage is recognized and the drug is discontinued, the better the prognosis for resolution of clinical and biochemical abnormalities. Improvement also may occur in dogs with irreversible hepatic cirrhosis.
- Phenobarbital is the drug of choice for long-term control of seizures in dogs. Adjust the dosage by determining the serum phenobarbital concentration (see sec. 10, ch. 3). A maximum serum concentration of 35 μg/liter rather than 40 μg/liter is recommended to decrease the likelihood of phenobarbital-associated hepatotoxicity.
- Gradually discontinue primidone or phenytoin over a 2- to 3-week period after initiating phenobarbital therapy.
- Potassium bromide is an investigational anticonvulsant drug that may be a useful alternative in dogs with anticonvulsant-induced hepatic disease because of its lack of hepatic metabolism or hepatotoxicity.
- Additional supportive measures are important in managing dogs with anticonvulsant-induced hepatic disease. Control complications such as ascites and hepatic encephalopathy, as discussed previously (see Table 1).

KEY POINT ▶ To detect early evidence of hepatic damage, routinely monitor liver enzymes (serum ALP and ALT), total serum bilirubin, cholesterol, albumin, and phenobarbital levels at least every 6–12 months in all dogs on chronic anticonvulsant therapy.

CORTICOSTEROID-INDUCED HEPATOPATHY (STEROID HEPATOPATHY)

Corticosteroid-induced, or steroid hepatopathy, is a commonly recognized sequela of glucocorticoid administration in dogs. Glucocorticoids cause hepatic glycogen accumulation and hepatomegaly (see Table 3). Steroid hepatopathy is a benign, reversible hepatic lesion that, with rare exceptions, is not associated with clinical liver dysfunction. The most important clinical significance of this disorder is not to mistake it for a more serious hepatic disease.

KEY POINT ▶ To avoid unnecessary diagnostic and therapeutic measures, be aware that increased serum ALP activity and hepatomegaly are commonly caused by glucocorticoid therapy in dogs.

Recognition of steroid hepatopathy often alerts the clinician to the presence of previously unsuspected spontaneous hyperadrenocorticism in dogs without a history of glucocorticoid therapy (see sec. 4, ch. 3). Cats are resistant to the hepatic effects of glucocorticoids and do not develop steroid hepatopathy.

Etiology

- Steroid hepatopathy has been associated with numerous glucocorticoids including cortisone, prednisone, prednisolone, dexamethasone, and triamcinolone. Lesions of steroid hepatopathy can develop within 2 days of corticosteroid administration.
- Endogenous production of excess glucocorticoids caused by spontaneous hyperadrenocorticism also results in steroid hepatopathy. Hepatic lesions are identical to those seen with exogenous administration of glucocorticoids.
- Individual variation and susceptibility to steroid hepatopathy also appears to play a role.

Clinical Signs

- Clinical signs reflect the systemic effects of hypercortisolism rather than hepatic disease and include PU/PD and polyphagia in an otherwise healthy dog.

Diagnosis

Suspect steroid hepatopathy in any dog with hepatomegaly and increased serum ALP activity that has a history of recent glucocorticoid therapy and/or clinical signs of hyperadrenocorticism.

History and Physical Examination

- Look for a history of previous glucocorticoid therapy within the past 3 months.
  - *Note*: Significant amounts of glucocorticoid can be absorbed from topical and ocular medications as well as from oral and injectable preparations.

- Hepatomegaly, which may be quite massive, frequently is detected.
- Other findings include abdominal distension and thinning of the hair coat.

Laboratory Evaluation

- Increased serum ALP activity is the most consistent biochemical abnormality detected in many (but not all) dogs with this hepatic lesion. In some dogs, this activity is attributed to the liver isoenzyme rather than the corticosteroid-induced isoenzyme (CIALP; see previous discussion). This increase can occur within 1–2 days of initiating glucocorticoid therapy and often is as high as 150 × normal.
- In contrast, ALT activity is normal or only mildly increased.
- Other biochemical tests that may be abnormal include serum GGT activity, BSP dye excretion, and SBA concentrations, which, however, generally are lower (<60 μmol/liter) than those obtained in dogs with other hepatic disorders.
- Total serum bilirubin, serum albumin, blood ammonia concentration, and hemostatic tests typically are normal.
- Other findings characteristic of hypercortisolism include neutrophilia, lymphopenia, eosinopenia, monocytosis, and hypercholesterolemia.

Radiography

- Hepatomegaly usually is detected on abdominal radiographs.
- Ultrasonography reveals hepatomegaly and diffusely increased liver echogenicity.

Liver Biopsy and Histopathologic Evaluation

- Grossly, the liver is enlarged, smooth, pale, and friable. Microscopically, hepatic lesions are characterized by severe, vacuolated ballooned hepatocytes in a patchy distribution.
- Periodic acid–Schiff (PAS) staining of alcohol- but not formalin-fixed tissue reveals that hepatic vacuoles contain glycogen granules. In most cases, special stains are not required for the experienced pathologist to diagnose this lesion.
- When hepatic biopsy suggests steroid hepatopathy and a history of glucocorticoid administration is lacking, perform diagnostic tests for endogenous hyperadrenocorticism (see sec. 4, ch. 3).

Treatment

- Steroid hepatopathy is reversible after withdrawal of exogenous glucocorticoids or treatment of spontaneous hyperadrenocorticism.
- The length of time required for complete resolution is unpredictable, varying from weeks to months.

CHRONIC HEPATITIS

Chronic hepatitis is a heterogeneous group of necrotizing inflammatory diseases of the liver. The clinical signs of chronic hepatitis initially are vague and nonspecific, such as anorexia, weight loss, and depression; however, as hepatitis becomes advanced, signs of liver failure develop, including jaundice, ascites, coagulopathy, or hepatic encephalopathy.

With few exceptions, the cause, pathogenesis, natural history, and optimal treatment of these disorders in dogs is unknown. Because the laboratory and histopathologic features often fail to determine the definitive etiology, combined clinical and histologic criteria rather than etiologic classifications generally are used to categorize patients with chronic hepatitis.

Idiopathic Chronic Hepatitis

Idiopathic chronic hepatitis is characterized by clinical signs and persistent laboratory indicators of hepatic disease in association with chronic portal inflammation, piecemeal hepatic necrosis, and fibrosis that frequently progresses to cirrhosis and liver failure.

Etiology

The disease must be considered idiopathic in most dogs; however, it is probable that after an initial inciting hepatocyte injury, immune mechanisms are involved in perpetuating the inflammation. Whether canine chronic hepatitis is comparable to the human disease, chronic active hepatitis, is controversial.

Signalment and Clinical Signs

- The incidence of idiopathic chronic hepatitis appears to be highest in female dogs.
- The mean age of onset is 5–6 years, but adult dogs of any age or breed can be affected.
- Common signs include anorexia, depression, weakness, PU/PD, ascites, jaundice, weight loss, and vomiting.

Diagnosis

The diagnosis is suggested by the clinical signs in conjunction with elevation of serum liver enzyme concentrations. The diagnosis can be confirmed only by liver biopsy. Historical and physical findings are consistent with chronic liver disease.

Laboratory Evaluation
- Serum ALT activity usually is >10 × normal, reflecting ongoing hepatic injury (inflammation); serum ALP activity is usually >5 × normal, reflecting intrahepatic cholestasis. Hyperbilirubinemia and bilirubinuria also are common.
- Liver function tests such as SBA concentration, BSP dye excretion, and ammonia tolerance frequently are abnormal, reflecting the degree of liver dysfunction.
- Less consistent findings include hypoalbuminemia, hyperglobulinemia, mild nonregenerative anemia, and abnormal hemostasis. Ascitic fluid, when present, typically is a transudate or modified transudate.

Radiography
- Radiographically the liver may appear small, and on ultrasonography the pattern of echogenicity may be abnormal.

Liver Biopsy

- Liver biopsy and histopathology confirm the diagnosis.
  - The liver often is small and nodular because of the fibrosis and nodular regeneration of cirrhosis.
  - The primary lesion is portal inflammation consisting primarily of lymphocytes and plasma cells and occasional neutrophils and macrophages. The inflammation extends into the hepatic lobule, causing piecemeal necrosis of hepatocytes. These lesions are essential criteria for categorization as idiopathic chronic hepatitis.
  - Fibrosis usually is present.

Differential Diagnosis

When chronic hepatitis has been confirmed histologically, look for potential inciting or perpetuating factors. If none are found, then idiopathic chronic hepatitis is the diagnosis. Recognized types of chronic hepatitis are listed in Table 6.

Treatment

Treatment includes drug therapy, discussed below, and supportive measures, previously described under Principles of Treatment for Liver Disease.

Prednisolone

- Give 1–2 mg/kg/day, PO, for immunosuppression until clinical remission occurs; then taper off to the lowest effective alternate-day maintenance dose.
- Monitor serum biochemistries every 1–2 weeks.
- A follow-up liver biopsy is required to ensure that the disease is in remission.

Azathioprine. When prednisolone alone is ineffective or side effects become objectionable, consider combination therapy using azathioprine (Imuran; Burroughs Wellcome) and prednisolone (at a lower dose if side effects are a problem).

- Give 2 mg/kg/day, PO, for induction therapy; for maintenance, give the same dose once every other day while giving prednisolone on the alternate days.
- Because azathioprine may cause bone marrow suppression, monitor periodically with a CBC.

Ursodeoxycholic Acid (UDCA). UDCA (Actigall; Summit Pharmaceutical) is a bile acid produced from chenodeoxycholic acid. UDCA has been useful in the treatment of humans with chronic hepatitis. Its use in

dogs is preliminary but promising. UDCA is believed to be beneficial by saturating the bile acid pool, thereby reducing synthesis of potentially toxic (hydrophobic) bile acids that may further perpetuate hepatic injury associated with cholestasis.

No signs of toxicity have been noted when UDCA is given to dogs at a dose of 5–15 mg/kg/day, PO, divided q12h. UDCA is used in conjunction with immunosuppressive therapy (described previously).

Prognosis

The response to treatment of idiopathic chronic hepatitis is variable, which is expected because it probably represents a heterogeneous group of diseases.

- Some dogs eventually can be taken off medication and remain in remission, but more often therapy must be continued indefinitely.
- Other dogs fail to respond, especially those that have advanced disease and cirrhosis (the treatment of cirrhosis and its complications is discussed elsewhere in this chapter).

Hepatic Copper Accumulation and Chronic Hepatitis

Copper accumulation in the liver can be associated with significant hepatic injury resulting in acute hepatitis, chronic hepatitis, and cirrhosis. The severity of hepatic injury is related to the amount of copper; when copper concentration exceeds 2000 μg/g dry weight (ppm), hepatic damage consistently occurs.

Hepatic copper concentration in normal dogs has been considered to be <400 μg/g; however, a recent study of 623 normal dogs (based on clinical signs and liver biopsy) suggests a wide continuum of normal hepatic copper concentrations, ranging from <100 μg/g to 2000 μg/g. Certain breeds including the West Highland white terrier, Doberman pinscher, cocker spaniel, keeshond, and Labrador retriever have higher mean values for hepatic copper than other breeds. Thus, in the individual dog, it is difficult to know the clinical significance of a copper concentration between 400 and 2000 μg/g.

Copper accumulation in the liver may be a cause or an effect of chronic hepatitis.

- Inherited metabolic defects in biliary copper excretion cause chronic hepatitis in Bedlington terriers and West Highland white terriers. Copper concentrations range from 850–12,000 μg/g in affected Bedlingtons and up to 3,500 μg/g in West Highland white terriers.
- Because copper normally is excreted in the bile, hepatic copper accumulation can also occur secondary to any cholestatic hepatobiliary disorder (such as idiopathic chronic hepatitis) that impairs bile flow.
  - Although not proven, Doberman pinschers with chronic hepatitis (copper concentration 300–2000 μg/g) probably have copper accumulation as an effect rather than a cause of chronic hepatitis. An alternative explanation is that these values may

---

TABLE 6. Types of Chronic Hepatitis in Dogs

Idiopathic chronic hepatitis
Copper-associated hepatitis of Bedlington terriers, West Highland white terriers, and Skye terriers
Chronic hepatitis of Doberman pinschers
Drug-induced chronic hepatitis (anticonvulsants, oxibendazole)
Leptospirosis-associated chronic hepatitis (*Leptospira interrogans* serovar *grippotyphosa*)
Infectious canine hepatitis virus–associated chronic hepatitis
Acidophil cell hepatitis
Lobular dissecting hepatitis
Idiopathic hepatoportal fibrosis

simply reflect "normal" copper concentrations in this breed.

- Whether secondary copper accumulation can further contribute to hepatic injury is unclear, but this is an important question since the role of copper chelator therapy in this situation is controversial.

■ Other breeds of dogs occasionally are diagnosed with chronic hepatitis and cirrhosis accompanied by increased hepatic copper concentrations. At this advanced stage of disease, it is difficult to know whether copper accumulation is a cause or an effect of the chronic hepatitis. As a general rule, the higher the copper content, the more likely it is to be a primary problem.

Copper-Associated Hepatitis in Bedlington Terriers

Etiology

■ Bedlington terriers have a hereditary (autosomal recessive) inability to excrete copper in the bile that is associated with progressive hepatic copper accumulation and chronic liver disease. Hepatic copper content increases with age. Because of extensive inbreeding, the prevalence within the breed is quite high.

■ Excess copper is stored in hepatic lysosomes. When hepatic copper accumulation is >2000 μg/g, progressive hepatic injury occurs including focal hepatic necrosis, chronic hepatitis, and eventually, cirrhosis. This disease is similar but not identical to Wilson's disease in humans.

Clinical Signs

Clinical signs and presentation vary widely, depending on the stage of disease.

■ Most affected dogs are presented as young or middle-aged adults of either sex with signs of hepatic failure of varying severity, including lethargy, depression, weight loss, vomiting, and jaundice. Acute fulminant hepatic failure with rapid deterioration and death occurs in rare instances.

■ Some middle-aged and older dogs are presented initially with end-stage liver disease and cirrhosis. In these animals there is a more chronic insidious clinical course, with similar but less severe signs. In the advanced stages of disease, cachexia, jaundice, ascites, and hepatic encephalopathy can occur.

■ Affected dogs may be asymptomatic, especially young dogs in which copper is accumulating but has not yet reached toxic hepatic concentrations.

Diagnosis

Suspect copper-associated hepatitis in any Bedlington terrier with historical, physical, or biochemical evidence of hepatic disease or with vague, unexplained illness. Asymptomatic dogs can be identified only by routine biochemical screening or liver biopsy. Definitive diagnosis requires liver biopsy.

History

■ Acute, recurrent episodes are common in many affected dogs. Stressful events such as whelping, showing, shipping, or a change in environment can precipitate these episodes.

■ Dogs initially presenting with end-stage cirrhosis often have no history of previous episodes of hepatitis.

Physical Examination

■ Findings in dogs with acute hepatitis include depression, lethargy, and dehydration. Hepatomegaly may occur. Jaundice may be detected within 48 hours of onset. Acute copper-induced hemolytic anemia may be a contributing factor.

■ With advanced disease, dehydration, emaciation, ascites, hepatic encephalopathy, and jaundice may be detected. The liver is small and not palpable.

■ Asymptomatic dogs are normal on physical examination.

Laboratory Evaluation

■ Biochemical findings vary with the stage of disease. Increased serum ALT activity is probably the most sensitive laboratory indicator of this disease, although up to a third of affected dogs will have normal ALT values. These are mostly younger dogs that are in the early stages of the disease.

■ Other serum biochemical abnormalities typical of hepatic dysfunction eventually develop, such as hyperbilirubinemia, bilirubinuria, hypoalbuminemia, increased SBA levels, and prolonged PT and APTT.

■ Acute release of copper from necrotic hepatocytes occasionally causes hemolytic anemia. Laboratory findings include low packed cell volume (PCV), hemoglobinemia, and hemoglobinuria. Plasma copper levels are increased during episodes of hemolysis.

Radiography

■ Abdominal radiographs are unremarkable except when advanced stages of disease are accompanied by microhepatica or ascites.

■ Ultrasonography of the liver may be normal in the early stages. As the disease progresses, findings are indicative of diffuse liver disease or microhepatica and cirrhosis.

Liver Biopsy and Histopathologic Evaluation. Liver biopsy is indicated for definitive diagnosis and staging of the disease. Perform liver biopsies in all dogs being considered for breeding. Dogs should be >1 year of age to ensure adequate time for copper accumulation. The spectrum of gross and microscopic features in the liver parallels the variable expression of the disease.

■ The liver can be grossly normal or swollen and smooth with accentuation of the lobules. As cirrhosis develops, the liver decreases in size and there is a mixture of fine and coarse nodules.

■ Histologically, H&E-stained hepatic tissue reveals dark granules in hepatocyte cytoplasm. In the early stages, centrilobular hepatocytes are most affected, but later the distribution is diffuse.

■ Histochemical stains for copper such as rhodanine and rubeanic acid are positive. These stains consistently detect copper in liver biopsies when amounts are >400 μg/g dry weight. Hepatic biopsies stored in formalin for >6 months lose their ability to pick up these stains.

■ Associated histologic hepatic damage is variable. In the most mildly affected animals, only centrilobular copper granules are detected. This progresses to focal hepatitis, lesions of chronic hepatitis, and eventually cirrhosis.

■ Perform quantitative copper analysis on fresh or formalin-fixed hepatic tissue (even tissue fixed >6 months). Affected dogs have hepatic copper concentrations of 850–12,000 μg/g dry weight.

Treatment

Management of the acute hepatic crisis involves symptomatic and supportive care to control electrolyte, acid-base, and fluid imbalances and hepatic encephalopathy (see Table 1).

■ Treatment of hemolytic anemia may require a blood transfusion.

■ Trientine hydrochloride (but not D-penicillamine) may be effective in chelating copper in the circulation.

■ Specific measures to control hepatic copper accu-mulation are summarized in Table 7. Base the choice of therapy for an individual patient on the severity of existing hepatic damage.

• Treat affected dogs with copper accumulation and chronic hepatitis with a copper chelator such as D-penicillamine (125 mg q12h, PO) or trientine hydrochloride (250 mg q12h, PO), which promotes urinary copper excretion (see Table 7).

• Lifelong therapy is necessary because copper reaccumulates if treatment is stopped.

■ Preliminary clinical evaluation suggests that hepatic copper concentrations decrease about 750–1000 μg/g dry weight per year with chelator therapy. There may be other protective effects of D-penicillamine besides depletion of hepatic copper, because many Bedlington terriers on long-term therapy do not develop hepatic failure despite continued elevated copper levels and ongoing hepatic damage. Additional effects that may be beneficial include inhibition of collagen deposition, stimulation of collagenase activity, immunosuppression, and immunomodulation.

■ Zinc acetate may be added to the chelator therapy

TABLE 7. Treatment of Hepatic Copper (Cu) Accumulation

Product	Formulation	Dose	Side Effects	Comments
Chelate Systemic Cu				
D-Penicillamine (Cuprimine, MSD; Depen, Wallace)	Cuprimine: 250-mg caps Depen: 250-mg tabs	10–15 mg/kg q12h, PO given on an empty stomach to improve absorption.	Anorexia and vomiting are common (start at reduced dose and increase to maintenance after a few days); dermatologic drug eruption (zinc deficiency?) or autoimmune-like vesicular lesions of mucocutaneous junctions;* reversible renal disease*	Causes systemic Cu chelation and urinary excretion; takes months to years to produce significant decrease in hepatic Cu concentration (750–1000 μg/g/year), but may produce subjective clinical improvement after a few weeks; not effective for treatment of Cu-associated hemolysis.
Trientine hydrochloride (Syprine, MSD; formerly Cuprid)	250-mg caps	15–30 mg/kg q12h, PO; give 1 hour before meals; do not give concurrently with any medication, including vitamin/mineral supplement	None noted as yet	Use as an alternative to D-penicillamine if vomiting occurs; may be useful for treatment of hemolysis by chelating Cu in blood; more expensive than penicillamine.
2,3,2-Tetramine	Not commercially available	15–30 mg/kg q12h, PO	None noted as yet	Derivative of trientine that is 4–9 × as potent; thus, lowers hepatic Cu concentrations more rapidly than D-penicillamine or trientine.
Decrease Intestinal Cu Absorption				
Ascorbic acid (vitamin C)	Many available	500–1000 mg/day, given with meals	None	Benefit in animals is unproven.
Zinc acetate, sulfate, or gluconate	Many available	5–10 mg elemental zinc/ kg q12h, use high end of dose initially, then lower dose for maintenance; separate administration from meals by 1–2 h.	Vomiting,† zinc-induced hemolysis	Induces intestinal metallothionein, which binds Cu and zinc and prevents absorption; six–week lag period for effect. Do not use zinc alone in dogs with active hepatitis (add Cu chelator). Monitor plasma zinc every 3–4 months to maintain level of >200 and <1000 μg/dl by adjusting dose.
Decrease Cu Intake				
Low copper diet	None commercially available	<0.5 ppm Cu in diet		Low Cu diet may slow further Cu accumulation but not "de-copper" the liver. Most commercial diets are high in Cu; even Cu-restricted diets such as Hill's Prescription Diet u/d (4 ppm) are not low enough. Therefore, feeding low-Cu diet is not required; but avoid high-Cu foods such as liver, shellfish, organ meats, chocolate, nuts, mushrooms, cereals, mineral supplements.

*Rare complications.
†Zinc gluconate may be less irritating to the stomach than other formulations. To minimize vomiting, open capsule and mix contents with small amount of tuna or hamburger.

but should not be used alone in dogs with active hepatitis. Whether zinc alone will be useful for long-term therapy is not known. A major advantage of zinc over D-penicillamine and trientine hydrochloride is that it is less expensive.

■ Low copper diets are of little value once hepatic copper accumulation has occurred (see Table 7).

Prognosis

■ Dogs with mild to moderate acute hepatic failure usually respond to supportive care.
■ If this disease is detected before severe hepatic failure occurs, many dogs can live out their lives with D-penicillamine therapy.
■ The prognosis is poor if there is fulminant hepatic failure or chronic end-stage cirrhosis and failure.

Prevention

■ Treatment of affected dogs with minimal hepatic injury is recommended in the hope of preventing acute hepatitis or progression to cirrhosis.
■ Zinc therapy is a promising and less expensive alternative to D-pencillamine in this setting.
■ Young dogs (< 1 year) may be less responsive to chelator therapy than older dogs.

Chronic Hepatitis in Doberman Pinschers

Chronic hepatitis in Doberman pinschers is associated with histologic features of chronic hepatitis and cirrhosis. Hepatic copper concentrations are increased in most but not all affected dogs.

Etiology

■ The underlying etiopathogenic mechanisms are unknown. The high frequency in this breed suggests a genetic basis. The wide age range (1.5–11 years) suggests that environmental influences modify a genetic predisposition.
■ The significance of the increased hepatic copper concentration has not been determined. Copper accumulation secondary to chronic hepatitis and cholestasis appears most likely because of the low magnitude (300–2000 μg/g) of copper detected. Alternatively, excess hepatic copper concentrations may make these dogs more susceptible to hepatic injury or these values may reflect normal values in Doberman pinschers.

Clinical Signs

■ Females are predominantly affected.
■ Clinical signs may be mild or absent when the disease is fortuitously diagnosed in the early stages. However, most dogs are diagnosed in the advanced stages of hepatic failure.
■ Signs include anorexia, weight loss, lethargy, PU/PD, vomiting, diarrhea, ascites, and jaundice.
■ Evidence of excessive bleeding (gingival bleeding, epistaxis, and melena) may be found.
■ Signs of hepatic encephalopathy often predominate in the terminal stages.

Diagnosis

Suspect chronic hepatitis in any Doberman pinscher (especially females) with clinical and biochemical evidence of hepatic disease. Definitive diagnosis requires liver biopsy. Consider concurrent von Willebrand's disease, because of its prevalence in this breed (see sec. 3, ch. 2), in affected dogs with a bleeding disorder.

■ Common physical examination findings include ascites, jaundice, weight loss, and encephalopathy. Splenomegaly (associated with portal hypertension) is common. The liver is small and not palpable.
■ Laboratory findings frequently include increased ALP and ALT activity, hyperbilirubinemia, bilirubinuria, hypoalbuminemia, increased SBA levels, hyperammonemia, and prolonged BSP retention. Coagulopathy and thrombocytopenia are common in the advanced stages.
■ Radiographic and ultrasonographic findings of microhepatica and ascites are consistent with chronic liver disease and cirrhosis.
■ Liver biopsy and Histopathologic Evaluation
  • Grossly the liver is small with micro- or macronodular cirrhosis.
  • Histologic lesions include a mixed inflammatory infiltrate in portal areas, piecemeal and bridging necrosis, and portal fibrosis. Intrahepatic cholestasis is a prominent feature.
  • Rhodanine and rubeanic acid stains usually are positive for copper, especially in periportal regions. Stains for hepatic iron usually are positive.
  • Quantitative copper analysis reveals mild to moderate copper accumulation (400–2000 μg/g).

Treatment

Effective treatment has not been established.

■ Institute, as needed, symptomatic and supportive therapy for complications of hepatic failure, including correction of fluid, electrolyte, and acid-base balance, and treatment of ascites, hepatic encephalopathy, and coagulopathies (see Table 1).
■ Therapy with immunosuppressant drugs such as prednisolone with or without azathioprine may be given, as described previously for idiopathic chronic hepatitis. The efficacy of this treatment remains to be determined, but generally the response is poor, possibly because most dogs are presented in advanced stages of liver failure. Whether ursodeoxycholic acid therapy is effective in this disease is unknown (see Idiopathic Chronic Hepatitis).
■ The use of copper chelating agents is controversial. Sporadic reports suggest that treatment of affected Dobermans with D-penicillamine decreases hepatic copper concentrations to <400 μg/g after 3–12 months of therapy (see Table 7). This is a notable difference from Bedlington terriers with copper accumulation, which may never achieve normal copper levels even with lifelong D-penicillamine therapy. Despite a decrease in hepatic copper content, it appears that hepatitis in Dobermans is progressive, suggesting that copper accumulation is secondary and not the cause of hepatic injury. D-Penicillamine

has not been found to be beneficial for humans with chronic liver disease unless they have hereditary copper storage disease.

Prognosis

- Treatment usually is unsuccessful. Most dogs die within weeks to months.
- The prognosis may be more favorable if the disease is detected in the early stages.

Copper-Associated Hepatitis in West Highland White Terriers

Etiology

Preliminary breeding studies suggest that excess hepatic copper accumulation in West Highland white terriers is inherited, but the mode of inheritance is unknown. Hepatic lesions include multifocal hepatitis and cirrhosis.

As with Bedlington terriers, evidence of hepatic damage is not noted until values are >2000 μg/g. However, there are notable differences from the disease in Bedlingtons, such as:

- West Highland white terriers do not accumulate copper continuously throughout life. Peak hepatic copper concentrations occur by 6 months of age and may even decrease after 1 year of age.
- The magnitude of copper increase generally is lower than in Bedlingtons. Hepatic copper concentrations in normal West Highland white terriers and in those with chronic hepatitis and cirrhosis form a continuum, with values of 400–3600 μg/g, making it difficult to establish a cut-off value to positively identify affected animals.

Clinical Signs

- Affected animals in the early stages of copper accumulation or those with focal hepatitis are usually asymptomatic.
- When widespread necrosis occurs, nonspecific signs of liver disease include anorexia, vomiting, diarrhea, lethargy, and jaundice.
- With advanced disease, jaundice and ascites are common.

Diagnosis

Episodes of hepatic necrosis may be precipitated by stressful events such as whelping or showing.

- The earliest biochemical abnormality associated with hepatic necrosis is increased ALT activity.
- With advanced disease, laboratory findings include increased liver enzyme activity, hyperbilirubinemia, increased SBA levels, impaired BSP excretion, hyperammonemia, and hypoalbuminemia. Hemolytic anemia has not been documented.
- Liver biopsy for histopathology and quantitative copper analysis are required for definitive diagnosis. Histologic features include copper granules (which are initially centrilobular but become diffusely distributed with time), multifocal hepatitis, and postnecrotic cirrhosis.

Treatment

- The principles of therapy are similar to those described for Bedlington terriers.
- Because hepatic copper accumulation is not continuous throughout life, mature dogs with <2000 μg/g may not require chelator therapy. Treatment for copper accumulation is indicated when copper concentrations are >2000 μg/g or when active hepatic necrosis is evident (see Table 7).
- Preliminary evidence suggests that both D-penicillamine and zinc acetate can decrease hepatic copper concentrations in West Highland white terriers, when given on a long-term basis.

Copper-Associated Hepatitis in Skye Terriers

Chronic hepatitis and cirrhosis associated with hepatic copper accumulation (800–2200 μg/g) has been described in genetically related Skye terriers.

- In the early stages, copper accumulation is absent, and biopsy findings indicate hepatocellular degeneration with cholestasis and mild inflammation.
- Chronic lesions are associated with intracanalicular cholestasis, chronic hepatitis, and cirrhosis.
- Skye terrier hepatitis is speculated to be a disorder of disturbed bile secretion with subsequent accumulation of copper.

Lobular Dissecting Hepatitis

- This form of chronic hepatitis has been reported in a few dogs, including three young male standard poodles. It is characterized histologically by lobular hepatitis; that is, inflammation and necrosis scattered in the hepatic lobule rather than concentrated in the periportal region as described for idiopathic chronic hepatitis. Bands of collagen and reticulin fibers subdivide and disrupt hepatic lobular architecture and progress to cirrhosis.
- It has been suggested that some previously described cases of idiopathic canine hepatitis and chronic active hepatitis may be more accurately described as lobular dissecting hepatitis.
- Clinical features are those of advanced hepatic failure and portal hypertension.
- Specific treatment has not been reported, but general measures for management of chronic liver failure are appropriate.

Acidophil Cell Hepatitis

Acidophil cell hepatitis has been described in Great Britain and is caused by an unidentified transmissable agent that is probably viral but distinct from canine adenovirus I (see sec. 2, ch. 9).

- It is characterized by acute or chronic hepatitis with slow progression to cirrhosis. Acidophils, which are a consistent histologic feature of the disease, represent dying hepatocytes.
- Signs usually are typical of chronic liver failure.
- Specific treatment has not been described, but general measures for management of chronic liver failure are appropriate.

HEPATIC CIRRHOSIS AND FIBROSIS

Cirrhosis is characterized by diffuse fibrosis and replacement of liver tissue with structurally abnormal regenerative nodules.

Etiology

- Cirrhosis is the irreversible end stage of chronic hepatic injury caused by infection, hepatotoxins (copper, anticonvulsants), immunologic injury (chronic hepatitis), chronic cholestasis (chronic cholangiohepatitis in cats), and hypoxia. The common denominator is hepatocyte death, which leads to repair by fibrosis and nodular regeneration.
- These processes further compromise adjacent normal hepatocytes, intrahepatic blood flow, and intrahepatic bile flow; thus, cirrhosis eventually reaches a point at which it is self-perpetuating.
- When cirrhosis is fully developed, the histologic features of the original inciting injury often are obscured by the cirrhotic changes.

Clinical Signs

Cirrhosis causes generalized hepatic dysfunction; thus, the clinical signs are those of chronic hepatic failure. A combination of jaundice, ascites, and hepatic encephalopathy is highly suggestive of cirrhosis.

Diagnosis

Laboratory Evaluation

Laboratory evidence of liver disease usually precedes the development of cirrhosis but may go undetected because signs at that stage may be insidious and vague.

- Serum liver enzymes usually are increased, although more modestly than during the active injury stage of liver disease.
- Circulating bilirubin, ammonia, and bile acids usually are increased, whereas serum albumin usually is decreased. Hyperglobulinemia is sometimes seen.
- Hemostatic abnormalities may reflect DIC, impaired hepatic synthesis of coagulation factors, or vitamin K deficiency due to cholestasis (least likely).

Radiography

- Microhepatica is common in dogs with cirrhosis, whereas most cats with biliary cirrhosis have hepatomegaly.
- Ultrasonography findings include microhepatica, irregular hepatic margins, focal lesions representing regenerative nodules, and increased parenchymal echogenicity associated with increased fibrous tissue. Splenomegaly and secondary portosystemic shunts also may be detected.

Liver Biopsy and Histopathologic Evaluation

Definitive diagnosis of cirrhosis requires liver biopsy.

- Laparotomy or laparoscopy provides a better appreciation for the gross nodularity of the liver than can be ascertained from blind percutaneous needle biopsy.
- Microscopic features include fibrosis, regenerative nodules, and disruption of normal hepatic architecture.
- Concurrent inflammation may be detected, especially when the inciting cause of cirrhosis is chronic inflammation.

Treatment

- Because cirrhosis is essentially irreversible, treatment is mainly supportive, emphasizing measures that control complications of severe generalized liver failure, such as ascites, encephalopathy, gastric ulcers, coagulopathies, and infection (see Table 1).
- If a probable cause or category of injury can be determined, specific treatment directed at preventing further injury may slow progression of cirrhosis. For example:
  - Adjust the drug regimen of dogs receiving anticonvulsants.
  - Treat dogs with copper-positive biopsies with a chelating agent such as D-penicillamine.
  - Treat dogs with histologic features of chronic hepatitis with immunosuppressive drugs.
- D-Penicillamine and prednisolone also have antifibrotic properties; however, the benefits of corticosteroids may be outweighed by the risk. These include a tendency for GI ulceration and bleeding, increased body catabolism that may exacerbate hepatic encephalopathy, and sodium retention that may exacerbate ascites and edema.
- Colchicine, an antifibrotic drug, has been used to treat humans with cirrhosis. Colchicine is a microtubule inhibitor, stimulant of collagenase activity, and inhibitor of collagen deposition. Its benefit in dogs with cirrhosis is unproven.
  - The recommended dose is 0.025–0.03 mg/kg/day, PO.
  - The major side effects in dogs are nausea, vomiting, and diarrhea. In humans, other side effects include bone marrow toxicity and myoneuropathy.

FELINE HEPATIC LIPIDOSIS

Hepatic lipidosis is an excessive accumulation of triglyceride in the liver that occurs when there is an imbalance between the rates of deposition and mobilization of fat from the liver. It is a common liver disease in cats and is associated with severe intrahepatic cholestasis and hepatic failure. Mortality is high if the disorder is untreated.

Etiology

General mechanisms of hepatic lipidosis include nutritional, metabolic, hormonal, toxic, and hypoxic liver injury. Diabetes mellitus is a well-recognized and easily diagnosed cause of hepatic lipidosis. Drug- (tetracycline) or toxin-induced injury can also cause histologic lesions of lipidosis. However, in most cats, severe hepatic lipidosis (>50% of hepatocytes involved within an acinar unit) is idiopathic.

The following mechanisms may be important in the development of idiopathic hepatic lipidosis:

- Anorexia and its effect on protein and lipid metabolism appear to be of key importance. Severe hepatic lipidosis most commonly develops in overweight cats that experience prolonged inappetence, usually lasting 2 weeks or longer.
- Accumulation of lipids in hepatocytes can result from disruption of normal fat metabolism at any of the following steps:
  - Excess mobilization of fat from peripheral stores, which may overwhelm hepatic fat dispersal and metabolism (may explain predilection in obese cats)
  - Increased hepatic synthesis of triglycerides (currently appears unlikely)
  - Inability of the liver to adequately oxidize fatty acids (possibly due to relative deficiency of carnitine)
  - Inability to synthesize or secrete lipoproteins (due to protein deficiency or build-up of orotic acid)
- Arginine deficiency may be important, because cats with lipidosis have decreased serum arginine concentrations and arginine is an essential amino acid in the cat that is required for normal urea cycle function and ammonia detoxification. Orotic acid build-up secondary to arginine deficiency can inhibit lipoprotein synthesis and exacerbate triglyceride accumulation.
- Taurine deficiency may contribute to intrahepatic cholestasis, because serum taurine concentrations are low and taurine is required for hepatic bile acid conjugation and normal bile acid metabolism in cats.

Clinical Signs

- Idiopathic hepatic lipidosis can develop in cats of any age. Females are affected more frequently than males. Many but not all affected cats are obese prior to the onset of disease.
- Prolonged anorexia, often of several weeks' duration, is the most consistent clinical sign.
- Other findings include lethargy, vomiting, constipation or diarrhea, and weight loss. Weight loss can be dramatic and may exceed 25% of the previous weight.
- Overt signs of hepatic encephalopathy such as hypersalivation, head pressing, dementia, and seizures are uncommon. However, nonspecific signs such as anorexia, lethargy and vomiting may be subtle signs of encephalopathy.
- Overt bleeding is uncommon.

Diagnosis

Clinical findings and laboratory evaluation in cats with idiopathic hepatic lipidosis suggest hepatic disease, but liver biopsy is required to distinguish hepatic lipidosis from other causes of hepatic disease such as cholangiohepatitis, FIP, and neoplasia.

History

- The history may reveal precipitating causes of anorexia such as stressful events (e.g., boarding, surgery, change in living arrangements), a diet change for weight reduction, and nonhepatic diseases associated with anorexia.

Physical Examination

- Findings include hepatomegaly, jaundice, muscle wasting, pallor, and seborrhea.

Laboratory Evaluation

- Hematologic findings are nonspecific and include a nonregenerative, normocytic, normochromic anemia with poikilocytosis and a normal WBC count.
- Serum ALP, ALT, and AST activities, fasting and postprandial SBA concentrations, and total serum bilirubin concentration usually are increased. Increases in liver enzymes precede increases in total bilirubin and bile acids. Serum ALP activity generally is higher in cats with lipidosis than with other hepatic diseases. Serum GGT activity, which usually parallels or exceeds serum ALP activity in most feline hepatic diseases, is normal or only mildly increased in hepatic lipidosis.
- Other potential findings include hypokalemia, prolonged BSP retention, hyperammonemia, hypoalbuminemia, and decreased BUN. Many affected cats have abnormal coagulation tests, especially prolonged PT and hypofibrinogenemia.

Radiography

- Radiographically, the liver is normal to increased in size.
- Ultrasonographic findings include hepatomegaly and diffuse increased echogenicity of the liver compared with falciform fat.

Liver Biopsy and Histopathologic Evaluation

Liver biopsy or fine-needle aspiration for cytology is required for definitive diagnosis.

- Grossly, the liver is enlarged, yellow, greasy, and friable with rounded edges. Biopsy specimens usually float in formalin.
- On routine H&E staining, severe vacuolization of hepatocytes in a micro- or macrovacuolar pattern is noted.
- Oil red O stain performed on nonparaffin embedded formalin-fixed tissue can confirm excess fat in the vacuoles.
- Inflammation or necrosis usually is absent.
- On cytologic evaluation, hepatocytes are foamy and vacuolated, and inflammatory cells are absent.

Treatment

Because of lack of information regarding the underlying cause, treatment is primarily supportive. The greatest success has been with aggressive nutritional support.

Nutritional Therapy

- Provide the daily caloric requirement (60 kcal/kg body weight/day) by force-feeding or nasogastric or gastrostomy tube. An endoscopically or surgically placed gastrostomy tube is preferable because long-term nutritional therapy (at least 3–6 weeks) usually is necessary (see sec. 1, ch. 3). Nasogastric tubes are adequate for short-term management and are preferable to force-feeding.
  - Oral appetite stimulants are usually inadequate to achieve the consistent caloric intake required for treatment of lipidosis. Avoid benzodiazepines, in particular, because they can exacerbate hepatic encephalopathy and are metabolized by the liver.
- Supplement a balanced, canned commercial cat food, such as Feline Prescription Diet p/d or c/d (Hill's Pet), with water to make a gruel that can be delivered through a tube in small feedings, 4–6 times daily. Commercial liquid diets such as CliniCare Feline Liquid Diet (Pet-Ag) or Feline Prescription Diet a/d (Hill's Pet) can also be used.
  - Use a restricted protein diet (Feline Prescription Diet k/d, Hill's Pet) only if hyperammonemia or overt signs of hepatic encephalopathy occur.
- A multiple vitamin supplement can be given at double the daily maintenance dose. Consider thiamine supplementation, in particular, because prolonged anorexia can result in thiamine deficiency. Initially, give 100 mg of thiamine q12h, IM, for several days; follow with 50–100 mg q12–24h, PO.
- Various dietary supplements have been recommended, based on the speculation that deficiencies may play a role in this disorder. However, feeding a balanced commercial cat food is usually adequate.
  - Taurine, 500 mg/day, has been recommended for the first month but is necessary only when taurine deficiency is strongly suspected.
  - Give arginine, 1 g/day, if a nonfeline liquid diet is used. Commercial feline diets are adequate in arginine.
  - L-Carnitine, 250–500 mg/day, has also been recommended empirically.

Fluid Therapy

- Intravenous fluid therapy with a balanced electrolyte solution supplemented with potassium chloride often is required in the initial stages of treatment (see Table 1).
- Avoid dextrose supplementation unless hypoglycemia is documented, because carbohydrate supplementation can stimulate hepatic fat synthesis and block fat oxidation for energy.

Control of Complications

- Abnormal blood coagulation test results and excess bleeding occasionally respond to vitamin K₁ therapy, suggesting severe cholestasis and vitamin K malabsorption (see Table 1). Fresh blood transfusion may be required for management of anemia.
- Hepatic encephalopathy is managed, as described in Table 1, with a low-protein diet, lactulose, and neomycin or metronidazole.

- Antibiotic therapy with amoxicillin is recommended to prevent infection secondary to compromised hepatic clearance of enteric organisms.
  - Avoid tetracycline because it can predispose to hepatic lipid accumulation.

Response to Treatment and Prognosis

- With aggressive nutritional and supportive care, approximately 65% of cats with lipidosis respond within 3–6 weeks. Biochemical parameters are often normal by 4 weeks. Recurrence is rare and there is no evidence of residual hepatic damage.
- The earlier treatment is initiated, the better the prognosis. Thus, institute nutritional support in any obese cat that becomes anorexic secondary to other disease processes.
- Consider the potential for lipidosis in any obese cat placed on a reducing diet. Monitor liver enzymes to evaluate for onset of lipidosis.

CONGENITAL PORTOSYSTEMIC SHUNT (PSS)

Portosystemic shunts (PSSs) are vascular communications between the portal and systemic venous systems that allow access of portal blood to the systemic circulation without first passing through the liver. Clinical signs of hepatic encephalopathy result from inadequate hepatic clearance of enterically derived toxins such as ammonia, mercaptans, short-chain fatty acids, and gamma aminobutyric acid. Decreased hepatic blood flow and lack of hepatotrophic factors result in hepatic atrophy. Urate urolithiasis is an important complication of PSS because of increased urinary excretion of ammonia and uric acid. Renal, cystic, and urethral calculi usually are green and contain an ammonia or uric acid component.

Etiology

PSS in dogs and cats can be congenital or acquired.

Congenital PSS

Congenital PSS is the most common and is categorized as single intrahepatic, single extrahepatic, or multiple extrahepatic.

- Single intrahepatic shunts provide a communication between the portal vein and the caudal vena cava, often via the left hepatic vein. Failure of the fetal ductus venosus to close results in an intrahepatic shunt. This type of shunt is most common in large-breed dogs.
- Single extrahepatic shunts usually connect the portal vein or one of its tributaries (left gastric or splenic vein) with the caudal vena cava cranial to the phrenicoabdominal veins. Less frequently, the anomalous vessel will enter the azygous vein. This type of shunt is most common in small-breed dogs and cats.
- Multiple extrahepatic shunts usually are acquired but occasionally are congenital. Multiple extrahepatic shunts detected in young dogs (<1 year) with no

evidence of severe hepatic disease on biopsy suggest a congenital mechanism.

Acquired PSS

Acquired shunts are collateral vessels that develop as a compensatory response to sustained portal hypertension caused by severe diffuse intrahepatic diseases such as chronic hepatitis and cirrhosis.

- These shunts usually appear as a tortuous plexus of vessels that communicate with the caudal vena cava in the area of the kidneys.
- Diagnosis and therapy are directed toward the underlying liver disease.

The following discussion focuses on congenital PSS.

Clinical Signs

Clinical signs of congenital PSS are referable to the CNS, GI system, or urinary tract.

- Signs of hepatic encephalopathy (HE) often predominate, including episodic weakness, ataxia, headpressing, disorientation, circling, pacing, behavioral changes, amaurotic blindness, seizures, and coma. Hypersalivation is a prominent clinical sign in cats.
  - Clinical signs of encephalopathy tend to wax and wane and are often interspersed with normal periods, reflecting the variable production and absorption of neurotoxic enteric products.
- GI signs of intermittent anorexia, vomiting, and diarrhea are common and are not necessarily accompanied by overt signs of HE.
- Psychogenic polydipsia and subsequent polyuria are frequent findings in dogs. If urolithiasis is a complicating feature, pollakiuria, dysuria, and hematuria may occur.

Diagnosis

Suspect congenital PSS in:

- Young dogs and cats with intermittent CNS, GI, or urinary tract signs.
- Dogs (except Dalmatians) or cats with urate urolithiasis.
- Dogs and cats of any age with clinical and biochemical evidence of hepatic insufficiency (especially hepatic encephalopathy) and absence of histologic evidence of severe intrahepatic disease.

Although congenital PSS may be suspected because of historical, physical, laboratory, and radiographic findings, a definitive diagnosis requires identification of a shunt by ultrasonography, contrast radiography, or exploratory laparotomy.

Signalment

- Congenital PSS is more common in purebred than mixed-breed dogs. Miniature schnauzers and Yorkshire terriers appear to be at increased risk. Domestic short-haired cats are affected more commonly than are purebred cats.
- No sex predilection has been noted. Affected male dogs commonly are cryptorchid.

- Age is an important diagnostic clue, because most animals develop signs by 6 months of age. Ductus venosus shunts often are recognized earlier than other types of shunts. A congenital PSS is also a diagnostic consideration in middle-aged and older dogs, because signs may be subtle and some cases go undiagnosed until the dog is 10 or 12 years of age.

History

- Many affected animals have a history of stunted growth or failure to gain weight compared with unaffected littermates.
- Prolonged recovery after general anesthesia or excessive sedation after treatment with tranquilizers, anticonvulsants, or organophosphates can be attributed to impaired hepatic metabolism of these substances. Signs of encephalopathy may be exacerbated by a protein-rich meal; GI bleeding associated with parasite infection, ulcers, or drug therapy; and administration of methionine-containing urinary acidifiers or lipotrophic agents.
- Clinical improvement after fluid therapy is common and most likely attributed to correction of dehydration and promotion of urinary excretion of ammonia and other toxins. Improvement with broad-spectrum antibiotic therapy reflects the effect of antibiotics on the toxin-producing intestinal flora.

Physical Examination

- Findings may be unremarkable except for small body stature or weight loss.
- The neurologic examination is normal or, if overt signs of HE are present, neurologic findings are consistent with diffuse cerebral disease.
- Ascites and edema are infrequent unless the shunt is complicated by portal hypertension or severe hypoalbuminemia.

Laboratory Evaluation

Routine hematologic and biochemical findings often are unremarkable. Although individual parameters might be only mildly abnormal, test results often reflect a pattern suggesting hepatocellular dysfunction in the absence of significant cholestasis or hepatocellular necrosis.

- Hematologic findings include microcytosis, target cells, poikilocytosis (especially in cats), and mild nonregenerative anemia. Microcytosis is not usually associated with iron deficiency. These RBC changes can be subtle but important diagnostic clues in an otherwise normal CBC.
- Urinalysis findings include dilute urine, ammonium biurate crystalluria, and mild bilirubinuria.
- Coagulation tests are normal. Mild thrombocytopenia occasionally is noted but does not appear to be clinically significant.
- Hepatocellular dysfunction is suggested by hypoproteinemia, hypoalbuminemia, hypoglobulinemia, hypoglycemia, decreased BUN, and mild hypocholesterolemia. Hypoalbuminemia is a consistent finding

in dogs, but not in cats. Total serum bilirubin concentration is normal.

- Liver enzyme (ALP and ALT) activity is normal to mildly (2–3 times) increased, consistent with a lesion of hepatic atrophy and minimal hepatocellular injury or intrahepatic cholestasis. Increases in ALP activity in these young animals may actually be due to the bone isoenzyme.
- Measure SBA concentrations to document hepatic dysfunction in dogs and cats suspected of having congenital PSS. Fasting SBA concentrations may be normal or increased, but PPSBA concentrations are consistently abnormal and usually exceed 100 μmol/liter. This pattern of normal FSBA concentrations with markedly increased PPSBA levels is characteristic of PSS. A consistently normal PPSBA concentration excludes a diagnosis of congenital PSS.
- Hyperammonemia is a common finding in animals with PSS, but fasting blood ammonia concentration may be normal. The ammonia tolerance test is consistently abnormal and is equal in sensitivity to PPSBA concentrations for detecting hepatic dysfunction associated with PSS (see Diagnostic Strategy for Liver Disease).

Radiography

- Microhepatica is a common radiographic finding in dogs, but not cats. Mild renomegaly of unknown clinical significance also is common. Intra-abdominal detail may be poor because of lack of abdominal fat. Ammonium urate urinary calculi may be visible on survey radiographs if they contain substantial amounts of magnesium and phosphate.
- Routine abdominal ultrasonography may demonstrate intrahepatic and extrahepatic shunts. Urinary calculi also can be identified.
- Rectal portal scintigraphy using technetium 99m pertechnetate is a noninvasive test (available at some referral institutions) that can confirm whether a shunt is present; however, it does not provide reliable anatomic information such as the type and location of the shunt.
- Positive-contrast portography is the procedure of choice to accurately characterize the type and location of a PSS. Techniques include splenoportography, mesenteric (or jejunal) portography, and cranial mesenteric or celiac arterial portography. An operative mesenteric portogram is preferred because it allows evaluation of the entire portal vein, does not require special equipment, and results in few complications.
- Institute therapy for hepatic encephalopathy prior to giving anesthesia for portography or for surgical correction (see below).

Technique

For Mesenteric Portography

1. Place the animal under general anesthesia (see sec. 1, ch. 2 for anesthesia of the patient with liver disease).
2. Isolate a loop of jejunum through a ventral midline incision.
3. Place two ligatures around a jejunal vein, and place an over-the-needle catheter (Abbocath, Abbott Hospitals) within the vessel. Tie the ligatures and secure the catheter to the vessel.
4. Temporarily close the abdominal incision.
5. Inject a water-soluble contrast agent (Conray, Mallinckrodt) as a bolus (2 ml/kg body weight) into the catheter.
6. If a rapid film changer is not available, take a lateral and ventrodorsal radiograph as the final milliliter is injected.

Interpretation

- If a single PSS is identified, it should be further characterized as intrahepatic or extrahepatic, because this has important surgical ramifications (see sec. 7, ch. 9).
- If multiple extrahepatic PSSs are identified, portal pressure determination and gross and microscopic findings of the liver are used to distinguish between congenital and acquired causes. An intrahepatic arteriovenous fistula should be considered in young dogs and cats with portal hypertension and secondary PSS (see next section).
- Identification of a patent intrahepatic portal system on portography is a favorable prognostic factor. Failure to visualize the intrahepatic portal system is not a reliable indicator of vascular atresia but may correlate with a greater occurrence of postoperative complications after complete or partial shunt ligation.
- In a young dog with hyperammonemia and hepatic encephalopathy, in which the liver biopsy and portogram are normal, suspect a rare congenital urea cycle enzyme deficiency.

Liver Biopsy and Histopathologic Evaluation

- The liver is grossly small but otherwise fairly normal in appearance.
- In some animals, biopsy findings are unremarkable.
- Liver biopsy most consistently reveals hepatocyte atrophy with small or absent portal veins. Varying degrees of sinusoidal congestion, biliary hyperplasia, arteriolar proliferation, lipogranulomata, and increased periportal connective tissue may be seen. Hepatocellular vacuolization is sometimes noted and may be severe.
- Microscopic CNS abnormalities include polymicrocavitation of the brain stem and cerebellum and an increased number of astrocytes in the cerebral cortex.

Treatment

Surgery

- The treatment of choice for dogs and cats with a single PSS is partial or total surgical ligation of the shunt (see sec. 7, ch. 9).
- Surgical ligation of multiple shunts is contraindicated. Suture attenuation (banding) of the abdominal vena cava has been recommended to raise the systemic venous pressure slightly above portal pressure,

thus increasing hepatic portal blood flow and improving hepatic function. Worsening of ascites and rear limb edema is a common complication.

Medical Therapy

Medical management of dogs and cats with PSS is palliative and is directed primarily at control of hepatic encephalopathy with a low-protein diet, lactulose, and neomycin (see Table 1).

- The short-term response to therapy for hepatic encephalopathy is often dramatic, and the animal usually is clinically normal even prior to surgical shunt ligation.
- If surgical shunt correction is not feasible or is declined by the owner, long-term medical management may control clinical signs for as long as 2–3 years. However, medical management of PSS does not reverse the progressive hepatic atrophy and alterations in carbohydrate, lipid, and protein metabolism.
- Acute decompensation of encephalopathy requires fluid therapy for correction of dehydration, electrolyte, and acid-base imbalances, and maintenance of blood glucose levels (see Table 1).
- When severe CNS depression or coma prevents the oral administration of lactulose and neomycin, administer these drugs via an enema (see Table 1).
- Identify and correct precipitating causes of encephalopathy whenever possible, such as hypoglycemia, GI bleeding from hookworm infection, and hypokalemia (see Table 1).
- Management of urate urolithiasis is discussed in sec. 8, ch. 3.

Complications

- Occasionally, seizures or status epilepticus is a complication of surgical shunt ligation. The pathogenesis is obscure, but seizures do not appear to be caused by simple hypoglycemia or hepatic encephalopathy.
- In addition to routine management of hepatic encephalopathy and correction of underlying metabolic imbalances such as hypoglycemia and hypocalcemia, manage seizures with intravenous phenobarbital. If seizures cannot be controlled with phenobarbital, consider general anesthesia with isoflurane.
- Mannitol may be indicated for control of cerebral edema and a respirator may be required to maintain pO_2 and pCO_2.
- The prognosis for recovery from this complication is poor.

Prognosis

The prognosis for resolution of signs after partial or total surgical ligation of the shunt is excellent if the animal survives the postoperative period. Most animals will remain clinically normal despite hepatic function tests that are improved but not completely normal.

HEPATIC ARTERIOVENOUS FISTULA

Intrahepatic arteriovenous (AV) fistulas are vascular communications between the hepatic artery and portal vein that result in portal hypertension, ascites, and secondary portosystemic shunts. They occur rarely in dogs and cats.

Etiology

Intrahepatic AV fistulas may be congenital, which is most common, or acquired as a result of abdominal trauma, hepatic surgery, hepatic neoplasia, cirrhosis, or rupture of a hepatic artery aneurysm.

Clinical Signs

Signs are similar to those of congenital PSS and include anorexia, lethargy, vomiting, diarrhea, PU/PD, and encephalopathy in a young animal (usually <1.5 years).

Diagnosis

History and Physical Examination

- Historical and physical findings are similar to those in congenital PSS, with the notable exception that marked ascites is a consistent finding with hepatic AV fistulas but is uncommon with congenital PSS.
- Other causes of ascites to be differentiated include hypoproteinemia and right-sided congestive heart failure.
- Auscultate the abdominal wall over the area of the liver for a continuous murmur (bruit) caused by runoff of arterial blood into the portal system.

Laboratory Evaluation

- Laboratory abnormalities are similar to those seen in congenital PSS and include hypoproteinemia, normal or mildly increased liver enzyme activity, and abnormal liver function tests including FSBA and PPSBA, blood ammonia and ATT, and BSP retention.
- Ascitic fluid typically is a transudate.

Radiography

- Survey radiographs show marked ascites.
- On abdominal ultrasonography, hepatic AV fistulas appear as tortuous, anechoic tubular structures in the liver. Multiple extrahepatic PSSs may also be identified.

Laparotomy

- The diagnosis is confirmed by celiac arteriography or exploratory laparotomy. Grossly, AV fistulas appear as thin-walled, tortuous, pulsating vascular channels that distort the hepatic parenchyma and elevate the overlying hepatic capsule.

Treatment

- Partial hepatectomy is indicated for treatment of hepatic AV fistulas involving one liver lobe (see sec. 7, ch. 9). Dearterialization is required if multiple lobes are involved.
- Despite resection of involved liver lobes, hepatic

function may not return to normal because of persistent shunting of portal blood through acquired PSS. Caudal vena cava banding has been recommended in this setting.

■ Medical management of hepatic encephalopathy with low-protein diet, lactulose, and neomycin is indicated (see Table 1).

HEPATOBILIARY NEOPLASIA

Primary and metastatic tumors are a significant cause of hepatic disease in dogs and cats. Metastatic tumors are more common than primary hepatic neoplasms. Lymphoma and pancreatic carcinoma are common secondary tumors.

Primary hepatic tumors of epithelial origin include:

■ Malignant tumors—hepatocellular carcinoma and cholangiocellular carcinoma (bile duct carcinoma). These tumors occur in three pathologic forms:
  • Massive—a single large mass in one liver lobe;
  • Nodular—discrete nodules in several liver lobes;
  • Diffuse—infiltration of large portions of the liver by nonencapsulated neoplastic tissue.
■ Benign tumors—hepatocellular adenoma (hepatoma) and cholangiocellular adenoma (bile duct adenoma).
  • Hepatocellular adenomas usually are single, large, pedunculated masses.
  • Bile duct adenomas usually are multilobular cystic structures containing clear mucinous fluid.

Primary hepatic tumors of mesodermal origin (sarcomas) are much less common and include fibroma, fibrosarcoma, hemangioma, hemangiosarcoma, leiomyosarcoma, and osteosarcoma.

Etiology

The cause of spontaneous primary hepatic neoplasms in dogs and cats is unknown.

Clinical Signs

Most affected animals are older and have vague, nonspecific signs of hepatic dysfunction that often do not appear until the more advanced stages of hepatic disease.

■ The most consistent signs are anorexia, lethargy, weight loss, vomiting, and abdominal distension.
■ Other signs include PU/PD, jaundice, diarrhea, and excessive bleeding.
■ Signs of CNS dysfunction such as depression, dementia, and seizures can be attributed to hepatic encephalopathy, hypoglycemia, or CNS metastases.

Diagnosis

Suspect hepatobiliary neoplasia in an older animal with clinical and biochemical evidence of hepatic disease accompanied by hepatomegaly.

Physical Examination

■ Findings often include a cranial abdominal mass or marked hepatomegaly. Abdominal effusion and hepatomegaly contribute to abdominal distension.
■ Other potential findings include pallor, jaundice, and cachexia.

Laboratory Evaluation

■ Potential hematologic findings include anemia and leukocytosis. Anemia usually is nonregenerative but may be regenerative if associated with excess bleeding or tumor rupture.
■ Biochemical findings are variable and nonspecific for liver disease. Increases in liver enzyme activity (ALT and ALP) usually are mild to marked but may be normal, especially with metastatic tumors. Other findings include hyperbilirubinemia, hypoalbuminemia, hyperglobulinemia, increased SBA concentrations, prolonged BSP dye retention, and abnormal coagulation tests.
■ Hypoglycemia, sometimes severe, occasionally is noted in dogs with hepatocellular carcinoma and less frequently with hepatocellular adenoma, leiomyosarcoma, and hemangiosarcoma. Serum insulin concentrations are normal to decreased.
  • Potential mechanisms of hypoglycemia include excess utilization of glucose by the tumor, release of insulin-like factors from the tumor, release of other factors such as somatostatin, and secondary hepatic parenchymal destruction with impaired glycogenolysis or gluconeogenesis.
■ Increased serum alpha-fetoprotein concentration (>250 ng/ml by enzymetry) may be an indicator of hepatocellular carcinoma and cholangiocellular carcinoma in dogs.
■ Analysis of abdominal effusion usually reveals a modified transudate, sometimes containing hemorrhage or neoplastic cells.

Radiography

■ Abdominal radiographic findings include symmetric or asymmetric hepatomegaly and ascites.
■ Perform thoracic radiographs to detect pulmonary metastases.
■ Ultrasonographic findings include focal, multifocal, or diffuse changes in hepatic echotexture.
  • Carcinomas appear as focal or multifocal hyperechoic, hypoechoic, or mixed echogenic lesions. Unfortunately, benign nodular hyperplasia, an aging change of minimal clinical significance, has a similar appearance.
  • Hepatocellular carcinoma usually appears as a focal hyperechoic mass.
  • Hepatic lymphoma may appear as a diffuse, mildly hyperechoic or multifocal hypoechoic pattern.
  • Ultrasonography may be unremarkable with diffuse hepatic involvement. The diagnosis of hepatic neoplasia cannot be made based on ultrasonographic findings alone.

Liver Biopsy/Histopathologic Evaluation

Definitive diagnosis of hepatic neoplasia requires liver biopsy and histopathologic evaluation.

- The procedure of choice for a single, large hepatic mass is laparotomy because excision of the mass can be performed concurrently.
- Ultrasound-guided biopsy is useful to diagnose focal or diffuse hepatic involvement.
- Blind percutaneous needle biopsy or fine-needle aspiration biopsy is most useful for diagnosis of diffuse hepatic neoplasia such as lymphoma, myeloproliferative disorders, and mastocytosis.

Treatment

Surgery

- Surgical removal of the affected liver lobe is the treatment of choice for primary hepatic neoplasms such as hepatocellular adenoma or carcinoma that involves a single lobe (see sec. 7, ch. 9). Early detection affords the best chance for success.
- Make a complete evaluation of the abdominal cavity for evidence of metastases and biopsy hepatic lymph nodes.
- When all lobes are affected, the prognosis is poor.

Chemotherapy

- Chemotherapy currently is not an effective means of control for primary liver tumors in dogs and cats.
- Secondary hepatic neoplasms such as lymphoma, mastocytosis, and myeloproliferative disease may temporarily respond to chemotherapeutic intervention (see sec. 3, chs. 5 and 6).

HEPATIC CYSTS

Single or multiple hepatic cysts occasionally are identified in the liver of dogs and cats, usually as incidental findings at necropsy but occasionally in the live animal.

Etiology

Hepatic cysts can be congenital or acquired, although this distinction is often difficult to make.

- Congenital polycystic disease of the liver and kidneys has been reported in Cairn terriers.
- Polycystic renal disease in cats has been associated with cystic dilation of the intrahepatic bile ducts (see sec. 8, ch. 1).
- Acquired cysts may represent benign bile duct adenomas.

Clinical Signs

- Most solitary hepatic cysts do not cause any clinical signs unless they compress or displace adjacent structures. Signs are more likely to occur when congenital polycystic disease is accompanied by dilation of the extrahepatic biliary tract.
- Affected Cairn terriers may be presented with abdominal distension caused by renomegaly and hepatomegaly.

Diagnosis and Treatment

Suspect a hepatic cyst whenever a cavitated hepatic mass lesion is detected by palpation, radiography, or ultrasonography.

- Surgery can confirm the diagnosis and allows excision of large solitary cysts.

CHOLELITHIASIS

Cholelithiasis occurs infrequently in dogs and cats. Choleliths may be present in the gallbladder (cholecystolithiasis), common bile duct (choledocholithiasis), or rarely, in the hepatic and lobar ducts. Most choleliths in dogs and cats consist of insoluble bile pigments. Minor components such as calcium, bile salts, protein, magnesium, phosphorus, iron, carbonate, and cholesterol also have been identified. Cholesterol choleliths, the most common type of stone in humans, are less likely to form in dogs because the cholesterol content of dog bile is lower than that in humans, and dogs have a better capacity for maintaining biliary cholesterol in solution. Little is known about the cholesterol content of cat bile, but cholesterol choleliths have been reported.

Etiology

The cause of spontaneous cholelithiasis in dogs and cats often cannot be determined. It is generally believed that gallstone formation requires initial nidus formation, retention of particles in the gallbladder, and then sustained growth of the cholelith. The following factors may be important in the development of pigment stones.

- Bile stasis and sludged bile is primarily composed of mucin, which subsequently binds calcium bilirubin pigments and cholesterol crystals.
- Increased gallbladder mucin acts as a nidus for cholelith formation.
- Cholecystitis and cholangitis can be associated with cholelithiasis, especially in cats. It is difficult to determine whether choleliths were formed as a consequence of bile stasis, inflammation, and bacterial infection, or whether cholelithiasis initiated the inflammation, which led to secondary biliary stasis and infection.
- Bacteria such as *E. coli* contain beta-glucuronidase, which can deconjugate bilirubin to a less soluble form that precipitates with calcium.
- Dietary factors are unlikely with balanced diets; however, dogs fed an experimental diet that is low in protein and fat, high in carbohydrates, and supplemented with cholesterol will form pigment stones. This diet is deficient in taurine, which may contribute to cholelithiasis by precipitating bile acids.

Clinical Signs

- Dogs and cats with cholelithiasis often are asymptomatic. Clinical signs are most likely when cholelithiasis is complicated by bacterial infection, extrahepatic bile duct obstruction, perforation of the gallbladder or bile ducts, or secondary hepatic involvement (cholangiohepatitis or biliary cirrhosis).
- Common signs include jaundice, vomiting, anorexia, weight loss, and dehydration.
- Signs may be acute or chronic, intermittent or persistent. An acute onset is most likely with sudden obstruction of the cystic or common bile duct by the cholelith or rupture of the gallbladder.

Diagnosis

Although it is uncommon, consider cholelithiasis in the differential diagnosis of any dog or cat with cholestatic hepatobiliary disease.

History and Physical Examination

- A long-standing history (months to years) of intermittent jaundice and vomiting is present in some affected animals.
- Physical examination may be unremarkable or findings may include jaundice, abdominal discomfort, hepatomegaly, fever, and abdominal distension. Fever is usually indicative of concurrent biliary bacterial infection or septic or bile peritonitis. Abdominal distension due to fluid accumulation is seen with secondary rupture of the biliary tract.
- Excessive bleeding may be noted with chronic common bile duct obstruction.
- Acholic feces are indicative of complete bile duct obstruction.

Laboratory Evaluation

- Laboratory findings may be unremarkable.
- Biochemical evaluation of symptomatic patients is not specific for cholelithiasis but is indicative of cholestatic hepatobiliary disease. Findings include moderate to marked increases in ALP and GGT activity and in cholesterol, SBA, and total serum bilirubin concentrations. Serum ALT activity usually is increased, indicating secondary hepatocyte damage associated with severe cholestasis.
- Potential hematologic findings include neutrophilia with a left shift, usually indicating bacterial cholangitis or cholecystitis or complications such as a ruptured gallbladder. A mild, nonregenerative anemia is common. With chronic extrahepatic bile duct obstruction, coagulation tests may be affected by vitamin K malabsorption.
- With biliary rupture, abdominocentesis reveals bile peritonitis.

Radiography

- On routine abdominal radiographs, choleliths may appear as radiopaque densities in the area of the gallbladder or bile ducts. However, pigment stones are usually radiolucent unless they contain calcium. Hepatomegaly is common.
- Other findings are determined by the presence of complications such as obstruction (a distended gallbladder), emphysematous cholecystitis (gas density in the area of the gallbladder), and peritonitis (loss of abdominal detail).

Ultrasonography

- Ultrasonography detects both radiolucent and radiopaque choleliths as hyperechoic densities in the gallbladder and bile ducts. Choleliths are differentiated from mural masses by the presence of acoustic shadowing and movement of the density with changes in position of the animal.
- Inspissated or sludged bile also appears in the gallbladder as an echogenic substance, but sludge does not cause acoustic shadowing. Sludged bile may indicate biliary stasis but can also be seen in sick, anorexic animals without clinical biliary tract disease.
- Complications of cholelithiasis can be identified ultrasonographically, such as distension of the gallbladder and bile ducts with cystic or common bile duct obstruction, thickening of the biliary tract associated with inflammation, abdominal fluid accumulation with rupture of the gallbladder, and absence of the gallbladder.

KEY POINT ▶ Because the majority of choleliths do not cause clinical signs, surgical removal may not always be warranted.

Laparotomy

Exploratory laparotomy generally is required for definitive diagnosis and treatment of cholelithiasis.

- Pigment choleliths usually are greenish-brown to black and may be single or multiple. Bile sludge appears grossly as viscous, greenish-black bile containing sandlike gritty material.
- Diagnostic and therapeutic procedures performed during exploratory laparotomy include:
  - Evaluation of the patency of the gallbladder and bile ducts
  - Removal of choleliths for chemical analysis and bacterial culture
  - Identification and repair of secondary biliary rupture
  - Collection of samples of affected tissue (liver, gallbladder) and bile for aerobic and anaerobic bacterial culture and biopsy.

Histopathologic Evaluation

- Histopathologic changes in the gallbladder, bile ducts, and liver may be absent with uncomplicated cholelithiasis. However, mild cholangitis and cholecystitis are common.

Treatment

- Institute supportive therapy to correct fluid, electrolyte, and acid-base imbalances prior to surgery.
- If a coagulopathy is detected, give vitamin K_1 for 24–48 hours prior to surgery (see Table 1).

- Administer systemic antibiotics in animals with inflammatory biliary tract disease and cholelithiasis. Ideally, base the choice of antibiotic on culture and sensitivity testing of bile and hepatic tissue obtained at surgery. See the discussion of antibiotic therapy of biliary infections under Cholangiohepatitis.
- Management of complications of cholelithiasis, such as ruptured gallbladder and biliary obstruction and rupture of the biliary tract, is discussed later in this chapter.
- Surgery of the biliary tract is discussed in sec. 7, ch. 9.

Prognosis

Little is known about the likelihood of recurrence of cholelithiasis in dogs and cats.

- If the underlying mechanism of cholelith formation is not reversed, recurrence is possible.
- A well-balanced commercial diet is recommended.
- Manage persistent cholangitis or cholangiohepatitis as described previously in this chapter.

EXTRAHEPATIC BILIARY OBSTRUCTION

Extrahepatic biliary obstruction of the common bile duct or large hepatic ducts interrupts bile flow into the intestine.

Etiology

Biliary obstruction can be a complication of primary biliary tract disorders such as cholelithiasis or biliary tumors or can be caused by extrahepatic disorders such as pancreatic fibrosis, and pancreatic or duodenal masses (Table 8).

Clinical Signs

- Signs of biliary obstruction include anorexia, vomiting, jaundice, weight loss, abdominal pain, diarrhea, acholic feces, and excessive bleeding.
- Diarrhea and steatorrhea are characterized by tan-colored feces and are attributed to failure to secrete bile acids, which results in malabsorption of fat and fat-soluble vitamins such as vitamin K.
  - With prolonged extrahepatic biliary obstruction, vitamin K malabsorption and the subsequent decreased synthesis of vitamin K–dependent factors results in a coagulopathy.

TABLE 8. Causes of Extrahepatic Biliary Obstruction

Cholelithiasis
Inspissated (sludged) bile
Cholangitis and cholecystitis
Acute pancreatitis, pancreatic abscess, pancreatic fibrosis
Biliary, hepatic, pancreatic, and duodenal neoplasia
Biliary stricture
Biliary hematoma
Liver flukes
Diaphragmatic hernia with entrapment of the gallbladder

- With complete biliary obstruction, the feces may become clay-colored because of a lack of bile pigments.

Diagnosis

The diagnostic strategy is to identify that biliary obstruction is present and, second, to identify the underlying cause of obstruction.

Physical Examination

- Findings include jaundice and hepatomegaly due to bile engorgement of the liver.
- A firm, distended gallbladder occasionally is palpated.
- Other findings are dependent on the underlying cause of obstruction, such as palpation of an abdominal mass (pancreatic or biliary neoplasia) and abdominal pain (acute pancreatitis, peritonitis).
- Fever may suggest bacterial cholangitis, biliary rupture with peritonitis, pancreatitis, or pancreatic abscess.

Laboratory Evaluation

- Biochemical findings reflect marked cholestasis, including increased serum concentrations of ALP, GGT, cholesterol, bile acids, and bilirubin. Unfortunately, biochemical findings cannot distinguish whether cholestasis is caused by intrahepatic or extrahepatic mechanisms. In general, values for total bilirubin and ALP activity tend to be higher with extrahepatic biliary obstruction. Serum ALT and AST activity are concurrently increased, due to secondary hepatic damage.
- On the CBC, a mild neutrophilia and mild, nonregenerative anemia are common. Neutrophilia with a left shift suggests the possibility of acute pancreatitis or abscess, bacterial cholangitis/cholecystitis, or biliary rupture.
- Findings on urinalysis include bilirubinuria and absence of urobilinogen.
- With vitamin K malabsorption, findings include prolonged PT, APTT, and activated clotting time (ACT). Platelet function defects have also been documented in dogs with biliary obstruction.

Radiography

Abdominal Radiography. Abdominal radiography is frequently nondiagnostic.

- Occasionally, a large, fluid-filled gallbladder can be seen superimposed over the liver. The liver may be normal to increased in size. Chronic biliary obstruction in dogs may lead to biliary cirrhosis and microhepatica.
- Other radiographic findings depend on the underlying cause of obstruction and may include cholelithiasis, emphysematous cholecystitis, pancreatitis, and mass lesions.

Ultrasonography. Ultrasonography is helpful to confirm extrahepatic biliary obstruction and to evaluate the underlying cause.

- In normal dogs, the cystic duct, common bile duct, and intrahepatic ducts are not visible. The cystic duct may be visible in some normal cats.
- With biliary obstruction, the biliary system, including the gallbladder, cystic duct, common bile duct, and intrahepatic ducts, becomes progressively dilated. The earliest detectable change is distension of the gallbladder and cystic duct, which occurs within 24 hours. By 48 hours, the common bile duct also is distended. Distension of intrahepatic ducts is not detected until 4–7 days after obstruction. Dilated hepatic biliary ducts are differentiated from hepatic and portal veins by their tortuosity and irregular branching patterns.
- Ultrasonographic evaluation of gallbladder emptying after cholecystokinin injection may be helpful to confirm biliary obstruction.
- Ultrasonography may identify underlying causes of biliary obstruction such as cholelithiasis, pancreatitis, or mass lesions.

Hepatobiliary Scintigraphy. Hepatobiliary scintigraphy may be used to confirm biliary obstruction but is available only at tertiary referral centers.

Laparotomy

Exploratory laparotomy usually is required to confirm extrahepatic biliary obstruction and to identify the underlying cause. The following diagnostic procedures are routinely performed:

- Evaluate bile duct and gallbladder patency.
- Identify location and cause of obstruction.
- Evaluate for evidence of secondary rupture of the biliary tract.
- Collect a sample of bile for aerobic and anaerobic bacterial cultures.
- Perform a liver biopsy.

Treatment
Surgery

Specific therapy requires surgery to correct the underlying cause of obstruction (see sec. 7, ch. 9).

- Prior to surgery, stabilize the patient with fluid therapy. Give vitamin K_1 parenterally for 24–48 hours prior to surgery to correct a coagulopathy.
- With complete biliary obstruction, no antibiotics are known to enter the bile.

Medical Therapy

If biliary obstruction occurs secondary to acute pancreatitis, manage the pancreatitis medically (see sec. 7, ch. 10) and reserve surgery for those patients in which biliary obstruction does not resolve with resolution of pancreatic inflammation.

BILIARY RUPTURE

Leakage of bile into the abdominal cavity results in chemical peritonitis that can be complicated by sepsis.

Etiology

- Biliary tract rupture is most frequently caused by blunt or sharp abdominal trauma from automobile-induced injuries, gunshot injuries, and bite wounds. Ductal rupture is most likely with blunt abdominal trauma.
- Other causes include cholelithiasis, cholecystitis, biliary neoplasms, and iatrogenic puncture during percutaneous liver biopsy. These usually cause gallbladder rupture.

Clinical Signs

- When gallbladder rupture occurs secondary to cholecystitis or cholelithiasis, acute onset of anorexia, vomiting, diarrhea, jaundice, abdominal pain, fever, and shock may occur.
- Signs of biliary duct rupture secondary to trauma tend to be chronic and develop more slowly than with rupture of the gallbladder. With traumatic biliary rupture, early signs such as abdominal pain and vomiting are frequently overshadowed by more immediate signs of shock, fractures, and other injuries. Other signs, such as anorexia, listlessness, weight loss, jaundice, ascites, and acholic feces, do not occur until days or weeks following the traumatic event.

Diagnosis
History and Physical Examination

- A history of recent abdominal trauma and progressive jaundice and abdominal distension suggests the possibility of biliary rupture.
- Physical examination findings consistent with biliary rupture include jaundice, abdominal distension, and acholic feces.
- Abdominal pain is most likely with acute rupture or septic peritonitis.
- Fever may occur with septic peritonitis or cholecystitis.

Laboratory Evaluation

- Laboratory findings include hyperbilirubinemia and increased ALP, ALT, and SBA concentrations.
- Abdominal fluid appears yellow or green. Chemical tests for bilirubin are positive and concentrations of bilirubin are higher in the abdominal fluid than in the serum.
- Cytologic examination reveals a mixed inflammatory infiltrate and bile-laden macrophages.
- Bacteria may be seen if bile peritonitis is complicated by sepsis.

Radiography

- Abdominal radiographs reveal poor abdominal contrast due to fluid accumulation.
- On ultrasonography, the gallbladder may not be visible, and even a small amount of abdominal fluid may be detected.
- Other radiographic and ultrasonographic findings

depend on the underlying cause of rupture, such as cholelithiasis, cholecystitis, and biliary neoplasia.

■ When trauma is suspected as the cause of biliary rupture, take thoracic films to detect other complications such as pneumothorax, diaphragmatic hernia, and bile pleuritis.

Laparotomy

Rupture of the biliary tract is confirmed at laparotomy.

■ Rupture of the gallbladder secondary to cholecystitis may be acute or chronic. With chronic gallbladder rupture, omental and hepatic adhesions are common. Biliary fistulas may develop from the gallbladder to other abdominal structures such as the diaphragm.

■ Submit abdominal fluid and affected biliary tissue for aerobic and anaerobic bacterial culture.

Treatment

Surgery is required to repair the biliary rupture and is discussed in sec. 7, ch. 9.

■ Prior to surgery, stabilize the patient with fluid therapy and give vitamin K_1 parenterally for 24–48 hours and antibiotics.

Supplemental Readings

Center SA: Pathophysiology and laboratory diagnosis of liver disease. *In* Ettinger SJ, ed.: *Textbook of Veterinary Internal Medicine*, Vol 2, 3rd Ed. Philadelphia: W. B. Saunders, 1989, p 1421.

Hardy RM: Diseases of the liver and their treatment. *In* Ettinger SJ, ed.: *Textbook of Veterinary Internal Medicine*, Vol 2, 3rd Ed. Philadelphia: W. B. Saunders, 1989, p 1479.

Johnson SE: Liver and biliary tract. *In* Anderson NV, ed.: *Veterinary Gastroenterology*, 2nd Ed. Philadelphia: Lea & Febiger, 1992, p 504.

Jones BD, Hitt M, Hurst T, et al.: Hepatic biopsy. Vet Clin North Am [Small Anim Pract] 15:39, 1985.

Strombeck DR, Guilford WG, eds.: *Small Animal Gastroenterology*, 2nd Ed. Davis CA: Stonegate, 1990.

Zawie DA, Shaker E: Diseases of the liver. *In* Sherding RG, ed.: *The Cat: Diseases and Clinical Management*, Vol. 2. New York: Churchill Livingstone, 1989, p 1015.

Liver and Biliary Surgery

Stephen Birchard

Surgery of the liver and biliary tract is commonly performed in small animals and can be very challenging. Animals frequently are presented with surgical diseases of these organs, such as liver tumors and obstruction or infection of the biliary system. Some of the procedures described below require specialized training and facilities. Others, such as liver biopsy, partial hepatectomy, and simple exploration of the biliary tract, can be performed in a standard veterinary practice. Regardless of the procedure, preparation for the surgery by reviewing anatomy, pathophysiology, and specific techniques is very important for a successful outcome. Preparation of the patient prior to surgery also is extremely important because most of these diseases have serious metabolic effects.

SURGERY OF THE LIVER

Anatomy

Liver Lobes

- The liver is divided into six lobes: the right lateral, right medial, caudate, quadrate, left lateral, and left medial.
- The caudate lobe is divided into the caudate process and the papillary process.

Liver Attachments

- The major liver attachments to other organs and the body wall are the triangular, hepatogastric, and hepatoduodenal ligaments.
- The falciform ligament extends from the liver to the diaphragm and ventral abdominal wall. This mesenteric remnant can be quite large and fat-filled in obese animals. Usually it is best to remove this structure during liver surgery to gain better visualization of important structures.
- The hepatorenal ligament is a thin fold of peritoneum that extends from the renal fossa of the caudate lobe to the ventral surface of the right kidney.

Blood Supply

Portal Vein

- The portal vein receives blood from the spleen, pancreas, and intestines.
- The major hepatic branches of the portal vein are the right lateral trunk, right medial branch, and left lateral trunk.
- The portal vein is the combination of the cranial and caudal mesenteric veins and the splenic vein.

- The portal vein can be seen at the base of the mesoduodenum. It forms the ventral boundary of the epiploic foramen.
- The portal vein eventually empties into the liver and supplies approximately 80% of the oxygenation of the liver. The remaining 20% comes from the hepatic arteries.
- In the fetus, the ductus venosus connects the portal vein to the caudal vena cava, allowing blood to bypass the liver. This vessel closes soon after birth in normal dogs. If it remains patent, it is called a patent ductus venosus and is one of the several types of portosystemic shunts.

Hepatic Arteries and Veins

- The hepatic artery is a branch of the celiac artery. Variable numbers of hepatic artery branches supply the liver lobes.
- Six to eight large hepatic veins drain the liver lobes to the caudal vena cava.
- The hepatic veins enter the vena cava at the hilus of the liver and are obscured by the liver parenchyma.

Preoperative Considerations

Liver diseases cause a variety of significant hematologic and metabolic disorders in animals. Prior to initiating surgery, perform appropriate diagnostics to confirm the disease and check for involvement of other organs. (See sec. 7, ch. 8 for diagnosis of liver problems.)

Of particular concern to the surgeon are the following potential problems:

- Hypoproteinemia—Evaluate serum proteins and consider administration of plasma or hyperalimentation if significantly low.
- Anemia—Evaluate the animal's hemogram and establish a baseline packed cell volume so that changes can be kept in perspective. Blood loss before, during, and after liver surgery is common and should be monitored closely.
- Coagulopathy—Analyze the animal's coagulation profile and correct abnormalities if possible (see sec. 3, ch. 2). Fresh whole blood transfusion before or during surgery may be necessary.
- Diffuse disease—Hepatic neoplasia may result in metastatic lesions. Thoracic and abdominal radiography and abdominal ultrasonography are helpful in determining the extent of disease.
- Impaired liver function—Manage hepatic encephalopathy, if present, medically (see sec. 7, ch. 8) to stabilize the animal prior to surgery.

761

■ Hypoglycemia—Consider giving the animal intravenous fluids supplemented with glucose before and during surgery (e.g., 5% dextrose in lactated Ringer's solution).

KEY POINT ▶ Diffuse hepatic disease may cause serious metabolic problems which can be compounded by anesthesia and surgery. Analyze liver function tests, such as serum bile acid and blood ammonia concentrations (see sec. 7, ch. 8) to determine the animal's ability to undergo anesthesia and surgery.

■ Liver trauma
  • Thoroughly evaluate all animals with a history of trauma to rule out thoracic trauma such as pneumothorax, pulmonary contusions, and other cardiopulmonary problems. Evaluate for damage to other organs such as the urinary tract, gastrointestinal tract, and neurologic and skeletal systems.
  • Animals with liver trauma usually have hemoperitoneum. Severe blood loss will cause clinical signs of shock and should be treated (see sec. 6, ch. 14 for treatment of hypovolemic shock).

KEY POINT ▶ Most animals with liver trauma can be treated conservatively (e.g., intravenous fluids or whole blood and autotransfusion of abdominal blood if not contaminated with bacteria or neoplastic cells).

Liver Biopsy and Partial Hepatectomy—Surgical Procedure

Objectives

■ Examine the entire liver for grossly evident abnormalities.
■ Obtain tissues for biopsy or completely remove the lesion by partial hepatectomy.
■ Minimize intraoperative blood loss.

Equipment

■ Standard general surgery pack and suture
■ Balfour and malleable retractors
■ Tru-Cut biopsy needle or skin punch biopsy instrument
■ Tissue stapling device (e.g., U.S. Surgical Autosuture TA) (optional)
■ Gelfoam

Technique

1. Place the animal in dorsal recumbency and prepare the entire ventral abdomen and caudal one-third of the sternum for aseptic surgery.
2. Perform a standard ventral midline abdominal approach. If additional exposure is necessary, also perform a left or right paracostal abdominal incision or a median sternotomy.
3. Use laparotomy sponges to protect the abdominal wall and place Balfour retractors to expose the liver and associated viscera.
4. Identify areas of liver to be removed or biopsied. If necessary, mobilize involved liver lobes by incising triangular ligaments. Greater exposure of the liver can be achieved by placing a laparotomy sponge between it and the diaphragm.
5. Liver biopsy can be achieved by a variety of techniques:
   a. Obtain tissue samples from the periphery of the lobe, using the "guillotine" technique.
   b. Use absorbable suture to surround a small segment of liver and tie the suture tight to cut through the parenchyma and strangulate the blood vessels and bile ducts (Fig. 1). Alternatively, place the suture in a horizontal mattress pattern.
   c. Excise the tissue distal to the ligature, using a scalpel or Metzenbaum scissors. Check for bleeding and, if necessary, place a small piece of Gelfoam over the cut surface.
   d. Alternatively, use the Tru-Cut needle or skin biopsy punch to obtain small pieces of liver tissue. These are especially helpful if the lesion is centrally located in the liver lobe rather than peripherally. Be sure to include some normal tissue in the biopsy specimen.
6. Remove large lesions by partial hepatectomy (Fig. 2):
   a. Divide the liver parenchyma proximal to the lesion, using large crushing clamps or finger fractionation. Ligate the ducts and vessels with absorbable sutures (e.g., 3–0 or 4–0 chromic catgut).
   b. Alternatively, use surgical staples to crush the tissue and ligate the vessels in one step.
   c. Complete removal of an entire liver lobe requires carefully placed ligatures to attenuate the large arteries and veins at the liver hilus. Oversew or transfix the vessels to prevent ligature slippage. Place large clamps on the vessels prior to resection of the lobe to prevent cranial retraction of the vessel.

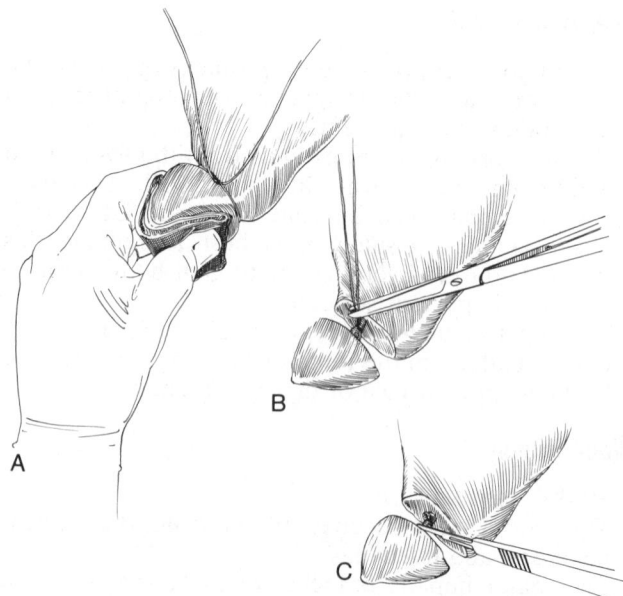

Figure 1. Guillotine method for intraoperative liver biopsy. Place a loop of absorbable suture around the tip of a liver lobe and tie tightly to cut through the liver parenchyma, ligating the vessels. Cut the suture ends and then cut the vessels to allow removal of the biopsy specimen.

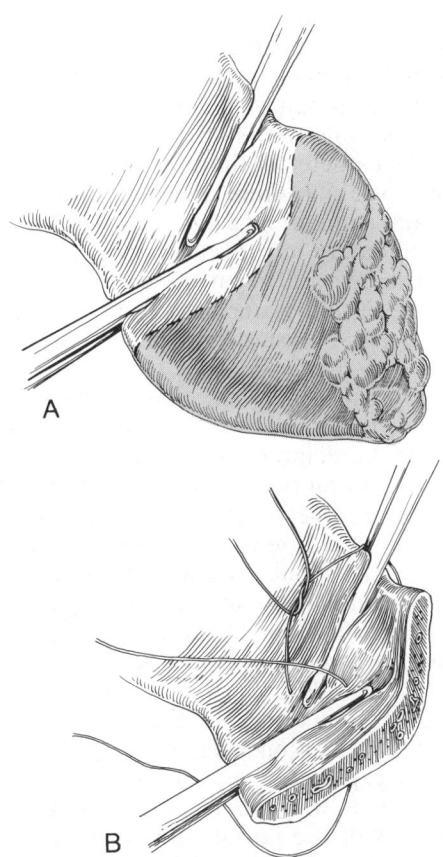

Figure 2. Partial hepatectomy. Lesions at the periphery of the liver lobe can be removed by placing crushing clamps across the lobe, proximal to the lesion, and then cutting distal to the clamps. Use absorbable sutures to ligate vessels proximal to the clamps. Tie these ligatures tightly as in the guillotine method for liver biopsy (see Fig. 1).

Postoperative Care and Complications

- Monitor for postoperative hemorrhage (oozing of blood from the incision, distension of the peritoneal cavity, pale mucous membranes). Administer blood transfusion if the hematocrit drops below 20%.
- Give supportive therapy with intravenous fluids and glucose until oral intake of food and water resumes.
- Monitor for evidence of pancreatitis (vomiting, increased serum amylase and lipase). Delay resuming oral intake and keep on intravenous fluid therapy until this resolves.

- After massive liver resection, monitor liver function by evaluating bilirubin and serum bile acid concentrations or the ammonia tolerance test. Liver function reportedly becomes abnormal after resection of 60% or more of the liver.

SURGERY FOR PORTOSYSTEMIC SHUNTS

Portosystemic shunts are abnormal vascular communications between the portal vein and a systemic vein. Diagnosis and medical treatment of this condition are discussed in sec. 7, ch. 8. Animals with portosystemic shunts can initially improve with medical management. However, the definitive and most effective therapy for long-term resolution of clinical signs is surgical attenuation of the shunt vessel. With recent advances in the intraoperative and postoperative management of these animals, morbidity and mortality rates associated with surgery have decreased to very acceptable levels.

Anatomy

Portosystemic shunts are divided anatomically into *extrahepatic* and *intrahepatic* (Fig. 3). Definition of shunt anatomy preoperatively is important because intrahepatic shunts are much more difficult to correct surgically than are extrahepatic shunts. Also, recognizing the anatomy prior to surgery helps decrease surgical time and patient morbidity.

Extrahepatic Shunts. Extrahepatic shunts are caudal to the liver. These are vascular communications between the portal vein and the caudal vena cava (portocaval shunt) or the azygos vein (portoazygos shunt). Extrahepatic portocaval shunts frequently join the caudal vena cava just adjacent to the epiploic foramen. Shunts involving the left gastric vein can be found near or on the lesser curvature of the stomach.

Intrahepatic Shunts. Intrahepatic shunts communicate with the caudal vena cava within or cranial to the liver parenchyma and can involve either the right or left branches of the hepatic portal vein.

Preoperative positive contrast portography helps differentiate between intrahepatic and extrahepatic shunts. Using these studies, the portal vein can be

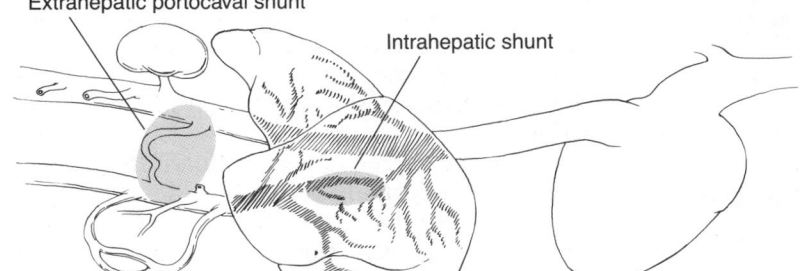

Extrahepatic portocaval shunt

Intrahepatic shunt

Figure 3. Schematic representation of an extrahepatic portocaval shunt and an intrahepatic portocaval shunt.

correlated to the thoracolumbar spine. The first branch of the hepatic portal vein (the right lateral trunk) is located at the 12th thoracic vertebra. If any part of the shunt is caudal to the 13th thoracic vertebra, it is probably extrahepatic.

Preoperative Considerations

- Stabilize the animal by medically treating the hepatic encephalopathy for 1–2 weeks (see sec. 7, ch. 8).
- Treat hypoglycemia, if present, with a 5% dextrose drip administered IV.
- If the animal is anorexic, consider giving nutritional support via nasogastric tube or some other feeding device.
- Avoid lactated Ringer's solution (LRS) for maintenance fluid administration. LRS can make the animal alkylotic and worsen the hepatic encephalopathy.

Anesthesia

KEY POINT ▶ Animals with portosystemic shunts have markedly reduced capacity to metabolize anesthetic drugs in the liver.

- Avoid using drugs such as the barbiturates and phenothiazine derivatives.
- Use diazepam (at a reduced dosage; see sec. 1, ch. 2) as a premedicant, if needed.
- Induce anesthesia via mask induction with isoflurane and oxygen or ketamine/diazepam combination (see sec. 1, ch. 2).
- Maintain anesthesia with isoflurane and oxygen via endotracheal tube.
- In addition to routine monitoring, monitor blood pressure because changes may occur during manipulation of the shunt.
- Administer a 5% dextrose drip IV during anesthesia and surgery to prevent severe hypoglycemia.

Surgical Procedure

Objectives

- Place a jejunal vein catheter to monitor portal pressures.
- Identify and attenuate the portosystemic shunt to redirect portal blood flow to the liver.
- Avoid causing portal hypertension.

Equipment*

- Standard general surgery pack and retractors (Balfour, malleable)
- Over-the-needle intravenous catheter (e.g., Jelco, Sureflo), water manometer, IV extension set, 3-way stopcock, heparinized saline
- Small and large right-angled forceps
- DeBakey tissue-holding forceps

Technique

1. Place the animal in dorsal recumbency and prepare the entire ventral abdomen and caudal one-third of the sternum for aseptic surgery.

*See equipment listed under Median Sternotomy, which may be needed if the shunt is intrahepatic (sec. 6, ch. 25).

2. Perform a routine ventral midline abdominal approach. If the shunt is intrahepatic, it also may be necessary to perform a caudal sternotomy.
3. Isolate a loop of jejunum and place two stay sutures (4–0 silk) around the jejunal vessels. Place an over-the-needle catheter in the jejunal vein and ligate in place with the silk suture. Place an additional suture around the catheter and either the intestinal serosa or the mesentery to prevent slippage.
4. After flushing with heparinized saline, connect an extension set and water manometer to the jejunal vein catheter. Measure preligation portal pressure (normal = 8–10 cm H_2O).
5. Explore the abdomen and identify the shunt.
   a. *Extrahepatic shunts* usually are found by retracting the duodenum ventrally and to the left, and then following the mesoduodenum cranially and dorsally to the level of the epiploic foramen. Ventral retraction of the lesser omentum usually exposes the shunt entering the caudal vena cava. Be careful not to injure the hepatic arteries, which lie adjacent to the shunts located in this position. Some shunts can be found by creating a small window in the lesser omentum and looking craniodorsal to the lesser curvature of the stomach. Shunts in other locations require careful exploration of the cranial abdomen for location. It may be necessary to locate other branches of the portal vein, such as the splenic vein or the left gastric vein, in order to find the shunt.
   b. The location of *intrahepatic shunts* varies. Exposure is facilitated by median sternotomy and ventral-to-dorsal division of the diaphragm. The intrahepatic shunt may be seen entering the caudal vena cava cranial to the liver. These shunts are usually closely adherent to the peritoneal surface of the diaphragm. Alternatively, the shunt or the branch of the portal vein entering the shunt may be seen and dissected caudal to the liver.
6. Carefully skeletonize a small portion of the shunt vessel and pass a silk ligature around it.

KEY POINT ▶ During shunt ligation, do not allow portal pressure to rise >10 cm above the preligation value or to reach an absolute value >20 cm H_2O.

7. Slowly ligate the shunt while monitoring portal pressure. Carefully observe the abdominal viscera, especially the pancreas and intestine, for evidence of portal hypertension (e.g., bluish color and congestion of venous vessels). Use both the portal pressure values and tissue appearance to be sure that portal hypertension is not developing during ligation.
   a. Reduce the degree of attenuation if there is any evidence of portal hypertension.
   b. Complete ligation is possible in rare cases; however, many animals respond well to only partial ligation of the shunt.
8. Remove the jejunal catheter and ligate the jejunal vein if necessary.

9. Close the abdominal incision in a routine fashion.

Postoperative Care and Complications

- Monitor for portal hypertension.
  - *Acute* portal hypertension is a life-threatening complication that may develop any time from immediately to several hours postoperatively. Watch for the following clinical signs of postoperative portal hypertension: acute collapse, severe abdominal pain, abdominal distension (ileus), pale mucous membranes, slow capillary refill, and diarrhea with frank blood.

KEY POINT ▶ If acute portal hypertension is suspected, reoperate immediately to remove the shunt ligature.

- - *Chronic* portal hypertension usually is manifested by ascites. Treatment generally is not necessary, and the ascites usually resolves in 1–3 weeks.
- Prevent hypoglycemia by giving 5% dextrose in saline until the animal resumes oral feeding.
- Add potassium to the fluid to prevent hypokalemia (see sec. 1, ch. 5 on fluid therapy).
- Continue medical management of hepatic encephalopathy (see sec. 7, ch. 8).
  - If the animal is doing well clinically, discontinue the lactulose and neomycin after 2–4 weeks.
  - Continue feeding a low-protein diet (e.g., Prescription Diet k/d [Hill's Pet]) until liver function improves significantly. Measure pre- and postprandial serum bile acid concentrations 3 and 6 months postoperatively to check for improvement in liver function. If no clinical improvement is seen, consider repeat portography and re-ligation of the shunt vessel if continued shunting of blood is seen.

SURGERY OF THE BILIARY SYSTEM

Anatomy

Gallbladder

- The gallbladder is a pear-shaped sac located between the quadrate and right medial lobes of the liver.
- In a medium-sized dog, it has a capacity of 15 ml.
- Bile drains from the gallbladder to the cystic duct, and then to the common bile duct.
- The gallbladder is divided anatomically into three parts: the fundus (blind end), body (middle portion), and neck.
- Histologically, the gallbladder wall consists of a mucosal lining, layer of smooth muscle fibers, submucosal layer, and serosal covering.
- Blood supply is via the cystic artery, a branch of the hepatic artery.

Bile Ducts

- Hepatic cells discharge bile into minute canaliculi, which coalesce to form interlobar ducts and then hepatic ducts.
- Hepatic ducts and the cystic duct drain into the bile duct (or common bile duct).

- The common bile duct is present in the lesser omentum, and the free portion is about 5 cm in length. It then travels through the duodenal wall (intramural portion is 1.5–2.0 cm in length), and empties into the major duodenal papilla. The minor pancreatic duct (in dogs) empties immediately adjacent to the opening of the bile duct. In cats, the common bile duct and pancreatic duct join and subsequently enter the duodenum at the major papillae as a common duct.

Preoperative Considerations

- Correct dehydration and serum electrolyte imbalances before surgery.
- If the animal is not already being treated for infection, administer prophylactic antibiotics (directed toward gram-negative and anaerobic bacteria) such as ampicillin, cephalosporins, and chloramphenicol.

KEY POINT ▶ If the bile duct is totally obstructed, coagulopathy may be present because of decreased absorption of vitamin K–dependent clotting factors (II, VII, IX, X).

- Give vitamin K_1 (Veda-K_1, Vedco), (1 mg/kg divided q8h, SC) 36 hours before surgery if necessary. If immediate surgery is required, give a fresh whole blood transfusion.

Cholecystectomy—Surgical Procedure

Cholecystectomy is indicated for severe diseases of the gallbladder, such as damage secondary to trauma, severe cholecystitis, neoplasia, and irreparable damage to the cystic duct.

Objectives

- Remove gallbladder while minimizing trauma to surrounding tissues.
- Prevent leakage of bile to the peritoneal cavity.
- Avoid damage to the remainder of the biliary duct system.

Equipment

- Standard general surgery pack and suture
- Small and large gallbladder and other right-angled forceps
- Hemostatic stainless steel clips
- Penrose drains (1/4 and 1/2 inch)
- Sterile cotton-tipped applicators

Technique

1. Prepare the animal as previously described for liver biopsy and hepatic surgery.
2. Isolate the gallbladder from the remainder of the peritoneal cavity with moistened laparotomy sponges.
3. Dissect the gallbladder from the fossa by blunt dissection. Sterile cotton-tipped applicators are helpful to separate the gallbladder from the surrounding hepatic tissue. Babcock forceps or stay sutures can be used to manipulate the gallbladder during this dissection.

4. Isolate and doubly ligate the cystic duct and cystic artery with absorbable sutures or hemostatic clips.
5. Place gallbladder forceps and incise the cystic duct and artery just distal to the forceps. Remove forceps and gallbladder.
6. Submit the gallbladder for culture and histopathology.
7. Place a Penrose drain in the area of the excised gallbladder (exiting the cranial abdominal wall) if bile leakage or other contamination occurred during surgery.
8. Close the abdominal incision in a routine fashion.

Cholecystotomy—Surgical Procedure

Cholecystotomy is indicated to remove biliary calculi or to flush the gallbladder of inspissated or infected bile. The gallbladder should be reasonably healthy and have a good blood supply to ensure satisfactory healing.

Objectives

- Open and inspect the gallbladder and its contents.
- Avoid spillage of bile into the peritoneal cavity.
- Provide a water-tight seal of the cholecystotomy incision.
- Submit samples of tissue, calculi, and/or bile for analysis and culture.
- Thoroughly flush the gallbladder and biliary ducts to remove stones and infected material.

Equipment

Equipment is the same as for cholecystectomy plus:

- Fine absorbable suture with taper or taper-cut needle (4–0, 5–0 polydioxanone or polyglactin 910).
- Infant feeding tube or small (#5 Fr) Brunswick rubber catheter.

Technique

1. Prepare and position the animal as previously described for liver biopsy and hepatic surgery. The surgical approach is the same as for a cholecystectomy.
2. Isolate the gallbladder from the remainder of the peritoneal cavity with laparotomy sponges.
3. Use stay sutures (5–0 silk) on the gallbladder on either side of the proposed incision.
4. Incise the gallbladder fundus, using a #11 scalpel blade and Metzenbaum or tenotomy scissors. Evacuate the contents and save samples of bile or calculi for analysis and culture.
5. Flush the gallbladder with warm, sterile saline.
6. To ensure patency, cannulate and flush the cystic and common bile ducts with an infant feeding tube or #5 Fr Brunswick catheter.
7. If necessary, perform a duodenotomy approximately 2–4 cm distal to the pylorus to pass a catheter retrograde into the common bile duct through the major duodenal papilla. Place a stent catheter if recurrent bile duct obstruction is expected or to stent a ruptured biliary duct (Fig. 4).

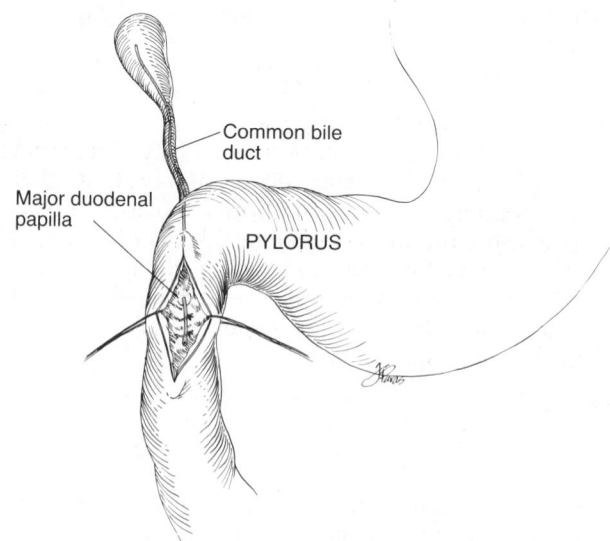

Figure 4. Placement of an indwelling stent catheter in the common bile duct. The catheter has been placed via a duodenotomy. Insert the catheter retrograde through the major duodenal papilla and into the gallbladder. Leave the end of the catheter in the duodenal lumen and ligate in place with 4–0 or 5–0 catgut; close the duodenotomy incision.

8. Close the gallbladder incision in a 1- or 2-layer inverting pattern (e.g., Cushing and/or Lembert), using 5–0 or 4–0 absorbable suture and a taper needle.
9. Place a Penrose drain in the cranial abdomen if bile leakage occurred during surgery.
10. Close the abdominal incision in a routine manner.

Cholecystoenterostomy—Surgical Procedure

Cholecystoenterostomy is surgical anastomosis of the gallbladder to the intestinal tract. The major objective is to bypass the cystic and common bile ducts when these ducts are irreversibly obstructed. Examples of indications are: severe scar tissue in the bile ducts (cholangitis), nonresectable neoplasia, severe cholangiohepatitis with sludged bile (in cats), and large bile duct calculi that cannot be dislodged. The gallbladder can be anastomosed to the duodenum (cholecystoduodenostomy) or to the jejunum (cholecystojejunostomy).

Objectives

- Diversion of bile from gallbladder directly to the duodenum or jejunum to bypass the cystic and common bile duct.
- Maintain sufficient lumen size to allow free flow of bile from the gallbladder to the intestine.
- Prevent bile or intestinal leakage.
- Provide a tension-free anastomosis.

Equipment

Equipment is the same as for cholecystotomy.

Technique

1. Prepare and position the animal as previously described for liver biopsy and hepatic surgery. The

surgical approach is identical to that for cholecystectomy.
2. Using blunt dissection, gently free the gallbladder from the surrounding liver tissue.
3. Bring a loop of duodenum or jejunum close to the gallbladder and place stay sutures in both structures.
4. Incise the gallbladder along the fundus and the intestine on its antimesenteric surface.
5. Perform a 2-layered anastomosis, using absorbable suture for the inner layer and a nonabsorbable monofilament suture for the outer layer. Make sure the anastomosis is at least 2.5 cm in diameter. This large opening helps prevent sequestration of intestinal contents in the gallbladder that could result in severe cholecystitis and cholangitis.
6. Close the abdominal incision in a routine manner.

Surgical Repair of Traumatic Biliary Rupture

Rupture of the biliary tract causes severe chemical and possibly septic peritonitis. Diagnosis and initial management of animals with bile peritonitis is discussed in sec. 7, ch. 13. Perform surgical correction of bile leakage promptly because metabolic consequences are serious and life-threatening.

Objectives

- Evaluate the entire liver and biliary tract for evidence of damage.
- Find the area of bile leakage and control it.
- Treat the peritonitis with copious lavage and abdominal drainage.
- Maintain competency of major biliary pathways.
- Provide nutritional access for hyperalimentation in patients in critical condition.

Equipment

Equipment is the same as for cholecystotomy, plus:

- Stent tubing (e.g., #5 Fr Brunswick catheter, infant feeding tube, Silastic tubing)

Technique

1. The preparation of the animal and surgical approach are the same as for cholecystectomy.
2. Evacuate fluid from the peritoneal cavity.
3. Examine the entire liver and biliary system for evidence of trauma and injury. Examine the remainder of the abdominal organs for abnormalities.
4. Find the source of bile leakage:
   a. If the gallbladder is intact, express it and look for leakage.
   b. If the above is unsuccessful, perform a duodenotomy over the major duodenal papilla and catheterize the common bile duct, using a #5 Fr Brunswick catheter or infant feeding tube. Flush the bile duct with sterile saline and look for leakage.
5. Correct the leakage.
   a. Suture the rent if it is in the gallbladder or a large bile duct. Use fine absorbable suture material (4–0 or 5–0 PDS).
   b. If primary closure is not possible, stent the torn duct by passing a soft catheter up the common bile duct through the major duodenal papilla. Make sure that the end of the catheter is at least 2–3 cm proximal to the rent. Secure the catheter to the duodenal mucosa by placing 1 or 2 ligatures of 5-0 catgut. Cut the catheter, leaving 2–3 cm in the lumen of the duodenum, and close the duodenal incision in a routine manner. In 1–2 weeks, the catheter will dislodge and be passed through the intestinal tract.
6. Lavage the abdomen with copious amounts of warm, sterile saline.
7. If peritonitis is present, leave the abdomen open for drainage (see sec. 7, ch. 13 on treatment of peritonitis). After several days, if drainage decreases and other parameters improve, close the abdomen.

Postoperative Care and Complications

- Maintain intravenous fluid therapy until oral intake resumes.
- Monitor for evidence of bile peritonitis: painful abdomen, fever, leukocytosis, icterus, and bile-stained fluid on abdominal tap.
- If cultures from the biliary tract are positive, administer long-term (6 weeks) antibiotic therapy.
- Monitor for evidence of pancreatitis; withhold food and water if it occurs (maintain the animal on intravenous fluids).
- Re-evaluate every 3–6 months for recurrence of biliary obstruction or ascending infection of the biliary tract after cholecystoenterostomy.

Supplemental Readings

Breznock EM, Whiting PG: Portacaval shunts and anomalies. *In* Slatter DH, ed.: *Textbook of Small Animal Surgery*. Philadelphia: W. B. Saunders, 1985, p 1156.
Evans HE, Christensen GC: *Miller's Anatomy of the Dog*, 2nd Ed. Philadelphia: W. B. Saunders, 1979, p 492.
Walshaw R: Surgical diseases of the liver and biliary system. *In* Slatter DH, ed.: *Textbook of Small Animal Surgery*. Philadelphia: W. B. Saunders, 1985, p 798.

10 Diseases and Surgery of the Exocrine Pancreas

Robert G. Sherding
Stephen J. Birchard
Susan E. Johnson

The pancreas is a V-shaped gland in the cranial abdomen comprised of an exocrine portion (the acinar cells) and an endocrine portion (the islets of Langerhans). The normal functions of the exocrine pancreas are summarized in Table 1. The principal disorders of the exocrine pancreas include pancreatitis, exocrine pancreatic insufficiency, and neoplasia. (Diseases of the endocrine pancreas are discussed in sec. 4, chs. 4 and 5.)

PANCREATITIS

Pancreatitis is an acute or chronic inflammatory condition of the pancreas that develops when intrapancreatic activation of enzymes results in progressive autodigestion of the gland. The clinical forms of pancreatitis are categorized in Table 2.

Etiology

In most animals with spontanous pancreatitis, an etiology is not identified and the pathogenesis is poorly understood. Based on clinical associations found in naturally occurring cases and on various experimental models for producing pancreatitis in dogs, the following have been proposed as etiologic or predisposing factors:

- Obesity and long-term intake of high-fat diets
- Ingestion of a fatty meal—e.g., meat trimmings
- Hyperlipidemia—e.g., as a result of intake of a fatty meal, hyperadrenocorticism, diabetes mellitus, hypothyroidism, or idiopathic hyperlipidemia of miniature schnauzers

TABLE 10–1. Functions of the Exocrine Pancreas

Secretory Products	Functions
Digestive enzymes*	
Trypsins	Protein digestion
Chymotrypsins	Protein digestion
Elastases	Protein digestion
Carboxypeptidases	Protein digestion
Amylase	Polysaccharide digestion
Phospholipase	Lipid digestion
Lipase	Lipid digestion
Colipase	Coenzyme facilitator of lipase
Bicarbonate†	Neutralization of gastric acid entering duodenum
Pancreatic trypsin inhibitor	Protection against autodigestion
Pancreatic intrinsic factor	Facilitation of cobalamin (vitamin B_{12}) absorption
Miscellaneous	Facilitation of zinc absorption Antibacterial (inhibits intestinal bacterial overgrowth) Trophic effect on intestinal mucosa

*Acinar cells secrete enzymes in response to cholecystokinin (CCK) which is released into the blood from the proximal intestine when partially digested food enters the duodenum from the stomach. Proteolytic enzymes are secreted as inactive precursors (zymogens) that are not activated until they enter the intestinal tract. Enteropeptidase from the duodenal mucosa activates trypsinogen to active trypsin; trypsin then activates the other proteases and phospholipase.

†Centroacinar and duct cells secrete bicarbonate-rich secretion in response to secretin released into the blood from the proximal intestine when acid enters the duodenum from the stomach.

TABLE 10–2. Categories of Pancreatitis

Acute Pancreatitis
(Abrupt onset; acute episodes may recur)

Mild (Edematous)
Self-limiting
No vascular compromise
No multisystem failure or complications
Uncomplicated recovery

Severe (Hemorrhagic)
Self-perpetuating (progressive)
Vascular compromise
Severe complications
Multisystem failure
Guarded prognosis

Chronic Pancreatitis
(May be continuous and "smoldering" or recurrent and episodic)

Mild
Minimal morphologic damage
Absence of complications

Severe
Progressive irreversible destruction of acinar and islet cells
Severe pancreatic fibrosis
Complications:
Exocrine pancreatic insufficiency
Diabetes mellitus
Extrahepatic bile duct obstruction

TABLE 10-3. Factors Involved in the Pathogenesis of Pancreatitis

Factor	Proposed Role in Pathogenesis
Pancreatic Enzymes	
Trypsin	Perpetuates proteolytic damage of pancreatic tissue (autodigestion)
	Perpetuates activation of more trypsin and other proteases
	Consumption of plasma protease inhibitors
	Coagulation/fibrinolysis (DIC)
	Activates kinin system and releases histamine from mast cells, contributing to edema and hemorrhage
Phospholipase A	Cell membrane damage (necrosis, noncardiogenic pulmonary edema)
	Liberation of toxins (e.g., myocardial depressant factor)
Elastase	Vascular damage (progression of edematous to hemorrhagic pancreatitis)
Chymotrypsin	Activation of xanthine oxidase (generation of oxygen-derived free radicals; see below)
Lipase	Local fat necrosis (peritonitis; "calcium soaps"; hypocalcemia)
Inflammatory Mediators	
Oxygen-derived free radicals	Damage of tissues by disrupting cell membranes through peroxidation of lipids in the membrane
	Endothelial cell injury (pancreatic edema and hemorrhage; DIC)
Kallikrein-kinin system	Vasodilation, hypotension, and shock
Complement	Local inflammation and aggregation of leukocytes; peritonitis
Coagulation/Fibrinolysis	DIC
	Thrombosis of pancreatic blood vessels
	Ischemic pancreatic necrosis

DIC = disseminated intravascular coagulopathy.

- Corticosteroid therapy and hyperadrenocorticism
- Reflux of duodenal contents (bile, activated enzymes, bacteria) into the pancreatic duct
- Pancreatic duct obstruction—e.g., as a result of duodenitis, edema, spasm, calculi, neoplasia, metaplasia, or aberrant parasite migration
- Biliary tract disease—e.g., pancreatitis associated with cholangiohepatitis in cats
- Infection—e.g., ascending enteric bacteria, parvovirus, and aberrant intestinal parasite migration; rarely feline infectious peritonitis virus, toxoplasmosis, and the pancreatic fluke *Eurytrema procyonis*
- Hypercalcemia—when total serum calcium exceeds 15 mg/dl, as can occur in hypercalcemia of malignancy, hyperparathyroidism, and vitamin D intoxication
- Abdominal trauma or surgery
- Hyperstimulation—by agents such as scorpion venom, cholinesterase inhibitors, cholinergic agonists, and caerulein
- Pancreatic ischemia—e.g., hypovolemia, thrombosis, local stasis of pancreas microvasculature
- Pancreatic neoplasia

Pathogenesis

The initiating events of pancreatitis are not fully understood, but acinar cell membrane damage (permeability) and intrapancreatic activation of trypsinogen are involved. Activated trypsin then activates other digestive enzymes, resulting in a progressive cascade of intrapancreatic enzyme activation and pancreatic autodigestion. Once initiated, amplification and progression of pancreatitis involves factors such as oxygen-derived free radicals, activated complement, the kallikrein-

kinin system, disseminated intravascular coagulopathy (DIC), bacterial endotoxins, and pancreatic ischemia (Table 3).

KEY POINT ▶ Activation of trypsin and other pancreatic enzymes is critical to the development of pancreatitis. Impaired pancreatic microcirculation is a key factor in the progression of mild edematous pancreatitis to severe necrotizing pancreatitis.

Clinical Signs and Manifestations

Clinical signs of acute pancreatitis are extremely variable, ranging from vague and nonspecific signs to obvious signs of an "acute abdomen" crisis. In chronic pancreatitis, episodic signs may correspond to periodic flare-ups of inflammation. In some cases, clinical signs are dominated by secondary complications (e.g., DIC) or sequelae (e.g., diabetes mellitus).

Canine Pancreatitis

- Vomiting (most consistent sign, but can be absent in some cases), anorexia, depression, and dehydration.
- Cranial abdominal pain, varying from mild to intense (manifested as restlessness, panting, trembling, hunched-up abdomen, praying position of relief, seeking of cool surfaces, and pain on palpation)
- Diarrhea (sometimes hemorrhagic)
- Fever (can be solely due to inflammation and does not necessarily imply infection)
- Weakness or, in severe cases, acute collapse from shock

Feline Pancreatitis

- Cats are more likely to have smoldering, low-grade chronic interstitial pancreatitis, manifested by vague, nonspecific signs of anorexia and weight loss, with or without vomiting. The disorder often goes unrecognized until discovered at necropsy.
- Concurrent cholangitis/cholangiohepatitis frequently is found; this may be related to the anatomic arrangement of the bile and pancreatic ducts that join and have a common opening into the duodenum in cats.

Acute Complications

- Shock, collapse, and hypothermia (due to hypovolemia and endotoxemia)
- Peritonitis (sterile exudate) and intra-abdominal fat necrosis
- Sepsis
- DIC—bleeding, thrombosis, infarction
- Jaundice (intrahepatic cholestasis, hepatocellular necrosis, biliary obstruction)
- Acute oliguric renal failure
- Intestinal hypomotility (ileus)
- Hypocalcemia (tetany is rare)
- Hyperglycemia (due to hyperglucagonemia and hypoinsulinemia)
- Cardiac arrhythmias (myocardial depressant factor; myocardial ischemia or necrosis)
- Respiratory distress (rarely, noncardiogenic pulmonary edema or pleural effusion)

Chronic Complications and Sequelae

- Pancreatic pseudocysts and abscesses, characterized by persistence or recurrence of signs associated with development of a cavitated pancreatic mass containing liquefied necrotic debris, which can be sterile (pseudocyst) or infected (abscess)
- Chronic relapsing pancreatitis, characterized by chronic smoldering disease with periodic flare-ups
- End-stage pancreatic fibrosis and atrophy, manifested as diabetes mellitus or exocrine pancreatic insufficiency or both
- Liver disease, resulting from common bile duct obstruction due to chronic fibrosing pancreatitis

Diagnosis

Clinical Signs and Physical Findings

- Suspect pancreatitis in animals presented for vomiting, depression, anorexia, and abdominal pain.
- Identifiable risk factors increase the index of suspicion (e.g., obesity, schnauzer breed, recent fatty meal, evidence of corticosteroid excess).
- A palpable right cranial abdominal mass or fluid suggests a pancreatic lesion.

Serum Pancreatic Enzymes

Dogs. The clinical diagnosis of acute pancreatitis usually is based on elevated serum concentrations of amylase and lipase. Serum enzyme concentrations often are normal in chronic pancreatitis except during acute flare-ups of inflammation. Although serum amylase and lipase concentrations are sensitive indicators of pancreatitis, they lack specificity because elevated enzyme levels are frequent in nonpancreatic diseases. However, nonpancreatic elevations do not usually exceed two to three times the upper limit of normal. There is an inconsistent correlation between the degree of enzyme elevation and the severity of the pancreatitis or the prognosis.

- Delayed renal clearance of enzymes combined with increased secretion due to hypergastrinemia can cause elevations in azotemic patients. This can be a diagnostic dilemma because acute pancreatitis often causes prerenal azotemia and sometimes overt oliguric renal failure. Urinalysis is helpful in these situations.
- Amylase and lipase may sometimes be increased in gastrointestinal, liver, and neoplastic disease. Normal circulating amylase originates from nonpancreatic sources, especially the intestinal mucosa; thus, enteritis can increase serum amylase.
- Corticosteroids in high doses can cause a significant increase (up to five-fold) in lipase concentrations in the absence of pancreatitis while amylase decreases or remains normal.
- Amylase and lipase usually increase in parallel, but not always; therefore, evaluation of both amylase and lipase together is more diagnostic than evaluating either one alone. One or both enzymes can be normal in the presence of severe pancreatitis, presumably due to depletion of stored enzymes in the pancreas.

Cats. Cats with pancreatitis generally develop smaller and less consistent enzyme elevations than dogs. In experimental pancreatitis in cats, serum lipase concentration increases while that of amylase decreases or remains within normal limits.

Amylase Assay Methods

- Catalytic methods—The amyloclastic method is valid for dogs, but the saccharogenic method is not.

KEY POINT ▶ Amylase cannot be measured by saccharogenic methods used for humans because dog serum contains high levels of maltase and glucoamylase that yield falsely elevated amylase values.

- Immunoassay methods are reliable but are also species-specific.

Other Tests for Pancreatic Enzymes and Enzyme inhibitors. These require further clinical evaluation before they can be recommended.

- Amylase isoenzyme analysis (for pancreas-specific isoenzyme)
- Assay for serum trypsin-like immunoreactivity
- Assay for serum phospholipase A_2
- Plasma protease inhibitor consumption (alpha$_1$-antitrypsin, alpha-macroglobulin)
- Assay for trypsin-antiprotease complexes in plasma

Ancillary Laboratory Findings

- Fasting hyperlipemia and icteric serum are common in patients with pancreatitis.

- The complete blood count (CBC) usually reveals neutrophilia, with or without a left shift. Severe necrosis, peritonitis, sepsis, or endotoxemia can sometimes cause neutropenia with a degenerative left shift. Hemoconcentration (elevated packed cell volume [PCV]) from dehydration is typical; occasionally anemia occurs. Red blood cell (RBC) fragments and macroplatelets are consistent with subclinical DIC.
- Elevated serum liver enzymes (alkaline phosphatase [ALP], alanine aminotransferase [ALT]), and bilirubin can result from hepatocellular injury (due to ischemia, sepsis, or toxins from the pancreas) and biliary obstruction.
- Azotemia (increased blood urea nitrogen [BUN] and creatinine) is common and can result from dehydration and hypovolemia (prerenal) or from renal damage and acute oliguric renal failure.

KEY POINT ▶ Because elevated levels of amylase, lipase, BUN, and creatinine are common in both renal failure and pancreatitis, assess the urine specific gravity (SG) as a reflection of renal concentrating ability; SG >1.025 indicates adequate tubular function.

- Hyperglycemia (usually transient, but some animals are diabetic after recovery)
- Hypocalcemia (usually subclinical; tetany is rare)
- Fasting hyperlipemia (hypertriglyceridemia and hypercholesterolemia)
- Hemostatic abnormalities consistent with DIC: prolonged activated partial thromboplastin time (APTT) and one-stage prothrombin time (OSPT), decreased platelets, decreased fibrinogen, and increased fibrinolytic products
- Abdominal fluid analysis (brownish red exudate; increased enzyme activity relative to blood; possible sepsis)
- Methemalbumin formation (human test not very applicable to dogs because hemin complexes with serum proteins other than albumin in dogs)

Radiography

- Increased density and loss of abdominal contrast and detail in the right cranial abdomen (localized peritonitis; ground-glass appearance)
- Displacement of the descending duodenum to the right and the pyloric antrum to the left, producing a widened angle or mass effect between the antrum and duodenum on ventrodorsal radiographs (on lateral views, the duodenum may be displaced ventrally)
- Gastric distension and static gas pattern (ileus) in the duodenum or transverse colon
- Delayed passage of barium from the stomach and through the duodenum; also, thickening, corrugation, or spasticity of the duodenum
- Possible complicating pulmonary edema or pleural effusion seen on thoracic radiography

Ultrasonography

- Irregular enlargement and decreased or mottled echogenicity of the pancreas suggest pancreatitis.

- Pancreatic pseudocysts and abscesses can be identified as pancreatic cavitations.

Medical Treatment

Mild acute pancreatitis often is self-limiting and may resolve spontaneously in a few days. Severe acute pancreatitis is a life-threatening multisystem crisis that requires intensive therapy. The goal of treatment is to rest the pancreas, provide supportive care, and control complications as they arise in order to allow time for the pancreatic inflammation to subside. Surgical intervention may be required when abscessation occurs.

KEY POINT ▶ Correction of hypovolemia by IV fluid therapy and prevention of pancreatic stimulation by temporary restriction of all oral intake are the most important therapeutic measures for acute pancreatitis.

Control Hypovolemia and Maintain Pancreatic Microcirculation

- Fluid Volume Replacement:
  - Administer a balanced electrolyte solution (e.g., lactated Ringers). To treat *shock,* give up to 85 ml/kg, IV, in the first hour (see sec. 6, ch. 14). To provide *rehydration* and *maintenance,* give 60 ml/kg/24h plus deficit plus extra losses (for a detailed discussion of fluid therapy, see sec. 1, ch. 5).
  - Monitor urine output (for oliguria) and respiratory function (for pulmonary edema).
  - Consider transfusion of plasma or whole blood (10–20 ml/kg) for maintenance of normoalbuminemia and plasma oncotic pressure in hypoproteinemic patients (when serum albumin is < 2.0 g/dl). This enhances pancreatic microcirculation and reduces pancreatic edema and helps to prevent renal failure, pulmonary edema, and pleural effusion. Plasma or whole blood can replace antiproteases (alpha-macroglobulins) that are consumed in pancreatitis. Use fresh whole blood plus heparin to treat overt DIC.
- Potassium supplementation: Add 20–30 mEq KCl per liter of maintenance fluids and frequently monitor serum K^+.
- Acid-base status is unpredictable in pancreatitis; avoid excessive bicarbonate administration if unwarranted, because this can precipitate hypocalcemia.
- Use glucocorticoids only in patients presented in shock and only short-term (1–2 doses, as described for treatment of shock in sec. 6, ch. 14). Glucocorticoids may impair clearance of circulating protease complexes.
- Control DIC to prevent pancreatic microthrombi (see sec. 3, ch. 2).
- Other unproven agents to promote pancreatic microcirculation include vasopressin (5 units in oil) and glucagon.

Prevent Stimulation of Pancreatic Secretion

- Restrict oral intake to place the pancreas at "rest."
  - Nothing per os usually is required for 3–4 days or

longer. Food (especially fats and proteins) stimulates pancreatic secretion through cholecystokinin (CCK) release. Even fluids can stimulate pancreatic secretion through gastric distension and release of gastrin.

- When vomiting has ceased for ≥ 24–48h, offer small amounts of water PO. If water is tolerated, then gradually reintroduce food, initially using a carbohydrate diet (e.g., rice, pasta) restricted in fat and protein to minimize pancreatic stimulation. Then gradually resume normal maintenance feeding of a balanced, moderately fat-restricted diet.
- Prolonged restriction of oral intake (1–2 weeks) is required for some patients, which may necessitate feeding of elemental nutrients by jejunostomy catheter or total parenteral nutrition, provided that an ICU facility is available.
■ Avoid anticholinergics; they are of questionable benefit and potentiate ileus of the intestinal tract.
■ Inhibition of gastric acid secretion with drugs like cimetidine is of unproven benefit.
■ Experimental treatment modalities include CCK inhibitors, glucagon, somatostatin, and enzyme inhibitors.

Promote Removal of Activated Enzymes

■ Promote plasma antiprotease activity.
- Alpha$_2$-macroglobulin binds circulating activated enzymes for removal by the mononuclear phagocyte system. Plasma or whole blood transfusion may benefit patients with fulminant pancreatitis by supplying macroglobulin (also supplies colloid in the form of albumin).
- Avoid glucocorticoids because they may have a detrimental effect on removal of macroglobulin-enzyme complexes.
■ Peritoneal lavage using a dialysis catheter can help to remove intraperitoneal enzymes, inflammatory mediators, and toxins. Although it is not practical to recommend as a routine method of treatment, it can be beneficial in cases of pancreatitis with abdominal effusion.

Control Abdominal Pain

■ Rest and confinement help to minimize pain.
■ If analgesia is needed, use meperidine HCl (Demerol, Winthrop) (5–10 mg/kg q8h, IM) or butorphanol (Torbugesic, Fort Dodge) (0.2–0.4 mg/kg q4–6h, SC, for dogs).
■ Oral pancreatic enzyme supplements (Viokase) and insulin have been beneficial for pain relief in humans with chronic pancreatitis, but this effect has not been evaluated in animal patients.

Control Acute Complications

■ Control sepsis (and prevent pancreatic abscessation):
- For prevention, administer ampicillin (20 mg/kg q8h, SC) or a cephalosporin (e.g., cephalothin, cephazolan) (20 mg/kg q6–8h, IV).
- If sepsis or peritonitis occurs or is suspected, add gentamicin (Gentocin; 2 mg/kg q8h, SC or IM) or amikacin (Amikin; 5 mg/kg q8h, IM or IV). However, if renal failure is present, adjust the aminoglycoside dosage or choose an alternative antibiotic.
■ Control DIC:
- Prevent by IV fluid therapy to promote perfusion of the microcirculation.
- To prevent microthrombi, give minidose heparin (10 units/kg q8h, SC)
- To treat overt DIC, see sec. 3, ch. 2.
■ Control oliguria:
- Prevent by vigorous IV fluid therapy to control hypovolemia.
- If oliguria occurs, give furosemide (Lasix; 1–2 mg/kg, IV; repeat once or twice).
■ Control hyperglycemia (if glucose exceeds 300 mg/dl) with short-acting regular crystalline zinc insulin (see sec. 4, ch. 4).
■ Control cardiac arrhythmias if they occur (see sec. 6, ch. 4).
■ Control noncardiogenic pulmonary edema if it occurs (see sec. 6, ch. 20).

Treat Chronic Complications and Sequelae

■ Surgical intervention is indicated for management of septic peritonitis (see sec. 7, ch. 13), for drainage or excision of pancreatic abscesses, and for cholecystoduodenostomy (after active pancreatitis is resolved) to relieve persistent biliary obstruction.
■ Insulin is indicated if persistent hyperglycemia consistent with diabetes mellitus occurs (see sec. 4, ch. 4).
■ Pancreatic enzyme supplementation is indicated for exocrine pancreatic insufficiency (see discussion in this chapter).

Prevent Recurrences

■ Identify and control underlying risk factors (see previous discussion under Etiology).
■ Feed a fat-restricted diet and avoid "treats."

Surgical Treatment of Pancreatitis

Medical treatment, as outlined in this chapter, is preferred for most animals with pancreatitis. However, surgery may be appropriate in certain situations. The decision to operate on an animal with pancreatitis is very difficult because such patients frequently are poor anesthetic and surgical risks. The surgical procedure may cause the animal's overall condition to worsen. Consider all options and thoroughly discuss the prognosis and potential complications with the owner prior to surgery.

Indications for Surgery

■ *Failure to respond to appropriate medical therapy*— Assuming an accurate diagnosis, consider an exploratory laparotomy if the patient's condition deteriorates or does not improve.
■ *Presence of a pancreatic abscess or other mass*— Consider surgery if repeated ultrasonographic examinations reveal persistence or enlargement of a

pancreatic abscess or other mass and if the patient's condition dictates aggressive action.

▪ *Severe icterus due to extrahepatic biliary obstruction*—As previously discussed, inflammation and tissue swelling associated with pancreatitis can cause biliary obstruction. Ultrasonography is helpful in making this diagnosis. If the obstruction and associated icterus does not improve with medical therapy, surgical exploration and biliary decompression may be necessary.

▪ *Severe pancreatitis and septic peritonitis*—Severe peritonitis may occur with pancreatitis (see sec. 7, ch. 13). Surgical lavage and drainage may be necessary.

Preoperative Considerations

▪ Thoroughly assess the animal and review the history and clinical course of events.
▪ Consider patient factors that may increase the complication rate, such as age, debilitation, sepsis, hypoproteinemia, DIC, diabetes mellitus, and disorders of other organ systems.
▪ Determine the coagulation status in animals with severe pancreatitis and possible DIC.

Surgical Procedure

Objectives

▪ Surgically expose the pancreas and determine type and extent of disease; remove devitalized tissue.
▪ Thoroughly explore the abdominal cavity for evidence of associated lesions or other problems.
▪ Lavage the peritoneal cavity to remove necrotic tissue debris, toxins, enzymes, and exudate.
▪ Provide drainage in cases of severe peritonitis.

Equipment

▪ Standard general surgery pack and suture
▪ 5 Fr. infant feeding tube or red rubber tube

Technique

1. Aseptically prepare the ventral abdomen.
2. Perform a standard ventral midline abdominal approach from the xyphoid to pubis.
3. Expose the pancreas by exteriorizing the small intestine and retracting the duodenum ventrally. Expose the left limb of the pancreas by retracting the transverse colon caudally.
4. Carefully and gently examine the pancreas for masses, abscesses, inflammation, and necrosis.
5. Gently open areas of abscessation digitally to establish ventral drainage. Obtain samples of fluid or tissue for bacterial culture. Carefully and judiciously debride necrotic pancreatic tissue and fat. Do not disrupt the pancreatic blood supply during dissection (see sec. 4, ch. 5 under description of partial pancreatectomy). Minimize trauma to normal or non-necrotic pancreatic tissues. Submit all tissues for histopathology.
6. Carefully examine the gallbladder and biliary ducts for evidence of obstruction.
   a. Gently squeeze the gallbladder to determine if bile is expressible through the common bile duct.
   b. Consider retrograde catheterization of the common bile duct, using an infant feeding tube, if complete obstruction is suspected (see sec. 7, ch. 9). A stent catheter can be left in the common bile duct if necessary (see sec. 7, ch. 9). This procedure is somewhat risky because a duodenotomy is necessary and duodenal healing may be impaired by the severe local inflammation created by the pancreatitis.
7. Thoroughly lavage the peritoneal cavity with warm sterile saline.
8. Establish abdominal drainage by leaving the abdomen open (see sec. 7, ch. 13) if severe peritonitis is present or if abscesses were opened during the pancreatic exploration. Otherwise, close the abdomen routinely.

Postoperative Care and Complications

▪ Maintain all aspects of medical therapy for pancreatitis (see previous discussion in this chapter). Consider plasma tranfusions for hypoproteinemia and whole blood transfusions for postoperative anemia (PCV <20%).
▪ See sec. 4, ch. 5 for postoperative care of the partial pancreatectomy patient.
▪ See sec. 7, ch. 13 for postoperative care of peritonitis.
▪ Consider total parenteral nutrition for animals with severe pancreatitis and open abdominal drainage.
▪ See under Medical Treatment in this chapter for dietary recommendations.
▪ Complications include septic shock, hypoproteinemia, worsening of pancreatitis and peritonitis, abdominal pain, and dehiscence of intestinal incisions.

Prognosis

Although most patients recover, pancreatitis is a life-threatening disease that frequently has a prolonged and unpredictable clinical course; thus, a guarded prognosis is warranted. The prognosis is poor when pancreatitis is complicated by septic shock, DIC, acute renal failure, or bowel infarction.

EXOCRINE PANCREATIC INSUFFICIENCY

Exocrine pancreatic insufficiency (EPI) occurs when severe progressive loss of acinar tissue from atrophy or inflammatory destruction results in insufficient secretion of digestive enzymes and clinical signs of malabsorption.

Etiology

Juvenile Pancreatic Acinar Atrophy

The most common cause of EPI is noninflammatory pancreatic acinar atrophy (PAA) of young dogs. The etiology of PAA is not known. Many breeds can be affected, especially large breeds. The highest incidence is in the German shepherd, in which the predisposition to PAA may be inherited as an autosomal recessive trait.

Chronic Relapsing Pancreatitis

The end stage of slowly progressive inflammatory destruction of the pancreas is fibrosis and atrophy which can result in EPI. Substantial islet destruction can result in concurrent diabetes mellitus. Any breed of dog can be affected, but most are smaller breeds and are middle-aged or older. Chronic pancreatitis or pancreatic duct occlusion can cause EPI in cats but is very rare.

Clinical Signs

The pathogenesis of malabsorption in EPI may involve not only impaired intraluminal digestion but also altered intestinal mucosal function and morphology, as well as overgrowth of bacteria within the lumen of the small intestine in many cases.

- Onset of signs in dogs with PAA is typically before 2 years of age, although occasionally it can occur later than this. Pancreatitis-induced EPI can occur at any age but most often is recognized in middle-aged and older dogs.
- Weight loss or failure to gain weight can occur despite a ravenous appetite and increased food intake. Intense hunger may cause pica and coprophagia in some dogs.
- Diarrhea from maldigestion and malabsorption of fat, carbohydrates, and protein is characterized by large volumes of soft, semi-formed or unformed, fatty feces with a rancid odor. The diarrhea may improve substantially with fasting or with feeding of a highly digestible or fat-restricted diet.
- Borborygmus and flatulence may occur.
- The hair coat is dull and poor in quality, with excessive shedding and greasy, oily hair around the perineum.

Diagnosis

- Diarrhea and weight loss are nonspecific signs that must be differentiated from other causes of intestinal malabsorption.
- Routine CBC, serum chemistries, urinalysis, and radiographs are generally unremarkable in EPI.
- For a discussion of the differential diagnosis of chronic diarrhea, see sec. 7, ch. 6.

Fecal Microscopy

The examination of Sudan and iodine-stained fecal smears for steatorrhea (excessive fat in the feces) and amylorrhea (excessive undigested starch in the feces) can be used as preliminary in-office screening procedures; however, sensitivity and specificity are fairly low.

- Direct Sudan stain—Detects excessive undigested fat (neutral, unsplit) as numerous large refractile orange droplets, indicating steatorrhea of pancreatic maldigestion.
- Indirect Sudan stain—The addition of acetic acid and heating renders fatty acids (split fat) stainable as well; thus, numerous droplets in a fecal specimen that is negative by direct Sudan staining suggest steatorrhea caused by malabsorption of fatty acids.
- Lugol's iodine stain—Detects undigested starch as blue-black granules, suggesting amylorrhea of pancreatic maldigestion.

Serum Trypsin-like Immunoreactivity (TLI) Assay

The serum TLI assay is highly sensitive and specific for detection of EPI. This test measures total circulating trypsinogen and trypsin in a single fasted serum sample and is available on a mail-out basis at selected veterinary laboratories (Table 4).

KEY POINT ▶ The serum TLI assay is the test of choice for confirmation of canine EPI. In normal dogs and in dogs with intestinal disease, serum TLI is 5 to 35 µg/L. In dogs with EPI, serum TLI is consistently < 2.5 µg/L.

Oral Bentiromide Digestion Test

The oral bentiromide (N-benzoyl-L-tyrosyl-P-aminobenzoic acid, or BT-PABA) test is fairly reliable for diagnosis of EPI in dogs, but it is not as accurate or easy to perform as the TLI assay. After administration of the bentiromide test substrate, a chymotrypsin-labile peptide (Chymex; Adria Labs.) (16.7 mg/kg, PO), serum samples are taken at 60 and 90 minutes and assayed for free PABA (see Table 4).

- Dogs with EPI, because they secrete very little chymotrypsin, develop a negligible rise in plasma PABA; however, false positive and false negative results sometimes occur.
- In cats, PABA levels are lower and less consistent than in dogs, but nevertheless a minimal rise in plasma PABA suggests EPI (see Table 4).

Assays of Fecal Proteolytic Activity

Assays of fecal proteolytic activity by azocasein hydrolysis or radial enzyme diffusion are indirect methods of evaluating pancreatic function.

TABLE 10–4. Normal Values for Pancreatic Function Tests

Test	Canine	Feline
Serum TLI assay*	5–35 µg/liter	31–115 µg/liter
Bentiromide test (peak PABA)	≥5.0 µg/ml	≥2.0 µg/ml
Radial enzyme diffusion (3-day mean)*	6–24 mm	6–17 mm
Azocasein hydrolysis (3-day mean)	19–200 ACU/g	29–207 ACU/g
Serum cobalamin*	225–660 ng/liter	200–1680 ng/liter
Serum folate*	6.7–17.4 µg/liter	13.4–38.0 µg/liter

*Available as mail-in test through Dr. David Williams, Dept. of Veterinary Clinical Sciences, 1248 Lynn Hall, Purdue University, West Lafayette, IN 47907 (Tel.: 317-494-0331).

TLI = trypsin-like immunoreactivity; PABA = para-aminobenzoic acid; ACU = azocasein units.

- Because the serum TLI assay is more reliable and practical, it is preferred over fecal proteolytic assays for diagnosis of canine EPI.
- A valid TLI assay for cats is not yet available, and the diagnostic accuracy of fecal proteolytic assays is acceptable if multiple fecal specimens are assayed.
- Fecal specimens are collected on each of 3 consecutive days and immediately frozen for shipment to the laboratory (see Table 4).

Measurement of Serum Folate and Cobalamin

Serum folate and cobalamin levels reflect intestinal absorptive function and the status of the intestinal flora. In addition, normal pancreatic secretions may have an influence. For normal values, see Table 4.

- Serum folate and cobalamin levels may be decreased in enteropathies that cause intestinal malabsorption.
- In small intestinal bacterial overgrowth, which commonly occurs in EPI, serum folate levels may be increased due to synthesis of folate by the overgrown bacteria, and cobalamin may be decreased because bacteria can utilize or bind the vitamin, making it unavailable for absorption.
- Deficiency of pancreatic intrinsic factor in EPI may contribute to the frequent finding of low cobalamin levels; enhanced folate absorption due to intestinal acidification may contribute to an increased serum folate.

Treatment

Pancreatic Enzyme Replacement

- Dried pancreatic extracts are available commercially as tablets, capsules, powders, granules, and enteric-coated preparations; enzyme content and bioavailability varies widely.
- Pancreatin powder preparations are recommended (Viokase-V, Fort Dodge; Pancrezyme, Daniels). Add 1 to 2 tsp per meal to the food just prior to feeding and divide the daily food intake into 2 to 3 meals per day.
- When the diarrhea is in remission and the animal is gaining weight, titrate to the minimum effective maintenance dose (1 tsp added to each of two meals daily is adequate for most dogs).

KEY POINT ▶ The effectiveness of enzyme supplementation is not increased by concurrent use of antacids, sodium bicarbonate, bile acids, or preincubation of enzymes with the food prior to feeding. Enteric-coated preparations and uncrushed tablets are less effective than powdered pancreatic extracts.

Diet

- Most dogs with EPI can be fed a maintenance diet; however, if the response to enzyme supplementation is incomplete, substitute a diet that is highly digestible, low in fiber, and restricted in fat (e.g., Prescription Diet i/d; Hill's Pet).
- In treated dogs that fail to gain desired weight,

provide supplemental calories in the form of medium chain triglycerides (MCT Oil, Mead Johnson; 1–2 ml/kg per day added to meals). Unlike conventional dietary fat, MCTs do not require lipolysis by pancreatic lipase for absorption.
- Consider multivitamin supplementation, especially the fat-soluble vitamins (A, D, E, and K). Cobalamin and tocopherol are often severely depleted in dogs with EPI; thus, give high dosages initially for repletion: cobalamin (vitamin B_{12}), 500 μg, SC once or twice per month for 2–3 months; and tocopherol (vitamin E), 500 units, PO, daily for the first month.

What to Do if There is Failure to Respond

- *Step 1:* Adjust diet and enzyme brand, form, and dosage according to the above recommendations; if there is no response, go to Step 2.
- *Step 2:* Administer antibiotics (e.g., tetracyclines, metronidazole, tylosin) for small intestinal bacterial overgrowth (see sec. 7, ch. 6). If there is no response, go to Step 3.
- *Step 3:* Administer an oral H_2-receptor blocker with meals, such as, cimetidine (Tagamet, 10 mg/kg) or ranitidine (Zantac, 2 mg/kg), to reduce acidic inactivation of enzymes. If there is no response, go to Step 4.
- *Step 4:* Reassess diagnosis and evaluate for intestinal mucosal disease via endoscopic biopsy.

PANCREATIC NEOPLASIA

Pancreatic neoplasms can be hormone-secreting tumors that arise from islet cells (insulinoma and gastrinoma are discussed in sec. 4, ch. 5), or they can arise from the exocrine pancreas as adenomas or adenocarcinomas of acinar or duct cell origin. Exocrine pancreatic adenomas are rare and usually unassociated with clinical signs. Exocrine pancreatic adenocarcinomas are more common and are discussed here. These are highly malignant and metastasize early to the liver, regional lymph nodes, mesentery, duodenum, stomach, and occasionally the lungs, often prior to the onset of clinical signs.

Clinical Signs

- Clinical signs are usually insidious and nonspecific, often mimicking chronic pancreatitis. Vomiting, anorexia, depression, and abdominal pain are usually noted first.
- Bile duct obstruction or extensive liver metastases may lead to jaundice.
- Duodenal invasion and obstruction may lead to persistent intractable vomiting.
- Peritoneal carcinomatosis may lead to peritoneal effusion.

Diagnosis

- Suspect pancreatic adenocarcinoma when a right cranial abdominal mass is identified by palpation, abdominal radiography, or abdominal ultrasonography in an animal with signs of chronic pancreatitis or obstructive hepatopathy. Serum bilirubin and liver enzymes usually are elevated.

■ Exploratory laparotomy and surgical biopsy are usually required for definitive diagnosis. Because chronic pancreatitis and pancreatic adenocarcinoma can have a similar gross appearance, histopathologic evaluation is necessary.

Treatment

Attempted surgical resection (pancreatectomy; see sec. 4, ch. 5) is sometimes palliative (e.g., for relief of bile duct or duodenal obstruction); however, in most cases surgery is not beneficial and virtually is never curative. Adjunctive chemotherapy can be used, but it also is of minimal benefit and efficacy.

Supplemental Readings

Hardy RM: Diseases of the exocrine pancreas. *In* Sherding RG, ed.: *The Cat: Diseases and Clinical Management.* New York: Churchill Livingstone, 1989, p 1007.

Strombeck DR, Guilford WG: The pancreas. *In Small Animal Gastroenterology,* 2nd Ed. Davis, CA: Stonegate Publishing, 1990, p 429.

Williams DA: Exocrine pancreatic disease. *In* Ettinger SJ, ed.: *Textbook of Veterinary Internal Medicine,* 3rd Ed. Philadelphia: W. B. Saunders, 1989, p 1528.

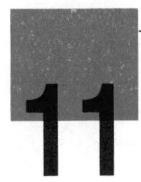

Anorectal Diseases

Robert G. Sherding

The presenting signs of anorectal disease can include any of the following: dyschezia, hematochezia, constipation, anal discomfort (licking, scooting), ribbon-like feces, fecal incontinence, anal discharge, foul perianal odor, matting of perianal hair, and perianal dermatitis. Physical examination establishes the diagnosis of anorectal disease in most cases. In many anorectal diseases, surgery is required for effective treatment.

CONSTIPATION

Constipation is a clinical sign characterized by absent, infrequent, or difficult defecation associated with retention of feces within the colon and rectum. When feces are retained for a prolonged period of time they become progressively harder and drier and, eventually, impacted as the mucosa continues to absorb water from the fecal mass. Terms associated with constipation are defined below.

Obstipation—A condition of intractable constipation in which the colon and rectum become so impacted with excessively hard feces that defecation cannot occur.

Dyschezia—A clinical sign often associated with constipation, characterized by difficult or painful evacuation of feces from the rectum and usually is associated with lesions in or near the anal region.

Tenesmus—A clinical sign characterized by straining to defecate, usually ineffectively or painfully; thus, it usually accompanies dyschezia.

Megacolon—A disorder (not a sign) in which the colon becomes severely and irreversibly dilated and hypomotile. Megacolon usually is idiopathic and is an important cause of chronic constipation and obstipation in cats.

Etiology

Underlying causes of or predisposing factors for constipation are listed in Table 1 and include dietary factors, environmental factors, painful defecation, anorectal or colonic obstruction, neuromuscular diseases, fluid and electrolyte disturbances, and drug-related effects.

- *Ingested foreign material,* such as indigestible fibrous material (especially hair in cats from their grooming behavior) and abrasives (especially bones in dogs), may become incorporated in the fecal mass and result

in the formation of hard fecal impactions that are difficult and painful to evacuate from the colon.

- *Environmental factors* that are not conducive to defecation or that vary from the daily routine to which the animal is accustomed may cause the animal to inhibit the urge to defecate, leading to constipation. For example, this may occur when an animal is kept in strange surroundings, such as in a kennel or veterinary hospital, or when its daily outdoor exercise routine is changed. Cats often suppress the urge to defecate when their litter box is dirty.
- *Painful defecation* caused by anorectal diseases (anal sacculitis, perianal fistulas) or orthopedic disorders that limit positioning for defecation (diseases of the pelvis, spine, or hips) often result in voluntary inhibition of defecation and lead to constipation.
- *Anorectal or colonic obstruction* that mechanically impedes the passage of feces may result from intraluminal causes, such as foreign bodies, perineal hernia, and stenosing neoplastic or inflammatory lesions, or from extraluminal causes, such as prostatic enlargement, compressive pelvic fractures, and pseudocoprostasis (feces matted in perianal hair).
- *Neuromuscular disorders* may lead to constipation by interfering with colonic innervation or smooth muscle function or the ability of the animal to assume the normal defecation stance. For example, this may occur in association with disease or injury of the lumbosacral spinal cord (canine intervertebral disc disease), spinal deformity (e.g., in Manx cats), endocrine disease (hypothyroidism), and dysautonomia, a progressively fatal autonomic polyneuropathy of young cats. When innervation of the anus is also impaired, fecal incontinence may be an associated clinical sign. The pathogenesis of idiopathic megacolon is poorly characterized but probably involves a primary or secondary neuromuscular dysfunction of the colon.
- *Fluid and electrolyte disorders* may predispose to constipation. Dehydration can cause the feces to become excessively dry and hard. Hypokalemia and hypercalcemia can affect colonic smooth muscle function.
- *Drug-induced constipation* may be a side effect of motility-modifying drugs (anticholinergics, opiates, opioids), antihistamines, barium sulfate, aluminum hydroxide, and diuretics.

Clinical Signs

- Constipated animals are usually presented because of failure to defecate over a period of days. The

TABLE 11–1. Classification and Causes of Constipation

Category	Cause
Dietary	Ingested foreign material mixed with feces (hair, bones, cloth, garbage, cat litter, rocks, plant material)
	Inadequate water intake
Environmental/psychological	Dirty litter box
	Prolonged inactivity
	Hospitalization
	Change in habitat or daily routine
Painful defecation	Anorectal disorders:
	Anal sac impaction or abscess
	Anorectal stricture, tumor or foreign body
	Myiasis
	Perianal fistula
	Perianal bite wound cellulitis or abscess
	Pseudocoprostasis
	Orthopedic disorders
	Spinal disease or injury
	Injuries of the pelvis, hip joints, or pelvic limbs
Rectocolonic obstruction	Extramural
	Prostatic hypertrophy, tumor, or prostatitis
	Paraprostatic cyst
	Pelvic fracture (malunion)
	Pelvic collapse due to nutritional bone disease
	Perianal tumor
	Pseudocoprostasis
	Intramural or intraluminal
	Rectocolonic stricture, tumor, or foreign body
	Rectal diverticulum or perineal hernia
Neuromuscular dysfunction	Lumbosacral spinal cord disease (injury, deformity, degeneration, neoplasia)
	Bilateral pelvic nerve injury
	Dysautonomia (Key-Gaskell syndrome)
	Hypothyroidism
	Idiopathic megacolon (?)
Fluid and electrolyte abnormalities	Dehydration
	Hypokalemia
	Hypercalcemia (hyperparathyroidism)
Drug-induced	Anticholinergics
	Adrenergic blockers and calcium channel blockers
	Phenothiazines and tricyclic antidepressants
	Opiates and opioids
	Diuretics
	Antihistamines
	Aluminum hydroxide
	Sucralfate
	Barium sulfate
	Iron
	Laxatives (overuse)

owner may notice tenesmus or frequent attempts to defecate with little or no passage of feces.

■ Dyschezia usually indicates anorectal disease. The animal first may cry out as it attempts to defecate, usually with straining (tenesmus) during the attempt; then it may cease the effort, walk around anxiously, and repeatedly try again.

■ Mucosal irritation caused by impacted feces may provoke a secretion of fluid and mucus, which bypasses the retained fecal mass and is expelled paradoxically as diarrhea during attempts to defecate.

■ Other signs may include anorexia, lethargy, vomiting, dehydration, and a hunched-up appearance caused by abdominal discomfort.

■ Constipation tends to be a recurrent problem.

Diagnosis

KEY POINT ▶ The presence of constipation usually is determined from the history and confirmed by rectal and abdominal palpation of colonic distension with hard feces. The goal of diagnosis is to identify predisposing factors.

History

Identify dietary, environmental, behavioral, psychological, and medication-related factors or predispositions.

Physical Examination

■ Perform a digital anorectal examination to detect painful or obstructive lesions of the anorectum.

■ Perform a neurologic examination (see sec. 10, ch. 1) to identify any underlying neurologic causes of constipation.

■ Evaluate the pelvic limbs, coxofemoral joints, pelvis, and lumbosacral spine for orthopedic problems that could cause difficulty maneuvering into the defecation stance or painful defecation.

■ In cats with constipation caused by dysautonomia (Key-Gaskell syndrome), additional manifestations of progressive autonomic failure that may be seen include urinary and fecal incontinence, megaesophagus, bradycardia, mydriasis, decreased lacrimation, and prolapse of the nictitating membranes.

Routine Laboratory Evaluations

Perform a serum biochemical profile, urinalysis, and complete blood count (CBC) to:

■ Evaluate animals with recurrent constipation to identify underlying systemic disease (e.g., chronic renal failure) that could cause constipation due to dehydration or electrolyte disturbances.

■ Evaluate severely constipated or obstipated animals, especially those that are vomiting or markedly depressed, in order to detect the metabolic consequences of prolonged fecal retention, such as, fluid and electrolyte imbalances, endotoxemia, and azotemia, and to guide supportive treatment.

Thyroid Function Testing

Evaluate thyroid function in dogs with recurrent constipation and other signs compatible with hypothyroidism (see sec. 4, ch. 1).

Abdominal Radiography

Perform abdominal radiography to:

■ Confirm the extent of colonic impaction with densely packed feces.

■ Identify the extreme dilatation of the colon that indicates megacolon.

■ Identify radiopaque foreign material (e.g., bone

chips) in the retained feces that indicates a dietary cause of constipation.

- Identify pelvic, coxofemoral, or spinal lesions that can cause constipation.
- Identify underlying prostatic enlargement that might cause constipation.

Barium Enema Contrast Radiography or Colonoscopy

Perform after removal of retained feces to evaluate the lumen of the colon when intraluminal obstructive lesions are suspected.

Myelographic and Electrodiagnostic Evaluation

Perform to evaluate the lumbosacral spinal cord and spinal nerves (see sec. 10, chs. 1 and 4) in selected patients in which impaired anorectal innervation is suspected.

Treatment

- Mild constipation resolves spontaneously or is treated on an outpatient basis by oral or suppository laxatives.
- Severe constipation initially may require evacuation of impacted feces from the colon (using enemas or manual extraction or both) along with correction of complicating dehydration and electrolyte imbalances.
- Additional therapeutic goals are to eliminate or control any underlying causes of constipation (see Table 1) that are identified and to prevent recurrences using dietary adjustments and laxative therapy as needed.
- Obstructing neoplasms, strictures and many anorectal disorders require surgical correction.
- Long-term management of megacolon or recurrent obstipation that is unresponsive to medical therapy in the cat may require subtotal colectomy (see sec. 7, ch. 7).

Oral Laxative Therapy

Oral laxative medications and dietary supplements can be prescribed as needed for control of constipation (Table 2). Laxatives act on intestinal mucosal fluid transport and colonic motility and are classified by their properties and mechanisms of action as bulk-forming, lubricant, emollient, osmotic, or stimulant. The use of an oral laxative often must be individualized by adjusting the dose until the desired frequency of defecation and fecal consistency is obtained.

High-Fiber Bulk-Forming Laxatives. These laxatives are added to food to promote soft feces and normal colonic motility as the initial approach for long-term control of constipation. These bulk-forming agents are nonabsorbable polysaccharide and cellulose derivatives that exhibit hydrophilic properties within the bowel. This method of treatment is available as a commercially prepared high-fiber diet (Prescription Diet w/d, Hills Pet Products) or as fiber additives for the regular diet, such as unprocessed wheat bran, pumpkin pie filling, or commercial sources of psyllium (see Table 2).

Lubricant Laxatives. Laxatives such as mineral oil and petrolatum products are used to soften and lubricate the feces to facilitate evacuation (see Table 2).

- Administer lubricants between meals so that they do not interfere with the absorption of fat-soluble vitamins.
- Avoid using mineral oil because its tastelessness can lead to inhalation lipid pneumonia; if necessary to use, always add flavoring and administer cautiously.

Emollient Laxatives. Docusate sodium (available in enema and oral forms), docusate calcium, and docusate potassium are mild laxatives that promote water penetration into the feces, thereby softening the feces (see Table 2).

- Do not mix docusate and mineral oil.

Osmotic Laxatives. These laxatives consist of poorly absorbed disaccharides (e.g., lactose or lactulose), ions (e.g., magnesium hydroxide, magnesium citrate), or inert osmotic agents (e.g., polyethylene glycol) that osmotically retain water in the bowel lumen to produce soft or fluid feces.

- A mild osmotic laxative effect can be produced in some animals by the addition of milk (lactose) to the diet in a quantity that exceeds the digestive capacity of small intestinal lactase, or by the administration of the nonabsorbable disaccharide lactulose (see Table 2). Excessive amounts of fermentable carbohydrates can cause abdominal discomfort and flatulence.

KEY POINT ▶ Lactulose is an excellent choice as a safe and effective all-purpose laxative for both dogs and cats. Lactulose can be expensive for long-term use in large-breed dogs.

- Magnesium hydroxide is available as an over-the-counter drug (see Table 2). Magnesium is contraindicated in patients with renal failure.
- Magnesium citrate and polyethylene glycol-electrolyte solutions (see Table 2) are used as cathartics for preparation of the bowel for colonoscopy. The large doses required depend on administration by orogastric intubation, which limits their use for routine treatment of constipation.

Stimulant Laxatives. Stimulant laxatives increase propulsive motility of the bowel. They are contraindicated in the presence of an obstructive lesion and are less appropriate for long-term use than other categories of laxatives.

- A useful stimulant laxative for dogs and cats is bisacodyl (see Table 2), which works by stimulating colonic smooth muscle and the myenteric plexus. Although beneficial on a short-term basis in conjunction with measures to soften the feces, long-term use may damage the myenteric plexus.
- Castor oil is hydrolyzed in the intestines to ricinoleic acid which stimulates colonic motility and secretion. Castor oil is not very useful for outpatient treatment because of poor patient acceptance, but it is effective

TABLE 11–2. Laxative Therapy for Constipation

Treatment	Product (Manufacturer)	Dose Regimen
Oral Cathartics		
Bulk-forming laxatives		
Coarse bran	All-Bran (Kellogg) and others	1–5 tbsp daily with food
Canned pumpkin	Pie filling (Libby)	1–5 tbsp daily with food
Psyllium	Metamucil (Procter & Gamble); Fiberall (CIBA)	1–5 tsp daily with food
High-fiber diet	W/d Prescription Diet (Hills)	Use as daily food source
Lubricant-laxatives		
White petrolatum	Laxatone (EVSCO)	1–5 ml daily PO
Mineral oil*	Many	5–25 ml daily (flavored)
Emollient laxatives		
Docusate sodium	Colace (Mead Johnson)	*Cat*: 50 mg daily PO *Dog*: 50–200 mg daily PO
Docusate calcium	Surfak (Hoechst-Roussel)	*Cat*: 50–100 mg daily PO *Dog*: 100–240 mg daily PO
Docusate potassium	Dialose (J & J–Merck)	100 mg daily PO
Saline laxative		
Magnesium hydroxide	Phillips Milk of Magnesia (Glenbrook)	2–8 tablets daily PO
Osmotic laxatives		
Lactose	Milk	Add to diet to effect
Lactulose	Duphalac Syrup (Reid-Powell); Cephulac (Marion Merrell Dow)	0.5–1 ml/kg; q8–12h PO
Polyethylene glycol and electrolytes†	Colyte (Reed & Carnick); GoLYTELY (Braintree)	25–40 ml/kg PO; repeat in 2–4 h (for bowel prep)
Stimulant laxatives		
Bisacodyl	Dulcolax (Boehringer Ingelheim)	*Cat*: 5 mg daily, orally *Dog*: 5–20 mg daily, orally
Castor oil†	Many	5–30 ml, orally (bowel prep)
Enemas and Suppositories		
Enemas		
Warm tap water		5–10 ml/kg
Isotonic saline solution		5–10 ml/kg
Docusate sodium	Colace (Mead Johnson)	5–30 ml
Mineral oil	Many	5–30 ml or 1–2 ml/kg
Sodium phosphate‡	Fleet Children's Enema (Fleet)	1–2 ml/kg or 1 enema unit
Bisacodyl	Fleet Bisacodyl Enema (Fleet)	1–2 ml/kg or 1 enema unit
Rectal suppositories		
Glycerin	Many	1–3 pediatric
Docusate sodium	Colace (Mead Johnson)	1–3 pediatric
Bisacodyl	Dulcolax (Boehringer Ingelheim)	1–3 pediatric

Caution: may cause lipid aspiration pneumonia and may interfere with absorption of fat-soluble vitamins; combination with docusate may cause undesirable absorption of mineral oil.
†Used mainly to prepare the colon for radiography or endoscopy.
‡Do *not* use in cats or small dogs.

for preparing the bowel for radiographic or endoscopic procedures.

Enema Therapy

Enema solutions are used to soften hard impacted feces and promote evacuation. Warm the enema solution prior to instillation and administer the calculated dose slowly so as not to induce vomiting. Commonly used enema solutions (see Table 2) include:

- Warm isotonic saline or tap water (5–10 ml/kg body weight), with or without the addition of a mild soap to stimulate defecation by an irritant effect (soap must not contain hexachlorophene because of its neurotoxicity)
- Docusate as an emollient
- Mineral oil as a lubricant

- Sodium phosphate solution, which has softening, bulk-producing, and irritant effects (safe to use only in medium-sized and large dogs with normal renal function)

KEY POINT ▶ Caution! Never use phosphate enemas in cats or small dogs because they may cause dangerous hypernatremia, hyperosmolality, hyperphosphatemia, and hypocalcemia. Do not mix mineral oil and docusate; docusate promotes mucosal absorption of mineral oil, whereas mineral oil coats the feces, reducing the emollient effect of docusate.

Manual Evacuation of Impacted Feces

- In severe constipation or obstipation, restore fluid and electrolyte balance parenterally and evacuate the colon manually under general anesthesia using a combination of:

- Colonic irrigation with warm isotonic saline as an enema solution to soften the impacted feces
- Extraction of retained fecal masses by gentle transabdominal manipulation to milk the feces into the distal rectum for digital or forceps removal (can use a sponge or whelping forceps)

■ To avoid excessive bowel trauma in animals with extensive fecal impaction, it may be advisable to evacuate the colon manually in stages over a period of 2–3 days.

Prevention/Ancillary Treatment

Following evacuation of retained feces from the colon, institute measures to prevent and control recurrences of constipation. Identify and eliminate or correct underlying causes or predisposing factors (see Table 1).

■ Prevent ingestion of constipating or abrasive materials such as bones.
■ Prevent hair ingestion by adopting a routine of regular grooming to remove loose hair from the animal's hair coat before it can be ingested.
■ Provide dogs a daily exercise routine and frequent opportunities to defecate.
■ Provide cats with clean litter at all times to encourage regular defecation.
■ Provide access to fresh water at all times to encourage water intake.
■ Adjust or discontinue the use of any medications that promote constipation.
■ Treat predisposing prostatic, endocrine (hypothyroidism), spinal, and orthopedic disorders.
■ Correct, whenever possible, painful or obstructing anorectal lesions, by surgery if necessary (see sec. 7, ch. 12).

KEY POINT ▶ For severe recurrent constipation, obstipation, or megacolon that is unresponsive to medical management in the cat, subtotal colectomy is an effective method of treatment.

PSEUDOCOPROSTASIS

Etiology

Pseudocoprostasis is a condition of obstruction of the anal opening when the surrounding hair becomes densely matted with feces. It occurs most often in long-haired breeds of dogs and cats, especially during bouts of diarrhea.

Clinical Signs

The anal obstruction leads to anal irritation, inability to pass feces, and constipation.

■ The animal usually is restless and attempts to bite or lick the anal region.
■ The owner may complain of an unexplained foul odor from the animal.

The matted hair often results in an underlying dermatitis and in warm weather attracts flies that may produce a maggot infestation (myiasis) of the anal area.

Diagnosis

Examination of the anal region is sufficient for diagnosis.

Treatment

■ Clip hair mats, cleanse the underlying irritated skin, and apply a topical antibiotic ointment. When the obstructing hair mats are removed, defecation should occur normally.
■ If the animal has severe colonic impaction of feces, measures to evacuate the colon may be required (see under Constipation).

PROCTITIS

Proctitis, or inflammation of the rectum, can cause tenesmus, diarrhea, and hematochezia. Therefore, it must be differentiated from other anorectal diseases. Because proctitis usually is a component of colitis, it is discussed under Colitis in sec. 7, ch. 6.

ANORECTAL PROLAPSE

Etiology

Anorectal prolapse usually is a consequence of an underlying disorder that produces persistent straining; thus it is associated with:

■ Intestinal diseases that cause diarrhea and tenesmus
■ Anorectal diseases that cause dyschezia
■ Lower urinary tract and prostatic diseases that cause stranguria
■ Dystocia

Clinical Signs

■ Partial prolapse involves only the rectal mucosa and appears as a red, swollen, doughnut-shaped ring of prolapsed mucosa.
■ Complete prolapse involves all layers of the rectal wall and appears as an edematous cylindrical-shaped mass. The prolapsed tissue may be viable (pink or red and moist) or necrotic (blackened and dry).

Diagnosis

Insert a thermometer or finger in the space between the prolapsed tissue and anal sphincter to probe for a cul-de-sac. If there is none and resistance is not met, the prolapsed tissue is an intussusception of ileum or colon (see sec. 7, ch. 6), rather than an anorectal prolapse.

Treatment

Successful management of anorectal prolapse includes repair of the prolapse and identification and treatment of the underlying cause. Evaluate the anus, rectum, intestines, and urogenital tract by palpation, urinalysis, fecal examinations, proctoscopy, and radiographic studies, as appropriate.

- Treat minor prolapse in which the tissue is viable by reduction and medical therapy to reduce tenesmus and prevent recurrence. Treatment may include:
  - Anticholinergic-antispasmodic drugs such as dicyclomine (Bentyl; Marion Merrell Dow), 0.15–0.20 mg/kg, q8–12h PO or SC
  - Hydrocortisone retention enema (Cortenema; Reid-Rowell), 10–60 ml q12–24h
  - Mesalamine retention enema (RowASA; Reid-Rowell) for dogs only, at an empirical dosage of 10–60 ml q12–24h
  - Mild sedation
- A temporary (2–3 days) anal purse-string suture may be required in animals with persistent straining that produces recurrence of the prolapse. Leave the pursestring suture loose enough to allow passage of feces.
- Perform amputation when the prolapsed tissue is nonviable.

Colopexy

Consider prophylactic colopexy for recurrent prolapse.

Technique

1. Perform colopexy via a ventral midline abdominal approach.
2. Place gentle traction on the descending colon to reduce the prolapse.
3. Perform the "pexy" by scarifying the serosa of the descending colon in 3 or 4 small areas (0.5–1.0 cm diameter) and scarifying corresponding areas of the peritoneal surface of the left body wall.
4. Appose the scarified areas of colonic serosa to the peritoneum using 2-0 or 3-0 monofilament nonabsorbable sutures.

PERINEAL HERNIA

Etiology

Perineal hernia occurs when weakness of the pelvic diaphragm muscles fails to support the rectal wall, resulting in persistent rectal distension and impaired defecation. The pathogenesis of the weakened pelvic diaphragm is poorly understood; male hormones have been implicated because the disease is extremely rare in castrated dogs. Aged, intact male dogs are almost exclusively affected, although perineal hernia has been reported in a few cats.

The hernia usually contains outpouched rectum and can be unilateral or bilateral; unilateral hernias are predominantly right-sided. The hernia sac may also contain retroperitoneal fat, prostate gland, and, rarely, abdominal organ such as the urinary bladder or intestine. The rectal defects associated with perineal hernia have been classified as follows:

Sacculation—Unilateral loss of support allows expansion of the rectal wall to one side.

Dilatation—Bilateral loss of support allows generalized distension of the rectum.

Deviation or flexure—The rectum curves or bends to one side within the hernia sac.

Diverticulum—An outpouching of mucosa through a defect in the rectal wall.

Clinical Signs

- Clinical signs include constipation, obstipation, dyschezia, and tenesmus.
- Stranguria may occur with herniation of the urinary bladder and associated urethral obstruction.

Diagnosis

Diagnosis is based on palpation of a reducible swelling ventrolateral to the anus and rectal palpation of the weakened pelvic diaphragm and rectal defect.

Treatment

The goal of initial treatment is evacuation of retained feces from the rectum (see under Constipation). Urethral catheterization or cystocentesis also may be necessary initially to relieve urinary obstruction.

- In some dogs with perineal hernia, normal defecations can be maintained by laxative therapy and stool-softening diets (see under Constipation).
- Castration of dogs with mild perineal hernia may prevent progression of the disorder.
- Perineal herniorrhaphy surgery combined with castration provides the best long-lasting results in most cases (see sec. 7, ch. 12).

KEY POINT ▶ Always perform castration as an adjunct to perineal hernia repair.

ANORECTAL FOREIGN BODIES AND FECOLITHS

Etiology

- Ingested foreign bodies such as bones, toys, sticks, and sewing needles can sometimes pass unobtrusively through the gastrointestinal tract and become lodged transversely within the rectum or at the anal sphincter.
- Foreign objects occasionally are inserted into the anus of an animal by a malicious or deranged person.
- Aged cats sometimes present because of inability to pass a firm lump of feces (fecolith) that is lodged in the anal canal between the internal and external sphincter.

Clinical Signs and Diagnosis

When a foreign body or fecolith is lodged in the anal canal or rectum, defecation becomes painful or impossible, and dyschezia, tenesmus, and secondary fecal impaction occur. Diagnosis is by rectal examination.

Treatment

- Most anorectal foreign bodies and fecoliths can be detected and removed by rectal palpation; sedation or anesthesia may be necessary. In some cases a proctoscope may facilitate foreign body extraction.
- There are two potentially serious complications of anorectal foreign bodies:
  - Rectal laceration resulting in retroperitoneal cellulitis
  - Anorectal stricture (see below).

ANORECTAL STRICTURE (STENOSIS)

Etiology

Strictures of the anus or rectum can result from the following causes:

- Trauma caused by passage of sharp foreign bodies (especially bones).
- Postsurgical scarring after anorectal surgery
- Chronic inflammation associated with anal sac disease, perianal fistulae, or proctitis.

Clinical Signs and Diagnosis

Anorectal strictures cause dyschezia, tenesmus, hematochezia, and secondary constipation. The stricture can usually be identified by digital rectal palpation, proctoscopy, or barium enema contrast radiography.

Treatment

Anorectal strictures usually require surgical correction (see sec. 7, ch. 12).

ANAL SPASM

Etiology

This rare idiopathic form of severe dyschezia occurs when the anal sphincter contracts in spasm when the animal attempts to defecate.

Clinical Signs

When attempting to defecate, the animal may cry out in pain, move about frantically before stopping to make another attempt to defecate, turn and stare at its hindquarters, and appear extremely anxious. There appears to be a cycle of painful defecation, leading to defensive contraction of the anal sphincter, leading to more pain.

Diagnosis

- Most affected dogs are German shepherds of temperamental disposition.
- Digital palpation of the rectum is vigorously resented, and the anal sphincter muscle feels hypertrophied and tightly contracted in spasm. Visually, the external sphincter muscle appears hypertrophied.
- To attribute dyschezia to anal spasm it is important to rule out structural causes of dyschezia (e.g., anal

sac disease, perianal fistulae) and to exclude anal stricture (stenosis) by thorough rectal examination under anesthesia.

Treatment

- Conservative treatment using anal sac evacuation, topical analgesics, antispasmodic-sedative drugs (Librax, Roche), and stool softeners has not been very successful.
- Resection of one or both anal branches of the pudendal nerve is required for palliation in most dogs. Fecal incontinence often is a postoperative problem.

IMPERFORATE ANUS AND RECTAL AGENESIS

Etiology

Imperforate anus and rectal agenesis are rare congenital malformations of cloacal development that result in an absence of a patent anal opening for defecation.

Clinical Signs

Within days or weeks of birth, the affected puppy or kitten develops signs of abdominal distension and discomfort, tenesmus, restlessness, vomiting, and loss of appetite.

Diagnosis

- The diagnosis is established by absence of an anal opening. Variations in the malformation range from an imperforate anal membrane covering the anal opening (atresia ani) to varying degrees of rectal agenesis (rectal atresia) in which the rectum ends in a blind pouch at some distance cranial to the anus.
- The terminal end of the rectum can be delineated radiographically by the intraluminal air when a lateral radiograph is exposed with the animal's hind end slightly elevated.
- In some animals, imperforate anus is associated with genitourinary defects such as rectovaginal fistula.

Treatment

The treatment for atresia ani is surgical opening and removal of the retained anal membrane, usually producing favorable results (see sec. 7, ch. 12). For rectal atresia, surgical correction is more difficult and requires combined abdominal surgery and rectal pull-through; thus, the prognosis is guarded.

RECTOVAGINAL FISTULA

Rectovaginal fistula is a rare congenital malformation of females characterized by passage of fecal material through the vaginal opening. In many cases there also is an imperforate anus. Persistent fecal incontinence through the vagina leads to perivulvar dermatitis. Colonic distension usually occurs when the puppy or kitten begins eating solid food. The defect can be surgically corrected but the prognosis is guarded (see sec. 8, ch. 17). Other related, rare anorectal anomalies include rectovestibular fistula, anovaginal cleft, and recto-urethral fistula.

ANAL SAC DISEASE

Anal sac disorders are the most common problem of the anal area in small animals, especially dogs. Anal sac disease has been classified as impaction, inflammation (sacculitis), infection, abscess, and rupture:

- *Impaction* usually is bilateral and indicated by a sac that is distended, mildly painful on palpation, and not readily expressed. The impacted contents are thick and pasty and dark brown or grayish brown.
- *Anal sacculitis* is associated with moderate or severe pain on palpation; the sacs contain a thinner-than-normal, yellowish or blood-tinged purulent fluid.
- *Anal sac abscess* usually is unilateral and characterized by marked distension of the sac with pus, cellulitis of surrounding tissues, erythema of the overlying skin, and fever.
- *Rupture*— Abscessed anal sacs may rupture through the adjacent skin, producing a draining fistulous tract.

These probably represent a continuum, in that impacted anal sacs tend to become inflamed and infected, and the infection may lead to abscessation and, finally, to rupture or fistulation.

All breeds of dogs can be affected. Anal sac disease is uncommon in cats and usually involves only impaction.

Etiology

The specific cause of anal sac disease is poorly understood. It is believed to be associated with conditions that promote inadequate emptying of the sacs, which should normally occur during defecation when feces of normal consistency are forced through a normally functioning anal sphincter. Abnormal retention of anal sac secretions leads to the impaction-inflammation-infection cycle.

Clinical Signs

- The most frequent clinical signs of anal sac disease are related to anal discomfort and include scooting, tenesmus, and licking and biting the anal area, perineum, or base of the tail.
- Chewing and licking may result in areas of self-inflicted (pyotraumatic) dermatitis.
- Tail chasing, malodorous perineal drainage, and change in temperament may be noted.

Diagnosis

The diagnosis of anal sac disease is based on the clinical signs and examination of the anal sacs. Examine the anal sacs by palpation with a gloved index finger inserted in the rectum and a thumb compressed against the skin ventrolateral to the anus.

Treatment

- *Anal sac impaction and sacculitis*—Manual evacuation of the sac contents to re-establish drainage may be all that is required in many animals.
  - Follow-up examination and expression of the anal sacs again in 1–2 weeks is advisable.
  - A high-fiber diet (see Table 2) may help to prevent recurrence.
- *Recurrence of impaction or sacculitis*—Irrigation with povidone-iodine solution using a lacrimal needle and instillation of an antibiotic (e.g., otic or ophthalmic antibiotic ointment) into the sac may be helpful, along with expression of the sacs every 3–4 days.
  - Consider culture and sensitivity testing of the sac contents for animals with troublesome recurrences.
- *Abscesses*—Drain, irrigate with povidone-iodine solution, and treat with systemic antibiotics.
  - Treat recurrent anal sacculitis or abscess by surgical excision of the sacs (see sec. 7, ch. 12). Delay anal sacculectomy until the severe inflammation associated with abscessation has resolved.

PERIANAL FISTULAE

This chronic progressive disease is characterized by deep ulcerating fistulous tracts and suppuration in the perianal tissues. Fistulae occur primarily in German shepherds, although it has been reported sporadically in Irish setters, Labrador retrievers, and various other breeds.

Etiology

The proposed pathogenesis includes infection and abscessation of the various glandular elements in and around the anus, promoted by the moist, contaminated environment of the area and a broad-based, low-slung tail conformation.

Clinical Signs

- Dogs with perianal fistulae usually present with signs of anal discomfort (licking the anal area, scooting, dyschezia, tenesmus).
- Hematochezia, constipation, fecal incontinence, and foul-smelling purulent perianal discharge may be present.

Diagnosis

Examination of the perianal area establishes the diagnosis.

- The fistulae first appear as small, draining puncture holes in the perianal skin; there is inflammation and hyperpigmentation of the surrounding skin.
- These small tracts enlarge and coalesce to form large, interconnecting fistulae and areas of ulceration and granulation tissue. The fistulous tracts may extend deep into the perirectal tissues, and the anal sacs may be infected or ruptured.
- Histopathological findings include hidradenitis, chronic necrotizing pyogranulomatous inflammation

of skin and hair follicles, cellulitis, necrosis, and fibrosis.

Treatment

Surgery is the most effective treatment for perianal fistulae (see sec. 7, ch. 12). Numerous surgical techniques have been advocated, including varying degrees of excision and debridement of diseased tissue, chemical and electrocautery, cryosurgery, and tail amputation. It is advisable to tailor the aggressiveness of the technique to the extensiveness of the lesions and to preserve as much normal tissue and anal function as possible.

Prognosis

- Postoperative complications such as fecal incontinence, anal stenosis, and recurrence of the lesions can lead to an unacceptable outcome.
- In general, early diagnosis and surgical intervention allows a less radical excision than required in advanced disease, which in turn means less risk of postoperative complications and a better prognosis.

PERIANAL DERMATITIS

Anal irritation, a common consequence of anal sac disease and other anorectal disorders, often causes licking and biting the anal area that leads to perianal dermatitis.

- Any pruritic skin condition (most notably from fleas) may cause local dermatitis in this area.
- The mucocutaneous junction of the perianal skin and anal mucosa may be severely inflamed and ulcerated like other mucocutaneous junctions of the body in any of the systemic mucocutaneous dermatologic disorders (e.g., pemphigus vulgaris, bullous pemphigoid, systemic lupus erythematosus, candidiasis, cutaneous drug eruption.
- Eosinophilic granuloma complex of cats may involve the perianal region.

Perianal dermatitis often can be treated topically; however, the key is to recognize that it is usually secondary to another anorectal or dermatologic disorder that must be identified and treated. For information regarding specific dermatologic disorders, see the respective chapters.

ANAL AND PERIANAL TUMORS

The most common tumor of the anal region is benign perianal (circumanal) gland adenoma of dogs. Other benign tumors of the anal area are rare and include lipoma and leiomyoma. The two most common anal malignancies are perianal (circumanal) gland adenocarcinoma and apocrine gland (anal sac, anal gland) adenocarcinoma. Other malignant tumors of the anal region include squamous cell carcinoma, melanoma, lymphoma, and mast cell neoplasia.

Perianal (Circumanal) Gland Adenoma
Etiology and Clinical Signs

- These androgen-dependent tumors occur most often in older, intact male dogs and they usually appear as small, firm well-circumscribed nodules in the skin surrounding the anus.
- Perianal gland adenomas may be incidental findings unassociated with clinical signs or they may cause anal irritation with scooting and licking at the anal area. In addition, they sometimes ulcerate and periodically bleed.

Treatment

- The treatment of choice is excision (see sec. 7, ch. 12) and adjunctive castration because of their hormone-dependency. Castration alone can produce regression of these tumors; however, excisional biopsy at the time of castration is necessary to rule out malignancy.
- Estrogens are inhibitory for perianal gland adenomas; however, they cannot be recommended for prolonged use because of their myelotoxic effects.

Perianal Gland Adenocarcinoma
Etiology and Clinical Signs

- These tumors occur most often in aged male dogs and may resemble an ulcerated perianal gland adenoma, except that they are locally invasive and may cause diffuse thickening of surrounding tissues.
- The tumors eventually metastasize to regional lymph nodes (sublumbar) and beyond.
- Their appearance can be confused with a perianal fistula lesion or a ruptured anal sac.

Diagnosis and Treatment

- For potentially malignant lesions of the perianal area, excisional biopsy is the diagnostic procedure of choice (see sec. 7, ch. 12). First perform thoracic and abdominal radiography and abdominal ultrasonography to evaluate for lung or lymph node metastasis.
- Early excision of malignant tumors of the anal region can be effective; however, when extensive local invasion or regional lymph node metastasis has occurred, the prognosis for a cure is poor.
- Repeated partial excisions, radiation therapy, cryosurgery, and chemotherapy have been used for palliative therapy in patients with inoperative malignancies of the anal region.

Apocrine Gland Adenocarcinoma
Etiology and Clinical Signs

- Apocrine gland adenocarcinoma arises in the anal sac and most often affects spayed older female dogs. These tumors are unique in that they can be an ectopic source of parathyroid hormone–like activity; thus, even very small apocrine gland adenocarcinoma nodules often produce a hypercalcemia of malignancy syndrome with polyuria and polydipsia.

■ Metastasis to lungs and/or regional lymph nodes (sublumbar) may occur.

Treatment

■ Surgical excision is the treatment of choice.
■ For medical treatment of associated hypercalcemia, see sec. 4, ch. 12.
■ Adjunctive chemotherapy may be necessary for incompletely excised or metastatic tumors (see sec. 3, ch. 5).

Supplemental Readings

Burrows CF: Constipation. *In* Kirk RW, ed.: *Current Veterinary Therapy IX.* Philadelphia: W. B. Saunders, 1986, p 904.
Johnston DE: Rectum and anus—surgical diseases. *In* Slatter DH, ed.: *Textbook of Small Animal Surgery.* Philadelphia: W. B. Saunders, 1985, p 770.
Sherding RG: Management of constipation and dyschezia. Comp Contin Educ Pract Vet 12:677, 1990.
Sherding RG: Diseases of the colon, rectum, and anus. *In* Tams TR, ed.: *Manual of Small Animal Gastroenterology.* Philadelphia: W. B. Saunders (in press).
Walshaw R: Removal of rectoanal neoplasms. *In* Bojrab MJ, ed.: *Current Techniques in Small Animal Surgery,* 3rd Ed. Philadelphia: Lea & Febiger, 1990, p 274.

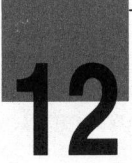 **Anorectal Surgery**

Ronald M. Bright

Surgery of the rectum and anus is associated with a high rate of complications. The high bacterial population of the rectum increases the risk of wound infection or dehiscence. Bowel preparation with multiple enemas can mechanically remove large numbers of bacteria; however, enemas should not be done within 8 hours of anorectal surgery. Synthetic absorbable sutures or monofilament nonabsorbable sutures should be used for surgery of the rectum and anus.

ANATOMY

The rectum begins at the brim of the pelvis and joins the anal canal just inside the anal opening. The anal canal is approximately 1–2 cm in length. The circumanal glands, anal glands and anal sacs are associated with the anus.

The rectum receives its blood supply from the caudal mesenteric artery and its branch coursing caudally, the cranial rectal artery. This artery forms anastomoses with the middle and caudal rectal arteries, which arise, in the male, from the prostatic artery, and in the female, from the internal pudendal arteries. At the caudal demarcation of the rectum are two anal sphincters (internal and external). Fecal continence is maintained by these sphincters, and surgery in this area always threatens their integrity.

RECTAL PROLAPSE

Rectal prolapse is almost exclusively limited to young dogs and cats. The most common cause is straining to defecate, associated with severe colitis or proctitis due to endoparasites. Other causes include foreign bodies, rectal neoplasia, dystocia, and, in the cat, persistent straining related to urethral obstruction or cystic calculi.

Differentiate this condition from prolapsed intussusception. In the latter condition, a probe can be inserted and advanced cranially into a space between the cylindrical mass and the edge of the anus. This cannot be done with a rectal prolapse.

Preoperative Considerations

- Treat underlying diseases (e.g., parasitism) while attempting conservative management of rectal prolapse.
- Initial management consists of manual reduction of the prolapsed tissue followed by a loose purse-string suture. The purse-string suture should be loose

enough to allow passage of loose feces, but tight enough to keep the prolapsed tissue reduced.
- Feed a low-residue (low-fiber) diet for 7–8 days while the purse-string suture is in place.
- Failure of conservative management may necessitate a surgical procedure.
- The preferred surgical procedure is colopexy unless there is nonviable tissue within the prolapsed segment of rectum.

Resection and Anastomosis

Objectives

- Remove devitalized tissue involved in the rectal prolapse.
- Remove excessive rectal tissue that continues to prolapse in spite of manual reduction or use of the purse-string suture technique alone or in conjunction with a colopexy.

Equipment

- General surgery pack
- A 3-cc syringe case

Technique

1. Place the animal in sternal recumbency in a perineal stand.
2. Insert a well lubricated 3-cc syringe case into the rectum.
3. Place three or four stay sutures around the circumference of the prolapsed tissue through all the layers of tissue. The needle should be against the syringe case at its deepest penetration (Fig. 1A).
4. Resect the prolapse around 180° of the circumference, caudal to the stay sutures (Fig. 1B).
5. Place synthetic absorbable sutures (3-0 or 4-0) through the full thickness of the incised bowel, being sure to incorporate the serosal layers. A simple interrupted appositional pattern is preferred (Fig. 1C).
6. Incise the remaining 180° and suture as described in step 5. Push the rectum cranially into the pelvic canal.

Postoperative Care and Complications

Short-Term

- Give a stool softener (see sec. 7, ch. 11) with food, which is introduced the day after surgery. Continue giving the stool softener for 2 weeks.
- Closely monitor for leakage from the anastomotic

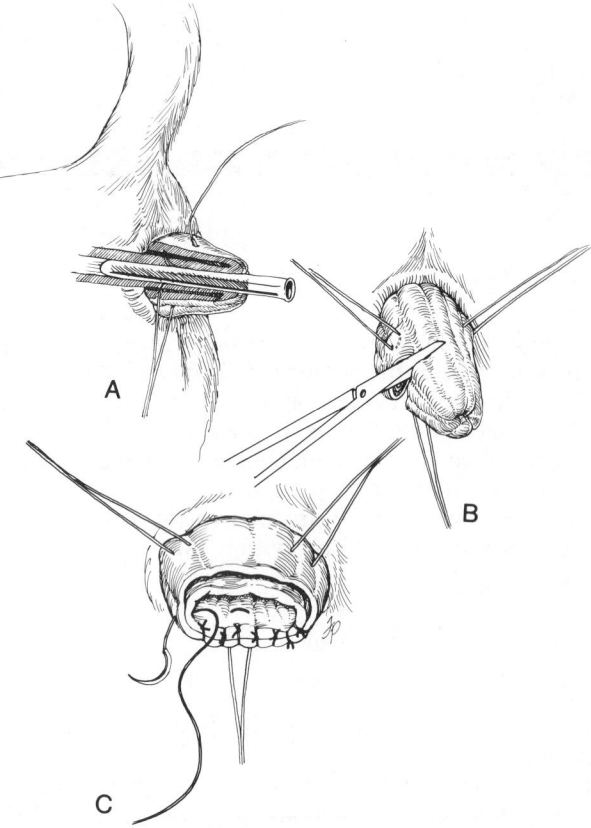

Figure 1. Resection and anastomosis of rectal prolapse.

site for at least 48 hours by observing the animal's temperature, level of activity, eating habits, and signs of excessive pain around the anorectal region. (Take care when placing a rectal thermometer.)
■ Recurrence of rectal prolapse may occur. A purse-string suture may have to be used again or a colopexy performed if it has not been done previously.

Long-Term

Long-term complications can include:

■ Recurrence of rectal prolapse
■ Fecal incontinence
■ Anorectal stricture

ANORECTAL STRICTURE

Causes of anorectal stricture can be benign (e.g., inflammation) or malignant (e.g., adenocarcinoma):

■ Inflammatory causes include perianal fistulae, prior anorectal surgery (including cryosurgery), and accidental trauma.
■ Adenocarcinoma of the rectum and anus is the most common cause of stricture, resulting in a scirrhous, annular ring-type lesion.

Preoperative Considerations

■ Simple, annular non-neoplastic lesions that are not too cranial in location may respond to a series of

bougienage or balloon dilations. During this therapy, give prednisolone for 10–14 days (1 mg/kg q12h).
■ For other lesions (e.g., adenocarcinoma), *resection/anastomosis* (described below) is the treatment of choice.

Surgical Procedure (Resection/Anastomosis with Rectal Pull-Through)

Objective

■ Restore bowel lumen size that will accommodate the aboral movement of feces with minimal resistance while preserving continence of the anorectal sphincter.

Equipment

■ General surgery pack
■ Senn retractors

Technique

1. Clip and aseptically prepare the perineal region.
2. Place a purse-string suture in the anus.
3. When the lesion is cranial to the anorectal junction, make an incision circumferentially around the anal ring.
4. Continue the perirectal dissection to normal tissue just cranial to the stricture ring. Avoid trauma to the sphincter muscles.
5. Place four stay sutures circumferentially through the normal rectal wall just ahead of the stricture.
6. Resect the diseased rectal tissue.
7. Pull the healthy tissue being held by the stay sutures caudally and appose to the anus. Avoid suturing under tension; mobilize more rectal tissue if necessary.

Postoperative Care and Complications

Short-Term

■ Feed the animal the following day.
■ Give stool softeners (see sec. 7, ch. 11) for 2 weeks following surgery.
■ Monitor for leakage from the anastomotic site, especially during the first 48 hours.
■ Fecal incontinence may occur.

Long-Term

■ A pelvic abscess due to earlier leakage from the anastomosis may be seen.
■ Postoperative stricture can occur, especially if tension was present at the suture line.

Prognosis

The prognosis is poor if the stricture was due to an adenocarcinoma. It is poor to guarded if the stricture is related to an inflammatory process.

ANAL STRICTURE LIMITED TO THE ANAL RING

Causes, preoperative considerations, and objectives are similar to those for anorectal strictures, as previously described.

Surgical Procedure

Technique

1. Cut the stricture in four places around the anal ring at 3, 6, 9, and 12 o'clock.
2. Make the incisions perpendicular to the ring. Extend one-half of each incision outward into the skin and the other half inward through the fibrotic mucosa.
3. Suture the incisions in the opposite direction to the edge of the anal ring.

ATRESIA ANI

This condition exists in several forms, the most common being type I (imperforate anus) and type II, in which the rectal pouch is located cranial to the membrane overlying the anus. Regardless of the type, the main problem is loss of continuity between the rectum and anus during embryonal development of the cloacal membrane.

Preoperative Considerations

■ Plain film radiography of the abdomen and pelvis with the animal standing helps to differentiate between type I and type II.
■ Because the patient usually is only days or weeks old, there is a relatively high anesthetic risk.

Surgical Procedure

Objective

■ Relieve the obstruction of feces in the rectum by opening the anus and reconstructing the anorectal junction.

Equipment

■ General surgery pack
■ Iris scissors
■ Fine mouse-tooth thumb forceps

Technique

Type I
1. Incise the skin overlying the anus in a cruciate pattern.
2. Protect the anal sphincter.
3. Incise the rectal pouch just under the incision in a cruciate pattern.
4. Suture the rectal circumference to the subcutaneous tissues and skin with 4-0 or 5-0 nylon in a one-layer simple interrupted appositional pattern using monofilament nonabsorbable suture.

Type II
1. Incise the membrane overlying the anus in a cruciate pattern.
2. Continue the perirectal dissection cranially until the rectal pouch is identified.
3. Incise the blind pouch as described in Step 3 for type I.

4. Rectocutaneous apposition is achieved as described in Step 4 for type I.

Postoperative Care and Complications

Short-Term

■ Monitor closely for suture line breakdown and infection of the surgical site.
■ Because of the young age of these patients, give aggressive fluid therapy (including dextrose to prevent hypoglycemia) during surgery and well into the postoperative period.
■ Initially, fecal incontinence often is a problem but resolves spontaneously in some animals.

Long-Term

■ Fecal incontinence may continue indefinitely.
■ Stricture is a possible sequela to anorectal surgery.
■ Megacolon that sometimes accompanies atresia ani may be permanent and constipation may be an ongoing problem.

PERIANAL FISTULAE

Perianal fistulae are multiple draining tracts that surround the anus and are chronic in nature. German shepherd and Irish setter breeds are affected most commonly (see sec. 7, ch. 11 for a complete description of this disease).

Preoperative Considerations

■ Consider conservative therapy, consisting of perianal cleansing with an antiseptic solution and application of hot packs.
■ Antibiotic therapy for 2–3 weeks may ameliorate the pain associated with this condition.
■ In most cases, some form of surgical intervention will be necessary. Regardless of the procedure, surgical excision of diseased tissue is a compromise between complete excision and minimization of trauma to spare the external anal sphincter.
■ An anal sacculectomy should accompany any excisional procedure.

Surgical Procedure

Objective

■ Remove diseased tissue around a portion of the anus and, if necessary, around its entire circumference.

Equipment

General surgery pack

Technique

1. Make a skin incision to incorporate all the diseased tissue surrounding the anus.
2. Dissect and continue into the deeper tissues until the cranial extent of the fistulous tracts is determined.

3. Take care to prevent damage to the external anal sphincter muscle or its innervation.
4. In some instances, a portion of the sphincter muscle may be removed coincidentally when attempting to excise the diseased tissue.
5. In severe cases, remove a doughnut-shaped piece of tissue, leaving healthy rectal tissue underneath.
6. Transversely incise the rectum to allow removal of the anus and diseased tissue.
7. Suture the rim of rectal mucosa directly to the skin, using 3-0 monofilament nonabsorbable suture.

Postoperative Care and Complications

- Keep the incision clean, using hydrotherapy twice a day.
- Give stool softeners for 1–2 weeks.
- Incisional dehiscence may occur but is usually treated conservatively (let heal by second intention).
- Fecal incontinence may occur after extensive resections.
- Recurrence of fistulas can occur. Treat by excision of affected tissues.

PERINEAL HERNIA

Perineal hernia results from weakening of the perineal muscles (i.e., the levator ani and lateral coccygeus) and external anal sphincter. Hernias may result in rectal sacculation and herniation of prostate, fat, bladder, or bowel (sec. 7, ch. 11). The exact cause is uncertain but is thought to be related to any condition that causes chronic tenesmus (constipation, prostatomegaly). Other possible causes include hormonal imbalance or degenerative changes to the levator ani musculature.

Preoperative Considerations

- Castration usually accompanies a herniorrhaphy. It is thought to help prevent recurrence by decreasing tenesmus related to prostatomegaly.
- Urethral obstruction secondary to bladder entrapment requires emergency treatment (cystocentesis and placement of a urethral catheter).

Surgical Procedure

Objectives

- Replace contents of hernial sac into peritoneal cavity.
- Reconstruct pelvic diagram.
- Prevent deviation of the rectum and retroflexion of the bladder and prostate gland.

Equipment

- General surgery pack.
- Self-retaining retractors.
- ¼″ Penrose drain.

Technique

1. Place the animal in sternal recumbency and secure the tail forward over the back.

2. Place a purse-string suture around the anus.
3. Make a half-curved or a curvilinear incision, beginning just lateral to the base of the tail and extending ventrally below the perineal bulge.
4. Using blunt dissection, remove the tissue overlying the hernial sac; open the sac with scissors.
5. Gently replace the herniated viscera into the abdominal cavity.
6. Dissect the tissue overlying the external anal sphincter, exposing the muscle striations.
7. Identify dorsolaterally the levator ani and lateral coccygeal muscles.
8. Palpate the sacrotuberous ligament and use as the lateral landmark.
9. Carefully isolate the neurovascular bundle, containing the pudendal nerve and the internal pudendal vessels and place a ¼″ Penrose drain around it to identify its presence as sutures are placed.
10. Repair the dorsal aspect of the hernia first by preplacing three or four sutures between the coccygeal musculature and the external anal sphincter. Monofilament nonabsorbable sutures or synthetic absorbable sutures such as PDS or Maxon are preferred (Fig. 2A).
11. The sacrotuberous ligament may be incorporated with the coccygeal muscle when insufficient musculature is present. The sutures are then tied.
12. Identify the obturator muscle and isolate by bluntly dissecting the overlying tissue.
13. Incise the caudal border of the internal obturator muscle and elevate the muscle with a periosteal elevator until the caudal border of the obturator foramen can be seen (Fig. 2B).
14. Partially or completely incise the tendon of the obturator muscle to allow the muscle to be drawn dorsomedially (Fig. 2C).
15. Preplace similar sutures between the obturator muscle and the external anal sphincter. Avoid penetrating the rectum. Knot the sutures after gently apposing the tissues.

Postoperative Care and Complications

Short-Term

- Straining to urinate or hematuria suggests iatrogenic trauma to the urethra by a misplaced suture.
- Rectal prolapse may occur, especially if a bilateral repair is done. Staging the repair several weeks apart will usually eliminate this complication.
- Fecal incontinence may result from damage to the pudendal or caudal rectal nerves or to the sphincter muscle itself. If damage to innervation is bilateral, the animal usually will not regain continence.
- Urinary incontinence sometimes occurs postoperatively but is infrequent. It appears to be associated with bladder retroflexion before surgery.
- Wound infection may result because of improper suture placement through the rectal wall, penetration of the anal sac, or contamination. This usually is seen in the first 48–72 hours postoperatively.

Long-Term

- Fecal or urinary incontinence may persist for weeks or months and sometimes indefinitely.

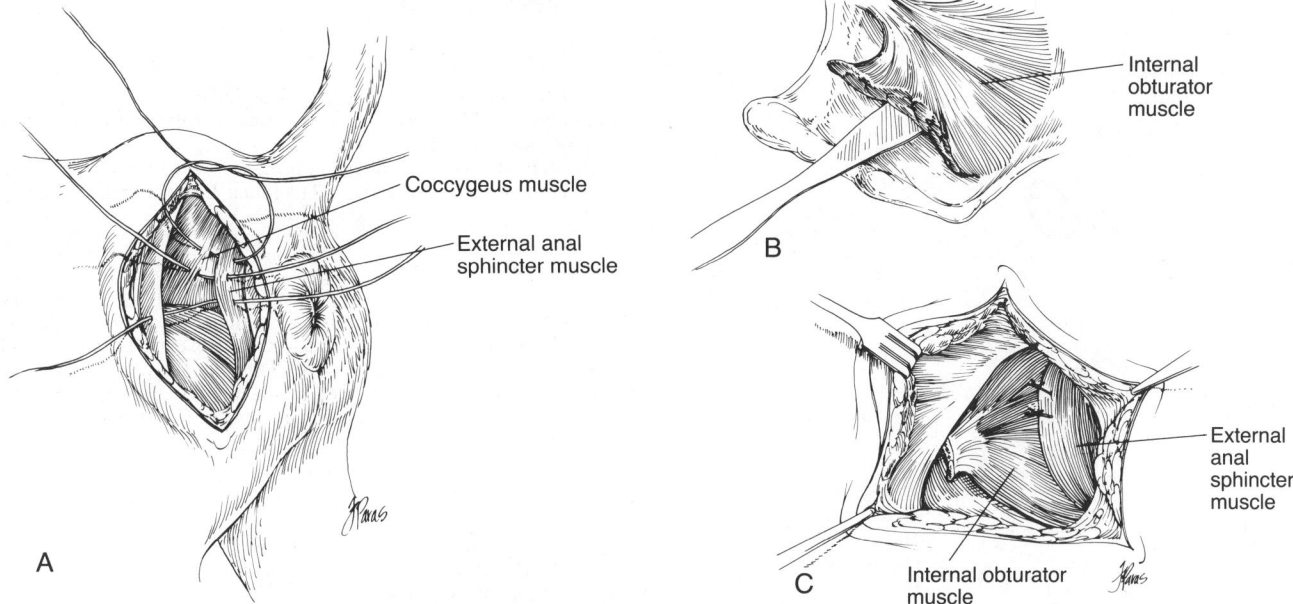

Figure 2. Repair of perineal hernia. Close the dorsal portion using the coccygeus and external anal sphincter muscles *(A)*. Close the remainder of the defect by elevating the internal obturator muscle *(B)* and suturing it to the external anal sphincter *(C)*.

- Recurrence is directly correlated with the skill of the surgeon and the severity of the hernia. Castration may help to decrease recurrence regardless of the skill level of the surgeon.
- Colopexy and vas deferens pexy can be performed on recurrent hernias or if initial hernia is severe.

Prognosis

- If the surgery is performed by an experienced surgeon, the prognosis is good.
- Use of the obturator flap technique is believed to be associated with fewer problems postoperatively and with a lower recurrence rate.

ANAL SACCULECTOMY

The primary goal of anal sac surgery is correction of longstanding anal sac infection (see sec. 7, ch. 11) that is refractory to conservative therapy.

Preoperative Considerations

- Do not perform anal sacculectomy during the acute inflammatory stage of infection.
- Administer antibacterial therapy, flush the anal sacs with antiseptic solutions, and use hot packs to control the sacculitis.
- Tumors of the apocrine glands of the anal sac are an indication for surgery.

Surgical Procedure

Objectives

- Remove the entire anal sac.
- Preserve anorectal function by carefully avoiding excessive trauma to the external anal sphincter muscle and its corresponding innervation.

Equipment

- General surgery pack
- Electrocautery
- Iris scissors (optional)

Technique

1. Place a scissors blade into the duct of each anal sac (Fig. 3*A*).
2. Use thumb forceps to place countertraction on the duct before cutting so that all structures can be exposed.
3. After incising the sac, identify the lining by its gray color.
4. Place mosquito forceps at opposite ends of the anal sac lining.
5. Use small Metzenbaum or iris scissors to bluntly dissect the sac free of its attachments, including the fibers of the external anal sphincter (Fig. 3*B*).
6. When dissecting medial to the anal sac duct, preserve the caudal rectal artery.
7. Use fine, nonabsorbable sutures to close the incision after flushing thoroughly with saline.

Postoperative Care and Complications

Short-Term

- Hemorrhage due to inadequate hemostasis may continue after closure of the skin.
- Rarely, temporary or permanent fecal incontinence may result.
- Wound infection is more likely because of the location of the surgical site.
- Tenesmus or dyschezia may occur for a few days but usually resolves spontaneously.

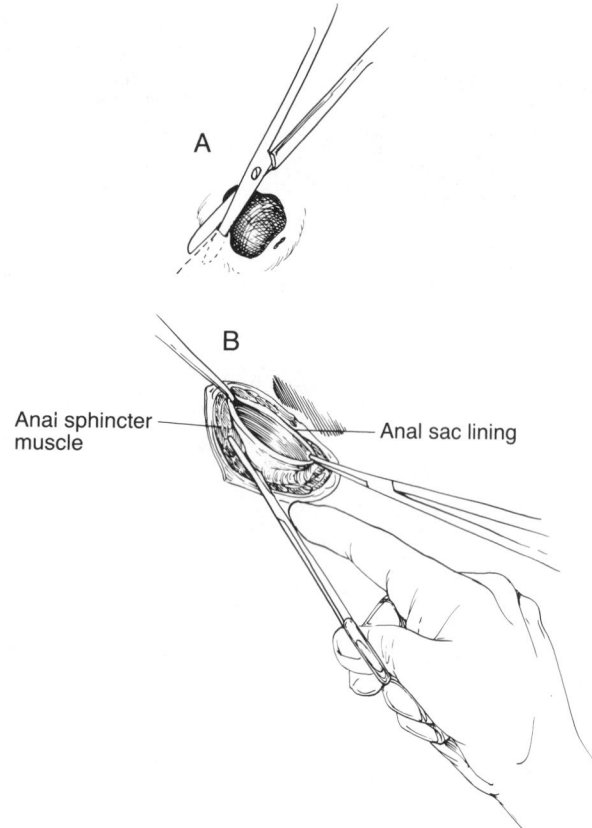

Figure 3. Surgical technique for resection of anal sac.

Long-Term

- Fistulous tracts may form after sacculectomy and are the result of incomplete excision of the anal sac lining.
- Wounds that do not heal after surgery may indicate a concurrent anal sac tumor.

Prognosis

The prognosis is good with complete excision of the sac lining and preservation of the external anal sphincter.

Supplemental Readings

RECTAL PROLAPSE

Bright RM: Diseases of the anus and perianal area. *In* Morgan R, ed.: *Handbook of Small Animal Practice*. New York: Churchill Livingstone, 1988, p 479.
Engen MH: Management of rectal prolapse. *In Current Techniques in Small Animal Surgery II*. Philadelphia: Lea & Febiger, 1983, p 184.

ANORECTAL STRICTURE

Bright RM: Diseases of the anus and perianal area. *In* Morgan R, ed.: *Handbook of Small Animal Practice*. New York: Churchill Livingstone, 1988, p 479.
Walshaw R: Rectoanal strictures in the dog. *In* Bojrab MJ, ed.: *Current Techniques in Small Animal Surgery II*. Philadelphia: Lea & Febiger, 1983, p 201.

ATRESIA ANI

Bright RM: Diseases of the anus and perianal area. *In* Morgan R, ed.: *Handbook of Small Animal Practice*. New York: Churchill Livingstone, 1988, p 479.
Grandage J: Rectum and anus. *In* Slatter DH, ed.: *Textbook of Small Animal Surgery*. Philadelphia: W. B. Saunders, 1984, p 768.

PERIANAL FISTULAE

Bloomberg MS: The clinical management of perianal fistulas in the dog. Comp Contin Educ Pract Vet 2:615, 1980.
vanEe RT: Tail amputation for treatment of perianal fistulas in dogs. J Am Anim Hosp 23:95, 1987.

PERINEAL HERNIA

Bilbrey SA, Smeak DD, DeHoff W: Fixation of the deferent ducts for retrodisplacement of the urinary bladder and prostate in canine perineal hernia. Vet Surg 19:24, 1990.
Early TD, Kolata RJ: Perineal hernia in the dog: An alternative method of correction. *In* Bojrab MJ, ed.: *Current Techniques in Small Animal Surgery II*. Philadelphia: Lea & Febiger, 1983, p 405.
Hardie EM, Kolata RJ, Early TD, et al.: Evaluation of internal obturator muscle transposition in treatment of perianal hernia in dogs. Vet Surg 12:69, 1983.

ANAL SACCULECTOMY

Walshaw R: Anal sac disease. *In* Bojrab MJ, ed.: *Current Techniques in Small Animal Surgery II*. Philadelphia: Lea & Febiger, 1983, p 196.

13 Peritonitis

Stephen J. Birchard

Peritonitis is a common problem in small animals. Primary peritonitis can occur in cats, but other forms of peritonitis in dogs and cats are usually secondary to other diseases or injuries. Advances in the diagnosis and treatment of peritonitis have lowered mortality rates.

KEY POINT ▶ The single most important recent advance in the surgical treatment of peritonitis is open abdominal drainage.

Open abdominal drainage allows more effective and complete drainage of the peritoneal cavity and has increased survival, even in cases of severe peritonitis. However, peritonitis continues to be a serious and life-threatening condition that requires aggressive management.

In this chapter the general topic of peritonitis is discussed. For more detailed information on the treatment of the specific causes of peritonitis, refer to appropriate chapters.

ANATOMY

The peritoneum is a serous membrane composed of mesothelial cells. It consists of the parietal peritoneum that lines the abdominal cavity and the visceral peritoneum that covers the abdominal viscera. The peritoneum has tremendous surface area (i.e., 50–100% of body surface area). The peritoneal cavity is closed in the male but open in the female through the reproductive tract. A small amount of fluid that lubricates the abdominal viscera is produced by the peritoneum.

ETIOLOGY

Viral

Feline infectious peritonitis is an example of primary peritonitis (see sec. 2, ch. 3).

Bacterial

Gastrointestinal Perforation or Leakage

KEY POINT ▶ Loss of bowel wall integrity accounts for the majority of cases of bacterial peritonitis in dogs and cats.

Leakage of bowel contents allows release of bacteria, predominantly anaerobes and gram-negative aerobes. Fluid and ingesta may also leak if gross bowel wall disruption occurs, resulting in a complex interaction of

bacterial, chemical, and foreign-body factors in the pathogenesis of peritonitis.

Bowel leakage can occur by a variety of mechanisms:

- Perforation—The bowel can be penetrated by external objects such as gunshot and a sharp object.
- Leakage from a necrotizing gastrointestinal neoplasm (carcinoma, lymphoma) can occur.
- Colonic perforation can occur secondary to the administration of high doses of corticosteroids in animals with spinal compression.
- Foreign bodies—Sharp intestinal or linear foreign bodies frequently cause perforation (see sec. 7, ch. 6). Also, intraluminal pressure on the intestinal wall by the foreign body can eventually lead to ischemic necrosis and leakage.
- Blunt trauma—Devitalization of the bowel can occur secondary to tearing of the mesenteric blood supply.
- Strangulation—Any process causing obstruction of the intestinal blood supply will cause loss of mucosal integrity and, eventually, full-thickness necrosis (see sec. 7, ch. 6). Loss of the so-called mucosal barrier can result in translocation of bacteria and/or endotoxins into the peritoneal cavity.
- Dehiscence—Unsatisfactory healing of a gastrointestinal incision may result in leakage through the wound and subsequent peritonitis.

Pyometra

Bacterial infection of the uterus can lead to peritonitis by leakage through the fallopian tubes or overt rupture of a pus-filled uterus (see sec. 8, ch. 14).

Prostatic or Liver Abscess

Abscesses of the prostate gland (see sec. 8, ch. 8) or liver (see sec. 7, ch. 8) may leak bacteria to the peritoneal cavity spontaneously or iatrogenically during surgical exploration.

Surgical Contamination

A breakdown in aseptic technique can result in contamination of the peritoneal cavity and peritonitis.

Chemical

Urinary Tract

Leakage of urine from any part of the urinary tract can cause chemical peritonitis. Disruption of the urinary system may occur as the result of spontaneous or iatrogenic trauma.

- Causes of urinary tract disruption include trauma

(blunt or penetrating), bladder or urethral rupture due to obstruction, and traumatic catheterization (see sec. 8, chs. 3 and 5). Urinary tract disruption frequently is associated with pelvic and sacral fractures or luxations.
- Bacterial peritonitis can complicate the chemical peritonitis from the urine leakage if urinary tract infection was present before the leakage occurred.

Biliary Tract

- Trauma to the biliary tract can cause leakage of bile due to rupture of the gallbladder or one of the bile ducts.
- Spontaneous leakage of bile can occur with necrotizing cholecystitis. Bacterial peritonitis may also complicate this situation.
- Bile is irritating to the peritoneum. However, several days may elapse before an affected animal is presented for clinical signs of peritonitis and biliary disease.

Gastrointestinal Tract

- Gastric fluid contains hydrochloric acid and therefore is very irritating to the peritoneum. Intestinal fluid contains bile and pancreatic enzymes that may cause chemical in addition to bacterial peritonitis.
- Leakage of gastric fluid may occur due to trauma or any of the other causes of tissue breakdown listed under Gastrointestinal Perforation or Leakage.
- Gastric fluid may leak secondary to perforating ulcers or necrotizing gastric neoplasms (see sec. 7, ch. 4).
- Tissue necrosis secondary to gastric dilatation volvulus can cause leakage of gastric contents.
- Gastric contents are not always sterile. Bacterial contamination associated with leakage of ingesta can complicate the peritonitis and result in a combination of chemical and septic peritonitis.

Chyle

- Disruption of the mesenteric lymphatics, lymph nodes, or cysterna chyli can cause leakage of chyle into the peritoneal cavity.
- Neoplasia or other diseases causing erosion or obstruction of the lymphatics are more likely causes than disruption due to trauma.
- Chyle is irritating to the peritoneum, although in some animals it is reabsorbed by the abdominal lymphatics.

Pancreatitis

- Leakage of pancreatic enzymes and various chemical mediators of inflammation from the inflamed pancreas causes peritonitis (see sec. 7, ch. 10).
- Local peritonitis is very common with pancreatitis. Severe, necrotizing pancreatitis or pancreatic abscess may cause generalized peritonitis.

Traumatic

Penetrating trauma that involves the peritoneal cavity, such as a gunshot or knife wound, will cause peritonitis even if the viscera are not injured.

Iatrogenic (Surgical)

- Varying degrees of peritonitis result from surgical manipulation of the peritoneum or abdominal structures.
- Analysis of peritoneal fluid after routine abdominal surgery shows increased neutrophils. Also, serum lipase concentrations significantly increase after abdominal exploration, suggesting pancreatic inflammation.
- Typically, peritonitis from routine visceral manipulation is clinically insignificant. Poor surgical technique, such as rough handling of tissues, allowing tissues to become desiccated, and lack of aseptic technique can result in more serious peritonitis.

Foreign Body
Sutures

- Implantation of excessive sutures or large sutures can result in focal peritonitis.
- Nonabsorbable braided sutures that are contaminated can cause chronic focal peritonitis and resultant sinus tracts and abscesses.

Surgical Sponges

- Failure to remove surgical sponges can result in focal or diffuse peritonitis. Even sponges considered to be sterile can cause a significant foreign body reaction. Contaminated sponges cause abscesses and possibly severe, septic peritonitis.
- Prevention of this complication is essential.
  - Count surgical sponges before and after surgery to be sure that none have been left in the abdomen.
  - Use sponges that contain a radiopaque marker to allow diagnosis of a sponge foreign body on abdominal radiography.

Other

- Failure to remove surgical instruments can cause a foreign-body reaction, irritation of viscera, and strangulation of blood supply to structures.
- Talc used on surgical gloves can cause a foreign-body, granulomatous, peritoneal reaction. After donning surgical gloves, rinse with sterile saline prior to opening the peritoneal cavity.
- Bacterial peritonitis is a complication of peritoneal dialysis caused by contamination during the procedure or ascending infection via the indwelling dialysis catheter.

DISTRIBUTION AND LETHAL FACTORS
Local Peritonitis

- Local peritonitis is common and usually does not require aggressive surgical management.
- The abdominal structures, such as the omentum and mesentery, are able to "wall off" inflammatory processes and prevent spread to the entire cavity.
- The production of fibrin by the peritoneum is also

an important process in confining bacteria and debris to an isolated area of the peritoneal cavity.

- Permanent adhesions can be a sequela of local peritonitis, but they rarely cause a significant clinical problem in small animals.

Diffuse Peritonitis

- Diffuse or generalized peritonitis occurs when the processes of confinement are overwhelmed and the entire cavity is affected.
- Diffuse peritonitis is a serious condition that requires aggressive medical and usually surgical therapy.
- Movement of the diaphragm, intestinal peristalsis, and gravity encourage dissemination of bacteria throughout the peritoneal cavity.
- Surgical manipulation of contaminated tissues can convert local to diffuse peritonitis.

Lethal Factors

Certain substances or combinations of substances have been shown to be especially devastating to the animal with peritonitis.

KEY POINT ▶ The addition of blood, fluid, or barium (or other foreign material) to bacterial contamination of the peritoneum can cause severe, frequently fatal peritonitis.

- Hemoglobin, in addition to bacteria, creates a lethal combination in peritonitis. Hemoglobin tends to reduce the ability of the neutrophils to phagocytize bacteria.
- Barium sulfate, in addition to bacteria, has the same effect as hemoglobin.
- Excessive peritoneal fluid acts as an adjuvant in peritonitis. Fluid causes dissemination of bacteria. Neutrophils phagocytize bacteria by migrating along visceral and peritoneal surfaces. Peritoneal fluid interferes with this process.
- Contamination of the peritoneal cavity with multiple species of bacteria, such as occurs with bowel leakage, causes a much more severe peritonitis than that due to one species.
- The combination of chemical and bacterial peritonitis is especially devastating. Proteolytic and lipolytic enzymes cause tissue necrosis, an ideal medium for bacterial growth.

CLINICAL SIGNS

Pain

The peritoneum is a very sensitive membrane. Irritation of the peritoneum can cause abdominal discomfort.

- The mildly affected animal is resistant to abdominal palpation.
- Signs of severe pain include reluctance to move and tachycardia and tachypnea.
- The animal may assume the "praying mantis" posture in an attempt to alleviate peritoneal pain.
- Peritoneal pain may cause the animal to contract the abdominal muscles, giving the abdomen a "tucked up" appearance.

Fever

- Pyrexia may or may not be present.
- Fever does not always imply the presence of sepsis but is more likely when bacterial contamination complicates the peritoneal inflammation.
- An animal with overwhelming peritonitis, dehydration, and shock may have a subnormal temperature.

Vomiting

Vomiting may occur due to irritation of serosal surfaces, ileus, or the primary disease causing the peritonitis.

Dehydration

- The peritoneum responds to inflammation by producing large amounts of protein-rich fluid.
- Loss of fluid from the peritoneum, inadequate intake of water and food, vomiting, and fever rapidly causes significant dehydration and hypovolemia.

Shock

- Hypovolemic shock can develop rapidly with peritonitis as a result of the processes described under Dehydration, as well as the sequence of events described in sec. 6, ch. 14 on shock.
- Septic shock also is possible with diffuse peritonitis owing to release of bacteria to the peritoneal cavity, followed by absorption to the systemic circulation. Lysis of gram-negative bacteria that have leaked from the bowel causes endotoxemia. These endotoxins have a direct cytotoxic effect, as well as causing many systemic changes such as vasodilation and blood pooling, hypoglycemia, and acidosis.

DIAGNOSIS

History

- Thoroughly review the animal's history to gain clues to the presence of peritonitis and possible etiologies.
- Give special attention to any history of trauma or prior abdominal surgery.
- Determine if the animal recently ate any foreign bodies that could have caused bowel perforation.
- Has the animal had any signs of gastric or colonic ulceration? A history of hematemesis, melena, or hematochezia is indicative of a more serious lesion of the gastrointestinal (GI) tract and increases the suspicion of perforation.
- Does the animal have the typical signalment or history of pancreatitis?

Physical Examination

- Look for the clinical signs listed previously.
- Carefully palpate the abdomen for evidence of pain, fluid, ileus, or masses.
- Check for fever.

Clinical Pathology

Fluid Analysis

Abdominocentesis. See sec. 1, ch. 3 for a description of the technique for abdominocentesis.

- Animals with peritonitis will have many neutrophils ($> 500/\mu l$) and may have bacteria on cytologic examination. Absence of bacteria suggests a sterile peritonitis, such as can occur with chemical peritonitis.
- The presence of bacteria within phagocytes confirms septic peritonitis. Bacteria within and outside phagocytes suggest that the infection is overwhelming the defense mechanisms. The presence of cocci and rods indicates mixed infection, such as can occur with GI perforation. Gram stain of the fluid can differentiate gram-negative rods (usually aerobes such as *Escherichia coli*) from gram-positive rods (usually anaerobes such as *Clostridium* spp.).
- Large numbers of red blood cells (RBCs) indicate hemorrhage associated with the peritonitis. This can occur with trauma, bleeding tumors, or development of disseminated intravascular coagulation.

Diagnostic Peritoneal Lavage (DPL). See sec. 1, ch. 3 for a description of the technique for DPL.

- Observe the gross appearance of the fluid. Opaque fluid is likely from animals with peritonitis.
- Analyze the fluid for neutrophils ($> 500/\mu l$ is considered a positive finding), toxic neutrophils, bacteria, bilirubin, creatinine higher than serum concentration, amylase > 200 IU, and vegetable fibers.
- Animals that have had recent surgery normally have a high number of nucleated cells in the peritoneal cavity ($> 6000/\mu l$).

Hematology

- Neutrophilia may be present with or without toxic neutrophils. A left shift (increase in number of band neutrophils) indicates more significant inflammation. A degenerative left shift (more bands than segmented neutrophils) indicates an overwhelming, life-threatening inflammatory process.
- Chronic blood loss or chronic infection may result in anemia.
- Hypoproteinemia due to loss of albumin is very common in peritonitis.

Serum Chemistry Profile

- Many parameters may be altered, depending on the type of peritonitis and the associated clinical signs.
- Electrolytes (sodium, potassium, and chloride) may be depleted in animals that are vomiting. Acidotic animals may be hyperkalemic. Dehydration can artificially elevate electrolyte concentrations.
- Hypoglycemia may be present in animals with septic peritonitis.
- Serum urea nitrogen is elevated in animals with uroperitoneum and in animals suffering from prerenal azotemia due to dehydration or shock.
- Serum pancreatic enzymes (amylase, lipase) frequently are mildly elevated in all types of peritonitis, and moderately to markedly elevated when underlying pancreatitis is the cause of peritonitis.
- Serum liver enzymes and bilirubin are variably increased in all types of peritonitis and may be markedly increased in sepsis, biliary tract rupture, liver abscess, and pancreatitis.

Radiography

Plain Radiography

- Plain abdominal radiography usually reveals lack of soft tissue detail either focally or throughout the abdomen. Fluid may be present in the peritoneal cavity.
- Pneumoperitoneum may be seen if any portion of the gastrointestinal tract has perforated or there has been penetrating abdominal trauma. Films obtained using horizontal projection can confirm air in the peritoneal space, because it rises to the dorsum of the cavity.
- Ileus may be present.

Contrast Studies

- Perform positive-contrast urethrography, cystography, and/or intravenous pyelography if uroperitoneum is suspected (see sec. 1, ch. 4).
- Perform positive-contrast gastrointestinal studies to diagnose perforation (see sec. 1, ch. 4). Avoid using barium as the contrast agent when perforation is suspected, because barium leakage into the peritoneal cavity can be devastating (treat with immediate laparotomy, peritoneal lavage and drainage).

Ultrasonography

- Ultrasonography can confirm the presence of peritoneal fluid. It is especially valuable for evaluating the pancreas as a potential cause of peritonitis.
- Soft tissue masses or abscesses may be seen (see sec. 1, ch. 4).

TREATMENT

Management of peritonitis consists of supportive care and definitive measures to eliminate or correct the cause. The decision to treat the animal medically or surgically depends on the cause and the animal's response to treatment. If a surgical disease is not suspected and the peritonitis is mild, medical treatment alone may suffice. However, promptly initiate surgical treatment if the peritonitis is moderate or severe, is not improving with medical treatment, or is due to a surgical lesion such as a perforated intestine, biliary or urinary rupture.

Medical Management

Fluids

Intravenous fluids are probably the most important supportive treatment. The type of fluids used depends on the type of peritonitis and the metabolic alterations present in the patient.

- In most cases, use lactated Ringer's solution supplemented with potassium to prevent or correct hypokalemia.
- After correcting the dehydration, give fluids at a maintenance rate, plus continuing losses, until the animal is able to maintain hydration with oral intake (See sec. 1, ch. 5 for fluid therapy details.)

Antibiotics

Systemic antibiotics are indicated in bacterial peritonitis. Choose antibiotics based on culture and sensitivity testing of peritoneal fluid.

- In the absence of culture results, use broad-spectrum bactericidal drugs. Results of Gram stain of abdominal fluid (see under Diagnosis) can be used to guide antibiotic choice.
- Combinations of antibiotics may be necessary if a mixed population of bacteria are present. For example, combine ampicillin or one of the cephalosporins (e.g., cephalothin) with an aminoglycoside (e.g., gentamicin) for peritonitis due to a mixed bacterial population.

Lavage and Drainage

KEY POINT ▶ One of the most important treatments for peritonitis is drainage of fluid and debris from the peritoneal cavity.

Abdominal drains such as Penrose drains or sump drains (e.g., a fenestrated Brunswick catheter inside a fenestrated Penrose drain) are ineffective for draining the entire peritoneal cavity for any longer than a few hours. However, these types of drains can be effective for the initial drainage of the abdomen or for animals that are producing large amounts of abdominal fluid.

- Open abdominal drainage has been used successfully in experimental and clinical peritonitis and is described under Surgical Management.
- Lavage of the peritoneal cavity has been recommended but is controversial. Addition of fluid to the peritoneal cavity may potentiate generalized peritonitis and should only be used when all of the lavage fluid can be drained. Therefore, lavage should be reserved for those patients that undergo surgical treatment of the problem.
- Addition of antibiotics or antiseptics to the lavage fluid has *not* been shown to have any benefit over the use of saline alone in conjunction with systemic antibiotics.
  - Do not use aminoglycosides in peritoneal lavage during anesthesia, especially if neuromuscular blocking agents are being used. Aminoglycosides can potentiate the effect of these agents. Also, they will be absorbed and can reach toxic blood levels if they also are being given parenterally.
  - Avoid using povidone-iodine (Betadine) in lavage fluid in animals with peritonitis, because it can also be absorbed and cause severe toxicity, possibly due to absorption of large amounts of iodine.

Surgical Management

Correction of lesions resulting in peritonitis is covered in the appropriate chapters. Open peritoneal drainage as a general treatment for peritonitis is discussed here.

Preoperative Considerations

- As discussed under Medical Treatment, correct fluid and electrolyte disorders, when possible, prior to surgery.
- Begin antibiotic treatment before surgery if contamination is present or is likely to occur during the surgery.

Technique for Open Peritoneal Drainage

1. After the laparotomy has been performed and the cause of the peritonitis has been corrected, lavage the abdominal cavity with warm, sterile saline. Use copious amounts of saline to flush bacteria and debris from the cavity. Discontinue flushing when the lavage solution appears clear on removal from the abdomen.
2. Partially close the abdominal incision. Use large horizontal mattress sutures of monofilament polypropylene or nylon (1, 0, or 2-0) in the linea alba to reduce the incisional gap to approximately 3–4 cm in width. Leave the remaining tissue layers open.
3. Cover the incision with a sterile dressing consisting of (from inside out) sterile Vaseline-impregnated gauze, sterile laparotomy sponges or towels, cotton, conforming gauze, and tape. Make the bandage large enough to extend several centimeters beyond the cranial and caudal aspect of the incision and construct it so that slippage will not occur.
   a. Large polypropylene sutures can be used as "laces" to hold the laparotomy pads or towels in place.
4. Change the bandage aseptically two or more times daily, depending on the quantity of fluid drainage. Omental or falciform ligament adhesions to the sutures can be gently broken down with a sterile-gloved hand between bandage changes. If necessary, obtain samples of peritoneal fluid periodically for cytology and culture.
   a. Weigh the bandage before and after placement on the animal to estimate fluid loss (500 ml = 1 lb). Use this information to help calculate fluid requirements and to monitor the trend of abdominal fluid production.
5. In most patients, the abdomen is closed within 5–7 days of the original surgery (see below). Perform abdominal closure by removing the original horizontal mattress sutures in the fascia and proceeding with a routine closure. Additional culture samples from the peritoneum may be obtained just before closure.

The decision on when to close the abdominal incision is subjective. I base this decision on several factors:

■ Overall progress of the patient
■ Quantity and character of fluid drainage from the abdomen
■ Persistence of fever or neutrophilia with a left shift on hemography

Postoperative Care and Complications

■ Keep the bandage as clean as possible. Urinary catheterization may be necessary in male dogs, or the animal can be kept on an elevated grate to prevent urine soaking of the bandage.
■ Open drainage of the abdomen can cause several complications:
  • Loss of fluids and proteins from the peritoneal cavity—Supportive care with IV fluids is very important. Hyperalimentation (or total parenteral nutrition) also is necessary if the animal is not eating adequately (see sec. 1, ch. 3 for nutritional management of the critical care patient).
  • Electrolyte depletion, especially potassium—Supplement IV fluids with potassium if necessary (see sec. 1, ch. 5).
  • Discomfort from the peritonitis and from open abdomen—Administer analgesics as necessary (e.g., morphine).
  • Herniation of abdominal viscera or omentum—This may occur if the bandage slips or is damaged by the animal. Gently lavage any tissue that becomes contaminated with sterile saline or remove surgically. Restrict exercise.

Supplemental Readings

Bjorling DE, Crowe DT, Kolata RJ, Rawlings CA: Penetrating abdominal wounds in dogs and cats. J Am Anim Hosp Assoc 18:742, 1982.

Bjorling DE, Latimer KS, Rawlings CA, et al.: Diagnostic peritoneal lavage before and after abdominal surgery in dogs. Am J Vet Res 44:816, 1983.

Crowe DT, Bjorling DE: Peritoneum and peritoneal cavity. *In* Slatter DH, ed.: *Textbook of Small Animal Surgery*. Philadelphia: W. B. Saunders, 1985, p 571.

MacCoy, D: Peritonitis. *In* Bojrab MJ, ed.: *Pathophysiology in Small Animal Surgery*. Philadelphia: Lea & Febiger, 1981, p 142.

Urogenital System

Daniel Smeak

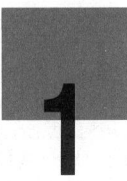

Diseases of the Kidney and Ureter

S. Dru Forrester
George E. Lees

ACUTE RENAL FAILURE

Acute renal failure (ARF) is a clinical syndrome associated with a rapid decline of renal function. It is characterized by abnormalities arising from the inability of the kidneys to adequately regulate fluid, electrolyte, and acid-base balance, and to adequately excrete metabolic waste products.

A laboratory abnormality of azotemia indicates retention of nitrogenous wastes. Causes of azotemia are categorized as prerenal, renal, and postrenal, depending upon the location of the lesion or the abnormality that limits renal function.

Prerenal azotemia occurs when glomerular filtration rate (GFR) is reduced by renal hypoperfusion that is caused by extrarenal circulatory impairment. Mild prerenal azotemia also may occur without reduction of GFR, because of excessive protein catabolism or increased fractional reabsorption of filtered urea (e.g., states of antidiuresis). Conditions that may reduce GFR causing prerenal azotemia include dehydration, hypovolemia, hypotension, congestive heart failure (see sec. 6, ch. 6) and hypoadrenocorticism (see sec. 4, ch. 3). Dogs and cats with prerenal azotemia concentrate urine to a specific gravity >1.035, unless concurrent disease (e.g., hypoadrenocorticism, hypercalcemia) or diuretic agents impair this ability. Prerenal azotemia resolves rapidly with appropriate treatment. Prolonged or severe hypoperfusion may cause ARF, however, particularly in predisposed patients (e.g., those with underlying renal disease).

Postrenal azotemia occurs when a lesion of the excretory pathway (e.g., renal pelves, ureters, urinary bladder, and urethra) causes obstruction to adequate urine flow or causes internal leakage of urine that is subsequently reabsorbed. Causes of postrenal azotemia include urolithiasis; urethral plugs; neoplasia; other space-occupying lesions; displacement or entrapment of the bladder (e.g., in a hernia); and traumatic rupture or perforation.

KEY POINT ▶ Clinical and pathophysiologic consequences of abrupt, complete obstruction of the urinary tract are similar to those of ARF; therefore, excluding postrenal causes of azotemia in the diagnosis of ARF is an important step.

Postrenal azotemia usually responds to correction of the underlying cause, although prolonged obstruction may cause irreversible renal damage. See subsequent discussions of postrenal azotemia in this chapter.

Renal azotemia occurs when lesions of renal tissues, such as vessels, glomeruli, tubules, or interstitium, cause a decreased GFR sufficient to elevate the plasma concentrations of nitrogenous wastes above normal. Correction of concomitant prerenal or postrenal abnormalities (e.g., dehydration, urinary obstruction) may reduce, but not resolve, renal azotemia.

KEY POINT ▶ When postrenal causes of azotemia are excluded from the diagnosis, evidence of an inadequate urine concentrating ability (urine specific gravity <1.017) is the hallmark of renal azotemia.

Etiology

In animals with ARF, the renal lesion is either nephrosis or nephritis. Causes of nephrosis, which is more common, are nephrotoxins and renal hypoperfusion (ischemia). The cause of nephritis is usually infection.

■ Nephrotoxins are the most common causes of ARF in small animals. Toxins that cause ARF are listed in Table 1 and include exogenous toxins, drugs, anesthetic agents, radiographic contrast dyes, and endogenous pigments.
■ Renal ischemia results from hypoperfusion and may be associated with severe dehydration, anesthetic procedures, hypovolemic shock (see sec. 6, ch. 14), disseminated intravascular coagulation (see sec. 3, ch. 2), or antiprostaglandin therapy (nonsteroidal anti-inflammatory drugs).
■ Infectious agents that can cause ARF include *Leptospira* spp. (see sec. 2, ch. 11), *Rickettsia rickettsii* (Rocky Mountain spotted fever; see sec. 2, ch. 10), *Ehrlichia canis* (see sec. 2, ch. 10), and any bacterial species that cause pyelonephritis (e.g., *E. coli*, *Proteus* spp., *Pseudomonas* spp., *Staphylococcus* spp., *Enterobacter* spp., and *Klebsiella* spp.). In general, acute pyelonephritis does not cause renal failure unless urine outflow is obstructed. Occasionally, ARF may occur secondary to septic embolization in patients with left-sided bacterial endocarditis (see sec. 6, ch. 7).

Clinical Signs

Clinical signs of ARF include anorexia, lethargy, depression, vomiting, diarrhea, and oliguria or anuria. Nonoliguric ARF (i.e., urine output remains normal or is increased) may occur in small animals (e.g., those with early or mild aminoglycoside nephrotoxicity).

Diagnosis

KEY POINT ▶ It is important to distinguish between acute and chronic renal failure because acute renal failure is a potentially reversible condition.

TABLE 1. Potential Toxic Causes of Renal Failure in Small Animals

Antibiotics	Endogenous Pigments
Aminoglycosides	Hemoglobin
Amphotericin B	Myoglobin
Tetracyclines	
Cephalosporins	**Radiographic Contrast Media**
	All iodinated contrast agents
Anesthetic Agents	
Methoxyflurane	**Nonsteroidal Anti-Inflammatory Drugs**
	Aspirin
Toxins	Ibuprofen
Ethylene glycol	Indomethacin
Heavy metals	Phenylbutazone

History

■ *History* identifies possible causes and predisposing factors for ARF (e.g., environmental toxins, drug therapy). A history of polyuria/polydipsia suggests chronic renal failure, although nonoliguric ARF can occur.

Physical Examination

■ *Physical examination* findings vary depending on the cause of ARF.
  • Nonspecific findings associated with ARF often include hypothermia, dehydration, depression, and oral ulceration.
  • Renal palpation usually reveals normal or enlarged kidneys in ARF. Chronic renal failure (CRF) is often characterized by small, firm, nodular kidneys. Painful, enlarged kidneys may occur with pyelonephritis, ARF, or obstructive uropathy.
  • Fever can be associated with the ARF that is caused by pyelonephritis or infectious disease.

Minimum Data Base

■ Depending upon the cause of ARF, the hemogram may be normal or it may demonstrate leukocytosis, with or without a left shift, and monocytosis. Hyperproteinemia and elevated hematocrit are associated with dehydration.
■ Anemia usually does not exist initially in ARF; however, with time it may occur owing to gastrointestinal hemorrhage, hemodilution, and hemolysis. Nonregenerative anemia is a frequent manifestation of CRF.
■ In addition to increased blood urea nitrogen (BUN) and creatinine concentrations, serum chemistry abnormalities may include hyperphosphatemia; hyperkalemia; and, infrequently, hypocalcemia.
■ Blood gas evaluations often show metabolic acidosis. Calculate the anion gap $[(Na + K) - (Cl + HCO_3)]$ to better characterize metabolic acidosis. Normal anion gap is 12–16 mEq/L. Although not specific for ethylene glycol toxicosis, this cause of ARF often is associated with a greatly increased anion gap, because of the accumulation of unmeasured anions.
■ Urinalysis includes evaluation of urine specific gravity, routine dipstick tests, and sediment examination.
  • In ARF, urine concentrating ability is inadequate (specific gravity, 1.007–1.017).
  • Urine sediment is evaluated for pyuria, bacteriuria, crystalluria, and casts.
    Pyuria and bacteriuria suggest urinary tract inflammation and infection.
    Hippurate and calcium oxalate crystals, especially in large numbers, suggest ethylene glycol toxicity. Calcium oxalate crystals may be found occasionally in normal animals and in cats with CRF.
    The presence of white and red blood cell casts indicates renal inflammation and hemorrhage, respectively.
    When leptospirosis is suspected, darkfield examination of urine for leptospires may be helpful.

Urine Culture

- *Culture urine* obtained by cystocentesis quantitatively in all patients with renal failure to rule out the possibility of urinary tract infection.

Serologic Evaluation

- *Serologic evaluation* is done when an underlying infectious disease, such as leptospirosis (see sec. 2, ch. 11, Rocky Mountain spotted fever (see sec. 2, ch. 10), or ehrlichiosis (see sec. 2, ch. 10), is suspected.

Abdominal Radiography

- Plain film abdominal radiography aids in evaluation of renal size and may help identify radiopaque uroliths associated with urinary tract obstruction and/or infection.
- Contrast procedures may help identify urinary tract rupture and/or obstruction to rule out postrenal azotemia and uremia. Excretory urography (intravenous urogram) is best for the evaluation of the upper urinary tract (renal pelves and ureters), whereas, urethrocystography is best for evaluation of the urinary bladder and urethra. In order to avoid additional renal injury, patients are well-hydrated prior to IV administration of contrast agents. See section 1, chapter 4, for description of these procedures.
- In animals with renal failure, excretory urography often is of limited value, because the kidneys cannot excrete contrast material well enough to produce diagnostically useful radiographic images.

Ultrasonography

- *Ultrasonography* may detect the presence and location of uroliths as well as evaluate renal parenchymal disease. Ultrasonography may substitute for contrast radiography—an important advantage in a patient with existing renal disease. See section 1, chapter 4 for ultrasonography technique and interpretation.

Renal Biopsy

- *Renal biopsy* (see sec. 8, ch. 2) generally is unnecessary in patients with well-defined historical, clinical, and laboratory evidence of ARF. However, renal biopsy may provide important diagnostic and prognostic information in certain instances.
  - When the cause of ARF is not apparent, especially when the mechanism of renal injury seems ongoing (e.g., active inflammation).
  - When response to therapy is not adequate or the clinical course does not progress as expected.
  - When very expensive forms of therapy (e.g., peritoneal dialysis, hemodialysis) are contemplated.
  - When distinction between ARF (reversible) and CRF (irreversible) is not otherwise possible.

Treatment of Acute Renal Failure

KEY POINT ▶ The objectives of treatment of ARF are to minimize further renal injury, promote diuresis if oliguria exists, and combat metabolic consequences of uremia.

With time, renal damage will be partially repaired and adequate function will be regained. Renal injury can be minimized by discontinuing administration of all nephrotoxic drugs, if possible, or by adjusting the dosage appropriately.

Correct all prerenal factors (e.g., dehydration, cardiac failure) so that renal perfusion is maintained.

Other treatments may be necessary to control vomiting, metabolic acidosis, hyperkalemia, hyperphosphatemia, and hypocalcemia.

In addition to general supportive measures, specific treatment of any underlying disease is indicated.

Fluid Therapy

See section 1, chapter 5.

- Initial Treatment
  - Calculate the dehydration deficit using the following formula to determine the volume of fluid (ml) to be administered initially:

  % dehydration × body weight (kg) × 1000

  - If cardiac function is normal, replace the dehydration deficit intravenously during a 2- to 6-hour period.
  - Choose the type of fluid on the basis of serum electrolyte concentrations, acid-base balance, and other factors. In most patients, lactated Ringer's solution can be used initially. In patients with severe hyperkalemia, 0.9% sodium chloride is more appropriate.
  - In some patients, clinical dehydration may not be evident. When vomiting or diarrhea exist, however, assume that the patient is subclinically dehydrated (3–5%) and treat accordingly. In most cases, slight overhydration is better than mild dehydration, because even mild hypovolemia can potentiate deterioration in renal function.
- Maintenance
  - After rehydration, the volume of fluid administered intravenously for daily maintenance equals the sum of continuing abnormal losses (e.g., from vomiting, diarrhea); insensible losses; and urine volume, using the guidelines and calculations in section 1, chapter 5.
  - Choose the appropriate fluid based on serum sodium concentration. Alternate lactated Ringer's solution with 5% dextrose to avoid hypernatremia during the maintenance and recovery phases of ARF.
  - Fluid therapy may be necessary throughout the maintenance phase and part of the recovery phase of ARF (usually 7–14 days).
- Discontinuing fluid therapy
  - Gradually taper fluid therapy in ARF patients, once the BUN and serum creatinine values return to normal or the oral fluid intake is tolerated without vomiting.
  - Provide unlimited access to water and reduce the patient's daily fluid infusion by half every 24 hours.
  - Monitor hydration (weight, skin turgor, other

signs) carefully and initially measure BUN, serum creatinine, and serum electrolyte values every 24 hours.

Correction of Oliguria

If oliguria persists after fluid deficits and other prerenal factors are corrected, additional treatment to increase urine production is indicated. Although increased urine formation does not necessarily indicate improved renal function, clinical improvement is generally facilitated by diuresis.

- *Volume expansion* by balanced electrolyte solutions promotes diuresis in normal animals and patients with nonoliguric forms of renal failure, but this approach is usually not effective in oliguric ARF patients. Because of the danger of fluid overload, fluid administration must not exceed actual losses once the patient becomes slightly (1–3%) overhydrated. Especially when cardiac function might be impaired, central venous pressure is monitored to guide the fluid administration rate and to minimize the risk of volume overload. Consider tailoring fluid therapy to sensible and insensible losses ("ins and outs," see sec. 1, ch. 5) to help avoid overhydration.
- *Osmotic Diuresis*
  - Mannitol (20 or 25% solution)
    Administer mannitol IV over 5–10 minutes at a dose of 0.25–0.5 gm/kg.
    Increased urine production should begin within 15 minutes; if adequate diuresis occurs, administer mannitol every 6–8 hours during the initial 24-hour treatment period.
    If diuresis does not occur, repeat the dose of mannitol every 15 minutes up to a total dose of 1.5 gm/kg. If urine still is not produced, do not give additional mannitol because vascular overload may occur.
  - Dextrose (20%) may be given in place of mannitol.
    Administer 25–65 ml/kg IV at a rate of 2 ml/min.
    After 10–15 minutes, reduce the rate to 1 ml/min.
    If adequate urine flow (i.e., 1–4 ml/min) is not observed by the time that half of the dextrose has been administered, discontinue the infusion.
    If adequate diuresis occurs, continue IV administration of a 10% dextrose solution to promote diuresis during the next 12–24 hours.

- *Loop diuretics,* such as furosemide, may be administered to promote diuresis.

KEY POINT ▶ Avoid using furosemide in animals with gentamicin-induced ARF, because it can potentiate toxicity.

- Administer furosemide at a dose of 2 mg/kg IV initially. If diuresis does not occur within 1–2 hours, give a second dose of 4 mg/kg.
- If again there is no response, administer 6 mg/kg. If there is still no response, other treatment is indicated (e.g., osmotic diuretic, vasodilator).
- If furosemide induces diuresis, administer it every 8 hours as needed. Monitor the patient for evidence of dehydration, hypokalemia, and other potential adverse effects.

- *Vasodilators*
  - Infusion of dopamine at low doses causes vasodilation of renal vasculature and increased renal blood flow.
  - See Table 2 for guidelines for the use of dopamine treatment. Monitor the ECG for arrhythmias.

If oliguria or anuria persists despite intensive medical therapy, alternative methods of supporting renal function (peritoneal dialysis, hemodialysis) must begin within 1–2 days or euthanasia is considered.

Managing Electrolyte Disturbances

KEY POINT ▶ Hyperkalemia is the most life-threatening electrolyte abnormality frequently associated with oliguric ARF.

- Serum potassium concentrations between 6 and 8 mEq/L usually do not cause severe clinical problems, and the patient responds to intravenous fluid therapy alone.
- If serum potassium concentration exceeds 8 mEq/L or signs of cardiotoxicity occur (e.g., tall and peaked T waves, widened QRS complexes, prolonged PR intervals, absent P waves, ventricular arrhythmias [see sec. 6, ch. 4]), hyperkalemia is treated.
- Administer sodium bicarbonate (0.5 to 1.0 mEq/kg IV) over 15–20 minutes to cause potassium to shift intracellularly. Sodium bicarbonate often is used first because these patients also demonstrate acidemia.
- Alternatively, administer dextrose 20% (0.5 to 1.0 g/kg IV) to stimulate endogenous insulin release, which causes serum potassium to shift intracellularly.
- Calcium may be provided to directly antagonize the cardiotoxic effects of potassium. Administer calcium gluconate (10%) IV to effect over a 10- to 15-minute period. Do not exceed a total calcium dose of 0.5–1.0 g/kg. Monitor the ECG concurrently and discontinue treatment if progressive bradycardia occurs.
- *Hypokalemia* may occur in ARF, especially during the diuretic phase. Hypokalemia results from increased urinary losses of potassium and decreased oral intake.
  - Add potassium to the IV fluids initially (see sec. 1, ch. 5 for dosage guidelines).

Table 2. Guidelines for Use of Dopamine to Increase Urine Production

1. Dilute 50 mg of dopamine in 500 ml of lactated Ringer's solution or 5% dextrose to make a final dopamine concentration of 100 μg/ml.
2. Infuse dopamine at a rate of 1–2 μg/kg/min using an infusion pump or a pediatric infusion set. Higher doses of dopamine may cause tachycardia, cardiac arrhythmias, and vasoconstriction of renal vessels.
3. If urine volume increases, continue dopamine until urine flow can be maintained by fluid therapy alone.
4. If urine volume does not increase within several hours, discontinue dopamine infusion.

KEY POINT ▶ In order to avoid iatrogenic hyperkalemia, the rate of IV administration of potassium must never exceed 0.5 mEq/kg/hr.

- Administer potassium orally if the patient is not vomiting and if the serum potassium concentration is >2.5 mEq/L.
■ *Hyperphosphatemia* may contribute to uremic signs in ARF patients.
  - Fluid therapy helps lower serum phosphorus concentration.
  - Other methods of lowering serum phosphorus (e.g., phosphate binders, low phosphate diets) are indicated once the patient tolerates oral feeding (see Chronic Renal Failure in this chapter).

Managing Acid/Base Disturbances

Metabolic acidosis is the most common acid/base disturbance associated with ARF. Most patients with mild acidosis respond to fluid therapy and do not require other specific treatment.

■ In general, metabolic acidosis need not be treated if blood pH is >7.2. When blood pH cannot be measured, use bicarbonate or total CO_2 values to determine need for treatment.
■ Administer bicarbonate for blood pH <7.2 (bicarbonate <14 mmol/L; total CO_2 <15 mmol/L).
  - Calculate the initial bicarbonate dosage (mEq) using the following formula:
    (base deficit) × (kg body weight) × (0.3).
  - Administer half the calculated amount by slow IV injection over 15 to 30 minutes.
  - Give the remainder of the calculated amount over the next 6 to 8 hours by adding to the IV fluid solution or by intermittent slow injections.
  - Base additional treatment on serial measurements of blood pH, bicarbonate, or total CO_2. The goal of treatment is to maintain values greater than the stated thresholds.

Control of Vomiting

Vomiting occurs in ARF for several reasons. Uremic toxins act centrally to stimulate the chemoreceptor trigger zone (CRTZ), which in turn, stimulates the vomiting center. Hypergastrinemia stimulates gastric H_2-receptors causing gastric hyperacidity and uremic gastritis.

■ Administer an H_2-receptor antagonist to help control uremic gastritis.
  - Administer cimetidine (Tagamet; SmithKline) IV during the uremic crisis at a dose of 10 mg/kg. Then, decrease the dosage to 5 mg/kg q12h.
  - Alternatively, administer ranitidine (Zantac; Glaxo) (2 mg/kg q12h PO).
■ If vomiting cannot be controlled by withholding all oral intake and giving H_2-receptor antagonists, consider administration of centrally acting antiemetics.
  - Trimethobenzamide (Tigan; Beecham) (3 mg/kg q8–12h IM) acts at the CRTZ; 100 mg rectal suppositories may be used in dogs over 6.8 kg.
  - Phenothiazine derivatives act at both the CRTZ

and vomiting center; therefore, they are very effective antiemetics.
  Chlorpromazine (Thorazine; SmithKline) (0.5 mg/kg q6–8h IM, IV)
  Hypotension is a potential disadvantage of these drugs, however.

Patient Monitoring

The primary objectives of patient monitoring are to evaluate response to therapy and to avoid potential complications. In general, monitoring is done more frequently early in the course of treatment and less often once the patient is stable or improving. Patient monitoring includes the subjective evaluation of clinical parameters, such as hydration status, and the collection of objective data, such as body weight, urine output, and laboratory test results.

■ Determine body weight and hydration status twice daily. Because clinical estimation of fluid losses can be inaccurate, changes in body weight are important aids in assessment of fluid balance. Rapid changes in body weight generally reflect net gains or losses of fluid and signal the need for changing the rate of fluid administration.
■ Determine hematocrit and total serum protein values daily to help evaluate hydration status more objectively.
■ Measure serum electrolytes, BUN, and serum creatinine concentrations daily in the initial management.
■ When severe hyperkalemia or metabolic acidemia exists, monitor the abnormality several times daily as needed to adjust treatment.
■ Monitor fluid therapy in any patient susceptible to overhydration (e.g., one with congestive heart failure) by measuring CVP and/or "ins and outs" (see sec. 1, ch. 5).
■ In an oliguric or anuric patient, urine output is best monitored by placing an indwelling urinary catheter. This placement helps to more accurately determine the volume of fluids to administer. However, because of the risk of urinary tract infection in an already compromised patient, connect the catheter to a closed drainage system and remove the catheter as soon as possible.

Treatment of Conditions Associated with Acute Renal Failure

Leptospirosis

■ Administer penicillin (25,000–40,000 units/kg IV q8h) for 2 weeks to eliminate leptospiremia.
■ Once BUN and creatinine concentrations return to normal, administer dihydrostreptomycin (10–15 mg/kg IM q12h) for 2 weeks to eliminate the carrier state and leptospiruria (for further details regarding leptospirosis, refer to sec. 2, ch. 11).

Ethylene Glycol (Antifreeze) Toxicity

■ If discovered promptly after ingestion (within 6 hours), induce emesis, lavage the stomach, and administer activated charcoal.

- Treatment to prevent metabolism of ethylene glycol to its toxic metabolites is most effective during the initial 24-hour period after ingestion.
  - Ethanol (20%) acts as a substrate for alcohol dehydrogenase and prevents metabolism of ethylene glycol to its toxic metabolites.

    In dogs, administer 5.5 ml/kg IV q4h for five treatments, then q6h for four additional treatments.

    In cats, administer 5.0 ml/kg IV q6h for five treatments, then q8h for four additional treatments.
  - 4-Methylpyrazole (5%) inhibits alcohol dehydrogenase and does not cause central nervous system depression like ethanol. This drug is not commercially available currently.

    Administer a loading dose of 20 mg/kg IV, followed by 15 mg/kg IV at 12 and 24 hours, and 5 mg/kg IV 36 hours after the first dose.

    4-Methylpyrazole is only recommended for dogs at this time.

Prevention

- Be careful when using nephrotoxic drugs.
  - Avoid them if another drug is also effective.
  - Maintain adequate hydration during treatment.
  - Avoid furosemide in combination with aminoglycosides.
- Keep fresh water available at all times for animals with CRF.
- Maintain adequate blood pressure during anesthesia.
- Advise owners to dispose of antifreeze where pets will not be exposed.

CHRONIC RENAL FAILURE

Chronic renal failure (CRF) is a syndrome characterized by an inability of the kidneys to perform adequately, owing to the progressive loss of function over a period of months to years. The pathophysiologic changes in CRF result from failure of the kidneys to perform normal excretory, regulatory, and synthetic functions. Loss of excretory function causes retention of nitrogenous substances (e.g., BUN, creatinine) that are eliminated by glomerular filtration. Inability to perform regulatory functions eventually leads to changes in electrolyte, acid/base, and water balance. Failure to synthesize erythropoietin leads to nonregenerative anemia. Decreased conversion of vitamin D to its active metabolite causes impaired intestinal calcium absorption and renal secondary hyperparathyroidism.

Etiology

Renal lesions that produce CRF may be either congenital or acquired. The occurrence of CRF in young animals of certain breeds prompts suspicion of congenital/familial disorders (Table 3). However, most animals with CRF have acquired disease. A variety of causes exist for acquired CRF, but in many cases, a specific underlying cause cannot be identified. Regard-

TABLE 3. Breeds with Congenital/Familial Renal Disease

Breed	Renal Disease
Abyssinian cat	Renal amyloidosis
Basenji	Renal tubular dysfunction
Beagle	Unilateral renal agenesis
Cairn terrier	Polycystic renal disease
Cocker spaniel	Tubulointerstitial fibrosis
	Renal cortical hypoplasia
Doberman pinscher	Glomerulosclerosis
Domestic longhaired and Persian cats	Idiopathic polycystic kidney disease
	Renal dysplasia
Lhasa apso	Tubulointerstitial fibrosis
Norwegian elkhound	Telangiectasia
Pembroke Welsh corgi	Glomerular atrophy
Samoyed	Renal dysplasia
Shih tzu	Renal dysplasia
Soft-coated Wheaten terrier	

less of the cause of nephron damage, CRF is an irreversible, usually progressive, condition.

- *Congenital and familial* diseases that cause CRF in dogs and cats are listed in Table 3.
- *Infectious and inflammatory conditions* are common acquired causes of CRF. Some primarily produce glomerular renal lesions. Others are primarily tubulointerstitial diseases. However, all components of the kidneys are affected once CRF develops. Infectious diseases that cause interstitial nephritis leading to CRF include leptospirosis (see sec. 2, ch. 11) pyelonephritis, and feline infectious peritonitis (FIP) (see sec. 2, ch. 3). Chronic glomerulonephritis also is a common cause of CRF in dogs and cats. This condition usually occurs secondary to disease in other organs. Glomerular lesions are caused by immune complex deposition (see sec. 3, ch. 3). Infectious and inflammatory diseases that may cause glomerulonephritis leading to CRF are numerous and diverse (see discussion of nephrotic syndrome).
- *Amyloidosis* is a frequent cause of CRF. In dogs, renal amyloidosis typically is a glomerular lesion that produces proteinuria leading to nephrotic syndrome and/or CRF. In cats, however, amyloid deposits form mainly in renal medullary interstitial tissue, eventually leading to CRF.
- *Neoplastic diseases* that may cause CRF include renal lymphosarcoma, especially in cats; renal carcinoma; and multiple myeloma.
- *Nephrotoxins*, such as ethylene glycol, aminoglycoside antibiotics, and hypercalcemia, can produce CRF because of subacute or chronic low-level exposure or acute renal failure aftermath.
- *Idiopathic* glomerular and/or tubulointerstitial disease is common in dogs and cats with acquired CRF. A specific underlying cause of renal disease cannot be identified.

Clinical Signs

The clinical signs of CRF vary with the degree of renal insufficiency and the underlying cause. Although animals of any age can be affected, younger dogs and cats most often develop CRF because of congenital/

familial, toxic, or infectious causes. Idiopathic CRF occurs most often in older dogs and cats.

- Lethargy, anorexia, and weight loss are nonspecific signs that often occur in patients with CRF.
- Gastrointestinal signs, including vomiting, diarrhea, and oral ulcerations, are common, especially in patients with uremia.
- Weakness and exercise intolerance may be observed, especially as anemia develops.
- Polyuria and polydipsia are frequent and often are the first signs.

Diagnosis

KEY POINT ▶ It is important to identify any active renal diseases that may contribute to progression of chronic renal failure. Treatable diseases that may be associated with CRF are listed in Table 4.

History

- *History* identifies factors that suggest a cause of CRF, including familial history, possibility of exposure to toxins and infectious diseases, and previous drugs administered.

Physical Examination

- Assess hydration status by evaluating skin turgor and moistness of mucous membranes.
- Examine the oral cavity for ulcerations that often occur with uremia. Pale mucous membranes suggest anemia.
- Evaluate the retinas for changes suggestive of systemic hypertension. Retinal hemorrhages, detachments, and vessel tortuosity occur with hypertension or hyperviscosity (see sec. 11, ch. 8).
- Palpate the abdomen to determine renal size. Small, firm, and "lumpy-bumpy" kidneys are typical of CRF. However, some diseases (e.g., lymphosarcoma, polycystic kidneys, FIP) may be associated with enlarged kidneys.
- Subcutaneous edema and/or ascites may occur in animals with nephrotic syndrome due to severe glomerular protein loss.
- Perform a rectal examination to evaluate the prostate gland, pelvic urethra, and trigonal area of the urinary bladder for abnormalities such as calculi, masses, and so forth.

Minimum Data Base

- Hemogram often reveals nonregenerative anemia. Hyperproteinemia occurs with some infectious (e.g.,

ehrlichiosis, FIP) and neoplastic (e.g., multiple myeloma) conditions.
- BUN and creatinine are elevated in CRF.

KEY POINT ▶ Approximately 75% of nephrons must be nonfunctional before BUN and serum creatinine concentrations increase; therefore, patients with renal insufficiency may have normal BUN and creatinine values.

- Hyperphosphatemia is usually present.
- Urinalysis shows inadequately concentrated urine, often in the isosthenuric range (1.008–1.013).
- Significant proteinuria may be observed in patients with glomerular disease.

Urine Culture

- *Perform quantitative urine culture* via cystocentesis to rule out urinary tract infection.

Abdominal Radiography

- Survey radiography is used to evaluate renal size and identify radiopaque uroliths.
- Excretory urography may be helpful for evaluation of conditions affecting the upper urinary tract (e.g., pyelonephritis, hydronephrosis, obstructive uropathy). However, reduced renal excretory function often limits this technique (see sec. 1, ch. 4).

Ultrasonography

- *Ultrasonography* may be employed to identify uroliths, hydronephrosis, and polycystic renal disease (see sec. 1, ch. 4).

Renal Biopsy

- *Renal biopsy* is considered when the information so obtained might alter treatment recommendations (e.g., in glomerulonephropathy) (see sec. 8, ch. 2).

Systemic Blood Pressure

Because of the prevalence of hypertension in small animals with renal disease (>50%), measure the blood pressure in all patients with CRF, especially those with glomerular disease. Direct measurement of blood pressure is more exact; however, indirect methods may provide useful information in the clinical setting (see sec. 6, ch. 11).

- Hypertension in dogs is defined as systolic and diastolic blood pressures >180 and 95 mm Hg, respectively.
- Systolic pressures >200 mm Hg and diastolic pressures >145 mm Hg are consistent with hypertension in cats.

Treatment of Chronic Renal Failure

Treat underlying causes if identified. However, because renal lesions that cause CRF are irreversible and usually progressive, no specific therapy is curative. Instead, the goals of conservative medical management

TABLE 4. Potentially Treatable Causes of Chronic Renal Failure

Pyelonephritis
Nephrolithiasis
Hypertension
Renal lymphosarcoma
Obstructive uropathy
Hypercalcemic nephropathy

of CRF are to control clinical signs of uremia; maintain adequate fluid, electrolyte, and acid/base balance; provide adequate nutrition; and minimize progression of renal failure.

Dietary Management

- *Dietary management* consists primarily of restricting the amount of protein, phosphorus, and sodium in the diet while providing adequate amounts of nonprotein calories, vitamins, and minerals.
  - Feeding a restricted amount of high-biologic value protein (e.g., Prescription Diet k/d; Hill's Pet Foods) decreases the amount of nitrogenous wastes and may delay the progression of renal failure, although this finding has not been proven in dogs and cats.

    Currently recommended protein levels for dogs are 2.0–2.2 gm/kg/day and 3.3–3.5 gm/kg/day for cats.

    Protein intake is individualized to prevent malnutrition, as evidenced by hypoalbuminemia, worsening anemia, and weight loss.
  - Phosphorus restriction may lessen signs of uremia and prevent progression of renal disease by blunting renal secondary hyperparathyroidism and decreasing renal mineralization. Protein-restricted diets are also phosphorus-restricted.
  - Dietary sodium restriction may decrease blood pressure in hypertensive animals. Sodium intake is restricted gradually (over 2–4 weeks) to allow the diseased kidneys sufficient time to adapt (see sec. 6, ch. 11). Avoid severely restricted sodium diets in patients with CRF, because they may cause volume depletion and renal hypoperfusion.

Management of Fluid, Electrolyte, Acid/Base Disorders

Fluid Therapy

Most patients with CRF have obligatory polyuria. Fluid balance is maintained by increased water consumption. Therefore, fresh water must be available at all times. If water intake is not adequate to maintain hydration, as often the case in cats, fluids are supplemented. Some owners are able to administer SC fluids at home.

Potassium Balance

- Hyperkalemia is uncommon in dogs and cats with mild-to-moderate CRF; however, it may occur in terminal CRF.
- Hypokalemia may occur presumably because of decreased oral intake and/or excessive urinary potassium loss.
  - Oral treatment is preferred except in cases of severe hypokalemia.
  - Dogs may be given potassium chloride (1–3 gm/day PO) or potassium gluconate elixir (5 mEq q8–12h PO).
  - Cats with severe hypokalemia (serum potassium <3 mEq/L) are given 5–8 mEq of potassium gluconate elixir per day in two divided doses. Once serum potassium returns to normal, a maintenance dose of 2–4 mEq/day is adequate.

See section 1, chapter 5, for a discussion of the treatment of hypokalemia.

Metabolic Acidosis

- Treat metabolic acidosis if plasma bicarbonate is <14 mmol/L or blood pH is <7.2.
- Start with oral sodium bicarbonate at a dose of 8–12 mg/kg q8–12h (1 teaspoon baking soda contains about 2000 mg of bicarbonate).
- Adjust the dose based on changes in blood pH, plasma bicarbonate, or total CO_2.
- The goal of treatment is to maintain blood pH >7.2, plasma bicarbonate >14 mmol/L, and total CO_2 >15 mmol/L.
- To prevent volume overload, avoid or minimize administration of sodium bicarbonate in patients with hypertension or congestive heart failure.

Management of Hyperphosphatemia

- Dietary phosphate restriction maintains normal serum phosphorus concentration in early CRF. In advanced CRF, however, additional treatment usually is needed to maintain serum phosphorus concentrations within the normal range.
- Intestinal phosphate binders are compounds that are given orally to reduce the absorption of phosphate from the intestine.
  - Maintain dietary phosphate restriction and administer intestinal phosphate binders (aluminum hydroxide, aluminum carbonate, calcium carbonate, calcium acetate) with meals.
  - Start with a dose of 30–90 mg/kg/day and adjust as needed to maintain normal serum phosphorus concentration.

Treatment of Nonregenerative Anemia

Specific treatment of anemia may be indicated when the hematocrit is <25% in cats and <30% in dogs.

- *Androgens* have been the mainstay of therapy for nonregenerative anemia associated with CRF; however, their efficacy has not been documented in small animals. In humans with CRF, androgens are more effective administered parenterally than orally. In general, androgens must be administered for several months before a beneficial effect occurs.
  - Stanozolol (Winstrol V; Winthrop) (1–4 mg PO q12–24h) and oxymetholone (Anadrol; Syntex) (1 mg/kg PO q12–24h) have been given in small animals with variable results.
  - Nandrolone decanoate (Deca-Durabolin; Organon) (1 mg/kg IM, SQ q7–10 days; up to 40 mg total dose in dogs, 20 mg in cats) appears to be more effective than oral androgens.
  - Potential side effects of androgen therapy include retention of sodium and water, hepatotoxicity, prostatomegaly, and worsening of pre-existing perianal adenomas. Hepatotoxicity occurs primarily with oral androgen therapy.
- *Transfusion therapy* is reserved for patients with clinical signs (e.g., weakness, lethargy, dyspnea) referable to anemia. Administer fresh whole blood

or packed red blood cells to raise hematocrit level to at least 25%.

- *Recombinant human erythropoietin* (rHuEPO) has replaced androgen and transfusion for treatment of nonregenerative anemia in humans with CRF. Preliminary trials that evaluate the safety and efficacy of rHuEPO administration for treatment of anemia in dogs and cats with CRF are in progress. Although some encouraging results have been obtained, recommendations for rHuEPO therapy for dogs or cats with CRF remains premature.

Management of Hypertension

Because of its potential consequences, hypertension is treated. Although not proved, it is possible that hypertension causes progression of CRF. The goal of treatment is to maintain systolic pressures of 120–160 mm Hg and diastolic pressures of 60–100 mm Hg. Avoid the pharmacologic management of hypertension unless systemic blood pressure changes can be monitored. See section 6, chapter 11, for more information about hypertension.

- *Dietary sodium restriction* is the initial step in the management of hypertension. Changes in dietary sodium are made gradually (2–4 weeks).
  - Feed dogs a diet with 0.1–0.3% sodium on a dry weight basis.
  - Feed cats a diet with 0.4% sodium on a dry weight basis.
- If hypertension is not controlled by dietary sodium restriction, *pharmacologic treatment* of hypertension is indicated. Use furosemide (1–2 mg/kg PO, q12–24h) initially. If necessary, add other antihypertensive drugs. See section 6, chapter 11, for a complete discussion of the management of hypertension.)

Patient Monitoring

Monitor patients with CRF to determine response to treatment and to detect signs of concurrent treatable disease. Evaluate animals with mild renal failure (e.g., azotemia, impaired concentrating ability) every 3–4 months and animals with moderate to advanced renal failure (e.g., azotemia, impaired concentrating ability, anemia, hyperphosphatemia, metabolic acidosis) every 1–2 months.

- Perform a physical examination to detect weight loss and evaluate hydration.
- Perform laboratory evaluation (hematocrit, serum chemistries, serum electrolytes, total CO_2, and urinalysis) to evaluate renal function and need for additional treatment or alteration of dosage.
- Measure blood pressure for detection and surveillance of systemic hypertension.

PYELONEPHRITIS

Pyelonephritis is a term that implies inflammation of the renal parenchyma and its pelvis; however, the term is often used to describe bacterial infection of the kidney. Altered host defense mechanisms (e.g., neph-

rolithiasis, ectopic ureter, immunodeficiency, hyperadrenocorticism, diabetes mellitus) may predispose patients to pyelonephritis; however, an identifiable underlying cause cannot be found in some patients. In general, the prevalence of urinary tract infections, including pyelonephritis, is higher in dogs compared with cats. For additional information on urinary tract infection, in general, and lower urinary tract infection, specifically, see section 8, chapter 3.

Etiology

KEY POINT ▶ Ascending infection from the lower urinary tract is the most common route of renal infection.

Although uncommon, microbial invasion may occur via the hematogenous route (e.g., septicemia). Organisms that cause pyelonephritis in dogs and cats include *Escherichia coli, Staphylococcus aureus, Streptococcus* spp., *Klebsiella pneumoniae, Pseudomonas aeruginosa,* and *Enterobacter* spp.

Clinical Signs

- Signs associated with acute pyelonephritis may include lethargy, anorexia, fever, vomiting, dehydration, lumbar pain, and polyuria/polydipsia.
- Chronic pyelonephritis often is subclinical or characterized by nonspecific findings, such as weight loss, decreased appetite, and polyuria/polydipsia.
- Many patients with pyelonephritis have concurrent signs of urethrocystitis (e.g., pollakiuria, stranguria, dysuria).
- Owners may notice discolored or malodorous urine.

Diagnosis

Because the clinical findings of pyelonephritis are often nonspecific, clinicians must maintain a high index of suspicion. In many cases, a presumptive diagnosis is made on the basis of clinical findings and positive urine culture findings.

History

- *History* helps identify clinical signs of pyelonephritis.

Physical Examination

- Palpate the kidneys to detect evidence of pain or renal enlargement, which may occur with acute pyelonephritis.
- Animals with chronic pyelonephritis may have normal physical examination findings.

Minimum Data Base

- *Serum biochemical profile* changes may include increased phosphorus, BUN, and creatinine due to associated renal failure.
- *Hemogram* changes may include a neutrophilic leukocytosis with a left shift in acute pyelonephritis, combined with nonregenerative anemia in chronic pyelonephritis.
- *Urinalysis* may show low urine specific gravity, py-

uria, bacteriuria, and white blood cell casts. The presence of white blood cell casts is a reliable indicator of renal involvement; however, they are frequently lacking in patients with renal infection. The absence of casts therefore, does not exclude the possibility of pyelonephritis.

Urine Culture

- *Quantitative urine culture* is done in all patients with suspected pyelonephritis. Although a positive urine culture result indicates urinary tract infection, it does not specify infection to the kidneys. Ideally, urine is collected by cystocentesis. Alternatively, samples obtained properly by catheterization may provide useful information.
  - In dogs and cats, bacterial growth from urine collected by cystocentesis indicates urinary tract infection.
  - In dogs, growth of $>10^5$ organisms/ml of urine collected by catheterization indicates urinary tract infection, whereas in cats, growth of $>10^3$ organisms/ml indicates infection.

Radiography

- Excretory urography may help support a diagnosis of pyelonephritis; however, changes are neither sensitive nor specific (see sec. 1, ch. 4).
- Dilatation of ureters and renal pelves and decreased opacity of contrast media in the collecting system may be observed in pyelonephritis.

Ultrasonography

- This can be used to identify dilatation of the renal pelves as well as nephrolithiasis (see sec. 1, ch. 4).

Treatment

The management of pyelonephritis includes correction of impaired host defenses, (if possible) and administration of appropriate antimicrobial therapy. Animals with acute pyelonephritis are treated with parenteral antimicrobials until systemic signs (e.g., fever, pain) subside, usually in 2–3 days. This therapy is followed by long-term oral antibiotic therapy.

- Because urinary pathogens have predictable susceptibility patterns, antimicrobial treatment is often based on identification of the infecting organism. See section 8, chapter 3, for treatment of infections affecting bladder and urethra.
- Administer the antimicrobial for 6–8 weeks (Table 5).
- Perform a urine culture 7–14 days after beginning treatment to determine the efficacy of the selected antimicrobial.
  - If urine culture results are negative, continue treatment.
  - If urine culture results are positive, select another antimicrobial based on results of culture and susceptibility.
- Perform a urine culture 5–7 days after discontinuation of antimicrobial treatment.

TABLE 5. Antimicrobial Dosages Used to Treat Pyelonephritis

Drug	Dosage (mg/kg)	Frequency
Ampicillin/amoxicillin	25	q8h
Cephalexin	18	q8h
Tetracycline	18	q8h
Trimethoprim sulfa	13	q12h
Amoxicillin/clavulanic acid	16.5	q8h
Enrofloxacin	2.5	q12h

- If infection is present, select a different antimicrobial and treat the patient for another 6–8 weeks.
- If there is no bacterial growth, perform urine cultures every 6–8 weeks until negative findings are obtained for three consecutive urine cultures. This approach detects recrudescence of infection that sometimes occurs, because antibiotics fail to completely eradicate the organism from the kidney, or new infection that occurs, because of host-kidney susceptibility factors.

NEPHROTIC SYNDROME

Nephrotic syndrome (NS) is caused by glomerular disease and is characterized by proteinuria, hypoalbuminemia, hypercholesterolemia, and edema. Dogs and cats with glomerular disease may not have all characteristics of NS, therefore, a more practical definition of NS may be proteinuria of sufficient magnitude to cause hypoalbuminemia.

Etiology

The major causes of NS in small animals are glomerulonephritis (GN) and amyloidosis. These lesions also are common causes of chronic renal failure.

- *Glomerulonephritis* may result from familial disorders or may be secondary to infectious/inflammatory

TABLE 6. Conditions Associated with Glomerulonephritis in Dogs and Cats

Familial	Neoplastic
Doberman pinscher	Lymphosarcoma
Samoyed	Mast cell tumor
Bull terrier	Many others
Infectious	**Inflammatory**
Bacterial endocarditis	Systemic lupus erythematosus
Infectious canine hepatitis	Chronic pancreatitis
Brucellosis	Chronic pyoderma
Dirofilariasis	Polyarthritis
Ehrlichiosis	
Borreliosis (Lyme disease)	
Systemic mycoses	
Pyometra	
Feline infectious peritonitis	
Feline leukemia virus infection	
Miscellaneous	
Hyperadrenocorticism	
Chronic glucocorticoid treatment	

diseases, neoplasia, and other causes (Table 6). In some cases, an underlying cause cannot be identified. Presumably, the pathogenesis of glomerulonephritis in most patients involves the deposition of antigen-antibody-complement complexes (immune complexes) in the glomeruli.

■ *Amyloidosis* is characterized by deposition of fibrillar proteins in various organs resulting in organ dysfunction.
  • In dogs, amyloid primarily affects glomeruli and causes a protein-losing glomerulonephropathy.
  • In cats, amyloid usually is deposited primarily in the renal medullary interstitium, causing chronic renal failure.
  • Amyloidosis may occur secondary to the same infectious/inflammatory processes as GN. In most cases, however, an underlying etiology is not found.

Clinical Signs

Clinical findings in dogs and cats with NS are often nonspecific and may reflect the underlying disease process.

■ Weight loss, edema, or ascites may occur as a result of hypoalbuminemia.
■ Signs of uremia (see previous discussions of ARF and CRF) may be observed in nephrotic patients with renal failure.
■ Some animals with proteinuria, of a nephrotic range, exhibit no clinical signs of illness.

Diagnosis

KEY POINT ▶ Look for historical, physical, and laboratory findings that might reveal an underlying cause of glomerular disease, such as evidence for infectious, parasitic, immune-mediated, or neoplastic disorders (see Table 6).

History

■ *History* can identify a familial predisposition to glomerular disease. Question the owners concerning health of littermates, dam, and sire.

Physical Examination

■ *Physical examination* findings may include peripheral edema, ascites, thin body condition, and poor haircoat.

Minimum Data Base

■ *Hematology* may reveal nonregenerative anemia hypoproteinemia (when hypoalbuminemia predominates) or hyperproteinemia (when hyperglobulinemia predominates), and leukocytosis.
■ *Serum biochemical findings* characteristic of NS include hypoalbuminemia and hypercholesterolemia. Other abnormalities may include hyperglobulinemia, and when glomerular filtration rate is also reduced, azotemia and hyperphosphatemia.
■ *Urinalysis*

KEY POINT ▶ The hallmark of glomerular disease is proteinuria in the absence of hematuria or pyuria.

Urine specific gravity values are variable. Animals with NS often retain the ability to concentrate urine.

Assessment of Proteinuria

Because semiquantitative test results for urine protein (e.g., dipstick) are affected by urine concentration, determine the significance of proteinuria by either measuring the protein in urine collected during a 24-hour period or calculating the urine protein-to-creatinine ratio (U Pr:Cr) in a spot sample.

24-Hour Protein Excretion

■ Collect and mix all the urine formed by the animal during a 24-hour period. Measure protein concentration in an aliquot of the mixed urine and multiply by urine volume to determine the amount of protein excreted during a 24-hour period.
■ Urine protein loss >30 mg/kg/day is abnormal in dogs; whereas, >35 mg/kg/day is abnormal in most cats.
■ Although collecting a 24-hour urine specimen usually is inconvenient, the procedure also can be carried out to determine endogenous creatinine clearance, which is an estimate of glomerular filtration rate (GFR).

Urine Protein-to-Creatinine Ratio

■ When renal function is stable (whether GFR is normal or reduced), determining the ratio between concentrations of protein and creatinine in a single urine specimen (U Pr:Cr) can be used to evaluate the magnitude of proteinuria.
■ U Pr:Cr >1 generally indicates an abnormal amount of daily urine protein loss. A U Pr:Cr of 1–5 is common with chronic interstitial nephritis; 3–40, with glomerulonephritis; and 10–40, with amyloidosis.
■ The U Pr:Cr also is proportional to the amount of daily urine protein loss. The average amount of urine protein loss in dogs with a particular U Pr:Cr can be estimated by the formula: (U Pr:Cr) × (20 mg/kg/day). Because the correlation of U Pr:Cr with daily urine protein loss is not exact, the calculated value is only an estimate of an individual animal's magnitude of proteinuria.

Ancillary Tests

KEY POINT ▶ Because glomerulonephritis may be associated with potentially treatable underlying conditions, perform ancillary diagnostic tests to rule out the possibility of these disorders.

See the appropriate chapters for more information about these conditions.
■ *Serology* to rule out the presence of ehrlichiosis, occult dirofilariasis, brucellosis, Lyme disease, feline leukemia virus, and systemic mycosis.
■ *Amylase and lipase* if pancreatitis is suspected.
■ *Immunology (antinuclear antibody, lupus erythema-*

tosus, and Coombs tests) to rule out the presence of systemic lupus erythematosus and immune-mediated hemolytic anemia.

- *Adrenocorticotropic hormone (ACTH) response test or low-dose dexamethasone suppression test* to rule out the possibility of hyperadrenocorticism.
- *Serum protein electrophoresis* to determine if hyperglobulinemia is polyclonal or monoclonal.
- *Thoracic and abdominal radiography* to detect occult dirofilariasis, systemic mycotic infection, pyometra, chronic pancreatitis, or neoplasia.
- *Fundic examination* to detect changes caused by feline infectious peritonitis, systemic mycosis, and hypertension.
- *Blood cultures* if bacterial endocarditis is suspected.
- *Abdominal ultrasonography* to detect pyometra, pancreatitis, and neoplastic or inflammatory masses.
- *Echocardiography* to detect vegetative valvular lesions consistent with bacterial endocarditis.

KEY POINT ▶ The only reliable way to distinguish between glomerulonephritis and amyloidosis is to obtain a renal biopsy for microscopic examination.

Renal Biopsy

Perform a renal biopsy (see sec. 8, ch. 2) if the results may alter the treatment. For example, GN and amyloidosis differ regarding treatment and prognosis. The decision to do a biopsy is made after the careful consideration of the risks involved, the need for an accurate prognosis, and the treatment goals of the owner.

Special preservative media (other than formalin) may be required for special studies of the tissue, such as immunofluorescence (e.g., Michel's solution) and electron microscopy (e.g., glutaraldehyde). Consult the laboratory for specific information.

- *Amyloidosis* is histologically characterized by extracellular deposition of fibrillar proteins with distinctive tinctorial properties. Among other features, amyloid deposits appear green when stained with alkaline Congo red and viewed under polarized light.
- *Glomerulonephritis* is a nonspecific term (analogous to dermatitis or enteritis) signifying the existence of glomerular changes due to inflammation. Although light microscopy is sufficient to distinguish amyloidosis from GN, complete characterization of GN requires immunofluorescent studies and sometimes electron microscopy, as well as light microscopy. With few exceptions, spontaneous GN in animals features the granular, discontinuous ("lumpy-bumpy") deposits of varying amounts of immunoglobulin and complement in glomeruli that are characteristic of immune-complex GN. Classification of GN based on light microscopic appearance includes four major categories:

Mesangioproliferative—glomerular hypercellularity due to proliferation of mesangial and/or endothelial cells.

Membranous—prominent changes in thickness and contour of glomerular basement membranes.

Membranoproliferative—combination of hypercellularity and glomerular basement membrane changes.

Sclerosis—end-stage glomerular collapse and fibrosis.

Treatment

Management of patients with NS includes specific treatment of the underlying glomerular disease and general supportive care of any associated complications.

Specific Treatment of Glomerulonephritis

- Eliminate any associated infectious, inflammatory, or neoplastic diseases. In some cases, glomerular lesions resolve when the underlying cause is eliminated (e.g., pyometra, heartworm). Unfortunately, a treatable underlying cause cannot be identified in all cases.
- *Immunosuppressive drugs* (e.g., prednisone, cyclophosphamide)
  - These have been used for treatment of GN on the premise that they suppress the formation of immune complexes and alter the inflammatory response.
  - Controlled studies documenting efficacy of immunosuppressive therapy in the management of GN in dogs and cats are lacking.
  - Potential adverse effects of using corticosteroids include protein catabolism and worsening azotemia; increased proteinuria and glomerular injury; increased risk of infection; and increased risk of thromboembolism.
  - Until appropriate studies demonstrate a benefit, routine corticosteroids for treatment of GN, unless specifically indicated for the underlying disease, is not recommended.
- *Antiplatelet therapy*
  - Platelet activation may contribute to the development of GN.
  - Platelet inhibition (e.g., by aspirin, dipyridamole) might delay end-stage renal disease; however, this effect remains to be proved in dogs and cats.
  - Until controlled studies demonstrate safety and efficacy, antiplatelet therapy probably is better restricted to aspirin administration. Standard aspirin dosage is 5 mg/kg q12h for dogs and q48–72h for cats. Some evidence suggests that an ultralow dosage (0.5 mg/kg) administered every 12 hours may be sufficient to control platelet aggregation.

Specific Treatment of Amyloidosis

As with GN, any associated inflammatory or infectious conditions are treated because it may lessen the severity of amyloid deposition.

KEY POINT ▶ No reliable treatment exists for amyloidosis, and most patients suffer terminal renal failure.

Various drugs have been recommended, and their

administration may have resulted in improvement in some cases.

- *Dimethyl sulfoxide (DMSO)*
  - DMSO administration has appeared to produce improvement in a few cases; however, its effectiveness is controversial.
  - Beneficial effects may be due to anti-inflammatory actions.
  - DMSO can be administered topically, orally, subcutaneously, or intravenously.
  - Dosage regimens in dogs have included 125 mg/kg, twice daily, and 80 mg/kg, three times weekly.
- Colchicine blocks hepatic secretion of the amyloid precursor.
  - It is most effective as a preventative.
  - It has not been evaluated in cats and dogs.
- Immunosuppressive agents are not given to patients with amyloidosis because these agents may potentiate amyloid deposition.

Supportive Treatment of Nephrotic Syndrome

- *Renal failure* may be a complicating factor of NS (see discussion of chronic renal failure treatment recommendations).
- *Proteinuria* contributes to many of the complications of nephrotic syndrome; therefore, an attempt to modify the degree of proteinuria is indicated.
  - Dietary protein supplementation has been recommended to offset urine protein loss and lessen the magnitude of hypoalbuminemia; however, some evidence has shown that increased protein intake may enhance progressive glomerular injury and actually worsen proteinuria.
  - Dietary recommendations are similar to those for patients with chronic renal failure (e.g., Prescription Diet k/d, Hill's Pet Foods).
    Feed dogs a diet containing 12–14% of its calories as protein.
    Feed cats a diet with 20% of its calories as protein.
  - Re-evaluate BUN, creatinine, and U Pr:Cr findings 2 weeks after changing diets. Continue dietary protein restriction if renal function has not deteriorated, magnitude of proteinuria is reduced or unchanged, and serum albumin concentration is increased or unchanged.
  - If the magnitude of proteinuria remains great and/or serum albumin concentration declines, consider supplementing the diet with protein up to the amount being lost daily in the urine.
    A boiled egg contains 6.5–7.0 gm of high-biologic value protein and can be given as a protein supplement.
    Discontinue protein supplementation if proteinuria or hypoalbuminemia worsens.
- *Excess fluid (edema)* may accumulate in interstitial compartments or in body cavities, secondary to hypoalbuminemia and decreased plasma oncotic pressure. Intravascular volume depletion stimulates renal retention of sodium and water, which potentiates the edematous state.
  - Avoid removing fluid from body cavities unless it causes respiratory distress. Excess fluid removal can potentiate hypovolemia and edema formation.
  - Begin by confining the animal and feeding a low-sodium diet.
  - Diuretics are given cautiously and only to patients with moderate-to-severe edema.
    Loop diuretics may be most effective in patients with a nephrotic disorder.
    Administer furosemide (2–4 mg/kg, q8–12h PO, SC, or IV) until edema resolves. Gradually taper the dose, and try to discontinue administration.
- *Hypertension* occurs in a high percentage of dogs with glomerular disease and may contribute to the progression of glomerular damage. (See chronic renal failure in this chapter for a discussion of the diagnosis and management of hypertension.)
- *Thromboembolism* of major vessels may occur in patients with a nephrotic disorder. Although any vessel can be involved, pulmonary artery thromboembolism occurs most often. It is characterized by the sudden onset of intractable dyspnea.
  - Factors that contribute to hypercoagulability in patients with NS include platelet hyperaggregability and glomerular loss of antithrombin III, a serum protease that inhibits several activated clotting factors (II, IX, X, XI, and XII).
  - Consider preventative measures to minimize the tendency towards thromboembolism.
    Reduce the magnitude of proteinuria.
    Treat any underlying inflammatory condition.
    Avoid intravenous catheters if possible.
    Maintain adequate hydration status.
    Avoid overzealous use of diuretics.
    Avoid corticosteroids.
  - Anticoagulant treatment
    Heparin is likely to be ineffective because its action requires adequate amounts of antithrombin III.
    Coumarin derivatives may be more effective; however, their use has not been critically evaluated in veterinary patients.
    Aspirin administration (see dosage under glomerulonephritis) prevents platelet aggregation and might reduce the incidence of thrombosis.
  - Thrombolytic drugs, such as streptokinase and urokinase, form a complex with plasminogen to form plasmin, a fibrinolytic factor. These drugs have not been evaluated in veterinary patients.

RENAL TUBULAR DISORDERS

Renal tubular disorders are caused by functional tubular defects that produce altered urine, and in some cases, plasma concentrations of various substances.

Etiology

- *Renal tubular acidosis* (RTA) may be acquired or congenital and is rarely observed in small animals.
  - *Proximal RTA (type II)* is characterized by bicarbonate wasting. It occurs as part of the Fanconi syndrome in certain breeds of dogs. Type II has

been observed subsequent to gentamicin nephrotoxicity in dogs.
- *Distal RTA (type I)* is characterized by an inability of the distal tubule to secrete hydrogen ions and to produce acid urine. It has been reported in one cat with pyelonephritis and in another cat with hepatic lipidosis
■ *Fanconi syndrome* is characterized by multiple proximal tubular dysfunctions, resulting in glucosuria, aminoaciduria, and phosphaturia. It is suspected to be an inherited disorder and has been observed in basenjis, Norwegian elkhounds, Shetland sheepdogs, and schnauzers. Acquired Fanconi syndrome has been reported in a dog treated with gentamicin and in two other dogs treated with streptozotocin.
■ *Renal glucosuria* is characterized by defective proximal tubular transport of glucose. It is an inherited defect in Norwegian elkhounds but has been observed in other breeds.
■ *Cystinuria* is characterized by defective tubular transport of the amino acid cystine and other dibasic amino acids. It occurs most often in dachshunds but has been observed in other breeds (e.g., English bulldogs). Cystine is sparingly soluble in urine, and animals with cystinuria are predisposed to cystine urolithiasis (see sec. 8, ch. 3, for further discussion of urolithiasis).
■ *Nephrogenic diabetes insipidus* is characterized by failure of the kidneys to concentrate urine because of a renal tubular inability to respond to normal amounts of antidiuretic hormone (ADH). It usually is an acquired disorder that occurs secondary to conditions that diminish renal tubular response to ADH (Table 7); however, it also is a rare congenital defect in dogs.

Clinical Signs

Clinical findings vary depending on the primary pathophysiologic process.

■ Stranguria, dysuria, or hematuria may occur with urolithiasis (e.g., cystinuria).
■ Polyuria/polydipsia may occur with glucosuria, Fanconi syndrome, or nephrogenic diabetes insipidus. Profound polyuria/polydipsia and nocturia occur with congenital nephrogenic diabetes insipidus.
■ Stunted growth and weight loss may be observed in

animals with glucosuria, congenital nephrogenic diabetes insipidus, and RTA.
■ Vomiting frequently occurs secondary to gastric distension with water due to polydipsia in animals with congenital nephrogenic diabetes insipidus.
■ Some metabolic disorders may be subclinical (e.g., renal glucosuria, cystinuria).

Diagnosis

History

■ *History* identifies the clinical findings and the signalment that may be associated with metabolic disorders.

Physical Examination

■ *Physical examination* findings are often nonspecific but may include decreased muscle mass, muscle weakness, distended urinary bladder, and palpable urocystoliths.

Minimum Data Base

■ *Hemogram* is usually normal.
■ *Serum chemical profile* data may be abnormal.
  • Hypokalemia may occur in RTA and Fanconi syndrome.
  • Hyperchloremia may be observed in RTA.
  • Hypophosphatemia may develop in Fanconi syndrome.
■ *Urinalysis*
  • Normoglycemic glucosuria occurs in renal glucosuria and Fanconi syndrome.
  • Proteinuria occurs in Fanconi syndrome.
  • Urine specific gravity indicates hyposthenuria (<1.008) in animals with congenital nephrogenic diabetes insipidus and ranges from 1.001–1.018 in dogs with Fanconi syndrome.
  • Cystine crystals may be observed in dogs with cystinuria; they are colorless and hexagonal and are more likely to form in concentrated acid urine.
  • Urine pH values >6.0 often occur in RTA. In the presence of metabolic acidosis, patients with proximal RTA can have an acid urine (<6.0), whereas patients with distal RTA cannot.
■ *Blood gas evaluation*

KEY POINT ▶ Hyperchloremic, metabolic acidosis with a normal anion gap is the hallmark of RTA.

■ *Ancillary tests*
  • Infuse sodium bicarbonate to help distinguish between proximal and distal RTA. Animals with proximal RTA respond with increased urine pH and fractional excretion of bicarbonate, whereas those with distal RTA do not.
  • Confirm the presence of Fanconi syndrome by performing renal clearance studies that show excess urinary losses of protein, amino acids, glucose, bicarbonate, phosphate, and potassium.
  • Perform a modified water deprivation test (as described by Feldman and Nelson) to confirm congenital nephrogenic diabetes insipidus. (See

TABLE 7. Conditions Associated with Acquired Nephrogenic Diabetes Insipidus

Infectious	Metabolic
Pyometra	Hypokalemia
Pyelonephritis	Hypercalcemia
Endocrine	**Drugs**
Hyperadrenocorticism	Corticosteroids
Hypoadrenocorticism	Anticonvulsants
Hyperthyroidism	Diuretics
Intrinsic Renal Disease	
Chronic renal failure	
Pyelonephritis	

sec. 4, ch. 6, for more details concerning water deprivation tests.)

Treatment

Renal Tubular Acidosis

- Identify and eliminate any underlying causes
- Administer sodium bicarbonate (1–2 mEq/kg PO) to control acidemia; higher doses may be needed for proximal RTA. Adjust the dosage based on response to therapy.
- Treat hypokalemia by supplementing potassium (see previous discussion in this chapter).

Fanconi Syndrome

- Discontinue any drugs that might cause acquired disease.
- Try to maintain a plasma bicarbonate concentration of 12–18 mEq/L by administering bicarbonate as needed.
- If hypokalemic, administer potassium to maintain normal serum concentrations (see sec. 1, ch. 5).
- Monitor the animal for development of severe acidosis, hypokalemia, or decline in renal function.
- Allow access to adequate supply of fresh water.

Renal Glucosuria

- Alone this is a benign condition and does not require treatment.

Cystinuria

- This predisposes the patient to the development of cystine urolithiasis.
- If cystine uroliths occur, remove them surgically (see sec. 8, ch. 2) or employ medical strategies to promote their dissolution (see sec. 8, ch. 3).

Nephrogenic Diabetes Insipidus

- If acquired, treat the underlying cause.
- For congenital nephrogenic diabetes insipidus
  - Feed a low sodium diet.
  - Administer chlorothiazide (Diuril, Merck Sharp & Dohme; 20–40 mg/kg, q12h PO). It enhances proximal tubular reabsorption of sodium, chloride, and water.

CYSTIC RENAL DISEASE

Cysts are epithelium-lined cavities that contain fluid. Renal cysts are dilated nephron segments that may be single or multiple (i.e., polycystic). Pseudocysts are accumulations of fluid that collect outside the renal parenchyma. They are not lined by epithelium, and, therefore, are not true cysts.

Etiology

- *Familial* polycystic disease has been reported in Cairn terriers and longhaired cats. This disease is inherited as an autosomal dominant trait in Persian cats.

- *Acquired* cystic disease may develop in animals with any type of chronic renal disease.
- *Perinephric pseudocyst* is an uncommon condition reported mainly in cats. Pathogenesis is unknown.

Clinical Signs

- Progressive abdominal enlargement is the most common clinical sign. This generally is the only sign in cats with perinephric pseudocysts.
- Vomiting, anorexia, weight loss, and polyuria/polydipsia occur secondary to renal failure in animals with familial polycystic renal disease.
- Solitary or multiple cysts that do not enlarge are usually of little clinical significance.

Diagnosis

History

- *History* identifies the clinical signs of cystic renal disease, especially in breeds with familial predispositions. Question the owner about an affected dam, sire, or sibling.

Physical Examination

- *Physical examination* findings include abdominal enlargement and nonpainful renomegaly.

Minimum Data Base

- *Hemogram* may show increased erythropoiesis in longhaired cats with idiopathic polycystic renal disease, possibly due to hypoxia-induced release of erythropoietin.
- *Serum chemistry profile* abnormalities include increased BUN and serum creatinine concentrations and hyperphosphatemia in renal failure.
- *Urinalysis*
  - Isosthenuria occurs in renal failure.
  - Bacteriuria and pyuria occur if secondary urinary tract infection is present.

Urine Culture

- *Culture urine* if urinary tract infection is suspected.

Excretory Urography

- *Excretory urography* (see sec. 1, ch. 4) confirms renomegaly in animals with polycystic renal disease and may show the cysts as multiple radiolucent areas in the renal parenchyma. In animals with perinephric pseudocyst, the kidney is demonstrated within the fluid-filled structure.

Ultrasonography

- *Ultrasonography* (see sec. 1, ch. 4) is quite useful for detection and characterization of fluid-filled renal lesions. Their number, size, and anatomic relationships can be assessed.

KEY POINT ▶ Ultrasonography is the procedure of choice for reliable diagnosis of polycystic kidneys and perinephric pseudocyst.

Aspiration

- *Aspirate the cyst* if necessary to confirm that it is a fluid-filled structure.

Treatment

- No specific treatment of cystic renal disease now exists. Bilateral polycystic kidneys result in CRF. A unilateral polycystic kidney can be treated by unilateral nephrectomy (see sec. 8, ch. 2), providing normal renal function is documented in the unaffected kidney.
- If renal failure exists, treat it medically (see CRF).
- Treatment for perinephric pseudocyst is surgical drainage and resection of the cyst walls. (See section 8, ch. 2, for a general discussion of renal surgery.)

Prognosis

The prognosis for animals with perinephric pseudocysts is good after surgical treatment; the prognosis for progressive bilateral polycystic kidney disease is poor. Advise the owner of the potential genetic aspects of the disease.

NEPHROLITHIASIS/URETEROLITHIASIS

Uroliths are polycrystalline concretions that are composed mainly of organic or inorganic crystalloids (90–95%) and a smaller but essential amount of organic matrix (5–10%). Uroliths form in the urinary space within the excretory pathway, and they usually are classified according to mineral composition.

KEY POINT ▶ In dogs and cats, the majority of uroliths are found in the urinary bladder or urethra (see sec. 8, ch. 3). Fewer than 10% are found in the renal pelvis.

Occasionally, nephroliths pass from the kidney and become ureteroliths.

Etiology

- *Urinary tract infection* (UTI) by bacteria that hydrolyze urea (e.g., *Staphylococcus, Proteus*) is the most common cause of magnesium ammonium phosphate (struvite) urolithiasis in dogs. UTI also may occur secondary to urolithiasis that initially developed in the absence of infection.
- *Metabolic disorders* that cause excessive urinary excretion of sparingly soluble compounds may predispose an animal to urolithiasis.
  - Inborn errors of metabolism predispose Dalmatians to urate urolithiasis, dogs with cystinuria to cystine urolithiasis, and animals with RTA to calcium phosphate urolithiasis.
  - Portal vascular anomalies predispose affected dogs and cats to the development of urate urolithiasis because of hepatic dysfunction.
  - Acquired metabolic disorders that predispose animals to urolithiasis include hyperparathyroidism (see sec. 4, ch. 2), which may lead to the formation of calcium phosphate uroliths.

- *Dietary factors*
  - High-magnesium alkalinizing diets promote struvite urolithiasis in cats.
  - Diets containing large amounts of corn gluten or soybean hulls have been associated with formation of silica uroliths.
  - Excessive dietary calcium or phosphorus intake may promote formation of calcium phosphate uroliths.
- *Idiopathic conditions* often cause urolithiasis. The pathogenic mechanisms of urolith formation in animals with calcium oxalate, sterile struvite, and silica urolithiasis are poorly understood.

Clinical Signs

- Clinical signs associated with renal and ureteral uroliths are diverse and primarily depend upon the following:
  - Size, number, and location of the stones.
  - Presence (degree and duration) or absence of obstruction to urine flow.
  - Presence or absence of UTI.
- Hematuria and signs of sublumbar or abdominal discomfort may be observed.
- Bilateral obstruction or unilateral obstruction with inadequate renal function in the contralateral kidney causes vomiting, anorexia, and depression, owing to postrenal azotemia/uremia.
- Urine may have a foul odor if UTI exists.
- An affected animal may have subclinical disease.

Diagnosis

History

- *History* identifies the breed predispositions (see sec. 8, ch. 3) and clinical signs associated with nephrolithiasis and ureterolithiasis.

Physical Examination

- *Physical examination* abnormalities may include sublumbar or abdominal pain and/or renomegaly. Fever may be found in a patient with UTI causing nephritis, especially with concurrent obstruction.

Minimum Data Base

- *Hemogram* usually is normal. Leukocytosis may be found when UTI causes pyelonephritis, especially with concurrent obstruction.
- *Serum Chemistry Panel*
  - Increased BUN, serum creatinine, and serum phosphorus concentrations accompany renal failure, bilateral ureteral obstruction, or unilateral obstruction of a single functioning kidney.
  - Hypokalemia, hyperchloremia, and metabolic acidosis may occur in cases of urolithiasis associated with renal tubular acidosis (see previous discussion).
  - Hypercalcemia occasionally is found in animals with calcium-containing uroliths; however, most of these animals are normocalcemic.
- *Urinalysis*

- Hematuria is a common finding.
- Suspect UTI when pyuria and/or bacteriuria are found.
- Urine pH tends to be alkaline with struvite uroliths and acidic with cystine uroliths. Urate and calcium oxalate uroliths may be associated with either alkaline or acidic urine.
- Examine sediment for struvite, ammonium urate, cystine, or calcium oxalate crystals. Crystalluria represents a risk factor for urolithiasis; however, do not presumptively identify the mineral content of uroliths solely on the type of crystalluria.

Urine Culture

- *Urine culture* is performed.

Radiography

- Confirm the presence, location, density, size, and number of uroliths with abdominal radiography.
- Urolith density is quite variable; however, oxalate, struvite, calcium phosphate, and silica uroliths usually are more radiodense than urate and cystine uroliths.
- Confirm the presence of nephrolithiasis and ureterolithiasis and the degree of urinary obstruction by excretory urography (see sec. 1, ch. 4). Consider cystourethrography to identify concomitant lower urinary tract uroliths (see sec. 1, ch. 4).

Ultrasonography

- *Ultrasonography* helps to confirm the presence and location of uroliths, identify radiolucent uroliths, and assess the degree of obstruction.

Urolith Analysis

- *Quantitative (crystallographic) urolith analysis* is required to accurately determine mineral composition of uroliths.

KEY POINT ▶ A tentative diagnosis of urolith composition often can be made using information from the clinical, laboratory, and radiographic findings.

Treatment

The goals of treatment are to correct any predisposing factors if possible, eliminate existing calculi by surgical or medical treatment, and prevent recurrence. Refer to section 8, chapter 3, for discussion of treatment for urolithiasis.

Nonobstructing, sterile nephroliths that do not increase in size, do not cause significant hematuria, and do not produce deterioration in renal function can be monitored without treatment. However, even for seemingly innocuous nephroliths, consider medical dissolution therapy if the mineral composition (struvite, urate, cystine) can be estimated with confidence.

Correct Underlying Causes

- When concomitant UTI exists, administer an appropriate antimicrobial drug and continue for 2–3 weeks after dissolution or removal of uroliths.

- Correct portosystemic shunts surgically, when possible (see sec. 7, ch. 9).
- Remove parathyroid adenoma in a patient with primary hyperparathyroidism (see sec. 4, ch. 2).

Medical Treatment

- This is not effective for calcium oxalate, calcium phosphate, or silica uroliths. Struvite, urate, and cystine uroliths may respond partially or completely to medical calculolytic therapy (see sec. 8, ch. 3, for description of protocols).
- *Monitor* the patient to determine efficacy of medical dissolution therapy efforts.
  - Reassess the size and location of uroliths using radiography and/or ultrasonography every 4–6 weeks.
  - Perform urinalysis periodically (every 4–6 weeks).
  - Crystalluria must be absent for medical dissolution therapy to be effective.
  - Perform urine culture periodically (every 4–6 weeks) to verify continuing control of UTI.
  - If uroliths enlarge or fail to steadily decrease in size, verify compliance with intended treatment instructions and based on that consider other treatment options. The original assessment of urolith mineral type might be incorrect, or the urolith might be composed of more than one mineral.
  - As nephroliths decrease in size, they may move into the ureter causing partial or complete obstruction.

Surgical Treatment

- *Surgical treatment* is required in some situations (see sec. 8, ch. 2).

KEY POINT ▶ Nephroliths or ureteroliths that obstruct urine flow to any substantial degree are surgically removed with little delay.

  - If treatment of uroliths composed of calcium oxalate, calcium phosphate, or silica is required, surgical removal is indicated.
  - Uroliths that fail to dissolve when treated with appropriate medical strategies may also require surgical removal.

Prevention

Prevention of recurrent urolithiasis depends upon the mineral type involved (see sec. 8, ch. 3).

RENAL PARASITISM

Etiology

Dioctophyma renale is the canine kidney worm. *D. renale* infection is a rare condition. Dogs become infected by ingesting the larvae or by ingesting a paratenic host, usually fish, that contains encysted larvae.

Clinical Signs

- Dogs often are asymptomatic. Signs of renal failure do not occur with unilateral involvement.

- Abdominal enlargement may occur if the worm migrates into the peritoneal cavity and causes peritonitis.
- Hematuria may be observed.

Diagnosis

History

- *History* identifies clinical findings and potential for exposure to a paratenic host.

Physical Examination

- *Physical examination* findings may be normal, or abdominal enlargement may be found.

Minimum Data Base

- Hemogram: eosinophilia, basophilia, and hyperproteinemia may be observed.
- Serum chemistries: azotemia does not occur unless both kidneys are affected or unless one kidney is affected and the other kidney is impaired owing to some other cause.

Urinalysis

- The diagnosis is confirmed by observing characteristic double operculated ova in urine sediment. Renal infestation is required for a patent infection.
- Hematuria, pyuria, and proteinuria may occur secondary to urinary tract inflammation.

Abdominal Fluid Analysis

- With peritoneal involvement, findings are consistent with peritonitis (see sec. 7, ch. 13).
- Look for parasitic ova in abdominal fluid.

Treatment

- No medical therapy is effective.
- Surgical Treatment
  - Perform a nephrectomy if severe unilateral renal infection exists and a nephrotomy if bilateral renal infection exists. (Surgical techniques for nephrectomy and nephrotomy are described in section 8, chapter 2).
  - If peritonitis is present, perform an exploratory procedure to identify and remove all parasites.

Prevention

Do not allow dogs to ingest paratenic hosts or infected water.

RENAL NEOPLASIA

Etiology

Primary Tumors

- Renal cell carcinoma, transitional cell carcinoma, and embryonal nephroblastoma are the most common primary renal tumors in dogs. A syndrome of dermatofibrosis and renal cystadenocarcinoma oc-

curs primarily in female German shepherd dogs and may be a heritable trait.
- Renal cell carcinoma is the most common primary renal tumor in cats.
- Renal tumors in dogs and cats are usually malignant.

Metastatic Tumors

- Metastatic neoplasia is more common than primary renal neoplasia.
- The kidneys are often involved in patients with lymphosarcoma, especially cats.
- Hemangiosarcomas, melanomas, mast cell tumors, and carcinomas also may metastasize to the kidneys.

Clinical Signs

- Clinical signs usually are vague and nonspecific. Lethargy, anorexia, and progressive weight loss may occur.
- Anorexia, vomiting, and polyuria/polydipsia may occur in patients that develop renal failure.
- Hematuria of renal origin may be observed.

Diagnosis

History

History identifies the clinical signs of renal neoplasia.

Physical Examination

- Palpate the kidneys for renomegaly.
- Examine for tumors or masses in other organ locations.

Minimum Data Base

- Hematology: polycythemia may occur with some renal tumors (e.g., carcinoma, fibrosarcoma) presumably owing to inappropriate production of erythropoietin.
- Serum chemistry profile: azotemia and hyperphosphatemia due to renal failure may occur with bilateral renal neoplasia, especially in cats with lymphosarcoma.
- Hematuria and proteinuria may be observed.

KEY POINT ▶ Feline leukemia virus status is determined in cats with renal lymphosarcoma. About 50% of affected cats are positive for FeLV by ELISA test (see sec. 2, ch. 1).

Radiography

- Survey abdominal radiographs may reveal unilateral or bilateral renomegaly. An abdominal mass that cannot be identified as kidney sometimes is seen.
- When a renal mass is suspected, perform excretory urography to confirm renal involvement (see sec. 1, ch. 4).
- Radiography of the thorax is needed to look for possible metastasis. This finding is most likely with renal cell carcinoma.

Ultrasonography

Ultrasonography of the abdomen helps confirm renal mass lesions.

Renal Biopsy

- In cats with bilateral renomegaly, cytologic examination of a fine-needle aspirate sample from a kidney often is diagnostic of lymphosarcoma and eliminates the need for renal biopsy.
- For other neoplasms, a kidney biopsy is performed. Tissue for histologic evaluation is submitted to determine definitive diagnosis. Surgical biopsy may be necessary to allow direct exposure of the neoplasm.

Treatment

Chemotherapy

- Treat lymphosarcoma with combination chemotherapy (see sec. 3, chs. 5 and 6).

Surgery

- Evaluate the function of the contralateral kidney prior to nephrectomy.
- With the exception of lymphosarcoma, surgical excision of the neoplastic kidney and its ureter is the treatment of choice (see sec. 8, ch. 2). Consider adjunctive treatment (see sec. 3, chs. 5 and 6).

Prognosis

The prognosis is guarded to poor for patients with malignant renal neoplasms.

RENAL/URETERAL TRAUMA

Because of their location in the abdominal cavity, traumatic injury to the kidneys and ureters is uncommon in small animal patients. See section 8, chapters 3 and 5, for discussion of bladder and urethral trauma.

Etiology

- *Blunt trauma* may be caused by vehicular injuries and falls from heights.
- *Penetrating trauma* may result from fight wounds, gunshot injuries, and other objects.

Clinical Signs

- In most cases, renal and ureteral trauma is mild and self-limiting.
- Rupture of the renal capsule, pelvis, or mid-to-upper ureter causes extravasation of urine into the retroperitoneal space, which is associated with vague nonspecific signs including abdominal pain and fever.
- Rupture of the distal ureter causes leakage of urine into the abdominal cavity. Clinical findings result from peritonitis and uremia and may include abdominal enlargement and pain.
- Macroscopic hematuria occurs frequently.
- Severe bruising to the ventral abdominal wall is often, but not always, seen with traumatically induced uroabdomen.
- Normal urination may be seen with unilateral ureteral rupture.

Diagnosis

KEY POINT ▶ Suspect renal/ureteral trauma when there are vague signs of abdominal discomfort; macroscopic hematuria; or fractures of the caudal ribs, vertebrae, or pelvis, particularly.

History

- Question the owner about the possibility of trauma.

Physical Examination

- Observe for any external signs of trauma.
- Palpate the abdomen to detect evidence of pain and fluid accumulation.

Minimum Data Base

- *Hemogram* is usually normal.
- *Serum chemistry panel* may reveal azotemia if the injury is not acute and significant urine leakage has occurred.
- *Urinalysis* may show hematuria.

Abdominal Fluid Analysis

Note: Urine leakage may remain confined to the retroperitoneal space and not result in uroabdomen.

- Perform cytologic evaluation. Nonseptic inflammation occurs most often with uroabdomen.
- Determine urea nitrogen and creatinine concentrations.
  - Urea is a small molecule; therefore, its concentration rapidly equilibrates with that of serum.
  - When urine leaks into the abdominal cavity, the creatinine concentration of the peritoneal fluid is greater than that of the serum initially.

Radiography

Radiography provides the most useful information regarding the location of ureteral rupture.
- *Survey abdominal radiographic* findings are rarely diagnostic of renal or ureteral trauma.
  - Signs suggestive of trauma include displacement, asymmetry, and inability to visualize one or both kidneys.
  - Urine leakage into the retroperitoneal space causes increased opacity and streaky, hazy areas in the retroperitoneum.
  - Loss of abdominal contrast occurs when urine leaks into the peritoneal space.
- *Contrast radiography*

KEY POINT ▶ Excretory urography is the diagnostic test of choice for renal and ureteral trauma.

- Look for an accumulation of contrast material in the area of suspected leakage.

- If a kidney is not visualized, perform renal arteriography to evaluate the kidney's vascular supply.
- Perform thoracic radiography in all trauma patients to evaluate for consequences of thoracic trauma.
- Ultrasonography may be helpful to deliniate the kidneys and retroperitoneal space.

Treatment
Supportive

- Stabilize the patient by administering fluids and employing other shock treatment measures as needed (see sec. 6, ch. 14).
- Observe the animal for evidence of a ruptured urinary tract. Other injuries may be self-limiting (e.g., renal contusions, hematoma).
- Provide abdominal drainage in animals with uroabdomen to stabilize them prior to surgery.

Surgery

- After stabilization and diagnostic evaluation, consider surgical treatment (see sec. 8, ch. 2).
- Indications for surgery include leakage of urine into the abdomen or retroperitoneal space, and crushing injury to the kidney or its vascular supply.

ECTOPIC URETER
Etiology

- Ureteral ectopia is a congenital abnormality whereby one or both ureters do not terminate in the trigone of the urinary bladder.
- In females, ectopic ureters may terminate in the vagina, urethra, or uterus. In males, ectopic ureters end in the pelvic urethra.

Clinical Signs

- Urinary incontinence is usually observed by the owner around the time of weaning. Incontinence can be continuous or intermittent.
- Animals with ureteral ectopia usually retain the ability to urinate normally. (See sec. 8, ch. 7, for discussion of micturition disorders.)
- Urine may have a foul odor if a urinary tract infection exists.
- Soiling of the perineal hair and skin with urine may cause dermatitis.

Diagnosis
History

- Identify urinary incontinence in a young animal (For a discussion of diagnostic approach and differential diagnosis for incontinence, see sec. 8, ch. 7.)
- Female dogs are affected most frequently; however, male dogs and cats may also be affected.

Physical Examination

- Verify urinary incontinence by urine-soaked vulva or hair or after observation during hospitalization.

- Look for other congenital defects.

Minimum Data Base

- This is usually normal with the exception of the urinalysis. Pyuria and bacteriuria often occur secondary to urinary tract infection.

Urine Culture

- *Perform urine culture* to rule out urinary tract infection.

Contrast Radiography

- Excretory urography (see sec. 1, ch. 4).
  - Usually confirms the diagnosis of ureteral ectopia.
  - Dilated ureters and hydronephrosis may occur secondary to urinary tract infection.
  - Inflating the bladder with CO_2 helps improve visualization of terminal ureters, and oblique films may be indicated to outline individual ureters.
- Retrograde contrast urethrography or vaginography may help to localize the site of ureteral termination.

Vaginoscopy and Cytoscopy

- Vaginoscopy or cytoscopy may be helpful to locate the terminal ureteral orifice and to evaluate for ureteral abnormalities.
- Surgical exploration occasionally is required to achieve a definitive diagnosis if cytoscopy is not available. Cytoscopy allows for evaluation of ureteral orifice location. Intramural ectopic ureter may enter the bladder in a normal trigonal position.

Treatment
Surgical Treatment

- *Surgical correction* is the treatment of choice (see sec. 8, ch. 2, for description of techniques).

KEY POINT ▶ Surgical correction cures about 50% of patients; incontinence continues in approximately 50%. One third of these animals respond to medical treatment.

Medical Treatment

- Treatment of urinary tract infection is indicated.
  - Culture urine to determine the species of infecting organism.
  - If pyelonephritis is suspected, administer an antimicrobial agent for 6–8 weeks.
  - Reculture urine 3–5 days after beginning treatment and again 5–7 days after discontinuing treatment.

Prevention

- Adrenergic stimulants (agonistic) may reduce incontinence following surgery (see sec. 8, ch. 7).
- Counsel the owners regarding possible inheritance of disease.
- Consider neutering the animal.

URETERAL OBSTRUCTION

Etiology

- *Neoplasia*
  - Primary ureteral tumors include leiomyosarcoma and leiomyoma.
  - Any abdominal tumor may compress a ureter causing extramural obstruction.
  - Extension of tumors from the bladder (e.g., transitional cell carcinoma, rhabdomyosarcoma) and prostate (e.g., adenocarcinoma) may obstruct the ureters.
- *Uroliths* formed in the kidney may enter a ureter, causing obstruction (see discussion of calculi of kidney and ureter).
- *Blood clots* may lodge in the ureter secondary to renal hematuria.
- *Strictures* may be congenital or occur secondary to inflammation or surgery.

Clinical Signs

- Partial and unilateral obstruction may be subclinical. Bilateral obstruction causes signs of renal failure (see previous discussion).
- Signs may result from the underlying disease.
  - Hematuria and stranguria may occur with urinary bladder neoplasia and prostatic disease.
  - Straining to defecate may be observed with prostatic disease.
  - Ureterolithiasis may cause pain and abdominal discomfort.

Diagnosis

History

- Look for clinical signs of ureteral obstruction.
- Determine the possible history of abdominal surgery or trauma, urolithiasis, and neoplasia.

Physical Examination

- Palpate the abdomen for evidence of pain and abdominal masses.
- Perform a rectal examination to evaluate the prostate gland, pelvic urethra, and sublumbar lymph nodes.
- Palpate the urinary bladder to detect a mass.

Minimum Data Base

- *Hemogram* may be normal or show an inflammatory response (e.g., pyelonephritis).
- *Serum chemistry panel* is usually normal. Azotemia may occur if both kidneys are affected.
- *Urinalysis* may show hematuria or pyuria associated with inflammation, neoplasia, or urolithiasis.

Radiography

- *Survey abdominal radiographs* may demonstrate radiopaque ureteroliths or compressing masses.
- *Excretory urography* confirms the presence and location of ureteral obstruction. Dilation of the ureter proximal to the obstruction and hydronephrosis often occur.

Ultrasonography

- Noninvasively detects changes (e.g., hydronephrosis) consistent with ureteral obstruction.
- Preferred over excretory urography in patients with compromised renal function.
- Normal findings do not rule out a diagnosis of obstruction.

Treatment

The goals of treatment are to provide supportive care and to remove the underlying cause, if possible.

Medical Treatment

- If the obstruction is partial, urine is sterile, and cause of obstruction may resolve spontaneously (e.g., blood clot), monitor the animal for a period of weeks to months.
- If partial obstruction occurs because of urolithiasis (e.g., struvite, urate), attempt dissolution of the urolith.

Surgical Treatment

- Indicated with evidence of progressive renal damage, persistent urinary tract infection, and no response to medical therapy.
- If ureteral neoplasia or stricture exists, surgical excision is the treatment of choice.
- If possible, remove extramural masses that compress the ureter. Severe renal damage from chronic obstruction and/or pyelonephritis with concurrent ureteral obstruction is treated by nephrectomy-ureterectomy, provided that the contralateral kidney is functioning adequately.

Supplemental Readings

ACUTE RENAL FAILURE

Brown SA, Barsanti JA: Gentamicin nephrotoxicosis in the dog. *In* Kirk RW, ed.: *Current Veterinary Therapy IX. Small Animal Practice.* Philadelphia: WB Saunders, 1986, p 1146.
Chew DJ: Acute renal failure. 7th Kal Kan Symp 1983, p 9.
DiBartola SP: Acute renal failure: pathophysiology and management. Compend Contin Educ Pract Vet 11:952, 1980.
Grauer GF, Thrall MAH: Ethylene glycol (antifreeze) poisoning. *In* Kirk RW, ed.: *Current Veterinary Therapy IX. Small Animal Practice.* Philadelphia: WB Saunders, 1986, p 206.
Greene CE, Shotts EB: Leptospirosis. *In* Greene CE, ed.: *Infectious Diseases of the Dog and Cat.* Philadelphia: WB Saunders, 1990, p 498.
Polzin D, Osborne C, O'Brien T: Diseases of the kidney and ureter. *In* Ettinger SJ, ed.: *Textbook of Veterinary Internal Medicine,* 2nd ed. Philadelphia: WB Saunders, 1989, p 1962.

CHRONIC RENAL FAILURE

Allen TA: Management of advanced chronic renal failure. *In* Kirk RW, ed.: *Current Veterinary Therapy X. Small Animal Practice.* Philadelphia: WB Saunders, 1989, p 1195.
Chew DJ, DiBartola SP: Diagnosis and pathophysiology of renal disease. *In* Ettinger SJ, ed.: *Textbook of Veterinary Internal Medicine,* 2nd ed. Philadelphia: WB Saunders, 1989, p 1893.
DiBartola SP, Davenport DJ, Chew DJ: Renal failure in young

dogs. *In* Kirk RW, ed.: *Current Veterinary Therapy X. Small Animal Practice.* Philadelphia: WB Saunders, 1989, p 1167.

Finco DR, Brown SA: New concepts and controversies on dietary management of renal failure. *In* Kirk RW, ed.: *Current Veterinary Therapy X. Small Animal Practice.* Philadelphia: WB Saunders, 1989, p 1198.

Polzin D, Osborne C, O'Brien T: Diseases of the kidneys and ureters. *In* Ettinger SJ, ed.: *Textbook of Veterinary Internal Medicine,* 2nd ed. Philadelphia: WB Saunders, 1989, p 1962.

Ross LA, Labato MA: Use of drugs to control hypertension in renal failure. *In* Kirk RW, ed.: *Current Veterinary Therapy X. Small Animal Practice.* Philadelphia: WB Saunders, 1989, p 1201.

PYELONEPHRITIS

Lees GE, Rogers KS: Diagnosis and localization of urinary tract infections. *In* Kirk RW, ed.: *Current Veterinary Therapy IX. Small Animal Practice.* Philadelphia: WB Saunders, 1986, p 1118.

Ling GV: Management of urinary tract infections. *In* Kirk RW, ed.: *Current Veterinary Therapy IX. Small Animal Practice.* Philadelphia: WB Saunders, 1986, p 1174.

NEPHROTIC SYNDROME

Barsanti JA, Finco DR, Vaden SL: Medical management of canine glomerulonephropathies. *In* Kirk RW, ed.: *Current Veterinary Therapy X. Small Animal Practice.* Philadelphia: WB Saunders, 1989, p 1174.

Center SA, Smith CA, Wilkinson E, et al: Clinicopathologic, renal immunofluorescent, and light microscopic features of glomerulonephritis in the dog: 41 cases (1975–1985). J Am Vet Med Assoc 190:81, 1987.

DiBartola SP, Chew DJ: Glomerular disease in the dog and cat. *In* Kirk RW, ed.: *Current Veterinary Therapy IX. Small Animal Practice.* Philadelphia: WB Saunders, 1986, p 1132.

Jergens AE: Glomerulonephritis in dogs and cats. Compend Contin Educ Pract Vet 9:903, 1987.

Polzin D, Osborne C, O'Brien T: Diseases of the kidneys and ureters. *In* Ettinger SJ, ed.: *Textbook of Veterinary Internal Medicine,* 2nd ed. Philadelphia: WB Saunders, 1989, p 1962.

Rackear D, Feldman B, Farver T, Lelong L: The effect of three different dosages of acetylsalicylic acid on canine platelet aggregation. J Am Anim Hosp Assoc 24:23, 1988.

Russo EA: Assessment of proteinuria in the dog and cat. *In* Kirk RW, ed.: *Current Veterinary Therapy IX. Small Animal Practice.* Philadelphia: WB Saunders, 1986, p 1111.

RENAL TUBULAR DISORDERS

Bovee KC: Canine cystine urolithiasis. *Vet Clin North Am (Sm Anim Pract)* 16:211, 1986.

Breitschwerdt EB: Nephrogenic diabetes insipidus. *In* Kirk RW, ed.: *Current Veterinary Therapy X. Small Animal Practice.* Philadelphia: WB Saunders, 1986, p 1140.

Brown SA: Fanconi's syndrome. *In* Kirk RW, ed.: *Current Veterinary Therapy X. Small Animal Practice.* Philadelphia: WB Saunders, 1989, p 1163.

Brown SA, Rakich PM, Barsanti JA, et al.: Fanconi syndrome and acute renal failure associated with gentamicin therapy in a dog. J Am Anim Hosp Assoc 22:635, 1986.

Feldman EC, Nelson RW: *Canine and Feline Endocrinology and Reproduction.* Philadelphia: WB Saunders, 2987, p 14.

Polzin D, Osborne C, O'Brien T: Diseases of the kidneys and ureters. *In* Ettinger SJ, ed.: *Textbook of Veterinary Internal Medicine,* 2nd ed. Philadelphia: WB Saunders, 1989, p 1962.

CYSTIC RENAL DISEASE

Crowell WA: Polycystic renal disease. *In* Kirk RW, ed.: *Current Veterinary Therapy IX. Small Animal Practice.* Philadelphia: WB Saunders, 1986, p 1138.

Lulich JP, Osborne CA, Walter PA, O'Brien TD: Feline idiopathic polycystic kidney disease. Compend Contin Educ Pract Vet 10:1030, 1988.

Polzin D, Osborne C, O'Brien T: Diseases of the kidneys and ureters. *In* Ettinger SJ, ed.: *Textbook of Veterinary Internal Medicine,* 2nd ed. Philadelphia: WB Saunders, 1989, p 1962.

NEPHROLITHIASIS/URETEROLITHIASIS

Osborne CA, Polzin DJ, Johnston GR, O'Brien TD: Canine urolithiasis. *In* Ettinger SJ, ed.: *Textbook of Veterinary Internal Medicine,* 2nd ed. Philadelphia: WB Saunders, 1989, p 2083.

Senior DF: Medical management of urate uroliths. *In* Kirk RW, ed.: *Current Veterinary Therapy X. Small Animal Practice.* Philadelphia: WB Saunders, 1989, p 1178.

Senior DF: Canine urolithiasis. *In* Brietschwerdt EB, ed.: *Nephrology and Urology.* New York: Churchill Livingstone, 1986, p 1.

RENAL PARASITISM

Brown SA, Prestwood AK: Parasites of the urinary tract. *In* Kirk RW, ed.: *Current Veterinary Therapy IX. Small Animal Practice.* Philadelphia: WB Saunders, 1986, p 1153.

RENAL NEOPLASIA

Klein MK, Cockerell GL, Harris CK, et al.: Canine primary renal neoplasms: a retrospective review of 54 cases. J Am Anim Hosp Assoc 24:443, 1988.

Mooney SC, Hayes AA, Matus RE, MacEwen EG: Renal lymphoma in cats: 28 cases (1977–1984). J Am Vet Med Assoc 191:1473, 1987.

RENAL/URETERAL TRAUMA

Pechman RD: Urinary tract trauma in dogs and cats. J Am Anim Hosp Assoc 18:33, 1982.

Zenoble RD, Pechman RD: Urinary tract trauma. *In* Kirk RW, ed.: *Current Veterinary Therapy IX. Small Animal Practice.* Philadelphia: WB Saunders, 1986, p 1155.

ECTOPIC URETERS

Faulkner RT, Osborne CA, Feeney DA: Canine and feline ureteral ectopia. *In* Kirk RW, ed.: *Current Veterinary Therapy VIII. Small Animal Practice.* Philadelphia: WB Saunders, 1983, p 1043.

URETERAL OBSTRUCTION

Polzin D, Osborne C, O'Brien T: Diseases of the kidneys and ureters. *In* Ettinger SJ, ed.: *Textbook of Veterinary Internal Medicine,* 2nd ed. Philadelphia: WB Saunders, 1989, p 1962.

2 Surgery of the Kidney and Ureter

Dale E. Bjorling

Biopsy of the kidney often gives the most reliable information regarding the presence of disease and the prognosis for improvement. When renal calculi are removed surgically, a nephrotomy is usually performed. When the renal pelvis and proximal ureter are dilated, a pyelolithotomy may be performed to remove calculi. Removal of the kidney (nephrectomy) is often considered because of severe damage due to trauma, neoplasia, infection, or obstruction of the ureter. Reattachment of the ureter to the renal pelvis is extremely difficult without magnification and is infrequently attempted in veterinary practice. This disorder is more commonly treated by unilateral nephrectomy and ureterectomy. A ureterotomy may be performed to remove calculi or other objects from the lumen of the ureter. Ureteral anastomosis is a challenge for the veterinarian in small dogs and in cats. Magnification is strongly encouraged during this procedure to improve outcome. Ureteroneocystostomy is a feasible treatment option for lesions of the distal ureter and is considered for ectopic ureter.

ANATOMY

Kidney

- The kidneys are normally found in the retroperitoneal space in a sublumbar location. The cranial pole of the right kidney may be in contact with the liver, and the left kidney may usually be found several centimeters caudal to the liver.
- The renal arteries divide into dorsal and ventral branches after arising from the aorta. Each branch divides into five to seven interlobar arteries. The interlobar arteries branch into arcuate arteries at the corticomedullary junction and ultimately give rise to the interlobular arteries. Multiple renal arteries may occur on the left side in up to 13% of all dogs but are rare on the right side. Multiple renal arteries are extremely uncommon in cats. The renal artery may give rise to the ovarian artery, and the ovarian vein occasionally drains into the renal vein.

Ureter

- The ureter is a muscular tube that lies within the retroperitoneal space. The ureter conveys urine to the bladder by coordinated peristaltic contractions.
- The arterial blood supply of the ureter is longitudinal and must not be disturbed during dissection of the ureter.
- The ureter approaches the bladder at an oblique angle and passes submucosally within the bladder wall towards the neck of the bladder. A valve-like function is provided by the submucosal location of the ureters, which decreases vesicoureteral reflux of urine.

RENAL BIOPSY

Preoperative Considerations

- Platelet count and coagulation function must be normal prior to undertaking renal biopsy.

KEY POINT ▶ Hemorrhage is a common occurrence after renal biopsy. Evaluate coagulation function prior to surgery. Apply pressure to the biopsy site until bleeding has stopped.

- If unilateral disease is present and if a percutaneous biopsy is to be performed, the site of disease is identified prior to performing the biopsy.

Surgical Procedure

Objectives

- Obtain a representative sample of renal tissue.
- Avoid damage to major vasculature or renal pelvis.
- Control hemorrhage.

Equipment

- Standard surgical instruments and suture
- Vim-Silverman or Tru-Cut biopsy needle (or other biopsy needle of surgeon's preference)
- Balfour self-retaining retractor for celiotomy approach.

Technique

The kidney may undergo biopsy through a percutaneous, or a "key-hole" approach, or a celiotomy. The celiotomy approach is described.

1. Place the animal in dorsal recumbency.
2. Aseptically prepare the ventral abdomen for a standard celiotomy incision.
3. Make a ventral midline approach to the abdominal

cavity and extend the incision cranially to the xiphoid process to facilitate exposure of the kidneys.
4. Place a self-retaining Balfour retractor to maintain exposure of the abdominal cavity.
5. Examine and palpate the kidneys. If an isolated lesion is present, select an appropriate biopsy site.
6. Obtain single or multiple biopsy samples using a biopsy needle, or perform a nephrotomy to collect a wedge or slice of renal tissue. The technique for biopsy during nephrectomy is discussed in this chapter under Nephrotomy.
7. When a biopsy needle is used, direct the needle away from the pelvis to avoid damaging this structure, and obtain at least two samples to be sure that a representative one has been taken. Apply pressure to the biopsy site for 5 minutes to promote hemostasis.
8. Close the body wall with synthetic absorbable or nonabsorbable suture in a simple continuous pattern, the subcutaneous tissues with absorbable suture in an interrupted or continuous pattern, and the skin with nonabsorbable suture in an interrupted or continuous pattern.

Postoperative Care and Complications

■ Establish diuresis by IV administration of a balanced electrolyte solution at a rate of 90 ml/kg/24 hr for 8 to 12 hours. This helps prevent the formation of blood clots within the renal pelvis.
■ Hematuria is occasionally observed after renal biopsy and is usually self-limiting.
■ Hemorrhage after renal biopsy can become life-threatening. If this occurs, surgically expose the kidneys via celiotomy, and place sutures in a mattress pattern through the capsule and superficial parenchyma to control hemorrhage. On rare occasions, uncontrollable hemorrhage necessitates nephrectomy.

NEPHROTOMY

Preoperative Considerations

■ Nephrotomy is most often performed for removal of renal calculi. Investigate the presence and location of other calculi within the urinary tract with excretory urography or ultrasonography prior to surgery.
■ Remove large solitary calculi that result in extensive dilation of the renal pelvis by pyelolithotomy (described elsewhere).
■ If possible, investigate coagulation function prior to surgery. Abnormal coagulation may result in prolonged hemorrhage after surgery. Correct fluid deficits and serum electrolyte abnormalities, if possible, prior to surgery.
■ If bilateral renal calculi are present, perform nephrotomy as a staged procedure. Perform the second surgery approximately 1 month after the first. Because of a transient decrease in renal function after nephrotomy, absent or decreased function of the contralateral kidney may preclude the performance of nephrotomy. In these instances, pyelolithotomy is greatly preferred.

Surgical Procedure

Objectives

■ Remove renal calculi.
■ Obtain renal biopsy or microbial culture sample.
■ Confirm patency of ureter.

Equipment

■ Standard surgical instruments and suture
■ Balfour self-retaining retractor
■ Catheters of appropriate diameter to pass into the ureter (3.5 Fr. or 5.0 Fr.)
■ Vascular forceps or Rommel tourniquet

Technique

1–4. Please see Renal Biopsy, Technique, 1–4.
5. The kidneys are examined and palpated. Free the affected kidney of its peritoneal attachments, and identify and isolate the renal vasculature.
6. Apply a Rommel tourniquet or vascular forceps to the renal artery and vein. The time the vasculature is occluded is noted, and ischemia of the kidney is limited to 30 minutes or less.
7. Make an incision through the renal capsule on the greater curvature of the kidney (Fig. 1A). The incision is of adequate length to allow exposure of the renal pelvis after the renal parenchyma has been divided or incised. Sharply incise the renal parenchyma with a scalpel.
8. Remove calculi from the pelvis and diverticula of the kidney. Submit the calculi for analysis.

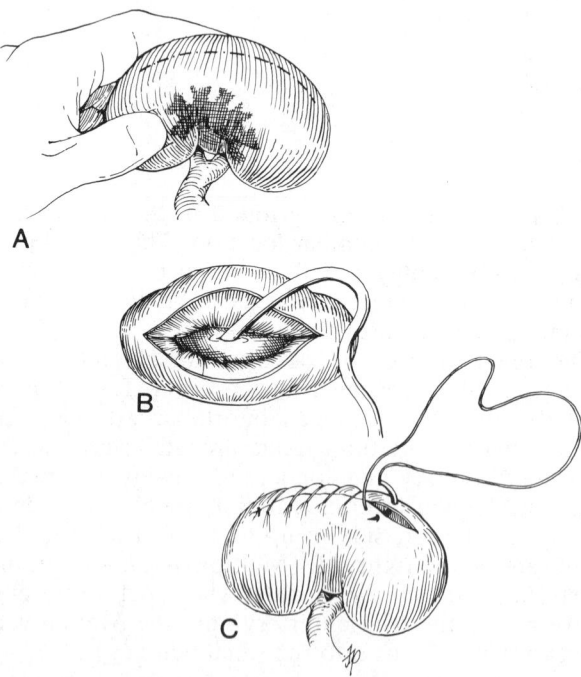

Figure 1. Nephrotomy. A, Make an incision through the renal capsule. Limit the length of the nephrotomy incision to the dimensions of the renal pelvis. B, Remove calculi from the renal pelvis, and pass a catheter through the ureter. C, Close the nephrotomy incision by placing sutures through the renal capsule and superficial parenchyma. (From Stone EA: Canine nephrotomy. Compend Contin Ed Pract Vet 9:883, 1987.)

Obtain samples for microbial culture. Pass a catheter into the ureter to assess patency (Fig. 1*B*).

9. If a biopsy is to be done, remove a wedge or slice of tissue 2 to 4 mm in thickness with a scalpel from the surface of the nephrotomy incision through the renal parenchyma. Take care to avoid damaging the pelvis or diverticula.
10. Appose the exposed surfaces of the renal parenchyma and hold them in this position with digital pressure, as the tourniquet or vascular forceps is removed. Maintain pressure for 5 minutes to allow clotting to occur.
11. Close the nephrotomy incision by placing a single layer of absorbable suture in a simple continuous pattern through the renal capsule and superficial parenchyma (Fig. 1*C*).
12. If calculi are present in the bladder, perform a cystotomy to remove them.
13. Return the kidney to its normal position within the abdominal cavity, and close the body wall, subcutaneous tissues, and skin in a routine manner.

Postoperative Care and Complications

- Initiate and maintain diuresis by IV administration of a balanced electrolyte solution at a rate of 90 ml/kg/24 hr. Continue this for at least 12 to 24 hours. Monitor the urine output to be sure that the kidneys are functioning satisfactorily.
- Hematuria is usually observed macroscopically for 1 to 3 days and microscopically for up to 1 week.
- Institute appropriate therapy to resolve infection and prevent reformation of the calculi.

NEPHRECTOMY

Preoperative Considerations

KEY POINT ▶ Function of the remaining kidney must be sufficient to support life.

- Preoperative evaluation of the function of a single kidney is often difficult. Common laboratory tests (determination of blood urea nitrogen, serum creatinine, serum potassium concentrations) are only relative indicators of renal function. Distinguish among prerenal, renal, and postrenal causes of azotemia. Concentration and excretion of a radiopaque dye on excretory urography demonstrates that the vascular supply to the kidneys is intact and that the kidneys are capable of extracting the dye from the blood stream and excreting it. This finding is only a relative indicator of renal function. Renal function can be determined only by the measurement of clearance of an indicator (e.g., creatinine, inulin, radioisotopes). Nuclear medicine allows determination of unilateral renal function, but determination of single kidney clearance of other indicators requires ureteral catheterization and collection of the urine from that kidney. In general practice, excretory urography and standard clinical pathologic testing

are routinely done and usually provide adequate information.
- If possible, correct metabolic and hydration imbalances prior to performing surgery.

Surgical Procedure

Indications are listed in the introduction to this chapter.

Objectives

- Remove the diseased kidney and associated ureter.
- Control hemorrhage.

Equipment

- Standard surgical instruments and suture
- Balfour retractor
- Vascular forceps (optional)

Technique

1–4. Please see Renal Biopsy, Technique, 1–4.
5. Examine and palpate the kidneys. Obtain biopsy samples of the kidney to be preserved to be sure that it is free of disease.
6. Release the diseased kidney of its attachments. Apply a vascular forceps or tourniquet to the renal vessels or ligate these vessels prior to dissection to minimize hemorrhage.
7. Ligate the renal vasculature with nonabsorbable suture or surgical staples or clips. Doubly ligate the renal vessels.
8. Remove the entire ureter as well. Leaving a segment of ureter may promote subsequent urinary tract infection by urine being retained within the ureteral remnant.
9. Examine the renal bed for hemorrhage prior to closure of the abdominal wall.
10. Close the abdominal wall, subcutaneous tissues, and skin in a routine manner.

Postoperative Care and Complications

- If the function of the remaining kidney is in doubt, initiate and maintain diuresis by IV administration of a balanced electrolyte solution at a rate of 90 ml/kg/24 hr until renal function and urine output appear satisfactory.
- Observe the patient for 24 hours for hemorrhage due to displacement of ligatures, vascular staples, or clips.
- Warn the owner that continued renal disease in the patient may result in irreversible injury to the remaining kidney.

URETEROTOMY AND URETERAL ANASTOMOSIS

Preoperative Considerations

- Ureterotomy is most often performed for removal of calculi that have lodged within the ureter and cannot be dislodged by flushing and/or catheterization. Prolonged obstruction of the ureter by calculi will result in necrosis of the ureteral wall and leakage of urine. Lesions of the distal ureter are best treated by ureteroneocystostomy.

■ Ureteral obstruction or disruption most often is diagnosed by excretory urography.
■ When ureteral calculi is the diagnosis, carefully examine the kidneys and bladder for the presence of additional calculi.
■ Warn the owner of the potential for stricture formation in the patient after ureteral surgery.

Surgical Procedure

Objectives

■ Relieve ureteral obstruction.
■ Insure patency and integrity of ureter.

Equipment

■ Standard surgical instruments and suture
■ Balfour retractor
■ Magnification loupes are highly desirable, and an operating microscope is optional.
■ Small (6–0 to 8–0) monofilament absorbable suture (polydioxanone [PDS; Ethicon] or polyglyconate [Maxon; Davis and Geck])
■ Catheters of appropriate size (3.5 or 5.0 Fr.)

Technique

1–4. Please see Renal Biopsy, Technique, 1–4. The incision is extended caudally to a few centimeters cranial to the pubis.
5. Examine and palpate the kidneys, ureters, and bladder.
6. To perform ureterotomy, identify the site of the ureterotomy and make a longitudinal incision over the area of obstruction. Remove the calculi, and pass a catheter through the ureterotomy site to the kidney and to the bladder to insure patency of the ureter. In extremely small patients, use a large suture (# 1 or 0) instead of a catheter. Close the ureterotomy incision transversely with small (6–0 to 8–0) absorbable suture in an interrupted or continuous pattern. The transverse configuration of the closure increases the ureteral diameter at the site of the ureterotomy. This maneuver is achieved by initially opposing the midpoint of the proximal and distal ends of the ureterotomy incision with a single suture.
7. Resect the devitalized portion of the ureter and identify the lumen of the proximal and distal remnants of the ureter. Make a linear incision 3 to 5 mm in length in the ends of the ureter to increase the circumference of the anastomosis. Perform the anastomosis with small, absorbable suture placed in an interrupted or a continuous pattern.
8. A catheter can be passed through the urethra, bladder, and ureter to divert the flow of urine past the ureterotomy or anastomotic site. The placement of a catheter (stent) following surgery is controversial, and some believe this practice

may predispose the patient to stricture formation in the ureter.
9. Close the abdominal wall, subcutaneous tissue, and skin in a routine manner.

Postoperative Care and Complications

■ Stricture formation is common, particularly in cats and small dogs. Re-evaluate the patient 3 to 4 weeks after surgery by excretory urography. If ureteral obstruction is observed, consider resecting the affected area of the ureter and performing an anastomosis or implanting the proximal portion of the ureter into the bladder (ureteroneocystostomy).

URETERONEOCYSTOSTOMY (URETERAL REIMPLANTATION)

Preoperative Considerations

■ This procedure is performed most often for treatment of ectopic ureter. Inform the owner that incontinence associated with the presence of an ectopic ureter may or may not resolve after performance of ureteroneocystostomy. Incontinence that persists after performance of this procedure may be the result of developmental abnormalities of the urethral sphincter.
■ Ureteroneocystostomy is preferable to resection and anastomosis of the distal ureter because a lower complication rate is observed after ureteroneocystostomy.

Surgical Procedure

Objectives

■ Restore flow of urine from ureter into the bladder.
■ Treat incontinence associated with ectopic ureter.

Equipment

■ Standard surgical instruments and suture
■ Balfour retractor
■ Magnification is extremely helpful with small patients but optional with large patients.
■ Fine-gauge (5–0 to 7–0) absorbable suture.

Technique

1–4. Please see Renal Biopsy, Technique, 1–4. The incision is continued caudally to the pubis.
5. Examine and palpate the kidneys, ureters, and bladder.
6. Identify the distal ureter and isolate it by dissection. Take care to preserve the longitudinal blood supply of the ureter. If the ureter is in an ectopic location, ligate the distal continuation (Fig. 2A). Preserve a sufficient length of ureter to allow implantation into the bladder under minimal tension.
7. Perform a ventral cystotomy and create a circular defect 5–10 mm in diameter in the cranial aspect of the mucosa of the dorsal wall of the bladder (Fig. 2B). Pass a forceps from the lumen

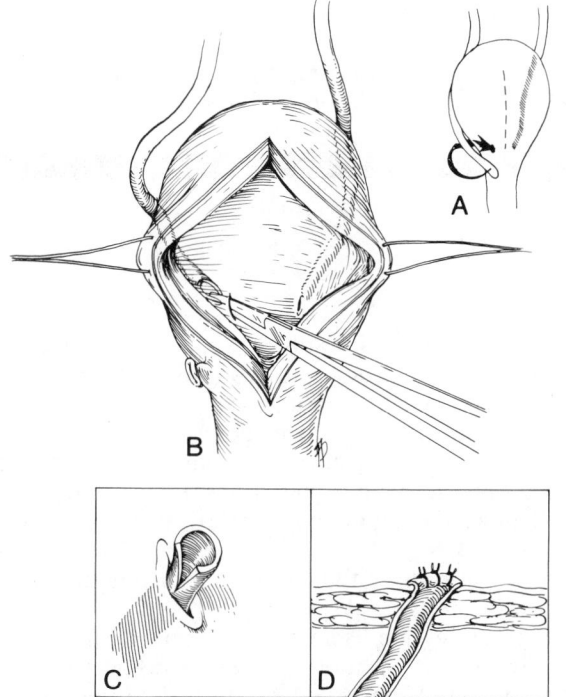

Figure 2. Ureteroneocystostomy. *A,* Isolate, ligate, and divide the distal ureter and perform a ventral cystotomy. *B,* Create a circular defect in the bladder mucosa, and pass forceps through the bladder wall. *C,* Debride and spatulate the end of the ureter. *D,* Suture the ureter to the bladder mucosa. (From Rawlings CA: Repaired ectopic ureter. *In* Bojrab MJ, ed.: *Current Techniques in Small Animal Surgery,* 3rd ed. Philadelphia: Lea & Febiger, 1990, p 374.)

of the bladder at an oblique angle in a caudal-to-cranial direction. Grasp the distal end of the proximal remnant of the ureter, or preferably a suture attached to this end of the ureter with the forceps, and draw the ureter through the bladder wall (Fig. 2*B*). As the ureter is drawn through the bladder wall, take care to avoid

twisting the ureter, because this may obstruct the ureter or its blood supply.

8. Make a longitudinal incision 5–10 mm in length in the ventral aspect of the end of the ureter (Fig. 2*C*). Secure the ureter to the edge of the defect created in the bladder mucosa with small (5–0 to 7–0) synthetic absorbable suture in an interrupted pattern (Fig. 2*D*). A ureteral catheter is not maintained after surgery.

9. Close the cystotomy incision in a standard manner (see sec. 8, ch. 4).

10. Close the abdominal wall, subcutaneous tissue, and skin in a routine manner.

Postoperative Care and Complications

■ Obstruction of the ureteroneocystostomy or leakage of urine from the site of ureteral reimplantation is extremely uncommon.

■ Treat urinary incontinence that persists after surgery by administration of alpha-agonists in an attempt to increase urethral sphincter tone. Warn the owner that incontinence due to ectopic ureter may or may not improve in the patient after surgery and medical therapy.

■ Perform excretory urography 4 weeks after surgery to assess the shape and function of the ureter.

Supplemental Readings

Christie BA: Kidneys. *In* Slatter DH, ed.: *Textbook of Small Animal Surgery.* Philadelphia: W. B. Saunders, 1985, p 1764.

Christie BA: Ureters. *In* Slatter DH, ed.: *Textbook of Small Animal Surgery.* Philadelphia: W. B. Saunders, 1985, p 1777.

Gahring DR, Crowe DT, Powers TE, et al.: Comparative renal function studies of nephrotomy closure with and without sutures in dogs. J Am Vet Med Assoc 171:537, 1977.

Mason LK, Stone EA, Biery DN, et al.: Surgery of ectopic ureters: Pre- and postoperative radiographic morphology. J Am Anim Hosp Assoc 26:73, 1990.

Stone EA, Mason AK: Surgery of ectopic ureters: Types, method of correction, and postoperative results. J Am Anim Hosp Assoc 26:81, 1990.

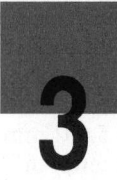

3 Diseases of the Urinary Bladder

Laine A. Cowan

INFECTION

Bacterial urinary tract infection is relatively common in the dog and much less common in the cat. Fungal, viral, and nematode infections occur, but they are rare. Infection can occur anywhere in the urinary tract, and the location within the urinary tract may effect prognosis, treatment, and diagnostic plan. Pyelonephritis refers to inflammation of the kidney due to infection (see sec. 8, ch. 1). Cystitis is inflammation of the urinary bladder of any cause. Bacterial cystitis is a urinary tract infection of the urinary bladder. A simple urinary tract infection (UTI) is the first episode of a bladder infection with no predisposing causes, such as calculi, prostatic disease, or anatomic abnormalities. A complex UTI includes chronic infections, recurring infections, infections that may involve the kidney or the prostate gland, and infections complicated by other problems (e.g., calculi, neoplasia, anatomic abnormalities, decreased host resistance). All UTIs in gonadally intact male dogs are considered complex because prostate gland involvement is assumed. For discussion of prostatic disease, see section 8, chapter 8.

Etiology

Usually, bacteria gain access to the urinary bladder by retrograde urethral migration. Although any bacterium has the potential to create a UTI, the mere presence of bacteria is insufficient to create an infection in a normal bladder. Rather, the organisms also must attach to the urothelium and overcome the urinary tract defense mechanisms in order to establish an infection.

Mechanisms in the host that resist infection include the following:

Urine flow
Inhibition of bacterial adhesion
Normal urethral flora
High urine osmolality
Other antibacterial factors.

Normal Mechanisms of Host Defense

- The normal complete emptying of the urinary bladder and expulsion of the urine washes bacterial pathogens out of the lower urinary tract. The high urethral pressure and the length of the male urethra may also help insure unidirectional urine flow.
- After bacteria gain access to the urinary tract, they must adhere to the mucosal surface. A uromucoid secretion coats the bladder mucosal surface, de-

creases the bacterial adherence to the bladder epithelium, and results in the expulsion of bacteria from the bladder during voiding.
- Commensal flora that are mostly gram positive inhabit the distal urethra. By binding to urothelial receptors, their adhesion to the surface of the urethra is thought to compete with pathogens for attachment to the receptors. The normal bacterial flora also may secrete substances that prevent attachment of other bacteria.
- The prostate gland secretes antibacterial factors into the urethra of the dog. Locally produced immunoglobulins (IgA) may contribute to limiting bacterial infection.

KEY POINT ▶ The high urine osmolality or the high urea content of cat urine inhibits bacterial growth and may play a role in limiting bacterial UTI in the cat.

Common Factors that Disrupt Host Defense Mechanisms

When any of the host defense mechanisms are compromised, UTI may result. Some predisposing factors include the following:

Inflammation
Catheterization
Glucocorticoids
Urine retention.

- Lower urinary tract inflammation of any cause (e.g., calculi, neoplasia) can disrupt the bladder mucosal defenses.
- Catheterization of the urinary bladder can cause mechanical irritation, or the catheter can serve as a scaffold for the bacteria to gain access to the urinary bladder.
- Increased systemic glucocorticoid levels (iatrogenic or hyperadrenocorticism) interfere with the host's resistance to infection and may cause polyuria. Both of these may compromise host defense.
- Any condition that results in an inability to completely empty bladder (e.g., functional or anatomic outflow obstruction, pain that prevents posturing to urinate, and various disorders of micturition described in sec. 8, ch. 7) may allow proliferation of any bacteria that reach the bladder.
- Polyuria may predispose an animal to a UTI by causing dilution of osmotic factors or prolonged urine retention and bladder distention.
- Diabetes mellitus predisposes an animal to UTI

because of glucosuria, polyuria, and decreased immunocompetency.

Clinical Signs

- UTI can result in urine that has an abnormal odor or appearance (hematuria, cloudy).
- UTI can result in dysuria. The animal has stranguria, pollakiuria, or less frequently urinary incontinence.
- Systemic signs are rare when the infection is limited to the urinary bladder.

KEY POINT ▶ An animal with UTI can be asymptomatic, especially if the UTI is secondary to increased glucocorticoid concentrations (e.g., hyperadrenocorticism, iatrogenically administered agents) or diabetes mellitus.

Diagnosis

History

- Consider UTI whenever any of the signs of cystitis (as previously listed) are observed.
- Consider UTI whenever there is a history of long-term corticosteroid administration, hyperadrenocorticism, or poorly controlled diabetes mellitus, even in the absence of any clinical signs.

Physical Examination

- Palpate the urinary bladder to detect distension; thickening; or any problems that may predispose the animal to a UTI, including cystic calculi and bladder masses.
- Palpate the kidneys for signs of pain, enlargement, asymmetry, and irregular surface contour (see sec. 8, ch. 1).
- Perform a digital rectal examination in dogs to detect urethral masses, calculi, or prostatic disease that may predispose to or complicate a bladder infection.
- Pass a urinary catheter if a urethral obstruction is suspected.
- If pain is observed during ambulation or physical examination, or if the animal cannot ambulate, neurologic and orthopedic examinations are indicated. These help determine whether the UTI is related to urinary retention associated with a reluctance or an inability to completely empty the urinary bladder.
- If a micturition disorder is suspected, watch the animal void and determine residual urine volume by bladder palpation or catheterization (see sec. 8, ch. 7).

Urine Analysis

- The UA is evaluated in animals with a history or signs suggestive of urinary tract inflammation. Collection of the urine by antepubic cystocentesis is preferred to eliminate the possibility of urethral or genital contamination.

KEY POINT ▶ The presence of bacteria in a urine specimen collected by antepubic cystocentesis is diagnostic of UTI. The presence of pyuria (>5 WBC/hpf*) is suggestive of UTI.

- Urease-producing bacteria (some species of *Staphylococcus, Proteus, Ureaplasma*) degrade urea, and the resulting hydroxyl ion production alkalinizes the urine. Because normal urine collected from dogs that have fasted is usually acidic, the presence of an alkaline urine from a dog that has fasted or from any cat may indicate the presence of a UTI with urease-producing bacteria. Weekly monitoring of first morning (fasting) urine pH by the owner may help detect the recurrence of UTI in a dog with a history of a chronic infection with urease-producing bacteria.

Urine Culture and Susceptibility

- These tests are indicated in all patients with pyuria, bacteriuria, and dysuria, and in patients with a history of glucocorticoid excess (hyperadrenocorticism or chronic exogenous administration).

Complete Blood Count, Serum Biochemical Profile

- In chronic or recurrent UTI, especially if the animal is systemically ill, use these tests to help identify underlying disease that may predispose the animal to UTI. Animals with infections confined to the urinary bladder rarely demonstrate abnormal laboratory test results.

Abdominal Radiography and Ultrasonography

- In chronic or recurrent UTI, use abdominal radiography and ultrasonography to rule out anatomic abnormalities and complicating factors (cystic calculi, bladder masses, urachal diverticula, prostatic disease, renal disease) from the differential diagnoses, which might cause UTI or prevent its resolution. Ultrasonographic evaluation or excretory urogram and double-contrast cystogram may be necessary to detect nonradiopaque calculi and renal, prostatic, or bladder structural abnormalities. These procedures are described in section 1, chapter 4. Urachal diverticula have been observed in dogs and cats with UTI, but in most cats the gross deformity of the bladder wall resolves with resolution of the UTI.

Prostatic Fluid Analysis

- Evaluation of prostatic fluid cytology and bacterial culture may be necessary to detect prostatic infections, which may complicate the management of bacterial cystitis.

Histologic Evaluation

- Although bladder biopsies are not routinely indicated to confirm a diagnosis of UTI, bladder masses (e.g., neoplasia) or anatomic abnormalities (e.g., diverticula) may predispose an animal to, or may be a result of, bladder infection (polypoid cystitis).

---

*White blood cells per high-power field.

■ If bladder masses are identified, or if anatomic abnormalities persist after resolution of the UTI, histologic evaluation of the tissue is indicated. Because cystoscopy equipment is not readily available, most bladder biopsy samples are obtained via laparotomy (see sec. 8, ch. 4).

KEY POINT ▶ Alterations in host defense mechanisms, predisposing factors, and other sites of infection must be investigated in animals with recurrent or chronic UTIs.

Treatment

Simple Urinary Tract Infection

■ Systemic oral antibiotics are administered for 2 to 3 weeks. Ideally, the antibiotic selected is based on the results of bacterial culture and susceptibility testing results. Alternatively, an antibiotic may be selected based on identification of the bacterium and likely susceptibility of that bacterium to antibiotics (Table 1).

■ Collect urine via cystocentesis for bacterial culture 5 to 7 days after discontinuing therapy to insure that the infection has been eliminated.

■ Repeat the first two steps if culture findings are positive.

Complicated Urinary Tract Infection

Refer to section 8, chapter 1, and section 8, chapter 8, for treatment of prostatic infections.

■ Eliminate any predisposing cause if possible.

■ Administer systemic antibiotics for a minimum of 10 to 14 days. The antibiotic selected is based on the results of bacterial culture and susceptibility testing.

■ Collect urine for bacterial culture 5 to 7 days and again 1 to 2 months after discontinuing therapy to insure that the infection has been eliminated.

■ If the same type of bacteria as originally cultured is present during either of the re-evaluations, administer antibiotics (choice based on recent susceptibility results) for an additional 6 to 8 weeks. To be certain that the chosen antimicrobial drug is effective, reculture the urine after 1 to 2 weeks of therapy.

■ If a urachal diverticulum persists after antimicrobial therapy, surgical resection of the defect may be indicated (see sec. 8, ch. 4).

■ If no bacteria are isolated while the animal is receiving antibiotics but the UTI recurs after their discontinuation, a once-daily dose of antibiotic at bedtime may be necessary for the long-term control of the infection. Before bedtime therapy is initiated, antimicrobial full-dose therapy is administered for 4 to 6 weeks. While the patient is on antimicrobial therapy, reculture the urine. If no bacterial growth is present, continue antimicrobial therapy by administering half of the daily dose at bedtime (after the dog has urinated). Monthly culturing of the urine is performed. If results are negative, continue therapy for 4 to 6 months. If bacteria are isolated, start the treatment and culture protocol again.

Prevention

■ Avoid or limit any predisposing factors, especially urethral catheterization, glucocorticoid administration, and incomplete bladder emptying. Prophylactic antibiotics are not effective in preventing UTI in an animal with an indwelling urinary catheter.

CYSTIC CALCULI

Macroscopic concretions in urine are calculi, which are named according to their location and mineral composition. Although calculi may occur anywhere in the urinary tract, they are found most commonly in the urinary bladder. Calculi in the urinary bladder are called cystic calculi or urocystoliths.

Cystic calculi occur much more frequently in dogs than in cats. Struvite (magnesium ammonium phosphate) calculi are the most common type of calculi in both species.

Etiology

Multiple factors are involved in the initiation and growth of calculi.

■ Calculi may form when urine becomes supersaturated with minerals. Supersaturation occurs because of the following:
  • Increased amount of mineral in the urine
  • Increased urine concentration of the minerals
  • Urine pH, which affects mineral solubility
  • Presence of stimulators and inhibitors of crystallization.

■ UTIs with urease-producing bacteria (*Staphylococcus, Proteus, Ureaplasma*) can cause struvite calculi by increasing the ammonium ions available and alkalinizing the urine. Conversely, urinary tract infections also can result from inflammation associated with the calculi.

■ Some types of calculi occur secondary to metabolic problems; for example, inherited alterations in urate metabolism in Dalmatian dogs and increased cystine excretion by the kidney in certain breeds.

■ Increased incidence of some types of calculi occur in specific breeds or in a specific gender (Table 2), but any breed can have any type of calculi.

KEY POINT ▶ Because the presence of urinary calculi may indicate the presence of a metabolic

TABLE 1. Predicted Antimicrobial Susceptibilities in Simple Urinary Tract Infections in Dogs

Bacteria	Antimicrobials*
Escherichia coli	Sulfonamide-trimethoprim, cephalexin
Staphylococcus	Ampicillin, penicillin
Streptococcus	Ampicillin, penicillin
Proteus	Ampicillin, cephalexin
Pseudomonas	Tetracycline
Klebsiella	Cephalexin

*See Appendix for dosages.

TABLE 2. Clinical Features of Canine Urocystoliths

Mineral Composition	Relative Incidence*	Relative Radiopacity†	Gender/Breed with Increased Incidence	Medical Dissolution
Magnesium ammonium phosphate	Common	Variable (usually radiopaque)	Miniature schnauzer	Low magnesium diet[a] Low protein diet High sodium intake pH <6.4
Uric acid and urates	Uncommon	Variable (usually nonradiopaque)	Dalmatian, English bulldog	Low purine diet[b] Allopurinol[c] pH = 7.0–7.5
Calcium oxalate	Uncommon	Very radiopaque	Male; miniature schnauzer, Lhasa apso, poodle, Shih Tzu, Yorkshire terrier	None available
Calcium phosphate	Uncommon	Very radiopaque	None	None available
Cystine	Uncommon	Variable (usually nonradiopaque)	Male; dachshund, English bulldog	Low sodium intake Low protein diet[b] +/− 2-MPG[d] pH = 7.5
Silica	Rare	Variable (usually radiopaque)	Male; German shepherd	None available

*Uncommon = 1 to 7%; rare = < 1% of uroliths analyzed.
†Depending on size and if additional minerals contribute to the urolith.
[a]Prescription Diet s/d; Hill's Pet Foods
[b]Prescription Diet u/d; Hill's Pet Foods
[c]Zyloprim (Burroughs Wellcome); 30 mg/kg/day divided into 2 or 3 doses.
[d]N-(2-mercaptopropionyl)-glycine (Sigma)

disease, determination of the pathogenesis of the calculi is important.

Clinical Signs

- Animals with calculi are commonly presented for signs of lower urinary tract inflammation, which include dysuria, stranguria, pollakiuria, and hematuria.
- If the calculi are the appropriate size, they may lodge in the urethra (most common in male dogs) and result in urethral obstruction. The dog may be presented with signs of straining to urinate and urinary incontinence, with or without accompanying systemic illness (see sec. 8, ch. 5).
- Because infection may accompany calculi, cloudy or urine with a foul odor may be present.
- In some animals, calculi may not cause any detectable clinical signs.

Diagnosis

KEY POINT ▶ Once calculi are diagnosed, the remainder of the urinary tract must be examined for the presence of additional calculi.

History

History of lower urinary tract inflammation, obstruction, or chronic urinary tract infections is common. Occasionally, dogs have histories of passing calculi in the urine.

Physical Examination

- A complete physical examination is essential to help identify problems that may predispose the animal to calculi formation or that may limit therapeutic options.
- Palpation of calculi may be easier when the bladder is not fully distended. Large calculi frequently are palpable as a firm masses in the bladder. If multiple calculi are present, a grating or sandy consistency may be palpable. Palpation of the bladder may elicit a pain response.
- A digital rectal examination of the urethra in all dogs and percutaneous palpation of the extrapelvic membranous urethra in male dogs may reveal additional calculi.

Urinalysis

- The pH, presence of bacteria, and presence of crystals may be helpful in estimating the composition of a calculus.

Urine Culture and Susceptibility

- Urine from animals with urinary calculi must be submitted for bacterial culture because urease-producing bacteria may cause struvite calculi, and UTIs may occur secondary to calculi-induced inflammation or obstruction.

Complete Blood Count, Serum Biochemical Profile

- These tests are evaluated to detect any predisposing factors that may contribute to the formation of calculi or may complicate therapy.
- When calculi cause urethral obstruction, the result may be progressive azotemia, dehydration, acidosis, and hyperkalemia.

Hepatic Function Tests

- Pre- and post-prandial serum bile acid or blood ammonia concentration tests are indicated in animals (except Dalmatian dogs) with ammonium urate calculi, because these calculi are frequently associated with portosystemic shunts (see sec. 7, ch. 8).

Abdominal Radiography and Ultrasonography

- Evaluate the entire urinary tract for calculi.
- The degree of radiopacity of calculi depends upon size, mineral composition, and number of the calculi (see Table 2 for radiographic appearance of calculi).
- An ultrasonographic evaluation or an excretory urogram and a double-contrast cystogram may be necessary to detect radiolucent calculi. These procedures are described in section 1, chapter 4.
- Vesicourachal diverticula may be present and are visualized with a positive or double-contrast cystogram in some cats with calculi.

Quantitative Stone Analysis and Bacterial Culture

- Calculi may be obtained after surgical removal (see sec. 8, ch. 4) or after having been passed in the urine. Once urolithiasis is diagnosed, retrieval of calculi by using a fine mesh fishnet or 4 × 4 gauze surgical sponge to strain the urine during voiding may increase the chances of obtaining a calculus for analysis.
- Send representative calculi to specialized laboratories for stone analysis, including quantitative mineral analysis. If collected sterilely, the layers of calculi can be cultured for bacterial growth.

KEY POINT ▶ Determination of the mineral composition of the calculi is needed for therapy and prevention.

Estimation of Urolith Composition

If a calculus is not obtained for analysis, the most likely mineral composition may be estimated based on signalment; results of serum biochemical profile; urine pH and crystalluria; radiographic appearance; urine culture results; and response to treatment.

Signalment

Some breeds of dogs have an increased incidence of specific types of calculi (see Table 2). In dogs less than 1 year old, infection-associated struvite calculi are the most common. In adult animals, age may not be helpful in estimating calculi composition.

Serum Biochemical Profile

If hypercalcemia or acidosis (associated with renal tubular disease) is present, consider calcium oxalate or calcium phosphate calculi.

Urine pH and Crystalluria

The crystals in a freshly collected urine specimen may reflect the type of mineral that is deposited on the surface of the calculus. Calculi may be heterogeneous, however, and the crystalluria may not represent the mineral composition of the interior of the calculi. Precipitation of minerals are pH dependent and in sterile urine, the pH may be helpful.

KEY POINT ▶ Struvite calculi usually form in alkaline urine; ammonium urate and silica calculi, in neutral-to-acid urine; cystine calculi, in acid urine; and calcium oxalate calculi, in urine of any pH.

Radiographic Appearance

The shape and relative radiopacity of calculi are variable and dependent upon size and other minerals in the calculi (see Table 2).

Urine Culture Results

Struvite calculi are often associated with UTIs.

If no dissolution occurs while on a strict calculolytic treatment regimen, the estimated composition of the urolith may not have been accurate.

Treatment

Medical dissolution and surgical removal are the potential therapeutic choices available to canine and feline patients with calculi. However, the therapeutic regimen varies with the mineral composition and not all types of calculi can be dissolved medically. Because the mineral composition governs the solubility of calculi, identification of the mineral composition is essential for determining the appropriate therapeutic regimen. Except for struvite calculi, calculolytic regimens are still being evaluated and their efficacy is controversial in animals.

- Medical management is most appropriate when the calculi are amenable to medical dissolution and no contraindications to medical management are present.
- Medical management might be contraindicated in a patient that cannot tolerate an increased sodium intake (e.g., those with heart failure, renal failure, hypertension, ascites); in a patient in which the risk of protracted calculi may be harmful (e.g., those with systemic infection, outflow (urethral) obstruction, renal insufficiency); or in a patient that does not respond to medical calculolytic management.
- Surgical removal of calculi is indicated when medical dissolution is contraindicated or not possible. Surgical removal of calculi may be indicated when quick resolution of the dysuria is preferred or when another abdominal surgical procedure is necessary.
- In general, medical dissolution protocols include inducing dilute urine; adjusting urine pH; decreasing renal excretion of the type of minerals constituting the calculi; controlling or eliminating UTIs; and, occasionally, increasing inhibitors of calculi formation.
- Medical therapy continues for 1 month after the calculi are no longer detected radiographically. Some of the regimens for calculi dissolution may be detrimental if continued indiscriminately for a protracted course.

In any of the following calculi, when a UTI is present, systemic antimicrobial therapy is continued until infection is eliminated and the calculi have dissolved or are removed.

Struvite Calculi

■ For dissolution, an acidifying diet, with limited magnesium and protein, that causes a diluted urine is recommended (e.g., Prescription Diet s/d; Hill's Pet Foods).

Ammonium Urate Calculi

■ If hepatic failure, portosystemic shunt, and renal failure have been ruled out from the diagnoses, allopurinol (Zyloprim; Burroughs Wellcome 30 mg/kg per day in two or three divided doses) and a nonacidifying (urine pH 7.0), purine-restricted diet (Prescription Diet u/d; Hill's Pet Foods) are recommended for calculi dissolution.

■ If a portosystemic shunt is present, therapy is directed to the correction of the shunt (see sec. 7, ch. 9).

Calcium Oxalate and Calcium Phosphate Calculi

■ No medical dissolution protocols are currently available.

■ If hypercalcemia is present, it is essential to identify and treat the underlying cause (see sec. 4, ch. 2).

Cystine Calculi

■ For dissolution, use a protein- and sodium-restricted, alkalinizing diet, such as Prescription Diet u/d; (optimal urine pH 7.5), and either *N*-(2-mercaptopropionyl)glycine (MPG) (30–40 mg/kg per day in two divided doses) or D-penicillamine (Cuprimine; Merck Sharp & Dohme) (30 mg/kg per day in two divided doses).

Silica Calculi

■ No medical dissolution protocols are currently available.

Prevention

Although calculi can be eliminated with medical dissolution or surgical removal, 5 to 47% of dogs have recurrence. Recurrence of cystic calculi can be reduced by eliminating the predisposing factors. Many of the same strategies employed for dissolution are utilized for prevention of recurrent urolithiasis. For prevention, the restrictions are not as severe and promoting the formation of dilute urine is always included. Strategies for prevention of recurrence are similar to but not the same as those for urolith therapy.

Struvite Calculi

■ In infection-associated struvite calculi, eliminating or controlling the infection is essential for prevention of recurrence. Instruct the owner to periodically monitor first morning urine pH to help indicate when the dog needs to be evaluated for urinary infection (see this chapter for management of urinary infection).

■ In sterile struvite calculi, maintaining a dilute, low-magnesium, acidic urine by feeding Prescription Diet c/d (Hill's Pet Foods) reduces recurrence of calculi.

Urate Calculi

■ Use a low-protein, alkalinizing diet (Prescription Diet u/d) with sodium bicarbonate added as needed to maintain an alkaline pH and to help prevent recurrence. If urate calculi recur while the animal is on this diet, administer allopurinol as a long-term preventative, at 10–20 mg/kg per day.

Calcium Oxalate and Calcium Phosphate Calculi

■ Avoid sodium and ascorbic acid supplementation.

■ Potassium citrate and/or thiazide diuretics in normocalcemic dogs may inhibit recurrence by decreasing urine calcium excretion.

Cystine Calculi

■ Promote alkalinization and dilution of the urine. For alkalinization, potassium citrate (Urocit-K) may be better than sodium-containing agents (sodium bicarbonate).

■ Restrict sodium to decrease the urinary excretion of cystine.

■ MPG (divided into two 30–40 mg/kg/day doses) may also decrease recurrence.

Silica Calculi

■ Because plant material contains more silica than meat does, feed a meat-based dog food.

■ Promote the formation of dilute urine by adding sodium chloride to the diet.

BLADDER NEOPLASIA

In the urinary tract of the dog, the bladder is the most common location for neoplasia. In the cat, bladder neoplasia is rare. Bladder neoplasms are usually malignant. They are more common in the female than in the male dog. Bladder neoplasms occur in older animals (mean age is 10 years). Bladder rhabdomyosarcoma is an exception, as it tends to occur in young dogs.

KEY POINT ▶ Transitional cell carcinoma is the most frequently diagnosed bladder neoplasm, occurring most often in older female dogs.

Malignant neoplasms include transitional cell carcinoma, rhabdomyosarcoma, fibrosarcoma, adenocarcinoma, and hemangiosarcoma; benign neoplasms include fibroma, papilloma, and leiomyoma. Bladder neoplasms tend to be diffuse infiltrating lesions rather than discrete masses. Although any portion of the bladder wall may be involved, transitional cell carcinomas usually affect the bladder trigone region.

Etiology

No etiologic agent has been identified in most dogs with bladder neoplasia. The prolonged contact of the bladder mucosa with carcinogens excreted by the kidneys may contribute to bladder carcinogenesis. Tryptophan metabolites are carcinogenic. Their low concentration in the urine of cats may partially explain the low incidence of bladder neoplasms in cats. Cyclophosphamide metabolites also have been implicated in bladder oncogenesis.

Clinical Signs

Dogs with bladder tumors usually have signs associated with lower urinary tract inflammation including stranguria, pollakiuria, and hematuria. Urinary tract neoplasia may also cause recurrent UTI, urinary incontinence, or anuria.

Diagnosis

KEY POINT ▶ Bladder neoplasia is indistinguishable from UTI and calculi on the basis of clinical signs alone.

History

The clinical signs are not specific for neoplasia. Most of the animals are therefore presented with a history of abnormal urination or hematuria partially responsive to antimicrobial therapy.

Physical Examination

- Abdominal palpation
  - Occasionally, the bladder may be distended from a mass occluding the bladder neck. If not distended, in rare instances, a mass may be palpable in the bladder.
- Rectal palpation
  - A thickened urethra or a mass may be palpable if the neoplastic or inflammatory tissue extends into the urethra or prostate gland. Palpable sublumbar lymphadenopathy can indicate metastasis.

Urinalysis

- The bladder may be inflamed or secondarily infected. Pyuria, hematuria, or bacteriuria may therefore be observed in dogs with bladder neoplasia.

Complete Blood Count, Serum Biochemical Profile

- If the animal is systemically ill or treatment of the neoplasm is anticipated, these tests are helpful for evaluating postrenal azotemia and for detecting associated problems.

Radiographic and Ultrasonographic Evaluation

- Contrast cystography or ultrasonography is usually necessary to identify the masses within the urinary bladder. Double-contrast cystography can help to rule out other causes of lower urinary tract inflammation (calculi, inflammatory polyps, blood clots).
- Radiographic examination of the sublumbar lymph nodes, pelvis, lumbar vertebrae, and lung is essential to detect metastatic disease.

KEY POINT ▶ Once a bladder mass is identified, an excretory urogram is indicated to detect any ureteral or trigonal invasion. A mass involving these areas decreases the likelihood of successful surgical excision.

Cytologic and Histologic Evaluation

- Cytologic or histologic evaluation is required for a definitive diagnosis. The signs and radiographic appearance are not pathognomonic for neoplasia.
- Urine submitted for cytologic evaluation may reveal neoplastic cells, although it can be difficult to differentiate reactive inflammation from neoplastic changes.
- To increase the likelihood of obtaining exfoliated cells, catheter cytology may yield additional information. A urethral catheter is aseptically placed in the urinary bladder, the urine is emptied, and the bladder is massaged (per abdomen). The catheter contents are aspirated and submitted for cytologic evaluation.
- If a mass is present, percutaneous (palpation or ultrasound-guided) fine needle aspirate specimens can be evaluated cytologically. A risk exists for seeding the peritoneum with neoplastic cells by this procedure.
- Bladder biopsy tissue can be obtained via cystoscopy or laparotomy.

Treatment

- If the neoplasm is confined to the bladder wall, sparing the trigone and bladder neck, the treatment of choice is surgical excision of the tumor and biopsy of the regional lymph nodes (see sec. 8, ch. 4).
- Chemotherapy, radiation, and surgical excision with reimplantation of the ureters in an intestinal segment have been attempted in dogs with trigonal involvement. These therapies are rarely indicated because they have not extended the symptom-free survival time and can cause severe complications.
- Current research using laser phototherapy has shown promising results. However, only a few dogs have been evaluated and this type of treatment is still experimental.

Prevention

- In animals receiving cyclophosphamide, limiting the duration of therapy and limiting the duration of contact of the metabolites with the bladder wall (inducing dilute urine and encouraging frequent voiding) may help prevent cyclophosphamide-induced cystitis and resulting neoplastic transformation (see subsequent discussion).

TRAUMA

Urinary bladder trauma most often is the result of motor vehicle accidents. When caudal abdominal or pelvic injuries are detected, concomitant trauma to the urinary bladder must be considered.

Etiology

When the bladder is distended, a sudden increase in abdominal pressure accompanying blunt trauma may cause urinary bladder contusions or rupture. Herniation of the bladder into an abdominal or, more rarely, a perineal hernia can also occur. Iatrogenic trauma from urethral catheterization, surgery, or rarely excessive abdominal palpation can also damage the urinary bladder.

Clinical Signs

- Clinical signs accompanying bladder trauma are nonspecific and may include hematuria, dysuria, and anuria.
- If the bladder is ruptured, abdominal distension, peritonitis, and uremia develop, depending upon the size and location of the tear and how quickly the problem is recognized and treated.

Diagnosis

History

- If the patient is evaluated within the first 12 hours after the trauma, signs referable to the lower urinary tract often are absent. Most commonly, the animal is presented following a motor vehicle accident because of lameness, abrasions, or shock. Owners are questioned if they have observed urination.

KEY POINT ▶ Normal micturition does not rule out a diagnosis of urinary bladder trauma.

Physical Examination

General Evaluation
- Evaluation and stabilization of the respiratory, circulatory, and neurologic status in a trauma patient must precede evaluation of the lower urinary tract.
- A patient with pelvic limb lameness, abrasions caudal to the thorax, or distended abdomen or perineal region may have had bladder trauma.
- Extensive bruising of the inguinal and caudal abdominal skin may indicate urine leakage into subcutaneous tissues.

Abdominal Palpation
- The abdomen is often painful on palpation if the bladder has ruptured.
- Uroperitoneum must be considered when abdominal distension develops following abdominal trauma.
- Absence of a palpable bladder, along with other typical findings, suggests, but does not definitely indicate, a ruptured bladder.

Rectal Palpation
- Palpation along the urethra may reveal hematomas or pelvic fragments that may lacerate the urethra or bladder or may impede complete bladder emptying.
- A perineal hernia containing the urinary bladder is usually apparent by palpation.

Observe Micturition
- If the animal has a history of dysuria or anuria following trauma, micturition must be observed. If

dysuria is confirmed, the urethra and urinary bladder are catheterized to rule out the possibility of an obstruction, bladder avulsion, or tears. A partial urethral tear may be worsened by catheter-induced trauma. Gentle handling and use of a soft flexible catheter are therefore mandatory.

Urinalysis

- Hematuria is the most common abnormality expected on urinalysis following bladder trauma.
- In an animal with azotemia following trauma, the urine specific gravity (collected before fluids are administered) is most helpful in ruling out a diagnosis of renal azotemia (see sec. 8, ch. 1).

Complete Blood Count, Serum Biochemical Profile

- If the animal is depressed 12 hours after trauma, these tests may help evaluate postrenal uremia. Increased serum urea nitrogen levels and hyperkalemia occur initially, followed by increased serum creatinine concentrations.

Radiographic Evaluation

- Abdominal survey radiograph findings may be normal or may demonstrate peritoneal or retroperitoneal effusion. A full urinary bladder may be present in an animal with a bladder or urethral laceration.
- A positive contrast cystogram is the best method to detect a bladder tear (see sec. 1, ch. 4). If the bladder is not adequately distended, small bladder rents may not be seen.
  - Irregular filling defects are likely to be blood clots in the bladder lumen.
  - Perineal hernias containing the urinary bladder are easily identified if a positive contrast cystogram is performed.

Abdominocentesis

- If fluid is detected in the peritoneal space by physical examination or radiography, the fluid is collected for evaluation.

KEY POINT ▶ Increased creatinine concentration in the abdominal fluid compared with the serum indicates uroperitoneum.

Treatment

- If mild hematuria or pollakiuria is present, and no tears in the urinary tract are identified, no therapy is indicated.
- If marked, persistent, gross hematuria is present, renal architecture is intact, and no rents in the urinary tract are present, atraumatically catheterize the bladder with a soft flexible catheter, and lavage the bladder with very cold water to help slow the hemorrhaging.
- If a small tear in the urinary bladder is present, urine escapes into the peritoneal space only with maximal bladder distension, and no peritoneal fluid is detected, an aseptically placed, soft flexible indwelling

urinary catheter may be placed for 3 to 7 days to keep the bladder empty while the rent heals.

■ If uroperitoneum is present and the animal is otherwise stable, surgical repair and lavage of the abdominal cavity is indicated.

■ If a uroperitoneum is present and the animal is unstable, removal of the urine is beneficial prior to the definitive repair. A urethral bladder catheter, Penrose drain, or peritoneal dialysis catheter may be used to help drain the peritoneal space. If hyperkalemic, give the patient fluid therapy using isotonic saline to decrease serum potassium level. Administer broad-spectrum antibiotics to help prevent septic peritonitis. (For a discussion of peritonitis and its treatment, refer to sec. 7, ch. 13).

■ If a perineal hernia containing a retroflexed urinary bladder occurs, decompressing the bladder via a urethral catheter or cystocentesis may facilitate returning the bladder to a more normal location. Surgery can be performed when the animal is stable.

Prevention

■ Minimizing the length of catheter that extends into the urinary bladder, using soft flexible catheters, and minimizing the duration of indwelling catheters will help limit iatrogenic trauma.

CYCLOPHOSPHAMIDE-INDUCED CYSTITIS

Cyclophosphamide is an alkylating drug commonly used in antineoplastic and immunosuppressive chemotherapeutic protocols (see sec. 3, ch. 5). Most commonly, cyclophosphamide induces sterile hemorrhagic cystitis after prolonged (greater than 8 weeks) administration, but adverse effects have occurred after a single injection.

KEY POINT ▶ Depending upon the severity of the bladder changes, cyclophosphamide-induced cystitis may resolve with discontinuation of the drug, or it may progress to chronic hemorrhagic, fibrosing cystitis, or rarely neoplasia.

Etiology

■ Cyclophosphamide is metabolized in the liver, and the metabolites are excreted in the urine. Chronic contact of the metabolites (acrolein) with the bladder mucosa causes hemorrhage, edema, and necrosis of the urinary bladder. These may ultimately result in fibrosis, necrosis, and rarely neoplasia.

Clinical Signs

■ The signs are typical of bladder inflammation and include hematuria and dysuria.

■ The signs may resolve after early discontinuation of the cyclophosphamide.

Diagnosis

History

■ A tentative diagnosis is made in a patient administered cyclophosphamide with a history of recent onset of lower urinary tract signs.

Physical Examination

■ A small thickened bladder may be palpable when chronic signs are present.

Urine Analysis and Culture

■ A sterile hemorrhagic inflammatory reaction usually is present.

Radiographic and Ultrasonographic Evaluation

■ If the clinical signs do not resolve after discontinuation of the cyclophosphamide, a double-contrast cystogram or ultrasonogram of the urinary bladder may help rule out the possibility of confounding problems, such as cystic calculi, necrotic (calcified) bladder mucosa, and neoplasia.

Histologic Evaluation

■ If the clinical signs do not improve after discontinuing the cyclophosphamide, a bladder wall biopsy sample may help confirm the diagnosis and rule out the diagnosis of secondary neoplasia.

Treatment

■ As soon as sterile cystitis is diagnosed, cyclophosphamide is discontinued.

■ If the animal's signs persist after 2 weeks, intravesicular instillation of dimethyl sulfoxide (DMSO) (10 ml of 50% DMSO diluted with 10 ml of sterile water, at weekly intervals to effect) may help relieve some of the inflammation.

■ If severe bladder hemorrhage persists, alum or 1% formalin, using general anesthesia, can be instilled into the urinary bladder to coagulate the mucosal surface and stop the hemorrhage.

■ Surgery may be necessary to excise necrotic mucosa or to obtain a biopsy sample to rule out the diagnosis of neoplasia.

Prevention

■ Restrict the duration of cyclophosphamide therapy when possible.

■ Decrease the urine concentration of the metabolites by promoting diuresis (add sodium chloride to the food to increase water intake).

■ Limit the contact of metabolites with the bladder mucosa by encouraging frequent urination after administration of the drug.

IDIOPATHIC LOWER URINARY TRACT DISEASE (ILUD) IN THE CAT

This is a heterogeneous group of lower urinary tract diseases in cats, induced by multiple factors. ILUD, also known as feline urologic syndrome (FUS), refers to the urethritis and cystitis usually associated with hematuria and struvite crystalluria in female and male cats, which can result in urethral obstruction in male cats (see sec. 8, ch. 5). ILUD is the most common category of lower urinary tract inflammation in the cat, and it affects approximately 1% of all cats. ILUD may occur in any age adult cat and has a high incidence of recurrence in the same cat (35%), especially if the first episode occurs when the cat is less than 4 years old. Division of ILUD into those cats with (male) and those cats without (male and female) urethral obstruction is helpful in diagnosis, treatment, and prognosis. Refer to the appropriate discussions of other causes of lower urinary tract inflammation, e.g., bacterial infections, cystic calculi, neoplasia, and urethral diseases.

Etiology

- By definition, the etiology of ILUD is unknown; however, more than one cause is likely.
- Several studies have implicated a viral etiology, and a cell-associated herpes virus has been identified in some cats with signs of ILUD.
- One hypothesis states that some abnormality, such as a viral infection, stimulates the formation of a mucoid matrix and that hematuria and dysuria occur concomitantly with matrix production.
- Struvite crystalluria is common in all cats, and it is hypothesized that the crystalluria in combination with the matrix formation may form "plugs" that obstruct the male urethra. If a male cat does not have a significant degree of concomitant crystalluria, or if a female cat with or without crystalluria is affected, the matrix passes through the urethral lumen and signs of hematuria and dysuria occur without urethral obstruction.
- Factors that have been associated with an increased occurrence of ILUD include the animal's access to the inside and outside of the house, obesity, and ingestion of a diet high in magnesium.

Clinical Signs

- Hematuria and dysuria and increased frequency of urination are the most common signs observed in cats with ILUD.

KEY POINT ▶ Cats with ILUD may urinate in inappropriate places, often using cool, smooth surfaces such as the bathtub, sink, or tile.

Diagnosis

History

- Consider ILUD in all cats with signs of lower urinary tract inflammation.
- Male cats may have a history of licking the perineal region, likely in response to the urethral inflammation.
- Cats may be presented with a history of "constipation" because prolonged periods in the litter box associated with stranguria may be mistaken for problems with defecation.

Physical Examination

- Palpate the urinary bladder to evaluate bladder size.
- A small, firm, or thickened bladder is usually palpable in cats without urethral obstruction. In these cats, gentle abdominal palpation often elicits urination.

Urine Analysis and Culture

- Hematuria and magnesium ammonium phosphate crystalluria usually are present.
- If pyuria, bacteriuria, or alkaline urine is detected in the urinalysis, submission of a urine sample collected by cystocentesis for aerobic bacterial culture is indicated.

Complete Blood Count, Serum Biochemical Profile

- If chronic or recurrent ILUD occurs, these tests are performed to help identify an underlying disease that might predispose the animal to lower urinary tract inflammation. Cats with inflammation confined to the urinary bladder or urethra rarely have any abnormal findings on these laboratory tests.

Radiographic and Ultrasonographic Evaluation

- If chronic or recurrent signs of lower urinary tract inflammation occur, abdominal radiography and ultrasonography are used to rule out the diagnoses of anatomic abnormalities or complicating factors (such as bladder, urethral, or periurethral masses, cystic calculi, urachal diverticula).

Treatment

Promote dilute, acid urine and allow time for recovery in cats without urethral obstruction. Antibiotics or corticosteroids do not enhance resolution of the clinical signs.

- Promotion of dilute urine
  - Feed canned cat food mixed with water
  - Add sodium chloride to food (¼ teaspoon/day). Do not add to cat food with a high sodium content.
  - Subcutaneous fluids may be helpful initially, because some cats remain in the litter box and neglect food and water requirements.
  - Recommend that fresh water be made available at all times.
- Urinary acidification
  - Administer DL-methionine (1000 mg/cat/day) or ammonium chloride (800 mg/cat/day) to effect, based on urine pH 4–6 hours postprandially, if alkaline urine persists while the cat is on an acidifying diet (e.g., Prescription Diet c/d, Hill's Pet Foods; Urological Diet, Purina).
- Magnesium restriction
  - Magnesium is a component of struvite crystals. Feeding a low magnesium diet (e.g., most canned cat foods) may help reduce this fraction.
- Time
  - ILUD is often self-limiting, 70% of cats get better within 5 days without treatment.

Prevention

- Avoid stress (e.g., new animals in household), because it may result in decreased water consumption.
- Encourage increased water intake by providing fresh water and moist food, and if necessary by adding water, broth, or bouillon plus water to food.
- Consider altering the urine with an acidifying diet or acidifying supplements.
- Feed a low magnesium diet.

Supplemental Readings

Brown SA, Barsanti JA: Diseases of the bladder and urethra. *In* Ettinger SJ, ed.: *Textbook of Veterinary Internal Medicine.* Philadelphia: WB Saunders, 1989, p 2108.

Burnie AG, Weaver A: Urinary bladder neoplasia in the dog: a review of seventy cases. J Small Anim Pract 24:129, 1983.

Johnston GR, Feeney DA, Osborne CA: Urethrography and cystography in cats. Part II. Abnormal radiographic anatomy and complication. Comp Cont Educ 4:931, 1982.

Laing EJ, Miller CW, Cochrane SM: Treatment of cyclophosphamide-induced hemorrhagic cystitis in five dogs. J Am Vet Med Assoc 193:233, 1988.

Osborne CA, Johnston GR, Kruger JM, et al.: Etiopathogenesis and biological behavior of feline vesicourachal diverticula. Vet Clin North Am [Sm Anim Pract] 17:697, 1987.

Osborne CA, Kruger JM, Johnston GR, Polzin DJ: Feline lower urinary tract disorders. *In* Ettinger SJ, ed.: *Textbook of Veterinary Internal Medicine.* Philadelphia: WB Saunders, 1989, p 2057.

Osborne CA, Polzin DJ, Johnston GR, O'Brien TD: Canine urolithiasis. *In* Ettinger SJ, ed.: *Textbook of Veterinary Internal Medicine.* Philadelphia: WB Saunders, 1989, p 2083.

Pechman RD: Urinary trauma in dogs and cats: a review. J Am Anim Hosp Assoc 18:33, 1982.

Schwarz PD, Willer RL: Urinary bladder neoplasia in the dog and cat. Probl Vet Med 1:128, 1989.

Stanton ME, Legendre AM: Effects of cyclophosphamide in dogs and cats. J Am Vet Med Assoc 188:1319, 1986.

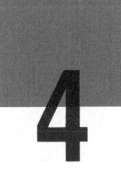

4 Surgery of the Urinary Bladder

Roger B. Fingland

Cystotomy is the most common surgical procedure on the urinary bladder in small animals. Subtotal or total cystectomy may be indicated for management of benign or malignant urinary bladder neoplasms. Incised bladder wall heals quickly and regains nearly 100% of original tissue strength after healing. The mucosal lining of the bladder is quite delicate and easily becomes edematous, necessitating meticulous tissue handling and proper suture placement. Intramural absorbable suture placement is ideal because material exposed to the bladder lumen may act as a nidus for calculi formation.

ANATOMY

- The urinary bladder is divided into three regions: (1) the cranial portion is the apex, (2) the caudal portion that joins the urethra is the neck, and (3) the segment between the apex and neck is the body.
- The ureteral openings and the urethral orifice form a triangular area on the dorsal aspect of the bladder called the trigone.
- The three ligaments of the bladder are composed of double layers of peritoneum. The ventral ligament extends from the ventral surface of the bladder along the ventral midline of the abdominal wall to the umbilicus. The ventral peritoneal ligament contains the urachus in the fetus. The urachus is an embryologic structure that connects the urinary bladder and the allantoic sac. The urachus closes and atrophies soon after birth, leaving a small scar at the apex of the urinary bladder. The lateral ligaments connect the lateral aspects of the bladder to the pelvic canal and enclose the ureters, deferent ducts, and umbilical arteries.
- The major blood supply to the bladder comes from the caudal vesical artery—a branch of the internal pudendal artery that lies in the pelvic fascia. The pelvic plexus of nerves is located dorsal to the bladder. The cranial vesical artery, present in only 50% of adult dogs, supplies the cranial aspect of the bladder. Venous blood drains into the internal pudendal veins. Bladder lymphatics drain into the hypogastric and lumbar lymph nodes.
- Sympathetic innervation to the bladder is via the hypogastric nerve, and parasympathetic innervation is via the pelvic nerves. The hypogastric and pelvic nerves reach the bladder through the lateral ligaments near the caudal vesical arteries.

ANOMALIES OF THE URACHUS

Preoperative Considerations

- Persistent urachus results when the entire urachal canal remains patent after birth. Urine is voided through the urachal opening at the umbilicus. Vesicourachal diverticulum results when the origin of the urachus at the bladder apex fails to close. The diverticulum forms a pocket of stationary urine, predisposing the animal to recurrent bacterial urinary tract infections (UTI).
- A persistent urachus is removed surgically.
- Vesicourachal diverticula often are diagnosed by contrast radiography in young animals with persistent UTI. Diverticula may be diagnosed fortuitously during abdominal surgery. Diverticulectomy is indicated in animals with persistent UTI. Diverticula discovered during abdominal surgery are removed to reduce the likelihood of recurrent UTI. Urachal scars commonly are observed at the dome of the bladder and seldom cause a problem. In contrast to urachal scars, diverticula are discrete pouch or sac openings from the bladder lumen.

Surgical Procedure—Persistent Urachus

Objectives

- Remove the patent urachus.
- Obtain specimens for bacterial culture and histopathologic analysis.

Equipment

- Standard general surgery instrument pack and suture
- Balfour retractor
- Laparotomy sponges

Technique

1. Place the animal in dorsal recumbency.
2. Prepare the ventral abdominal region for aseptic surgery.
3. Perform a routine ventral midline celiotomy from approximately 3 cm cranial to 3 cm caudal to the umbilicus.
4. Make an elliptic incision around the umbilical opening, and dissect the urachus free to the urinary bladder.
5. Place a Balfour retractor and isolate the urinary bladder with moistened laparotomy sponges.
6. Place stay sutures in the bladder to facilitate retraction.

7. Create a full-thickness elliptic incision in the bladder around the origin of the patent urachus.
8. Submit the patent urachus for histologic analysis.

KEY POINT ▶ Do not ligate the urachus at the bladder apex. This may result in a vesicourachal diverticulum and predispose the animal to persistent urinary tract infection.

8. Remove a 4-mm by 1-cm section of the bladder wall from the edge of the incision. Divide the section in half, and submit samples for bacterial culture and susceptibility testing and histologic analysis. Alternatively, portions of the excised vesicourachal junction may be submitted.
9. Remove the stay sutures and laparotomy sponges, and close the bladder as described in the Cystotomy discussion to follow.
10. Close the abdominal wall routinely.

Postoperative Care and Complications

- Postoperative complications are rare.
- Administer antibiotics based on the results of bacterial culture and sensitivity testing. Prolonged (>4 weeks) antibiotic therapy may be necessary to reduce the risk of recurrent UTI.
- See the Cystotomy, Postoperative Care and Complications discussion.

Surgical Procedure—Vesicourachal Diverticulum Excision

Objective

- Remove the vesicourachal diverticulum.
- Obtain samples for bacterial culture and sensitivity testing and histologic analysis.

Equipment

- Standard general surgery instrument pack and suture
- Balfour retractor
- Laparotomy sponges

Technique

1. Patient positioning and surgical approach are the same as those described for persistent urachus.
2. Do not make an elliptic incision around the umbilicus.
3. Isolate the urinary bladder with moistened laparotomy sponges.
4. Place stay sutures to facilitate retraction.
5. Make a full-thickness elliptic incision in the bladder wall around and approximately 5 mm from the edge of the diverticulum.
6. Divide the excised diverticulum in half.
7. Submit samples for histologic analysis and bacterial culture and susceptibility testing.
8. Remove stay sutures and laparotomy sponges.
9. Close the bladder as described in Cystotomy.
10. Close the abdominal incision routinely.

Postoperative Care and Complications

- Postoperative complications are rare. Recurrent infections after removal of the diverticulum are uncommon.
- Administer antibiotics based on the results of bacterial culture and susceptibility testing. Prolonged antibiotic therapy (>4 weeks) may be necessary.
- See Cystotomy, Postoperative Care and Complications.

CYSTOTOMY

Preoperative Considerations

- Cystotomy in small animals is indicated most commonly for removal of cystic calculi.
- Neoplasia of the urinary bladder and ureteral reimplantation also may require cystotomy.
- Antibiotics are not administered preoperatively. If indicated, administer antibiotics intraoperatively after specimens for culture and susceptibility testing have been obtained.

Surgical Procedure

Objectives

- Open the urinary bladder to remove calculi, reimplant ureters, or explore the bladder lumen.
- Obtain samples for bacterial culture and susceptibility testing and histologic analysis.
- Prevent urine leakage into the peritoneal cavity.

Equipment

- Standard general surgery pack and suture
- Balfour retractor
- Laparotomy sponges
- Urinary catheter (male dogs)
- Human gallbladder scoop or sterile teaspoon to aid in stone removal
- 12-ml syringe
- 22-gauge needle

Technique

1. Place the animal in dorsal recumbency.
2. Prepare the ventral abdominal region and vulvar area in the female for aseptic surgery.
3. Incise the skin and subcutaneous tissue on the ventral abdominal midline.
4. In male dogs, incise the skin and subcutaneous tissue parallel and adjacent to the prepuce.
5. Identify and ligate the preputial branches of the caudal superficial epigastric vessels in the subcutis.
6. Incise the linea alba from the umbilicus to the pubis. The paramedian approach can be used in male dogs.
7. Position the Balfour retractor. Explore the abdomen for associated abnormalities of the kidneys, ureters, prostate, urethra, and iliac lymph nodes.
8. Isolate the urinary bladder with moistened laparotomy sponges.

9. Place stay sutures at either end of the proposed cystotomy incision to facilitate retraction and atraumatic manipulation (Fig. 1A).
10. Remove urine from the bladder by cystocentesis.
11. Orient the cystotomy incision to avoid major vessels and provide optimal exposure for the procedure. Dorsal or ventral cystotomy incisions are equally acceptable for removal of calculi. A ventral incision is preferred for exposure of the ureteral openings.

KEY POINT ▶ A ventral cystotomy incision has no greater risk of leakage or adhesion formation than does a dorsal incision.

12. Make a stab incision into the bladder with a scalpel (Fig. 1B).
13. Extend the incision proximally and distally with Metzenbaum scissors.
14. Avoid "corkscrewing" the incision around the bladder.
15. Avoid the trigone.
16. Remove uroliths with the gallbladder scoop or sterile teaspoon.

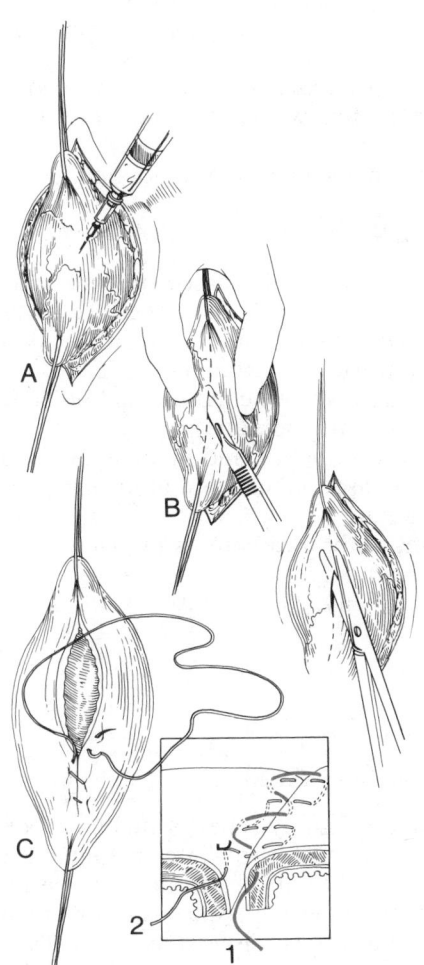

Figure 1. Cystotomy. *A*, With stay sutures in place, remove urine from bladder. *B*, Make stab incision with scalpel and extend with Metzenbaum scissors. *C*, After uroliths are removed and biopsy material taken, close with a two-layer inverting pattern.

KEY POINT ▶ Always submit uroliths to the laboratory for stone analysis.

17. Retrograde flushing may be required to remove small calculi from the proximal urethra in male dogs. Pass a sterile urinary catheter retrograde (from outside the penis) to the level of the os penis, occlude the end of the penis, and flush vigorously with sterile saline.
18. Feel for grit or roughness as the catheter is passed.
19. Do not close the bladder until absolutely certain that all stones have been removed.
20. Incise a 4-mm by 1-cm full-thickness wedge of bladder wall from the edge of the cystotomy incision.
21. Submit half the wedge for histologic analysis and half for bacterial culture and susceptibility testing.

KEY POINT ▶ A full-thickness wedge of bladder wall is submitted for bacterial culture and susceptibility testing even if urine has been submitted for culture.

22. Vesicourachal diverticula are removed if present.
23. In a female dog that requires an indwelling urinary catheter postoperatively, place it before bladder closure.
24. Pass a catheter normograde through the urethra and out the vulva.
25. Attach the end of a Foley catheter to this catheter.
26. Pull the Foley catheter retrograde into the bladder lumen.

KEY POINT ▶ Avoid incorporating the ureters in the bladder closure, especially with dorsal incisions.

27. Close the cystotomy (see subsequent description).
28. Remove stay sutures and laparotomy sponges.
29. Close the abdominal wall routinely.

Classically, cystotomy incisions are closed with a two-layer continuous inverting pattern. Coated synthetic absorbable suture material (3–0) with a swaged-on urogenital tapered needle is an ideal choice. A Cushing pattern, incorporating all tissue layers except the mucosa, is used for the first row of sutures, followed by a Lembert pattern (Fig. 1C). The bladder wall may be quite thick in animals with chronic cystitis, making inversion of the wall difficult.

Single-layer and double-layer continuous or interrupted appositional suture patterns can be utilized successfully for closure of cystotomy incisions. Appositional patterns are preferred when the bladder wall is thick and friable. An appositional pattern is necessary when the cystotomy incision extends so far distally that inversion might result in occlusion of the ureters or urethra.

Postoperative Care and Complications

■ Hematuria for 12 to 36 hours after surgery is common.
■ If a transurethral catheter was placed, connect it to a closed collection system.
  • Remove 1–2 days postoperatively.
■ Long-term (≥4 weeks) antibiotic and dietary ther-

apy, based on results of bacterial culture and susceptibility testing and stone analysis findings, is necessary in animals with urolithiasis.

- Although rare, urine leakage from inadequate bladder closure may occur, particularly if obstruction develops distally. Monitor urine production.
- Observe for stranguria.
- Obtain abdominal radiographs after surgery, if multiple radiopaque stones were present, to confirm that all stones were removed.

BLADDER TRAUMA

Preoperative Considerations

- See *Diseases of the Urinary Bladder* (sec. 8, ch. 3) for a discussion of the etiology, pathophysiology, clinical signs, laboratory abnormalities, and diagnosis of ruptured bladder.
- Contusions, partial-thickness lacerations, and iatrogenic ruptures during catheterization usually heal spontaneously and are managed medically. Urinary diversion (transurethral catheterization or tube cystostomy) and antibiotic therapy are considered.
- Intraperitoneal ruptures of the urinary bladder may heal spontaneously. This outcome is inconsistent and unpredictable.
- Surgical repair is the treatment of choice.

KEY POINT ▶ Fluid, electrolyte, and acid-base disorders (dehydration, hyperkalemia, acidosis, azotemia) must be managed prior to anesthetizing an animal for repair of a ruptured bladder.

- Animals with a ruptured bladder that cannot be anesthetized because of fluid, electrolyte, and acid-base abnormalities may be treated initially by temporary urinary diversion. Place large Penrose drains transabdominally to drain urine from the peritoneal cavity.
- Administer intravenous fluid therapy with isotonic saline, antibiotics, and sodium bicarbonate therapy if necessary.

Surgical Procedure

Objective

- Remove urine from the peritoneal cavity.
- Repair ruptured bladder.
- Identify and treat other intra-abdominal injuries.

Equipment

- Standard general surgery instrument pack and suture
- Balfour retractor
- Laparotomy pads
- Suction device
- Foley catheter (if tube cystostomy is indicated).

Technique

1. Place the animal in dorsal recumbency.
2. Prepare the ventral abdominal region for aseptic surgery.
3. Perform a routine ventral midline celiotomy from the umbilicus to the pubis.
4. Perform an abdominal exploratory.
5. Isolate the urinary bladder with moistened laparotomy sponges.
6. Locate the rupture in the urinary bladder.
7. Place stay sutures to facilitate exposure of the rupture.
8. Debride nonviable tissue from the edges of the rent.
9. Approximate the edges of the rent with 3–0 synthetic absorbable suture material using an inverting or approximating suture pattern.
10. Remove the stay sutures.
11. If the viability of the bladder wall is questionable, resect the nonviable region if possible. Alternatively, cover the area with omentum or, preferably, a serosal patch using jejunum.
12. Manage other intra-abdominal injuries.
13. Lavage the peritoneal cavity with copious amounts of warm physiologic saline solution.
14. Remove residual flush solution.
15. Swab the peritoneal cavity, and submit the sample for bacteriologic culture and susceptibility testing.
16. A sterile transurethral catheter may be placed to keep the bladder decompressed particularly if the repair is tenuous or the viability of the bladder wall is questionable. Urinary diversion seldom is necessary following proper repair of ruptured bladder.
17. Abdominal wall closure is routine.

Postoperative Care and Complications

- Administer antibiotics based on culture and susceptibility testing results. Therapeutic administration of broad-spectrum antibiotics is indicated in animals with extensive tissue trauma.
- The animal may be hematuric and pollakiuric for 12 to 48 hours after surgery.
- Continue to monitor and manage fluid, electrolyte, and acid-base imbalances after surgery. Monitor urine output.
- If a transurethral catheter is in place, remove it 2 to 3 days after surgery.
- See Cystotomy, Postoperative Care and Complications.

SUBTOTAL CYSTECTOMY

Preoperative Considerations

- Subtotal cystectomy is performed most commonly in an attempt to cure or palliate an animal with bladder neoplasia. Subtotal cystectomy may be indicated to remove benign lesions, such as traumatic or congenital diverticula (see discussion of urachal anomaly), polyps, intramural granulomas, and devascularized areas of bladder wall.
- Therapeutic results are related to the size and location of the bladder neoplasm and the presence or

absence of metastasis. Animals with bladder neoplasia must undergo thorough diagnostic testing, including contrast radiographic studies and cytologic evaluation, prior to surgical intervention.

- Neoplasms located in accessible areas of the bladder can be removed by partial cystectomy. Subtotal cystectomy is not considered when there is extensive involvement of the neck or trigone of the bladder or when a large portion of the bladder wall is affected.
- A substantial portion of the nontrigone bladder, perhaps greater than 75%, can be excised with few untoward effects.

Surgical Procedure

Objective

- Remove abnormal section of bladder wall.
- Biopsy a bladder mass.
- Maintain reservoir function of bladder.

Equipment

- Standard general surgery instrument pack and suture
- Balfour retractor
- Sterile urinary catheter

Technique

1. Patient positioning, surgical approach, and isolation of the bladder are as described previously in Cystotomy.
2. Locate the area to be removed by gentle palpation.
3. Excise the abnormal bladder wall, including approximately 1 cm of normal-appearing tissue on all sides.
4. Wide surgical margins (>3 cm) are not necessary if the disease process is benign.
5. Ureteral transplantation may be necessary. Refer to section 8, chapter 2.
6. Close the bladder with 3–0 synthetic absorbable suture material in an appositional or inverting pattern (see Cystotomy).
7. If neoplasia is suspected, explore the entire abdomen for metastasis. Biopsy regional lymph nodes.
8. Close the abdomen routinely.

Postoperative Care and Complications

- Adjunct radiotherapy or chemotherapy may be beneficial following subtotal cystectomy for bladder neoplasia.
- Hematuria and pollakiuria are observed commonly after subtotal cystectomy.
- Frequent voiding may persist due to loss of reservoir volume.
- The reservoir function of the bladder returns, at least partially, by 3 months.
- See Cystotomy, Postoperative Care and Complications.

TUBE CYSTOSTOMY

Preoperative Considerations

- Tube cystostomy is indicated for temporary diversion of urine from the urethra.

- Male dogs with metabolic alterations resulting from obstruction to urine outflow frequently are unable to tolerate general anesthesia.
- Temporary diversion of urine via tube cystostomy permits delay of definitive repair of urethral trauma or removal of urethral calculi until metabolic alterations are corrected.
- Tube cystostomy is a practical means of temporary urine diversion when the bladder has lost contractile function.
- General anesthesia usually is not needed for tube cystostomy. Narcotic analgesics, such as oxymorphone combined with local infiltration of lidocaine, are adequate.

Surgical Procedure

Objective

- Divert the flow of urine from the urethra via a Foley catheter placed into the bladder.

Equipment

- Standard general surgery instrument pack and suture
- 8 Fr. Foley catheter with intact balloon
- Small Gelpi or Weitlaner retractor

Technique

1. Administer oxymorphone (0.1 to 0.3 mg/kg IV).
2. Position the animal in dorsal recumbency.
3. Prepare the ventral abdominal region for aseptic surgery.
4. Infiltrate the abdominal wall with lidocaine in the area of the planned paramedian incision—approximately 3 cm lateral to the midline at the level of the prepuce.
5. Make a 4-cm paramedian incision through the abdominal wall. Avoid incising the distended urinary bladder. Place the self-retaining retractor.
6. Pass the Foley catheter through the abdominal wall via a paramedian stab incision made adjacent to the celiotomy incision.
7. Place a pursestring suture in the wall of the bladder on the ventral side near the apex. Use 3–0 synthetic absorbable suture material with a swaged-on taper needle.
8. Pass the Foley catheter into the bladder through a stab incision in the center of the pursestring suture.
9. Tighten and tie the pursestring suture. Do not occlude the catheter.
10. Inflate the balloon of the Foley catheter with sterile saline.
11. Preplace four sutures of 2–0 or 3–0 synthetic absorbable material between the bladder and the abdominal wall, where the Foley catheter exits.
12. Secure the bladder to the body wall by tying the preplaced sutures.
13. The potential for intraperitoneal leakage of urine may be lessened by placing omentum around the catheter between the bladder and body wall prior to tying the preplaced sutures (Fig. 2).
14. Close the paramedian incision routinely.

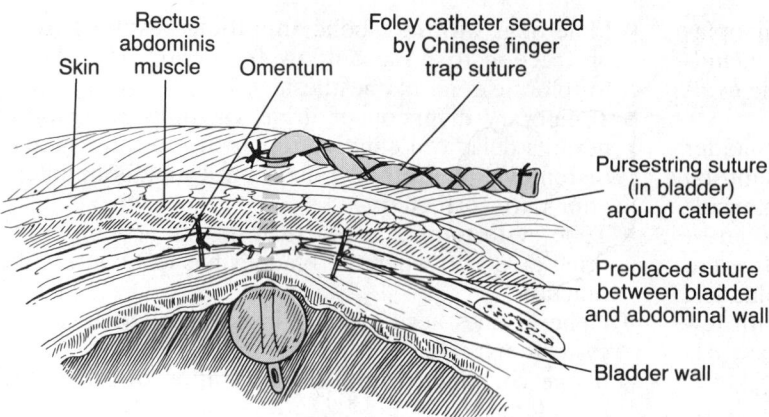

Figure 2. Suture and tube placement for tube cystotomy.

15. Secure the Foley catheter to the body wall using the Chinese finger trap knot (see sec. 1, ch. 3).

Postoperative Care and Complications

- The Foley catheter can be attached to a closed sterile urine collection system (preferred) or capped and drained intermittently.
- Place an Elizabethan collar or side-brace on the animal to prevent mutilation of the system.
- Therapeutic administration of a broad-spectrum antibiotic is advisable.
- Deflate the balloon and withdraw the catheter when it is no longer needed. If the catheter has been in place for approximately 7 days, the stoma will heal spontaneously. Earlier removal may require surgical closure of the bladder and abdominal wall.
- Rarely, adhesions between the bladder and peritoneum from tube cystotomy can inhibit complete bladder emptying. Placement of the Foley catheter in the body of the bladder rather than the apex helps prevent this problem.

Supplemental Readings

Osuna DJ: Postoperative management of urinary tract surgical patients. Compend Cont Ed 9:873, 1987.

Stone EA: Surgical therapy for urolithiasis. Vet Clin North Am [Sm Anim Pract] 14:77, 1984.

URETHRAL CALCULI

Urethral calculi are macroscopic mineral concretions lodged within the urethra. In dogs and cats, urethral calculi occur less frequently than bladder calculi; however, the former may be life-threatening if they cause complete obstruction of urine outflow. Calculi rarely lodge in the female urethra because of its diameter, distensibility, and length. In dogs, urethral calculi most commonly lodge just caudal to the os penis or at the ischial arch where the urethra narrows.

Etiology

- Urethral calculi usually form in the urinary bladder. If the diameter of the calculi is smaller than the proximal urethral diameter, they may migrate into the urethra.
- Causes of the initial formation of urethral calculi are variable, depending on their mineral composition (see sec. 8, ch. 3).

Clinical Signs

- Clinical signs can be acute, intermittent, or undetectable.
- Dysuria, urinary incontinence, and hematuria are common signs when calculi do not completely occlude the urethral lumen.
- Stranguria, distended abdomen, and severe depression from postrenal azotemia occur when calculi cause complete urethral obstruction.

Diagnosis

History

- Consider calculi in male dogs and cats with signs of dysuria, especially in male dogs with stranguria and anuria.
- Some animals with urethral calculi have a prior history of bladder calculi, but many animals have no previous history of urinary tract problems.

Physical Examination

- Suspect an obstruction to urine flow when there is a large, firm urinary bladder.
- If the bladder is not distended, gently palpate the abdomen to detect bladder calculi, which may accompany urethral calculi.
- Examine the urethra by:
  - Digital palpation per rectum
  - Palpation of the perineal region in male dogs
  - Inspection of the external urethral orifice

Observation of Urination

- The character and color of the urine stream may be helpful in localizing the problem to the lower urinary tract or specifically to the urethra.
- If hematuria occurs only at the beginning of the urine stream, the bleeding may originate in the urethra.

Urethral Catheterization

- Gentle aseptic catheterization of the urethra may help localize the problem to the urethra (if resistance is encountered).
- A grating or gritty sensation may be felt as the catheter encounters urethral calculi.

Urinalysis

- Collect urine by cytocentesis before allowing the dog to urinate.
- Urine pH and the presence of bacteria and crystals may help to determine the composition of calculi (see Table 2, sec. 8, ch. 3).

Radiographic Evaluation

- Urethral calculi often can be identified and dislodged without the aid of radiography; however, radiographs are useful for documenting the size, number, and location of calculi before and after urethral backflushing.
- A positive-contrast cystourethrogram allows localization of nonradiopaque calculi and detection of predisposing or subsequent abnormalities of the urethra (e.g., stricture, blood clot) (see sec. 1, ch. 4).

Serum Biochemical Profile

- The presence of hypercalcemia or decreased hepatic function may help identify the underlying etiology and mineral composition of the calculi (see sec. 4, ch. 2 and sec. 7, ch. 8).
- If urethral obstruction is present, evaluate for hyperkalemia, metabolic acidosis, and azotemia.

Treatment

KEY POINT ▶ The first goal of therapy is to restore urethral patency.

Establishing Urethral Patency

Urethral obstruction usually is relieved by retrograde catheterization alone or by propulsion of the calculi into the urinary bladder, via catheterization and back-flushing of the urethra. If conservative methods fail, surgery is indicated.

Method 1—If the urethral calculi are recently detected and the obstruction is incomplete, the urethral calculi may be pushed into the urinary bladder as a urethral catheter is gently advanced.

Method 2—Urethrohydropropulsion. If Method 1 fails and the calculi are proximal to the os penis, attempt urethrohydropropulsion. Before starting this procedure, assess the size of the urinary bladder. Careful administration of a sedative or an analgesic may help avoid patient distress and promote relaxation of the urethral skeletal muscles.

KEY POINT ▶ If the bladder is distended, remove most of the urine by cystocentesis to help decrease the hydrostatic pressure, which will oppose the retrograde movement of the calculi.

Technique

1. Aseptically pass a soft flexible catheter proximally until the calculus is contacted.
2. Attach a syringe (12–20 ml) of sterile saline to the end of the catheter. Occlude the urethral orifice while injecting saline into the urethra as the assistant compresses the urethra by digital pressure proximal to the obstruction (rectal palpation).
3. As the urethra is dilated by the hydrostatic force of the saline, the assistant quickly releases the urethral compression. If successful, this will cause a gradual retropulsion of the calculus into the bladder.

Method 3—**Surgery.** If Methods 1 and 2 fail, surgery is indicated to remove or bypass the calculi (see sec. 8, ch. 6). In severely depressed patients, perform surgical diversion of urine flow (e.g., tube cystostomy) utilizing local anesthesia if possible (see sec. 8, ch. 4).

■ After urethral patency is restored, maintain an indwelling urethral catheter and monitor urine output until the animal is stable.

Management of Fluid, Electrolyte, and Acid-Base Status

■ Avoid potassium-containing IV fluids and medications in severely hyperkalemic patients (see sec. 1, ch. 5).
■ Correct any fluid deficit with isotonic saline administered IV or SC, depending on the severity of the deficit. Lactated Ringer's solution may be used after correction of hyperkalemia.
■ Usually, relief of the obstruction and fluid therapy rapidly corrects acidosis and hyperkalemia.
■ See discussion of hyperkalemia in this chapter under Urethral Obstruction in Cats with Idiopathic Lower Urinary Tract Disease.

Treatment of Cystic Calculi

■ When it is determined that all calculi are within the urinary bladder, surgically remove as described for bladder calculi (see sec. 8, ch. 4) to prevent recurrence of obstruction.

KEY POINT ▶ Urethral obstruction may recur after urethral calculi are retropulsed into the urinary bladder. Not all calculi are susceptible to medical dissolution.

Prevention

The frequency of recurrence and the recommended protocols to prevent recurrence of calculi are variable and are dependent on the mineral composition of the calculi and the presence of bacterial infection (see sec. 8, ch. 3).

Permanent urethrostomy usually can prevent recurrence of life-threatening urethral obstructions. However, the urethrostomy may allow pathogenic bacteria to bypass the urethral high-pressure zone, resulting in an increased incidence of ascending urinary tract infections. If a permanent urethrostomy is performed, periodically culture the urine (collected by cystocentesis) for bacteria.

URETHRAL OBSTRUCTION IN CATS WITH IDIOPATHIC LOWER URINARY TRACT DISEASE (ILUTD)

ILUTD, also called feline urologic syndrome (FUS) is a common problem of unknown etiology. In male cats with ILUTD a conglomerate of struvite crystals, mucus, and debris may form and may obstruct or "plug" the outflow of urine with potential life-threatening consequences. See sec. 8, ch. 3 for discussion of cystitis associated with ILUTD.

KEY POINT ▶ Treat urethral obstruction in a male cat as a medical emergency.

Etiology

Formation of mucoid matrix is thought to be secondary to an abnormality of the urinary tract such as viral infection. Hematuria and dysuria results. If the matrix is produced in sufficient quantity, it forms a gel in the urethral lumen. If a male cat has a significant amount of crystalluria, the crystals combine with the gel and result in formation of a plug that obstructs the normally small diameter urethral lumen.

Clinical Signs

Affected male cats may have pollakiuria, stranguria, and hematuria. The owner usually reports that the cat constantly licks the perineum.

Diagnosis

History

■ Suspect urethral obstruction in any male cat with the clinical signs previously described.

- The owner reports a history of:
  - "Constipation," because prolonged periods in the litter box associated with stranguria may be mistaken as a problem with defecation.
  - "Suspected trauma" or "intoxication," when the cat actually is moribund owing to uremia or hyperkalemia.

Physical Examination

- In early urethral obstruction, the only abnormality is a large, firm urinary bladder that is tender on palpation.
- A cat with long-standing urethral obstruction will be depressed, bradycardic, and recumbent, with a firm, overdistended bladder.
- This is a medical emergency, and an abbreviated physical examination may be warranted to expedite medical treatment.
  - Diagnostic tests discussed later may have to be delayed until the animal is stable.
  - In male cats with a large firm bladder, gently palpate the penile urethra to locate and possibly dislodge the obstruction.

Urine Analysis and Culture

- Hematuria and magnesium ammonium phosphate crystalluria usually are present.
- If pyuria, bacteriuria, or alkaline urine is detected in the urinalysis, submit a urine sample (collected by cystocentesis prior to catheterizing the urethra) for aerobic bacterial culture.

KEY POINT ▶ Exercise extreme care when performing cystocentesis in a cat with a turgid bladder. Accidental bladder rupture may cause acute uroperitoneum and rapid deterioration of the patient.

Serum Biochemical Profile

- In cats with long-standing obstruction, perform a serum biochemical profile to assess azotemia, hyperkalemia, and acidosis.

Electrocardiography

- In cats with long-standing obstruction and bradycardia or arrhythmia, monitor the heart rate and rhythm with an electrocardiogram (ECG) during the initial treatment period to avoid hyperkalemia-induced cardiogenic and anesthesia-related death (see sec. 6, ch. 4 on arrhythmias).

Radiographic Evaluation

- If the obstruction cannot be alleviated using a urethral catheter, a positive-contrast urethrogram may help identify the location and cause of the problem (e.g., stricture, extraluminal compression); however, completion of the procedure or interpretation of the results may be difficult if the obstruction is acute.
- Recurrent obstructions always warrant a survey abdominal radiograph to rule out cystic calculi, which usually are radiopaque in cats. Frequent episodes of recurrence may also warrant urethrography, although perineal urethrostomy is preferred because usually it prevents further recurrences.

Treatment

In cats with urethral obstruction, the therapeutic goals are to relieve the obstruction and to normalize the fluid, electrolyte (e.g., treat hyperkalemia), and acid-base balance of the patient. Cats that are bradycardic and collapsed or moribund with urethral obstruction require emergency treatment.

If medical management fails to prevent recurrence of urethral obstruction, perineal urethrostomy surgery may be necessary (see sec. 8, ch. 6).

Management of Hyperkalemia

Hyperkalemia-induced cardiac dysfunction and atrial standstill is the principal life-threatening complication of long-standing urethral obstruction.

- Monitor the ECG during emergency management. Hyperkalemic cardiac effects can be antagonized (calcium gluconate), or the plasma potassium concentrations can be decreased (sodium bicarbonate or glucose and insulin).
- Sodium bicarbonate usually is the initial choice for treatment. It has the advantage of treating both the hyperkalemia (by driving the potassium intracellularly) and the severe acidosis that typically accompanies advanced urethral obstruction.
  - For severe (symptomatic) hyperkalemia, administer 1 mEq/kg of sodium bicarbonate by slow IV injection over 1–2 minutes; then infuse an additional 1–2 mEq/kg slowly over 30–60 minutes.
- An alternative method for lowering potassium levels by driving it intracellularly is to administer glucose (0.5–1.0 g/kg of 20% dextrose IV) with or without regular insulin (0.5 units/kg).
- Calcium gluconate (10% solution) can be administered to effect (over 15 minutes, IV) to temporarily antagonize the hyperkalemia when urgent control of life-threatening cardiac effects is needed. Fortunately, this usually is not necessary.
- As soon as possible after (or during) these treatments and initiation of intravenous fluid administration, establish urethral patency.

Establishing Urethral Patency

Although urethral catheterization usually is required, attempt initially to relieve the obstruction by gently massaging the penis. The site of obstruction usually is in the penile urethra a few millimeters to 2 centimeters proximal to the urethral orifice.

Catheterization. To relieve the obstruction by catheterization, anesthesia is often required; use only the minimal amount needed and closely monitor the animal (see sec. 1, ch. 2).

Technique

1. Carefully perform cystocentesis to relieve some of the bladder distension and the accompanying increased hydrostatic pressure.

2. To facilitate insertion of the urethral catheter, place the cat in dorsal recumbency and straighten the urethra by extending the penis caudally and ventrally.

3. Use aseptic technique and gentle handling to backflush the urethra by pulse-injecting sterile saline from a syringe (10–20 ml diameter) through an open-ended urethral catheter.

4. Advance the catheter into the bladder and drain the urine. Gently rinse the bladder with chilled saline until the fluid is clear. If severe hematuria is present, chilled saline may control hemorrhage.

5. Maintain urethral patency with a soft flexible urethral catheter and a closed collection system if a narrow urine stream persists after relieving the obstruction, if marked bladder hemorrhage is present, or if the cat was severely depressed (indicating long-standing obstruction and severe metabolic derangement).

Alternative Methods

- When urethral patency cannot be established with atraumatic insertion of a urethral catheter, perform tube cystotomy or multiple cystocenteses to keep the bladder decompressed until the animal is stable enough for surgery.
- Perineal urethrostomy is indicated for animals that cannot be catheterized or animals with recurrent urethral obstruction (see sec. 8, ch. 6).

Management of Uremia, Acidosis, and Dehydration

- Correct fluid deficits with an isotonic electrolyte solution administered parenterally. Isotonic saline is preferred initially if acidosis and hyperkalemia are severe; otherwise, Ringer's lactate can be used. The route of administration depends on the severity of the abnormalities.
- Usually relief of the obstruction in combination with fluid therapy rapidly corrects the acidosis and azotemia.
- IV fluids may have to be administered well above maintenance requirements because obstructive urine output generally is above normal. Monitor urine output and hydration status closely.

Management of Polyuric Renal Failure

Polyuric renal failure often ensues if the urethral obstruction is long-standing. The polyuria may lead to hypokalemia, hyponatremia, and dehydration. The amount of urine produced and the duration of the diuresis phase is variable and can last 2–5 days.

KEY POINT ▶ In cats, closely monitor; if the urine output is voluminous, supplemental parenteral fluid and electrolyte administration may be necessary to maintain normal hydration and eukalemia.

- If the cat is azotemic, monitor blood urea nitrogen (BUN) and creatinine levels and calculate parenteral fluid volume input to match the measured output. Renal function parameters should progressively improve.

- The fluid administration can be gradually tapered as renal function improves (see sec. 8, ch. 1).

Management of Urinary Incontinence

After correction of obstruction, there may be a period of inability to urinate, bladder overdistension, and urinary incontinence due to impaired detrusor contraction. The most effective treatment for this problem is to keep the bladder empty by frequent manual expression of the bladder or by an indwelling closed urine collection system until detrusor function recovers (usually 1 to 3 days).

Prevention

Measures for prevention of urethral obstruction in cats with ILUTD are similar to those recommended for all cats with ILUTD (see sec. 8, ch. 3):

- Encourage increased water intake to keep the urine dilute
- Acidify the urine (with an acidifying diet or urinary acidifiers)
- Maintain a low magnesium intake

URETHRAL TRAUMA

Motor vehicle accidents are the most common cause of urinary tract trauma. Pelvic fractures may cause urethral rupture near the vesiculourethral junction. This type of injury occurs almost exclusively in males. Iatrogenic trauma during catheterization of the urethra probably is more common but less severe than that caused by motor vehicular accidents. Postrenal azotemia, urethral stricture, and periurethral hematoma are the most common potentially serious sequelae to urethral trauma. Uncommonly, urethral laceration or necrosis can result in cutaneous or rectal fistulas.

Etiology

Urethral lacerations, abrasions, and compressions may occur secondary to fractures of the pelvis or the os penis. Iatrogenic urethral trauma may result from overzealous attempts to advance a urethral catheter when the animal is inadequately restrained, the urethra is abnormal (e.g., calculi, inflammation), or the catheter is rigid and inflexible. Occasionally, bite wounds, gunshot wounds, and foreign body penetration can cause trauma to the extrapelvic urethra.

Clinical Signs

- Dysuria, hematuria, and urinary incontinence are common signs of lower urinary tract trauma; however, urethral injury can be asymptomatic.
- Anuria, depression (from uremia), and abdominal, inguinal, or perineal swelling and bruising can occur with large urethral lacerations.

Diagnosis

History

Often there is a recent history of:

- Trauma (motor vehicle accident)

- Urethral catheterization

Physical Examination

- Although identification of a urethral laceration by palpation is difficult, associated pelvic fractures may be readily apparent on digital palpation per rectum.
- Abdominal, inguinal, or perineal swelling and bruising may be detected during physical examination, depending on the duration of the laceration and the location and volume of extravasated urine.
- Stranguria or hematuria after trauma suggest urinary tract injury, but these signs do not localize the problem to the urethra.
- Pass a urethral catheter to help determine if a rupture has occurred.

Abdominal Radiographs

- Peritoneal and retroperitoneal effusion may be observed on plain radiographs in some animals with urethral lacerations.
- Usually a positive-contrast urethrogram is necessary to document the presence and severity of a urethral laceration (see sec. 1, ch. 4). In most cases, if a posttraumatic urethral laceration is documented, a positive-contrast cystogram is indicated to rule out accompanying bladder trauma (see sec. 1, ch. 4).

Abdominocentesis

If peritoneal effusion is present and radiography is inconclusive, perform a cytologic examination of the abdominal fluid (i.e., determine if the concentration of creatinine in effusion is greater than in serum) to rule out uroperitoneum.

Complete Blood Count (CBC) and Serum Biochemical Profile

These tests are indicated if the animal is systemically ill or does not respond to treatment. Metabolic alterations are similar to those seen with ruptured bladder (see sec. 8, ch. 3).

Treatment

- If urethral laceration is complete, surgical repair is necessary (see sec. 8, ch. 6).
- In small urethral (i.e., transected urethra) deficits, stenting of the defect with a urinary catheter or urinary diversion via tube cystostomy for 10–14 days usually is effective (see sec. 8, ch. 4).
- If a contaminated wound or urinary tract infection is present, antimicrobial therapy is indicated.
- Urethral stricture is a potential complication of urethral trauma.

Prevention

- Catheter-associated iatrogenic urethral trauma can be minimized by use of soft, flexible catheters, gentle manipulation, and aseptic technique. Avoid urethral catheterization when it is not needed.
- Fracture-associated urethral lacerations usually occur at the time of the initial trauma; immobilization of pelvic fracture fragments can minimize further urethral and periurethral trauma.

URETHRAL NEOPLASIA

Primary urethral neoplasia is uncommon in dogs and very rare in cats. Urethral tumors usually are malignant, epithelial (transitional cell and, less frequently, squamous cell) carcinomas and occur most frequently in older female dogs. Benign urethral mass lesions such as urethral polyps and granulomatous urethritis, although rare, need to be distinguished from neoplasms.

Etiology

No specific etiology has been recognized that induces urethral tumors in dogs. Carcinogenic factors involved in bladder cancer may predispose dogs to urethral neoplasia.

Clinical Signs

Signs of urethral neoplasia cannot be differentiated from other causes of lower urinary tract inflammation and obstruction. Signs may be absent or unrecognized early in the course of the disease.

- Dysuria, hematuria, and urinary incontinence are the most common signs in dogs with urethral neoplasia.
- Occasionally the signs may be temporarily responsive to antimicrobial therapy.

Diagnosis

History

Consider urethral neoplasia in old female dogs with recurrent urinary tract infections or intermittent or chronic stranguria, pollakiuria, or hematuria.

Physical Examination

KEY POINT ▶ Palpation of a thickened or irregular urethra by rectal or vaginal digital examination is highly suggestive of urethral neoplasia.

- In some dogs, metastatic sublumbar lymphadenopathy may be palpable, depending on the size of dog and of the lymph nodes.
- Determining the bladder size after the dog urinates may be helpful in assessing the degree of urine outflow obstruction.

Cytologic Examination

- Cytologic examination of voided urine or urine collected by catheterization may reveal neoplastic cells.
- Cells for cytologic examination also may be collected by aseptically advancing a urethral catheter to the center of the diseased urethra and massaging the urethra while aspirating through the catheter.
- Reactive urothelial proliferation may resemble neoplastic transformed cells cytologically; therefore, his-

tologic confirmation of the diagnosis may be necessary before initiating aggressive therapy.

Urinalysis and Culture

Bacterial urinary tract infections (pyuria, hematuria, and bacteriuria) are common in dogs with urethral neoplasia because local host defenses are compromised.

Complete Blood Count (CBC) and Serum Biochemical Profile

If the animal is systemically ill or if treatment of the neoplasm is anticipated, perform these tests to help rule out postrenal azotemia and evaluate the animal's general health.

Vaginal Examination

- Because the neoplastic cells usually involve the entire length of the urethra, the distal urethra may appear grossly abnormal.
- Fine-needle aspirates can be collected for cytologic evaluation and punch biopsies can be used for histologic examination with minimal discomfort to the patient if local anesthesia is used.

Radiologic Evaluation

- Evaluate survey abdominal and thoracic radiographs for the presence of metastasis. Potential sites of metastasis include the sublumbar lymph nodes, lumbar vertebrae, pelvis, and lungs.
- An excretory urogram and a positive-contrast urethrocystogram can assess the extent of urinary tract involvement.

Urethral Endoscopy

The extent of urethral mucosal involvement can be determined and a guided biopsy can be procured, using an appropriate-size cystoscope or endoscope.

Histologic Evaluation

Because chronic inflammation of the urothelium may resemble neoplastic infiltration cytologically and radiographically, histologic evaluation is recommended. Methods for obtaining tissue for histologic evaluation include:

- Vaginoscopic or endoscopic biopsy
- Catheter biopsy (see the discussion of bladder neoplasia in sec. 8, ch. 3)
- Surgery

Treatment

Medical Management

No prospective or retrospective studies of medical management of canine urethral tumors have been reported. However, a poor response is expected because similar types of bladder tumors respond poorly to current chemotherapeutic and radiation protocols.

Surgery

Surgical salvage procedures rarely are feasible.

- Do not consider surgery when there is:
  - Distant metastasis
  - Local extension beyond the urethra
  - Involvement of more than 85% of the urethral length
- Consider antepubic urethrostomy (see sec. 8, ch. 6) if only the distal urethra is involved.
- Ureteral transplantation procedures are not recommended because of severe complications.

Supplemental Readings

Davies JV, Read HM: Urethral tumours in dogs. J Small Anim Pract 31:131, 1990.

Kruger JM, Osborne CA: The role of viruses in feline urinary tract disease. J Vet Intern Med 4:71, 1990.

Osborne CA, Kruger JM, Johnston GR, Polzin DJ: Feline lower urinary tract disorders. *In* Ettinger SJ, ed.; *Textbook of Veterinary Internal Medicine.* Philadelphia: W. B. Saunders, 1989, p 2057.

Pechman RD: Urinary trauma in dogs and cats: A review. J Am Anim Hosp Assoc 18:33, 1982.

6 Surgery of the Urethra

Dale E. Bjorling

Urethral disorders in dogs and cats frequently result in partial or complete obstruction. Emergency care may be required to restore the flow of urine and to treat metabolic imbalance. The presence of calculi within the urethra is often accompanied by urinary tract infection (UTI) and cystic calculi. Aggressive medical and dietary management is required after surgery to prevent recurrence. Care is taken during surgical manipulation of the urethra to minimize the potential for postoperative scar tissue formation and subsequent urethral obstruction.

KEY POINT ▶ Metabolic imbalance in an animal with urethral obstruction is corrected prior to performing general anesthesia and prolonged operative procedures.

ANATOMY
Male Canine Urethra

- The urethra in the male canine is divided into three parts: the prostatic, membranous, and cavernous or penile portions.
- The urethral sphincter is not a discrete structure in the dog. Urethral pressure profiles demonstrate a zone of increased pressure that extends from the prostatic urethra into the membranous urethra. Of the components of the urethral sphincter closure mechanism (fibroelastic tissue, smooth muscle, striated muscle), smooth muscle is probably primarily responsible for maintaining tone in the resting state. Therefore, alpha-adrenergic agonists may be successful in the treatment of sphincter incompetence.
- The smooth muscle of the urethra is innervated by autonomic nerves arising from the pelvic plexus. The striated musculature receives innervation from branches of the pudendal nerve.
- The distal portion of the penile urethra lies within the os penis. Dilation of the urethra is limited within the os penis and in the perineal portion of the urethra, as it curves around the ischium. These are common locations for calculi to become lodged within the urethra.

Male Feline Urethra

- The male feline urethra consists of three parts: (1) the preprostatic, which lies between the bladder and the prostate gland and is relatively longer than the corresponding portion of the male canine urethra; (2) the prostatic part, which extends from the prostate to the bulbourethral glands; and (3) the penile urethra. Immediately caudal to the bulbourethral glands, the urethral lumen rapidly narrows from approximately 4 mm in diameter to 1 mm. This diameter is maintained through the remainder of the penile urethra. When the penis is retracted, the prostatic and proximal penile urethra may assume the appearance of a flattened or gentle "s," which complicates urethral catheterization unless the penis is manually extended.
- An area of increased pressure thought to correspond to the sphincter mechanism is found in the urethra caudal to the prostate. Despite a decrease in intraurethral electromyographic activity after perineal urethrostomy in male cats, urinary incontinence is an uncommon finding. This may be due to the contribution of smooth muscle fibers as well as the remaining striated fibers of the urethral sphincter, which results in resting urethral pressure greater than intravesicular pressure during bladder distension.
- The urethra is innervated by branches of the pudendal nerve and receives autonomic fibers from the pelvic plexus.

Female Canine and Feline Urethra

- The urethra in the female dog and cat is relatively short in comparison to the male and corresponds to the portion of the male urethra found cranial to the level of the mid prostate. The female urethra is also relatively larger in diameter and more distensible than the corresponding male urethra.
- It appears unlikely that a discrete urethral sphincter is present in either dogs or cats. The urethral pressure profile does not demonstrate a discrete increase in pressure, but the major increase in urethral pressure develops in the mid urethra of the female dog. A discrete area of increase in urethral pressure has been observed in female cats associated with striated musculature near the external urethral orifice.
- The female urethra is innervated by autonomic fibers of the hypogastric and pelvic nerves and sensory and motor fibers from the pudendal nerve.
- Obstruction of the female urethra is extremely uncommon because of the short length, wide diameter, and relative distensibility of the urethra.

URETHRAL ANASTOMOSIS
Preoperative Considerations

- Perform urethral anastomosis for treatment of urethral disruption, prostatectomy, stricture formation, or removal of granulomatous or neoplastic masses.

849

- Perform retrograde positive contrast urethrocystography to identify the location of obstruction or disruption.
- Treat animals that are uremic as a result of urethral obstruction or leakage of urine into the periurethral tissues prior to inducing anesthesia and performing surgery.

KEY POINT ▶ Incomplete lacerations or defects (discussed later in this chapter) may be satisfactorily treated by maintenance of a urethral catheter to divert the flow of urine for 2 to 3 weeks. This form of treatment will be successful only when an intact urethral mucosa bridges a portion of the injured area.

Surgical Procedure

Objectives

- Remove diseased tissue.
- Restore urethral continuity.
- Minimize the potential for postoperative stricture formation.

Equipment

- Standard surgical instruments and suture
- Urinary catheters of appropriate diameter and length
- Gelpi or Weitlaner self-retaining retractors
- Monofilament nonabsorbable suture (4–0 or 5–0) or synthetic absorbable suture (4–0 or 5–0)
- Magnification (optional)
- Penrose drains, if cellulitis or tissue necrosis due to extravasation of urine has occurred.

Technique

1. The positioning of the animal depends upon the portion of the urethra to be operated upon.
2. With the animal positioned appropriately, prepare the overlying skin for aseptic surgery.
3. Pass a sterile urethral catheter from the external urethral orifice in a retrograde direction to facilitate identification of the proximal end of the distal portion of the urethra.
4. If the distal end of the proximal portion of the urethra cannot be identified, perform a cystotomy and pass a urethral catheter in an antegrade direction.
5. Excise the damaged portions of the urethra. Although it is critical that a tension-free anastomosis be performed, do not be reluctant to debride and resect an adequate amount of urethra to properly treat the disease process.
6. If the urethra cannot be reconstructed without undue tension across the anastomotic site, consider alternatives, such as prepubic urethrostomy.
7. With the urethral catheter in place, perform the anastomosis by placing full-thickness sutures in a simple interrupted pattern.
8. Place the first suture through the dorsal aspect of the urethra.
9. Cut the ends of the suture at a sufficient length so that they may be grasped by a forceps.

10. Gently rotate the urethra to facilitate placement of subsequent sutures.
11. Place sutures evenly; six to eight sutures are usually sufficient to perform a satisfactory anastomosis.
12. Maintain a urethral catheter connected to a sterile urine collection bag for 7–10 days after surgery.
13. Displacement of the catheter can be discouraged by use of an Elizabethan collar or a body brace. Alternatively, a cystostomy catheter can be placed to divert the flow of urine from the urethra (see sec. 8, ch. 4).
14. Close the wound in a standard manner.

Postoperative Care and Complications

- If the urethral catheter is removed prematurely, a decision must be made regarding whether or not to replace the catheter. If resistance is encountered during attempts to pass the urethral catheter, this is abandoned.
- Monitor the animal carefully for evidence of urine leakage.
- Warn the owners of the potential development of stricture, and advise them to carefully observe the animal during urination for evidence of urethral obstruction.
- Perform a retrograde positive contrast urethrocystogram 2–3 months after surgery to evaluate the urethral diameter at the anastomotic site.
- Treat infection or the presence of urinary calculi appropriately.

URETHROTOMY IN THE DOG

Preoperative Considerations

- Perform this procedure to remove calculi lodged caudal to the os penis or in the perineal urethra and to temporarily divert the flow of urine.
- If the animal is azotemic and depressed, perform this procedure without sedation by infiltrating the tissue overlying the urethra with local anesthetic.
- If calculi remain in the kidneys, ureters, bladder, or urethra after performance of a urethrotomy, perform definitive surgery to remove the calculi after the animal is stabilized.
- Perform urethrotomy only after attempts to pass a urethral catheter or to flush calculi in a retrograde direction into the bladder have failed.

Surgical Procedure

Objectives

- Relieve urethral obstruction.
- Remove urethral calculi.
- Pass urethral catheter.
- Allow treatment of azotemia prior to definitive repair.

Equipment

- Scalpel, hemostats, thumb forceps, Metzenbaum scissors

- Urethral catheter
- Suture to secure urethral catheter

Technique

1. Restrain the dog in dorsal (prescrotal urethrotomy) or lateral recumbency (perineal urethrotomy).
2. Infiltrate the skin and subcutaneous tissues overlying the urethra with local anesthetic.
3. Prepare the skin overlying the intended site of urethrotomy for aseptic surgery.
4. Make an incision 3–4 cm in length over the urethra at the level of obstruction.
5. Using a combination of blunt and sharp dissection, expose the appropriate area of the urethra.
6. In the prescrotal location, identify the retractor penis muscles and retract them laterally. The urethra appears as a purple structure on the midline flanked on either side by the white penile tunic.

KEY POINT ▶ Take care to incise the urethra on the ventral or caudal midline. The urethra is a highly vascular structure and will bleed briskly when incised.

7. Remove calculi from the urethra with forceps.
8. Pass a urethral catheter from the urethrotomy site into the bladder.
9. Maintain the urethral catheter after surgery to monitor urine output and diminish the likelihood of subsequent urethral obstruction prior to surgical removal of cystic calculi.
10. Leave the urethrotomy open to heal by second intention or suture with 4–0 monofilament non-absorbable or synthetic absorbable suture in a simple interrupted or simple continuous pattern.

Postoperative Care and Complications

- Hemorrhage may be observed intermittently, usually associated with urination. The flow of urine dislodges clots, and urokinase (a plasminogen activator found in urine) interferes with clot formation. This complication may be minimized by suturing the urethrotomy site.
- If the urethrotomy site is sutured, seroma or abscess formation may occur.
- On rare occasion, a stricture may form at the urethrotomy site. This is more likely when the urethral mucosa has sustained significant damage.
- Treat UTI and calculi with appropriate antibiotic and dietary therapy and other interventions to prevent reformation of calculi. Inform the owner that surgery will not cure this problem, and appropriate medical therapy is critical to a satisfactory outcome.
- If large calculi from the bladder pass into the urethra, urethral obstruction may recur despite the presence of the urethrotomy.
- If the skin incision is made too close to the scrotum, the testes may prolapse through the skin incision. Treat this prolapse by suturing the caudal aspect of the incision.
- Swelling and edema of the scrotum and testes may be observed because of the inflammation associated with performance of the urethrotomy or subcuta-

neous accumulation of urine. Subcutaneous accumulation of urine occurs infrequently if the urethrotomy incision is appropriately positioned near the caudal end of the os penis.
- Prolonged urethral obstruction and distension of the bladder may result in a loss of detrusor function of the bladder resulting in loss of contractile function of the bladder.

URETHROSTOMY IN THE MALE DOG

Preoperative Considerations

- Urethrostomy creates a permanent opening for the urethra and is performed proximal to the site of narrowing, obstruction, or destruction of the urethra. Perform a urethrostomy in the male dog in the perineal, scrotal, prescrotal, and prepubic positions.
- Urethrostomy is most often performed in the scrotal position, because the urethra is wide and superficial at this location. Minimal hemorrhage occurs, and a cosmetic result is achieved. Urethrostomy in the perineal position is usually avoided because of the potential for urine scalding of the caudal surface of the thighs. Prepubic urethrostomy is discussed further in this chapter.

KEY POINT ▶ Inform the owner that the performance of a urethrostomy will not cure urinary tract infection or urinary calculi. In fact, performance of a urethrostomy may predispose the animal to the development of urinary tract infection. The overall incidence of urinary tract infection after urethrostomy in male dogs is low, however.

- Urethrostomy decreases the potential for urethral obstruction due to passage of calculi but does not eliminate it. Calculi of sufficient diameter may still become lodged in the urethra proximal to the site of urethrostomy.

KEY POINT ▶ Performance of scrotal urethrostomy necessitates castration of the animal. Inform the owner prior to undertaking surgery.

- Animals that have azotemia because of urethral obstruction are treated prior to undertaking a prolonged anesthetic and operative procedure.

Surgical Procedure—Scrotal Urethrostomy

Objectives

- Allow the discharge of urine proximal to the site of urethral obstruction or destruction.
- Diminish the possibility of urethral obstruction due to urinary calculi.

Equipment

- Standard surgical instruments and suture
- Monofilament nonabsorbable suture (4–0 or 5–0) or synthetic absorbable suture (4–0 or 5–0) with swaged taper or taper-cut needle.

- Urethral catheter
- Delicate forceps for grasping and holding the urethra (optional)
- Magnification (optional)

Technique*

1. Place the dog in dorsal recumbency.
2. Prepare the caudal ventral abdomen, prepuce, scrotum, and ventral perineal region for aseptic surgery.
3. Make a circumferential incision around the scrotum at the point of reflection of the skin from the ventral body wall (Fig. 1A). Preserve enough skin to minimize tension on the suture line.
4. Isolate, ligate, and divide the spermatic cords and vessels by a combination of sharp and blunt dissection.
5. Free the scrotum and testes of their attachments to the ventral abdomen and penis and remove them (Fig. 1B).
6. Retract the paired retractor penis muscles laterally.
7. Secure the tunic of the penis to the subcutaneous tissues with four to six interrupted sutures of absorbable material (2–0 or 3–0) (Fig. 1C).
8. Place these sutures in such a manner that an adequate amount of skin is available to be sutured with minimal tension to the site of incision in the ventral urethra.
9. Make an incision in the ventral surface of the urethra for the length of the urethrostomy site (approximately 5 cm) (Fig. 1D).
10. If tension is encountered as the skin is drawn towards the edge of the urethra, abduct the stifles. This usually diminishes the amount of tension placed on the skin in this position.
11. Suture the skin to the edge of the urethra with 3–0 or 4–0 monofilament nonabsorbable suture in an interrupted or continuous pattern (Fig. 1E and F). The distal continuation of the urethra into the os penis remains open.

Postoperative Care and Complications

- Apply an Elizabethan collar or a body brace to prevent postoperative self-mutilation.
- Hemorrhage may be observed intermittently from the urethrostomy site. This is particularly noticeable when the animal urinates. In the immediate postoperative period, treat this by application of pressure or a cold compress. Sedation of the animal, particularly with acepromazine (which may decrease the systemic blood pressure), may also decrease the incidence of hemorrhage. Warn the owner that hemorrhage may occur for up to 2 weeks after the surgery.
- Remove sutures 2 weeks after surgery. Sedate animals that are difficult to handle for suture removal.

KEY POINT ▶ Inform the owner that the removal of the sutures may result in intermittent

---

*The procedure for scrotal urethrostomy is described. The technique may be applied to urethrostomy in the perineal or prescrotal position.

hemorrhage from the urethrostomy site for 2 to 3 days.

- Treat the presence of UTI and urinary calculi by appropriate antibiotic, dietary, and medical therapy. Inform the owner that performance of urethrostomy will not treat UTI or prevent calculi formation and that urethral obstruction may recur if calculi form.
- Leakage of urine into the subcutaneous tissues is uncommon.
- Stricture formation is extremely uncommon but may occur. If this happens, repeat the surgery.
- Scalding of the inner surface of the thighs by contact of the skin with urine is extremely uncommon.
- Prolonged urethral obstruction and distension of the bladder may result in a loss of detrusor function of the bladder.
- Urinary incontinence is uncommon.

PERINEAL URETHROSTOMY IN THE MALE CAT

Preoperative Considerations

- This procedure is performed most often in cats that suffer recurrent urethral obstruction because of feline urologic syndrome (FUS). Improved dietary management of this disorder has greatly decreased the frequency with which this procedure is performed.

KEY POINT ▶ Performance of perineal urethrostomy will not cure FUS, and signs of this disorder may persist after surgery. Inform the owner that the surgery is performed to diminish the probability of urethral obstruction and not to cure FUS.

- This procedure can be used to treat any form of urethral obstruction due to lesions of the urethra distal to the bulbourethral glands.
- Performance of this procedure necessitates castration of the cat and amputation of the distal penis. Inform the owner of these procedures.

Surgical Procedure

Objectives

- Create a cutaneous opening of the urethra near the bulbourethral glands.
- Create a urethral opening of satisfactory diameter.
- Minimize tension across the suture line to decrease the potential for stricture formation.
- Preserve urethral sphincter function.

Equipment

- Standard surgical instruments and suture
- Delicate instruments to handle urethra
- 3.5 Fr. catheter
- Fine periosteal elevator (Freer)
- Monofilament suture (4–0 or 5–0)

Technique

1. Place the cat in ventral recumbency with the hindquarters slightly elevated.

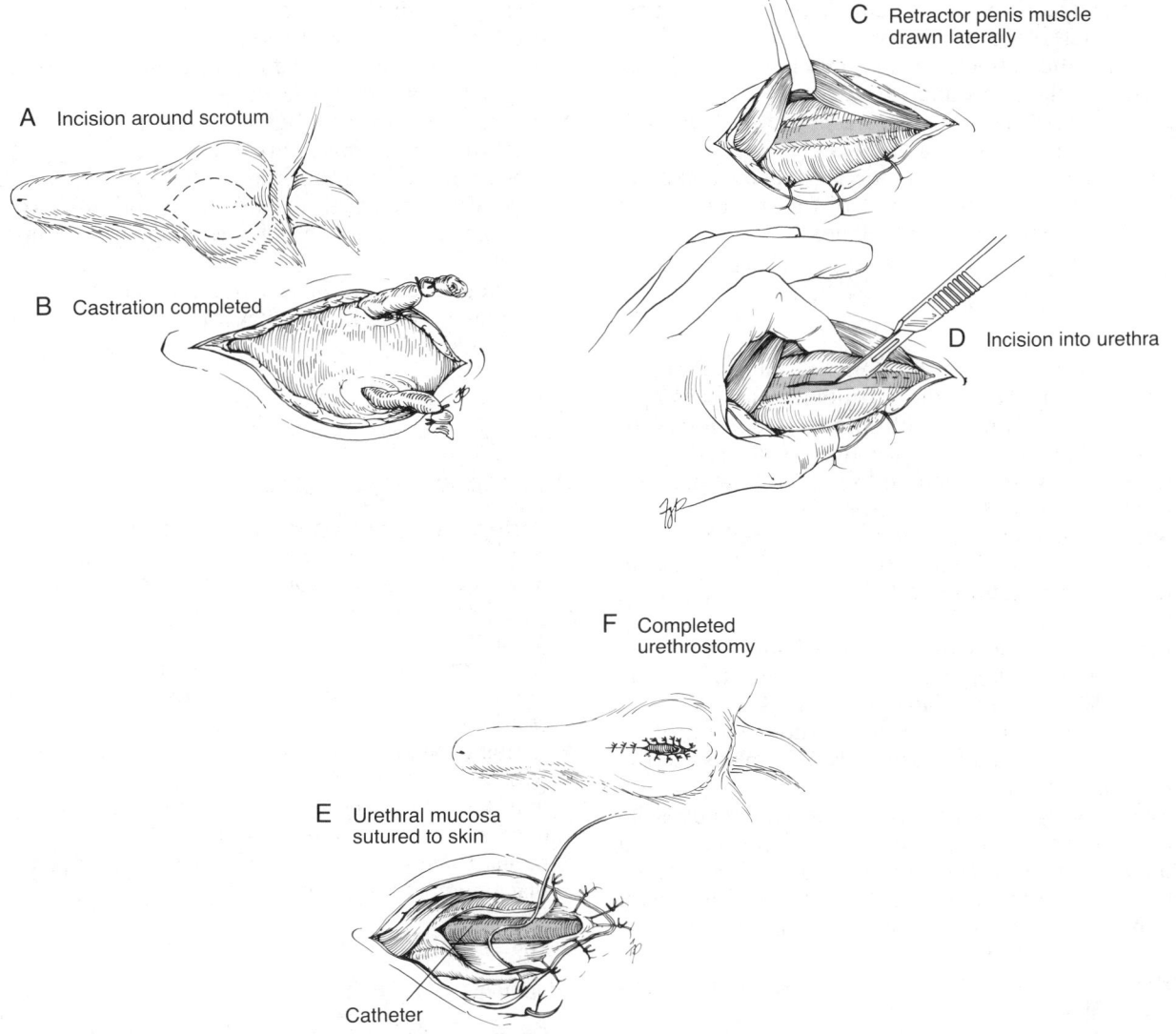

Figure 1. Scrotal urethrostomy. *A,* An incision is made encircling the scrotum. *B,* The spermatic cord and vessels are ligated and severed, and the scrotum and testes are removed. *C,* The retractor penis muscles are drawn laterally, and the subcutaneous tissues are secured to the corpora cavernosa. *D,* An incision is made on the ventral midline of the urethra. Placement of a catheter facilitates identification of the urethra. *E,* The urethra is sutured to the skin. *F,* The cranial opening of the urethra at the urethrostomy site remains open. (From Smeak DD, Fingeroth JM: Scrotal urethrostomy. *In* Bojrab MJ, ed.: *Current Techniques in Small Animal Surgery,* 3rd ed. Philadelphia: Lea & Febiger, 1990, p 381.)

2. Secure the tail in a forward position.
3. Place a pursestring suture around the anus.
4. Completely evacuate urine from the bladder.
5. Prepare the perineal area surrounding the scrotum and prepuce for aseptic surgery.
6. If the cat is intact, make an incision at the reflection of the scrotum from the surrounding skin. This incision encircles the scrotum and continues ventrally along the line of reflection of the prepuce from the skin.
7. If the cat has previously been castrated, make an incision encircling the prepuce and scrotal remnant. Ventrally, the incision comes to a point.
8. Isolate, ligate, and divide the spermatic cords and vessels.
9. Sharply divide the ventral attachments of the penis to the pelvic floor near their attachment to the penis.
10. Continue sharp and blunt dissection circumferen-

tially adjacent to the penis until the ischiocavernous muscles are identified. Take care to restrict dissection to the area immediately adjacent to the penis.
11. Divide or free the ischiocavernous muscles and penile ligament of their attachments to the ischium to allow the penis to be drawn caudally. The muscles will bleed profusely if incised.
12. Incise the fascia overlying the attachment of the ischiocavernous muscles to the ischium.
13. Sever the attachment of the ischiocavernous muscles to the ischium with a periosteal elevator. This usually results in minimal hemorrhage.
14. Continue dissection in a cranial direction until the penis is freed of its ventral attachments and the caudal aspect of the bulbourethral glands lies at the level of the skin incision.
15. Limit dorsal dissection to minimize the potential for incontinence.

16. Retract the penis in a caudal direction, and pass the catheter into the urethra.
17. Identify the retractor penis muscle on the dorsal aspect of the penis and excise it.
18. Excise the distal penis and prepuce and discard, along with the scrotum and testes.
19. With the urethral catheter in place, make an incision in the dorsal aspect of the urethra to the level of the bulbourethral glands.

KEY POINT ▶ Continue the incision cranially until the portion of the urethra that enlarges in diameter is reached.

20. Secure the tunic of the penis distal to the bulbourethral glands to the subcutaneous tissues by a few (two to four total) interrupted sutures of absorbable material. Place these sutures so that the skin may be brought to the edge of the urethral incision without tension across the suture line.
21. Suture the skin to the edge of the urethra. Place the first suture through the apex of the incision through the urethra and the most dorsal aspect of the skin incision.
22. Place interrupted sutures on either side from dorsal to ventral to create a satisfactory urethrostomy opening. Use monofilament suture (4–0 or 5–0).
23. After sutures have been placed along the urethra for a distance of approximately 1.5 cm, excise the remaining penis.
24. Place and tighten an encircling suture submucosally around the exposed end of the penis. This will diminish hemorrhage from the body of the penis.
25. Close the remainder of the skin incision with nonabsorbable suture in an interrupted or continuous pattern.
26. Remove the urethral catheter upon completion of the surgery.
27. Remove the pursestring suture around the anus.

Postoperative Care and Complications

- An Elizabethan collar is often used to prevent self-inflicted damage of the urethrostomy site. Many surgeons, however, prefer to allow the cat access to the operative site to keep it clean.
- Hemorrhage is frequently observed after surgery. In the early postoperative period, control is by application of pressure or cold compresses (ice packs). Tranquilization of the animal may be helpful in controlling prolonged hemorrhage.
- Stricture of the urethrostomy site is one of the more commonly observed complications.
  - This complication most often results from failure to satisfactorily free the penis from its attachments within the pelvic canal, causing tension on the suture line; poor mucosa-to-skin apposition; or failure to continue the urethral incision far enough cranially.
- Subcutaneous leakage of urine may result in cellulitis and abscessation. This leakage usually results from poor mucosa-to-skin apposition, especially at the proximal aspect of the urethrostomy.
- Urinary or fecal incontinence is infrequently observed after perineal urethrostomy in cats.

- The overall incidence of UTI in cats after perineal urethrostomy is low; however, it is more commonly observed in these cats than in male cats that have not undergone the procedure.
- Perineal hernia has been reported after perineal urethrostomy in male cats but is rare.
- Obstruction of the urethra may occur after performance of a perineal urethrostomy because of the persistence of FUS or the development of urinary calculi.
- Prolonged urethral obstruction and distension of the bladder may result in a loss of detrusor function of the bladder.

PREPUBIC URETHROSTOMY

Preoperative Considerations

- Perform this procedure for treatment of diseases resulting in the loss of urethral function distal to the prostatic and pelvic portions of the urethra.
- This procedure can be performed in male or female animals.
- If a sufficient length of urethra and the associated innervation remain intact, the animal retains urinary continence.
- If this procedure is to be performed in a male dog with an enlarged prostate, a partial prostatectomy may have to be performed. This prevents the presence of the enlarged prostate within the subcutaneous tissues from interfering with the appropriate placement of the stoma.

Surgical Procedure

Objectives

- Create a new urethral opening on the ventral abdominal surface using the remaining length of urethra.
- Retain urinary continence.

Equipment

- Standard surgical instruments and suture
- Balfour retractors
- Monofilament nonabsorbable suture (4–0 or 5–0)
- Urethral catheter
- Magnification (optional)

Technique

1. Place the animal in dorsal recumbency.
2. Prepare the caudal surface of the ventral abdomen for aseptic surgery.
3. Make an incision on the ventral midline of the abdomen from the umbilicus to the pubis in female dogs and cats and male cats and in a parapreputial position in male dogs.
4. Examine the bladder, prostate (in male dogs), and urethra.
5. Identify the diseased portion of the urethra.
6. Transect the urethra, retaining the maximal amount of normal proximal urethra.
7. Resect the affected urethra if neoplasia is present.

8. Ligate vessels leading to the distal portion of the urethra and associated tissues.

KEY POINT ▶ Take care during dissection to preserve the innervation and vascular supply of the bladder neck and proximal urethra.

9. If difficulty is encountered in identifying the lumen of the proximal urethra, pass a catheter in a retrograde direction or perform a cystotomy to allow passage in an antegrade direction.
10. Bring the proximal urethra and adjacent structures to the level of the skin incision, and select an appropriate site to create the stoma.
11. The stoma is created on the ventral midline in female dogs and cats and male cats and in a parapreputial position in male dogs. The stoma can be placed in the incision through which the abdominal cavity was entered. Position the stoma to allow the urethra to curve in a gentle arc through the ventral abdominal wall to avoid kinking or obstructing the urethra (Fig. 2).
12. Avoid twisting the urethra when passing it through the abdominal wall.
13. Close the abdominal wall in a standard manner leaving 1.5–2.0 cm of the distal end of the proximal urethra exposed. The abdominal wall is not tightly closed in the area through which the urethra passes.
14. Secure the adventitia surrounding the urethra to the subcutaneous tissues with two absorbable sutures.
15. Make an incision 1.5–2.0 cm in length on the ventral surface of the distal end of the proximal urethra. This is done to increase the diameter of the stoma.
16. Close the subcutaneous tissues in a standard manner.
17. Partially close the skin incision.
18. Suture the end of the urethra to the skin with monofilament nonabsorbable suture (4–0 or 5–0) in an interrupted pattern to create the urethrostomy opening.
19. Close the remainder of the skin incision in a standard manner.
20. Passage of a catheter into the urethra may facilitate accurate placement of sutures through the wall of the urethra.
21. Do not leave the catheter in place after surgery unless monitoring of urine output is necessary.

Postoperative Care and Complications

■ Use an Elizabethan collar or a body brace to prevent trauma after surgery.
■ Leakage of urine into the subcutaneous space or abdominal cavity will result in cellulitis or peritonitis. Prevent this by accurate suture placement during the operative procedure.
■ Stricture formation is an unusual complication of this procedure. When stricture occurs, repeat the surgery or revise the opening.
■ If the procedure is performed appropriately and a satisfactory length of proximal urethra is available, urinary continence is retained. If urinary continence is lost, treatment with alpha-agonists (see sec. 8, ch. 7) can be instituted to increase urethral tone. This therapy may or may not be successful if nerve or muscle function is lost.
■ Performance of prepubic urethrostomy predisposes an animal to the development of ascending UTI.
■ Loss of urinary continence predisposes an animal to scalding of the ventral abdominal surface with urine.
■ In obese animals or animals with redundant skin in the area of the urethral stomas, resection of skin and fat may be required to prevent obstruction of the stoma by adjacent skin folds.
■ Urethral obstruction may occur because of the placement of the stoma in a position that results in the development of an acute angle in the urethra.

URETHRAL PROLAPSE IN THE MALE DOG

Preoperative Considerations

■ This prolapse occurs most often in young brachycephalic dogs.
■ The most common complaint of the owner is that the dog develops hematuria when it urinates or becomes excited. Hemorrhage is usually self-limiting.
■ After the exposed urethral tissue has been traumatized, hemorrhage may recur during or following urination because of dislodgement of blood clots by the flow of urine.
■ Diagnosis of urethral prolapse is made by direct observation of exposed urethral tissue that appears as a ring surrounding the external urethral orifice. In this diagnosis, the penis must be extruded from the prepuce.
■ If the animal is not to be used for breeding, castration may help control urethral prolapse.

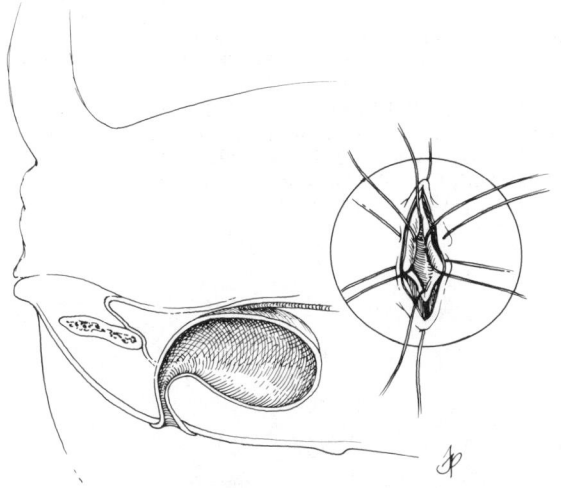

Figure 2. Prepubic urethrostomy. The urethra is brought across the body wall at a "gentle angle" to prevent urethral obstruction. An incision is made on the ventral surface of the urethra, and the urethra is sutured to the skin. (From Bjorling DE: Traumatic injuries of the urogenital system. Vet Clin North Am [Sm Anim Pract] 14:61, 1984.)

Surgical Procedure

Objectives

■ Prevent hemorrhage from the tip of the penis.
■ Excise exposed urethral tissue and prevent recurrence.
■ Maintain an adequate urethral lumen.

Equipment

■ Standard surgical instruments and suture
■ Tourniquet or Penrose drain
■ Urethral catheter
■ Monofilament nonabsorbable suture (4–0 or 5–0)

Technique

1. Place the dog in dorsal recumbency.
2. Prepare the interior of the prepuce and the penis for aseptic surgery.
3. Extrude the penis from the prepuce.
4. Pass a urethral catheter into the urethra until the tip lies approximately at the level of the scrotum.
5. Apply a tourniquet to the penis caudal to the os penis. Application of the tourniquet will maintain the penis in an exteriorized position. Use a commercial tourniquet or a tourniquet created with a forceps and Penrose drain.
6. Partially excise the exposed urethral mucosa by making an incision through the distal extent of the penile tunic and urethra, extending around half the circumference of the distal penis. This incision is proximal to damaged urethral mucosa and provides an exposed edge of the penile tunic, which is subsequently sutured to the urethra.
7. Suture the cut edge of the urethra to the tunic of the penis with monofilament nonabsorbable suture (4–0 to 5–0) in an interrupted pattern.
8. After the incision that has been made is partially closed, excise the remainder of the exposed urethral tissue by continuing the incision circumferentially.
9. Close the remainder of the defect with monofilament nonabsorbable suture in a similar interrupted pattern.

KEY POINT ▶ The purpose of initiating closure prior to complete excision of the urethral tissue is to prevent retraction of the urethral tissue within the penis and to facilitate accurate suture placement.

10. Remove the tourniquet and urethral catheter.

Postoperative Care and Complications

■ Intermittent hemorrhage may persist for 2–3 days (or longer) after surgery. This is usually associated with urination or excitement. If hemorrhage is excessive, re-examine the tip of the penis. Make a decision regarding placement of additional sutures. Tranquilization (e.g., with acepromazine) of the dog may decrease the occurrence of hemorrhage.
■ Recurrence of urethral prolapse is uncommon. If this occurs, repeat the surgery.
■ Mutilation may occur and is discouraged by the use of an Elizabethan collar, a body brace, or sedation.
■ Sedate the dog for suture removal.
■ Urethral prolapse rarely occurs in older animals. If observed in older animals, give consideration to the presence of a tumor at the tip of the penis. If the surgeon has any concern that the tissue excised may be neoplastic, submit this tissue for histologic evaluation. Tumors of the distal urethra and penis are extremely uncommon.

Supplemental Readings

Anson Al W: Urethral trauma and principles of urethral surgery. Compend Cont Ed Pract Vet 9:981, 1987.

Bjorling DE: Traumatic injuries of the urogenital system. Vet Clin North Am [Sm Anim Pract] 14:61, 1984.

Bradley RL: Prepubic urethrostomy: An acceptable urinary diversion technique. Probl Vet Med 1:120, 1989.

Gregory CR, Holliday TA, Vasseur PB, et al.: Electromyographic and urethral pressure profilometry: Assessment of urethral function before and after perineal urethrostomy in cats. Am J Vet Res 45:2062, 1984.

Gregory CR, Willits NH: Electromyographic and urethral pressure evaluations: Assessment of urethral function in female and ovariohysterectomized female cats. Am J Vet Res 47:1472, 1986.

Layton CE, Ferguson HR, Cook JE, Guffy MM: Intrapelvic urethral anastomosis: A comparison of three techniques. Vet Surg 16:175, 1987.

Poogird W, Wood AKW: Radiologic study of the canine urethra. Am J Vet Res 47:2491, 1986.

Smith CW: Surgical diseases of the urethra. *In* Slatter D, ed.: *Textbook of Small Animal Surgery.* Philadelphia: W. B. Saunders, 1985, p 1799.

Weber WJ, Boothe HW, Brassard JA, Hobson HP: Comparison of the healing of prescrotal urethrotomy incisions in the dog: Sutured vs. nonsutured. Am J Vet Res 46:1309, 1985.

Yoshioka MM, Carb A: Antepubic urethrostomy in the dog. J Am Anim Hosp Assoc 18:290, 1982.

7 Micturition Disorders

Mary Anna Labato

Micturition is a two-stage process involving the passive storage and the active voiding of urine. Processes that interfere with the storage and voiding of urine are termed micturition disorders. The loss of voluntary control of micturition is defined as urinary incontinence.

Most cases of micturition disorders have been reported in middle-aged and geriatric dogs. The clinical importance of these disorders is twofold:

- Incontinence is unacceptable to most owners; if not adequately treated, this disorder may result in euthanasia of the pet.
- Micturition disorders may lead to unresponsive urinary tract infection, resulting in an ascending pyelonephritis.

It is critical that the etiology of micturition disorders is diagnosed correctly in order to implement proper treatment.

NORMAL ANATOMY AND PHYSIOLOGY OF THE URINARY BLADDER

In order to recognize the many possible manifestations of micturition disorders, it is imperative to understand the anatomy of the bladder, its functional composition, and the neurophysiology of micturition.

Bladder Function

Bladder function is primarily under the influence of smooth muscle. The body of the bladder contains smooth muscle, referred to as the detrusor muscle. The outlet conduit is composed of the trigone and proximal urethra. The smooth muscle fibers of the detrusor continue into the proximal urethra, forming a functional internal urethral sphincter. The distal urethra is composed of striated skeletal muscle and functions as an external sphincter.

During the storage phase of micturition, the bladder functions as a low-resistance, high-capacity vessel. The urethra functions as a high-resistance barrier. The reverse is true during the voiding phase. The bladder acts as a muscular pump, and the urethra is a low-resistance vessel.

Nervous Control

Nervous control of the bladder and urethra is a combination of autonomic and somatic interactions. The micturition reflex is integrated by numerous inter-neurons and synapses between the sympathetic and parasympathetic systems.

Parasympathetic Innervation

Parasympathetic innervation is supplied to the detrusor by the pelvic nerve, which arises from sacral spinal cord segments (S1–S3). Stimulation of the pelvic nerve results in detrusor contraction.

Sympathetic Innervation

Sympathetic innervation is supplied via the hypogastric nerve, which is composed of preganglionic fibers exiting the lumbar spinal cord (L1–L2) and synapses in the caudal mesenteric ganglion. Sympathetic innervation is supplied to both the detrusor and urethral smooth muscles and facilitates the storage phase of micturition. Alpha-adrenergic fibers synapse in smooth muscle in both the trigone and urethra. Stimulation results in contraction of these muscles and forms a functional internal urethral sphincter. There are also alpha-adrenergic fibers that have a modulating effect on the external urethral sphincter. Beta-adrenergic fibers synapse in the detrusor muscle; stimulation results in relaxation.

Somatic Innervation

The pudendal nerve, which arises from sacral spinal cord segments (S1–S3), provides somatic stimulation of the striated urethral musculature.

Higher Centers of Innervation

For voluntary control of micturition to occur there must be integration between the cerebral cortex, pons, and the spinoreticular tract. A second pathway from the cerebral cortex to the sacral nuclei coordinates voluntary sphincter control. Additionally, cerebellar neurons inhibit nervous transmission to the reticulo-spinal pathway in the pons.

ETIOLOGY OF MICTURITION DISORDERS AND INCONTINENCE

Disorders of micturition and continence can be divided broadly into two types: neurogenic and non-neurogenic (Table 1).

Neurogenic Disorders

There are three types of neurogenic disorders: lower motor neuron, upper motor neuron, and detrusor-urethral dyssynergia.

TABLE 1. Disorders of Micturition

Type of Disorder	Diagnostic Features	Treatment
Neurogenic		
Lower motor neuron bladder	1. Distended, easily expressed bladder 2. Continuous incontinence—dribbling of urine 3. No perineal or bulbospongiosus reflex 4. No detrusor reflex	1. No effective therapy 2. Manual expression q8h 3. Trial with bethanechol chloride 4. Concurrent antibiotics
Upper motor neuron bladder	1. Large, turgid bladder 2. Difficult manual expression 3. Increased sphincter tone 4. ± detrusor reflex	1. Aseptic intermittent catheterization initially 2. Concurrent antibiotics 3. Long-term management usually frustrating
Detrusor-urethral dyssynergia	1. Large, nonexpressible bladder 2. Initiation of urine stream with abrupt disruption of urination 3. Intact spinal reflexes 4. Bladder easily catheterized	1. Phenoxybenzamine 2. Baclofen 3. Diazepam 4. Dantrolene
Non-neurogenic		
Hormone-responsive incontinence	1. Older, neutered animal 2. Voluntary control of urination with intermittent incontinence 3. Incontinence usually when relaxed or asleep	1. Diethylstilbestrol (females) 2. Testosterone (males) 3. Phenylpropanolamine
Urethral incompetence	1. Loss of voluntary control when placed in a stressful situation or at rest 2. Ability to urinate voluntarily	1. Phenylpropanolamine 2. Ephedrine 3. Imipramine
Urge incontinence (detrusor hyperreflexia)	1. Frequent small urinations 2. Urine spraying 3. Stranguria 4. Hyperreflexive detrusor	1. Treat cystitis 2. Propantheline bromide 3. Flavoxate 4. Oxybutynin 5. Dicyclomine
Atony from overdistension	1. Large, flaccid bladder 2. Large residual urine volume 3. Continuous incontinence 4. Intact perineal and bulbospongiosus reflex 5. No detrusor reflex	1. Remove mechanical obstruction 2. Indwelling catheterization 3. Bethanechol chloride
Paradoxical incontinence	1. Stranguria 2. Persistent urine dribbling 3. Large, turgid bladder that is difficult to express	1. Remove obstruction 2. Indwelling catheterization 3. Surgical exploration
Ectopic ureter(s)	1. Continuous dribbling of urine 2. Ability to urinate voluntarily	1. Surgical transposition of ureters 2. Phenylpropanolamine

From Handbook of Small Animal Practice. New York: Churchill Livingstone, 1988. Reprinted with permission from Churchill Livingstone.

Lower Motor Neuron Disorders

Lower motor neuron, or atonic, bladder results from lesions involving the sacral spinal cord segments or pelvic nerve, including intervertebral disc disease, cauda equina syndrome, sacroiliac luxations, sacrococcygeal fracture/separation, and tumors (e.g., spinal lymphoma). This type of disorder causes both detrusor and sphincter areflexia. Dribbling of urine with the bladder remaining full often is referred to as overflow incontinence.

Upper Motor Neuron Disorders

Upper motor neuron, or automatic, bladder results from a lesion involving the spinal cord above the sacral spinal cord segments, such as intervertebral disc disease, tumor, or trauma. This disorder causes incomplete reflex detrusor contraction and spasticity of the urethral sphincter with resulting incomplete emptying of the bladder.

Voluntary control is lost and manual expression is difficult if not impossible. After a period of days to weeks the spinal reflexes resume. Nonvoluntary micturition is initiated when the threshold capacity of the bladder is reached (automatic bladder).

Detrusor-Urethral Dyssynergia

In this condition, the initiation of the detrusor reflex resulting in voiding is followed by an involuntary contraction of the urethral sphincter. It results from lesions or partial lesions (masses, degeneration) of the reticulospinal tract. Increased sympathetic activity of both the smooth and striated urethral musculatures may result from a lesion cranial to or involving the caudal mesenteric ganglion.

Non-neurogenic Disorders

A number of disorders resulting in urinary incontinence are non-neurogenic in origin. A brief description of each disorder follows.

Hormone-Responsive Incontinence

Hormone-responsive incontinence is one of the most frequently diagnosed disorders. It is a disorder of older animals (mean age of occurrence is 8 years); however, it has been documented in animals as young as 8–9 months.

Hormone-responsive incontinence is seen primarily in spayed female dogs, who may be predisposed because of decreased sex hormone production believed to contribute to the maintenance of normal urethral muscle tone and mucosal integrity.

Occasionally hormone-responsive incontinence occurs in castrated male dogs, and it has been reported infrequently in neutered male and female cats.

Urethral Incompetence (Stress Incontinence)

This is the most common nonhormonal cause of urinary incontinence in small animals. Stress incontinence is a syndrome reported in women that consists of involuntary release of urine secondary to an increase in intra-abdominal pressure without detrusor atony or detrusor hyperreflexia. Urethral incompetence is the veterinary counterpart of stress incontinence. The cause is thought to be urethral smooth muscle incompetence or urethral malposition.

Urge Incontinence (Detrusor Hyperreflexia)

Urge incontinence is the result of involuntary detrusor contractions resulting in frequent voiding of small volumes of urine. The condition may result from an inflamed or irritated bladder or occasionally from partial spinal long tract or cerebellar involvement. The syndrome commonly is seen in cats that suffer from cystitis or "feline urologic syndrome." However, an idiopathic form has been documented in cats and dogs without any evidence of cystitis.

Detrusor Atony From Overdistension

This condition results from a mechanical or functional outflow obstruction, causing separation of the tight junctions of the detrusor muscle. Subsequent contractions of the detrusor muscle are weak and ineffectual. A functional outflow obstruction may have a neurogenic component. It usually is the result of excessive sympathetic stimulation to the urethra, resulting in increased urethral tone. Common examples of mechanical obstruction are:

■ Urethral obstruction (especially in cats)
■ Cystic and urethral calculi
■ Neoplasia of the trigone or urethra
■ Severe urethritis
■ Stricture of the urethra
■ Prostate disease

As a result of a functional or mechanical obstruction, there is an increase in urine volume until the intravesicular pressure can overcome the urethral resistance. Once the urethral pressure has been overcome, dribbling of urine occurs because of ineffectual detrusor contractions.

Paradoxical Incontinence

This is similar to overflow incontinence from detrusor atony. It is an involuntary dribbling of urine associated with an outflow obstruction. It often results from a partial urethral obstruction caused by urethral calculi, neoplasia, or urethritis. The difference between the two conditions is a matter of duration and whether the atony is temporary or permanent. Paradoxical incontinence is of a shorter duration. When the partial obstruction is relieved, normal function returns, and the detrusor contracts effectively.

Ectopic Ureter(s)

Ectopic ureter and other congenital urethral malformations are a common cause of urinary incontinence. The abnormal entry of the ureter(s) into the distal urethra or vagina from a congenital malformation results in continuous or intermittent dribbling of urine.

CLINICAL SIGNS

■ Incontinence—dribbling of urine, loss of voluntary control, and urine-scald dermatitis
■ Abnormal micturition—inability to urinate, disruption of the urine stream, stranguria, dysuria, and abdominal pain or discomfort
■ Lower motor neuron bladder—dribbling of urine and a large distended bladder that is easily expressed by manual compression.
■ Upper motor neuron bladder:
  • A full bladder that is difficult to express initially.
  • Voluntary control is lost.
  • After a period of days to weeks, the spinal reflexes resume and nonvoluntary micturition is initiated when the threshold capacity of the bladder is reached.
  • Incomplete and inappropriate urination is the result.
■ Detrusor-urethral dyssynergia (differentiate from mechanical obstruction):
  • Initiation of voiding, often after a period of hesitation, which then is abruptly disrupted.
  • Stranguria
■ Hormone-responsive incontinence—normal voluntary urination with involuntary dribbling when the animal is relaxed or asleep.
■ Urethral incompetence (stress incontinence)—signs similar to hormone-responsive incontinence; also involuntary loss of urine when placed in a stressful or new situation
■ Detrusor hyperreflexia—frequent small urinations, stranguria, and urine spraying in cats; small bladder (compare detrusor atony from overdistension)
■ Detrusor atony from overdistension—stranguria, dysuria, persistent urine dribbling; large distended bladder
■ Paradoxical incontinence—same clinical signs as detrusor atony
■ Ectopic ureter(s):
  • Continuous or intermittent dribbling of urine usu-

ally with ability to urinate appropriately and voluntarily.
- Most commonly diagnosed in young dogs and cats

DIAGNOSIS

History

The history is of the utmost importance; include the following items:

- Reproductive status
- If animal was neutered, age at neutering
- Age at onset of problem
- Previous medical problems, especially those involving the urogenital system
- Previous history of trauma
- Description of abnormality
- If the problem is incontinence, ask:
  - Is it continuous or intermittent?
  - What is the amount of urine passed?
  - Is the animal aware that urine is being passed?
- If the animal has difficulty urinating, ask:
  - How frequent is urination?
  - Is there nocturia, dysuria, or hematuria?

Physical Examination

Perform a general examination with particular attention to the urogenital system, and perform a neurologic examination.

- Palpate the bladder carefully prior to and immediately following voiding to evaluate the extent of distension, tone, and ease with which the bladder may be expressed manually.
  - Lower motor neuron lesions generally are associated with easy manual expression and reduced sphincter tone.
  - Upper motor neuron lesions generally are associated with difficult manual expression and increased sphincter tone.
- In the neurologic examination, evaluate the innervation of the urogenital system.
  - The perineal reflex evaluates the pudendal nerve. Pricking or pinching the skin of the perineum results in contraction of the anal sphincter.
  - The bulbospongiosus reflex evaluates the integrity of both the pudendal nerve and sacral spinal segments. Squeezing the distal portion of the penis or the edges of the vulva will cause the anal sphincter to contract.
- Perform a rectal examination to evaluate the prostate gland, the pelvic diaphragm, and anal tone.

KEY POINT ▶ Observe the animal when urinating to verify the micturition abnormality.

- Measure the residual urine volume. Allow the animal to void until urine is no longer passed; catheterize the bladder and collect and measure any residual urine. In a normal animal, the residual urine volume should not exceed 0.4 ml/kg.
- Perform vaginoscopy if ectopic ureters are suspected; however, this is often a low-yield procedure. Ure-

throscopy is often diagnostic for ectopic ureter but requires specialized equipment.

Laboratory Evaluation

- Evaluate renal function by determining blood urea nitrogen and serum creatinine concentration.
- To evaluate for associated urinary tract infection, perform a urinalysis and urine culture and sensitivity test via cystocentesis, if possible, before any bladder catheterization.

Radiographic Examination

Both survey and specialized studies may be useful.

- Use survey radiographs to evaluate any obvious abnormalities in the bladder, urethra, pelvis, or spine.
- Use contrast radiographic studies (intravenous urography, retrograde urethrocystography, and vaginourethrography; see sec. 1, ch. 4) to evaluate for:
  - Ectopic ureters
  - Bladder wall thickening
  - Calculi
  - Urachal diverticulum
  - Prostatic enlargement
  - Urethral strictures
  - Skeletal abnormalities in the pelvis

Urodynamic Studies

Urodynamic studies to evaluate micturition disorders routinely consist of the cystometrogram and urethral pressure profile; electromyography also may be a part of the study. These specialized modalities are readily available at most veterinary institutions and are becoming increasingly common in private referral practices.

- The cystometrogram is a pressure-volume recording that measures bladder tone and volume, threshold volume and pressure, maximum contraction pressure, and the detrusor reflex.
- The urethral pressure profile measures intra-urethral resistance and identifies and localizes areas of increased or decreased resistance.
- Electromyography can evaluate coordination of muscular activity between the detrusor and urethral sphincter. Electromyography is usually performed on the anal sphincter; however, with specialized catheters that incorporate electrodes it can also be performed directly on the urethral sphincter.

Diagnosis of Individual Disorders
Lower Motor Neuron Bladder

- The bladder typically is large, distended, and easily expressed.
- The incontinence is continuous.
- There is a loss of perineal, bulbospongiosus, and detrusor reflexes.

Upper Motor Neuron Bladder

- The bladder is large, turgid, and initially extremely difficult to express.

- There is a history of an inability to urinate.
- Frequently there is concomitant hindquarter paresis or paralysis.

Detrusor-Urethral Dyssynergia

- Diagnosis is made by observation; commonly there is stranguria, initiation of voiding, and then abrupt disruption of the urine stream.
- Palpation often reveals a large, nonexpressible bladder.
- The bladder is easily catheterized.
- There is no evidence of stricture or obstruction when a retrograde contrast cystourethrogram is performed. A cystometrogram reveals an intact pelvic nerve; however, the urethral pressure profile reveals increased resistance.

Hormone-Responsive Incontinence

- There is a history of neutering and the development of intermittent incontinence.
- Palpation commonly reveals a small bladder.
- Urinalysis may or may not show evidence of cystitis.
- Typically there is response to sex hormone supplementation.

KEY POINT ▶ Urinary tract infection results in an exaggeration of the incontinence; if infection is present, resolve it before making a diagnosis of hormone-responsive incontinence.

Urethral Incompetence (Stress Incontinence)

- There is a history of intermittent incontinence when the animal is at rest or placed in a stressful situation.
- Palpation reveals a small bladder.
- The animal is able to urinate voluntarily.
- There is no evidence of infection on urinalysis.
- There are no radiographic abnormalities.

Urge Incontinence or Detrusor Hyperreflexia

- On physical examination the bladder is found to be small.
- Cystometrography reveals involuntary smooth muscle contractions during the filling phase of micturition. Contractions can be spontaneous or provoked but cannot be suppressed.
- Urodynamically, detrusor instability usually appears as a rapid, involuntary increase of >15 cm of water pressure during the filling phase of the cystometrogram. However, there is voluntary control of urination.
- In cases associated with cystitis, there may be a history of urine spraying or infection, and there is evidence of inflammation on urinalysis. A urine culture may be positive or negative.
- With cystitis, the bladder may be thickened on palpation, and a contrast cystourethrogram may reveal bladder wall thickening.
- In idiopathic detrusor hyperreflexia there is no evidence of cystitis and no abnormalities on contrast cystourethrograms.

Detrusor Atony from Overdistension

- There is a history of continuous incontinence and urine outflow obstruction.
- Abdominal palpation reveals a large, flaccid bladder.
- Neurologic examination reveals intact perineal and bulbospongiosus reflexes; yet there is an absent or weak detrusor reflex.
- There is a large residual urine volume.
- Urodynamic studies may help rule out a neurogenic component.

Paradoxical Incontinence

- Base the diagnosis on the results of an urinalysis, plain, and often contrast, radiographs.

Ectopic Ureters

- Definitive diagnosis made by intravenous urography and retrograde cystourethrography.
- There usually is a history of continuous incontinence with ability to urinate voluntarily. Usually a small bladder is revealed on abdominal palpation.
- In the physical examination urine-soaked fur often is seen along the rear legs.
- The animal typically is young when the diagnosis is made.

TREATMENT

Individual Disorders

Individual disorders are discussed in terms of their treatment modalities. See Table 2 for details of treatment, including drug dosages.

KEY POINT ▶ Remember that urocystitis commonly is associated with micturition disorders. Proper treatment of the underlying infection is equally as important as the treatments recommended for individual disorders.

Lower Motor Neuron Bladders

- Manually express the bladder three or four times daily.
- Long-term therapy for this disorder has not been successful.
- Bethanechol may be administered to increase detrusor contractions. Side effects such as vomiting, diarrhea, salivation, and anorexia may limit the drug's usefulness.
- Complications include urine scalding, decubital ulcers, and recurrent urinary tract infections.
- Agents that have been used experimentally to treat an atonic or hypocontractile bladder include metoclopramide, which has been reported to directly stimulate detrusor contractions in humans and dogs, and prostaglandins E_2 and F_2, which have been shown to stimulate both detrusor and urethral smooth muscle.

TABLE 2. Pharmacologic Management of Micturition Disorders

Agent	Class	Indications	Dosages	Side Effects	Contraindications
Baclofen (Lioresal; Geigy)	Skeletal muscle relaxant	Detrusor-urethral dyssynergia	Dogs: 1–2 mg/kg q8h PO	General muscle weakness Gastrointestinal upset	
Bethanechol chloride (Urecholine; Merck Sharp & Dohme)	Parasympathomimetic	Detrusor atony	Dogs: 2.5–10.0 mg q8h SC Cats: 2.5–5.0 mg q8h PO	Vomiting Diarrhea Salivation Anorexia	Urethral obstruction
Dantrolene (Dantrium; Norwich Eaton)	Skeletal muscle relaxant	Functional urethral obstruction due to increased external urethral tone	Dogs: 3–15 mg divided q8–12h PO	Generalized muscle weakness Hepatotoxicity	
Diazepam (Valium; Roche Products)	Skeletal muscle relaxant	Functional urethral obstruction due to increased external urethral tone	Dogs: 2–10 mg q8h PO	Sedation	
Dicyclomine (Bentyl; Marion Merrell Dow)	Anticholinergic, direct-acting smooth muscle relaxant	Detrusor hyperreflexia Urge incontinence	Dogs/Cats: 10 mg q6–8h PO	Diarrhea Sedation	Obstructive uropathy Hyperthyroidism Cardiac disease Prostatic hypertrophy
Ephedrine (various brand names and manufacturers)	Alpha-adrenergic agonist	Urethral sphincter incompetence	Dogs: 5–15 mg q8h PO Cats: 2–4 mg q8h PO	Restlessness Excitability Hypertension	Hypertension
Estrogens (Diethylstilbestrol; Lilly)	Female sex hormone	Hormone-responsive incontinence	Dogs: 0.1–1.0 mg/day for 3 days, then 1.0 mg once weekly PO	Induce signs of estrus Bone marrow toxicity	
Flavoxate (Urispas; Smith Kline & French)	Anticholinergic, smooth muscle relaxant	Detrusor hyperreflexia Urge incontinence	Dogs/Cats: 100–200 mg q6–8h PO	Vomiting Increased intraocular pressure Tachycardia	Glaucoma
Imipramine (Tofranil; Geigy)	Tricyclic antidepressant	Urethral incompetence	Dogs: 5–15 mg q12h PO Cats: 2.5–5.0 mg q12h PO	Tachycardia Tremors Hyperexcitability Seizures	
Oxybutynin (Ditropan; Marion Merrell Dow)	Anticholinergic, smooth muscle relaxant	Detrusor hyperreflexia	Dogs/Cats: 5 mg q8–12h PO	Diarrhea Sedation	Hyperthyroidism Cardiac disease Prostatic disease
Phenoxybenzamine (Dibenzyline; Smith Kline & French)	Alpha-adrenergic blocker	Functional outflow obstruction	Dogs/Cats: 0.25–0.5 mg/kg q8h PO Dogs (alternate): 2.5–20.0 mg/day PO	Nausea Hypertension Increased intraocular pressure	Glaucoma Diabetes mellitus
Phenylpropanolamine (various brand names and manufacturers)	Alpha-adrenergic agonist	Urethral sphincter incompetence Hormone responsive incontinence	Dogs: 1–2 mg/kg q12h PO Cats: 1 mg/kg q12h PO	Restlessness Excitability Hypertension	Hypertension
Propantheline bromide (Pro-Banthine; Schiapparelli Searle)	Anticholinergic	Detrusor hyperreflexia Urge incontinence	Dogs: 7.5–30 mg q8–24h PO start low Cats: 7.5 mg q24–72h PO	Vomiting Xerostomia Sedation Constipation Increased intraocular pressure	Glaucoma
Testosterone					
Testosterone cypionate (DEPO-testosterone; Upjohn)	Male sex hormone	Hormone-responsive incontinence	Dogs: 1–2 mg/kg q2–4 wk IM		
Testosterone propionate			Dogs: 0.5–1 mg/kg, 2–3× per week, SC or IM		

From Handbook of Small Animal Practice. New York: Churchill Livingstone, 1988. Reprinted with permission from Churchill Livingstone.

Upper Motor Neuron Bladders

- Initially it is difficult to express the bladder manually. Because of the risk of bladder rupture, do not attempt this until manual evacuation of the bladder is tolerable.
- Instead, aseptically catheterize the patient at least three times daily to completely empty the bladder. Avoid using an indwelling catheter because of the risk of urinary tract infections.
- Perform frequent urinalyses with culture and sensitivity testing.
- Concurrent antibacterial agents may be indicated, especially with long-term intermittent catheterization.

Detrusor-Urethral Dyssynergia

Treat by decreasing sympathetic tone or with muscle relaxants (see Table 2):

- Phenoxybenzamine is an alpha-adrenergic blocking agent used to decrease internal sphincter resistance.
- Diazepam and dantrolene can be used as skeletal muscle relaxants to decrease external sphincter resistance.
- Baclofen is a skeletal muscle relaxant that decreases muscle tone by a depressive effect on the central nervous system (CNS). The drug inhibits medullary interneurons and spinal reflexes.

Hormone-Responsive Incontinence

Replacement of the sex hormone is necessary for successful treatment (see Table 2).

- Treat female dogs with diethylstilbestrol.

KEY POINT ▶ Estradiol cypionate is not recommended because of the potential for bone marrow suppression.

- Testosterone cypionate may be used in male dogs. No side effects have been noted.
- In some instances, animals develop a tolerance for hormonal replacement. Additional therapy with a sympathetic alpha-agonist that increases urethral tone is then indicated (see Table 2).

Urethral Incompetence (Stress Incontinence)

Treat with drugs that increase urethral tone (see Table 2).

- The most successful drugs are the sympathomimetic alpha-adrenergic agonists, which directly increase urethral smooth muscle tone. The drug of choice is phenylpropanolamine; an alternate drug is ephedrine.
- Imipramine is a tricyclic antidepressant agent that causes inhibition of norepinephrine re-uptake at the synaptic level and results in increased urethral tone.

Urge Incontinence (Detrusor Hyperreflexia)

Treat with drugs that reduce detrusor hyperspasticity and relax smooth muscle (see Table 2).

- Propantheline bromide is an anticholinergic drug which decreases detrusor hyperspasticity. Start with the lowest possible dosage and slowly increase until signs are alleviated or side effects are encountered.
- Direct-acting smooth muscle relaxants are promising in the treatment of this syndrome. These drugs also have a mild anticholinergic effect. Recommended drugs include flavoxate, oxybutynin, and dicyclomine.

Detrusor Atony From Overdistension

This is the single disorder in which indwelling urinary catheterization for up to 7–14 days is indicated to keep the bladder as small as possible in order to re-establish tight junction connections in the detrusor muscle.

- It is imperative to remove the obstruction or primary cause. Occasionally anti-inflammatory therapy (corticosteroids) is indicated.

- Perform frequent urinalyses and administer appropriate antibiotics, based upon susceptibility results.
- The cholinergic drug bethanechol has been used successfully to stimulate detrusor contractions in both neurogenic and non-neurogenic atonic bladders (see Table 2). It is effective for postobstructive atony; however, be careful to ensure urethral patency.
- When the overdistension is caused by increased urethral resistance, administer an alpha-adrenergic blocker prior to giving bethanechol chloride. Phenoxybenzamine is the drug of choice (see Table 2).

Paradoxical Incontinence

Treat by relieving the obstruction. Retropulsion of calculi or urethrostomy (e.g., urethritis) or surgical exploration (e.g., neoplasia) (see sec. 8, ch. 6) may be required.

- In some instances indwelling catheterization may be indicated (e.g., severe urethritis) until the inflammation is brought under control.

Ectopic Ureter(s)

Treat by surgical transposition of the ureter(s) to the trigonal area (see sec. 8, ch. 2).

- Ectopic ureters are often associated with other urinary tract abnormalities (urethral incompetence) that may be treated with alpha-adrenergic agonists.

Teflon Injections

Teflon injections have been used experimentally for the treatment of urethral sphincter incompetence in dogs (Arnold et al., 1989). A Teflon paste is injected cystoscopically into urethral and periurethral tissues. This procedure inflates the tissues and compresses the urethral lumen at the site of injection. Good results were achieved, and Teflon injection has been used in the treatment of urinary incontinence of diverse causes in human patients. This treatment holds promise for dogs that are resistant to pharmacologic management, but additional long-term studies are needed.

Surgical Techniques

Surgery for disorders of the urinary system and micturition are discussed elsewhere in this text (see sec. 8, chs. 2, 4, and 6).

Initial studies with a prosthetic sphincter made of Silastic (a polymeric silicone product) have been promising. This surgical technique possibly may be used as a last-resort therapy when medical management has failed, or when owners are unable or unwilling to administer medications indefinitely.

Supplemental Readings

Anderson K: Current concepts in the treatment of disorders of micturition. Drugs 35:477, 1988.

Arnold S, Jager P, DiBartola SP, et al.: Treatment of urinary incontinence in dogs by endoscopic injection of Teflon. J Am Vet Med Assoc 195:1369, 1989.

Dean PW, Novotny MJ, O'Brien DP: Prosthetic sphincter for urinary incontinence: Results in three cases. J Am Anim Hosp Assoc 25:447, 1989.

Labato MA: Disorders of micturition. *In* Morgan RV, ed.: *Handbook of Small Animal Practice.* New York: Churchill Livingstone, 1988, p 621.

Lappin MR, Barsanti JA: Urinary incontinence secondary to idiopathic detrusor instability: Cystometrographic diagnosis and pharmacologic management in two dogs and a cat. J Am Vet Med Assoc 191:1439, 1987.

Lovering JS, Tallett SE, McKendry JBJ: Oxybutynin efficacy in the treatment of primary enuresis. Pediatrics 82:104, 1988.

Moreau PM: Neurogenic disorders of micturition diagnosis and therapy. *In* Proceedings of Fourth Annual Veterinary Medical Forum. Washington D.C., 1986, p 4.

Moreau PM, Lappin MR: Pharmacologic management of urinary incontinence. *In* Kirk, RW, ed.: *Current Veterinary Therapy X.* Philadelphia: W. B. Saunders, 1989, p 1214.

Resnick NM, Subbarao VY, Laurino E: The pathophysiology of urinary incontinence among institutionalized elderly persons. N Engl J Med 320:1, 1989.

Ruffmann R: A review of flavoxate hydrochloride in the treatment of urge incontinence. J Int Med Res 16:317, 1988.

Sackman JE, Sims MH: Electromyographic evaluation of the external urethral sphincter during cystometry in male cats. Am J Vet Res 51:1237, 1990.

Zorzitto ML, Holliday PJ, Jewett MAS, Herschorn S, et al.: Oxybutynin chloride for geriatric urinary dysfunction: A double-blind placebo-controlled study. Age Aging 18:195, 1989.

8 Diseases of the Prostate Gland

Nancy D. Kay

Diseases of the prostate gland are common in middle-aged and older dogs. Large breed dogs (especially Doberman pinschers) are more commonly affected. Although cats have prostate glands, for unknown reasons feline prostatic disease is extremely rare. This chapter discusses canine prostatic disease only.

ETIOLOGY

Several types of prostatic disease exist and some may occur simultaneously (e.g., prostatic cyst with abscessation, prostatic neoplasia with bacterial prostatitis).

Benign Prostatic Hyperplasia

To some degree, both hypertrophy (increased size) and hyperplasia (increased numbers) of prostatic cells account for enlargement of the gland in all middle-aged and older noncastrated dogs.

KEY POINT ▶ Benign prostatic hyperplasia is the most common disorder of the prostate gland.

- Causes of benign prostatic hyperplasia include an imbalance in the ratio of androgens to estrogens, increased numbers of androgen receptors, and increased tissue sensitivity to androgens.
- Dihydrotestosterone is the main androgen that promotes prostatic hyperplasia.

Squamous Metaplasia

This morphologic alteration of prostatic epithelial cells is caused by estrogen stimulation arising from an exogenous or endogenous (e.g., Sertoli cell tumor) source.

Cystic Hyperplasia

This condition refers to the presence of multiple fluid-filled cavities within the prostatic parenchyma that result from the obstruction of glandular excretory ducts.

- Cystic hyperplasia commonly is associated with benign prostatic hyperplasia and squamous metaplasia.

Paraprostatic Cysts

These fluid-filled structures develop adjacent to the prostate gland and result from fluid accumulation within embryologic vestiges (uterus masculinis). The cystic lining may become calcified.

Bacterial Prostatitis

Bacterial prostatitis occurs when normal host resistance is altered.

- Predisposing causes include disruption of normal glandular architecture (benign hyperplasia, squamous metaplasia, neoplasia), urethral diseases, urinary tract infections, alterations in urine flow, altered prostatic secretions, and host immune dysfunction.
- Infection usually occurs by an ascending route, although hematogenous spread of bacteria also may occur.
- The most common pathogens are *Escherichia coli*, *Staphylococcus*, *Proteus mirabilis*, *Streptococcus*, and *Mycoplasma*. Less common isolates include *Klebsiella*, *Brucella canis*, *Pseudomonas*, and *Ureaplasma*. Anaerobic infections are rare.

Nonbacterial Prostatitis

Nonbacterial prostatitis has been documented in dogs.

- Clinical signs are similar to those associated with chronic bacterial prostatitis.
- The etiology of the inflammation is uncertain.

Prostatic Abscesses

Prostatic abscesses are extensions of bacterial prostatitis in which obstruction of an excretory duct has occurred.

- A pre-existing cyst may become an abscess when it becomes infected secondarily.

Prostatic Neoplasia

Neoplasia is relatively rare compared with other forms of canine prostatic disease.

- Prostatic adenocarcinoma and transitional cell carcinomas are most common.
- Previously, castration was thought to prevent the development of prostatic cancer. In one study (Obradovich et al., 1987), 19 of 43 dogs were castrated at least 3 years prior to the development of prostatic disease. It was concluded that castration at any age has no sparing effect on the development of prostate cancer.
- Development of prostatic cancer in dogs may not be hormonally mediated or may be influenced by nontesticular hormones. Hormones produced by the adrenal and pituitary glands may play a significant role.

CLINICAL SIGNS

Clinical signs associated with canine prostatic disease are variable. Depression, anorexia, and vomiting are systemic manifestations of bacterial prostatitis or prostatic abscessation. Other clinical signs do not correlate well with etiology (Table 1). Hematuria and blood dripping from the prepuce are the most frequent signs seen with most types of prostatic disease. In animals with uncomplicated benign prostatic hyperplasia, however, clinical signs frequently are absent until prostatomegaly becomes marked.

- *Hematuria* is caused by reflux of blood from the prostatic urethra into the bladder. It also may be associated with a concurrent bacterial cystitis.
- *Urethral discharge* results from the exudation of blood, pus, and/or prostatic fluid into the prostatic urethra. This fluid drips passively from the penile urethra and is often blood-tinged.
- *Stranguria* is present if partial or complete urethral obstruction results from prostatic enlargement.
- *Fecal tenesmus* or a *change in stool diameter* occurs when prostatic gland enlargement encroaches on the rectum. *Constipation* may be secondary to avoidance of pain associated with defecation.
- *Fever, depression, anorexia, vomiting,* and *diarrhea* are signs of systemic involvement and are most commonly associated with bacterial prostatitis or prostatic abscessation.
- *Recurrent urinary tract infection* in a male dog may be associated with nonresolving or recurrent bacterial prostatitis.
- *Abdominal distension* may be caused by a paraprostatic cyst or prostatic abscess.
- *Caudal abdominal pain, lumbar pain,* and/or *hindlimb stiffness* may be associated with metastasis of prostatic neoplasia to bone or muscle or with peritonitis associated with prostatic abscess.
- *Hypertrophic osteopathy* may occur secondary to prostatic disease such as tumors.
- *Hindlimb pitting edema* may occur secondary to lymphatic invasion by metastatic tumors.
- *Urinary incontinence* can be caused by impingement on the pelvic nerves by an adjacent prostatic mass (tumor or abscess).
- Other clinical conditions that may be associated with prostatic disease include *impaired libido, infertility, sepsis, ketoacidotic diabetes mellitus, perineal hernia,* and *testicular tumor.*

DIAGNOSIS

Localizing and defining the etiology of diseases of the prostate gland can be a challenging task. Until recently, few diagnostic techniques have combined reliability and specificity of results with safety and ease of application. The ideal method for the diagnosis of prostatic disease should localize the disease to the prostate gland and eliminate other parts of the urinary and reproductive tracts as sources of the disease.

Physical Examination

Abdominal palpation in dogs with prostatic disease may reveal abdominal pain, abdominal distension, or the presence of an abdominal mass.

KEY POINT ▶ A rectal examination is essential in the diagnosis of prostatic disease.

- In rectal examination, include palpation ventrally for assessment of the prostate gland and palpation dorsally for assessment of iliac lymph node enlargement or lumbar pain.
- Evaluate the prostate gland for location, size, symmetry, surface contour, consistency, movability, and pain. The normal prostate gland is intrapelvic symmetric, smooth, movable, and nonpainful.
- As the prostate gland enlarges with disease, it may move cranially over the pelvic brim. Therefore, simultaneous rectal and caudal abdominal palpation may be helpful.

KEY POINT ▶ The prostate gland of a normal Scottish terrier may be up to four times larger than those of other breeds.

TABLE 1. Incidence of Clinical Signs Associated with Prostatic Disease

Prostatic Disease (No. of Cases)*	Hematuria	Blood Dripping from Prepuce	Stranguria	Tenesmus	Depression/ Anorexia	Vomiting	Diarrhea	Abdominal Pain	Hindlimb Deficit	Chronic UTI
Bacterial prostatitis (12)	4	3	2	2	3	2	2	1	0	2
Nonbacterial prostatitis (7)	1	2	0	0	0	0	0	1	0	3
Hyperplasia (16)	7	6	1	1	0	0	1	0	0	4
Neoplasia (4)	3	3	2	3	0	0	0	0	1	0
Squamous metaplasia (2)	2	0	1	0	0	0	0	0	0	1

UTI = urinary tract infection.
*Some prostate glands were affected by more than one disease process.
From J Am Anim Hosp Assoc.

Imaging Studies

Abdominal Radiography

Abdominal radiography rarely determines the specific etiology of prostatic disease, but it can reveal various associated abnormalities, including:

- Prostatomegaly
- Prostate gland asymmetry
- Abnormal fluid-filled mass in the caudal abdomen
- Prostate gland mineralization
- Iliac lymph node enlargement
- Vertebral or pelvic bone periosteal reactions
- Decreased soft tissue detail in the caudal abdomen due to tissue inflammation
- Urinary or fecal retention

KEY POINT ▶ Prostate gland mineralization and iliac lymph node enlargement are often but not always associated with prostatic neoplasia.

Urethrography

Positive-contrast retrograde urethrography may help to localize the disease process. However, there is no correlation between the presence of urethroprostatic reflux and the type of prostatic disease. Reflux may be observed in some dogs without prostatic disease.

Ultrasonography

Ultrasonography can be used to evaluate the prostate and to guide percutaneous needle aspiration or needle core biopsy. Ultrasound observations may include:

- Prostatomegaly
- Intraprostatic cyst or abscess (appears as focally hypoechoic or anechoic)
- Paraprostatic cyst
- Focal or multifocal areas of increased echogenicity (may represent bacterial prostatitis or neoplasia)
- Shadowing (may represent bacterial prostatitis or neoplasia)
- Prostatic calculi
- Iliac lymphadenopathy

Laboratory Studies

Complete Blood Count (CBC)

- Hemogram abnormalities do not consistently correlate with the occurrence of infectious or noninfectious prostatic diseases. An exception is neutrophilic leukocytosis, which is consistently associated with acute, fulminant bacterial prostatitis.
- A mild to moderate nonregenerative anemia may occur in chronic inflammatory prostatic disease.

Urinalysis and Urine Culture

- Bacterial cystitis and bacterial prostatitis may occur independently.
- Urinalysis and urine culture are always indicated for animals with signs of urinary tract disease. However, they may not be useful in the diagnosis of prostatic disease.

- For example, urine sediment examination is not reliable for the diagnosis of prostatic neoplasia, and urine cultures can be negative in dogs with bacterial prostatitis or prostatic abscess.
- For this reason, in addition to urine, evaluate prostatic fluid or tissue or both in dogs suspected of prostatic disease.

Prostatic Fluid or Tissue Culture

This procedure is necessary for documentation of bacterial prostatitis. *Mycoplasma* organisms require specialized culture media (PPLO agar); therefore, it is necessary to specifically request this culture (see Tables 2–4 for techniques for collection of microbiology specimens).

Prostatic Fluid Cytology

Cytologic studies may identify benign prostatic hyperplasia, squamous metaplasia, bacterial prostatitis, nonbacterial prostatitis, and prostatic neoplasia (see Tables 2–4 for techniques for collection of cytology specimens).

Specimen Collection

Ejaculate Specimen

For purposes of ejaculate collection, handle the dog in a quiet environment. Many dogs are more responsive if exposed to a female in estrus or to vaginal swabs obtained from a female in estrus (see Table 2 for technique).

Advantages of this technique:

- It is relatively easy to perform.
- It is safe.
- It can be done without chemical restraint.
- It is inexpensive.
- It provides specimens for bacterial culture.

Disadvantages of this technique:

- Success depends on the animal's compliance, which may be diminished if the animal is old, ill, weak, or nervous and overexcited.
- It is difficult to effectively separate the prostatic fluid component from the presperm and sperm components.

TABLE 2. Technique for Collection of Ejaculate Specimen

1. Retract the prepuce and gently cleanse the tip of the glans penis with a sterile gauze sponge.
2. Apply digital pressure with one hand at the base of the penis proximal to the bulbus glandis.
3. With the other hand, manipulate the penis within the sheath.
4. Collect the specimen in a sterile container.
5. The first two components of the ejaculate (presperm and sperm) are milky in appearance. Separate these from the third component, which is clear prostatic fluid, by collecting into two different sterile containers.
6. Perform a bacterial culture on the prostatic fluid.

■ A positive bacterial culture fails to localize the disease process. Potential sources of infection include the testes, epididymi, deferent ducts, prostate gland, and urethra. A distal urethral culture with quantitation of organisms is useful in interpreting ejaculate specimen culture results.

■ The ejaculate specimen is not useful for cytology.

Prostatic Wash Specimen

A prostatic wash specimen has potential microbiologic and cytologic applications (see Table 3 for technique).

Advantages of this technique are similar to those of ejaculate specimen collection.

Disadvantages of this technique:

■ Results may be inaccurate due to urine and urethral contamination as well as volume dilution by urine. Microbiology results are noninterpretable in cases with concurrent bacterial cystitis.

■ The prostate gland may not be within reach for effective rectal massage (abdominal prostatic massage may be effective).

■ Overzealous massage can rupture a prostatic abscess or cause sepsis in dogs with acute bacterial prostatitis.

Urethral Brush Specimen

This technique utilizes a 90-cm microbiology specimen brush designed for bronchoscopic use (Microbiology Specimen Brush; Microvasive) (see Table 4 for technique).

Advantages of this technique are similar to those of ejaculate specimen collection and prostate wash, *plus:*

■ The disease process is localized to the prostate gland; urethral contamination is minimized because of the plug in the tip of the catheter.

■ Useful cytologic and microbiologic information is obtained.

Disadvantages of this technique:

■ The specimen brush cannot be reused, which makes the procedure relatively expensive.

TABLE 3. Technique for Performing Prostatic Massage

1. Pass urethral catheter into the bladder and remove all urine.

2. Flush bladder with 5 ml sterile physiologic saline solution and save fluid. Label this specimen Sample 1.

3. Retract catheter tip and align it with the caudal pole of prostate gland (positioning is determined via rectal palpation).

4. Massage prostate gland for 1 minute.

5. Flush 5 ml sterile physiologic saline solution slowly through catheter while the urethral orifice is occluded around catheter to prevent retrograde loss of sample.

6. Advance catheter into bladder as fluid is aspirated. Save fluid and label Sample 2.

7. Quantitate bacterial numbers in both specimens to ascertain significance of bacterial growth in prostatic fluid specimen (Sample 2).

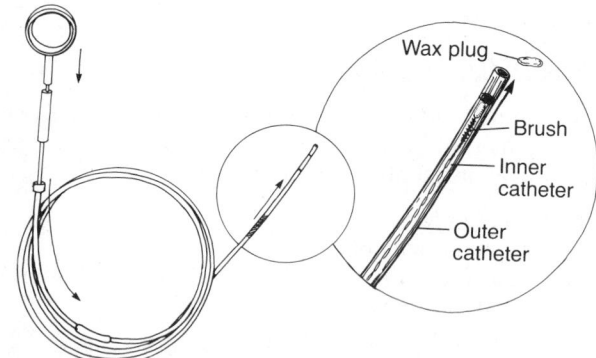

Figure 1. The microbiologic specimen brush used for obtaining prostatic urethral specimens.

■ The prostate gland may not be within reach for effective rectal massage (abdominal massage may be effective).

■ Overzealous massage can rupture a prostatic abscess or cause sepsis in dogs with acute bacterial prostatitis.

Ultrasound-Guided Prostatic Aspirate

This technique utilizes ultrasonography to guide the insertion of a needle into the prostate gland. Its documented use is for the diagnosis of bacterial infection and possibly neoplasia. Usefulness is limited to diagnosis of paraprostatic cysts.

Advantages of this technique:

■ It is a safe procedure in noninfectious conditions.

■ It accurately localizes the source of bacterial infection to the prostate gland.

Disadvantages of this technique:

■ Specialized equipment and skills are required.

■ Chemical restraint usually is necessary.

■ Aspiration of a prostatic abscess has the potential to result in peritonitis.

Prostate Gland Biopsy

■ Prior to performing biopsy, evaluate the animal for normal coagulation status.

■ Several techniques have been described for prostate biopsy, including transperineal, transrectal, transabdominal, ultrasound-guided, and biopsy via laparotomy (see sec. 8, ch. 9).

■ Ultrasound-guided prostate gland biopsy utilizes ultrasonography to assist in directing the biopsy instrument into the gland.

  • The frequency of complications is less than with some other biopsy techniques, and the success of obtaining a definitive diagnosis is enhanced because focal lesions can be visualized ultrasonographically.

  • Chemical restraint as well as specialized skill and equipment are necessary.

■ If ultrasonography is not available, biopsy via laparotomy is the most accurate, although the most invasive, technique.

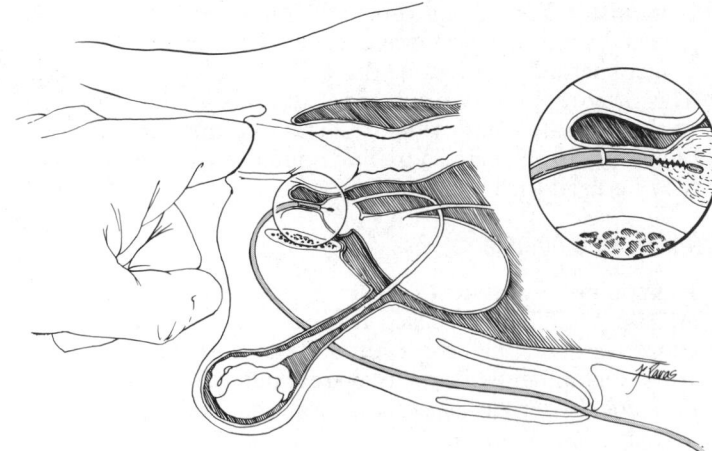

Figure 2. With the catheter positioned in the prostatic urethra, advance and retract the brush five or six times (inset).

■ Several complications from prostate gland biopsy are possible (Table 5).

TREATMENT

Treatment of canine prostatic disease is based on the specific disease process. Conservative management (castration and drug therapy) of canine prostatic disease is discussed in this chapter. Surgical management of prostatic disease is discussed in sec. 8, ch. 9.

Benign Prostatic Hyperplasia and Sterile Cystic Hyperplasia

Therapy may not be indicated if clinical signs are absent. However, it is advisable to caution owners that problems associated with prostatomegaly may develop.

TABLE 4. Technique for Obtaining Urethral Brush Specimen

1. Place animal in lateral recumbency.
2. Retract prepuce and cleanse end of glans penis with sterile swab.
3. Advance a sterile, 90-cm microbiologic specimen brush (Microbiology Specimen Brush, Microvasive) into urethra (Fig. 1).
4. Direct an assistant to use rectal palpation to align tip of catheter with the caudal pole of prostate gland (Fig. 2). The catheter is then held in this position.
5. Have the assistant massage prostate gland per rectum for 1 minute.
6. Advance the inner catheter approximately 1 cm within the urethra, thereby dislodging the absorbable catheter plug (see Fig. 1).
7. Advance and retract microbiologic brush five or six times within prostatic urethra for sample collection (see Fig. 2).
8. Following sample collection, retract brush and inner catheter and remove apparatus from urethra.
9. Expel any fluid within catheter into a test tube containing 3 ml sterile lactated Ringer's solution.
10. Extend brush, remove with sterile scissors, and drop into the same test tube.

A description of various treatment modalities follows.

Castration

■ Castration is the treatment of choice in dogs not intended for breeding.
■ A significant decrease in prostate gland size occurs within 1–4 weeks following castration.

Estrogen Therapy

■ Theoretically, estrogen acts to decrease prostatic tissue mass by decreasing the concentration of gonadotropin-releasing hormone which, in turn, decreases the concentration of testosterone. In fact, however, estrogen may act directly on the prostate gland to cause stromal hypertrophy and squamous metaplasia.
■ It also may alter prostatic secretions and increase the gland's susceptibility to infection.
■ Bone marrow suppression is a potential serious side effect.

KEY POINT ▶ Because of potentially serious side effects, estrogen is contraindicated for the treatment of benign prostatic hyperplasia.

Megestrol Acetate

KEY POINT ▶ Megestrol acetate effectively decreases the size of the prostate gland without impairing fertility in cases of benign prostatic hyperplasia.

■ Megestrol acetate interferes with the conversion of testosterone to dihydrotestosterone, the main androgen that promotes prostatic hyperplasia.

TABLE 5. Complications Associated with Prostate Gland Biopsy

Periprostatic hemorrhage	Hematuria
Perineal hematoma	Septicemia
Urethral perforation	Fever
Perineal abscessation	Peritonitis
Dissemination of neoplastic cells	Urethral fistula formation

■ Administer 0.55 mg/kg q24h, PO, for 4 weeks; then give the same dosage once a week. Do not use for longer than 32 consecutive days.
■ This drug reportedly produces a decrease in the size of the prostate gland without decreasing the number of spermatozoa. Thus, a treated animal subsequently may be used for breeding purposes.

Delmadinone Acetate

■ Delmadinone acetate (Tardak; Syntex Labs.) is an androgen inhibitor licensed for use in dogs in some countries other than the United States and Canada.
■ It is recommended for the treatment of benign prostatic hyperplasia, perianal tumors, and hypersexuality.
■ Delmadinone acetate is administered at 1.5–2.0 mg/kg for dogs <10 kg, 1.0–1.5 mg/kg for dogs 10–20 kg, and 1.0 mg/kg for dogs >20 kg; SC or IM; subsequent dosages at 3- to 4-week intervals usually are necessary.
■ Effects are observed within 2–4 days. A second treatment is recommended at 8 days if no improvement is noted.
■ Concurrent use of other steroid drugs should be avoided, and this drug is contraindicated in dogs with a history of decreased fertility or lack of libido if they are to be used for breeding.

Squamous Metaplasia

■ Discontinue any source of exogenous estrogen.
■ Castration is the treatment of choice. Examine the testicles histopathologically for the presence of an estrogen-secreting Sertoli cell tumor.

Bacterial Prostatitis

Principles of Antibiotic Therapy (see Table 6 for specific drugs and dosages)

■ Select an antibiotic based on urine or prostatic fluid culture and susceptibility results.

KEY POINT ▶ The ideal antibiotic for bacterial prostatitis is lipid-soluble and therefore capable of penetrating the blood–prostate gland barrier. Antibiotics of choice include erythromycin, chloramphenicol, trimethoprim-sulfa, clindamycin, oleandomycin, and enrofloxacin.

■ The ideal antibiotic has a relatively low degree of protein binding, which allows greater drug availability for diffusion into the prostate gland. Chloramphenicol is highly protein bound; therefore, it should be used at the higher end of the recommended dosage range (see Table 6).
■ In cases of bacterial prostatitis, the pH of the prostatic fluid is usually acidic. Antibiotics that work best in an acidic environment are erythromycin, enrofloxacin, clindamycin, trimethoprim-sulfa, and chloramphenicol.
■ Continue antibiotic therapy for a minimum of 4 weeks. Re-culture the prostatic fluid 5–7 days after the onset of therapy to document the *in vivo* effec-

TABLE 6. Antibiotics Recommended for the Treatment of Bacterial Prostatitis

Drug	Dosage
Trimethoprim-sulfa (Tribrissen; Coopers)	2.2 mg/kg (based on trimethoprim fraction) q12h PO or SC
Chloramphenicol (multiple manufacturers)	50 mg/kg q8h PO, IV, SC, or IM
Erythromycin (multiple manufacturers)	10 mg/kg q8h PO
Clindamycin (Antirobe; Upjohn)	5–10 mg/kg q8h PO, IV, or IM
Enrofloxacin (Baytril; Haver)	5 mg/kg q12h PO*

*This is twice the manufacturer's current recommended dosage.

tiveness of the antibiotic, and again in 2–3 weeks following discontinuation of therapy.
■ If initial culture and susceptibility results cannot be obtained, a good initial treatment choice is trimethoprim-sulfa, chloramphenicol, or enrofloxacin.

Treatment of Concurrent Septicemia or Peritonitis

■ Obtain abdominal fluid and/or blood for bacterial culture and susceptibility testing and select an appropriate antibiotic.
■ Obtain a blood specimen for bacterial culture and susceptibility.
■ Monitor the patient for hypoglycemia.
■ Administer IV fluids and parenteral antibiotics.
■ If a prostatic abscess is thought to be the source of septicemia, surgical drainage is indicated (see sec. 8, ch. 9).

Castration

Castration diminishes the potential for recurrence of bacterial prostatitis. It should not be performed until the patient is clinically stable and has been on antibiotic therapy for at least 1–2 weeks. Rule out the presence of a prostatic abscess or paraprostatic cyst, because castration alone typically is not curative for these conditions.

Nonbacterial Prostatitis

■ Because nonbacterial prostatitis in dogs has only recently been described and the etiology is unknown, effective therapy has not been reported. Castration is likely to be beneficial.
■ Treatment of nonbacterial prostatitis in humans has included tetracycline, corticosteroids, anticholinergic drugs, and muscle relaxants. No consistently positive results have been reported.

Paraprostatic Cysts and Prostatic Abscesses

■ Medical therapy consists of antibiotics if infection is present and treatment of concurrent septicemia, peritonitis, or hypoglycemia.
■ Paraprostatic cysts and moderate to severe prostatic

abscesses are indications for surgical therapy (see sec. 8, ch. 9).

Prostatic Neoplasia

Multiple therapeutic modalities exist; however, the prognosis in cases of prostatic neoplasia is poor.

Radiation Therapy

▪ Intra-operative radiation therapy is currently the treatment of choice. It is well tolerated by the patient and has few side effects.
▪ Radiation therapy is not indicated if metastasis is detected. The most common sites of metastasis are the iliac lymph nodes. Other sites include the lungs, omentum, mesentery, pelvis, and lumbar vertebrae.

Prostatectomy

Prostatectomy (sec. 8, ch. 9) is associated with complications, especially urinary incontinence, but can be offered if the tumor is small and has not metastasized.

Chemotherapy

No known protocols have any documented efficacy.

Castration

Castration is of questionable benefit. The cancer growth may not be hormonally mediated or it may be affected by nontesticular hormones (adrenal androgens or estrogens, luteinizing hormone [LH], follicle-stimulating hormone [FSH], prolactin, growth hormone).

Estrogen Therapy

Estrogen therapy suppresses gonadotropin secretion by the pituitary gland which, in turn, decreases the level of testicular testosterone secretion. As with castration, nontesticular hormones are unaffected.

Hormone Therapy

Hormonal manipulation is currently being investigated. The advantage of a total androgen blockade over castration is that all sources of androgen production are affected rather than just testicular androgens.

▪ Luteinizing hormone–releasing hormone (LH-RH)

agonists cause a transient rise followed by a paradoxical decrease in FSH, LH, and testosterone release. This decrease may be due to downregulation of, or a decrease in, the number of pituitary LH-RH receptors.
▪ Ketoconazole (see sec. 4, ch. 3, for details of ketoconazole therapy) inhibits testicular and adrenal testosterone synthesis and decreases the testosterone level to that of a castrated dog in 24–48 hours. The dosage range in humans is 400–1200 mg/day. Currently, a dosage for the treatment of canine prostatic neoplasia has not been determined.
  • Ketoconazole has been shown to have a significant effect on hormonal production by the adrenal gland in the treatment of canine hyperadrenocorticism at an oral dose of 9.7 to 13.4 mg/kg/day, PO. A similar dosage may be effective in the treatment of canine prostatic neoplasia.
  • Dosages of 10–30 mg/kg/day are tolerated by most dogs when used for antifungal therapy.

Supplemental Readings

Eichenberger T, Trachtenberg J: Effects of high-dose ketoconazole in patients with androgen-independent prostatic cancer. Am J Clin Oncol 11:S104, 1988.

Feeney DA, Johnston GR, Klausner JS, et al.: Canine prostatic disease—comparison of ultrasonographic appearance with morphologic and microbiologic findings: 30 cases (1981–1985). J Am Vet Med Assoc 190:1027, 1987.

Feeney DA, Johnston GR, Osborne CA, et al.: Maximum-distention retrograde urethrocystography in healthy male dogs: Occurrence and radiographic appearance of urethroprostatic reflux. Am J Vet Res 45:948, 1984.

Hargis AM, Miller LM: Prostatic carcinoma in dogs. Compend Contin Educ 5:647, 1983.

Kay ND, Ling GV, Nyland TG, et al.: Cytological diagnosis of canine prostatic disease using a urethral brush technique. J Am Anim Hosp Assoc 25:517, 1989.

Kay ND, Ling GV, Johnson DL: A urethral brush technique for the diagnosis of canine bacterial prostatitis. J Am Anim Hosp Assoc 25:527, 1989.

Moffat EF, Kirk D, Tolley DA, et al.: Ketoconazole as primary treatment of prostatic cancer. Br J Urol 61:439, 1988.

Obradovich J, Walshaw R, Goullaud E: The influence of castration on the development of prostatic carcinoma in the dog. J Vet Int Med 1:183, 1987.

Olsen PN, Wrigley RH, Thrall MA, et al.: Disorders of the canine prostate gland: Pathogenesis, diagnosis, and medical therapy. Compend Contin Educ 9:613, 1987.

Turrel JM: Intraoperative radiotherapy of carcinoma of the prostate gland in ten dogs. J Am Vet Med Assoc 190:48, 1987.

Wolfson JS, Hooper DC: Treatment of genitourinary tract infections with fluoroquinolones: Activity in vitro, pharmacokinetics, and clinical efficacy in urinary tract infections and prostatitis. Antimicrob Agents Chemother 33:1655, 1989.

Surgery of the Prostate Gland

Harry W. Boothe

Surgical procedures of the prostate gland include biopsy, drainage procedures (including drain tube placement and marsupialization), and prostatectomy (partial or complete). Orchidectomy of the patient with prostatic disease is recommended either prior to or at the time of prostatic surgery (see sec. 8, ch. 11 for castration technique). Prostatic disorders that may require surgery include hyperplasia, trauma, infection (abscess), cyst formation, and neoplasia. A thorough understanding of prostatic anatomy is necessary prior to performing surgery. Information in this chapter refers only to the dog because prostatic disease is extremely rare in cats.

ANATOMY

- The prostate gland completely encompasses the proximal portion of the male urethra at the neck of the bladder.
- The craniocaudal position of the prostate is age-dependent; the prostate is confined to the pelvic cavity until about 4 years of age and is essentially totally within the abdomen by 10 years of age.
- The dorsal prostatic surface is flattened and has a mid-dorsal sulcus. The gland has a relatively thick capsule and is divided into right and left lobes by a prominent median septum.
- The two deferent ducts enter the craniodorsal surface of the prostate.
- The blood supply is closely allied to the nerve supply, with both being located in the lateral pedicles. The prostatic artery gives off branches to the ductus deferens, urethra, urinary bladder, ureters, and rectum. Damage to branches of the prostatic artery may result in devascularization of surrounding structures.
- The hypogastric (sympathetic) and pelvic (parasympathetic) nerves follow the vasculature.

KEY POINT ▶ The hypogastric and pelvic nerves are required for micturition and continence. Avoid iatrogenic trauma to these structures.

- The prostatic lymph vessels empty into the iliac lymph nodes.

BIOPSY

Preoperative Considerations

- Accurate preoperative assessment of prostatic size, consistency, and location is important. Palpation (both rectal and abdominal), radiography (including contrast radiography), and ultrasonography are helpful in gaining this information.
- Adequate immobilization of the prostate gland during biopsy is indicated, particularly when using needle biopsy techniques.

KEY POINT ▶ Aspiration of the prostate should be performed prior to needle biopsy to exclude abscessation.

Surgical Procedures

Objectives

- Obtain a representative sample of the prostate gland for histologic and microbiologic evaluation.
- Avoid entering the prostatic urethra.
- Minimize blood loss and potential dissemination of infection.

Equipment

- Tru-Cut biopsy needle (one-handed model) or Franklin-Silverman needle
- Scalpel blade and handle

Technique

1. Place dog in sternal recumbency with the tail positioned over the back.
2. Prepare perineal region from the base of tail to ventral to the level of the ischial tuberosities.
3. Direct an assistant to exert gentle pressure on the caudal abdomen to position prostate gland into the pelvic inlet.
4. Perform rectal examination to define the position of prostate gland.
5. Incise the perineal skin (5 mm long) just off the midline midway between the anus and ischial tuberosity.
6. Insert biopsy needle in the closed position through the prostatic capsule under digital control within rectum by the other hand.
7. Fully insert the inner cannula into prostate gland and, while holding the inner cannula stationary in its extended position, sharply advance the outer cannula over the inner rod.
8. Remove biopsy needle in a closed position.
9. Verify that an adequate biopsy has been obtained by extending the inner cannula and seeing prostatic tissue in the specimen notch.
10. Place biopsy sample in the appropriate transfer containers for histologic and microbiologic testing.

Procedure for Wedge Biopsy

Equipment

- Standard general surgical pack and suture.
- Laparotomy sponges.

Technique

1. Place dog in dorsal recumbency on a level surgery table.
2. Aseptically prepare ventral abdominal region from the xiphoid process to caudal to the pubic brim.
3. Incise skin and ventral abdominal wall from the umbilicus to the pubis while avoiding the prepuce. Use a midline or abdominal approach.
4. Gently retract urinary bladder cranially using a stay suture. Isolate prostate gland with moistened laparotomy sponges.
5. Excise a representative wedge of prostatic tissue, using scalpel blade.
6. Close the prostatic defect (simple continuous pattern, absorbable suture).
7. Routinely close ventral abdominal wall (simple interrupted or continuous pattern, synthetic absorbable suture), subcutaneous tissue (simple continuous pattern, absorbable suture), and skin (simple interrupted pattern, nonabsorbable suture).

Postoperative Care and Complications

Short-Term

- Closely monitor for hemorrhage, including hematuria, infection, and urine leakage.
- Monitor for postoperative orchitis and scrotal edema.

Prognosis

- The prognosis depends on disease process(es) present.
- Prostatic biopsy is usually associated with minimal patient morbidity.

DRAINAGE PROCEDURES

Preoperative Considerations

- Distinguish between infectious and noninfectious causes of fluid retention within or near the prostate gland.
- Microbiologic testing of prostatic fluid is indicated to assist in selection of antimicrobial agent.
- Ultrasonography is helpful to determine the degree and location of cavitation within the prostatic parenchyma.
- When prostatic abscessation is present, drainage or resection of diseased parenchyma is indicated.
- Perform orchidectomy prior to or at the time of a prostatic drainage procedure.

KEY POINT ▶ Always biopsy the prostate gland as part of the drainage procedure.

- Choice of drainage procedure (i.e., placement of drain tubes or marsupialization) depends on the size and location of prostatic cavitation. Large cystic lesions often are more amenable to marsupialization.

Surgical Procedure

Objectives

- Create a common cavity to provide ventral drainage.
- Thoroughly lavage cavity at the time of drainage.
- Avoid entering the prostatic urethra if possible.
- Minimize blood loss and dissemination of infection.

Placement of Drain Tube(s)

Equipment

- Standard general surgical pack and suture
- Red rubber urethral catheter(s) or Penrose drain(s)
- Suction apparatus, tubing, and tip
- Laparotomy sponges

Technique

1. Place dog in dorsal recumbency. Catheterize the urethra.
2. Aseptically prepare ventral abdominal region from the xiphoid process to caudal to the pubic brim.
3. Incise skin and ventral abdominal wall from the umbilicus to the pubis while avoiding the prepuce.
4. Isolate the prostate from the rest of the peritoneal cavity, using laparotomy sponges.
5. Incise the ventrolateral aspect of the prostatic lobe(s) containing the fluid. Avoid vessels and nerves contained in the lateral pedicles.
6. Remove accumulations of fluid, using suction and lavage after digitally creating a common cavity.

KEY POINT ▶ Creation of a common prostatic cavity during any drainage procedure improves drainage and decreases the probability of recurrence.

7. Place one or more drains into the prostatic cavity while avoiding the urethra as follows:
   a. Pass Penrose drain(s) (¼″) through the cavity to exit on the ventrolateral aspect of each lobe (Fig. 1), or
   b. Position a single red rubber catheter to permit continuous drainage of the prostatic cavity.
8. Exteriorize the end(s) of the drain tube(s) through the body wall approximately 2 cm lateral to the prepuce, and suture the drain to the skin.
9. Routinely close ventral abdominal wall (see Wedge Biopsy).

Procedure for Marsupialization

Equipment

- Standard general surgical pack and suture
- Suction apparatus, tubing, and tip
- Laparotomy sponges

Technique

1. See steps 1–4 under Technique for Placement of Drain Tube(s).

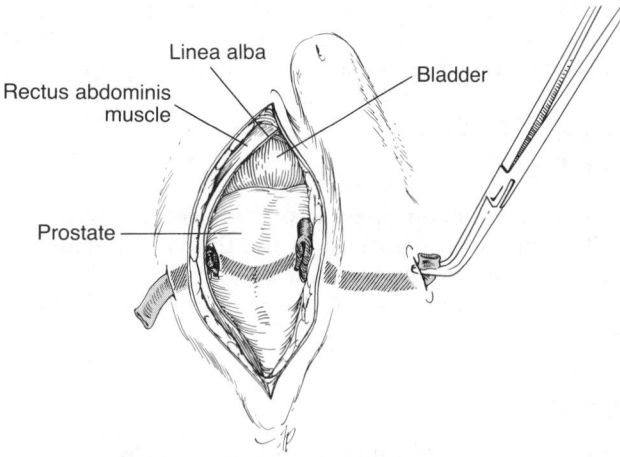

Figure 1. Prostatic drainage procedure. A single Penrose drain has been placed within the abscess cavity of the prostate and exits on the ventrolateral aspects of the gland. The ends of the drain are placed through the body wall and skin on each side of the prepuce.

2. Incise the ventrolateral aspect of the fluid-filled prostate and evacuate fluid, using suction and lavage after digitally creating a common cavity.
3. Incise skin (5 cm long), subcutaneous tissue, and abdominal musculature just lateral to the prepuce on the side opposite the original skin incision.
4. Place the walls of the prostatic cavity near the skin incision and appose the prostatic wall adjacent to the incision to the external fascia of the rectus abdominis muscle (simple continuous pattern, absorbable suture) and the incised prostatic edges to the skin (simple interrupted pattern, nonabsorbable suture).
5. If a paraprostatic cyst is present and can be dissected free from surrounding tissues, resection of all or most of the cyst is indicated. This eliminates the complications associated with marsupialization.
6. Routinely close the ventral abdominal wall (see Wedge Biopsy).

Postoperative Care and Complications

Short-Term

- Prevent self-inflicted trauma to the drain(s) or the stoma site by using a side brace until the drain tubes are removed.
- Continuous suction drainage using a single red rubber catheter and a suction reservoir may be more effective in evacuating prostatic cavities than simple gravity drainage; however, such drainage requires more conscientious postoperative patient observation and care.
- Passage of urine through the drainage tubes may occur but usually resolves in a few days.
- Prostatic abscessation requires aggressive medical therapy to eliminate infection and usually responds better to drain tube placement than to marsupialization.
- Remove drains at about 3 weeks after surgery.
- Administer an appropriate antibiotic (see sec. 8, ch. 8) to patients with prostatic abscessation for 2–4 weeks after the hospitalized period.

Long-Term

- Long-term complications of prostatic drainage procedures include urinary incontinence (46% incidence), recurrent urinary tract infection (30% incidence), recurrence of prostatic abscessation (18% incidence), and urethrocutaneous fistula formation (2% incidence).
- Carefully monitor response to therapy through urine or prostatic fluid culture and susceptibility testing, as well as ultrasonography, if available, for several days after discontinuing antibiotics.

Prognosis

- Paraprostatic cysts respond best to complete or partial surgical removal, because recurrence following drainage is relatively common.
- Prostatic abscessation has potential for significant morbidity and mortality, and immediate postoperative mortality may approach 25%.
- The incidence of postoperative sepsis and shock approximates 33%. Rupture of a prostatic abscess results in a mortality rate of approximately 50%.
- Patients with prostatic abscessation that survive the initial 2 weeks after surgery will likely make a satisfactory recovery.

PARTIAL (SUBTOTAL) PROSTATECTOMY

Preoperative Considerations

- The surgeon should be familiar with the vascular anatomy of the diseased prostate.
- Partial prostatectomy is indicated for stable patients with recurrent abscessation and for dogs with cystic disease that have not responded to more conservative methods (i.e., orchidectomy).

KEY POINT ▶ Prostatic neoplasia is *not* an indication for performing a partial prostatectomy.

- Place a urethral catheter in urinary bladder to aid in identification of the urethra.

Surgical Procedure

Objectives

- Remove as much diseased prostatic tissue as possible while maintaining urinary continence.
- Avoid traumatizing the prostatic urethra.
- Maintain the blood supply to the prostatic urethra and adjacent organs.

Equipment

- Standard general surgical pack and suture
- Electrocoagulation unit with both coagulation and cutting capabilities
- Laparotomy sponges

Technique

1. See steps 1–4 under Technique for Placement of Drain Tube(s).

2. Isolate and ligate all major vessels leading to the prostate, while staying immediately adjacent to the prostate gland.
3. Incise and remove the prostate to within approximately 5 mm of the lateral aspect of the prostatic urethra, using either scissors and electrocoagulation or cutting electrocoagulation (Fig. 2).
4. Routinely close the ventral abdominal wall.

Postoperative Care and Complications

Short-Term

- Submit excised tissue for histologic and microbiologic testing.
- Maintain urinary diversion (i.e., indwelling urethral catheter) for approximately 5 days.
- Prevent self-inflicted trauma to urinary catheter by using a side brace until catheter is removed.
- Shock, urine leakage, and urinary incontinence are potential short-term complications of partial prostatectomy.

Long-Term

- Nocturnal urinary incontinence has been identified as a long-term complication of partial prostatectomy in approximately 50% of patients.

Prognosis

- The prognosis depends on the disease process(es) present.
- Resolution of prostatic and urinary tract infection is likely following partial prostatectomy.

TOTAL PROSTATECTOMY

Preoperative Considerations

- Indications for total prostatectomy include severe trauma, neoplasia with no apparent metastasis, and recurrent prostatic abscessation unresponsive to other less invasive surgical procedures.

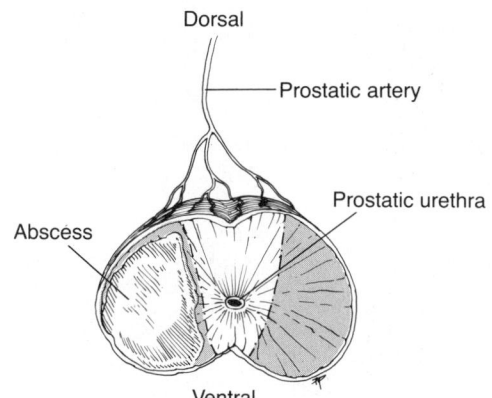

Figure 2. Partial (subtotal) prostatectomy technique. The shaded area denotes the prostatic parenchyma to be removed to within approximately 5 mm of the prostatic urethra using sharp dissection and selected or cutting electrocoagulation.

KEY POINT ▶ Urinary incontinence is a common complication of total prostatectomy.

Surgical Procedure

Objectives

- Remove the entire prostate gland.
- Preserve the blood supply to the urinary bladder and urethra.
- Preserve as much urethra as possible.
- Perform an accurate urethral anastomosis.

Equipment

- Standard general surgical pack and suture
- Electrocoagulation unit
- Laparotomy sponges
- Urethral catheter

Technique

1. Place a urethral catheter to aid in identification of the urethral lumen.
2. See steps 1–4 under Technique for Placement of Drain Tube(s).
3. Expose the prostate by careful dissection through the periprostatic fat as close to the prostate as possible.
4. Ligate and divide the prostatic vessels and ductus deferens close to the gland.
5. Carefully dissect the prostatic tissue from the urinary bladder and urethra, using sharp and blunt dissection.
6. Transect the urethra as close to the prostate gland and as far from the bladder neck as possible.
7. Transect the urethra as close to the caudal extent of the prostate as possible.
8. Remove the prostate gland by slipping it off the urinary catheter, and reposition the catheter into the urinary bladder.
9. Approximate the urethral ends in an end-to-end fashion (simple interrupted pattern, synthetic absorbable suture), starting at the dorsal aspect of the urethra.
10. Thoroughly lavage the abdomen prior to closure.
11. Provide urinary diversion by performing a prepubic tube cystostomy (see sec. 8, ch. 4) or maintaining placement of the urethral catheter.
12. Routinely close the ventral abdominal wall.

Postoperative Care and Complications

Short-Term

- Prevent self-inflicted trauma to the catheter by using a side brace.
- Complications include urine leakage at the urethral anastomosis, urinary incontinence, and urethral stricture.

Long-Term

- Urinary incontinence may be a long-term complication. Attempt control using drugs to increase proximal urethral tone (see sec. 8, ch. 5)

Prognosis

- Prostatic neoplasia in the dog is most commonly malignant (adenocarcinoma or transitional cell carcinoma), metastasis is most common to the iliac lymph nodes, periprostatic tissue, urinary bladder, pelvic structures, and lung.
- Successful treatment of prostatic neoplasia is difficult because of its aggressive biologic behavior; micrometastasis to adjacent tissues is probable when no gross evidence of metastasis exists.

Supplemental Readings

Basinger RR: Surgical management of prostatic diseases. Compend Contin Educ Pract Vet 9:993, 1987.

Evans HE, Christensen GC: *Miller's Anatomy of the Dog.* Philadelphia: W. B. Saunders, 1979, p 565.

Hardie EM, Barsanti JA, Rawlings CA: Complications of prostatic surgery. J Am Anim Hosp Assoc 20:50, 1984.

Hardie EM, Stone EA, Spaulding KA, Cullen JM: Subtotal canine prostatectomy with the neodymium:yttrium-aluminum-garnet laser. Vet Surg 19:348, 1990.

Johnston DE: Prostate. *In* Slatter DH, ed.: *Textbook of Small Animal Surgery.* Philadelphia: W. B. Saunders, 1985, p 1635.

Mullen HS, Matthiesen DT, Scavelli TD: Results of surgery and postoperative complications in 92 dogs treated for prostatic abscessation by a multiple Penrose drain technique. J Am Anim Hosp Assoc 26:369, 1990.

Weaver AD: Transperineal punch biopsy of the canine prostate gland. J Small Anim Pract 18:573, 1977.

10 Diseases of the Scrotum and Testes

Susan F. Soderberg

Diseases of the testes and scrotum may cause discomfort with an acute injury or infection or may cause systemic effects with an endocrinopathy. Most dogs with testicular diseases have no clinical signs. Expect infertility, with or without testicular atrophy, if the disease is chronic.

KEY POINT ▶ Early diagnosis and therapy of testicular disease are critical to preserving reproductive function.

ETIOLOGY

Congenital Diseases

Congenital diseases of the testicles are detectable prior to puberty.

- Cryptorchidism is the failure of one or both testes to descend into the scrotum. Normal descent of the testes into the scrotum is complete by 6 to 8 weeks of age but occasionally is delayed to as late as 6 months of age.
  - The undescended testis may be found within the abdominal cavity or the inguinal canal or lateral to the penis.
  - This defect is considered hereditary in most breeds and is a sex-linked, autosomal recessive trait.
- Testicular hypoplasia results from abnormal development of the seminiferous tubular germinal epithelium. This development leads to significant reduction in sperm number and infertility. A significant decrease in the size of one or both testicles is present at the time of puberty.
- Aplasia of the testicular duct system results in impaired transport of sperm to the urethra, accumulation of sperm proximal to the obstruction, potential development of sperm granuloma, and subsequent testicular degeneration. This defect is commonly unilateral.
- A female pseudohermaphrodite has the external genitalia of a male but generally has more than a single X chromosome. These individuals frequently have an XXY karyotype. Male pseudohermaphrodites have testicular hypoplasia, cryptorchidism, or abnormal development of the penis or prepuce.
- Scrotal hernia (herniation of abdominal organs or omentum through the inguinal canal into the scrotum) may be congenital or traumatic in origin.

Infectious or Inflammatory Diseases

Infections of the testes and scrotum are often detected with swelling, pain, and enlargement of the affected area.

- Scrotal dermatitis
  - Local irritation can be an acute reaction from chemical irritants, such as soaps, dips, or disinfectants, or from insect bites, such as fly strike.
  - Acute orchitis causes dermatitis by stimulating excessive licking of the scrotum.
  - Abrasions and other traumatic insults, such as surgical preparation can also initiate scrotal dermatitis.
  - The scrotum can be involved in any generalized dermatitis.
- Acute orchiepididymitis may develop from several routes.
  - Direct trauma, especially a puncture wound, can initiate bacterial infection in the testis.
  - Bacterial septicemias, originating in other organ systems, may spread to the testicles via the lymphatics.
  - Bacterial prostatitis or cystitis may initiate infection by descent down the vas deferens.
  - *Brucella canis* or distemper virus may be the causative agent in some cases of orchiepididymitis.
  - Bacterial infections can cause suppurative inflammation that results in abscess formation, which may rupture and drain through the scrotal skin.
- Chronic orchiepididymitis may develop secondary to acute infection.
  - Orchiepididymitis may appear in an animal with no previous history of or owner's awareness of an inflammatory testicular problem.
  - Slow, progressive, low-grade, nonsuppurative inflammation with fibrosis may be caused by *B. canis, Escherichia coli,* or canine distemper virus.

Trauma

Traumatic injury to the testes and scrotum can result in abrasion, contusion, hematoma, laceration, or edema. All such lesions require prompt treatment to avoid acute or chronic orchiepididymitis.

Adverse Drug Reactions

Many drugs, toxins (e.g., lead), and irradiation are capable of causing damage to the seminiferous epithelium and subsequent deterioration in semen quality. Some of the agents that can adversely affect semen quality include amphotericin B, anticancer drugs, and cimetidine. Deleterious drugs are withdrawn as soon as possible to allow recovery of the seminiferous epithelium before severe or permanent damage occurs.

Endocrine Diseases

Endocrinopathies, such as hypothyroidism and diabetes mellitus, or abnormally high or low concentrations of glucocorticoid, estrogen, androgen, or gonadotropin alter spermatogenesis. Such conditions alter the metabolism of the gonadal hormones and gradually cause deterioration of the seminiferous epithelium.

Immune-mediated Diseases

Immune-mediated orchitis develops subsequent to exposure of spermatozoal antigens to the immune system. Normally, a blood-testis barrier prevents such exposure. Traumatic and infectious diseases of the epididymis or testis can damage this barrier and result in exposure of spermatozoal antigens to the general circulation and immune system. Invasion of the interstitial tissues of the testes and epididymis with lymphocytes and plasma cells follows. This infiltrate results in deterioration of the seminiferous epithelium.

Neoplasia

- Scrotal tumors most commonly include mast cell tumors (see sec. 3, ch. 7) and melanomas (see sec. 3, ch. 9). These tumors have a high potential for malignant behavior and require radical therapy.
- Primary testicular neoplasias include the Sertoli cell tumors, interstitial cell tumors, and seminomas.
  - When these tumors occur in scrotal testes, they are most often benign.
  - If the Sertoli cell tumors and seminomas are located within the abdominal cavity they may be malignant.
  - These tumors compromise testicular integrity and function by invading or compressing seminiferous tubules or by producing abnormally elevated levels of estrogen or testosterone.
  - Elevations in testosterone levels (interstitial cell tumors) can contribute to the development of benign prostatic hyperplasia, perineal hernia, or perineal adenoma.
  - Elevations in estrogen levels by Sertoli cell tumors can contribute to the development of squamous metaplasia of the prostate gland, feminization, and myelotoxicity.

Idiopathic Diseases

- Testicular torsion occurs most often in an enlarged, neoplastic abdominal testis. Rarely, testicular torsion occurs in a scrotal testis and, usually, after a traumatic incident. It is more common in a cryptorchid testicle located in the abdomen. The testis rotates on its horizontal axis resulting in torsion of the spermatic cord. Occlusion of venous and lymphatic drainage from the testis causes testicular engorgement and eventual necrosis.
- A spermatocele is a cystic distension in the testicular duct system that contains sperm.
- A sperm granuloma is an accumulation of sperm in the duct system that generates a chronic, inflammatory process. These granulomas develop slowly; fertility is maintained until total obstruction occurs. The degree of compromise in semen quality depends upon whether the obstruction is in a major duct or is unilateral or bilateral and whether an immune-mediated disease develops.
- A varicocele is a dilation and subsequent thrombosis of a spermatic vein. This condition results in disruption of normal blood flow and thermoregulation of the testis.

CLINICAL SIGNS

Acute, inflammatory diseases of the testes and scrotum are most commonly characterized by pain, swelling, and licking of the scrotum. Anorexia, listlessness, fever, reluctance to walk, or a stiff and stilted gait is intermittently reported. Acute abdominal pain may occur with testicular torsion. Changes in testicular size, testicular consistency, or semen quality is more commonly detected with chronic disease.

DIAGNOSIS

History and Physical Examination

Historical information, including duration of clinical disease, is important to an accurate diagnosis.

- Determine the disorders of other organ systems and previous systemic illnesses.
- Determine whether exogenous administration of drugs has occurred that could adversely affect testicular function.
- Determine whether traumatic episodes or periods of serious stress are involved.
- Determine the breeding management practices and housing facilities.

Perform complete physical examination in order to recognize underlying problems in other organ systems.

- The scrotum should be uniform in thickness.
  - Chronic or severe scrotal inflammation may alter normal thermoregulatory processes which can thereby alter spermatogenesis and/or spermatozoal storage in the epididymis.
  - Scrotal swelling may be the result of diffuse thickening of the scrotum; edema from local inflammation; testicular or epididymal enlargement; inguinoscrotal hernia; or systemic edematous conditions, such as hypoalbuminemia or vasculitis.
- The location of the two testicles is noted. Both testicles should be located within the scrotum by 4 to 6 months of age. The testicles are then palpated for size, shape, and consistency.
  - The normal testicle is oval with a smooth, regular outline.

- The two testicles should be approximately the same size, comfortably filling the scrotal cavity.
- An irregular surface, nodule, or adhesion to the scrotum may be the result of chronic inflammation, infection, or neoplasia.
- Soft, spongy, or doughy testicles are indicative of a degenerative process.
- Firm, hard testicles result from neoplasia or acute orchitis.
- Testicular pain upon palpation suggests acute orchitis or testicular torsion, especially if the testis is enlarged.

Ultrasound

Testicular and scrotal ultrasound may help delineate testicular neoplasia, abscess, testicular torsion, and scrotal hernia.

Semen Evaluation

A semen evaluation is performed as part of the reproductive examination to determine the male's fertility status and to provide samples for cytology and culture. The technique for collection of ejaculate is described in section 8, chapter 8. Perform the microscopic examination of sperm immediately after collection. Semen evaluation determines the following.

- Color
  - Semen is normally white to opalescent and opaque.
  - Semen that has a green tint, with or without clumps, clots, or flakes, is found with infection in the reproductive tract.
  - Red semen is generally the result of hemorrhage from the prostate gland or from a traumatized engorged penis.
  - Any agent (urine, purulent debris, blood) that contaminates the semen can affect the concentration, motility, and life of the sperm.
- Motility
  - A normal semen sample contains greater than 70% of the sperm's progressing in a forward direction.
  - Spermatozoa moving in circles or in a side-to-side motion, without forward progress, are not normal.
  - The percentage of actively motile sperm is reduced when the semen is exposed to temperature extremes, water, urine, purulent debris, blood, or lubricants.
- Sperm number
  - The number of sperm in an ejaculate varies, depending in part upon the age, testicular weight, sexual activity, and possibly season of the year. Sperm are counted using a hemocytometer.
  - Normal fertility is thought to be possible when the sperm count is over 200 million in an ejaculate.
  - When damage occurs to the seminiferous tubules from scrotal or testicular disease, the sperm count drops for a period from weeks to months.
- Interpretation
  - No single characteristic is an accurate measure of fertility.
  - For a male to be considered acceptable for breeding, the semen evaluation exceeds the minimum criteria suggested for percentage of progressive motile sperm, sperm concentration per ejaculate, and sperm morphology.
  - Re-evaluation of several samples is performed over 6 months before permanent infertility is diagnosed.

Suspected infections can be determined as follows.

- Bacterial cultures and susceptibility tests are performed.
  - Bacterial cultures from deep draining wounds will identify the causative organism. Superficial wounds are often contaminated with organisms from the environment.
  - Culture of the sperm-rich fraction of the ejaculate identifies the organisms that originate in the testes and prostate.
  - Culture of the prostatic fraction is more specific for prostatic organisms (see sec. 8, ch. 8).
  - If each fraction is cultured separately, the sperm-rich fraction and prostatic fraction yield less than 100 bacteria/ml in normal dogs.

KEY POINT ▶ Test all males presented for reproductive failure, chronic scrotal dermatitis, or orchitis for *B. canis.*

- *B. canis* infections may cause orchitis, epididymitis, testicular atrophy, discospondylitis, generalized lymphadenopathy, or fever of unknown origin.
- Use serum agglutination tests for screening. False-positive findings are possible with this test.
- Diagnosis is confirmed with the agar-gel immunodiffusion test.

Cytology

Fine needle aspiration along with cytology of the testes and scrotum is a rapid and inexpensive method for diagnosis.

- Impression smears of scrotal lesions can uncover fungal elements, neoplastic cells, or other infiltrates.
- Fine needle aspiration of the epididymis is indicated when palpation of the epididymis is abnormal or when azoospermia is present. The aspirate is evaluated for live motile sperm, inflammatory cells, and bacteria.
- Fine needle aspiration of the testicle should demonstrate mature spermatozoa and all phases of maturing seminiferous epithelium. Inflammatory cells, bacteria, or neoplastic cells might also be detected.

Biopsy

A testicular biopsy is indicated to assess histology when reduction or lack of sperm in the ejaculate persists. The purpose of the biopsy is to identify the etiology of the problem, to formulate a rational therapeutic plan, and to provide a prognosis. The technique for testicular biopsy is described in section 8, chapter 11. Complications as the result of a testicular biopsy are uncommon but include immune-mediated orchitis or testicular atrophy.

Other Tests

When testicular atrophy is discovered, endocrinopathy due to testicular neoplasia or hormone-producing organs may be responsible.

- Hypothyroidism adversely affects reproductive function. Thyroid hormone levels are measured in any male showing poor libido and lethargy (see sec. 4, ch. 1).
- Abnormal cortisol levels (excessive or deficient) also adversely affect reproductive function (see sec. 4, ch. 3).
- Testosterone levels can become elevated with interstitial cell tumors. Testosterone deficiency may be detected in a female pseudohermaphrodite.
- Estradiol elevations may be detected with Sertoli cell tumors or with seminomas.
- Variation in luteinizing hormone (LH) levels have not been correlated with specific changes in testicular function or disease.
- Follicle-stimulating hormone (FSH) concentrations have been found to become elevated in direct proportion to the amount of histologic damage to the seminiferous epithelium. The highest levels are found when the seminiferous tubules contain only the Sertoli cells.

Karyotyping is used to determine the chromosomal composition of a suspected intersex abnormality (XXY) (sec. 8, ch. 19).

TREATMENT

Remove the causative agent of disease whenever possible.

- Exposure to all drugs is discontinued whenever they are not required for the long-term well-being of the individual.
- Soaps, detergents, and disinfectants that are used in the cages and kennels must be diluted and rinsed well after use.
- Topical insecticide sprays, dips, or grooming products must not be applied to the scrotum.

If an endocrinopathy has been identified in the diagnostic workup, appropriate therapy is instituted. The semen quality does not show improvement for several months after control of these endocrinopathies has been achieved.

Cryptorchidism

Hormone therapy has been successful in treating certain individuals with cryptorchidism, when various criteria are met.

- Individuals that may benefit from treatment need to be younger than 16 weeks of age and have both testes palpable outside the inguinal ring.
- Testes that can be physically manipulated near the scrotal opening have a better chance of responding to therapy. It is possible that some cases that respond to medical management of cryptorchidism would have eventually resolved without treatment.

- The ethics of medical management, because of strong genetic implications, is dependent upon the opinions of the veterinarian and the owner.
- Surgical therapy to place a retained testis into the scrotum is an unethical practice and is not offered as an option.
- The most commonly used medical therapy for cryptorchidism is serial injections of human chorionic gonadrotropin (hCG). Intramuscular administration of 100 to 1000 IU of hCG is given four times in a 2-week period. Those animals that respond to treatment generally do so within 1 month of therapy.

Superficial Scrotal Lesions

Topical therapy can prove beneficial for superficial scrotal lesions.

- Careful daily rinsing and cleansing along with judicious use of topical ointments (e.g., Panolog) prove most helpful.
- An Elizabethan collar is often necessary to prevent further irritation caused by licking.
- Scrotal swelling and inflammation are reduced as rapidly as possible with cold water or ice to minimize heat damage to the testes.

Septic Orchiepididymitis

Systemic therapy is required for septic orchiepididymitis.

- In dogs with acute orchiepididymitis—when maintaining fertility is not a concern—treatment is aimed at stabilization with IV fluids and broad-spectrum antibiotics. The antibiotic of choice, before culture results are available, is trimethoprim-sulfadiazine, most commonly, or aminoglycoside. Resistant *Staphylococcus* infections may require treatment with cephalosporin or oxacillin. Orchiectomy is performed once stabilization has been achieved.
- If the owner desires reproductive function maintained in the animal with acute orchiepididymitis, therapy is expanded beyond supportive care with IV fluids and systemic antibiotics. Cold compresses are placed on the scrotum to minimize thermal damage to the germinal epithelium. An anti-inflammatory agent, such as corticosteroid or aspirin, may be used to control inflammation, local hyperthermia, and exposure of the immune system to spermatozoal antigens following disruption of the blood-testis barrier. Unilateral orchiectomy may be necessary to prevent damage to an unaffected testis. The prognosis for maintaining normal fertility is guarded.
- If chronic orchiepididymitis is diagnosed, the prognosis for fertility is guarded to poor. When a positive culture occurs, administer appropriate antibiotic therapy for a minimum of 3 weeks. If plasmacytic lymphocytic infiltration is identified histologically, immunosuppressive drugs (e.g., prednisone, Cytoxan, Imuran) may be beneficial.
- A dog positively diagnosed with *B. canis* is not used as a breeding animal, because it is a potential source of infection for other dogs and for humans. Affected animals are neutered or euthanized. Treatment at-

tempts can be expensive and offer little hope for cure. Persistent bacteremia may be eliminated during antibiotic therapy but often recurs in 1 to 3 months after therapy. Antibiotics that have been recommended are minocycline, which is very expensive and doxycycline or tetracycline, in combination with an aminoglycoside, such as gentamicin.

Other Diseases

Orchiectomy is indicated for conditions that have no treatment protocol or for which treatment has failed (see sec. 8, ch. 11). Orchiectomy is indicated with testicular torsion, testicular hypoplasia, and testicular ductular aplasia or for cryptorchid dogs over 6 months of age. Orchiectomy may also be necessary to correct scrotal hernias. After removal of the testicle and spermatic cord, the hernial sac is ligated with a transfixing ligature. Unilateral orchiectomy may be performed when there is unilateral trauma, infection, or tumor in a male that the owner desires to continue breeding. Testicles of infertile males are removed to reduce the risk of androgen-induced conditions (prostatitis, neoplasia, perineal hernia). Submit abnormal testicles for histopathologic evaluation following surgery.

Supplemental Readings

Barsanti JA: Abnormalities of the external genitalia. *In* Lorenz MD, Cornelius LM, eds.: *Small Animal Medical Diagnosis.* Philadelphia: J. B. Lippincott, 1987, p 366.

Cox VS: Cryptorchidism in the dog. *In* Morrow DA, ed.: *Current Therapy in Theriogenology 2.* Philadelphia: W. B. Saunders, 1986, p 541.

Feldman EC, Nelson RW: Disorders of the canine male reproductive tract. *In* Feldman EC, Nelson RW, eds.: *Canine and Feline Endocrinology and Reproduction.* Philadelphia: W. B. Saunders, 1987, p 481.

Johnson CA: Disorders of the canine testicles and epididymides. *In* Morrow DA, ed.: *Current Therapy in Theriogenology 2.* Philadelphia: W. B. Saunders, 1986, p 551.

Seager SWJ: Semen collection and evaluation in the dog. *In* Morrow DA, ed.: *Current Therapy in Theriogenology 2.* Philadelphia: W. B. Saunders, 1986, p 539.

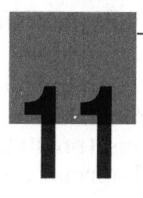

11 Surgery of the Testis and Scrotum

Harry W. Boothe

Orchidectomy is the most commonly performed surgical procedure of the testis. The technique depends, in part, on species and location of the testes (i.e., ectopic or scrotal). Indications for performing orchidectomy are listed in Table 1. Testicular biopsy may be part of a fertility examination. Scrotal ablation may be part of a routine orchidectomy or for neoplasia resection, especially in older dogs. It is also performed at the time of scrotal urethrostomy and feline perineal urethrostomy.

KEY POINT ▶ Obtain owner consent prior to performing orchidectomy as a primary procedure or concurrently with another surgical procedure.

ANATOMY

- The testes are positioned obliquely within the scrotum, with their long axis directed dorsocaudally.
- The scrotal testis is covered by peritoneum (parietal and visceral vaginal tunics) and a dense, white, fibrous capsule (tunica albuginea).
- The testis and epididymis are connected to the parietal vaginal tunic by the caudal ligament of the epididymis.
- The arterial and venous patterns are similar, with the right testicular artery originating from the abdominal aorta cranial to the left and the veins forming an extensive pampiniform plexus in the spermatic cord.
- The right testicular vein empties into the caudal vena cava, whereas the left terminates in the left renal vein; testicular lymphatics drain into the iliac lymph nodes.
- The canine scrotum is located more ventrally than the feline.
- The scrotal wall consists of the skin and dartos, a layer of smooth muscle and elastic fibers.

TABLE 1. Indications for Performing Orchidectomy in the Dog and Cat

Reproductive neutering	Benign prostatic hyperplasia
Modification of behavior patterns	Perianal adenoma
Testicular neoplasia	Perineal hernia
Severe testicular or scrotal trauma	Scrotal urethrostomy (canine)
Refractory orchitis/epididymitis	Perineal urethrostomy (feline)

- The external spermatic fascia attaches to the caudal aspect of the scrotum as the scrotal ligament.
- Blood supply to the scrotum is principally via branches of the external pudendal artery; lymphatic drainage is to the inguinal lymph nodes.

TESTICULAR BIOPSY

See also section 8, chapter 18.

Preoperative Considerations

- Usually only one testis is sampled.
- Incisional techniques usually provide the most architectural information.
- Fixation of specimens in Bouin's, Zenker's, or Stieve's fixative is preferable to formalin fixation because of better preservation of architectural detail.

Surgical Procedure

Objectives

- Obtain a representative sample of the testis for histologic evaluation.
- Minimally disrupt the testicular architecture.

Equipment

- Standard general surgical pack and suture
- Sterile, thin razor blade
- Bouin's, Zenker's, or Stieve's fixative

Technique

1. Place animal in dorsal recumbency and aseptically prepare the prescrotal area.
2. Incise skin just cranial to the scrotum and place the testis with the epididymis away from incision.
3. Incise the tunics with scalpel blade and the tunica albuginea with sterile, thin razor blade, while avoiding blood vessels.
4. Excise the bulging testicular tissue using the razor blade, or, if testicular tissue does not bulge, excise a wedge of testicular parenchyma. The razor blade's sharp, flat blade makes it ideal for this procedure.
5. Close the tunica albuginea and the tunics separately (simple interrupted pattern, 4–0 absorbable suture).
6. Routinely close skin (simple interrupted pattern, nonabsorbable suture).

Postoperative Care and Complications

- Uncommon complications include hemorrhage, infection, local hyperthermia, scarring, adhesions, and atrophy.
- A temporary slight decrease in sperm count may occur.

Prognosis

- The prognosis depends on the disease process(es) present.
- Minimal patient morbidity is expected.

ORCHIDECTOMY IN THE DOG

Preoperative Considerations

- Determine the location of the testes prior to surgery.
- Remove scrotal testes using either the closed or open method (choice of technique is surgeon's preference).
- Approach an abdominal testis through a parapreputial skin incision, and an extra-abdominal ectopic testis by incising directly over the testis.
- Histologically examine all ectopic and grossly abnormal testes.

Surgical Procedures

Objectives

- Remove both testes.
- Minimize postoperative complications and patient morbidity.

Equipment

- Standard general surgical pack and suture

Technique for Scrotal Testis (Closed Technique)

1. Place dog in dorsal recumbency and aseptically prepare the prescrotal area. Avoid clipping and scrubbing scrotal skin to minimize dermal irritation.
2. Incise prescrotal skin on the midline while gently pushing one testis toward the skin incision.
3. Incise the subcutaneous tissue and spermatic fascia over the testis to expose the parietal vaginal tunic.
4. Exteriorize the tunic-covered testis and, using scissors, incise the spermatic fascia and scrotal ligament close to the testis.
5. Reflect the fat and fascia surrounding the parietal vaginal tunic using a gauze sponge to enable maximal exteriorization of the spermatic cord.
6. Double-ligate the intact spermatic cord and vaginal tunics using transfixation ligatures of absorbable suture material (Fig. 1).
7. Transect the spermatic cord and cremaster muscle distal to the ligatures and return them to the inguinal region.
8. Routinely close the subcutaneous tissue (simple interrupted pattern, absorbable suture) and skin (simple continuous subcuticular pattern, absorbable suture or routine skin closure with monofilament nonabsorbable suture).

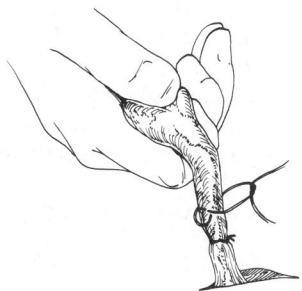

Figure 1. Transfixation (double) ligation of the intact spermatic cord. The suture needle is carefully passed through the spermatic cord between the cremaster muscle and the ductus deferens. The entire spermatic cord is enclosed in the ligature.

Technique for Scrotal Testis (Open Technique)

1. Exteriorize the testis as described for closed technique.
2. Incise the parietal vaginal tunic where ligatures are to be placed.
3. Double-ligate the spermatic cord using transfixation ligatures of absorbable material.
4. Alternatively, incise the parietal vaginal tunic over the testis, and then double-ligate the spermatic cord using transfixation ligatures of absorbable material.
5. Ligate the parietal vaginal tunic and cremaster muscle using an encircling ligature; transect the spermatic cord and cremaster muscle, and return them to the inguinal region.
6. Routinely close the subcutaneous tissue (simple interrupted pattern, absorbable suture) and skin (simple continuous subcuticular pattern, absorbable suture or routine skin closure with monofilament suture).

Technique for Abdominal Ectopic Testis

1. Place dog in dorsal recumbency and aseptically prepare the ventral abdominal region from the xiphoid process to caudal to the pubic brim.
2. Incise skin and ventral abdominal wall from the umbilicus to the pubis while avoiding the prepuce. A midline or abdominal approach is used.
3. Locate the ectopic testis by tracing one of the following:
   The ductus deferens from its prostatic termination
   The testicular artery from its aortic origin
   The testicular vein from its termination in the caudal vena cava (or left renal vein)
   The gubernaculum testis to the testis
4. Double-ligate the testicular vessels and ductus deferens.
5. Transect the vessels and ductus deferens; remove the testis and submit it for biopsy.
6. Routinely close the ventral abdominal wall.

Technique for Extra-abdominal Ectopic Testis

1. Place dog in dorsal recumbency and prepare the pubic region.
2. Incise skin and subcutaneous tissue directly over the testis.
3. Double-ligate and transect the spermatic cord.

4. If the testis is not found subcutaneously, extend the incision into the abdomen and find the testis as previously described.
5. Routinely close the subcutaneous tissue (simple interrupted pattern, absorbable suture) and skin (simple interrupted pattern, nonabsorbable suture).

Postoperative Care and Complications

Short-Term

- Scrotal bruising and inflammation, particularly following the open technique.
- Hemorrhage, which may be serious. Severe scrotal swelling from hemorrhage may necessitate scrotal ablation.
- Scrotal infection which may require drainage or scrotal ablation
- Use an Elizabethan collar to help prevent self-inflicted trauma. Subcuticular skin closure also helps to prevent self-trauma to the incision.

Prognosis

- Prognosis following orchidectomy of the cryptorchid dog is generally favorable even with testicular neoplasia, which usually is benign.

ORCHIDECTOMY IN THE CAT

Preoperative Considerations

- There are no special preoperative considerations (see Orchidectomy in the Dog).

Surgical Procedure

Objectives

- See Orchidectomy in the Dog.

Equipment

- Standard minor surgical pack

Technique

1. Position cat in dorsal recumbency with the rear limbs pulled cranially and aseptically prepare the perineal region.
2. Incise the scrotum over each testis and expose the testis.
3. Grasp the parietal vaginal tunic with hemostats, separate it from the testis, and excise it.
4. Separate the ductus deferens from the rest of the spermatic cord and separate it from the testis.
5. Tie two square knots in the spermatic cord using the ductus deferens and spermatic vessels as separate strands and transect the spermatic cord distal to the knots.
6. Alternatively, ligate the spermatic cord with absorbable suture material.
7. Do not suture the scrotal incision.

KEY POINT ▶ The traction avulsion technique of feline orchidectomy is *not* advisable because of

the potential for significant postoperative complications.

Postoperative Care and Complications

- See Orchidectomy in the Dog.

Prognosis

- See Orchidectomy in the Dog.

SCROTAL ABLATION

Preoperative Considerations

- Indications include severe trauma, neoplasia, ischemia, scrotal abscess, orchidectomy in old dogs with pendulous scrotums, scrotal urethrostomy, and feline perineal urethrostomy.
- Plan the skin incisions to leave sufficient skin for tension-free closure.

Surgical Procedure

Objectives

- Reduce postoperative problems following orchidectomy in the dog.
- Allow incision into the urethra and subsequent urethrostomy.
- Remove redundant scrotal tissue.

Equipment

- Standard general surgical pack and suture

Technique

1. Place animal in dorsal recumbency and prepare the periscrotal region.
2. Incise skin in a curvilinear fashion near the base of the scrotum, with the incisions curved toward the scrotum (Fig. 2).
3. Transect the scrotal septum after orchidectomy and routinely close subcutaneous tissue (simple interrupted pattern, absorbable suture) and skin (simple interrupted pattern, nonabsorbable suture).

Postoperative Care and Complications

Short-Term

- Prevent self-inflicted patient trauma (an Elizabethan collar may be indicated).

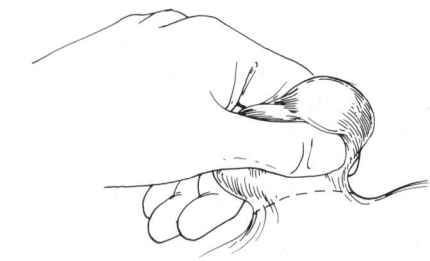

Figure 2. Ablation of the scrotum in the dog. The curved scrotal skin incision curves towards the scrotum to ensure tension-free closure of the incision. (From Harvey CE: Scrotal ablation and castration in the dog. J Am Anim Hosp Assoc 9:170, 1973.)

Common complications include hemorrhage, particularly associated with urethrostomy procedures (see sec. 8, ch. 6), infection, and dehiscence.

Prognosis

■ Minimal patient morbidity is expected.

Supplemental Readings

Boothe HW: Testis, epididymis, and spermatic cord. *In* Slatter DH, ed.: *Textbook of Small Animal Surgery.* Philadelphia: W. B. Saunders, 1985, p 1620.

Boothe HW: Scrotum. *In* Slatter DH, ed.: *Textbook of Small Animal Surgery.* Philadelphia: W. B. Saunders, 1985, p 1649.

Crane SW: Orchidectomy of descended and retained testes in the dog and cat. *In* Bojrab MJ, ed.: *Current Techniques in Small Animal Surgery,* 3rd ed. Philadelphia: Lea & Febiger, 1990, p 416.

Evans HE, Christensen GC: *Miller's Anatomy of the Dog.* Philadelphia: W. B. Saunders, 1979, p 554.

Harvey CE: Scrotal ablation and castration in the dog. J Am Anim Hosp Assoc 9:170, 1973.

Larsen RE: Testicular biopsy in the dog. Vet Clin North Am [Small Anim Pract] 7:747, 1977.

Pettit GD: There's more than one way to castrate a cat. Modern Vet Pract 62:713, 1981.

Phillips JT, Leeds EB: A closed technique for canine orchiectomy. Canine Pract 3:23, 1976.

12 Diseases of the Penis and Prepuce

Susan F. Soderberg

Diseases of the penis and prepuce are most commonly characterized by abnormal discharges at the preputial orifice. Alternatively, defects may be present which do not allow for the normal movement of the prepuce over the penis. These defects may not allow the penis to be extended from the prepuce, causing pain and inability to breed, or the penis may become trapped outside the prepuce, resulting in compromised venous return and traumatic injury from exposure.

ETIOLOGY

Underlying causes of disease found in the penis and prepuce include:

- Congenital defects
- Balanoposthitis
- Traumatic injuries
- Foreign material
- Neoplasia

Congenital Defects

Congenital diseases of the penis and prepuce include hypospadias, penile hypoplasia, persistent penile frenulum, preputial stenosis, and phimosis. These defects are responsible for compromising the normal movement of the penis in or out of the prepuce.

Hypospadias. Hypospadias and/or failure of preputial closure is the result of failure of the genital folds and/or genital swellings to fuse during fetal development. This failure results in abnormal development of the penile urethra, penis, prepuce, or scrotum.

- Most commonly, the urethral opening is found to be abnormally positioned ventral and caudal to its normal opening at the tip of the penis.
- Occasionally, the urethral opening will be found in the perineal region.
- The penis commonly is underdeveloped, and the prepuce is incomplete ventrally.

Penile Hypoplasia. Penile hypoplasia is an underdevelopment of the penis such that it is much shorter than the prepuce. Urine may pool within the prepuce, often causing irritation of the preputial lining and infection.

- This defect is most frequently found in the Great Dane, collie, Doberman pinscher, and cocker spaniel.

- Penile hypoplasia may be an indication of female pseudohermaphrodism.

Persistent Penile Frenulum. This is a band of connective tissue extending from the ventral tip of the penis to the prepuce. The band unites the penis and prepuce during fetal development.

- Normally the penile frenulum ruptures before puberty as a result of normal mechanical stress.
- When the connective tissue persists, it hinders extrusion of the penis from the prepuce and causes deviation of the penile tip in a ventral or lateral direction.

Preputial Stenosis. In this condition, the preputial opening is extremely small, compromising the extrusion of the penis (phimosis) and/or the flow of urine. If urine cannot escape, infection is a common sequela.

- In neonates, septicemia may result and cause death by 10 days of age.
- This severe neonatal defect is most frequently found in the German shepherd and golden retriever.

Os Penis Deformity. Deformity of the os penis results in deviation of the penis, occasionally causing inability to retract the penis fully into the prepuce.

- A congenitally shortened os penis may result in excessive flaccidity of the penile tip, causing impaired copulation.

Balanoposthitis

Balanoposthitis is inflammation of the penile and preputial mucosa.

- The most common cause is bacterial infection. Other sporadic infectious causes include herpesvirus (HV) and fungi such as *Candida* and *Blastomyces*.
- Mild infection causing a small amount of yellow-green discharge from the preputial opening is so common that it generally is considered normal.
- Copious amounts of purulent discharge require further investigation and treatment.

Trauma

Causes of trauma to the penis and prepuce include a fall, a blow to the inguinal region, or injuries inflicted by fighting.

- Traumatic injury may result in contusion, hematoma formation, laceration, or fracture of the os penis.

Foreign Body

Foreign bodies may be accidentally or maliciously lodged within the prepuce or around the penis.

■ Grass awns, other plant material, or small objects may be entrapped in the preputial cavity, often causing balanoposthitis.
■ Preputial hair or rubber bands may be wrapped around the penis, causing venous engorgement that prevents the penis from retracting back into the prepuce (paraphimosis).

KEY POINT ▶ If the penis becomes trapped outside the prepuce, severe injury, desiccation, and necrosis of the penis may rapidly occur.

■ Urethral obstruction can occur secondary to paraphimosis.

Neoplasms

Neoplasms involving the mucosa of the prepuce and penile surface include transmissible venereal tumors, papillomas, and carcinomas.

■ Urethral neoplasms such as transitional cell carcinoma, squamous cell carcinoma, and rhabdomyosarcoma occasionally extend to the penis.
■ Transmissible venereal tumor (TVT) is a contagious tumor found on the external genitalia of male and female dogs.
  • It is spread primarily by sexual contact but can also spread by licking and other forms of contact.
  • In the male, it is most often found as a fleshy, friable mass at the base of the penis.

CLINICAL SIGNS

■ Purulent preputial discharge in copious amounts occurs with balanoposthitis, urine pooling in the prepuce, foreign bodies, and occasionally neoplasms. Discomfort and excessive licking often are exhibited when purulent discharges are present.
■ Hemorrhagic discharge can occur with traumatic injuries, neoplasms, and bleeding in the urinary tract. Lesions of the urinary tract that may cause hemorrhage from the prepuce include prostatitis, urethral prolapse, calculi, trauma, and neoplasia. Clinical signs when hemorrhagic discharge is present include excessive licking and discomfort.
■ Urinary incontinence and/or urine scalding of the abdomen and perineum are commonly detected with hypospadias and penile hypoplasia.
■ Urinating in unexpected directions (e.g., on the rear feet) may be noticed with a persistent penile frenulum, causing deviation of the penile tip.
■ Unwillingness or inability to copulate due to pain when attempting an erection or the inability to extend the penis can be signs of persistent penile frenulum, deformity of the os penis, or preputial stenosis.
■ Many dogs have no clinical signs despite the presence of disease.

DIAGNOSIS

History

Obtain a complete history and determine the duration of events associated with the onset of signs.

KEY POINT ▶ It is important to determine if there is a history of systemic illness, traumatic episodes, and breeding problems in animals with penile diseases.

Physical Examination

Perform a complete physical examination before investigating the source of the complaint.

■ Visually inspect the prepuce, penis, and urethral orifice.
■ Normal findings include the following:
  • The prepuce is complete ventrally and completely covers the penis in its normal position.
  • A small amount of yellow-green discharge is found at the preputial orifice.
  • The prepuce moves freely over the penis and the penis is easily exposed by pulling the prepuce caudally over the bulbus glandis.
  • The penile mucosa is pinkish white, smooth, and nonpainful to the touch.
  • The urethral orifice is located at the tip of the penis.
■ Hyperplasia of the lymphoid follicles in the area of the bulbus glandis and preputial mucosa is common in many male dogs.
■ Palpate the penis and os penis to the brim of the pelvis. Swellings may be caused by a urolith, foreign body, hematoma, fracture of the os penis, or neoplasm.
■ Perform a rectal examination to rule out prostatic disease and diseases of the pelvic urethra.

Imaging Studies

■ Radiography may be used to detect congenital defects of the os penis, fractures of the os penis, and defects of the pelvis and pelvic canal.
■ Contrast urethrography may be performed to identify obstructive lesions, diverticulae, and traumatic damage of the urethra.

Laboratory Studies

Cytology

Cytology of preputial discharges and masses can help to determine their etiology.

■ Cytology of the normal preputial discharge contains variable numbers of epithelial cells, inflammatory cells (primarily neutrophils), and extracellular bacteria.
■ Balanoposthitis is characterized by large numbers of toxic neutrophils, often engulfing bacteria.
■ Causative agents (foreign material or fungi) may also be detected by cytologic inspection of the discharge.
■ Cytology of TVT reveals large round cells with

numerous mitotic figures. The cells resemble lymphoblasts.
- Perform histopathologic diagnosis of all neoplasms in order to formulate the best therapeutic plan.

Culture and Sensitivity Testing

To determine the most effective therapy for bacterial infections, perform culture and sensitivity testing of all preputial discharges.

Culture of HV usually is unsuccessful; however, a fourfold rise in serum neutralization titers may indicate a diagnosis of HV. HV infection usually has no clinical signs in adult dogs (see sec. 2, ch. 9).

Cytogenetic Evaluation

- To detect female pseudohermaphrodites, perform cytogenetic karyotype evaluation in dogs with hypospadias or penile hypoplasia.

TREATMENT

The objectives of medical therapy are:

- Elimination or prevention of infection
- Prevention of adhesion formation
- Reduction of inflammation

Medical Therapy

Trauma

- In animals with traumatic injury to the penis and prepuce, apply local pressure to control hemorrhage, and then cleanse and debride the wounds.
- Sutures may be necessary, depending on the nature of the wound.
- After the wounds are repaired, extrude the penis from the prepuce twice daily in order to apply an antibiotic ointment and prevent adhesions.

Balanthoposthitis

- Administer specific local and systemic antimicrobial drugs, such as trimethoprim-sulfadiazine after foreign bodies or other predisposing factors are eliminated.
- Remove copious preputial discharges and foreign debris with a douche of 10% povidine-iodine.

Paraphimosis

- Treat paraphimosis promptly to prevent further trauma and vascular compromise to the exposed penis.
- Heavy sedation or anesthesia may be necessary to provide adequate therapy.
- Thoroughly cleanse, lubricate, and replace the penis into the prepuce. Cool water soaks or dextrose solutions may be applied to reduce edema.
- Remove any foreign material such as preputial hair constricting the penis.
- If the penis cannot be replaced into the prepuce, the preputial orifice may need to be enlarged (see sec. 8, ch. 13).
- If severe necrosis of the penis has developed from prolonged exposure and vascular compromise, amputation of the penis may be necessary (see sec. 8, ch. 13).

TVT

- TVTs are treated most successfully with chemotherapeutic regimens. Vincristine (Oncovin; Lilly) is effective administered at a dosage of 0.5 mg/m^2, IV, once a week for 3–6 weeks.

Surgical Therapy

- Surgical correction of congenital or acquired conformational defects is indicated if the dog has clinical signs.
- Conditions that require surgical consideration include hypospadias, penile hypoplasia, preputial stenosis, deviation or fractures of the os penis, or a persistent penile frenulum. (Specific reconstructive techniques are discussed in sec. 8, ch. 13.)
- Surgical resection of carcinomas should be radical whenever possible. Amputation of the penis and sheath may be necessary for complete tumor removal (see sec. 8, ch. 13).

Supplemental Readings

Barsanti JA: Vaginal and preputial discharges. *In* Lorenz MD, Cornelius LM, eds.: *Small Animal Medical Diagnosis.* Philadelphia: J. B. Lippincott, 1987, p 359.

Feldman EC, Nelson RW: Disorders of the canine male reproductive tract. *In* Feldman EC, Nelson RW, eds.: *Canine and Feline Endocrinology and Reproduction.* Philadelphia: W. B. Saunders, 1987, p 481.

Hornbuckle WE, White ME: Preputial discharge in the dog. *In* Kirk RW, ed.: *Current Veterinary Therapy X.* Philadelphia: W. B. Saunders, 1989, p 1259.

Johnston SD: Disorders of the canine penis and prepuce. *In* Morrow DA, ed.: *Current Therapy in Theriogenology 2.* Philadelphia: W. B. Saunders, 1986, p 549.

13 Surgery of the Penis and Prepuce

Harry W. Boothe

Surgical procedures of the penis and prepuce include:

Penile amputation to treat traumatic or neoplastic lesions

Enlargement of the preputial orifice to treat phimosis or paraphimosis

Cranial advancement of the prepuce to treat minor deficiency in preputial length

Severance of persistent penile frenulum

Diagnosis and medical treatment of penile problems are discussed in sec. 8, ch. 12.

ANATOMY

Penis

- The feline penis is shorter, directed caudally and covered with small papillae compared to its canine counterpart, but both species have three principal penile divisions: root, body, and distal portion (glans).
- The penile corpora contain enlarged venous spaces and have two principal divisions: corpora cavernosa and corpus spongiosum.
- Each corpus cavernosum (right and left) arises from the ischial tuberosity, continues distally in the dorsolateral part of the penile body as far as the os penis, and is covered by the tunica albuginea.
- The corpus spongiosum originates within the pelvic cavity, surrounds the penile urethra throughout its course, and supplies both the bulbus glandis and pars longa glandis in the distal penis.
- The os penis is located in the penile body and is attached to the bulbus glandis, pars longa glandis, and tunica albuginea.
- The four paired extrinsic penile muscles in the dog are retractor penis, ischiocavernosus, bulbospongiosus, and ischiourethralis.
- The principal blood supply to the penis is from three branches of the artery of the penis, which is a continuation of the internal pudendal artery: artery of the bulb, deep artery of the penis, and dorsal artery of the penis.
- Venous drainage occurs via the internal and external pudendal veins; lymphatic drainage is into the inguinal lymph nodes.
- See sec. 8, ch. 6 for penile anatomy associated with perineal urethrostomy in cats.

Prepuce

- The canine and feline prepuce covers the nonerect penis.

- Paired preputial muscles extend from the xiphoid cartilage to the dorsal preputial wall.
- Blood supply is via the caudal superficial epigastric artery and dorsal artery of the penis; lymphatic drainage is into the inguinal lymph nodes.

PENILE AMPUTATION

Preoperative Considerations

- The location and extensiveness of traumatic or neoplastic penile lesions determine the site of penile amputation. Animals with urethral prolapse that recurs after attempts to resect urethral mucosa may require partial penile amputation. Nonsurgical management of certain neoplasms of the penis (e.g., transmissible venereal tumor) may be preferable (see sec. 8, ch. 12).
- Preputial shortening may be indicated after partial penile amputation.
- Bilateral orchidectomy, scrotal ablation, and either scrotal (preferred) or perineal urethrostomy are indicated following extensive penile amputation.

Surgical Procedure

Objectives

- Provide hemostasis by ligation and closure of the tunica albuginea.
- Create a permanent urethrostomy by suturing urethral mucosa to either penile mucosa or skin.
- Avoid an osteotomy by positioning the amputation site either cranial or caudal to the os penis.

Equipment

- Standard general surgical pack and suture
- Penrose drain tubing for temporary tourniquet application

Technique—Partial Amputation

1. Place dog in dorsal recumbency, prepare the preputial cavity by multiple flushes with chlorhexidene solution (Nolvasan; Fort Dodge), and catheterize the urethra.
2. Maintain penile exteriorization from the prepuce by placing Penrose drain tubing around the penis as far caudally as possible. Place a tourniquet around the penis proximal to the site of excision.
3. Create bilateral flaps of the tunic and cavernous tissue, using sharp dissection, proximal to the os penis while leaving the urethra intact.

889

4. Dissect the urethra and transect it just distal to the proposed amputation site.
5. Transect the os penis, if necessary, with bone-cutting forceps at the base of the flap.
6. Identify and ligate blood vessels after loosening the tourniquet and appose the tunica albuginea and flaps of erectile tissue (simple interrupted pattern, absorbable suture).
7. Suture urethral mucosa to penile mucosa over the ventral portion of the end of the penile stump (simple interrupted, absorbable suture) after incising the urethra along its dorsal midline (Fig. 1).

Technique—Subtotal Penile Amputation

1. Place dog in dorsal recumbency and prepare ventral abdominal and perineal regions.
2. Incise skin in a curvilinear fashion along each side of the prepuce to an appropriate level on the perineal midline (Fig. 2).
3. Isolate and temporarily encircle the penis cranial to the scrotum, using a heavy ligature proximal to the initial transection site.
4. Transect and remove the penis, prepuce, testes, and scrotum.
5. Exteriorize the proximal portion of the penis through a separate midline perineal skin incision; remove the temporary ligature, provide definitive hemostasis, and close the tunica albuginea over the end of the penis (simple interrupted pattern, absorbable suture).
6. Perform a perineal urethrostomy proximal to the penile amputation site (simple interrupted pattern, nonabsorbable sutures) (see sec. 8, ch. 6).
7. Routinely close the ventral abdominal incision.

Postoperative Care and Complications

■ Hemorrhage and/or hematoma formation may occur at the penile amputation or urethrostomy site.

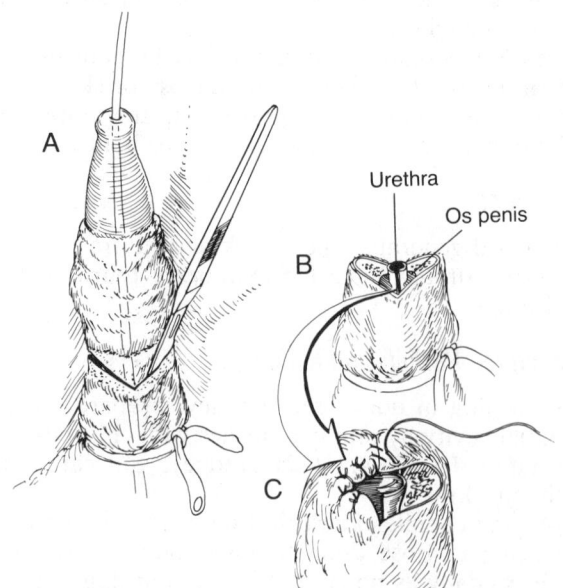

Figure 1. Closure of the end of the penis following partial penile amputation. The urethral mucosa is sutured to penile mucosa near the ventrum of the incision, while the remainder of the end of the penis is closed.

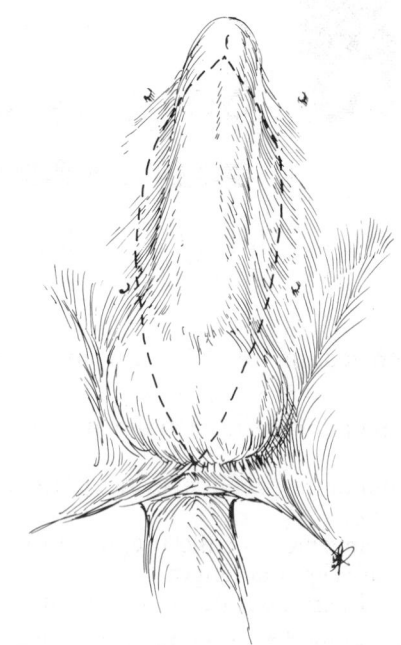

Figure 2. Skin incision for a subtotal penile amputation. The skin incision extends from cranial to the prepuce to the perineal midline.

■ Prevent self-inflicted trauma.

Prognosis

■ The prognosis depends on the disease process(es) present.
■ Urethral stricture may occur if healing is complicated (e.g., urethral mucosal dehiscence occurs).
■ Minimal long-term patient morbidity is expected.

ENLARGEMENT OF THE PREPUTIAL ORIFICE

Preoperative Considerations

■ Use this procedure to correct phimosis (multiple attempts may be necessary). Position the incision on the dorsal aspect of the prepuce to avoid persistent exposure of the distal portion of the penis.

Surgical Procedure

Objectives

■ Enlarge the preputial orifice to allow unrestricted movement of the penis in and out of the prepuce.
■ Minimize fibrous tissue formation by accurately apposing tissues.
■ Completely excise neoplasms, if present.

Equipment

■ Standard general surgical pack and suture

Technique

1. Position dog in dorsal recumbency and aseptically prepare the parapreputial area.
2. Excise a wedge-shaped segment of skin, subcutaneous tissue, and preputial mucosa on the dorsal

surface of the prepuce to enable exteriorization of the end of the penis.

3. Appose the preputial mucosa to the skin (simple interrupted pattern, nonabsorbable sutures).

Postoperative Care and Complications

- Prevent self-inflicted trauma to the surgical site (an Elizabethan collar may be necessary).
- Postoperative fibrosis may create an insufficient preputial orifice.
- Patient growth may necessitate another surgical procedure.

Prognosis

- The prognosis generally is good, provided there is complete excision of tumor.

CRANIAL ADVANCEMENT OF THE PREPUCE

Preoperative Consideration

- This procedure is indicated in dogs with incomplete preputial coverage of the penis in order to prevent desiccation and irritation. Only minor deficiencies (<1–2 cm) in preputial length can be corrected by advancing the prepuce cranially along the abdominal wall.

Surgical Procedure

Objective

- Achieve complete coverage of the distal penis.

Equipment

- Standard general surgical pack and suture

Technique

1. Place dog in dorsal recumbency and aseptically prepare the ventral abdomen.
2. Make a U-shaped incision in the skin immediately cranial to the prepuce.
3. Dissect this part of the prepuce from the abdominal skin, advance the prepuce cranially until the penis is covered, and mark this point on the skin.
4. Make a U-shaped incision in the skin at the mark and excise the skin between the two incisions.
5. Suture the prepuce to its cranial position (simple interrupted pattern, absorbable and nonabsorbable sutures).

Postoperative Care and Complications

- Although adequate penile coverage may be achieved at surgery, exposure of the distal penis may return postoperatively.

- Prevent self-inflicted trauma.

Prognosis

- Repair of congenital preputial defects has a guarded prognosis.
- An extensive preputial deficiency may require partial or subtotal penile amputation or preputial reconstruction.

SEVERANCE OF PERSISTENT PENILE FRENULUM

Preoperative Considerations

- The penile frenulum normally ruptures by puberty.
- The persistent penile frenulum usually is composed of minimally vascular connective tissue.

Surgical Procedure

Objective

- Sever the persistent penile frenulum to enable painless extrusion of the penis from the prepuce.

Equipment

- Standard minor surgical pack

Technique

1. Place dog in lateral recumbency and aseptically prepare the preputial cavity.
2. Exteriorize the penis and sever the penile frenulum with scissors. Control hemorrhage with local pressure.

Postoperative Care and Complications

- Prevent self-inflicted trauma.

Prognosis

- The prognosis is good.

Supplemental Readings

Boothe HW: Penis. In Slatter DH, ed.: Textbook of Small Animal Surgery. Philadelphia: W. B. Saunders, 1985, p 1628.
Boothe HW: Prepuce. In Slatter DH, ed.: Textbook of Small Animal Surgery. Philadelphia: W. B. Saunders, 1985, p 1633.
Christie TR: Phimosis and paraphimosis. In Bojrab MJ, ed.: Pathophysiology in Small Animal Surgery. Philadelphia: Lea & Febiger, 1981, p 442.
Evans HE, Christensen GC: Miller's Anatomy of the Dog. Philadelphia: W. B. Saunders, 1979, p 554.
Hobson HP: Surgical procedures of the penis. In Bojrab MJ, ed.: Current Techniques in Small Animal Surgery, 3rd Ed. Philadelphia: Lea & Febiger, 1990, p 423.
Smith MM, Gourley IM: Preputial reconstruction in a dog. J Am Vet Med Assoc 196:1493, 1990.

14 Diseases of the Ovaries and Uterus

Amy M. Grooters

DISEASES OF THE OVARIES

Primary ovarian disease is uncommon in the dog and cat and includes ovarian cysts and ovarian neoplasia. For information concerning infertility in the bitch and queen, see sec. 8, ch. 18.

Cystic Ovarian Disease

Ovarian cysts may be normal structures, including vesicular follicles and cavities within immature corpora lutea, or abnormal structures, including follicular cysts and luteinized cysts. Remnant ovarian tissue resulting from incomplete ovariohysterectomy may also become cystic.

Clinical Signs

Signs associated with abnormal ovarian cysts are due to excess sex hormone secretion by the cystic structure or decreased function of the remaining ovarian tissue.

Persistent Anestrus. Persistent anestrus or an increased interestrous interval is the most common clinical sign associated with follicular and luteinized cysts.

- When associated with nonfunctional follicular cysts, this is probably the result of a mass effect of the cystic structure, causing a decrease in the surrounding functional ovarian tissue.
- Luteinized cysts prolong anestrus through persistent progesterone secretion.

Persistent Estrus. The duration of estrus in the bitch usually is 5–9 days and is considered abnormal if it lasts more than 3 weeks.

- Persistent estrus can be caused by continued secretion of estrogen by follicular cysts, or it can be caused by functional ovarian tumors.
- Persistent estrus may be identified by the owner as behavior consistent with estrus or as persistent hemorrhagic vaginal discharge.
- Differentiate this condition from *split estrus*, which may be seen in young bitches. Split estrus occurs when follicular development is followed by follicular regression instead of progressing to ovulation, resulting in clinical signs of proestrus that are not followed by signs of estrus until the bitch enters estrus during a subsequent cycle (usually 2–12 weeks later).

Diagnosis

- Perform *vaginal cytology* to confirm estrogen influence in a bitch displaying signs consistent with persistent estrus. A majority of superficial cells is expected (see sec. 8, ch. 16 for vaginal cytology techniques).
- Measure *plasma estrogen concentrations* to confirm excess estrogen secretion; however, normal concentrations do not rule out functional ovarian cysts.
- *Abdominal ultrasonography* may be used to identify cystic ovarian structures; however, this modality cannot definitively differentiate normal from abnormal cystic structures.
- *Surgical exploration* provides a definitive diagnosis.

Treatment

Ovariohysterectomy. Ovariohysterectomy (see sec. 8, ch. 15) is the treatment of choice for nonbreeding animals and is curative.

Medical Therapy. Pharmacologic agents to induce luteinization of the cysts may be attempted in breeding bitches. The following drugs have been used:

- Gonadotropin-releasing hormone (Cystorelin, Sanofi), given once at a dose of 50 μg/bitch, IM.
- Human chorionic gonadotropin (HCG; Steris), given once at a dose of 22 units/kg, IM.
- Poor response to treatment and recurrence of cystic disease are possible following medical therapy. Insufficient information is available to evaluate response and recurrence rates or to predict fertility following treatment.
- When medical therapy is successful, response is expected in 2–3 weeks and indicated by a change in vaginal cytology from cornified to noncornified cells.

Ovarian Neoplasia

Tumors of the ovary are uncommon in the bitch and queen and are classified according to their embryologic origin as epithelial, germ cell, or sex-cord stromal tumors. The most common ovarian tumors in the bitch are epithelial and granulosa cell tumors.

Classification

Epithelial Tumors
- *Papillary adenoma* is a benign tumor that often occurs bilaterally and is one of the most common ovarian neoplasms seen in the bitch.

- *Papillary adenocarcinoma* is a malignant tumor that frequently is bilateral. Metastasis is common through the ovarian bursa to the abdominal cavity, as well as to regional lymphatics and distant sites. Abdominal cavity metastasis may result in peritoneal effusion. Adenocarcinoma is the most common malignant tumor of the ovary in the bitch.
- *Cystadenoma* is a less common benign epithelial tumor that consists of multiple thin-walled cysts.

Sex-Cord Stromal Tumors

KEY POINT ▶ Granulosa cell tumors occur frequently in the bitch and are the most common ovarian tumor in the queen.

- Granulosa cell tumors are usually large unilateral tumors that are often palpable, can cause abdominal distension, and may produce signs of hyperestrogenism including persistent estrus.
  - These tumors commonly are malignant in the cat but often are benign in the dog, with metastasis occurring in only 10–25% of cases.
- *Thecomas* and *luteomas* are rare, but these cell types may be found in combination with granulosa cell tumors.

Germ Cell Tumors

- *Dysgerminomas* are uncommon. These large unilateral tumors have a metastatic rate of 10–20%.
- *Teratomas,* which develop as multiple tissue types such as epithelium, cartilage, and bone, are large benign unilateral tumors and may cause a palpable abdominal mass or abdominal enlargement.

Diagnosis

Many ovarian tumors cause no symptoms and may be incidental findings at necropsy or surgery.

- Most signs associated with ovarian neoplasia are related to a large abdominal mass, peritoneal effusion, local or distant metastasis, or hyperestrogenism.
- Abdominal radiography or ultrasonography can be used to confirm the presence of a mass but rarely allows determination of its origin.
- Definitive diagnosis is made through exploratory laparotomy.

Treatment

Ovariohysterectomy. The treatment of choice for ovarian neoplasia is ovariohysterectomy, which is often curative if metastasis has not occurred. Avoid rupture of the tumor during removal.

- Exploration of the abdomen allows staging of the tumor, and biopsy of local lymph nodes is indicated if they are enlarged.
- Chemotherapy may be used in addition to surgery for metastatic tumors, but this is only palliative. Cyclophosphamide (50 mg/m^2, PO, given three times a week) has been used in dogs for granulosa cell tumors and carcinomas.

DISEASES OF THE UTERUS

Pyometra

Pyometra in dogs and cats is the result of hormonally induced changes in the uterus that allow secondary infection to occur. The patency of the cervix (closed or open pyometra) is an important influence on the severity of the disease, its prognosis, and the treatment options that can be offered.

Etiology

Cystic Endometrial Hyperplasia. The first step in the development of pyometra is cystic endometrial hyperplasia (CEH), which is an exaggerated response of the endometrium to progesterone. The mechanism is as follows:

- Following ovulation, the intact female enters a luteal phase (diestrus) that is characterized by elevated plasma progesterone concentrations for 8–10 weeks.
- In preparation for a possible pregnancy, the uterus responds to increases in progesterone with glandular hypertrophy and increased endometrial secretory activity.
  - Prolonged progesterone influence causes this glandular tissue to become cystic, edematous, and grossly thickened.
- Excessive secretions may accumulate within the uterus, providing an ideal environment for bacterial growth. This is complicated by the inhibition of myometrial contractility by progesterone, which decreases uterine drainage.

Exogenously administered progestins, such as megestrol acetate (Ovaban; Shering), result in similar endometrial changes that are especially severe with higher doses or prolonged administration.

Bacterial Infection. Secondary bacterial infections usually originate from contamination through the cervix, and may be facilitated by a progesterone-mediated inhibition of leukocyte function.

- *Escherichia coli,* the most common organism isolated, has a specific affinity for progesterone-sensitized endometrium, and can bind to the endometrium and myometrium through a specific antigen.

Exogenous Estrogens. Exogenous estrogens alone do not cause cystic endometrial hyperplasia, but they do potentiate the effects of progesterone on the uterus, thereby predisposing to pyometra.

KEY POINT ▶ The use of estrogen to prevent pregnancy greatly increases the risk of developing pyometra and is a common cause of pyometra in young bitches.

Clinical Signs

Signalment. Pyometra occurs in older intact bitches and queens except when exogenous estrogens or progestins are given, in which case younger animals may be affected.

History

- Signs of pyometra usually occur 1–2 months after estrus or exogenous progesterone administration.
- Lethargy, depression, and anorexia are common; these signs are more severe in cases of closed-cervix pyometra. Vomiting and diarrhea also occur more often with closed pyometra.
- Vaginal discharge is present in most animals with pyometra and typically is purulent but may contain blood or mucus.
- Polyuria and compensatory polydypsia may occur because of impairment of renal tubular concentrating ability. This is probably due to unresponsiveness of the tubules to antidiuretic hormone (ADH) mediated by *E. coli* endotoxin, although the exact mechanism is unknown.
- Cats with pyometra are sometimes presented primarily for evaluation of abdominal distension.

KEY POINT ▶ Because pyometra is such a common disease, a high index of suspicion is warranted when an intact female animal is presented with nonspecific signs of illness.

Physical Examination

- Common findings in open-cervix pyometra include lethargy, dehydration, a palpable uterus, and vaginal discharge.
- Closed-cervix pyometra is more likely to result in septicemia, which may cause shock, hypothermia, and collapse.
- Fever is a variable finding and often is absent.

Diagnosis

Clinical Pathology

- *Hematology* typically shows an inflammatory leukogram characterized by extreme neutrophilia with a left shift. In more severe cases, sepsis results in toxic changes in the neutrophils and a degenerative left shift. However, a normal leukogram can also occur with pyometra, and is usually associated with an open cervix. A mild nonregenerative anemia and hyperproteinemia are common.
- *Serum chemistry abnormalities* include hyperglobulinemia due to chronic antigenic stimulation and azotemia that usually is prerenal.
- Electrolyte abnormalities may be present if vomiting has been severe.
- *Urinalysis* may reveal isosthenuria caused by decreased concentrating ability, and proteinuria caused by immune complex glomerular damage or preexisting renal disease.
- Do not attempt cystocentesis when pyometra is suspected because of the possibility of damage to the friable uterus and subsequent abdominal contamination.

Radiography and Ultrasonography

- Perform *abdominal radiography* to confirm the presence of an enlarged uterus and to evaluate for the possibility of uterine rupture and peritonitis. A normal nongravid uterus cannot be detected on abdominal radiographs.
- Pyometra results in a fluid-dense tubular structure in the caudal abdomen that often displaces bowel loops cranially and dorsally. However, this is also the appearance of a gravid uterus before fetal skeletal calcification (<42 days of gestation). Therefore, pyometra must be differentiated from pregnancy, which may also be associated with a vaginal discharge.

KEY POINT ▶ Open-cervix pyometra may allow enough drainage to prevent radiographically detectable uterine enlargement; therefore, the inability to visualize the uterus on abdominal radiographs does not rule out the possibility of pyometra.

- Perform *abdominal ultrasonography* to differentiate pyometra from pregnancy.

Cytology and Culture

- Vaginal cytology and culture may be helpful in the diagnosis of pyometra but do not provide a definitive diagnosis.
- Cranial vaginal cultures may be used to choose an appropriate antibiotic if medical therapy is employed.

Treatment

- *Ovariohysterectomy* is the treatment of choice for pyometra.
- Medical management may be attempted in stable animals whose breeding potential is of utmost importance.
- The decision to treat pyometra surgically or medically depends on the condition of the animal at the time of presentation, its age, and the importance to the owner of preserving the animal's reproductive capacity.

Surgical Management

Preoperative Considerations

- Institute fluid and antibiotic therapy before surgery in all cases. Animals with signs of sepsis or shock require very aggressive fluid therapy. Immediately administer broad-spectrum antibiotics intravenously, such as cephalothin (Keflin; Lilly) (22 mg/kg q8h) and amikacin (Amiglyde-V; Fort Dodge) (5–10 mg/kg q12h).

KEY POINT ▶ Because of their nephrotoxicity, use aminoglycosides such as amikacin cautiously in dehydrated animals or in those with questionable renal function.

- Surgically remove the uterus as soon as the animal is stable enough for anesthesia.

Surgical Procedure. For a discussion of ovariohysterectomy, see sec. 8, ch. 15.

Postoperative Considerations

- Continue supportive care with fluids and injectable antibiotics postoperatively, if necessary. However, most animals show great improvement following removal of the uterus if abdominal contamination has not occurred.

- Continue oral antibiotic therapy (e.g., cephalosporin or trimethoprim-sulfa) for 10–14 days after surgery.
- The prognosis is good if there is no uterine rupture or other cause of abdominal contamination, with mortality rates below 10%.
- In animals with gross peritoneal contamination and resultant peritonitis, treat with open abdominal drainage (see sec. 7, ch. 13).

Medical Management. The basis of medical treatment of pyometra in the bitch and queen is the use of pharmacologic agents to reduce the plasma progesterone concentration, relax the cervix, and promote myometrial contraction, resulting in evacuation of the uterus. Several different drugs, including ecbolic and hormonal compounds, have been used in the past in an attempt to treat pyometra. However, only prostaglandins produce a consistent response. Concomitant systemic antibiotics are used to prevent bacteremia during uterine evacuation.

Indications
- Reserve medical management for younger, breeding animals without signs of sepsis or severe illness at the time of presentation.
- Both open- and closed-cervix pyometra can be treated with prostaglandins. However, medical treatment of closed-cervix pyometra carries a guarded prognosis because of a low response rate and the potential for uterine rupture or retrograde movement of uterine contents through the oviducts into the abdominal cavity, causing peritonitis.

Prostaglandin Therapy. Prostaglandin $F_{2\alpha}$ ($PGF_{2\alpha}$) acts by causing cervical dilation, myometrial contraction, and, at higher dosages, luteolysis.

- Naturally occurring and synthetic analogs of $PGF_{2\alpha}$ are available. However, only the natural product (Lutalyse; Upjohn) should be used because the synthetic analogs are highly potent compounds whose efficacy for pyometra in small animals has not yet been investigated. None of the prostaglandins currently are approved for use in small animals.
- *Protocol* (for bitches and queens): Administer 0.25 mg/kg $PGF_{2\alpha}$ SC once daily for 3–5 days. The duration of therapy is dictated by the response as measured by resolution of uterine discharge and decreased uterine size. The character of the vaginal discharge will usually change to serous or serosanguineous before it disappears.
- Clinical improvement is not apparent until 48 hours following the first prostaglandin injection. For this reason, medical therapy is a poor option for animals presented with evidence of sepsis or toxemia. If these signs occur during the course of prostaglandin treatment, ovariohysterectomy may be needed.
- Monitor all animals treated with prostaglandins, especially those with closed-cervix pyometra, for signs of abdominal contamination and peritonitis, necessitating surgery.
- Recheck the animal 2 weeks after prostaglandin therapy. If purulent vaginal discharge or uterine enlargement is still present, a second series of injections can be administered.

- *Side effects* of prostaglandin therapy are encountered routinely, especially with initial administration. They include restlessness, panting, vomiting, defecation, tachycardia, fever, abdominal pain, and salivation. These effects occur within 15–120 minutes after SC injection of $PGF_{2\alpha}$.
  - The severity of the reaction is dose-dependent and decreases with subsequent injections, so that side effects are usually minimal by the fourth and fifth administrations.
  - Empirically, side effects may be reduced by walking the animal for 30 minutes after each injection.

Antibiotic Therapy
- Administer systemic broad spectrum bactericidal antibiotics such as trimethoprim-sulfa (Tribrissen; Burroughs Wellcome), 15 mg/kg q12h, PO, concurrent with prostaglandin therapy to prevent bacteremia during uterine evacuation. Base the choice of antibiotics on sensitivity testing results of cranial vaginal cultures. Continue oral antibiotics for 1–3 weeks following evacuation of the uterus.

Complications. Complications of medical therapy include uterine rupture, contamination of the peritoneal cavity, sepsis, and the side effects of the prostaglandin itself as previously described.

- Evaluate animals treated with $PGF_{2\alpha}$ daily for signs of peritonitis and sepsis.

Prognosis

- Success rates for clinical resolution of open-cervix pyometra following prostaglandin treatment range from 76% to 93%. Approximately one-third of bitches treated successfully for open-cervix pyometra require two series of prostaglandin injections.
- The response of closed-cervix pyometra to medical therapy is poor, with 25–40% of bitches treated obtaining clinical resolution. The percentage of bitches with closed-cervix pyometra requiring two series of injections is higher than for those with open-cervix pyometra.
- Recurrence of pyometra after medical therapy is fairly common and is reported to be as high as 77% in bitches followed long-term. This may indicate that prostaglandin therapy does not totally resolve the uterine pathology but simply reduces it to a subclinical level. For these reasons, animals treated successfully with prostaglandins should be bred during the first subsequent estrus to maximize the chances of obtaining a litter.
- The percentage of successfully treated bitches that go on to produce at least one normal litter is reported to be 40–74%. Data concerning the response and recurrence rates in the queen are not available.

Acute Metritis

Metritis is a severe postpartum bacterial infection of the uterus that may progress rapidly to sepsis and toxemia.

Etiology

The onset of metritis is almost always in the immediate postpartum period, although it may also occur after artificial insemination, natural breeding, or abortion.

- Ascending bacterial infection occurs secondary to a predisposing factor such as a retained placenta, retained fetus, or trauma from dystocia or obstetrical manipulations.
- *Escherichia coli* is the most common invading organism, but gram-positive bacterial infections also occur.

Clinical Signs

Acute metritis can occur in any postpartum bitch but most often is associated with a predisposing complication of parturition.

- The onset of clinical signs is acute and occurs within 1 week of parturition.
- Abnormalities reported in the history are consistent with systemic illness and include lethargy, anorexia, loss of maternal instinct, poor milk production, and vomiting.
- A foul-smelling vaginal discharge is typical.
- Physical examination reveals depression, dehydration, tachycardia, fever, and an enlarged turgid uterus.
- Metritis may progress rapidly to sepsis and subsequent shock and hypothermia.

Diagnosis

The diagnosis of acute metritis is usually based on the history and physical examination alone. Further diagnostics are useful to confirm the diagnosis and assess the severity of the accompanying sepsis.

Clinical Pathology. The hemogram reflects a severe bacterial infection with a neutrophilia with a left shift or leukopenia with a degenerative left shift in septic animals. Serum chemistries usually are normal with the exception of prerenal azotemia.

Radiology and Ultrasonography. Perform abdominal radiographs or ultrasonography to confirm uterine enlargement and to check for the presence of retained fetuses. Ultrasonography may be useful to identify a retained placenta.

Cytology and Culture. Evaluation of the vaginal discharge can help to differentiate acute metritis from other causes of postpartum vaginal discharge such as hemorrhage and normal lochia.

- The discharge of acute metritis is septic, containing neutrophils, bacteria, and sometimes endometrial cells.
- Cranial vaginal cultures are not diagnostic for metritis but are useful in guiding antibiotic therapy.

Treatment

Because of its acute progressive nature, metritis necessitates immediate therapy. Administer IV fluids and antibiotics in conjunction with removal of the uterine contents through pharmacologic evacuation or ovariohysterectomy, depending on whether the animal will be used for breeding. Because of the debilitating nature of this disease and its effect on milk production, most bitches with acute metritis are unable to nurse their pups, necessitating bottle-feeding of the litter.

Medical Management

Fluid Therapy. Initiate fluid therapy on presentation. Septic animals may require shock doses of IV fluids (see sec. 6, ch. 14).

Antibiotic Therapy. Administer broad-spectrum bactericidal intravenous antibiotics immediately.

- A combination of amikacin (Amiglyde-V; Fort Dodge) (5–10 mg/kg q12h, IV) with cephalothin (Keflin; Lilly) (22 mg/kg, q8h, IV) or amikacin with sodium penicillin G (25,000 units/kg, q6h, IV) is often used if sepsis is suspected.
- *Note:* Because of their nephrotoxicity, use aminoglycosides such as amikacin cautiously in dehydrated animals or those with questionable renal function.
- Base the choice of antibiotic on sensitivity results from cranial vaginal cultures, once these are available.
- Continue oral antibiotics for 1–2 weeks following removal of the uterine contents.

Uterine Evacuation. This is accomplished pharmacologically with ecbolic agents to stimulate myometrial contraction and promote uterine involution. Uterine rupture is a potential complication of initiating contractions in a friable or obstructed uterus.

- Administer oxytocin, 0.5–1.0 units/kg (maximum 20 units), IM; repeat in 1–2 hours if needed.
- Administer prostaglandin $F_{2\alpha}$ (Lutalyse; Upjohn) once daily for 3–5 days at a dose of 0.25 mg/kg, SC (see discussion of pyometra for details of prostaglandin therapy).

Uterine Infusion. If the cervix can be cannulated, an intrauterine infusion of 2% povidone-iodine solution or sterile saline may be helpful.

- Because of the friable state of the diseased uterus, uterine rupture is a potential complication, and catheterization should be done cautiously.

Surgical Management. Indications for ovariohysterectomy (see sec. 8, ch. 15) in the treatment of acute metritis include uterine rupture, retained fetuses, poor response to medical management, and animals not intended for future breeding.

Prognosis

- Acute metritis carries a guarded prognosis because progression to sepsis and toxemia can rapidly cause life-threatening illness.
- Chronic metritis may result in infertility.

Subinvolution of Placental Sites

Normal uterine involution occurs to a large degree in the 4–6 weeks following parturition and is fully complete by 12 weeks post partum. During this time, sloughing of collagenous masses from placental sites and reconstruction of the endometrium result in a hemorrhagic vaginal discharge called lochia. This discharge is normally present for up to 6 weeks after parturition. Subinvolution of placental sites (SIPS) is a delay in the normal involution process that results in a persistent hemorrhagic postpartum discharge.

Etiology

- The cause of the failure of normal involution in SIPS is unknown.
- Histopathologically, SIPS is characterized by the invasion of trophoblast-like cells into the endometrium and myometrium, which may prevent involution.
- Lack of thrombosis in endometrial blood vessels results in persistent hemorrhage from the uterus.
- SIPS may involve all placental sites in the uterus, or only a portion of them, with the remaining sites showing normal involution.

Clinical Signs

- SIPS occurs most often in young (<3 years) female dogs of any breed which may be either primiparous or multiparous.
- Persistent hemorrhagic vaginal discharge lasting longer than 6 weeks post partum is usually the only sign associated with SIPS, and affected bitches appear otherwise healthy on physical examination.
- Abdominal palpation may reveal distinct, firm round masses within the uterus.
- Very rarely is the amount of hemorrhage from the uterus enough to produce signs of anemia.

Diagnosis

- The diagnosis of SIPS usually is based simply on the presence of a persistent hemorrhagic postpartum discharge in an otherwise healthy bitch. Rule out other causes of hemorrhagic discharge following parturition, including metritis, retained fetal or placental tissues, coagulopathy, trauma to the genital tract, and chronic vaginitis.
- Abdominal palpation, radiography, and ultrasonography can aid in the differential diagnosis of SIPS.
- Vaginal cytology consists of erythrocytes, neutrophils, and parabasal cells. Occasionally, trophoblast-like cells are present in the discharge, suggesting SIPS.
- A definitive diagnosis of SIPS of placental sites can be made only on histopathology.

Treatment

- Most bitches with SIPS do not require treatment because spontaneous resolution of the discharge usually occurs.
- Ovariohysterectomy is the treatment of choice in nonbreeding animals.
- Monitor breeding animals with SIPS for potential complications, including perforation of the uterine wall, ascending metritis, and anemia.

Prognosis

- Because the disease is self-limiting and complications are infrequent, the prognosis is good.
- There does not seem to be any decrease in fertility in bitches following spontaneous resolution of SIPS, and there is no predisposition for recurrence of subinvolution with future litters.

Uterine Prolapse

Uterine prolapse is a rare problem in the bitch and queen that usually occurs during or immediately after parturition but also can be seen following abortion.

- Prolapse may be associated with dystocia, forced fetal or placental extraction, or excessive straining due to retained tissues, metritis, or other causes. However, it may also occur with normal parturition.
- The diagnosis is made by identification of the prolapsed uterine tissue, which must be differentiated from vaginal hyperplasia and neoplasia (see sec. 8, ch. 16).
- Treatment of uterine prolapse includes supportive fluid therapy and either reduction or amputation of the prolapsed tissue. If prolapse occurs as a complication of excessive straining, eliminate the cause of the straining.
  - For a discussion of manual reduction and surgical amputation for uterine prolapse, see sec. 8, ch. 15.
  - If the uterus is re-placed, administer systemic antibiotic therapy to treat metritis.

Uterine Torsion

Torsion of the uterus is uncommon in small animals and usually occurs near the end of gestation (although it can occur without pregnancy), resulting in dystocia.

- Clinical signs include abdominal distension, abdominal pain, and hemorrhagic vaginal discharge.
- Abdominal radiographs are consistent with either a gravid or fluid-filled uterus.
- Treatment of uterine torsion is ovariohysterectomy because the ischemic uterine tissue usually is devitalized.

Uterine Neoplasia

Tumors of the uterus are very rare in dogs and cats.

- Leiomyomas, which are benign tumors arising from the myometrium, account for the majority of uterine tumors.
- Leiomyosarcoma is the most common malignant neoplasia in the bitch, whereas endometrial adenocarcinoma is most common in the queen.
- Other tumor types include fibrosarcoma, fibroma, lipoma, and adenoma.

Clinical Signs

- Many uterine tumors are not associated with clinical signs and are discovered as incidental findings at necropsy or during elective ovariohysterectomy.

- Large tumors may cause abdominal distension or compression of the gastrointestinal or urinary tracts, resulting in tenesmus and dysuria.
- If vaginal discharge is present, it typically is hemorrhagic.

Diagnosis

- The diagnosis of uterine neoplasia is supported by identification of a mass lesion on abdominal radiographs or ultrasonography.
- Vaginal cytology is rarely helpful because leiomyomas and leiomyosarcomas do not readily exfoliate neoplastic cells.
- Exploratory laparotomy is often necessary for definitive diagnosis.

Treatment

- Ovariohysterectomy is the only recommended treatment for uterine neoplasia. It is usually curative unless metastasis has occurred.

Abortion

Etiology

Abortion may be the result of fetal, maternal, or placental disorders. These disorders represent a variety of etiologies, including systemic or reproductive tract disease in the bitch or queen, fetal maldevelopment, and infectious agents.

Maternal Disorders. Maternal disorders that result in abortion may be systemic or may be confined to the reproductive tract. Any serious systemic illness potentially can result in abortion through secondary effects on the uterus and/or fetus. Disorders of the reproductive tract that result in abortion may be uterine or ovarian in origin.

- Uterine diseases that can cause abortion include chronic endometritis, cystic endometrial hyperplasia, and uterine adhesions.
- Ovarian diseases may result in abortion if the corpus luteum fails to secrete progesterone in amounts sufficient to maintain pregnancy, which is termed hypoluteoidism. Cases of primary hypoluteoidism in the bitch and queen have not been well documented.

Fetal Maldevelopment. Maldevelopment resulting in fetal death causes resorption or abortion, depending on the stage of gestation.

Infectious Agents. Organisms that can cause abortion in the bitch include *Brucella canis, Campylobacter, Streptococcus, Leptospira, Escherichia coli, Toxoplasma,* canine herpesvirus, canine distemper virus, and *Mycoplasma.* Of these, *B. canis* and canine herpesvirus are probably the most important because of their impact on breeding programs. In the queen, viral agents such as feline leukemia virus, feline infectious peritonitis, and feline rhinotracheitis are most important.

Brucellosis

Brucella canis infection usually causes abortion in the third trimester of gestation, but it may also cause embryonic death and subsequent resorption early in pregnancy.

- Most dogs with brucellosis are not seriously ill, and many are asymptomatic carriers.
- In addition to abortion and resorption, *B. canis* infection is associated with infertility and pups which may be stillborn or bacteremic.
- *B. canis* infection is important because of its impact on breeding populations; it can have devastating results because it is a highly contagious organism for which there is no vaccine or effective treatment (see sec. 2, ch. 11 for more information).

Canine Herpesvirus

Infection with canine herpesvirus has been reported to cause late gestation abortion, stillbirth, mummified fetuses, a decrease in the number of pups per litter, and infertility in the bitch.

- In addition, it causes an acute hemorrhagic septicemia in neonatal puppies of affected bitches (see sec. 2, ch. 9 for more information).

Drugs. Drugs that have been associated with abortion in the bitch include glucocorticoids and chloramphenicol.

Clinical Signs

- Observable signs of abortion vary according to the etiology and time of gestation.
  - Early fetal resorption may occur without any clinical signs or may be associated with a vaginal discharge.
  - Bitches aborting late in gestation may show signs consistent with normal parturition, such as restlessness and abdominal contractions.
- Signs of systemic illness such as anorexia, lethargy, vomiting, or diarrhea at any time during pregnancy may be an indication of recent or impending abortion and are an indication for thorough evaluation of the bitch.
- Bitches with canine herpesvirus may develop vesicular or follicular lesions of the vaginal mucosa soon after they are infected. These lesions are transient and often recur during proestrus.

Diagnosis

A definitive diagnosis of abortion is difficult to make unless expulsion of fetuses is actually observed. Documentation of early pregnancy is difficult, so that early embryonic resorption may be clinically indistinguishable from infertility. Ultrasonography can be used to consistently demonstrate pregnancy in the bitch after 16 days of gestation. Radiographic detection is dependent on fetal skeletal calcification, which can be seen after 42 days of gestation.

General Diagnostics

- Give all animals suspected of aborting a pregnancy a thorough physical examination to evaluate for systemic illness.
- If signs of illness are detected, a hemogram, biochemical profile, and urinalysis are indicated.

■ Thoroughly evaluate the possibility of pyometra in any diestral animal with systemic signs of illness.
■ Abdominal palpation may allow assessment of pregnancy status if the animal is in mid or late gestation.

KEY POINT ▶ Ultrasonography is an invaluable tool for assessing the status of pregnancy in the bitch and queen and is especially helpful in early gestation.

■ In addition to evaluating the presence and viability of any fetuses in the uterus, ultrasonography may indicate uterine pathology in some cases. It is also useful for the identification of retained pups (either alive or dead) in an animal which is known to have aborted.
■ If an aborted fetus and/or placenta is available, perform necropsy, histopathology, and culture.
■ Samples from a cranial vaginal swab or from post-abortion vaginal discharge may also be useful for culture.

Specific Diagnostics

Serology. Serologic tests for *B. canis* are indicated in any bitch suspected of abortion or fetal resorption. Several serologic tests are available for evaluation of canine brucellosis (see also sec. 2, ch. 11).

■ The rapid slide agglutination test (RSAT) is an excellent screening test because it gives very few false-negative results, and thus an animal with a negative RSAT is almost certainly free from infection.
■ However, because false-positive results are fairly common, retest bitches with positive RSAT results with the more specific tube agglutination test (TAT), which has a low incidence of false-positive results.
■ An agar gel immunodiffusion (AGID) test is available for retesting of samples that were positive on the RSAT or TAT.

Plasma Progesterone. Plasma progesterone concentrations can be measured to document hypoluteoidism as a cause of abortion.

■ Progesterone concentrations <2 ng/ml are inadequate to maintain pregnancy and are consistent with luteal failure.
■ In some cases luteal regression and low progesterone levels may occur secondary to another primary disorder; therefore, a low plasma progesterone level does not definitively indicate primary hypoluteoidism.

Treatment

The objective of therapy for abortion is identification and treatment of the underlying etiology. Supportive care such as fluid therapy may be necessary in animals with signs of systemic illness.

Uterine Infections. For a detailed discussion of the management of uterine infections, see previous sections in this chapter.

■ Pyometra is best treated with ovariohysterectomy, but may be managed medically in some bitches without severe illness.

■ Retained fetal or placental tissues are best treated surgically but may respond to medical evacuation of the uterus in some cases.

Brucellosis

Medical Therapy. Currently no effective treatment protocols are available for the cure of canine brucellosis. Although treatment with combinations of tetracycline, dihydrostreptomycin, trimethoprim-sulfadiazine, and demeclocycline have been somewhat effective in transiently eliminating bacteremia, none have been able to completely eliminate the infection, and bacteremia can recur after therapy is discontinued.

■ The most effective therapeutic regimen has been the combination of minocycline (12.5 mg/lb q12h, PO) given for 2 weeks and streptomycin (10 mg/lb q12h, PO) given for the first week. Unfortunately, minocycline administered at this extremely high dose is prohibitively expensive.

Prevention. Because no vaccine is available, prevention of canine brucellosis can be accomplished only through identification and elimination of infected animals.

■ In kennels that are free of brucellosis, isolate all new animals until they are brucellosis-negative on two tube agglutination tests at least 1 month apart.
■ Include an RSAT for brucellosis screening in pre-breeding examinations. Do not use any brucellosis-positive animal for breeding because of the likelihood of spread of the disease to other breeding animals and because pups born to that bitch are likely to be stillborn or bacteremic.

Hypoluteoidism
■ Decreased luteal function because of primary ovarian failure can be treated with exogenous progesterone in some cases. This must be done with caution, however, for the following reasons:
  ● Hypoluteoidism is not well understood in the bitch.
  ● Low plasma progesterone concentrations may be a complication of an underlying disorder and may not always be an indication for progesterone therapy.
  ● Progesterone administration predisposes to the development of pyometra in the bitch and queen.
■ Despite these problems, exogenous progesterone has been used successfully in a few bitches with recurrent fetal resorption associated with consistently low plasma progesterone levels.

PREGNANCY TERMINATION

Unwanted pregnancy is a common problem presented to the small animal practitioner. The first step in evaluating the bitch presented for mismating is confirmation that mating has actually occurred. This assessment is based on a careful history and a vaginal smear. Vaginal cytology is used to identify the stage of estrus and to check for the presence of sperm.

■ If a bitch presented for recent mating is found to be

in proestrus or diestrus, it is unlikely that conception has occurred.

■ Sperm or sperm heads will be present for 24 hours in the vaginal cytology of 65% of bitches that have been mated, and for 48 hours in 50%. The presence of sperm confirms breeding, but lack of sperm does not rule it out.

Ovariohysterectomy

Ovariohysterectomy is the treatment of choice for bitches not intended for future breeding. Because a uniformly safe and effective medical alternative for termination of pregnancy is not currently available, ovariohysterectomy is recommended for an older bitch or one whose reproductive importance is questionable.

Medical Methods

None of the protocols discussed here are consistently effective, and most are associated with significant side effects. Therefore, advise owners wishing to pursue medical treatment of unwanted pregnancy of the possibility of failure and the risks of potentially serious side effects. In some cases, it may be safer for the bitch to allow her to carry the litter to term instead of attempting medical termination of the pregnancy.

Estrogens

Estrogenic compounds traditionally have been used for termination of pregnancy in the dog and cat. However, the serious side effects produced by these agents severely limit their usefulness.

Mechanism. Exogenous estrogens delay the transport of fertilized ova through the oviducts and may stimulate contraction of the uterotubular junction. This prevents migration of the embryo into the uterus, where implantation normally occurs in the bitch on the twelfth day of diestrus. Estrogens may also act by interfering with implantation or through a direct embryotoxic effect.

Protocols
Estradiol Cypionate (ECP)
■ ECP, an injectable estrogen, is not approved for pregnancy termination in dogs or cats.
■ ECP is used in the bitch at a dose of 0.022–0.044 mg/kg (not to exceed 1 mg total dose), IM, given once within 3 days of mating. This protocol has been shown to be 50–100% effective in terminating pregnancy.
■ Cats are given a single dose of 0.25 mg, IM, within 3 days of mating.

KEY POINT ▶ Never give ECP more than once in the same estrus or in total doses exceeding 1 mg (dog) or 0.25 mg (cat).

Estradiol Benzoate or Valerate
■ Administer a single dose of 0.1 mg/kg (not to exceed 3 mg total dose), IM, within 3–5 days of mating.

Diethylstilbestrol (DES). DES has been used in both injectable and oral forms. However, the injectable product is no longer available, and the oral form has demonstrated poor efficacy.

■ Protocols for the oral preparation include 1 mg/30 lb (or 75 μg/kg) q24h, PO, for 7 days following mating.
■ The success of this protocol has been reported to be as low as 8%.

Side Effects. Because of their serious side effects, including bone marrow suppression and pyometra, even at recommended doses, estrogens are not recommended for pregnancy termination in the bitch.

KEY POINT ▶ Bone marrow suppression and increased incidence of pyometra are serious potentially life-threatening side effects that severely limit the use of estrogens for pregnancy termination.

Bone Marrow Suppression
■ Bone marrow suppression results in aplastic anemia, thrombocytopenia, and sometimes leukopenia, usually within 2–8 weeks of estrogen administration.
■ The susceptibility of individual dogs to bone marrow suppression is extremely variable.
■ Although most occurrences are associated with doses above the recommended range or with multiple repeated doses, suppression has been documented in dogs given proper doses.
■ Cats may be affected by bone marrow suppression but appear to be somewhat more resistant than dogs.

Pyometra
■ Although estrogens do not cause pyometra directly, they do potentiate the effects of progesterone on the uterus, which may result in cystic endometrial hyperplasia and pyometra.
■ The administration of estrogen for pregnancy termination is the most common cause of pyometra in young bitches (see previous discussion of pyometra).

Prognosis for Future Reproduction. Estrogen administration may be associated with future infertility problems in the bitch. The mechanism of this effect is not well understood.

Prostaglandins

Although not approved for use in companion animals, prostaglandins increasingly have been advocated in recent years for pregnancy termination in dogs. Despite problems with side effects and resistance to luteolysis in early diestrus, prostaglandins may offer the practicing veterinarian the best option for medical pregnancy interruption. Prostaglandins should only be used in young healthy bitches and are contraindicated in animals with pre-existing cardiovascular or respiratory problems.

Mechanism. The secretion of progesterone by the corpus luteum is required throughout gestation for the maintenance of pregnancy in the bitch. Prostaglandins terminate pregnancy through luteolysis and subsequent decrease in plasma progesterone concentration. The corpus luteum of the bitch is not sensitive to the luteolytic action of prostaglandin throughout pregnancy; the immature corpus luteum is resistant to luteolysis for the first 2–3 weeks of gestation. Prostaglandins administered during this time often cause a transient fall in plasma progesterone concentrations, which then return to a normal gestational level, allowing maintenance of pregnancy. However, when administered after 25–30 days of gestation, prostaglandins can cause complete luteolysis, although this response is not consistent. In addition to luteolysis, prostaglandins also have an ecbolic and possibly a direct embryotoxic effect, which may add to their effectiveness as abortifacients.

Protocols
Natural PGF$_{2\alpha}$

- In bitches, administer PGF$_{2\alpha}$ (Lutalyse; Upjohn), 30–250 μg/kg, q12h, SC, for 4–7 days (to effect), after day 25–30 of gestation. This protocol has been reported to be 50–100% effective in terminating pregnancy. The higher dosages are more consistent in causing luteolysis, but also result in more severe side effects.
- The use of PGF$_{2\alpha}$ for pregnancy termination in cats has not been extensively studied. However, a dosage of 0.5–1 mg/kg, SC, given twice, has been reported to cause luteolysis in the cat when administered after day 40 of gestation.

Prostaglandin Analogs.
Analogs such as fluprostenol (Equimate; Haver/Diamond) and cloprostenol (Estrumate; Haver/Diamond) have been studied as abortifacients in the bitch because they cause luteolysis at much lower doses than natural prostaglandins and may be associated with fewer side effects. However, until these compounds have been more extensively evaluated in the bitch and queen, protocols for pregnancy termination cannot be recommended.

- Hospitalize animals during prostaglandin therapy.
- Nesting behavior may be observed 1–2 days before abortion occurs, which is usually within 4 days after the initiation of treatment.
- Because of decreasing plasma progesterone concentrations, a temperature drop similar to that seen with normal parturition occurs within 24 hours of abortion. Prostaglandin therapy may result in abortion of only part of a litter.
- Evaluate the bitch or queen after abortion to ensure that no fetuses remain in the uterus that might be carried to term. This is accomplished through palpation or ultrasonography.

Side Effects.
See discussion of pyometra under Diseases of the Uterus.

Prognosis for Future Reproduction
- Prostaglandin therapy does not seem to alter future reproductive capability in the bitch. However, this assessment is based on a small number of cases and needs to be further evaluated.
- A shortening of the interestrous interval following prostaglandin-induced luteolysis has been noted consistently in bitches treated with PGF$_{2\alpha}$ for pregnancy termination. The normal anestrous period in the dog is 4–10 months. However, following PGF$_{2\alpha}$ therapy, it may be as short as 40 days.

Nonhormonal Compounds

Several derivatives of triazole isoquinoline have been shown to be effective in terminating pregnancy in the bitch. The most widely studied of these experimental agents is DL 717-IT. Interruption of pregnancy is accomplished through a direct toxic effect on the uteroplacental complex, causing degeneration and subsequent resorption. These drugs are administered after 15–20 days of gestation in the bitch to allow time for implantation to occur. Although these compounds currently have had very limited clinical application, experimental studies have demonstrated consistent results with minimal side effects.

Glucocorticoids

Dexamethasone may cause termination of pregnancy in mid to late gestation; however, specific protocols for dose and duration of treatment have not been developed. In one group of bitches, a dose of 0.5 mg/kg dexamethasone q12h, IM, for 10 days starting on day 30 of gestation resulted in interruption of pregnancy. The mechanism through which glucocorticoids act to terminate pregnancy has not been documented.

DYSTOCIA

Abnormalities of parturition are common in veterinary medicine. Base the decision to intervene with parturition on historical, physical, and diagnostic information and a familiarity with the numerous causes of dystocia. Understanding the pattern of gestation and changes occurring during the stages of labor can help to determine whether a problem in parturition is imminent.

Normal Parturition

The length of gestation in the bitch and queen is 63 days from the time of ovulation. However, the time to parturition from any single breeding date may vary from 58 days to as long as 70 days because the signs of estrus (i.e., receptivity) may occur both before and after ovulation actually takes place. A more accurate whelping date can be calculated as 57 days after the onset of diestrus, which is marked by a change in the vaginal cytology to mostly noncornified cells. Parturition often occurs earlier in animals with large litters and later in those with small or single pup litters. A transient temperature drop occurs within 24 hours of the onset of parturition and may be detected with twice-daily monitoring.

Although the following description of parturition refers specifically to the bitch, normal parturition in the queen is very similar. Parturition in the bitch and queen consists of three stages:

Stage I Labor. Stage I is characterized by prepartum behavior changes including anxiety or restlessness, panting, anorexia, shivering, and sometimes vomiting. Nesting behavior is also evident. Uterine contractions begin during this stage but are not detectable externally. Stage I labor usually lasts 6–12 hours in the bitch and ends with complete dilation of the cervix.

Stage II Labor. This is the segment of parturition during which the fetus is expelled. It is characterized by visible uterine contractions and straining. The first fetus should be delivered within 1–2 hours of the onset of stage II labor. Following delivery of the fetus, the bitch will often enter a resting phase which may last up to 4 hours. Active straining returns for 5–30 minutes before the expulsion of the next fetus. Two or more pups may be delivered in rapid succession, especially in bitches with large litters. A problem should be suspected if the resting phase lasts longer than 4 hours or if the bitch is actively straining for more than 30–60 minutes without producing a pup.

Stage III Labor. Stage III includes the expulsion of the placenta. This usually occurs within 5–15 minutes of the delivery of the fetus. Multiple placentas may follow the delivery of several pups if they are whelped within a short period of time. A greenish vaginal discharge is associated with placental separation and is a normal finding during and after delivery.

Etiology

The causes of dystocia can be classified as maternal, including uterine inertia and anatomic abnormalities, or fetal, due to malformation, malposition, or fetal death. In some cases, dystocia is caused by a combination of maternal and fetal factors.

Maternal Causes

Anatomic Abnormalities

■ A narrow pelvic canal may be a congenital lesion in brachycephalic breeds and terriers or an acquired problem in the case of previous pelvic fractures or neoplasia within the pelvic canal.

■ Uterine malposition can occur with a uterine torsion or from prolapse of the uterus through an inguinal hernia.

■ Developmental abnormalities of the genital canal that result in dystocia include vaginal stenosis, vulvar hypoplasia, and persistent hymen in the form of a vertical band or annular fibrotic stricture.

■ Insufficient strength of the abdominal muscles may prevent fetal expulsion in English bulldogs.

Uterine Inertia. Primary uterine inertia may be complete, resulting in a total absence of the signs of stage II labor, or partial, which occurs after part of a litter has been delivered. The primary types must be differentiated from secondary uterine inertia, which is the result of exhaustion from persistent straining against an obstruction. Secondary uterine inertia frequently is seen in small breeds of dogs.

■ Primary uterine inertia is characterized by a gestation length of greater than 68–70 days in a bitch that has shown a temperature drop or has entered stage I labor and then fails to exhibit signs of stage II labor within 24–36 hours.
  • Causes of primary uterine inertia include insufficient stimulation for uterine contraction due to a small litter (especially single fetus litters), overstretching of the uterus due to a large litter, stress and anxiety in first-litter bitches, and underlying systemic diseases (e.g., hypocalcemia, hypoglycemia, sepsis).

■ Secondary uterine inertia, which is secondary to persistent straining against an obstruction, can complicate obstructive dystocia and result in failure of the bitch to resume stage II labor after the obstruction has been corrected.
  • Diagnosis is made by identifying a loss of uterine contractions in association with an obstruction.
  • Secondary uterine inertia is never the only cause of dystocia.

Fetal Causes

■ *Fetal oversize* may be absolute or relative to the size of the birth canal. Causes of a large fetus include a large sire, a single fetus litter, and prolonged gestation.

■ *Fetal malposition* can result in obstructive dystocia. The orientation of the fetus during delivery is described in terms of presentation, position, and posture.
  • *Presentation* is cranial, caudal, or transverse, depending on which part of the fetus is delivered first. Cranial and caudal presentations are both normal in the bitch.
  • *Position* describes the area of the uterus which is adjacent to the dorsal surface of the fetus. A dorsal position is normal.
  • *Posture* describes the relationship of the pup's head and limbs to its body. Extended and flexed postures are both normal.

■ *Fetal developmental abnormalities* such as severe hydrocephalus can cause obstruction.

■ *Fetal death* can result in malpositioning of the fetus and may cause dystocia through secondary effects on the uterus.

Diagnosis

The diagnosis of dystocia can be difficult and necessitates a thorough history. It is based on the recognition of one or more of the following:

■ Obvious structural abnormalities that prevent parturition, such as vaginal stenosis or previous pelvic fractures that have narrowed the pelvic canal

■ Prolonged gestation >70 days from the first breeding or >60 days from the onset of diestrus (a gestation length >65 days from first breeding, especially with a large litter, is questionable)

■ Active straining for more than 30–60 minutes without expulsion of a fetus

■ A resting phase without signs of straining for more than 4 hours between deliveries, with known retained pups

■ Intermittent weak contractions for more than 2 hours without delivery of a fetus

■ Systemic signs of illness such as fever, profound weakness, and vomiting

■ Signs of pain during parturition such as crying out or biting at the vulvar area

■ Purulent or hemorrhagic vaginal discharge

■ Evidence of fetal death characterized radiographically by intrafetal gas patterns, collapse of the spinal column, or overlapping of the skull bones

Treatment

Once the diagnosis of abnormal parturition has been made, the first step in management is to rule out obstructive dystocia. Perform a physical examination including vaginal palpation. Clip and cleanse the perineum before vaginal examination, which is done with sterile gloves and lubrication. Abdominal radiographs are used to help determine fetal number, position, and viability. If available, abdominal ultrasonography is an excellent tool for determining fetal viability. Evidence of systemic illness such as sepsis or hypoglycemia warrants appropriate treatment for the underlying problem. If uterine contractions are not present, medical or surgical treatment for uterine inertia is indicated. However, attempt medical therapy only if the possibility of obstruction has been eliminated. Base the decision to manage the dystocia medically, through manipulation, or with surgical intervention on information gathered from the history, physical examination, and radiography.

Medical Management

Tranquilization. Relief of stress may allow progression of stage II labor in a nervous first-litter bitch. Acepromazine at low doses (0.05 mg/kg, IM) can be used safely in an otherwise healthy bitch.

Ecbolic Agents. These drugs stimulate uterine contractions. They may decrease postpartum hemorrhage, prevent retained fetal membranes, and facilitate uterine involution.

KEY POINT ▶ Rule out the presence of an obstruction before administering ecbolic agents.

- *Oxytocin* is the agent used most commonly to stimulate uterine contraction. Because it may also cause cervical contractions, it should only be used if the cervix is dilated.
  - Give oxytocin initially at 5–20 units (bitch) or 3–5 units (queen), IM.
  - If there is no response to the first dose, repeat at intervals of 30–40 minutes for a total of up to three doses.
- *Ergonovine maleate* is a more potent ecbolic agent with a longer half-life than oxytocin. Because of the possibility of inducing uterine rupture, this drug is not recommended for routine use in the treatment of uterine inertia, but it may be used to help control postpartum hemorrhage.
- *Calcium gluconate* given intravenously is indicated when hypocalcemia can be documented in a bitch with uterine inertia. It may also be helpful in animals with a normal serum calcium level and is often given 5–15 minutes before the second or third dose of oxytocin.
  - Give 2–10 ml of 10% calcium gluconate slowly IV.
  - Monitor for cardiac arrhythmias and stop administration if they occur.
- *Dextrose* is indicated for any animal with uterine inertia and confirmed hypoglycemia. It is more commonly used in conjunction with oxytocin therapy or after oxytocin has failed to stimulate uterine contractions.
  - Give 5–10 ml of 50% dextrose slowly IV.

Manipulation

Manual manipulation is used to assist the delivery of a fetus through the vaginal canal. It is useful in some cases of obstructive dystocia due to fetal malposition, slight fetal oversize, or fetal death, but is not indicated in obstructive dystocia once secondary inertia has occurred. Manual delivery may also be necessary to retrieve the last pup of a litter in cases of partial primary uterine inertia.

- Digital manipulation, when possible, is preferable to instrumental manipulation.
- Place the bitch in a standing position and use adequate sterile lubrication and sterile gloves.
- Attempt to determine the position of the fetus and correct any malposition through repulsion and repositioning.
- Once proper positioning is established, use gentle traction on the fetus in a caudoventral direction. Gentle rotation or side-to-side motion may aid in delivery. Do not place traction on the fetal extremities.
- Use instrumental manipulation only when necessary. Do not use instrumentation on a fetus that cannot be palpated digitally.
  - Guide the instrument into place with a finger and palpate the area after placement to ensure that the vaginal mucosa is not included in the grasp of the forceps.

Surgical Management

Perform cesarean section to manage dystocia in cases of uterine inertia (especially those unresponsive to medical treatment), obstructive dystocia that cannot be corrected through manipulation, and fetal death associated with putrefaction. For a discussion of the surgical management of dystocia, see sec. 8, ch. 15.

Supplemental Readings

Feldman EC, Nelson RW: Diagnosis and treatment alternatives for pyometra in dogs and cats. *In* Kirk RW, ed.: *Current Veterinary Therapy X.* Philadelphia: W. B. Saunders, 1989, p 1305.

Feldman EC, Nelson RW: *Canine and Feline Endocrinology and Reproduction.* Philadelphia: W. B. Saunders, 1987, p 430.

Gaudet DA, Kitchell BE: Canine dystocia. Compend Contin Educ 7:406, 1985.

Herron MA: Tumors of the canine genital system. J Am Anim Hosp Assoc 19:981, 1983.

Johnston SD: Subinvolution of placental sites. *In* Kirk RW, ed.: *Current Veterinary Therapy IX.* Philadelphia: W. B. Saunders, 1986, p 1231.

Kenney KJ, Matthiesen DT, Brown NO, Bradley RL: Pyometra in cats: 183 cases (1979–1984). J Am Vet Med Assoc 191:1130, 1987.

Magne ML: Acute metritis in the bitch. *In* Morrow DA, ed.: *Current Therapy in Theriogenology 2.* Philadelphia, W. B. Saunders, 1986, p 505.

Pollock RVH: Canine brucellosis: Current status. Compend Contin Educ 1:255, 1979.

Romagnoli SE, Cela M, Camillo F: Use of prostaglandin $F_{2\alpha}$ for early pregnancy termination in the mismated bitch. Vet Clin North Am [Small Anim Pract] 21:487, 1991.

15

Surgery of the Ovaries and Uterus

Roger B. Fingland

Surgical procedures performed on the uterus and ovaries include ovariohysterectomy, cesarean section, and, rarely, ovariectomy. Uterine surgery usually is straightforward but requires sound basic surgery skills and a thorough understanding of the anatomy and physiology of the reproductive tract.

ANATOMY (Fig. 1)

Ovaries

- The ovaries are located 1–3 cm caudal to the kidneys.
- The ovaries are attached to the abdominal wall by the mesovarium, a part of the broad ligament.
- The suspensory ligament is the cranial continuation of the broad ligament and extends between the ventral third of the last two ribs and the ventral surface of the ovary.
- The proper ligament is a continuation of the suspensory ligament and extends from the caudal end of the ovary to the cranial end of the uterine horn.
- The ovarian arteriovenous complex (OAVC) lies on the medial side of the broad ligament and supplies the ovaries and the cranial portion of the uterine tube. The distal two-thirds of the OAVC is convoluted in the dog, similar to the pampiniform plexus in males.
- The left ovarian vein drains into the left renal vein; the right ovarian vein drains into the caudal vena cava.

Uterus

- The uterus consists of the cervix, body, and two uterine horns. The oviducts (uterine tubes) connect the uterine horns and the ovaries.
- The uterus is attached to the dorsolateral wall of the abdominal cavity and the lateral wall of the pelvic cavity by paired double folds of peritoneum called broad ligaments.
- The round ligament is the caudal continuation of the proper ligament. The round ligament extends caudally and ventrally in the broad ligament and, in most bitches, passes through the inguinal canal terminating subcutaneously near the vulva.
- The uterine branch of the internal iliac artery is the main artery to the uterus. The uterine branch of the urogenital artery supplies the caudal portion of the uterus, the cervix, and part of the vagina. The uterine branch of the ovarian artery supplies the cranial part of the uterine horns.

OVARIOHYSTERECTOMY

Objective

- To remove the uterus and ovaries.

Preoperative Considerations

- Elective sterilization is the most common indication for ovariohysterectomy. Ovariohysterectomy is the

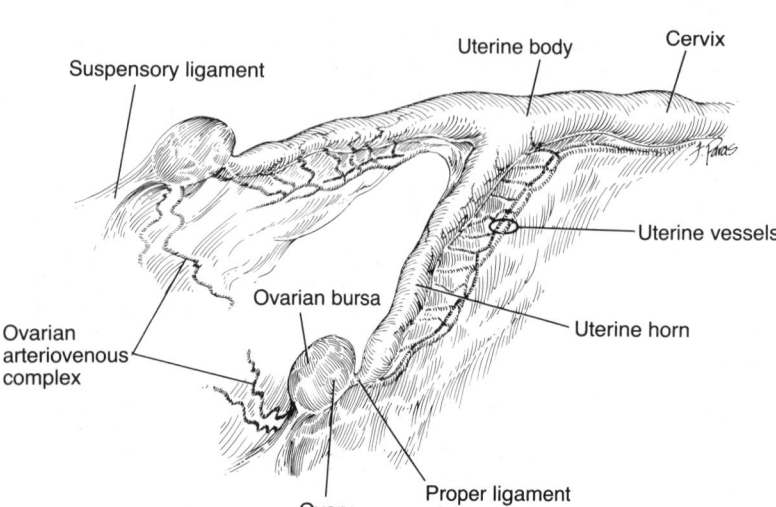

Figure 1. Anatomy of the uterus and ovaries.

Suspensory ligament

Uterine body

Cervix

Uterine vessels

Ovarian arteriovenous complex

Ovarian bursa

Uterine horn

Ovary

Proper ligament of the ovary

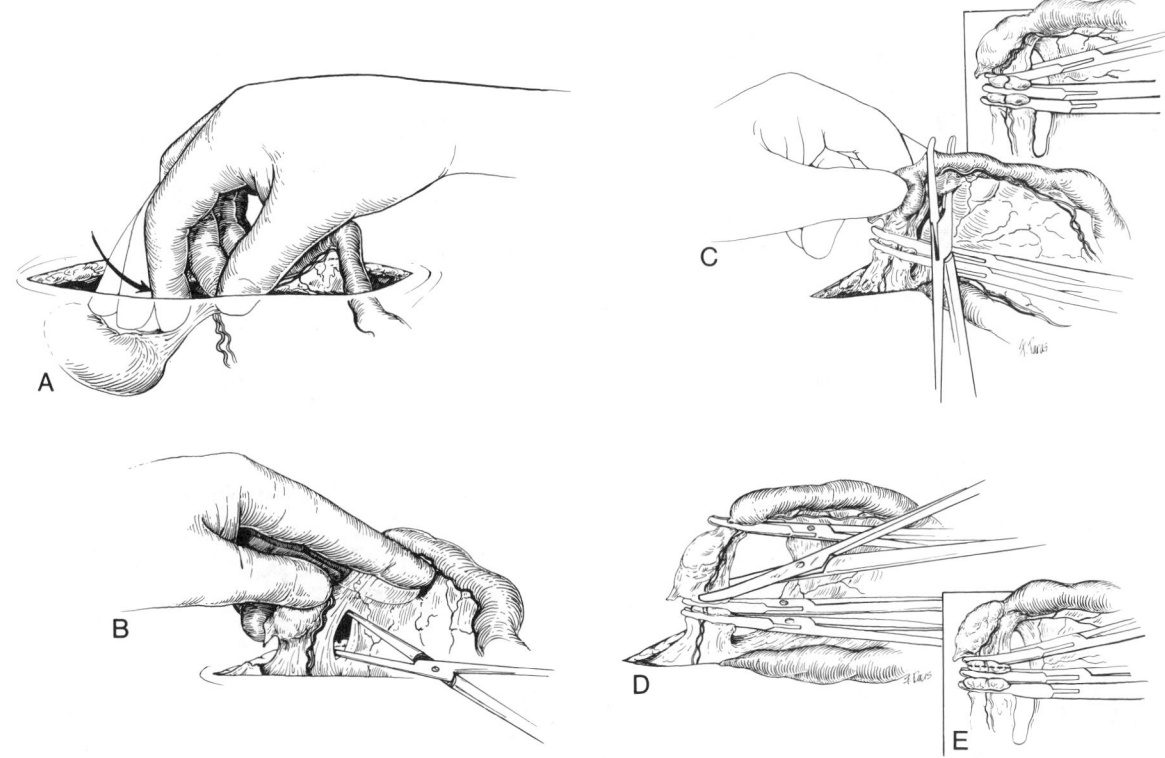

Figure 2. Ovariohysterectomy. *A*, Separate the suspensory ligament; *B*, open the mesovarium immediately caudal to the OAVC; *C*, triple-clamp the OAVC; *D*, transect the OAVC between the ovary and the clamp; *E*, alternative clamp and transection method.

Illustration continued on following page

treatment of choice for most uterine diseases including pyometra, uterine torsion, cystic endometrial hyperplasia, uterine rupture, and uterine neoplasia (see sec. 8, ch. 14 for description of these diseases).

KEY POINT ▶ Ovariohysterectomy before the first estrus provides a definitive protective factor against development of mammary neoplasia.

Whether the procedure is elective or not, appropriate preoperative evaluation, including a complete history, physical examination, and complete blood count (CBC) is recommended.

Surgical Procedure

Equipment

- Standard general surgery instrument pack and suture
- Ovariohysterectomy (Snook) hook (optional)
- Chromic catgut (2–0 or 3–0) or synthetic absorbable suture material for all ligatures

Technique

1. After anesthetizing the animal, manually express the urinary bladder.
2. Position animal in dorsal recumbency.
3. Prepare the entire ventral abdominal region for aseptic surgery.
4. Skin incision:
   a. *Dog:* Make a ventral midline incision extending from the umbilicus to a point half-way between the umbilicus and the brim of the pubis.
   b. *Cat:* Begin the ventral midline incision approximately 1 cm caudal to the umbilicus and extend the incision caudally 3–5 cm.
   c. A longer abdominal incision is required to remove an enlarged uterus (e.g., pyometra).
   d. Attempt to incise exactly on the midline in lactating bitches to avoid trauma to the mammary glands.
5. Enter the abdominal cavity through the linea alba.
6. Locate the left uterine horn using the ovariohysterectomy hook or index finger. Displace the omentum and bowel cranially if necessary to find the uterus.
7. Place a small hemostat across the proper ligament to aid in caudal retraction of the ovary.
8. Grasp the ovary between the thumb and middle finger. Place the index finger as far proximal as possible on the suspensory ligament (Fig. 2A).
9. Place tension on the suspensory ligament by rotating the index finger caudally. Gradually increase tension on the suspensory ligament until the ligament breaks.

KEY POINT ▶ Avoid placing tension on the ovarian arteriovenous complex (OAVC) during manipulation of the suspensory ligament or when placing ligatures.

10. Identify the OAVC. Using a Rochester-Carmalt hemostatic forceps (clamp), make an opening in the mesovarium immediately caudal to the OAVC in an area clear of vessels and fat (Fig. 2B).
11. Triple-clamp and transect the OAVC (Fig. 2C).

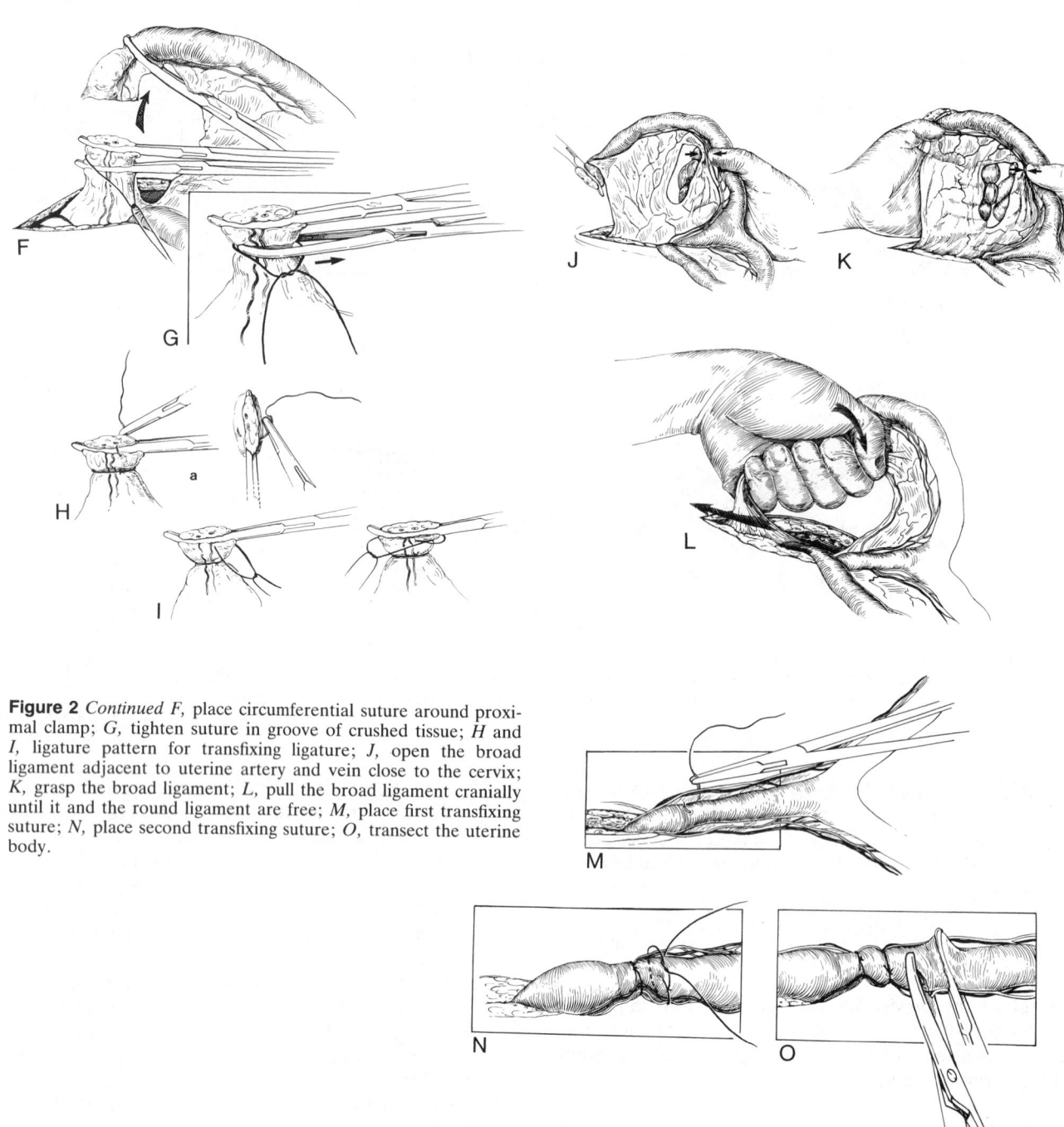

Figure 2 *Continued F,* place circumferential suture around proximal clamp; *G,* tighten suture in groove of crushed tissue; *H* and *I,* ligature pattern for transfixing ligature; *J,* open the broad ligament adjacent to uterine artery and vein close to the cervix; *K,* grasp the broad ligament; *L,* pull the broad ligament cranially until it and the round ligament are free; *M,* place first transfixing suture; *N,* place second transfixing suture; *O,* transect the uterine body.

a. Double-clamp the OAVC with Rochester-Carmalt hemostatic forceps. Place the first clamp immediately proximal (toward the aorta) to the ovary and the second clamp approximately 5 mm proximal to the first. Place a third clamp across the proper ligament between the ovary and the uterine horn. Transect the OAVC between the middle clamp and the ovary (Fig. 2*D*).

b. Alternatively, place all three clamps across the OAVC proximal to the ovary. Transect the OAVC between the middle clamp and the clamp adjacent to the ovary (Fig. 2*E*).

KEY POINT ▶ Place the hemostatic forceps on the OAVC as close as possible to the ovary to prevent accidental inclusion of the ureter.

12. Loosely place a circumferential suture around the proximal clamp. Tighten the suture as the clamp is removed (Fig. 2*F*). In this manner, the circumferential suture is tightened in the groove of crushed tissue created by the clamp (Fig. 2*G*).

KEY POINT ▶ The clamp adjacent to the ligature may need to be loosened before knotting to ensure proper tightness of the knot.

13. Place a transfixing ligature between the circumferential suture and the transected end of the OAVC (Fig. 2*H* and *I*). A full ligature (circumferential) may be used instead of a transfixing ligature in young cats.

KEY POINT ▶ Do not include ovarian tissue in the ligatures.

14. Grasp the OAVC (without grasping a ligature) with thumb forceps, remove the middle clamp, and inspect the OAVC for bleeding. If bleeding occurs, place a second circumferential suture on the OAVC proximal to the first.
15. Follow the left uterine horn distally to the bifurcation, locate the right uterine horn, and follow the right uterine horn proximally to the right OAVC.
16. Ligate and transect the right OAVC as described previously.
17. Transect the broad ligament.
    a. Mass ligation of the broad and round ligaments seldom is necessary. Individually ligate large vessels in the broad ligament.
    b. In most preparturient animals, the broad ligament can be manually separated. Make an opening in the broad ligament adjacent to the uterine artery and vein close to the cervix (Fig. 2*J*). Place four fingers through the opening in the broad ligament and grasp the entire broad ligament, including the round ligament (Fig. 2*K*). Pull the broad ligament cranially (not ventrally) until the broad ligament and the round ligament are free (Fig. 2*L*).
18. Exteriorize the uterine body and locate the cervix.
19. Divide the uterine body. The entire uterus proximal to the cervix should be removed during routine ovariohysterectomy. The circumference of the uterine body and the surgeon's preference determine which technique is used. Three of these techniques are described later.
20. Evaluate the OAVC pedicles and the uterine body prior to abdominal closure. The left and right OAVC are located immediately caudal to the caudal pole of the respective kidney.
    a. Locate the left OAVC pedicle by retracting the descending colon medially, exposing the left paralumbar gutter.
    b. Locate the right OAVC pedicle by retracting the duodenum medially, exposing the right paralumbar gutter.
    c. Retroflex the bladder. The ligated uterine body lies ventral to the descending colon and dorsal to the bladder.
21. Close the abdominal incision routinely.

Triple Clamp Technique for Dividing the Uterine Body

1. Place three clamps immediately proximal to the cervix. Transect the uterine body between the middle and the proximal clamp.

2. Individually ligate the uterine artery and vein bilaterally between the distal clamp and the cervix.
3. Loosely place a circumferential suture around the distal clamp and tighten the suture as the clamp is slowly withdrawn.
4. Place a transfixing ligature between the circumferential ligature and the remaining clamp. Hold the uterus with thumb forceps and remove the remaining clamp.
5. Evaluate the uterine stump for bleeding.
6. Place an additional circumferential suture if needed.

Double Transfixing Suture Technique for Dividing the Uterine Body

1. Exteriorize and retroflex the uterus.
2. Place a transfixing ligature around the uterine body immediately proximal to the cervix. The initial pass of the suture should encompass the left uterine artery and vein and one-third the width of the uterine body (Fig. 2*M*).
3. Place a second transfixing ligature 5 mm proximal to the first. The initial pass of the second transfixing suture should encompass the right uterine artery and vein and one-third the width of the uterine body (Fig. 2*N*).
4. Place a clamp proximal to the transfixing sutures to prevent backflow of blood and uterine contents. Transect the uterine body between the clamp and the proximal transfixing suture (Fig. 2*O*).

This technique is advantageous because clamps are not placed on the section of the uterine body that is ligated thus eliminating the potential for inadvertently tearing the uterine body with the clamp. The author uses this technique in cats and most dogs for routine ovariohysterectomy.

Parker-Kerr Suture Pattern Technique for Dividing the Uterine Body

The Parker-Kerr suture pattern occasionally is used when the uterine body is quite large. This suture pattern is time-consuming and results in inversion and occlusion of the uterine body remnant, which may predispose the animal to uterine stump pyometra or vaginal bleeding. This ligation technique seldom is indicated, even in animals with pyometra.

Postoperative Care

■ Postoperative care following elective ovariohysterectomy is routine.
■ Postoperative care following ovariohysterectomy for pyometra:
  • Dogs with pyometra frequently have renal dysfunction without associated morphologic abnormalities, and they may be azotemic, oliguric, or anuric. Monitor renal function and maintain hydration after surgery. Diuresis with crystalloid fluids administered intravenously for 24–36 hours after surgery is advisable.
  • Dogs with pyometra may be toxemic or septicemic (see sec. 8, ch. 14). Administer broad-spectrum antibiotics during surgery, and continue antibiotics

after surgery if the animal is toxemic or septicemic or if peritonitis was present at surgery.

Postoperative Complications

Complications following elective ovariohysterectomy are rare and may include the following:

Hemorrhage

- Hemorrhage is the most common complication following ovariohysterectomy in dogs weighing more than 25 kg.
- Common causes of hemorrhage include tearing of the OAVC while breaking the suspensory ligament, failure to ligate large vessels in the broad ligament, tearing of the uterine artery due to excessive traction on the uterine body, premature removal of a clamp during ligation, failure to adequately tighten circumferential or transfixion sutures, or coagulation defects.
- The incidence of hemorrhage can be reduced by maintaining meticulous surgical technique. Avoid becoming complacent during routine ovariohysterectomy.

Uterine Stump Pyometra

Uterine stump pyometra can occur if a portion of the uterine body or uterine horn is not removed and the animal has an elevated serum progesterone level. The source of elevated serum progesterone can be endogenous from residual ovarian tissue or exogenous from progestational compounds administered for treatment of dermatitis.

KEY POINT ▶ Complete excision of the uterine body and ovaries reduces the incidence of uterine stump pyometra.

Ovarian Remnant Syndrome (Recurrent Estrus)

- This condition results from functional residual ovarian tissue.
- Treatment is removal of residual ovarian tissue.

KEY POINT ▶ To increase the likelihood of identifying residual ovarian tissue, perform exploratory celiotomy to find ovarian remnants when the dog is showing signs of recurrent estrus.

- If ovarian tissue is not located, identify both ureters and resect remnants of the OAVC pedicles bilaterally.

Ligation of Ureter

- This condition is most likely to occur when the urinary bladder is distended and the trigone and ureterovesical junction are displaced cranially.
- Hydronephrosis and occasionally pyelonephritis can result.
- Ureteronephrectomy may be required.
- Avoid by careful placement of ligatures on the OAVC and uterine body.

Urinary Incontinence

- Causes include low systemic estrogen level, adhesions or granulomas of the uterine stump that interfere with urinary bladder sphincter function, and vaginoureteral fistula from common ligation of the vagina and ureter (very uncommon).
- Estrogen-responsive urinary incontinence in older bitches spayed at an early age is uncommon and poorly understood. Prudent administration of exogenous estrogens or alpha-adrenergic drugs may be indicated (see sec. 8, ch. 7).

Fistulous Tracts and Granulomas

- Sublumbar fistulous tracts in spayed bitches may develop when nonabsorbable multifilament suture material, such as polymerized caprolactam (Braunamid, Jorgensen) is used for ligating the OAVC or uterine body.
- Treatment is exploratory celiotomy and removal of suture material.

KEY POINT ▶ Do not use nonabsorbable multifilament suture material for ligation of the OAVC or uterine body.

Body Weight Gain

Weight gain is a common complication; the cause is poorly understood.

Eunuchoid Syndrome

This is a rare complication identified in working dogs after ovariohysterectomy. Clinical signs include decreased aggression, loss of interest in work, and decreased stamina.

Complications Related to Celiotomy

The most common complications associated with celiotomy are:

- Laceration of the spleen or urinary bladder
- Failure to remove gauze sponges from the abdominal cavity
- Dehiscence
- Seroma formation
- Self-mutilation of the abdominal wound

CESAREAN SECTION

Objective

- Remove all fetuses from the gravid uterus as quickly as possible.

Preoperative Considerations

Indications for Cesarean Section

- Dystocia from primary uterine inertia
- Protracted dystocia resulting in secondary uterine inertia
- Obstructive dystocia (oversized fetus or narrow pelvic canal)

Prolonged gestation
Dystocia from fetal malpositioning
Fetal death with putrefaction

Certain breeds (chihuahuas, English bulldogs) frequently require cesarean section because of a high incidence of dystocia.

Anesthesia

■ Animals that require cesarean section often have fluid and metabolic disturbances that make them poor candidates for general anesthesia.
■ Correction of fluid and metabolic abnormalities should be well underway prior to induction of anesthesia. Intravenous fluid therapy and prophylactic administration of a broad-spectrum antibiotic such as cefazolin (Lyphomed) (25 mg/kg, IV) are recommended.
  • Various regimens for induction and maintenance of anesthesia (see sec. 1, ch. 2 for general principles of anesthesia) have been recommended.
  • Intravenous narcotics combined with local anesthesia may be used in dogs.
  • Ketamine and local anesthesia may be used in cats.
  • Administer standard inhalation anesthesia after the puppies or kittens are removed.

KEY POINT ▶ Minimize time from induction to delivery by fully preparing the animal prior to anesthesia.

■ Induce anesthesia and intubate the animal on the surgery table, preferably after the initial skin preparation.

KEY POINT ▶ Inform the owner prior to surgery that ovariohysterectomy may be necessary if the uterus is not viable.

Surgical Procedure

Objective

■ To remove all fetuses from the gravid uterus as quickly as possible.

Equipment

■ Standard general surgery instrument pack and suture
■ Laparotomy sponges
■ Clean towels
■ Doxapram (Dopram; A.H. Robins) and naloxone (Narcan; Elkins-Sinn) (if narcotics are used for induction)
■ Incubator or heat lamp

Technique

1. Position the animal in standard dorsal recumbency. A 20° lateral tilt from dorsal recumbency is not necessary because supine hypotension syndrome does not occur in the parturient bitch.
2. Perform the final skin preparation rapidly.
3. Incise skin, subcutaneous tissue, and linea alba on the ventral midline beginning cranial to the umbilicus and extending as far caudally as necessary to exteriorize the uterus.

KEY POINT ▶ Avoid incising mammary tissue when making the initial skin incision. Enter the abdominal cavity cautiously to avoid lacerating the gravid uterus.

4. Exteriorize the uterus.
5. Isolate the uterus from the abdominal viscera with moist laparotomy sponges.
6. Identify an avascular area on the dorsal or ventral midline of the uterine body. Make a small incision in the uterine body with a scalpel. Do not inadvertently lacerate a fetus with the scalpel.
   a. Extend the incision with Metzenbaum scissors to a sufficient length to accommodate the largest fetus. The uterus may tear during extraction of a fetus if the length of the incision is not adequate.
7. Move a fetus to the incision by gently squeezing the uterine horn (Fig. 3A).
8. Grasp the fetus and gently pull it from the uterus.
9. Break the amnionic sac as the fetus is removed. Direct fetal fluids away from the operative field to minimize contamination (Fig. 3B).
10. Clamp and transect the umbilical vessels approximately 2 cm from the fetal abdominal wall (Fig. 3C).
11. Place the neonate on a sterile towel and pass it to an assistant. Alternatively, the neonate can be passed to the assistant before the umbilical vessels are transected, leaving this responsibility to nonsterile individuals in the OR.
12. Remove the placenta by gently pulling it from the endometrium. To decrease the potential for severe postoperative uterine hemorrhage, do not remove the placenta if placental separation is difficult.
13. Extract the remaining fetuses.
14. Palpate the uterus from the pelvic canal to the ovaries to make certain that no fetuses remain.
15. The uterus will contract rapidly after all fetuses have been removed, and occasionally during extraction of the last few fetuses. Administration of oxytocin rarely is necessary to initiate uterine involution.
16. Uterine closure
    a. Use 2–0 or 3–0 chromic catgut or synthetic absorbable suture material.
    b. Close the uterine incision with a one- or two-layer inverting suture pattern (e.g., Cushing and Lembert).
17. Locally rinse the uterus with warmed physiologic saline solution prior to returning it to the abdominal cavity.
18. Lavage the abdominal cavity with warm physiologic saline solution if contamination or spillage of uterine contents occurred.

Postoperative Care and Complications

Care of Neonates

KEY POINT ▶ Remove the fetal membranes from the neonate's mouth and nose immediately after delivery.

■ Clamp the umbilical vessels and remove the fetal membranes if this was not done by the surgeon.

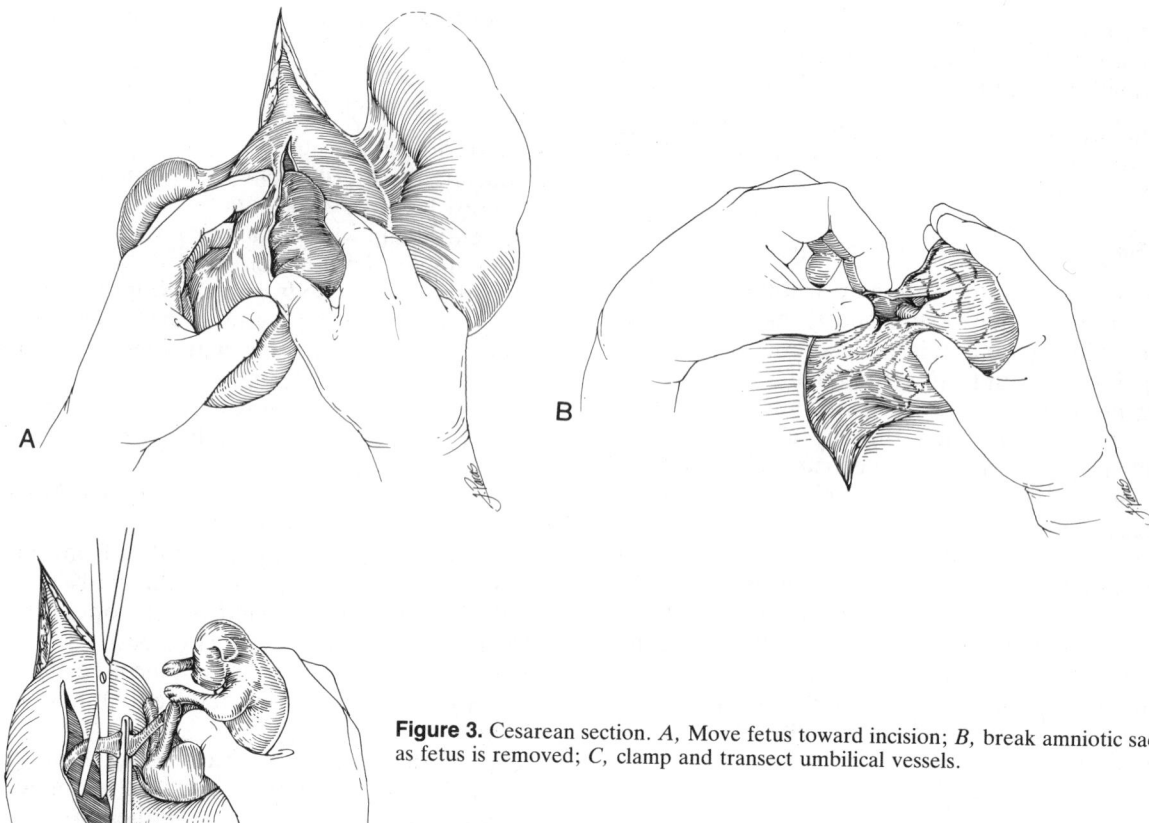

Figure 3. Cesarean section. *A,* Move fetus toward incision; *B,* break amniotic sac as fetus is removed; *C,* clamp and transect umbilical vessels.

- Clear mucus from the mouth and nares with gentle suction or cotton swabs.
- Assess the viability of the neonate. Neonates often are bradycardiac and apneic.
  - Dry the neonate briskly with a soft towel because skin stimulation reflexly stimulates respiration.
  - Mucus can be cleared from the upper airway by grasping the neonate firmly and slowly swinging it downward.
- Administer a respiratory stimulant such as doxapram (Dopram; A.H. Robins) (0.25 to 1.0 mg, PO or IM) if the neonate does not respond to mechanical stimulation.
- Poor neonatal viability can be due to anesthetic agents administered to the dam for induction of anesthesia. Administer a narcotic antagonist such as naloxone (Narcan; Elkins-Sinn) (0.01 mg/kg, PO or IM) if the dam was given a narcotic for induction of anesthesia.
- Medications can be dropped on the neonate's tongue.
- Some neonates may not breathe spontaneously for 30–60 minutes after delivery. Be persistent with resuscitation efforts. Neonates that do not breathe spontaneously can be intubated with a sterile puppy feeding tube.
- Place neonates in an environmental temperature of approximately 32°C.

- Examine neonates for congenital abnormalities such as cleft palate, imperforate anus, hernias, and limb deformities.

Care of the Dam

- Clean residual antiseptic solution, blood, and fetal fluids from the dam's mammary glands prior to allowing the neonates to nurse.
- Place the dam with neonates after anesthetic recovery so that neonates receive colostrum as soon as possible after birth.
- Make certain that the dam has adequate milk and that each neonate nurses.
  - Oxytocin (Anthony) (0.5 units/kg, IV or IM) can be administered to stimulate milk production.

KEY POINT ▶ Ovariohysterectomy performed in conjunction with cesarean section should not interfere with the dam's mothering instincts or ability to produce milk. Ovarian hormones are not important for maintenance of lactation.

- Consider discharging the dam and neonates as soon as the dam has recovered from anesthesia and has demonstrated appropriate behavior toward the neonates.

Complications

- Potential short-term complications include hemorrhage, hypovolemia, and hypothermia.
  - Place the dam in a warm, quiet environment and administer crystalloid or colloid fluids, if indicated.
- Potential long-term complications include peritonitis, wound dehiscence, agalactia, and uterine hemorrhage.
  - Prolonged severe uterine hemorrhage may require administration of oxytocin or, in nonresponsive cases, emergency ovariohysterectomy.
- Monitor serum calcium levels if hypocalcemia is suspected.
- Although multiple cesarean sections can be performed on a dam, uterine scarring may prevent future placentation and peritoneal adhesions may complicate subsequent celiotomies.

UTERINE PROLAPSE

Preoperative Considerations

- Uterine prolapse can occur any time during or up to several days after parturition.
- Animals presented with uterine prolapse may be clinically stable or may have mild to severe metabolic imbalances. Treat disturbances in fluid, electrolyte, or acid-base balance before managing the uterine prolapse.
- Access the viability of the prolapsed uterus.
- Treatment options include manual reduction, manual reduction with immediate ovariohysterectomy, internal reduction via celiotomy, and amputation of the uterus externally.
  - Manual reduction of the prolapsed uterus is the treatment of choice, although an episiotomy may be required.
  - Ovariohysterectomy may be necessary after manual reduction if the uterus is devitalized.
  - Consider external amputation only if the uterus cannot be reduced.

Manual Reduction

Technique

1. Epidural anesthesia is preferred, but standard general anesthesia can be used.
2. Clean the uterus and wrap it with sterile gauze sponges soaked in physiologic saline. Soaking the sponges with a hypertonic dextrose solution may help to reduce swelling.
3. Apply sterile water-soluble lubricating jelly to the uterus and attempt gentle reduction with a gloved finger or with a sterile smooth syringe case.
4. If manual reduction is unsuccessful, prepare the perineum and the prolapsed uterus for aseptic surgery and perform an episiotomy (see sec. 8, ch. 17 for technique). Reduction should be facilitated by

episiotomy. If manual reduction still is not possible, consider external amputation.

Surgical Procedure for External Amputation of Prolapsed Uterus

Objectives

- Resect the prolapsed uterine horns and, if possible, the ovaries.
- Avoid contamination of the abdominal cavity.
- Minimize uterine hemorrhage.

Equipment

- Standard general surgical instrument pack.

Technique

1. Administer epidural or general anesthesia.
2. Position animal in dorsal recumbency with the rear limbs tied forward.
3. Prepare the ventral abdominal and perineal areas for aseptic surgery. Place a purse-string suture in the anus.
4. Incise the uterine body near the vulva. Place stay sutures in the incised proximal wall of the uterine body to prevent retraction into the vagina.
5. Identify the uterine horns.
6. Apply gentle caudal traction on the uterine horns to expose the ovaries. Ligate the right and left ovarian arteriovenous complex.
7. If the ovaries cannot be exposed, place two circumferential ligatures around each uterine horn as far cranial as possible. Transect the uterine horns between the two ligatures.
8. Double-ligate and transect the uterine vessels.
9. Close the proximal stump of the uterine body with a synthetic absorbable suture material in a simple interrupted pattern and reduce the remaining tissue into the abdomen.
10. If the ovaries remain, perform a ventral midline celiotomy and bilateral ovariectomy.

Postoperative Care and Complications

- Recurrence after successful manual reduction of a uterine prolapse is rare.
- Complications seldom occur after manual reduction or external amputation of the uterus. Life-threatening hemorrhage may occur after external amputation.

Supplemental Readings

Berzon JL: Complication of elective ovariohysterectomies in the dog and cat at a teaching institution: Clinical review of 853 cases. Vet Surg 8:89, 1979.
Gaudet DA: Retrospective study of 128 cases of canine dystocia. J Am Anim Hosp Assoc 21:813, 1985.
Gaudet DA: Canine dystocia. Compend Contin Educ 7:406, 1985.
Roberts DD, Straw RC: Uterine prolapse in a cat. Compend Contin Educ 10:1295, 1988.

16

Diseases of the Vagina and Vulva

Amy M. Grooters

DISEASES OF THE VULVA

The vulva or female external genitalia consists of the labia, clitoris, and vestibule (for a review of vulvar anatomy see sec. 8, ch. 17). The vestibule, which connects the vagina to the external genital orifice, embryologically arises from the caudal portion of the urogenital sinus and fuses with the müllerian ducts to form the vestibulovaginal junction. The clitoris develops from the genital tubercle, whereas the labia are formed from the genital swellings.

Developmental Abnormalities

Vulvar anomalies usually are detected because of the secondary problems they cause. Diagnosis of these abnormalities often is made on the basis of physical examination and digital palpation.

Vulvar Hypoplasia

Etiology. A small vulva usually is the result of hypoplastic development in bitches spayed before reaching sexual maturity. The juvenile vulva often is recessed, resulting in urine pooling and moist dermatitis in the skin folds of the perivulvar region. This is a particular problem in obese, older animals.

Clinical Signs. Most signs of vulvar hypoplasia are related to secondary urine pooling and perivulvar dermatitis and include excessive licking of the vulva and malodor. Severe perivulvar dermatitis results in ulcerative lesions that can be very painful, making cleaning of the area difficult. Secondary vaginitis is common, and urine pooling also predisposes the animal to ascending urinary tract infection. Recurrent cystitis occurs in some cases.

Treatment. Medical therapy for the secondary dermatitis (see sec. 5, ch. 1) and vaginitis (see later in this chapter) has limited success without concurrent surgical correction of the underlying anatomic abnormalities. Episioplasty is used to remove excessive perivulvar skin and to elevate the recessed vulva (see sec. 5, ch. 16). Weight reduction is important in obese animals.

Vulvar Stenosis

Etiology. Abnormal fusion of the genital folds and genital swellings results in stenosis of the vulva. This usually occurs at the vestibulolabial junction and is manifested as a narrowing of the canal in that region.

Clinical Signs. Affected animals may show signs of pain when mating is attempted.

If pregnancy does occur (either through natural breeding or artificial insemination), the stenosis may cause dystocia.

Treatment. Perform an episiotomy (see sec. 8, ch. 17) to enlarge the canal temporarily to relieve dystocia.

Permanent vulvar canal enlargement (episiostomy) may be indicated in breeding animals. In episiostomy, an episiotomy incision is made and, instead of closing the midline incision in three layers, the mucosa is sutured to the skin along both sides of the incision, thereby enlarging the canal.

Acquired Abnormalities

Clitoral Hypertrophy

Etiology
- Enlargement of the clitoris is associated with intersex abnormalities, in which case it is a developmental abnormality (see sec. 8, ch. 19), with hyperadrenocorticism (see sec. 4, ch. 3), and rarely with the use of anabolic steroids.

Clinical Signs
- The clitoris normally lies within the vestibule, but with hypertrophy may protrude through the vulvar cleft.
- Vaginitis results from irritation and poor drainage caused by the enlarged clitoris, and abrasion and drying from chronic protrusion causes clitoritis.
- Affected animals may be asymptomatic or may show signs related to inflammation, including excessive licking and, infrequently, vaginal discharge.

Treatment
- Nonspecific therapy includes treatment of the secondary vaginitis and protection of the exposed clitoris with lubricants and topical antibiotic ointments. However, this will rarely eliminate clinical signs without correction of the underlying cause.
- Withdrawal of anabolic steroids or treatment of hyperadrenocorticism will often cause regression of the enlargement.
- Clitoral resection is indicated in hermaphrodites and pseudohermaphrodites with persistent clinical signs and may also be necessary in some animals with clitoral hypertrophy secondary to anabolic steroid administration or hyperadrenocorticism (if conservative treatment fails), especially if an os clitoris is present.

- Remove the enlarged clitoris via an episiotomy. Incise sharply around the base of the clitoris and control hemorrhage (usually profuse) with electrocoagulation. Appose the remaining vestibular mucosa with absorbable suture.
- Dogs with intersex abnormalities may have large "phalluses" containing a urethra. In this situation the urethra is spared during clitoral resection and spatulated to the remaining vestibular mucosa.

Vulvar Enlargement

- Edema and swelling of the vulva occur in response to estrogenic stimulation. This is a normal finding in bitches in estrus, but if it is present for more than 14 days it may indicate persistent estrus due to estrogen-secreting ovarian neoplasia or cystic ovarian disease.
- Vulvar enlargement associated with estrus resolves when the bitch enters diestrus, although older intact females with numerous recurrent episodes may have chronic hypertrophy and thickening. Ovariohysterectomy (see sec. 8, ch. 15) is the treatment of choice for vulvar enlargement caused by ovarian hormone imbalance.

Vulvar Neoplasia

For a discussion of tumors of the vulva, see Vaginal Neoplasia.

DISEASES OF THE VAGINA

The vagina develops from the complete fusion of the caudal portions of the paired müllerian ducts. These ducts unite with the caudal segment of the urogenital sinus to form the hymen at the vestibulovaginal junction. This membrane is gone by birth in the normal canine (for a review of vaginal anatomy, see sec. 8, ch. 17).

Developmental Abnormalities

Vaginal Stenosis and Persistent Hymen

Vaginal stenosis and persistent hymen are discussed together because clinical signs, diagnosis and treatment of both disorders are similar.

Etiology

- *Vaginal stenosis* secondary to segmental hypoplasia or aplasia of the genital canal can occur at any point in the vagina or vestibule, but it is most common at the vestibulovaginal junction.
- *Persistent hymen* occurs as an incomplete perforation of the hymen (imperforate hymen) or as an incomplete fusion of the müllerian ducts resulting in a residual vertical membrane that divides the vagina sagittally.
  - *Incomplete perforation of the hymen* is caused by inadequate union of the müllerian ducts with the urogenital sinus. This results in hymal remnant tissue at the vestibulovaginal junction in the form of either a vertical band or an annular fibrotic stricture.

- An *elongated vertical vaginal septum* results in partial or complete partitioning of the vagina along its long axis. If the partition is complete, a double vagina is formed.

Clinical Signs

Many animals with congenital vaginal defects do not show any clinical signs. When present, clinical signs associated with vaginal stenosis and the various forms of persistent hymen are similar and include breeding difficulty, chronic vaginitis, and intermittent positional dribbling of urine.

Dyspareunia

- Dyspareunia, or pain and difficulty during mating, may be the first indication of vaginal stenosis or persistent hymen. The bitch usually allows mounting, but the vaginal anomaly prevents intromission, causing signs of pain in the bitch and often in the sire as well.
- Hymal remnants or stenosis may result in dystocia if an affected bitch is able to mate normally or is artificially inseminated.

Chronic Vaginitis

- Chronic inflammation causes excessive licking of the vulva and occasionally a persistent vaginal discharge.

KEY POINT ▶ Chronic vaginitis is a common complication of persistent hymen and responds poorly to medical therapy without surgical correction of the underlying anomaly.

Urine Pooling

- Urine pooling cranial to the vestibulovaginal junction occurs with annular fibrotic strictures, vertical bands, and vaginal stenosis. Chronic vaginitis as well as positional dribbling of urine that resembles incontinence may result (for differential diagnosis of urinary incontinence, see sec. 8, ch. 7).
- The owner typically reports that the animal leaks urine when lying down.
- The static urine in the vagina predisposes to ascending urinary tract infection, a potential source of recurrent cystitis.
- Retention of fluids in the uterus and cranial vagina occurs with complete obstruction caused by vaginal aplasia and may be confused with pyometra.

Diagnosis
Digital Palpation

KEY POINT ▶ Digital palpation is the most useful tool for diagnosis of congenital vaginal defects.

- The most common location for vaginal anomalies is the vestibulovaginal junction, which is just cranial to the external urethral orifice and is easily reached digitally.
  - A single small central opening cranial to the vestibule is suggestive of an annular fibrotic stricture or vestibulovaginal stenosis. Often this opening is too small to allow digital penetration into the vagina.
  - Two small openings, each lateral to a central

membrane, are suggestive of a vertical band, elongated sagittal septum, or double vagina. Occasionally the band is so tense that it can be "strummed" with a finger.

- Do not confuse muscular contraction or spasm during palpation with stenosis.
- Because of the relaxation of the vestibulovaginal tissues that occurs during estrus, digital palpation at this time may reveal an increased diameter compared to that during diestrus.

Other Diagnostic Procedures

- Vaginoscopy with a speculum or fiberoptic equipment is helpful in evaluating the cranial vaginal mucosa but often bypasses abnormalities at the vestibulovaginal junction.
- A vaginogram performed by infusing radiographic contrast through a Foley catheter may help to identify an elongated vaginal septum or to delineate the extent of segmental stenosis.

Treatment

- *Manual dilation* of the stenotic area under general anesthesia can be attempted in animals with segmental hypoplasia or imperforate hymen. Results with digital dilation or bougienage are inconsistent, and recurrence of a stricture or inadequate dilation is common.
- *Surgical excision* of remnant membranes is the treatment of choice for clinically affected breeding animals with persistent hymen (see sec. 8, ch. 17).

Acquired Abnormalities

Acquired disorders of the vagina include vaginal hyperplasia, vaginal prolapse, vaginal neoplasia, and vaginitis.

Vaginal Hyperplasia

Etiology

- Estrogenic stimulation normally causes some degree of swelling and edema in the vulvar and vaginal tissues of the bitch.
- Vaginal hyperplasia is an exaggerated response to estrogen that results in excessive edema and enlargement of the mucosal folds of the vaginal floor.

Clinical Signs

- Vaginal hyperplasia occurs most often in young, intact, large-breed female dogs during proestrus or estrus.
- Rarely, it may be associated with parturition.
- Affected bitches often are presented because of the owner's observation of a mass at the vulva.
- Other signs include dysuria, excessive licking of the vulva, painful mating, and a bulging perineum. The protruding tissue has a mass-like appearance and may be traumatized.
- The clinical appearance of vaginal hyperplasia varies in severity.
  - In mild disease, the swelling is confined to the folds of the ventral vaginal floor cranial to the urethral orifice.
  - More severe hyperplasia may cause protrusion of these tissues as a tongue-shaped mass through the

labia. It may also progress to a vaginal prolapse involving the full circumference of the vaginal wall.
- Vaginal hyperplasia begins during proestrus, enlarges throughout estrus, and subsides during diestrus. It tends to recur with each estrus.

Diagnosis

- The primary differential diagnosis for vaginal hyperplasia is vaginal neoplasia.
- Diagnosis of hyperplasia usually can be made based on the signalment, the appearance and origin of the protruding tissue, and stage of the estrous cycle.
- Vaginal cytology is useful to confirm the stage of estrus.
- Vaginal biopsy can be performed to definitively differentiate hyperplasia from neoplasia in questionable cases.

Treatment

Spontaneous Regression. Regression of the hyperplasia typically occurs when the bitch enters diestrus. Recurrence is common in subsequent estrus periods and can be prevented by ovariohysterectomy.

KEY POINT ▶ Ovariohysterectomy is the treatment of choice for vaginal hyperplasia in nonbreeding animals.

Medical Therapy. Medical therapy for breeding bitches involves conservative management of the exposed tissue until spontaneous resolution occurs or attempts to eliminate the estrogenic stimulation with hormonal manipulation. Because it interferes with natural breeding, vaginal hyperplasia is a standard indication for artificial insemination in breeding bitches.

- Conservative management includes topical antibiotic ointment to minimize drying of mucous membranes and prevention of further trauma. The everted tissue can be lubricated and reduced, if possible, and then kept in place with stay sutures until it regresses during diestrus.
- Hormonal treatment is aimed at shortening the time to diestrus by inducing ovulation.
  - Gonadotropin-releasing hormone (Gn–RH) (Cystoreline; Abbott) (2.2 µg/kg, IM) induces ovulation during the follicular phase. However, many bitches have already ovulated by the time vaginal hyperplasia is diagnosed, in which case Gn-RH will not shorten the clinical course. Gn-RH may cause ovarian cysts or luteinization of immature follicles.
  - Megestrol acetate (Ovaban; Schering) has been used to prevent vaginal hyperplasia through estrogen antagonism; however, because ovulation is prevented through the same mechanism, it cannot be used in bitches intended to be bred during that cycle.

Surgical Excision

- Surgical excision of exposed vaginal tissue is indicated to:
  - Remove devitalized or severely traumatized tissue

- Attempt to prevent recurrence of vaginal hyperplasia in subsequent cycles
■ Surgical resection is often the best option for managing hyperplasia in breeding animals, but recurrence may continue to be a problem despite previous resection. Only ovariohysterectomy offers a permanent cure.

Vaginal Prolapse

■ Prolapse of the vagina may occur as a consequence of severe vaginal hyperplasia, or may be associated with mechanical factors without any underlying vaginal pathology.
■ Severe vaginal hyperplasia is the most common cause of vaginal prolapse and results in a "doughnut-shaped" mass protruding from the vulva.
■ Vaginal prolapse without vaginal hyperplasia is rare and may be associated with dystocia, tenesmus, or forced separation during mating.
■ Management of vaginal prolapse associated with vaginal hyperplasia consists of supportive care and treatment of the underlying disorder (see Vaginal Hyperplasia).
■ Vaginal prolapse that is not associated with vaginal hyperplasia may be treated successfully with manual reduction of the vaginal tissue and placement of temporary retention suture in the vulva (see sec. 8, ch. 17).

Vaginal Neoplasia

The most common neoplasms of the canine vagina and vulva are leiomyomas and fibromas, which are benign tumors originating from smooth muscle or connective tissue. Other tumors include transmissible venereal tumors, leiomyosarcomas, and lipomas. Most vaginal and vulvar tumors in dogs and cats are benign.

Benign Tumors
Etiology
■ *Leiomyomas* arise from the smooth muscle of the vaginal or vestibular wall. They are often pedunculated and do not readily exfoliate neoplastic cells. These tumors are noninvasive and do not metastasize, but may recur following surgical resection. Leiomyomas may be either intraluminal or extraluminal.
■ *Lipomas* may occur in the vagina but are much less common.

Signalment. Older intact female dogs are most often affected.

Clinical Signs
■ Clinical signs include vaginal discharge or bleeding, protrusion of a mass through the vulvar cleft, excessive licking of the vulva, dysuria, dyschezia, and constipation due to rectal compromise if masses are extensive.
■ Extraluminal leiomyomas and lipomas often cause perineal swelling.

Diagnosis
■ Most vaginal tumors are identified by visual or digital examination (rectal and vaginal).

■ Vaginoscopy may be useful for diagnosis of cranial vaginal tumors and can also facilitate biopsy.
■ Vaginal cytology generally is not useful in the diagnosis of vaginal neoplasia because of the failure of these tumors to shed cells. However, fine-needle aspiration may be attempted with masses that are externally accessible.
■ Definitive diagnosis of vaginal and vulvar tumors is usually made by excisional biopsy.

Treatment
■ *Surgical resection* is the treatment of choice for benign vaginal and vulvar tumors. Adequate surgical exposure often requires an episiotomy (see sec. 8, ch. 17). Recurrence of the tumor may follow resection.
■ Consider *ovariohysterectomy* as an adjunct to surgical resection to lower the incidence of recurrence of benign vaginal tumors. This recommendation is based on the possibility that leiomyomas are estrogen-dependent tumors.

Malignant Tumors
■ *Leiomyosarcoma* is the most common malignant tumor of the canine vagina. Others include squamous cell carcinoma, hemangiosarcoma, adenocarcinoma, and mast cell tumor.
■ These tumors are less often pedunculated than benign tumors and have a greater tendency to recur following resection. There is no evidence for hormonal dependency of malignant vaginal tumors.

Transmissible Venereal Tumors
Canine transmissible venereal tumor (TVT) is a proliferative tumor of the vagina and vulva that is transmitted during sexual or social contact by the direct transplantation of neoplastic cells. (see sec. 8, ch. 12).

Signalment. TVT occurs in younger (mean age 4 years) sexually active male and female dogs. Incidence is higher in crowded urban populations.

Clinical Signs
■ TVTs may be solitary or multiple and are friable, hemorrhagic, cauliflower-like masses that may be necrotic or traumatized.
■ The most common site in the bitch is the caudal vagina or vestibulovaginal junction.
■ Extragenital sites include the skin, oral cavity, nasal cavity, and perineum.
■ Metastasis is rare but usually occurs in regional lymph nodes. Distant metastasis is possible.

Treatment
■ *Surgical excision* is effective in some animals in which total resection is possible. However, the frequency of recurrence after surgery and the difficulty in obtaining complete excision in some locations make surgery a poor option in many cases. Surgery is not useful for metastatic TVT.
■ *Radiation* is effective, and may be used either as the sole means of treatment or as an adjunct to surgery. Most dogs show a total response following a single dose.
■ *Chemotherapy* is the treatment of choice for multiple or metastatic TVT and can also be used as a first-

line treatment for solitary local tumors. Both single and multi-agent protocols are effective.

- Combination chemotherapy agents include vincristine, cyclophosphamide, and methotrexate.
- Single agent therapy with vincristine at 0.025 mg/kg (maximum 1 mg), IV, once weekly for 3–7 weeks appears to be as effective as combination therapy, with the advantage of having fewer side effects.

Vaginitis

Etiology

Juvenile Vaginitis. This occurs commonly in female dogs less than 1 year of age. The cause of the vaginal inflammation is nonspecific, and it usually resolves spontaneously after the first estrous cycle.

Bacterial Vaginitis. Bacterial vaginitis is rarely a primary disorder but is commonly seen secondary to abnormalities of the genital or urinary tracts.

- Predisposing genital abnormalities may be congenital or acquired.
  - Developmental abnormalities include vaginal stenosis, persistent hymen, and vulvar hypoplasia.
  - Acquired abnormalities include clitoral hypertrophy, vaginal or vestibular foreign body, vaginal neoplasia, and vaginal trauma.
- Urinary tract disorders that may cause a secondary vaginitis are urinary tract infection and urinary incontinence.

Viral Vaginitis. Vaginitis caused by canine herpesvirus infection (see sec. 2, ch. 9) may cause vesicular or follicular mucosal lesions in the vagina and vestibule of the bitch.

- Lesions are usually transient and may recur, often during proestrus.
- Bitches infected with herpesvirus may manifest infertility, abortion, and stillbirth.

Clinical Signs

- Animals with vaginitis are usually presented for vaginal discharge and/or excessive licking of the vulva. Other signs may include pollakiuria and increased attention from male dogs.
- Vaginitis must be distinguished from other causes of vaginal discharge.
  - Nonpathologic reasons for vaginal discharge include proestral discharge (serosanguineous), early diestral discharge (mucoid), and postpartum discharge (dark brown or green), which may normally persist for 4–6 weeks following parturition.
  - Abnormal discharge may be the result of vaginal neoplasia or uterine disease such as open pyometra, subinvolution of placental sites, acute metritis (see sec. 8, ch. 14), and brucellosis (see sec. 2, ch. 11).

Diagnosis

Digital Examination. Digital examination of the vulva and vagina is indicated in all cases of vaginitis to identify underlying anatomic anomalies.

Vaginal Cytology. Cytology is important in the differentiation of vaginitis from other causes of vaginal discharge.

- Perform vaginal cytology by placing a cotton-tipped applicator in the vagina and then rolling it on a slide. Stain the smear with Diff-Quick or Wright's stain.
- Cytology consistent with vaginal inflammation shows large numbers of neutrophils that range from healthy to toxic in appearance and may contain phagocytized bacteria.
- Do not confuse vaginitis with the normal discharge of diestrus, which is characterized by moderate numbers of healthy neutrophils. Proestral discharge contains red blood cells and increasing numbers of keratinized squamous epithelial cells.

Bacterial Culture and Sensitivity Testing. Culture and sensitivity testing of the cranial vagina is indicated in cases of chronic vaginitis.

- Bacteria are found in the cranial vagina of 60% of normal bitches. The most common isolates include *Staphylococci, Streptococci, Escherichia coli,* and *Pasteurella.*
- Because these organisms cultured from bitches with chronic vaginitis are qualitatively the same as those found in normal bitches, culture results cannot be the sole basis for a diagnosis of bacterial vaginitis. However, they may be helpful in choosing a course of treatment.

Urinalysis. Urinalysis obtained by cystocentesis followed by urine culture and sensitivity testing, if indicated, is useful for identifying a predisposing or secondary urinary tract infection.

Abdominal Radiography and Ultrasonography. These modalities may help to distinguish vaginitis from uterine causes of vaginal discharge (see sec. 1, ch. 4).

Treatment

Juvenile Vaginitis

- Usually no specific treatment is required; the condition resolves after the first estrus. Medical therapy does not appear to shorten the clinical course and therefore is not routinely indicated.
- Nonspecific vaginitis in young bitches that becomes chronic indicates the need for further diagnostics including careful digital palpation for congenital anomalies. If no underlying problems are detected, institute medical management of the vaginitis with systemic and topical antimicrobials, as described for bacterial vaginitis.

Bacterial Vaginitis

- Ideally, treat through detection and resolution of the underlying primary genital or urinary abnormality.
- Most cases of secondary vaginitis resolve quickly with conservative medical therapy once the primary problem is corrected.
- Chronic vaginitis with no apparent predisposing cause is a frustrating problem and often is poorly responsive to medical management.
- Medical treatment consists of systemic antibiotic therapy and local (topical) therapy.
  - Base systemic antibiotic therapy on culture and sensitivity results, and continue treatment for 2–4 weeks. A good empirical choice is trimethoprim-sulfa (Tribrissen; Burroughs Wellcome), 15 mg/kg q 12 h, PO.

KEY POINT ▶ Because trimethoprim-sulfa can cause keratoconjunctivitis sicca in some dogs, monitor tear production in bitches treated with this agent for prolonged periods.

- Local therapy includes topical antibiotics, antiseptic douches, and sometimes glucocorticoids (when antibiotic therapy is unsuccessful). Place 10–30 ml of a douche solution of 1:10 diluted chlorhexidine (Nolvasan; Fort Dodge), or povidone-iodine solution (Betadine Douche; Purdue Frederick) in the vagina with a bulb syringe, disposable enema bottle, or soft large diameter catheter. Administer 1–3 times daily for 2–4 weeks.

Viral Vaginitis
- Treat viral vaginitis due to canine herpesvirus infection with nonspecific therapy, as no vaccine is available.
- Isolate bitches with evidence of infection. Instruct owners not to use these animals for breeding.

Supplemental Readings

Calvert C, Leifer CE, MacEwen EG: Vincristine for treatment of transmissible venereal tumor in the dog. J Am Vet Med Assoc 181:163, 1982.

Johnson CA: Diagnosis and treatment of chronic vaginitis in the bitch. Vet Clin North Am [Small Anim Pract] 21:523, 1991.

Thacher C, Bradley RL: Vulvar and vaginal tumors in the dog: A retrospective study. J Am Vet Med Assoc 183:690, 1983.

Wykes PM: Diseases of the vagina and vulva in the bitch. *In* Morrow DA, ed.: *Current Therapy in Theriogenology 2.* Philadelphia: W. B. Saunders, 1986, p 476.

17

Surgery of the Vagina and Vulva

Roger B. Fingland

The surgical procedures performed most commonly on the vagina and vulva are episiotomy, episioplasty, and excision of hyperplastic vaginal tissue. Episiotomy is performed to increase exposure to the vagina for excision of vaginal masses. Vaginal neoplasia is uncommon, and the majority of vaginal tumors are benign. Vaginal hyperplasia and vaginal prolapse are more common in intact females during estrus. Diseases of the external genitalia that require surgical intervention are rare in neutered females. See sec. 8, ch. 16 for discussion of diseases of the vagina and vulva.

ANATOMY

Vagina

- The vagina is a musculomembranous distensible canal that extends from the uterus to the vulva.
- The caudal boundary of the vagina is located cranial to the urethral opening, a point demarcated from the vestibule by a transverse mucosal ridge. A hymen normally is not present at the vestibulovaginal junction in the adult, although a vestige is retained in some females.
- The vagina is quite long in dogs, necessitating episiotomy for adequate surgical exposure of the cranial aspect.
- The longitudinal folds (rugae) of the vaginal mucosa allow significant expansion in diameter during pregnancy and whelping.
- The dorsal median postcervical fold extends from the cervix and terminates caudally by blending with longitudinal folds of vaginal mucosa. This fold can be mistaken for the cervical os during vaginoscopy.
- Blood supply to the vagina is via the vaginal artery, a branch of the urogenital artery.

Vulva

The vulva (external genitalia) consists of three parts:

- The *vestibule* is the space between the vagina and the labia.
  - The urethral tubercle (papilla), a ridge-like projection on the ventral floor of the vestibule caudal to the vestibulovaginal junction, contains the external urethral orifice.
  - The vestibulovaginal junction is readily identified because the vestibular mucosa is smooth, unlike the vaginal mucosa, which is thrown into distinct ridges.
- The *labia* form the external boundary of the vulva.

- The right and left labia join dorsally and ventrally at the commissures.
- The labia open to form the vulvar cleft.
- The *clitoris* is the homologue of the penis.
  - The clitoris normally does not contain structures comparable to the os penis or the urethra of the male.
  - An os clitoris may develop in response to altered hormone balance.

The vulva is surrounded by two striated circular muscles.

- The constrictor vestibule muscle fuses along its caudal surface to the external anal sphincter.
- The thinner constrictor vulvae muscle lies immediately caudal to the constrictor vestibule muscle.

Blood supply to the vestibule, labia, and clitoris is via branches of the urogenital arteries and the internal and external pudendal arteries.

EPISIOTOMY

Preoperative Considerations

- Episiotomy temporarily enlarges the vulvar cleft, increasing exposure to the vestibule and vagina.

Indications

- To resect benign or malignant vaginal masses
- To reduce a vaginal prolapse
- To resect vaginal strictures
- To manage dystocia resulting from inadequate vulvar diameter
- To suture vaginal lacerations
- To expose urethral papilla for catheterization if unable to visualize

Surgical Procedure

Objective

- Temporarily enlarge the vulvar cleft to enhance exposure of the vestibule and vagina.

Equipment

- Standard general surgery instrument pack and suture
- Gelpi or Weitlaner retractor
- Sterile Foley catheter

Technique

1. Episiotomy can be performed under general, epidural, or local anesthesia.

2. Position dog in ventral recumbency, preferably in a perineal stand.

KEY POINT ▶ To avoid femoral nerve palsy, make certain the edge of the table or perineal stand is well-padded when placing animals in the perineal position.

3. Place a pursestring suture in the anus.
4. Prepare the perineal region for aseptic surgery.
5. Flush the vestibule and vagina with dilute antiseptic solution (e.g., chlorhexidene)
6. Place a Foley catheter in the urinary bladder, using sterile technique.
7. Place surgical drapes so that the vulvar cleft and dorsal commissure are exposed. Exclude the anus from the surgical field.
8. Insert a finger in the vestibule and identify the caudodorsal aspect of the vaginal canal. This point represents the dorsal extent of the episiotomy incision (Fig. 1 A).
9. Make a median skin incision, beginning at the point described above and extending ventrally to include the dorsal commissure of the vulvar cleft (Fig. 1B).
10. Using Metzenbaum scissors, complete the episiotomy by incising the muscular layer and the mucosa in the same plane as the skin incision (Fig. 1C).
11. Complete the procedure for which the episiotomy was performed (Fig. 1D).
12. Closure—three layers (Fig. 1E).
    a. Appose the mucosal edges with 3–0 absorbable suture material in a simple continuous pattern with knots exposed to the lumen.
    b. Appose the muscular layer and subcutaneous tissue together with 3–0 absorbable suture material in a simple continuous pattern.
    c. Appose the skin edges with 4–0 absorbable suture material, using a continuous subcuticular suture pattern.
13. Remove the pursestring suture from the anus.

Postoperative Care and Complications

■ A side brace or Elizabethan collar may be necessary to prevent self-trauma.
■ Clean the incision if it becomes soiled.
■ Postoperative complications are uncommon and usually are related to poor surgical technique (e.g., carrying the incision too far dorsally or improper suture placement).

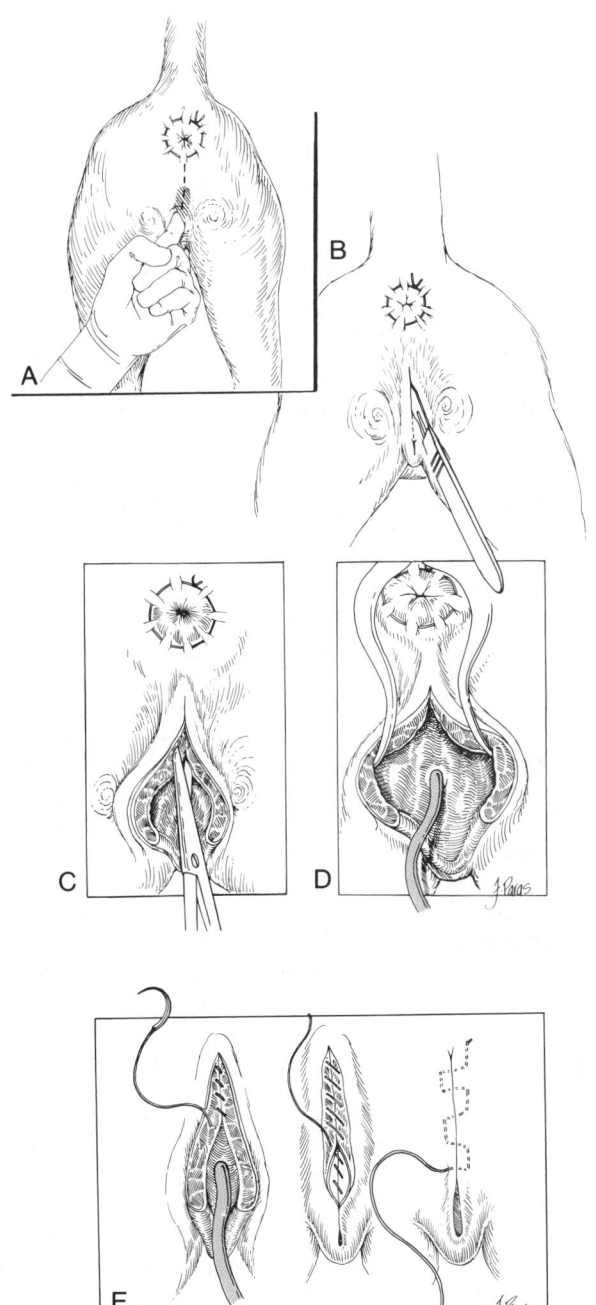

Figure 1. Episiotomy. *A,* After pursestring suture is placed around anus, insert finger in the vestibule to identify the caudodorsal aspect of the vaginal canal. *B,* Incise medially, from the caudodorsal aspect of the vaginal canal to the dorsal commissure of the vulvar cleft. *C,* Extend the depth of the incision with Metzenbaum scissors. *D,* Complete the procedure for which episiotomy is needed (in this case, bladder catheterization). *E,* Close in three layers.

EPISIOPLASTY

Preoperative Considerations

■ Episioplasty is indicated for aged, obese dogs with chronic perivulvular pyoderma resulting from redundant perivulvular skin and a recessed juvenile vulva. Juvenile vulva is common in dogs spayed prior to reaching sexual maturity.
■ Manage severe perivulvular pyoderma medically prior to performing episioplasty (see sec. 5, ch. 1).

Administer systemic antibiotics based on culture and sensitivity testing.

Surgical Procedure

Objective

■ Remove redundant perivulvular skin to reduce the incidence of skinfold pyoderma.

Equipment

■ Standard general surgery instrument pack and suture

Technique

1. Episioplasty can be performed under general or epidural anesthesia. General anesthesia is preferred.
2. Position dog in ventral recumbency in a perineal stand. (Pad the edge of the perineal stand.)
3. Place a pursestring suture in the anus.
4. Prepare the perineal region for aseptic surgery.
5. Determine the amount of perivulvular skin to be removed by plicating the redundant skin between the thumb and finger.
6. Make a crescent-shape incision around the vulva, beginning lateral to the ventral commissure of the vulva, curving laterally and then dorsally to a point 1 cm dorsal to the dorsal commissure of the vulva. Complete the crescent-shape incision by making a mirror-image incision on the contralateral side.
7. Make a second crescent-shape incision around the vulva. This incision begins and ends at the same points as the first incision. The second incision extends more dorsally than the first, creating a wider arc and including the redundant perivulvular skin.
8. Remove the perivulvular skin isolated by the two crescent-shape incisions.
9. Remove excessive subcutaneous tissue dorsal to the vulva.
10. Temporarily approximate the skin edges dorsal to the vulva. Remove additional skin dorsally if the skin folds are not eliminated or the vulva remains recessed. Do not alter the shape of the skin defect.
11. Control hemorrhage with ligation and electrocoagulation.
12. Closure may not be uniform because the incision nearest the vulva is shorter than the more dorsally placed incision. Follow these steps to avoid formation of "dog ears."
    a. Place an absorbable suture (simple interrupted pattern) in the subcutaneous tissue at the dorsal midpoint of the defect.
    b. Place additional subcutaneous sutures (simple interrupted pattern) at the midpoints of the remaining defects until the skin edges are apposed. (Bury all knots.)
    c. Place monofilament nonabsorbable skin sutures (simple interrupted pattern) at the 9, 12, and 3 o'clock positions. If there are discrepancies in the skin edges, place simple interrupted skin sutures closer together on the shorter (ventral) side of the defect than the longer (dorsal) side.
13. Remove the pursestring suture from the anus.

Postoperative Care and Complications

■ See Episiotomy.
■ Continue systemic antibiotic therapy after surgery, as needed (usually 7–10 days), to manage residual pyoderma. Topical antibacterial therapy may be required to control pyoderma.
■ Place obese dogs on a weight-reducing diet.
■ Complications are rare with proper technique.
  • Perivulvular pyoderma may persist if skin excision was insufficient.
  • Overzealous excision may result in excessive tension on the suture line and dehiscence. Ideally, dehiscence should be managed by wound debridement and primary closure. Keep the wound open if primary closure is not a viable option.

PERSISTENT HYMEN EXCISION

Preoperative Considerations

■ A number of congenital abnormalities that obstruct or constrict the vestibulovaginal opening occur in animals, but not all represent persistent hymen. Incomplete perforation of the hymen in dogs usually is observed as a vertical septum or an annular fibrous constriction at the vestibulovaginal junction.
■ Most animals with persistent hymen are asymptomatic. Symptomatic animals usually present for breeding or whelping problems or chronic vaginitis. Vaginitis results from inadequate drainage of vaginal or uterine secretions or urine pooling. Positional incontinence occasionally is observed in animals that pool urine.
■ A digital vaginal examination usually is adequate to obtain a diagnosis of persistent hymen. Vaginal septa are palpated as firm central bands with small stoma on either side. A small central stoma that does not allow penetration of the finger represents an annular constriction. Vaginal examinations with specula or fiberoptic equipment are helpful but can be difficult to interpret, leading to misdiagnosis. A vaginogram seldom is necessary.
■ Per vagina resection or digital breakdown is possible when the persistent membrane is thin and located distally in the vaginal vault. More frequently the membrane is located at the vestibulovaginal junction, necessitating an episiotomy for adequate surgical exposure.

Surgical Procedure

Objective

Excise the persistent hymen.

Equipment

■ Standard general surgery instrument pack and suture
■ Gelpi or Weitlaner retractor
■ Sterile Foley catheter

Technique

1. Perform an episiotomy as described previously.
2. Expose the vestibulovaginal junction and place a self-retaining retractor.
3. Place a Foley catheter in the urethra to avoid inadvertent damage to the urethral papilla.
4. Identify and excise the vertical band or annular constriction.

a. *Vertical band*: Place a curved instrument cranial to the band and retract the band caudally. Superficially transect the band at the dorsal and ventral attachments. Close the mucosal defects with 4–0 absorbable suture material in a simple continuous pattern.

b. *Annular constriction*: Thin membranes can be circumferentially excised at the mucosal attachment. When submucosal fibrous tissue exists, make a circumferential incision in the mucosa adjacent to the membrane and submucosally dissect and excise the fibrous tissue band. Close the mucosal defect with 4–0 absorbable suture material in a simple interrupted pattern. Alternatively, suture the mucosal defect with short runs of a simple continuous pattern.

KEY POINT ▶ Rarely, dogs have both a vertical band and annular constriction. Evaluate the diameter of the vaginal opening after resecting a vertical band and prior to closure.

5. Close the episiotomy incision as described previously.
6. Remove the pursestring suture from the anus.

Postoperative Care and Complications

■ A side brace or Elizabethan collar may be necessary to prevent self-trauma.
■ Excision of persistent hymen often is curative.
■ Rarely, dogs may require intermittent digital dilation to prevent fibrous narrowing after excision of annular constrictions. Permanent stenosis is possible in animals with this complication.

VAGINAL HYPERPLASIA EXCISION

Preoperative Considerations

■ Vaginal hyperplasia occurs when there is an exaggerated response by the vaginal mucosa to estrogen during the follicular phase of the estrous cycle. The mucosa of the vaginal floor cranial to the urethral papilla is redundant and may protrude through the labia. In contrast to vaginal prolapse, the urethra does not become exteriorized and can easily be catheterized. Most dogs are asymptomatic and are presented because the mass is aesthetically displeasing. Self-trauma or desiccation can lead to ulceration and infection of the redundant mucosa. Breeding bitches may be unable to copulate.
■ The redundant vaginal mucosa spontaneously regresses during diestrus but frequently recurs during subsequent periods of estrus.
■ Brachycephalic dogs are affected most commonly. A hereditary predisposition is suspected but not proven.
■ Application of a petroleum-based ointment or temporary labial closure with horizontal mattress sutures provides temporary relief. Resection of the redundant mucosa may be necessary in severe cases or in bitches used for breeding. Recurrence after resection may occur.
■ Ovariohysterectomy prevents recurrence and can be used as the sole means of treatment if the vaginal prolapse is small and not devitalized.

Surgical Procedure

Objective

■ Excise redundant vaginal mucosa.
■ Excise benign vaginal tumors (e.g., fibroma).

Equipment

■ See Episiotomy.

Technique

1. Perform an episiotomy as described previously (Fig. 2 *A* and *B*).
2. Identify the margins of the redundant mucosa on the floor of the vagina.
3. Elevate the *mucosal* mass and identify the urethral papilla on the floor of the vagina caudal to the mass.

KEY POINT ▶ Identify the urethral orifice and catheterize the urethra with a Foley catheter prior to excising the mucosal mass.

4. Make an elliptical superficial incision around the base of the mucosal mass.
5. Excise the mucosal mass. Electrocoagulate bleeding submucosal vessels. Do not extend the excision deeper than the mucosa (Fig. 2*C*).
6. Suture the mucosal defect with 3–0 absorbable suture material in a simple continuous pattern (Fig. 2*D*).
7. Close the episiotomy incision as described previously.
8. Remove the pursestring suture from the anus.

Postoperative Care and Considerations

■ A side brace or Elizabethan collar may be necessary to prevent self-trauma.
■ Owners of breeding animals should be informed that vaginal hyperplasia may recur after redundant mucosa has been excised. Excision should be considered palliative rather than curative.

VAGINAL PROLAPSE EXCISION

Preoperative Considerations

■ Vaginal prolapse is observed most commonly during estrus. Hyperplasia of vaginal mucosa and weakness of perivaginal supportive tissues are thought to be causative factors. Excessive straining may be contributory. Rarely, vaginal prolapse results from forced separation after mating. Vaginal prolapse may regress during diestrus.
■ Vaginal prolapse is more common in certain family lines and may be hereditary.

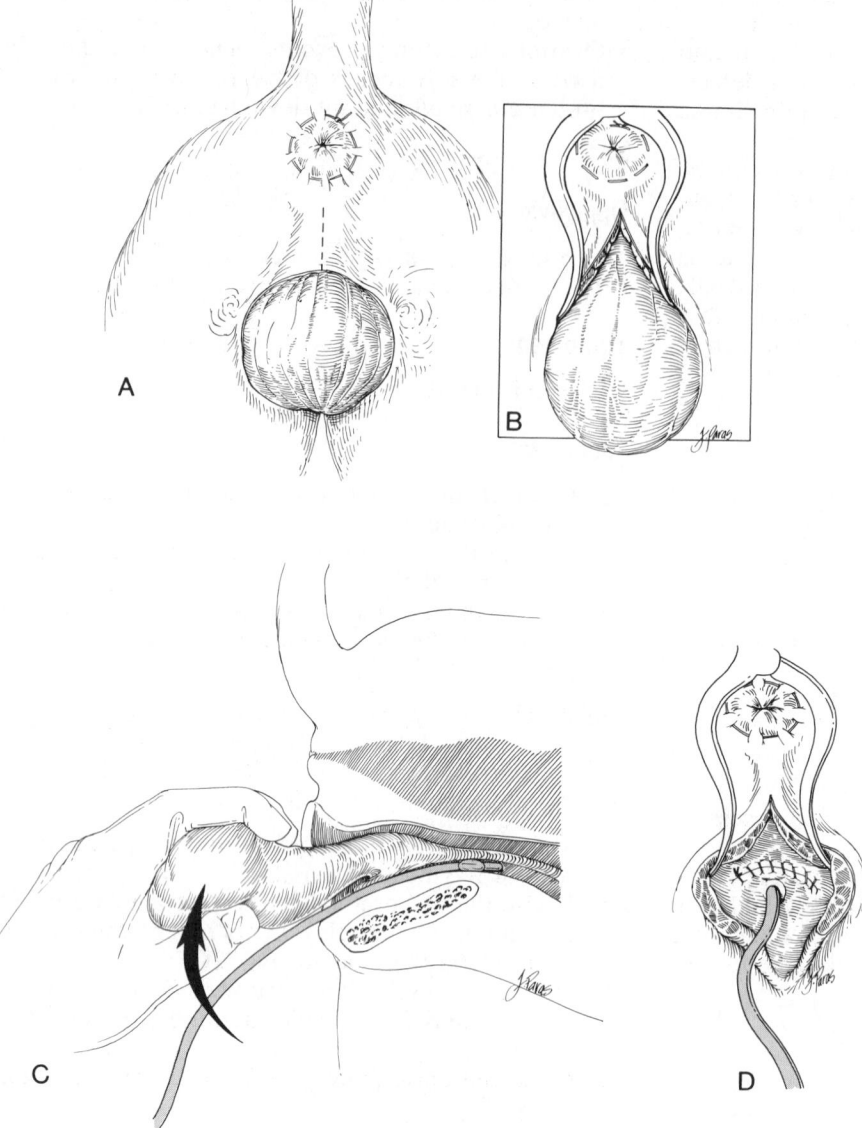

Figure 2. Excision of vaginal hyperplasia. *A*, Perform episiotomy as described previously. *B*, Retract skin to expose hyperplastic tissue. *C*, Elevate mass and identify urethral papilla. *D*, Suture mucosal defect in a simple continuous pattern.

- Vaginal prolapse may be partial or complete. Prolapse of the complete vaginal circumference through the labia results in the appearance of a doughnut-shaped mass ventral to the anus. This is in contrast to vaginal hyperplasia, in which redundant mucosa arises from the ventral aspect of the vagina. The urethral papilla may be observed on the prolapsed vaginal mucosa.
- Venous congestion can result in engorgement and discoloration of the prolapsed vaginal mucosa. Desiccation and self-trauma lead to ulceration and infection of the mass.
- After a thorough cleaning, coat the mass with sterile lubricating jelly and gently replace the mass with a finger or appropriately sized syringe case. Place temporary nonabsorbable sutures (mattress pattern) across the vulva if the vagina tends to reprolapse.
- Consider general anesthesia followed by episiotomy if the prolapse cannot be replaced digitally in the awake dog. Manual replacement still may not be possible if a large part of the vagina is prolapsed or if there is extensive mucosal edema.

- Repositioning by cranial traction on the uterine body through a ventral midline celiotomy may be considered when repositioning via the vulvular approach is unsuccessful and the mucosa is healthy. Permanent hysteropexy is accomplished by suturing the uterine body or horns to the abdominal wall.
- Excision of the prolapsed portion of the vagina is indicated when repositioning is not possible because of extensive venous engorgement or ulceration and necrosis of the vaginal mucosa.
- As in vaginal hyperplasia, ovariohysterectomy is helpful in reducing recurrence.

Surgical Procedure

Objective

- Excise the prolapsed portion of the vagina.

Equipment

- Standard general surgery instrument pack and suture
- Sterile Foley catheter

Technique

1. Position dog in dorsal recumbency with the rear legs tied forward (Fig. 3*A*).
2. Place a pursestring suture in the anus.
3. Gently clean the prolapsed vagina. Prepare the perineal region for aseptic surgery.

KEY POINT ▶ Perform an episiotomy only if necessary to expose the base of the prolapsed vaginal tissue.

4. Identify the urethral papilla and place a Foley catheter in the urethra.
5. Identify the proposed line of excision at the base of the prolapsed portion of the vagina. Identify the urethra by palpating the Foley catheter through the vaginal wall.
6. Incise the outer mucosal layer for approximately 4 cm along the proposed line of excision. Carry the incision through all layers of the vaginal wall to the inner mucosal layer. Insert index finger or sterile syringe case into the prolapsed vaginal opening to identify the inner mucosal layer (Fig. 3*B*). Carefully incise the inner mucosal layer, exposing the finger or syringe case.

7. Control hemorrhage with electrocoagulation or ligation.
8. Using 2–0 absorbable suture material, place horizontal mattress sutures in the vaginal wall between the mucosal surfaces, approximately 5 mm from the cut edge.
9. Continue this incision/suture technique in approximately 4-cm increments until the prolapsed tissue is excised (Fig. 3*C*).
10. Appose the cut edges of the inner and outer mucosal layers with 4–0 absorbable suture material in either a simple interrupted pattern or short runs of a simple continuous pattern (Fig. 3*D*).
11. Remove the pursestring suture from the anus.

Postoperative Care and Complications

- A side brace or Elizabethan collar may be necessary to prevent self-trauma.
- Mild vaginal bleeding may occur for 24 hours after surgery.
- Future breeding and whelping will not be impaired by this procedure. Breeding females prone to vaginal

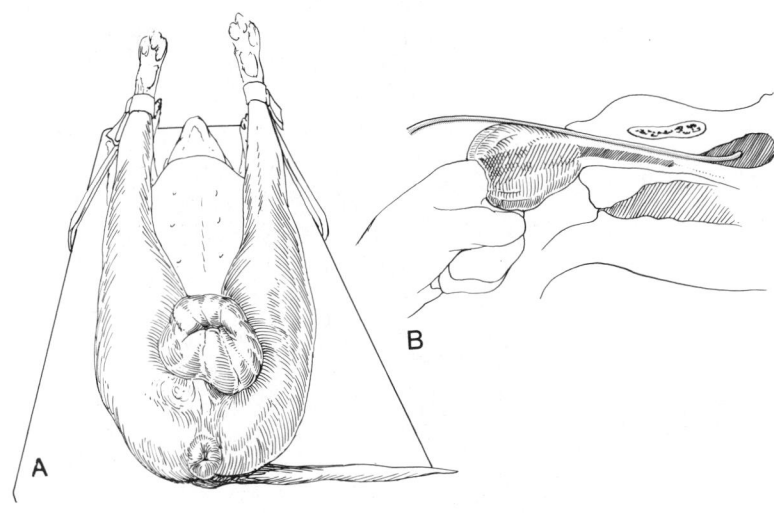
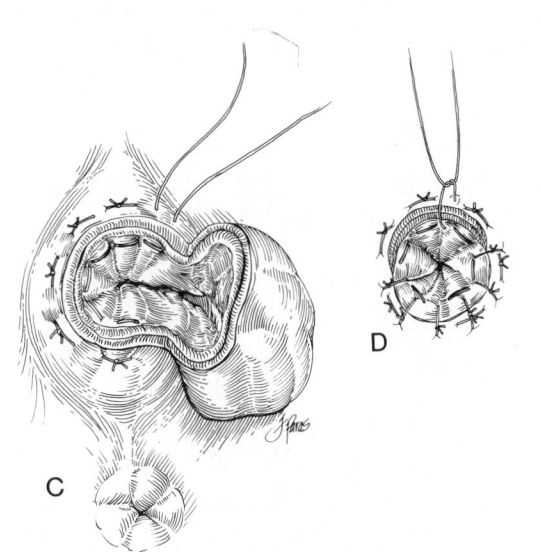

Figure 3. Correction of vaginal prolapse. *A*, Position dog in dorsal recumbency. *B*, Insert index finger or sterile syringe case into prolapsed opening to identify inner mucosal layer. *C*, Suture and incise around the prolapsed tissue. *D*, Suture together the cut edges.

prolapse is ill-advised because the condition may be heritable.

■ If labial sutures are placed, make certain that the animal is able to urinate spontaneously after surgery. Swelling around the urethral papilla may necessitate catheterization for several days after surgery.

Supplemental Readings

Bilbrey SA, Withrow SJ, Klein MK, et al.: Vulvovaginectomy and perineal urethrostomy for neoplasms of the vulva and vagina. Vet Surg 18:450, 1989.

Wykes PM, Soderberg SF: Congenital abnormalities of the canine vagina and vulva. J Am Anim Hosp Assoc 19:995, 1983.

18 Infertility

Nigel R. Perkins
Walter R. Threlfall

Infertility is defined as a temporary or permanently reduced ability to conceive and produce a normal number of viable offspring. It may be manifested as failure to breed, reduced conception rate, small litter size, abortion, stillbirths, or nonviable offspring. Causes may be infectious or noninfectious. Assessment of both male and female animals for breeding potential and evaluation of the breeding management is important in any fertility evaluation.

Poor reproductive management of breeding animals is considered to be one of the major causes of poor reproductive performance. Advances in knowledge and technology have allowed more intensive efforts to diagnose and manage problems associated with reproductive failure. In addition, the rising value of purebred animals for show and sale purposes and the availability of semen shipping and freezing have increased the demand for reproductive evaluation and treatment.

FEMALE INFERTILITY

Etiology

In this discussion, the fertility of the male is presumed to be satisfactory. Causes and factors associated with infertility are listed in Table 1.

Clinical Signs

The infertile animal commonly is presented with a history of an unsuccessful breeding. However, some animals are presented with signs pertaining to genitourinary tract disease without a specific history of an unsuccessful breeding.

Common clinical signs include:

- Failure to become pregnant or failure to whelp after a known mating
- Refusal to breed when presented to a male
- Failure to show pubertal estrus by 24 months of age or prolonged anestrus (>10 months) in an adult bitch
- Abnormal cyclic behavior in a postpubertal bitch, including prolonged estrus, split heats, short interestrous interval, and anestrus
- Palpable enlargement of the uterus in a non-pregnant bitch
- Abortion or pregnancy loss with or without vulvar discharge
- Physical anomalies involving the external genitalia

such as enlargement of the clitoris or presence of abnormally developed external genitalia
- Abnormal or persistent vulvar discharge or a mass protruding from the vulvar lips
- Small litter size and reduced conception rate

Diagnosis

History

- Infertility usually is identified by historical assessment of the bitch's general health, cyclicity, previous

TABLE 1. Causes of Infertility in the Bitch

Abnormal Cycles	Normal Cycles
Failure to Cycle	**Refusal to Breed**
Prepubertal	Vaginal/vulvar strictures
OHE	Vaginal prolapse/hyperplasia
Ovarian hypoplasia/aplasia	Psychological/territorial
Androgens/progestogens	Musculoskeletal
Intersex	
Ovarian neoplasia	**Occlusive Lesions**
Cushing's disease	Segmental aplasia/hypoplasia
Hypothyroidism	Inflammation
	Neoplasia
Prolonged Anestrus	
Ovarian senility	**Cystic Endometrial Hyperplasia**
Androgens/progestogens	
Ovarian neoplasia	**Reproductive Tract Neoplasia**
Cushing's disease	
Hypothyroidism	**Infection**
	Brucella canis
Prolonged Proestrus/Estrus	Canine herpesvirus
Cystic ovarian disease	*Mycoplasma*
Ovarian neoplasia	*Ureaplasma*
Estrogen administration	Miscellaneous bacteria
Short Interestrous Interval	**Immunologic**
Split estrus	Anti-sperm antibodies
Unknown	Anti-zona antibodies
	Abortion
	Brucellosis
	Herpesvirus infection
	Toxoplasmosis
	Mycoplasma/ureaplasma infection
	Parvovirus infection
	Distemper
	Miscellaneous bacterial infections
	Iatrogenic
	Inherent Infertility
	Old age
	Hypoluteoidism
	Failure of ovulation
	Failure of CL function
	Improper Breeding Management

TABLE 2. Vaginal Cytology

	Early Proestrus	Late Proestrus	Estrus	Day 1 Diestrus
Superficial cells	10–15%	80%	80–100%	< 80%
Intermediate/parabasal cells	85–90%	< 20%	Few	20–50%
Debris	+	–	–	+
White blood cells	+/–	–	–	+
Red blood cells	+	+/–	–	–
Foam/metestrus cells	–	–	–	–

Adapted from Feldman and Nelson, 1987 and Burke, 1984.
+ = Present; – = absent.

conceptions, pregnancy termination, delivery of non-viable offspring, and failure of neonates to survive.

■ Diagnostic evaluation is used in conjunction with the history to identify the cause and to determine the treatment and prognosis.

■ Evaluate breeding management practices historically and prospectively because a significant number of infertility cases are resolved simply by initiating good reproductive management practices.

KEY POINT ▶ Recommendations made in this chapter regarding the approach to the infertile bitch are confined to the *Brucella*-negative animal. Due to the poor success rates obtained with medical therapy and the risk of zoonosis, the authors currently recommend that animals whose sole purpose is for breeding that are positive on tube agglutination test (TAT) for brucellosis be euthanized.

Physical Examination

Physical examination (including rectal examination) objectives:

■ Identify systemic diseases or defects that may have an effect on reproductive performance.

■ Detect the presence and nature of vulvar discharge and swelling.

■ Evaluate the pelvic canal and vulva, vestibule, and caudal vagina for abnormalities such as strictures, adhesions, foreign bodies, and space-occupying lesions.

■ Determine the presence of diffuse or discrete enlargement or secretions in the mammary glands.

■ Assess size, consistency, and tone of the uterine horns, body, and cervix and look for the presence of uterine distension with fluid, fetuses, or gas.

Laboratory Evaluation

Routine Studies. Complete blood count (CBC), biochemistry profile, and urinalysis to aid in the diagnosis of underlying systemic disease and specific diseases of the genitourinary tract.

Brucella canis Serology

■ Screen serum from all breeding animals for *B. canis* antibodies using the 2-mercaptoethanol rapid slide agglutination test (RSAT).

■ Retest animals testing positive, using a test of higher specificity such as the tube agglutination test (TAT) or blood culture.

■ Test animals routinely every 6 months.

■ Breed animals only to a tested negative animal.

Thyroid Function Testing. Always evaluate thyroid function of dogs presented for infertility (see sec. 4, ch. 1).

Vaginal Cytology. Vaginal cytology provides information regarding:

■ Stage of the cycle
■ Whether estrus is progressing normally
■ Presence or absence of vaginitis or vaginal neoplasia
■ Diagnosis of vulvar discharge originating from the uterus (e.g., metritis, pyometra)

Technique

Vaginal Cytology
1. Cleanse the perineal area and clip long hair.
2. Pass a sterile cotton swab, moistened with bacteriostatic sterile saline, into the cranial vagina and roll to obtain sample.
3. Roll the swab onto a glass slide, fix with alcohol, and stain with a commercial rapid stain such as Diff-Quik, new methylene blue, or Wright's stain.

Interpretation (Table 2)
■ Evaluate the stained slide for relative numbers of superficial, intermediate, and parabasal epithelial cells and for background debris, mucus, leukocytes, and erythrocytes.

■ Foam and metestrous cells may be visible in bitches in early diestrus.

■ Bacteria may be visible on slides from normal bitches. The presence of large numbers of degenerate neutrophils with intracellular and extracellular bacteria is indicative of vaginitis, urinary tract disease, or uterine infection or inflammation.

■ The presence of degenerating muscle fibers in a specimen from a postpartum bitch is suggestive of a retained nonviable fetus.

■ Spermatozoa are visible in 65% of vaginal cytology smears taken within 24 hours of breeding; therefore, vaginal cytology provides valuable information in the evaluation of a bitch suspected of having been inadvertently bred.

■ Vaginal cytology may contain cells suggestive of

neoplasia in bitches with vaginal or urinary tract neoplasia.

Vaginal Culture

■ Use a guarded culture rod.
■ Interpret positive cultures with caution and in combination with the results of other aspects of the examination.
  • A heavy growth of a pure culture in the presence of signs of inflammation on vaginal cytology is indicative of vaginitis.
  • Light, mixed bacterial cultures and growth in the absence of any inflammatory infiltrate on vaginal cytology may be indicative of contamination rather than a significant bacterial vaginitis.

Vaginoscopy. Vaginoscopy can provide additional information on the state of the mucosa lining the vagina, vestibule, and vulva. It allows:

■ Determination of the origin of vulvar discharges
■ Visualization of space occupying lesions within the vulva and vagina
■ Determination of the stage of the estrous cycle

Technique

Vaginoscopy

1. Pass a rigid or flexible endoscope into the vagina aseptically.
2. Slightly distend the vagina with air to allow visualization of the mucosa cranially to the level of the dorsal vaginal fold, which lies caudal to the cervix. Often, the cervix is not visible because of narrowing of the vaginal lumen in the area of the dorsal vaginal fold.

Interpretation

■ Proestrus is associated with enlargement and edema of vaginal folds.
■ Declining estrogen and rising progesterone concentrations at the time of the luteinizing hormone (LH) surge result in progressive loss of edema and the development of an increasingly wrinkled vaginal mucosa.
■ Maximum wrinkling and angulated mucosal folds are observed 1–2 days after ovulation.
■ Toward the end of estrus, the appearance of the vaginal mucosa changes abruptly to a flattened, thin surface. This appearance persists into anestrus.

Imaging Studies

■ Abdominal radiographic and ultrasonographic examination (also see chs. 1–4) can be helpful.
■ They aid in determining size, shape, and nature of contents of the uterus and surrounding abdominal structures.
■ Utilization of a 7.5 MHz ultrasound probe allows visualization of the ovaries for the presence of follicles, corpora lutea, and cystic ovarian disease.
■ Contrast radiography can outline vaginal lesions and congenital anomalies.

Canine Herpesvirus Culture

■ A presumptive diagnosis of acute neonatal herpesvirus (HV) infection can be made based on the clinical signs and history and confirmed by submission of samples of liver, kidney, and spleen chilled for virus culture and additional samples placed in 10% formalin for histopathologic examination and serum from the dam for serum neutralizing antibody concentrations (see sec. 2, ch. 9).
■ Other clinical forms of HV infection may be more difficult to diagnose than the acute neonatal type.
■ In abortion cases, include fresh, chilled, formalinized placenta samples in addition to the samples listed above.
■ Samples from adult animals with upper respiratory signs, conjunctivitis, or urogenital vesicular lesions include nasal, transtracheal, conjunctival, vaginal, and preputial swabs for virus isolation and serum for neutralizing antibody concentrations.
■ In animals suspected of being inapparent carriers, perform vaginal/preputial and nasal conjunctival swabs in addition to serum neutralizing antibody levels.

Mycoplasma/Ureaplasma Cultures

■ A presumptive diagnosis is based on a kennel history of infertility with reduced conceptions, vaginal discharge, early embryonic and fetal deaths, abortion, stillbirths, fading pups, and neonatal deaths.
■ Diagnosis is made by isolation of the organism from a guarded vaginal culture of the cranial vagina when a vaginal discharge is present. (Not all laboratories have the capability to culture these fastidious organisms.)
■ Examine aborted fetuses, placenta and any postabortion discharge for a possible bacterial, viral, or mycoplasmal cause. Include histopathologic and culture samples.
■ A pure culture of high numbers of organisms is significant if associated with inflammation as determined by vaginal cytology or with a clinical history of infertility in the kennel.

Toxoplasmosis Serology

See sec. 2, ch. 13.

Endocrine Testing

■ *Serum progesterone* concentration is indicative of luteinization within ovarian granulosa and thecal cells. During proestrus and early estrus, progesterone levels remain low (<1.0 ng/ml). Levels rise to about 2 ng/ml at the time of the LH surge and to 5 ng/ml (range, 3–8 ng/ml) at the time of ovulation.
  • Serial progesterone assays may be used in conjunction with vaginal cytology and estrus behavior to aid in determining the time of ovulation and to recommend a time for breeding. A progesterone concentration of >2 ng/ml at 15–30 days after the end of estrus indicates the presence of normal functional corpora lutea.
■ *Serum estradiol* concentrations are of little diagnostic

use because of the wide variation in normal animals. Serum concentrations are lowest during diestrus and anestrus (<15 pg/ml), rise during proestrus to a peak in late proestrus (60–100 pg/ml), and fall during estrus and early diestrus.

- Levels may be grossly elevated in some animals with cystic ovarian follicles and steroid-producing tumors such as the granulosa-thecal cell tumor.
- The degree of cornification of vaginal epithelial cells on vaginal cytology is a relatively sensitive bioassay for serum estrogen levels.

■ *Testosterone* concentrations are low in diestrus and anestrus and rise in proestrus to a peak during estrus of about 500 pg/ml. Testosterone levels have little diagnostic value in reproductive disorders in the bitch.

■ *Luteinizing hormone* (LH) is secreted in a pulsatile manner, with peaks as high as 30 ng/ml in a normal intact bitch. Ovariectomized animals and animals with ovarian aplasia/hypoplasia may have constantly high LH concentrations (30 ng/ml) due to the lack of negative feedback from ovarian steroids.

- Three serum samples taken 20 minutes apart are necessary to differentiate a pulsatile peak in a normal animal from consistently elevated levels in animals with ovarian hypoplasia/aplasia or after bilateral ovariectomy.
- A commercial urinary LH assay has been recently made available (International Genetics Inc., 271 Great Valley Parkway, Malvern, PA 19355) for use in managing breeding bitches. This assay allows identification of the optimal time to breed a bitch based on detection of the LH surge.

■ *Follicle-stimulating hormone* concentrations vary considerably in intact bitches and are of little diagnostic value.

■ *Serum relaxin* concentration is low in nonpregnant bitches and rises significantly in pregnant bitches after day 21 of pregnancy. A commercial assay, if available, may be a sensitive and accurate method of pregnancy diagnosis.

■ *Challenge testing* may be utilized in animals suspected of having remnants of ovarian tissue present after ovariohysterectomy. Administration of human chorionic gonadotropin (hCG) or gonadotropin releasing hormone (Gn-RH) to a bitch or queen showing vulvar swelling and cornification of vaginal cytology may result in resolution of vulvar swelling, decrease in cornification, and a rise in serum progesterone concentration.

Karyotyping

■ Karyotype examination is indicated when an intersex condition is suspected (see sec. 8, ch. 19). Such animals may have abnormalities in the external or internal genital organs and/or a history of failure to cycle or infertility.

■ Draw a heparinized blood sample in an aseptic manner and submit rapidly to a laboratory for lymphocyte culture, mount preparation, and chromosomal examination.

Exploratory Laparotomy and Uterine Biopsy

This technique provides information in the diagnosis of oophoritis, salpingitis, endometritis, cystic endometrial hyperplasia, subinvolution of placental sites, adenomyosis, segment aplasia/hypoplasia, adhesions involving the reproductive tract, and neoplasia involving the ovaries, uterine tubes, uterus, and cervix.

Technique

1. Perform a ventral midline laparotomy under general anesthesia to expose the reproductive tract (sec. 8, ch. 15).
2. Inspect the tract for the presence of abnormalities, evidence of ovarian follicular or luteal activity, and patency of the uterine tubes.
3. Make an incision in the antimesenteric surface of the uterus and pass a sterile, moistened culture swab into the uterine lumen for a uterine culture.
4. Remove a sample of endometrium from the area of the incision and fix for histopathologic examination.
5. Repeat procedure at a site in the opposite horn.
6. Close the abdominal incision routinely.

Infertility in Bitches with Abnormal Cycles

Failure to Cycle

Diagnosis
History

■ Determine methods and frequency of estrus detection.
■ Rule out prior ovariohysterectomy.
■ Animals younger than 24 months of age may be prepubertal.
■ Rule out the possibility of prior treatment with progestogens or androgens that could suppress signs of cyclicity, usually for the duration of treatment and a variable time afterward.

Physical Examination

■ Perform a general physical examination to determine if animal's general health status is compatible with cyclicity (adequate body condition) for signs of estrus or proestrus.
■ Examine for any systemic disease which may interfere with cyclicity.
■ Examine for evidence of intersex conditions (see sec. 8, ch. 19).
■ Examine for clinical evidence of endocrine dysfunctions such as hyperadrenocorticism, hypothyroidism, and pituitary dwarfism.

Laboratory Evaluations

■ Perform a CBC, biochemistry profile, and urinalysis, if indicated.
■ Vaginal cytology results (weekly for 6 months) provide information regarding the stage of the estrous cycle, whether the cycle is normal or abnormal, and the presence of metritis or pyometra if the cervix is relaxed or of cervicitis or vaginitis.
■ Screen for *B. canis* using the RSAT. Confirm positive RSAT results using a test of higher specificity such as the TAT or blood culture (see sec. 2, ch. 11).
■ Measure basal T_3 and T_4 concentrations and/or per-

form a thyroid-stimulating hormone (TSH) stimulation test (see sec. 4, ch. 1).
■ Endocrine testing:
  • Perform serum progesterone assays every 1–2 weeks. Progesterone concentration of >2 ng/ml is suggestive of functional corpora lutea.
  • LH concentration >30 ng/ml in three successive samples 20 minutes apart suggests ovariectomy or ovarian hypoplasia/aplasia.
■ Karyotyping is recommended in animals:
  • With evidence of abnormal external genitalia
  • With a history of never having cycled
  • Over 18 months of age with no evidence of cyclicity after 6 months of weekly vaginal cytologic smears.

Ultrasonography. Ultrasonographic evaluation of the reproductive tract provides information on the presence or absence of uterine enlargement and/or accumulation of fluid and abnormalities such as ovarian masses. (See sec. 1, ch. 4 for more information on ultrasonography.)

Laparoscopy/Laparotomy. Consider laparoscopy or exploratory laparotomy to evaluate the reproductive tract.

Treatment
Karyotypically Abnormal Animals. Neuter animals with abnormal karyotypes.

Karyotypically Normal Animals. Animals with normal karyotypes that have not cycled by 30 months of age are candidates for estrus induction. The authors use the following various regimens:

■ Administer follicle-stimulating hormone (FSH), 1–2 mg, SC or IM, on days 1, 3, 6, and 9, performing vaginal cytology on each of these days. When vaginal cytology shows 80% superficial cells, breed the bitch and administer human chorionic gonadotropin (hCG), 500–1000 units, IM or IV.
■ Administer FSH, 2 mg/day for 5–10 days, followed by hCG as above.
■ Administer FSH, 25 mg weekly for up to 5 doses. When the bitch enters proestrus, discontinue FSH and perform vaginal cytology. Administer hCG as above and breed.
  • If the bitch shows signs of proestrus and then begins to regress to anestrus, give 25 mg, 10 mg, and 5 mg FSH on successive days and follow with breeding and hCG.

Neoplasia. Surgically remove neoplastic ovaries (see sec. 8, ch. 15).

Endocrine Disorders. Treatment schedules for endocrine disorders such as hyperadrenocorticism, pituitary dwarfism, hypothyroidism, and hyperthyroidism are detailed in their respective chapters.

Prolonged Anestrus in a Previously Cycling Bitch

Diagnosis
History
■ Old age (>6–8 years) may be associated with a reduction in fertility and irregular cyclicity. Some breeds such as wolf breeds and basenjis may cycle only once a year.

■ Evaluate the accuracy of observations for estrus behavior signs.
■ Evaluate for evidence of severe stress such as disease, malnutrition, debilitation, and even temperature extremes, which may suppress signs of proestrus/estrus or may prolong anestrus.
■ Rule out the possibility of treatment with progestogens or androgens.

Physical Examination
■ Perform a general physical examination to evaluate for systemic disease.
■ Examine for clinical evidence of endocrine dysfunction such as hypothyroidism and hyperadrenocorticism.

Laboratory Evaluations
■ Perform vaginal cytology weekly.
■ Screen for *B. canis,* using the RSAT.
■ Measure basal T_3 and T_4 concentrations and/or perform TSH stimulation test.
■ Perform endocrine testing (see previous discussion in Failure to Cycle).
■ Perform CBC, biochemistry profile, and urinalysis, if indicated.

Ultrasonography
Ultrasonographic evaluation of the reproductive tract with a 7.5 MHz transducer provides information regarding increased ovarian size.

■ Karyotype animals >18 months of age that fail to cycle after 6 months of exposure to other cycling females and males.

Laparoscopy/Laparotomy
Consider laparoscopic examination or exploratory laparotomy.

Treatment
■ Place bitch with other cycling females and expose regularly to male.
■ Induce estrus, as described previously in treatment of Failure to Cycle.
■ Surgically remove neoplastic ovaries (see sec. 8, ch. 15).
■ No effective treatment exists for the decline in fertility seen in aging bitches.

Prolonged Proestrus/Estrus

Diagnosis
History
■ Obtain information on method of estrus detection (i.e., what were the signs?).
■ Ensure that the length of proestrus and estrus was >21 days.
■ Rule out the possibility of treatment with estrogenic products.

Physical Examination
■ Perform a general physical examination.
■ Examine the external genitalia for evidence of estrogenic influence (enlarged, edematous vulva and vulvar discharge) and abdominal masses such as ovarian tumors.

Laboratory Evaluations

- Vaginal cytology can demonstrate the presence of estrogenic influence as determined by the degree of cornification and the presence or absence of white blood cells, red blood cells, and background debris.
- Endocrine testing: Estrogen concentrations greater than 15 pg/ml (often as high as 60–100 pg/ml) are suggestive of proestrus or estrus.

Imaging Studies

- Ultrasonographic examination of the reproductive tract can rule out enlarged ovaries and follicular structures on the ovaries.
- Radiographs of the abdomen may provide information about the presence of enlarged ovaries and ovarian masses.

Treatment

- Induce ovulation or luteal tissue with hCG (500–1000 units, IV or IM) or Gn-RH (50–100 μg, IV or IM). Check animals using ultrasonography, vaginal cytology, and serum progesterone assay prior to treatment and 14 days post-treatment to monitor response.
- Administer androgen therapy (Cheque Drops; Upjohn) for 3–4 months and then breed on the subsequent estrus.
- Recommend ovariohysterectomy for bitches that are not intended for breeding purposes.
- Surgically remove neoplastic ovaries (see sec. 8, ch. 15).

Shortened Interestrus Interval

Diagnosis
History

- Determine methods and frequency of estrus determination.
- Determine that interestrus interval is <4 months.
- Rule out possibility of treatment with hormonal compounds such as estrogens.

Physical Examination

- Perform general physical examination.
- Observe behavior of female in presence of intact male.

Laboratory Evaluations

- Perform vaginal cytology to confirm that the bitch is in estrus.
- Consider endocrine testing, including estrogen concentration and progesterone concentration assays.

Treatment

- Induce ovulation (as described previously in Treatment for Prolonged Anestrus) when animal is in estrus as determined by vaginal cytology and progesterone assays; followed with breeding.
- Administer androgen therapy (Cheque Drops; Upjohn) for 3–4 months and then breed on subsequent estrus.
- Ovariohysterectomy is recommended for animals not intended for breeding.

Infertility in Bitches with Normal Cycles
Refusal to Breed

Diagnosis
History

- Determine the duration of interestrus interval, proestrus and estrus, and when attempts were made to breed the animal with respect to these stages in the estrus cycle.
- Obtain information on methods of estrus detection and determination of the time to breed.
- Ascertain age and experience of the breeding animal.
- Consider the possibility of psychological and dominance interactions interfering with successful breeding.

Physical Examination

- Perform a general physical examination.
- Examine the musculoskeletal system to diagnose painful conditions interfering with libido. Evaluate for evidence of musculoskeletal problems such as arthritis, hip dysplasia, and neural dysfunctions resulting in pain on physical movement when animal is mounted by male.
- Perform digital and vaginoscopic examination of the vulva and vagina to diagnose neoplastic lesions and congenital/acquired stenotic lesions involving the genitourinary tract that may produce pain and aversion behavior on attempted copulation.
- Observe attempted breedings.

Laboratory Evaluations

- Perform vaginal cytology to determine whether the bitch is in estrus.
- Progesterone serum concentration assays can help to determine the stage of the cycle.

Treatment

- Stenotic and space-occupying lesions affecting the vulva and vagina are discussed in sec. 8, chs. 16 and 17.
- Ensure that the potential breeding pair is psychologically compatible. Transport the bitch to the male to ensure that the male remains within his own domain where he is likely to remain dominant.
- Separate animals housed together prior to or at the onset of proestrus to enhance the probability of mating.
- Artificial insemination is recommended when the animal refuses to breed or when either animal is physically incapable of breeding because of musculoskeletal problems.

Occlusive Lesions

Occlusive lesions resulting in obstruction to passage of semen and/or ova may occur due to congenital or acquired defects involving the female reproductive tract.

Diagnosis
History

- Obtain evidence of normal cyclicity, estral behavior, and acceptance of male.
- Ascertain if artificial insemination technique has been used with failure to conceive.

Physical Examination
- Perform a general physical examination.
- Perform digital and vaginoscopic examination of the vulva and vagina to rule out the possibility of a stenotic or aplastic lesion.

Laboratory Evaluations
- Monitor the bitch throughout estrus with vaginal cytology and progesterone concentrations to assure that insemination is occurring at the correct time followed by ovulation and corpora lutea development.
- Perform uterine culture and biopsy.
- Measure basal T_3 and T_4 concentration and/or perform TSH stimulation tests.

Ultrasonography
Ultrasonographic examination of the reproductive tract will provide information regarding the presence of abnormalities.

Laparotomy/Laparoscopy. Consider laparoscopic surgery and/or exploratory laparotomy:

- To determine the presence of a normal reproductive tract
- To examine for occlusive lesions in the oviducts or uterine horns

Treatment
- Treatment of conditions involving the vulva and vagina, uterus and ovaries, and ovarian bursae is discussed in sec. 8, chs. 14–17.
- Surgical reconstruction of affected areas may be attempted to allow breeding and fertilization to occur.
- Alternatives are artificial insemination and embryo transfer.

Cystic Endometrial Hyperplasia

Diagnosis
History. The history usually shows failure to conceive, despite evidence of normal cyclicity and estral behavior, after acceptance of male or satisfactory artificial insemination technique.

Physical Examination
- Perform a general physical examination.

Laboratory Evaluation. The diagnosis usually is based on uterine biopsy.

Treatment
- Perform ovariohysterectomy (see sec. 8, ch. 15).

Tumors of the Uterus or Cervix
(Also see sec. 8, ch. 14)

Diagnosis
History
The owner may have observed abdominal enlargement and abnormal vulvar discharge.

Physical Examination
- Perform a general physical examination.
- Palpate the abdomen and examine the rectum for uterine or cervical enlargement.

Imaging Studies. Ultrasonographic or radiological examination of the abdomen to detect the presence of a mass associated with the uterus or cervix.

Laparoscopy/Laparotomy. Laparoscopic surgery, exploratory laparotomy, and excisional biopsy can accurately diagnose the type and extent of the tumor.

Treatment
- Perform ovariohysterectomy if both uterine horns or ovaries are involved or if the tumor is malignant.
  - Consider unilateral removal if only one side is involved, depending on the type of tumor.

Infections

Infections involving the female reproductive tract (also see sec. 8, ch. 14) may interfere with fertilization and pregnancy maintenance by directly affecting sperm, ovum, or embryo or indirectly as a result of the mediators and by-products of the inflammatory response.

Diagnosis
History
- Obtain details of breeding management and hygiene.
- Look for evidence of pyometra, such as fever, depression, anorexia, dehydration, polyuria, polydipsia, and vulvar discharge.
- Look for evidence of endometritis, metritis or cervicitis, such as abnormal vulvar discharge.

Physical Examination
- Perform a general physical examination. Results depend on the extent and type of infection, (e.g., pyometra, cervicitis).
- Examine the external genitalia for evidence of vulvar discharge.
- Palpate the abdomen to detect uterine enlargement.
- Perform vaginoscopy to determine the origin of a vaginal discharge.

Laboratory Evaluations
- Take specimens for vaginal culture and susceptibility testing to determine choice of drugs in therapy.
- Vaginal cytology can help in staging the estrous cycle and evaluating evidence of inflammation or infection with increased WBC numbers.
- CBC, biochemistry profile, and urinalysis aid in the diagnosis of systemic diseases such as pyometra and in selection of treatment.

Imaging Studies. Perform abdominal radiography or ultrasonography to detect uterine enlargement and to determine the nature of uterine contents.

Treatment
Pyometra
- After stabilizing the animal, perform ovariohysterectomy if the animal is not to be used for breeding or is severely ill systemically (see sec. 8, ch. 15).
- Use medical supportive therapy and administer prostaglandin in selected bitches <6 years of age that are used primarily for breeding (see sec. 8, ch. 14).

Endometritis and Metritis
- Perform ovariohysterectomy.
- Alternatively, administer intrauterine and/or systemic antibiotics and prostaglandin.

Vaginitis
- Remove inciting causes (see sec. 8, ch. 16).
- Local therapy usually consists of vaginal douches.

Canine Herpesvirus (HV)
See section 2, chapter 9.

- Isolate animal until acute lesions heal.
- Consider culling breeding animals in kennel situations since infected animals may remain as a source of infection for other animals in the kennel.

Mycoplasma *and* Ureaplasma *Infections*
- Administer systemic antibiotics based on culture and sensitivity tests. Drugs currently considered effective include tetracycline, tylosin, chloramphenicol, and ampicillin. Continue treatment for 2–3 weeks and combine with vaginal douches of 1% povidone-iodine (Betadine).
- Isolate infected animals.
- Reduce population density in kennel situations.
- Monitor hygiene and ventilation.
- Monitor levels of infection with periodic cultures of vagina in bitches and prepuce in males.

Immunologic Causes

Immunologic causes of infertility in the dog are uncommon.

Diagnosis
History. There usually is a history of repeated unsuccessful breedings to the same male, with no evidence of abnormalities in previous female reproductive examinations.
Physical Examination. Perform a thorough physical examination (usually normal).
Laboratory Evaluation. Definitive diagnosis depends on demonstration of anti-sperm antibodies in the vaginal mucus of the bitch.

Treatment
- Breed bitch to a different male.
- Consider the empirical use of corticosteroids.

Abortion

Abortion may result from infectious or noninfectious causes.

Diagnosis
History. Record when pregnancy was diagnosed, stage of pregnancy when abortion occurred, and clinical signs prior to and at time of abortion.

Physical Examination
- Perform a general physical examination.
- Perform a complete necropsy of any aborted fetuses and placentas.

Laboratory Evaluations
- Submit samples from aborted fetuses and placentas for gross, histopathologic, and microbiologic evaluation.
- Take samples for guarded cultures of the cranial vagina at the time of or as soon as possible following abortion.

- Submit paired serum sample for canine HV serum neutralizing antibodies.

Treatment
- Euthanize animals testing positive (TAT) for *B. canis.*
- Cull animals testing positive for canine HV from the breeding program.
- Treat incidental bacterial infections resulting in abortion with specific antibiotics as determined by culture and sensitivity tests.
- Combine all treatments with proper kennel hygiene and isolation of pregnant animals to prevent the risk of disease spread.
- Treatment of animals with infectious diseases, such as toxoplasmosis, distemper, feline infectious peritonitis, feline leukemia, and parvovirus and HV infection, is discussed in detail in their respective chapters.

Advanced Age

Bitches older than 6 years of age may have a decline in fertility associated with age. No treatment exists for the age-associated decline in fertility.

Hypoluteoidism

Evidence of hypoluteoidism has not been substantiated in the dog and is considered to be an unlikely cause of infertility.

Diagnosis
- Diagnosis depends on endocrine testing:
  - Progesterone concentrations of 2–5 ng/ml 10–30 days after ovulation suggest inadequate luteal function.
  - Concentrations <2 ng/ml indicate failure of ovulation and/or normal luteinization with inadequate luteal function.

Treatment
- Progesterone supplementation to maintain serum progesterone levels is a potential treatment.
- The authors know of no scientific reports detailing doses or treatment regimes in the dog and currently do not routinely prescribe treatment because of the risk of complications such as pyometra and diabetes mellitus.

Breeding Management

Although not a direct cause of female infertility, often improper breeding management is an indirect cause. Be sure to obtain an accurate and complete history. In assessing and implementing breeding management, it is essential to evaluate:

- Kennel hygiene and evidence of overcrowding
- Methods of estrus detection, timing of breeding, and the number of breedings per bitch per cycle
- The use of natural breeding or artificial insemination
- General health factors such as nutrition, vaccination schedule, and parasite control

Treatment

- Perform a breeding soundness examination of the proposed male prior to breeding.
- Perform vaginal smears on the bitch every 2 days from the first day of proestrus as an aid in determining the best time to breed the bitch.
- Consider a vaginal culture during early proestrus if the bitch has a history of vaginitis or if vaginal cytology suggests infection.
- Serum progesterone assays aid in determining the time of ovulation. Serum progesterone concentrations of 2 ng/ml are associated with the occurrence of the LH surge, and 5 ng/ml with the time of ovulation.
- Urinary or serum luteinizing hormone concentrations may be monitored as an aid in determining the time of ovulation.
- Breed the bitch every 2–3 days during estrus beginning on the second or third day as determined by vaginal cytology, rising progesterone concentrations, and behavioral response to the presence of the male.
- Continue breeding until 2–3 days after ovulation or until the bitch demonstrates signs of diestrus, including refusal of the male and vaginal cytology showing an abrupt increase in the proportion of parabasal and intermediate cells and a decrease in superficial epithelial cells (see Table 2).
  - Serum progesterone concentrations >5 ng/ml suggest recent ovulation and may be used as an indicator to stop breeding.
- Bitches may be bred by vaginal insemination or uterine deposition of chilled fresh or thawed frozen semen via laparotomy or laparoscopy.
  - Perform daily vaginal cytology and progesterone assays every 1–3 days to allow more accurate staging of the cycle, breed when cytology is consistent with estrus and progesterone concentration is 2–5 ng/ml. This should reduce the number of breedings required.
- Ovulation induction agents such as Gn-RH and hCG may be used prior to or at the time of insemination to induce ovulation. One or more additional breedings may be required after the injection of hCG or Gn-RH because of the lag time between injection and ovulation.
  - Dose rates vary but are commonly in the range of 500–1000 units hCG, IM or IV, and 50–100 µg, IM or IV, for Gn-RH.

Examination for Pregnancy

Examine the bitch for pregnancy using ultrasonography at 15–30 days postbreeding.

- If diagnosed pregnant, monitor the bitch by palpation and ultrasonography to ensure that normal fetal development occurs.
  - Determine serum progesterone concentrations on samples taken during pregnancy to monitor development and function of corpora lutea (although progesterone insufficiency has not been documented in the bitch).
  - If diagnosed nonpregnant, examine the bitch by palpation and ultrasonography to ensure that there is no uterine fluid accumulation with the subsequent risk of pyometra.
  - An ultrasonographic examination, utilizing a 7.5 MHz transducer, may provide information on the presence of corpora lutea.
  - Perform a progesterone assay between 20–30 days after the bitch enters diestrus to determine if functional corpora lutea are present.
- Consider further procedures in the evaluation of the infertile bitch that fails to conceive after optimal management, including laparoscopic surgery, exploratory laparotomy, karyotype examination and evaluation for immunologic causes of infertility.

Prevention of Infertility

Prevention of fertility problems depends primarily on optimal reproductive management and early diagnosis and therapy of reproductive problems.

- Breed animals when young (2–6 years), as fertility is maximal during this time and declines with advancing age.
- Screen all breeding animals for *B. canis*, using the RSAT, every 6 months. Breed bitches only with tested negative males.
- Remove animals infected with canine HV from the breeding kennel because of the risk of latent infection and spread of disease to other animals.
- Perform a breeding soundness examination on all potential sires prior to use; use only fertile males as sires.
- Perform vaginal cytology routinely during periods of proestrus and estrus to aid in breeding management. Progesterone and luteinizing hormone assays taken during proestrus and estrus also aid in breeding management of the bitch.
- Perform routine health procedures such as deworming treatments, vaccinations, and regular physical examinations.
- Avoid hormonal treatments that may have adverse effects on cyclicity and normal uterine function.
- Ensure optimal neonatal survival with adequate management of the bitch during pregnancy, whelping, and the neonatal period.
- Recommend ovariohysterectomy for all nonbreeding bitches.

MALE INFERTILITY

Etiology

Causes associated with infertility are listed in Table 3.

Clinical Signs

Signs suggesting canine male infertility or disorders affecting the male reproductive tract include:

- Lack of interest in estral bitches
- Failure of conception after breeding reproductively normal bitches
- Reduced litter size

TABLE 3. Causes of Male Infertility

Failure of Erection
Prepubertal/delayed puberty
Congenital anomalies
    Intersex
    Penile hypoplasia
    Hypospadias
    Preputial stenosis
    Persistent penile frenulum
    Congenital shortened penis
Behavioral/psychological
Testicular hypoplasia/degeneration
Pain
    Orchitis/periorchitis
    Prostatitis
    Musculoskeletal
Systemic disease

Erection and No Ejaculation
Retrograde ejaculation
Penile analgesia
Pain
Segmental aplasia or outflow obstruction

Ejaculation and Normal Semen Quality
Physical inability to breed
Behavioral/psychological
Improper breeding management
Female infertility
Venereal disease

Ejaculation and Abnormal Spermatozoa
Testicular hypoplasia
Testicular degeneration
Orchitis/epididymitis
Testicular neoplasia
Prostate abnormalities
Autoimmune infertility
Obstructive lesion
Poor semen handling technique
Kartagener's syndrome

Abnormal Scrotal Contents
Inguinal/scrotal hernia
Cryptorchidism
Ectopic testis(es)
Testicular torsion
Testicular neoplasia
Orchitis/periorchitis/epididymitis
Sperm granuloma
Testicular hypoplasia/degeneration
Intersex conditions

Penile and Preputial Abnormalities
Preputial discharge
Congenital anomalies of penis/prepuce
    Hypospadias
    Penile hypoplasia
    Persistent penile frenulum
    Preputial stenosis
Preputial mass/tumor
Urethral prolapse
Posthitis/balanoposthitis
Fracture of the os penis
Paraphimosis
Priapism

- Abortions
- Heritable defects in offspring
- Abnormal ejaculate (e.g., reduced sperm motility, increased morphological abnormalities, brown or red coloration)
- Reluctance or refusal to breed
- Preputial discharge

- Underdeveloped external genitalia (small penis, prepuce, or scrotum)
- Cryptorchidism
- Signs of feminization
- Scrotal enlargement, heat, or pain
- Abdominal mass or abdominal pain
- Pain on urination or defecation

Diagnosis

Precede diagnostic examination with a complete history. Use the history to assess general health and management, breeding practices, past breeding performances, and any previous diseases and administered medications. In this discussion, diagnostic, management, and treatment approaches are combined in a prospective method aimed at resolving problems associated with infertility. The recommendations made apply only to *Brucella*-negative dogs; the authors recommend that all *Brucella*-positive animals be euthanized because of the public health risk and the poor success with medical therapy.

Physical Examination

- Perform a complete physical examination to identify disorders of nonreproductive body systems.
- Palpate the scrotum to ensure the presence of two normal scrotal testes. Note the size, symmetry, and consistency of the testes. In addition, palpate the epididymides, vas deferens, and spermatic cords to detect abnormalities.
- Initially examine the penis and prepuce by palpating through the sheath in the unstimulated dog. The dog may then be restrained in dorsal recumbency if necessary and the penis gently manipulated out of the sheath in order to examine the penis and prepuce more closely. Examine the penis and prepuce in the erect state at the time of semen collection. Look for signs of inflammation, trauma, and foreign bodies or masses.
- Examine the os penis by palpation through the penis for signs of irregularities that may be caused by fracture of the os and congenital abnormalities in shape.
- Perform digital rectal palpation of the pelvis, pelvic urethra, and prostate gland. Palpation of the prostate gland may be facilitated by elevating the chest of the dog and using the free hand under the abdomen to elevate the prostate toward the finger inserted within the rectum. Examine for changes in size, consistency, and symmetry of the two lobes of the gland.
- Examine the mammary chain by palpation.

Laboratory Evaluations

CBC, Biochemistry Profile, and Urinalysis. These basic laboratory studies aid in the diagnosis of underlying systemic diseases and of specific diseases affecting the reproductive tract.

Brucella canis Testing. See previous discussion of *B. canis* in Female Infertility.

Thyroid Function Testing. Test thyroid function of all dogs presented for infertility (see sec. 4, ch. 1).

Semen Collection and Evaluation

Collection. Collect semen via manual stimulation, in a warm (37° C) sterile latex or plastic cone connected to a sterile semen collection vessel.

Evaluation. Evaluate semen sample immediately after collection. Store semen at 37° C until motility is evaluated and morphologic slides are made. The sample then may be permitted to come to room temperature.

- *Color* should be milky white. Abnormal coloration usually is due to contamination with urine or blood or the presence of WBCs.
- Record *volume* in order to calculate the total sperm numbers in the ejaculate.
- Assess *motility and debris* by microscopic examination of a drop of ejaculate. Estimate and record the percentage of cells showing linear, progressive motility.
- Determine *sperm concentration* by hemocytometer, spectrophotometer, or Coulter counter. This value is then used in combination with volume to calculate the total sperm number in the ejaculate. The expected total sperm number is $300–1000 \times 10^6$ per ejaculate and is dependent on breed.
- Evaluate *semen morphology* by mixing one drop of semen with nigrosin-eosin stain on one end of a slide and using another slide to make an even smear of stained cells. Air-dry the smear and examine under oil immersion; evaluate the proportion of normal cells and primary and secondary abnormalities by counting 100–200 cells. A wet mount of a mixture of sperm and 10% buffered formalin can also be used with phase-contrast microscopy.
- *Cytologic examination* of an air-dried semen smear, stained with a rapid commercial stain such as Diff-Quik, Wright's, or new methylene blue, provides information about the presence and identification of epithelial and inflammatory cells.
- Perform *quantitative aerobic bacterial culture*. A bacterial count >10,000/ml suggests genital infection, whereas <10,000/ml suggests urethral contamination.
- The role of *anaerobes* in male genital tract infection is thought to be minor and anaerobic cultures are not routinely performed. A semen sample may be placed in Ames transport medium and sent to a microbiologic laboratory capable of performing *Mycoplasma/Ureaplasma* cultures.
- *Virus isolation* for canine herpesvirus may be performed.
- *Semen pH* normally is 6.3–7.0. Semen pH does not change dramatically, even in animals with semen abnormalities, but this information is useful in monitoring and choosing antibiotics for dogs with chronic prostatitis (see sec. 8, ch. 8) because antibiotic trapping within the prostate gland is facilitated. For example, choose a basic antibiotic for an animal with acidic prostatic fluid or ejaculate.
- *Seminal alkaline phosphatase concentration* is used as a marker of the completeness of ejaculation. Alkaline phosphatase originates within the epididymis and is normally present at concentrations of 5,000–40,000 units/liter within the ejaculate. Azoo-

spermic patients with seminal alkaline phosphatase concentrations less than 5,000 IU/l may have not ejaculated completely or may have bilateral outflow obstruction of the tubular tract distal to the epididymis.

- *Scanning and transmission electron microscopy* may be performed on semen samples from animals with suspected ultrastructural sperm defects resulting in defects in sperm motility or enzyme release.

Epididymal Aspiration

- Aspiration aids in the diagnosis of obstructive lesions involving the outflow tract, neoplasia, sperm granuloma, and epididymitis.
- Indications include the presence of a palpable abnormality affecting one or both epididymides and azoospermic ejaculate.

Technique

Epididymal Aspiration

1. The animal may be sedated, standing, or anesthetized.
2. Prepare the area over the tail of the epididymis aseptically, and pass a 23- to 25-gauge syringe needle through the skin and into the epididymis.
3. Aspirate a small amount of contents into the needle and syringe.
4. Stain slides and evaluate for the presence of spermatozoa, inflammatory cells, and bacteria.
5. A sample may be submitted for microbiologic culture and susceptibility examination.

Testicular Biopsy

- Biopsy provides information regarding the etiology and severity of a testicular lesion and prognosticating a return to normal function.
- Indications include the presence of oligospermia, azoospermia, high percentages of primary abnormalities in the ejaculate, and abnormalities in size, shape, or consistency of a testicle.
- Methods for obtaining tissue samples include excisional wedge resection (see sec. 8, ch. 11), fine-needle aspiration and split-needle biopsy. The authors prefer the split-needle biopsy technique.

Technique

Testicular Biopsy

1. Place animal under general anesthesia in lateral recumbency.
2. Clip the scrotum and prepare aseptically.
3. Make a small incision in the scrotal skin over the ventral surface of the testis, taking care not to involve the area of the head of the epididymis.
4. Pass a Tru-Cut biopsy punch into the testicular parenchyma, angling toward the caudal aspect of the testis, and take sample.
5. Place sample in 10% formalin or Bouin's solution for analysis.
6. Evaluate samples microscopically for the presence of germ and Sertoli cells, proliferation and maturation of germinal epithelium, spermatids within seminiferous tubule lumens, Leydig cells, and evidence of lesions.

Karyotyping. Indications include:

- Testicular hypoplasia/aplasia
- Abnormal external phenotype (e.g., small penis, ambiguous genitalia)
- Suspected congenital lesions associated with infertility (see sec. 8, ch. 19)

Imaging Studies. Pelvic and abdominal radiographic and ultrasonographic examination provide information regarding:

- Testicular lesions and tumors
- Presence and abnormalities of retained testicles
- Prostate gland abnormalities

Canine Herpesvirus (HV) Culture. Culture for HV is indicated in animals suspected of being clinically infected or subclinical carriers of the virus (see previous discussion in Diagnosis of Female Infertility; also see sec. 2, ch. 9).

Mycoplasma and *Ureaplasma* Cultures
- Diagnosis depends on isolation of the organism from the ejaculate or from preputial swabs or urethral swabs.
  - A pure culture may be interpreted as significant if isolated in association with inflammatory cytologic findings and clinical signs suggesting the disease.
  - Recovery of the organism in the absence of cytologic signs of inflammation or clinical signs consistent with infection (early embryonic death, fetal death, reduced conception rate, abortion, stillbirths, fading pups, and neonatal deaths), is likely to be caused by contamination.

Endocrine Testing
- Basal testosterone levels are difficult to interpret because of the wide variation in normal serum concentrations (0.5–10 ng/m). The use of a Gn-RH or hCG stimulation test may provide more information regarding testosterone concentrations. Testosterone concentrations in intact and cryptorchid animals may be expected to rise to 3.7–7.5 ng/ml 1–4 hours after administration of Gn-RH (2 μg/kg, IM, for dogs; 25 μg total dose for cats) or hCG (40 units/kg, IM, for dogs; 250 units total dose for cats).
- Serum follicle-stimulating hormone (FSH) concentration levels have been used as an indicator of spermatogenesis. In the presence of testicular lesions and reduced spermatogenesis, testicular inhibin production declines and FSH concentration rises. Guidelines for FSH concentrations are as follows:
  - Normal dog, 20–130 ng/ml
  - Active acute testicular degeneration, 130–250 ng/ml
  - Severe testicular damage and depletion of seminiferous tubules, >250 ng/ml
- Luteinizing hormone (LH) concentrations provide information regarding the presence of lesions in the testes. In the presence of testicular dysfunction, LH concentrations tend to rise, probably due to:
  - Increased Gn-RH release associated with increased stimulation of FSH production
  - Decreased Leydig cell testosterone production associated with testicular damage

Failure of Erection

Diagnosis

History
- Ensure that bitch is in heat.
- Rule out prior castration.
- Animals younger than 24 months of age may be prepubertal.
- Timid and socially inexperienced dogs may fail to attain an erection.

Physical Examination
- Examine for:
  - Severe testicular atrophy or degeneration
  - Evidence of intersex conditions (see sec. 8, ch. 19)
  - Congenital disorders such as penile hypoplasia, hypospadias, persistent frenulum, and preputial stenosis (see sec. 8, chs. 5, 12)
  - Painful conditions such as acute orchitis, prostatitis, fracture of the os penis
  - Musculoskeletal conditions such as vertebral osteoarthritis and hip dysplasia
- Evaluate for neural lesions involving pelvic nerve branches necessary for penile innervation and erection that may result in failure of erection (see sec. 10, ch. 1).

Laboratory Evaluations
- Endocrine testing includes measurement of serum testosterone concentrations.
- Karyotyping is indicated when an intersex condition is suspected. Affected animals may have abnormal or ambiguous external genitalia and azoospermia or oligospermia.
- Testicular biopsy provides information regarding the presence of testicular degeneration or atrophy (see sec. 8, ch. 11 and previous discussion in this chapter).

Treatment

- Ensure that dog is mature.
- Ensure that breeding animals are physically and psychologically compatible.
- Do not breed animals with congenital anomalies.
- Alleviate painful conditions preventing erection by judicious use of analgesics or surgical correction.

Erection with Failure to Ejaculate

Diagnosis

History. The history usually includes pain resulting in loss of erection and loss of interest in an estral bitch.

Physical Examination
- Rule out the possibility of penile analgesia and os penis fracture.
- Perform testicular biopsy on azoospermic animals to assess the degree of function within the seminiferous tubules.

Laboratory Evaluation. Examine urine after breeding for the presence of spermatozoa (indicating retrograde ejaculation) or elevated alkaline phosphatase (suggesting blockage of vas deferens).

Treatment

- Some cases of outflow obstructive lesions that prevent flow of sperm from testicles to penile urethra may be alleviated by surgical reconstruction.
- Retrograde ejaculation may be treated within 1–3 hours before mating with sympathomimetic agents such as pseudoephedrine (5–7 mg/kg, q12h, PO) or phenylpropanolamine (3 mg/kg, q12h, PO). Little data are available about the success of this treatment.

Ejaculation with Normal Semen Quality

Diagnosis

History
- Assess reproductive management.
- Evaluate the possibility of psychological incompatibility.
- Evaluate prior reproductive performance of the male and female.

Physical Examination
- Perform a general physical examination.
- Evaluate the genitalia.

Laboratory Evaluations. Useful studies include:

- Collect and examine semen.
- Thyroid function testing
- HV titers and isolation of positive animal.
- *Mycoplasma* and *Ureaplasma* cultures

Treatment

- Ensure optimal reproductive management.
- Ensure that bitch is in estrus and reproductively normal.

Ejaculation with Abnormal Spermatozoa

Diagnosis

History
- Evaluate prior reproductive performance.
- Consider the presence of paraneoplastic syndromes (hyperestrogenism) such as gynecomastia, attractiveness to other males.
- To prevent detrimental results, ensure optimal technique in collection and handling of semen.

Physical Examination
- Perform a general physical examination.
- Examine the reproductive tract, including the prostate.
- Collect and examine semen.

Laboratory Evaluations. Useful studies include:

- Aerobic and anaerobic culture of the ejaculate
- Seminal plasma evaluation
- Testicular biopsy

Treatment

- No effective treatment exists for testicular hypoplasia.
- Treat testicular degeneration by removing the inciting cause and, if possible, allowing time for recovery. See Table 4 for causes of testicular degeneration.

- Treat acute orchitis and epididymitis with medical supportive therapy, including specific antibiotics as determined by culture and sensitivity testing. Combinations of cold therapy, anti-inflammatory treatment, and antibiotics may be used in an attempt to salvage a valuable breeding animal; however, castration usually is necessary.
- Determine the condition of the prostate and prostatic fluid.

Abnormal Scrotal Contents

Also see sec. 8, chs. 10 and 11.

Diagnosis

History
- Inquire about change in the size or shape of the scrotum.
- Check previous medication administration.

Physical Examination
- Scrotal enlargement may be due to inguinal hernia, testicular torsion, testicular neoplasia, orchitis, periorchitis, epididymitis, sperm granuloma, hydrocele, hematocele, or scrotal abscess.
- Reduction in the size of the scrotum occurs with cryptorchidism, testicular hypoplasia, testicular degeneration, and intersex conditions.

Laboratory Evaluations. Useful studies include:

- CBC
- Karyotyping
- Thyroid screening or stimulation tests
- Semen collection and examination
- Ultrasonographic examination of the scrotum and abdomen

TABLE 4. Causes of Testicular Degeneration

Heat
    Inflammation
    Fever
    Environmental temperature
    Cryptorchidism
Cold
Radiation
Vascular ischemia
Zinc and vitamin A deficiency
Toxicities
    Heavy metals
    Rare earth salts
Androgenic or estrogenic compounds
Efferent ductule obstruction
Neoplasia
Old age
Trauma
Orchitis
    Brucella canis
    Escherichia coli
    Proteus vulgaris
    Miscellaneous bacteria
    Canine distemper virus
    Immune-mediated
Parasitic lesions
Debilitating disease
Diabetes

- Radiography of the abdomen
- Testicular biopsy (see sec. 8, ch. 11 and previous discussion in this chapter)

Penile and Preputial Abnormalities

Also see sec. 8, chs. 12 and 13.

Diagnosis

History. The owner usually reports preputial discharge and swelling or enlargement.

Physical Examination
- Perform a general physical examination.
- Examine the reproductive tract.
- Evaluate the nature of preputial discharge and possible causes:
  - Serous—urinary tract disease, ectopic ureter, HV infection, prostatic cyst
  - Purulent—posthitis, balanoposthitis, prostatitis, preputial foreign body, urethritis, paraphimosis, preputial stenosis, genitourinary neoplasia
  - Hemorrhagic—prostatic disease, trauma, urinary tract disease, neoplasia, bleeding disorders, preputial foreign body
- Examine for the presence of penile or preputial tissue at preputial orifice, which may indicate:
  - Transmissible venereal tumor
  - Paraphimosis
  - Urethral prolapse
  - Priapism (spinal cord disease is a common cause)
- Rule out os penis fracture
- Examine for penile and/or preputial abnormalities

Laboratory Evaluations. Useful studies include:

- Urinalysis
- Cytology
- Semen collection and examination

- Impression smears and biopsy of abnormal-appearing tissue

Prevention of Infertility

Prevention of infertility problems depends primarily on optimal reproductive management and early diagnosis and therapy of reproductive disorders.

- Perform routine *B. canis* screening tests every 6 months. Use only *brucella*-negative animals as breeding sires.
- Follow routine vaccination and deworming programs.
- Ensure adequate socialization of young animals.
- Regular monitoring of semen quality and physical examination of the internal and external genitalia provide information regarding the dynamic nature of the reproductive tract.
- Castrate young animals not intended primarily for breeding and older animals past their breeding age.

Supplemental Readings

Burke TJ: *Small Animal Reproduction and Infertility: A Clinical Approach to Diagnosis and Treatment.* Philadelphia: Lea & Febiger, 1986.

Ettinger SJ: *Textbook of Veterinary Internal Medicine: Diseases of the Dog and Cat,* 3rd Ed. Philadelphia: W. B. Saunders, 1989.

Feldman EC, Nelson RW: *Canine and Feline Endocrinology and Reproduction.* Philadelphia: W. B. Saunders, 1987.

Lein DH: Infertility and reproductive diseases in bitches and queens. *In* Roberts SJ, ed.: *Veterinary Obstetrics and Genital Diseases (Theriogenology),* 3rd Ed. Woodstock, VT: Published by the author, 1986.

Shille VM: Management of reproductive disorders in the bitch and queen. *In* Kirk RW, ed.: *Current Veterinary Therapy IX. Small Animal Practice.* Philadelphia: W. B. Saunders, 1986, p 1225.

Shille VM, Olson PN: Dynamic testing in reproductive endocrinology. *In* Kirk RW, ed.: *Current Veterinary Therapy X. Small Animal Practice.* Philadelphia: W. B. Saunders, 1989, p 1282.

Thrall MA, Olson PN: The vagina. *In* Cowell RL, Tyler RD, eds.: *Diagnostic Cytology of the Dog and Cat.* Goleta, CA: American Veterinary Publications, Inc., 1989.

19 Intersex Abnormalities

Nigel R. Perkins
Walter R. Threlfall

Intersexuality is an uncommon cause of reduced fertility in the dog and cat and may be congenital or inherited. The term *intersex* traditionally has meant an animal having genital organs with some characteristics of both sexes. In this chapter, the term intersex is used to describe animals with abnormalities in chromosomal, gonadal, or phenotypic sex, regardless of whether observable characteristics of both sexes are present. Other frequently used terms for these abnormalities are hermaphroditism (presence of male and female gonads) and pseudohermaphroditism (presence of one type of gonad with one or more characteristics of the opposite sex in the external genitalia).

Normal sexual differentiation depends on a chronological sequence of events, beginning with determination of the chromosomal sex at fertilization, followed by development of gonadal sex, and finally by phenotypic sex. The presence of a Y-chromosome, or part thereof, is the primary determinant of chromosomal and gonadal sex. Differentiation of the fetal testes is followed by production of müllerian inhibiting substance (MIS) by Sertoli cells and of testosterone by Leydig cells. The production of MIS results in regression of the müllerian duct system; the presence of testosterone results in development of the wolffian duct system into the epididymides and vas deferens. Testosterone is converted to dihydrotestosterone (DHT) in the external genitalia, which stimulates the development of the prostate gland, urethra, penis, prepuce, and scrotum.

The female karyotype (XX) results in the development of the müllerian duct system, which forms the female genital tract, and in the regression of the wolffian duct system.

ETIOLOGY

Many intersex conditions occur without any apparent cause. Factors known to induce intersex conditions include:

- Inherited defects
- Abnormal sex chromosome constitution
- Fetal exposure to androgenic or progestational hormones

Inherited Defects

Inherited defects result in a number of intersex conditions, including XX sex reversal, XX true hermaphroditism, persistent müllerian duct syndrome, and defective steroid synthesis or action.

Abnormal Sex Chromosome Constitution

This condition is caused by errors in chromosome replication, fertilization, or early cleavage divisions of the embryo.

Fetal Exposure to Androgens or Progestogens

Fetal exposure to androgens or progestogens results in masculinization of female offspring. Effects include increased anogenital distance, clitoral hypertrophy, and development of a rudimentary prepuce or scrotum.

CLINICAL SIGNS

Clinical signs associated with intersex conditions vary.

External Appearance

- Masculinization of female external phenotype with clitoral enlargement, development of an os penis, increased anogenital distance, vaginal hypoplasia, development of a rudimentary prepuce and scrotum, and gonads either within the scrotum or subcutaneously
- Feminization of the male external phenotype with incomplete development or complete lack of a scrotum; subcutaneous, inguinal, or abdominal gonads; penile, preputial, and testicular hypoplasia and hypospadias (incomplete urethral fusion).

Phenotypic Animals

- Phenotypic males with hypoplastic testes incapable of spermatogenesis are associated with an XXY sex chromosome constitution, as seen in the majority of tortoise-shell, male cats.
- Phenotypic males may show signs of estrus, including intermittent hematuria, preputial swelling, and attractiveness to other males.
- Phenotypic females with small body stature, infantile reproductive tract, and failure of cyclicity are associated with an XO chromosome constitution

Infertility

- Infertility in phenotypic females, characterized by irregular cyclicity, failure of conception, small litter sizes, abortions, or complete failure of cyclicity, is associated with many intersex conditions.

- Infertility in phenotypic male intersex animals is characterized by azoospermia, oligospermia, high percentages of abnormal or nonmotile sperm, testicular hypoplasia, cryptorchidism, and lack of libido. Some phenotypic males show intermittent hematuria and pyometra associated with changes in the female portion of the reproductive tract.

DIAGNOSIS

The diagnosis of intersex abnormalities depends on classification of chromosomal, gonadal, and phenotypic sex. Most animals with intersex abnormalities are presented because of abnormal external genitalia or problems related to infertility.

History

Identify management, environmental, behavioral and medication-related influences on fertility and estrus behavior.

Physical Examination

- Examine and evaluate the appearance of the external genitalia (vulva or prepuce, clitoris or penis, position of the urinary orifice, presence of scrotum and testes).
- Perform a digital rectal examination to evaluate the pelvic canal for the presence or absence of a prostate gland and caudal vagina.
- Note coat color, which is important as an aid in the diagnosis of cats with an XXY chromosome (the majority have a tortoise-shell or calico coat color).

Exploratory Laparotomy

Laparotomy is a useful diagnostic procedure.

- It facilitates examination of the internal genitalia and degree of development or regression of the male and female reproductive tracts (wolffian and müllerian duct derivatives).
- It allows gonadectomy and hysterectomy to minimize risks of gonadal tumors and the development of pyometra in endometrial tissues.

Histology

- Perform histologic examination of the gonads and excised reproductive tracts to identify ovarian or testicular tissue and the müllerian or wolffian duct derivatives.
- Perform serial sections through an entire gonad in order to diagnose cases of ovotestes.

Karyotyping

- Karyotype examination of cultured somatic cells or blood lymphocytes provides an accurate representation of the sex chromosome constitution of an animal.
- A blood sample is drawn aseptically and transported by overnight express at room temperature to a cytogenetics laboratory for lymphocyte culture and chromosome analysis.

Other Laboratory Tests

- Other tests include:
  - Male histocompatibility (H-Y) antigen assays to detect the presence of H-Y antigen on white blood cells from suspected intersex animals
  - Androgen receptor assays to determine the presence or absence of androgen receptors in target tissues of intersex animals
- These tests provide additional information regarding specific defects in some intersex conditions. However, such tests are not readily available and therefore have limited application in small animal practice.

TREATMENT AND MANAGEMENT

There is no curative treatment for intersex conditions. Therapy is symptomatic and is aimed at ensuring that affected animals are comfortable and can urinate normally.

Medical

- Use topical cleansing and application of ointment for urine scalding in cases of hypospadias.
- Treat urinary tract infections with appropriate antibiotics.

Surgical

- Surgically correct minor abnormalities in the urethra and prepuce if urine scalding is a problem.
- Perform penile amputation and scrotal urethrostomy in more severe cases of distal urethral anomalies.
- Perform clitoridectomy if clitoris is enlarged, traumatized, or exposed and causing discomfort.
  - Take care to minimize hemorrhage associated with the highly vascular clitoris and to locate the urethral opening prior to surgery, because occasionally it will involve the clitoris.
- Remove abdominal gonads and uterus, if present, to minimize risks of neoplastic changes in retained gonads and cystic endometrial hyperplasia/pyometra.

Supplemental Readings

Chastain CB, Guilford WG, Schmidt D: The 38,XX/39,XXY genotype in cats. Compend Contin Educ 10:17, 1988.

Marshall LS, Oehlert ML, Haskins ME, et al: Persistent müllerian duct syndrome in miniature schnauzers. J Am Vet Med Assoc 181:798, 1982.

Myers-Wallen VN, Patterson DF: Disorders of sexual development in dogs and cats. In Kirk RW, ed.: Current Veterinary Therapy X: Small Animal Practice. Philadelphia: W. B. Saunders, 1989, p 1261.

Randolph JF, Center SA, McEntee M, Goldberg EH: H-Y antigen positive XX true bilateral hermaphroditism in a German shorthaired pointer. J Am Anim Hosp Assoc 24:417, 1988.

Winter H, Pfeffer A: Pathogenic classification of intersex. Vet Rec 100:307, 1977.

Skeletal System

Paul A. Manley

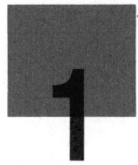

Fractures of the Skull

Mark M. Smith

Fractures of the zygomatic arch require surgery if they interfere with mastication or compress ocular structures. The most common extracranial fracture requiring surgery is a depression fracture of the frontal sinus. Intracranial fractures that require surgery are those that depress into brain parenchyma, causing significant compromise of cerebral function. Most skull fractures are amenable to conservative management.

Weigh the complications of general anesthesia in a neurologically compromised patient against the positive effects of surgical intervention. Fine motor movement is not necessarily required of small animal pets; therefore, intracranial surgery rarely is performed.

ANATOMY

Zygomatic Arch

- The cranial portion of the zygomatic arch is formed by the zygomatic bone and the caudal portion by the zygomatic process of the temporal bone.
- The zygomatic arch forms the ventral and lateral rim of the orbit.

Calvarium

- The dorsal sagittal crest courses craniocaudal over the calvarium.
- The nuchal crest courses mediolateral over the caudal edge of the skull.
- The frontal sinus of the frontal bone comprises the frontal encasement of the brain.
- The diploic calvarium has two distinct cortical bone layers between which is an interstitial layer of honeycombed bone and vessels.

- The brain is encased by the frontal, parietal, temporal, and occipital bones.
- The temporalis muscles cover almost the entire calvarium.

ZYGOMATIC ARCH FRACTURE
Preoperative Considerations

- Prior to anesthesia and surgery, perform a complete neurologic examination on all head trauma patients.
- General anesthesia may alter intracranial pressure (ICP), leading to exacerbation of intracranial edema and/or hemorrhage.
- To reduce ICP, consider hyperventilation (to reduce $Paco_2$), osmotic agents, corticosteroids, and an anesthetic protocol including barbiturates.
- Obtain skull radiographs to document fracture displacement and to screen for other, less apparent fractures. If possible, perform radiography immediately before surgery, thus avoiding the necessity for, and risk of, two separate anesthetic procedures.
- Confirm the presence of an intact optic nerve and vision prior to surgery. Surgery for a zygomatic arch fracture may be contraindicated if ocular function is irreversibly impaired.

KEY POINT ▶ Acepromazine may lower the central nervous system (CNS) seizure threshold, and ketamine increases cerebral blood flow. Do not use these drugs in patients with a history of brain trauma.

Surgical Procedure
Objectives

- Reduce fractures that can cause compression of the eye or cosmetic deformity.

- Avoid trauma to the zygomaticotemporal and zygomaticofacial nerves.

KEY POINT ▶ Nondisplaced fractures of the zygomatic arch have a good prognosis for uncomplicated healing with conservative management.

Equipment

- Standard general surgical pack and sutures
- Gelpi or Weitlaner self-retaining retractors
- Sharp periosteal elevator
- Small Steinmann pins and orthopedic wire (multiple sizes, 18–24 gauge)
- Small malleable retractor

Technique

1. Place the patient in ventral recumbency with the head supported. Attach tape to the mandibular canines and the table to secure head position.
2. Prepare the periocular area for aseptic surgery. Ocular lubricating ointment will avoid corneal damage from antiseptic agents.
3. Incise the skin directly over the zygomatic arch.
4. Incise and elevate the periosteum using a sharp periosteal elevator. Be careful to avoid the zygomaticotemporal and zygomaticofacial nerves (medial to the zygomatic bone).
5. Use a small malleable retractor to protect the orbit.
6. Reduce and secure fracture fragments using orthopedic wire (18–24 gauge, depending on the size of the animal). Small pins may be used to make holes in the bone for wire placement. Small orthopedic plates may be required to maintain reduction in extremely comminuted fractures or when cosmesis is of paramount importance.

KEY POINT ▶ Do not use small pins as a component of the definitive repair, because pin migration following surgery may cause ocular and intracranial trauma.

7. Closure:
   a. Appose subcutaneous tissues in a simple interrupted pattern (absorbable suture).
   b. Subcuticular sutures (absorbable suture) provide skin apposition and avoid suture irritation of ocular structures.

Postoperative Care and Complications
Short-Term

- Perform serial neurologic examinations to monitor changes in neurologic status.
- Monitor for clinical signs of seroma and infection.

Long-Term

- Excessive bony callus may compress ocular structures and interfere with mastication.
- Periarticular fractures may lead to degenerative joint disease of the temporomandibular joint (TMJ) and bony anklyosis.
- If normal function is inhibited or pain persists,

resection of the affected segment of the zygomatic arch is indicated. Reconstruction of the muscle tissue provides acceptable appearance and function.

Prognosis

- The prognosis is good with conservative management.
- With operative management, the prognosis is good to excellent.

EXTRACRANIAL FRACTURES

Extracranial fractures include fractures of the nuchal crest, sagittal crest, and frontal sinus.

Preoperative Considerations

- See Zygomatic Arch Fracture.

Surgical Procedure
Objective

- Maintain reduction of severely displaced fractures of the nuchal crest, sagittal crest, and frontal sinus.

KEY POINT ▶ The cranial muscle mass usually prevents severe fracture displacement and provides enough fracture stability to allow conservative management of most extracranial fractures.

Equipment

- Standard general surgical pack and sutures
- Gelpi or Weitlaner self-retaining retractors
- Sharp periosteal elevator
- Small Steinmann pins and orthopedic wire (multiple sizes, 20–24 gauge)

Technique

1. Place the patient in ventral recumbency with the head supported. Attach tape to the mandibular canines and table to secure the head position.
2. Prepare the fracture area for aseptic surgery.
3. Make a skin incision directly over the fractured bony prominence.
4. Elevate the periosteum to allow anatomic reduction.
5. Frontal sinus fractures usually are depressed, requiring elevation and fixation with orthopedic wire.
6. Reduce and fix nuchal and sagittal crest fractures with orthopedic wire.

KEY POINT ▶ Do not use small pins as a component of the definitive repair because pin migration following surgery may cause ocular or intracranial trauma.

7. Appose muscle fascia and subcutaneous tissues in individual layers, using absorbable suture in a simple interrupted pattern.
8. Close the skin similarly, using nonabsorbable suture.

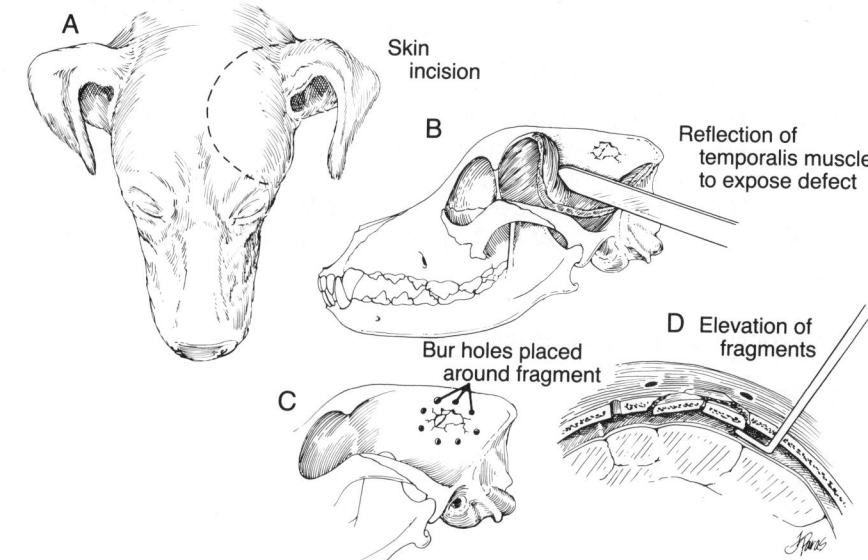

Figure 1. Procedure for repairing intracranial fracture. See text for explanation.

Postoperative Care and Complications

Short-Term

- Perform serial neurologic examination to monitor for change in neurologic status.
- Monitor for clinical signs of seroma and infection.
- Subcutaneous emphysema may occur secondary to frontal sinus fracture. Whether management of the fracture is surgical or conservative, a compressive bandage will minimize continued formation of subcutaneous emphysema until organized hematoma and fibrin deposition provide a functional barrier to air migration from the frontal sinus. Thus, bandaging is recommended for 2–4 days.

Long-Term

- Fractures usually heal without complications, providing acceptable cosmesis.
- Most complications are related to CNS trauma, such as seizures (see sec. 10, ch. 3).

INTRACRANIAL FRACTURES

Preoperative Considerations

- Preoperative anesthetic and neurologic concerns are similar to those for zygomatic arch fractures.
- Fractures may be linear cracks, depressed bony fragments, or comminuted separate bony fragments.
- Intracranial fractures are usually closed fractures.
- Comminuted calvarial fractures may lacerate meninges, venous sinuses, or the cerebral cortex.
- Calvarial fractures usually are associated with CNS compromise. Medical management of CNS trauma is indicated prior to diagnostic procedures requiring anesthesia.
- Progressive deterioration in CNS status despite intensive medical management is an indication for skull radiography to determine fracture severity.

Surgical Procedure

Objectives

- Elevate depressed calvarial fractures that may cause extensive functional loss of cerebral mass.
- Remove large comminuted fragments of the calvarium that may cause cerebral laceration.

KEY POINT ▶ Linear and minor depressed intracranial fractures are best managed conservatively.

Equipment

- Standard general surgical pack and sutures
- Gelpi or Weitlaner self-retaining retractors
- Sharp periosteal elevator
- Pneumatic or electric bur drill

Technique

1. Place the patient in ventral recumbency with the head supported. Attach tape to the mandibular canines and table to secure the head position.
2. Prepare the dorsal skull area for aseptic surgery.
3. Make a dorsal incision (Fig. 1A).
4. Incise the superficial temporal fascia and elevate the temporalis muscle ventrally to expose the fracture area (Fig. 1B).
5. Drill multiple small bur holes through the calvarium around the periphery of the fracture area to allow elevation of the fracture fragments (Fig. 1C).
6. Elevation is accomplished with a small, blunt elevator.
7. Remove any large comminuted fragments that may cause laceration. Despite the potential for large calvarial defects, replacement of the temporalis muscle provides adequate coverage.
8. Closure:
   a. Replace the temporalis muscle and appose the superficial fascia using absorbable suture in a simple interrupted pattern.

b. Close the subcutaneous layers similarly, followed by skin closure using nonabsorbable suture in a simple interrupted pattern.

KEY POINT ▶ Meticulous, atraumatic surgical technique, prevention of cerebral edema, and removal of hematoma if calvarial fragments are removed are of the highest priority when operating upon intracranial fractures.

Postoperative Care and Complications

Short-Term

- Perform serial neurologic examinations to monitor for change in neurologic status.
- Monitor for clinical signs of seroma and infection.

Long-Term

- Bony healing occurs without complication; however, neurologic recovery depends on the location and severity of the original traumatic incident.

Prognosis

- The prognosis for cranial fracture repair is good.
- The prognosis for neurologic recovery is guarded.

Supplemental Readings

Dulisch ML: Skull and mandibular fractures. *In* Slatter DH, ed.: *Textbook of Small Animal Surgery*. Philadelphia: W. B. Saunders, 1985, p 2286.

Newton CD: Fractures of the skull. *In* Newton CD, Nunamaker DM, eds.: *Textbook of Small Animal Orthopaedics*. Philadelphia: J.B. Lippincott, 1985, p 287.

Oliver JE. Craniotomy, craniectomy, and skull fractures. *In* Bojrab MJ, ed.: *Current Techniques in Small Animal Surgery*. Philadelphia: Lea & Febiger, 1975, p 359.

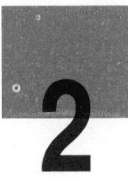

2 Fractures and Dislocations of the Mandible

Paul E. Howard

Mandibular fractures are encountered commonly in small animal practice and can present a unique set of challenges to the veterinarian. Dislocations of the mandible are uncommon but can occur alone or in conjunction with a fracture. Many surgical and non-surgical techniques have been described for mandibular fracture repair. Certain principles must be followed if clinical success is to be achieved on a consistent basis.

Anatomy

The mandible is composed of two halves, divided into a horizontal component (body) and a vertical component (ramus). The two halves of the mandible, joined rostrally at the mandibular symphysis, compose the lower jaw.

- The alveolar border is that part of the body into which the tooth roots insert.
- The dorsal half of the ramus is the coronoid process.
- The mandibular foramen, located on the medial side of the ramus, is the caudal opening of the mandibular canal through which traverses the mandibular alveolar artery and vein and the mandibular alveolar nerve.
  - The mandibular canal opens cranially at the three mental foramina.
  - The mandibular alveolar nerve is a branch of the trigeminal nerve supplying motor and sensory innervation to the mandible.

The condyloid processes of the hemimandibles articulate with the mandibular fossae of the temporal bones to form the temporomandibular joints (TMJ), which permits considerable dorsal-ventral motion.

Mandibular fractures can be divided into three broad groups, based on anatomic location of the fracture:

- Mandibular symphysis—most common area fractured in cats, often an open fracture
- Mandibular body—most common area fractured in dogs, usually an open fracture
- Ramus—least common area fractured, owing to its protection by an adjacent muscle mass (masseter muscle).

Etiology

The primary cause of mandibular fractures is trauma, including:

- Being struck by motor vehicle
- Fighting
- Gunshot injury
- Falling from excessive heights (cat falling from high-rise building window)

Iatrogenic fracture of the mandible may occur during overzealous attempts at tooth extraction in animals with severe periodontal disease and/or metabolic disease causing osteoporosis.

Clinical Signs

Clinical signs are variable, and include:

- Crepitus on manipulation of the mandible
- Asymmetry of the jaw
- Nasal or oral hemorrhage
- Nasal obstruction

Diagnosis

- Diagnosis usually is not difficult and is based upon a recent history of trauma, malocclusion, and, frequently, a palpable fracture.
- Oblique radiographs of the skull are helpful in identifying the fracture site and demonstrating the degree of fracture displacement.
  - Examine radiographs carefully for associated maxillary and other skull fractures.
  - When an animal presents with a mandibular symphyseal separation, evaluate the condyloid process radiographically for the presence of a fracture.

Complications

- The most common complication when considering all types of mandibular fractures is dental malocclusion.
- Other complications are osteomyelitis, nonunion, malunion, implant failure, and infection of soft tissues.
- Complications are more likly to occur in open fractures and in fractures requiring the removal of teeth at the time of fixation.

Surgical Procedures

Principles applicable to all fractures and dislocations of the mandible are discussed here. Techniques for the repairs of specific problems are discussed with each condition further in the chapter.

Preoperative Considerations

- Because mandibular fractures are primarily an orthopedic problem, consider the following principles of orthopedic repair:
  - Anatomic reduction of the fracture ensures proper dental occlusion.
  - Rigid fixation of the fracture permits the earliest return to function.
  - Placement of fixation devices can be impeded by tooth roots.

KEY POINT ▶ Avoid perforation of tooth roots and invasion of the mandibular canal.

- Perforation of tooth roots ultimately will require endodontic therapy or extraction of the involved tooth.
- Treat fractures of the mandibular body as open fractures; thus, antibiotic therapy is indicated. Fractures of the caudal aspect of the body are sometimes closed.
- Osteomyelitis is encountered infrequently, but, when present, can be very difficult to eliminate.
- The presence of a tooth in a fracture line will not prevent fracture healing. In an experimental study, teeth adjacent to mandibular osteotomy sites retained their viability, were encased in new woven bone, and did not loosen.

KEY POINT ▶ Do not remove a tooth in a fracture line if it aids in the reduction and stabilization of the fracture.

- Loss of teeth often makes anatomic reduction of the fracture more difficult. If indicated, extract the tooth when no longer needed for fracture repair.
- Provide means of delivering proper nutrition to the animal during the healing phase.
  - If the animal cannot receive food and water per os, consider placement of a pharyngotomy or gastrostomy tube. The latter is preferred for long-term feeding.
- Intubate animals during anesthesia and fracture repair to prevent aspiration of blood and irrigating solution.
  - In repair of severe mandibular fractures, the endotracheal tube is exited from the side of the pharynx to permit unobstructed evaluation of occlusion during surgery.

Objectives

- Reduce the bone fragments and maintain this position until adequate bone healing occurs. Determine if the mandible requires surgical reduction or if the fracture is sufficiently aligned to permit conservative treatment.
- Allow early return to normal function, primarily mastication, with the use of rigid fixation.
- Maintain the animal's nutritional status at an optimal level.

Equipment

- Standard general surgical pack
- Wire twisters and wire cutters
- Orthopedic wire (18–24 gauge)
- Bone plates and screws
- External fixation devices
- K-wires and intramedullary pins

Postoperative Care and Complications

- Feed animals a gruel for 2 weeks. Feed canned food or dry food softened with water for an additional 4 weeks before returning to the usual diet.
- Prevent dogs from chewing bones, sticks, balls, and other hard objects that may disrupt the fracture repair during the healing phase.
- Daily oral flushing with chlorhexidine preparations may be beneficial in the immediate postoperative period in reducing oral bacteria in animals with open fractures.
- Evaluate animals no later than 2 weeks postoperatively to ensure that proper occlusion has been maintained.

MANDIBULAR SYMPHYSEAL FRACTURES

A mandibular symphyseal fracture is a commonly encountered unstable fracture that prevents normal mastication. This type of fracture is repaired easily with minimal equipment, most frequently with wire, although pins and screws can be used with equal success.

Wire Stabilization

Technique

1. Place the animal in dorsal recumbency and prepare the chin for aseptic surgery.
2. Make a midline stab incision in the skin slightly rostral to the caudal extent of the mandibular symphysis.
3. Insert a hypodermic needle (larger than the anticipated wire size) through the skin incision, lateral to one hemimandible, and exit in the oral cavity immediately caudal to the canine tooth (Fig. 1A).
4. Insert a strand of orthopedic wire of appropriate size (24 gauge for cats and small dogs; 20 or 18 gauge for large dogs) through the distal end of the needle and remove the needle, leaving the strand in place (Fig. 1B).
5. Through the same stab incision in the skin, insert the needle lateral to the contralateral hemimandible and exit the needle caudal to the canine tooth (Fig. 1C).
6. Pass the end of wire *that is in the mouth* into the end of the needle until it exits the needle hub. Remove the needle, leaving both wire ends exiting the stab incision in the chin.
7. Maintain proper alignment of the rostral ends of the hemimandibles, with digital pressure, and twist-tighten the wire to maintain anatomic reduction of the symphysis. Cut off the twisted wire, leaving at least 3 twists (Fig. 1D).

Postoperative Care and Complications

- Leave the wire ends exposed, and clean the area with warm water as necessary.

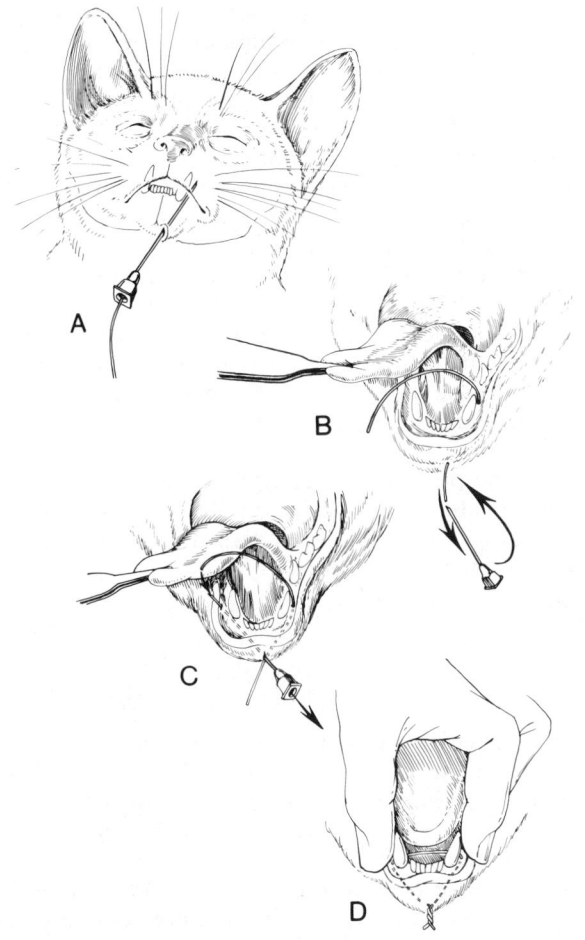

Figure 1. Wire stabilization for manibular symphyseal fracture. See text for details.

- Feed a soft diet until the wire is removed.
- Leave wire in place for 6 to 8 weeks. Remove by cutting the exposed wire in the animal's mouth; extract the cut ends through the skin incision by pulling on the twisted end. A short-acting general anesthetic facilitates the procedure and eliminates animal discomfort.

Alternative Techniques

- A noninvasive technique involves placing a piece of orthopedic wire around the base of the canine or incisor teeth and tightening the wire so that the wire twists are rostral to the incisor teeth.
- Interdental wiring techniques can be used instead of the wire loop technique.

ROSTRAL MANDIBULAR BODY FRACTURES

Repair of fractures behind the canine teeth or between the rostral premolar teeth is complicated because only a small amount of bone is available for implant insertion. The majority of the rostral mandible is composed of tooth root structure. Frequently this type of fracture occurs bilaterally, complicating the repair.

Tape Muzzle

Unilateral fractures of the rostral mandible often can be repaired satisfactorily with a tape muzzle. Tape muzzles are tolerated well by most dogs. Brachycephalic breeds and cats are less tolerant of the muzzle (see sec. 9, ch. 3).

Figure-Eight Wire

This procedure is indicated in bilateral fractures.

Technique

1. Pass orthopedic wire around the canine teeth and between the roots of the first premolar teeth in the caudal fracture segments. Wire passage under the furcation of the tooth is facilitated if a pathway is first established with a K-wire. When stabilizing bilateral fractures, tighten the wires in unison to maintain equal compressive forces.
2. A secondary wire may be required through holes drilled in the ventral aspect of the mandible to prevent distraction of the fracture line due to the pull of the figure-eight wires.
3. To keep the wire passed around the canine teeth from slipping, cover the wire with composite material (see sec. 7, ch. 1).
4. Alternatively, drill a hole in the mandible rostral to the canine tooth and pass the wire through this hole. Similarly, a hole can be drilled in the mandible rather than passing the wire through the premolar tooth furcation.

KEY POINT ▶ When drilling holes in the mandible, avoid tooth roots.

Cross-Pinning

- Use large K-wires or small intramedullary (IM) pins to stabilize bilateral fractures in selected cases. Avoiding tooth roots is often difficult using this technique.

CENTRAL MANDIBULAR BODY FRACTURES

These fractures offer the greatest number of repair options, including internal and external fixation, splinting devices, and muzzles. The choice of repair depends upon a number of factors including available equipment, expertise of the veterinarian, and cost.

Plate Fixation

The method of choice is plate fixation because it provides rigid, anatomic reduction and maintains normal occlusion. This permits an early return to function without the need of external fixation devices or intraoral splints. The major drawbacks are the requirement for technical proficiency in the use of plating equipment and the expense of the implants.

Technique

1. Place the animal in dorsolateral recumbency (dorsal recumbency if the fractures are bilateral).

2. Make a skin incision along the ventrolateral margin of the mandibular body.
3. Elevate the subcutaneous tissues with a periosteal elevator to expose the fracture site.
4. Conform the plate to fit as ventral as possible on the lateral aspect of the mandibular body to avoid placing screws through adjacent tooth roots and the mandibular canal. The plate should be long enough to permit the placement of two screws on each side of the fracture site.
   a. In complicated mandibular fractures, mandibular reduction forceps (Synthes) can aid in maintaining fracture reduction while the plate is being applied.
   b. Placement of plates on the dorsolateral surface of the mandible is not recommended as it can result in gingival erosion, damage to tooth roots, and osteomyelitis.
5. Following plate application, close the subcutaneous tissues and skin. Intraoral approaches are recommended by some surgeons to avoid possible contamination and infection that may result from an approach through the skin. The author, however, prefers exposure through a skin incision because infection with this approach is uncommon, and the restricted access via an intraoral approach makes it less desirable.

External Pin Fixation

In cases of severely comminuted body fractures, external pin fixation is an excellent method for maintaining spatial relationships and occlusion during fracture healing.

- Fixation can be accomplished with conventional pins, clamps, and connecting bars, with screws and acrylic (bi-phase external fixation), or with IM pins and acrylic (modified bi-phase external fixation).
- Advantage:
  - Dissection of soft tissue for the placement of the pins is minimal.
  - Fracture reduction can be fine-tuned without the need for removing pins previously placed into the bone.
  - Occlusion is maintained in the repair of fractures in which bone loss is present.
  - Bi-phase or modified bi-phase splints can be contoured around the rostral end of the mandible.
- Disadvantages:
  - The protruding device can be dislodged.
  - Pin loosening can result in loss of fracture reduction.

Technique

KEY POINT ▶ Do not insert pins rostral to the third mandibular premolar tooth or the root of the canine tooth may be penetrated.

1. Make small stab incisions in the skin over the intended site of pin or screw placement. Bluntly dissect to the bone surface with a periosteal elevator.

2. After determining the number of pins to be used in the fracture repair (a minimum of three pins in each fracture segment is desirable), insert one pin in each fracture segment. Accurate pin placement can be facilitated by predrilling with a pin or drill bit that is smaller than the final pin.
3. After loosely joining the pins with clamps and a connecting bar, reduce the fracture achieving normal occlusion, and tighten the clamps.
4. Insert additional pins into the mandible by first passing the pin through a clamp previously placed on the connecting bar. (Inserting pins in this manner ensures that all pins are placed in the same plane, negating the need for additional connecting bars that would add unnecessary weight to the fixation device.)
5. After the pins are placed and the clamps are tightened, evaluate the occlusion. If necessary, loosen the clamps to permit better reduction of the fracture and to improve occlusion.

KEY POINT ▶ Although this is sometimes recommended, do not cover the clamps and connecting bar with tape, but leave them exposed to facilitate cleaning.

6. An alternative to the use of clamps and connecting bar is dental acrylic (see sec. 7, ch. 1). Silastic tubing or other suitable material is impaled on the pins. The acrylic is injected into the tubing and, once hardened, fracture reduction is maintained. A disadvantage of acrylic is that, once the acrylic has hardened, adjustment of the fracture reduction and improvement of occlusion is not possible.

Postoperative Care and Complications

- Clean the sites where the pins or screws exit the skin daily with a disinfectant. This is facilitated if the external fixation device is not covered with tape or other material.
- Once a week, evaluate fixation devices that use clamps to be sure that the nuts are secure.
- The major complication is premature dislodging or loosening of the implant.

Interdental Wiring

- This technique works best when the teeth abutting the fracture line are not loose and the fracture is inherently stable.
- Wire configurations vary from the simple loop around the tooth on each side of the fracture to more complex configurations involving multiple teeth (see sec. 9, ch. 3).

Intrafragmentary Wiring

Interfragmentary wiring is used in combination with interdental wiring (Fig. 2).

Technique

1. Make a skin incision over the ventral surface of the mandible and reflect the underlying subcutaneous tissues.

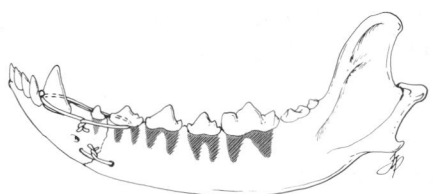

Figure 2. Interfragmentary and interdental wiring for fracture repair.

2. Pass the wire through drill holes in the fragments.
3. When stabilizing oblique fractures, wire placement must neutralize the overriding of the fragments.

Intramedullary Pinning

■ The use of IM pins for the repair of mandibular body fractures is not recommended, although there are reports of its successful use in the treatment of such fractures. The normal mandibular curvature makes it difficult to insert an IM pin into the mandibular body without invasion of the mandibular canal or damage to the tooth roots.
■ Placement of IM pins into the mandibular canal has been done without apparent detrimental effects. Nevertheless, pin placement in this area is discouraged.
■ Fractures repaired with IM pins have a high risk of nonunion or malunion with resultant malocclusion. This is because most IM pins have a tendency to resist bending to conform to the curved portion of the mandibular canal, resulting in distraction of the fracture.

Tape Muzzle

■ A tape muzzle can be used as the sole means of stabilizing minimally displaced or nondisplaced fractures (see sec. 9, ch. 3).
■ Stresses on internal fixation devices can be reduced when used in combination with a tape muzzle.

CAUDAL MANDIBULAR BODY FRACTURES

■ Treat minimally displaced fractures in this region with a tape muzzle (see sec. 9, ch. 3).
■ Stabilize displaced and unstable fractures with internal fixation methods such as bone plates and interfragmentary wiring.
■ Some methods of fracture fixation are not suitable for caudal body fractures.
  • External fixation pins are difficult to position properly in the caudal fracture segment.
  • Insufficient-size teeth or lack of a suitable number of teeth in the caudal fracture segment prevent use of interdental wiring techniques.

MANDIBULAR RAMUS FRACTURES

The ramus is a thin bone in which improperly placed implants will loosen prematurely. Complete surgical exposure of the ramus is difficult because of muscle attachment. The higher the location of the fracture on the ramus, the less critical is the need for surgical intervention.

■ Fractures of the ramus often are minimally displaced owing to the adjacent musculature, which aids in maintaining reduction and stability during fracture healing. Many of these fractures will respond favorably if jaw motion is restricted with a tape muzzle.
■ Animals with fractures of the lower ramus, especially when bilateral, benefit from fracture stabilization. Various methods can be used, including small plates, interfragmentary wiring, and K-wire fixation in combination with orthopedic wire.

Technique

Two approaches can be combined to provide greater exposure of the angular portion of the ramus and the TMJ.

1. Expose the angular portion of the ramus by making a skin incision along the ventrolateral border of the caudal mandible.
   a. Incise the platysma muscle to expose the digastricus muscle.
   b. Continue deeper dissection to expose the mandible and the masseter muscle, which is subperiosteally reflected dorsally to expose the masseteric fossa and the condyloid and angular processes.
2. Alternatively, expose the dorsal aspect of the ramus by making a skin incision along the caudoventral margin of the zygomatic arch.
   a. Incise the platysma muscle and reflect it ventrally, exposing the lateral surface of the TMJ and the condyloid process.
3. Apply the selected implant after fracture reduction.
4. Pin and wire combinations or interfragmentary wiring techniques work well in the lower part of the ramus, in which the bone is thicker than the dorsal aspect of the ramus.
5. Bone plates are the preferred method of stabilization of the ramus because of the thinness of the bone.
   a. Reconstruction plates (Synthes) can be contoured in multiple planes and are well suited for use in this area.
   b. Use of a T-plate reduces the amount of surgical exposure required for plate application.

CONDYLOID PROCESS FRACTURES

Fractures of the condyloid process of the mandible occur infrequently and usually are minimally or nondisplaced. They usually occur in association with other mandibular fractures.

■ Evaluate the TMJ radiographically when an animal with other mandibular fractures is presented.
■ In younger animals, fractures of the condyloid process are more likely to heal and remodel without

surgical intervention. For displaced fractures or condylar fractures in older animals, internal fixation may be of benefit.

Condylectomy

Condylectomy is recommended in animals with a nonreducible condyloid process fracture. This technique has several advantages:

- Normal dental occlusion and range of jaw motion is maintained and problems with mastication or degeneration of the contralateral TMJ are not encountered.
- Degenerative joint disease of the TMJ can develop subsequent to condyloid process fractures. In severe cases, a condylectomy can alleviate the discomfort or pain caused by degeneration of the joint.

Bilateral condylectomies should be avoided.

Technique

1. The approach to the TMJ is as previously described for mandibular ramus fractures.
2. Insert a K-wire or small IM pin from the ventral surface of the mandible to a sufficient depth to maintain reduction. Avoid penetration of the articular surface of the condyloid process.

MANDIBULAR (TMJ) LUXATIONS

Luxation of the mandible occurs infrequently and can be an isolated injury or found in association with mandibular or maxillary fractures. Evaluate cats presented for mandibular symphyseal separations for possible luxation of the TMJ.

Etiology

Temporomandibular dysplasia is a nontraumatic cause of TMJ luxation and has been reported in American cocker spaniels, Basset hounds, Irish setters, and St. Bernards. This can result in open mouth jaw locking, requiring manual reduction.

Diagnosis

Suspect TMJ luxation when malocclusion of the mandible exists without an identifiable fracture.

- TMJ luxation can be rostral or caudal as well as unilateral or bilateral. The direction often can be determined on physical examination. The mandible can deviate toward the normal side (rostral luxation) or the luxated side (caudal luxation).
- The diagnosis and direction of luxation is confirmed radiographically.

Preoperative Considerations

- If the luxation is of traumatic origin, ensure a patent airway and identify potentially life-threatening associated injuries.
- Mandibular or maxillary fractures may hinder efforts to reduce the mandibular luxation.

- Evaluate the TMJ radiographically for the presence of fractures that may prevent reduction of the luxation.

Surgical Procedure

Objectives

- Reduce the mandibular luxation atraumatically to reestablish normal jaw motion and occlusion.
- In cases of open mouth jaw locking, provide unrestricted movement of the ramus.

Equipment

- No special equipment is needed.

Technique—TMJ Luxation

1. Place the animal, under general anesthesia, in dorsal recumbency.
2. Place a small dowel or pencil across the last molars to act as a fulcrum.
3. Close the animal's mouth over the pencil and move the mandible in the appropriate direction to reduce the luxation.
   a. When reducing the luxation, open reduction may rarely be required. Exposure for open reduction is as previously described for the approach to the dorsal aspect of the ramus.
4. After reduction, apply a tape muzzle (as previously described) to minimize reluxation and limit mouth opening during the healing phase.
5. Interarch wiring has been used as an alternative to the tape muzzle for preventing reluxation but has the following disadvantages:
   a. A pharyngostomy tube is required.
   b. Wire stretching and breaking can occur.
   c. Aspiration pneumonia is possible.

Technique—Jaw Locking

Jaw locking occurs when the condyloid process of the ramus is trapped lateral to the zygomatic arch. This can occur when the mouth is opened widely, often when dogs yawn. While some dogs are able to effect reduction unassisted by exaggerated jaw movements, many dogs require assistance in unlocking the jaw.

1. When the jaw is locked, there is a prominent bulge below the zygomatic arch on the locked side. Unlock the jaw by opening the jaw as far as possible and applying pressure over the prominent bulge.
2. While continuing to apply pressure, close the jaw.
3. In chronic cases, partially resect the zygomatic arch or condyloid process to prevent lateral fixation of the ramus.

Postoperative Care and Complications

TMJ Luxation

- Maintain the tape muzzle for 2–3 weeks.
- Feed soft diet for 4–6 weeks with gradual reintroduction of a dry diet.

■ Reluxation is possible. If reduction cannot be maintained, a mandibular condylectomy is indicated.

Jaw Locking

■ No special care is necessary regarding feeding or activity.

■ Complications are not reported.

Recommended Reading

Taylor RA: Mandibular fractures. *In*: Bojrak MJ, ed.: *Current Techniques in Small Animal Surgery*. Philadelphia: Lea & Febiger, 1990, p 890.

3 Fractures of the Maxilla

Paul E. Howard

Maxillary fractures generally refer to any fracture of the upper jaw and adjacent bone.

ANATOMY

- The upper jaw is composed of paired maxilla and incisive bone (also called premaxilla) jointed along the midline by their contralateral counterparts.
  - The maxilla contains the canine, premolar, and molar teeth. It varies greatly in form among different breeds of dogs (i.e., brachycephalic, mesocephalic, dolichocephalic).
  - The incisive bone joins caudally with the maxilla and contains the incisor teeth. The portion between the teeth and nasal cavity is very thin and can be damaged easily from trauma or during dental procedures involving the incisor teeth.
- The palatine bone is located caudomedial to the maxilla and forms the caudal part of the hard palate. Along its lateral suture, it joins with the maxilla to form the major palatine foramen.
  - The major palatine foramen is at the level of the distal margin of the maxillary fourth premolars.
  - The minor palatine foramen (occasionally two or more) is found caudal to the major palatine foramen.
- The bones of the upper jaw are covered with gingiva (the gums), which is composed of dense fibrous tissue covered by smooth vascularized mucosa. The gingiva extends around the necks of the teeth and into the alveolar sockets. It is continuous externally with the mucosa, and internally with the hard palate.
- The major blood supply to the upper jaw is provided by the pterygopalatine portion of the maxillary artery.
  - The minor palatine artery arises from the ventral surface of the maxillary or one of its terminal branches dorsal to the last maxillary molar tooth and supplies the adjacent soft and hard palate.
  - The major palatine artery arises rostral to the minor palatine artery from a common trunk with the sphenopalatine artery, exits through the major palatine foramen, and supplies the mucosa overlying the hard palate. This artery frequently anastomoses with its contralateral counterpart.

GENERAL PRINCIPLES OF FRACTURE FIXATION
Preoperative Considerations

- Diagnosis of maxillary and incisive bone fractures is usually not difficult. Direct observation and palpation often are sufficient for definitive diagnosis.

- Consider any fracture of the maxilla in which the integrity of the gingiva is disrupted an open fracture. Antibiotic therapy is appropriate.
- Evaluate maxillary fractures radiographically to assess the extent and severity of the injury.
- Maintenance of a patent and functioning airway is of primary importance. Respiratory distress can result from hemorrhage, edema, and soft-tissue obstruction secondary to associated trauma.
- When the animal's condition is stabilized, evaluate the dental occlusion. The site of malocclusion and its severity can identify the location and severity of the fracture.

KEY POINT ▶ Restoration of normal anatomic alignment of the fracture ensures restoration of dental occlusion unless the teeth are traumatized.

- Stable fixation of the teeth often provides suitable stabilization of the fractured bone.
- Stabilization of bone fragments can be difficult, owing to thinness of bone or the presence of tooth roots.
- Noninvasive methods of fracture fixation often result in satisfactory healing of the fracture and are preferred to invasive surgical procedures.
- Indications for open reduction of fractures:
  - Airway obstruction due to depression fractures (unreduced fractures of the nasal or maxillary bones can result in callus formation and later obstruction of the nasal passages)
  - Lack of alternative measures for acceptable dental occlusion or fracture stabilization
  - Presence of an oronasal defect, either from trauma or tooth loss
  - Severe facial deformity

Objectives

- Ensure a patent airway.
- Establish and maintain acceptable dental occlusion.
- Correct severe facial deformities.

Equipment

Specialized equipment is not required. Equipment needed varies, depending on the method of repair selected, and may include:

- Wire twisters and cutters
- Orthopedic wire of various sizes (18–24 gauge)
- Bone plates and screws

- External fixation devices
- K-wires and small intramedullary (IM) pins
- Adhesive tape

POSTOPERATIVE CARE AND COMPLICATIONS

- Feed a soft diet (gruel or liquid) until fractures are healed. Adherence to this principle will ensure that the client administers the altered diet as long as temporary implants are in place.
- Deny access to bones, balls, chew toys, and other hard objects to prevent dislodging the fixation device.
- Instruct the owner to examine the oral cavity once daily to ensure that proper dental occlusion is being maintained and that any external implants used are still in place. Instruct the owner to avoid excessive manipulation of the jaw.
- Radiographically evaluate fracture healing in 4–6 weeks. Remove exposed fixation devices when there is radiographic evidence of bony union.
- Continue postoperative restrictions for 3–4 weeks following radiographic evidence of bony union to ensure sufficient osseous healing before allowing resumption of normal activities and return to a normal diet.

Complications

Complications are infrequently encountered but may include the following:

- Infection—Severe periodontal disease can compromise fracture healing due to the large numbers of bacteria in the area of the fracture.
- Oronasal fistula
  - Chronic fistulas may lead to respiratory infection due to aspiration of food particles and saliva.
  - Although usually located at the site of a missing tooth, traumatically induced fistulas can exist anywhere between the oral and nasal cavities.
  - Conservative treatment usually is not successful and surgical intervention is required (see sec. 7, ch. 1).
- Bone sequestration—rare due to the good vascular supply to the area.
- Chronic respiratory obstruction
  - Causes include malalignment of fracture fragments and callus produced as fracture healing progresses occluding normal air flow.
  - Depending on the severity of the obstruction, surgical intervention to reestablish a patent air passage may be necessary (see sec. 1, ch. 3).
- Malocclusion or tooth loss
  - Trauma to the maxilla can damage tooth structure resulting in loss of tooth vitality.
  - Treat nonviable teeth endodontically to eliminate the potential for abscess formation (see sec. 7, ch. 1).
  - Extract excessively loose or irreparably damaged teeth after they are no longer needed for fracture stabilization.
- Altered normal growth in young animals (<6 months of age).

PROCEDURES

Tape Muzzle

Indications

- Repair of nondisplaced or minimally displaced fractures involving the hard palate or teeth, in which normal dental occlusion can be established and maintained without other means of fixation
- An adjunct to fixation, used in combination with internal fixation, in which the purpose is to limit postoperative jaw motion
- Temporary means of reducing motion at the fracture site until definitive methods of repair are employed

Preapplication Considerations

- To properly evaluate alignment and stability, general anesthesia or heavy sedation may be required.
- If proper occlusion is present, maintain a 1-cm gap between the incisors as the tape muzzle is applied.
- If occlusion can be maintained only by holding the mouth completely closed with interdigitation of the teeth, apply the muzzle with the mouth closed.
  - Provide alimentation by pharyngostomy tube or gastrostomy tube (see sec. 1, ch. 3).
  - Be sure that the animal can breathe through its nose.

KEY POINT ▶ If possible, avoid muzzling with the animal's mouth completely closed, because open-mouthed breathing and evaporation of saliva from the tongue play an important role in thermoregulation.

Technique

1. Place the first piece of tape is around the posterior muzzle with the sticky side of the tape facing out. When the circle is complete, double back the tape on itself to cover the adhesive and prevent it from sticking to the dog.
2. Place a second ring of tape in the same manner and secure it snugly around the neck, immediately behind the ears (Fig. 1).

KEY POINT ▶ An unanesthetized animal may resist attempts to apply the tape around the nose. Premeasure the animal's muzzle with your hands and make a tape ring based on this measurement. Slip the ring over the animal's muzzle while an assistant holds the animal's mouth closed.

3. Join the two rings of tape with lateral straps, made by folding a piece of tape on itself with the adhesive side inward. Secure these to the rings by an additional layer of tape wrapped around the nose and neck rings. Excess tape is trimmed away.
4. Remove the muzzle by cutting the neck ring and slipping off the nose ring.

Postoperative Care and Complications

- If necessary use an Elizabethan collar to prevent attempts by the dog to remove the muzzle.

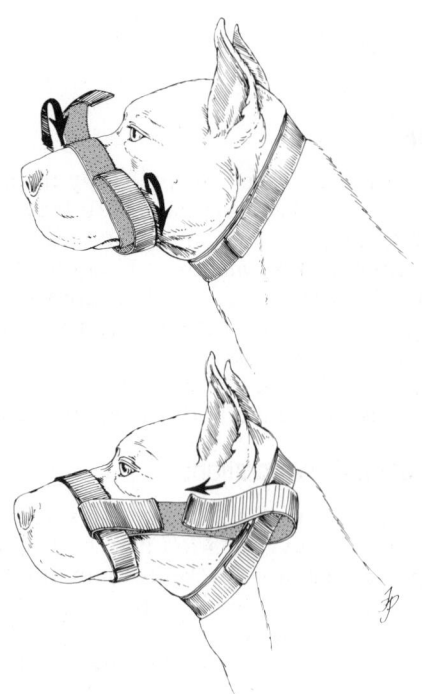

Figure 1. Procedure for creating a tape muzzle. See text for explanation.

- Restrict diet to soft food; do not allow chewing of hard objects.
- Instruct owner to examine the skin around the tape daily for signs of redness or discharge. Moist dermatitis has been encountered under the tape around the muzzle. The condition resolves rapidly once the muzzle is removed.
- Muzzles used long-term may need to be replaced periodically.
  - Muzzles soiled from feed and water can cause irritation to the skin.
  - The tape rings will stretch slightly, permitting excessive jaw motion and requiring replacement of the tape.
- Leave muzzle on until fracture is stable (usually 4–8 weeks).
- Jaw motion following removal of the tape muzzle often is restricted. Normal range of motion return in 1–3 weeks without the need for physical therapy.

Interdental Wiring

Interdental wiring is used as a primary method of fracture stabilization of fractures of the hard palate and alveolar bone or in conjunction with other fixation procedures. It is an excellent method for maintaining dental occlusion.

Technique

1. Use the largest-size orthopedic wire (usually 22- or 24-gauge) that can be passed between the involved teeth without distorting occlusion and that can be conformed intimately to the surface of the teeth.

KEY POINT ▶ Wire not closely conformed to the teeth will not provide adequate stability.

2. Place the wire as close to the gingival margin as possible. Wire that tends to slip off owing to the conical shape of the tooth (e.g., canine tooth) can be kept in position by securing the wire in place with a small amount of composite material (see discussion of oral cavities in sec. 7, ch. 1). In multirooted teeth, the wire can be placed through the furcation in preference to around the tooth.
3. Place wire twists on the buccal side of the teeth and bend the twisted end parallel to the long axis of the tooth to minimize soft tissue irritation.
   a. Twists covered with composite resin or brace wax reduce soft tissue irritation.
4. Incorporate teeth on each side of the fracture site in the wire pattern until the first tooth solidly embedded in alveolar bone can be included. Including additional teeth in the repair does not provide added stability.

Ivy Loop

This is a simple wiring pattern for stabilizing a fracture between two teeth that have remained firmly embedded in their respective alveolar sockets (Fig. 2).

Technique

1. Make a loop in the middle of the wire and place the wire between the two involved teeth, with the loop on the buccal surface of the teeth and the wire tails on the lingual aspect.
2. Pull one wire tail tightly around the distal aspect of the caudal tooth to the buccal surface where it is threaded through the wire loop.
3. Draw the other tail around the mesial aspect of the rostral tooth to the buccal surface of the tooth.
4. Cross and twist the two ends of wire on each other while applying firm traction to the wires, ensuring an even twist.
5. Cut the twisted wire, leaving three twists to prevent separation of the wire ends.

Stout Continuous Loop

This wiring pattern is indicated for the stabilization of alveolar and palate fractures in which teeth adjacent

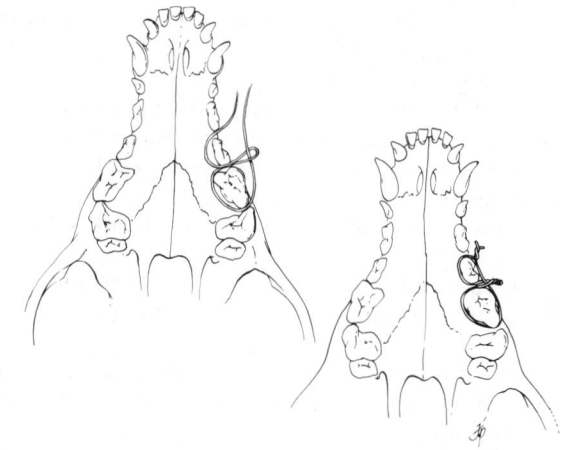

Figure 2. Initial *(left)* and final *(right)* appearance of Ivy loop wiring pattern.

to the fracture are loose. The pattern is continued until solidly embedded teeth are encountered on both sides of the fracture (Fig. 3).

Technique

1. Identify the teeth to be wired and place a piece of wire along the buccal aspect of the teeth. Measure and cut a small length of wire beyond the last tooth at one end, and a working length of wire at least 1½ times the distance between the teeth being wired.
2. Bring the working end of wire around the tooth to the lingual side and pass it through the interproximal space and under the wire lying on the buccal surface of the tooth. Bring the working wire over the stationary wire and pass it back through the interproximal space. Before pulling the wire tight, twist a single loop in the working wire where it passes over the stationary wire.
3. Continue this pattern the entire length of the teeth until the last solidly embedded tooth is encountered. Pull the wire around the last tooth to the buccal surface of the tooth.
4. Before twisting the wire ends together, apply traction to the stationary wire and twist each loop in the working wire tightly, beginning at the far end and working toward the free ends of wire.
5. After tightening all the working loops, twist the two ends of wire evenly on each other until tight and cut off the excess wire, leaving three twists.
6. In a modification of this technique, place the loops through the interproximal spaces and thread the stationary wire through the loops. Tighten the wire as previously described.

Interfragmentary Wiring

This is a potentially useful method for repairing comminuted fractures of the maxilla or incisive bone. Multiple wire can be used to stabilize hard palate fractures or transverse fractures of the maxilla. Small-diameter wire (22 or 24 gauge) is preferred because it conforms better to the thin bone than does heaver gauge wires.

Technique

1. Drill small holes in the fragments and preplace the wire through drill holes in adjacent fragments. Each fragment requires a minimum of two wires to provide sufficient stability. In some cases, three or more wires may be placed through a single fragment.
2. Preplace all wires before tightening them to ensure proper positioning of all wires.
3. Discard very small pieces of bone rather than attempting to replace them. The resultant osseous defect will be covered with soft tissue and new bone formation can be expected if the periosteum is preserved.

Pin and Wire Fixation

The primary indication for pin and wire fixation is the stabilization of palate fractures in which interdental or interfragmentary wiring techiques alone do not provide adequate fracture stabilization.

Technique

1. Insert K-wires or small IM pins, determined by the size of the animal involved, from the alveolar margin across the fracture, and exit on the opposite side. The pin actually traverses the floor of the nasal cavity.
2. Exercise care during pin placement to avoid penetrating tooth roots.
3. Orthopedic wire is placed in figure-eight fashion around the ends of the pin and tightened. As the wire is tightened, compression is applied at the fracture site. The wire twists are positioned so as to minimize subsequent trauma to adjacent soft tissues.

EXTERNAL PIN FIXATION

This often described but infrequently used method of fixation uses external pins and acrylic to stabilize comminuted fractures of the nasal and maxillary bones. External pin fixation has the following disadvantages:

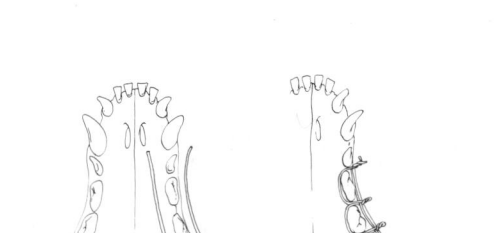

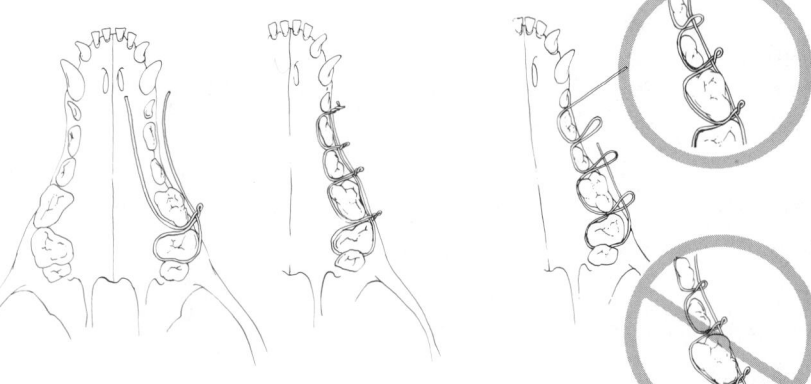

Figure 3. Initial *(left)* and final *(center and right)* appearance of Stout, continuous loop wiring pattern. Note that the working wire is *not* twisted lingual to the stationary wire.

- The thinness of the bone makes it difficult to achieve secure retention of the pins long enough for fracture healing to occur.
- The external apparatus can be dislodged, resulting in loss of fracture reduction.

Technique

The principles of standard external fixation for stabilization of long bone fractures apply to this method.

1. Insert pins through stab incisions in the skin, minimizing the need for extensive soft tissue dissection.
2. When possible, place a minimum of 2 pins in each fracture fragment, to avoid rotation of the fragments.
3. Keep pin entry sites clean to minimize pin tract infections.
4. Connect the external pins with acrylic rather than external metal bars because the reduced weight is advantageous, and the use of acrylic permits the incorporation of pins of various sizes in multiple planes.

KEY POINT ▶ Use an Elizabethan collar to protect the apparatus.

Plate and Screw Fixation

Plating maxillary fractures is seldom necessary, but this method of fracture fixation is employed in selected cases.

- Comminuted fractures with a bony defect can be effectively stabilized with a plate.
- Transverse fractures of the premaxilla, which are difficult to stabilize with interfragmentary wires, are amenable to plate and screw fixation.

Technique

1. Because of the minimal soft tissue overlying the maxilla, use small, thin bone plates.
2. The thinness of the bone necessitates the use of short screws.
3. Because the maxilla has only a single cortex, maximize plate length and the number of screws.
4. Avoid tooth roots and the infraorbital foramen.
5. Reconstruction plates (Synthes) and plastic plates (Lubra) can be more easily contoured to the maxilla than can conventional plates.

Supplemental Readings

Bone DL: Maxillary fractures. *In* Bojrab MJ, ed.: *Current Techniques in Small Animal Surgery*. Philadelphia: Lea & Febiger, 1990, p 883.

Dulisch ML: Skull and mandibular fractures. *In* Slatter DH, ed.: *Textbook of Small Animal Surgery*. Philadelphia: W. B. Saunders, 1985, p 2286.

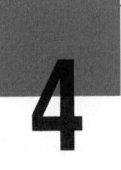

4 Neoplasms of the Maxilla and Mandible

Paul E. Howard

Neoplasms of the oral cavity and associated structures are encountered commonly in dogs and cats. The oral cavity is the fourth most common site of neoplasms, accounting for approximately 5% and 7% of malignant tumors in dogs and cats, respectively. Oral neoplasms in dogs often are malignant; in cats they are nearly always malignant.

KEY POINT ▶ Squamous cell carcinoma is the most frequently identified neoplasm in cats; malignant melanoma, squamous cell carcinoma and fibrosarcoma are the neoplasms diagnosed most often in dogs.

- Certain breeds of dogs appear to be predisposed to oral tumors, including boxers, German shepherds, German shorthaired pointers, golden retrievers, cocker spaniels, and Weimaraners.
- When oral tumors are considered collectively, male dogs are affected more frequently than female dogs.
- Small-breed dogs have a greater tendency to develop malignant melanoma; large-breed dogs are more prone to develop squamous cell carcinoma and fibrosarcoma.
- Dogs with heavily pigmented oral mucosa are predisposed to malignant melanomas.

TUMOR TYPES

Benign Nonodontogenic Neoplasms

Epulis

Epulides are fibromatous tumors of the periodontal ligament, differentiating them from odontogenic tumors. They are rarely seen in the cat but are among the most frequently observed oral tumors in the dog.

- There is an equal distribution between sexes.
- A familial predisposition has been noted in boxers.

Epulides are categorized into three different types based upon histologic appearance.

Fibromatous Epulis

- These are benign, noninvasive growths in which the periodontal ligament stroma is the dominant cell type.
- They appear as pedunculated masses that are usually multiple and grow by expansion.
- The enveloping nature of the lesion can cause interference with mastication. Treatment is necessary only if the lesion is causing clinical signs.

Treatment

- Surgical excision of only the visible portion of an epulis usually results in recurrence.
- Because the origin of the lesion is the periodontal ligament, prevention of recurrence requires extraction of the involved tooth and curettage of the associated periodontal ligament.
- An alternative procedure is en bloc resection of the bone and involved tooth.

Ossifying Epulis

- Biologic behavior is similar to that of fibromatous epulis, except that the tumor has an osteoid component.
- Malignant transformation to osteosarcoma has been reported.

Treatment

- Treatment, as described for fibromatous epulides, is necessary only if the tumor is causing clinical signs.

Acanthomatous Epulis

This locally invasive neoplasm causes destruction of adjacent alveolar bone and is found most often on the rostral mandible. It does not metastasize.

Treatment

A variety of treatment modalities can be used.

- Simple local excision results in a high rate of recurrence.
- Wide surgical excision of affected bone (partial mandibulectomy or partial maxillectomy) is effective.
- Radiation therapy is effective and can be curative.
- Radiation often is combined with surgical excision of large tumors.
- Epulides rarely undergo malignant transformation and recur as squamous cell carcinoma, fibrosarcoma, or osteosarcoma.

Other Benign Nonodontogenic Neoplasms

These include fibroma, lipoma, hemangioma, chondroma, osteoma, and histiocytoma. They are seen less frequently than epulides. However, because of their similar clinical appearance to other tumors, biopsy and histopathological evaluation are necessary.

Malignant Nonodontogenic Neoplasms
Malignant Melanoma (MM)

- MM is the most commonly diagnosed oral tumor in dogs but is rare in cats.

- The incidence in male and female dogs is 4:1.
- Animals with darkly pigmented oral mucosa may be at greater risk for the disease.

■ MM is noted for its rapid local infiltration, frequent recurrence rate, and high likelihood of metastasis to regional lymph nodes and the lungs.

- Amelanotic melanoma can be mistaken on gross observation for other oral neoplasms, indicating the necessity for histologic diagnosis.

Treatment

■ Wide surgical excision (partial maxillectomies and mandibulectomies) currently appears to be the most effective method of treatment.

■ Radiation therapy is followed by high rate of recurrence. In one study, a complete response was obtained in 21% of patients, and 1-year disease-free interval occurred in 8%. When radiation therapy was combined with hyperthermia, there was an improved disease-free interval.

■ Chemotherapy and immunotherapy have been used to a minimal degree, and their efficacy is unknown at this time.

Prognosis

KEY POINT ▶ The prognosis for malignant melanoma is poor; the 1-year survival rate is <10%.

Squamous Cell Carcinoma (SCC)

■ SCC is the most common malignant tumor of the oral cavity in cats and the second-most common malignant oral tumor in dogs.

- In cats, differentiate SCC from inflammatory lesions such as eosinophilic granuloma and nasopharyngeal polyp.

■ SCC can be classified as tonsillar and nontonsillar.

- Both types occur with equal frequency in dogs.
- In dogs, nontonsillar SCC occurs with equal frequency in males and females; tonsillar SCC occurs more frequently in males.

■ Nontonsillar SCC is locally invasive but slow to metastasize to regional lymph nodes and lungs. It often invades bone, causing lysis of bone and loosening of teeth; the radiographic appearance can be confused with osteosarcoma and osteomyelitis.

■ Tonsillar SCC is very aggressive and has a poor prognosis (see sec. 7, ch. 1).

Treatment

■ Wide surgical excision is the treatment of choice.

■ Nontonsillar SCC is potentially sensitive to radiation therapy if treated aggressively.

Prognosis

■ The prognosis in cats is poor, because local recurrence is common.

■ The prognosis in dogs is better; about 50% of treated dogs live for 1 year.

Fibrosarcoma (FS)

■ In dogs, FS is diagnosed third most frequently after MM and SCC. It is the second most frequent malignant tumor in cats, but much less common than SCC.

■ FS is seen twice as often in canine males as in females.

■ It is more common in large-breed dogs than in small breeds.

■ The FS tends to invade local tissues rapidly, causing bony destruction.

■ Metastasis occurs late in the course of the disease, but local recurrence is very common.

Treatment

■ Effective treatment of FS can be difficult, especially of tumors involving the hard palate.

■ Wide surgical incision is the treatment of choice.

■ Fibrosarcomas respond poorly to orthovoltage radiation, chemotherapy, and immunotherapy.

■ Cryosurgery is not recommended because it is believed to stimulate recurrence.

Prognosis

■ The prognosis is poor, owing to local recurrence and eventual metastasis.

■ The 1-year survival time is less than 20%.

Osteosarcoma

■ Osteosarcoma is uncommon in dogs and cats.

■ The initial presenting complaint is jaw pain, and radiographs obtained early in the course of the disease may be nondiagnostic.

Treatment

■ Wide surgical excision of the involved bone in combination with chemotherapy is currently recommended, but the prognosis is poor.

Other Malignant Nonodontogenic Neoplasms

Other types of these tumors less commonly seen include adenocarcinoma, undifferentiated carcinoma, transmissible venereal tumor, mast cell tumor, hemangiosarcoma, and tonsillar lymphosarcoma.

Odontogenic Neoplasms

■ Odontoma, a rare tumor of dental origin, can invade all of the dental tissues (enamel, cementum, dentin, and pulp).

■ Ameloblastoma is a benign, slow-growing, invasive neoplasm of epithelial origin. It occurs most commonly in the mandible, grows by expansion, and metastasizes infrequently.

Treatment

■ Because these tumors arise from deep alveolar bone, local, nonaggressive therapy often results in recurrence.

■ Wide surgical excision usually is curative.

■ Radiation can be used, but recurrence is likely.

CLINICAL SIGNS

■ Clinical signs of benign and malignant oral neoplasms are similar and include excessive salivation, oral hemorrhage, reluctance to eat or difficulty eating, jaw pain, loose teeth, and facial asymmetry.

■ Weight loss can occur secondary to the above clinical signs.

KEY POINT ▶ Consider neoplasia in an animal that requires dental extraction because of excessive tooth mobility.

DIAGNOSIS

- Base a tentative diagnosis on the age, sex, and breed of the animal and the gross appearance and location of the lesion.
- Make a definitive diagnosis by histopathologic evaluation of a representative lesion specimen.
  - Obtain a specimen by incisional or excisional biopsy, depending on the nature and extent of the lesion.
  - Perform fine-needle aspiration of regional lymph nodes to evaluate for metastasis.
- Radiology
  - Radiographs of the skull can assess the extent of bony involvement.
  - Multiple projections may be necessary to adequately assess bony changes.
  - Obtain thoracic radiographs in all cases of malignant oral neoplasia to examine distant metastatic lesions. Ideally, perform thoracic radiography before the animal is anesthetized for biopsy.
  - Inform owners that false-negative thoracic radiographs can occur.

PRINCIPLES OF THERAPY

- The goal of therapy is the elimination of neoplastic tissue while preserving function and, if possible, cosmetic appearance.
  - The severity of the lesion at the time of treatment may permit only palliative measures.
  - Slowly progressing, noninvasive neoplasms are more responsive to therapy than are rapidly growing, invasive tumors.
- No single treatment protocol is effective for all oral tumors (see Treatment in preceding discussion of specific neoplasms). Adapt protocols to the animal being treated, based on the following factors:
  - Tumor type and primary site
  - Age and overall health of the animal
  - Extent of tissue involvement
  - Presence of lung metastasis
  - Expertise of the veternarian
  - Cost of treatment and owner preference

KEY POINT ▶ Early, aggressive therapy of malignant oral tumors offers the best chance of success.

- In selected tumors, combination of treatment modalities may be more effective than individual modalities.
- Aggressive surgical management improves success rates. Table 1 compares the responsiveness of various tumor types to surgery and radiation therapy.
- Cryotherapy (freezing of tissue to destroy tumor cells) is not recommended because of associated complications and poor results compared with surgery.

TABLE 1. Responsiveness of Common Oral Tumors to Aggressive Surgical Excision and Radiation Therapy

Tumor Type	Surgery	Radiation
Epulis		
Fibromatous	+ + +	NI
Ossifying	+ + +	NI
Acanthomatous	+ +	+ + +
Malignant melanoma	+	+
Squamous cell	+ + + (dogs)	+ + + (rostral tumors)
carcinoma	+ (cats)	+ + (caudal tumors)
Fibrosarcoma	+ +	+ +
Osteosarcoma	+ +	+

NI = not indicated; + = poor; + + = fair; + + + = good.

SURGICAL EXCISION

- Surgical procedures range from simple local excision to mandibulectomy and maxillectomy.
  - Hemimandibulectomy is partial or total removal of bone and associated teeth from one side of the mandible.
  - Hemimaxillectomy is the en bloc removal of the portion of the maxilla between the 2nd and 1st premolars that is confined to one side of the maxilla (see Fig. 3).
  - Caudal hemimaxillectomy is the en bloc resection of the maxilla from the 4th premolar caudally.
- Local excision often is unsuccessful, owing to tumor recurrence at the primary surgical site.
- En bloc resection (mandibulectomy, maxillectomy) of the affected bone is recommended to prevent local tumor recurrence.
- Stabilization of the hemimandibles using pins, screws, or bone grafts is unnecessary and is not recommended.

Anatomy

- The masseter muscle lies on the lateral surface of the ramus with some fibers of the superficial layer projecting around the ventral and caudal borders of the mandible to insert on the ventromedial surface.
- The temporalis muscle inserts on the coronoid process of the mandible, with some fibers inserting further down on the ventral margin of the masseteric fossa.
- The lateral pterygoid muscle inserts on the medial surface of the mandibular condyle.
- The medial pterygoid muscle inserts on the medial and caudal surfaces of the angular process of the mandible.
- The inferior alveolar artery and vein enter the mandibular foramen located on the medial side of the ramus at approximately the level of the last molar, midway between the cranial and caudal edges of the ramus. The artery exits at the mental foramen of the mandible.
- The blood supply to the maxilla is via the major and minor palatine arteries (which lie just deep to the mucosa of the hard palate) and the infraorbital artery

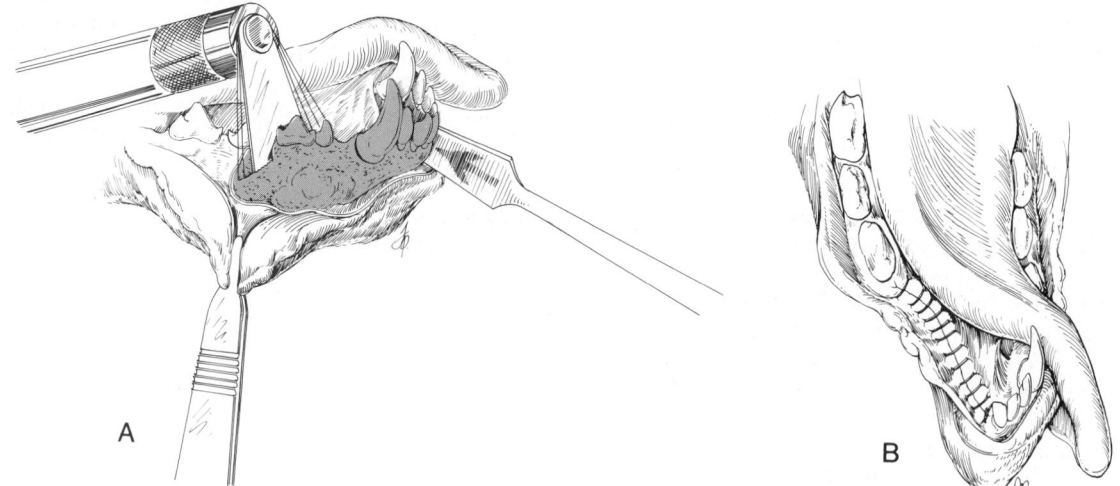

Figure 1. Unilateral hemimandibulectomy. *A*, Incise the gingiva around the lesion, keeping at least 1 cm of normal tissue around it. Separate the mandibular symphysis and continue the original incision through the bone. *B*, Cover the bone and close the incision.

(exits through the infraorbital foramen dorsal to the upper third premolar tooth). The infraorbital vein and nerve parallel this artery.

Preoperative Considerations

- Indications:
  - Evidence of malignancy or local invasiveness (bone involvment) in the absence of distant metastasis
  - Tumor recurrence
  - Radiation effective (fibrosarcoma, malignant melanoma)
  - Small, mobile, and easily resectable mass
  - Palliation in tumors that are not resectable

KEY POINT ▶ The first attempt at surgery offers the best chance at success. Local recurrence of the neoplasm often is due to an insufficiently aggressive approach to the initial removal of the lesion.

- When performing excision of mass lesions, include a margin of at least 1 cm of normal-appearing tissue.
- Show owners pictures of animals that have undergone mandibulectomy and maxillectomy to prepare them for the animal's postoperative appearance and to reassure them that gross deformities do not result.
- Reserve electrocautery for coagulation, and use sparingly. Incisions made with electrocautery heal slowly and have a tendency toward dehiscence.
- The suture material of choice is a synthetic absorbable suture used with a cutting needle (e.g., polyglactin, polydioxanone [PDS])
- Drape the surgical site as well as possible; recognize that the procedure is not being performed in a sterile field.
- Administer intravenous broad-spectrum antibiotics at the time of anesthetic induction. It is rarely necessary to continue them postoperatively.

Positioning of the Animal

Good exposure is important, especially when considering surgery of the caudal aspect of the oral cavity.

Maxillectomy

- Surgery of the maxilla and premaxilla usually is best accommodated by placing the animal in dorsal recumbency.
- The use of sterile tongue depressors to keep the mouth open will cause minimal obstruction for the surgeon.
- Alternatively, use a sterile mouth speculum or tape the dog's mouth open to an anesthetic screen or to IV stands placed on each side of the operating table.
- Tie the endotracheal tube to the mandible.

Mandibulectomy

- Surgery of the mandible is best accomplished with the dog in lateral recumbency or, when operating on the caudal mandible per os, in sternal recumbency.
- When the animal is placed in sternal recumbency, hold the jaw open by taping the maxilla to IV stands on both sides of the operating table.
- Rostral mandibulectomy is best performed in dorsal recumbency with the animal's mouth held open by an oral speculum.

Surgical Procedures

Objectives

- Excise all neoplastic tissue.
- Reconstruct oral soft tissues to preserve function.

Equipment

- Standard surgical pack and sutures
- Oral speculum
- Electrocautery
- Bone saw and/or osteotome and mallet
- Bone wax

Technique

Unilateral Rostral Hemimandibulectomy

1. Incise the gingiva around the lesion while attempting to include a minimum of 1 cm of normal tissue (Fig. 1*A*). Reflect the lip ventrally.

2. Continue the dissection around the entire bone, incising the soft tissue attachments on the lingual side of the mandible.
3. Separate the mandibular symphysis with an osteotome and mallet. Use an oscillating saw to facilitate separation and osteotomy of the mandible.
4. The inferior alveolar artery and vein will be severed. Control resultant hemorrhage with electrocautery or, preferably, bone wax.
5. Do not attempt to stabilize the hemimandibles.
6. Cover the bone and close the defect by suturing the labial gingival mucosa to the lingual mucosa in a single layer, using absorbable suture material (Fig. 1*B*).

Technique

Bilateral Rostral Hemimandibulectomy

1. Perform the same procedure as that described for unilateral hemimandibulectomy.
2. Resection of the mandibles caudal to the second premolar teeth necessitates the resection of skin to effect a cosmetic closure.

Technique

Central Hemimandibulectomy

1. The procedure is similar to that for unilateral rostral hemimandibulectomy, except that a central portion of the mandible is removed, preserving the symphysis and temporomandibular joint (TMJ).
2. When covering the osteotomized ends of the mandible, osteotomize the bone slightly beyond "normal" limits. This allows normal gingival and oral mucosa to be pulled over the bone ends and sutured without tension.

Technique

Caudal Hemimandibulectomy

1. Make a skin incision paralleling the zygomatic arch.
2. Incise the periosteum and elevate the temporalis muscle subperiosteally from the zygomatic bone dorsally and medially.
3. Elevate the masseter muscles subperiosteally from their origin on the ventral zygomatic arch. Continue subperiosteal dissection until the zygomatic bone is freed completely of all muscle attachments.
4. Using an oscillating saw, transect the zygomatic arch at its rostral and caudal margins. Alternatively, resect the zygomatic bone with Gigli wire or a hobby saw.
   a. Use of an osteotome and mallet is not recommended because of the potential for splintering the bone.
   b. Wrap the zygomatic bone in a blood-soaked sponge in anticipation of replacing it during closure of the surgical wound.
5. Elevate the masseter muscle ventrally from the ramus and incise and elevate the temporalis muscle to expose the ramus.
6. Osteotomize the ramus with an oscillating saw.
   a. The location of the tumor will determine whether the TMJ can be preserved.

b. If disarticulation of the TMJ is necessary, use sharp dissection to incise the joint capsule and soft tissue attachments. Avoid trauma to the maxillary artery located just medial to the TMJ. Ligate this vessel if necessary to remove the section of mandible.
7. Close the incision by securing the osteotomized zygomatic bone with orthopedic wire at each end.
8. Suture the masseter muscle to the zygomatic bone with nonabsorbable sutures passed through the muscle fascia and encircling the bone.
9. Appose and suture the subcutaneous tissues and skin using accepted surgical techniques.

Technique

Premaxillectomy (for Lesions Rostral to the Second Premolar)

1. Make an incision at least 1 cm around the lesion (Fig. 2*A*).
2. Control hemorrhage, which often is profuse when the palate is incised, with temporary direct pressure or electrocoagulation.
3. Elevate the mucoperiosteum outward from the lesion in preparation for excising the diseased bone.
4. Using the incision line as a guide, cut the bone with an oscillating saw or side-cutting bur and free it from remaining soft tissue attachments.
5. Remove the mobilized section of bone en bloc, creating an oronasal defect.
   a. Exercise care when removing the bone to minimize damage to normal turbinate tissue. Remove diseased or damaged turbinates.

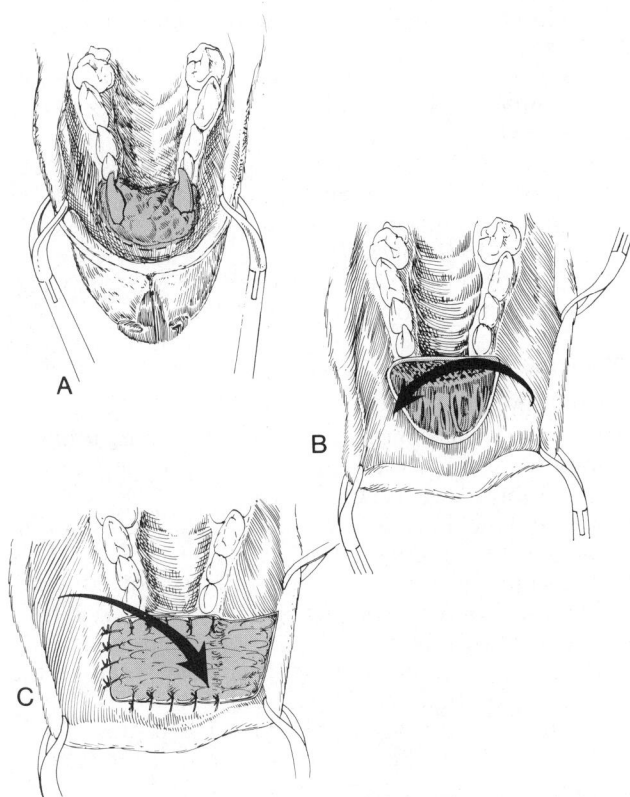

Figure 2. Bilateral premaxillectomy, double flap technique. *A*, Site of incision. *B*, First flap parallel to excised dental arch. *C*, Second flap from opposite side of premaxilla.

6. Create a labial flap adjacent to the defect of sufficient size to allow suturing the flap to the palatal mucosa without tension.
   a. The labial flap can be a sliding flap or a reversed flap in which the mucosal surface is flipped over to form the floor of the nasal cavity.
   b. The sliding flap is less likely to fail because of vascular compromise. The length of the flap should not exceed three times the width of the flap base.
   c. Create a labial flap by undermining the tissue adjacent to the defect to include the mucosa, submucosa, and subcutaneous tissue.
   d. Allow the exposed surface to heal by epithelialization, which usually is complete in 3–4 weeks.
7. Suture the labial flap to the palatal mucosa in two layers, using absorbable synthetic suture material on a cutting needle.
   a. Suturing the deep layer is facilitated by passing the suture through small drill holes (made with a K-wire) in the hard palate.
   b. Suture the outer layer in a simple interrupted pattern. Alternatively, intersperse a far-far-near-near suture pattern to disperse any tension on the suture line.
8. Large defects may require labial flaps on both sides that are sutured on the midline (problems with healing may be encountered).
9. To improve the postoperative cosmetic appearance of the nose, use a double flap technique in which the flaps overlap each other to provide additional soft tissue to support the nose.
   a. Create the first flap with the base of the flap paralleling the just-removed dental arch (Fig. 2B).
   b. Create a second, rostrally based, labial flap of similar size on the opposite side of the premaxilla (Fig. 2C).
   c. Reverse the first flap to place the mucosa on the floor of the nasal cavity, and suture this flap to the nasal mucosa and through holes previously drilled in the hard palate.
   d. Rotate the second flap over the first flap and suture in place as previously described.

Technique

Hemimaxillectomy

1. Make a mucosal incision around the lesion, attempting to leave at least 1 cm of normal tissue between the lesion and the incision (Fig. 3A).
2. Elevate the mucosa with a periosteal elevator to expose the underlying bone.
3. Excise the mass by ostectomy of the involved bone. The ostectomy can be performed with an oscillating saw, side-cutting bur, or osteotome and mallet.
   a. If this equipment is not available, remove the diseased bone with bone rongeurs.
4. Control hemorrhage, which often is profuse when the palate is incised, with ligation or cautery after removal of the section of bone.
   a. Occlusion of the carotid arteries before performing surgery will reduce the amount of hemorrhage during ostectomy of the diseased portion

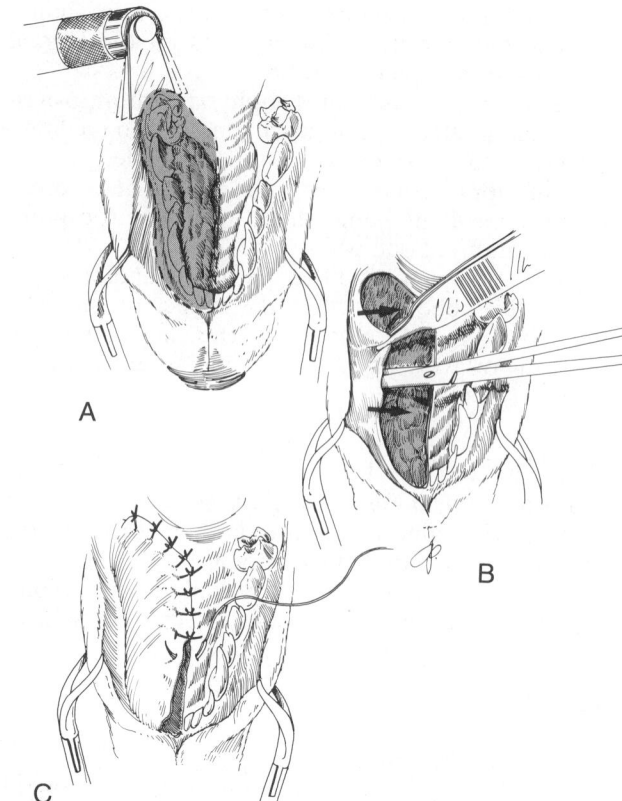

Figure 3. Hemimaxillectomy. *A,* Incise around lesion, then remove mass by ostectomy. Create *(B)* and close *(C)* labial flap.

of the maxilla. This usually is not necessary, but may be beneficial in dogs with a low preoperative packed cell volume (PCV) (see sec. 6, ch. 18 for details of temporary carotid artery occlusion).
5. After mobilizing the bone, sever soft tissue attachments and remove the bone en bloc, exposing the nasal cavity.
   a. Remove nasal turbinates involved in the disease process or damaged severely during ostectomy via sharp dissection.
   b. Control hemorrhage with direct pressure, ligation, cautery, or placement of Gelfoam.
6. Base the labial flap created to close the defect (Fig. 3B and C) rostrally or caudally, with the flap rotated into position, along what was the mucogingival border, with the flap flipped over so the mucosa becomes the floor of the nasal cavity; or along the tip margin, with the mucosa undermined sufficiently to be pulled over the defect.
   a. Flaps based along the lip margins tend to have a poor cosmetic appearance during the initial postoperative period. However, after healing is complete there is little noticeable cosmetic differences among the various techniques.
7. An alternative technique for small lesions is to mobilize the palatal mucosa and slide the mucosa to the incised buccal margin where the tissues are sutured. The exposed hard palate heals by epithelialization. The advantage of this technique is that the operated area is still covered with the normally thicker palatal mucosa.

a. The major palatine artery may have to be ligated. Alternatively, the major palatine foramen can be enlarged with bone rongeurs or a bur, and the major palatine artery can be mobilized and preserved.

Technique

Caudal Hemimaxillectomy

1. The proximity of the palatine, lacrimal, and zygomatic bones may require their resection, depending on the extent of the disease process.
2. Ligate major vessels encountered during the resection.
3. Create labial flaps as described to close the defect.
4. When extensive disease in the caudal maxilla necessitates removal of the bone supporting the globe, postoperative sinking of the globe can be encountered.
   a. Procedures to support the globe, using synthetic materials or adjacent musculature, can be attempted.

Postoperative Care and Complications

■ If necessary, give analgesics during the initial postoperative period for relief of pain.
■ Elizabethan collars are necessary occasionally to prevent self-mutilation or disruption of skin incisions.
■ Feed a liquid diet (water and gruel) on the day following surgery.
   • Intravenous maintenance fluids may be necessary until the animal adapts to the loss of the rostral portion of the mandible or maxilla (1–3 days).
   • Consider pharyngotomy or gastrostomy tubes (see sec. 1, ch. 3) in those rare cases where oral intake is likely to be delayed for a considerable period (e.g., severe debilitation, lingual dysfunction).
■ Evaluate animals as necessary for the first month following surgery. If there are no complications, the initial postoperative evaluation can be delayed until the end of the first month.
   • Subsequently, examine the animal every 3–4 months for evidence of tumor recurrence. If a mass is seen at the site of the previous surgery or elsewhere, obtain a biopsy immediately.
■ Thoracic radiography is recommended every 6 months for evidence of tumor metastasis.
■ Transient edema and ranula can occur following mandibulectomies but usually do not require treatment. Dehiscence of suture lines can be due to excessive tension on the excisional line, excessive use of electrocautery, constant licking by the animal, necrosis of the labial mucosa flap, animal debilitation, and tumor necrosis.
   • Examine the oral cavity to monitor incision line healing.
   • Postoperative nasal discharge is presumptive evidence of maxillary suture line dehiscence.
■ Allow minor wound dehiscence to heal by second intention. Resuture more severe breakdowns (e.g., where bone is exposed). Eliminate tension on the suture line.

• In some instances, extraction of the tooth adjacent to the margin of the ostectomy site and elevation of the palatal and buccal mucosa will provide adequate mobility of sufficient tissue to achieve healing at the ends of the ostectomy site.
■ The cosmetic appearance of dogs and cats usually is good, even after major resection of bone and soft tissue.
■ Tissue swelling, inversion of the upper lips, and drooling may occur for several days. These problems improve markedly in a few weeks.
■ Protrusion of the tongue often is temporary following unilateral rostral partial hemimandibulectomy but may be permanent following bilateral rostral partial mandibulectomy.
■ Removal of the TMJ in conjunction with the ramus will cause some medial displacement of the mandible. Infrequently, it is necessary to lower the crown height of the lower canine tooth on the unoperated side to prevent chronic impaction into the oral mucosa of the hard palate, which could result in an oronasal fistula.
   • If the pulp canal is entered during this procedure, seal the pulp canal using a vital pulp canal procedure (see sec. 7, ch. 1). Nasal discharge, noisy respirations, inappetence, and facial swelling may occur after premaxillectomy. With general medical support, these conditions improve in 5–7 days.

RADIATION THERAPY

Radiation therapy is efficacious in treatment of certain oral tumors. Major limitations are the limited number of radiation centers available and the cost.

Indications

■ Radiosensitive neoplasms such as SCC and acanthomatous epulis.
■ Cases in which surgical excision is:
   • Very difficult or impossible
   • Unsuccessful in removing all the neoplastic tissue
■ Combined with surgical excision:
   • To kill residual tumors postoperatively
   • When radiation alone is not effective in treating the neoplasm

Complications

In most cases there is a narrow range between the radiation dose that is curative and one that can cause serious side effects.

■ Common side effects include moist desquamation and mucositis. These problems resolve with supportive care.
■ Hair loss is expected and often is permanent. Hair regrowth of a different color and texture sometimes occurs.
■ Ocular pathology, including corneal ulcers, keratoconjunctivitis sicca, and cataracts, can occur when the irradiated area includes the eye.

- Improper dosing can cause radiation burns resulting in severe tissue sloughing and bone necrosis.
  - This complication in the maxilla can result in an oronasal fistula that may respond poorly to aggressive surgical therapy.
- A long-term complication is recurrence of the tumor in the irradiated field.

Supplemental Readings

Bradley RL, MacEwen EG: Mandibular resection for removal of oral tumors in 30 dogs and 6 cats. J Am Vet Med Assoc 184:460, 1984.

Salisbury SK, Lantz GC: Long-term results of partial mandibulectomy for treatment of oral tumors in 30 dogs. J Am Anim Hosp Assoc 24:285, 1988.

Salisbury SK, Thacker HL, Pantzer EE, et al.: Partial maxillectomy in the dog. Comparison of suture material and closure techniques. Vet Surg 14:265, 1985.

Salisbury SK, Richardson DC, Lantz GC: Partial maxillectomy and premaxillectomy in the treatment of oral neoplasia in the dog and cat. Vet Surg 15:16, 1986.

Withrow SJ, Holmber DL: Mandibulectomy in the treatment of oral cancer. J Am Anim Hosp Assoc 19:273, 1983.

5 Fractures and Dislocation of the Spine

S. D. Wagner

ATLANTOAXIAL INSTABILITY

Atlantoaxial instability can result in varying degrees of compression to the cervical spinal cord. Miniature and small-breed dogs are most often affected by absence, malformation, failure to ossify, and insufficient ligamentous support of the odontoid process. Fractures of the odontoid process or between the process and body of C2 can occur in dogs of all breeds.

Surgical Anatomy of the Atlantoaxial Area

- The atlantoaxial joint is a pivot joint that permits the head and atlas to rotate around a longitudinal axis.
- The dens or odontoid process is a peglike eminence along the ventral surface of C2 (axis) which projects rostrally to lie on the floor of C1 (atlas) in the spinal canal.
- The dens is secured to the ventral arch of the atlas by the transverse atlantal ligament, to the occipital condyles by the paired alar ligaments, and to the ventral aspect of the foramen magnum by the apical dental ligament. The dorsal arches of the atlas and axis are stabilized by the dorsal atlantoaxial ligament.

KEY POINT ▶ Luxation with an intact dens, luxation resulting from congenital dens malformation, and fractures through the dens or body of the axis result in dorsal displacement of the axis and compression of the spinal cord (Fig. 1).

Clinical Signs and Diagnosis

- Clinical signs range from cervical pain to motor dysfunction in all four limbs.

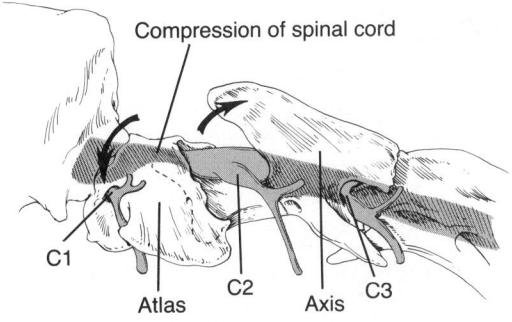

Figure 1. Dorsal displacement of the axis.

- Lateral cervical radiography under general anesthesia may show widening of the atlantoaxial space (i.e., the space between the dorsal spine of the axis and the dorsal arch of the atlas). Ventrodorsal and open mouth radiography can outline the dens.

Surgical Procedures

Preoperative Considerations

- Be cautious when manipulating the neck, especially in flexion, to minimize further damage to the spinal cord.
- Ventilator assistance may be indicated if acute cord edema affects respiratory centers.
- The surgical procedures described here require advanced skills; therefore, these cases should be referred to a surgical specialist.

Objectives

- Stabilize the dorsal arch of the atlas to the dorsal spine of the axis with a prosthetic ligament.
- Stabilize fractures and/or remove malformed dens.
- Avoid further damage to the spinal cord.

Equipment

- Standard orthopedic and neurologic packs
- Gelpi or Weitlaner self-retaining retractors
- Lempert rongeurs or high-speed pneumatic drill and small round bur
- Bipolar cautery and suction setup
- Large-gauge (0–2) monofilament synthetic suture material
- K-wires or small Steinmann pins
- Rigid vacuum-type apparatus* for patient stabilization on operating room table

Technique

Dorsal Approach
1. Place the animal in sternal recumbency with the front legs tied cranially and the head supported in a slightly flexed position.
2. Prepare the skin from the middle of the cranium to C7 for aseptic surgery.
3. Incise the skin on the dorsal midline from the external occipital protubance to C3 or C4.

*Vac-pac, Olympic Medical, Seattle, WA 98108.

965

4. Palpate the transverse processes of C1 and the spinous process of C2.
5. Reflect the paravertebral muscles from the arches of C1 and the spinous process of C2 from the midline, and retract with self-retaining retractors. These muscles are the cervicoscutularis, cervicoauricularis superficialis, and platysma. Separate the paired cervicoscutularis and cervicoauricularis muscles, which join at a fibrous raphe.
6. With deeper dissection, separate the paired bellies of the biventor cervicis, and elevate the rectus capitis dorsalis major muscle to expose the dorsal spinous process of the axis. Reflect the caudal capitis muscle from one side of the spinous process of the axis.
7. If dissection is to extend laterally, identify and preserve the paravertebral and cerebrospinal arteries and the first and second cervical nerves.
8. The spinal cord can be decompressed by hemilaminectomy, but this usually is not indicated. Perform decompression by removing the caudal arch of the atlas and cranial dorsolateral lamina of axis with Lempert rongeurs or high-speed drill.

KEY POINT ▶ Removal of too much dorsal arch will compromise dorsal fixation.

a. Continuous downward pressure on the spine of the axis will reduce the luxation.
9. Drill two transverse holes (cranial and caudal) into the dorsal spine of the axis.
10. Insert a reversed swedged-on needle of adequate length, extradurally, starting at the caudal edge and under the dorsal arch of the atlas.
11. When the needle is visualized at the atlanto-occipital space, form a retrieval loop from the accompanying suture material (Fig. 2).
12. Pass the prosthetic suture material through the retrieval loop and pull the loop under the dorsal atlas arch.
13. Fashion the prosthetic ligament from nonmetallic, heavy-gauge monofilament suture material. Divide the prosthetic ligament suture, pass the ends through the holes in the axis, and tie secure.
14. Routinely close the incision with interrupted absorbable suture material in an interrupted pattern.

Technique

Ventral Approach

This approach is indicated when damaged dorsal structures cannot support a fixation device or when dorsal repair has failed.

KEY POINT ▶ Arthrodesis of the C1–C2 joint space is described but is technically difficult to perform.

1. Place the animal in dorsal recumbency with the front legs tied caudally.
2. Prepare the ventral cervical region, from the caudal mandibles to the manubrium, for aseptic surgery; include an area on the proximal humerus for bone graft.
3. Incise the skin on the ventral cervical midline from the larynx to vertebra C4.

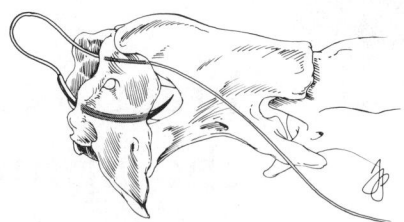

Figure 2. Swedged-on needle technique for prosthetic ligament.

4. Separate the paired sternohyoideus muscles and retract with self-retaining retractors. Elevate the longus colli muscle from vertebral bodies.
5. Identify, protect, and retract the trachea, esophagus, carotid sheath, and vagus nerve (away from the surgeon).
6. Identify the C1–C2 joint caudal to the pointed ventral tubercle of C1.
7. If indicated, excise a malformed or fractured odontoid process through a burred slot made in the ventral arch of the atlas.
8. Remove the cartilage from the articular surfaces of the C1–C2 joint; drive transarticular pins from the ventral surface of the axis across the atlantoaxial joint into the atlas, medial to the alar notch.
9. Collect cancellous bone from the proximal humerus and implant at the arthrodesis site.
10. Using absorbable suture material, close muscles and subcutaneous tissue routinely in a simple interrupted pattern.

Postoperative Care and Complications

- The respiratory center may be damaged at the time of injury or intraoperatively. Provide ventilatory assistance, gradually weaning from the ventilator by serial monitoring of arterial blood gases when the animal is exposed to short periods of room air.
- Support the surgical site with neck and body braces.
- Restrict exercise for 3–4 weeks.
- Complications of the dorsal approach:
  - Suture breakage and reluxation
  - Insufficient bone to support the fixation device
  - Insufficient reduction
  - Suture material pulled out of bone
- Complications of the ventral approach:
  - Iatrogenic damage to the spinal cord with orthopedic pins
  - Inadequate pin placement
  - Pin migration before bony fusion occurs

SPINAL FRACTURES AND DISLOCATIONS

Repair of spinal fractures and dislocations depends on the area of spinal cord involvement, neurologic signs, size of patient, the surgeon's expertise, amount of vertebral displacement, ventral stability, concurrent injuries, and continued neurologic deterioration despite medical management.

- Consider surgical stabilization for animals with spinal fractures or luxations that are unstable and are not responding to medical therapy.

KEY POINT ▶ The thoracolumbar and lumbosacral junctions are prone to fracture and luxation because they are the sites of marked transition between the stiff and the mobile sections of the spine.

Surgical Anatomy

- Vertebrae vary in size and shape and consist of:
  - Body
  - Dorsal arch that forms the spinal canal
  - Paired lateral invertebral foramina through which the spinal nerves, arteries, and veins pass
  - Single dorsal spines (other than C1) that vary in size
  - Cranial and caudal articular facets
  - Transverse, accessory, and mammillary processes for muscle attachment
  - Fibrocartilaginous disc interposed between vertebral endplates
- The ratio of vertebral canal diameter to spinal cord diameter is greater in the cervical area than other areas.
- The cervical dorsal spinous processes are poorly formed (short and thin) whereas the thoracic and mid-lumbar vertebrae have large uniform dorsal spinous processes that can support orthopedic devices. The dorsal spinous processes of L7 and S1 are reduced or nonfunctional.
- The cervical vertebral bodies are flat ventrally and are suitable for the application of orthopedic appliances. Surgical exposure of the ventral cervical region generally is easier than with the dorsal approach.
- The lumbar vertebral bodies are long, allowing orthopedic appliance fixation on the dorsolateral surface if major nerve roots from L4–5 through L7–S1 can be avoided. The ventral approach to lumbar vertebrae for internal stabilization generally is not recommended.
- Lateral surgical exposure to the thoracic vertebrae is hindered by the rib head and the potential for entrance into the thoracic cavity. Hemilaminectomy or laminectomy of the caudal thoracic vertebrae can be performed.

Surgical Procedures

Preoperative Considerations

- Recognition of clinical neurologic signs exhibited by the awake animal on physical examination is important for lesion location. Intact cerebral recognition of deep pain is important for the prognosis (see sec. 10, ch. 4 for more information on spinal cord diseases).

KEY POINT ▶ If cerebral recognition of pain is absent for 24 hours, the prognosis is poor.

- Take care that physical manipulation does not worsen compression of the spinal cord, especially in a sedated or anesthetized animal.
- Immobilize the animal to prevent additional spinal cord damage prior to surgery; use a small cage or body cast or strap the animal to a rigid board.

- Preoperative radiographs may not show the extent of spinal cord injury due to the fracture luxation.
- Myelography may be indicated to evaluate spinal cord compression at the fracture luxation site and to evaluate areas cranial and caudal to the traumatized area (see sec. 1, ch. 4).

KEY POINT ▶ Localize the lesion by neurologic examination prior to analgesics, sedation, or general anesthesia. Make a complete assessment of body systems (cardiovascular, urogenital, etc.) especially in cases of automobile accidents.

- Spinal fractures or luxations should be repaired by a surgical specialist.

Objectives

- Decompress the spinal cord, if indicated.
- Evaluate spinal cord integrity by durotomy, if indicated.
- Minimize additional trauma to spinal cord by fracture reduction and stabilization.

KEY POINT ▶ No single internal fixation technique or surgical approach is adequate for all vertebral fracture luxations in small animals. Anatomy and lesion location dictate the choice of orthopedic implant.

Equipment

- Orthopedic and neurologic packs
- 2.7 mm and 3.5 mm bone plating sets and Lubra Plates
- Assorted size intramedullary (IM) pins
- Methylmethacrylate
- Gelpi or Weitlaner self-retaining retractors
- Curved, sharp-point Lempert or Cicherelli rongeurs (6½″)
- Power drill
- Bipolar electrocautery and suction setup
- Scalpel blades (#10, 11, 15)
- High-speed pneumatic drill and associated bur sizes
- Gelfoam
- External fixator clamps (medium size)

Technique

Dorsal Approach to Midcervical Vertebrae

1. Place the animal in sternal recumbency, with the cervical neck supported in flexion.
2. Prepare the area from the external occipital protuberance to the first thoracic vertebrae for sterile surgery.
3. Make a midline skin incision.
4. Make a dorsal midline incision in the fibrous median raphe, from the aponeurosis of the platysma, cleidocervicalis, and trapezius muscles.
5. Expose the longitudinal yellow elastic fibers of the nuchal ligament, running from the axis to the first thoracic vertebrae along the dorsal spinous processes.
6. Make an incision in the rectus capitis, spinalis and

semispinalis cervicis, and multifidus cervicis muscles along one side of the nuchal ligament.

7. Control hemorrhage by direct pressure or bipolar cautery or cover the area with a free piece of skeletal muscle or Gelfoam.

8. Spinal cord decompression by laminectomy or hemilaminectomy can be achieved through the dorsal approach.

KEY POINT ▶ Dorsal stabilization of cervical fractures or luxations is difficult because the thin and inconsistent spinous processes in this area may not support dorsal spinous plates; vascular and neurologic structures also make dorsolateral plating difficult.

Technique

Dorsal Approach to the Caudal Cervical Vertebrae

1. Place the animal in sternal recumbency, with the cervical neck supported in flexion.

2. Prepare the dorsal cervical region from the external occipital protuberance to the fifth thoracic vertebrae for aseptic surgery.

3. Incise the skin on the midline from C2 to T1.

4. Incise and retract the midline raphe, which is composed of the aponeurosis of the trapezius muscle cranially and rhomboideus muscle caudally.

5. Expose the subscapularis laterally, the splenius cranially, and serratus dorsalis muscle caudally.

6. Incise the splenius and serratus dorsalis muscles to expose the semispinalis capitis and longissimus cervicis muscles, along with the nuchal ligament.

7. Dissect the semispinalis capitis, longissimus cervicis, and multifidus muscles to expose the dorsal spinous processes.

8. Spinal cord decompression of the affected area is achieved by dorsal laminectomy.

Technique

Ventral Approach

1. Place the animal in dorsal recumbency, with the front legs tied caudally and the neck extended.

2. Prepare the ventral cervical region from the caudal mandibles to the manubrium for aseptic surgery.

3. Incise the skin on the ventral cervical midline from the larynx to the manubrium.

4. Separate and retract the paired sternohyoideus and sternothyroideus muscles with self-retaining retractors.

5. Identify and retract the following structures: esophagus, carotid artery, jugular vein, vagosympathetic trunk, and recurrent laryngeal nerve.

6. Elevate the longus colli muscle from the ventral surface of the vertebral body.

7. If indicated, place a bone plate ventrally so that at least two screw holes engage on either side of the fracture luxation after the ventral spinous processes have been burred to provide a flat surface.
   a. Angle the screws in the plate away from spinal cord.
   b. Plastic plates placed in this area are flexible so that the cancellous screws do not pull out of the bone, although the plate may break.

c. If necessary, add cancellous bone graft from the proximal humerus to the fracture site to increase the chances of fusion.

8. If the plate cannot be applied ventrally, place two Steinmann IM pins or bone screws in each vertebra on either side of the fracture luxation at angles of 25–30° to the midline and directed into the dorsolateral vertebral cortex.
   a. Align the fracture and apply methylmethacrylate in a circular mass to incorporate the Steinmann pins or screws.
   b. Be sure that the size of bone cement on the orthopedic implants does not interfere with normal tracheal position when closing the wound.

9. Close the ventral muscles and subcutaneous tissue routinely with absorbable suture material in a simple interrupted pattern.

Technique

Thoracolumbar Fracture Luxation

1. Place the animal in sternal recumbency and use a vacuum positioner (see Vac-pac previously) to stabilize in this position.

2. Prepare the area T8 through L7 for sterile surgery.

3. Make a midline to slightly lateral dorsal midline skin incision.

4. Expose the dense lumbodorsal fascia after incision of the fat.

5. Incise the supraspinous ligament around and between the tip of each dorsal spinous process.

6. Elevate the multifidus lumborum muscle from the spinous processes and vertebral arches laterally to the mammillary processes.

7. Incise the muscular aponeurosis on each mammillary and accessory process. Blood vessels will be encountered at each process.

8. Be careful to identify the dorsal branches of the spinal nerves at the intervertebral foramina.

9. Palpate rib 13 to use as a landmark to locate the area of trauma.

10. Perform laminectomy or hemilaminectomy if decompression is indicated. Avoid placing rongeur jaws into spinal canal.

Technique

Internal Fixation for Thoracolumbar Fracture Luxation
Dorsolateral Vertebral Body Plate (Fig. 3)

1. Position the metal bone plate dorsal to the transverse process so that hemilaminectomy of the spinal cord can be performed without loss of fixation. Hemilaminectomy can also be done before applying the plate.

2. Limit plate application to the caudal thoracic and cranial lumbar region to avoid severing the femoral, sciatic, and pudendal nerves as they exit the caudal lumbar region.

3. Place bone screws into the vertebral bodies angled away from the spinal cord, but not in a ventral direction, to avoid vascular structures.

4. Plate application to caudal thoracic vertebrae requires dislocation of rib heads.

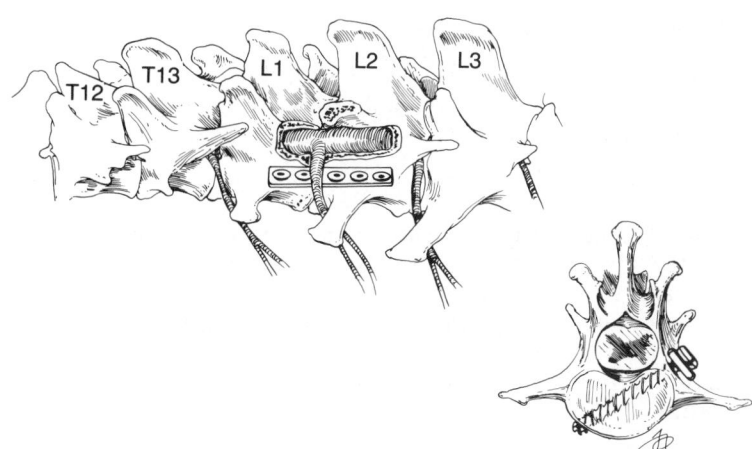

Figure 3. Dorsolateral vertebral body plate. Inset shows correct angle of body screws.

Dorsal Spinous Process Stabilization

Use this method to stabilize comminuted vertebral body fractures or fractures of the caudal lumbar spine when the major nerve roots do not allow vertebral body plating. The dorsal spinous processes must be present and intact.

1. "Sandwich" the dorsal spinous processes between two polyvinylidine fluoride plates (Lubra Plate) by a bolt, with washer and nut, that passes between the processes.
2. Distal to L4, the dorsal spinous processes may not be prominent enough to support this manner of fixation.
   a. Attach the caudal end of the plate to transilial pins.
   b. Use a combined dorsal spinal plate fixation and a type II external fixator (Kirschner-Ehmer).
   c. Repair fracture luxation of L7–S1 with transilial pins alone.

KEY POINT ▶ In biomechanical studies applied to isolated canine lumbar spines, the combination of a dorsal spinous process plate and a dorsolateral vertebral body plate provided the most rigid stabilization.

Other Fixation Methods

Other methods of fixation, in decreasing order of stability and strength, are dorsolateral vertebral body plate, dorsal spinous process plate, polymethylmethacrylate-pin technique, and vertebral body cross-pins. Spinal stapling has not been biomechanically evaluated.

Postoperative Care and Complications

- Turn recumbent animals to avoid pressure sores. Use water bed or air mattress.
- Use manual urinary bladder expression or intermittent catheterization q8h for dogs unable to urinate. If using an indwelling catheter with closed drainage system, culture urine q48–72h.
- Administer broad-spectrum antibiotic, based on urine bacterial culture and sensitivity tests.
- To maintain hygiene and lessen muscle atrophy, give a whirlpool bath for 20 minutes q12h.
- Avoid gastrointestinal hemorrhage by avoidance or

judicious use of glucocorticoids and minimize hospital stress. An oral H_2 antagonist (e.g., cimetidine) may be indicated to prevent gastrointestinal hemorrhage (see sec. 7, ch. 4).
- Monitor for breakage or loosening of orthopedic implants before fracture luxation heals. Plastic plates may fail owing to fracture of plates or dorsal spinal process. A methylmethacrylate collar can fracture.
  - Wound drainage and seroma formation will be evident if plate loosens.
  - Reluxation or fracture failure can occur if orthopedic implants fail; at least 6 weeks is necessary for healing to occur.
  - If reduction is unstable, proliferative callus formation will encroach on the spinal cord, with subsequent worsening of clinical signs.

CAUDAL CERVICAL SPONDYLOMYELOPATHY

Caudal cervical spondylomyelopathy (wobbler syndrome) is a condition characterized by extradural spinal cord compression due to malformation of bony or ligamentous structures that react to instability or chronic disc disease. Affected animals have an abnormal gait most noticeable in the rear legs. Great Danes and Doberman pinschers are most commonly affected, but the disorder may occur in other breeds. Great Danes are usually affected at a young age, Dobermans may not exhibit clinical signs until middle age. The compressive lesions can be static (constant pressure) or dynamic (intermittent pressure).

KEY POINT ▶ The compressive lesion of caudal cervical spondylomyelopathy is usually hypertrophy of the annulus fibrosus secondary to chronic disc disease, vertebral malformation, or instability.

Anatomy
Cervical Spinal Canal

- Articular facets and joint capsule
- Vertebral canal
- Ligamentum flavum located dorsal to the canal
- Dorsal longitudinal ligament and dorsal annulus fibrosus, located ventral to the canal
- Cervical vertebral bodies (rectangular in shape)

Clinical Signs

■ Signs include varying degrees of neurologic deficit, including pain, paraparesis, ambulatory tetraparesis, and nonambulatory tetraparesis.

Diagnosis

■ Lateral radiography may show bony vertebral body changes, but myelogram is necessary to demonstrate sites and type of cord compression.
■ Stress radiography (mild flexion, mild extension, or linear traction) during myelogram may differentiate static compression from dynamic compression on the cord.

KEY POINT ▶ *Caution:* Flexion and tension stress radiography can worsen clinical signs.

■ Myelography findings:
  • Ventral spinal cord compression from hypertrophied dorsal annulus fibrosus secondary to chronic type II disc disease (i.e., gradual protrusion of a disc into the spinal canal)
  • Dorsal spinal cord compression from hypertrophied ligamentum flavum
  • Dorsolateral compression from malformed articular processes
  • Compression from tipping of the craniodorsal edge of the caudal vertebral body and the caudodorsal lamina of the cranial vertebra

Preoperative Considerations

■ Prior to surgery, wean animals from antiprostaglandins (e.g., Banamine) and nonsteroidal anti-inflammatory drugs (NSAIDs).
  • Aspirin can cause platelet dysfunction for the life of the circulating platelet (10 days).
  • Prolonged bleeding time due to platelet dysfunction makes surgery more difficult.

Surgical Procedures

No single operative procedure can be recommended for all dogs. The procedures described should be performed by a surgical specialist. Because hypertrophy of the dorsal annulus fibrosus at C5–C6 and C6–C7 is relatively common, two methods of treatment for this condition are described in detail: ventral decompression alone and ventral distraction with vertebral fusion.

Objectives and Indications

■ Base the decision for surgery and choice of technique on stress myelography (flexion-extension) and on linear traction radiographic findings.
■ Dorsal laminectomy with fat graft is indicated for static lesions such as ligamentum flavum hypertrophy, malformed articular processes, and vertebral canal stenosis.
  • Disadvantages include the requirement for extensive muscle dissection, especially in large breeds, and the potential for fracture through the articular facets.

• An advantage is that compression can be done at multiple sites through a single surgical approach.
■ Ventral decompression alone is indicated when a single disc space is involved, to remove disc material and the dorsal annulus fibrosus for decompression of the spinal cord.
■ Ventral vertebral distraction and fusion is indicated for a compressive lesion that can be resolved by linear traction. Advantages include:
  • The dorsal annulus fibrosus is preserved.
  • The spinal canal is not entered.
  • Distraction can be maintained with a tibial cortical allograft held in position with a plastic plate, with Steinmann pins and a methylmethacrylate collar, or with a Harrington rod that hooks into the ventral aspect of the vertebral end plates.

Equipment

■ Orthopedic and neurologic packs
■ Scalpel blades (# 10, 11, 15)
■ Gelpi retractors
■ Suction and electrocautery setup
■ Gelfoam or bone wax
■ High-speed air drill and burs
■ Lubra Plates, drill bits, screw taps, and bone screws
■ Power drill

Technique

Ventral Decompression

1. Place the animal in dorsal recumbency, with the front legs tied caudally and the neck slightly hyperextended.
2. Prepare the ventral cervical region from caudal mandible to manubrium for aseptic surgery.
3. Incise the skin from the wing of C1 to the manubrium.
4. Separate the paired sternohyoideus muscles.
5. Retract the trachea and esophagus to the left of the midline. To prevent tracheal collapse, be sure that the endotracheal tube extends to the thoracic inlet.
6. Elevate the longus colli muscles from the ventral aspects of the involved intervertebral space.
7. Use the transverse processes of C6 as landmarks to locate the involved disc space.
8. Bur out the disc space initially to visualize its cranial slope.
9. Outline the proposed slot with the bur: the slot should be one-half the length and width of the adjacent vertebral body; an oval or rectangular slot works well.
10. Remove the bone in three uniform layers, observing color changes to recognize when approaching the spinal canal.
11. Control bleeding from cancelleous bone by packing with gauze sponges, Gelfoam, muscle, or bone wax.
12. Remove the dorsal part of the annulus fibrosus, using blunt tartar scrapers, a #11 surgical blade, fine hemostats, or a small curet.

13. Avoid laceration of the vertebral sinus, which has been displaced. When suction is used, especially in small dogs, be careful that exsanguination does not occur from a lacerated sinus.
14. Flush the area with saline solution.
15. Close the muscle, including the longus colli, with absorbable suture material in an interrupted pattern.

Technique

Ventral Distraction with Vertebral Fusion

1. Make a ventral slot, using an approach similar to that described previously for ventral decompression, with the following exceptions:
   a. The spinal cord is not invaded.
   b. The depth of the slot is approximately three-fourths of the vertebral body width, measured radiographically.
2. Place a cortical allograft in the slot while applying linear traction on the animal's head and limbs.
   a. Alternatively, autogenous cancellous bone can be used to fill the slot.
   b. Gelpi retractors can be used as a vertebral spreader.
3. Hold the graft in place with a plastic bone plate and four screws that engage the vertebral bone on either side of the slot (Fig. 4).
   a. Steinmann pins and a methylmethacrylate collar can be used instead of a plastic plate.
4. Close the soft tissue as previously described for ventral decompression.

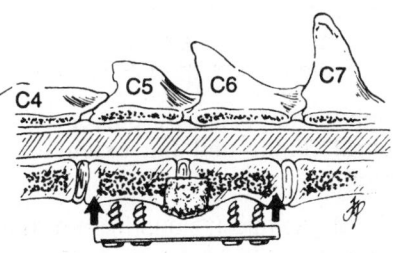

Figure 4. Ventral distraction and fusion of cervical vertebrae.

KEY POINT ▶ Ventral vertebral fusion is used for dynamic lesions in which traction will reduce ligamentous redundancy.

Postoperative Care and Complications

- Nursing problems in large dogs that are not ambulatory are common. Avoid pressure sores.
- Neck braces that extend to thorax can be used for support.
- The condition may worsen as a result of surgical trauma, hemorrhage, inadequate tissue removal, inadequate reduction, and improper placement of orthopedic equipment.
- Long-term problems include:
  - Movement of the orthopedic implant
  - Failure of distraction devices
  - Collapse of the disc space
- Accelerated degenerative changes in the disc spaces adjacent to the surgically fused area may cause recurrence of clinical signs (domino effect).

Prognosis

- The prognosis is better in animals presenting with pain alone, paraparesis, or ambulatory tetraparesis.
- Nonambulatory tetraparetic patients have a poor prognosis.

Supplemental Readings

Bruecker KA, Seim HB, Withrow SJ: Clinical evaluation of three surgical methods for treatment of caudal cervical spondylomyelopathy of dogs. Vet Surg 18:197, 1989.

Cook JR, Oliver JE: Atlantoaxial luxation in the dog. Compend Contin Educ Pract Vet 3(3):242, 1981.

Lewis DD, Stampley A, Bellah JR, et al.: Repair of sixth lumbar vertebral fracture-luxations, using transilial pins and plastic spinous-process plates in six dogs. J Am Vet Med Assoc 194:538, 1989.

Lyman R: Continuous dorsal laminectomy for the treatment of caudal cervical vertebral instability and malformation. Proceedings 13th Kal Kan Symposium, The Ohio State University Press, 1989.

VanGundy TE: Disc-associated wobbler syndrome in the Doberman pinscher. Vet Clin North Am 18:667, 1988.

Walter MC, Smith GK, Newton CD: Canine lumbar spinal internal fixation techniques: A comparative biomechanical study. Vet Surg 15:191, 1986.

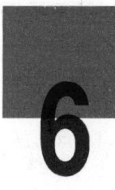

6 Neoplasia of the Axial Skeleton

Mark M. Smith

Osteosarcoma and chondrosarcoma are the two most common primary neoplasms affecting the axial skeleton. These neoplasms have a similar radiographic appearance, with osteolytic, osteoblastic, or mixed osteoblastic/osteolytic characteristics. Hemangiosarcoma and fibrosarcoma are other primary bone tumors that must be considered. Overall, these tumors more commonly affect the ribs and pelvis than the vertebrae. Multilobular osteoma (chondroma rodens) is the most common tumor of the skull.

Early recognition and accurate diagnosis are of paramount importance for client education and rationale for surgical intervention. Surgery may be diagnostic (vertebrae), palliative (pelvis), or curative (rib), depending on tumor invasiveness and location of axial skeletal involvement. Tumors of the mandible, maxilla, and nasal cavity are discussed in other chapters in this section. The types of neoplasms and principles of treatment discussed in this chapter are similar to those for tumors of the cranium. Removal of cranial tumors requires specialized equipment and skills and therefore is best handled by a surgical specialist. Tumors of the appendicular skeleton are discussed in sec. 9, ch. 22.

HISTORY AND CLINICAL SIGNS

- Patients usually are presented for swelling over a bony prominence.
- Intrathoracic extension of neoplasia of the rib may cause respiratory compromise.
- Pain or an unusual gait secondary to neurologic dysfunction (transverse myelopathy) may be related to neoplasms of the vertebrae.
- Animals with skull tumors usually present because of a palpable mass. Neurologic signs may develop if brain impingement occurs.
- Constipation may result from pelvic tumors.

DIAGNOSIS

Pelvis and Ribs

- Include two radiographic projections of the lesion.
- Radiographic signs of primary bone neoplasms (e.g., osteosarcoma, chondrosarcoma) may range from primarily lytic to proliferative lesions.
- Polyostotic lytic lesions are seen with malignant lymphoma and multiple myeloma (see sec. 3, ch. 6).

KEY POINT ▶ Do not use radiography as the sole basis for determining tumor type.

- Determine the presence of metastatic disease.
  - Perform palpation, and fine-needle aspiration of regional lymph nodes, if enlarged.
  - Evaluate three-projection thoracic radiographs (ventrodorsal, left, and right lateral) to detect pulmonary metastasis.
  - Perform abdominal palpation for mass lesions, vertebral palpation for metastasis-related pain, and a rectal examination for intrapelvic masses.

Skull and Vertebrae

- Survey radiographs of the spine often show osteolysis secondary to primary bone neoplasia or to invasion of soft tissue neoplasia.
- Osteosarcoma or multilobular osteoma of the cranium appears radiographically as a proliferative bony lesion of the flat bones.
- Perform cerebral spinal fluid (CSF) analysis to rule out infection and inflammation (see sec. 10, ch. 1). CSF of patients with vertebral neoplasia may have increased levels of protein and elevated pressure.

KEY POINT ▶ Because most tumors affecting the spinal cord are extradural, cytologic examination of the CSF may be normal.

- Myelography is important to detect the exact site of the vertebral tumor and the extent of spinal cord compression.

KEY POINT ▶ Metastatic lesions from remote malignant tumors may mimic primary neoplasms of the axial skeleton. Histopathologic examination of biopsy tissue is required for differentiation.

- Computed tomography (CT) is useful to evaluate intracranial effects of skull tumors.

Bone Biopsy

Objectives

- Obtain multiple tissue samples of the tumor for histopathologic diagnosis.
- Avoid causing iatrogenic trauma to the vertebrae or skull, if they are involved.

Equipment

- Small suture pack and suture material
- Jamshidi-type biopsy needle or bone trephine
- Sterile ruler

Technique

1. Prepare the cutaneous area over the tumor site for aseptic surgery.
2. Make a skin incision large enough to introduce the biopsy instrument over the center of the lesion.
3. Measure the center of the tumor from the nearest prominent anatomic landmark.
4. Take a minimum of two biopsies: one from the center of the tumor and one from the center directed to the periphery. Use extreme caution when performing biopsy of tumors of the cranium.
5. Using a horizontal mattress pattern, place sutures of absorbable material in the subcutaneous or fascial layers to minimize hemorrhage from the biopsy site.
6. Close the skin with nonabsorbable suture material in a simple interrupted pattern.

KEY POINT ▶ Biopsy of vertebral lesions is best performed during decompressive laminectomy or with the aid of fluoroscopy to guide biopsy needle placement.

TREATMENT

Surgical Procedures for Rib Neoplasia: Resection and Thoracic Wall Reconstruction

Objectives

- Completely remove the thoracic wall mass.
- Attempt to obtain wide tumor-free margins.
- Minimize hemorrhage.
- Provide rigid reconstruction to prevent abnormal chest wall movement.
- Perform airtight closure to prevent pneumothorax.

Equipment

- Standard general surgical pack and suture material
- Two large Gelpi or Beckman self-retaining retractors
- Gigli wire or Liston bone cutters
- Chest tube, 3-way stopcock, and large syringe
- Polypropylene mesh

Technique

1. Place the animal in lateral recumbency with the hindlimbs extended caudally and the forelimbs extended cranially.
2. Prepare the lateral chest wall for aseptic surgery.
3. Incise the skin over the mass. If the tumor is adhered to the dermis, make a large, elliptical skin incision around the tumor.
4. Incise or, preferably, reflect the latissimus dorsi muscle if it is not adhered to the tumor.
5. Incise all remaining muscle layers one intercostal space cranial and caudal to the mass.
6. Cut all involved ribs and intercostal muscles 2 cm dorsal and ventral to the tumor, using Liston bone cutters and Metzenbaum scissors.
7. Clamp and ligate the intercostal arteries and veins.
8. Place a chest tube a minimum of two intercostal spaces cranial or caudal to the resection site.

KEY POINT ▶ Consider giving an intraoperative lidocaine intercostal nerve block to decrease pain during the acute postoperative period (see sec. 6, ch. 25, Principles of Thoracic Surgery).

9. Use polypropylene mesh to reconstruct large thoracic wall defects.
10. Place polydioxanone or polypropylene sutures, using an interrupted horizontal mattress pattern, in a paracostal location to secure the mesh.
    a. A slight fold may be created along all borders of the mesh to provide a double-thickness layer for holding sutures.
11. Secure the mesh to the cut ribs with sutures of similar material, using a circumferential simple interrupted pattern. Create slight tension on the mesh to provide rigidity.
12. Suture the latissimus dorsi and external abdominal oblique muscles over the defect with absorbable suture material in an interrupted pattern to provide a tissue seal.
13. Close subcutaneous tissues with absorbable suture material in an interrupted pattern to minimize dead space.
14. Appose the skin routinely, using nonabsorbable suture material.
15. Use the chest tube system to reestablish negative intrathoracic pressure.

KEY POINT ▶ Small thoracic wall defects may be closed using adjacent latissimus dorsi and external abdominal oblique muscles without the need for a mesh implant.

Postoperative Care and Complications

Short-Term
- Closely monitor for hemorrhage, seroma formation, and pneumothorax.
- Apply a light chest bandage to minimize seroma formation and air migration along the chest tube.

KEY POINT ▶ Place the bandage to allow normal chest excursion and optimal pulmonary function.

- Analgesics that minimally affect pulmonary function (butorphanol, 0.4 mg/kg q6h IM) may be required in the acute postoperative period.

Long-Term
- Repeat physical and radiographic examination every 4–6 months to monitor for recurrence or metastasis.
- Consider adjuvant chemotherapy if the tumor is malignant or if tumor cells are present in resected tissue margins (see discussion of chemotherapy in sec. 3, ch. 5).

Prognosis

- Chest wall neoplasms usually are malignant and carry a poor prognosis if incompletely excised.
- The prognosis is guarded even if the tumor is com-

pletely resected because subclinical distant metastasis may have occurred before surgery.

Surgical Procedure for Pelvic Neoplasia: Resection of the Ilial Wing

Objectives

- Completely remove the pelvic mass.
- Obtain wide, tumor-free margins.
- Minimize hemorrhage.
- Avoid damage to major pelvic limb nerve tracts in order to maintain limb function.

Equipment

- Standard general surgical pack and suture
- Two large Gelpi or Beckman self-retaining retractors
- Gigli wire or osteotome and mallet

Technique

1. Place the animal in lateral recumbency.
2. Prepare the lateral pelvic area and proximal hindlimb for aseptic surgery.
3. Incise the skin over the mass. If the tumor is adhered to the dermis, make a large elliptical incision around the tumor.
4. Incise through the superficial, middle, and deep gluteal muscles cranial to the acetabulum.
5. Incise the sartorius and tensor fascia lata muscles prior to their insertion on the ilium.
6. Incise the iliocostalis and longissimus muscles cranial to the pelvic mass.
7. Incise the quadratus lumborum and iliacus muscles prior to their insertion on the medial aspect of the ilium.
8. Cut the sacroiliac joint and ilial body using a Gigli wire or osteotome and mallet.
9. Elevate the other fascial attachments to free the proximal ilial segment.
10. Control hemorrhage with electrocoagulation or individual vessel ligation.

KEY POINT ▶ Maintain wide margins of excision with no gross evidence of tumor.

11. Closure:
    a. Appose the resected muscle ends by simple interrupted sutures of absorbable material placed in the fascia.
    b. Extensive resection may require Penrose drain placement to minimize potential dead space.

KEY POINT ▶ Make separate small incisions in the surgical area for entrance and exit of drains, avoiding the primary wound incision.

    c. Close subcutaneous tissues with absorbable sutures in a simple interrupted pattern.
    d. Appose the skin similarly, using nonabsorbable sutures.

Postoperative Care and Complications

Short-Term

- Use a modified Robert Jones bandage to decrease the incidence of seroma. Bandage application and maintenance is more cumbersome in male dogs.
- Monitor the wound for signs of seroma and infection.
- Administer analgesic therapy (butorphanol, 0.4-mg/kg, IM, q6h) during the acute postoperative period.

Long-Term

- Repeat physical and radiographic examination every 4–6 months to monitor for recurrence and metastasis.
- Consider adjuvant chemotherapy if the tumor was malignant or if tumor cells are present in resected tissue margins (see discussion of chemotherapy, sec. 3, ch. 5.)

Prognosis

- Same as for rib neoplasia.

Surgical Procedure for Vertebral Neoplasia: Dorsal Laminectomy

Because laminectomy is a difficult surgical procedure that should be performed only by surgical specialists, only an overview of the procedure is given here. (See sec. 10, ch. 4 for more information on principles of surgery of the spinal cord.)

Objectives

- Debulk the tumor.
- Decompress the spinal cord.
- Obtain tissue for histopathologic diagnosis.

Equipment

- Standard general surgical pack and suture material
- Two large Gelpi or Beckman self-retaining retractors
- Pneumatic or electric power equipment for laminectomy
- Kerrison or Lempert bone rongeurs
- Iris scissors

General Procedure

- Preoperatively administer dexamethasone (0.5 mg/kg, IV) to decrease edema of the spinal cord related to surgical manipulation.
- Save adequate amounts of tumor tissue in 10% buffered formalin for histopathologic evaluation.
- The laminectomy procedure ends when the spinal cord is relieved of the compression effect of the tumor.
- Dorsal laminectomy can be combined with hemilaminectomy if additional lateral exposure is required.

KEY POINT ▶ Iatrogenic vertebral fracture/luxation is unlikely, because reactive bone and scar tissue secondary to the neoplasm compensates for the destabilizing sequelae of laminectomy and tumor debulking.

Postoperative Care and Complications

Short-Term

- Monitor for seroma formation and infection at the wound site.
- Perform serial neurologic examinations to monitor neurologic status.
- Administer prednisolone (0.5 mg/kg q12h, PO) for anti-inflammatory therapy (if necessary) until neurologic status is improved.
- Urine retention requires frequent manual decompression of the bladder or maintenance of a closed indwelling catheter system. Monitor for development of urinary tract infection.
- Turn the patient every 4 hours to prevent decubital ulcers secondary to prolonged recumbency.

Long-Term

- Supportive therapy and good nursing care are mandatory during the neurologic recovery period.
- Consider adjuvant chemotherapy and/or radiation therapy (see sec. 3, ch. 5, based on the histopathologic diagnosis, because complete resection of the tumor is not possible.

PROGNOSIS

- The prognosis for malignant tumors of the vertebral axial skeleton is poor.
- Neoplasms secondarily affecting vertebrae (e.g., lymphoma) may warrant a guarded prognosis, based on responsiveness to chemotherapy.

Supplemental Readings

Holiday TA, Higgins RJ, Turrel JM: Tumors of the nervous system. *In* Theilen GH, Madewell BR, eds.: *Veterinary Cancer Medicine.* Philadelphia: Lea & Febiger, 1987, p 601.

LaRue SM, Withrow SJ: Tumors of the skeletal system. *In* Withrow SJ, MacEwen EG, eds.: *Clinical Veterinary Oncology.* Philadelphia: J. B. Lippincott, 1989, p 234.

Orton C.: Thoracic wall. *In* Slatter DH, ed.: *Textbook of Small Animal Surgery.* Philadelphia: W. B. Saunders, 1985, p 536.

7 Fractures of the Shoulder

Thomas M. Turner

Fractures of the shoulder, and particularly of the scapula, may be associated with concurrent thoracic trauma. This may range from nondisplaced rib fractures to more severe internal thoracic trauma such as lung contusions, pneumothorax, and hemothorax (see sec. 6, ch. 24). Damage to neurologic structures such as the brachial plexus and peripheral nerve components, particularly the suprascapular nerve, may also occur with shoulder fractures. Therefore, a thorough preoperative evaluation of the thorax and neurologic function is mandatory before proceeding with definitive fixation.

ANATOMY

- The shoulder is a diarthrodial joint that is dependent on the surrounding supportive soft tissue structures.
  - The primary stabilizing structures are the medial and lateral glenohumeral ligaments and the joint capsule.
  - The more "active" ligaments are the biceps tendon, supraspinatus tendon, infraspinatus tendon, subscapularis tendon, and teres minor tendon.
- The scapula is a broad, thin, expansive bone with a prominent spine along the central aspect of the scapular body.
- The greatest density of bone stock occurs along the line of reflection of the scapular spine from the body and in the region of the scapular neck and glenoid.
- The weakest area of the scapula is at the scapular neck.
- The suprascapular nerve lies along the cranial and lateral aspect of the scapular neck. Identify and protect this structure during the surgical approach and repair of fractures in this area.

FRACTURES OF THE SCAPULA

Preoperative Considerations

- Manage minimally displaced or nondisplaced fractures of the scapula by strict cage confinement or alternatively by placing the animal's limb in a modified Velpeau sling.
- Frequently, fractures involving the scapula tend to override, resulting in relative limb shortening and the potential for impingement on the brachial plexus and other neurovascular structures. Internal fixation of scapula fractures provides rigid stability, thus allowing a very rapid return to function.
- Because of the thinness of the scapula, stabilization of fractures generally is achieved with bone plates. In some fracture types, hemicerclage wires also may be advantageous.
- Assess the integrity of the ligamentous supporting structures and if damaged, repair them to maintain normal shoulder function.

Surgical Procedures

Objectives

- To stabilize the fracture fragments in an anatomic position in order to prevent limb shortening, malalignment, and support of the glenoid, allowing joint function.
- To restore the articular surface of the glenoid to allow return of normal joint range of motion and function.

Equipment

- Standard orthopedic pack, periosteal elevators, bone fragment clamps and plate benders
- Orthopedic wire (0.8 mm and 1.0 mm in diameter) and wire twister (useful in some fractures)
- A wide variety of bone plates, including the 2.0-mm dynamic compression plate (DCP) or cuttable plate, 2.7-mm DCP standard plate and finger plate series (rarely, the 3.5-mm standard plate series may be used)

Technique

Preliminary Procedures

1. Place the animal in lateral recumbency with the limb prepared for aseptic surgery.
2. Use a standard lateral or craniolateral approach to the scapula for exposure of the specific area of the fracture.
3. Select an appropriate bone plate and contour with a plate bender to the specific area to be stabilized.

Technique

Scapular Spine Fractures (Fig. 1)

1. Contour a small finger plate (2.0 mm or 2.7 mm) to 90°, attach to the scapular spine, and then attach to the scapular body with appropriate screws.
2. Alternatively, apply a series of two or more hemicerclage wires to stabilize the spine to the body.

Technique

Fractures or Osteotomy of the Acromion

1. If the fragment is of sufficient size, reattach to the scapular body using a lag screw (2.0 mm, 2.7 mm, or 4.0 mm) (see Fig. 1).

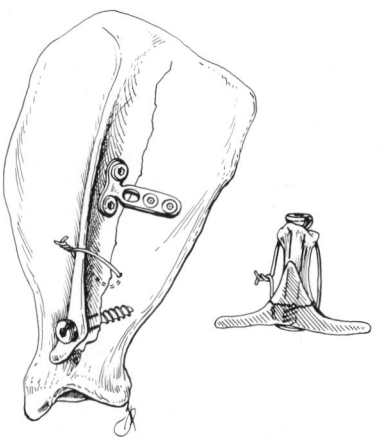

Figure 1. A fracture of the scapular spine can be stabilized using a T-plate and a lag screw through the acromion process into the body. Alternative fixation may be achieved using hemicerclage wires.

2. Alternatively, apply two or more hemicerclage wires to reattach the fragment.
3. As another alternative, stabilize the fracture with a figure-eight cerclage wire, with or without Kirschner pins, using a tension band technique (Fig. 2).

Technique

Fractures of the Scapular Body
▪ Anatomic reduction of the fracture fragments involving the body is important to restore proper anatomic length.

1. To achieve fixation of the fracture fragments, apply a bone plate either cranial or caudal to the scapular spine.
2. Preferably, use three or more screws on either side of the fracture line.

KEY POINT ▶ To obtain maximum thread purchase, direct screws obliquely into the region of the reflection of the scapular spine from the body.

3. Stabilize multiple fractures individually with a combination of small plates and hemicerclage wires.
4. Alternatively, place the fracture fragments in anatomic position and bridge the entire area with the plate serving as a buttress.

Technique

Scapular Neck Fractures (Fig. 3)
▪ Scapular neck fractures tend to override, owing to the distal pull of the deltoid muscles and the medial and proximal pull of the pectoralis muscles.
▪ Displacement of these fractures may result in impingement on the adjacent brachial plexus as well as limb shortening and compromise of the range of motion of the shoulder.

1. Identify and protect the suprascapular nerve.
2. Use fingerplate or mini-fingerplate series and standard plates (2.0 mm and 2.7 mm) for stabilizing fractures in this area.
3. Alternatively, stabilize these fractures with two Kirschner pins inserted in a crosspin technique.
   a. It may be difficult to insert the pins at a proper angle to achieve maximum purchase on either side of the fracture line.

Technique

Glenoid Fractures (Fig. 4)
1. Approach via an osteotomy of the acromion.

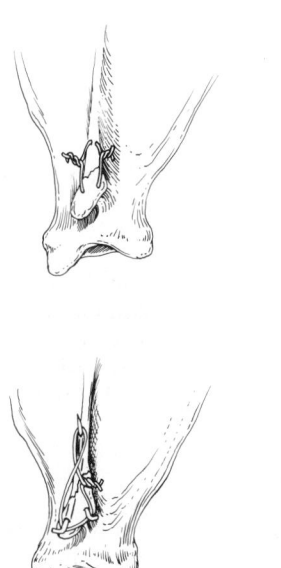

Figure 2. A fracture of the acromion process may be stabilized with two interfragmentary wires *(top)* or with a Kirschner wire and a figure-eight wire *(bottom)*.

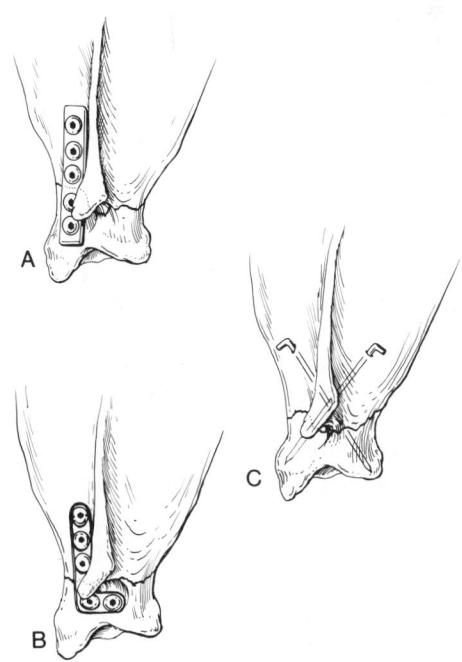

Figure 3. *A*, A scapular neck fracture may be stabilized with a 2.7 mm or 2.0 mm standard plate if at least two screws of purchase can be obtained in the glenoid fragment. Alternatively, the fracture may be stabilized using *(B)* a finger plate, which allows for two screws of purchase parallel to the articular surface, or *(C)* two crossed Kirschner wires.

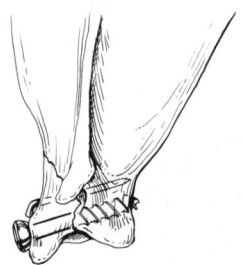

Figure 4. Stabilized glenoid fractures with a lag screw to compress the fracture site, obtaining supplementary fixation with a Kirschner wire.

KEY POINT ▶ Because they are intra-articular fractures, glenoid fractures always require open reduction and internal fixation. Accurate alignment of the articular surface is imperative to restore normal joint function.

2. Identify and protect the suprascapular nerve.
3. When the fracture fragments are anatomically repositioned and the articular surface is congruous, achieve fixation with a Kirschner pin inserted parallel to the articular surface.
4. Insert a lag screw parallel to the articular surface to obtain compression of the fracture site. The Kirschner pin may be retained to serve as supplemental fixation or, if sufficient bone stock allows, may be replaced with an additional lag screw.

Scapular Tuberosity Avulsions

■ This fracture is an avulsion of the cranial aspect of the glenoid rim. The tuberosity is the site of attachment of the tendon of origin of the biceps muscle.
■ This fracture occurs most frequently in immature animals.
■ The fracture fragment usually is small, composed primarily of metaphyseal bone, and is distracted distally, owing to contracture of the biceps muscle.

Technique

1. Osteotomy of the greater tubercle of the humerus provides the best exposure for repair of this fracture (see description later in this chapter of osteotomy repair).
2. When anatomic reduction is achieved, stabilize the fracture using a single lag screw (2.7 mm or 4.0 mm).
3. Alternatively, stabilize the fracture with a tension band wire technique, using 1–2 Kirschner pins and a figure-eight wire.

KEY POINT ▶ The avulsed fragment of bone usually is small and soft. Therefore, avoid overtightening the screw, which can result in iatrogenic fragmentation of the scapular tuberosity.

T Fractures

■ These fractures are a combination of a scapular neck fracture and a glenoid fracture. They are difficult to repair and generally require an acromion osteotomy.

Technique

1. Direct attention initially to reestablishing the articular surface of the glenoid fragments (see previous discussion of glenoid fractures).
2. Re-attach the reconstructed glenoid fragment to the scapular body, using a standard plate or fingerplate series (2.0 mm, 2.7 mm) (see previous discussion of scapular neck fractures).

Postoperative Care

■ Restrict activity for 6 weeks or longer, depending on the healing of the fracture as well as the degree of comminution of the fracture fragments.
■ Evaluate the fracture radiographically at 4–6 week intervals until it has healed.
■ If pending failure is evident radiographically (e.g., loosened screws), institute one or more of the following measures:
  • Restrict the animal's activity further.
  • Apply coaptation splint support.
  • Place the limb in a non–weight bearing sling.
  • Perform an additional internal stabilization procedure.

Complications

■ Malalignment at the articular surface is an important potential complication.
■ Malalignment of the scapular body may lead to a valgus or varus position of the limb. Nonunion of fractures in these locations is rare.
■ A more commonly encountered complication is injury to the suprascapular nerve, which can result in atrophy of the infraspinatus muscles.

Prognosis

■ The prognosis is good provided technical principles of bone plate application are followed.
■ The potential for restoration of shoulder joint range of motion is good.

PROXIMAL HUMERAL FRACTURES

See also sec. 9, ch. 9, Fractures of the Humerus.

Preoperative Considerations

■ Fractures of the proximal humerus occur with much less frequency than scapular fractures.
■ Generally, these fractures occur in skeletally immature animals in the form of a Salter type I or II fracture (see sec. 9, ch. 25) with involvement of the growth plate.

Surgical Procedures

■ Physeal fractures generally require only a craniolateral approach to the shoulder.
■ Complex fractures involving the humeral head require osteotomy of the acromion and a shoulder joint capsulotomy.
■ Fractures involving the humeral head necessitate

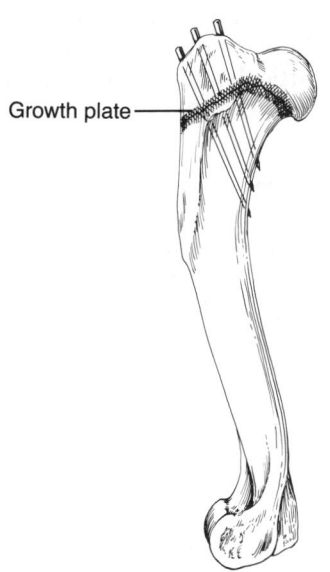

Figure 5. A Salter physeal fracture of the proximal humerus may be stabilized using two or three small-diameter pins or Kirschner wires.

reestablishment of the articular surface in order to be congruent with the opposite glenoid cavity.

Objectives

- Restore anatomic alignment of the articular surface.
- Restore function by reestablishing joint congruency and stability.

Equipment

- Standard orthopedic pack and bone reduction forceps
- A selection of Kirschner and Steinmann pins

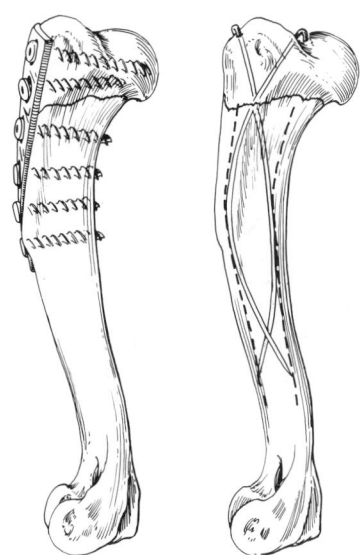

Figure 6. A fracture of the humeral neck may be stabilized with a standard dynamic compression plate (DCP) or T-plate, obtaining a minimum of two screws of purchase in the proximal fragment *(left)*, or with Rush pins or smooth pins inserted using a Rush pin technique *(right)*.

- Bone plate sets including 2.7-mm and 3.5-mm series (occasionally a 4.5-mm series)

Technique

Preliminary Procedures

1. Place the animal in lateral recumbency with the limb prepared for aseptic surgery.
2. Use a standard lateral or craniolateral approach for exposure of the specific area of the humeral fracture.

Technique

Fractures of the Proximal Epiphysis (Fig. 5)

1. In immature animals, stabilize the fracture using two or more smooth Kirschner or Steinmann pins inserted from the proximal aspect of the greater tubercle into the caudal cortex of the metaphyseal region.
2. Alternatively, stabilize the fracture fragment with Rush pins or pins inserted in a Rush pin technique.

Technique

Fractures or Osteotomy of the Greater Tubercle

1. In immature animals, stabilize the tubercle with two or more smooth Kirschner or Steinmann pins. Insert the pins through the tubercle into the caudal cortex.
2. In mature animals, stabilize the tubercle with two or more lag screws or pins.

Technique

Fractures of the Humeral Head

1. If only one fracture line is present, anatomically align and stabilize the fracture fragment with three smooth Kirschner pins; in mature animals, use lag screws.
   a. Avoid penetrating the articular surface of the humeral head.
2. If multiple fragments of the humeral head are present, reconstruct and stabilize them with appropriate Kirschner pins or lag screws, and then reattach to the proximal humeral metaphyseal region. If necessary, use a bone plate to support the reconstructed fragments.

Lesser Tubercle Fractures

- These fractures occur most frequently in immature animals.
- Use lag screw fixation for stabilization.

Technique

Fractures of the Humeral Neck (Fig. 6)

1. Anatomically align the fracture fragment and then stabilize it using a T-plate, with the horizontal aspect of the plate directed proximally, or a standard DCP plate, with at least two screws of purchase in the proximal fragment.
2. Alternatively, stabilize the fracture using smooth Kirschner pins or small-diameter Steinmann pins inserted in a Rush pin technique.

Postoperative Care

- Obtain appropriate radiographs immediately postoperatively and at intervals of 4–6 weeks until the fracture is healed.

- Assess the shoulder joint by placing the shoulder through a range-of-motion exercise to be certain that metal does not protrude into the articular surface and that the shoulder is stable.

Complications

- Nonunion or malunion in this region occurs rarely.
- Premature closure of the proximal humeral growth occurs infrequently.

Prognosis

- Owing to the high density of cancellous bone and the large cross-sectional area present, these fractures usually heal consistently and rapidly.

- The prognosis is good for maintaining a normal range of motion of the shoulder, provided accurate alignment of the articular surface is achieved at the time of fracture stabilization.

Supplemental Readings

Brinker WO, Hohn RB, Prieur WD: *Manual of Internal Fixation in Small Animals*. New York: Springer-Verlag, 1984, p 129.
Newton CD, Nunamaker DM: *Textbook of Small Animal Orthopedics*. Philadelphia: JB Lippincott, 1985, pp 333–343, 357.
Piermattei DL, Greely RG: *An Atlas of Surgical Approaches to the Bones of the Dog and Cat*, 2nd Ed. Philadelphia: W. B. Saunders, 1980, p 59.

8 Scapulohumeral Luxation

Robert A. Taylor

Scapulohumeral luxation is an infrequent clinical condition. Congenital and traumatic luxations occur; the latter is more common.

Medial luxation of the humeral head is most common, especially in smaller breed dogs. Lateral luxation of the humeral head, while less common, usually occurs in larger dogs (Fig. 1). Cranial and caudal luxations are rare.

Clinical Signs

- The principal signs are varying degrees of lameness, depending on the severity of the luxation.

Diagnosis

- Diagnosis is made by physical examination and confirmed by radiography.
- Careful palpation of the area between the acromion of the scapula and greater tubercle can be helpful.
  - In medial luxations, hold the elbow in a flexed position and abduct the lower limb.
  - In lateral luxations, hold the elbow in a flexed position and adduct the lower limb.
- Examine both shoulders simultaneously and use the normal limb for comparison.

ANATOMY

- The shoulder joint is a ball-and-socket joint. The articular surface of the scapula forms the concave glenoid and the convex humeral head articulates within. Although the joint is capable of movement

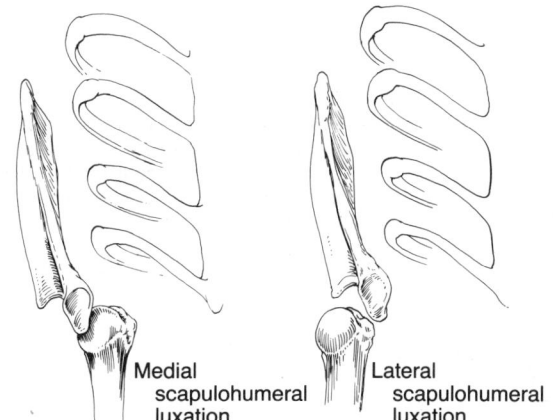

Figure 1. Medial *(left)* and lateral *(right)* luxations of the scapulo-humeral joint.

Medial scapulohumeral luxation

Lateral scapulohumeral luxation

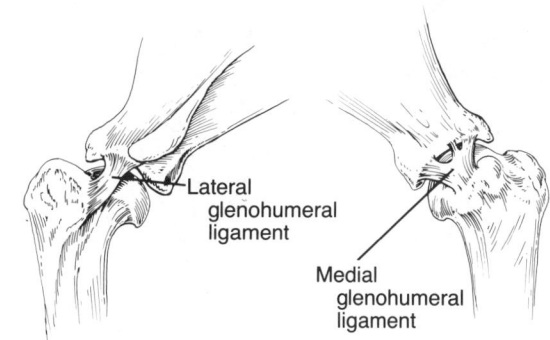

Figure 2. The glenohumeral ligaments.

Lateral glenohumeral ligament

Medial glenohumeral ligament

in any direction, its major actions are flexion and extension.
- The joint capsule is continuous and blends with the medial and lateral glenohumeral ligaments (Fig. 2). These ligaments help to support the joint and may be 2.0 mm or greater in thickness.
- The subscapularis, supraspinatus, infraspinatus, and teres minor muscles provide periarticular support.
- The tendon of origin of the biceps brachii and its sheath join with the joint capsule on its cranial medial aspect and provide additional stability. The bicipital tendon is held in the bicipital groove by the small but sturdy transverse humeral ligament.
- Luxation is not possible unless the glenohumeral ligaments and joint capsule have been ruptured.

PREOPERATIVE CONSIDERATIONS

- Radiograph the shoulder to rule out intra-articular fractures.
- General anesthesia is recommended for both procedures versus no anesthetic for closed reduction.
- Closed reduction is a nonsurgical event.

CLOSED REDUCTION

Procedure for Medial Luxation

1. Flex the elbow and pull the limb laterall, exerting digital pressure on the scapular s
2. Gently rotate the limb downward to luxation.
3. Place the limb in a Velpeau sling fo
4. If the joint is stable upon remo begin passive range-of-motion ex sible, encourage swimming as a therapy, but restrict exercise for 1 .

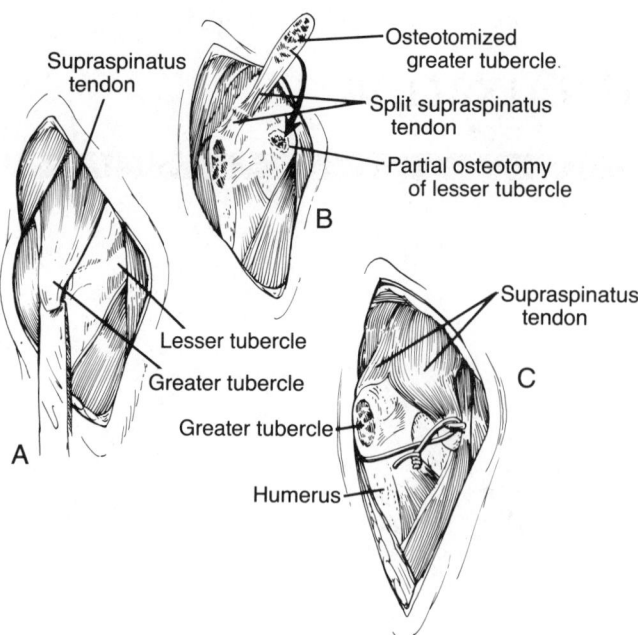

Figure 3. *A,* An oscillating bone saw or osteotome is used to partially osteotomize the greater tubercle. *B,* The supraspinatus tendon is split with a scalpel blade. *C,* The split portion of the supraspinatus tendon is attached to the region of the lesser tubercle.

Procedure for Lateral Luxation

1. Flex the elbow and extend the shoulder to reduce the luxation.
2. Gently rotate the humeral head upward to facilitate reduction.
3. Use a spica splint to support the joint for 10–14 days.

KEY POINT ▶ Open reduction and stabilization are indicated for recurrent luxations or when closed reduction fails owing to interposed soft tissue or hematoma.

SURGICAL PROCEDURES—OPEN REDUCTION

Objectives

■ Surgically repair the ruptured glenohumeral ligament and joint capsule.
■ Stabilize the shoulder joint and prevent recurrent luxations.

Equipment

■ Standard general surgical pack and suture material
■ Standard orthopedic set
■ Oscillating bone saw
■ Osteotomes and mallet
■ Kirschner wires and pin chuck
■ Appropriate retractors

Technique

Surgical Repair of Medial Luxation

1. Place the dog in lateral recumbency with the affected leg up. After preparing the limb for aseptic surgery, place the distal extremity in a sterile stockinette so that it is accessible to intraoperative manipulation. Make an incision on the craniomedial aspect of the joint.
2. Reflect the skin and subcutaneous tissue and incise the brachiocephalicus muscle along its medial edge and retract it.
3. Incise the superficial and deep pectoral muscles near their point of insertion on the humerus. Be sure to separate the supraspinatus muscle from the deep pectoral muscle.
4. Using an osteotome or oscillating saw (Fig. 3*A*), partially osteotomize the greater tubercle of the humerus. Hold the osteotome on the crest of the greater tubercle and make the medial line of the cut parallel to the humeral border of the transverse humeral ligament. Avoid cutting the infraspinatus tendon.

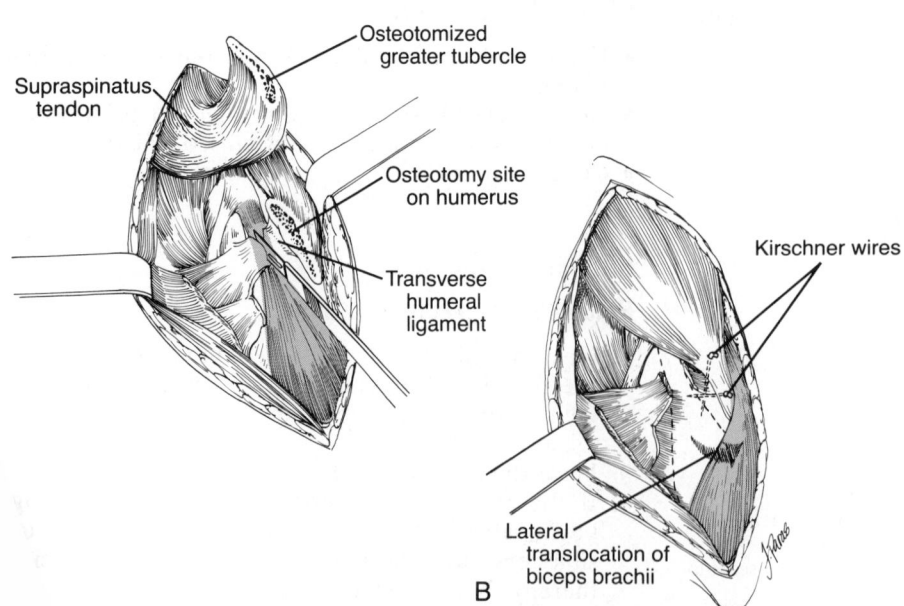

Figure 4. *A,* Transection of the transverse humeral ligament. *B,* Lateral translocation of the bicipital tendon. Kirschner wires stabilize the greater trochanter back to its origin.

5. Using sharp dissection, carefully split the supraspinatus tendon (Fig. 3B).
6. Partially osteotomize the lesser tubercle and prepare it to accept the bony fragment of the greater tubercle. Secure the greater tubercle fragment (with the attached portion of the supraspinatous tendon) in place with two Kirschner wires (Fig. 3C).
7. Suture the deep pectoral muscle over the lesser tubercle. Advance the superficial pectoral muscle over the proximal cranial border of the humerus and suture it to the deltoideus muscle. Suture the brachiocephalicus muscle to the brachial fascia.
8. Close the subcutaneous tissue and skin routinely.

Monitor for signs of seroma formation, hemorrhage, and infection.

Technique

Repair of Lateral Luxation
1. Positioning and draping is similar to that for surgical repair of medial luxation.
2. Skin incision and tissue retraction are the same as for medial luxation repair.
3. Incise the superficial and deep pectoral muscles. Incise the deltoideus muscle near the point of insertion on the cranial lateral aspect of the proximal humerus.
4. Transect the transverse humeral ligament and free the bicipital tendon from the surrounding tissue (Fig. 4A).
5. Completely osteotomize the greater tubercle to allow reflection of the intact tendon.
6. Translocate the bicipital tendon laterally on the opposite side of the osteotomized greater tubercle

(Fig. 4B). Secure the greater tubercle with several Kirschner wires.
7. Reattach the muscles and close the skin and subcutaneous tissue routinely.

Postoperative Care

■ Following medial luxation repair:
  • Support the limb in a Velpeau sling for 7–10 days; if the repair is stable, this may be unnecessary.
■ Following lateral luxation repair:
  • If necessary, place the limb in a Spica splint for additional support.
  • Strict cage rest for 7–10 days is advised, especially if the limb is not bandaged.
■ Monitor for seroma formation, hemorrhage, and signs of infection.
■ Begin physical therapy the first postoperative week with passive range-of-motion exercises. After suture removal, swimming and partial weight bearing can begin.

Prognosis

The prognosis good with adequate stabilization.

Supplemental Readings

Craig E, Hohn RB, Anderson WD: Surgical stabilization of traumatic medial shoulder dislocation. J Am Anim Hosp Assoc 16:93, 1980.
Hohn RB, Rosen H, Bohning RH, et al.: Surgical stabilization of recurrent shoulder luxation. Vet Clin North Am 1:537, 1971.
Vasseur PB: Clinical results of surgical correction of shoulder luxation in dogs. JAVMA 182:5, 1983.
Vasseur PB, Moore D, Brown SA: Stability of the canine shoulder joint: An in vitro analysis. Am J Vet Res 43:2, 1982.
Vasseur PB, Pool RR, Klein K: Effects of tendon transfer on the canine scapulohumeral joint. Am J Vet Res 44:5, 1983.

9 Fractures of the Humerus

Robert B. Parker

ANATOMY

- The proximal portion of the humerus is fairly strong and thick cranially and extends to the large deltoid tuberosity. The musculospiral groove starts posteriorly and twists cranially over the lateral aspect of the bone. The brachialis muscle and the neurovascular structures, including the clinically significant radial nerve, lie within the musculospiral groove.
- When viewed cranially, the bone is essentially straight; however, the medullary canal runs slightly lateral to medial from proximal to distal. Distally, the medial condyle is larger than the lateral condyle, and is in a more direct line with the medullary canal. The lateral condyle has a thinner epicondylar attachment to the bone, and is the main weight-bearing surface for the radial head.
- Important muscles to identify laterally are the lateral head of the triceps, the brachialis with the radial nerve, the brachiocephalicus, and the acromial head of the deltoid.
- Important medial soft tissue structures include the medial head of the triceps, the biceps brachii, and the median and ulnar nerves.

ETIOLOGY

- Most humeral fractures occur secondary to motor vehicle trauma or are caused by a fall from excessive heights.

Diagnosis

- Rule out injuries associated with thoracic trauma. Perform a complete clinical and radiographic examination to rule out pneumothorax, hemothorax, diaphragmatic hernia, rib fractures, chylothorax, and traumatic myocarditis.
- The neurovascular integrity of the limb is of paramount importance. Fully assess the injured forelimb. Consider thoracic radiography for all animals with humeral fractures.
- Obtain radiograms of the involved humerus to characterize the fracture(s). If necessary (e.g., prebending bone plates), obtain radiograms of the normal humerus.

Treatment

Because it is difficult to immobilize the shoulder joint with closed reduction and external fixation, most humeral fractures are treated by open reduction and internal fixation.

Equipment

- General surgical instrument pack
- Jacob's pin chuck and a complete assortment of Steinmann pins and Kirschner wires
- Bone-holding forceps
- Small and large reduction forceps with points
- Cerclage wire equipment
- Periosteal elevator
- Kirschner apparatus (external pin fixators)
- Additional (AO) type equipment* for plate and screw fixation (for selected fractures)

PROXIMAL HUMERAL PHYSEAL FRACTURES

Preoperative Considerations

- This type of fracture is seen infrequently in young dogs prior to physeal closure (10–13 months).
- The fracture typically is complete, but incomplete and impaction fractures can also occur.
- Except for incomplete fractures, closed reduction is very difficult. Open reduction of complete fractures is recommended.
- In selected cases, use a Velpeau sling or spica cast to immobilize the shoulder joint.

Surgical Procedure

Objectives

- Provide stable fixation while allowing continued physeal growth.
- Provide early range of motion.

Technique

Open Reduction

1. After preparing the limb for aseptic surgery, use a cranial approach with cranial retraction of the brachiocephalicus muscle to elevate and expose the fragments.
2. Use small pointed forceps to carefully grasp the epiphysis and use the elevator to lever the fragments into reduction.
3. Achieve fixation with double Kirschner wires or Steinmann pins, beginning at the greater tubercle. To prevent compression of the physis, do not use a figure-eight tension band.
4. Cancellous lag screws have been used by some

*Assoc. Study Int. Fixation, Synthes Ltd., Wayne, PA 19087.

surgeons, but they can cause interfragmentary compression and premature physeal closure (see sec. 9, ch. 7 for additional information on shoulder fractures).

Postoperative Care

- Encourage early range of motion exercise by allowing restricted activity.
- Remove fixation devices when healing is complete.

KEY POINT ▶ Premature closure of the physeal plate may occur as a result of the initial or surgical trauma; however, this is rarely a clinical problem.

PROXIMAL DIAPHYSEAL FRACTURES

Preoperative Considerations

- Proximal fractures are the least common diaphyseal fractures owing to the comparative strength of the humerus in this area.
- Most proximal diaphyseal fractures occur just proximal to the deltoid tuberosity. The distal fragment is displaced cranially due to the pull of the deltoid muscle, and medially due to the pull of the pectoral muscle.
- Evaluate the brachial plexus and the radial nerve. Accurate reduction is important because excessive callus production can produce postoperative pressure on these neural structures.
- Many of these fractures occur secondary to pathologic metabolic bone disease. Carefully evaluate radiographs of the fracture for evidence of bone disease. Perform appropriate tests if metabolic disease is suspected.

Surgical Procedure

Objective

- Because closed reduction with external fixation probably is not an option, stable open reduction with internal fixation is recommended.

Technique

Open Reduction

1. For open reduction, use a cranial approach, incise the skin along the craniolateral aspect of the humerus, beginning at the scapular tuberosity. Incise the fascial attachment of the brachiocephalicus muscle on the cranial aspect of the humerus to allow cranial retraction of the muscle. Elevate the deltoid muscle and retract it caudally to gain access to the fracture site.
2. Place single or double Steinmann pins retrograde from the fracture site into the proximal fragment (Fig. 1).
3. Because the fractures often are transverse, a single intramedullary (IM) pin may not provide rotational stability. Use a type I external fixator (see sec. 9, ch. 17) or hemicerclage wires to provide rotational stability.

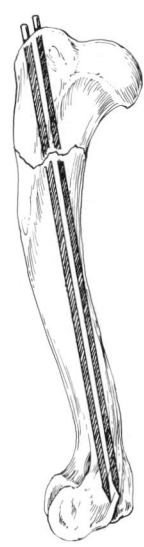

Figure 1. Steinmann pin placement for repair of a proximal diaphyseal fracture.

4. Alternatively, double rush pins provide excellent rotational stability in fractures of this type.
5. In very large dogs, a bone plate applied to the cranial surface of the humerus is an excellent method of fixation. The basic principle of three screws (6 cortices) above and three screws below the fracture site applies.

Postoperative Care

- External fixation is not desirable following internal fixation; however, if necessary, use a Velpeau sling or shoulder spica cast.
- Encourage early range of motion by allowing restricted exercise.

DIAPHYSEAL FRACTURES

Preoperative Considerations

- Muscle contracture causes overriding of the fragments.
- The fractures often are spiral or oblique and may entrap the radial nerve.
- Consider early closed reduction and closed normograde pinning. Attempt this only within the first few days following the injury.

Surgical Procedure

Objective

- Provide stable fixation without jeopardizing important neurovascular structures.

Technique

1. For open reduction, make a lateral approach to expose mid-shaft to distal fractures. Incise the fascia cranial to the lateral head of the triceps muscle to allow cranial retraction of the brachiocephalicus and superficial pectoral muscles, and caudal retraction

of the triceps. At the distal one-third of the incision, use extreme care to identify the radial nerve as it crosses from caudal to cranial between the brachialis and lateral head of the triceps. Use the brachialis muscle as a cushion to protect the radial nerve. Retract the brachialis either proximally or distally to expose the fracture site.

2. Many humeral fractures in small to medium-sized dogs can be successfully repaired with a combination of pins, stacked pins, full or hemicerclage wires, or Kirschner apparatus. This is particularly valid with oblique or spiral fractures.

   a. When using pin fixation, retrograde the pins into the proximal fragment from the fracture site. When the fracture is reduced, the pin should enter the medial condyle when driven into the distal fragment. Correct pin placement is slightly lateral to medial to engage the medial condyle (Fig. 2, *left*).

KEY POINT ▶ It is important to try to direct the pin slightly laterally when retrograding into the proximal humeral fragment.

   b. Rotational stability may not be achieved without additional pin, orthopedic wire, or a Kirschner apparatus support.

3. Because the humerus is difficult to expose and is anatomically a complex bone, the exposure for plate fixation can be difficult; however, cranial, lateral, or medial plate fixation can produce excellent results.

   a. Cranial plate placement is preferred for midshaft fractures. After exposure and reduction, contour an appropriately sized plate to fit the cranial aspect of the bone (Fig. 2, *right*). Protect the radial nerve distally. Freeing the origin of the extensor carpi radialis muscle may enhance distal exposure; however, the supratrochlear foramen may limit the distal extent of the plate.

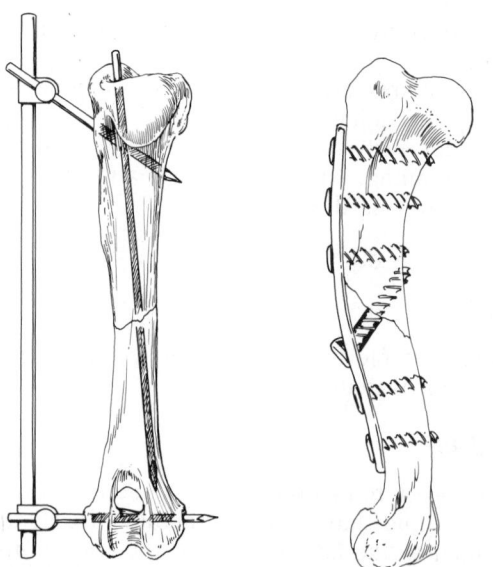

Figure 2. Fixation of diaphyseal fracture. *Left*, External pin fixation. *Right*, Internal cranial plate placement.

   b. Lateral plate placement is difficult because of the contours of the musculospiral groove.

   c. Medial plate placement affords a fairly flat bony surface, and the plate can be contoured onto the medial condyle. Medial placement is especially useful for distal diaphyseal fractures. The medial approach involves a medial skin incision and careful division between neurovascular structures. Retract the biceps brachii muscle and the median nerve cranially, and retract the medial head of the triceps and ulnar nerve caudally. The pectoral muscles limit exposure proximally.

Postoperative Care

- Restrict activity, but encourage early range of motion.
- If a Kirschner apparatus is used to supplement rotational or axial stability, remove in 4–6 weeks.
- Remove IM pins following fracture healing; supplemental cerclage or Kirschner wires are usually left in place.
- Do not remove bone plates unless they are causing a problem.

SUPRACONDYLAR FRACTURES

Preoperative Considerations

- The supratrochlear foramen creates a weak point in the distal humeral metaphysis.
- The medial condyle is on a straight line with the diaphysis of the humerus. Additionally, the majority of the forces are transmitted through the lateral condyle, which articulates with the radial head. The lateral condyle junction with the shaft in the area of the supratrochlear foramen is smaller and weaker than the medial side.
- Rigid internal fixation generally is indicated. Excessive callus formation from inadequate immobilization can result in impairment of normal elbow function.

Surgical Procedure

Objective

- Provide stable internal fixation to allow early weight bearing and range of motion.

Technique

1. The surgical approach is similar to the previously described lateral and medial approaches.

   a. The caudal approach to the elbow joint by olecranon osteotomy also provides excellent exposure to the supracondylar area. This approach is particularly useful for comminuted fractures in this area in large-breed dogs, when plating is anticipated.

2. Steinmann pin(s) placed well into the medial condyle, with an additional cross pin from the lateral condyle to produce rotational stability, may provide adequate stability. A type I external fixator, using a transcondylar distal fixation pin, can provide additional fixation and rotational stability.

a. To seat the Steinmann pin adequately in the medial condyle, initially retrograde the pin distally into the medial condyle from the fracture site. The pin exits the condyle medial to the ulna and can be withdrawn until the tip is flush with the fracture site. After reduction, advance the pin proximally to exit the humerus at the greater tubercle. Withdraw the pin proximally until the distal tip is flush with the medial condyle.

3. Alternatively, double Rush pins can provide excellent stability.

4. Because of the propensity for nonunion in medium and large-sized dogs and in dogs with severely comminuted fractures, small bone plates have been applied to the caudal medial or lateral ridges of the epicondyles. This is usually done through a caudal approach (osteotomy of the olecranon).

Postoperative Care

KEY POINT ▶ Physical therapy (e.g., active or passive elbow flexion and extension) is critical to prevent postoperative limitation of elbow function.

■ See the previous discussion of diaphyseal fractures postoperative care suggestions.

CONDYLAR FRACTURES

Preoperative Considerations

■ About 90% of condylar fractures involve the lateral condyle.

KEY POINT ▶ The lateral condyle, which carries most of the force through the elbow joint, anatomically is not as rigidly attached to the humeral diaphysis as the medial condyle.

■ Anatomic reduction is necessary to prevent secondary degenerative joint disease.
■ The lateral condyle generally is displaced distally owing to the pull of the extensor carpi radialis muscle.
■ For some unknown reason, spaniel-type dogs are prone to this injury.

Surgical Procedure

Objectives

■ Achieve perfect anatomic alignment and interfragmentary compression because the joint surface is involved.
■ Restore range of motion of the elbow joint as quickly as possible.

Technique

1. Open reduction and internal fixation usually are necessary. However, closed reduction maintained with a condyle clamp and fixation with a percutaneously applied transarticular lag screw have been described.

2. For open reduction, use a lateral or craniolateral approach.
3. Align intercondylar and supracondylar fracture lines perfectly and hold with a Vulsellum or AO pointed reduction forceps.
4. Use a transcondylar lag screw with an antirotation Kirschner wire to achieve interfragmentary compression (Fig. 3, *left*).
   a. The starting point for the drill bit is slightly distal and cranial to the most prominent point of the lateral condyle. Aim the drill at the corresponding point on the medial side. After measuring and tapping, place an appropriate screw.
   b. When using a fully threaded screw, overdrill the lateral cortex to achieve interfragmentary compression ("lag" effect).
   c. As an alternative method of achieving precise screw location with a fully threaded screw, use the overdrill bit to make the gliding hole in the lateral condyle. Rotate the condyle laterally to expose the intercondylar fracture surface of the lateral condyle. Center the drill at the fracture surface and direct it laterally to exit the bone just distal and cranial to the lateral prominence. Then reduce the fracture and use a drill sleeve insert (in the drill hole in the lateral condyle) to direct the smaller drill into the medial condyle. Place the screw routinely.
   d. Place an antirotational Kirscher wire across the condyles or across the supracondylar ridge (Fig. 3, *left*).
   e. If the supracondylar portion of the fracture is oblique enough, place additional screws along this aspect for additional stability (Fig. 3, *right*).
   f. Using crossed Kirschner wires to achieve intercondylar stability has not been successful in my experience.

Postoperative Care and Complications

■ Encourage early range of motion.
■ The lag screws usually are not removed.
■ Reduced range of motion and arthritis of the elbow joint are the most common complications. Accurate alignment and apposition of fracture fragments reduces the incidence of these problems.

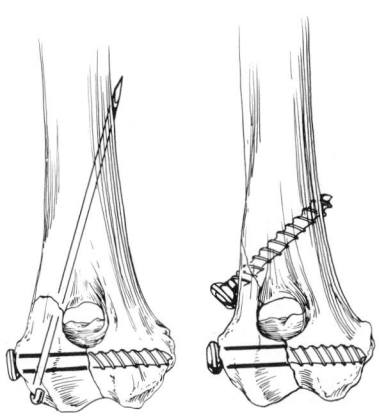

Figure 3. Fixation of condylar fractures. *Left*, Transcondylar lag screw and anti-rotation K-wire. *Right*, With oblique fractures, use two lag screws for increased stability.

T OR Y (INTERCONDYLAR) FRACTURES OF THE HUMERAL CONDYLES

Preoperative Considerations

- In this type of fracture, both the lateral and medial condyles are fractured from the humeral metaphysis; in addition, an intra-articular fracture occurs between the condyles.
- The basic principles of repair are the same as for supracondylar and single condylar fractures.
- These usually are very difficult to repair adequately. Consider referring these cases to an orthopedic specialist.

Surgical Procedure

Objective

- Achieve accurate anatomic reduction and stability in an unstable area.

Technique

1. Expose the fracture through a caudal approach via olecranon osteotomy.
2. Lag the condyles together initially to create a "two-piece fracture" (now similar to a supracondylar fracture) which is attached to the humeral diaphysis; or attach the medial condyle to the humerus; follow with lag-screw fixation of the lateral condyle to the medial condyle (Fig. 4, *left and center*).
   a. For more rigid stability, stabilize the supracondylar portion of the fracture with two small caudally placed bone plates (Fig. 4, *right*).

Postoperative Care and Complications

- Encourage early function or passive range of motion exercises.
- In one series, 46% of dogs regained moderate to normal limb function; 18% had severe lameness as a result of deformity and osteoarthritis.

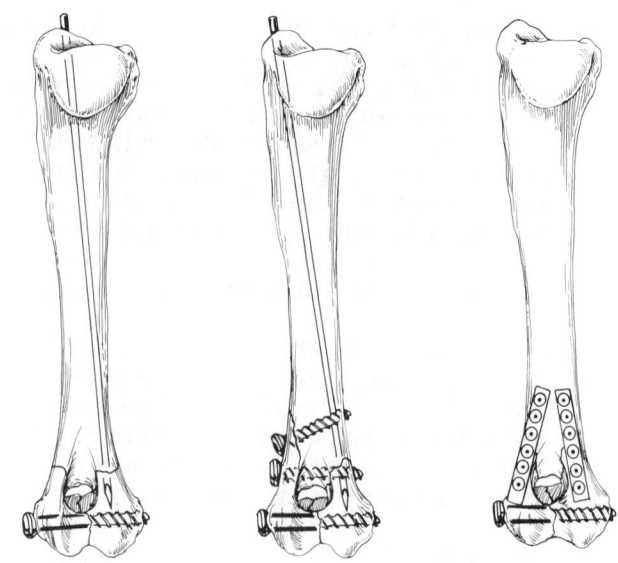

Figure 4. Fixation methods for intercondylar fractures. *Left*, Attach condyles with lag screw, then secure to humeral diaphysis with Steinmann pins. *Center*, Attach medial condyle to humerus with lag screw; then attach lateral condyle with lag screws and pin. *Right*, Caudal bone plates provide further stability.

Supplemental Readings

Berzon JL: Humeral fractures. *In* Slatter DH, ed.: *Textbook of Small Animal Surgery*. Philadelphia: W. B. Saunders, 1985, p 2061.

Brinker WO, Piermattei DL, Flo GL: *Handbook of Small Animal Orthopedics and Fracture Treatment*. Philadelphia: W. B. Saunders, 1990, p 175.

Denny HR: Pectoral limb fractures. *In* Whittick WG, ed.: *Canine Orthopedics*. Philadelphia: Lea & Febiger, 1990, p 357.

Nunamaker DM: Fractures of the humerus. *In* Newton CD, Nunamaker DM, eds.: *Textbook of Small Animal Orthopedics*. Philadelphia: JB Lippincott, 1985, p 357.

10 Traumatic Luxation of the Elbow Joint

Larry J. Wallace

The elbow joint is a reasonably stable joint and therefore excessive force is required for a luxation to occur. As a result, a significant injury to the ligament and periarticular soft tissue injury can occur. The severity of soft tissue injury is directly related to the intensity of the trauma causing the luxation.

ANATOMY

- The biomechanical stability of the elbow joint is directly related to its unique bony anatomy and the anatomy of the ligaments, joint capsule, and periarticular soft tissue attached to the three bones composing the joint.
- The elbow is a compound joint (i.e., several bones articulate) formed by the articulation of the humeral condyles, the head of the radius, and the ulnar semilunar notch. It is classified as a hinge joint (Fig. 1).
- The humeral radial articulation provides for 90° of supination of the distal extremity.

KEY POINT ▶ The bony stability of the elbow joint is maintained by the large medial humeral condyle, which prevents medial displacement of the radial head and the anconeal process, located in the olecranon fossa medial and deep to the lateral humeral epicondyloid crest.

- The primary soft tissue support of the elbow joint comes from the medial and lateral collateral ligaments. These ligaments originate from their respective humeral epicondyles and insert on both the radius and ulna by caudal and cranial crura that divide from the major ligament near their insertion.
- The olecranon ligament is very small; it originates just proximal to the anconeal process and attaches proximal to the inner surface of the medial condyle.
- A small oblique ligament originates on the cranial-dorsal surface of the supratrochlear foramen and obliquely crosses the cranial surface of the joint. At the level of the annular ligament, the oblique ligament divides into two branches. The shorter branch merges with the cranial crus of the medial collateral ligament; the longer branch attaches to the proximal medial border of the radius near the tendons of insertion of the brachialis and biceps brachii muscles.
- The annular ligament runs transversely around the head of the radius attaching the radius to the ulna.

- The joint capsule provides additional support for the elbow joint.

LUXATION OF THE ELBOW JOINT

Etiology

- In the absence of a fracture, traumatic luxations of the elbow are generally caudolateral or lateral. The majority of luxations are lateral with respect to the displacement of the radius and ulna.

KEY POINT ▶ The elbow joint is more likely to luxate laterally because the larger medial humeral condyle, with its slight downward bevel, helps to prevent medial displacement of the radius and ulna. In hyperflexion of the elbow, the entire anconeal process can slip over the lateral epicondyloid crest but is unable to slip over the larger caudal aspect of the medial condyle.

Clinical Signs

- In all cases of traumatic luxation of the elbow joint there is an acute onset of lameness.

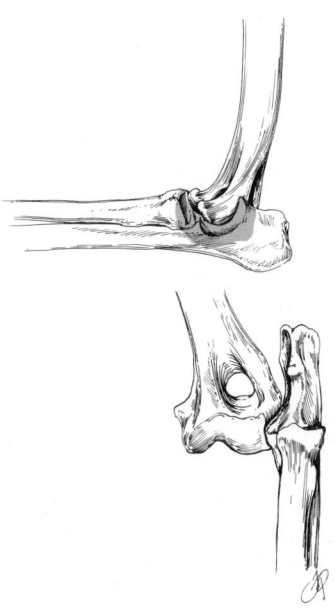

Figure 1. The luxated left elbow. *Top*, Lateral view; *bottom*, anterior view.

- The radius and ulna dislocate lateral to the distal humerus. Spasm of the muscles of the brachium pull the radius and ulna up proximal and lateral to the lateral humeral condyle (Fig. 1). The antebrachium and foot are abducted. Flexion and extension of the elbow joint are prevented because the joint surfaces are no longer in apposition.
- In an occasional patient, as the radius and ulna dislocate laterally the anconeal process may stay locked in position on the lateral epicondyloid crest. In these cases the luxation remains in a caudolateral position.

Diagnosis

The definitive diagnosis is based on lateral and anteroposterior radiographic evaluation of the elbow joint.

KEY POINT ▶ Radiographic examination is essential to determine if any fractures are present within the elbow and if there has been any avulsion fracture associated with either of the collateral ligaments.

Preoperative Considerations

- The majority of elbow luxations can be repaired with closed reduction if this is performed within the first 3 days following the injury.
- After 3 days, the muscle contracture and adhesions that develop between muscles make closed reduction difficult if not impossible. In such cases, open reduction is necessary.

KEY POINT ▶ Open reduction of traumatic elbow luxations is indicated in all cases of chronic elbow luxation in which closed reduction is impossible, and in all cases in which bone fragments are present in the elbow joint, regardless of whether the luxation is acute or chronic.

Surgical Procedures

Objectives

- Reestablish normal elbow function.
- Minimize degenerative changes in the elbow joint.

Equipment

- Standard orthopedic pack
- Bandage material

Technique

Closed Reduction
1. Position the animal in lateral recumbency with the affected leg up.
2. Place a sandbag on the examination table so that it supports the medial side of the elbow joint and elevates the elbow from the table at about the same level as the shoulder joint (Fig. 2).
3. Maximally flex the luxated elbow joint by placing one hand around the distal one-half of the ante-

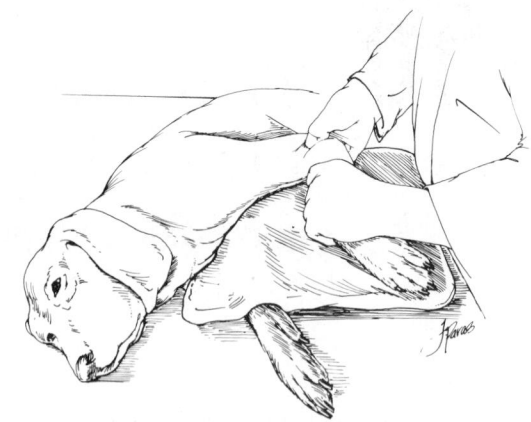

Figure 2. Position of patient and sandbag for closed reduction of elbow luxation.

brachium and placing the thumb of the opposite hand over the top of the olecranon process.
4. With the elbow joint maximally flexed, force the olecranon and proximal radius distally along the lateral aspect of the humerus (Fig. 3A).
5. When the anconeal process is at the level of the lateral epicondyloid crest of the humerus, abduct and rotate the antebrachium inward while continuing to force the olecranon and proximal radius distally. This will bring the tip of the anconeal

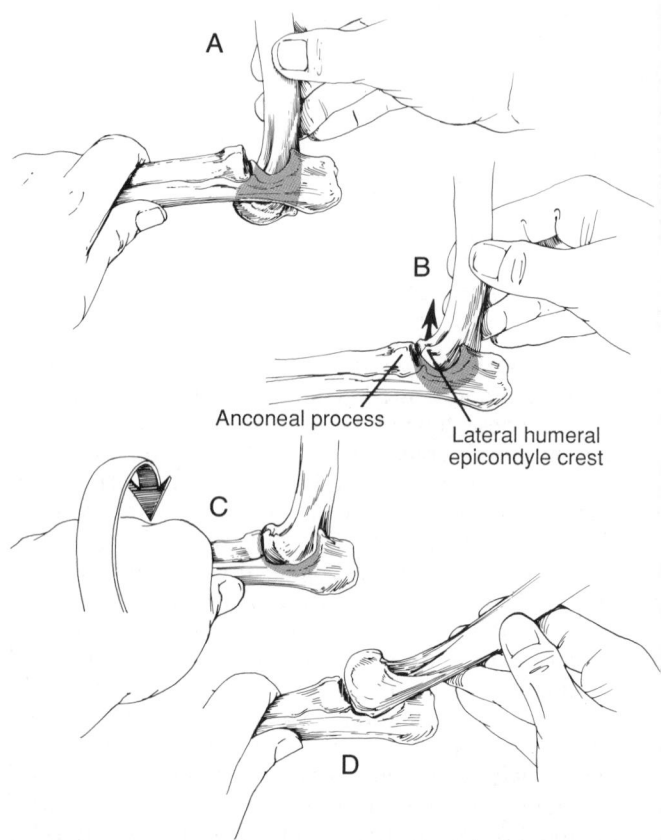

Anconeal process

Lateral humeral epicondyle crest

Figure 3. Reduction of the elbow. *A*, Hold the limb in traction. *B*, Pull radius and ulna distally. *C*, Internally rotate the ulna and radius. *D*, Extend the elbow.

process over the lateral humeral epicondyloid crest (Fig. 3*B*).

6. When the anconeal process is positioned over the lateral epicondyloid crest, with the thumb of one hand maintain a distal lateral-to-medial force on the olecranon process while, with the opposite hand, slowly extend the antebrachium, while internally rotating it. During this procedure, the anconeal process acts as a fulcrum to assist in bringing the radial head down to the level of the lateral humeral condyle (Fig. 3*C*).

7. When the radial head is at the level of the lateral humeral condyle, reduction of the elbow joint is achieved as a result of the combination of lateral-to-medial force on the olecranon and the proximal radius, slight adduction of the antebrachium, and continued extension of the elbow (Fig. 3*D*).

8. Following reduction, keep the elbow joint in the extended position. The anconeal process will thus be fully within the olecranon fossa of the distal humerus, and its tip may extend into the supratrochlear foramen.

9. Evaluate the integrity of the collateral ligaments. If severe instability is present, consider surgical repair of the damaged ligament. In most cases, this is unnecessary.

10. Immobilization of the elbow joint generally allows some healing of damaged soft tissue, especially in smaller animals. Surgical repair of damaged soft tissue is more frequently necessary in large dogs that are very active.

11. If necessary, repair ruptured ligaments with nonabsorbable suture material (see sec. 9, ch. 21 for discussion of tendon and ligament repair).

12. If a ligament is severely damaged and cannot be sutured, place a bone screw at the origin and insertion of the ligament and place nonabsorbable suture material around the screws in a figure-eight pattern.

13. If an avulsion fracture is present, surgery is necessary to reattach the avulsed origin or insertion of the ligament. This is readily accomplished using a lag screw and a ligament washer.

Technique

Open Reduction

1. Position the animal in lateral recumbency with the affected limb up. Perform routine surgical preparation and free-draping of the limb.

2. Use a lateral approach to the elbow joint. Incise the skin, subcutaneous tissue, anconeal muscle, and joint capsule.

KEY POINT ▶ To avoid additional injury to soft tissues and articular cartilage, lavage the joint frequently with lactated Ringer's solution.

3. Carefully remove fibrous and granulation tissue and debris from the joint.

4. Inspect the joint surfaces for articular cartilage damage.

5. Perform reduction as described above for closed reduction.

6. Do not insert instruments into the joint to act as a lever in reducing the luxation, as this may cause further damage to the articular cartilage.

7. If reduction is impossible with this approach and greater exposure is needed, use a transolecranon approach (see sec. 9, ch. 9).

8. Following reduction, evaluate the ligamentous stability of the joint. If ligamentous repair is necessary, follow the procedure described for closed reduction.

9. Close the joint routinely. If the transolecranon approach was used, fix the olecranon process of the ulna in place using two Kirschner wires and a tension band (see sec. 9, ch. 11).

KEY POINT ▶ Chronic elbow luxations can be very difficult to maintain in complete reduction after open reduction, owing to muscle tension on the radius and ulna. The radius and ulna may tend to subluxate laterally even when the elbow is placed in extension and placed in a splint.

10. If it is difficult to maintain reduction, place a small IM pin or Kirschner wire (depending on the size of the patient) through the proximal ulna and advance it into the distal humerus.

11. Bend over the end of the pin protruding from the proximal ulna to prevent it from migrating cranially. Remove the splint and pin in about 3 weeks.

Postoperative Care and Complications

Cases with Minimal Ligament Damage

- Most of these cases are acute and are treated by closed reduction.
- Obtain postreduction lateral and anteroposterior radiographs.
- Apply a splint to maintain the elbow in extension during the radiographic procedures and for 2 weeks postoperatively (e.g., Schroeder-Thomas or shoulder spica splints) (Fig. 4).
- Restrict activity to leash walking for at least 2 weeks after the splint is removed.
- Examine at 2, 4, and 6 weeks. Reevaluate elbow function.

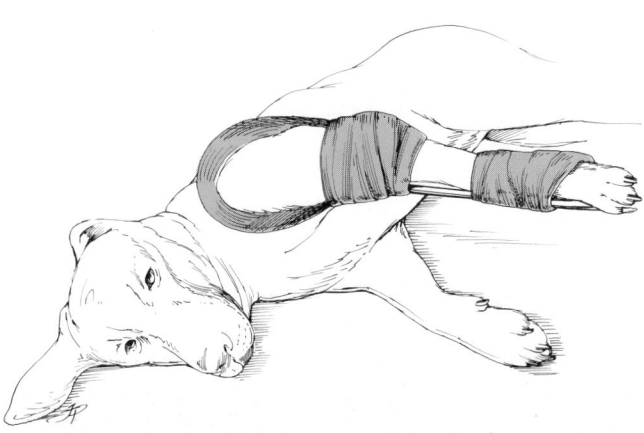

Figure 4. Schroeder-Thomas splint maintains the elbow in extension after reduction.

- Repeat lateral and anteroposterior radiography at postoperative week 4.
- Gradually increase the exercise program after post-operative week 4.
- Physical therapy of the elbow joint usually is not needed in these cases.

Cases with Surgical Repair of Ligaments and Chronic Cases with or without Severe Ligament Damage

- Patients with injuries in this category require a longer convalescent period.
- Obtain postreduction lateral and anteroposterior radiographs. Apply a splint to maintain the elbow in extension during radiography and for 3 weeks post-operatively.
- Instruct the owner to keep the animal quiet and confined, except for walks on a short, hand-held leash.
  - After 3 weeks, allow restricted activity (e.g., no running and leash walks only) for an additional 5 weeks.
  - Gentle flexion and extension physical therapy exercises of the elbow may be necessary in these cases.
- Reevaluate elbow function at 2, 4, 6, and 8 weeks.

- Obtain lateral and anteroposterior radiographic views at postoperative weeks 4 and 8.
- Gradually increase exercise after postoperative week 8.

Prognosis

- The prognosis is good for acute uncomplicated elbow luxations that are properly treated soon after the injury.
- Acute cases in which surgical repair of a ligament is needed generally have a good prognosis.
- The prognosis is guarded in chronic cases in which there is severe cartilage damage.

Supplemental Readings

Brinker W, Piermattei D, Flo G: Traumatic luxation of the elbow. *In Handbook of Small Animal Orthopedics and Fracture Treatment*. 2nd Ed. Philadelphia: W. B. Saunders, 1990, p 496.

Campbell JR: Luxation and ligamentous injuries of the elbow of the dog. Vet Clin North Am 1:429, 1971.

Nunamaker DM: Fractures and dislocations of the elbow. *In* Newton C, Nunamaker D, eds.: *Textbook of Small Animal Orthopedics*. Philadelphia: JB Lippincott, 1985, p 369.

Piermattei DL, Greeley RG: *Atlas of Surgical Approaches to the Bones of the Dog and Cat*, 2nd Ed. Philadelphia: W. B. Saunders, 1979.

Taylor RA: Treatment of elbow luxations. *In* Bojrab MJ, ed.: *Current Techniques in Small Animal Surgery*, 3rd Ed. Philadelphia: Lea & Febiger, 1990 p 772.

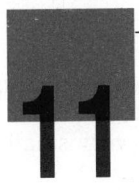

11 Fractures and Growth Deformities of the Radius and Ulna

James Tomlinson

FRACTURES OF THE RADIUS AND ULNA

Fractures of the radius and ulna are commonly seen in small animal practice. Although most of these fractures occur as a result of automobile accidents, they also result from falling or jumping. Fractures of one or both bones and a wide variety of fracture types are seen. Open fractures of the distal one-half of the radius and ulna are common, owing to minimal soft tissue coverage. Complications include delayed union, nonunion, joint stiffness, and arthritis.

Anatomy

Radius

- The radius is the main weight-bearing bone of the forelimb and is shorter than the ulna. The radius is composed of the head, neck, body, and distal extremity. The medullary canal is elliptical in shape owing to flattening of the radius. In smaller dogs, the medullary canal is nonfunctional, although it can be seen radiographically.
- The radius is attached to the ulna by an interosseous ligament that helps to maintain their spatial relationship following fracture. The short radial collateral ligament runs from the styloid process of the radius to the radial carpal bone and provides medial support to the joint.
- The cranial surface of the distal radius contains three grooves that contain (from medial to lateral) the tendons of abductor pollicis longus, extensor carpi radialis, and common digital extensor muscles.

Ulna

- The ulna is the longest bone in the body and is composed of the olecranon, trochlear notch, anconeus, and body and the distal extremity called the styloid process.
- The olecranon has a strong muscular attachment, the triceps muscle.
- The ulnar body tapers as it crosses caudal to the radius to articulate with the carpus. The medullary canal of the ulna functionally ends about one-third from the distal end.
- The strong, short ulnar collateral ligament runs from the tip of the styloid process of the ulna to the ulnar carpal bone, giving lateral support to the carpal joint.

Vascular Supply

- The radial and interosseous arteries provide the main arterial supply to the antebrachium and are subject to injury from trauma or surgery.
- The radial artery travels along the palmaromedial aspect of the radius just under the flexor carpi radialis muscle.
- The interosseous artery branches into other interosseous arteries that run in the space between the radius and ulna.

Nerve Supply

- The radial, median, and ulnar nerves supply the antebrachium and manus.

General Preoperative Considerations

- Evaluate the thorax for pulmonary contusions, pneumothorax, diaphragmatic hernia, and traumatic myocarditis with thoracic radiography and electrocardiography.
- Examine the animal for concurrent injuries; inspect other limbs for fractures or other significant injury.
- Inspect the antebrachium for evidence of wounds indicating an open fracture.
- Evaluate nerve function of the affected limb by testing reaction to a painful stimulus to the skin of the various dermatomes and by withdrawal of the limb.
- Initially place the limb in a Robert Jones bandage or splint to prevent further soft tissue damage and to prevent the fracture from becoming an open fracture.
- Take two radiographic views of the fractured limb, including the elbow and carpus.

General Objectives of Surgical Procedures

- Align and stabilize the fracture(s) to permit uncomplicated healing with normal joint and limb function.

KEY POINT ▶ Exact anatomical alignment and rigid fixation (compression) of articular fractures is imperative.

- Allow an early return to weight bearing.
- Preserve neurovascular structures during repair.

General Postoperative Care and Complications for Radial and Ulnar Fractures

- Place the limb in a soft padded bandage for 3–10 days to reduce postoperative swelling. Provide more rigid external support if needed.
- Reevaluate the fracture radiographically every 3–4 weeks until the fracture has healed.
- Restrict activity until the fracture has healed.

Complications

- Delayed and nonunion healing (see sec. 9, ch. 28), osteomyelitis (see sec. 9, ch. 27), and implant failure may occur.
- Joint fractures are prone to the development of degenerative joint disease and the formation of callus that interferes with joint mobility if anatomic alignment and rigid stability have not been achieved.
- Joint stiffness can develop with articular fractures. Rigid stability of the fracture allows early, controlled use of the joint.

KEY POINT ▶ Radius and ulna fractures in immature animals may cause premature closure of the growth plates and synostosis of the radius and ulna. Both conditions cause growth deformities of the limb. Early recognition and intervention is necessary to minimize growth deformities.

Olecranon Fractures

Objective

- Counteract the distractive force of the triceps and convert it into a compressive force by use of the tension band principle.

Equipment

- General surgery pack and standard suture material
- Monofilament stainless steel surgical wire (20 and 18 gauge)
- Intramedullary (IM) pins and Kirschner wires
- Jacobs chuck or power drill
- Wire-tightening device (vise grips or wire twister)
- Pin and wire cutter
- Bone reduction forceps

Technique

1. Place the animal in lateral recumbency, with the affected leg up, and prepare the limb for aseptic surgery.
2. Make a caudolateral skin incision centered over the olecranon.
3. Reflect the skin and subcutaneous tissue to expose the olecranon and proximal shaft of the ulna. Subperiosteally elevate the extensor and flexor carpi ulnaris muscles from the proximal shaft of the ulna.
4. Reduce the fracture and hold it in reduction with bone reduction forceps.

5. Drive two IM pins parallel from the tip of the olecranon across the fracture line and into the distal segment of the ulna (in very small animals, drive only one Kirschner wire).
6. Drill a hole (perpendicular to the ulnar long axis) in the distal ulnar segment 1½–2 times distance from the olecranon to the fracture line.
8. Insert surgical wire in the hole and place the wire around the pins in a figure eight fashion.
9. Twist the wire in two places, medially and laterally, to achieve equal tension on both arms of the wire.
10. Bend the pins over and cut them off short. Cut the wires leaving two to four twists and bend the wire tips over (Fig. 1).
11. Close the subcutaneous tissue and skin routinely.

Trochlear Notch Fractures

Objectives

- Maintain precise anatomic alignment of the fracture (because it is an articular fracture).
- Perform rigid fixation of the fracture to minimize periosteal callus.
- Counteract the distractive forces of the triceps muscle by use of the tension band principle.

Equipment

- Equipment is the same as for olecranon fractures with the addition of bone plating equipment.

Technique

Small and Medium-Sized Dogs; Cats; No Fracture Comminution Present

1. Repair the fracture with a tension band wiring technique, as described previously for olecranon fractures.
2. Maintain anatomic alignment of the fracture while driving the pins and tightening the wire in a figure-eight configuration.

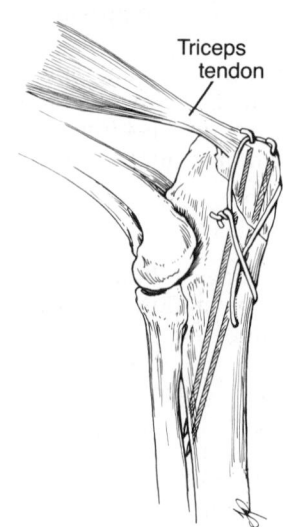

Figure 1. Pin and wire placement for olecranon fracture repair.

Large Dogs; Fractures with Comminution

1. Expose the trochlear notch, as described for olecranon fractures.
2. Reattach butterfly segments of bone with lag screws and Kirschner wires.
3. Contour a bone plate to the caudal or caudolateral side of the ulna and secure it to the ulna with bone screws (Fig. 2).
4. If comminution is not present, apply the plate with a compression technique. If comminution is present, apply the plate in a neutralization manner (e.g., no compression).

Radial Head Fractures

Objectives

- Perform precise anatomic reduction of the fracture and rigid fixation.

Equipment

- General surgery pack and standard suture material
- Hohmann retractor
- Bone screws and bone screw insertion equipment
- Power drill and Jacobs pin chuck
- Kirschner wires

Technique

1. Place the animal in lateral recumbency, with the affected limb up, and prepare the limb for aseptic surgery.
2. Incise the skin, beginning at the proximal end of the lateral epicondyle of the humerus and continuing distally over the radial head to the proximal one-fourth of the radius.
3. Incise the subcutaneous tissue and the antebrachial fascia along the same line to expose the extensor muscles of the antebrachium.
4. Dissect between the ulnaris lateralis muscle and the lateral digital extensor. Tenotomize the ulnaris lateralis, leaving sufficient tendon for suturing. If necessary, incise the anconeus muscle from the lateral epicondyle of the humerus.
5. Reflect the lateral digital extensor muscle cranially with a Hohmann retractor to expose the fracture.

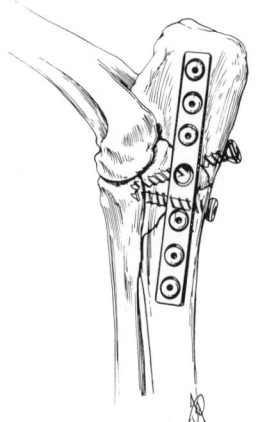

Figure 2. Bone plate and screw replacement for trochlear notch fracture repair.

6. Drive a Kirschner wire across the fracture line to hold the fracture in reduction.
7. Insert a screw in "lag screw" fashion to compress the fracture line.
8. For small fragments, place two or three Kirschner wires in a divergent pattern.
9. Reattach the ulnaris lateralis tendon with nonabsorbable monofilament suture material in a horizontal mattress pattern. Suture the muscle fascia and subcutaneous tissue in a simple continuous pattern, using absorbable suture material. Close the skin routinely.

Radial Neck and Proximal Physeal Fractures

Objectives

- Stabilize the fracture in immature animals without fracture compression to help prevent premature closure of the growth plate.
- Stabilize and align radial head so that it articulates properly with the humeral condyle.

Equipment

- General surgery pack and standard suture material
- Jacobs pin chuck
- Kirschner wires

Technique

1. Approach the fracture as described for radial head fractures, and reduce the fracture.
2. Stabilize the fracture with two Kirschner wires placed in crosspin fashion from the lateral side. Start one pin just below the articular surface of the radius and drive it distomedial. Start the second pin distal to the fracture and drive it proximomedial.
3. Bend the pins over and cut them off short.
4. Take care not to penetrate the articular surface of the radius.
5. Close the tissue as described for radial head fractures.

Postoperative Care

- Remove the Kirschner wires in 3–4 weeks and monitor for premature closure of the growth plate.

Monteggia Fractures

This is a fracture of the ulna that can occur at various levels, with a radial head luxation.

Objectives

- Reduce and stabilize the radial head luxation.
- Align and stabilize the ulnar fracture.

Equipment

- General surgery pack and standard suture material
- Bone plating equipment
- Power drill
- Bone reduction forceps

Technique

1. Expose the ulnar fracture, as described for olecranon and trochlear notch fractures. Expose the ulna as far distally as needed.
2. Expose the radial head, as described for radial head fractures, if the luxation cannot be reduced closed.
3. Reduce the ulnar fracture and hold it in reduction with bone reduction forceps.
4. If the annular ligament is ruptured, contour and apply a bone plate to the caudal aspect of the ulna. Insert a screw in "lag screw" fashion into the radius from the ulna through the plate to secure the radial head in position (Fig. 3).
5. If the annular ligament is intact, contour and apply a bone plate to the caudolateral aspect of the ulna.

Midshaft Radial and Ulnar Fractures

Objective

- Achieve healing of the fracture with proper angulation, rotation and length of the limb.
- Prevent synostosis of the radius and ulna in immature animals.

Equipment

- Fiberglass casting tape, stockinette, 1″-wide medical tape
- General surgery pack and standard suture material
- Bone reduction forceps
- Jacobs pin chuck and power drill
- Kirschner-Ehmer apparatus
- Bone plating equipment

Technique

Closed Reduction and Cast Fixation for Minimally Displaced Transverse Fractures
1. Place 1″-wide medical tape stirrups on the dorsal and plantar surface of the foot.
2. Apply a snug-fitting double layer of stockinette

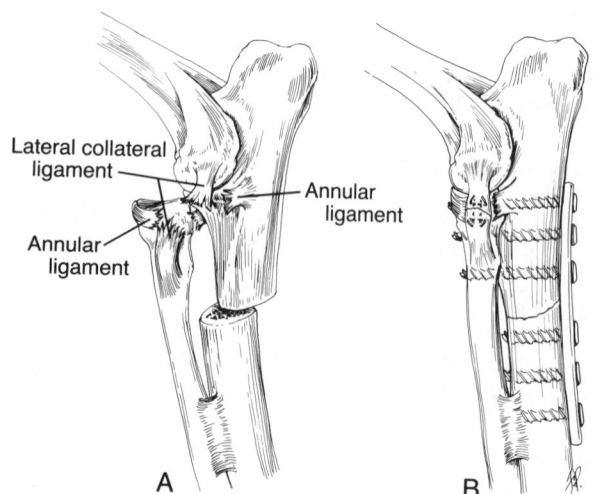

Figure 3. Monteggia fracture repair. *A*, Anatomy of fracture and ligament damage; *B*, plate placement and ligament repair. See text for details.

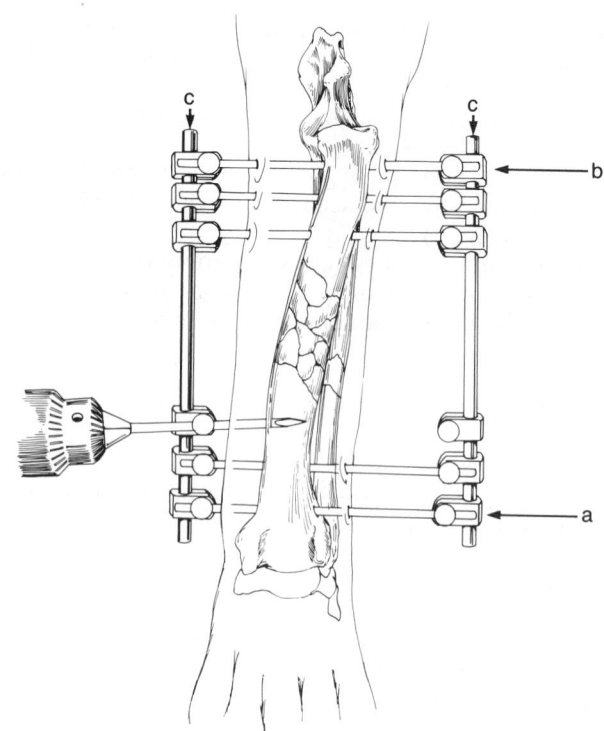

Figure 4. External skeletal fixation. See text for explanation.

over the limb. Make the stockinette long enough to extend 1″ past the tip of the toes and as far proximal above the elbow as possible.
3. Reduce the fracture and position the limb for correct angular and rotational alignment.
4. Place the carpus in a slight varus position, flexed 5–10°.
5. Flex the elbow to a functional angle (approximately 140°).
6. After wetting, apply the fiberglass casting tape, starting at the tip of the 2nd and 5th nails.
7. Overlap the casting tape 50% with each wrap, working from distal to as far proximal as possible above the elbow.
8. Apply four or five layers of fiberglass casting tape.
9. Reflect the stockinette and stirrups over the end of the cast and incorporate them into the final layer of cast material.
10. Hold the limb in the proper position until the cast has set.

External Skeletal Fixation for Comminuted Fractures and Simple Fractures
1. Reduce comminuted fractures closed.
2. Use a limited open approach if the fracture cannot be reduced closed.
3. Make small stab incisions in the skin before driving the transfixation pins.
4. Drive the most distal transfixation pin across the radius perpendicular to the long axis of the radius from medial to lateral and parallel to the radial carpal joint (Fig. 4, a). Drive the transfixation pins through the skin on both sides of the limb.
5. Drive the most proximal transfixation pin (Fig. 4, b) in a similar manner, parallel to the articular surface of the radial head.

6. Apply connecting bars (Fig. 4, c) to the transfixation pins on both the lateral and medial sides.
7. Place the appropriate number of single connecting clamps on the connecting bar.
8. Align the fracture and tighten the end connecting clamps to maintain reduction of the fracture.
9. Drive the remaining transfixation pins through the connecting clamps and tighten them.
10. If possible, place three or four transfixation pins on each side of the fracture line.
11. Cover the external skeletal fixation device with gauze and tape to protect the fixator and furniture surfaces.

Plate Fixation for Distal Metaphyseal Fractures

These fractures occur primarily in small dogs. There is a high incidence of nonunion if these fractures are not treated correctly.

Objectives

■ Achieve anatomic alignment with compression of the fracture.
■ Insert a cancellous bone graft.

Equipment

■ General surgery pack and standard suture material
■ Mini-bone plating equipment (1.5 mm and 2.0 mm screws and plates)
■ Power drill
■ Curet (Brun, 3–0)
■ Small bone reduction forceps

Technique

1. Place the dog in lateral recumbency, with the affected leg up, and prepare the limb for aseptic surgery.
2. Make a skin incision on the dorsal aspect of the leg, starting at the cephalic vein and extending distally to the mid-metacarpus. Make the incision lateral to the cephalic vein.
3. Incise the subcutaneous tissue and fascia along the same line.
4. Identify the extensor carpi radialis and the common digital extensor tendons and subperiosteally elevate them from their grooves in the radius.
5. Incise the abductor pollicis muscle for additional proximal exposure.
6. Reduce the fracture and hold it in reduction with bone reduction forceps.
7. Contour a bone plate to the cranial surface of the radius and apply the plate. In small dogs, use a 1.5 mm or 2.0 mm bone plate.
8. Make a 2-cm long incision over the craniolateral aspect of the greater tubercle of the humerus.
9. Incise the subcutaneous tissue along the same line. Drill a small hole in the greater tubercle.
10. Use a #3–0 Brun curet to collect a cancellous bone graft from the greater trochanter. During the collection process, place the graft on a bloody sponge.
11. Pack the bone graft around the fracture site.
12. Close the subcutaneous tissue and the skin incisions routinely.
13. After surgery, apply a soft padded bandage to the leg.

Fractured Styloid Process of Ulna

Objective

■ Reduce and stabilize the fracture to reestablish lateral support to the carpus.

Equipment

■ General surgery pack and standard suture material
■ Surgical stainless steel wire (20 and 18 gauge)
■ Kirschner wires
■ Jacobs pin chuck
■ Wire tightening device (vise grips, wire twister)
■ Pin and wire cutter
■ Bone reduction forceps

Technique

1. Place the animal in lateral recumbency with the affected leg up and aseptically prepare the limb.
2. Make a skin incision over the lateral aspect of the styloid process. Incise the subcutaneous tissue along the same line.
3. Dissect between and elevate the tendons of the lateral digital extensor and the extensor carpi ulnaris.
4. Reduce the fracture and drive a Kirschner wire from the distal tip of the ulna just above the ulnar collateral ligament into the proximal segment.
5. Drill a hole in the proximal segment of the ulna and pass a wire through the hole.
6. Place the wire around the tip of the pin in a figure-eight configuration, and tighten the wire on both arms of the figure-eight.
7. Close the deep fascia and subcutaneous tissue with absorbable suture in a simple continuous pattern. Close the skin routinely.
8. Splint the fracture for 3–4 weeks postoperatively.

GROWTH DEFORMITIES OF THE RADIUS AND ULNA

Growth deformities of the radius and ulna result from trauma and disruption of the blood supply to the physis; retained cartilaginous cores (see sec. 9, ch. 23); and synostosis (bony bridging) of the radius and ulna. Specific treatment depends on the physis injured, the extent of deformity, and the age of the animal.

Anatomy

■ The radius and ulna form the largest paired bones of the body. Abnormal growth of one bone may affect the other bone, elbow or carpus.
■ In dogs, the growth plates (physes) of the radius and ulna close about 7–9 months of age (see sec. 9, ch. 25 for more information about physeal structure).
■ The distal ulnar physis is conical in shape, making it

vulnerable to crushing during trauma. The two radial physes are relatively flat.

- The distal ulnar physis contributes 85% to the longitudinal growth of the ulna; the proximal physis (olecranon) contributes 15%.
- The proximal and distal radial physes contribute 40% and 60%, respectively, to the longitudinal growth of the radius.
- The radius and ulna must grow in a synchronous manner to retain a normal shape and joint congruity. As the radius and ulna grow, they normally slide past each other.

Preoperative Considerations

- Early recognition and treatment of physeal injury of the radius and ulna is the key to prevention or minimization of deformities.
- Base treatment of a growth deformity on whether the dog is mature or immature (whether physes are still growing) and on the specific deformity.

KEY POINT ▶ The general principles of treatment of growth deformities are prevention or correction of angular deformities and joint abnormalities and maintenance of acceptable leg length.

- Obtain lateral and craniocaudal radiographs of the affected and normal forelimbs. Include both the elbow and carpus.
- Preplan corrective procedures on paper or cleared radiographic film by making tracings and cutouts copied from the radiographs.

General Postoperative Care and Complications for Growth Deformities

- In immature dogs, splint the limb when ostectomy has been performed. The other intact bone will hypertrophy to withstand the added stress.
- Reevaluate the leg radiographically at least every 3 weeks until the dog has stopped growing.
- If bone bridges the ostectomized gap before growth has ceased, repeat the original surgery.
- If the procedure for immature dogs does not correct the deformity, perform the procedure recommended for mature dogs after bone growth stops.

General Prognosis

- The prognosis is guarded, especially for mature dogs with severe deformities.

Surgical Procedure to Correct Premature Closure of the Distal Ulnar Physis

Immature Dogs

Objectives

- Remove a section of the ulna to allow unrestrained growth of the radius.
- Prevent regrowth of the ulna by placement of a free fat graft.

Equipment

- General surgery pack and standard suture material
- Gigli wire saw or oscillating bone saw
- Gelpi retractor

Technique

1. Place the animal in lateral recumbency, with the affected leg up, and prepare the limb for aseptic surgery.
2. Make a 6-cm incision over the lateral aspect of the distal third of the ulna. Incise the subcutaneous tissue and antebrachial fascia along the same line.
3. Dissect between the extensor carpi ulnaris and the lateral digital extensor muscles to expose the ulna. Elevate the muscles and tendons from the ulna on top of the periosteum all the way around the bone.
4. Using the Gigli wire saw or the oscillating saw, ostectomize at least 2 cm of the ulna at the junction of the distal one-third and middle one-third of the bone.
5. Remove all the periosteum to prevent rapid bone regrowth.
6. Make a 3-cm incision over the flank just in front of the wing of the ilium.
7. Dissect down to the subcutaneous fat and collect a piece of fat large enough to completely fill the defect in the ulna.
8. Place the fat graft in the ulnar defect and close the antebrachial fascia in a simple continuous fashion with absorbable suture material.
9. Close the subcutaneous tissue and skin routinely.
10. Place the limb in a splint for the first month following surgery.

Mature Dogs

Deformities

- Cranial and/or medial bowing with lateral torsion of the radius
- Carpal valgus with external rotation
- Limb shortening
- Malalignment of radius and/or ulna in the elbow joint

Objectives

- Correct angular and rotational deformity
- Correct joint incongruity
- Maintain as much leg length as possible

Equipment

- General surgery pack and standard suture material
- Gigli wire saw or oscillating bone saw
- Kirschner-Ehmer fixation device
- Jacobs pin chuck or power drill

Technique

1. Place the animal in lateral recumbency, with the affected leg up, and prepare the limb for aseptic surgery.
2. Drive a transfixation pin across the most distal

aspect of the radius, aligned parallel with the craniocaudal plane and mediolateral plane of the articular surface of the radius (Fig. 5).

3. Drive a second transfixation pin in the same manner as the first pin, except as far proximal as possible and parallel to the articular surface of the proximal radius.
4. Approach the radius as described previously for fractures of the distal radius.
5. Perform an osteotomy of the radius at the point of maximal curvature of the radius.
6. Fracture the ulna at the same level, either manually or with a saw.
7. Connect the transfixation pins on the lateral and medial sides with single connecting clamps and connecting bars. Place the appropriate number of single connecting clamps on the connecting bars.
8. Manually align the proximal and distal transfixation pins so that they are parallel to each other in both planes. Tighten the connecting clamps to hold the proper alignment (Fig. 6).
9. If there is any concern over the alignment, obtain radiographs of the leg at this point.
10. Drive the remaining transfixation pins through the open single connecting clamps.
11. Close the incisions routinely.
12. Cover the Kirschner device with gauze and tape.
13. If elbow incongruity is not severe, it will resolve with weight bearing after the ulna is cut.

Surgical Procedure to Correct Premature Closure of the Proximal Radial Physis

Generally this deformity is recognized after the bone growth of the radius is finished. If it occurs in an immature dog, use the technique described for complete premature closure of the distal radial physis in immature dogs.

Deformities

- There is distal luxation of the radial head from the humerus.
- Leg is straight.

Objective (Mature Dogs)

- Reposition the radial head into the elbow joint so that it articulates properly with the humerus and ulna.

Equipment

- General surgery pack and standard suture material
- Bone plating equipment
- Power drill
- Oscillating saw

Technique

1. Place the animal in lateral recumbency, with the affected leg up and prepare the limb for aseptic surgery.
2. Approach the radial head as described previously for radial head fractures.

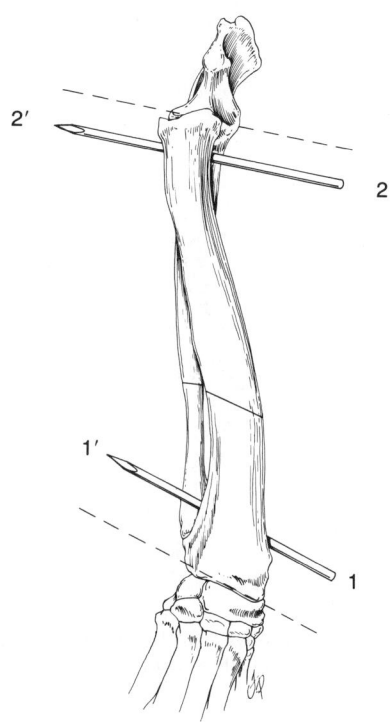

Figure 5. Pin placement for repair of premature closure of the distal ulnar physis. Place the first pin (1–1′) parallel to the cranial-caudal and medial-lateral plane of the articular surface of the radius. The second pin (2–2′) is parallel to the articular surface of the proximal radius.

3. Approach the midshaft of the radius as described previously for midshaft radial fractures.
4. Perform a stepped radial osteotomy. Make the longitudinal arm of the osteotomy long enough to accept two bone screws (Fig. 7).

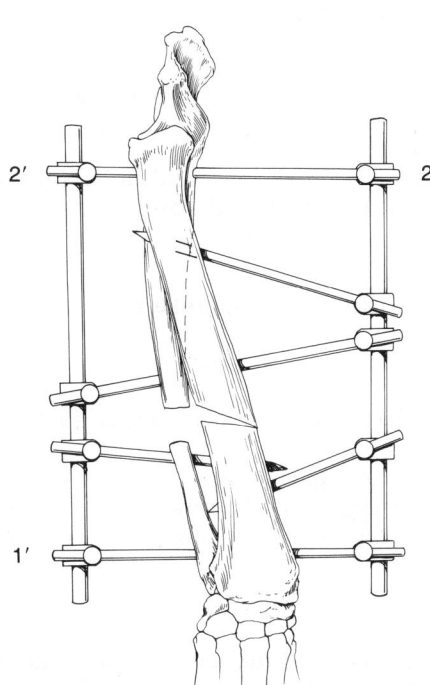

Figure 6. Final pin placement (see Fig. 5), osteotomy, and ulnar fracture for repair of premature closure of the distal ulnar physis.

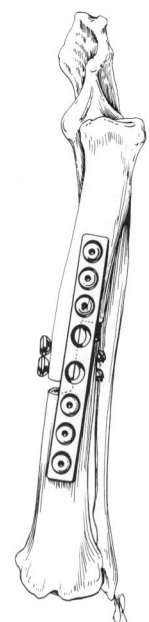

Figure 7. Plate and screw placement for stepped radial osteotomy performed for repair of premature closure of the proximal radial physis.

5. Slide the radial head proximally so that it articulates correctly with the humeral condyle and the ulna.
6. Place two screws, from medial to lateral, in "lag screw" fashion across the osteotomy site.
7. Apply a bone plate on the cranial aspect of the radius to further stabilize the osteotomy.
8. Collect a cancellous bone graft from the proximal humerus.
9. Place the bone graft in the defect in the radius.
10. Close the incisions routinely.
11. Place the leg in a soft padded bandage for 10–14 days postoperatively.

Surgical Procedure to Correct Premature Closure of the Distal Radial Physis

Premature closure of the distal radial physis can be complete or partial. If partial closure occurs, the lateral aspect of the physis usually is affected.

Complete Closure (Immature Dog)

Deformities

- Distal radial head luxation and elbow joint incongruity occurs.
- The limb is shortened.
- Usually the leg remains straight.
- Bowing of the radius and ulna occurs rarely.

Objectives

- Remove a section of the radius to allow unrestricted growth of the ulna.
- Prevent regrowth of the radius until the other growth plates have stopped growing.

Equipment

- General surgery pack and standard suture material
- Gigli wire saw or oscillating saw

Technique

1. Place the animal in lateral recumbency, with the affected leg down, and prepare the limb for aseptic surgery.
2. Approach the midshaft radius as described previously for midshaft radial fractures.
3. Ostectomize a 2-cm section of radius, including the periosteum. Protect the interosseous artery.
4. Collect a free fat graft from the flank, as described previously for premature closure of the distal ulnar physis in immature dogs.
5. Place the fat graft in the radial defect and close the antebrachial fascia with absorbable suture material in a continuous pattern.
6. Close the incision routinely.
7. Place the leg in a splint (distal humerus) postoperatively.
8. When the dog has stopped growing, reconstruct the defect in the radius with a cancellous bone graft.

Partial Lateral Closure (Immature Dog)

Deformities

- Carpal valgus with external rotation
- Cranial and medial bowing of the forelimb
- Shortening of the limb
- Elbow joint incongruity

Objectives

- Remove the closed portion of the distal radial physis
- Prevent bony bridging of the removed physis with a fat graft.

Equipment

- General surgery pack and standard suture material
- Curets

Technique

1. Place the animal in lateral recumbency, with the affected leg up, and prepare the limb for aseptic surgery.
2. Approach the distal radius as described previously for distal radial fractures.
3. Carefully expose the physis to minimize damage.
4. Probe the physis with a 25-gauge needle to determine the extent of the closure.
5. Use a curet to remove the closed section of the physis.
6. Place a free fat graft collected from the flank in the defect.
7. Close the incision routinely.
8. Splint the leg until bone growth is complete.
9. When bone growth is complete, remove the fat graft, if necessary, and graft the defect with cancellous bone.

Mature Dogs

Deformities

The deformities are the same as described for complete and incomplete closure in immature dogs.

Objectives

■ Reestablish congruity to the elbow joint.
■ Correct angular deformity of the limb.

Equipment

■ Equipment is same as listed for premature closure of the proximal radius and distal ulna in mature dogs.

Technique

■ If the radial head is luxated distally and the limb is straight, use the technique described previously for correction of premature closure of the proximal radius in mature dogs.

■ If angular and rotation deformity is present, use the techniques described previously for correction of premature closure of the distal ulna in mature dogs.

Supplemental Readings

Brinker WO, Hohn RB, Prieur WD: *Manual of Internal Fixation of Fractures*. New York: Springer-Verlag, 1984, p 144.

Brinker WO, Piermattei DL, Flo GL: Fractures of the radius and ulna. *In* Brinker WO, Piermattei DL, Flo GL, eds: *Handbook of Small Animal Orthopedics and Fracture Treatment*. Philadelphia: W. B. Saunders, 1990, p 195.

Brinker WO, Piermattei DL, Flo GL: Fractures and corrective surgery in young growing animals. *In* Brinker WO, Piermattei DL, Flo GL, eds: *Handbook of Small Animal Orthopedics and Fracture Treatment*. Philadelphia: W. B. Saunders, 1990, p 244.

Johnson AL: Correction of radial and ulnar growth deformities resulting from premature physeal closure. *In* Bojrab MJ, ed.: *Current Techniques in Small Animal Surgery*. Philadelphia: Lea & Febiger, 1990, p 793.

Piermattei DL, Greeley RG: *An Atlas of Surgical Approaches to the Bones of the Dog and Cat*. Philadelphia: W. B. Saunders, 1979, p 108.

Probst CW: Stabilization of fractures of the radius and ulna. *In* Bojrab MJ, ed.: *Current Techniques in Small Animal Surgery*. Philadelphia: Lea & Febiger, 1990, p 783.

12 Fractures and Dislocations of the Carpus

Kurt J. Matushek

Injuries to the carpus consist of fractures, ligamentous damage due to luxations or subluxations, and combinations of the two.

Fractures of the carpus are rare and are seen most often in racing greyhounds and working dogs.

KEY POINT ▶ Remember that almost all fractures of the carpus involve articular surfaces when managing these fractures and when giving a prognosis.

Equipment

- General surgery pack and standard suture material
- Bone-holding forceps
- Lag screws (1.5 mm or 2 mm)

ANATOMY

Osseous Structures (Fig. 1)

- The carpus consists of seven bones arranged in two rows and a small sesamoid bone located in the tendon of insertion of the abductor pollicis longus muscle.
- The bones of the proximal row are the radial, ulnar, and accessory carpal bones.
  - The radial carpal bone, the largest of the carpal bones, is located on the medial aspect of the proximal row. It articulates proximally with the radius and distally with the four distal carpal bones.

- The ulnar carpal bone is the lateral bone of the proximal row. It articulates proximally with the radius and ulna, distally with the fourth carpal bone and fifth metacarpal bone, and with the accessory carpal bone on the palmar aspect.
  - The accessory carpal bone is located on the palmar surface of the carpus. It articulates with the ulnar carpal bone and the styloid process of the ulna.
- The first, second, third, and fourth carpal bones make up the distal row.
  - The fourth carpal bone is the largest bone in the distal row. It articulates distally with the fourth and fifth metacarpals.

Articulations

- The carpal joints include the antebrachiocarpal, the middle carpal, and the carpometacarpal joints. The joints between the carpal bones of each row are called intercarpal joints.
- As a group, the carpal joints act to permit flexion and extension, with a small amount of medial and lateral movement.
- The greatest amount of motion occurs in the antebrachiocarpal joint. The middle carpal joint accounts for approximately 10–15% of carpal motion. Very little motion occurs in the carpometacarpal and intercarpal joints.

Ligamentous Structures

- No long collateral ligaments span all three joints of the carpus.
- Support to the carpus is provided by two sleeves of collagenous tissue with the tendons in between.
  - The superficial sleeve is a thickening of the deep carpal fascia.
  - The deep sleeve is a thickened fibrous layer of the joint capsule.
  - The two sleeves fuse laterally and medially to form short collateral ligaments.
- The flexor retinaculum, formerly called the transverse palmar carpal ligament, provides support to the palmaroproximal aspect of the carpus.
  - The flexor retinaculum attaches laterally to the accessory carpal bone and medially to the styloid process of the radius, the radial carpal bone, and the first carpal bone.
- The palmar carpal fibrocartilage crosses the palmar surface of the carpus and attaches to all the carpal bones except the accessory carpal bone.

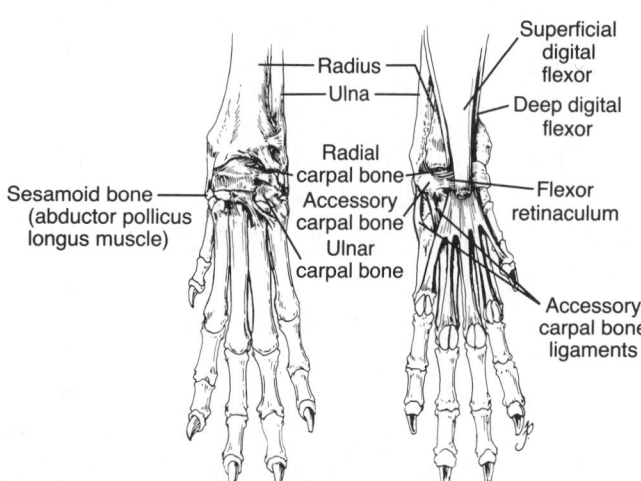

Figure 1. Anatomy of the carpus. *Left*, Dorsal view; *right*, palmar view.

- The palmar carpal fibrocartilage is particularly heavy distally and attaches to the proximal ends of the third, fourth, and fifth metacarpals.
■ The short radial collateral ligament consists of two parts, both originating from the styloid process of the radius: the straight portion, which inserts on the medial surface, and the oblique portion, which inserts on the palmaromedial surface of the radial carpal bone.
■ The short ulnar collateral ligament originates on the ulnar styloid process and inserts on the ulnar carpal bone.
■ The accessory carpal bone is stabilized distally by two ligaments, both of which originate from the free end of the accessory carpal bone. One ligament attaches to the fifth metacarpal, and the other to the fourth metacarpal.
■ Other multiple small ligaments attach the carpal bones to each other and to the metacarpals.

FRACTURES OF THE RADIAL CARPAL BONE

Preoperative Considerations

■ Fractures occur because of:
  • Hyperextension injuries, resulting in chip fractures of the proximal dorsal border.
  • A fall, resulting in slab fractures.
■ Lameness usually is acutely severe; however, with chronic injuries, the injured limb may become partially weight-bearing.
■ Diagnosis may be difficult because the fragments usually are only minimally displaced.
  • High-detail radiographs are essential for diagnosis.
  • Oblique radiographic views often are necessary.
■ Bone fragments tend not to reattach, resulting in synovitis and degenerative joint disease.

Surgical Procedure

Objectives

■ Remove small chips that cannot be reduced and stabilized adequately.
■ Stabilize larger fragments with lag screws or multiple Kirschner wires.

Equipment

■ General surgery pack and standard suture material
■ Bone-holding forceps
■ Lag screws or Kirschner wires
■ Esmarch bandage and tourniquet

Technique

1. Surgery is most often performed with a tourniquet in place; most fractures can be exposed through a dorsal approach (see description under Pancarpal Arthrodesis).
2. Alignment and reduction is achieved with small, pointed bone-holding forceps.
3. If lag screws are used, countersink the screw head to avoid interference with the movement of other structures.

Postoperative Care and Complications

■ Place the limb in a splint for 1–3 weeks postoperatively.
■ Restrict exercise for 6–8 weeks or until there is radiographic evidence of union.
■ Secondary degenerative joint disease is common, and intermittent lameness can occur.

FRACTURES OF THE ACCESSORY CARPAL BONE

Preoperative Considerations

■ This type of fracture is common in racing greyhounds; it is rare in other breeds.
■ When possible, internal fixation of fragments is preferable.

Surgical Procedure

Technique

1. Use a palmarolateral approach to the accessory carpal bone.
2. Reduce and stabilize fracture using screws placed in a "lag screw" fashion.

Postoperative Care and Complications

■ Maintain the limb postoperatively in a splint for 4–6 weeks.
■ Resume training (in athletic dogs) in 12–16 weeks.

FRACTURES OF THE ULNAR CARPAL BONE AND CARPAL BONES 1–4

■ Fractures of these bones are very rare.
■ Most often these are small chip fractures of the dorsal surface, resulting from hyperextension injuries.
■ Treatment consists of removal of the fragments followed by splintage for 2 weeks. Restrict exercise for 8 weeks.

LUXATIONS AND SUBLUXATIONS OF THE CARPUS—HYPEREXTENSION INJURIES

Luxations and subluxations are most commonly seen as a result of hyperextension injuries resulting from falling or jumping from a height. The hyperextension force causes tearing and rupture of the palmar joint capsule and ligaments and results in loss of support of any or all of the three carpal joints.

Clinical Signs and Diagnosis

■ The injured limb usually is non–weight bearing if the animal is presented immediately after the injury. However, most animals begin walking on the leg in a relatively short period, although a limp is present.
■ Mild tenderness and swelling of the carpus usually is present.

- A plantigrade stance is characteristic of a hyperextension injury. Most dogs walk on their carpal pads.
- Occasionally, the injury is bilateral. When this occurs, perform bilateral surgery.
- Standard radiographic views may not always demonstrate the lesion. A lateral-to-medial projection taken with stress applied to the toes to create carpal hyperextension is necessary to determine which carpal joint is involved.
- In general, the antebrachiocarpal joint is injured 5–10% of the time; the middle carpal joint, 50–70%; and the carpometacarpal joint, 25–40%.

KEY POINT ▶ External coaptation (splints or casts) is rarely if ever successful in treating hyperextension injuries. Many injuries appear improved immediately after the cast is removed but are worse in 1–2 weeks.

Preoperative Considerations

- Panarthrodesis has been advocated for all hyperextension injuries regardless of the specific carpal joint involved.
  - Results have generally been good, with 74% of owners in one series of cases reporting normal use of the limb.
- Selective arthrodesis of the involved joints is probably a better approach. Because 90% of the motion in the carpus occurs in the antebrachiocarpal joint, if this joint can be saved, very little alteration in gait would be expected.

Surgical Procedure

Objectives

- Follow the basic principles of joint fusion:
  - Remove all articular cartilage from the joint surfaces.
  - Use a cancellous bone graft.
  - Provide rigid internal or external fixation for a sufficient time to allow complete union of the fusion.

Equipment

- General surgery pack and standard suture material
- Esmarch bandage and tourniquet
- Air-powered drill
- Bone curets
- Steinmann pins
- Compression plates and screws
- Type II Kirschner-Ehmer device

Technique

Pancarpal Arthrodesis
Dorsal Approach

1. Place the animal in lateral recumbency, with the affected limb up, and prepare the limb for aseptic surgery.
2. Apply an Esmarch bandage and tourniquet to the limb to provide hemostasis.

3. Make a skin incision on the dorsal midline, extending from the junction of the cephalic and accessory cephalic veins to the mid-metacarpus (Fig. 2).
4. Incise the fascia between the tendons of the extensor carpi radialis and common digital extensor muscles and retract to expose the joint capsule.
5. Make incisions in the synovial membranes of the carpal joints to expose the articular surfaces.
6. Remove all articular cartilage, using an air-powered drill or bone curets.
7. Use autogenous cancellous bone graft from the proximal humerus or the wing of the ilium to pack all joint spaces.
8. Achieve rigid internal fixation with a 7-hole compression plate.
   a. Bend the plate to provide 5–10° of hyperextension.
   b. Place three screws in the distal radius, one screw in the radial carpal bone, and three screws in the third (or fourth) metacarpal (Fig. 3, *top*).
9. Alternatively, stabilize the joint with a type II Kirschner-Ehmer device, placing 2 pins in the distal radius and 2 pins in the third and fourth metacarpal (Fig. 3, *bottom*).

Postoperative Care

- Place the limb in a caudal splint for 6–8 weeks postoperatively, or until radiographic union is evident.

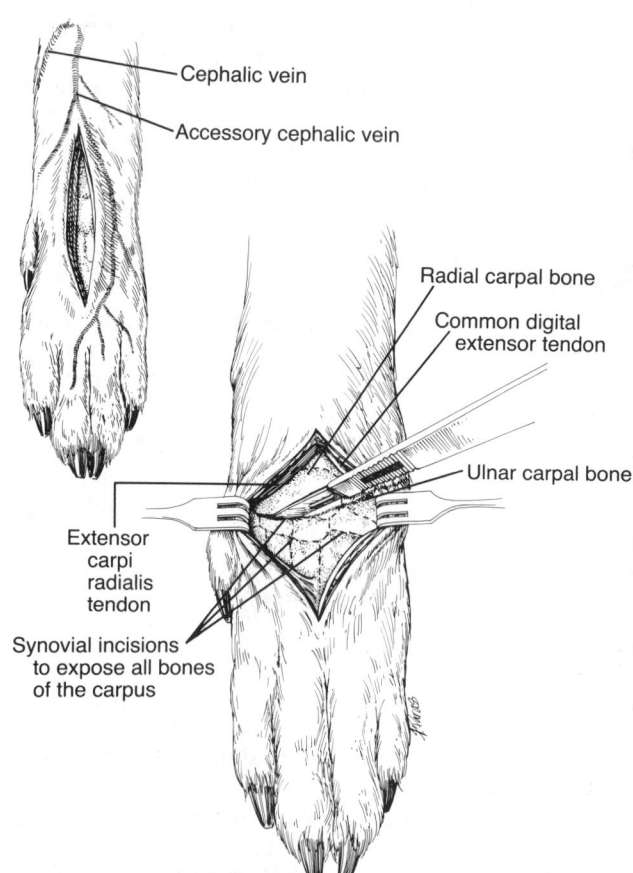

Figure 2. Dorsal surgical approach to the carpus. Avoid incising venous drainage *(top left)*.

Cephalic vein
Accessory cephalic vein
Radial carpal bone
Common digital extensor tendon
Ulnar carpal bone
Extensor carpi radialis tendon
Synovial incisions to expose all bones of the carpus

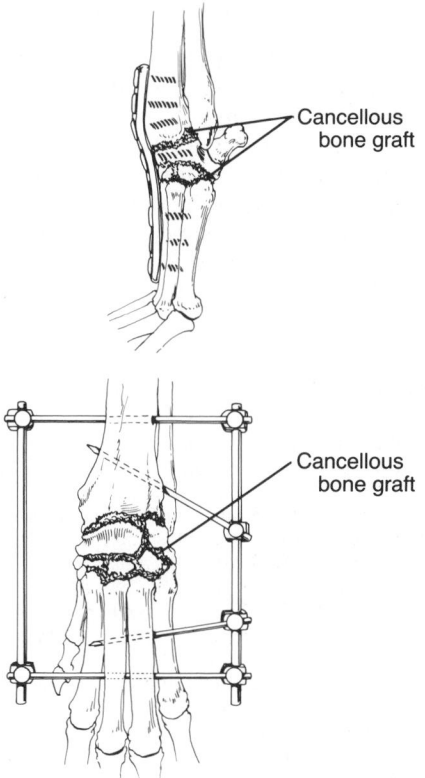

Figure 3. Pan-carpal arthrodesis, dorsal approach. *Top*, Plate stabilization; *bottom*, stabilization with K-E apparatus.

Palmar Approach

KEY POINT ▶ Palmar surface plating appears to be biomechanically superior to dorsal surface plating; however, surgical exposure is somewhat more difficult.

1. Place the animal in lateral recumbency, with the affected limb down, and prepare the limb for aseptic surgery.
2. Apply an Esmarch bandage and tourniquet to provide hemostasis.
3. Make a caudomedial skin incision extending from the medial aspect of the distal radius to a point midway between the base of the first digit and the carpal pad and then along the medial side of the metacarpus.
4. Dissect the cephalic vein free and retract medially. Bluntly dissect the subcutaneous tissue to expose the deep antebrachial and carpal fascia.
5. Make a sharp incision through the periosteum and antebrachial fascia on the medial border of the radius and continue distally through the flexor retinaculum where it attaches to the styloid process of the radius and the radial and first carpal bones.
6. Transect the tendons of the deep flexor of the first digit and the flexor carpi radialis.
7. Continue the dissection distally through the periosteum of the second metacarpal.
8. Free the entire flexor tendon, vascular, and neural bundle from the underlying bone and retract them laterally.

9. Using an air-powered drill, remove all accessible articular cartilage.
10. Contour a compression plate to the palmar surface with the joint in 5–10° of hyperextension.
11. Place three screws in the distal radius and 3 screws in the third metacarpal. If possible, place additional screws in the radial carpal and third carpal bones.
12. Pack all joint surfaces with a cancellous bone graft.
13. Close the deep tissues and skin routinely.

Postoperative Care

■ Apply a soft bandage until swelling has subsided; then place the limb in a splint for 4–5 weeks.

Technique

Partial Carpal Arthrodesis

KEY POINT ▶ Partial carpal arthrodesis is indicated when the antebrachiocarpal joint and its ligaments and the ligaments of the accessory carpal bone are intact.

1. Use a dorsal approach to the carpus, as described previously for pancarpal arthrodesis. However, remove the articular cartilage from the middle carpal and carpometacarpal joints only.
2. Pack a cancellous bone graft into the joint spaces.
3. Several techniques can be used to achieve stabilization.

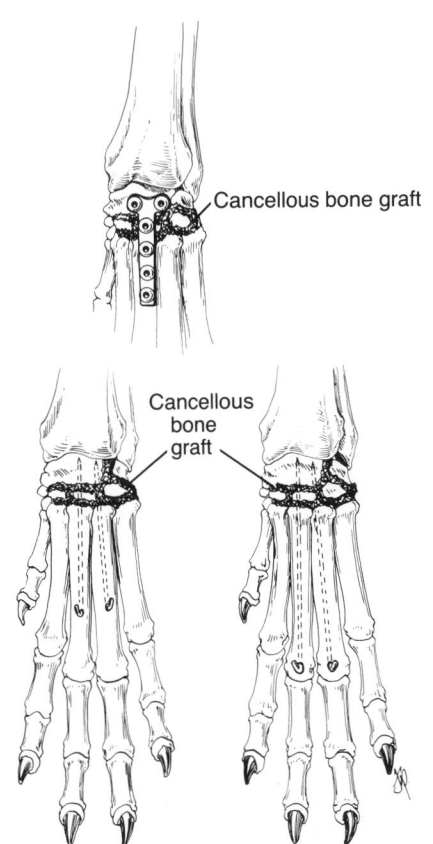

Figure 4. Partial carpal arthrodesis. *Top*, Plate stabilization; *bottom*, stabilization with intramedullary pins.

a. Apply a T- or L-plate to the dorsal aspect of the third or fourth metacarpal with the T or L portion attached to the radial carpal bone (Fig. 4, *top*). During extension, do not allow the plate to overlap the antebrachiocarpal joint. Place the limb in a palmar splint for 6 weeks postoperatively, or until there is radiographic evidence of union.

b. Alternatively, place Steinmann pins normograde from the third and fourth metacarpals and embed the pins in the radial carpal and ulnar carpal bones (Fig. 4, *bottom*). The pins originate from slots drilled into the dorsal surfaces of the metacarpals. Bend the pins upward to prevent pin migration and soft tissue trauma. Place the limb in a palmar splint for 6–12 weeks postoperatively, or until there is radiographic evidence of union. Remove the pins after healing is complete.

c. For partial carpal fusion without the use of metallic implants, prepare the articular surfaces as described previously and pack a cancellous bone graft into the joint spaces. Place the limb in a splint immediately postoperatively. When swelling from the surgery has decreased (approximately 3 days) apply a full cast to the limb from the elbow distally with the carpus in 5–10° of hyperextension. Change the cast every 4 weeks until union is evident radiographically (usually about 12 weeks).

Postoperative Complications

■ Postoperative swelling because of impairment of lymphatic or venous drainage is common and usually subsides within a few days.
■ If fusion occurs, complications are rare.
■ The most common reasons for arthrodesis failure are any one or a combination of the following:
  • Incomplete removal of articular cartilage
  • Inadequate bone grafting
  • Inadequate internal or external support for a sufficient period of time.

Supplemental Readings

Brinker WO, Piermattei DL, Flo GL: *Handbook of Small Animal Orthopedics and Fracture Treatment*. Philadelphia: W. B. Saunders, 1983, p 386.
Chambers JN, Bjorling DE: Palmar surface plating for arthrodesis of the canine carpus. J Am Anim Hosp Assoc 18:875, 1982.
Evans HE, Christensen GC: *Miller's Anatomy of the Dog*, 2nd ed. Philadelphia: W. B. Saunders, 1979, pp 190, 248.
Gambardella PC, Griffiths RC: Treatment of hyperextension injuries of the canine carpus. Compend Contin Educ Pract Vet 4:127, 1982.
Johnson KA: Accessory carpal bone fractures in the racing greyhound: Classifications and pathology. Vet Surg 16:60, 1987.
Johnson KA, Dee JF, Piermattei DL: Screw fixation of accessory carpal bone fractures in racing greyhounds: 12 cases (1981–1986). J Am Vet Med Assoc 194:1618, 1989.
Slocum B, Devine T: Partial carpal fusion in the dog. J Am Vet Med Assoc 180:1204, 1982.

13 Pelvic Fractures

Peter Muir

Kenneth A. Johnson

Paul A. Manley

Pelvic fractures in dogs and cats occur most often as a consequence of severe trauma and are frequently associated with other orthopedic injuries as well as injuries to other body systems. Decisions regarding management of pelvic fractures can be assisted by recognizing the types of pelvic fractures that have a higher priority for surgical treatment and by diagnosing concurrent injuries of other body systems.

SURGICAL ANATOMY

- Each half of the pelvis is composed of the ilium, ischium, pubis, and acetabulum, which are fused as the os coxae or hip bone.
- The sacroiliac joint has a limited range of motion and is composed of a synchondrosis craniodorsally and a synovial articulation ventrally.
- The sacrotuberous ligament extends from the caudolateral part of the apex of the sacrum and the transverse processes of the first caudal vertebra to the lateral part of the ischiatic tuberosity. The sacrotuberous ligament is absent in the cat.
- The sacrum and pelvic bones form a complete bony canal. Therefore, pelvic fractures usually are multiple, or a pelvic fracture may be accompanied by sacroiliac fracture or luxation. If a pelvic fracture appears to be single, examine radiographs carefully for evidence of additional, undisplaced fractures.
- The major weight-bearing regions of the pelvis are the sacroiliac joint, body of the ilium, and acetabulum.

DIAGNOSIS AND EVALUATION OF PELVIC FRACTURES

- Thorough physical examination may be difficult in injured animals that are in pain or shock. After giving emergency treatment, complete the general physical examination as soon as possible.
- Management of cardiopulmonary, neurologic, and soft tissue injuries may have a higher priority than that of orthopedic injury. Obtain thoracic radiographs routinely in animals with suspected pelvic fractures.
- Injury to intra-abdominal and intrapelvic organs such as the liver, spleen, urinary bladder, and urethra commonly accompany pelvic fractures. Surgical treatment of soft tissue injuries may take priority over pelvic fracture repair.
- When the patient is in stable condition, perform an orthopedic examination.
  - Carefully palpate the pelvic bones, manipulate the hip joints, and perform a rectal examination to detect pelvic fractures.
  - Obtain radiographs of the pelvis in at least two projections to fully evaluate bone injury. Further radiographs, including contrast studies, may be necessary to evaluate soft tissue injury. It may be necessary to sedate or anesthetize the patient to obtain high-quality diagnostic radiographs.
- Perform a neurologic examination to detect damage to the spinal cord, cauda equina nerve roots, and peripheral nerves.

CONSERVATIVE TREATMENT

In many animals with pelvic fractures, conservative treatment is all that is needed for successful fracture healing and normal pelvic limb function. However, careful nursing is required for several weeks, because multiple injuries commonly are present. Patient size is an important consideration in making the decision to manage pelvic fractures without surgery. Small dogs and cats are much easier to manage for extended periods of time.

The following measures are helpful in conservative therapy.

- Dogs and cats with pelvic fractures often are reluctant to stand and may be unable to turn over. Turn these animals regularly and use a padded bed to help prevent decubital ulcers.
  - Give analgesics as needed.
- Pain, bone instability, and neurologic injury may make it difficult for animals with pelvic fractures to urinate and defecate normally.
  - Empty the urinary bladder regularly by manual expression or catheter drainage, to prevent excessive distension, overflow incontinence, and urine soiling.
  - If necessary, give a mild laxative or stool softener for constipation.
- Some patients are able to stand and walk within a few days; however, restrict activity to a cage for 4–6 weeks.
- If limb adduction is weak as a consequence of ventral pelvic fractures or muscle trauma, place tape-hobbles

between the pelvic limbs for 5–10 days to assist recovery.
- To monitor fracture healing, obtain radiographs every 4–6 weeks during recovery.

INDICATIONS FOR SURGERY

The chief advantages of surgical treatment of pelvic fractures are reduced pain, early return to normal function, avoidance of fracture-associated disease, and minimal hospitalization time. Pelvic fractures may result in marked narrowing of the pelvic canal if left untreated, with the risk of consequent obstipation, dystocia, dysuria, or sciatic nerve entrapment. If operative treatment of pelvic fractures is delayed beyond 5 days, muscle spasm and fibrosis may make reduction of the fracture fragments difficult, because of the large muscle mass surrounding the pelvis.

Surgical treatment may be indicated for the following injuries:

- Fracture of the ilium with ipsilateral fracture of the pubis and ischium creating an unstable acetabulum
- Intra-articular fractures (acetabulum)
- Markedly displaced, unstable, or painful sacroiliac fracture or luxation
- Severe bilateral fractures of the pelvis or displaced pelvic fracture associated with an additional major orthopedic injury of a pelvic limb, such as hip luxation or fracture of the femur
- Fracture of the ischium associated with the caudal aspect of the acetabulum
- Fracture of the pubis or separation of the pubic symphysis associated with abdominal wall rupture and herniation of abdominal organs

FRACTURES OF THE ILIUM

Preoperative Considerations

- Fractures of the ilium are usually oblique and are often accompanied by fractures of other regions of the pelvis.

KEY POINT ▶ If fracture displacement is present, the caudal fragment usually is displaced medially, and thus the pelvic canal is narrowed.

- A thorough neurologic examination is important, particularly with markedly displaced fractures, as damage to the sciatic nerve may be present.
- Surgical repair of fractures of the ilium is recommended if there are multiple pelvic fractures or an additional major pelvic limb injury. Surgical treatment may consist of more than one operation.
- Precontouring the bone plate to the ilium of an intact pelvic specimen from an animal of a similar size reduces operating time.
- Administer prophylactic antibiotics at the time of anesthetic induction.

Surgical Procedure

Objectives

- Anatomically reduce and stabilize the ilium.
- Relieve pain.
- Provide early restoration of pelvic limb function.
- Avoid iatrogenic sciatic nerve damage.

Equipment

- Standard general surgical pack and suture material
- Gelpi or Weitlaner self-retaining retractors
- Orthopedic surgical pack with AO-ASIF and Kern bone-holding forceps and Hohmann retractors
- Bone-plating equipment
- Periosteal elevator
- Suction and electrocautery setups

Technique

1. Place the animal in lateral recumbency and stabilize the pelvis by placing sandbags under the animal and securing the animal to the table.
2. Place a gauze sponge in the rectum, and place a pursestring suture in the anus.
3. Prepare the skin for aseptic surgery on either side of the body of the ilium, from the midlumbar area to the base of the tail.
4. Use a ventrolateral (gluteal roll-up) approach to the ilium.
5. Make a skin incision from the iliac crest to the greater trochanter.
6. Incise and retract the cutaneous trunci muscle and subcutaneous fat to expose the pelvic musculature.
7. Maintain hemostasis by careful electrocoagulation.
8. Dissection and fracture stabilization:
   a. Identify and separate the sartorius, the tensor fasciae latae, and middle gluteal muscles. Retract the sartorius muscle and the tensor fasciae latae muscle ventrally, and retract the middle gluteal muscle dorsally to expose the ilium. Subperiosteal reflection of the middle and deep gluteal muscles dorsally exposes the lateral surface of the body of the ilium.
   b. During exposure of the body of the ilium, it may be necessary to retract branches of the cranial gluteal vein, artery, and nerve that supply the tensor fasciae latae muscle.
   c. Preserve the lateral circumflex femoral vessels immediately cranial to the acetabulum.

KEY POINT ▶ Avoid damage to the sciatic nerve, which lies dorsomedial to the ilium, during dissection and reduction of the fracture.

   d. After exposing the fracture, use ASIF bone-holding forceps to manipulate and reduce the caudal fragment. Attaching bone-holding forceps to the greater trochanter or ischium is helpful in reduction of the caudal ilial fragment.
   e. After reducing the fracture, contour a bone plate to the body of the ilium. Position the plate so that one screw in the cranial fragment can be placed in the body of the sacrum to engage more bone. The cranial part of the wing of the ilium

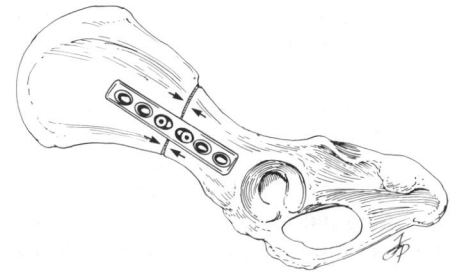

Figure 1. Slightly oblique fracture of the body of the ilium that has been reduced and stabilized with a six-hole dynamic compression plate. The screws have been loaded to produce compression of the fracture.

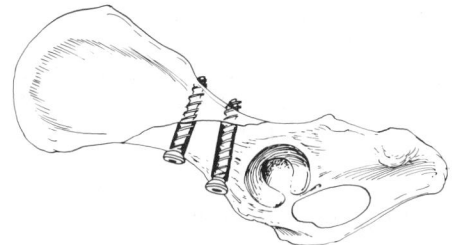

Figure 2. A long oblique fracture of the body of the ilium that has been stabilized with two fully threaded screws. The near cortex has been overdrilled to produce interfragmentary compression of the fracture as the screws are tightened.

is thin and screws may strip easily if the sacrum is not used.

f. Initially, attach the plate to the caudal fragment. Lateral traction on the caudal fragment assists final reduction of the fracture and aids the reduction of accompanying fractures in other regions of the pelvis.

g. If a dynamic compression plate is used to stabilize a transverse fracture, compress the fracture by using the drill guide in the load position before screw placement (Fig. 1). If a bone plate is used, place at least two screws on both sides of the fracture. Select all implant sizes according to the guidelines in Table 1.

h. If fracture comminution is present, smaller fracture fragments may be stabilized with Kirschner wires to further assist fracture reduction.

i. It may be possible to stabilize oblique fractures of the body of the ilium with bone screws alone, particularly in large dogs. Use the screws for lag effect by overdrilling the cortex closest to the head of the screw, or use partially threaded screws. The fracture will be compressed as the screws are tightened (Fig. 2).

9. Closure:

a. Close the muscle and fascia (absorbable suture, interrupted pattern), subcutaneous tissue (absorbable suture, simple continuous pattern), and skin (nonabsorbable suture, interrupted pattern; or intradermal absorbable suture, simple continuous pattern).

b. Remove the pursestring suture from the anus.

Postoperative Care and Complications
Short-Term

■ Evaluate immediate postoperative radiographs for plate contouring and screw placement, particularly any screws inserted into the body of the sacrum.

TABLE 1. Guidelines for Implant Sizes for Fractures of the Ilium in Dogs and Cats

Body Weight (kg)	Plate Size (mm)
<10	2.0 DCP or VCP
10–20	2.7 DCP or PRP
>20	3.5 DCP or PRP

DCP = dynamic compression plate; VCP = veterinary cuttable plate; PRP = pelvic reconstruction plate.

■ Closely monitor for hemorrhage and seroma formation.

■ Good patient care is essential to encourage early mobility and return to normal function (see Conservative Treatment).

■ Reassess the neurologic status of the patient.

Long-Term

■ Restrict activity for 6–8 weeks to minimize the risk of fixation failure.

■ If neurologic deficits are present, reevaluate these regularly.

■ Obtain radiographs every 4–6 weeks to monitor fracture healing.

■ As a rule, do not remove the plate and bone screws. Stress protection by the plate is not a recognized complication.

Prognosis

■ The prognosis is good with anatomic reduction, stable fixation, and no neurologic damage. Pelvic fractures usually heal in 6–10 weeks. Delayed union or nonunion is uncommon because the pelvic bones have a large proportion of cancellous bone, and their extensive soft tissue coverage maintains a good blood supply to the fractured bone and also provides some degree of fracture stabilization.

■ If neurologic deficits are present after surgery, the prognosis is fair to poor, and recovery of normal function may be delayed by several weeks or may not occur.

■ If the implant is too small or if insufficient screws are placed on both sides of the fracture, plate breakage or screw loosening may occur.

FRACTURES OF THE ACETABULUM

Preoperative Considerations

■ Fractures of the acetabulum usually are accompanied by fractures of other regions of the pelvis. If other major weight-bearing regions of the pelvis are fractured, multiple surgical procedures may be necessary.

■ Fractures of the acetabulum are classified by the anatomic location (cranial, central, or caudal acetabulum), the degree of comminution, and the degree of displacement.

■ Conservative management has been advocated for undisplaced and caudal fractures of the acetabulum. However, the treatment of choice for all intra-articular fractures of the acetabulum is surgical stabilization, because this minimizes the severity of subsequent degenerative joint disease.

KEY POINT ▶ When it is not possible to reconstruct comminuted acetabular fractures anatomically, conservative management or stabilization of the major fragments, followed by an immediate or delayed femoral head and neck ostectomy, is indicated.

■ Damage to the joint capsule may be associated with fractures of the acetabulum, especially if the hip is luxated.
■ A thorough neurologic examination is important, particularly with displaced fractures of the caudal acetabulum, because damage to the sciatic nerve may be present.
■ Administer prophylactic antibiotics at the time of anesthetic induction.

Surgical Procedure

Objectives

■ Anatomically reduce and stabilize the acetabulum to restore joint congruity and limb function.
■ Relieve pain.
■ Provide early restoration of pelvic limb function.
■ Avoid iatrogenic sciatic nerve damage.

Equipment

■ Standard general surgical pack and suture material
■ Gelpi or Weitlaner self-retaining retractors
■ Orthopedic surgical pack with ASIF and Kern bone-holding forceps and Hohmann retractors
■ Bone-plating equipment including acetabular plates
■ Periosteal elevator
■ Suction and electrocautery setups

Technique

1. Place the animal in lateral recumbency and stabilize the pelvis by placing sandbags under the animal. Secure the animal to the table.
2. Place a gauze sponge in the rectum, and place a pursestring suture in the anus.
3. Prepare the skin for aseptic surgery on both sides of the hip joint, from the midlumbar area to the base of the tail.
4. Make a caudolateral approach to the hip joint for dorsal and caudal fractures, because this minimizes damage to the gluteal musculature. If further surgical exposure is needed during surgery, extend the approach to a dorsal one by gluteal tenotomy or osteotomy of the greater trochanter.
5. Make a curved skin incision, centered over the caudal surface of the greater trochanter, beginning

close to the dorsal midline, and ending at the junction of the proximal and middle thirds of the femur.
6. Incise and retract the subcutaneous tissues to expose the underlying musculature.
7. Dissection and fracture stabilization:
   a. Incise the fascia of the biceps femoris muscle along its cranial border.
   b. Free the cranial part of the origin of the biceps femoris muscle from the sacrotuberous ligament. Transect the insertion of the superficial gluteal muscle on the third trochanter, and retract this muscle dorsomedially. Retract the biceps femoris muscle caudally.
   c. Identify and avoid the caudal gluteal vein and artery and the sciatic nerve.
   d. Transect the combined tendons of the internal obturator and gemelus muscles close to their insertion in the trochanteric fossa. Retract these muscles caudomedially, along with the sciatic nerve, by the use of a stay suture in the tendons.
   e. Retract the middle and deep gluteal muscles cranially. It may be necessary to transect the deep gluteal tendon to expose the cranial portion of the acetabulum.
   f. Preserve the joint capsule; do not elevate it from the acetabular bone. To observe the joint surface, perform a small arthrotomy.
   g. After exposing the fracture, use ASIF small reduction forceps to manipulate and reduce the fracture fragments. Place Kern bone-holding forceps on the ischium to aid in elevation of the caudal fragment. Bone-holding forceps placed on the greater trochanter also will provide lateral traction and aid in manipulation of the femoral head for better identification of the fracture.
   h. Fractures of the acetabulum rarely are stable when reduced. Maintain reduction of the fracture by placing point-to-point bone-holding forceps craniocaudally across the acetabulum (Fig. 3). If necessary, place shallow drill holes (1.1 or 1.5 mm) in each fragment to prevent the point-to-point forceps from slipping.

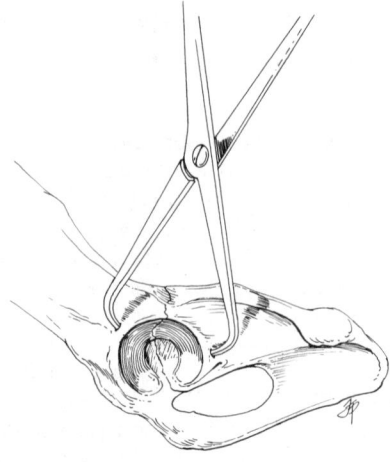

Figure 3. Two-piece fracture of the acetabulum that has been reduced with the aid of point-to-point bone-holding forceps, placed in a cranial-to-caudal direction in predrilled (1.5 mm) drill holes.

i. When the fracture has been reduced, apply a precontoured bone plate. If interfragmentary compression is applied, slightly overbend the plate.

j. Stabilize fractures of the acetabulum with an acetabular plate, a small dynamic compression plate, or a pelvic reconstruction plate. Engage at least four cortices on both sides of the fracture. Because of the thin cortical bone that is present in the pelvis, carefully drill and tap the screw holes. Select implants according to the guidelines in Table 2.

8. Closure:

a. If the joint capsule has been torn or incised, appose it with sutures in a simple interrupted pattern. Reattach the tendon of the internal obturator and gemellus muscles.

b. Close the fascia (absorbable suture, continuous pattern), subcutaneous tissue (absorbable suture, simple continuous pattern), and skin (nonabsorbable suture, interrupted pattern or intradermal absorbable suture, simple continuous pattern).

c. Remove the pursestring suture from the anus.

Postoperative Care and Complications

■ See Fractures of the Ilium.

Prognosis

■ The prognosis is good if anatomic reduction of the acetabulum is achieved, hip stability is maintained, and no neurologic damage is present.

■ If anatomic reduction is not achieved, the prognosis is fair to poor. Degenerative joint disease is likely to develop, and further surgical or medical treatment may be necessary.

■ The prognosis is fair to poor if femoral head excision is performed to repair a comminuted acetabular fractures.

SACROILIAC FRACTURE OR LUXATION

Preoperative Considerations

■ If luxation of the sacroiliac joint has occurred, craniodorsal displacement of the ilium usually is present, and there are fractures in other regions of the pelvis. Less frequently, bilateral sacroiliac joint separation may occur.

TABLE 2. Guidelines for Implant Sizes for Fractures of the Acetabulum in Dogs and Cats

Body Weight (kg)	Plate Size (mm)
<10	2.0 AP, 2.0 DCP
10–20	2.0 or 2.7 AP, 2.7 DCP or PRP
20–30	2.7 AP, 2.7 DCP or PRP
>30	2.7 AP, 3.5 DCP or PRP

AP = acetabular plate; DCP = dynamic compression plate; PRP = pelvic reconstruction plate.

■ Perform a thorough neurologic examination, particularly when displacement of the fracture is marked or luxation is severe, because damage to the cauda equina nerve roots may be present.

■ Surgery often is recommended for animals with severe injury, particularly if neurologic deficits are present, because lameness may persist for a prolonged period with conservative management.

■ Because surgical treatment of sacroiliac fracture or luxation is technically difficult, undertake surgical treatment only after careful consideration of other options, including conservative management and referral.

KEY POINT ▶ In many animals with sacroiliac luxation or fracture, the displacement is not severe and the injury will respond well to conservative management. However, successful reduction and stabilization of the sacroiliac joint alleviates pain more quickly, allowing more rapid return to normal function.

■ Administer prophylactic antibiotics at the time of anesthetic induction.

Surgical Procedure

Objectives

■ Anatomically reduce and stabilize the sacrum and sacroiliac joints.

■ Relieve pain.

■ Provide early restoration of pelvic limb function.

■ Avoid iatrogenic damage to the cauda equina nerve roots and sciatic nerve.

Equipment

■ Standard general surgical pack and suture material

■ Gelpi or Weitlaner self-retaining retractors

■ Orthopedic surgical pack with ASIF and Kern bone-holding forceps and Hohmann retractors

■ Bone-plating equipment

■ Periosteal elevator

■ Suction and electrocautery setups

Technique

1. Place the animal in lateral or ventral recumbency, and stabilize the pelvis by placing sandbags under the animal. Secure the animal to the table.

2. Place a gauze sponge in the rectum, and place a pursestring suture in the anus.

3. Prepare the skin for aseptic surgery on both sides of the dorsal midline, from the midlumbar area to the base of the tail. With bilateral fracture or luxation, bilateral incisions may be necessary.

4. Use a dorsolateral or ventrolateral approach to the sacroiliac joint. (For the ventrolateral approach, see Fractures of the Ilium.) A dorsal approach may be used for bilateral sacroiliac fractures or luxations.

5. Make a skin incision for the dorsolateral approach over the crest of the ilium.

6. Incise and retract the cutaneous trunci muscle and the subcutaneous fat to expose the pelvic musculature.

7. Maintain hemostasis by careful electrocoagulation.

8. Dissection and fracture stabilization:
   a. Incise the middle gluteal muscle along its origin at the cranial and dorsal borders of the wing of the ilium, and subperiosteally elevate it, beginning cranially.
   b. During dissection, protect the cranial gluteal artery, vein, and nerve, which cross medially to laterally over the caudal iliac spine and enters the middle and deep gluteal muscles. The sacrospinalis muscle and dorsal sacroiliac ligament usually are disrupted and therefore require little additional dissection.
   c. Maneuver the ilium using Kern bone-holding forceps. Initially, displace the ilium ventrally and laterally to expose the articular surface of the sacrum.
   d. Place a drill hole in the body of the sacrum (Fig. 4). Align the drill hole perpendicular to the midsagittal plane, rather than perpendicular to the articular surface of the sacrum, in order to avoid misdirection of the screw dorsally or ventrally. Make the depth of the drill hole two-thirds of the width of the sacral body, and measure the hole with a depth gauge and tap the hole.
   e. The site on the medial surface of the ilium that corresponds to the drill hole in the sacrum determines the exact location of the drill hole on the lateral surface of the ilium. Overdrill the hole to allow compression of the sacroiliac joint with a fully threaded lag screw.
   f. Determine the length of the screw by adding the thickness of the ilium to the depth of the sacral drill hole. Select the size of the bone screw from the guidelines in Table 3.
   g. Place the screw into the ilium until the tip of the screw just protrudes from the medial surface. Reduce the sacroiliac joint and insert the screw to stabilize and compress the joint.

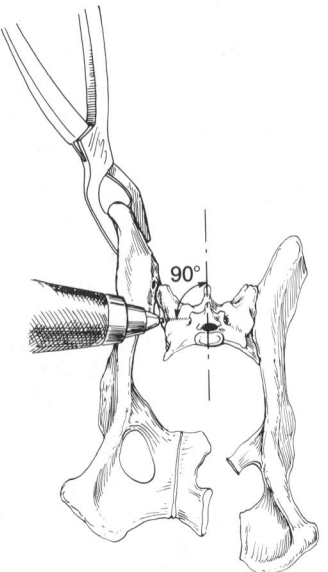

Figure 4. Surgical approach to sacroiliac luxation. Bone-holding forceps have been placed on the wing of the ilium to assist reduction. A hole has been drilled into the body of the sacrum in preparation for reduction of the luxation.

TABLE 3. Guidelines for Screw Sizes in Repair of Sacroiliac Fracture or Luxation in Dogs and Cats

Body Weight (kg)	Single Screw (mm)	Two Screws (mm)*
<10	2.7	2.7 and 2.0
10–20	3.5 or 4.0	3.5 and 2.7
20–30	4.5	4.5 and 3.5
>30	6.5	6.5 and 3.5

*Place the smaller screw craniodorsal to the larger screw, which is inserted into the body of the sacrum.

   h. If indicated, place a second screw just cranial and dorsal to the first to give two-point fixation. Determine the screw length by measurement from dorsoventral radiographs, so that it does not penetrate the neural canal. A second screw may be necessary if the patient is a large dog, the sacrum is fractured, or the first screw is not ideally placed in the body of the sacrum.
   i. With bilateral fractures or luxations, screw(s) may be placed bilaterally, or a single screw may be placed through both ilial wings and the sacral body. In the latter instance, use an aiming device to ensure that the drill hole is placed in the correct plane.
9. Closure: See Fractures of the Ilium.

Postoperative Care and Complications

Short-Term

- Because errors in screw placement are common, carefully evaluate immediate postoperative radiographs for screw placement.
- Closely monitor for hemorrhage and seroma formation.
- Good patient care is essential to encourage early mobility and return to normal function (see Conservative Treatment).

Long-Term

- If neurologic deficits are present, reevaluate the animal regularly for improvement in function. Intensive patient care may be necessary for a number of weeks after surgery.
- Obtain postoperative radiographs to monitor joint and fracture healing.
- As a rule, do not remove the bone screws.

Prognosis

- The prognosis is good with correct positioning of the bone screws and no neurologic damage.
- If the bone screws do not correctly engage the sacral body, fixation failure is more likely.
- If neurologic deficits are present after surgery, the prognosis is fair to poor.

FRACTURES OF THE ISCHIUM
Preoperative Considerations

- Fractures of the ischium usually are associated with fractures of other major weight-bearing regions of the pelvis. If appropriate surgery is performed to anatomically reduce and stabilize other, functionally more important fractures, additional fixation of ischial fractures usually is unnecessary.

- Fractures of the ischium usually are displaced ventrally as a consequence of tension created by the caudal thigh muscles (the biceps femoris, semitendinosus, and semimembranous muscles).
- Occasionally, isolated fractures of the ischium may be encountered. If severe pain is associated with the fracture(s) or if displacement of the fracture fragments is such that the function of the hip joint is impaired, internal fixation may be indicated (see Acetabular Fractures).

KEY POINT ▶ Surgical repair of fractures of the ischium usually is unnecessary.

FRACTURES OF THE PUBIS

- Fractures of the pelvic symphysis, which is composed of the pubic and ischial symphyses, may be associated with fractures of other regions of the pelvis. This problem is more common in young animals in which bony union of the symphysis has not yet occurred.
- Anatomic reduction and stabilization of the other, more functionally important pelvic fracture(s) usually makes surgical treatment of the pubic fracture unnecessary. However, internal fixation of pubic fractures may occasionally be indicated.
- If pubic fractures are associated with a caudal abdominal wall rupture and herniation of abdominal or pelvic organs, surgical repair of the hernia may be assisted by internal fixation of the fractures. Cerclage wire is usually the preferred method for fixation.

KEY POINT ▶ Surgical repair of fractures of the pubis usually is unnecessary.

HEALED PELVIC FRACTURES ASSOCIATED WITH A NARROWED PELVIC CANAL

- Obstipation and dystocia occasionally are associated with healed pelvic fractures and a narrowed pelvic canal. This problem is most commonly encountered in cats and small dogs whose pelvic fractures are more likely to be managed conservatively.
- Manage dystocia by cesarean section or ovariohysterectomy.
- Operations designed to widen the pelvic canal have been described. Osteotomy of the ilium, the ischium, and the pubis, and lateralization of the caudal fragment with a plate is the preferred method.
- In dogs and cats with obstipation, a subtotal colectomy may be necessary (see sec. 7, ch. 7), because colonic dysfunction is not always relieved by corrective osteotomy and widening of the pelvic canal.

KEY POINT ▶ If obstipation has been present for several months, normal colonic motility does not always return after the bony pelvic canal has been widened, and obstipation can continue to be a problem.

Supplemental Readings

Brinker WO, Piermattei DL, Flo GL: *Handbook of Small Animal Orthopedics and Fracture Treatment*, 2nd Ed. Philadelphia: W. B. Saunders, 1990.

DeCamp CE, Braden TD: The surgical anatomy of the canine sacrum for lag screw fixation of the sacroiliac joint. Vet Surg 14(2):131, 1985.

14 Coxofemoral Joint

Marvin L. Olmstead

The coxofemoral joint is the most proximal of the free-moving joints of the pelvic limb. Surgery frequently is performed on or near this joint to treat conditions such as coxofemoral luxations and hip dysplasia. Avascular necrosis of the femoral head, which is not as common as hip dysplasia or coxofemoral luxations, also can be successfully treated surgically.

Anatomic considerations, pathophysiology, and treatment of these conditions of the coxofemoral joint are discussed in this chapter.

ANATOMY

- The coxofemoral joint is a ball-and-socket joint made up of the femoral head (ball) and the acetabulum (socket).
- In a normal animal, the joint capsule fits tightly around the rim of the acetabulum and attaches around the circumference of the femoral neck just distal to the junction of the head and neck. When the limb is taken through range-of-motion exercises, the tight fit of the joint capsule helps maintain joint congruency.
- The ligament of the head of the femur runs between the acetabular fossa and the fovea capitis of the femoral head.
  - The fovea and the fossa are sometimes mistakenly identified as radiographic abnormalities.

KEY POINT ▶ The fovea causes a natural flattened area on the femoral head that can be mistaken for the flattening associated with hip dysplasia. The fossa creates a shadow that can be mistaken for a fracture line.

- The blood supply to the femoral head is extensive.
  - Small arterial loops arise from the iliolumbar artery cranially; the lateral circumflex femoral artery dorsally, cranially, and ventrally; and the medial circumflex femoral artery dorsally, caudally, and ventrally. They all penetrate the femoral head at the joint capsule attachment.
  - No significant blood vessels penetrate the ligament of the head of the femur.
- Several surgically important muscles have their insertions or origins close to the coxofemoral joint, either on the proximal femur or the pelvis.
  - The middle and deep gluteal muscles originate on the wing of the ilium and insert on the cranial and dorsal border of the greater trochanter.
  - The superficial gluteal muscle originates on the sacrum and the first coccygeal vertebra and inserts on the lateral face of the third trochanter.
  - The internal and external obturator and gemelli all insert in the caudal trochanteric fossa.
  - The vastus lateralis and intermedius muscles insert on the cranial face of the femur, whereas the rectus femoris inserts on the pelvis cranial to the acetabulum.
  - The tensor fascia lata muscle inserts along the caudal lateral edge of the femur, covering the vastus lateralis muscle, and along the cranial edge of the biceps femoris muscle via three or more tissue slips.
  - The origin of the pectineus muscle is just ventral to the acetabulum.
- Two angles of surgical significance have been described in the proximal femur:
  - With the femur viewed from a cranial position, the *angle of inclination* is the angle formed between a line that bisects the long axis of the femur and a line that bisects the femoral neck. In the normal dog, this angle is 135–145°.
  - With the femur viewed from a straight lateral position, part of the femoral head is displaced forward of the femoral shaft owing to the anteversion angle of the femoral neck. One method of measuring this angle involves taking radiographs of the femur with the dog on its back with the long axis of the femur positioned 90° to the radiographic plate and the stifle flexed 90°. The radiographic beam must pass directly down the center of the femur, parallel to its long axis. One line is drawn parallel to the caudal edge of the femoral condyles, and a second bisects the femoral head and neck. The angle created by the intersection of these two lines is the *anteversion angle*, which, in normal dogs is 20–27°.
  - Abnormal alterations can occur in these angles during hip development, resulting in pathology in the hip or further down the limb.

COXOFEMORAL LUXATIONS

Most coxofemoral luxations are craniodorsal displacements of the femoral head; almost all others are caudoventrally displaced. Usually these are associated with motor vehicle accidents; thus, full evaluation of other organ systems for trauma (see sec. 6, ch. 24 and sec. 1, ch. 3), as well as coxofemoral joint evaluation, is indicated in these patients.

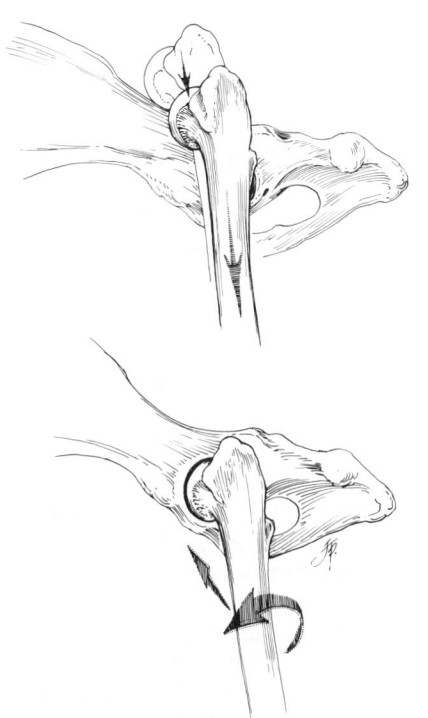

Figure 1. Closed reduction of the coxofemoral joint. External rotation and distal traction of the limb *(top)* is followed by internal rotation of the femoral head *(bottom)*.

Diagnosis

KEY POINT ▶ In the evaluation of the coxofemoral joint for luxation, include gait analysis, manipulation of the hip, comparison of hind limb lengths, and two radiographic views of the pelvis.

- Limbs with a luxated hip usually will not bear weight; if a cranial dorsal luxation is present, the limb may be externally rotated and adducted.
- Range-of-motion evaluation of the hip may reveal grating and/or pain in the area of the coxofemoral joint.
- Evaluate the relation between the caudal edge of the greater trochanter and the cranial edge of the ischiatic tuberosity to determine the position of the proximal femur:

- If a caudoventral luxation is present, there will be no space between these two structures.
- If a craniodorsal luxation is present, there will be space that does not close (as in the normal animal) when the limb is externally rotated.
- When both hind limbs are pulled directly caudally, they will be equal length in a normal animal. If they are uneven in length, this is a strong indication that the coxofemoral joint is dislocated.
- The primary method of diagnosis is radiography of the coxofemoral joint. This can:
  - Rule out fractures of the proximal femur which can mimic a luxation on physical examination.
  - Evaluate the acetabulum for the presence of an avulsion fracture from the femoral head (an absolute indication for surgery).

Treatment
Closed Reduction

If there is no avulsion fracture, an early attempt at closed reduction of the joint under general anesthesia is recommended.

- To perform reduction for a craniodorsal luxation:
  - Externally rotate the femoral head.
  - Apply distal traction to the limb until the head is even with the acetabulum; and then rotate the femoral head internally, causing it to drop into the acetabulum (Fig. 1).
- Reduction of a caudoventral luxation is accomplished by abducting and externally rotating the limb.
- The longer the femoral head is out of position, the more damage is done to the dorsal joint capsule. An intact joint capsule is helpful in maintaining reduction.
- If the reduced hip easily luxates again, perform open reduction.
- If the reduced hip snaps solidly into position, place the hip in a flexion sling for a craniodorsal luxation; alternatively for a caudoventral luxation (Fig. 2) place the legs in hobbles. Apply these restriction bandages for 10–14 days in the adult and 7–10 days in the immature animal.
- Examine any reduced hip physically on a daily basis or instruct the owner to do this, until the restriction bandage is removed.
  - If there is any question about the hip's position,

Figure 2. After reduction, use a flexion (Ehmer) sling for a craniodorsal luxation *(left)* and hobbles for a caudoventral luxation *(right)*.

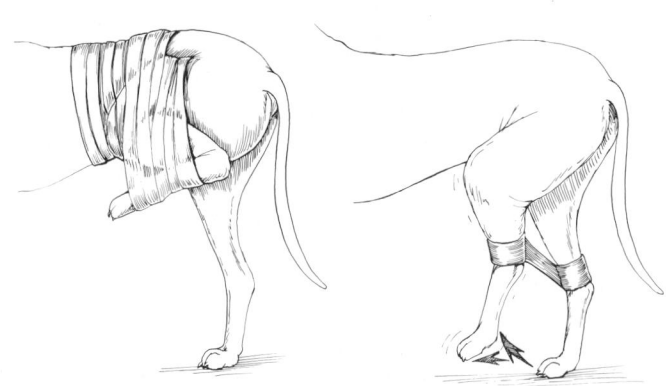

reevaluate with lateral pelvic radiographs. If the hip is reluxated, perform open reduction.

Open Reduction—Surgical Procedures

Objectives

- Reduce the luxated coxofemoral joint.
- Reconstruct as much stabilizing soft tissue as possible.
- Remove fibrous tissue from the acetabulum, remnants of the ligament of the head of the femur, and avulsed bone fragments that cannot be stabilized.

Equipment

- Standard surgery pack and suture material
- Special equipment as needed for specific procedures (noted in following text)

Techniques

1. The standard approaches used for surgical repair of luxations are the cranial lateral approach to the hip and the trochanteric osteotomy approach. Occasionally a caudal approach (caudal to the greater trochanter of the femur) to the coxofemoral joint may be used.
2. Initially, assess the overall damage and the status of supporting tissues, clean out the acetabular cup, and reduce the femoral head into the cup.
3. Once the head is reduced, use one or more stabilization techniques to secure the femoral head into the acetabulum.
4. If the joint capsule is minimally damaged and adequate capsular tissue is present on either side of the tear, suture the capsule (this may be the only support necessary).
   a. Use an absorbable monofilament suture of significant size (2–0, 0, or 1, depending on the animal's size), placed in a cruciate pattern.
   b. If adequate capsule is attached to the acetabular rim but not enough solid capsule is attached to the femoral neck, drill an anchor hole with lateral to cranial orientation in the proximal femur. Pass one-half of the suture strands through the hole and tie them tightly to the other half of the strands (Fig. 3).

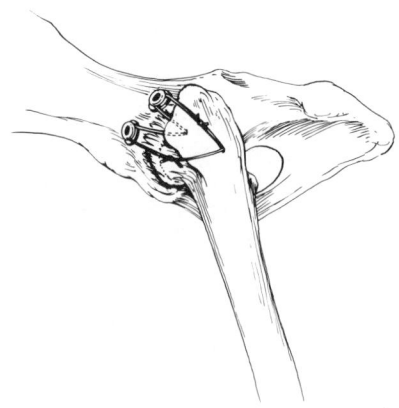

Figure 4. Suture support for a damaged capsule.

5. The capsule may be so severely damaged that it cannot hold a conventionally placed suture. (This may occur if there is a long delay between the time of injury and repair.)
   a. In these cases suture support can be provided by making anchor points for the sutures. Drill a hole (as described in 4b above) for an anchor site in the femur. Place one to three bone screws (usually a 3.5 mm cortical screw) in the dorsal rim over the acetabulum as anchor points on the pelvis. String the suture support between these to form a dorsal reinforcement (Fig. 4).
   b. Alternatively place a temporary intramedullary pin in the proximal femur, parallel with the neck axis, and through the acetabular fossa. Be sure that the pin does not extend too far into the pelvic canal (Fig. 5). Keep the limb immobile with a flexion sling until the pin is removed, 7–10 days after surgery.
   c. Another alternative is to place a toggle pin through a hole in the acetabular fossa with suture attached to it. This creates an artificial ligament between the head of the femur and the acetabulum. Pass the suture through a hole drilled, from lateral to medial, in the proximal femur. The hole enters the femur just dorsal to the third trochanter and exits at the insertion point of the ligament of the head of the femur on the femoral head. Pull all the suture strands through this hole, and then pass half the suture strands

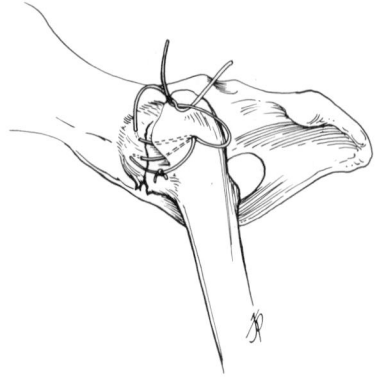

Figure 3. Surgical repair of luxation if adequate capsule remains attached to the acetabular rim.

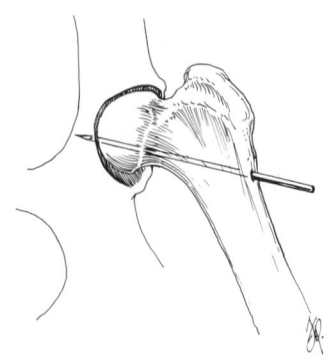

Figure 5. Temporary intramedullary pin for open reduction of coxofemoral joint.

through a second hole in the femur drilled in a cranial to caudal direction. Tie the two sets of suture strands together.

6. Rotate the femoral head inwardly, and tighten the gluteal muscle pull on the femur by moving the greater trochanter to a position caudal and distal to its original location. This technique can be used with a trochanteric osteotomy approach.

    a. Do not depend on this technique as the sole means of stabilization.

    b. Any positional changes in gait caused by this relocation are temporary, because the gluteal muscles eventually will stretch.

7. If the femoral head does not remain in the acetabulum even with the application of support techniques, consider the use of a primary salvage procedure such as excision arthroplasty or total hip replacement.

Postoperative Care and Complications

- If there is any doubt about the strength or security of the stabilization, place the limb in an immobilization sling or bandage for 7–14 days.
- Examine the sling or bandage and the visible parts of the limb daily for odor, chewing, swelling, pressure sore development, and slippage.
- Check the spacial relationship between the greater trochanter and the ischiatic tuberosity daily. If this changes, evaluate the position of the femur with lateral radiography of the pelvis. This can be accomplished without removing the sling.
- Restrict the animal's activity (leash walking only) for 1 month after the surgery.
- The most common complication following surgery or closed reduction is reluxation. If reluxation occurs after open reduction, consider excision arthroplasty or total hip replacement.

AVASCULAR NECROSIS OF THE FEMORAL HEAD

- This condition (also known as Legg-Perthes or Legg-Calvé-Perthes disease, osteochondritis juvenilis, and coxa plana) is most commonly found in adolescent, small-breed dogs of either sex; occasionally it occurs in large breeds.
- Trauma is not usually associated with the onset of lameness, and the lameness can progress to non–weight bearing.
- The condition occurs bilaterally in about 15% of the animals.
- Changes in the proximal femur seen radiographically and grossly are the result of collapse and remodeling of the trabecular bone of the femoral head following the avascular episode.
  - It is not clear what causes the femoral head to become avascular; following this, the bone revascularizes and remodels as the dead bone undergoes resorption.
- Weight bearing causes the weakened subchondral bone to collapse, which, in turn, leads to fracture of the cartilage.

Diagnosis

- Base the diagnosis on physical examination and radiographic findings. Abduction of the limb often elicits a pain response, even before radiographic signs are evident. Crepitus is sometimes observed with flexion and extension of the joint.
- The limb may be shortened and the muscles atrophied.
- Radiographs are needed for a definitive diagnosis. The ventrodorsal straight-leg view of the pelvis is the most helpful in assessing the femoral heads.
  - The joint space may be widened, and numerous foci of decreased bone density may be seen in the femoral head and neck.
  - In advanced stages, these may be irregular indentations, flattening, and possibly fragmentation of the femoral head. Osteophytes on the acetabular rim and secondary osteoarthritis in the joint may also be seen.

Supportive Treatment

Some dogs will respond to nonsurgical treatment including limited activity and analgesics. However, in most cases surgery is ultimately necessary.

KEY POINT ▶ Surgical treatment of avascular necrosis of the femoral head has a much higher success rate than nonsurgical treatment.

Surgical Procedures

Objectives

- Eliminate painful bone-to-bone contact.
- Preserve hip motion as close to normal as possible.

Equipment

- Standard surgical pack and suture material
- Specialized equipment, depending on the specific procedure

Preoperative Considerations

- Because most of the dogs with this condition are small breeds, excision arthroplasty (see later in this chapter) is the most common procedure performed for this disease.
- In large dogs, consider total hip replacement (see below) as an option.

HIP DYSPLASIA

Hip dysplasia is a faulty development of the hip joint characterized by varying degrees of joint laxity that permit subluxation early in life. As the condition progresses, deformation of the architecture of the acetabulum and femoral head is accompanied by the development of degenerative joint disease.

KEY POINT ▶ Hip dysplasia is the most prevalent disorder of the canine hip and the most important cause of osteoarthritis in that joint.

- Although almost all breeds are at risk, hip dysplasia most commonly affects large- and giant-breed dogs, and its mode of inheritance is polygenetic.
- Joint instability occurs as muscle development and maturation lag behind the rate of skeletal growth.
  - The first 60 days of life are the most critical period for the developing soft tissue structures.
  - When the stress and weight exerted at the hip joint exceed the strength limits of the supporting soft tissues, joint instability results.

Diagnosis

Base the diagnosis of hip dysplasia on the history, physical examination, and radiographic evaluation of the coxofemoral joints.

Physical Examination

- Lameness of the hind limb and gait abnormalities frequently are seen, especially after exercise periods, motion of the coxofemoral joint often is limited because of joint pain.
- Joint laxity and pain may be elicited by examination of the range of motion of the coxofemoral joint. Joint laxity will be present in mild to moderately dysplastic animals.
- Ortolani sign: With a hand placed on the knee of the affected limb, apply dorsal pressure to the femur while moving the limb from an adducted to an abducted position.
  - The click or pop that is heard or felt as the femoral head enters or exits the acetabulum is a positive Ortolani sign and an indication of joint laxity.
  - If the hip is normal or if changes in the acetabulum preclude movement of the femoral head in and out of the acetabulum, the Ortolani sign will be negative.

Radiography

Radiographs are needed for a positive diagnosis of hip dysplasia.

- In early cases, proper positioning of the ventrodorsal view is extremely critical; in advanced stages, the changes are pronounced and positioning is less important.
- Radiographic changes associated with hip dysplasia range from subluxation of the femoral head to severe degenerative joint disease, with marked alterations in the architecture of the femoral head and the acetabulum.

Nonsurgical Therapy

Nonsurgical therapy is recommended for animals mildly affected by hip dysplasia and those with an initial episode of lameness.

- Restrict activity to allow the inflammatory response within the joint capsule to subside.
- Give medication to relieve pain and reduce the inflammation associated with the degenerative joint disease. Aspirin (20 mg/kg q12h)is sometimes adequate.

KEY POINT ▶ When nonsurgical therapy is no longer effective or if the patient is constantly disabled over an extended period, consider one of the following surgical therapies.

Surgical Procedures—Overview

Various surgical procedures that have been effective in the treatment of hip dysplasia are discussed. An improved quality of life for the patient is the ultimate goal. The procedures are not listed in any order of preference.

Triple Pelvic Osteotomy

Preoperative Considerations

- In the ideal candidate for this procedure, there is some coverage of the femoral head by the acetabulum and there are no signs of degenerative joint disease in the hip.
- Most dogs with pathologic changes that meet the above criteria are 5–13 months of age.

Objective

- Increase the amount of acetabular coverage over the femoral head by rotating the acetabular portion of the pelvis.
- Maintain the normal architecture and congruency of the femoral head and acetabulum.
- Prevent the development of degenerative joint disease.

Equipment

- Standard surgical pack and suture material
- Equipment necessary to insert bone screws
- Bone plates designed for pelvic osteotomy (e.g., pelvic osteotomy plate; Synthes, Slocum Ent., Inc.)
- Orthopedic wire
- Oscillating bone saw
- Osteotomes

Technique

1. Expose the ilium, pubis, and ischium
   a. Make a lateral approach to the wing of the ilium with dorsal elevation of the middle and deep gluteal muscles (see sec. 9, ch. 13).
   b. Approach the pubis through a second incision over the pectineus muscle or through the lateral approach to the ilium by retracting the vastus muscles caudally and the rectus femoris muscle cranially.
   c. The approach to the ischium depends on the site of the osteotomy. If the osteotomy is performed from the ischial tuberosity cranial to the obturator foramen, make an approach directly over the tuberosity. If the osteotomy is performed

just caudal to the acetabulum, extend the lateral incision and reflect the biceps femoris muscle caudally.

2. Perform osteotomies at the ilium, pubis, and ischium so that the acetabulum can be rotated in a manner that provides more dorsal coverage of the femoral head. Rotate the acetabulum until the femoral head can no longer be dislocated by the Ortolani manipulation.

3. Hold the tilt on the acetabulum in place with bone plates if a transverse osteotomy has been performed, or with screws and orthopedic wire if a stair-step osteotomy is done.

4. Some surgeons also stabilize osteotomy of the ischium with orthopedic wire.

5. Close the incisions routinely.

Postoperative Care and Complications

■ Restrict activity for 8 weeks.
■ Immediate postoperative radiographs may indicate no apparent change in the acetabular coverage of the femoral head. In some cases, subsequent radiographic evaluations reveal improved acetabular coverage and a femoral head well seated in the acetabulum.
■ Occasionally, the desired amount of femoral head coverage is never achieved. This most often occurs when a patient has a totally luxated hip or when many degenerative changes are present at the time of surgery.
■ If the acetabulum is rotated too far at the time of surgery, extension of the coxofemoral joint will be limited and result in a gait alteration.

Femoral Head and Neck Excision Arthroplasty

Preoperative Considerations

This salvage procedure can be performed in dogs of all ages; it is most successful in dogs weighing <18 kg.

Objectives

■ Remove the femoral head and neck.
■ Eliminate painful contact points in the joint.
■ Allow a fibrous tissue joint to replace the ball and socket joint.

Equipment

■ Standard surgical pack and suture material
■ Mallet and osteotome, oscillating bone saw, Gigli wire, or bone cutter
■ Rongeur or rasp

Technique

1. Use a cranial lateral approach or a ventral approach (pectineal myotomy near its origin on the prepubic tendon).

2. Perform osteotomy of the femoral neck by cutting the bone from the lateral-most edge of the trochanteric fossa to a point just dorsal to the lesser trochanter (Fig. 6).

3. Remove the femoral head and neck. It may be

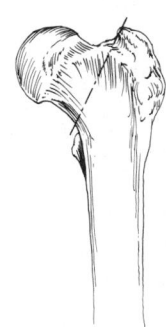

Figure 6. Site of osteotomy for femoral head and neck excision arthroplasty.

necessary to incise the ligament of the head of the femur. If using a ventral approach, this is done following osteotomy of the femoral neck. If using cranial lateral approach, this is done before osteotomy so that the head and neck can be better exposed by rotating the femur externally.

4. Examine the remaining portion of the proximal femur for rough areas or bone spurs and remove any, if present.

5. It is sometimes advisable to remove a portion of the dorsal acetabular rim to ensure that no bone-to-bone rubbing occurs during locomotion.

6. Close the incision routinely.

Postoperative Care and Complications

■ Encourage use of the operated limb 3–7 days postoperatively. Use passive range-of-motion exercise on patients that do not willingly use the limb.
■ Obtain radiographs to document the amount and configuration of the remaining bone.
■ On the average it will take 2–3 months for the limb to reach its ultimate postoperative functional level. In some animals the gait will be indistinguishable from normal; in others an obvious gait abnormality will be present.
■ Because a scar tissue joint is formed after surgery, all animals will have a limited range of motion. The clinical significance of this limitation depends on the activity of the animal, the animal's size, and the amount of restrictive scar tissue that is present.
■ Because normal muscle mass is not regained there may be marked atrophy of the limb.
■ The femur may displace dorsally relative to the pelvis. If the displacement is large, a post-legged gait with the stifle at nearly full extension can result.

Pectineal Myectomy

Preoperative Considerations

■ This procedure can be done on dogs of all ages.
■ Performance of this procedure does not exclude attempting other procedures, should this be unsuccessful.
■ This procedure does not alter the progression or intensity of changes in the joint caused by hip dysplasia, but may palliate joint pain.

Objectives

- Remove all of the belly of the pectineus muscle bilaterally.
- Alter the muscle pull on the hip, thus changing the articular contact points within the hip.

Equipment

Standard surgical pack and suture material

Technique

1. Place the dog in a dorsal recumbent frog-leg position.
2. Make an incision 10–16 cm long over the pectineus muscle on the medial aspect of the thigh.
3. Isolate and incise the muscle at its origin proximally and its muscle-tendon junction distally. Take care to avoid the femoral artery and vein that pass just lateral to the middle of the muscle belly.
4. Close the dead space tightly by meticulous suture of the fascia and subcutaneous layers.

Postoperative Care and Complications

- Restrict activity for 2 weeks.
- The most common postoperative complication is seroma formation. This requires aspiration or drainage only if the seromas become very large. Usually the fluid is absorbed and no treatment is needed.
- In some dogs, the gait is noticeably improved and there seems to be marked pain relief. The length of time for which this relief persists varies.

Intertrochanteric Osteotomy
Preoperative Considerations

- Patient selection is important. Qualifications include:
  - A marked increase in the angle of anteversion and/or inclination (see previous discussion under Anatomy)
  - Minimal degenerative changes in the joint
  - Age close to skeletal maturity (6–8 months)

Objectives

- Decrease the angles of inclination and anteversion.
- Position the femoral head more deeply in the acetabular cup.

Equipment

- Standard surgical pack and suture material
- Intertrochanteric osteotomy bone plates and 3.5-mm cortex screws (Synthes)
- Intertrochanteric osteotomy instrument set (Synthes)
- Oscillating bone saw

Technique

1. Approach the femur craniolaterally, exposing the cranial surface of the femoral neck.
2. Perform a transverse intertrochanteric osteotomy.
3. Perform a second osteotomy along a preplanned line that will allow removal of a wedge of bone and a decrease in the angle of inclination to less than normal, thus creating a coxa vara position.
4. Decrease the angle of anteversion to normal by rotating the proximal femur caudally.
5. Rigidly fix the bone segments in position with a 3.5-mm hook plate (Synthes) or with standard bone plates.
6. Close the incision routinely.

Postoperative Care and Complications

- Restrict activity for 8 weeks.
- A significant number of patients are pain-free and function with normal mobility.
- Some patients develop degenerative joint disease.

Total Hip Replacement

This procedure, which provides an artificial femoral head and artificial acetabular cup, demands a high degree of technical proficiency and strict adherence to good aseptic and surgical techniques. Referral to an experienced specialist is recommended.

Preoperative Considerations

- The growth plates must be closed before this procedure can be performed; thus, the animal must be at least 9 months of age. There is no upper age limit, but older animals should be fully evaluated for systemic disease.
- Depending on the size of the femur and the depth of the acetabular cup, the minimum weight of the animal is 13–18 kg.
- Consider total hip replacement when a disabling condition of the hip exists with no other systemic or hind limb pathology. The dog must be totally free of infection anywhere in the body.

Objectives

- Replace the degenerative coxofemoral joint with a high density polyethylene cup and a cobalt chrome or titanium ally femoral prosthesis.
- Provide a mechanically sound, pain-free joint that will last the dog's life.

Equipment

- Standard surgical pack and suture material
- Reaming and implantation instruments designed specifically for canine total hip replacements (Bio-Medtrix Ltd.)
- High-density polyethylene cup, a cobalt chrome femoral head, and titanium alloy femoral stem (Bio-Medtrix Ltd.)
- Oscillating bone saw
- Power drill

Technique

1. Approach the coxofemoral joint through a craniolateral approach.
2. Remove the femoral head and a portion of the neck

along an osteotomy line that parallels the collar of the prosthesis, and ream the acetabular cup to the medial pelvic wall.

3. Cement the prosthetic acetabular cup and the femoral stem into position with polymethylmethacrylate (Howemedica).

4. After the femoral head is secured onto the stem, reduce it into the cup.

5. Close the joint capsule tightly; close the remaining tissues in layers.

Postoperative Care and Complications

■ Restrict activity to leash walking for 2 months, after which the dog can return to full activity, even if it includes vigorous work.

■ Over 95% of dogs treated with this procedure have satisfactory function if established techniques are followed. Increased muscle mass, extended exercise tolerance and improved hip motion commonly are observed.

■ Although degenerative joint disease usually is present in both hips, 80% of dogs receive sufficient relief that the other hip does not need to be replaced. The limb with the hip replacement becomes dominant, thus reducing the unoperated limb's weight-bearing load.

■ Complications include infection, implant loosening, luxations, fractures, and neuropraxia. The majority of these can be successfully treated.

Supplemental Readings

Brinker WO, Piermattei DL, Flo GL: Diagnosis and treatment of orthopedic conditions of the hindlimb. *In* Brinker WO, Piermattei D, Gretchen F: *Handbook of Small Animal Orthopedics* and *Fracture Treatment*, 2nd ed. Philadelphia: W. B. Saunders, 1990, p 341.

Hauptman J: The hip joint. *In* Slatter D, ed.: *Textbook of Small Animal Surgery*. Philadelphia: W. B. Saunders, 1985, p 2135.

Olmstead ML: Total hip replacement. Vet Clin North Am [Sm Anim Pract] 17:943, 1987.

Riser WH, et al.: Hip dysplasia: Perspectives of the eighties. Seminars Vet Med [Sm Anim] 2:87, 1987.

Schrader SC: Triple pelvic osteotomy of the pelvis as a treatment for canine hip dysplasia. J Am Vet Assoc: 178:39, 1981.

15 Fractures of the Femur and Patella

Peter Shires

Surgery of the femur usually is performed to repair fractures. Biopsy of tumors or cysts or obtaining samples for bone cultures are less common reasons for femoral surgery. The femur is the bone most commonly associated with traumatic fractures in the dog. Surgical repair of femoral injuries may be divided into surgery of the proximal, diaphyseal, and distal femur.

PROXIMAL FEMUR

Anatomy

- The proximal femur includes the femoral head, the femoral neck, the trochanters, and their attachments to the femoral shaft.
- The ligament of the head of the femur connects the fovea capitis of the femoral head to the acetabular fossa.
- The articular surface and epiphysis of the femoral head are separated from the femoral neck by the capital physis.
- The joint capsule of the hip joint inserts at about the midpoint of the femoral neck.
- The primary blood supply to the epiphysis of the femoral head is through four vessels running longitudinally in folds of the joint capsule (Fig. 1).
- The greater trochanter is the point of attachment for the deep and middle gluteal muscles and the piriformis muscle.
- The trochanteric fossa is the site of insertion of the internal obturator, external obturator, and the gemellus muscles.
- The articularis coxae inserts on the cranial aspect of the femoral neck.
- The lesser trochanter is the site of insertion of the iliopsoas muscle on the medial aspect of the proximal femur.
- The third trochanter is lateral and is the site of indentation of the superficial gluteal muscle and the origin of the quadratus femoris muscle and part of the vastus lateralis muscle.
- The proximal femur is the site of origin of the vastus lateralis, vastus medialis, vastus intermedius, quadratus femoris, and adductor longis muscles and of the proximal part of the adductor magnus et brevis muscles.
- The deep muscles of the femur are covered by the tensor fasciae latae and biceps femoris muscle confluence.
- The sciatic nerve runs caudal to the hip on top of the gemellus, internal obturator, and quadratus femoris muscles. It is covered by the biceps femoris and the superficial gluteal muscles.
- The femoral artery, nerve, and vein are very superficial in the femoral triangle on the medial aspect of the proximal to mid-femur.
- The nutrient artery for the femur enters caudally just distal to the major trochanter as a branch of the medial circumflex femoral artery.

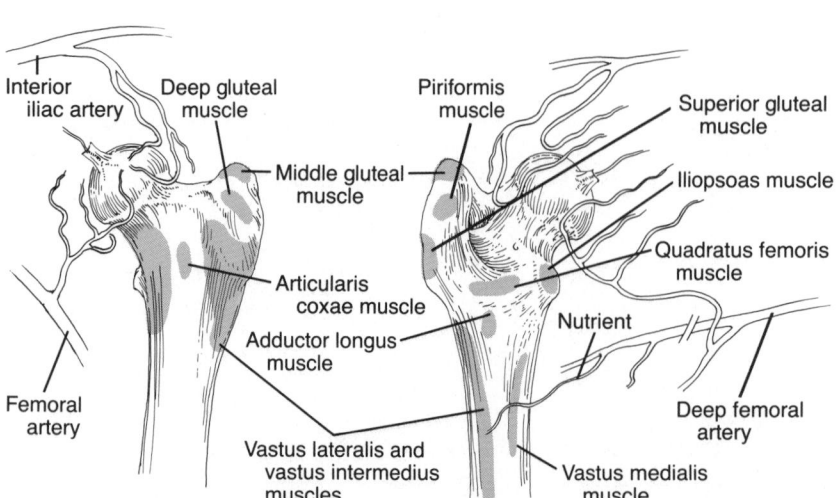

Figure 1. *Left*, Cranial view; *right*, caudal view. Proximal femur showing the muscle attachments and main blood supply.

Preoperative Considerations

KEY POINT ▶ Evaluate the entire patient for trauma-related problems; neurologic, urologic, and intrathoracic injuries are common in impact situations.

- Stabilize the patient before considering surgery.
- Take a minimum of two radiographic views to evaluate the proximal femur.
- Give intraoperative broad-spectrum antibiotics IV (at induction of anesthesia; repeat if necessary) if the surgery will take longer than 2 hours.
- Continue treatment with systemic antibiotics if the fracture is open (see sec. 9, ch. 27).

Surgical Procedure

Objectives (for all proximal femoral injuries)

- Expose the femoral neck.
- Osteotomize the femoral neck.
- Repair fractures of the femoral neck.
- Expose the greater trochanter for osteotomy and fixation.
- Expose the proximal femur for fracture repair.

Equipment

- Standard general instrument pack and suture material
- Orthopedic instruments, as required (e.g., for fracture fixation, ostectomy, subtrochanteric derotational osteotomy), including:
  - Intramedullary (IM) pins
  - Orthopedic and Kirschner wires
  - Osteotomes and mallet or oscillating bone saw
  - Plates and screws
  - Bone reduction forceps
- Self-retaining retractors (e.g., Gelpi, Weitlaner)
- Hohmann retractors (for femoral head ostectomy)

Technique

Techniques are similar for all objectives listed. Increased exposure is necessary to accomplish more complicated procedures. Techniques are described in order of procedure completion.

Common (Craniolateral) Approach

1. Prepare the affected leg for aseptic surgery.
2. Make a linear or slightly curved skin incision centered over the cranial aspect of the greater trochanter, starting near the dorsal mid-line and ending on the cranial aspect of the proximal one-third of the femur.
3. Incise the subcutaneous tissue to expose the tensor fasciae latae muscle. Incise two layers of the fasciae latae muscle along the cranial border of the biceps femoris muscle to expose the underlying vastus lateralis muscle.
4. Extend the fascial incision proximally through the gluteal fascia along the cranial border of the superficial gluteal muscle.
5. Bluntly dissect the loose connective tissue between the vastus lateralis muscle and the gluteal muscles to allow insertion of self-retaining retractors to expose the joint capsule (Fig. 2).

KEY POINT ▶ Several vessels, including the cranial femoral artery and vein and the branches of the femoral nerve, criss-cross the connective tissue and will be significantly damaged if dissection is rough.

6. Using a scalpel, incise through the joint capsule from the acetabulum, longitudinally along the femoral neck, to the proximal femur at the insertion of the vastus lateralis muscle.
7. If necessary, partially incise the tendon of insertion of the deep gluteal muscle and the origin of the vastus lateralis muscle to increase exposure of the femoral neck.

Femoral Head and Neck Ostectomy. See sec. 9, ch. 14.

Femoral Neck/Capital Physeal Fracture Repair

1. Rotate the femur outward to expose the fractured surface.
2. Retrograde a Kirschner wire of appropriate size through the femoral neck fracture surface to exit the lateral surface of the proximal femur.
3. If a compression (lag) screw is used, drill a gliding hole through the center of the femoral neck to exit the lateral surface of the proximal femur.
4. If multiple Kirschner wires are used, preplace them all through the femoral neck, using the same technique as described in (2) above.
5. Withdraw the wires from the lateral surface until the pinpoints are flush with the fracture surface.
6. Rotate the femur inward to reduce the fracture.
7. Rotate the femoral head until the fracture is anatomically aligned.
8. Advance one Kirschner wire into the femoral head without penetrating the articular surface (Fig. 3, *left*).
9. If a compression screw is used, insert a drill sleeve into the gliding hole and drill through the femoral head. The articular cartilage should preferably not be penetrated. Measure and tap the hole and place a screw of suitable length. Compress the fracture without penetrating the articular surface with the screw (Fig. 3, *right*).
10. Kirschner wires are used and drive these individually into the head without penetrating the cartilage.

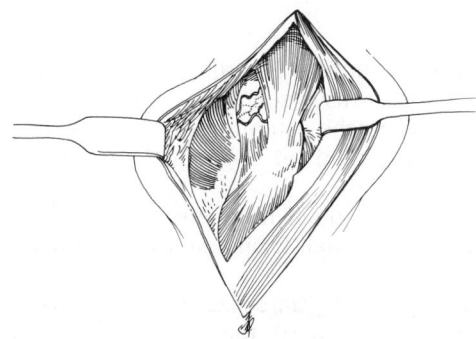

Figure 2. Craniolateral approach to the hip joint.

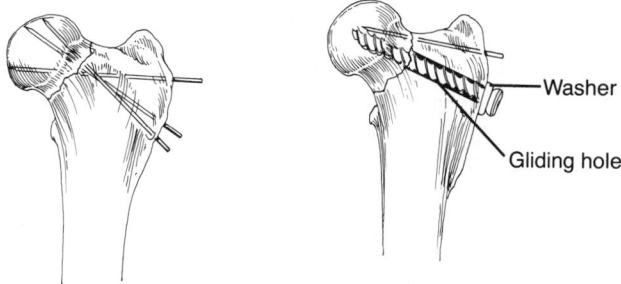

Figure 3. Fixation of femoral neck fractures. *Left,* Multiple Kirschner wires; *right,* compression screw and Kirschner wire.

KEY POINT ▶ Lifting and rotating the proximal femur allows limited examination of the femoral head surface to check for penetration by the implants. Movement of the femur should be unrestricted and smooth and should not produce crepitation.

11. After adjustments have been made to ensure that have not penetrated the articular surface, bend the lateral aspect of the Kirschner wires over and cut off close to the trochanter.

Trochanteric Osteotomy

This technique is used for exposure of the hip joint or as part of open reduction of coxofemoral luxation (see sec. 9, ch. 14).

1. Incise the tendon of the superficial gluteal muscle near the third trochanter.
2. Retract the belly of the superficial gluteal muscle proximally.
3. Incise the proximal origin of the vastus lateralis muscle and elevate the muscle to expose the osteotomy (or fracture) site, along the femoral neck.
4. If necessary for exposure, incise and elevate the adductor muscle origin caudally.
5. If an osteotomy is planned, pass a curved Kelly forceps under the deep gluteal insertion.
6. Using the curved Kelly forceps as a guide, direct the osteotome (or pull the Gigli wire through), and osteotomize the trochanter off the proximal femur, leaving the medial and deep gluteal muscles attached to the osteotomized bone.

KEY POINT ▶ Identify and protect the sciatic nerve, which is caudal to the femur and can be traumatized by excessive manipulations.

Trochanter Fracture Repair

1. Drill a hole transversely through the femur at least 1 cm distal to the osteotomy (fracture) site.
2. Thread a strand of 18-gauge orthopedic wire through the hole.
3. Clamp the proximal fragment in its anatomic position with a small-fragment bone reduction forceps.
4. Drive two appropriate-size Kirschner wires from the proximal end of the trochanter, across the osteotomy (fracture) line, and down the femur until they seat in compact bone.

5. Pass one free end of the orthopedic wire proximal to the pins and under the gluteal tendons (Fig. 4).

KEY POINT ▶ Form a figure-of-eight configuration (tension band wire) around the pin ends and through the hole.

6. Twist the free ends of wire together and twist a loop of wire on the other cross-over strand.
7. Tighten both twists evenly until the osteotomy (fracture) is securely closed.
8. Bend the pin ends over laterally and cut off the excess.
9. Cut the twisted wire, leaving two twists in place.

Proximal Femoral Shaft Fracture Repair

1. Extend the subperiosteal/subvastus lateralis dissection distally and elevate the adductor caudally until the fracture is adequately exposed.

KEY POINT ▶ Both muscles (vastus lateralis and adductor) can be entirely released if necessary, but they must be reattached.

2. Repair the fracture(s) with appropriate orthopedic techniques and implants.
3. Use cerclage wires, hemi-cerclage wires, pins, Kirschner wires, skewers, and lag screws to rebuild the fragments into a two-piece fracture.
4. Stabilize the fracture with a plate and screws.

KEY POINT ▶ The femoral neck and trochanters provide excellent anchors for screw fixation.

5. Place an autogenous cancellous bone graft harvested from another site (e.g., proximal tibia or wing of ileum) around the fracture to aid in healing.
6. Reattach the vastus lateralis and adductor muscles to their origins with absorbable sutures.
   a. If necessary, elevate the periosteum to obtain enough tissue for suturing.
   b. Alternatively, use surrounding musculature or drill holes in the femur to anchor the proximal ends of these muscles.

Closure

1. Close the incised tendon of the superficial gluteal muscle with several mattress sutures using absorbable suture material.
2. Close the fascia of the gluteal muscles to the cranial edge of the superficial gluteal muscle with a simple continuous absorbable suture.

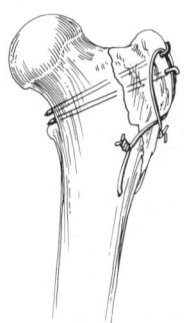

Figure 4. Tension band fixation of trochanter fracture or osteotomy.

3. Close the fascia of the tensor fasciae latae muscle to the cranial edge of the biceps femoris muscle with a simple continuous absorbable suture.
4. Close the subcutaneous tissue with a simple continuous absorbable suture.
5. Close the skin with simple interrupted, monofilament, nonabsorbable sutures.

Postoperative Care

Femoral Head and Neck Osteotomy

■ See sec. 9, ch. 14.

Femoral Neck/Physeal Fracture Repair

■ Take two postoperative radiographic views of the repair.
■ Restrict activity (cage rest) for 3 days, and then allow leash walking only for 2–3 weeks.
■ Perform non-weight bearing physical therapies (swimming, passive flexion-extension exercises).
■ Repeat radiographs of the fracture at 4 weeks to evaluate healing.
■ If healed, start a gradual return to full function.
■ Remove pins (Kirschner wires) if palpable, any time after 6 weeks if the bone has healed radiographically.
■ Remove screws and plate only if causing a problem and only after 6 months.

Trochanteric Osteotomy/Fracture

■ Measures are the same as for femoral neck/physeal fracture repair, except:
  • Restrict activity (cage rest) for at least 24 hours.
  • Repeat radiographs at 6 weeks to evaluate healing.

Proximal Femur Fracture

■ General measures are the same as for femoral neck/physeal fracture repair, except:
  • Remove implants, if indicated, after 3–6 months.
■ The proximal femur is subject to considerable and variable stresses that jeopardize all fixations. If any doubt exists as to the stability of a fracture fixation, a conservative postoperative approach is recommended.
  • Apply an Ehmer sling (see sec. 9, ch. 14) to prevent weight bearing during the initial 1–2 weeks of healing.
  • Start physical therapy (non–weight bearing) and gradually increase controlled activity from week 2 to week 4.
  • After week 4 obtain repeat radiographs before starting significant activity levels.

Postoperative Complications

■ Femoral neck/physeal fracture healing includes a period during which increased vascularity causes bone demineralization of the femoral neck. This "apple coring" effect is transient and of no significance unless the fracture is unstable or infected. Monitor with serial radiographs if necessary.
■ Implant failure and improper selection or application

of orthopedic techniques can lead to failure of healing.

FEMUR DIAPHYSIS

Anatomy

■ The shaft of the femur has muscle attachments on its caudal and medial aspects. Proximally and laterally, the adductor muscles are attached to most of the length of the femur. The origin of the vastus medialis muscle is found medial and proximal, whereas the insertion of the pectineus muscle is medial and distal. The insertion of the semimembranous muscle is distal and medial.
■ The femoral shaft is encased in a sheath of muscles including the vastus medialis, lateralis, and intermedius; rectus femoris; semimembranous; semitendinosus; and pectineus muscles.
  • On the lateral aspect, this muscle mass is surrounded by a fascial compartment made up of the tensor fasciae latae and biceps femoris muscle sheaths. Medially the sartorius muscle continues this fascial sheath.
  • The femoral artery and nerve pass medially down the length of the shaft within this compartment.
■ The sciatic nerve is lateral to the semimembranous muscle and caudal to the vastus lateralis muscle.

Preoperative Considerations

■ See under Proximal Femur.

Surgical Procedure

Objectives

■ Expose the femoral shaft.
■ Repair fractures of the femoral shaft.

Equipment

■ Standard general instrument pack and suture material
■ Orthopedic instruments as required for pinning, wiring, and plating.
■ Self-retaining retractors (e.g., Gelpi, Weitlaner) or an assistant with hand-held retractors (e.g., Army-Navy).
■ Several bone-holding forceps (e.g., Speedlock, Lane, Kirschner).

Technique

1. Prepare the leg for aseptic surgery.
2. Incise the skin from the trochanter to the patella on the cranial lateral aspect of the femoral shaft.
3. Expose the tensor fasciae latae muscle where it joins the biceps femoris muscle aponeurosis.
4. Incise both fascial layers, from the trochanter to the patella.
5. Retract the biceps femoris muscle caudally and the vastus lateralis muscle cranially.
6. Incise the intermuscular septum between the vastus lateralis and the biceps femoris muscles to expose the femoral shaft.

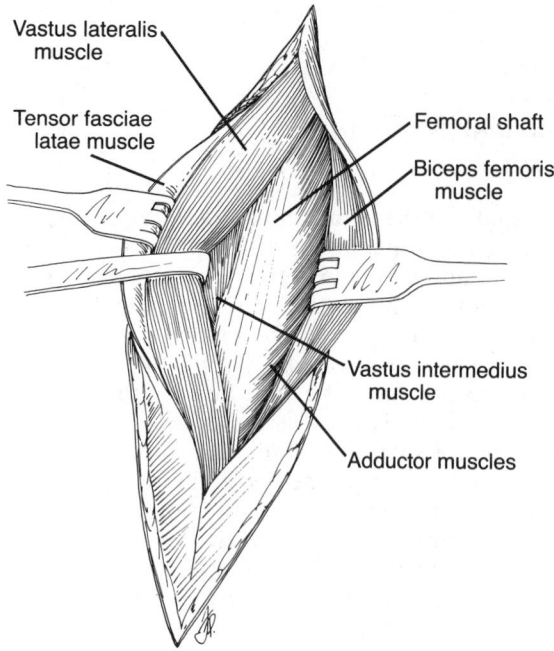

Figure 5. Lateral approach to the midshaft of the femur.

7. Bluntly separate the vastus intermedius muscle from the cranial aspect of the femur (Fig. 5).
8. Elevate (only as much as necessary) the adductor muscles subperiosteally on the caudal aspect of the femur; minimal elevation helps to preserve the blood supply to the bone.
9. Isolate the bone fragments and clean the fracture surfaces carefully.

KEY POINT ▶ Remove fragments without muscle attachments and wrap them in blood-soaked sponges; maintain all soft tissue attachments to the remaining fragments.

10. Rebuild the proximal and distal fragments with the appropriate orthopedic devices until a two-piece fracture remains. A combination of cerclage, hemi-cerclage, and Kirschner wires and interfragmentary screws, skewer pins, and figure-of-eight wire can be used to achieve a stable, two-piece fracture.
11. Use avascular bone fragments only if they are necessary to obtain stability in the fracture. These fragments must be securely fixed in order to be incorporated into the healing callus.
12. Reduce and align the two major fragments and apply the appropriate orthopedic fixation device to maintain these in alignment under stable conditions.
13. In general, a two- or three-piece fracture with long oblique fracture lines can be rebuilt with cerclage wire and supported with one or more normograded (driven proximal to distal) IM pins. IM pins also can be driven retrograde from the fracture site to the proximal femur.
    a. Extend and adduct the hip joint while driving the IM pin through the proximal femur to avoid trauma to the sciatic nerve. Reduce the fracture and drive the pin into the distal fragment.

b. Highly comminuted fractures are relatively unstable after being rebuilt and require added fixation devices to maintain alignment and stability. In these less stable situations, plating techniques or a combination of intramedullary and Kirschner-Ehmer devices may be necessary to achieve stability (Fig. 6).

KEY POINT ▶ All implants should lie directly against the bone; hence limited local muscle elevation is necessary to attach wires and plates.

14. Harvest autogenous cancellous bone graft from another site and pack around the fracture before closure. This is especially prudent if defects are present after reconstruction.
15. Flush the area copiously with warm normal saline solution *before* placing the cancellous bone graft in defects.

Closure
1. Close the fascia of the tensor fasciae latae to the biceps femoris with absorbable sutures in a simple interrupted pattern.
2. Close the subcutaneous tissue and skin routinely.

Postoperative Care

- General measures are the same as for femoral neck/physeal fracture except:
  - Use a non–weight-bearing sling if the fixation is unstable in any respect.
  - Start leash walking at 3–5 days if the fixation is stable. Increase exercise slowly over a 4-week period.
  - Repeat radiographs at 6 weeks to evaluate fracture healing.
  - Remove implants, if indicated (e.g., IM pins usually are removed), when there is radiographic evidence of healing; with IM pins this is generally 6–8 weeks postoperatively.

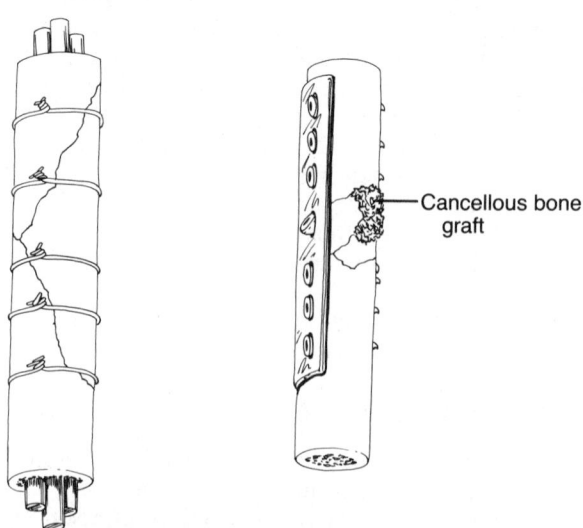

Figure 6. Diaphyseal femoral fracture fixation. *Left,* Simple long oblique fracture repaired with cerclage wires and intramedullary pins; *right,* comminuted transverse fracture repaired with a plate, screws, and cancellous bone graft.

Postoperative Complications

- Orthopedic implant failure, improper implant selection, and improper use of implants are the most common causes of fracture collapse, malunion, and nonunion (see sec. 9, ch. 28). Osteomyelitis may result from contamination.
- Large devitalized bone fragments that are not stabilized can lead to the development of chronic draining tracts and osteomyelitis.
- Extensive subperiosteal dissection and rough handling of bone can produce an excessive periosteal reaction and large callus formation.

DISTAL FEMUR

Anatomy

- The distal femur includes the metaphysis, condyles, trochlea, and patella.
- The quadriceps muscle group inserts on the proximal tibia through the patellar tendon, which includes the patella within it.
- The two heads of the gastrocnemius muscle originate on the distal, caudal aspects of the medial and lateral metaphyses, and include the fabellae in their tendons of origin.
- The superficial digital flexor muscle originates just medial to the lateral head of the gastrocnemius muscle next to the fabella.
- The long digital extensor muscle originates in a fossa on the distal lateral condyle.
- The popliteus muscle originates on the caudal lateral condyle.
- The joint capsule on the stifle joint extends from above the trochlea, around both condyles, and underneath the fabellae bilaterally.
- The aponeuroses of the biceps femoris muscle laterally and the sartorius muscle medially blend with the fibrous joint capsule over the distal femur.
- The femoral artery divides into the popliteus and saphenous arteries, which run laterally and medially, respectively, on the caudal aspect of the distal femur.
- Several small branches of these two arteries supply the femur, the patella, and the vastus lateralis muscle.
- The muscular branch of the caudal femoral artery bridges the fascial separation between the biceps femoris muscle and the vastus lateralis muscle just above the lateral fabella.
- The peroneal and saphenous nerves supply the lateral and medial aspects of the distal femur, respectively, and run caudal to the femur.

Preoperative Considerations

- Obtain a minimum of two radiographic views for evaluation of the distal femur.
- Palpate joint stability with the animal under sedation or anesthesia to investigate the possibility of simultaneous ligamentous injuries in the stifle.
- The age of the patient influences choice of implant for repair of distal femoral fractures. In young animals, bone is softer, and healing is more rapid than in older animals (see sec. 9, ch. 25).
- The majority of distal femoral fractures are physeal fractures; warn owners of the consequences of physeal closure in younger animals.

Surgical Procedure

Objectives

- Expose the distal femur and repair fractures of the metaphysis and epiphyses of the distal femur.
- Expose the articular surface of both distal femoral condyles for accurate intra-articular fracture reconstruction.
- Expose the patella and repair fractures of the patella.

Equipment

- Standard general instrument pack and suture material
- Orthopedic instruments as required for specific procedures, including pinning, wiring, and screw fixation.

Technique

1. Prepare the leg for sterile surgery.
2. Expose the distal femur and patella using a lateral, medial, or cranial approach. For patient positioning convenience, the lateral approach is most frequently used.
3. Extensive reconstruction of the articular surface may require an osteotomy of the tibial crest for added exposure of the distal femur.

Lateral Approach

1. Make a slightly curved skin incision from the distal one-third of the femur to the tibial crest just lateral to the patella.
2. Incise the subcutaneous tissue to expose the fascial layer.
3. Incise the fibrous joint capsule and fascia starting at the tibial plateau just lateral to the patella tendon and extending proximally, parallel to the patellar tendon and the patella.
4. Follow the border of the vastus lateralis muscle caudally to the septum between the biceps femoris and the vastus lateralis muscles. Separate these two muscles, double-ligating the muscular branch of the caudal femoral artery that bridges them distally.
5. Bluntly elevate the quadriceps muscles from the distal femur and luxate the patella medially to expose the distal femur (Fig. 7).
6. Expose and gently clean the fracture ends.

KEY POINT ▶ Handle the metaphyseal bone gently, especially in young animals.

7. Apply the appropriate orthopedic implants as indicated by the fracture type. For simple physeal fractures, cross-pinning, multiple pinning, and modified Rush pinning techniques are appropriate.
    a. Start the pins from the fracture line and retrograde distally out through the epiphysis, avoiding the articular surface; or start from the caudola-

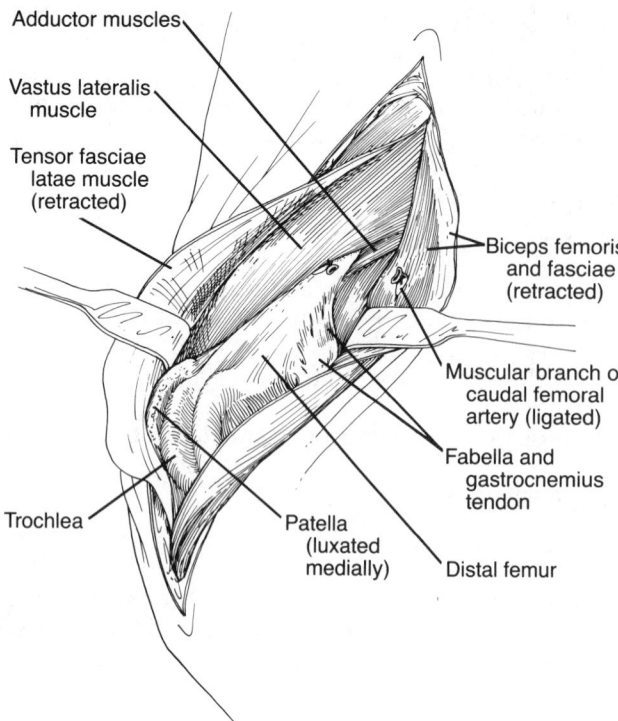

Adductor muscles

Vastus lateralis muscle

Tensor fasciae latae muscle (retracted)

Biceps femoris and fasciae (retracted)

Muscular branch of caudal femoral artery (ligated)

Fabella and gastrocnemius tendon

Trochlea

Patella (luxated medially)

Distal femur

Figure 7. Lateral approach to the distal femur.

teral and caudomedial aspect of the epiphysis and drive (normograde) to the fracture line.

b. Adjust the pins until the pinpoint is flush with the fracture line, realign the fracture anatomically, and drive the pins proximally up the shaft of the femur in one of the previously mentioned configurations.

c. Cut off the pins flush with the condyles and lavage the joint copiously with saline solution before closure (Fig. 8).

Medial Approach

1. The technique is basically identical to that for the lateral approach except it is made on the medial aspect of the distal femur. Also:

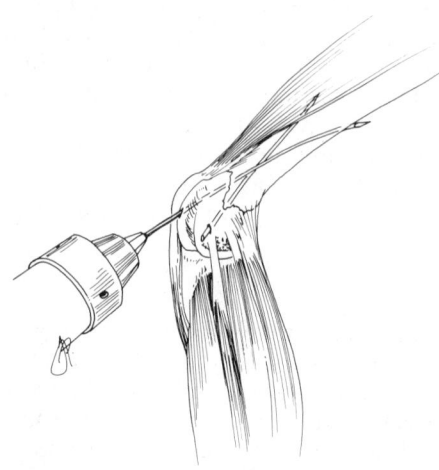

Figure 8. Cross-pinning of a distal femoral physeal fracture using a lateral approach.

2. Substitute medial for lateral (vastus medialis muscle for vastus lateralis muscle, and cranial sartorius muscle for biceps femoris muscle) to achieve medial exposure of the distal femur.

Cranial Approach

1. Incise the skin from the lateral distal one-third of the femur to the medial aspect of the proximal tibia.
2. Separate the fascia as described for the medial and the lateral approaches, which are combined to give wider bilateral exposure of both condyles.

Tibial Crest Osteotomy

1. A tibial osteotomy can be combined with any of the previously described approaches to achieve additional exposure for complicated fractures.
2. Isolate the patellar tendon through the original skin incision.
3. Place an osteotome under the patellar tendon, aimed distally, and osteotomize the tibial crest free from the proximal tibia.

KEY POINT ▶ Be sure to remove enough bone to facilitate fixation when reattaching the tibial crest.

4. Retract the quadriceps muscle proximally to fully expose the joint.
5. Repair intra-articular fractures with good visibility of the critical articular surface.
6. Compression (lag) screw fixation of intra-articular fracture fragments is recommended to allow accurate reconstruction and avoid movement, thus reducing the potential for arthritis.
7. Repair the osteotomy by pinning the tibial crest into position with two large Kirschner wires transversely placed through the osteotomized bone fragment and into the proximal tibia. Place a figure-of-eight tension band wire around the base of the pins and through a hole in the cranial tibia, distal to the osteotomy site.

Patellar Fracture Repair

1. Expose the patella via the lateral approach as previously described. Visualize the patella by rotating the distal quadriceps muscle.
2. Pass two Kirschner wires lengthwise through the patella across the fracture line.
3. Rotate the quadriceps muscle back to its normal position and loop a figure-of-eight orthopedic wire around the pin ends on the cranial surface of the patella.
4. Twist both long strands of the figure-of-eight wire to tighten the tension band apparatus and close the fracture line of the patella.
5. Cut the pin ends as short as possible. Cut the twisted wire, leaving two twists.

Closure

1. Close the joint capsule with monofilament absorbable suture in a simple continuous pattern.
2. Close the fascial layer with absorbable sutures in a simple interrupted pattern.
3. Close the subcutaneous tissue and skin routinely.

Postoperative Care

- General measures are the same as for femoral neck/physeal fracture except:
  - Restrict activity (cage rest) for at least 24 hours.
  - If fixation is judged to be stable start leash walking 1–2 days postoperatively.
  - If fixation is unstable, support the leg in a flexion sling.

Postoperative Complications

- Quadriceps tie-down (contracture) occurs when adhesions form between the healing fracture callus and the overlying quadriceps muscle and patellar tendon. This is most likely to happen if the leg is fixed in an extended position (e.g., with a Thomas splint). Tie-down can be prevented by early mobilization and/or a flexion sling for support.

KEY POINT ▶ Help to avoid quadriceps tie-down, do not apply splints that place the stifle in extension.

- If intra-articular fractures are not reduced anatomically, degenerative joint disease and hence postoperative joint pain can result. Accurate reduction and fixation is essential.

- If the animal is very young at the time of the physeal fracture, femoral shortening is to be expected. If shortening is less than 20% compared with the normal leg, clinical signs are unlikely.

Supplemental Readings

Aron JN, Kaddatz LA, Dueland R: A review of reduction and internal fixation of proximal femoral fractures in the dog and man. J Am Anim Hosp Assoc 15:455, 1979.

Berg JR, Egger EL, Konde LJ, et al.: Evaluation of prognostic factors for growth following distal femoral physeal injuries in 14 dogs. Vet Surg 13:142, 1984.

Brinker WO, Piermattei DO, Flo GL: *Handbook of Small Animal Orthopedics and Fracture Treatment.* Philadelphia: W. B. Saunders, 1983.

Evans HE, Christensen JC: *Miller's Anatomy of the Dog,* 2nd Ed. Philadelphia: W. B. Saunders, 1979.

Newton CD, Nunamaker DM: *Textbook of Small Animal Orthopedics.* Philadelphia: J. B. Lippincott, 1985.

Piermattei DO, Greeley RG: *An Atlas of Surgical Approaches to the Bones of the Dog and Cat,* 2nd Ed. Philadelphia: W. B. Saunders, 1979.

Shires PK, Hulse DA: Internal fixation of physeal fractures using the distal femur as an example. Compend Contin Educ Small Anim Pract 2(11):854, 1980.

Slatter DH: *Textbook of Small Animal Surgery,* Vols. 1 and 2, 2nd Ed., Philadelphia: W. B. Saunders, 1993.

Sumner-Smith G: *Decision Making in Small Animal Orthopedic Surgery.* Toronto: B. C. Decker, 1988.

16 Orthopedic Disorders of the Stifle

R. Tass Dueland

Common traumatic and congenital/developmental conditions of the stifle include patella luxation, cruciate disruptions, meniscal problems, collateral ligament injuries, and stifle luxation. The first three listed (and excluding fractures) compose 95% of stifle disorders in dogs and cats.

ANATOMY

Cranial Stifle

- The quadricep muscle components, patella, trochlear groove and notch, patella tendon, and tibial tuberosity are aligned linearly with the coxofemoral joint, talocrural joint, and paw. Normally there is no medial or lateral deviation of these structures.
- Craniomedial and caudolateral ligamentous bundles compose the cranial cruciate ligament, which originates on the caudomedial aspect of the lateral femoral condyle and inserts centrally on the tibial plateau caudal to the cranial intermeniscal ligament (Fig. 1).
- The caudal cruciate ligament originates in the craniodistal trochlear notch and inserts on the caudocentral tibial plateau and medial popliteal notch.
- The fat pad lies caudal to the patella tendon and helps to supply its vascularity.
- The long digital extensor tendon originates on the lateral femoral condyle cranial to the lateral collateral ligament and popliteus muscle.
- Retinacular fibrous tissue overlies the craniolateral and craniomedial aspect of the stifle joint.

- The trochlear notch is the more distal non–weight-bearing portion of the trochlear groove.

Caudal Stifle

- Medial and lateral fabellae articulate intracapsularly with the femoral condyles and have strong fabello-femoral ligaments (Fig. 2).
- The medial meniscus is attached to the tibia and to the medial collateral ligament. The lateral meniscus has femoral and tibial attachments.
- Note the caudocentral insertion of the caudal cruciate ligament on the tibia and the caudolateral origin of the cranial cruciate.
- The popliteus muscle courses under the lateral collateral ligament.
- Neurovascular structures run longitudinally and centrally close to the caudal joint capsule.

GENERAL PREOPERATIVE CONSIDERATIONS

- Accurate client communication and a successful return to function by the patient are enhanced by meticulous evaluation of the stifle joint preoperatively and intraoperatively. This facilitates an accurate diagnosis and selection of the appropriate procedure(s).
- Radiography is useful:
  - To confirm the diagnosis
  - To determine the animal's age
  - For comparison with the opposite joint
  - For legal documentation
- Perform a thorough orthopedic examination, including the joints, bones, and muscles of the affected extremity.

Orthopedic Evaluation

Include the following maneuvers in palpation of the stifle:

- Perform gentle full range-of-motion exercises in normal flexion and extension; then repeat with internal and external rotation.
  - Often, clicks caused by meniscal pathology and crepitation from osteoarthritis can be detected.
- With the femur held motionless with one hand and the proximal tibia held securely by the other hand, attempt cranial movement of the tibia after placing

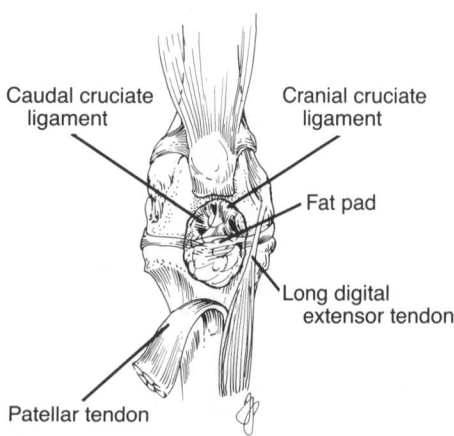

Figure 1. Anatomy of the cranial stifle.

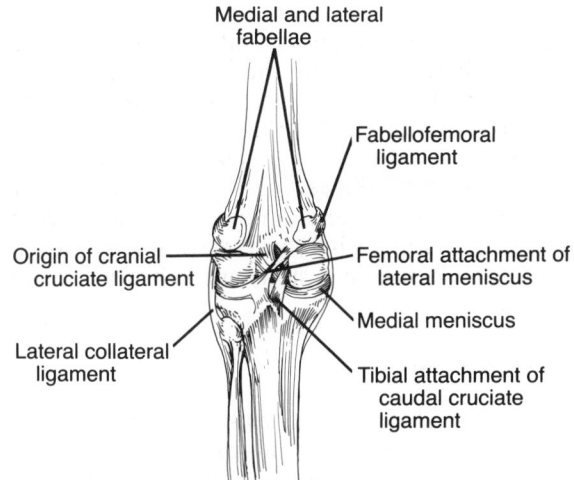

Figure 2. Anatomy of the caudal stifle.

Medial and lateral fabellae

Fabellofemoral ligament

Origin of cranial cruciate ligament

Femoral attachment of lateral meniscus

Medial meniscus

Lateral collateral ligament

Tibial attachment of caudal cruciate ligament

the stifle in slight to moderate flexion (drawer sign or Lachman test).

■ With a finger held over the tibial tuberosity and the femur held securely, flex the hock to detect cranial movement of the tibia (tibial compression test).
  • This test (and the Lachman test) indicates laxity of the cranial cruciate ligament (see later in this chapter).
■ With the femur held motionless, determine internal and external movement of the tibia on the femur by grasping the hock and rotating the tibia. Normal range of motion is 20–30° of internal rotation and 5–10° of external rotation with the stifle in flexion.
■ To detect any luxation tendencies, exert medial and lateral digital pressure on the patella while putting the stifle through range of motion.
■ Exert pressure with the thumbs on the lateral side of the femoral condyle and proximal tibia, and then repeat on the medial side. Laxity of the collateral ligaments is detected by increased laxity of the joint space.
■ Exert deep pressure of the stifle area with a fingertip to ascertain focal points of pain from soft tissue tears and bone bruises.

KEY POINT ▶ Perform the tests sequentially while the animal is conscious, and repeat when the animal is sedated or anesthetized. Plan appropriate surgical procedures based on this diagnostic information.

GENERAL PRINCIPLES OF STIFLE SURGERY

1. For the majority of the surgical procedure, place the dog in dorsal recumbency with the forelegs and unaffected rear limb secured. This gives good access to both sides of the stifle in a comfortable operating position. Place the instrument table over the dog's trunk.
2. Perform an arthrotomy of sufficient length to facilitate luxation of the patella and, using flexion and retraction, identify, inspect, and assess the articular surfaces of the patella, trochlear groove, tibial plateau, pericondylar, and supracondylar areas of the

femur, patellar tendon, fat pad, and long digital extensor tendon.
  a. When operating alone, place the sterile, covered paw on your (gowned) abdomen.
  b. By moving your body forward and backward you can adjust the amount of flexion of the stifle.
3. Place a small, sharp rake retractor (Senn) deeply behind the fat pad; retract it and inspect both cruciates.
4. Place a second retractor on either side of the first to examine the menisci.
  a. To see the caudal horns well, place the tip of a narrow Hohmann retractor (Synthes 399.18) or curved hemostat just behind the tibial plateau. Positioning the instrument against the trochlear notch acts as a lever to move the tibia forward and increase exposure.

PATELLAR LUXATION

Medial patellar luxations often affect miniature breeds; lateral luxations are more common in large and giant breeds. Patellar luxations generally are congenital or developmental. Contributing factors include structural abnormalities such as coxa vara and coxa valgus (decrease and increase, respectively, in the angle formed by the head and neck of the femur and the axis of its shaft), bowing or torsion of the distal portion of the femur, shallow trochlear groove, increased internal or external tibial rotation, and a malpositioned tibial tuberosity.

Patellar luxations are classified as:

■ Grade I: The patella lies in the trochlear groove but can be manually subluxated or luxated.
■ Grade II: Spontaneous luxation occurs clinically. The patella can be luxated manually but reduces spontaneously or with gentle manipulation.
■ Grade III: The patella is luxated most of the time but can be reduced manually.
■ Grade IV: The patella luxation cannot be reduced manually. Often, flexure contracture has occurred and limb use is minimal.

Diagnosis

■ History usually reveals intermittent rear leg lameness. The lameness classically is characterized by rapidly alternating use and disuse of the limb, particularly during exercise.
■ Definitive diagnosis is based on physical examination. Palpate the patella while placing the stifle through full range of motion.

Preoperative Considerations

■ Evaluate the maximum internal and external rotation of the tibia on the femur. An increase in internal rotation >30° (often occurring in miniature breeds) indicates lateral retinacular laxity and the need for lateral imbrication.
■ Patellar luxation procedures vary; some animals require only one step whereas others need combined procedures.

- In some cases combined parapatellar arthrotomy/release is necessary (to release means to diminish the pull or tension on tissue, often accomplished by incising perpendicularly to the line of tension).
- In other cases, combined arthrotomy/imbrication is needed (to imbricate means to tighten, either by suturing alone or by excision and subsequent closure of tissue.

Surgical Procedures

Objective

- Stabilize the patella anatomically in the trochlea while maintaining full range of pain-free motion.

Equipment

- Standard orthopedic surgical pack and suture material
- Preferably, power-burring, oscillating saw, and drill *or*
- Double-action large rongeurs, bone curets, and fine hand saw (hacksaw or Exacto saw #236).
- Sharp osteotomes and mallet

Basic Principles

- Reduce the patella luxation and determine whether the tissues are tight on the side toward which the patella luxates or whether the tissues opposite the luxated side are very lax.
  - If the former is present, perform combined parapatella arthrotomy/release to diminish the pull of the tissues.
  - If the latter is present, combined arthrotomy/imbrication is indicated to tighten the lax side.
- With an adequately deep trochlear groove and no excessive tibial rotation, a release may be the only step needed to maintain the patella in its anatomic position.
- With a shallow trochlea, deepening can be accomplished by trochleoplasty, chondroplasty, or wedge recession
- Correct medial rotation of the tibia with translocation of the tibial tuberosity.

Technique

Trochleoplasty

1. Following arthrotomy and inspection of the stifle, mark the medial and lateral boundaries of the planned trochlear groove by longitudinal cuts in the trochlear cartilage, using a scalpel blade. To prevent fracture, try to obtain as much width and height as possible without weakening the remaining condylar bone.
2. Remove the articular cartilage within the marked lines by power burring or with a rongeur.
3. Reduce the luxated patella for a trial fit and, if necessary, smooth the new surface with a fine half-round file or rasp. The depth of the new trochlea should accommodate the patella so that one half to two-thirds of the patella's height is in the groove.

4. Verify depth, smoothness, and stability by palpating the patella while putting the joint through its range of motion (flexion and extension with internal and external rotation of the tibia).
5. Close the synovia and joint capsule with appropriately sized monofilament nylon sutures in an interrupted cruciate pattern. If possible, perform partial-thickness closure whereby the suture is not within the joint. Remaining skin and subcutis closure is routine.

Postoperative Care

- Begin physical therapy, consisting of hot packs and gentle, passive flexion and extension to half the normal range of motion on the day of surgery. Twenty repetitions, four to six times daily is recommended. Swimming after suture removal is permitted.
- Restricted activity (leash walking only, no stairs, no ball playing, etc.) for 1 month.
- Give analgesics (e.g., butorphanol, 0.2 mg/kg, IM; Bufferin, 1 tablet/15 kg, bid with food) as needed.

Technique

Chondroplasty

1. Make a trochlear outline, as described for trochleoplasty, down to subchondral bone (Fig. 3).
2. Using a thin, sharp curved osteotome (Zimmer #2881–00–01, #2881–00–02) perform an osteotomy and create a rectangular cartilage flap with the hinge either proximally or distally. Include 1–2 mm of bone in the thickness of the flap.
3. Remove underlying bone with power burring, a bone curet, or rongeurs.
4. After adequate depth is obtained, press the flap manually into the new groove. Pressure from the patella helps keep the flap in position.
5. Close the skin and subcutis routinely.

KEY POINT ▶ This technique is best used in dogs less than 6 months of age in which the mineralized tissue is relatively soft and pliable for creating a flap.

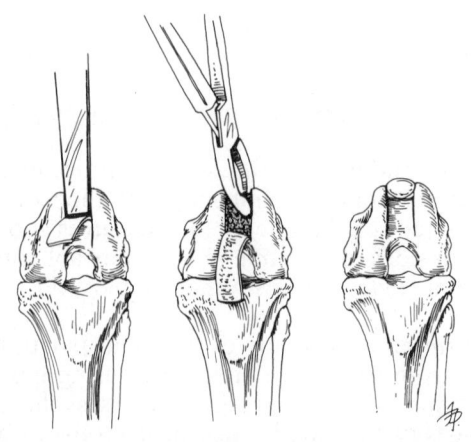

Figure 3. Chondroplasty procedure. See text for details.

Postoperative Care

■ Perform physical therapy and administer analgesics, as described previously for trochleoplasty.

Technique

Wedge Recession

1. Make a trochlear outline as described for trochleoplasty.
2. With a power saw or fine hand saw, make two pie-shaped cuts at the peripheral borders previously outlined. Medial and lateral condylar osteotomies should meet centrally. Remove this central piece of bone and articular cartilage and place it in a blood-soaked sponge.
3. The shallowness of the trochlea determines the width of the next two saw cuts, which are parallel and peripheral to the first cuts. Remove these two pieces of bone. Place the trochlear segment with its intact cartilage into the recess; this results in a deeper trochlea with preservation of most of the articular surface.
4. Pressure of the articulating patella ensures good contact of the osteotomized segment. If stability of the segment is questionable, drive small Kirschner wires horizontally through the condyles into the reinserted segment.
5. Close the skin and subcutis routinely.

Postoperative Care

■ Perform physical therapy and administer analgesics, as described for trochleoplasty.

KEY POINT ▶ Use caution with this technique in immature animals with open physes. Premature closure may occur; therefore it is better suited for animals >8 months of age.

Technique

Patelloplasty

1. Occasionally, after deepening and widening of the trochlea, the patella is still too large for the groove. Pivot the patella on edge.
2. With a power bur or rongeurs, remove bone from the medial and lateral surfaces of the patella until it fits well into the trochlear groove.

Postoperative Care

■ Perform physical therapy and administer analgesics, as described previously for trochleoplasty.

Imbrication

After the depth of the trochlear groove is reestablished, reevaluate the status of tibial rotation. If there is medial or lateral rotary instability, perform imbrication of the lax side, using one of several techniques.

Technique

1. DeAngelis Technique (fabella to patella tendon): Using nonabsorbable monofilament suture, place mattress pattern sutures around the medial and lateral fabellae or into the fabellofemoral ligament and running under the retinaculum, engaging the distal pole of the patella tendon.
2. Flo Technique: Place the proximal aspect of the sutures similarly, but distally engage the proximal tibia through a transverse drill hole in the tibial tuberosity.
3. Place additional sutures, if needed, in a fanlike pattern, originating at the fabella and engaging the parapatella tissue.
4. Alternatively, scarify the retinacular tissue with the scalpel blade and use a Lembert suture pattern to place several bilateral parapatella sutures.
5. If there is redundant tissue on one side of the patella after reduction, make two elliptical incisions through retinaculum, capsule, and synovia. Remove the redundant tissue and imbricate using routine closure or a vest-over-pants pattern.
6. Fibular head transposition technique (discussed later in this chapter): Use to correct rotational instability for medial patella luxation. A disadvantage is that the procedure is technically difficult in miniature dogs.

KEY POINT ▶ As a rule, when suturing is the main component of imbrication, physical therapy should be gentle to diminish stress upon the suture material, avoid creep and failure of the suture, and allow adequate time for tissue healing.

Tibial Tuberosity Translocation

Equipment

■ Osteotome and mallet or a dental molar cutter
■ Kirschner wires or orthopedic wire

Technique

1. Perform medial and lateral parapatellar arthrotomies.
2. With an osteotome/mallet or molar cutter, make an osteotomy of the tibial tuberosity, leaving the soft tissue still attached distally if possible (Fig. 4, *left*).
3. Hold the osteotomized tibial tuberosity in position with a bone clamp (Synthes 399.07), after creating a bed in the tibia by roughening the site with a rongeur or curet.
4. Using a power or hand drill, make two small holes through the newly positioned osteotomized segment and through the base of the tibial tuberosity (Fig. 4, *right*).
5. Place an appropriately sized (20–22 gauge) orthopedic wire through the holes in a mattress pattern and twist tightly medially to secure the bone in the new site. Cut the wire, leaving 2–3 twists. The new location of the insertion of the patella tendon should realign the forces to maintain the patella in position, assuming other disruptive forces have been corrected.
6. If the new position is not closely adjacent to the osteotomy site, insert Kirschner wires, a tension band, or lag screws obliquely for stable fixation.

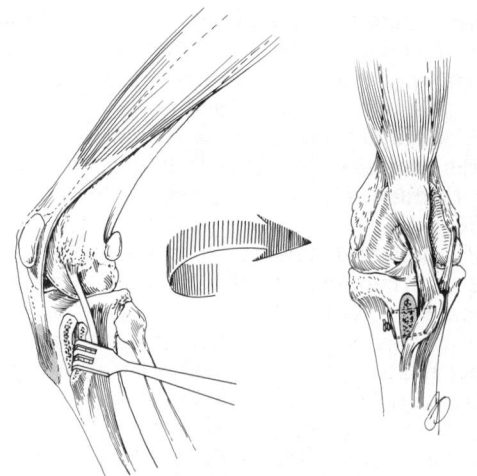

Figure 4. Tibial tuberosity transposition. *Left,* Area of partial osteotomy of tibial tuberosity is shown in color; the cranial tibial muscle is reflected. *Right,* The newly positioned segment is pinned in place.

KEY POINT ▶ Exercise great care in young animals not to cause physeal growth arrest by inappropriate placement of Kirschner wires or lag screws through the physes.

a. If the wire ends cause skin irritation, they may be removed after bony union has occurred.

KEY POINT ▶ Because medial and lateral rotary instability/laxity contributes significantly to malalignment of the tibial tuberosity, correction of the laxity by imbrication (Flo) may eliminate the need for transposition of the tuberosity.

CRANIAL CRUCIATE LIGAMENT (CL) RUPTURE

Diagnosis

- The history usually reveals an acute onset of rear limb lameness, particularly during exercise. Lameness may partially or completely resolve, then recur with exercise.
- Chronic and persistent lameness may also be seen, especially in older, overweight dogs.

Diagnostic Manipulations

Two diagnostic manipulations can confirm abnormal cranial movement of the tibia at the stifle.

First Maneuver

- Position the thumbs on the caudolateral aspect of the limb so that the lower thumb engages the head of the fibula while the upper thumb is placed in the region of the lateral fabella or the edge of the lateral femoral condyle.
- Wrap the other fingers of the upper hand around the cranial aspect of the lower thigh, keeping the femur motionless and the patella in the trochlea groove.
- Test the cranial laxity of the stifle joint is with the tibia in full extension, in modest flexion (15–30°)

(Lachman test), and in 45–90° (or more) of flexion (cranial drawer sign).
- With complete rupture of both bands of the cranial CL, cranial laxity is detectable at each position.
- With partial rupture, laxity may be detectable at only one of these positions.
- Severity of laxity is subjectively ranked in 2-mm increments (e.g., 1+ = 2 mm; 2+ = 4 mm; 3+ = 6 mm; 4+ = 8 mm) of cranial displacement (translation) of the tibia on the femur.

Second Maneuver (Tibial Compression)

- Use one hand to hold the femur motionless, with the index finger resting on the tibial tuberosity; gently dorsoflex the hock with the other hand.
- The gastrocnemius muscle will tighten and, when cranial CL laxity is present, the tibia can be felt to move cranially under the index finger.

In the author's experience the cranial drawer/Lachman test is more consistent than the tibial compression test. However, both tests should be done. A diagnostic impression is obtainable in 90% of unanesthetized dogs if proper positioning and a calm approach is used.

Preoperative Considerations

- Preoperative stifle radiographs are useful to document the extent of the degenerative joint disease, presence of normal fabellae, and avulsions of ligamentous attachments.
- To rule out predisposing or concurrent diseases, consider obtaining a routine laboratory database of complete blood count (CBC), serum chemistry profile, and urinalysis.

Surgical Procedures

Objectives

- Visually assess the extent of joint damage.
- Arrest the progression of degenerative joint disease by stabilizing the joint.
- Reduce or eliminate cranial translation (drawer sign) of the tibia relative to the femur.
- Debride the joint and replace the damaged cranial CL with an autogenous graft.

Patellar Tendon Procedure (For Dogs Weighing 25–175 lb)

Equipment

- Standard orthopedic pack including 2 Senn retractors (1 each, sharp and dull)
- C-clamp drill guide (Synthes #312.47), with 3.2-mm and 4.5-mm drills and drill sleeve inserts (312.45, 312.32)
- Alligator forcep or suture passer
- Power saw/drill (e.g., 3M minidriver) or Steinmann pin/hand chuck, Exacto saw #236 (1.25″) or hack saw*
- Osteotomes 1.0″ and 0.75″ and mallet

*Government surplus rotary dental saws are reasonably priced and serve well for this procedure.

Technique

1. Place the dog in dorsal recumbency and prepare the stifle for aseptic surgery.
2. Make a cranial skin incision extending from 2 inches above the patella to the tibial crest. Suture a sterile stockinette to the incision.
3. Incise the superficial fascia and fatty layers longitudinally on the midline, exposing the deeper fascia, the cranial head of the sartorius muscle, the patella, and the patellar tendon (Fig. 5).

KEY POINT ▶ If the cranial CL rupture diagnosis is uncertain preoperatively, perform arthrotomy and joint inspection before creating a new ligament.

4. Make two parallel incisions through the first layer of the fascia lata/quadriceps fascia starting 2–3 mm lateral to the cranial head of the sartorius muscle and continuing distally over the patella, through the patellar tendon, to the tibial tuberosity. Make the width of these incisions uniform and equal to the middle third of the patellar tendon (generally 4–6 mm in a 40 to 70 lb dog) (Fig. 5A).
5. Free the fascial and patellar tendon portions of the graft from the underlying tissue. Cut the most proximal (fascial) end of the graft transversely, leaving the distal (patellar tendon portion) graft still attached to the tibial tuberosity. Be careful to cut through the full thickness of the patellar tendon, but do not cut into the underlying fat pad, to avoid unnecessary bleeding.
6. Make converging saw cuts into the patella from the previous guiding incisions made over the patella. The bone cuts join in the outer third of the patella and do not reach the articular surface of the patella (Fig. 5B). If these pie-shaped cuts are made properly, one or two taps with an osteotome and mallet will dislodge the bony segment of the graft. To ensure preservation of insertions of the fascia proximally and patellar tendon distally to the patellar wedge, make the saw cut 2–3 mm deep.
7. Using a scalpel, make a final dissection to free up the graft. Use Metzenbaum scissors to trim the soft tissue of the graft to uniform dimensions. If the patellar wedge is oversized, reduce it with rongeurs or a power bur.
8. Perform a lateral parapatellar arthrotomy and luxate the patella medially to expose the stifle joint. Perform a thorough inspection of the stifle, as previously described. Remove the remnants of the ruptured cranial CL with sharp dissection, using a #15 scalpel blade. If necessary, perform corrective surgery for meniscal problems (see later in this chapter), cartilaginous defects, and exostosis removal to complete the joint debridement.
9. Place the C-clamp drill guide at the anatomic origin of the cranial CL, drilling a tunnel through the lateral femoral condyle from exterior to interior. For dogs 25–60 lb, use a 3.2-mm drill; for larger dogs, use a 4.5-mm drill. Make the tunnel longitudinally oblique to prevent bony edges from eroding the graft (Fig. 5C).
10. Reduce the patella, with a curved hemostat placed through the void made in the patella tendon, create a tunnel through the fat pad. Grasp the proximal end of the graft with a hemostat and bring it through the patellar tendon defect and into the stifle via the fat pad tunnel. Place an alligator forceps into the stifle joint via the lateral condylar tunnel. With the jaws grasping the proximal (fascial) end of the graft, pull the graft through the condylar tunnel without twisting it. A small thumb forceps may be needed to guide the patellar portion of the graft into the bony tunnel. Occasionally, enlargement of the tunnel with bone curets or redrilling is necessary. During the following weeks, the patellar portion of the graft lies entirely in the

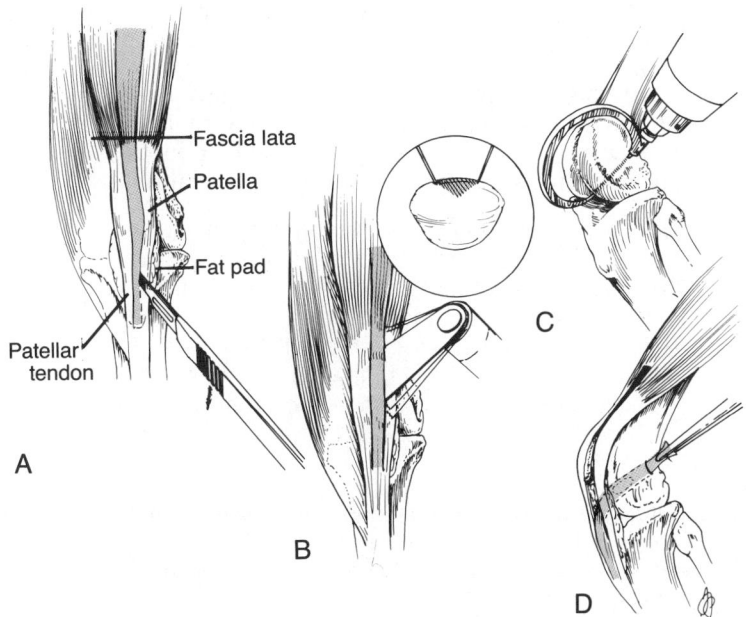

Figure 5. Patellar tendon technique for repair of cranial cruciate rupture. See text for details.

Fascia lata
Patella
Fat pad
Patellar tendon

condylar tunnel and is firmly incorporated in the tunnel, providing permanent stability of the cruciate graft (Fig. 5D).

11. After thorough lavage of the joint, suture the fascial defect, patellar tendon defect, and arthrotomy incisions using 00 to 1 monofilament nylon in a cruciate pattern. Secure the graft last, after adjusting tension as necessary by incorporating the proximal fascial portion of the graft into the arthrotomy closure with 3–4 nylon sutures. A very minimal drawer sign (trace to 1+) is acceptable at closure because the joint usually tightens in the postoperative period. Routinely close the subcutaneous tissue and skin.

   a. Supplemental imbrication (Flo or DeAngelis technique) sutures are unnecessary.

12. If a power saw/drill and a C-clamp drill guide are not available, the procedure can be performed with minor modification of the above technique:

   a. Make a medial (not lateral) arthrotomy in order to drill the tunnel with a Steinmann pin and hand chuck. If a C-clamp drill is not available, it is easier and more accurate to make the tunnel from the interior of the stifle to the exterior.

   b. Luxate the patella laterally; this makes it possible to line up the drill hole without interference from the reflected soft tissue. Make a small separate lateral incision to accept the passage of the graft and facilitate suturing of the graft.

   c. Patellar osteotomies can be made with an Exacto saw or a hacksaw. Other aspects of the surgery are the same.

Postoperative Care

Apply a sterile Robert Jones bandage (RJB), supplemented with a 3–4″-wide, full-length cranial fiberglass slab and secure the bandage to the body with a belly band.

KEY POINT ▶ The RJB cannot be removed prematurely; it can be replaced but not removed!

■ Replace the bandage as necessary but use for 1 month to prevent stifle motion in order to allow bony incorporation of the patellar segment in the condylar tunnel with resultant strong graft fixation.

KEY POINT ▶ Inform owners that autogenous tissue graft used to replace the cranial cruciate ligament is biomechanically weaker than the original ligament, and that during the first 3 months after surgery the graft is undergoing revascularization and needs protection from stress. Recommend restricted, leash-only exercise and no use of stairs.

■ Gradually increase exercise after 3 months, with return to full function in 6–9 months.

■ Excess graft tension diminishes revascularization and normal healing of the graft.

Prognosis

■ The author has been very satisfied with the results of this technique, having used and refined it for more than 25 years. On the few occasions where the stifle was later operated, the graft appeared strong and stable.

Fibular Head Transposition Procedure

Initial experience with this recently developed technique for cranial CL stabilization has been varied. (A complete description is available in the literature.)

■ The head of the fibula is freed from its ligamentous attachments to the tibia and advanced cranially. This allows the lateral collateral ligament (which attaches to the fibular head) to counteract internal rotation of the tibia and cranial drawer of the stifle.

■ The main advantages are that exercise restriction is minimal, no splints are used, and weight bearing resumes rapidly compared with other techniques.

■ In the author's experience, dogs weighing >30 lb are better candidates than smaller dogs in which the fibula may fracture.

KEY POINT ▶ A fracture reduction forceps (Synthes #399.07) is useful to hold the fibular head in position while placing Kirschner and tension band wires.

Fascial Strip Over-The-Top Procedure (for Dogs Weighing 15–25 lb)

Equipment

■ Standard orthopedic pack and suture material

Technique

1. Place the dog in dorsal or lateral recumbency and prepare the stifle for aseptic surgery.

2. Make a craniolateral skin incision similar to that in the patellar tendon technique but slightly more lateral.

3. Perform a craniolateral arthrotomy with formation of a distally based fascial strip. For adequate biomechanical strength, make the width of the strip 2–3 times the width of the patellar tendon. The length needed is twice the distance from the proximal patella to the tibial tuberosity. The base of the strip is at the level of the joint line.

4. Cut the fascial strip proximally and insert it, cranial to caudal, through a fat pad tunnel made with a hemostat (Fig. 6). Using a hemostat, enter the caudolateral joint capsule caudal to the lateral fabella, grasping the proximal end of the graft in the joint and pulling it through the intercondylar notch lateral to the caudal CL and over the top of the lateral condyle. Make a small incision through the joint capsule, pull the fascial strip through it, and secure it to the capsule/periosteum with six–eight monofilament nylon sutures (2–0) with the appropriate tension to achieve a minimal drawer sign.

5. Close the arthrotomy incision with nonabsorbable nylon suture. Complete closure may not be possible

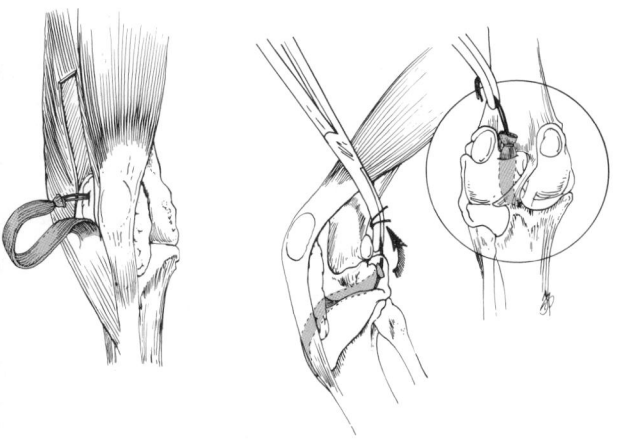

Figure 6. Fascial strip over-the-top technique for repair of cranial cruciate rupture. See text for details.

distally, depending on the width of graft harvested. Use a lateral imbrication suture of No. 1 polyglyconate (Maxon; Davis & Geck) from fabella to distal patellar tendon for temporary stabilization of the joint until healing occurs.

6. Routinely close the remaining tissues.

Imbrication Procedure
(for Dogs Weighing <15 lb)

■ An alternative is the fascial strip over-the-top procedure described previously.

Equipment

■ Standard orthopedic pack and suture material

Technique

1. Place the dog in dorsal recumbency and prepare the stifle for aseptic surgery.
2. Make a medial or lateral parapatellar skin incision.
3. Perform a medial or lateral arthrotomy.
4. Debride the joint and close the arthrotomy incision as previously described for the fascial strip over-the-top procedure.
5. Anchor extracapsular medial and lateral imbrication nylon sutures (0, 1, or 2) around the medial and lateral fabellae or through the fabellofemoral ligament. (Sterilized 50-, 80-, and 100-lb test monofilament nylon has provided good results.)
6. In a closed technique, the author finds it easier to place the suture needle around the fabella using a caudal to cranial motion, "walking" the tip of the needle up the caudal aspect of the femur until the proper angle is attained and the needle can be brought through the tissue. A sturdy needle assists the maneuver.
   a. Pull firmly on the suture to confirm that suture placement is correct and that the fabella has been properly engaged.
   b. If the fixation feels inadequate, the tissue may be incised to visualize the fabella (open technique).
7. After proper fabella placement, run the suture distally under the retinaculum and anchor it into the distal portion of the patellar tendon (DeAngelis

technique) or through a transverse drill hole (Flo technique) placed in the tibial tuberosity (Fig. 7). With the stifle flexed slightly, tighten the mattress pattern sutures until the drawer sign is eliminated.

Postoperative Care

■ No bandage or splint is required.
■ Restrict exercise as for previously described techniques for several months until adequate fibrosis and healing occurs.

CAUDAL (POSTERIOR) CRUCIATE LIGAMENT (CL) RUPTURE

The importance of the caudal CL is controversial in both dogs and humans. A large series in humans (Clancy et al., 1983) indicated severe pathology results with time. In dogs, isolated rupture of the caudal CL without bony avulsion is, in the author's 35-year experience, extremely rare.

Diagnosis

Diagnosis is based on:

■ A history of acute lameness and caudal drawer sign tested at 90° of stifle flexion
■ A caudal sag of the proximal tibia, compared with the normal, opposite side, viewed on a lateral radiographic projection
■ Avulsion of the bony attachment

Surgical Procedure

Objectives

■ Similar to those for cranial CL except rupture repair

Equipment

■ Similar to that for the patellar tendon procedure for cranial CL rupture

Technique

1. Make a cranial skin incision extending from 4 cm above the patella to 4 cm below the tibial tuberosity.

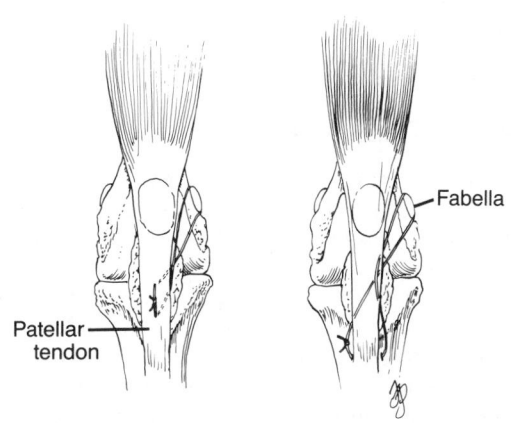

Figure 7. Imbrication techniques of DeAngelis *(left)* and Flo *(right)*.

2. Perform a medial arthrotomy and debridement of the caudal CL.
3. Drill two tunnels. Extend one tunnel from the origin of the caudal CL at the nonarticulating portion of the trochlear groove, exiting on the medial side of the medial femoral condyle. Extend the second tunnel from a point approximately 2 cm below the tibial plateau just medial of the midline, directed caudally to exit just below the centromedial portion of the tibial plateau.
4. Harvest a patellar tendon graft as in the cranial CL patellar tendon procedure; in addition, obtain a piece of tibial tuberosity bone (4 mm wide × 6 mm long × 2 mm thick), including its patellar tendon insertion (i.e., making a free graft). Drill holes in each of the patellar and tuberosity pieces of bone and pass long nylon suture strands through the holes.
5. Using a suture passer, introduce the sutures that are attached to the patellar segment into the tibial tunnel in a cranial to caudal direction, and pull the patellar portion of the graft through, leaving the tibial graft segment in the tibial tunnel. Similarly, draw the patellar piece into the femoral tunnel.
6. Insert partially threaded 4.0 mm Synthes screws, with the far cortex engaged, near the cranial tibial tunnel and at the exit of the femoral tunnel. Use these to anchor the tuberosity and patellar sutures after adjusting the graft to its proper tension.
7. Close the incision and tissues routinely. Place the limb in a Robert Jones bandage for 1 month, as described in the patellar tendon procedure for cranial CL rupture repair.
8. For bony avulsion injuries, if the bony portion is large enough, drill holes in the *bony* segment (lag screws or a Bunnell suture pattern can be used). The suture can be passed through the ligament using a Bunnell pattern, and the suture ends passed through the bony drill holes. This gives firm fixation of the sutures to the ligament.
   a. Make two drill holes through the avulsion site, exiting on the medial side of the femur or on the cranial surface of the tibia.
   b. Using a suture passer, pass the sutures through the drill holes and tie them securely; this anatomically reduces the avulsion fracture and restabilizes the caudal CL.

MENISCAL PROBLEMS

Preoperative Considerations

■ An isolated meniscal tear or laxity is rare in dogs, compared with humans. More commonly, meniscal pathology is associated with an acute partial, or a complete cruciate tear.
   • Secondary meniscal damage can occur in the weeks and months following an unrecognized or untreated cruciate injury.
■ The resultant craniocaudal and rotational laxity allows the femoral condyles to traumatize the caudal horn of the medial meniscus (Fig. 8*A*). A common

lesion is a folding cranially of the caudal horn of the medial meniscus.
■ This can be diagnosed by palpating a click or clunk during range of motion as the femoral condyle slips over the double thickness of the folded meniscus.
■ Total (complete) meniscectomy is not advised unless there is severe damage of both caudal and cranial horns.

Surgical Procedure

Objectives

■ Remove or repair damaged portions of the menisci

Equipment

■ Standard orthopedic pack and suture material
■ Narrow Hohmann retractor (Synthes #399.18)
■ Scalpel blade (#15)

Technique

1. Place the dog in dorsal recumbency with the forelegs and unaffected rear limb secured. Perform sterile preparation, stockinette, draping, and suturing in of stockinette to the skin incision.
2. Because meniscectomy usually is performed in conjunction with CL reconstruction, use the arthrotomy approach (medial or lateral) appropriate for the cruciate technique. Make the arthrotomy of sufficient length to permit adequate retraction and exposure of both menisci.
3. After dislocating the patella from the trochlea, insert a small, sharp Senn retractor behind the fat pad and exert traction cranially. Keep the retractor in position until all internal joint manipulation is completed.
   a. Avoid trauma to the fat pad with retractors to prevent damage to the vascular supply.
4. Debride cruciate and meniscal remnants, as necessary, and evaluate all joint structures for damage.
5. Place a second, dull Senn retractor on the medial side of the central Senn retractor to visualize the medial meniscus, and then place it laterally to visualize the lateral meniscus.
6. To facilitate visualization of the caudal horns, insert a narrow Hohmann retractor or hemostat to pry the tibial plateau forward (see General Principles of Stifle Surgery in this chapter).
7. Use a probe to determine laxity of the menisci and the extent of any tears.
8. Grasp the partially detached, forward-displaced caudal horn with a hemostat at the midportion. Often, the medial caudal horn is still attached peripherally to the medial collateral ligament and to the caudal tibial insertion.
9. With traction on the caudal horn a #15 scalpel blade is used to make a perpendicular cut to sever the caudal horn from the normally attached cranial horn. The meniscal-medial collateral attachment is usually cranial to the folded caudal horn.
10. Cut the remaining attachment (to the tibia) by placing the blade horizontally under the remaining caudal horn, and remove the caudal horn.

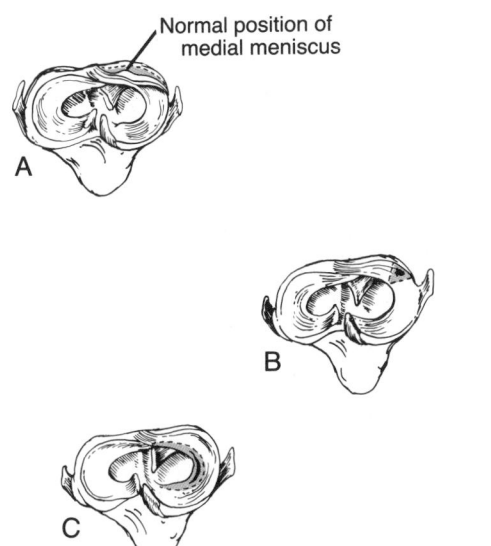

Figure 8. Repair of medial meniscus injuries. See text for details.

a. Be careful to avoid cutting into the cartilage of the condyle or tibial plateau or lacerating the caudal CL or popliteal vessels caudal to the meniscus.
11. Flush the joint well with Ringer's lactate solution, reposition the patella and run the joint through a range of motion. No crepitation or clicks should be felt.
12. Remove any areas of localized injury or tears with a scalpel and create a vascular access channel running from the peripheral synovium (Fig. 8*B*). In "bucket handle" tears (Fig. 8*C*), the vascularity of central area (shaded area, Fig. 8*C*) is compromised and therefore is removed by sharp dissection.

COLLATERAL LIGAMENT DISRUPTIONS

Preoperative Considerations

- Collateral ligament injuries usually occur as a result of severe medial (varus) or lateral (valgus) stress to the stifle by blunt force to the joint with the paw fixed during weight bearing.
- Collateral ligament strains are graded as to severity:
  - First degree—stretching and minor disruption of collagen fibers
  - Second degree—partial tearing
  - Third degree—complete discontinuity of the substance of the ligament or avulsion of a bony attachment.
- Animals usually are presented with acute lameness.
- Verify joint instability with stress radiographs.
- First- and second-degree injuries respond well to rest and restricted exercise.
- Third-degree injuries require surgical repair and partial immobilization for a few weeks, using a modified Robert Jones bandage before allowing early mobilization.

Surgical Procedure

Objectives

- Restore the integrity of the injured ligament and the stability of the stifle.

Equipment

- Standard orthopedic pack and suture material
- Power drill
- Spiked washers/screw

Technique

1. Surgical approach is directly over the damaged ligament.
2. For complete ligament tears, use a Bunnell locking loop, or triple pulley suture pattern (see sec. 9, ch. 21) for primary repair.
3. For bony avulsion, use a screw and spiked washer (Synthes #219.9, 219.93–95) if the bony portion is large enough to accept a screw. When the bony portion is small, use a ligament fixation plate (Synthes #65.00.1, 65.00.10, 65.00.11).
4. Reinforce a severely traumatized ligament by forming a supplemental fascial strip with two parallel incisions cranial and caudal to the involved collateral ligament: then suture the fascial strip to the repaired collateral ligament; or a fascial strip can be folded down and sutured to the ligament to reinforce the primary repair.
5. Alternatively, place screws at the origin and insertion of the collateral ligament and make a prosthetic ligament by looping wire (18 or 20 gauge) in a figure-eight pattern around the screws. This wire or #1 to 3 nylon usually breaks with time, but enough scar tissue forms to stabilize the joint.

STIFLE LUXATION

Preoperative Considerations

- Severe trauma is necessary for complete stifle luxation to occur. The condition is more common in cats.
- Physical examination reveals total laxity in all directions: cranial, caudal, and rotational; the medial and lateral aspects of the stifle joint open up excessively.
- Usually, the patellar tendon is not disrupted; however, the popliteus and long digital extensor tendons may be torn, as well as both cruciates, both collaterals, and, in varying degrees, the meniscal attachments.

Surgical Procedure

Objectives

- Repair ligaments and tendons to reestablish joint stability.

Equipment

- Standard orthopedic pack and suture material
- Power drill/drill bits
- Kirschner-Ehmer pins and clamps

Technique

1. Make a long lateral parapatellar skin and arthrotomy incision and assess the damage to ligaments, tendons, menisci, and cartilage.
2. If possible, stabilize the menisci by suturing peripheral attachments; otherwise, perform meniscectomy.
3. Repair the long digital extensor tendon, popliteus, and collateral ligaments with locking tendon loop, pulley, or Bunnell suture patterns; spiked washer and screw; or fascial reinforcement as described previously under collateral ligament repair.
4. Cruciate stabilization may be done by intracapsular replacement or extracapsular imbrication techniques.

Postoperative Care

- To allow adequate unstressed healing, immobilize the repaired stifle for 3–4 weeks with a Kirschner-Ehmer device or a cast. Allow gradual return of motion by using a Robert Jones bandage for 2 weeks and then a light wrap.
  - With any form of immobilization of the stifle, the joint should be in a functional (partially flexed) position.
- Some limitation of joint range of motion is acceptable and preferable to instability.

KEY POINT ▶ For complete, multiple, midsubstance ligament disruptions, apposition of ligament ends is important for healing to occur; however, early mobilization also is important for complete biomechanical recovery.

Supplemental Readings

Arnoczky SP, Marshall JL: The cruciate ligaments of the canine stifle: An anatomical and functional analysis. Am J Vet Res 38:1807, 1977.

Brinker WO, Piermattei DL, Flo GL: *Handbook of Small Animal Orthopedics and Fracture Treatment*, 2nd Ed. Philadelphia: W. B. Saunders, 1990, p 403.

Chiroff RT: Experimental replacement of the anterior cruciate ligament: A histological and microradiographic study. J Bone Joint Surg 57-A:1124, 1975.

Clancy WG, Narechania RG, Rosenberg TD, et al.: Anterior and posterior cruciate ligament reconstruction in Rhesus monkeys. J Bone Joint Surg 63-A:1270, 1981.

Clancy WG, Thomsen E, Dueland RT, et al.: Anterior cruciate and posterior cruciate ligament reconstruction with patella tendon utilizing a medial vascular graft, lateral vascular graft, and free patella tendon graft. Trans ORS 12:70, 1987.

Clancy WG, Shelbourne KD, Zoellner GB, et al.: Treatment of knee joint instability secondary to rupture of the posterior cruciate ligament. J Bone Joint Surg 65-A:310, 1983.

Dueland RT: A recent technique for reconstruction of the anterior cruciate ligament. J Am Anim Hosp Assoc 2:1, 1966.

Noyes FR, Butler DL, Grood ES, et al.: Biomechanical analysis of human ligament grafts used in knee-ligament repairs and reconstructions. J Bone Joint Surg 66-A:344, 1984.

Patterson RH, Smith GK, Gregor TP, Newton CD: Biomechanical stability of four cranial cruciate ligament repair techniques in the dog. Vet Surg 20:85, 1991.

Smith GK, Torg JS: Fibular head transposition for repair of the cruciate deficient stifle in the dog. J Am Vet Med Assoc 187:375, 1985.

Torg JS, Conrad W, Kalen V: Clinical diagnosis of anterior cruciate ligament instability in the athlete. Am J Sports Med 4:84, 1976.

Woo SL-Y, Inoue M, McGurk-Burleson E, Gomez MA: Treatment of the medial collateral ligament injury. II: Structure and function of canine knees in response to differing treatment regimens. Am J Sports Med 15:22, 1987.

Yoshiya S, Audrish JT, Manley MT, Bauer TW: Initial graft tension on the outcome of ACL reconstruction: An in vivo study in dogs. Trans ORS 12:102, 1987.

17 Fractures of the Tibia and Fibula

Erick L. Egger

Fractures of the tibia and fibula compose a significant proportion (15–20%) of all long bone fractures in small animals. In addition, the minimal soft tissue coverage of these bones increases the incidence of contamination of open fractures which may result in infection and healing complications. Proper treatment of tibial and fibular fractures requires:

- An understanding of the disruptive biochemical forces that must be controlled to promote the healing process
- Selection of a fixation technique that will control these forces
  - Application of fixation without damaging the fracture healing process or compromising the function of the limb.

ANATOMY, FUNCTION, AND BIOMECHANICS OF THE TIBIA AND FIBULA

The anatomy of the tibia and fibula can be divided into regions based on their location, function, architecture, and the forces acting on them.

Epiphysis

Location and Function

Proximally the epiphysis consists of:

- The tibial plateau, which provides support for the articular cartilage of the distal stifle joint (for information concerning the stifle joint, see sec. 9, ch. 16)
- The fibular head, which serves as the distal attachment for the lateral collateral ligament
- The tibial tubercle, which is the insertion point of the patellar tendon of the quadriceps muscle

Distally, the epiphyseal region consists of:

- The cochlea tibiae, which supports the distal articular cartilage
- The medial malleolus, which is the proximal attachment of the medial collateral tarsal ligaments
- The fibular epiphysis, which acts as the proximal attachment of the lateral collateral tarsal ligaments

Biomechanics

- The epiphyseal regions of the tibia and fibula are primarily composed of loosely woven, trabecular bone surrounded by a thin shell of dense cortex. This architecture limits the holding power of fixation implants, requiring extra care in their application.

- The epiphyseal regions that serve as ligament and tendon attachments are subjected to distractive forces. Consequently, repair of avulsion fractures of these areas must control these tensile forces.
- The epiphyseal regions that support articular cartilage are subjected to compressive loads that tend to separate the fragments, resulting in articular incongruity, instability, and eventually degenerative arthritis. Fixation of these fractures must provide anatomic reduction and rigid immobilization so that the fracture will heal with minimal callus formation, and so that early joint motion can be initiated to avoid joint stiffness.

Physis

- The physeal regions of the tibia and fibula are located adjacent to the epiphysis and exist only in growing immature animals.
- The hypertrophied layer and calcifying layers of the physis are relatively fragile. Consequently, these layers are commonly the site of fracture with trauma.
- Because the cartilage layers are irregular and transverse, fractures tend to interdigitate well when reduced and require only control of bending forces.

Metaphysis

- The metaphysis is an indistinct region of bone located between the physis and the diaphysis (central shaft).
- The function of the metaphysis is the gradual alteration of the general construction of the bone from the wide-diameter thin cortex of the epiphysis to the narrow-diameter thick cortex of the diaphysis. The biomechanics and architecture of these regions change along their length.

Diaphysis

- The diaphysis is the central portion of the tibia and makes up the majority of its length.
- The tibial diaphysis is subjected to severe bending and torsional forces, in addition to axial compressive loads. Its hollow tubular construction of relatively thick cortical bone maximizes its effectiveness in resisting these forces.

PREOPERATIVE CONSIDERATIONS

General Considerations

- Examine the animal carefully for nonorthopedic injuries.

- Evaluate cardiovascular status. If cardiopulmonary problems are suspected, radiograph the thorax.
- Evaluate neurologic status. Determine deep pain perception in the fractured limb for local nerve damage, and proprioceptive and sensory perception in the other limbs for evidence of nerve or spinal cord trauma.
■ Examine the animal carefully for concurrent muscoskeletal injuries.

KEY POINT ▶ Nearly all small animals with tibial and/or fibular fractures are able to support themselves on the remaining three limbs. If not, suspect additional injuries.

■ Determine the extent of soft tissue injury and fracture contamination.
- Cover all open fractures with sterile bandages to prevent further contamination, and debride as soon as possible.
- Broad-spectrum antibiotics are indicated if the fracture is open. Obtain samples for culture and sensitivity testing from the fracture site before beginning antibiotic therapy.
- Until definitive treatment is possible, support all tibial fractures with a compressive wrap or splint to prevent additional soft tissue injury.

Specific Considerations in Selecting a Fracture Fixation Technique

■ Determine the potential axial stability of the reduced fracture based on preoperative fracture radiographs.
- Stable fractures generally are simple transverse or short oblique. They tend to impact and become more stable upon weight bearing.
- Unstable fractures have patterns, such as long oblique or comminuted, which tend to override or collapse upon axial loading.
■ Perform rigid fixation of extensively contaminated open fractures. However, avoid placing large implants in the fracture site.
■ Fractures in immature animals heal quickly, but:
■ Premature physeal closure can occur with internal fixation.
■ Immature animals rapidly develop joint stiffness with limb immobilization.
■ Implants quickly loosen in the soft bone of immature animals.
■ Fractures in very old animals heal slowly.
- Brittle bone in older animals often splinters when implants are applied.

SURGICAL PROCEDURES

Objectives

■ Provide adequate stability for fracture healing to occur while causing minimal damage to the biologic healing process.
■ Restore normal limb function by minimizing joint stiffness and muscle atrophy and avoiding the development of degenerative joint disease.

Pin and Tension Band Wire Fixation
Indications

■ Avulsion fractures of the fibular head
■ Avulsion fractures of the lateral (fibular) malleolus and medial (tibial) malleolus (Fig. 1)
■ Avulsion fractures of the tibial tubercle

Equipment

■ General orthopedic pack:
- Standard surgical pack
- Bone and fracture reduction forceps
- Periosteal elevator
- Jacob's hand chuck
- Wire pliers and cutters
■ Stainless steel monofilament orthopedic wire (18–22 gauge)
■ Kirschner wires (0.035–0.062 in)

Technique

1. Incise the skin directly over the affected bone.
2. Reduce and stabilize fracture with small fragment reduction forceps.
3. Create a transverse hole through the intact tibia approximately equidistant from the fracture line with the hand chuck and a Kirschner wire.
4. Insert two parallel Kirschner wires through the fragment, across the fracture, and into the parent bone.

KEY POINT ▶ In the treatment of malleolar fractures, avoid penetrating the articular surface of the distal cochlea.

5. Pass orthopedic wire (18 gauge for most dogs, 20–22 gauge for small dogs and cats) through the transverse hole, cross the wire over the fracture site, and pass one end under the ligament or tendon attachment.
6. Twist both ends of wire together to form a figure eight. Tighten the wire just enough to compress the fracture (see Fig. 1).

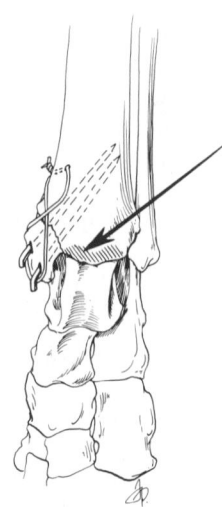

Figure 1. Pin and tension wire fixation of a medial malleolar avulsion fracture. Do not violate the cochlear articular surface with the Kirschner (K) wire *(arrow)*.

7. Cut off excess orthopedic and Kirschner wires. Bend the Kirschner wires over and embed them in the soft tissues to trap the orthopedic wire loop and minimize soft tissue irritation.
   a. In the treatment of tibial tubercle fractures, if the animal still has significant growth potential, do not use tension band wires because this procedure can induce premature physeal closure. If necessary, use additional Kirschner wires oriented perpendicular to the physis for fixation stability.
8. Close soft tissues routinely.

Interfragmentary Lag Screw Fixation

Indications

- Intra-articular fractures of the proximal epiphysis (tibial plateau) and distal epiphysis (tibial cochlea)
- Reconstruction of comminuted shaft fractures prior to neutralization plating (see Fig. 6)

Equipment

- General orthopedic pack
- Bone screws and application instrumentation
- Power drill
- Kirschner wires

Technique

1. Manipulate fragments to obtain anatomic reduction of the intra-articular portion of the fracture and temporarily stabilize with fracture forceps.
2. Insert an interfragmentary screw and compress the intra-articular fracture line, using either a partially threaded screw or over-drilling the near fragment to create a gliding hole for fully threaded screws. Orient the screw perpendicular to the fracture line.
3. Insert additional screws or cross pins, depending on the fragment size, to prevent rotation around the first screw and to provide additional support.

Cross Pin and Rush Pin Fixation

Indications

- Transverse fractures of the epiphysis (may be combined with interfragmentary lag screw technique if the fracture extends into a joint)
- Axially stable fractures of the metaphysis (Fig. 2)
- Salter I and II fractures of the proximal and distal physis

Equipment

- General orthopedic pack
- Kirschner wires or small Steinmann pins (1/16–1/8" in diameter)
- Pin cutter

Technique

1. Manipulate the fracture and reduce through an open approach. Medial approach to the tibial shaft is preferred owing to relative lack of soft tissues.

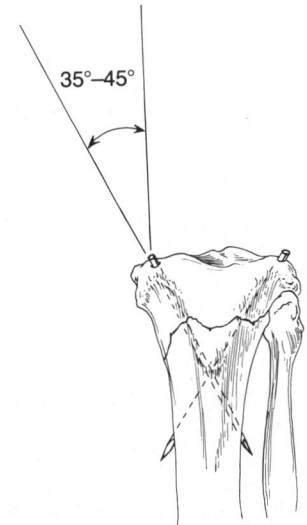

Figure 2. Fracture of the proximal tibial metaphysis fixed with cross pins. Note the angle of pin insertion and penetration of the parent diaphyseal cortex.

2. Select the proper pin diameter (approximately 15% of bone diameter for cross pins, 10% for pins placed in the Rush technique).
3. With a hand chuck (a power drill can be used for cross pins), insert pins from the medial and lateral aspect of the fragment across the fracture into the medullary canal of the parent bone.
4. Orient cross pins obliquely to the long axis (35–45°) so that they penetrate the far cortex (parent bone) when inserted (see Fig. 2).

KEY POINT ▶ Cross pins provide excellent fracture fixation, but because they can interfere with normal function of the growth plate, use them with caution in immature animals.

5. Orient rush pins placed in the Rush technique more parallel (25–35°) to the long axis. During insertion they bounce off the inner cortex of the medullary canal and are driven in to impact into the trabecular bone of the distant metaphysis.
   a. Pins placed in the Rush technique may be preferable for physeal fractures because of their smaller diameter (resulting in less damage to the germinal tissue) and because of their more perpendicular orientation to the physis (allowing sliding of the physis along the pins as it grows).
   b. Prebend the pins to facilitate reflection of the pins off the inner cortical wall as they are inserted.
6. Cut off excess pin length and countersink the ends below bone level (if the pins will not be removed) or bend the ends over to avoid soft tissue interference.

Intramedullary (IM) Pin and Wire Fixation

Indications

- Simple, axially stable fractures of the tibial diaphysis
- Other selected reducible tibial diaphyseal fractures

Contraindications

- Infected or significantly contaminated open (grade 3) fractures (see sec. 9, ch. 26)
- Fractures that cannot be reconstructed

Equipment

- General orthopedic pack
- Steinmann pins
- Pin cutter

Technique

IM Pinning Technique for Simple, Axially Stable Tibial Fractures

1. Select a pin diameter 50–60% of the smallest medullary canal diameter.
2. Reduce the fracture, usually by manipulation through a medial open approach.
3. Insert the pin at a point midway between the tibial tubercle and medial collateral ligament along the edge of the tibial plateau (about 1 cm distal to the articular surface).
4. Drive the pin distally (normograde) down the proximal fragment and across the fracture to impact into the distal metaphyseal bone.
5. Determine the pin insertion length by comparison with a second pin, identical in length, held outside the limb.

KEY POINT ▶ Avoid driving IM pins through the articular cartilage of the cochlea, because this can result in development of significant arthritis.

6. Remove excess pin length with a pin cutter.
7. Determine rotational stability. If significant rotational motion persists, apply interfragmentary wire or a two-pin external fixator.
   a. Two-pin fixation is similar to type I external skeletal fixation (described later) but uses only two pins, one above and one below the fracture.

Technique

Wiring Techniques for Fracture Reconstruction Prior to IM Pinning
With Cerclage Wires

Cerclage wires can only be used on long oblique fracture lines (fracture line length ≥ 2 × bone diameter) (Fig. 3).

1. Use large (18 gauge for medium and larger dogs; 22 gauge for toy breeds and cats) monofilament wire.
2. To control motion, at least two wires must cross the complete fracture line.
3. Orient wires perpendicular to the long bone axis, space apart at least one-half bone diameter, and twist to tighten.
4. Use cerclage wires to protect fissure fractures as necessary.
5. Always use an IM pin in addition to the cerclage wires to control bending forces.

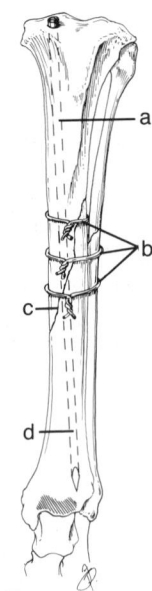

Figure 3. Use of cerclage wire to prevent axial collapse of a long oblique fracture stabilized with an intramedullary (IM) pin. (a) Pin diameter equals 50–60% of medullary canal; (b) wires must be perpendicular to bone axis and ½ bone diameter apart; (c) fracture length must be ≤2 × bone diameter; (d) stop pin insertion short of cochlea.

With Interfragmentary Wires

Use interfragmentary wires to stabilize short oblique patterns (fracture length <2 × bone diameter) when only wire can be applied.

1. Create holes in each bone fragment with a hand chuck and Kirschner wire. Position the holes so the wire crosses the fracture perpendicular to the fracture line, thus providing maximum interfragmentary compression when the wire is tightly twisted.
2. Thread the wire through the holes and incorporate the IM pin that has been inserted to the level of the fracture as described previously.
3. Reduce the fracture, complete the IM pin insertion, and tighten the interfragmentary wire.

External Skeletal Fixation

Indications

- Stable, reducible, and nonreducible fracture patterns depending on ESF frame configuration:
  - Type I (unilateral) frames are relatively flexible in axial bending. Therefore, they are appropriate for relatively stable fractures (Fig. 4).
  - Type II (bilateral) and type III (trilateral) configurations (Fig. 5) have axial rigidity comparable to that of plates.
- Open fractures with significant soft tissue damage or infected fractures, because rigid fixation can be obtained without large implants (e.g., IM pins, plates) in the fracture site.
- Contraindications
- Intra-articular fractures
- Avulsion fractures of ligament and tendon epiphyseal attachments

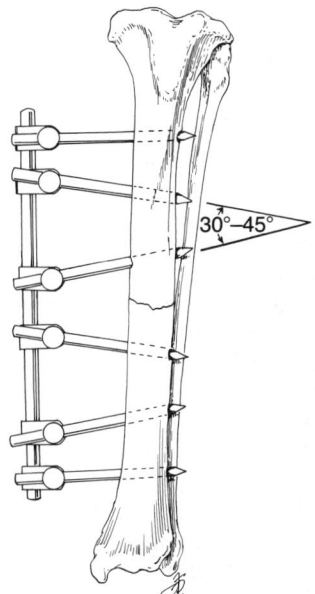

Figure 4. A six-pin type I (unilateral) external skeletal fixator applied to the medial side of a relatively stable tibial fracture. Addition of a lateral connecting bar would convert this to a type II (bilateral) fixator.

Equipment

- General orthopedic pack
- Low-speed power drill
- Kirschner apparatus is available in three sizes for small animal application
- Methylmethacrylate (can be used instead of connecting clamps and bar).

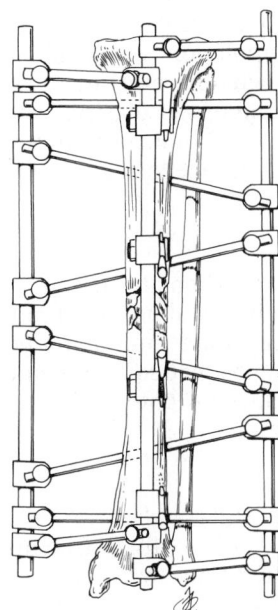

Figure 5. A very rigid type III (trilateral) external skeletal fixation (ESF) configuration applied to a nonreconstructible diaphyseal fracture.

Technique

1. Fixation usually is placed on the medial side of the tibia. However, it can be oriented laterally or cranially to avoid soft tissue injuries.
2. Hold the fracture in approximate reduction, and insert the most proximal and distal fixation pins though small skin incisions into each fragment, using a low-speed power drill.
3. Slide a connecting bar with the appropriate number of clamps onto the end fixation pins. Place at least three pins in each fragment.
4. Reduce the fracture, using closed manipulation or a limited open approach, and tighten the end clamps.
5. Insert fixation pins through the remaining open clamps into the bone and tighten each connecting clamp when placing the pin. Obtain a 30° angle between at least two of the pins in each fragment. Threaded pins reduce the incidence of loosening of pins.
6. For unstable fractures, insert additional pins and bars in other planes to create more rigid frame configurations.
7. Collect autogenous cancellous bone graft from the proximal medial tibial tuberosity and place it in any bony defects remaining after fracture reduction.
8. Do not completely close incisions or wounds of open or infected fractures (see Postoperative Care and Complications).

Plate and Screw Fixation

Indications

- The stabilized limb is needed for immediate weight bearing because of orthopedic or neurologic injuries to the other limbs.
- Restricted activity or adequate postoperative care is not possible.
- Rigid fixation is necessary (e.g., in large, very active dogs).

Equipment

- General orthopedic pack
- Plates, screws, and specialized instrumentation for their implantation
- Power drill

Technique

1. Contour an appropriate-size plate to the shape of the intact bone and apply the plate to the medial (tensile) side of the tibia.
2. If the fracture pattern is axially stable, compress the fracture by applying the plate in the compression mode. When using dynamic compression plates, compression is achieved by drilling screw holes such that the screw slides toward the fracture line.
3. Initially, rebuild long, oblique, and reducible comminuted fractures with interfragmentary lag screws and/or wires. Apply a plate to the tibia without compression to protect the interfragmentary fixation

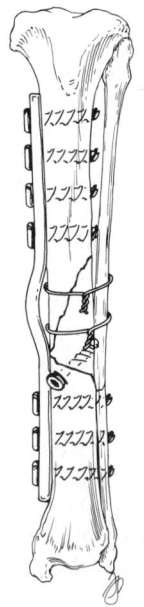

Figure 6. Use of a plate to protect a reconstructed comminuted tibial fracture from excessive bending forces. The screw and wires maintain reduction, and the plate "neutralizes" the weight-bearing forces.

from bending forces (i.e., neutralization mode) (Fig. 6).

4. To prevent collapse under loading, apply a heavy plate in the buttress mode for nonreducible fractures.
   a. Add cancellous autograft to the fracture to stimulate rapid formation of load-sharing callus.
   b. Alternatively, remove detached bone fragments (break into small pieces and add to bone graft), transversely osteotomize fragment ends, and collapse the fracture to reestablish good cortical contact and a stable repair. As much as 20% of the tibial length may be removed without causing permanent dysfunction.

POSTOPERATIVE CARE AND COMPLICATIONS

Immediate Postoperative Care

■ Apply a compressive wrap (Robert Jones bandage) for 3–5 days to prevent soft tissue swelling and to protect the incision.
■ Use gauze and tape to cover the connecting bars and clamps of external fixators. This decreases the incidence of the fixator "hanging up" on objects in the environment and protects the opposite limb.

KEY POINT ▶ Do not primarily close infected and severely open fractures. Lavage and debride the wound q 24–48 h until healthy granulation tissue covers the wound (7–10 days). Complete wound closure at that time or allow complete healing by second intention if there is tension at the wound margins.

Implant Removal

■ Do not routinely remove small implants such as cross pins, cerclage wires, lag screws, and tension band wires unless they cause problems such as joint interference and chronic drainage.
■ Remove large IM pins unless the proximal pin end has been buried by tibial growth.
■ Partially disassemble (destabilize or dynamize) rigid external fixation frames to a flexible configuration after early osseous bridging has occurred (about 6 weeks postoperatively). This increases fracture loading, stimulating callus hypertrophy and remodeling while protecting the fracture from excessive forces that might cause refracture. Remove the balance of the fixator when fracture healing is complete.
■ Remove bone plates in the following situations;
   • Animal with short hair coat develops pain in limb when exposed to cold ambient temperatures.
   • Stiff plate design induces bone atrophy due to stress protection.
   • Chronic infection and drainage does not resolve.

Complications

Nonunion

■ Hypertrophic nonunion:
   • There is exuberant callus proliferation without fracture bridging because of inadequate fracture immobilization. These fractures are biologically active and require only adequate immobilization.
   • Augment existing fixation or replace with a more rigid fixation technique to allow the fracture to heal.
■ Atrophic nonunion:
   • There is lack of callus production, bone sclerosis, and bone resportion, reflecting a loss of biologic healing potential. These nonunions usually result from significant vascular damage from the trauma, surgical manipulation, or unstable fixation.
   • Treatment includes resection of nonviable bone, reestablishment of vascularity, control of infection, rigid fixation, and induction of new bone proliferation with an autogenous cancellous bone graft.

Malunion

■ Malunion occurs when the fracture heals but poor alignment results in abnormal limb function. This may reflect inadequate initial reduction or loss of reduction owing to inadequate fixation.
■ Treatment includes osteotomy, realignment, and adequate fixation.

Infection

■ Acute infection of a tibial fracture occurs when bacterial proliferation overwhelms the body's defense mechanisms.
■ Clinical signs include pain, swelling, and erythema that reflect the underlying accumulation of exudate and necrotic tissue.

- Immediate aggressive treatment is indicated to avoid progression to chronic osteomyelitis and nonunion:
  - Open the incision and extend the margins, if necessary, to ensure adequate drainage.
  - Culture the wound for aerobic and anaerobic organisms to determine specific antibiotic sensitivity.
  - Repeatedly lavage and debride the fracture site to remove exudate and necrotic soft tissue.
  - Initiate systemic broad-spectrum antibiotic therapy (e.g., cephalothins) until culture and sensitivity testing indicate specific therapy.
- See sec. 9, ch. 27 for management of chronic osteomyelitis.

Growth Deformities

Growth deformities can result from trauma to the germinal layer of one of the physes, or from application of fracture fixation that limits physeal elongation. Angular deformities become apparent about 3 weeks after physeal injury; arthritic changes follow if the condition is not corrected. Treatment depends on the cause of physeal dysfunction and the animal's maturity.

- In actively growing animals:
  - Resect the osseous bridge crossing the physis and replace with autogenous fat graft.
  - Remove fixation implants that might be inhibiting physeal growth.
- In mature animals:
  - Perform corrective osteotomy and articular realignment.

Supplemental Readings

Aron DN: External skeletal fixation. Vet Med Report 1:181, 1989.

Chan KL, Leung YK, Cheng JC, Leung PC: The management of Type III open tibial fractures. Injury 16:157, 1984.

Coombs R, Green SA, Sarmiento A: *External Fixation and Functional Bracing.* London: Orthotext, 1989, p 13.

Egger EL: Static strength evaluation of six external skeletal fixation configurations. Vet Surg 12:130, 1986.

Johnson AL, Kneller SK, Weigel RM: Radial and tibial fracture repair with external skeletal fixation. Effects of fracture type, reduction, and complications on healing. Vet Surg 18:367, 1989.

Piermattei DL, Greeley RG: *An Atlas of Surgical Approaches to the Bones of the Dog and Cat,* 2nd Ed. Philadelphia: W. B. Saunders, 1979, p 176.

Robertson WW: Newest knowledge of the growth plate. Clin Orthoped Rel Res 253:270, 1990.

Vandewater AL, Olmstead ML: Premature closure of the distal radial physis in the dog: A review of eleven cases. Vet Surg 12:7, 1983.

18 Luxation, Subluxation, and Shearing Injuries of the Tarsal Joint

Dennis N. Aron

Luxation, subluxation, and shearing injuries of the tarsus involve damage to the supporting ligaments of the joint. Treatment and prognosis of these injuries depend on the location of the ligament damage and subsequent joint instability. Subluxations can be caused by spontaneous overstress or external trauma. Vehicular trauma usually causes luxations and shear injuries. Conservative treatment of most of these injuries with external coaptation is not advised, because continued instability and the development of degenerative joint disease are the likely outcome.

KEY POINT ▶ Surgical stabilization gives the most consistent results in repair of luxation, subluxation, and shearing injuries of the tarsus.

SURGICAL ANATOMY AND SPECIAL CONSIDERATIONS

General

- The tarsus consists of the tibia, fibula, metatarsal bones, and seven specific tarsal bones orderly stacked in levels (Fig. 1).
- A multiple complex arrangement of ligaments connects the bones of the joint and helps to prevent luxation (Fig. 2).
- The *tarsocrural* joint is formed by the tibia and fibula

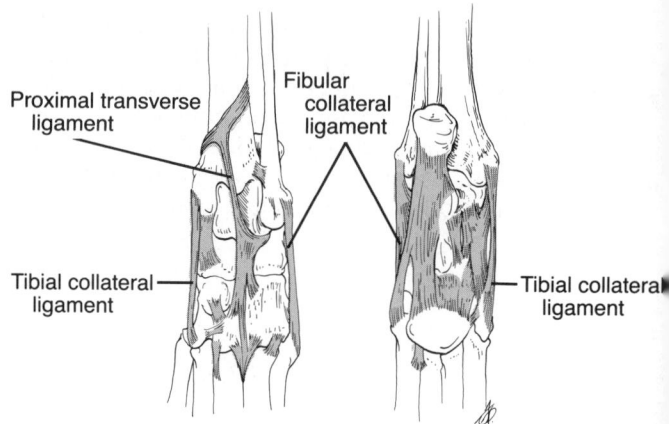

Figure 2. Cranial *(left)* and caudal *(right)* views of the ligamentous anatomy of the tarsus.

at the proximal level and by the talus and calcaneus at the distal level.

- The *intertarsal* joints are all the articulations between the tarsal bones. Several of these joints are named and include the:
  - Talocalcaneal joint—between the talus and calcaneus
  - Talocalcaneocentral joint—between the talus and central tarsal bone (includes a small communication with the calcaneus)
  - Calcaneoquartal joint (proximal intertarsal joint)—between the calcaneus and fourth tarsal bone
  - Centrodistal joint (distal intertarsal joint)—between the central tarsal bone and distal numbered tarsal bones
  - Tarsometatarsal joints—between the distal tarsal and metatarsal bones

Tarsocrural Joint

- Synonyms for this joint are the tibiotarsal, talocrural, and hock joint.
- Most luxations, subluxations, and shear injuries directly involve this joint.
- The major ligaments providing stability on the medial side of the joint are the long medial ligament and the tibiocentral and tibiotalar short component ligaments (Fig. 3A).

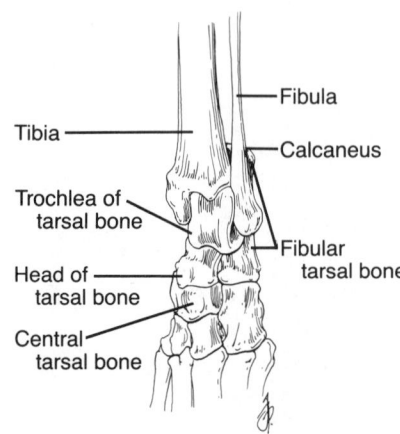

Figure 1. Anatomy of the bones of the tarsus.

Labels in Figure 1: Tibia, Fibula, Calcaneus, Trochlea of tarsal bone, Head of tarsal bone, Fibular tarsal bone, Central tarsal bone

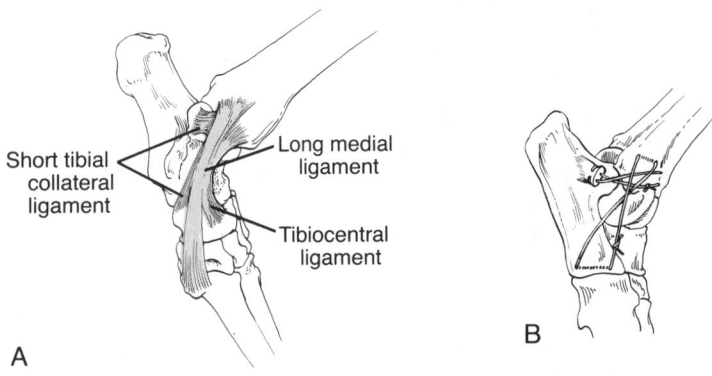

Figure 3. *A*, Medial ligamentous anatomy of the tarsus; *B*, suture prosthesis repair of medial ligament injury. Sutures are tunneled through the bones at points where the ligaments attach. Alternatively, bone screws can be placed at these points and sutures passed around them.

- The major ligaments providing stability on the lateral side of the joint are the long lateral ligament and the calcaneofibular short component ligament (Fig. 4).
- The components of the medial and lateral ligaments complement each other in maintaining the talus in the mortise provided by the tibia and fibula.
- Certain parts of the ligament complexes are tighter in extension (long lateral and medial ligaments and tibiocentral short component ligament) or flexion (calcaneofibular and tibiotalar short component ligaments).
- The tibiotalar and calcaneofibular short component ligaments of the medial and lateral sides, respectively, are especially important for maintaining stability of the joint. The joint capsule and malleoli also contribute to joint stability.
- The gross anatomy of the medial and lateral collateral ligament complexes are similar (see Figs. 3 and 4). The components cross each other at the tarsocrural joint space, providing the greatest amount of ligament and an advantageous spatial arrangement directly over the joint.

KEY POINT ▶ In the reconstruction of the collateral ligamentous supporting structures of the tarsocrural joint, consider the complementary nature of ligamentous structure and function.

Intertarsal and Tarsometatarsal Joints

- The most common injury is damage to the plantar ligaments and tarsal fibrocartilage (see Fig. 2).
- The plantar ligaments and tarsal fibrocartilage limit extension of the intertarsal joints.
- Most of the intertarsal joint stability is provided by three distinct plantar ligaments. These ligaments fuse, with a thickening of the joint capsule (the tarsal fibrocartilage) at the tarsometatarsal joint.
  - The first ligament originates from the plantar surface of the sustentaculum tali and attaches to the central tarsal bone and tarsometatarsal joint capsule.
  - The second ligament originates from the plantar-lateral surface of the calcaneus. It joins with the long component of the lateral collateral ligament complex and attaches to the base of the fifth metatarsal bone.
  - The third ligament originates from the body of the calcaneus and attaches to the fourth tarsal bone and the base of the fourth and fifth metatarsal bones.

TARSOCRURAL LUXATION AND SUBLUXATION

Surgical methods are recommended for treatment of luxation or subluxation injuries of the tarsocrural joint.

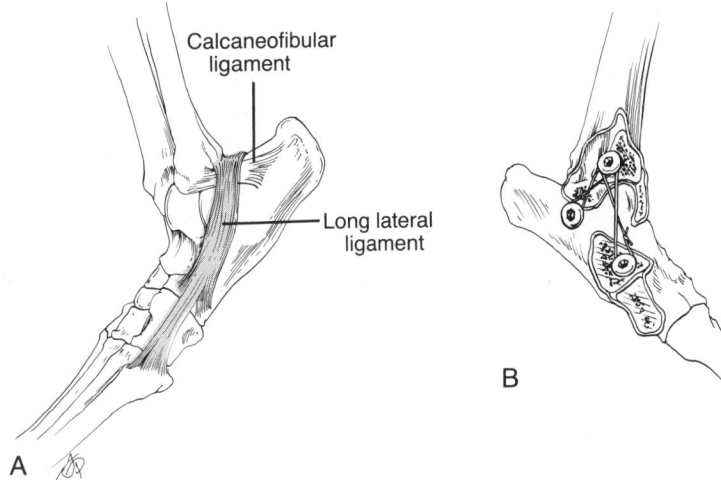

Figure 4. *A*, Lateral ligamentous anatomy of the tarsus; *B*, suture prosthesis repair of lateral ligament injury. Sutures are tunneled through the bones at points where the ligaments attach. Alternatively, bone screws can be placed at these points and sutures passed around them.

Luxation and subluxation usually are the result of rupture of the medial or lateral collateral ligament complex.

Double-Prosthesis Replacement

■ Double-prosthesis replacement (described later) closely reproduces the components of the intact medial and lateral collateral ligament complexes, thus allowing nearly normal joint stability to be maintained throughout a functional range of motion.
■ Similar to the components of the normal collateral ligaments, double-suture prostheses become taut and lax with flexion and extension. Because of this, wire is not useful. Certain sutures (see later) give more successful results, most likely owing to the retention of elasticity upon cyclic loading.
■ Clinically, double-ligament replacement gives results superior to conservative management with splints or nonanatomic single ligament replacement methods. The prognosis is good for long-term function with most closed luxation and subluxation injuries, depending on timely repair (within 5 days of injury) and absence of articular damage.

Preoperative Considerations

■ Tarsocrural luxation results from different combinations of injuries including:
  • Fractures of both malleoli
  • Fracture of one malleolus and damage to the contralateral ligament complex
  • Fracture of the fibula and damage to the medial ligament complex
  • Uncommonly, damage to both the lateral and medial collateral ligament complexes and no fractures
■ Tarsocrural subluxation usually results from complete rupture or avulsion of either the lateral or medial collateral ligament complex.
  • In medial ruptures, the paw tilts abnormally toward the lateral direction with a laterally (valgus) applied force.
  • In lateral ruptures, the tilt is in a medial direction with a medially (varus) applied force.
■ Occasionally, there is rupture of only the long or short components of the medial or lateral ligament complexes. Less joint laxity makes these subluxation injuries more difficult to diagnose. Determine joint laxity using the following methods:
  • Place lateral and medial tilt forces on the hock at different joint angles: Laxity in extension but not flexion suggests major damage to the long medial ligament and tibiocentral short component, or long lateral ligament; laxity in flexion only suggests that most damage is isolated to the tibiotalar or calcaneofibular short components.
  • Make a dorsoplantar (stress) radiograph while applying lateral and medial tilt forces on the hock: Take the stress radiograph at the tarsocrural joint angle that produces the subluxation; for subtle subluxations, compare this radiograph with a similar radiograph of the contralateral (normal) hock.

KEY POINT ▶ Routine dorsoplantar and lateral radiographic views are always needed to check for concomitant tarsal injuries. Stress radiographs are useful to confirm the diagnosis but are not always necessary.

Surgical Procedure

Objectives

■ Stabilize the joint.
■ Maintain an adequate range of motion.
■ Avoid trauma to the articular surfaces.
■ Achieve pain-free weight bearing.
■ Minimize patient morbidity and owner expense.

Equipment

■ Standard orthopedic instrument pack and suture material
■ Gelpi self-retaining retractors
■ Small periosteal elevator
■ Orthopedic drill (power drill preferred)
■ Orthopedic screws, washers, and insertion equipment
■ Kirschner wires
■ Assortment of straight and curved needles
■ Coaptation splint
■ Braided polyester* or monofilament polybutester† suture material

Technique

1. Clip the injured limb from the level of the proximal femur, extending distally to include the paw. Include the paw in the sterile field to allow direct manipulation.
2. Place the animal in lateral recumbency, with the injured limb up for lateral replacement or down for medial replacement, and prepare the limb for aseptic surgery.
3. Expose the subluxation through a curved skin incision centered over the medial or lateral malleolus.
   a. Begin from the distal one-fourth of the tibia and continue to the proximal metatarsal bones.
   b. Locate the medial or lateral collateral ligament complex along the same line by incising the subcutaneous tissue and deep fascia.
4. Inspect the components of the ligament complexes for damage.
   a. To help assess the damage, stress the ligament components with a varus or valgus tilt in both flexion and extension.
   b. It is unlikely that there will be a totally isolated injury to only one component of the ligament complex. The ligaments can appear intact but may have lost considerable function owing to internal derangement of the collagen fibers.

KEY POINT ▶ Usually, the ligament components are too badly damaged to allow primary suturing of the torn ends or reattachment to bone. Replace irreparable ligaments

---

*Polydek or Tevdek; Deknatel, Inc., Queens Village, NY 11429
†Novafil, Davis + Geck, Manati, PR 00701

and protect repaired ligaments with prosthetic sutures.

5. Replace or protect the medial or lateral ligament complexes with two figure-of-eight heavy sutures anchored to the bone directly or with bone screws.
   a. Drill bone tunnels in the malleolus in locations similar to the origins of the components of the ligament complex (see Figs. 3*B* and 4*B*). Bone tunnels serve as anchors for the suture prostheses.
   b. Secure the suture prosthesis that mimics the lateral or medial short components to tags of the torn ligament at the insertion site. Use a locking loop suture pattern to grip the torn ligament (see sec. 9, ch. 21). A bone screw (see Shear Injury) may be needed to fix the prosthesis to the insertion site (see Fig. 4*B*).
   c. Secure the suture prosthesis that mimics the lateral or medial long components and tibiocentral short components to a drill hole in the tubercle of the distal talus or distal calcaneus (see Fig. 3*B* and 4*B*). A bone screw (see Shear Injury) may be used to fix the prosthesis (see Fig. 4*B*).
6. Use one or two for (large patients) strands of #1–5 braided polyester or monofilament polybutester sutures for prosthetic replacement or protection.
   a. Set the sutures in a figure-of-eight pattern.
   b. Do not use absorbable sutures.
   c. Do *not use* monofilament nylon and monofilament polypropylene for sutures. They tend to stretch permanently and are better suited for primary repair of torn ligaments.
7. Tie the long and short suture prostheses.
   a. Tie the short prosthesis with the tarsocrural joint held in approximately 90° flexion for dogs and 70° for cats.
   b. Tie the long suture prosthesis with the joint in a functional standing angle of 135° for dogs (varies with breed) and 120° for cats.
   c. After the sutures are tied, tighten the screws against the bone.
8. Expose the luxation injury through separate surgical incisions on the medial and lateral sides of the joint.
   a. Fix the malleolar fracture with a tension band technique.
   b. Replace or protect the contralateral ligaments.
9. To manage luxations due to fracture of the fibula and damage to the contralateral ligament complex:
   a. Replace or protect the medial ligaments.
   b. Stabilize the fibula by fixing the limb in a long, rigid coaptation splint. Extend the splint from above the stifle to the paw and position the stifle and hock joints in a functional angle. Maintain for 4–6 weeks.

Postoperative Care

■ Immobilize the tarsocrural joints with a short, rigid coaptation splint.
  • Extend the splint from just below the stifle distally to include the digits.
  • Place the hock in a functional standing angle.

  • Provide rigid coaptation with a full circular cast or a padded soft wrap reinforced with an orthopedic splint. Materials for the splint can vary (e.g., fiberglass slab, aluminum rods).
■ Maintain the coaptation splint for 2–6 weeks; the length of time depends on the amount of initial trauma and joint instability. A longer time is required for luxation and major subluxation injuries, a shorter time for incomplete tears and partial injuries.
■ After the rigid splint is removed, carefully allow weight bearing to resume.
  • To control the amount of movement in the tarsocrural joint, apply progressively weaker soft wraps for 4–8 weeks.

KEY POINT ▶ Do not allow an animal to bear full weight on an unprotected limb after removal of rigid coaptation.

SHEAR INJURY

Preoperative Considerations

■ Shear injury usually occurs when an animal is trapped by a moving vehicle, resulting in shearing by the road surface of supporting ligaments, joint capsule, and malleolus.
■ The medial joint is injured more commonly than the lateral joint.
■ Perform wound management and ligament replacement when the bone and cartilage damage is mostly isolated to the malleolus. Severe soft tissue damage makes stabilization difficult and prolongs healing.
■ Although a successful ligament replacement gives better results than a tarsocrural joint arthrodesis, consider joint arthrodesis if there is extensive bone and cartilage damage.

Surgical Procedure

Objectives

■ Prevent infection.
■ Anatomically stabilize the tarsocrural joint, eliminate pain, and maintain a functional range of motion.
■ Avoid trauma to the articular surfaces.
■ Attain wound coverage with full-thickness skin.
■ Minimize patient morbidity and owner expense.

Equipment

■ Equipment is the same as for tarsocrural luxation and subluxation plus:
  • External skeletal fixator
  • Wound dressing materials

Technique

Wound Management and Debridement
1. Prior to debridement and ligament replacement, cover the shear wound with a temporary sterile dressing and apply a temporary splint to prevent further damage to the unstable joint. Exteriorized

material will contaminate deeper recesses if replacement into the wound is attempted.

   a. Do not push or "stuff" extruded soft tissue, bone, or cartilage back into the wound.

   b. Do not soak the wound.

2. Perform debridement as soon as the animal is a stable candidate for surgery, ideally within 6 hours from the time of injury, and preferably sooner.

KEY POINT ▶ Ligament reconstruction and wound closure can be delayed but do not delay wound debridement.

   a. Anesthetize the animal and remove the temporary splint.

   b. Keeping the wound covered, clip the limb, and cleanse with an appropriate antiseptic.

   c. Remove the dressing and thoroughly irrigate the wound with copious amounts of a prewarmed balanced electrolyte solution (see sec. 5, ch. 18).

   d. Obtain cultures of the joint surface for identification of contaminating organisms and their sensitivity to antibiotics. A Gram stain may be helpful in identifying bacteria type.

3. After moving the animal to the operating area, perform a final surgical scrub and drape the limb.

4. Debride the wound of all visible necrotic tissue and road dirt and other foreign material. Be careful to avoid damage to articular surfaces.

   a. During the debridement process, lavage continuously with copious amounts (1 liter or more) of a balanced electrolyte solution such as lactated Ringer's, using a moderate amount of pressure, through a 30- to 60-ml syringe and 18- or 19-gauge needle or catheter.

5. Perform ligament replacement at this time or delay for repeat wound debridement or orthopedic referral. If delaying replacement:

   a. Cover the wound with an absorbent dressing to keep the wound moist (e.g., wet-to-dry dressing; see sec. 5, ch. 18).

   b. Stabilize the joint with a rigid coaptation splint.

   c. Change the dressing once a day or more frequently if necessary.

6. Repeat wound debridement when questionably viable or necrotic tissue is left in the wound after the first procedure. Continue this process until only viable tissue is present in the wound.

Ligament Replacement

The ligament replacement technique usually requires three bone screws and two figure-of-eight heavy sutures.

1. Use 4.0-mm partially threaded cancellous screws or 2.7-mm cortical screws with 2.7-mm spiked washers,* depending on the size of the animal. Place the screws as close as possible to the origin and insertion of the components of the ligament complex (see Figs. 3A and 4A).

2. Position the origin screw in the distal tibia for the medial ligament or the distal fibula and tibia for the lateral ligament. Direct this screw slightly proximal

---

*Synthes Ltd., Wayne, PA 19087.

to avoid penetrating joint cartilage and to obtain maximum bony purchase.

3. Position the insertion screw for the medial tibiotalar short ligament in the proximoplantar quadrant of the medial trochlear facies of the talus.

4. Position the screw corresponding to the insertion of the medial long and tibiocentral short ligaments through the tubercle at the plantar base of the talus. Direct this screw slightly proximodorsally.

5. Position the screw corresponding to the insertion of the calcaneofibular short ligament proximoplantar to the base of the lateral articular facies of the tuber calcis.

6. Position the insertion screw for the long ligament through the tubercle at the dorsal extent of the base of the calcaneus. Direct this screw slightly proximoplantar.

7. Using one or two (for large patients) strands of #1–5 polyester or monofilament polybutester sutures as prosthetic replacements, place suture(s) around the origin screw and the short insertion screw, and separate suture(s) around the origin screw and long insertion screw.

   a. Set the sutures in a figure-of-eight pattern.

   b. Tie taut the tibiotalar or calcaneofibular short suture prosthesis with the tarsocrural joint held in approximately 90° flexion for dogs and 70° for cats. Tie taut the medial long or lateral long suture prosthesis with the tarsocrural joint in a functional standing angle of 135° for dogs (varies for some breeds) and 120° for cats.

   c. Tighten the screws against the bone.

KEY POINT ▶ Never perform primary soft tissue closure over a shear injury.

8. If possible, allow second intention healing; alternatively, perform delayed closure or apply a skin graft (see sec. 5, chs. 18 and 19) after all surfaces of the wound and prosthetic sutures are covered with healthy granulation tissue.

Postoperative Care

■ Immobilize the tarsocrural joint for 2–4 weeks, using transarticular external skeletal fixation.

   • Use the fixator to provide consistent stability during serial debridement and general wound management and following prosthetic replacement.

   • Remove the fixator when the wound appears healthy and the prosthetic sutures are sufficiently covered by granulation tissue and wound contraction.

■ After the fixator is removed, immobilize the hock for an additional 2–4 weeks with a short rigid coaptation splint. This gives less stability than the fixator but does not risk failure of the prosthetic sutures.

■ After removal of the rigid splint, allow progressive weight bearing with the aid of decreasingly padded soft splints for an additional 4–8 weeks.

Prognosis

The prognosis is good to guarded for long-term pain-free function if there is no damage to the articular surfaces other than the malleolus.

TARSOCRURAL JOINT ARTHRODESIS

Tarsocrural joint arthrodesis can be done by tarsocrural joint fusion or pantarsal fusion.

- Pantarsal arthrodesis includes fusion not only of the tarsocrural joint but also of the intertarsal and tarsometatarsal joints.
- Pantarsal arthrodesis gives more consistent functional results and there is less patient morbidity.

Preoperative Considerations

Indications for performing tarsocrural joint arthrodesis instead of ligament replacement include:

- Moderate to severe osteochondral damage to the joint mortise
- Prolonged tarsocrural joint subluxation or luxation causing moderate to severe degenerative joint disease
- Failure of reconstructive surgery or postoperative development of painful degenerative joint disease

Surgical Procedure (Pantarsal Arthrodesis)

Objectives

- Fuse the tarsocrural, intertarsal, and tarsometatarsal joints.
- Fuse the hock at a functional angle.
- Allow pain-free use of the limb.
- Minimize patient morbidity and owner expense.

Equipment

- Standard orthopedic instrument pack and suture material
- Gelpi self-retaining retractors
- Power drill
- Power saw or osteotome and mallet
- Pneumatic surgical bur (optional)
- Bone curets
- Kirschner wires
- Bone plates, screws, and application equipment
- Coaptation splint

Technique

1. Approach the joint dorsally from the distal one-third of the tibia, extending over the tarsal bones and ending at the proximal one-third of the third metatarsal bone.
2. Using a power saw or osteotome, cut the articular cartilage from the distal tibia and trochlea of the talus.
   a. Cut the distal tibia perpendicular to the longitudinal axis.
   b. Cut the trochlea of the talus at an appropriate angle, allowing the distal tibia to rest flush on the talus and form the proper weight-bearing angle at the hock. Prior to surgery, use the animal's contralateral limb to determine the correct weight-bearing angle (approximately 140° for dogs (varies with certain breeds) and 120° for cats).

3. Match the tibia to the talus at the appropriate angle and temporarily fix the two bones with Kirschner wires.
4. With a bone curet or pneumatic bur, remove as much cartilage as possible from the intertarsal and tarsometatarsal joints.
5. Obtain autogenous cancellous bone from the ipsilateral greater tubercle of the humerus and proximal tibia. Pack cancellous bone into the intertarsal and tarsometatarsal joints and around the tarsocrural joint.
6. Apply a bone plate to the dorsal surface of the distal tibia, tarsus, and third metatarsal bone (Fig. 5).
   a. Bend an appropriately sized eight- to ten-hole plate to the proper fit.
   b. Fix three cortical screws and the plate to the tibia, two or three screws to the tarsal bones, and three screws to the third metatarsal bone.
   c. Alternatively, do not place screws in the tarsal bones, and pack this area with cancellous bone.
7. Remove the temporary Kirschner wires, pack more cancellous bone around the tarsocrural joint, and perform routine closure.

Postoperative Care

- Apply a short, rigid coaptation splint or full cylinder cast below the stifle until there is radiographic evidence of bone fusion.
- Remove the bone plate after there is complete bone union, usually in 6–9 months.
- Protect the arthrodesis for 6 weeks following plate removal with a splint or padded bandage; restrict exercise.

OVERVIEW OF INTERTARSAL LUXATION AND SUBLUXATION INJURIES

- Many intertarsal ligament injuries are a result of daily activity and occur without known trauma.
- Acute loading (e.g., with jumping) can damage plantar ligaments and cause a hyperextension injury.

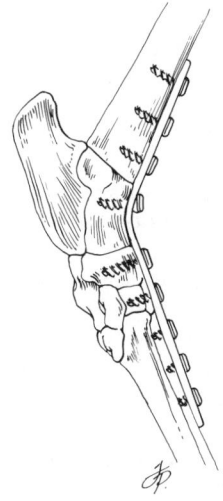

Figure 5. Plantarsal arthrodesis by dorsal application of a bone plate.

- Affected animals usually are non–weight bearing or walk plantigrade, have variable swelling in the tarsal region, and have instability of the tarsus.
- Palpation and stress radiographs (see sec. 1, ch. 4) usually can localize the area of injury.
- Hyperextension injuries are repaired by arthrodesis or tension band wire stabilization.
- Because surgery is performed only on the low-motion intertarsal or tarsometatarsal joints, the prognosis usually is excellent for pain-free normal function.

PROXIMAL INTERTARSAL SUBLUXATION WITH PLANTAR INSTABILITY

Preoperative Considerations

- Injury to the plantar ligaments of the calcaneoquartal and talocalcaneocentral joints results from excessive dorsiflexion; the hock collapses and the animal walks plantigrade.
- A traumatic episode usually is not identified.
- Diagnose by palpation and stress radiographs (see sec. 1, ch. 4).
- This condition does not respond to conservative management with coaptation splints. Treat surgically by arthrodesis of the calcaneoquartal joint.

Surgical Procedure

Objectives

- Fuse the calcaneoquartal joint.
- Avoid trauma to the tarsocrural joint.
- Achieve pain-free, normal weight bearing.
- Minimize patient morbidity and owner expense.

Equipment

- Standard orthopedic instrument pack and suture material
- Gelpi self-retaining retractors
- Intramedullary (IM) pins
- Bone curets or pneumatic bur
- Bone drill and assorted drill bits
- Kirschner wires
- Orthopedic wire (18 or 20 gauge)
- External coaptation devices

Technique

1. Expose the joint plantar-laterally with medial retraction of the tendon of the superficial digital flexor.
2. Using a bone curet or pneumatic bur, remove articular cartilage from the surfaces of the calcaneus and fourth tarsal bone.
3. Insert an appropriate-size single IM pin ($^5/_{64}''$–$^1/_8''$) from the proximal calcaneus down the shaft.
   a. Drill a pilot hole in the (very hard) calcaneus before inserting the IM pin.
   b. Position the pin in the dorsal medullary canal.
4. Obtain autogenous cancellous bone from the proximal tibia and pack it into the joint space.

5. Reduce the joint, drive the IM pin across the joint, and fix the pin in the distal end of the fourth tarsal bone (Fig. 6).
6. Retract the IM pin slightly, cut it short, and countersink it beneath the cartilage of the tuber calcis.
7. Drill a transverse hole across the distal portion of the fourth tarsal bone and the middle section of the calcaneus.
8. Place an orthopedic tension band wire (18 or 20 gauge) in a figure-of-eight pattern through the drilled holes (see Fig. 6).
   a. Set the wire directly against the bone under all soft tissue.
   b. Tighten the wire evenly with a double-twist method and bend the twists over to rest against bone.
9. Reduce the superficial digital flexor tendon and suture the lateral retinaculum to stabilize the tendon.
10. Close the subcutaneous tissue and skin routinely.

Postoperative Care

- Place a short (from the proximal tibia to the paw) rigid coaptation splint for 2 weeks. Follow with a soft coaptation splint for 2 more weeks.
- Restrict activity until bony fusion of the joint is evident on radiographs (usually 6–8 weeks).

PROXIMAL INTERTARSAL LUXATION WITH PLANTAR INSTABILITY

Preoperative Considerations

- This condition occurs infrequently, compared with subluxation injury.
- Trauma results in a high-energy hyperextension injury. There is more joint displacement and instability than with subluxation injury.
- Because of the severe instability in this condition, perform arthrodesis of the intertarsal joint with a bone plate rather than with a less rigid pin and wire tension band technique.

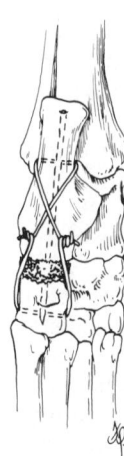

Figure 6. Fusion of the calcaneoquartal joint via pin and tension band wire fixation and cancellous bone graft.

Surgical Procedure

Objectives

■ Fuse the proximal intertarsal joint. Otherwise, objectives are the same as for proximal intertarsal subluxation.

Equipment

■ Standard orthopedic instrument pack and suture material
■ Gelpi self-retaining retractors
■ Bone curets or pneumatic bur
■ Power drill
■ Bone plates, screws, and application equipment
■ External coaptation devices

Technique

1. Make a lateral approach from the tuber calcis, extending over the calcaneus and fourth tarsal bone and ending over the proximal one-third of the fifth metatarsal bone.
2. Using a bone curet or pneumatic bur, remove articular cartilage from the bones of the proximal intertarsal joint.
3. Place autogenous cancellous bone in the joint space. Reduce the joint.
4. Place a bone plate on the lateral aspect of the calcaneus, fourth tarsal bone, and proximal fifth metatarsal bone (Fig. 7).
   a. Shape the bones slightly to accommodate the plate.
   b. Secure an appropriate-size seven-hole plate with two screws in the calcaneus, one in the calcaneus and talus, one in the fourth and central tarsal bones, and three in the fourth and fifth metatarsal bones.
   c. Alternatively, do not place the screw in the fourth and central tarsal bones, and pack this area with cancellous bone.
5. Close the tissue and skin routinely.

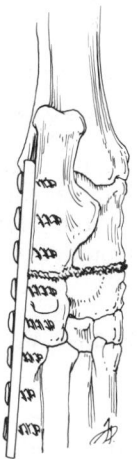

Figure 7. Proximal intertarsal joint fusion via lateral application of a bone plate and cancellous bone graft.

Postoperative Care

■ Protect the arthrodesis with a short rigid coaptation splint or cylinder cast. Remove the splint when there is radiographic evidence of bony fusion.
■ Remove the bone plate after the arthrodesis is complete. If retained, the plate usually loosens, causing pain and lameness.

DISTAL INTERTARSAL (TARSOMETATARSAL) SUBLUXATION WITH PLANTAR INSTABILITY

Preoperative Considerations

■ This condition is less common than proximal subluxation injury.
■ The cause is tearing of the plantar tarsal fibrocartilage and usually is associated with trauma.
■ A few days after the injury the animal attempts weight-bearing and walks plantigrade.
■ Consistent with hyperextension injuries, surgical arthrodesis is the treatment of choice.

Surgical Procedure

Objectives

■ Fuse the distal intertarsal joint. Otherwise, objectives are the same as for proximal intertarsal subluxation.

Equipment

■ See Proximal Intertarsal Subluxation with Plantar Instability.

Technique

1. Expose the injury by an incision over the plantar-lateral calcaneus, fourth tarsal bone, and metatarsal bones.
2. Retract the superficial and deep digital flexor tendons medially and laterally to expose the joints.
3. Remove articular cartilage from the distal intertarsal joint surfaces.
4. Pack autogenous cancellous bone into the joint space.
5. Use a pin and tension band wire technique similar to that described for proximal intertarsal subluxation with plantar instability, but slightly modified.
   a. Insert an appropriate size IM pin ($\frac{5}{64}"$–$\frac{1}{8}"$) down through the calcaneus; extend through the fourth tarsal bone and continue into the distal one-half of the fourth metatarsal bone.
   b. Drill transverse holes for the tension-band wire (18 or 20 gauge) in the distal one-third of the calcaneus and the bases of two or three of the metatarsal bones.
   c. Place the wire in a figure-of-eight pattern under the superficial digital flexor tendon.
6. Alternatively, perform the tarsometatarsal arthrodesis with a bone plate. Use bone screws to secure two holes of a five-hole plate to the fourth and central tarsal bones and distal tarsal bones proxi-

mal to the subluxation, and three holes to the metatarsal bones distal to the subluxation.

Postoperative Care

Maintain a short rigid coaptation splint until there is radiographic evidence of bony fusion.

OTHER INTERTARSAL-TARSOMETATARSAL SUBLUXATION INJURIES

Proximal Intertarsal Subluxations with Dorsal Instability

- Physical examination findings include:
  - Primary damage of the dorsal ligaments and dorsal joint capsule
  - Frequently, concurrent lateral or medial instability
  - Usually, no evidence of external trauma
- The animal places full weight on the limb with only periodic lameness, which is made worse by coincident lateral or medial instability.
- Diagnose by palpation and stress radiographs.
  - Slight dorsal swelling and increased flexion and opening of the dorsal joints are seen.
  - Lateral or medial instability may be concurrent with dorsal laxity.

Treatment

- If possible, manage the instability with rigid coaptation splints.
- Surgical repair may be necessary if:
  - Injuries are severe.
  - The instability does not respond to splinting.
  - Dorsal ligament damage is associated with lateral or medial damage.
  - The affected animal is a large, athletic dog.

Surgical Technique and Postoperative Management

1. Fix the dorsal instability with a neutralization bone screw placed from the medial side of the head of the talus, diagonally into the distal tarsal bones.
2. Remove articular cartilage prior to screw placement.
3. Supplement with an appropriately positioned figure-of-eight tension band wire for concurrent lateral or medial instability; a neutralization screw may not be needed.
4. Postoperatively, maintain a rigid coaptation splint for 3 weeks.
   a. Use soft splints an additional 3 weeks.
   b. Remove the screw or tension band wire if it loosens.

Distal Intertarsal Subluxation with Dorsomedial Instability

- This type of subluxation can occur alone or combined with other areas of instability involving the tarsus.
- Diagnose by palpation and stress radiographs.

- Valgus deformity and dorsomedial instability are seen.
- Stabilize with a medially positioned tension band wire.

Stabilization Technique and Postoperative Management

1. Place a bone screw in the central and fourth tarsal bones proximally, and a second screw in the second, third, and fourth tarsal bones distally.
2. Secure a figure-of-eight-wire (20 or 22 gauge) around the screws.
3. Postoperatively, maintain a rigid coaptation splint below the stifle for 3 weeks. After this, use soft splints an additional 3 weeks.

Tarsometatarsal Subluxation with Dorsomedial Instability

- Stabilize with a medially positioned tension band.

Stabilization Technique and Postoperative Management

1. Place a bone screw in the central and fourth tarsal bones proximally, and a second screw in the second and fourth metatarsal bones distally.
2. Secure a figure-of-eight wire around the screws.
3. Postoperatively, maintain a rigid coaptation splint below the stifle for 3 weeks. Use soft splints an additional 3 weeks.

Tarsometatarsal Subluxation with Dorsal Instability

- This is a subtle injury that requires stress radiographs to confirm the diagnosis.
- If possible, stabilize with rigid coaptation splints.
- Injury in a large dog or chronic injury may require surgical arthrodesis, using a pin and tension band wire or bone plate technique.
- Alternatively, the arthrodesis can be done by inserting cross-pins from the proximal metatarsal bones into the distal tarsal bones.
- Postoperatively, maintain a rigid coaptation splint below the stifle for 3 weeks. Use soft splints for an additional 3 weeks.

Luxation of The Head of the Talus, the Central Tarsal Bone, and the Talocalcaneus

- These types of luxation occur as an isolated injury or with concomitant tarsal joint instability. Usually, luxation of the head of the talus and the talocalcaneal luxation are the result of relatively high-energy trauma.

Technique and Postoperative Management

1. Reduce the luxated tarsal bone(s) and stabilize with a cortical bone screw.
   a. For luxation of the head of the talus or talocalcaneal luxation, insert a neutralization screw from the talus to the calcaneus.

b. For the central tarsal bone luxation, insert a neutralization screw from the central tarsal bone to the fourth tarsal bone.

c. Place the screw so that the luxated bones are held in position (neutralized). Do not compress the bones.

2. Postoperatively, maintain a rigid coaptation splint below the stifle for 3 weeks. Use soft splints an additional 3 weeks.

Supplemental Readings

Aron DN: Management of open musculoskeletal injuries. Semin Vet Med Surg 3:290, 1988.

Aron DN: Prosthetic ligament replacement for severe tarsocrural joint instability. J Am Anim Hosp Assoc 23:41, 1987.

Aron DN: Tendons. *In* Bojrab MJ, ed.: *Current Techniques in Small Animal Surgery,* 3rd ed. Philadelphia: Lea & Febiger, 1990, p 549.

Aron DN, Purinton PT: Collateral ligaments of the tarsocrural joint: An anatomic and functional study. Vet Surg 14:173, 1985.

Aron DN, Purinton PT: Replacement of the collateral ligaments of the canine tarsocrural joint: A proposed technique. Vet Surg 14:178, 1985.

Brinker WO, Piermattei DL, Flo, GL: *Handbook of Small Animal Orthopedics and Fracture Treatment,* 2nd Ed. Philadelphia: W. B. Saunders, 1990, p 435.

Matthiesen DT: Tarsal injuries in the dog and cat. Compend Contin Educ Small Anim Pract 5:548, 1983.

Swaim SF, Henderson RA: *Small Animal Wound Management.* Philadelphia: Lea & Febiger, 1990.

19 Orthopedic Disorders of the Distal Extremities

Steven C. Budsberg

Disorders of the extremities distal to the carpus and tarsus usually result from direct trauma. Most abnormalities involve bone fracture and/or ligament damage associated with joint instability. The majority of fractures involve the metacarpal and metatarsal bones. Animals are usually presented with acute, non–weight-bearing lameness. Regardless of the bone being managed, internal fixation, external coaptation, or a combination of both can be used. If fractures are open, proper open wound management is required and indicate the method of fixation. It is essential to follow the generally accepted principles of fracture repair, including adequate reduction, alignment, and proper fixation, for the successful management of these injuries.

METACARPAL AND METATARSAL FRACTURES

Anatomy

The metacarpal and metatarsal bones are numbered 2 to 5, from medial to lateral. There are usually five metacarpal and four metatarsal bones. The third and fourth bones bear most of the forces transmitted through the limb.

Each bone is divided into the proximal base, middle body, and distal head.

Body Fractures

Body fractures may involve one or more bones. Racing animals may develop stress fractures of these bones. External reduction and coaptation usually are effective, but internal fixation may be required in cases involving multiple limb trauma, multiple bone fractures, and comminuted, severely displaced, or unstable fractures.

Preoperative Considerations

- Rule out associated injuries with a thorough physical examination and appropriate diagnostic tests.
- Identify the bone and region involved.
- Determine the type of injury (e.g., soft tissue, open or closed fracture, degloving injury).
- The number of bones involved affects treatment.
- Indications for external coaptation include:
  - Single bone fractures
  - Multiple, nondisplaced fractures without other limb trauma

  - In combination with appropriate internal fixation (e.g., intramedullary pins, screws, plates)
- Indications for internal fixation include:
  - Multiple bone fractures with severe displacement
  - Combined fractures of the third and fourth bones
  - Additional limb injury
  - Fracture in working or show dogs
  - Open fractures

Surgical Procedure

Objectives

- Reduce, align, and stabilize the fractures.
- Maintain healthy soft tissues.
- Preserve joint function.

Equipment

- Standard surgical pack and suture material
- Kirschner wire (various sizes)
- Minifragment plates and screws (1.5, 2.0, and 2.7 mm)
- Small self-retaining retractors
- Small bone-holding forceps

Technique

1. Place the animal in dorsal recumbency, clip the hair, and prepare the extremity for aseptic surgery.

KEY POINT ▶ Because of the central and digital pads, surgical approach via the palmar or plantar surfaces of the metacarpal and metatarsal bones is contraindicated.

2. Make a dorsal incision directly over the affected bone or joint.
   a. To approach a single bone, make a longitudinal incision directly over the bone. To expose adjacent bones, make an incision between them, if necessary.
   b. To approach multiple bones, make two parallel longitudinal incisions or a curved incision incorporating the entire dorsal region (Fig. 1).
3. Incise the deep fascia directly over the bone.
   a. In the metacarpus, identify and retract the major tendons (i.e., the tendons of the common digital extensor and lateral digital extensor muscles).
   b. In the metatarsal region, take care to protect the tendon of the long digital extensor muscle (Fig. 2).
4. Intramedullary (IM) pinning for fracture repair:

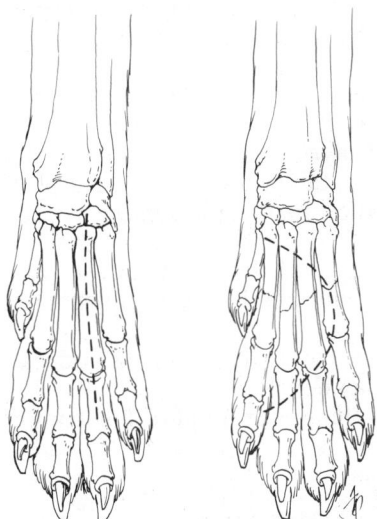

Figure 1. Dorsal incision lines for metacarpal fractures of a single bone *(left)* or multiple bones *(right)*.

a. Antegrade the pins from distal to proximal through a predrilled hole in the dorsal surface (Fig. 3). (Make the predrilled guide hole with a pin one size larger than the intended IM pin.) Bend the pin ends slightly to facilitate removal and to avoid entering the metacarpotarsophalangeal (MP) joint.

KEY POINT ▶ When passing pins in an antegrade fashion, it is preferable to use a hand drill rather than a power drill to allow the pins to "bounce off" (instead of penetrating) the palmar/plantar cortex.

b. Alternatively, retrograde the pins from the fracture site to the predrilled hole in the dorsal cortex, reduce the fracture, and seat the pins in the proximal segment (Fig. 4).

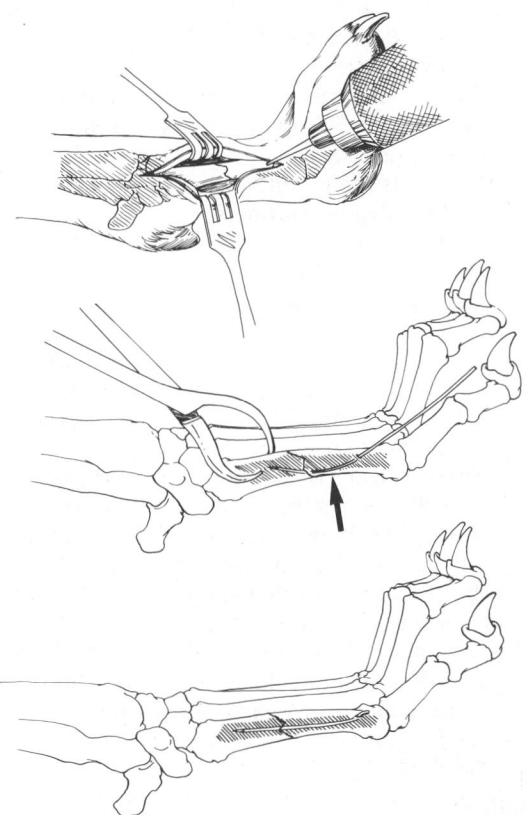

Figure 3. Placement of an intramedullary pin for repair of a metacarpal fracture. The center view shows how the pin is "bounced off" the palmar cortex *(arrow)*.

KEY POINT ▶ Fixation with single IM pins can accomplish reduction and alignment; however, this procedure does not adequately stabilize the fracture.

c. Use supplementary external coaptation of fiberglass (molded half-circumference cast) or metal (palmar/plantar splint).

5. Plate fixation:
   a. For fixation of the third and fourth bones, place the plates on the dorsal surface. For fixation of the second and fifth bones, place the plates on the medial and lateral surfaces, respectively, or dorsally.
   b. A minimum of four cortices of screw purchase above and below the fracture is required.

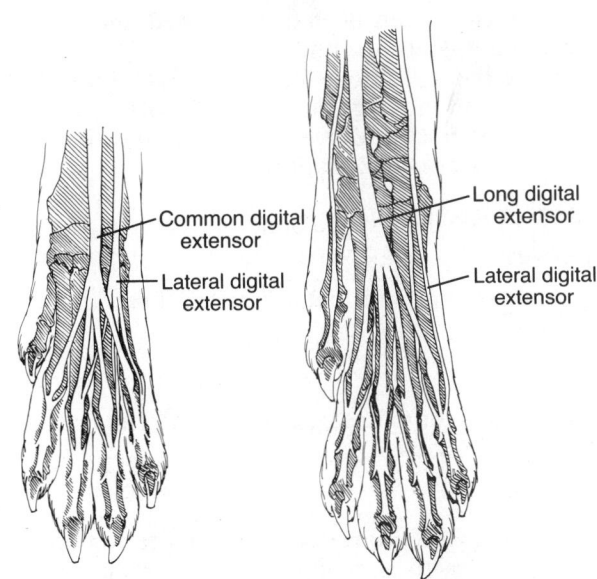

Common digital extensor

Lateral digital extensor

Long digital extensor

Lateral digital extensor

Figure 2. Important tendons of the metacarpus *(left)* and metatarsus *(right)*.

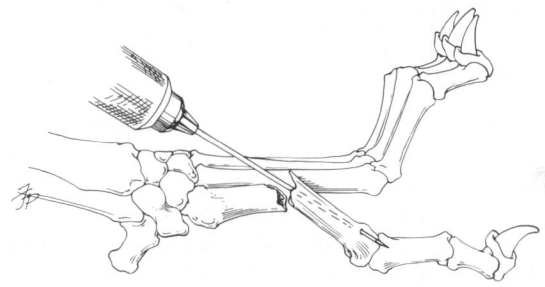

Figure 4. Retrograde placement of an intramedullary pin from the fracture site to a predrilled hole in the dorsal cortex.

c. Perform supplementary external coaptation, as described previously.
6. Lag screw fixation:
   a. Use in oblique fractures, primarily the first, second, and fifth metacarpals and the second and fifth metatarsals.
   b. Perform supplementary external coaptation.
7. Close the incision routinely.

Base and Head Fractures

Preoperative Considerations

■ Base fractures usually involve the second and fifth metacarpals, owing to ligamentous attachment; avulsion fractures commonly are seen. Valgus and varus displacement often is noted.
   • Internal fixation is strongly recommended.
   • Nondisplaced fractures may be treated with a palmar splint; however, some displacement usually occurs. Delayed union may be a problem because of the motion from ligamentous attachment.
■ Head (articular) fractures usually have concurrent subluxation or complete luxation of the MP joint owing to the collateral ligament attachment.
   • Reconstruction of the articular surface is required.

Surgical Procedure

Objective

■ Reduce, align, and stabilize the fracture.
■ Repair or reconstruct ligament instability of the joint.
■ Reconstruct the articular surface, if necessary.

Equipment

■ Same as for body fractures, described previously

Technique

1. The approach is the same as for body fractures, described previously.
2. In base fractures, accomplish fixation with lag screws or a tension band technique. Supplementary external coaptation is required.
3. In head fractures, use Kirschner and cerclage wires or a combination Kirschner wire and hemicerclage technique. Supplementary external coaptation is required.
4. Close the incision routinely.

Postoperative Care and Complications

KEY POINT ▶ Management of soft tissue injuries in open fractures is as important as internal fixation.

■ Maintain external coaptation in combination with IM pins and lag screw fixation until there is clinical union of the fracture. Animals with plate fixation require coaptation for approximately 4 weeks.
■ Remove IM pins following clinical bone union. In working dogs, also remove plates. Lag screws and plates in nonworking animals may be left in permanently.

■ If postoperative bleeding is anticipated, apply a pressure bandage for 48–72 hours to minimize hemorrhage.
■ In all cases, control and limit exercise until clinical bone union (usually 6–10 weeks).
■ Rarely, delayed union and nonunion may result from inadequate stabilization. Excessive proliferative callus formation may cause tendon entrapment and/or pain.
■ Valgus or varus deviation may result from undetected or untreated concurrent collateral ligament damage.
■ If joint surfaces are involved, degenerative joint disease may develop.
■ Tissue swelling may require hot compresses or hydrotherapy.

PHALANGEAL FRACTURES

Phalangeal fractures are similar to metacarpal and metatarsal fractures. They usually are single injuries; however, they may occur in association with other, more severe multiple injuries to the paw.

Anatomy

■ Each digit consists of a proximal phalanx and a distal phalanx. The phalanges are numbered similar to the metacarpals and metatarsals.
■ The proximal and middle phalanges are divided into a proximal base, middle body, and distal head.
■ The distal phalanges are approximately the same size in all digits and are partially covered by the nails.
■ *Dewclaw* is the term applied to the variably developed first digit of the hind paw.
■ Polydactyly (extra digits) is common in cats.

Preoperative Considerations

■ Same considerations as metacarpal and metatarsal fractures
■ Open, severely comminuted fractures may require digit amputation.
■ Most fractures can be reduced closed and immobilized in a fiberglass splint.
■ Some of the indications for internal fixation include:
   • Large working dogs or racing animals
   • Articular fractures involving the base or head
   • Failed external coaptation

Surgical Procedure
Objectives

■ See metacarpal and metatarsal fractures, discussed previously.

Equipment

■ The same as for metacarpal and metatarsal fractures, discussed previously

Technique

1. Make an incision directly over the affected bone.
2. Articular fractures require anatomic reduction and fixation with lag screws, orthopedic wire sutures, Kirschner wire, or a combination of these.

3. Treat body fractures with miniplates or (for oblique fractures) cross-pins and lag screws.

Postoperative Care and Complications

■ See metacarpal and metatarsal fractures, described previously.
■ External coaptation is required until clinical bone union.

PALMAR AND PLANTAR SESAMOID INJURIES

Fractures of the sesamoid bones of the MP joints usually are seen in racing greyhounds. However, they can cause lameness in any dog, particularly large-breed animals. Signs include sudden lameness with swelling and pain on palpation. Injuries of the second and seventh sesamoids are reported to be the most common.

Anatomy

■ The sesamoid bones are numbered 1 to 8 medial to lateral (two for each MP joint).
■ The sesamoid bone articulates primarily with the head of the metacarpal/metatarsal bone and secondarily with the palmar tubercles of each proximal phalanx.
■ Occasionally, bipartite sesamoid bones are present and may be mistaken for fractures.

KEY POINT ▶ Old sesamoid fractures or bipartite sesamoid bones may be mistaken in the cause of lameness.

Indications

■ An acute injury requires external coaptation. The foot is splinted in slight flexion.
■ Recurrent lameness requires internal intervention.

Surgical Procedure

Objective

■ Remove the damaged sesamoid.

Technique

1. Make an incision adjacent to the metacarpal/metatarsal pad, with the middle of the incision directly over the MP joint.
2. Slightly undermine the pad to allow retraction and further deep dissection of the affected sesamoid bone.
3. Identify the distal venous arch on the proximal aspect of the incision.
4. Dissect directly over the sesamoid bone and move the flexor tendon to the side if necessary.
5. Transect the sesamoid ligaments and remove the offending fragments.
6. If less than one-third of the total bone is fragmented, leave the larger fragment and remove the smaller one.
7. Close each incised fascial plane with simple interrupted sutures of an absorbable suture material.
8. Close the remainder of the incision routinely.

Postoperative Care and Complications

■ Place a snug padded bandage on the paw for 7–10 days.
■ Limit exercise for 2 weeks and gradually increase to normal by 6 weeks.
■ Complications are rare.

Supplemental Readings

Benedetti LT, Berry K, Bloomberg M: A technique for intramedullary pinning of metatarsals and metacarpals in cats and dogs. J Am Anim Hosp Assoc 22:149, 1986.

Bennett D, Kelly DF: Sesamoid disease as a cause of lameness in young dogs. J Small Anim Pract 26:567, 1985.

Dee JF, Dee LG, Early TD: *Manual for Internal Fixation in Small Animals*. Berlin: Springer-Verlag, 1984, p 206.

Evans HE, Christensen GC: *Miller's Anatomy of the Dog*. Philadelphia: W. B. Saunders, 1979, p 192.

20 Amputation of the Digit and Claw

Paul A. Manley

ANATOMY

Distal Phalanx (Cats)

- The distal phalanx (P3) in the cat is made up of a bony component and the claw (Fig. 1).
- The distal end of P3 is composed of an ungual crest and an ungual process.
- The ungual crest encircles the base of the third phalanx and projects into the claw.
- The stratum basale contains the germinal cells of the claw and extends into the ungual crest.

Dewclaw (Dogs)

- The dewclaw is the medial or first digit of the rear limb in the dog. Often, the P1 and P2 are missing, and P3 and the claw are attached only by skin and fibrous tissue.
- In some breeds, there are multiple dewclaws.
- The dewclaw articulates with metatarsal bone I, which is often small and may be fused to tarsal bone I.
- If two dewclaws are present, there may be complete duplication of the phalanges and metatarsal bone I.
- Blood supply to the first digit is via the dorsal metatarsal artery and the lateral dorsal proper digital artery (a branch of the dorsal pedal artery).

Digits (Dogs and Cats)

- The digits consist of three phalanges (P1, P2, and P3) and a nail or claw. The first digit in the front foot does not have a middle phalanx (P2); the first digit in the rear foot is the dewclaw.
- The superficial digital flexor tendon attaches to the proximal end of P2; the deep digital flexor attaches to P3; the common digital extensor tendon attaches to the extensor process of P3.
- A digital pad is located on the palmar and plantar aspect of the distal interphalangeal joint of each digit, except for the first one. Metacarpal and metatarsal pads are located on the palmar and plantar aspects, respectively, of the metacarpophalangeal and metatarsophalangeal joints.
- Blood supply is via dorsal and palmar (or plantar) digital arteries; venous drainage is via dorsal and palmar (or plantar) digital veins.

ONYCHECTOMY (CATS)

Onychectomy often is performed on house cats as an elective procedure; however, it may be necessary to perform this procedure when a claw is severely traumatized or infected.

Preoperative Considerations

- Avoid damage to the digital pad when removing the claw.
- Inform owners that most cats should be kept indoors as house pets after declawing.
- It is seldom necessary to remove the claws of the rear limbs.

KEY POINT ▶ The germinal cells of the claw extend into the ungual crest. To prevent claw regrowth, completely remove the ungual crest.

Surgical Procedure

Objectives

- Completely remove the claw(s).
- Prevent regrowth of a deformed claw.
- Protect the digital pad.
- Prevent excessive blood loss.

Equipment

- Penrose drain or appropriate tourniquet
- Scalpel blade (#12)
- Curved Kelly forceps
- Nail trimmers (Resco or White)

Technique

1. Place a tourniquet above the elbow.
2. Prepare the entire foot with a germicidal soap and solution.
3. Extend the claw by grasping the tip with forceps or by pushing up on the digital pad.

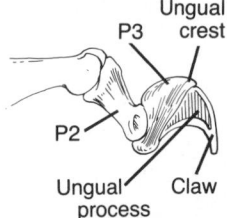

Figure 1. Distal phalanx of the cat. Note the position of the ungual crest relative to the claw.

4. Position the nail trimmer so that one blade rests dorsally at the distal interphalangeal joint and the other blade rests at the distal margin of the digital pad (see Fig. 2). Close the blades and, with a slight twisting motion of the wrist, remove the claw and P3.
   a. Alternatively a #12 scalpel blade may be used to disarticulate the distal interphalangeal joint.
5. When using nail trimmers, it is common to leave a small portion of the palmar aspect of P3. Grasp this with forceps and remove with a scalpel. If the piece is very small, removal is unnecessary (Fig. 2).
6. Following de-clawing, apply a snug-fitting bandage to the level of the distal antebrachium. Avoid excessive tightness of the proximal portion of the bandage to ensure adequate blood supply to the paw.
7. Remove the tourniquet.

Postoperative Care and Complications

Short-term

- Bleeding after bandage removal occasionally is a problem. If necessary, replace the bandage, removing in 2–3 days.
- Use shredded paper as cat litter for two weeks after surgery.
- Commercial cat litter may work its way into the wound and irritate the declawed area.

Long-Term

- Treat infection by establishing drainage at the distal extremity and administering systemic antibiotics.
- Regrowth of a deformed nail can result from incomplete removal of the ungual crest. Disarticulation of the distal interphalangeal joint via scalpel is indicated.
- Chronic lameness may result from incomplete removal of the ungual crest or trauma to the digital pad.

DEWCLAW REMOVAL (DOGS)

Dewclaw removal is usually an elective procedure, although the claw may become traumatized, especially if it is only loosely attached to the skin.

Preoperative Considerations

- Removal of the dewclaw for cosmetic reasons is best performed in the neonate.

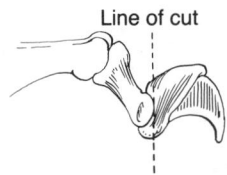

Line of cut

Figure 2. Distal phalanx of the cat (see Fig. 1). This line of excision ensures complete removal of the ungual crest, although a small piece of P3 is left behind.

Surgical Procedure

Objectives

- Remove dewclaw and minimize scarring on the medial aspect of the foot.

Equipment

- Standard surgical pack and suture material
- Bone cutters

Technique

Neonates
1. Surgically scrub the dewclaw.
2. Grasp the nail with small forceps and abduct it from the metatarsus.
3. With scissors, cut the dewclaw from its attachment to the metatarsal bone.
4. Use a single absorbable suture to close the skin.

Older Animals
1. Anesthetize the animal and prepare the foot for aseptic surgery.
2. Make an elliptical incision around the base of the dewclaw.
3. Ligate the metatarsal and the dorsal proper digital arteries.
4. If only soft tissue attachment exists from the dewclaw to the metatarsal bone, remove the dewclaw and close the skin. If a bony attachment exists, disarticulate P1 from metatarsal bone I.
5. Alternatively, use bone cutters to transect P1 close to its base.
6. Close the skin routinely.

Postoperative Care and Complications

- In neonates, a bandage is not necessary. In older dogs, place a bandage over the foot for 5–7 days.
- Scar formation at the site may be caused by the animal's removing sutures prematurely, leading to wound dehiscence. The use of stainless steel sutures or a bandage may prevent this complication.

DIGIT REMOVAL (DOGS AND CATS)

Digit amputation in dogs and cats usually is performed because of severe trauma, osteomyelitis, or neoplasia. The level of amputation depends on the condition and the site of involvement. The digit may be removed at the metacarpophalangeal joint, metatarsophalangeal joint, proximal interphalangeal joint, or distal interphalangeal joint or by transecting the bones of the digit.

Preoperative Considerations

- Digit amputation proximal to the distal interphalangeal joint may necessitate digital pad removal. In performance animals, it may be preferable to maintain the digital pad.
- The primary weight-bearing digits are the third and fourth.

Surgical Procedure

Objectives

- Remove the digit.
- Minimize blood loss.

Equipment

- Same as for dewclaw removal

Technique

1. Prepare the limb for aseptic surgery and free-drape the foot.
2. For digit removal distal to mid-P2, make a transverse incision on the dorsal aspect of the digit around to the digital pad.
   a. Ligate the digital arteries and veins.
   b. Disarticulate the digit at the distal interphalangeal joint, after transecting the flexor and extensor tendons. Alternatively, use bone cutters and transect P2.
   c. Suture the subcutaneous tissue of the pad to the extensor tendon with absorbable suture material and close the skin routinely.
3. For digit removal proximal to mid-P2, make an elliptical incision at the base of the digit.
   a. Ligate the vessels and disarticulate the digit with a scalpel or bone cutters (see step 2b previously).
   b. A proximal extension of the elliptical skin incision usually facilitates cosmetic closure of the skin (Fig. 3).
   c. Close the subcutaneous and skin layers routinely.

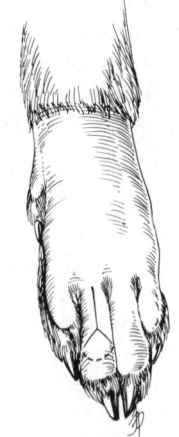

Figure 3. Skin incision *(arrow)* for digit removal proximal to mid-P2.

Postoperative Care

- Apply a bandage to the foot for 7–10 days. Keep the bandage clean and dry.
- Maintain skin sutures for 10–14 days.

Supplemental Readings

Dee JF, Dee LG, Earon-Wells RD: Injuries of high performance dogs. *In* Whittick WG, ed.: *Canine Orthopedics*. Philadelphia: Lea & Febiger, 1990, p 519.

Krahwinkel DJ, Bone DL. Surgical management of specific skin disorders. *In* Slatter DH, ed.: *Textbook of Small Animal Surgery*. Philadelphia: W. B. Saunders, 1985, p 509.

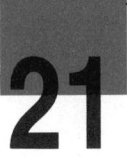

21 Surgery of Skeletal Muscle and Tendons

Steven W. Petersen

Surgery of skeletal muscle usually is directed at repair of injuries such as muscle belly rupture and laceration. Accordingly, the decision for surgery depends upon the chronicity or acuteness of the injury and the potential for lost function with scar tissue healing. Occasionally, an orthopedic approach necessitates the transection of a muscle belly to gain improved exposure to a long bone fracture or joint.

Primary suture apposition of severed tendons is termed tenorrhaphy. Indications for tenorrhaphy are similar to those described for skeletal muscle repair. Tendon lacerations are common; tendon ruptures are seen less frequently. Several orthopedic surgical approaches utilize tendon transection to achieve exposure to various joints.

ANATOMY

Skeletal Muscle

- Skeletal muscle is composed of bundles or fascicles of muscle fibers, each enveloped in their own connective tissue sheath. Each muscle fiber consists of multiple individual myofibrils, the fundamental subunit of skeletal muscle.
- Muscle fibers gradually terminate at the proximal and distal ends of most muscle bellies, and connective tissue continues on as the tendon of origin or insertion, respectively. Some muscles attach directly to bone periosteum without this connective tissue interface.
- The vascular supply of muscle is well developed in order to provide for its high metabolic needs. Arteries branch from neighboring vessels and enter the muscle belly at distinct locations. Veins and nerves accompany arteries. Locations for entrance of these neurovascular bundles remain relatively constant in different animals.

Tendons

- Tendon superstructure resembles that of muscle. Collagen fibers are arranged in bundles and surrounded by a loose connective tissue sheath, the endotenon. Intrinsic blood vessels, nerves, and lymphatics are carried within the endotenon.
- The epitenon is a connective tissue sheath that surrounds the entire tendon and is, in turn, enveloped by the paratenon, which is the outer connective tissue layer that covers the tendon.
- Tendon vascularity is sparse compared with that of muscle. Vessels entering at the musculotendinous junction are the predominant blood supply. Distally, the tendon is supplied by vessels that enter at the osseous tendon insertion. Extrinsic vessels that travel along the paratenon supply the middle portion of the tendon.

SURGERY OF SKELETAL MUSCLE

Preoperative Considerations

- Muscle injuries in which wound edges are not apposed heal by deposition of fibrous scar tissue.
  - Myofibrils cannot penetrate the thick band of scar tissue that forms between unapposed muscle wound edges.
  - As interposed scar tissue remodels and elongates, muscle function is lost because the muscle belly is no longer able to fully contract.
- Myofibril regeneration can occur to a limited extent with direct wound edge apposition.
  - Small numbers of myofibrils are able to penetrate the smaller connective tissue scar that forms at the junction of apposed muscle edges.

KEY POINT ▶ Complete muscle tissue regeneration does not occur across the scar.

  - Experimentally, complete muscle belly lacerations that have been surgically repaired regain only 50% of their ability to produce tension and only about 80% of their ability to shorten.

Surgical Procedure

Objective

- To provide muscle-to-muscle appositional anastomosis
- To thoroughly excise all preexisting scar tissue
- To delicately handle tissues, because muscle regeneration is dependent upon an intact blood supply

Equipment

- Standard instrument pack
- Self-retaining and hand-held retractors
- Synthetic nonabsorbable monofilament suture
- Penrose drains, rubber tubing, Silastic buttons

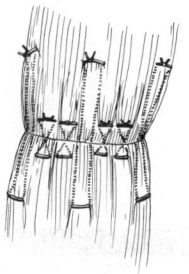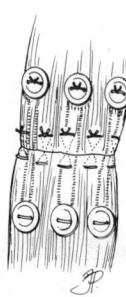

Figure 1. Suture patterns for muscle apposition. *Left*, Interrupted cruciate sutures with interposed deeper horizontal mattress sutures. *Right*, Silastic buttons prevent deep tension sutures from pulling out.

Technique

KEY POINT ▶ When incising muscles, make incisions parallel to the muscle fibers.

1. Thoroughly debride wound edges to remove scar tissue and hematomas.
2. Place sutures within the dense outer fascial sheath and/or deeper, inner belly fascial layers, using simple interrupted cruciate or horizontal mattress patterns (Fig. 1, *left*).
3. Use sections of Penrose drains, rubber tubing, or Silastic buttons as stents to prevent deeper tension sutures from pulling out (Fig. 1, *right*).

Postoperative Care and Complications

- Completely immobilize affected limb and muscle for 2–3 weeks.
- Gradually return the animal to normal activity over the ensuing 4–6 weeks.
- Use active physiotherapy (passive range of motion with progressively increased flexion/extension) as the animal is allowed to return to activity.
- The primary complication is loss of function resulting from muscle atrophy and/or excessive scar tissue deposition.

SURGERY OF TENDONS

Preoperative Considerations

- Selection of correct suture pattern and material is fundamental to the success of the repair.
- Manage deep tendon lacerations with a contaminated wound with delayed primary tenorrhaphy:
  - Tag severed tendon ends with small-diameter nonabsorbable sutures.
  - Immobilize the limb to prevent further tendon segment distraction (e.g., transarticular external fixator).
  - Treat contaminated wounds in an "open" manner with sterile dressings, daily wound debridement, and lavage.
  - Proceed with tenorrhaphy, as described subsequently, and delay wound closure until healthy granulation tissue is present.

Surgical Procedure

Objectives

- Anatomically align the tendon ends.
- Delicately manipulate tissues to avoid iatrogenic injury to the tendon ends.
- When planning the surgical approach, allow ample space for identification and debridement of the tendon ends.

KEY POINT ▶ Minimize gap formation at the tenorrhaphy site.

- In contrast to muscle, make incisions in tendons perpendicular to tendon fibers.

Equipment

- Same as for muscle, described previously

Technique

1. Meticulously debride traumatized edges, scar tissue, and hematoma at severed tendon ends.

KEY POINT ▶ Use synthetic, nonabsorbable, monofilament, nonreactive suture material such as nylon or polypropylene for anastomosis.

2. Select the largest-diameter suture that will pass atraumatically through the tendon.
3. The suture pattern of choice is the three-loop pulley tenorrhaphy (Fig. 2):
   a. Place each loop of the pattern in a different plane of tissue, rotating approximately 120°.
   b. Place sutures alternately in a near-far (loop #1), middle-middle (loop #2), and far-near (loop #3) manner.
   c. Minor alteration in the degree of rotation between loops allows use of this pattern for tenorrhaphy in tendons of all shapes and diameters.
4. In the common calcaneal and triceps tendons, which are composed of several smaller tendons, suture each tendon individually, using the three-loop pulley pattern.

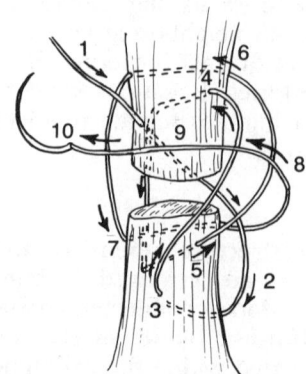

Figure 2. Three-loop pulley tenorrhaphy suture pattern. Needle passes follow numbered sequence and alternate in a near-far, middle-middle, and far-near pattern. Loops are oriented in separate planes of tissue and rotate approximately 120° from each other.

5. Anastomose the paratenon of larger composite tendons with fine sutures in an interrupted pattern.
6. If necessary, use adjoining fascia to reinforce the tenorrhaphy in large-diameter tendons.

Postoperative Care and Complications

KEY POINT ▶ Staged return to activity is critical for a successful repair.

- Restrict activity, allowing gradual return to normal function:
  - Completely immobilize the limb with a full cast or transarticular external fixator (no stress across the tenorrhaphy) for the first 3 to 4 weeks.
  - During the second 3–4 weeks, use a partial cast to allow minimal weight bearing (limited longitudinal stress across the tenorrhaphy will allow collagen fibers to realign along lines of tension).
  - Place a padded bandage (modified Robert Jones) to allow increased weight bearing (permiting increased stress across the tenorrhaphy and tendon axis) for the final 3–4 weeks.
- A bivalved cast allows the suture line to be inspected during the extended healing/immobilization period without having to apply a new cast.

- Premature weight bearing with excessive stress across the tenorrhaphy may result in suture pullout or failure with secondary disruption of the repair.
- Manage failed tenorrhaphy as described for the initial procedure.

Supplemental Readings

Aron DN: Tendons. *In* Bojrab JM, ed.: *Current Techniques in Small Animal Surgery*, 3rd Ed. Philadelphia: Lea & Febiger, 1990, p 549.

Berg JR, Egger EL: In vitro comparison of the three loop pulley and locking loop suture patterns for repair of canine weightbearing tendons and collateral ligaments. Vet Surg 15:107, 1986.

Bloomberg M: Muscles and tendons. *In* Slatter DH, ed.: *Textbook of Small Animal Surgery*. Philadelphia: W. B. Saunders, 1985, p 2331.

Chaplan A, Carlson B, Faulkner J, et al.: Skeletal muscle. *In* Woo SLY, Buckwalter JA, eds.: *Injury and Repair of the Musculoskeletal Soft Tissues*. Park Ridge, IL: Am Acad Orthopaed Surgeon, 1988, p 213.

Easley KJ, Stashak TS, Smith FW, Vanslyke G: Mechanical properties of four suture patterns for transected equine tendon repair. Vet Surg 19:102, 1990.

Jann HW, Stein LE, Good JK: Strength characteristics and failure modes of locking loop and three loop pulley suture patterns in equine tendons. Vet Surg 19:28, 1990.

Morshead D, Leeds EB: Kirschner-Ehmer apparatus immobilization following Achilles tendon repair in six dogs. Vet Surg 13:11, 1984.

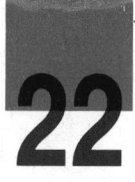

22 Neoplasia of Thoracic and Pelvic Limbs

Bernard M. Bouvy

ETIOLOGY

Neoplasia of the appendicular skeleton can affect bones primarily or secondarily. Tumors that arise from bone include osteosarcoma (intraosseous or parosteal), osteoma, chondrosarcoma, chondroma, osteochondroma (including multiple cartilaginous exostoses), enchondroma, fibrosarcoma, hemangiosarcoma, malignant mesenchymoma, liposarcoma, plasma cell myeloma (multiple myeloma), lymphosarcoma, and giant cell tumor (osteoclastoma).

In the dog, the most common primary bone tumor is osteosarcoma, with the highest incidence in the distal radius and proximal humerus. Osteosarcomas are aggressive tumors that rapidly metastasize to the lungs.

Soft tissue tumors may infiltrate underlying bone; these include squamous cell carcinoma, malignant melanoma, and connective tissue tumors such as synovial cell sarcoma (malignant synovioma), rhabdomyosarcoma, and fibrosarcoma. On rare occasions, metastases to bone from primary neoplasia elsewhere in the body occur. Carcinomas are most likely to metastasize to limb bones. Tumors that metastasize to bone usually are diaphyseal, whereas primary bone tumors usually are metaphyseal.

CLINICAL SIGNS

- Clinical signs can vary from a nonpainful swelling to non–weight-bearing lameness.
- Conditions that are most often mistaken on radiography for bone neoplasia are hypertrophic osteodystrophy, osteomyelitis (bacterial or mycotic), and traumatic injury.

DIAGNOSIS

- The definitive diagnosis cannot be substantiated by radiography alone. A representative biopsy for histopathologic and microbiologic evaluation often is necessary for distinction.
- Obtain biopsies by wedge resection (soft tissue tumor) or by using a bone trephine.
- Obtain multiple samples to increase accuracy.

TREATMENT

- In rare instances, benign tumors and soft tissue tumors not involving bone can be treated successfully by local resection.
- In most cases, local control of the tumor requires partial or complete amputation of the affected limb.
- Despite the poor long-term survival associated with most limb malignancies, amputation has important immediate advantages, including relief of pain, improvement of attitude and mobility, and improved quality of life.

SURGICAL ANATOMY

Anatomy relevant to limb amputation includes the major blood vessels to be ligated. Accurate identification of these vessels can limit significant blood loss.

Thoracic Limb
- The axillary artery extends from the cranial border of the first rib to the joint tendinous insertion of the teres major and latissimus dorsi muscles. It lies deep to the brachial plexus.
- Major veins include the cephalic vein (deep to the cleidobrachialis muscle), the brachial vein, and the axillary vein (caudal and cranial to the axillary artery, respectively).

Pelvic Limb
- The femoral artery lies superficially in the femoral triangle between the caudal belly of the sartorius muscle and the pectineus muscle.
- The femoral vein lies caudal to its satellite artery.

LIMB AMPUTATION

Preoperative Considerations
- Radiograph the thorax to rule out gross metastasis to the lungs.
- Perform a thorough evaluation of the lymph nodes (including cytology, if they are enlarged), all extremities (including bone radiologic survey, if indicated), spine, and abdominal cavity for spread of the disease.
- Perform a complete blood count (CBC), serum biochemical panel, and urinalysis to assess the animal's overall condition.
- Obtain a representative biopsy to confirm neoplasia.

Osteosarcoma can sometimes be an exception to this rule when radiologic features of involved bone do not support other pathologies.

KEY POINT ▶ Using a bone trephine or bone marrow biopsy needles, obtain bone core biopsies *from the center and margin* of the suspected area to ensure diagnostic sampling.

- Base indications for partial or total amputation on location and biological behavior of the tumor or on poor prognosis for a functional limb because of uncontrollable pain or irreversible damage.
- Assess gross margins of bone involvement on fine-detail radiographs to determine the extent of surgery necessary to excise the neoplasm.

KEY POINT ▶ Perform the amputation at least one joint above involved bone.

- Amputation of a limb is difficult for an owner to accept. Prior to surgery, explain the functional and cosmetic changes resulting from amputation.
- Palpate the other legs to assess their potential for function under superloading conditions. Radiograph the pelvis before rear leg amputation in dogs predisposed to hip dysplasia.
  - In the case of aggressive neoplasms, amputate the affected limb regardless of these findings.
- In animals with malignant tumors, especially osteosarcoma, be sure that owners have a realistic view of the treatment objectives and realize that cure is unlikely.

Surgical Procedures

Objectives

- Achieve local tumor control by complete resection of tumor with wide margins of normal tissue.
- Minimize blood loss.

KEY POINT ▶ To avoid pooling of large amount of blood in the limb, double-ligate arteries before veins (use reverse procedure if dissemination of disease is concern). Achieve systematic hemostasis throughout the procedure.

- Preplan skin and soft tissue incisions to allow cosmetic closure of wound after amputation.
- Preserve the vascular supply to the remaining skin and muscles.
- Eliminate dead spaces during closure and do not close tissues under tension.

KEY POINT ▶ Close in multiple layers using "walking" suture patterns. Place Penrose drains in wound if significant dead space remains.

- Obtain a short amputation stump to avoid trauma resulting from attempted use.

Equipment

- Standard general surgical pack and silk suture material for vascular ligation
- Electrocautery unit
- Bone-cutting device (saw, Gigli wire, or osteotome)
- Elastic compression bandage

Technique

Thoracic Limb Amputation with Removal of the Scapula

Use this technique when the tumor involves the humerus or scapula. Disarticulation of the shoulder is sometimes performed when the scapula is not involved but is not recommended because it is technically more difficult than removal of the scapula.

1. Place the dog in lateral recumbency and aseptically prepare the entire leg and chest wall for surgery.
2. Incise the skin along the spine of the scapula to the greater tubercle of the humerus. Carry the incision circumferentially to the medial side of the shoulder joint.
3. Ligate and divide the cephalic vein as it runs deep to the cleidobrachialis muscle.
4. Sharply separate the omotransversarius and the cervical and thoracic trapezius muscles from the scapular spine.
5. Subperiosteally elevate the rhomboideus and serratus ventralis muscles from the medial aspect of the scapula, and abduct the latter from the chest wall.
6. Sever the common insertion of the latissimus dorsi, teres major, and cutaneous trunci muscles from the teres tubercle of the humerus.
7. Ligate and divide the thoracodorsal artery and vein and cut their satellite nerve. Further abduct the scapula and rotate it medially.
8. Ligate and divide the axillary and lateral thoracic arteries and the brachial and axillary veins.
9. Transect the brachial plexus of nerves with scissors or scalpel.
10. Complete the amputation by cutting the pectoral and cleidobrachialis muscles away from the humerus.
11. Routinely close the muscles, subcutaneous tissues, and skin.

KEY POINT ▶ In all amputation procedures, eliminate dead space during closure and do not close tissues under tension.

12. Apply a soft padded compressive bandage around the chest.

Technique

Thoracic Limb Amputation at the Midhumerus

Use this method when there is no tumor involvement of the humerus or scapula. This technique is faster and causes less blood loss than removal of the scapula because it requires transection of insertions of only three muscles and requires no major muscle belly transections.

1. Place the dog in lateral recumbency and aseptically prepare the entire leg for surgery.
2. Incise the skin circumferentially at the junction of the middle and distal thirds of the humerus, curving laterally as low as the epicondylar ridge.

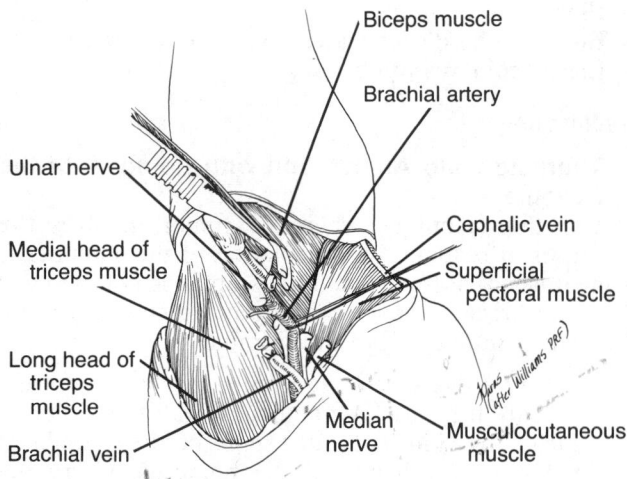

Figure 1. Medial dissection of vessels and nerves for thoracic limb amputation at midhumerus.

3. Expose, ligate, and divide the brachial artery and vein (Fig. 1).
4. Sever the median, ulnar, and musculocutaneous nerves.
5. Isolate and transect the triceps tendon at the level of the olecranon (Fig. 2).
6. Tenotomize the biceps and brachialis muscles at their distal insertion on the medial aspect of the radius and ulna.
7. Ligate and transect the cephalic vein at the distal one-third of the humerus. Sever the radial nerve at the same level.
8. Reflect the three severed tendons proximally to subperiosteally elevate the brachiocephalic muscle from the humerus.
9. Complete the amputation with osteotomy of the humerus, leaving the proximal one-third of this bone.
10. Cover the humeral stump by suturing the three cut muscles together.
11. Routinely close subcutaneous tissues and skin.

Technique

Pelvic Limb Amputation at the Midfemur

Use this technique when the tumor does not involve the femur. This method has the advantage of lateral protection of the genitalia in males.

1. Place the dog in lateral recumbency and aseptically prepare the entire leg and hemipelvis for surgery.
2. Incise the skin in two connected semicircles; ventrolaterally from the tuber ischii down to the patella and up to the flank and ventromedially from the ends of the lateral incision down to midthigh.
3. Transect the caudal belly of the sartorius and gracilis muscles at midthigh.
4. Isolate, ligate, and divide the saphenous nerve and the femoral artery and vein.
5. Transect the pectineus muscle at its insertion on the femur, and the cranial sartorius and quadriceps muscles proximal to the patella.

6. Incise the tensor fasciae latae and biceps femoris muscles along the skin incision.
7. Isolate the sciatic nerve trunk and sever it at the greater trochanter.
8. Transect the abductor cruris caudalis, semitendinosus, semimembranosus, and adductor magnus et brevis muscles at midthigh.
9. Complete the amputation by osteotomy of the femur, leaving the proximal one-third of this bone.
10. Routinely close the muscles, subcutaneous tissues, and skin.

Technique

Pelvic Limb Amputation by Hip Disarticulation

Use this technique when there is "tumor" involvement of the femur. Tumors of the proximal femur may require en bloc resection of the acetabulum (subtotal hemipelvectomy) with the femur to ensure complete removal.

1. Place the dog in lateral recumbency and aseptically prepare the entire leg and pelvis for surgery.
2. Incise the skin in two connected semicircles, ventrolaterally from the tuber ischii down to midthigh and up to flank, and ventromedially from the ends of the lateral incision down to the inguinal fold.
3. Isolate, ligate, and divide the femoral and superficial circumflex femoral arteries and femoral vein.
4. Transect the sartorius, pectineus, gracilis, and adductor magnus et brevis muscles 2 cm from their origin (Fig. 3A and B).
5. Ligate and divide the medial circumflex femoral artery and vein.
6. Elevate the iliopsoas muscle from the lesser trochanter of the femur.
7. Sever the saphenous and femoral nerves.
8. Cut the medial coxofemoral joint capsule and round ligament.
9. Transect the tensor fasciae latae, biceps femoris, abductor cruris caudalis, semitendinosus, and semimembranosus muscles in their proximal one-third.

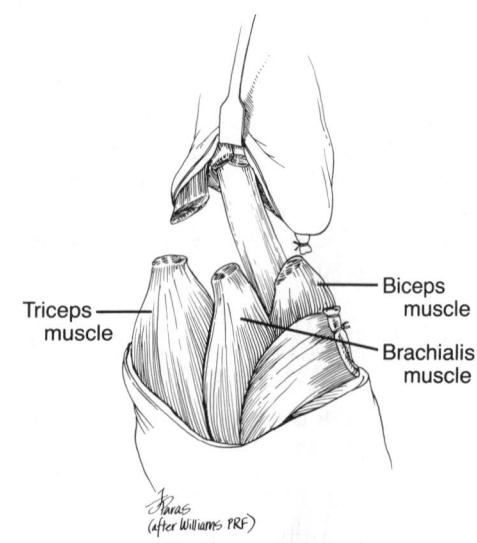

Figure 2. Transection of muscles for thoracic limb amputation at midhumerus.

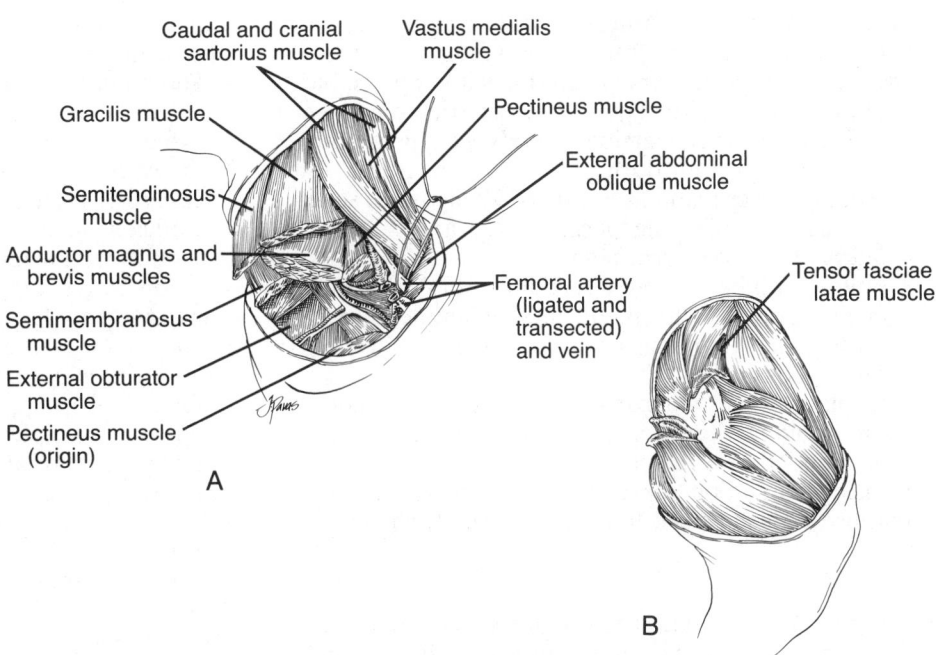

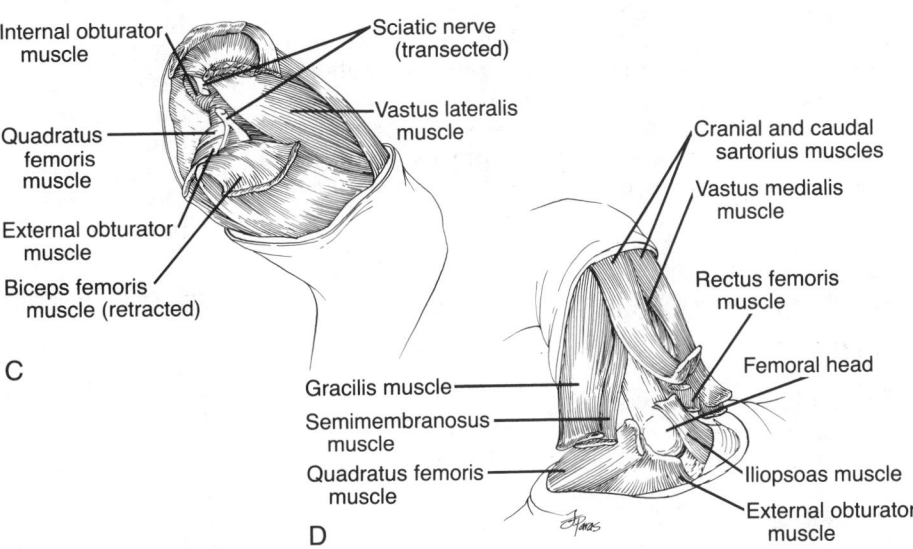

Figure 3. Dissection of muscles, vessels, and nerves for pelvic limb amputation by hip disarticulation. *A* and *D,* medial views; *B* and *C,* lateral views.

10. Sever the sciatic nerve distal to its branches to the upper thigh muscles (Fig. 3*C*).
11. With the leg in flexion and abduction, sever the hip rotator muscles, including the internal and external obturator and the gemellus muscles.
12. Complete the amputation by severing the three gluteal muscles (superficial, middle, and deep), and the lateral joint capsule and by elevating the rectus femoris muscle from the iliopubic eminence (Fig. 3*D*).
13. Routinely close the muscles, subcutaneous tissue, and skin.

Postoperative Care and Complications

Short-Term

■ Submit the amputated limb or the entire diseased area for histopathologic confirmation of the preoperative diagnosis. On the basis of preoperative biopsy alone, osteosarcoma can be confused with other primary bone tumors.
■ Closely monitor for hemorrhage and hypovolemic shock.
■ Treat seroma formation by pressure bandages, and treat infection with antibiotic therapy. Drain large seromas or abscesses by opening part of the incision or placing a Penrose drain.
■ Beginning 24 hours after surgery, apply hot packs to the surgical site 3–4 times daily until suture removal.
■ Assist walking with towel support until dog has adapted to amputation.

Long-Term

■ Frequently (every 8 weeks) reevaluate the dog clinically and radiographically for detection of tumor at the amputation stump and in the chest.
■ Advise strict weight control for large dogs, especially after forelimb amputation.

- Use adjunctive chemotherapy and immunotherapy for malignancies. The following investigative protocol is used at the authors' institution with appreciable prolongation of survival period for osteosarcoma (see sec. 3, ch. 5) for conversion of body weight to body surface area (m^2) for dosing).
  - Administer cisplatin at a dose of 70 mg/m^2 as soon as possible following surgery; repeat at 28-day intervals for four treatments.
  - Follow with liposome-encapsulated MTP-PE (muramyl tripeptide-phosphatidylethanolamine; a macrophage activator) at a dose of 2 mg/m^2 biweekly for 8 weeks.
  - Cisplatin given alone for two to four treatments can prolong the disease-free interval and is recommended in a clinical setting.
- Consider radiation therapy for radiosensitive neoplasms (e.g., mast cell tumors; see sec. 3, ch. 7).

Prognosis

- The prognosis is good if the tumor was benign.
- The prognosis is fair if the tumor was malignant and completely excised and there is no preoperative evidence of distant metastasis. With adjunctive chemotherapy, the average survival time for patients with osteosarcoma is approximately 10–12 months.
- If the tumor is biologically aggressive, incompletely excised, or has spread to distant organs, the prognosis is poor. Survival time usually is less than 6 months.

LIMB-SPARING PROCEDURES

Objectives

- Obtain local tumor control.
- Provide a pain-free and functional limb.
- Enhance long-term survival.

Chemotherapy and Radiation

Chemotherapy and radiation usually are administered before surgical debulking.

Bone Allograft

Bone allograft techniques should be performed by a surgical specialist. Most referral centers possess banks of frozen or gas-sterilized bones.

- Consider bone allograft in cases of limb neoplasm if one or more of the following conditions apply:
  - The tumor is confined to less than 50% of the length of a long bone, with minimal or no soft tissue involvement.
  - No evidence of metastasis, infection, or concurrent disease is present.
  - Sufficient healthy bone stock remains for internal fixation with screws and plate.
  - Preoperative biopsy reveals a benign or nonaggressive neoplasm.
  - The owner refuses limb amputation.
  - A sterile allograft from a healthy animal is available.
- Technical principles are similar to those for the use of allografts in treatment of noninfected comminuted long bone fractures.
  - Expose the involved long bone from one epiphysis to the other.
  - Resect all abnormal-appearing soft tissue.
  - Osteotomize the neoplastic area with wide normal cortex margins, as assessed grossly and from fine-detail radiographs.
  - Insert a cortical bone allograft of appropriate diameter and length in the bone defect and stabilize with plate and screws.
- Postoperative complications may include infection, sequestration, fracture, fixation failure, and tumor recurrence either locally or from metastases.
  - Monitor for complications by frequent reevaluation.

Supplemental Readings

Bone DL, Aberman HM: Forelimb amputation in the dog using humeral osteotomy. J Am Anim Hosp Assoc 24:525, 1988.

Evans HE, Christensen GC: *Miller's Anatomy of the Dog.* Philadelphia: W. B. Saunders, 1979.

LaRue SM, Withrow SJ, Power BE, et al.: Limb-sparing treatment for osteosarcoma in dogs. J Am Vet Med Assoc 195:1734, 1989.

MacEwen EG, Kurzman ID, Rosenthael RC, et al.: Therapy for osteosarcoma in dogs with intravenous injection of liposome-encapsulated muramyl tripeptide. J Natl Cancer Inst 81:935, 1989.

Newton CD, Nunamaker DM: *Textbook of Small Animal Orthopaedics.* Philadelphia: J. B. Lippincott, 1985.

Slatter DH: *Textbook of Small Animal Surgery,* Philadelphia, W. B. Saunders, 1985.

Shapiro W, Fossum TW, Kitchell BE, et al.: Use of cisplatin for treatment of appendicular osteosarcoma in dogs. J Am Vet Med Assoc 192:507, 1988.

Straw RC, Withrow SJ, Richter SL, et al.: Amputation and cisplatin for treatment of canine osteosarcoma. J Vet Int Med. In press.

23 Diseases Affecting Developing Bone

James K. Roush

Some of the diseases affecting developing bone are discussed in this chapter. See respective chapters for other developmental bone diseases, such as hip dysplasia, avascular necrosis of the femoral head, and osteochondrosis.

PANOSTEITIS

Panosteitis is a disease of young large-breed dogs manifested by intermittent lameness of one or more limbs. Onset occurs in the first year of life. The disease is self-limiting but clinical signs may persist in one or more limbs for months. Differentiate panosteitis from other causes of lameness in young dogs, such as hip dysplasia and osteochondritis dissecans.

Etiology/Histopathology

- The etiology of panosteitis is unknown.
- Panosteitis may have a polygenetic origin, because German shepherd dogs are commonly affected.
- Contributing causes include stress, transient vascular abnormalities, metabolic disorders, allergies, hyperestrogenism, and autoimmune reaction following viral infection.
- The characteristic histopathologic lesion is degeneration of medullary adipocytes, followed by stromal cell proliferation, intramembranous ossification, and regeneration of the adipose bone marrow.

Clinical Signs

Signalment

- Panosteitis usually is seen in large and giant-breed dogs, most often 5–12 months of age; however, it has been reported in dogs up to 5 years of age.
- Male dogs are affected more frequently than females (4:1 ratio). In females, the first episode of the disease often occurs in association with the first estrus.
- Panosteitis has been reported in the German shepherd, Great Dane, Irish setter, St. Bernard, Doberman pinscher, Airedale, basset hound, and miniature schnauzer.

Lameness

- There is acute onset of weight-bearing lameness without a history of recent trauma.

KEY POINT ▶ Lesions often resolve in one bone and develop in another, resulting in the classic history of "shifting leg" lameness.

- Pain due to the disease is of intermittent duration and severity, but the dog rarely, if ever, is completely non–weight bearing on the affected limb or limbs.
- Lameness or radiographic lesions may occur simultaneously in multiple limbs or bones, or lameness may resolve for a period of time, only to recur in another limb. After a bone passes through the lesion cycle, it is unlikely that it will be affected again, but this may occur if the disease affects another bone in the limb.
- Clinical signs often continue for several months and usually resolve by 18–20 months of age.

Diagnosis

KEY POINT ▶ Diagnosis of panosteitis is established by eliciting pain on firm palpation of a long bone and by characteristic radiographic lesions.

Physical Examination

- Applying firm pressure to the diaphyses of the affected bone results in clinical signs of discomfort.

Laboratory Evaluation

- Hematology and serum chemistry profiles usually are normal.
- Eosinophilia occurs inconsistently (this disease was previously referred to as eosinophilic panosteitis).

Radiography

Confirm suspected cases by survey radiography of the affected bone(s).

- Early radiographic lesions are characterized by areas of increased density and accentuated trabecular pattern within the medullary cavity (Table 1).
  - These areas may be focal or multifocal and commonly occur first near the nutrient foramen.
  - Bone cortices may be thickened, and progressive mottling and opacification of the medullary cavity occur.
  - A smooth, linear periosteal proliferation may develop.
- During resolution, sclerotic areas gradually decrease in size and density. Radiographic signs may persist for several months after lameness resolves.

TABLE 1. Characteristic Radiographic Lesions Seen in Diseases Affecting Developing Bone

Disease	Lesion
Panosteitis	Medullary density in diaphyseal region
Hypertrophic osteodystrophy	Radiolucent metaphyseal line adjacent to physis
Hypertrophic osteopathy	Periosteal reaction beginning on metacarpals or metatarsals, bilaterally symmetric
Craniomandibular osteopathy	Bony proliferation on ventral mandible and skull
Cartilaginous exostosis	Large, smooth bony protuberance in metaphyseal area
Bone cyst	Well-circumscribed, radiolucent metaphyseal defect
Retained enchondral cartilaginous core	Longitudinal, linear radiolucent defect in distal ulna

- There is no correlation between the radiographic lesions and severity of clinical signs.

Differential Diagnoses

- Differentiate panosteitis as a cause of lameness from other diseases that are characterized by onset during or shortly after the rapid-growth phase in large-breed dogs.
  - In particular, eliminate hypertrophic osteodystrophy, osteochondritis dissecans of the shoulder or elbow (see sec. 9, ch. 24), ununited anconeal process (see sec. 9, ch. 24), and hip dysplasia (see sec. 9, ch. 14) as a cause of lameness before ascribing clinical signs to panosteitis.

Treatment

KEY POINT ▶ Panosteitis is a self-limiting disease.

- No specific therapy for panosteitis exists.
- Administer buffered aspirin (10–25 mg/kg q8h, PO), as needed, to alleviate pain.
- Restrict exercise in severely affected animals.
- Inform clients that the lameness may shift to other limbs and that the animal may be intermittently lame for 6–18 months.

HYPERTROPHIC OSTEODYSTROPHY

Hypertrophic osteodystrophy (HOD) is a developmental disease of young, rapidly growing large and giant-breed dogs. Dogs with HOD exhibit lameness in one or more limbs in association with swelling and inflammation of the metaphyseal regions of long bones. The incidence of the disease has declined in recent years. Complications related to prolonged recumbency, anorexia, and hyperthermia have been reported in severely affected animals. The overall prognosis for HOD is guarded. Although many dogs recover spontaneously, permanent bone changes and physical deformities may develop.

Etiology

- The etiology of HOD is unknown.
- Historically, the disease has been attributed to vitamin C deficiency, but decreased levels of ascorbic acid in the serum or urine do not appear to be related to the disease.
- Skeletal lesions similar to those of HOD have been produced experimentally by feeding a free-choice diet abnormally high in protein, calories, and calcium.

Clinical Signs

Signalment

KEY POINT ▶ HOD occurs only in growing animals with open physes.

- Onset of clinical signs usually occurs at 3–4 months of age (range, 2–8 months).
- HOD has been reported in the Great Dane, Irish wolfhound, St. Bernard, Irish setter, Labrador retriever, basset hound, greyhound, German shepherd, German short-haired pointer, borzoi, boxer, Dalmatian, Weimaraner, Doberman pinscher, and collie.

Systemic Signs

- The severity of HOD varies, ranging from an absence of systemic signs to severe anorexia, weight loss, fever, and depression.
- Clinical signs are episodic in nature, and lameness often is bilaterally symmetric.

Lameness

- Lameness varies from a mild limp in minimally affected dogs to non–weight-bearing lameness in severely affected animals.
- Affected long-bone metaphyses are extremely swollen, warm, and painful in animals with severe disease.
- Multiple long bones and limbs are affected, and, in extreme cases, dogs are reluctant to stand or move.

Diagnosis

Physical Examination/History

- Affected metaphyses are warm and swollen on palpation.
- Signs of pain may be elicited on palpation of the metaphyseal areas.
- Pyrexia of up to 106°F may be present.
- The history may include recent weight loss, reluctance to move, and anorexia.

Laboratory Evaluation

- Laboratory data are normal or mild abnormalities related to anorexia and stress may be present.

Radiography

- Radiographic changes usually occur in the metaphyses of the long bones and are bilaterally symmetric. Other bones, including the mandible, ribs, and scapula, may be affected.
- The characteristic radiographic lesion is generalized sclerosis and enlargement of the metaphysis.

KEY POINT ▶ Radiolucent areas form in the metaphysis and coalesce to form an area of low density parallel to the growth plate, called a double physeal line (Fig. 1).

- Radiopaque deposition of bone in the soft tissue outside the periosteum may occur.
- Irregular widening of the physis may be seen in later stages of the disease.
- Subperiosteal or extraperiosteal bone formation is seen in metaphyseal regions and may involve the diaphysis.

Differential Diagnoses

- Differentiate HOD from other causes of lameness in immature large or giant-breed dogs.
  - Other diseases that result in metaphyseal swelling or in signs of pain during palpation of long bones include panosteitis, bone-associated neoplasms, and hypertrophic osteopathy. Radiographic lesions in these diseases are distinct and allow easy differentiation; the last two diseases are unlikely to be the cause of lameness in young dogs.

Treatment

KEY POINT ▶ There is no specific treatment for HOD.

- In mild or moderately affected dogs, there is often spontaneous remission.
- Correction of dietary imbalances and decreased caloric intake may be beneficial.

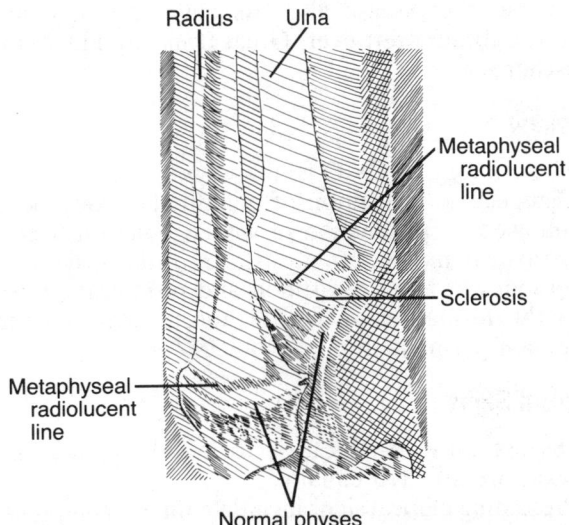

Figure 1. Metaphyseal radiolucent lines and metaphyseal sclerosis proximal to distal radial and ulnar physis in a dog with hypertrophic osteodystrophy.

- Good supportive care of severely affected dogs is essential to prevent decubital ulcers, provide nutrition (see sec. 1, ch. 3), and maintain hydration (see sec. 1, ch. 5).
- Give nonsteroidal analgesics, as needed, to relieve discomfort (buffered aspirin, 10–25 mg/kg q8h, PO).
- Severely affected animals may require nutritional intake via force-feeding or pharyngostomy or gastrostomy tube (see sec. 1, ch. 3). Parenteral fluids may be needed to prevent dehydration in these animals (see sec. 1, ch. 5).
- There is no evidence that mineral, vitamin C, or vitamin D supplements are beneficial; these substances actually may accelerate the rate of dystrophic calcification.

HYPERTROPHIC OSTEOPATHY

Hypertrophic osteopathy (HO) is a pathologic disease process secondary to a space-occupying mass in the abdominal or thoracic cavities. The disease has been reported in many species, including dogs, cats, and humans. HO is characterized by bilateral symmetric swelling of the distal limbs accompanied by the development of smooth periosteal bone formation. HO has been referred to as hypertrophic pulmonary osteoarthropathy, pulmonary osteoarthropathy, and hypertrophic pulmonary osteopathy. Hypertrophic osteopathy is the term that most accurately reflects the rare joint involvement and the variable site of the primary space-occupying lesion.

Etiology

- Hypertrophic osteopathy occurs secondary to a variety of diseases and occurs in dogs and cats of all breeds and ages.
- HOP is most often secondary to metastatic pulmonary neoplasia, although it has been reported with primary pulmonary neoplasia, pulmonary abscesses, pulmonary tuberculosis, chronic bronchopneumonia, spirocercosis, dirofilariasis, rib tumors, bacterial endocarditis, liver adenocarcinoma, and various primary bladder neoplasms (neurofibrosarcoma, botryoid rhabdomyosarcoma, and transitional cell sarcoma).
- The pathogenic mechanisms underlying the bone pathology are unknown. Recent evidence points to an increased peripheral vascular supply secondary to the pulmonary lesion. This increased peripheral blood flow has been observed both in dogs and humans and may be related to an unknown nervous reflex.

Clinical Signs

KEY POINT ▶ Signs of HO often are present months before onset of clinical signs relating to the underlying disease; early recognition is important for diagnosis and treatment of the primary disease.

Signalment

- Dogs and cats with HO may be of any breed and usually are affected late in life.
- A reported increased incidence of the disease in female and large-breed dogs may be due to the increased incidence of mammary tumor metastasis in female dogs, and of primary bone tumors in large-breed dogs.

Lameness

- Most animals present with acute or gradual lameness of all four limbs and with reluctance to move.

Diagnosis

Physical Examination

- The distal limbs are swollen, firm, and warm.
- Signs of pain may be elicited on deep palpation of the long bones.

Laboratory Evaluation

- Laboratory findings reflect the underlying disease process and are not characteristic of HOP.

Radiography

- Survey radiographs demonstrate a bilateral, symmetric, generalized periosteal proliferative reaction affecting the long bones of the appendicular skeleton (Fig. 2). Endosteal bone proliferation does not occur.
- Distal portions of the limbs, especially the metatarsals and metacarpals, are involved first, but periosteal proliferation eventually may involve the mandible, pelvis, ribs, and vertebrae.
- In very early cases, periosteal new-bone formation is not evident, but symmetric soft tissue swelling is present.
- If the primary disease resolves, the bony and soft tissue radiographic abnormalities regress.

KEY POINT ▶ Thoracic and abdominal radiographs

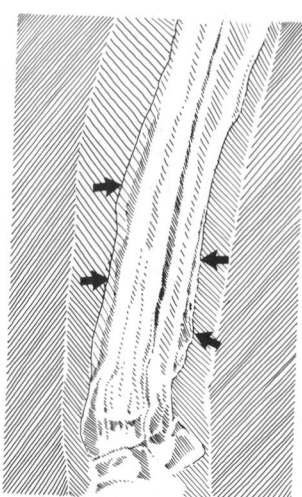

Figure 2. Smooth periosteal proliferation *(arrows)* on radius and ulna characteristic of hypertrophic osteopathy.

are essential to evaluate the underlying disease process and to confirm the diagnosis of HO.

Differential Diagnoses

The bony periosteal reactions of hypertrophic osteopathy are similar to those of panosteitis and hypertrophic osteodystrophy, but HO will not exhibit the increased medullary opacities of panosteitis, nor the radiolucent metaphyseal line characteristic of HOD.

Treatment

KEY POINT ▶ Removal of the underlying primary lesion usually results in regression of the lameness and distal limb lesions.

- Resection of primary or metastatic pulmonary neoplasms provides temporary relief of signs related to HO, but long-term survival is limited.
  - Appropriate treatment of dirofilariasis, spirocercosis, and primary lung disease may increase the chances for long-term survival.
- Inflammation and clinical signs of pain resolve 1–2 weeks after removal of the thoracic or abdominal mass. Periosteal reactions regress in 3–4 months, but residual radiographic changes may persist in severe cases. Lameness may persist in some animals even after removal of the mass.
- When resection of the primary mass is not feasible, unilateral vagotomy (on the side of the lesion) may provide temporary regression of clinical signs.

CRANIOMANDIBULAR OSTEOPATHY

Craniomandibular osteopathy (CMO) is a non-neoplastic, noninflammatory proliferative bony disease in growing dogs that affects bones of endochondral origin, most commonly the mandibles, occipital bones, or temporal bones. Bony lesions are bilateral and symmetric. CMO occurs predominantly in terriers, especially Scottish, West Highland white, and Cairn terriers, but the disease also has been reported in the boxer, Labrador retriever, Great Dane, and Doberman pinscher.

Etiology

- The etiology of CMO is unknown.
- Osteoclastic resorption of mandibular bone occurs, followed by production of woven bone on both the periosteal and endosteal surfaces of the bone. Cyclic episodes of bone resorption and proliferation result in the formation of mature fibrous bone that may remain permanently.

Clinical Signs

- Disease onset occurs at 4–10 months of age. Both sexes are affected equally.
- Presenting clinical signs include pain on manipulation or opening of the mouth, mandibular swelling, ptyalism, inability to open the mouth, intermittent fever, and lethargy.

Diagnosis

Physical Examination

Signs of pain are elicited during direct palpation of the swelling or attempts to open the mouth. In advanced cases, the clinician may be unable to open the mouth more than 1 or 2 cm. Dogs may be febrile during the period of bone proliferation. Lymphadenopathy or temporal muscle atrophy may be present.

Radiography

Diagnosis of CMO is confirmed by radiographic evidence of the bony proliferative lesions.

- Obtain survey radiographs of the skull and mandible, including oblique, dorsoventral, and lateral views, to assess the extent of the disease.
- A non-neoplastic, bilateral symmetric bony proliferation is seen projecting from the periosteal surfaces of the mandible or other bones of the cranium (Fig. 3).
- Angular processes of the mandible and bullae may fuse and obstruct jaw motion. Lesions may also involve the occipital bone, parietal bone, frontal bone, maxilla, and appendicular bones.
- The proliferation of new bone decreases as growth slows, and becomes radiographically static when the animal is approximately 1 year old. Partial or complete regression of bony lesions occurs, but moderate or severe cases result in permanent bone proliferation to varying degrees.
- The prognosis is poor for dogs with radiographic evidence of partial or complete bony ankylosis of the temporomandibular joints (TMJs).

Differential Diagnoses

- Lesions of CMO in the appendicular skeleton may appear radiographically similar to HOD, but CMO lacks the metaphyseal radiolucent line of HOD.
- Radiographic appearance differentiates CMO from bony neoplasia and osteomyelitis.

Treatment

- There is no specific therapy for CMO.
- Administer analgesic therapy (buffered aspirin, 10–25 mg/kg q8h, PO), as needed.
- Nutritional support by gastrostomy or enterostomy tube or parenteral supplementation may be necessary. As the condition stabilizes, most animals have impaired mouth function but are capable of maintaining normal nutritional status.
- Surgical intervention to reduce new bone mass and increase TMJ range of motion has not been beneficial.

MULTIPLE CARTILAGINOUS EXOSTOSIS

Multiple cartilaginous exostosis (MCE) is a disease of dogs and cats in which multiple ossified protuberances arise from the bone cortex in metaphyseal regions. The lesions are a cylinder of cortical bone surrounding a core of cancellous tissue that is covered with a layer of cartilage. Vertebrae, ribs, and long bones commonly are affected. The exostosis ceases to grow when the physis nearest the exostosis ossifies.

Etiology

MCE probably is hereditary in dogs, horses, and humans.

The accepted pathogenesis is that the exostosis is derived from cartilage that separates from the physis during development.

Clinical Signs

- The animal often is presented with a firm, distinct swelling on the involved bone.
- Lameness or limb dysfunction develops only when adjacent structures such as the tendons or nerves are compressed or mechanically distorted by the exostoses.
- Other clinical signs, including pain, lameness, mechanical dysfunction, and neurologic deficits, depend on the structure affected.

Diagnosis

Physical Examination

- A smooth, immovable bony swelling is visible and palpable near a metaphysis.
- Pain may be elicited on palpation of the mass or surrounding soft tissues.

Radiography

- Obtain skeletal survey radiographs of animals with suspected cartilaginous exostosis.
  - Radiographic lesions are radiopaque osseous metaphyseal densities of variable size.
  - Large, scattered radiolucent areas of hyaline cartilage may be present within the exostosis. The exostotic growths may involve any bone except the skull.
- Surgical biopsy of the lesion confirms the diagnosis.

Treatment

KEY POINT ▶ Removal of the exostosis relieves associated pain, mechanical dysfunction, and neurologic deficits.

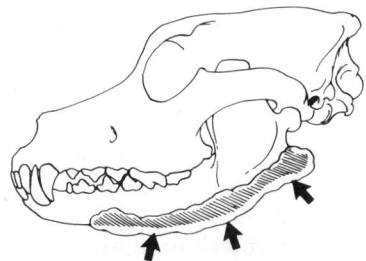

Figure 3. Bony proliferation *(arrows)* on the ventral mandible of a dog with craniomandibular osteopathy.

- Removal of MCE sometimes is requested to improve cosmetic appearance.
- Malignant transformation of exostoses to chondrosarcomas or osteosarcomas has been reported. Continued growth of the exostosis after the animal is mature suggests malignant transformation.
- In general, the diagnosis is good after removal of uncomplicated MCE.

BONE CYSTS

Bone cysts are smooth radiolucent cavities found rarely in the long bones of dogs. Flat bones (e.g., mandible, ribs) also may be affected. Four types of bone cysts have been described in dogs:

- Monostotic (affecting one bone)
- Polyostotic (affecting more than one bone)
- Aneurysmal
- Subchondral

Aneurysmal bone cysts are extremely rare in dogs and are locally aggressive. Bone cysts, found in young, large-breed dogs, do not produce clinical signs until they attain a large size.

Etiology

- The etiology of monostotic, polyostotic, and aneurysmal bone cysts is unknown.
- Subchondral bone cysts often are not primary lesions and usually are the result of chronic degenerative joint disease or diseases leading to degenerative joint disease (e.g., rheumatoid arthritis, systemic lupus erythematosus).

Clinical Signs

Signalment

- The age of affected animals ranges from 4 to 30 months, but most animals are less than 1 year of age.
- Breeds reported to develop bone cysts include the German shepherd, Weimaraner, Irish wolfhound, Afghan, saluki, Great Dane, and Doberman pinscher.

Presentation

- Pain, swelling, and stiffness of the nearest joint may be present.
- Acute lameness or swelling may occur at the site of the cyst owing to a pathologic fracture.

Diagnosis

Radiography

- Survey radiographs establish a diagnosis of bone cysts. A benign, expansive, radiolucent area in the metaphysis is characteristic.
- The metaphyseal cortex may be thinned by expanding cysts.
- Pathologic fractures will be evident radiographically.

Histopathology

- The cyst is lined by fibrous connective tissue.
- Aneurysmal bone cysts are filled with blood, and the blood spaces are lined by connective tissue trabeculae. Multinucleate giant cells and mature bone may be present in these cysts.
- Monostotic and polyostotic cysts may fill with blood after pathologic fracture.

Differential Diagnoses

- Differentiate bone cysts from more aggressive lesions such as chondrosarcoma, osteosarcoma, and giant cell tumors.

Treatment

- Curettage of the walls and filling of the defect with cancellous bone is the definitive treatment in most animals.
- Treat pathologic fractures through cysts by debridement of the cyst wall, cancellous graft, and fracture fixation.
- Cyst resection may be indicated if the lesion is located in flat bones (e.g., rib resection or mandibulectomy).

RETAINED ENCHONDRAL CARTILAGINOUS CORES

Retained enchondral cartilaginous cores occur in the distal ulnar metaphysis of young, large-breed dogs. Radiographically, the retained enchondral cartilage is seen as a central, longitudinal radiolucent cone in the distal ulnar metaphysis and usually is an incidental finding of no clinical significance. These lesions, however, may interfere with normal growth of the ulna, resulting in forelimb deformities.

Etiology

- The etiology is unknown.

Clinical Signs

- Signs may include valgus deviation, external rotation of the carpus, and cranial bowing of the radius.

Diagnosis

- Survey radiographs establish the diagnosis in animals with appropriate forelimb deformities.
- The lesion also may be an incidental finding unrelated to clinical lameness if normal growth of the ulna is apparent.

Treatment

- No treatment is necessary for animals without forelimb deformity.
- Immature animals with forelimb deformities may benefit from distal ulnectomy, which allows spontaneous correction of radial and ulnar deformities during continued growth (see sec. 9, ch. 11).

■ Mature animals require ulnar and radial osteotomy to correct forelimb deformity (see sec. 9, ch. 11).

Supplemental Readings

Alexander JW: Orthopedic diseases. *In* Slatter DH, ed.: *Textbook of Small Animal Surgery,* 1st Ed. Philadelphia: W. B. Saunders, 1985, p 2312.

Alexander JW: Selected skeletal dysplasias: Craniomandibular osteopathy, multiple cartilaginous exostoses, and hypertrophic osteodystrophy. Vet Clin North Am [Sm Anim Pract] 13:55, 1983.

Goldschmidt MH, Biery DN: Bone cysts in the dog. *In* Newton CD, Nunamaker DM, eds.: *Textbook of Small Animal Orthopaedics,* 1st Ed. Philadelphia: J. B. Lippincott, 1985, p 611.

Lenehan TM, Fetter AW: Hypertrophic osteopathy. *In* Newton CD, Nunamaker DM, eds.: *Textbook of Small Animal Orthopaedics,* 1st Ed. Philadelphia: J. B. Lippincott, 1985, p 603.

Lenehan TM, Fetter AW: Hypertrophic osteodystrophy. *In* Newton CD, Nunamaker DM, eds.: *Textbook of Small Animal Orthopaedics,* 1st Ed. Philadelphia: J. B. Lippincott, 1985, p 597.

Lenehan TM, Van Sickle DC, Biery DN: Canine panosteitis. *In* Newton CD, Nunamaker DM, eds.: *Textbook of Small Animal Orthopaedics,* 1st Ed. Philadelphia: J. B. Lippincott, 1985, p 591.

Riser WH, Newton CD: Craniomandibular osteopathy. *In* Newton CD, Nunamaker DM, eds.: *Textbook of Small Animal Orthopaedics,* 1st Ed. Philadelphia: J. B. Lippincott, 1985, p 603.

24 Osteochondrosis

Timothy M. Lenehan

Osteochondrosis is seen in young, rapidly growing animals of many species. It is characterized by a defect in endochondral ossification.

- Disruption of endochondral ossification in the articuloepiphyseal complex results in osteochondritis dissecans (OCD), which is most commonly reported in the caudal aspect of the humeral head, the medial humeral condyle, and the medial and lateral femoral condyles and trochlear ridges of the talus.
- Disturbances of endochondral ossification in the metaphyseal growth plate can result in focal growth plate thickening (retained endochondral cartilage cores of the distal ulna), cartilage retention nests (femoral epiphyses), physeal slowing (radius curvus), and "slippage" of metaphyseal growth plates (ununited anconeal process [UAP]; proximal calcaneus).

In the elbow joint, three disorders are believed to be related to osteochondrosis: UAP, fragmented coronoid process (FCP), and OCD.

- Dogs with FCP and OCD of the distal medial humeral condyle present with similar clinical symptoms; their diagnosis and treatment can be approached identically. However, these two entities can occur alone, together, individually with UAP, or both together with UAP.
- UAP describes a radiologic diagnosis pertaining to the failure of a specific growth plate in the elbow to close completely. When presented with a dog with forelimb pain and UAP, do not immediately assume that the elbow pain is directly related to the UAP and that surgical removal of the process is the solution; rather, give further consideration to other potential causes of elbow pain.

UAP

Anatomy and Pathophysiology

- In the dog, the anconeal process develops from a separate center of ossification and unites with the proximal ulna at 20–24 weeks of age (physeal closure). Therefore, diagnosis of UAP prior to 24 weeks of age may be premature.
  - If in doubt, radiograph the contralateral elbow for comparison (the incidence of bilateral UAP is approximately 30% in dogs).
- Union of the anconeal process to the ulna initially occurs at the distal aspect of the physis and then progresses proximally along the growth plate.
- Incomplete endochondral ossification can result in foci of retained cartilage within an otherwise closed physis; such retention nests can mimic UAP.
- An intact anconeal process provides stability to the elbow joint, particularly in extension (weight-bearing phase). Failure of union of this process results in foreign body irritation, mild to moderate elbow instability (depending on the size of the UAP), and subsequent osteoarthritic production.
- Blood supply to the anconeal process is via the dorsal periosteal capsular attachments; the bone can remain viable and capable of endosteal callus formation unless completely separated from these attachments.
- In chondrodystrophic breeds, UAP may accompany (or result from) premature closure of the distal ulna and asynchronous growth of the radius and ulna.

UAP in Immature Dogs (<1 Year)

Clinical Signs

- Dogs with UAP present with varying degrees of lameness that usually worsens with exercise.

Diagnosis

- Detailed preoperative radiographs of the elbow are mandatory. The following views are helpful:
  - *Straight lateral*—to evaluate all compartments of the joint, assess relative bone lengths (radius/ulna), and observe for panosteitis lesions.
  - *Flexed lateral*—facilitates detailed evaluation of the region between the anconeal process and the ulna.
  - *Craniocaudal*—to examine the medial joint compartment for concurrent arthritis, FCP, and OCD of the medial aspect of the humeral condyle.
  - *Craniocaudal medial oblique*—to evaluate for FCP not visible on a standard craniocaudal view.
- Assess the elbow for:
  - Panosteitis in adjacent bones
  - Coexistent FCP or OCD lesions in the elbow joint
  - The degree of osteoarthritis present in the elbow
  - The type of UAP
  - Incongruities indicating a radioulnar growth inequity

KEY POINT ▶ If panosteitis is present, a "radiographic" UAP may be clinically silent; alternatively, there may be two (or more) clinically significant problems.

Preoperative Considerations

- Concomitant FCP, OCD of the medial aspect of the humeral condyle, or both may dramatically change the prognosis, both with and without surgical intervention.

- Factors determining the surgical approach include the number of lesions present and the type of UAP. Four categories can be defined:
  - *Cartilage retention nest*—In this lesion (usually an incidental finding), the anconeal process is united. It is unlikely to be the cause of the lameness.
  - *Delayed union*—A normal union proceeds distoproximally. Confine/rest animals with a delayed union and radiograph the elbow monthly until there is evidence of union.
  - *Nondisplaced nonunion*—The anconeal process is apposed to the proximal ulna by collagenous tissue or fibrocartilaginous interface. Such fragments may be successfully reconstructed, depending on the bone density (screw-holding power), viability of the tissue interface, degree of compression achieved with the lag screw, and postoperative care taken by the owner.
  - *Displaced nonunion*—The anconeal process is physiologically (lack of blood supply or viable interface tissue) or anatomically separated from the proximal ulna and acts as a foreign body that interferes with normal joint function. Optimally, these "joint mice" should be removed. In some cases, the anconeal process becomes lodged in the supratrochlear foramen, thus minimizing the irritant effect.

KEY POINT ▶ Theoretically, surgical reconstruction is preferable to removal because reconstruction maintains elbow stability, thereby diminishing the potential for subsequent arthritic development.

- An elbow with a displaced, free-floating nonunion benefits from surgery, as the "joint mouse" is removed. However, joint incongruity, and subsequent arthritic progression, will remain.

Surgical Procedures

Objectives
- Remove or reconstruct the UAP.
- Address concurrent disease in the medial elbow compartment (OCD/FCP).

Equipment
- Standard surgical pack and suture material
- Gelpi self-retaining retractors
- Suction and cautery set up
- Bone elevator (Sayre) and rongeurs (medium)
- Drill, bits, taps, and screws
- Small bone curet

Technique

1. Place the dog in lateral recumbency, with the affected limb up, suspended, and prepared from carpus to shoulder for aseptic surgery.
2. Make a routine lateral approach to the elbow, placing the incision in the anconeus muscle closer to the ulna than to the humeral condyle.
3. Using the Gelpi retractor, retract the lateral head of the triceps and anconeus muscles.

4. Slightly flex the elbow and externally rotate the antebrachium for the best visualization of the anconeal process and its tissue interface with the ulna.
5. If a displaced nonunion is present, remove the process.
6. If the nonunion is not displaced, determine the chances for successful reconstruction:
   a. Assess the vascular supply to the process.
   b. Assess mobility at the nonunion site.
   c. Assess the shape of the anconeal process for elbow congruency.
7. If in doubt, attempt lag screw fixation of the UAP.
   a. Drill the thread hole either free-hand, entering at the apex of the anconeal process and exiting at the caudal ulna; or with a drill, entering at the caudal ulna and exiting at the apex of the anconeal process (the latter may require a C-clamp drill guide).
   b. Over-drill the ulnar hole.
   c. Tap the anconeal drill hole.
   d. Place the lag screw from caudal to cranial and observe the degree of compression (Fig. 1).
   e. Do not let the screw tip protrude beyond the tip of the process.
8. Do not hesitate to remove the process if:
   a. Technical difficulties prevent successful reconstruction.
   b. Bone quality (screw purchase) is poor and the nonunion site will not compress.
   c. Joint congruency is disrupted by the repaired process.
9. Lavage the joint thoroughly and routinely close the muscle, fascia and subcutaneous tissues (absorbable sutures; simple interrupted pattern), and skin.
10. If radioulnar growth disparity is suggested radiographically, a proximal diaphyseal ulnar osteotomy repaired with pins and a figure-eight tension band wire releases pressure on the anconeus in the trochlear groove and may facilitate union.

Postoperative Care and Complications

Short-Term
- Apply light, modified Robert Jones bandage from the digits to above the incision site and leave in place

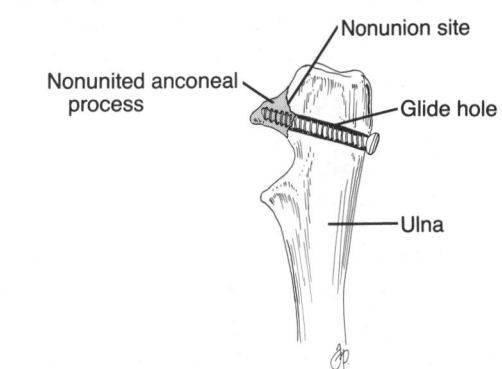

Figure 1. The lag screw is placed in a caudo-cranial direction across the nonunion site and compresses the nonunion. Placement in this direction facilitates removal at a later date and keeps metal out of the joint.

for 10–14 days to minimize swelling and seroma formation and to discourage excessive use of the limb.

- Remove sutures in 10–14 days.
- If the anconeal process has been removed, no further restriction is necessary.

Long-Term

- Confine the dog to house and leash walking only for 6–8 weeks.
- Obtain follow-up radiographs at 4 and 8 weeks to assess process union.
- Surgical nonunions require subsequent screw and anconeal process removal.
- Animals with union may experience low-grade lameness until the screw is removed.

Prognosis

- The prognosis is excellent if surgical reconstruction is successful.
- In animals with process removal, the prognosis is good to fair; most animals will begin to show lameness related to osteoarthritis at 6–7 years of age.

UAP in Mature Dogs (>1 Year)

Diagnosis

- Detailed preoperative radiographs of the elbow are mandatory. Use the radiographic views and guidelines to assess the elbow listed previously under UAP in Immature Dogs. Determine whether the anconeal process is lodged in the olecranon fossa (and hence immobile) or whether the UAP is free-floating.
- In animals >1 year of age, cartilage retention nests, delayed union, and nondisplaced nonunion are rare. Displaced nonunion is commonly seen. The UAP may be free-floating or lodged in the olecranon fossa. It is unlikely that a UAP lodged or ankylosed in the olecranon fossa is the cause of lameness.
- Differential diagnoses include:
  - Hyperextension/flexion injury resulting in fractured osteophytes and inflamed capsular tissue; signs include pain in the elbow and with mild to moderate joint effusion.
  - Displaced nonunion; signs include pain in the elbow and mild joint effusion.
  - Covert septic arthritis; elbow is painful with mild to moderate joint effusion. Diagnostically, the majority of cells are mature neutrophils with rare intracytoplasmic bacteria/degenerate neutrophils. Culture and sensitivity are usually negative. Treat with rest, NSAID therapy, and cephalosporins for 3 to 4 weeks.
  - Overt septic arthritis; elbow is warm, painful, and swollen. Diagnostically, joint fluid is turbid with mature, degenerate neutrophils and many intracytoplasmic bacteria. Culture is positive, and treatment is joint lavage or surgical drainage.

OSTEOCHONDROSIS (OCD/FCP) OF THE ELBOW
Anatomy and Pathophysiology

- OCD and FCP affect the medial joint compartment of the elbow; UAP affects the caudal joint compart-

ment (Fig. 2). All three problems eventually lead to arthritic changes in all joint compartments.

- Joint congruency hinges on uniform growth of the humeral, radial, and ulnar bony components.
- A defect in endochondral ossification, uneven joint loading due to asymmetric growth of the radius and ulna, or both, can cause two problems:
  - Joint mice (FCP, OCD)
  - Incongruent joint surfaces
- In young dogs, the age at closure for growth plates around the elbow varies:
  - Anconeal process—5–6 months
  - Proximal radius—8–9 months
  - Olecranon—8–9 months
  - Distal humeral condyles—7–8 months
- The lateral aspect of the joint is relatively free of major neurovascular structures. The medial aspect of the elbow, however, is rich in major nerves (median and ulnar) and vascular structures (brachial artery and vein).

KEY POINT ▶ Clinical diagnosis of OCD/FCP often is made prior to growth plate closure; therefore, avoid surgical approaches requiring osteotomies.

OCD/FCP in Immature Dogs (<1 Year)

Diagnosis

For accurate preoperative diagnosis, detailed preoperative radiographs are mandatory. Table 1 lists typical radiographic changes seen in OCD/FCP.

- Using the radiographic views and guidelines described previously (see UAP in Immature Dogs), perform the following evaluations:
  - Rule out panosteitis, UAP, and radioulnar growth disparities.
  - Assess the degree of arthritis present.
  - Attempt to differentiate FCP and OCD (Fig. 2).
- FCP and OCD can be difficult to differentiate radiographically in young dogs. Radiographic changes usually are not evident before the animal is 7–8 months old.

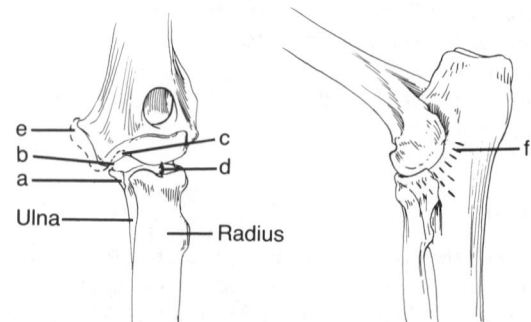

Figure 2. Anteroposterior *(left)* and lateral *(right)* views of the elbow demonstrate fragmented coronoid process (FCP) fragment (a), osteochondritis dissecans (OCD) flaps (b), OCD flap bed (or FCP kissing lesion) (c), increased humeroradial joint space (d), elongated medial humeral condyle (e), and increased radioulnar sclerosis (f) seen in dogs with FCP/OCD.

TABLE 1. Radiographic Findings Seen in Animals with OCD/FCP

Findings Typical of FCP
Fragment in medial joint compartment (A-P view)
Widened humeroradial joint space (A-P view)

Findings Typical of OCD
Flap in medial humeral joint compartment (A-P view)
"Divot" or flap bed in medial humeral condyle (A-P view)
Flattened, elongated medial humeral condylar joint surface (A-P view)

Findings Common to OCD and FCP
Fuzziness and periosteal proliferation on the dorsal anconeal process (flexed lateral view) and in the medial joint compartment (cranial-caudal view)
Increased radioulnar interface sclerosis (lateral view)

OCD = osteochondritis dissecans; FCP = fragmented coronoid process; A-P = anteroposterior.

- Diagnosis also can be difficult because both conditions may occur concurrently. For example:
  - Osteophytes on the medial coronoid process may mimic FCP fragments.
  - A radiographically indistinct FCP may appear as a humeral condylar "kissing lesion" that mimics an OCD lesion.

Preoperative Considerations

KEY POINT ▶ Often an accurate diagnosis of OCD or FCP is made only during surgery.

- A similar surgical approach can be used for OCD and FCP.

Surgical Procedure

Objectives
- Remove the fragment and/or flap of the OCD/FCP lesion, while minimizing trauma to the young, growing joint.
- Curet the flap bed (or kissing lesion) to stimulate neochondrogenesis.

Equipment
- Same as for UAP in the Immature Dog

Technique

KEY POINT ▶ There is no easy method for visualization of all joint compartments using a single surgical approach.

1. Place the dog in lateral recumbency, with the affected limb down, suspended and prepared from the carpus to the axillar for aseptic surgery.
2. Make a medial approach to the elbow through the skin and deep antebrachial fascia. Separate the pronator teres from the flexor carpi radialis at their origins on the medial epicondyle, holding them apart with Gelpi retractors (Fig. 3).
3. Make a transverse cut in the joint capsule caudal and cranial to the collateral ligament. Carry this incision as far cranial as practical, taking care not to damage the median nerve or brachial vessels.

4. Using the edge of the table as a fulcrum and the antebrachium as a lever, open the medial joint compartment.
5. Locate the coronoid process and, if it is fragmented, remove it.
   a. FCP removal can usually be accomplished through a capsulotomy, with or without a partial desmotomy (division of the ligaments).
6. Alternatively, remove the OCD flap.
   a. If further exposure is needed, a medial collateral desmotomy may be followed by a pronator teres tenotomy.
   b. OCD flap removal and curettage generally necessitate a complete desmotomy. Curettage the OCD flap to healthy, bleeding bone so that a clot forms a base for neochondrogenesis.
7. Thoroughly lavage the joint with sterile saline solution.
8. Close the desmotomy and tenotomy with a locking loop or horizontal mattress suture pattern (0, 1–0 Prolene/Nylon), followed by 2–0 Vicryl/gut closure of the capsule, and all other tissue planes.

Postoperative Care and Complications

- Apply a light, modified Robert Jones bandage from the digits to above the incision site and leave in place for 7 days (capsulotomy) to 14–21 days (desmotomy).
- Remove sutures in 10–14 days.
- Confine the dog to house and restrict activity to leash walking for 4 weeks; allow access to yard through weeks 4–8 prior to resumption of full activity.

Prognosis

- The degree of elbow incongruity, arthritis at the time of surgery, the size of the flap/fragment, and the surgical technique determine outcome.

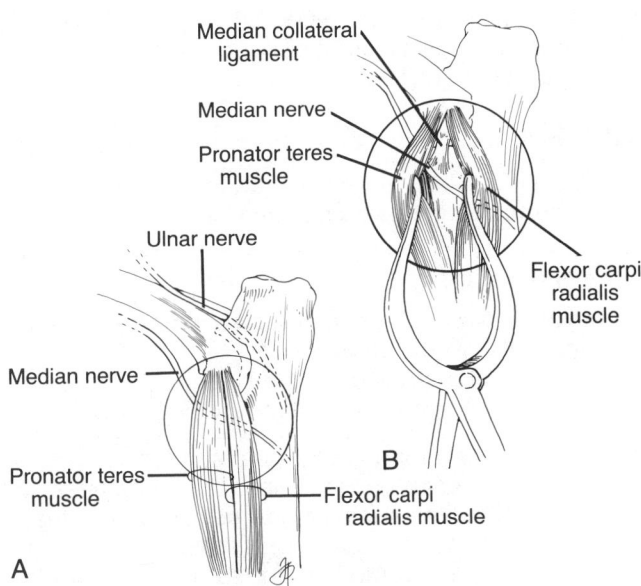

Figure 3. Medial approach to the elbow. *Left,* Pronator teres and flexor carpi radialis muscles and the median nerve visualized. *Right,* In separation of the flexor carpi radialis and pronator teres muscles with a Gelpi retractor, a transverse cut is made in the joint capsule to expose the medial aspect of the elbow joint.

KEY POINT ▶ It is unrealistic to expect dogs with advanced arthritis and large lesions to benefit significantly from surgery.

OCD/FCP in Mature Dogs (>1 Year)

Anatomy

■ See OCD/FCP in Immature Dogs.

Treatment

■ Surgical procedures are generally not warranted in older animals for uncomplicated FCP/OCD lesions. In most animals with FCP/OCD that are >1 year of age arthritic changes are too extensive to warrant surgical intervention.
■ Differential diagnosis for acute lameness is similar to that for older animals with UAP, and includes hyperextension/flexion injury and septic arthritis.
■ Diagnosis and treatment are similar to that described for UAP in Mature Dogs.

OCD/FCP/UAP IN THE SAME ELBOW

Anatomy

See UAP and Osteochondrosis (FCP/OCD).

Preoperative Considerations

■ The diagnosis is based on detailed preoperative radiographs (as described previously).

KEY POINT ▶ Multiple lesions in the elbow reduce the likelihood of surgical success.

Surgical Procedure

Objectives

■ Remove or reconstruct the UAP.
■ Address any concurrent disease in the medial elbow compartment (FCP/OCD).

Equipment

■ Same as for UAP in The Immature Dog *plus*
■ Osteotome/mallet or oscillating saw

Technique

1. In young dogs with open physes, make two separate approaches to the elbow:
   a. A lateral approach for the UAP.
   b. A medial approach to treat the FCP/OCD.

KEY POINT ▶ Advantages of a dual surgical approach include minimal invasiveness; disadvantages include having to turn the animal and repeat preparation and draping of the limb for surgery.

2. If the physes around the elbow are closed, make an approach to the elbow using a proximal ulnar diaphyseal osteotomy (Fig. 4).

   a. Make a lateral approach to the elbow carried down the caudolateral surface of the ulna through the skin and superficial fascia.
   b. Following incision of the anconeus and lateral triceps muscles, reflect the extensor carpi ulnaris and abductor pollicis longus muscles laterally, while elevating the flexor carpi ulnaris and deep digital flexors from the medial aspect of the ulna, exposing the annular and interosseous ligaments.
   c. Perform a transverse osteotomy of the ulna below the level of the radial head, followed by transection of the lateral annular ligament, and caudal crus of the ulnar collateral ligament.
   d. Externally rotate the proximal ulna to allow exposure of the entire elbow joint.

3. Following correction of the UAP/FCP/OCD, thoroughly lavage the joint with sterile saline solution and realign the ulna.

4. Close the osteotomy incision using two pins and a figure-8 tension band wire. Suture the annular ligament, and close all muscle and fascial planes in layers.

Postoperative Care and Complications

■ Apply a light, modified Robert Jones bandage from the digits to above the incision site and leave in place for 10–14 days.
■ Remove suture in 10–14 days.
■ Restrict activity to the house and leash walking only for 6–8 weeks.
■ Obtain follow-up radiographs at 4 and 8 weeks to assess osteotomy healing.
■ Ulnar nonunions most commonly result from use of small pins or wires of inadequate strength.

Prognosis

■ The greater the number of problems and the more radical the surgical technique, the more guarded is the prognosis.

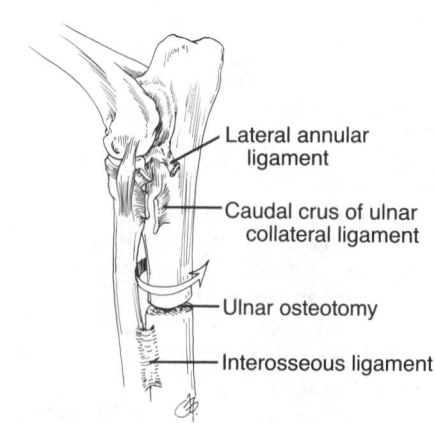

Figure 4. A proximal ulnar diaphyseal osteotomy allows full visualization of all compartments of the elbow in the mature dog.

OCD OF THE SHOULDER, STIFLE, AND HOCK

In dogs, OCD can occur not only in the elbow but also in the shoulder, stifle, and hocks.

Anatomy

▪ See respective chapters on shoulder, stifle, and hock injuries.

Pathophysiology

▪ A basic defect in endochondral ossification results in abnormal subchondral bony development and often results in formation of a cartilage flap in the overlying area.
▪ The size of the flap can be quite variable, and in some joints the flap has, as a component, some underlying bone (OCD tarsus). Thus, OCD results in two distinct joint abnormalities: a joint mouse and a resultant joint incongruity. Neither problem can be "cured."
▪ Removal of the flap/fragment removes the source of irritation.
▪ Curettage of flap bed results in neochondrogenesis, but the material properties of the resulting fibrocartilage are not equal to those of hyaline cartilage, and the new cartilage rarely grows to a height or density that reestablishes full joint congruency (particularly in the hock).
▪ In a complex joint such as the elbow, the existence of a flap/concave bed may inhibit or modify normal development of impinging structures (opposing joint surfaces). Hence, while surgery can remove the joint mouse and stimulate some neochondrogenesis, it cannot fully resolve the residual joint incongruity.
▪ Removal of the joint mouse may significantly slow down *but not completely arrest* arthritic progression. This has been demonstrated clinically and scientifically in the shoulder of the dog.

Preoperative Considerations

▪ As the size of the flap/fragment increases in relation to joint surface area, the residual joint incongruity following fragment removal similarly increases. Hence, a small OCD lesion has less impact on a simple, large surface area joint (shoulder) than on a smaller (tarsus) or more complex joint (stifle, elbow).
▪ Clinically, dogs with OCD of the hock seem to fare equally well with or without surgery; this may be related to the small joint/large fragment ratio.
▪ Surgical intervention typically helps but does not entirely alleviate clinical symptoms in dogs with OCD of the stifle and elbow (complex joints, variably sized fragments). Optimal results can be expected in a large joint with a small lesion; suboptimal results in a complex, small joint with a large lesion.
▪ The degree of osteoarthritis present at the time of diagnosis is important. As the degree of arthritis progresses, the benefits of surgical intervention diminish.
▪ Ideal surgical candidates are young dogs with small flaps/fragments and no arthritis.
▪ Old (and young) dogs with severe arthritis and large fragments/flaps are unlikely to benefit from surgical intervention.

Surgical Procedures

▪ Surgical objectives are similar to those described for OCD of the elbow.
▪ See respective chapters on shoulder, stifle, and hock injuries for description of surgical approaches.

Postoperative Care and Complications

▪ See respective chapters on shoulder, stifle, and hock injuries.
▪ Also see postoperative care for OCD of the elbow.

Supplemental Readings

Lenehan TM, Nunamaker DM: Lateral approach to the canine elbow by proximal ulnar diaphyseal osteotomy. J Am Vet Med Assoc 180:523, 1982.

Lenehan TM, van Sickle DC: Ununited anconeal process, ununited medial coronoid process, ununited medial epicondyle, patella cubiti, and sesamoidal fragments of the elbow. *In* Newton CD, Nunamaker DM, eds.: *Textbook of Small Animal Orthopaedics.* Philadelphia: J. B. Lippincott, 1985, p 999.

Probst CW, Flo G, McLaughlin M, DeCamp C: A simple medial approach to the canine elbow for treatment of fragmented coronoid process and osteochondritis dissecans. J Am Anim Hosp Assoc 25:331, 1989.

Pediatric Fractures

Paul A. Manley

The majority of fractures in immature animals involve the metaphyseal area of the long bones. The metaphyseal area is the site of the growth plate, which is weaker than the surrounding bones and supporting ligaments. Occasionally, the diaphysis of the long bones is fractured in immature animals. Principles for management of these diaphyseal fractures are the same as for adult animals.

ANATOMY

Metaphyseal Growth Plate (Physis)

- The metaphyseal growth plate (MGP) (also called the physis) separates the epiphysis from the metaphysis and is the major site of longitudinal bone growth.
- The MGP has a cartilage component composed of developmental zones, a bony component composed of trabecular bone, and a fibrous component composed of fibroblasts and fiber bundles.
- Blood supply to the metaphysis and epiphysis is separated by the MGP until closure of the growth plate occurs. The epiphyseal vessels supply the germinal cells; the metaphyseal vessels supply the metaphyseal side of the MGP.
- The zones of the MGP, from superficial to deep, are reserve, proliferative, hypertrophic, ossification, and metaphyseal.
  - The *reserve zone* contains several layers of randomly arranged chondrocytes. These chondrocytes function to store nutrients.
  - The *proliferative zone* is the growth zone of the MGP. The chondrocytes divide and form palisades of cells at right angles to the long axis of the bone. Longitudinal growth occurs as a result of active cell division and matrix production by these chondrocytes.
  - The chondrocytes enlarge in the *hypertrophic zone* by storing calcium and increasing their fluid intake. It is more appropriate to refer to this area as the zone of cellular swelling, because the cells swell rather than hypertrophy. As the cells enlarge, the matrix is squeezed into longitudinal septae. Near the bottom or deep portion of this zone, the cells begin to degrade and deposit calcium in the matrix.
  - Vessels from the metaphyseal capillaries invade the deep portion of the hypertrophic zone and result in mineralization of the matrix. This results in the formation of primary and secondary spongiosa in the *ossification zone*.
  - The *metaphyseal zone* is characterized by remodeling of the primary and secondary spongiosa.

- Although most of the longitudinal growth of long bones comes from the MGP, the epiphysis of immature animals has an epiphyseal growth plate that gives rise to some increase in bone length.

Classification of Injuries

KEY POINT ▶ Physeal fractures usually occur through the hypertrophic zone of the physis, because the cells are large and there is very little supporting matrix.

- A large number of fractures in the immature animal involve the metaphyseal growth plate. These fractures have been classified into five types by Salter and Harris (Fig. 1):
  - Type I is a separation of the epiphysis from the metaphysis through the hypertrophic zone of the physis.
  - Type II is a fracture through the hypertrophic zone with fracture of a portion of the metaphysis.

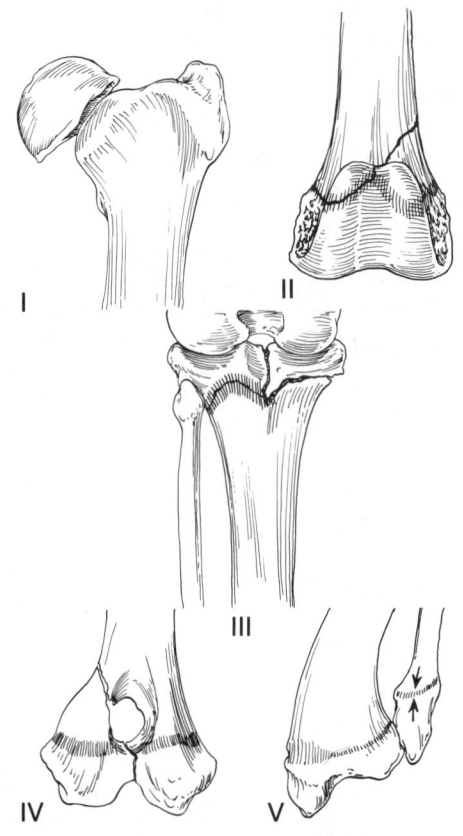

Figure 1. Five different types of growth plate fractures. See text for explanations.

- Type III is a fracture that extends from the joint surface to the hypertrophic zone of the physis and along the hypertrophic zone to the periphery.
- Type IV is a fracture that extends from the joint surface to the hypertrophic zone and through a portion of the metaphysis.
- Type V is a crushing injury to some or all of the MGP. In this injury there is a high incidence of premature physeal closure because the germinal cells of the physis are injured.

PREOPERATIVE CONSIDERATIONS

Tissue Handling

The bone of immature animals is very soft and can be fractured easily during reduction attempts.
In fractures of the MGP, the germinal cells are usually with the epiphyseal fragment; be careful when manipulating this segment of bone.
Early treatment of the fracture usually facilitates easy reduction.

Growth Potential

The prognosis depends on the type of injury, location of the fracture, type of repair, and growth potential remaining in the MGP at the time of injury.
Premature physeal closure of a single bone may result in limb shortening or an angular limb deformity if only a portion of the physis is affected.
Premature physeal closure of one of a pair of bones (e.g., radius and ulna; see sec. 9, ch. 11) may result in angular limb deformity and joint subluxation.

SURGICAL PROCEDURES

General Considerations

If the fracture is less than 48 hours old, and is a type I or II growth plate fracture, it may be reduced and held in place with a cast.
If internal fixation is necessary in a growth plate fracture, the method chosen should provide adequate stabilization and minimize further damage to the physis.

- Regardless of the location of the fracture, the method of internal fixation should not span the MGP if there is growth potential left.
- Single or paired pins or Kirschner wires are the implants of choice for fractures involving the MGP.
- Pins, cerclage wires, external fixators, plates, and screws are appropriate methods of internal fixation for diaphyseal fractures in immature animals. (See appropriate chapters for details on surgical management of specific diaphyseal fractures.

POSTOPERATIVE CARE AND COMPLICATIONS

- Obtain follow-up radiographs at 2- to 3-week intervals for signs of premature growth arrest.
- Remove implants that cross the growth plate in 3–4 weeks to decrease their effects on potential growth.
- Loss of bone length may result in altered gait; however, most animals have the ability to compensate fairly well unless >25% of the bone length is lost.
- Premature closure of the physis of one of a pair of bones (e.g., radius and ulna) usually results in significant angular deformity and joint incongruity. Single or multiple osteotomies may be necessary to correct the deformities.
- It may be necessary to perform multiple osteotomies in young animals to allow for continuous growth.

Supplemental Readings

Brinker WO, Piermattei DL, Flo GL: *Handbook of Small Animal Orthopedics and Fracture Treatment*, 2nd Ed. Philadelphia: W. B. Saunders, 1990.
Manley PA, Henry WB, Wilson JW: Diseases of the epiphysis. *In* Whittick WG, ed.: *Canine Orthopedics*, 2nd Ed. Philadelphia: Lea & Febiger, 1990.
Rang ME: *The Growth Plate and Its Disorders*. Edinburgh: Livingstone, Ltd, 1969.
Salter RB, Harris WR: Injuries involving the epiphyseal plate. J Bone Joint Surg 45A:487, 1963.

Charles E. DeCamp

An open fracture is a broken bone that has been exposed to the environment and contaminated by or infected with bacteria. The soft tissue injury that accompanies an open fracture may be a simple puncture wound or a complex injury with vascular compromise and tissue necrosis. Successful management of open fractures depends upon proper treatment of soft tissue wounds and fracture fixation. If soft tissue wounds are properly managed, the morbidity of wound infection is reduced and fracture healing can proceed at a normal rate.

CLASSIFICATION OF OPEN FRACTURES

Open fractures are classified as types I, II, or III, based upon the mechanism and severity of soft tissue injury (Fig. 1). The purpose of classification is to determine the likelihood of serious infection. The type of wound management and the choice of fracture fixation partly depend on the classification.

- Type I develops when a fracture fragment penetrates the skin, exposing the fracture to bacterial contami-

nation. Soft tissue injury is minor, and wound infection is unlikely with proper care.
- Type II develops when an external object forcefull[y] penetrates the skin and soft tissues, creating a fracture and contaminating the wound. Fracture severit[y] is highly variable, but soft tissue injury is relativel[y] minimal and usually is not complicated by vascula[r] compromise and tissue necrosis. Bacterial contamination generally is more extensive than for type [I] injuries.
- Type III develops when an external object forcefull[y] penetrates the skin and soft tissues, creating a fracture, contaminating the wound, and severely damaging the soft tissues. The ability of the body t[o] combat soft tissue infection commonly is complicate[d] by vascular compromise and necrosis. The risk o[f] bacterial infection is very high.

KEY POINT ▶ Type I open fractures are least likely t[o] develop wound infections; type III open fractures almost always have some level of infection.

- In all fracture types, if the wound has been neglecte[d] and infection develops, manage the injury as thoug[h] it were a type III injury.

PREOPERATIVE CONSIDERATIONS

- The diagnosis of an open fracture may be made b[y] direct inspection, palpation, and radiography.
- If skin penetration, laceration, or avulsion is presen[t] assume that the fracture is open and contaminate[d] until proven otherwise.
- Cover all open wounds with a sterile dressing.
- Obtain radiographs after dressing placement.
  - Radiographic signs of air within the soft tissue[s] adjacent to a fracture is diagnostic of an ope[n] fracture.
- Use aseptic technique when manipulating the woun[d]

KEY POINT ▶ Violating the rules of strict asepsis during early wound management increases the probability of nosocomial infection.

- If preparation of the wound cannot proceed immediately, use external coaptation for temporary sta[] bilization of the fracture. Apply a reinforced Robe[rt] Jones bandage for injuries below the stifle or elbow[.] Use a spica splint for open fractures of the femur o[r] humerus.
- To prepare the wound, remove the sterile bandag[e]

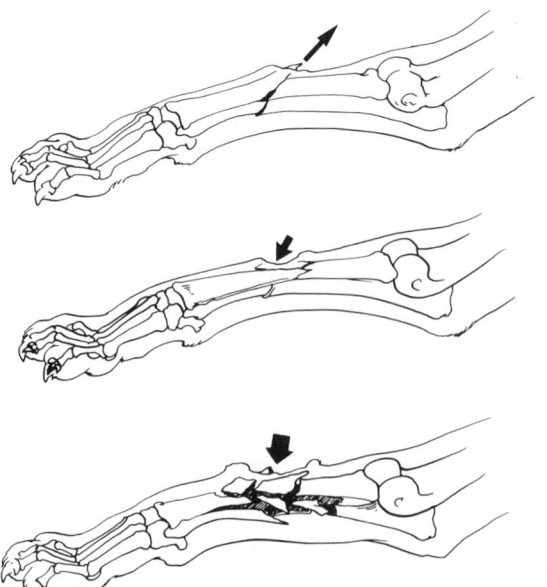

Figure 1. Types of open fractures. *Top,* Type I: fracture fragment penetrates skin. *Center,* Type II: penetrating object causes minor injury to soft tissue. *Bottom,* Type III: penetrating object causes extensive damage to soft tissue.

and carefully clip surrounding hair to avoid contamination. If necessary, cover the wound with sterile gauze sponges moistened with sterile saline to prevent introduction of the clipped hair into the wound.

- Lavage the wound with copious amounts of sterile saline or lactated Ringer's solution to wash small particulate matter from the wound interstices (see sec. 5, ch. 18).
- Betadine and alcohol may be used on the skin surrounding the wound; however, avoid contact of detergents or alcohol with the open wound.
- Remove a sample of fluid from the fracture site for laboratory tests, using a swab if the size and type of wound permit its introduction. Base definitive antibiotic treatment on culture and sensitivity tests. A Gram stain may reveal the organism type and aid in the initial choice of antibiotics.
- Consider giving broad-spectrum systemic antibiotics; however, this is less important than proper wound management in preventing infection.

SURGICAL DEBRIDEMENT, FRACTURE FIXATION, AND SOFT TISSUE RECONSTRUCTION

Objectives

- Improve wound environment to reduce the risk of infection.
- Reconstruct soft tissue to cover bone and provide limb function. It may be necessary to defer this aspect if severe tissue defect or necrosis is present.
- Provide temporary or definitive fracture fixation.

Equipment

- Two standard general orthopedic packs and suture material
- Bone curet and brush
- Scalpel blades
- Sterile saline or lactated Ringer's solution
- Fracture fixation equipment:
  - Materials for external coaptation
  - External skeletal fixation pins and clamps
  - Power drills
  - Bone plating equipment

Surgical Debridement

Technique

Type I Open Fracture

1. Little or no surgical debridement is required.
2. If the bone is not visibly exposed and the wound is small, copiously lavage the wound with sterile lactated Ringer's solution.
3. Sharply excise necrotic tissue, if present, from the wound before fracture fixation.

Technique

Type II Open Fracture

1. Surgical debridement generally is not extensive; however, be careful to remove all nonviable tissue.

2. Copiously lavage the wound with sterile lactated Ringer's solution before fracture fixation.

Technique

Type III Open Fracture (Extensive Debridement and Lavage)

1. Prepare the limb and wound for aseptic surgery. If a surgical approach to a bone is anticipated, extend the skin preparation to the appropriate anatomic field.
2. Drape the limb using standard aseptic technique, using water-impermeable drapes.
3. Sharply excise necrotic skin, fat, fascia, and muscle from the wound.
4. When extensive debridement is required, to avoid tissue maceration be sure to discard scalpel blades as they become dull.
5. Remove any loose, dirty, small fragments of bone.
6. To preserve the blood supply and prevent development of bone sequestra, maintain tissue attachments to bone fragments. Do not remove the fragments if this will disrupt the blood supply for the surgical exposure.

KEY POINT ▶ Clean large, attached bone fragments with a bone curet or brush if necessary. *Do not remove them.*

7. Clean, but do not debride, tendons, ligaments, intact blood vessels, and nerves unless they are necrotic.
8. If necessary, extend access to the bone by a surgical approach for fracture fixation. If severe contamination or infection is present, apply external fixation with minimal or no surgical approach.

Fracture Fixation

- Do not carry out fracture fixation until initial wound management is complete, as described previously.
- If the fracture is stable and nonarticular and involves a bone distal to the stifle or elbow joint, external coaptation may be effective. Most other fractures require surgically applied orthopedic fixation.

Technique

1. If a surgical approach is made, take a swab from the fracture site and submit for culture and sensitivity testing.

KEY POINT ▶ To avoid bacterial contamination from debrided tissues, use a new, sterile pack for the surgical approach and fracture fixation.

2. *Type I open fractures*—Repair with the appropriate method of external or internal fixation.
   a. If a surgical approach is made to the bone, avoid contact with the traumatic wound to prevent bacterial contamination. Skin drapes may be used.
   b. After fracture fixation, close the wound routinely. Penrose drains or delayed wound closure techniques usually are not necessary.

3. *Type II open fractures*—Repair with the appropriate method of external or internal fixation.
   a. If a surgical approach is made to the bone, avoid contact with the traumatic wound. Skin drapes may be used.
   b. Because bacterial contamination of the wound can be more severe than for type I fractures, provide proper drainage of exudates.
   c. If the surgical wound is closed, place Penrose drains to exit the wound at a site ventral to the surgical incision.
   d. If bacterial contamination is severe, perform delayed (see sec. 5, chs. 17 and 18) or partial wound closure to ensure proper drainage.

KEY POINT ▶ Treatment of most type III open fractures proceeds in the following order: wound care, fracture fixation, and skin reconstruction.

4. *Type III open fractures*—Carefully choose a method that reduces the risk and severity of wound infection.
   a. In general, do not use metallic implants unless adequate wound drainage is assured. Intramedullary (IM) pins are not recommended because of the difficulty in providing surgical drainage from the medullary canal.
   b. Bone plates may be used in conjunction with delayed or secondary wound closure techniques, unless severe infection is present.
   c. External skeletal fixation (see sec. 9, ch. 17) is recommended because a fixator may be constructed that avoids placement of metallic implants directly in the fracture site. However, anatomic considerations may contraindicate their use.

KEY POINT ▶ Regardless of the type of orthopedic implant, rigid fixation is mandatory for definitive treatment of the fracture.

   d. If an external fixator cannot be used, type I external fixator, transarticular external fixator, or external coaptation may be used as temporary fixation so that local wound care and resolution of infection may proceed. When the wound environment has improved, other methods of internal fixation such as bone plates and lag screws may be applied with less risk of infection.

RECONSTRUCTIVE SOFT TISSUE SURGERY

- Primary, delayed primary, or secondary closure techniques (see sec. 5, chs. 17 and 18) may be used to treat traumatic wounds in open fractures.
- Wounds may be allowed to heal by second intention.
- Some wounds may not heal because of their large size, or because they are located at a site of active motion or pressure point (e.g., elbow). In these cases, reconstruct the skin wound with a skin flap or graft (see sec. 5, ch. 19).

- Skin flaps or grafts may be constructed at the time of fracture fixation but often are delayed until a healthy bed of granulation tissue indicates that wound infection is resolved.
- If arthrodesis is the primary method of orthopedic fixation for the carpus or tarsus, skin reconstruction should *precede* the arthrodesis by approximately 1 month. This allows full resolution of soft tissue infection and good soft tissue cover over the proposed arthrodesis site.

Postoperative Care

- Proper postoperative wound care is mandatory to prevent and control infection.
- Keep open wounds bandaged, and replace the bandage daily to prevent accumulation of exudates at the wound site.
- Lavage open wounds daily with sterile saline or lactated Ringer's solution, until the development of healthy granulation tissue indicates resolution of infection.
- Restrict activity, depending on the fracture type and method of fixation.
- Use an Elizabethan collar, if necessary, to prevent the animal from licking its wounds or removing the bandages.
- Stage implant removal to provide optimal bone healing and minimize risk of long-term wound or bone infection.
- Perform a physical examination and obtain radiographs at appropriate intervals to evaluate proper bone healing and resolution of infection.

Complications

- Continued infection suggests the presence of necrotic soft tissue or bone, an unstable fracture site, or unstable orthopedic implants.
- Delayed healing of a fracture may develop from prolonged infection at the fracture site, poor reduction, unstable fixation, or bone loss due to trauma or infection.

KEY POINT ▶ Most complications can be avoided with proper wound management, orthopedic fixation, and postoperative care. Serial examinations to assess progress are essential to avoid development of major problems.

Supplemental Readings

Brinker WO, Piermattei DL, Flo GL: *Handbook of Small Animal Orthopedics and Fracture Treatment*. Philadelphia: W. B. Saunders, 1990, p 50.
Dueland RT: Open (compound) fractures. *In* Brinker WO, Hohr RB, Prieur WD, eds.: *Manual of Internal Fixation in Small Animals*. Berlin: Springer-Verlag, 1984, p 108.
Nunamaker DM: Open fractures and gunshot injuries. *In* Newton CD, Nunamaker DM, eds.: *Textbook of Small Animal Orthopaedics*. Philadelphia: J. B. Lippincott, 1985, p 481.
Richardson DC: Fracture first aid: The open (compound) fracture. *In* Slatter DH, ed.: *Textbook of Small Animal Surgery*. Philadelphia: W. B. Saunders, 1985, p 1945.

27 Osteomyelitis

Kenneth A. Johnson

Osteomyelitis implies inflammation of bone and the soft tissue elements of marrow, endosteum, periosteum, and vascular channels. It is caused most often by infectious organisms. Bacterial osteomyelitis is classified as:

- Acute, with systemic illness and no radiographic alteration in the bone in the first 5–10 days *or*
- Chronic, with progressive destruction and proliferative osseous change beyond 10–20 days.

Traditionally, osteomyelitis has been considered to have a poor prognosis; however, with improved understanding of pathophysiology and proper surgical treatment, it is sometimes curable. Osteomyelitis can mimic panosteitis (see sec. 9, ch. 23), hypertrophic osteopathy (see sec. 9, ch. 23), and neoplasia (see sec. 9, ch. 22); complicate a fracture; or cause nonunion (see sec. 9, ch. 28). It must be differentiated from these diseases.

ETIOLOGY

Bacteria

- Bacterial infections are acquired by direct inoculation, by extension of existing infection, and hematogenously (Table 1).

KEY POINT ▶ Although the type, virulence, and quantity of bacteria are important, bacteria alone will not necessarily cause osteomyelitis. Initiating factors include altered blood flow, soft tissue injury, impaired host tissue defenses, bone necrosis, fracture instability, foreign material, and radiation necrosis of bone (Fig. 1).

- Infections with β-lactamase–producing *Staphylococ-*

TABLE 1. Routes of Infection in Osteomyelitis

Open reduction and internal fixation of fractures; other orthopedic intervention
Open fractures
Extension from soft tissue infection (periodontal disease, rhinitis, otitis media)
Traumatic injuries and bite wounds
Penetrating foreign bodies including sticks and grass awns
Gunshot injury
Hematogenous
Prosthetic joint replacement surgery

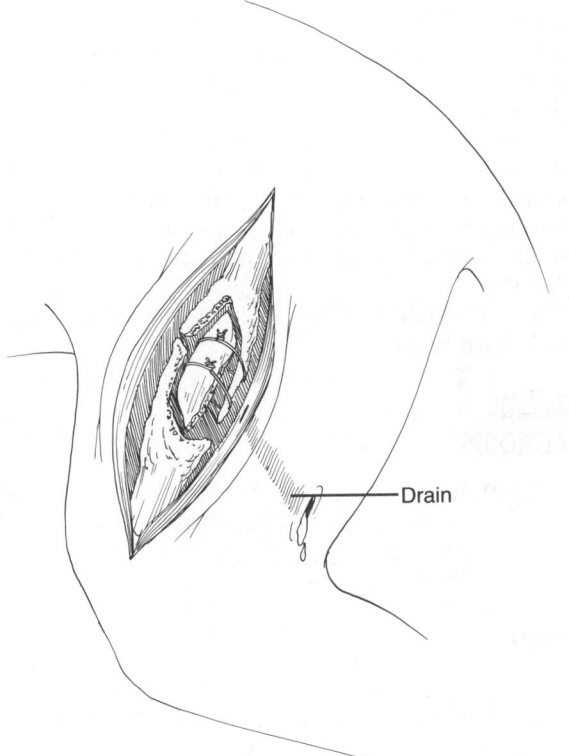

Figure 1. Chronic osteomyelitis with sequestrum, loose unstable implants, and involucrum walling off the focus of infection. These conditions favor chronic bacterial infection, and purulent exudate drains through a dependent sinus.

cus organisms predominate. Other organisms include *Streptococcus* spp., *Brucella canis*, Gram-negative bacteria *(Escherichia coli, Proteus* spp., *Klebsiella)*, and anaerobic bacteria *(Bacteroides* spp., *Actinomyces viscosus, Clostridium* spp.).
- Bacteria colonize the surface of implants and sequestra, producing a coating of mucopolysaccharide called glycocalyx. Glycocalyx prevents resolution of chronic osteomyelitis by protecting bacteria from the actions of phagocytes, antibiotics, and antibodies.

Fungi

- Fungal infections often are multicentric and disseminate hematogenously after pulmonary inoculation (see sec. 2, ch. 12). Most infections involve the metaphyses, flat bones, vertebral bodies, and discs.
- *Coccidioides immitis, Blastomyces dermatitidis, Histoplasma capsulatum, Cryptococcus neoformans,* and *Aspergillus* spp. can cause fungal osteomyelitis.

1091

Corrosion of Implants

■ Corrosion occurs in implants composed of dissimilar metals, such as spring-loaded intramedullary (IM) Jonas pins and vitallium plates with stainless steel screws. A sterile inflammatory response occurs, with localized bone lysis and a draining tract. Secondary bacterial infection subsequently develops.

CLINICAL SIGNS

■ Osteomyelitic lesions invariably are painful and cause lameness, disuse atrophy, and occasional neurologic deficits. Bone fractures may contribute to these signs.
■ Excessive pain, inflammation, or exudation may be the first sign of acute osteomyelitis in the first week following orthopedic surgery or trauma.
■ In chronic osteomyelitis, single or multiple sinus tracts intermittently open and drain mucopurulent exudate.
■ Other nonspecific signs include anorexia, lethargy, and depression.

DIAGNOSIS

KEY POINT ▶ The diagnosis of osteomyelitis usually is based on history, radiology, or microbiology findings or a combination of these.

History

■ Findings may include trauma, open fracture, orthopedic surgery, or travel in an endemic fungal region.

Physical Examination

■ Palpate the musculoskeletal system to localize the involved bone(s).
  • Heat, swelling, redness, and tenderness are present in the acute phase.
  • Muscle atrophy, fibrosis, and contracture are features of chronic disease. Enlarged regional lymph nodes may be palpable.
  • Limb angulation, shortening, instability, and crepitus are present when fracture or nonunion (see sec. 9, ch. 28) coexists with osteomyelitis.
■ Perform a neurologic examination (see sec. 10, ch. 1) to identify concomitant involvement of spinal cord or peripheral nerves.
■ Sinus tracts follow fascial planes and emerge distal or dependent to chronically infected bone (see Fig. 1). Yellow-brown mucopurulent exudate drains intermittently. Inactive tracts are closed with scar tissue.
■ Scarring of the skin and underlying tissues is evidence of previous incisions, drainage, open fracture, trauma, foreign body penetration, fracture surgery, or bone fixation by IM pins or external fixators.
■ Thoracic auscultation and radiography are essential if pulmonary involvement is a possibility.

Hematology

■ Results may be consistent with systemic infection (neutrophilic leukocytosis) in acute osteomyelitis but usually are unremarkable in patients with chronic osteomyelitis.

Radiography and Radionuclide Imaging

Radiography is an important means of evaluating the extent of osteomyelitis, sequestra (dead, avascular bone that has become separated from the viable bone), involucrum (bony proliferation around a sequestrum), and concomitant fracture.

Survey Radiography

■ In acute osteomyelitis, only soft tissue swelling is seen initially.
■ Depending on age of the animal, bone resorption, sclerosis, and periosteal new bone are seen after 5–10 days.
■ Bone sequestra are diagnostic of chronic osteomyelitis.
■ Fracture nonunion due to instability (see sec. 9, ch. 28) can be difficult to distinguish from nonunion due to infection.
■ Fungal osteomyelitis lesions tend to affect the metaphyses and may be multiple, with a lytic, proliferative, or mixed appearance.
■ Deep postoperative wound infections are indistinguishable from acute osteomyelitis because there are no radiographic changes.

Contrast Radiography

■ This modality is useful in some animals for delineation of the course and extent of sinuses and radiolucent foreign bodies.
■ Perform a sinogram (or fistulogram) with water-soluble contrast media (e.g., Urografin 76%) injected slowly through a Foley catheter inserted in the sinus. Inflate the balloon to prevent leakage.

Radionuclide Imaging

■ Imaging of the bone after indium-111 labeling of leukocytes is the most sensitive and specific noninvasive means of detecting osteomyelitis; however, it rarely is needed in routine cases.
■ Indium-111 imaging is indicated in the diagnosis of acute osteomyelitis and when radiographic signs of chronic osteomyelitis are equivocal. Specialized equipment is necessary.

Laboratory Evaluation

Cytology

■ Sterile aspiration centesis can detect and drain fluid accumulations.
■ Stain smears of fluid with Difco Quick to look for toxic neutrophils, phagocytized bacteria, and fungal organisms.

Bacteriology

KEY POINT ▶ Results of tests of cultures from externally draining tracts are an inaccurate representation of causative organisms, as these tracts are often colonized by skin organisms.

■ Obtain aerobic and anaerobic cultures of fluid collected by sterile aspiration from deep within the wound or, preferably, on samples of fluid, necrotic tissue, and sequestra collected at the time of surgical debridement.

Histopathology

■ Histopathologic examination of tissue and bone biopsies is essential if neoplasia (see sec. 9, ch. 22) is suspected.
■ Analysis of methenamine silver and periodic acid–Schiff stained tissue sections can demonstrate fungal hyphae.

TREATMENT

Plan the treatment regimen according to the etiology, chronicity, location, and severity of the osteomyelitis lesion. The majority of osteomyelitis cases are bacterial in origin and chronic. Acute osteomyelitis is diagnosed much less frequently. However, treat soft tissue infections associated with open fractures, trauma, bites, and surgery as if acute osteomyelitis exists, because delays in appropriate treatment invariably lead to chronic osteomyelitis. Manage fungal osteomyelitis as a part of the overall systemic mycotic disease (see sec. 2, ch. 12).

Surgical Procedures

Objectives

■ Identify pathogenic organisms.
■ Determine antibiotic sensitivity.
■ Drain infected tissue.
■ Remove avascular bone (sequestrectomy).
■ Stabilize the fracture.
■ Implant a bone graft to aid osseous union of fractures.

Equipment

■ Standard surgical pack and suture material
■ Volkmann curet
■ Gelpi or Volkmann retractors
■ Silver probe
■ Fracture instruments (external fixator or plate and screws)
■ Bone graft collection instruments

Acute Osteomyelitis

The major objectives of surgery are to debride infected tissue, provide drainage, and stabilize fractures.

Preoperative Considerations

■ Commence antibiotic therapy immediately. The initial choice of antibiotic is empirical.
  • Administer cloxacillin (30 mg/kg q6h) or amoxicillin-clavulanate (20 mg/kg q8h) for suspected β-lactamase–producing *Staphylococcus* infections.
  • Give metronidazole (15 mg/kg q12h) for suspected anaerobic infections.
  • Give Ciprofloxacin (5–11 mg/kg q12h) for suspected gram-negative infection.

KEY POINT ▶ The ultimate choice of an antibiotic depends on results of microbiologic tests.

Technique

1. Aseptically prepare the region for surgery and drape with water–impervious material.
2. Expose focal osteomyelitic lesions by removal of overlying normal cortical bone with a drill or Volkmann curet, to allow drainage.
3. Open infected surgical wounds extensively by removal of sutures. Debride necrotic muscle, fascia, hematoma, foreign material, and nonfunctional sutures. Collect samples for microbiologic tests.
4. Open and drain traumatic wounds (e.g., bites) and open fractures, making a surgical incision to allow dependent drainage.
5. Keep wounds open to permit adequate drainage and irrigation.
6. Cover exposed bone with viable muscle.
7. Metallic implants can be left exposed, but cover with a sterile dressing.

KEY POINT ▶ Closed suction drainage systems and Penrose drains are contraindicated because they provide ineffective drainage and potentiate ascending infections and abscessation.

8. If the fracture fixation is stable, treat osteomyelitis without removal of the implants, until healing or loosening of implants occurs.

KEY POINT ▶ Bone can heal in the presence of infection, provided there is stable fixation.

9. Loose implants lead to the unfortunate triad of fracture instability, persistence of infection, and bone resorption (Fig. 2). Remove loose implants immediately, and stabilize the fracture with another device.

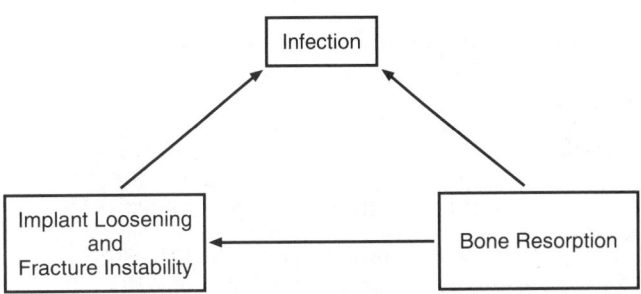

Figure 2. The unhappy triad of osteomyelitis.

10. External skeletal fixation is the preferred method for providing both temporary and definitive fracture stability in the tibia, mandible, and radius-ulna, where active osteomyelitis exists.
    a. The large muscle groups surrounding the femur and humerus allow application of only type I or biplanar (pins placed laterally and cranially) external fixation. These configurations may not provide sufficient stability for healing, owing to excessive pin-bone stress, soft tissue necrosis around pins, pin tract osteomyelitis, and premature pin loosening.
    b. Use plates only secondarily, after the infection becomes quiescent, and when an external fixator is no longer effective.
11. Irrigate wounds intraoperatively with 1–2 liters of sterile physiologic saline, under pressure with a 60-ml syringe.

Postoperative Care and Complications

- Repeat daily irrigation, using sterile technique, until infection is controlled.
- After 3–5 days, wound closure with granulation tissue begins to occur. Reopen the wound if drainage and irrigation are not possible.
- Pack dressings of sterile, dry gauze or paraffin-impregnated gauze into the wound. Cover this with a layer of viscose-cast padding and conforming cotton bandage and adhesive elastic bandage.
- Protect incisions on the trunk or upper limbs with a tie-over bandage (extend over the dorsum of the animal).
- Elizabethan collars provide further wound protection until healing is complete.
- Select antibiotics on the basis of bacteriologic findings, and administer for 4–6 weeks.
- Obtain radiographs at intervals of 7–14 days to evaluate fracture fixation and healing, and progress of osteomyelitis.

Chronic Osteomyelitis

Preoperative Considerations

Assess soft tissue in regard to vascularity, peripheral nerve injury, muscle contracture, joint stiffness, and pain to determine if a cure is feasible or if amputation is indicated. In animals with phalangeal osteomyelitis, immediate digit amputation (see sec. 9, ch. 20) is an acceptable treatment.

Technique

1. Expose the infected bone, using an appropriate approach, to remove sequestra and debride necrotic tissue and bone.

KEY POINT ▶ Careful search for and removal of sequestra is crucial for success of surgical treatment of osteomyelitis.

  a. Sequestra may migrate and become trapped in a draining sinus some distance from the original infection.

  b. Elevate extensive involucrum with a chisel to reach sequestra and establish drainage.
2. To prevent a pathologic fracture, support bone weakened by extensive debridement with external fixation (see sec. 9, ch. 17) or a splint.
3. Chronic osteomyelitis often is a sequela of fracture repair by internal fixation. Stabilize these fractures to allow healing of the fracture (see Acute Osteomyelitis).
4. Remove implants composed of dissimilar metals that are responsible for corrosion and osteomyelitis. Provide alternative stable fixation if the fracture is ununited.
5. Keep wounds open and irrigate with sterile saline solution (see Acute Osteomyelitis).
6. After 7–10 days, graft bone defects caused by debridement, osteomyelitis, or fracture with autologous cancellous bone, when granulation tissue permits rapid vascularization and incorporation of the graft (Fig. 3). Cancellous bone grafts are not at risk of sequestration.

Postoperative Care and Complications

- Select antibiotics on the basis of the bacteriology and administer for 4–6 weeks.

KEY POINT ▶ It is useless to proceed with treatment of chronic osteomyelitis with antibiotics, unless microbiologic culturing, surgical drainage, sequestrectomy, and fracture stabilization are meticulously performed.

- Obtain radiographs at intervals of 7–21 days to assess progression of healing and resolution of infection.
- If there is lack of response to treatment or recurrence of osteomyelitis, one or more of the following may be necessary:
  • Re-examine for sequestra.
  • Repeat debridement.
  • Reestablish drainage.

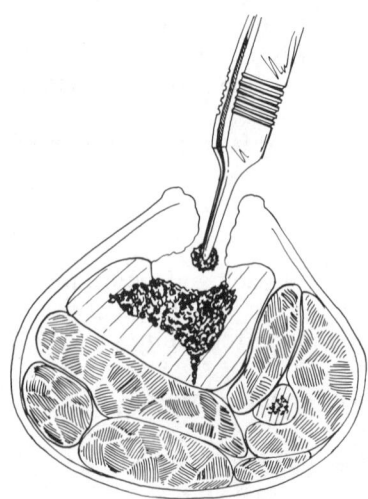

Figure 3. Autologous cancellous bone grafting of fractures and bone deficits in chronic osteomyelitis after the infection is controlled and healthy granulation tissue fills the wound. The graft is inserted by elevation of granulation tissue or via a separate approach through normal tissues.

- Reevaluate fracture stability.
- Perform a bone graft.
- Repeat microbiology tests.
- Change the type of antibiotic.
▪ Use skin grafts (see sec. 5, ch. 19) or myocutaneous flaps to cover extensive open wounds on the distal limbs that fail to close by second intention healing.
▪ Implant removal is necessary after healing of fractures.

Supplemental Readings

Brinker WO, Hohn RB, Prieur WD: *Manual of Internal Fixation in Small Animals*. Berlin: Springer-Verlag, 1984, p 112.

Newton CD, Nunamaker DM: *Textbook of Small Animal Orthopaedics*. Philadelphia: J. B. Lippincott, 1985, p 499.

Weber BG, Cech O: *Pseudarthrosis, Pathophysiology, Biomechanics, Therapy, Results*. Bern: Hans Huber, 1976.

28 Delayed Union, Nonunion, and Malunion

Randy J. Boudrieau

DELAYED UNION AND NONUNION

Healing times for similar fractures in any single group of patients are fairly uniform; however, a small number will have longer than "normal" healing times, or may fail to heal. The particular type of fracture (comminuted or simple), the bone involved and location (distal radius/ulna or midshaft humerus), the age of the animal, and the type of fixation utilized all influence normal healing times.

- Classification:
  - When the fracture requires longer than normal time to heal but shows definitive signs of progression in healing, it is classified as a *delayed union*.
  - A fracture that does not heal over a similar period and that has no tendency toward further healing is classified as a *nonunion* (Table 1).

Other classifications are based on fracture site, fragment displacement, and presence or absence of infection.

Delayed Union. Delayed union usually needs no other therapy than continuation of ongoing treatment of the fracture. Continued immobilization (assuming stable fixation) allows healing to eventually occur in the majority of cases. A delayed union, however, may be preliminary to a nonunion.

Nonunion. Nonunion results from local factors at the fracture site, because most fractures unite within a reasonable time despite systemic factors such as malnutrition, generalized metabolic or endocrine abnormalities, and acute or chronic generalized disease states. In most cases, these local factors can be identified (Table 2). Nonunion requires some form of surgical intervention in order for healing to progress.

KEY POINT ▶ The most common cause of delayed or nonunion is inadequate fixation and resulting instability at the fracture site.

Problems Related to Nonhealing Fracture. Patients with nonhealing fractures may have additional problems related to function, such as disuse muscle atrophy, decreased range of joint motion and stiffness related to scar tissue contraction, neurovascular dysfunction, and limb angulation and/or shortening.

Anatomy

Bone Healing

- Bone heals by either primary (haversian remodeling) or secondary (periosteal callus) union.
- Secondary bone healing, with formation of visible periosteal callus, begins with connective tissue formation that progresses to form fibrocartilage and finally bone.
- Primary bone healing occurs without formation of connective tissue; bone deposition occurs directly (fracture gaps <0.8 mm) without any visible callus. Familiarity with these concepts allows accurate sequential evaluation of the healing process.

Histology

- The most notable histologic feature is increased periosteal cartilage in the callus in lieu of bone formation.
- Persistent fracture gaps at the bone ends (sometimes greater than that present at the time of the original fracture) are filled with cartilage/fibrocartilage callus.
- Sclerosis of the bone ends at the fracture site may occur, effectively sealing the medullary cavity.

Preoperative Considerations

Clinical Signs

- Pain usually is present at the level of the fracture, and movement of this area may be detected clinically (occasionally these areas are relatively stable and are pain-free).
- Palpable enlargement of the fracture area is present.

TABLE 1. Expected Approximate Healing Times of Uncomplicated Diaphyseal Fractures with Minimal Loss of Cortical Bone

Age of Animal	External Skeletal and Intramedullary Pin Fixation	Bone Plate Fixation*
<3 mo	2–3 wk	4 wk
3–6 mo	4–6 wk	2–3 mo
6–12 mo	5–8 wk	3–4 mo
>1 yr	7–12 wk	5–8 mo

*Fractures stabilized by this method may not be considered clinically healed (have sufficient strength) as early as fractures stabilized by other means of fixation, because direct cortical union (primary bone healing by haversian remodeling) is not supported by periosteal callus. This is of primary importance when considering timing of implant removal. Clinical function is not adversely affected by this method of fixation because plates provide rigid fixation.

TABLE 2. Factors Associated with Delayed Union and Nonunion

Local Factors*
Fracture location
Fracture gap
    Soft tissue interposition
    Bone loss secondary to trauma
Soft tissue trauma
    Loss of blood supply as a result of initial trauma
Contamination, infection
Neoplasia

Treatment Factors†
Malposition (inadequate reduction)
Fracture gap
    Soft tissue interposition
    Distraction (by implants or external fixation devices)
    Bone loss due to intraoperative removal
Soft tissue trauma
    Loss of blood supply due to surgical trauma
Inadequate fixation (internal or external)‡
    Instability
Postoperative infection

*Related to the fracture.
†Related to reduction and fixation.
‡Most common factor.

- Muscle atrophy and joint stiffness are likely sequelae to limb disuse.
- The affected limb usually is non–weight bearing.

Diagnosis

Radiographic Evaluation

- Radiographic signs vary, depending on the extent of healing (delayed union versus nonunion) and the type of delayed or lack of healing observed; classification of these events is the basis for treatment.
- Radiography allows sequential evaluation of healing:
  - *Delayed union*: There is continued healing, albeit slow, as indicated by progressive callus formation and resorption of dead bone. A persistent fracture line with evidence of some nonbridging callus is characteristic. The marrow cavity remains open without evidence of significant sclerosis of the bone ends.
  - *Nonunion*: There is no evidence of progression of fracture healing (i.e., little or no change on sequential radiographic evaluation). Smooth fracture surfaces (no periosteal "irritation") are typical, with evidence of sclerosis at the bone ends and sealed marrow cavities.
- Assess treatment factors relating to the fracture fixation. For example, a small, radiolucent halo visible around a loose device (screws, wires, etc.) or a change in the position of the implants on serial radiographs indicates implant instability.

KEY POINT ▶ Base differentiation of a delayed union from a nonunion not only on time but, more specifically, on serial radiographic evaluation.

Surgical Plan

- Always prepare for at least one autogenous cancellous graft donor site.

- Obtain tissue from the fracture site for aerobic and anaerobic bacterial culture and sensitivity testing.
- Administer perioperative antibiotics (Keflin, 40 mg/kg, IV, once before or during surgery). Continuation of antibiotic therapy depends on culture results.
- If infection is present (see sec. 5, ch. 18) consider open wound management (and secondary wound closure with an autogenous cancellous bone graft at a later date).
- If primary closure is performed, consider closed suction drainage of the fracture site.
- Decide whether to increase the stability of the fixation without disturbing the fracture site (delayed union or viable nonunion) or to debride the fracture site and add an autogenous cancellous bone graft in addition to increasing the stability of the fixation (nonviable nonunion).

KEY POINT ▶ If necessary, change the fixation to obtain rigid stability.

- Rigid stability is best achieved with screw and plate fixation. Place the plate under tension in order to compress the fracture fragments together and thus use the frictional forces generated at the point of fragment contact to increase stability.
- Consider options for treatment of soft tissue complications (e.g., joint stiffness, contracture).

Surgical Procedure

Objectives

- Increase the stability of the reduction by increasing or changing the fixation (consider plating the fragments under tension).
- Debride the fracture site as necessary to provide restimulation for fracture healing.
- Perform autogenous cancellous bone grafting if necessary to promote osseous union.
- Restore satisfactory function of the affected bone and joint.

Equipment

- Standard orthopedic pack and suture material
- Implants, preferably screw and plate fixation (may require a separate tension device in order to obtain greater compression at the fracture site)
- Oscillating saw (for making osteotomy cuts)
- Bur set or rongeurs (for debriding fragment ends)
- Curets for procurement of cancellous grafts
- Closed suction drainage system

Technique

1. Prepare the affected limb for aseptic surgery. Aseptically prepare a suitable donor site for harvest of autogenous cancellous bone. Usually the wing of the ilium and the proximal humerus yield a large amount of bone graft.
2. Make a standard anatomic approach to the affected bone, preserving all soft tissue structures. A large amount of fibrous connective tissue probably is adhered to the overlying muscle bellies; identifica-

tion of the various tissue planes is generally difficult and requires sharp dissection. Exercise caution when approaching sites of major neurovascular structures.

3. Obtain samples for aerobic and anaerobic bacterial culture and sensitivity testing of the fracture site.

4. *Delayed union or viable nonunion*: Increase the stability of the fixation with implants such as additional IM pins or application of an external skeletal fixator (see sec. 9, ch. 17), or change the implant device (e.g., type III external skeletal fixator or bone plate placed under tension).

5. *Nonviable nonunion*:
   a. Debride the fracture site. Remove any loose metal, dead bone, sequestra, and infected tissue.
   b. Remove the fibrous connective tissue in the fragment gap by local debridement (bur or rongeurs) or transverse ostectomy (1.0–2.0 cm) of the entire nonunion site (Fig. 1). *Note*: the latter technique creates a small amount of limb shortening, but this is generally not a functional problem in animals, owing to their flexed joint stance.
   c. Reestablish medullary continuity (and therefore the medullary circulation) by drilling the sclerotic bones (Fig. 2).
   d. "Shingle" or decorticate as shown in Figure 3 (Judet technique).
   e. Place an autogenous cancellous bone graft around the debrided fracture site. To prevent possible contamination, use separate sterile instruments to procure and place the graft. Bone grafts may not be necessary in cases in which the nonunion site has been ostectomized back to healthy bone, and circumferential fragment contact is ensured under stable, compression plate fixation. Add a cancellous graft if any doubt concerning healing exists.
   f. When utilizing plate fixation, a separate tension device may be required in order to achieve adequate fragment compression if >4.0 mm of compression is desired.

6. If the tissues appear healthy, routinely close the incision. Place closed suction drains if any question

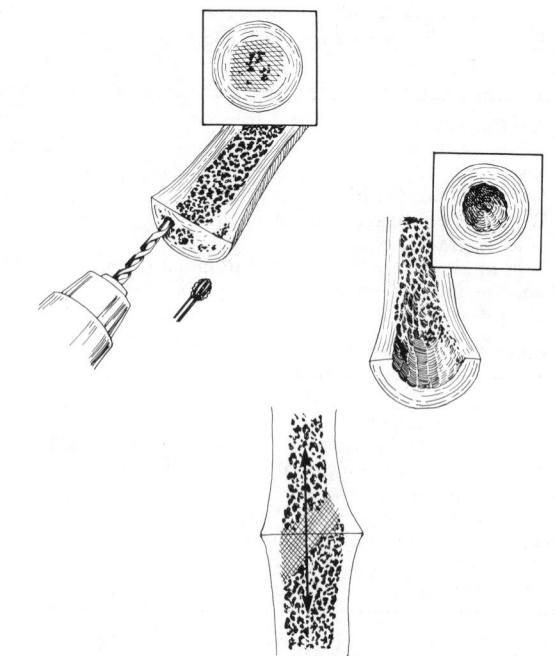

Figure 2. Following an osteotomy or debridement of the fracture site, the medullary canal may remain sealed by the remaining sclerotic bone at this level. *Top, left*, Medullary continuity is reestablished by drilling from the fracture site into the medullary canal or by using a bur. *Center, right*, the end of this process is shown. *Bottom*, Both fracture fragments are reapposed and medullary continuity is reestablished *(arrow)*. Insets show cross sections of bone. Hatched areas depict removed sclerotic bone.

of contamination/infection exists or if dead space with continued diffuse bleeding is present.

7. Open wound management is indicated if tissues appear grossly infected; perform delayed primary

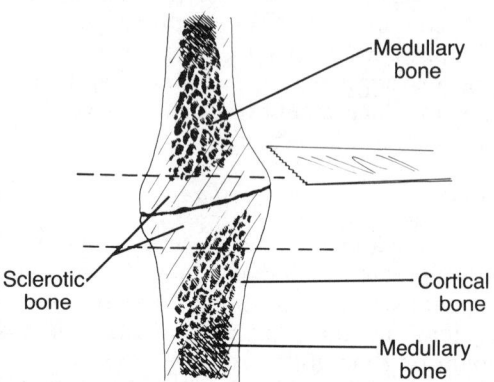

Figure 1. Nonviable nonunion with sealed medullary cavity (sclerotic bone at fracture margin). Dotted lines indicate level of osteotomy cuts made to remove 1.0–2.0 cm of bone, essentially ostectomizing the entire nonunion site.

Medullary bone

Sclerotic bone

Cortical bone

Medullary bone

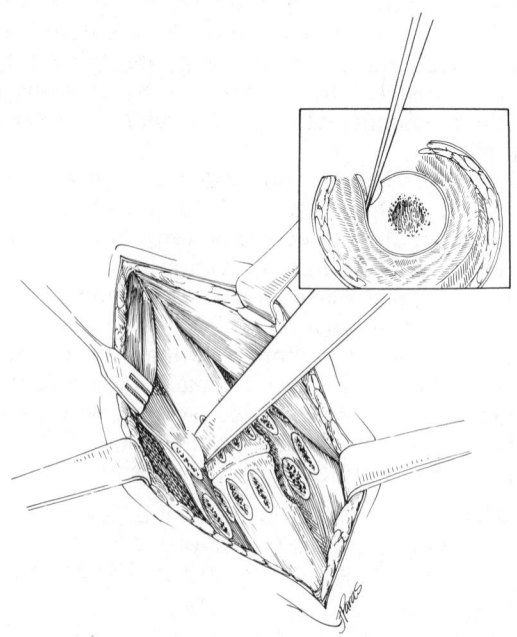

Figure 3. Small cortical chips of bone are elevated from the shaft but remain attached to the surrounding soft tissues (Judet technique). A chisel *(inset)* is used to elevate these fragments of bone after the periosteum is split longitudinally with a scalpel.

closure and autogenous cancellous bone grafting, at a later date, when a healthy granulation tissue bed has developed (see sec. 9, ch. 17).

8. Healing proceeds provided fixation is stable in presence of infection.

Postoperative Care and Complications
Physical Therapy

▪ Perform passive range of motion of joints adjacent to the surgical site.
▪ Perform or encourage active range of motion exercises (controlled) such as short walks and swimming.
▪ Encourage weight bearing (controlled). Limb use favors improved circulation and exercise of the musculature, which in turn improves the local fracture environment.

Open Wound Management

▪ Change bandage(s) at least once daily (pack entire wound with wet-to-dry gauze). Keep the soft tissues and (more important) bone moist. The goal is establishment of a healthy granulation tissue bed to cover both bone and implant (may be difficult owing to the physical size of the plate).
▪ Perform delayed primary closure, usually with the addition of an autogenous cancellous bone graft. Consider using closed suction drains and a compression bandage if dead space is present.
▪ Following apparently successful open wound management of infected wounds, persistent drainage and local or diffuse incisional dehiscence (usually over the implant) may occur. Continued wound management is required during fracture healing, and the implants are left in position if stability can be maintained. Subsequent implant removal is necessary to finally eliminate the infection.

Prognosis

▪ The prognosis generally is good, provided a severe functional deficit (joint contraction, etc.) or overwhelming infection is not present at the onset of treatment.
▪ Limb shortening usually does not result in a major functional abnormality if not more than 20–30% of length is lost; however, the gait will be altered due to mechanical lameness.

MALUNION

Many fractures heal with some degree of deformity without significant effect on function or appearance. These are not considered true malunions. Malunion implies a union with deformity sufficient to cause a functional and/or cosmetic defect. Malunion can occur as a result of untreated or improperly treated fractures.

Malunion may result in angular and rotational deformities, limb shortening, and soft tissue adhesions. These problems may directly affect adjacent joint function by alteration of the articular surfaces and/or supporting ligamentous structures. They also may affect the adjacent joints indirectly through changes in the functional angles placed on the joint and the abnormal stresses thus placed on the ligaments and joint capsule. Joint involvement, either direct or indirect, may result in decreased range of joint motion and degenerative joint disease (see sec. 9, ch. 29). Correction of the malunion is accomplished by osteotomy through the area of greatest deformity, followed by realignment with stable skeletal fixation.

Precise fracture management can prevent malunion. Serial radiographic evaluation of the fracture throughout the healing period is essential to ensure continued appropriate fragment apposition and alignment. If a deformity is identified early, immediate corrective measures may prevent further complications.

Preoperative Considerations
Diagnosis

▪ Carefully evaluate the entire limb for bone and joint problems. Define the area of the long bone with the greatest amount of deformity: bowing of the bone in the cranial-caudal aspect, varus/valgus angulation, or rotational abnormalities along the axis of the bone. For example, a distal radial malunion resulting from premature distal ulnar physeal growth arrest (see sec. 9, ch. 11) results in cranial bowing, carpal valgus, and external rotation of the distal radius.
▪ Define the orientation of the adjacent joints. All axes of joint rotation should be parallel to the weight-bearing surface (e.g., a distal radial malunion resulting from premature distal ulnar physeal growth arrest results in angling of the radiocarpal joint surface cranially and medially). Depending on the duration of the deformity, severe derangements of the intercarpal joints also may be present.
▪ Assess adjacent structures to the malunion for abnormalities of orientation and function (e.g., degenerative joint disease, joint contraction, altered range of motion).

KEY POINT ▶ Undertake surgical therapy for malunion only when the procedure is justified by the impairment of function or cosmetic defect.

Surgical Plan

▪ Determine the amount of angulation present in the awake, weight-bearing animal and compare with that in the opposite normal limb.
▪ Determine the amount of angulation observed on radiographic evaluation of the involved limb and compare with radiographs of the opposite normal limb. Carefully determine joint axis orientation.
▪ Compare and collate information derived from the physical examination and the radiographic evaluation to determine the amount of correction (angle) of osteotomy required.
▪ Using a duplicate radiograph of the involved limb, draw the limb and joint axes and plot the angle of correction at the area of greatest deformity.
  • Cut the radiograph along the predrawn lines and place in the corrected position to evaluate the planned osteotomy cut and the expected result, making adjustments as necessary.

- This two-dimensional radiograph allows correction to be planned in only *two* planes: cranial-caudal and medial-lateral. Determine the remaining rotational deformity by observation at the time of surgery. (See sec. 9, ch. 11 for more information about growth deformities of the radius and ulna.)

Surgical Procedure

Objectives

- Straighten the limb by corrective osteotomy.
  - The closing wedge osteotomy is the most versatile and easy to use technique. The loss of bone length is approximately equal to the width of wedge removed.
  - Other osteotomy techniques (reverse wedge, oblique, and dome) are more difficult to perform and/or less precise in the correction of the malunion.
- Provide stable fixation.
  - Apply a plate with bone fragments placed under tension for maximal stability.
  - Alternatively, apply Kirschner-Ehmer external skeleton fixation (see sec. 9, ch. 17) when a very short fragment must be stabilized adjacent to a joint.

Equipment

- Standard orthopedic pack and suture material
- Implants (preferably screw and plate fixation, external skeletal fixator, Kirschner wires)
- Oscillating saw
- Goniometer (for measuring angles)

Technique (Closing Wedge Osteotomy)

1. Determine the angle of correction, based on the previously evaluated radiographs and physical examination.
2. Prepare the affected limb for aseptic surgery. Consider aseptic preparation and full draping of the opposite normal limb in the operative field for use as a comparison (especially important with chondrodystrophic-breed dogs).
3. Perform a standard surgical exposure of the bone at the level of greatest deformity.
4. Use Kirschner wires as marker pins to define:
   a. The axis of rotation of the adjacent joint at both ends of the bone
   b. Perpendicular to the long axis of the bone (parallel to the adjacent joints) at the level of the greatest deformity
5. Make the first osteotomy cut parallel to the Kirschner wire that is defining the axis of rotation of adjacent joint (this takes into consideration the rotational correction in addition to the cranial-caudal correction).

6. Make the second osteotomy cut parallel to the second Kirschner wire. Cut so that the width at the apex of the wedge is minimal, thereby removing the least amount of bone.
7. Reduce both bone fragments (full contact with both osteotomy surfaces) and temporarily secure with two small crosspins (Kirschner wires). Make any necessary adjustments further at this time.
8. Apply plate fixation to both bone fragments under tension (standard ASIF, i.e., Association for the Study of Internal Fixation, technique, including prestressing of the implant), and then remove crosspins.
9. Close the surgical wound routinely.

Postoperative Care and Complications

- Provide standard postoperative care as for any fracture fixation, including exercise restriction and physical therapy. Evaluate the postoperative conformation and gait.
- Persistent, mild cosmetic disfiguration requires no further therapy.
- Continued functional problems require further, more precise surgical correction.
- Complications include:
  - Inadequate or over-correction of the deformity
  - Continued functional problems due to other, previously unrecognized abnormalities (e.g., degenerative joint disease, abnormal range of motion)
  - Slightly decreased range of joint motion when the fixation device is placed immediately adjacent to the joint (generally not a functional limitation)
  - Slight limb shortening (generally not a functional limitation)
  - Infection (as can occur after any surgical procedure)
  - Delayed union or nonunion

Prognosis

- The prognosis generally is good with proper case selection.

Supplemental Readings

Binnington AG: Delayed union and nonunion. *In* Slatter DH, ed.: *Textbook of Small Animal Surgery*. Philadelphia: W. B. Saunders, 1985.

Brinker WO, Hohn RB, Prieur WD, eds.: *Manual of Internal Fixation in Small Animals*. Berlin: Springer-Verlag, 1984.

Newton CD: Principles and techniques of osteotomy. *In* Newton CD, Nunamaker DM, eds.: *Textbook of Small Animal Orthopaedics*. Philadelphia: J. B. Lippincott, 1985.

Piermattei DL, Greeley RG: *An Atlas of Surgical Approaches to the Bones of the Dog and Cat*, 2nd Ed. Philadelphia: W. B. Saunders, 1979.

Rudy RL: Corrective osteotomy for angular deformities. Vet Clin North Am 1:549, 1971.

Weber BG, Cech O: *Pseudoarthrosis: Pathology, Biomechanics, Therapy, Results*. Bern: Hans Huber, 1976.

29 Degenerative Joint Disease

David M. Clark

Degenerative joint disease (DJD), a debilitating condition commonly seen in small animals, is characterized by loss of hyaline cartilage matrix and death of chondrocytes. It is more common in dogs than cats, although both species can be affected.

KEY POINT ▶ Although normal aging results in articular cartilage changes, it does not usually produce DJD.

Because it is presently very difficult, perhaps impossible, to cure DJD, prevention is the best treatment. Most therapy for animals affected by DJD is palliative and aimed at alleviating clinical signs.

Osteoarthritis is commonly used as a synonym for DJD but is somewhat inaccurate since it implies an inflammatory process.

ANATOMY AND PHYSIOLOGY

- Diarthrodial joints possess hyaline cartilage tightly bound to the cortical end plates of the bones composing the joint. This cartilage is made up of chondrocytes embedded in a matrix of proteoglycan, collagen, and water that provides load-bearing properties to the tissue.
- Chondrocytes are responsible for the synthesis and maintenance of the matrix in which they are embedded.
- Chondrocytes exist in an environment isolated from the rest of the body by the matrix they generate; they lack innervation and an intrinsic blood supply and are limited in their repair response to injury.
- The joint is enclosed by a well-vascularized joint capsule, which has a deep synovial layer and a superficial fibrous (supporting) layer. A small amount of joint fluid, a derivative of serum, is contained within the normal joint.
- Articular cartilage is nourished primarily by diffusion of nutrients from the joint fluid, assisted by normal motion of the joint (the synovial pump).

ETIOLOGY

- Degenerative joint disease may occur after a joint sustains an injury such as an intra-articular fracture or infection, following prolonged immobilization, when instability (e.g., hip dysplasia) or malarticulation are present, or as a sequela to developmental joint diseases such as osteochondrosis.
- Disruption of normal biomechanics, interference of cartilage nourishment by diffusion from synovial fluid, or alteration of normal intra- or extracellular environments can stimulate the formation and release of degradative enzymes from chondrocytes, and later from synoviocytes and leukocytes, that cause loss of cartilage matrix.
- Loss of matrix decreases the ability of the tissue to withstand the stress of use, leading to further insult, cartilage breakdown, and eventually death of chondrocytes.
- Cartilage breakdown products and prostaglandins from the above processes irritate the synovial membrane, causing pain when the affected joint is moved.

CLINICAL SIGNS

- In most cases, animals affected by DJD are presented with a history of episodic lameness or dysfunction that is made worse by extended periods of inactivity, such as sleeping overnight or cage confinement.
  - The lameness may improve after light activity; the owner may observe that the animal tends to "warm out" of the lameness.
  - Unusually strenuous activity often results in an increase in severity of the lameness after a rest period.
  - Mild to complete non–weight-bearing lameness may be seen.
- The frequency and severity of the discomfort and dysfunction may increase as the disease progresses.

DIAGNOSIS

Diagnosis of DJD is usually suggested by the history and physical examination, supported by radiographic findings, and occasionally confirmed by analysis of joint fluid. Eliminate septic, infectious, and immune-mediated joint disease from the list of differential diagnoses; these joint problems are relatively uncommon in small animals.

History

KEY POINT ▶ Carefully question the client to obtain any history of previous injury, disease, or dysfunction of the affected joint.

Physical Examination

- Physical examination reveals one or more joints that evoke pain reactions when manipulated. Such joints may not be obviously swollen.

- In many cases, movement of the affected joint produces *crepitus*, a grinding sensation felt by the examiner that is comparable to that perceived by rubbing coarse sand on a smooth, hard surface. This is due to loss of cartilage from joint surfaces and/or the presence of osteophytes (see below).
- Joint laxity may be present on palpation.

Radiographic Examination

Evaluation of radiographs of the affected joint can reveal:

- *Osteophytes* (new bone formation) at the points of joint capsule attachments—these are a hallmark of DJD.
- *Subchondral sclerosis*—this is probably due to biomechanical changes within the joint as it loses cartilage.
- In severe or long-standing cases, *the joint space may appear to be narrowed*. Employ careful radiographic techniques and be cautious in evaluation, because this appearance can be an artifact caused by malpositioning. Radiography of the affected joint *while it is bearing weight* is the most reliable method for evaluating joint space collapse.
- Evidence of predisposing disease or injury is seen.

KEY POINT ▶ The early pathophysiologic processes of DJD take place before radiographic evidence of the disease is present. Radiographic signs of DJD indicate that the problem is chronic.

Evaluation of Joint Fluid

- Perform aspiration of joint fluid, using sterile technique, with a 20–22 gauge hypodermic needle and a 3- to 6-ml syringe.
- In cases of DJD, cytologic and biochemical analyses usually indicate that the pathologic process in the joint is *nonseptic* and *noninflammatory*.
- This test is useful for differentiating DJD from the bacterial, rickettsial, and autoimmune arthritides (see appropriate chapters). See sec. 9, ch. 30, for a comparison of joint fluid composition in various joint diseases.

TREATMENT

The goal of medical treatment is to minimize clinical signs and discomfort so as to maximize comfortable function. In most instances this is possible, but the condition of many animals tends to worsen over time and become unresponsive to therapy. New drugs currently under evaluation may prove to be effective in halting the degenerative process.

KEY POINT ▶ The accepted therapies for DJD are directed at pain relief (palliation); treatment cannot alleviate the primary physiologic processes in affected cartilage.

Drug Therapy

Nonsteroidal Anti-Inflammatory Drugs (NSAIDs)

Buffered Aspirin (Acetylsalicylic Acid)
- Aspirin is the mainstay of therapy in animals with DJD. It is commonly given with a small meal at a dose of 20–25 mg/kg q8h, PO; smaller doses may be tried initially.
  - Its desired effect is the analgesia it provides, because in most cases of DJD inflammation is minimal.
  - In severe cases in which synovial inflammation is more prominent, the anti-inflammatory effects at the above doses may be helpful.
- In dogs, side effects are few and usually are limited to gastric irritation. This side effect can be controlled with H_2-receptor blockers that inhibit gastric acid secretion (see sec. 7, ch. 4).
- Use aspirin with caution in cats; a dose of 10 mg/kg q52h, PO, has been suggested, but experience with aspirin therapy in cats with DJD is relatively limited.

Phenylbutazone
- Phenylbutazone often is administered in animals in which buffered aspirin is not tolerated, although some prefer to use it as the first treatment.
- Give at a dose of 0.5–1.0 mg/kg q8h, PO; the effects are similar but not identical to those of aspirin.
- In dogs, side effects may include gastric irritation and bone marrow depression.
- Do not use phenylbutazone in cats.

Ibuprofen
- Ibuprofen occasionally is used at a dose of 5 mg/kg q8h, PO, in dogs. This drug may have superior analgesic properties to the aforementioned drugs, in that response is sometimes seen after all else has failed; however, several cases of secondary perforating gastric ulcers have been observed (by the author).
- Use extreme caution if giving this drug; it is not generally recommended. Control gastric acidity with H_2-receptor blockers (e.g., cimetidine), as described in sec. 7, ch. 4.

Other NSAIDs
- A plethora of other NSAIDs is available.
- Few, if any, have been rigorously evaluated for animal use, and therefore these drugs are not recommended.
- Fatalities have resulted from the use of some NSAIDs in dogs and cats.

Corticosteroids

- Systemic corticosteroids, in varying dosages and regimens, have been used for alleviation in severe cases of DJD.
- Because of known serious systemic side effects, use corticosteroids such as prednisone (1–2 mg/kg q12h, PO; then decrease dose) only as a last attempt to control discomfort and dysfunction.
- There are no known evaluated protocols for intra-articular corticosteroid therapy for DJD in small animals, although corticosteroids occasionally are used in this manner.

KEY POINT ▶ Corticosteroids and NSAIDs are known to have deleterious effects on articular cartilage. NSAIDs exert this effect on degenerating cartilage only, but corticosteroids affect *normal* cartilage. Design therapeutic regimens to administer the minimum amount of drug necessary to control signs.

Other Anti-Inflammatory Medications

- Drugs such as orgotein and dimethyl sulfoxide (DMSO) have been employed to reduce the discomfort of DJD.
- Rigorous evaluation of these protocols is lacking; use of these compounds should be minimal until more information is available concerning their safety and efficacy.

Chondroprotective Agents

- Compounds such as polysulfated glycosaminoglycans have shown promise as chondroprotective agents in treatment of DJD. Apparently, they inhibit the generation or action of the chondrodestructive enzymes responsible for matrix breakdown.
- Treatment regimens remain to be established, and controlled clinical trials are necessary before use of these drugs in small animals can be recommended.

Surgery

No surgical procedure can arrest the progression of DJD. However, various procedures can be employed to salvage limb function.

Resection Arthroplasty

- The best example of arthroplasty is excision of the femoral head and neck for DJD affecting the hip joint (see sec. 9, ch. 14). Removal of the joint eliminates pain and in most cases returns acceptable function.
- Such procedures have been successfully used on the scapulohumeral joint as well.

Joint Replacement

- Replacement of a degenerating joint with an artificial one is largely limited to the canine hip (see sec. 9, ch. 14), although a human finger joint prosthesis has been used to replace the feline stifle joint.

Arthrodesis

- Arthrodesis, or the surgical fusion of a joint, is an effective way of eliminating the discomfort from a degenerating joint. Obviously, because complete loss of normal range of motion of the joint results, function is affected.
- Generally, arthrodesis of joints below the elbow and stifle in the dog allows acceptable function; arthrodesis performed above these levels results in significant gait alterations and may not be as successful (see appropriate chapters for discussion of arthrodesis of specific joints).

Supportive Care

Nearly all patients affected by DJD in the appendicular skeleton will benefit from:

- Body weight reduction—These patients should carry as little body weight as is practical and consistent with good health. Initiate reducing diets for obese animals. The results of body weight reduction can be very rewarding.
- Exercise—Encourage *moderate and consistent* exercise. Periods of heavy exercise followed by periods of little activity generally exacerbate the signs of DJD.

PREVENTION

KEY POINT ▶ By far, the most effective method of treating DJD is to prevent it.

- Accurate and timely diagnosis of joint disease and effective early treatment of articular fractures, disorders of cartilage maturation, ligamentous injury, and primary joint infections will minimize the chances of development of DJD.
- The use of newer agents such as polysulfated glycosaminoglycans early in the course of treatment may allow cartilage preservation by arresting the cycle of cartilage degeneration.

Supplemental Readings

Clark DM: The biochemistry of degenerative joint disease and its treatment. Compend Contin Educ Pract Vet 13:275, 1991.

Hammerman D: The biology of osteoarthritis. N Engl J Med 320:1322, 1989.

Howell DS: Etiopathogenesis of osteoarthritis. *In* McCarty DL, ed.: Arthritis and Allied Conditions: A Textbook of Rheumatology. Philadelphia: Lea & Febiger, 1990, p 1595.

30 Immune-Mediated Joint Disease

David M. Clark

Immune-mediated joint disease is an uncommon but important cause of lameness in dogs. It is one of a class of diseases in which the immune system inappropriately attacks normal structures, leading to discomfort, dysfunction, and in some cases destruction of the affected joints. Like similar diseases in humans, these diseases currently are not curable, but treatment may result in remission of signs and improved quality of life for varying periods of time.

In the dog, the immune-mediated arthropathies often are classified as:

- *Erosive*—There is destruction of cartilage, subchondral bone and ligaments or tendons.
- *Non-erosive*—Connective tissue destruction is not a primary feature of the disease.

In this chapter, the etiology, clinical signs, diagnosis and treatment of these two forms of arthritis are compared and contrasted. (See sec. 3, ch. 3 for information on systemic immune-mediated diseases.)

ETIOLOGY

Despite extensive investigation, the exact etiology of immune-mediated joint disease is not known.

Erosive Forms

- The erosive forms (including rheumatoid arthritis) arise from an alteration in host IgG molecules that become antigenic. IgM antibody (rheumatoid factor) is then formed in response, and complexes with the altered IgG. Phagocytosis of these immune complexes and activation of complement trigger an inflammatory response in the synovial membrane and periarticular tissues that ultimately results in the clinical and pathologic signs of the disease.
- Canine erosive joint disease is very similar to the disease described as rheumatoid arthritis in humans.

Nonerosive Forms

- The nonerosive forms are most commonly seen in small animals and are characterized by deposition of immune complexes in synovial tissue as well as many other tissues, again inciting an inflammatory reaction. When such immune complexes involve *antinuclear antibodies*, this disease is termed systemic lupus erythematosus (SLE) in animals and humans (see sec. 3, ch. 3) but is rarely recognized in dogs.
- Most canine cases of immune complex–mediated arthritis are *idiopathic*.

- In cats, a chronic progressive polyarthritis with a predilection for distal joints has been presumed to be immune-mediated, although infectious agents (feline leukemia virus (FLV), feline syncytium-forming virus, *Mycoplasma* spp.) also may play a role.

KEY POINT ▶ In contrast to degenerative joint disease, the initial site of pathophysiology in immune-mediated joint disease is the synovial membrane, not the articular cartilage.

CLINICAL SIGNS

Erosive Form

- This form primarily affects toy- and small-breed dogs; the average age of onset of signs is approximately 4 years, although all ages may be affected.
- The onset often is insidious. Initial signs of shifting limb lameness, joint swelling, and episodic fever/lethargy frequently progress to more severe multijoint involvement.
- As joint destruction occurs, angular deformities in the affected limbs may be seen. In general, the most distal joints on the limb are affected first, but all diarthrodial joints are susceptible.

Nonerosive Form

- This form primarily affects medium-size and large-breed dogs, with an average age of onset of 5–6 years.
- Common signs are an acute onset of episodic fever/lethargy, swelling in more than one joint (the distal joints are at greater risk of involvement) and joint capsular/periarticular swelling. Affected dogs ambulate with short strides and may appear to be "walking on eggshells."
- Range of motion of affected joints may be decreased initially, but animals with long-standing disease may experience ligamentous damage with resultant instability.

DIAGNOSIS

- Diagnosis of immune-mediated joint disease is suggested by the history and physical examination, supported by radiographic examination, and confirmed by nonspecific and specific clinical laboratory tests, joint fluid analysis, results of histologic evaluation of synovial biopsies, and response to therapy.

KEY POINT ▶ In the differential diagnosis of immune-mediated joint disease, eliminate degenerative joint disease, infectious/septic arthritis, and diffuse muscular/neuromuscular or metabolic disease as potential causes of similar clinical signs.

Physical Examination

- Physical examination confirms the presence of the lameness and detects swollen joints, joint laxity, and/or angular deformities.
- Evaluate all joints to determine the extent of involvement.
- About 30% of dogs with the nonerosive form have some type of dermatopathy (see sec. 5, ch. 9).
- Lymphadenopathy and splenomegaly occasionally are noted as extra-articular signs of rheumatoid arthritis.

Radiographic Evaluation

Erosive Form

- Early in the disease, periarticular swelling, joint capsular swelling, and osteoporosis of juxta-articular bone are evident. As the disease progresses, subchondral bone cysts are seen and articular cartilage is lost, beginning at joint margins.
- The joint space eventually may collapse and, as capsular and ligamentous support of the joint is lost, deformity, especially in the carpal and tarsal areas, becomes evident.
- Signs of secondary degenerative joint disease (see sec. 9, ch. 29) may be seen and may complicate radiographic diagnosis.

Nonerosive Form

- In contrast to the erosive form, radiographic findings are limited to joint capsule distension and periarticular soft tissue swelling.
- Occasionally secondary changes consistent with degenerative joint disease are seen, particularly in long-standing cases in which joint instability is present.

Laboratory Evaluation

- A complete blood count (CBC) in immune-mediated joint disease generally indicates the presence of nonseptic inflammation.
- SLE-associated polyarthritis can occur with autoimmune hemolytic anemia and thrombocytopenia.
- Routine serum chemistry evaluations usually are normal, but over 50% of patients with the nonerosive form have a persistent proteinuria due to glomerular involvement in this disease (see sec. 3, ch. 3).
- Some specific laboratory tests may be useful in documenting the existence of immune-mediated joint disease. These tests involve the detection of rheumatoid factor (an antibody of the IgM class), antinuclear antibodies, and neutrophils that have engulfed antibody-coated nuclear debris of another cell (LE cells).

- Table 1 illustrates the results seen in both forms of immune-mediated joint disease; these tests substantiate but do not establish definitive diagnosis. Differences in laboratory techniques may further cloud the issue; clinicians should familiarize themselves with their laboratory's protocols and interpret results received accordingly.

KEY POINT ▶ Negative serologic tests do not rule out immune-mediated arthropathies and are consistent with the idiopathic form of the disease.

Joint Fluid Analysis

Analysis of joint fluid aspirated from an affected joint is a critical step in the diagnosis of immune-mediated joint disease and will usually reveal a marked inflammatory response.

- White cell counts per cubic millimeter range from 2000–3000 to 100,000, but most will be in the range of 10,000–30,000.
- The predominant cell type is the nondegenerative neutrophil; lymphocytes, plasmacytes, monocytes and macrophages also can be seen. No microorganisms should be evident cytologically or upon culture of the fluid obtained.
- See Table 2 for a comparison of joint fluid analysis in various arthropathies.

KEY POINT ▶ Joint fluid analysis documents the presence of inflammation but may not distinguish inflammation from infection.

Synovial Biopsy

In cases in which the diagnosis of immune-mediated joint disease is elusive, histologic evaluation of synovial tissues may prove useful when such findings are correlated with clinical data.

- Perform open biopsy using strict sterile technique.
- Harvest synovial tissue and if possible a section of the cartilage–bone margin from the edge of the joint for examination. If an infectious or septic etiology is suspected, submit these tissues for culture to identify the causative agent.

TABLE 1. Comparison of Clinical Laboratory Findings of Tests to Detect Immune-Mediated Disease

Test*	Results	
	Erosive	Nonerosive
Rheumatoid factor	+ in 25% of cases	−
Antinuclear antibody	Occasionally detected	+ in some cases
LE cells	Rarely detected	+ in some cases

*Recall that all tests may be negative in idiopathic immune-mediated arthritides.

+ = positive; − = negative.

TABLE 2. Comparison of Results of Joint Fluid Analysis in Different Classes of Joint Disease*

Disease	Mucin Clot	Appearance	WBC Count (mm³)
Normal	+	Clear	0–2900
DJD	+	Clear	<3000
Immune-mediated	±	Turbid	>5000; neutrophils are well preserved
Septic arthritis	−	Very turbid	Usually >60,000; degenerate neutrophils

*Isolation or observation of significant numbers of any microorganism from joint fluid is highly supportive of an infectious or septic etiology, regardless of cell count. Cell counts in immune-mediated and septic joints may be similar in many cases.

WBC = white blood cell; DJD = degenerative joint disease; + = positive; ± = can be positive or negative; − = negative.

Erosive Form

■ The joint capsule is thickened, with hypertrophy of the villi. Fibrovascular granulation tissue (pannus) can be seen invading from the joint margins and destroying cartilage and bone in its path.
■ Histologically, many plasma cells, lymphocytes, and small blood vessels can be observed in the subsynovial area of the joint capsule. Cartilage and subchondral bone loss often is apparent.

Nonerosive Form

■ Pannus formation and destruction of articular cartilage and bone are not prominent.
■ The joint capsule is thickened, and there is accumulation of plasma cells, lymphocytes and neutrophils in the subsynovial region.

KEY POINT ▶ It is more important to distinguish immune-mediated joint disease from other arthropathies than it is to determine the form of immune-mediated joint disease. Treatment is similar for most cases of immune-mediated joint disease.

TREATMENT

The immune-mediated arthritides are difficult to cure; rheumatoid arthritis currently is considered incurable and relatively unresponsive to therapy.

■ Inform the client that treatment is aimed at control-

ling autoimmune processes while minimizing clinical signs. In some cases, therapy must be carried out for the life of the animal, although animals with the idiopathic form may experience extended remission of signs after therapy is tapered and discontinued.

Anti-inflammatory Drug Therapy

■ Steroidal and nonsteroidal anti-inflammatory medications are used to decrease the inflammatory reaction resulting from antigen-antibody complex stimulation. Additionally, immunosuppression with corticosteroids and other potent chemotherapeutic agents is used to control destructive autoimmune reactions. Such therapy is fraught with potential complications (see sec. 3, ch. 5).
■ Frequent adjustments of therapeutic regimens often are necessary, and accurate patient monitoring is critical for optimal results.
■ It is common to try several drugs or drug combinations before discovering which is best for the patient.
  • Warn the client that recurrence or worsening of signs may occur.
■ Table 3 lists several drugs and regimens that have been used with some success. In general, when remission of signs is achieved, gradually decrease dosage to lowest effective maintenance dose.

KEY POINT ▶ Prior to initiating any immunosuppressive therapy, be sure that infectious or septic diseases such as pyometra, bacterial endocarditis, and septic arthritis are not present.

TABLE 3. Drug Regimens Used for Control of Immune-Mediated Arthritis*

Drug	Dose	Action	Comments
Acetylsalicylic acid (aspirin)	20–25 mg/kg q8h PO	Analgesic; anti-inflammatory	Generally more effective for degenerative joint disease
Glucocorticoids (Prednisone, prednisolone)	1–2 mg/kg q12h until remission achieved; then decrease to lowest effective maintenance dose	Anti-inflammatory; immunosuppressive	First choice for nonerosive forms; can be used alone or in combination with other drugs
Cyclophosphamide* (Cytoxan; Mead Johnson)	1.5–2.5 mg/kg PO, q24h 4 days/week	Immunosuppressive	Monitor WBC count; watch for hemorrhagic cystitis (see sec. 3, ch. 5)
Azathioprine* (Imuran; Burroughs Wellcome)	*Dogs:* 2 mg/kg, q24h PO *Cats:* 0.5 mg/kg, q24–48h PO	Immunosuppressive	Monitor WBC count; relatively toxic in cats
Gold sodium thiomalate (Solganal; Schering)	1 mg/kg IM once weekly	Unknown	Used in erosive forms; limited clinical experience

*Glucocorticoids are commonly administered with this drug.

Surgery

Surgery generally plays a minor role in the treatment of immune-mediated joint disease.

- In erosive forms, arthrodesis of badly damaged joints has been advocated to preserve limb function; however, the processes that originally destroyed the joint are still ongoing in the postarthrodesis patient.
  - Unless the joint capsule can be completely removed (difficult to accomplish), immune-mediated destruction of the healing arthrodesis may occur.
- In the nonerosive forms, subtotal synovectomy may provide a period of relief for the patient. This technique has not been widely adopted by veterinarians.

Supportive Care

Nearly all patients will benefit from:

- Body weight reduction—Body weight should be as minimal as is practical and consistent with good health. Institute reducing diets for obese animals.
- Exercise—Encourage light to moderate exercise. Heavy exercise even during periods of minimal clinical signs can injure the affected joints.

Supplemental Readings

Hulse DA: Diseases affecting the joints. *In* Harvey CE, Newton CD, Schwartz A, eds.: *Small Animal Surgery*. Philadelphia: J. B. Lippincott, 1990, p 627.

Lipowitz AJ: Immune-mediated arthropathies. *In* Newton CD, Nunamaker DM, eds.: *Textbook of Small Animal Orthopaedics*. Philadelphia: J. B. Lippincott, 1985, p 1055.

Rosenthal RC: Chemotherapy. *In* Slatter DH, ed.: *Textbook of Small Animal Surgery*. Philadelphia: W. B. Saunders, 1985, p 2405.

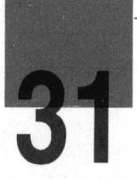

31 Lyme Disease

Paul A. Manley

Lyme disease (borreliosis) is a polysystemic disease caused by the spirochete *Borrelia burgdorferi*. The disease has been associated with polyarthritis in dogs, cattle, horses, and human beings. In Wisconsin, Minnesota, and in eastern coastal states, borreliosis is transmitted to animals and people by the bite of the deer tick, which acts as a host of the spirochete. *Borrelia* species belong to the eubacterial phylum of spirochetes (as do *Leptospira* and *Treponema*). *B. burgdorferi* is easy to isolate from ticks but is difficult to isolate from clinically affected patients. The outer membrane of the spirochete can undergo antigenic variation during the course of infection, which may limit the effectiveness of a vaccine.

ETIOLOGY

Borrelia burgdorferi is carried by the deer tick, *Ixodes dammini*. In California and other western states, *I. pacificus* is believed to be the carrier; in the southeastern states, *I. scapularis* has been implicated. Other species of ticks, including *Amblyomma americanum* and *Dermacentor variabilis* (the dog tick), and insects such as horse flies, deer flies, and mosquitoes can carry *B. burgdorferi*; however, only ticks have been linked with disease transmission. The route of infection is via the bite of an infected tick.

Borreliosis commonly affects hunting dogs, but they are incidental hosts. Deer support the adult population of *I. dammini* but are not believed to become infected by the spirochete. Mice are the main reservoirs of borreliosis because they maintain the larval and nymphal stages of *I. dammini* and can become infected with the spirochete. Birds may be important reservoirs because they have the ability to transmit ticks and spirochetes over long distances.

CLINICAL SIGNS

- Polyarthritis is the most common clinical sign reported in dogs. The arthritis is usually subclinical but may be septic or immune-mediated because of the presence of the spirochete in the synovium and/or synovial fluid.
- Systemic signs include anorexia, weight loss, lethargy, lymphadenopathy, and pyrexia; however, the animal may show no systemic signs other than lameness.

DIAGNOSIS

History

- Lameness can be acute or chronic and progressive.
- Often systemic signs may be traced to exposure of the animal to a wooded environment or a tick-infested area.

Physical Examination

- Swelling of one or more joints may be evident.
- There may be signs of considerable pain on palpation of the joints with no evidence of joint instability.

Laboratory Evaluation

- Immunofluorescent antibody (IFA) tests and enzyme-linked immunosorbent assays (ELISA) are the most accurate diagnostic test; serums titers <1:128 = negative; 1:128–1:256 = low positive; 1:512 and up = highly positive.
  - In an endemic area, a positive titer can be an incidental finding.
- Evaluate animals with a negative titer and clinical signs suggesting borreliosis for immune-mediated causes of polyarthritis (see sec. 9, ch. 30); retest in 1 month for Lyme disease.
- Animals with a high titer and no clinical signs suggesting disease may have been exposed recently to *B. burgdorferi*. Retest in 1 month; a rising titer indicates active infection.
- Joint fluid analysis for titers may help to establish a diagnosis; also joint fluid of dogs with Lyme disease may show neutrophilic inflammation.

Radiographic Evaluation

- Radiographically, there is evidence of joint effusion, but usually little or no evidence of degenerative joint disease.

TREATMENT

- Treat all dogs with clinical signs suggestive of borreliosis and a positive titer antibiotics for 14–21 days. Appropriate choices are tetracycline (15–25 mg/kg q8h), doxycycline (10 mg/kg q12h), and cephalexin (22 mg/kg q8h).
- Animals with active infection should show a rapid response to antibiotic therapy. If the therapy is effective, retest in 1–3 months to confirm the diagnosis (rising titer).

- If the initial response to therapy is poor, consider alternative antibiotics and other diagnoses.
- Prolonged antibiotic therapy is sometimes required.

PREVENTION

- A vaccine for Lyme disease in dogs has been conditionally licensed and marketed. The vaccine is a killed bacterin, which has been tested for efficacy on experimental animals challenged with *B. burgdorferi*.
  - Little information exists about the vaccine's ability to protect against natural infection with *B. burgdorferi*, and safety of the vaccine has not been confirmed in infected and serologically positive dogs that are asymptomatic. For these reasons, this vaccine currently cannot be recommended.

- Reduce the risk of exposure of animals by limiting access to tick-infested areas.
- Use of tick repellents, such as dips, sprays, and powders, and reduction of the tick population in the environment may help to reduce the incidence of Lyme disease.
- Periodically check animals for ticks and promptly remove them to decrease exposure to *B. burgdorferi*.

Supplemental Readings

Cohen ND, Cohen D: Borreliosis in horses: A comparative review. Compend Contin Educ Pract Vet 12:1449, 1990.

Kimminau KM: Lyme disease in pets and people: An update. Compend Contin Educ Pract Vet 10:385, 1989.

Roush JK, Manley PA, Dueland RT: Rheumatoid arthritis subsequent to *Borrelia burgdorferi* in two dogs. J Am Vet Med Assoc 195:951, 1989.

Neuromuscular System

William R. Fenner

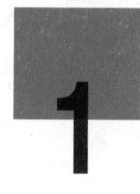

1 Diagnostic Approach to Neurologic Disease

William R. Fenner

PRINCIPLES OF NEUROLOGIC EXAMINATION

Objectives

- Confirm that neurologic disease is present.
- Localize the site of any lesion(s).
- Determine the extent to which the nervous system is involved.
- Assist in the choice of diagnostic aids.
- Determine the prognosis.

Approach

As you perform the examination, try to be logical, methodical, and consistent.

- Develop a consistent sequence and follow it with all patients.
- Begin with the general and advance to the specific.
- Perform painful portions of the examination last.

PROCEDURES FOR THE NEUROLOGIC EXAMINATION

General Observations

Mental Status

Mental status is regulated by the brain stem and cerebrum and consists of level and content of consciousness.

- Begin by evaluating the level of consciousness. A normal animal is alert; an abnormal animal is de- pressed, stuporous, or comatose, depending on the severity of the mental depression. Abnormal levels of consciousness may result from lesions of the brain stem or cerebrum.
- In addition to the level of consciousness, evaluate the patient for mentational disorders. Behavior of a normal animal is described as appropriate; an animal with abnormal behavior is considered demented.
  - A demented animal is unaware and unconcerned with its surroundings. It may head-press, walk off tables, and in other ways show a complete disre- gard for its own safety and well-being.
  - Dementia is a sign of a cerebral disorder.

Head Posture

Head posture is regulated by the vestibular system.

- A normal animal holds its head in a plane parallel to the ground.
- If an animal holds one ear closer to the ground than the other ear, it is described as having a head tilt.
- In some animals, the chin is tucked under or pulled tightly toward the sternum; this postural abnormality (ventroflexion) may be seen in cats with polymyopa- thies (e.g., hypokalemia) or thiamine deficiency and in dogs with atlanto-axial-occipital malformations.

Coordination of Head Movement

This is regulated primarily by the cerebellum. Disturbances of head coordination appear as head tremors.

Circling

Circling is a nonspecific finding in animals with brain disease.

- A lesion in any part of the brain may cause circling; the animal usually circles toward the diseased side.
- Circling in brain stem and cerebellar injury usually is a result of a vestibular injury, therefore, circling is accompanied by a head tilt.
- It is not known why animals with cerebral injury circle, but they rarely have head tilts.

Gait and Stance

Gait

A normal gait requires the integration of almost the entire nervous system; therefore, an abnormal gait may be the result of injury to almost any part of the nervous system.

- Sensory disturbances, such as loss of proprioception, usually result in ataxia or loss of coordination of limb movements. Signs of loss of coordination of the limbs include swaying, veering, crossing over of the limbs, and scuffing of the toes.

KEY POINT ▶ Ataxia may be seen with disease or injury of the cerebellum, brain stem, spinal cord, and peripheral nervous system (PNS) injuries to the spinal nerves or to cranial nerve 8 (vestibular nerve). A cerebral lesion rarely causes ataxia.

- Cerebellar lesions cause ataxia in most patients.
- Cerebral lesions produce weakness characterized by stumbling, falling, tripping, and inability to initiate or sustain activity. Weakness may be caused by an injury to the cerebrum, brain stem, spinal cord, and peripheral spinal nerves. When classifying the weakness, also consider the resting muscle tone in the limbs.
- Spasticity is an increase in muscle tone resulting in decreased flexion of the limbs during movement. As a result, the gait is rigid and choppy.
  - Spasticity implies a lesion of the upper motor neuron (UMN), and may be seen with injuries to cerebrum, brain stem, and some levels of the spinal cord.

Stance

Normal animals stand with their limbs at about shoulder or hip width, with the weight equally distributed on all four limbs.

- Abnormal posture may be caused by a diminished sense of position (proprioception), weakness, or pain.
- Many animals present with abnormal posture as the result of pain from orthopedic disorders rather than neurologic disturbances.

Tests of Postural Reactions

Attitudinal and postural (A-P) reactions test the integrity of the interconnecting pathways that regulate posture and movement as an extension of the evaluation of gait and stance. These tests evaluate the proprioceptive fibers of peripheral nerve, spinal cord, brain stem, cerebrum, and cerebellum. Some tests also evaluate special proprioception. The upper motor neurons and their connections to lower motor neurons are also evaluated.

Because so many portions of the nervous system are evaluated, A-P reactions are good screening tools for detecting nervous system disorders, but are not very helpful with specific localization.

- With lesions of the cerebrum, the clinical deficit normally is seen in the limbs on the opposite side of the body (contralateral) from the diseased hemisphere.
- With brain stem lesions, the clinical signs usually are bilateral but are worse on the same side (ipsilateral) as the brain stem injury.
- With lesions of the cerebellum, spinal cord, and peripheral nerves, the clinical signs are almost always on the same side of the body as the nervous system injury.
- With cerebellar injuries, A-P reactions usually are present but are ataxic.
- With peripheral vestibular injuries, A-P reactions are preserved, but the animal tends to lean, fall, and roll to the diseased side when the maneuvers are performed.
- With lesions in other regions in the nervous system, A-P reactions generally are lost or absent.

Proprioceptive Positioning

A limb is abnormally abducted or adducted, or the paw is turned so that the animal bears weight on the dorsal surface of its paw (stands knuckled over). If A-P reactions are intact, the animal briskly brings the limb back to a normal resting position.

Hemihopping

The limbs on one side are held off the ground while the patient is hopped sideways on its other two limbs. A normal animal has no trouble maintaining itself during this test.

Wheelbarrowing

The thoracic or the pelvic limbs are held off the ground while the patient is walked forward and then backward on its other two limbs. A normal animal has no trouble maintaining itself and walking normally during this test.

Other A-P Reactions

Additional A-P reactions include the extensor postural thrust reaction, righting reaction, visual placing reactions, tactile placing reactions, and tonic neck reactions. All these tests evaluate the same basic pathway, although each may test one portion of the nervous system more completely than another. These tests are well described in standard neurology texts.

Cranial Nerve (CN) Examination

The CN examination involves testing the function of each CN. In most cases, the presence of a CN deficit confirms the presence of a lesion above the foramen magnum. The CN examination allows precise localization of intracranial diseases in many cases. Because many CNs supply only the motor or the sensory component of CN reflex, but not both, the testing of a CN reflex generally involves testing more than one nerve. This is unlike spinal reflexes in which generally the sensory and motor components of a reflex are both carried by the same nerve.

Many of the CN reflexes also are under higher control. Therefore, a CN reflex evaluates:

- two peripheral CNs (one motor and one sensory)
- a central connection (usually the brain stem)
- a higher regulatory center (usually the cerebrum)

A lesion in any one of these sites may cause loss of the reflex being tested. For a more complete review of the neuroanatomy of CNs, consult a neuroanatomy textbook.

Menace Response
(Also see sec. 11, ch. 11)

The menace response tests CN2 (sensory) and CN7 (motor) and their central connections in the brain stem and cerebrum. The test is performed by making a menacing gesture toward an animal. The normal response is an avoidance response (for example, an eye blink or turning of the head).

- Loss of the menace response normally indicates a lesion in one of the following sites: retina (ipsilateral), optic nerve (ipsilateral), optic tract (contralateral), cerebrum (contralateral), brain stem (ipsilateral), or facial nerve (CN7) (ipsilateral).
- Some animals with cerebellar disorders may have an ipsilateral loss of the menace response as well.
- False-positive menace responses also occur, most commonly when the movement of the hand produces air currents that stimulate the corneal reflex.
- Sounds and other distractions may make the menace response difficult to evaluate.

Pupillary Light Reflex (PLR)
(Also see sec. 11, ch. 11)

This tests the reflex portion of the optic nerve (CN2) and the visceral function of the oculomotor nerves (CN3). The test is performed by illuminating the eye with a bright light source. The normal response is rapid constriction of both pupils.

The pupillary constriction in the eye being illuminated is called the *direct pupillary response,* the constriction in the opposite pupil (the one being illuminated indirectly) is called the *consensual response.* Failure of one or both pupils to constrict is an abnormal PLR.

- A lesion of CN2 produces loss of constriction in both pupils when the affected eye is illuminated; however,

when the normal eye is illuminated, both pupils constrict.
- If the lesion is in CN3 or the brain stem, the affected pupil fails to constrict regardless of which eye is being illuminated, but the unaffected eye constricts normally when each eye is illuminated.
- Because ophthalmic diseases such as posterior synechia or severe iris atrophy may also produce loss of pupillary responsiveness, a thorough eye examination is essential in any patient with abnormal pupils (see sec. 11).
- Other causes of a misleading PLR are increases in sympathetic tone and a weak light source, both of which will slow the PLR.

Pupillary Symmetry

In this test the eyes are observed for equal pupils.

- If CN3 and the sympathetic nerve to the eye are normal, the two pupils will be equal in size.
- If the pupils are unequal (anisocoria), this indicates possible damage to one of these two nerves.
  - If CN3 is abnormal, the large pupil is denervated and the PLR will be absent in that eye.
  - If the sympathetic nerve is abnormal, the small pupil is abnormal and the PLR will be normal in both eyes.
- Cats may have mild, physiologic anisocoria if one eye is receiving more light than the other. For this reason, ensure that both eyes receive equal illumination when evaluating for anisocoria.
- A number of ophthalmic disorders may produce anisocoria, including glaucoma, iritis, uveitis, and synechia (see sec. 11). Because of this, all patients with anisocoria should have a complete ophthalmic examination.

Pupillary Size

The size of the pupil is determined by the amount of ambient light (CN2) and the integrity of the innervation of the pupillary muscles (CN3 and sympathetic nerve).

- Abnormally large pupils may be caused by excitement (sympathetic stimulation), bilateral optic nerve injury, CN3 paralysis, or ophthalmic disease.
- Abnormally small pupils may be associated with loss of sympathetic tone, excess parasympathetic tone, or ophthalmic disease.

Ocular Position

In normal dogs and cats, both eyes look in the same direction at any given time (normally straight ahead). This normal resting position is determined by the influence of the cerebrum and CN8 on the extraocular muscles (CNs 3, 4, and 6). If one of these portions of the nervous system is not functioning, deviation of one or both of the eyeballs may occur.

Strabismus is the term used to describe deviation of only one globe.

- Medial strabismus may result from an injury to CN6 (abducens nerve).
- Ventrolateral strabismus may result from injury to CN3 or CN8 (vestibulocochlear nerve).
- A lesion to CN4 (trochlear nerve) results in intorsion (a form of rotation) of the eye, which can be recognized only in animals with oval pupils or on ophthalmic examination.
- Passive deviation of both eyes in the same direction (gaze paresis) is sometimes seen in cerebral injuries.

Ocular Motility

Voluntary Eye Movement. Voluntary eye movement is initiated by cerebral stimulation of (CNs 3, 4, and 6). As the animal looks around the examination room, it is observed to see if it appears unable to move the eyes in one or more directions.

- With a cerebral lesion, both eyes are involved, and there is a tendency for the eyes to look toward the diseased cerebral hemisphere.
- With a lesion of the cranial nerves, only one eye is involved. The involved eye will tend to have strabismus at rest and totally lack the ability to move.

Involuntary Eye Movements—Nystagmus. Involuntary rhythmic oscillations of the eyes, termed nystagmus, can be induced by turning the head. This maneuver stimulates CN 8, which in turn stimulates CNs 3, 4, and 6, which innervate the extraocular muscles. This involuntary eye movement is called physiologic nystagmus.

Physiologic Nystagmus. Physiologic nystagmus is characterized by rhythmic oscillation of both eyes, first moving slowly away from the direction in which the head is turning, and then moving rapidly in the same direction. This recurring slow-fast, slow-fast oscillation continues as long as the head is moving.

- A lesion of CN 8 or its central connections may result in loss of the ability to initiate physiologic nystagmus, so that neither eye will move.
- A lesion of one or more of the cranial nerves that innervate the eyeball itself (CN 3, 4, or 6) paralyzes only that eye, resulting in loss of physiologic nystagmus in the paralyzed eye.

Pathologic Nystagmus. When a normal animal's head is not moving, it does not display any involuntary eye movements. If nystagmus is present when the head is at rest, this is a sign of nervous system disease and is called pathologic nystagmus. This usually is the result of an imbalance in the special proprioceptive system, which includes the inner ear, brain stem, cerebellum, and CN8. A lesion of any of these structures can cause pathologic nystagmus. Features of pathologic nystagmus that may help localize its origin include the *direction, method of induction,* and *persistence* of the nystagmus.

- Direction of nystagmus:
  - In *horizontal nystagmus,* the eyes move in a plane parallel to the head (i.e., the eyes move from side to side).

KEY POINT ▶ Horizontal nystagmus is most commonly seen in peripheral vestibular disease (see sec. 5, ch. 23). The "fast" component of the nystagmus usually is away from the diseased side.

- In *vertical nystagmus,* the eyes move in a plane perpendicular to the head (e.g., the eyes move up and down).

KEY POINT ▶ Vertical nystagmus is most commonly seen in central vestibular disease. The fast component of the nystagmus is usually away from the diseased side; therefore, brain stem disease causes upgoing nystagmus, and cerebellar disease causes downgoing nystagmus.

- In *rotatory nystagmus,* the eyes rotate in a clockwise or counterclockwise direction in the orbit, with components of both horizontal and vertical movement. This type of nystagmus is not localizing; it may occur with a lesion anywhere in the special proprioceptive system.
- Method of induction of nystagmus:
  - *Resting nystagmus* occurs when the head is at rest and in a normal position. This type of nystagmus is most characteristic of peripheral vestibular disease.
  - *Positional or induced nystagmus* occurs when the head is still but is in an abnormal position (e.g., on its side or upside down). Positional nystagmus is most characteristic of central vestibular dysfunction (e.g., brain stem and cerebellar lesions). It is also seen during the recovery phase of peripheral vestibular diseases.
- Persistence of nystagmus:
  - *Permanent nystagmus* persists over time. It may have any direction and method of induction, but it is consistently present. Permanent nystagmus is characteristic of all brain stem diseases and of progressive peripheral vestibular and cerebellar diseases.
  - *Resolving nystagmus* disappears over a period of 10–14 days. It does not recur unless there is new damage to the vestibular system. Resolving nystagmus is characteristic of nonprogressive peripheral vestibular and cerebellar diseases. In this period, nystagmus may become positional (recovery phase).

Facial Symmetry

Facial paralysis (CN7) may result from injury to the contralateral cerebrum, ipsilateral brain stem, and ipsilateral peripheral nerve.

- Clinical signs include drooping of the lip, deviation of the nasal philtrum, increases in palpebral fissure (pseudoptosis), and in some animals true ptosis (drooping of the eyelid).
- Confirm the diminished muscle function by testing the palpebral and/or corneal reflexes.

Palpebral Reflex

This reflex tests CN5 and its brain stem connection to CN7.

- Initiate the reflex by touching the palpebral margins, which produces an eye blink. Generally complete loss of the eye blink occurs.
- In some animals with incomplete paresis of CN5 or 7 lagophthalmos or incomplete closure of the palpebral margins is observed.

Corneal Reflex

Like the palpebral reflex, this reflex tests CN5 and its brain stem connection to CN7.

- Initiate the reflex by lightly touching the cornea, which produces an eye blink.

Retractor Oculi Reflex

This reflex tests CN5 and its brain stem connection to CN6 (abducens nerve).

- Initiate the reflex by lightly touching the cornea, which produces retraction of the eye into the orbit.
- Lack of the reflex usually is a sign of neurologic dysfunction.
- In some animals with loss of the retrobulbar fat pad, the eye may be enophthalmic and incapable of retraction, whereas in others, a retrobulbar mass may prevent retraction.

Facial Sensory Examination

This tests CN5 and its cerebral connections.
Lightly stimulate the nasal mucosa, which should produce an avoidance response such as head turning.

- The nasal mucosa is a more reliable site for stimulation than the lips, which are relatively insensate in some animals.

Gag Reflex

The gag reflex, which is easier to test in dogs than in cats, tests CN9 (glossopharyngeal nerve) and CN10 (vagus nerve) and their brain stem connections.

- To initiate the test, lightly stimulate the oropharynx, which should produce a swallowing reflex. Loss of the reflex usually indicates brain stem or peripheral nerve dysfunction.
- Examine the pharynx for evidence of paralysis of the soft palate, and look at the larynx for evidence of laryngeal paralysis. (may be difficult in an awake animal) Either conditions may result from brain stem injuries or peripheral nerve injuries to CN9 or CN10.

Tongue Examination

- Look for atrophy of the tongue, which can be produced by brain stem or peripheral nerve injury to CN12.
- Also look for deviation of the tongue, which can be caused by cerebral injuries as well as brain stem and peripheral nerve injuries.

Spinal Reflex Examination

The spinal segmental reflexes directly test the reflex arcs of the spinal cord. They also indirectly test the higher centers in the brain that regulate the spinal reflexes.

KEY POINT ▶ If an injury occurs within the reflex arc, it will cause loss of the reflex. Such a reflex loss allows precise localization of a nervous system injury. Because a lesion in the lower motor neuron (LMN) is involved, loss of reflexes is called an LMN sign of an LMN reflex change.

KEY POINT ▶ If a lesion occurs cranial to a reflex arc, it disconnects the reflex from its higher (brain) regulation. This regulation tends to be inhibitory, and thus loss of regulation results in exaggeration of reflexes. Because this exaggeration reflects a lesion in the CNS, involving upper motor neuron (UMN) pathways, these reflex changes are called UMN signs or UMN reflexes.

UMN changes are not as precisely localizing as LMN reflexes. Spinal reflexes are classified into three groups:

- Proprioceptive reflexes
- Nociceptive reflexes
- Special (released) reflexes

This division is based on the type of sensory stimulation required to elicit the first two reflexes and on the special conditions required to elicit the third reflex.

Proprioceptive Reflexes

These myotatic reflexes are initiated by stretch of tendons or muscle spindles. They have a strong influence from the UMN and therefore are likely to be exaggerated with UMN lesions. Increases and decreases in the force of reflex activity are both components of proprioceptive reflexes; thus, it is important to grade the strength of these reflexes. A standard grading scale is:

0 = absent reflex
1 = diminished reflex
2 = normal reflex
3 = increased reflex
4 = increased reflexes with clonus

Thoracic Limb Proprioceptive Reflexes

Triceps reflex. This tests the radial nerve and arises from spinal cord segments C7-T2.

- Elicit by striking the tendon of insertion of the triceps muscle. A normal response is a slight extension of the elbow.
- Often it is difficult to obtain and, when present, to interpret this reflex in normal animals.

Extensor Carpi Radialis Reflex. Like the triceps reflex, this tests the radial nerve and spinal cord segments C7-T2.

- Elicit by striking the muscle belly of the extensor carpi radialis muscle, which results in extension of the carpus.
- This reflex is easier to elicit than the triceps reflex.

Biceps Reflex. This reflex evaluates the musculocutaneous nerve, which arises from spinal cord segments C6-C7.

- Initiate by striking the tendon of insertion of the biceps tendon, causing a slight flexion of the elbow.
- This reflex is more difficult to obtain than the triceps reflex and is difficult to interpret.

Pelvic Limb Proprioceptive Reflexes

Patellar Reflex. This reflex tests the femoral nerve and its cord segments (L4-L6).

- Elicit by striking the patellar tendon, producing extension of the stifle.
- When testing this reflex, a phenomenon known as a *false localizing sign* sometimes occurs, because paralysis of the sciatic nerve results in a hyperactive patellar reflex. It may be due to functional loss of the antagonist muscles that oppose the extensors of the stifle.

Cranial Tibialis Reflex. This reflex tests the peroneal branch of the sciatic nerve, which originates from spinal cord segments L2-S2.

- Initiate by striking the belly of the cranial tibial muscle. The normal response is flexion of the tarsus.

Gastrocnemius Reflex. This reflex tests the tibial branch of the sciatic nerve, which originates from spinal cord segments L6-S2.

- Elicit by striking the belly of the gastrocnemius muscle or its tendon of insertion. The expected normal response is extension of the tarsus; however, many patients have flexion of the tarsus.

Nociceptive Spinal Reflexes

The nociceptive reflexes are initiated by nociceptive (painful) stimuli, such as pinching, compression, and pin pricks, that induce withdrawal of the limb or some other reflex action. It is important to realize these reflexes only test the integrity of a spinal reflex arc.

KEY POINT ▶ The fact that reflex withdrawal is present tells nothing about the health of the nociceptive pathways traveling cranially to the brain. The most significant change seen is loss of a nociceptive reflex, which indicates an LMN lesion.

These reflexes do not have a large UMN influence; therefore, they do not normally become exaggerated with UMN lesions.

Thoracic Flexor Reflex. This reflex utilizes all the peripheral nerves of the thoracic limb and tests spinal cord segments C6-T2.

- Elicit by digital compression. The normal response is withdrawal of the limb from the source of the stimulus.
- Loss of the reflex indicates a lesion in the reflex arc.

Pelvic Limb Flexor Reflexes. These reflexes test the sciatic nerve and its branches and L6-S2 nerve roots, the fibers go to form the sciatic.

- Initiate by digital compression. The normal response is withdrawal of the limb from the source of the stimulus.
- Loss of this reflex indicates a lesion in the reflex arc.

Perineal reflexes. The most commonly used is the *anal reflex*, which tests the perineal and pudendal nerves, spinal cord segments S1-S3, and the cauda equina.

- Initiate by lightly pricking or stroking the perianal skin. The expected response is constriction of the anal sphincter and flexion of the tail.
- If a mild weakness is suspected, it is best to test the reflex during a digital rectal examination, in order to estimate the strength of contracture of the sphincter.

Special (Released) Reflexes

These are reflexes that are suppressed by the UMN in normal animals. When disconnection between the reflex arc and the UMN occurs, these reflexes become released or uninhibited. Thus, the presence of these reflexes indicates loss of UMN inhibition to a reflex arc.

Babinski Reflex. This occurs only in the pelvic limbs.

- Elicit by lightly stroking the plantar aspect of the metatarsus. In a normal animal, the toes either are unaffected or flex slightly.
- In the presence of UMN disease, the toes spread apart and elevate (dorsiflex), which is known as a positive Babinski reflex.

Crossed Extensor Reflex. This abnormal reflex may be seen in any limb.

- Initiate by eliciting a flexor response in an animal in lateral recumbency. In a normal animal, the limb being stimulated flexes and the contralateral, paired limb is unaffected.
- In the presence of UMN disease, when the stimulated limb flexes, the contralateral paired limb will involuntarily extend.

KEY POINT ▶ The crossed extension reflex is a consistent sign of UMN dysfunction.

Nociceptive Evaluation

Nociceptive evaluation (testing pain responses) is a logical continuation of the flexor reflexes that tests for more than simple reflex withdrawal of the limbs. Cerebral recognition of pain perception is essential for a positive response to these tests.

Decreased Pain Perception

A mild loss in pain perception is called *hypalgesia* or *hypesthesia*. If the loss is total it is referred to as *analgesia* or *anesthesia*.

- Loss of pain perception is tested by producing enough pain so that cerebral recognition occurs and a reaction is produced.

- To elicit reaction, compress the digits vigorously. The expected response is turning of the head and/or vocalization.

This evaluation tests peripheral nerves, spinal cord, brain stem, and cerebrum. The cerebellum is not involved in the nociceptive pathways.

KEY POINT ▶ Peripheral nerve lesions usually cause focal sensory loss, confined to the distribution of the involved nerve(s), Spinal cord lesions cause a bilateral, symmetric sensory loss proceeding caudally from the approximate level of the injury.

- Brain stem lesions rarely produce detectable analgesia, because a lesion of that severity would result in the death of the animal.
- Cerebral lesions produce only hypalgesia.
- The sensory deficit with a cerebral lesion is unilateral and is contralateral to the diseased hemisphere.

Increased Sensitivity or Exaggerated Response to Pain

Hyperesthesia refers to increased sensitivity; *hyperpathia* is an exaggerated response to pain. In veterinary medicine these two terms are used interchangeably.

Exaggerated responsiveness to pain is tested by digital manipulation of the paraspinal muscles, stimulation of the paraspinal region with a hemostat or safety pin, or a similar maneuver.

- The objective is to produce a recognizable stimulus that is not normally bothersome to the patient.
- This stimulus is applied up and down the spine, looking for an area where the patient shows an unusually acute response to the stimulus.
- An exaggerated response usually is an indication of a nerve root or meningeal lesion (e.g., herniated disc or meningitis).

KEY POINT ▶ Paraspinal stimulation is valuable for localizing spinal cord lesions, because a hyperpathic response indicates that the problem is extramedullary and establishes the location of the lesion.

INTERPRETATION OF THE NEUROLOGIC EXAMINATION

Make a list of abnormal findings, along with a list of the anatomic regions of the nervous system. Mark each anatomic region where a lesion could produce the listed findings (Fig. 1), and then ask yourself the following questions:

Does the patient have a neurologic disease?

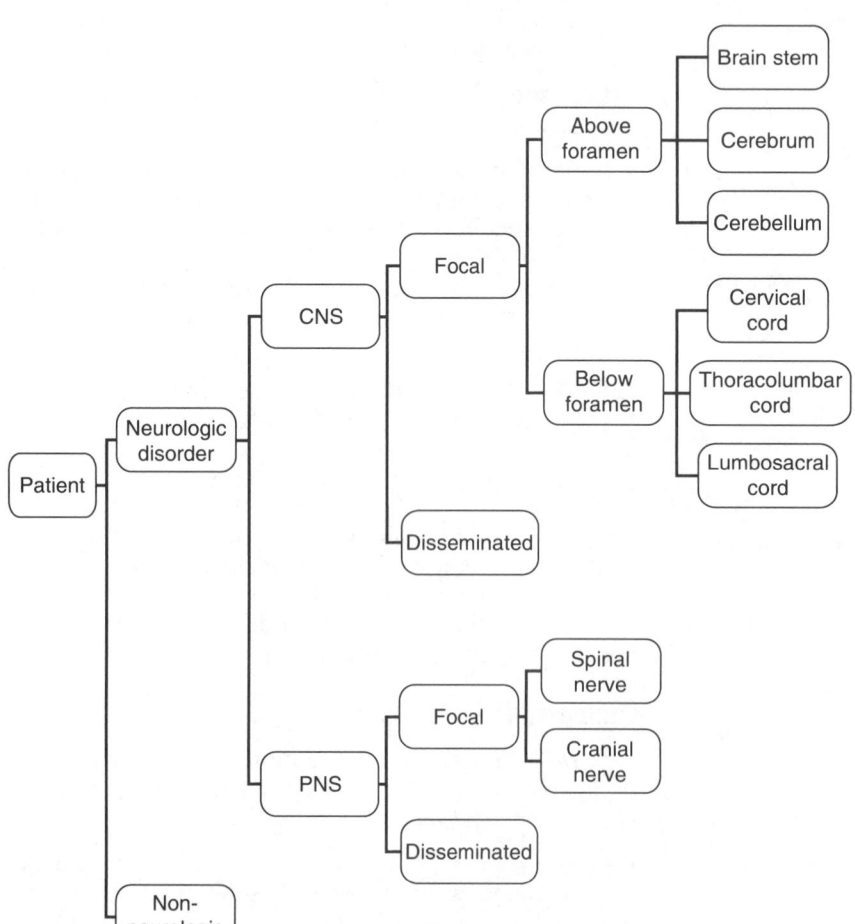

Figure 1. Localization flow chart. (CNS = central nervous system; PNS = peripheral nervous system.)

- If there are pluses after any of the listed findings, answer this question in the affirmative.
- Is the disease in the CNS or PNS?
- If the animal has CN deficits, use your evaluation of the limbs and mental status to answer this question.
- If there are only isolated cranial nerve deficits with no other signs, the lesion probably is in the PNS.
- If there are CN deficits, plus the presence of limb signs, the lesion probably is in the CNS.
- If the disease is below the foramen magnum and UMN reflex changes are present, the lesion probably is in the CNS.
- If all spinal reflexes are LMN reflexes, the lesion probably is in the PNS.
- Is the disease above or below the foramen magnum?
- If the animal has a CN abnormality, historical seizures, abnormal head posture, abnormal head coordination, or abnormal level of consciousness, the lesion is likely to be above the foramen magnum.
- If the lesion involves the limbs alone, the lesion is most likely below the foramen.
- At this point in the interpretation of the neurologic examination, negative findings become as important as positive findings.
- For example, an UMN tetraparetic patient may have a cerebral, brain stem, or cervical cord injury.
- If the patient has no head signs, look for a cord lesion based on the negative head findings combined with the positive limb findings.
- After you have localized the lesion (above or below the foramen; CNS or PNS), try to localize the lesion more precisely.
- What do you gain by localizing the disease?
- You will know whether the problem is focal or disseminated and this knowledge is useful because the probable etiologies are different for each class.
  - Disseminated diseases usually are caused by inflammations, metabolic diseases, and degenerations.
  - Focal diseases usually are caused by masses, trauma, and vascular lesions.
- Localization automatically eliminates some differentials from the diagnosis.
  - For example, a cat with signs suggesting a focal cerebral mass would not have an intervertebral disc extrusion as the cause of the problem.
- Localization also helps in choosing diagnostic aids because certain diagnostic tools are only of value with lesions in certain anatomic regions.
  - An example is the electroencephalogram, which is helpful only in patients with cerebral injuries. Using this tool in a patient with peripheral nerve disease is a misdirected effort and a waste of the client's money.

Selection of Diagnostic Aids

Diagnostic aids are laboratory tests and procedures that help to determine which differential diagnosis is the most likely cause of the patient's signs. The primary purpose of a diagnostic aid is to provide etiologic information. As a consequence of establishing a diagnosis, these tests may also provide prognostic information. In addition, some tests provide anatomic information, allowing "fine-tuning" of the results of the neurologic examination.

Diagnostic aids used in evaluation of the nervous system include general screening tests such as routine serum biochemistries and blood counts, that identify metabolic and toxic injuries to the nervous system. Also included are specific tests of nervous system anatomy (e.g., neuroradiology), function (e.g., cerebrospinal fluid analysis, electrodiagnostic tests), or both (e.g., electromyography).

To select the most appropriate diagnostic aids, combine historical information with neurologic examination findings. After interpreting results of the diagnostic aids, the diagnosis should be evident. This approach is summarized in Figure 2.

GENERAL SCREENING TESTS

Hematology

Limitations

In the majority of patients with nervous system disease, there are minimal hematologic changes. There are exceptions, such as encephalitis and patients with systemic disease that secondarily affects the nervous system (e.g., lead poisoning).

Positive Results

White Blood Cell (WBC) Changes. Elevation of WBC numbers often is an indication of an inflammatory disease process; however, a low WBC count may be seen in viral infections.

Red Blood Cell (RBC) Changes. Anemia, if profound, may result in hypoxia with secondary cerebral signs. An abnormally high RBC count (polycythemia) may result in increased serum viscosity. This can cause diminished blood flow to muscles and produce a my-

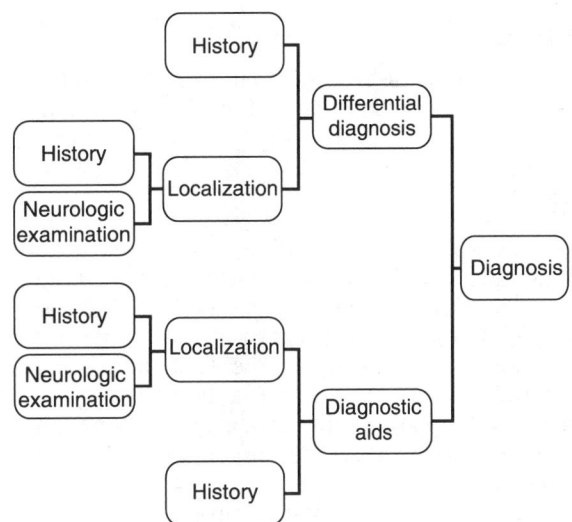

Figure 2. Diagnostic approach flow chart.

asthenia-like syndrome; it also may result in sludging of cerebral blood flow with subsequent CNS infarction.

Biochemical Tests

These tests are helpful in evaluating animals for metabolic illness. Because the cerebrum has very high metabolic demands, it is affected by many generalized metabolic disorders. The motor unit also appears susceptible to a wide variety of generalized metabolic insults. Examples of biochemical abnormalities that impact on the nervous system include hypo- and hyperglycemia, hypo- and hypercalcemia, hypo- and hyperkalemia, hypo- and hypernatremia, acidosis and alkalosis, uremia, hyperamnonemia, hyperlipidemia, and hyperviscosity from dysproteinemia.

Urinalysis

Many of the metabolic diseases that affect the nervous system produce changes in the urine. In addition, many CNS infections affect the urinary system, therefore, evaluation of urinalysis may be helpful in CNS infections.

Fecal Analysis

Severe parasitism has been reported as a cause of CNS disease in young animals.

Serology

Many viral, fungal, and protozoal infections of the nervous system result in the development of antibodies. These antibodies may be assayed in the patient's serum or in CSF (refer to the chapters on infectious diseases in section 2 for specific information).

Immunofluorescence

Some of the viral infections that affect the nervous system may be tested for directly by using immunofluorescent techniques to test for antigen in CSF or nervous tissue (the latter is reserved for postmortem examination).

Toxicology

Blood can be assayed for many of the toxins known to affect the nervous system (e.g., lead poisoning).

NEURORADIOLOGY

Radiography, with or without the use of enhancing techniques, can be used to visualize the supporting structures of the nervous system and in some cases the nervous system itself. These studies provide information about the anatomy of the CNS and can reveal structural abnormalities, but generally they do not provide information about neurologic function (see sec. 1, ch. 4 for additional information about neuroradiology)

Positioning of the animal, proper exposure techniques, and choice of contrast, when appropriate, are important when performing neuroradiology.

Positioning

At least two views at 90° angles are required for proper identification of abnormalities. Because of the irregularity of the shape of most structures evaluated in neuroradiology, proper positioning is critical, and, most radiographs that evaluate the nervous system are taken with the patient under anesthesia.

Radiographic Density

The spinal cord and discs appear less dense because they are surrounded by bone; thus, in many cases disc and cord evaluation depend on the visualization of accompanying changes in the supporting structures. A short scale of contrast is preferred for spinal radiographs (see sec. 1, ch. 4).

Plain Radiography of the Spine

- Indications: To localize surgical lesions and to diagnose nonsurgical lesions of bone tissue.
- Advantages: Noninvasive and allows diagnosis of bony lesions.
- Disadvantages: Requires anesthesia; false-negative results are common.

Myelography

- In myelography of the spine, positive (radiopaque) contrast material is injected into the subarachnoid space to outline the spinal cord before taking radiographs (see sec. 1, ch. 4).
- Indications. To localize surgical lesions and to diagnose nonsurgical lesions of soft tissue, such as intramedullary tumors or vascular lesions.
- Advantage: Allows diagnosis of soft tissue lesions.
- Disadvantages: Requires anesthesia; causes mild meningitis, and may worsen underlying cord injury; false-negative (degenerations and small mass lesions) and false-positive (air bubbles in dye column, extradural dye) results can occur.

Choice of Contrast Materials

Metrizamide and Iohexol are currently being used.

- They are less irritating and more radiopaque than previously used contrast materials but are relatively expensive.
- Because they appear to inhibit the uptake of glucose into the CNS, seizures may occur on recovery from anesthesia.
  - To prevent this complication, a dextrose-containing solution is given intravenously during and immediately following myelography.

Interpretation (Location of Lesions)

- Extradural—most common; a lesion involving the discs or vertebrae
- Intramedullary—cord swelling from any cause (e.g., edema, tumor, or hemorrhage)
- Intradural and extramedullary—quite rare; usually a tumor of the meninges

Skull Radiography

The skull is a complex structure composed of about 40 different bones. There are three basic head shapes in dogs: brachiocephalic (short-head), mesaticephalic (intermediate head), and dolicocephalic (long-head).

Positioning

The normal, bilateral symmetry of the skull is helpful in radiographic evaluation. Because good positioning is extremely important, radiographs should be taken with the animal under anesthesia.

- On lateral views, elevate the nose to keep the skull parallel to the x-ray plate.
- Routine views of the skull include lateral and either ventrodorsal (VD) or dorsoventral (DV).
- Special views are taken for the tympanic bullae, foramen magnum, nasal passages, and teeth.

Normal Findings

The dorsal calvaria are of uniform thickness, with the thickness appropriate for the breed.

- Convolutional markings can be seen on the inside of the skull, which represent the normal indentations of the sulci and gyri of the brain.
- The nasal passages and frontal sinuses contain air outlining delicate bone turbinates.

Abnormal Findings

See Table 1.

Computerized Tomography (CT)

See section 10, chapter 2.

TABLE 1. Radiographic Lesions of the Skull and Spine seen on Radiography

---

Congenital Lesions of the Skull
  Hydrocephalus
  Occipital dysplasia

Congenital lesions of the spine
  Cervical vertebral instability (canine wobbler syndrome, spondylolisthesis)
  Cervical vertebral stenosis
  Atlantoaxial malformation

Traumatic lesions
  Skull: fractures
  Spine: fractures, fracture-luxation

Infectious lesions
  Skull: middle ear infections, rhinosinusitis
  Spine: discospondylitis

Neoplasia of the skull or spine

Degenerative lesions of the spine
  Spondylosis
  Spinal arthritis (spondylitis)
  Degenerative intervertebral disc disease

Lesions seen on myelography
  Intervertebral disc disease
  Spinal vertebral body lesions (tumors or abscesses)
  Spinal cord tumors
  Spinal cord hemorrhage or edema

Magnetic Resonance Imaging (MRI)

See section 10, chapter 2.

CEREBROSPINAL FLUID (CSF) COLLECTION AND ANALYSIS

Factors Affecting CSF Production

- Drugs: Furosemide decreases the rate of production by 50%. Furosemide dosages of 0.9–2.0 mg/kg have been reported to be effective.
- Hydrostatic pressure: Increases in CSF pressure have little effect on the rate or volume of CSF production.
- Osmolality: Acute serum hyperosmolality lowers production, whereas acute serum hypo-osmolality raises production. A 1% change in osmolality results in a 6.7% change in CSF production, either up or down.

Effects of Elevated Intracranial Pressure

Elevations of intracranial pressure, which produce elevations of CSF pressure, can have devastating effects both on the nervous system and systemically.

- Nervous system effect: The most serious sequela to increased CSF pressure is the tendency for herniation of brain contents; this is generally fatal.
- Systemic effects: Cardiac arrhythmias, subendocardial hemorrhage, pulmonary edema, gastrointestinal hemorrhage, and gastrointestinal ulceration may occur with elevations of intracranial pressure.

CSF Collection

- *Purpose*
  - To obtain fluid for diagnostic evaluation
  - To introduce contrast agents into the spinal fluid
  - To introduce therapeutic agents into the spinal fluid
- *Indications:* CSF collection and analysis are indicated in patients with:
  - An abnormal neurologic examination
  - Recurring fevers, epilepsy
  - Chronic pain
- *Contraindications:*
  - Recent CNS trauma
  - Rapidly declining level of consciousness
- *Advantages:* CSF taps are generally safe, inexpensive, and, when positive, very helpful.
- *Disadvantages:*
  - Anesthesia usually is required in small animals.
  - In spinal cord diseases, a lumbosacral tap is needed because of the flow of CSF, which is technically more difficult than a cerebellomedullary cistern tap.
  - CSF taps often are nondiagnostic except in inflammations.

Technique

1. Collect CSF for analysis at the cerebellomedullary cistern or by lumbar puncture.

a. In small animals, the lumbar space is more difficult to enter, yields smaller volumes of fluid, and has a higher rate of blood contamination.

b. The cerebellomedullary cistern is easier to enter in small animals, yields larger volumes of generally less contaminated fluid, but may not evaluate the spinal cord.

2. The average distance between the skin and subarachnoid space in the cervical spine varies with the size of the patient. Reported distances for dogs and cats are ½ inch for cats and dogs < 4.5 kg; ¾ inch for dogs 4.5 to 9.1 kg; 1 inch for dogs 9.1 to 22.7 kg; 1½ inches for dogs 22.7 to 50.9 kg; and 2 inches for dogs > 50.9 kg.

3. After measuring pressures, collect the CSF by allowing it to drip into a container.

4. If the fluid is going to be stored for any length of time keep it in a plastic container, as WBCs adhere to glass. If the CSF is to be stored, it is essential to refrigerate it immediately to slow degradation of cells.

Complications

- The most common complication is blood contamination.
- The most serious complication is brain herniation. In the face of elevated intracranial pressure, the pressure shift created by the removal of CSF may precipitate a shift in intracranial contents. This sudden movement of intracranial contents (brain herniation) generally results in death.

CSF Analysis

Analysis includes measuring CSF pressure and gross visual examination, cytologic analysis, biochemical analysis, and culture of CSF. In addition, serologic procedures may be indicated. Because as there are slightly different normal values for fluid collected from cerebellomedullary and lumbar spaces, note where the fluid was collected. Fluid from the cerebellomedullary cistern tends to have slightly more cells and lower protein than the fluid from the lumbar space.

Pressure

Opening pressure (OP) is measured at the beginning of collection, using a manometer. Simpson showed that normal values for the dog are dependent on body weight (BW). The published formula for calculation of normal values for a given patient based on body size is:

$$OP = 46.5 + 3.83(BW) - 0.048(BW)^2$$

with BW measured in kilograms. Normal pressures using this formula are 50–140 mm H_2O.

When measuring CSF pressure, only elevations of pressure above normal are considered significant.

- Severe elevations are considered diagnostic of a mass effect such as a tumor.
- Mild to moderate elevations may be seen with encephalitis, meningitis, and hydrocephalus.
- Normal CSF pressure doesn't exclude the possibility

of any of the aforementioned diseases, because it i only one piece of the diagnostic puzzle.

Gross Visual Examination

Normal CSF is clear and colorless.

- In the presence of inflammation, CSF generall becomes turbid and assumes an off-white to grayis color.
- Pink discoloration is usually caused by blood contam ination.

Spin the CSF sample down to remove the influenc of RBCs and examine the supernatant.

- Yellow-orange colored CSF (xanthochromic) gener ally indicates either breakdown of hemoglobin fron previous hemorrhage or severe elevations of CSI protein (>100 mg/dl).

Cytologic Evaluation

Cytologic evaluation consists of a total cell count o unconcentrated CSF and preparation of a slide from concentrated CSF sample for evaluation of cell type and differential numbers.

- Perform the total cell count quickly because cell from CSF begin to degenerate rapidly following collection.
- If the slides cannot be prepared immediately refrig erate the sample.
- The type and number of cells present reflect the cause of the inflammation and thus provide etiologi information.
- Normally there are <5 WBCs/µl.
- The presence of 5–10 WBCs/µl suggests pathologi disease; >10 WBCs/µl are definitive.
- The presence of 5–50 WBCs/µl suggests a mil inflammatory process as seen with viral diseases an some forms of trauma and vascular disease.
- The presence of 50–200 WBCs/µl suggests a mod erate inflammation, as seen with fungal, protozoal and immune diseases.
- The presence of >200 WBCs/µl indicates a marke inflammatory process, as seen with bacterial menin gitis and some immune diseases.

Diagnostic Interpretation

Suppurative Meningitis. Suppurative meningitis i diagnosed if the number of cells in the CSF ar increased and are predominantly neutrophils. Suppu rative meningitis is the most common pathologic re sponse to bacterial encephalitis, although it is als characteristic of acute, severe viral infections of th nervous system, idiopathic vasculitis/meningitis i young dogs, and some tumors.

Mixed (Granulomatous) Inflammation. Mixed in flammation is diagnosed when the increased numbe of cells in the CSF are composed of multiple cell type including macrophages, lymphocytes, neutrophils, an sometimes plasma cells. Although a mixed cytology i generally the result of a granulomatous encephalitis such as fungal, protozoal, and idiopathic diseases, thi cytologic change may also be seen in chronic bacterial infections that are being inadequately treated.

Nonsuppurative Inflammation. Nonsuppurative inflammation is diagnosed when the numbers of cells in the spinal fluid are increased and are composed primarily of mononuclear cells, especially lymphocytes. It is most characteristic of viral and rickettsial infections. Although this type of CSF abnormality is least likely to be the result of an acute bacterial infection of the nervous system, it may occur.

Prognostic Value of CSF Cytology. In humans and in experimental studies in animals with bacterial meningitis, there appears to be a correlation between the numbers of WBCs in pretreatment CSF cytology and prognosis. High initial WBC counts were associated with a favorable prognosis. Animals with continued high WBC counts after therapy had a poor prognosis.

Biochemical Evaluation

When evaluating the chemical contents of the CSF, remember that CSF is produced both by active transport and by ultrafiltration. As a result, CSF contains essentially the same constituents as plasma, but they are present in different concentrations. Generally the levels of CSF constituents are lower than the serum levels. The two constituents measured most commonly for diagnostic purposes are *protein* and *glucose*.

Protein Levels. The concentration of protein is generally quite low in CSF compared to plasma. In dogs and cats, protein from a cerebellomedullary cisternal tap is generally less than 25 mg/dl, whereas that from a lumbar puncture may be as high as 45 mg/dl. This elevation may be the result of an increase in the permeability of the blood-brain barrier, production of immunoglobulins in the intrathecal space, or a combination of both. Conditions known to elevate CSF protein include encephalitis, meningitis, neoplasms, CNS infarctions, and trauma. The spinal fluid protein should be qualitatively as well as quantitatively analyzed, which is best done by electrophoresis or immunoelectrophoresis. In normal CSF, albumin composes about 75% of the protein, and most of the remainder is globulin.

Glucose. Normal CSF glucose levels are about 60–80% of those in blood. In humans, the ratio between blood glucose and CSF glucose is routinely lower in bacterial infections. There does not appear to be a similar relationship between bacterial encephalitis and decreased spinal fluid glucose in dogs. Plasma glucose can decrease dramatically in the presence of septicemia and bacteremia. A meningitic patient that is also bacteremic will likely have a drop in CSF glucose.

CSF Serologic Examination

The CSF may be examined serologically for antibodies against infectious agents (as well as for bacterial antigens as mentioned above). The presence of antibodies may be helpful in the diagnosis of viral, fungal, and rickettsial diseases, but are less helpful in bacterial encephalitis. Little or no antibody is present in normal animals. In most circumstances, the presence of antibodies is an indication of local immunoglobulin production, indicating that the organism against which the antibodies are found is the cause of the encephalitis.

A limitation of serology is that paired titers are required for greatest accuracy.

False-Positive Antibody Levels

■ False-positive antibody levels can be caused by leakage of plasma proteins into the CSF. For example, in encephalitis, fever may transiently open the blood-brain barrier, resulting in some leakage of antibodies. Those antibodies present may be the result of previous infections.
■ Increased albumin on CSF electrophoresis supports a false-positive diagnosis, as does simultaneous serum antibody titer measurement.

ELECTROENCEPHALOGRAPHY

Electroencephalography (EEG) is the graphic recording of shifts in resting membrane potential of the dendritic network in the superficial layers of cerebral cortex. This network is influenced and modulated by the activity of subcortical nuclear centers such as the reticular formation.

The goals when evaluating an EEG are to recognize the presence of abnormal patterns and to determine the area of the brain where these patterns originate. This information can be used to differentiate between possible etiologies.

■ *Indications:* EEG evaluation is indicated for patients suspected of having:
  • Any type of cerebral dysfunction
  • A multifocal disease, in order to discern if the cerebrum is involved.
■ *Advantages:* EEG is noninvasive, relatively inexpensive, and frequently can be performed without chemical restraint.
■ *Disadvantages:*
  • EEG tracings often are artifact-laden and difficult to interpret.
  • Tracings may be affected by the patient's age, drugs, and normal variations in wakefulness.

Evaluation

The EEG can be a valuable tool if carefully performed. However, there is only a small body of hard data about veterinary EEG, and there is a high level of artifact in veterinary EEG. These two facts suggest caution when interpreting electroencephalograms. Consider them as a piece of data with no more significance than other laboratory tests.

Diagnostic Interpretation

■ *Metabolic diseases*—diffuse slowing, decreased background frequency, and possible triphasic waves
■ *Toxic injuries*—diffuse slowing with a decrease in background frequency
■ *CNS inflammation*—diffuse slowing, decreased background frequency, and sometimes fast transients
■ *Vascular disorders*—focal slowing with sharp waves

and spikes if hemorrhage into parenchyma has occurred
- *Abscess*—focal slowing
- *Neoplasms*—focal slowing; focal fast transients also seen, especially with rapidly growing neoplasm

BRAIN STEM AUDITORY EVOKED RESPONSE (BAER)

- *Indication:* This procedure is used to test the nervous system pathways for hearing.

Technique

1. Recording electrodes are placed over the ear and the cerebrum and connected to an amplifier.
2. A sound made in the ear is a stimulus that triggers EEG recording of all brain activity that occurs during the 100 msec following the stimulus.
3. About 1000 stimuli are recorded, and the waveform patterns are compared by a data processor.
4. All random occurrences of waveforms are deleted, leaving only responses that appear consistently in every tracing. This "averaged response" is the BAER.

Diagnostic Interpretation

Conduction Deafness. There is loss of all waveforms on the BAER. This is the most common type of congenital deafness, and the BAER is widely used for screening in puppies.

Peripheral Vestibular Disease

- With otitis media/interna, there usually is loss of all waveforms.
- With idiopathic vestibular disease, the BSAER may not be affected, because it tests hearing but not balance.
- With brain stem vestibular diseases, often there are increased latencies, and sometimes actual loss, of later waveforms.

ELECTRODIAGNOSTIC EXAMINATION OF THE MOTOR UNIT

The electrodiagnostic examination of the motor unit consists of three parts:

- Needle electromyography (EMG)
- Nerve conduction studies (NCS)
- Repetitive nerve stimulation (RNS)

Each test evaluates different aspects of the motor unit. Interpretation of abnormal electrodiagnostic findings is summarized in Table 2 (also see Table 3).

Needle EMG

- *Indications:* EMG provides information about the functional status of motor unit innervation.
- *Advantage:* EMG is used primarily as a localizing tool, but it may indirectly provide etiologic information (e.g., in a suspected case of botulism, a positive EMG would exclude this disorder from further consideration).
- *Disadvantage:* False-negative results are common, and positive test results may be contradictory, confusing, or difficult to interpret.
- *Procedure:* A needle is inserted into a muscle and the muscle potentials are recorded and evaluated.

Diagnostic Interpretation

Motor Unit Action Potentials (MUAPs)
Acute Neurogenic Lesions. With acute lesions, there is a reduction in the number of available motor units; this reduction leads to reduced recruitment. Those MUAPs seen are normal in amplitude and duration.
Chronic Neurogenic Lesions. When the lesions become chronic, there is axon sprouting of the terminal branches of surviving neurons. These axon sprouts reinnervate some of the denervated muscle fibers. The MUAPs of the recruited muscles will then have a prolonged duration (temporal dispersion) and may become polyphasic.

TABLE 2. Interpretation of the Abnormal Electrodiagnostic Examination

Procedure	Abnormal Finding	Interpretation
Electromyography	Increased insertional activity	Neuropathies Myopathies Myotonia Cramps Electrolyte disorders
	Spontaneous activity	Myopathies Neuropathies (axon or cell body) Electrolyte disorders
Motor unit action potentials	Diminished size	Myopathies Acute denervation
	Increased size	Reinnervation Myopathies
Nerve conduction studies	Decreased velocity	Myelinopathies
Repetitive nerve stimulation	Incremental or decremental response	Junctionopathies

Myopathic Lesions. With myopathic lesions (e.g., polymyositis), the recruitment pattern is normal but all MUAPs are reduced in size. In most neuromuscular junction (NMJ) disorders, MUAPs are normal or reduced in amplitude if they can be elicited. However, some myopathies (e.g., myotonia congenita) are characterized by bizarre discharges called myotonic discharges. These are high-frequency repetitive discharges that wax and wane in frequency and amplitude, causing a characteristic "dive-bomber" sound.

Spontaneous Activity. Spontaneous resting activity requires denervation. Denervation may be seen with motor neuron destruction, axonal transection, and inflammatory myopathies that produce segmental necrosis of muscle. Spontaneous depolarizations are known as fibrillation potentials or positive sharp waves (PSWs), depending on their size and shape.

Fibrillation Potentials. Fibrillation potentials reflect denervation hypersensitivity. They are 1–5 msec in duration, have an initial positive deflection, and may be biphasic or triphasic, with fibrillation amplitudes of 25–200 μV. Fibrillation potentials may be abolished by the use of curare.

PSW. PSWs are biphasic, with an initial positive deflection, 10–100 msec in duration, and amplitudes of 50–1000 μV. Because PSWs may be induced by needle movement in normal muscle, they are considered pathologic only if they persist after the needle has come to rest.

Nerve Conduction Studies

Nerve conduction studies measure latency or two-point nerve conduction velocities. Latency is the amount of time that elapses between stimulus and response.

■ *Indications:* The speed of conduction primarily evaluates the health of the myelin sheath. The size and duration of MUAPs are indicative of the number of healthy fibers. This also evaluates the NMJ, because some junctionopathies may result in complete conduction blockade.

Procedures

Motor Nerve Conduction Testing. The M wave, also called the direct evoked compound muscle action potential, is the potential measured from a distal muscle after proximal stimulation of a nerve. This is best elicited with a supramaximal stimulus. It tests demyelination and the number of healthy axons.

Sensory Nerve Conduction. This procedure tests the sensory nerve and the dorsal root ganglion. The procedure is similar to motor nerve conduction testing, except that the stimuli are applied distally and the recordings are made directly from the nerve proximal to the site of stimulation.

Diagnostic Interpretation

Myelin Injuries. With injury to myelin, there is an increase in intranodal conduction time, leading to slowing of conduction velocities. Because not all fibers conduct at the same rate, there is temporal dispersion (prolonged duration) of the evoked potential as well. Because the NMJ remains intact in demyelination, needle EMG should be normal.

Axonal Injuries. With axonal injury that spares the myelin sheath, the nerve conduction may be normal or mildly decreased. There is a reduction in the number of available motor units; this reduction leads to reduced size of the evoked potential. As the neurogenic lesion becomes chronic, there is axon sprouting of the terminal branches of surviving neurons. These axon sprouts reinnervate some of the denervated muscle fibers. The evoked potential will then have a prolonged duration (temporal dispersion) and may become polyphasic. This occurs because the axon sprouts conduct more slowly than the normal fibers, so that the muscle fibers receive their impulses at different times. In addition, because the motor unit now has more fibers, the evoked potential will be increased in amplitude. Because the axon must be healthy in order for the NMJ to remain intact, there will be denervation of the muscle and the EMG will be abnormal.

Combined Injuries. There will be abnormalities in conduction velocity and in the amplitude of the evoked response. This occurs as a result of wallerian degeneration.

Repetitive Nerve Stimulation

Repetitive nerve stimulation (RNS) measures the amplitude of the motor unit potential during a supramaximal stimulus. RNS tests the health of the NMJ. If there is a progressive change in the amplitude during the first five stimuli, it is abnormal. An increase in amplitude is called an *incremental response;* a decrease in amplitude is called a *decremental response.* For a complete evaluation, RNS should be performed at both fast and slow rates.

Incremental Response. An incremental response is best seen on fast stimulation. It suggests a presynaptic disease such as botulism, myasthenic syndrome, aminoglycoside intoxication, hypocalcemia, and hypermagnesemia. Most of the disorders that result in incremental responses appear to involve the role of calcium in the release of acetylcholine.

Decremental Response. A decremental response, especially to slow repetitions, suggests a postsynaptic disease, especially myasthenia gravis. Other conditions that may cause this response include myasthenic syndrome and botulism.

OTHER MOTOR UNIT TESTS

Tensilon Test

In myasthenia gravis, where the disorder is in the postsynaptic NMJ, anticholinesterase drugs can reverse the clinical symptoms. The most widely used of these drugs is Tensilon (edrophonium HCl), which has the advantage of a short (10 minutes) duration of action (see sec. 10, ch. 5 for more information).

TABLE 3. Diagnostic Study Findings in Various Diseases Categories

Disease Category	Diagnostic Modality	Findings
Degeneration		
	Radiography	
	Plain	Usually normal; degeneration of supportive structures (i.e., discs) may be seen.
	Contrast	Usually not affected; may be decreased in size of NS with NS degeneration; may be compression with supportive structure (disc) degeneration.
	CSF analysis	Usually not affected; in future, may detect enzyme abnormalities.
	Electrodiagnostics	
	EEG	In cerebral degeneration: diffuse slowing of waves.
	EMG	In spinal gray matter degeneration: diffuse denervation.
	NCS	In PNS degeneration: slowed conduction and abnormal waveforms.
	RNS	In NMJ degeneration: delayed transmission and small-amplitude waveforms.
Anomalies		
	Radiography	
	Plain	Bony anomalies can be seen (e.g., hemivertebrae, occipital dysplasia); NS anomalies cannot be seen (e.g., hydrocephalus, spinal dysraphism).
	Contrast	Can reveal anomalies that change size of NS or its components (e.g., hydrocephalus causes increased size of ventricle).
	CSF analysis	Usually normal.
	Electrodiagnostics	
	EEG	In cerebral anomalies: slowing of waves over site of anomaly (e.g., diffuse with hydrocephalus).
	EMG	In spinal gray matter anomalies: denervation at site of gray matter destruction.
	NCS and RNS	Usually normal; PNS anomalies occur rarely.
Metabolic		
	Radiography	
	Plain	Not affected.
	Contrast	Usually normal.
	CSF analysis	Usually normal; in future, may detect chemical abnormalities (e.g., changes in neurotransmitter levels).
	Electrodiagnostics	
	EEG	In cerebral dysfunction: diffuse slowing of waves; abnormalities wax and wane.
	EMG	Usually normal; diffuse denervation can be seen if PNS is involved.
	NCS	In PNS dysfunction: slowed conduction and abnormal waveforms.
	RNS	In NMJ dysfunction: delayed transmission and small-amplitude waveforms.
	Blood testing	Most helpful diagnostic tool.
Neoplasia		
	Radiography	
	Plain	Usually normal, unless tumor involves bone.
	Contrast	May show NS swelling and/or compression at tumor site, injury to vascular supply, leakage from vessel due to blood-brain barrier injury.
	CSF analysis	Increased cells are seen only if tumor invades ventricles/subarachnoid space (e.g., lymphoma, choroid plexus tumor); protein increases due to blood-brain barrier injury.
	Electrodiagnostics	
	EEG	In cerebral neoplasia: focal slowing of waves over tumor; epileptic spikes due to irritation may be seen.
	EMG	In spinal cord neoplasia: focal denervation in muscle innervated by affected spinal segment.
	NCS and RNS	Usually normal.
Nutritional		
	Radiography	
	Plain	Usually normal; secondary bone changes may be seen.
	Contrast	Usually normal.
	CSF analysis	Usually normal; may be abnormal metabolite levels in some cases.
	Electrodiagnostics	
	EEG	In cerebral dysfunction: diffuse slowing of waves; abnormalities wax and wane.
	EMG	Usually normal; if PNS is involved, diffuse denervation may be seen.
	NCS	In PNS dysfunction: slowed conduction and abnormal waveforms.
	RNS	In NMJ dysfunction: delayed transmission and small-amplitude waveforms.
	Blood testing	May be helpful in some cases.

Muscle Enzymes

Any disease process that results in necrosis of the muscle cell membrane releases muscle enzymes into the systemic circulation. The most significant of these conditions is polymyositis. Because many incidental conditions (e.g., muscle trauma from an intramuscular injection), also release these enzymes, the use of muscle enzymes for diagnostic purposes must be done cautiously.

TABLE 3. Diagnostic Study Findings in Various Diseases Categories *Continued*

Disease Category	Diagnostic Modality	Findings
Inflammation	Radiography	
	Plain	Rarely helpful, unless there is bone infection.
	Contrast	Usually not helpful; may show spinal cord swelling at site of granuloma/abscess.
	CSF analysis	Usually increased WBCs; type (neutrophils, lymphocytes, eosinophils, etc.) reflects nature of etiology; protein is elevated as result of blood-brain barrier injury and also due to production of immunoglobulins.
	Electrodiagnostics	
	EEG	If cerebrum is involved: diffuse multifocal changes; seizure discharges also may be seen.
	EMG	If spinal cord is involved: multifocal areas of denervation.
	NCS	If PNS is involved: slowed conduction and abnormal waveforms.
	RNS	NMJ rarely is involved.
Infarct	Radiography	
	Plain	Usually normal.
	Contrast	Can show NS swelling and/or compression at infarct site; may show injury to vascular supply and leakage from vessels due to blood-brain barrier injury.
	CFS analysis	Cells are sometimes seen with hemorrhage; protein is increased due to blood-brain barrier injury.
	Electrodiagnostics	
	EEG	In cerebral infarcts: focal slowing of waves over infarct; epileptic spikes due to irritation may be seen.
	EMG	In spinal cord infarcts: focal denervation in muscle innervated by affected spinal segment.
	NCS and RNS	Usually normal.
Toxic	Radiography	
	Plain	Usually normal.
	Contrast	Usually normal.
	CSF analysis	Usually normal; may be abnormal metabolite levels in some cases.
	Electrodiagnostics	
	EEG	In cerebral dysfunction: diffuse slowing of waves; abnormalities wax and wane.
	EMG	Usually normal; if PNS is involved, diffuse denervation can be seen.
	NCS	In PNS dysfunction: slowed conduction and abnormal waveforms.
	RNS	In NMJ dysfunction: delayed transmission and small-amplitude waveforms.
	Blood testing	May be helpful in some cases.
Trauma	Radiography	
	Plain	Can show fractures and dislocations and evidence of joint instability (see sec. 9, ch. 5).
	Contrast	Can show compression and areas of edema; may show vascular injury.
	CSF analysis	Cells usually are increased (especially RBCs); protein usually is increased due to blood-brain barrier injury.
	Electrodiagnostics	
	EEG	In cerebral injury: focal slowing of waves; epileptic spikes due to irritation may be seen.
	EMG	In spinal cord injury: focal denervation in muscle innervated by affected spinal segment.
	NCS	In PNS injury: slowed or blocked conduction resulting from focal/multifocal nerve damage.
	RNS	Rarely affected.

NS = nervous system; CSF = cerebrospinal fluid; EEG = electroencephalography; EMG = electromyography; NCS = nerve conduction studies; PNS = peripheral nervous system; NMJ = neuromuscular junction; RNS = repetitive nerve stimulation; WBCs = white blood cells; RBCs = red blood cells.

MUSCLE AND NERVE BIOPSY

Inflammatory and degenerative diseases of nerve and muscle are best diagnosed by biopsy (also see sec. 10, chs. 5 and 6). These procedures can now be done safely with minimal complications. The tissues require special handling and processing; therefore, arrangements should be made with the laboratory prior to collection of the samples. Analysis by a laboratory that is experienced in handling these biopsies will avoid overinterpretation of results.

RESULTS OF DIAGNOSTIC STUDIES IN VARIOUS DISEASE CATEGORIES

Diagnostic study findings are listed by disease category in Table 3.

Supplemental Readings

Chrisman CL: *Problems in Small Animal Neurology,* 2nd Ed. Philadelphia: Lea & Febiger, 1991.
Oliver JE, Lorenz MD: *Handbook of Veterinary Neurologic Diagnosis.* Philadelphia: W. B. Saunders, 1983.

2

Diseases of the Brain

William R. Fenner

Diseases of the brain stem, cerebellum, and cerebrum each cause different signs because of the different functions of each region. However, the disease processes that affect each region often are the same. For this reason, the clinical presentation of lesions in each region is discussed first, followed by a discussion of specific diseases according to pathogenesis. If a disease is limited in its effects to a specific region, it is noted in the discussion of that disease process.

CLINICAL SIGNS AND NEUROLOGIC EXAMINATION

Brain Stem Lesions

Clinical Signs

- Deficits of the cranial nerves (CNN): CNN III–XII arise from the brain stem. Dysfunction of more than one cranial nerve usually is seen in patients with brain stem lesions, and the dysfunction often is partial.
- Vestibular signs are common and include loss of balance, head tilt, pathologic nystagmus, and circling.
- Ataxia of gait and abnormal postural reactions are common owing to involvement of proprioceptive pathways and the vestibular system.
- Limb weakness results from injury to motor pathways. This will produce upper motor neuron (UMN) signs (e.g., increased reflexes, rigidity) in affected limbs.
- Abnormal levels of consciousness are manifested as depression, stupor, or coma. The abnormalities result from injury to the reticular activating system (RAS).
- Altered heart rate and rhythm or altered respiratory patterns are less frequent signs, but they often indicate a more life-threatening injury.

Anatomic Localization

- Midbrain: Primary signs involve the eyes (CNN III and IV) and the level of consciousness (RAS).
- Pons: Primary signs involve the face (CNN V and VII), gait and balance (vestibular system), and further abnormalities of gait (cerebellar tracts).
- Medulla: Primary signs involve swallowing and prehension or tongue function (CNN IX, X, and XII), balance and gait (the vestibular system), and heart rate, heart rhythm, and respiration (reticular formations).

Intramedullary versus extramedullary:
- If cranial nerve signs are more significant than limb signs, consider an extramedullary location.
- If long tract signs are more significant than cranial nerve signs, consider an intramedullary location.

Neurologic Examination

General Observations
- Mental status: Depressed in many cases; depressed consciousness usually indicates a lesion rostral to CN V.
- Head Posture: Tilted, usually toward the side of the lesion; head tilts indicate that CN VIII or the medial longitudinal fasciculus is involved.
- Circling: Usually toward the side of the lesion.

Cranial Nerve Examination
- Midbrain: The eyes are the principal portion of the head involved in midbrain diseases.
  - Internal ophthalmoplegia: The pupil is paralyzed.
  - External ophthalmoplegia: The extraocular muscles are paralyzed.
- Pons: The muscles of facial expression (CN VII), sensation to the face and head (CN V), and the vestibular system (CN VIII) are the primary targets of pontine diseases.
- Medulla: The pharynx, tongue, respiration, and vestibular system are the primary targets of medullary diseases.

Gait and Stance (Generally Abnormal)
- Limb ataxia usually is present, owing to unconscious and special proprioceptive involvement. Ataxia is most commonly seen with lesions caudal to the midbrain.
- Limb weakness usually is present and often is severe and asymmetric. Because the weakness results from injury to UMN pathways, the limbs will be hypertonic with normal to exaggerated spinal reflexes.
- Abnormal postural reactions are common. Depression of postural reactions results from involvement of the conscious proprioceptive pathways, as well as from UMN injury.

Spinal Reflexes
- Spinal reflexes are preserved. When reflexes are abnormal, they are generally exaggerated because of damage to UMN pathways.

Sensory Examination
- Pain perception in the limbs usually is normal, although some patients have mild decreases in pain perception (hypalgesia).

■ Loss of facial pain perception is common because of CN V damage. Facial hyperesthesia resulting from damage to CN V may occur, although this is uncommon.

Cerebellar Lesions

Clinical Signs

■ Gait and Stance Abnormalities: Cerebellar lesions produce abnormal rate, range, and force of voluntary movement. Typically the degree of movement is exaggerated. Over- or undershooting of objects occurs, followed by correction movements (intention tremor). Abnormalities include:
  - Wide-based stance
  - Irregular, deviating gait
  - Ataxia accentuated by circling or turning
  - Veering when attempting to walk in a straight line
  - Hypermetria
■ Ataxia of head and trunk: The patient over- or undershoots when trying to reach food or water. There may be swaying of the trunk while standing.
■ Titubation: If the lesion is in the spinocerebellum, arrhythmic forward and backward movements of the trunk, known as titubation, occur. The patient cannot sit or stand without assistance.
■ Strength and reflexes: Most patients have normal strength and reflexes. Some patients will be hypotonic and may appear to have slightly diminished reflexes.
■ Preservation of postural reactions: Although correction movements usually are hypermetric, the ability to initiate correction movements for abnormal posture is preserved.
■ Vestibular signs (head tilt, pathologic nystagmus, circling): The presence of these signs indicates a lesion in the vestibulocerebellum. This portion is rarely injured in congenital diseases; therefore, the presence of vestibular signs is a reliable indicator of acquired cerebellar disease.
■ Menace deficit: Some (rare) patients have a menace deficit in the presence of normal vision and normal CN VII (facial) function. The mechanism is not well understood.
■ Tremor: Tremor is a regular, rhythmic, oscillating movement, usually involving alternating contraction and relaxation of agonist and antagonist muscles.
  - Intention tremor: A tremor that develops during, and is markedly worsened by, voluntary movement. It is especially prominent in highly controlled movements (e.g., eating).
  - Postural tremor: Usually a fine tremor that involves the head, trunk, and upper extremities and disappears when the animal is not supporting itself. Postural tremor may be physiologic and thus often is seen with metabolic diseases.
■ Anisocoria: Some patients may have unequal pupil size. The pupillary changes seen with cerebellar disease are unpredictable and include both miosis and mydriasis. The mechanism is incompletely understood.

Neurologic Examination

■ Mental status generally is normal.
■ Ataxia, hypermetria, broad-based stance, normal postural reactions.
■ Spinal reflexes are generally normal.
■ Sensory examination findings usually are normal.
■ Head tilts may be seen with asymmetric lesions.
■ Circling may be seen in some cerebellar patients.
■ Cranial Nerve Evaluation:
  - Menace may be absent (unknown mechanism).
  - Pathologic nystagmus may be present; it is usually positional and vertical.

Cerebral Disorders

Clinical Signs

Cerebral disease of any etiology tends to cause similar signs. These signs include:

■ Seizures: Although true seizures are always a reflection of cerebral dysfunction, some clinical signs not of cerebral origin can be confused with seizures, such as vestibular disturbances, syncope, neck pain spasms, and myasthenic collapse.
  - Narcolepsy, another cerebral dysfunction, may be confused with a seizure disorder.
■ Personality changes: These can include changes in sleeping and eating habits, urination and defecation habits, and changes in affection. Loss of discipline or training may be a manifestation of personality change.
  - Personality changes also are a common side effect of anticonvulsant drugs.
■ Abnormal mentation: Dementia (i.e., loss of the ability to respond correctly to stimuli) may be seen with any cerebral disease. When dementia is associated with agitation, the patient is described as delirious.
  - Stupor and coma generally indicate bilateral cerebral disease
■ Visual abnormalities: Decreased vision, with normal pupillary light reflexes, is a common sign.
■ Circling: Patients may walk in large aimless circles, usually toward the affected hemisphere.
■ Proprioceptive deficits: Many patients display proprioceptive deficits. When unilateral deficits are seen, the clinical abnormality is usually on the side opposite to the diseased hemisphere.
■ Cranial nerve deficits: Occasional cranial nerve weakness, especially of CN VII, is seen. Clinical manifestation of the deficit will be opposite the diseased hemisphere.
■ Sensory deficits: Abnormal pain perception in the limbs and face (CN V) may occur. The clinical manifestation of the sensory deficit will be opposite the diseased hemisphere.

The signs described above may occur in any combination, and not all signs will be present in every patient. Cerebral diseases are further classified by etiology, as *extracranial* and *intracranial*.

Extracranial Origin. These cerebral disorders result from systemic, metabolic, nutritional, and toxic processes; as such they may be classified as secondary cerebral disorders.

- The cerebrum is not the primary target in most of these conditions; rather, it is an innocent bystander. As a result, there is usually minimal to no anatomic damage to the cerebrum.
- The predominant clinical signs frequently are referable to other organs, and the general physical examination often is abnormal.
- The neurologic signs most commonly include seizures, personality changes, and waxing and waning dementia. The neurologic examination is frequently normal except for the mental status examination.
- The underlying disease processes are diagnosed by laboratory evaluation of blood, urine, and body tissue and by radiographic evaluation.

Intracranial Origin. These disorders, in which the central nervous system (CNS) is the primary target, may be further subdivided into *structural* and *functional*.

- Structural (organic) disorders are characterized by anatomic abnormalities of the CNS.
  - The predominant clinical signs include seizures, visual loss, circling, weakness, personality changes, and other neural deficits.
  - Neurologic examination findings are abnormal, even between seizures.
  - Diagnosis requires specific neurologic diagnostic aids such as cerebrospinal fluid (CSF) analysis, electroencephalography (EEG), and skull radiographs.
- In functional disorders (idiopathic epilepsy), seizures are the only clinical abnormality, and all laboratory tests are normal.
  - The diagnosis is one of exclusion.

Neurologic Examination

- Mental status usually is abnormal in both extracranial and structural disorders but frequently is normal in idiopathic epilepsy, except during the immediate postictal period.
- Head posture generally is normal. Head tilt is not seen in cerebral lesions.
- Circling frequently is seen. Usually the circling is in wide, aimless circles in the direction of the lesion.
- Gait and stance
  - The gait generally is normal, but postural reactions usually are depressed. Most patients will have mild weakness.
- Spinal reflexes are preserved or exaggerated, which is consistent with injury to the UMN.
- Sensory examination results often are abnormal. Generally, the animal is aware of the noxious stimulus, but is unable to localize its source.
- Generalized hyperesthesia may be seen, but is uncommon.
- Cranial nerve examination findings often are abnormal. Cerebrally produced cranial nerve deficits are referred to as *supranuclear dysfunctions*.

- Menace: The menace reflex often is depressed, but the pupillary light reflex is not affected.
- Facial reflexes: Often there is depression of the facial reflexes and weakness of the muscles of facial expression (CN VII).
- Facial sensation: Many patients are unable to properly integrate sensory information from the face, and some patients will have marked analgesia, reflecting dysfunction of CN V.

DIAGNOSIS

Differential diagnoses for brain disorders are listed in Table 1.

Blood Tests

- *Principle:* Because the cerebrum is more susceptible to the effects of metabolic processes than any other part of the CNS, include a careful screening for metabolic disease in the diagnostic evaluation of any patient with cerebral dysfunction. It is unusual for brain stem or cerebellar lesions to be caused by metabolic processes, except for conditions producing coma (e.g., hypoglycemia) or diffuse demyelination (e.g., over-rapid correction of hyponatremia).
- *Use:* Standard tests include a hemogram, serum or plasma biochemistries, and (if infections are suspected) serology for those infections most likely to occur in the species being evaluated.

Radiography

Plain Skull Radiography

Obtain skull radiographs in patients with suspected lesions of bone or cartilage, hydrocephalus, tumors, and head trauma. Each of these processes has the capacity to alter or produce bone density resulting in radiographic abnormalities. In most other brain disorders there are no radiographic changes.

Contrast Radiography

- *Principle:* This technique involves the injection of a positive or negative contrast agent into the ventricular or vascular system of the brain.

TABLE 1. Differential Diagnoses for Brain Disorders

Acute Onset
Stable/improving course
  Trauma
  Inflammations
  Vascular malformations
Progressive course
  Neoplasia
  Inflammations

Subacute/Chronic Onset
Progressive course
  Degenerations
  Neoplasia
  Inflammations
  Malformations

- *Use and Limitations:* Contrast radiography is performed when hydrocephalus, tumors, or vascular injury is suspected. Noninvasive imaging techniques (CT, MRI), which are safer and less difficult, are preferred.

Computerized Tomography (CT)

- *Principle:* A computer enhances the image generated by radiography, using a two-dimensional format, to create a cross-sectional image (see sec. 1, ch. 4). A dye can be injected IV to further test the integrity of the blood-brain barrier.
- *Use:* CT is valuable in the diagnosis of mass lesions and is indicated for all patients with brain stem disease. It can:
  - Detect a mass
  - Assess its vascularity and any secondary effects (e.g., edema, ventricular obstruction)
  - Determine whether it is intramedullary or extramedullary
- *Limitations:*
  - CT may not detect degenerations and inflammations.
  - It is fairly expensive.
  - It requires anesthetization of the patient for several hours.

Magnetic Resonance Imaging (MRI)

- *Principle:* A computer-enhanced signal is generated by protons in various tissues of the CNS (see sec. 1, ch. 4). The resulting image can be displayed in a two-dimensional format, giving the appearance of a cross-section of the area being viewed.
- *Use:* MRI is potentially the most valuable diagnostic aid for CNS disorders. It can:
  - Localize lesions to specific tissues and distinguish between specific types (e.g., blood and CSF, gray matter and white matter)
  - Distinguish secondary from primary effects and, in some cases, inflammation from edema
  - Test the integrity of the blood-brain barrier and evaluate the metabolic status of specific tissues, by means of labeled compounds that have been injected as tracers
- *Limitations:* At present, MRI is prohibitively expensive and is available only at human hospitals and research institutions.

Electrodiagnostic Tests

Brain Stem Evoked Response (BSER)

- *Principle:* In response to sound, a computer-enhanced electronic signal is generated by various parts of the auditory pathway. The signal consists of a series of waves, with each peak corresponding to the transmission of the signal through a known portion of the nervous system. By measuring the latency, amplitude, and duration of the wave forms, information about the health of the brain stem can be obtained.
- *Use:* BSER is valuable as a localizing aid. It is helpful in confirming the presence of brain stem involvement but does not provide etiologic information.
- *Limitations:* Because BSER utilizes sound, the peripheral organs responsible for hearing must be normal. External ear infections, wax in the ear canal, or injury to the tympanic membrane can produce invalid test results.

Visual Evoked Response (VER)

- *Principle:* A computer-enhanced electronic signal is generated by light pathways in response to a series of light flashes. The resulting signal consists of a series of waves, with each peak corresponding to the transmission of the signal through a known portion of the nervous system. By measuring the latency, amplitude, and duration of the wave forms, information about the health of the visual pathways can be obtained.
- *Use:* VER is valuable as a localizing aid. It is helpful in confirming the presence of cerebral involvement but, as with BSER, does not provide etiologic information.
  - VER can aid in the diagnosis of blindness.
  - Limitations: Because VER utilizes light, the peripheral organs responsible for vision must be normal. Cataracts, retinal degenerations, retinal detachment, and ocular inflammation can produce invalid test results.

Electroencephalography (EEG)

- *Principle:* EEG provides a graphic recording of the changes in threshold potential of the subcortical dendritic network of the cerebral cortex, which in theory provides information about the state of cerebral function.
- *Use:* EEG is indicated for all patients with a history of cerebral disease. It can:
  - Distinguish between extracranial and intracranial diseases.
  - Confirm that the cerebrum is involved in diffuse disease processes.
  - Aid in the diagnosis of epilepsy.
- *Limitations:*
  - There is a lack of standardized methods for interpretation.
  - EEG is affected by many external factors, including the age of the subject, drugs, level of arousal, type and placement of electrodes used for the recording, and filter settings.

Cerebrospinal Fluid (CSF) Analysis

This procedure is the most easily performed, universally available, and reliable test for brain diseases in veterinary medicine. CSF taps are relatively safe and inexpensive.

- *Indications:*
  - Structural and idiopathic brain disorders
  - Fever of unknown origin
- *Use:* CSF analysis is helpful in the diagnosis of disseminated disorders, suspected mass lesions, and certain metabolic diseases.

Collection Procedure

- Following anesthetization and intubation of the animal, the CSF is collected from the cerebellomedullary cistern (cisterna magna) at the occipito-atlantal junction. The only equipment required is a needle with a stylet.
- Submit the fluid sample to a laboratory equipped to handle the sample rapidly; timing is less crucial if samples have been properly prepared and refrigerated.
- The procedure for CSF collection is described in detail in sec. 10, ch. 1.

Analysis

Evaluation includes both gross and laboratory examinations.

Color/Clarity
- Normal CSF is clear and colorless.
- Cloudy fluid often indicates pleocytosis, or an increase in the number of white blood cells (WBCs) (>200 WBCs/μl).
- A yellowish discoloration of CSF (xanthochromia) may indicate previous hemorrhage or protein elevations >150 mg/dl.
- Pink or red CSF indicates the presence of red blood cells (RBCs) or hemoglobin.

Cytology
- The upper limit of normal for both RBCs and WBCs in CSF is 5 cells/μl. Generally, 5–10 WBCs/μl suggests pathology, and >10 WBCs/μl are definite evidence of a pathologic process.
  - A range of 5–50 WBCs/μl is considered a mild elevation, 50–200 WBCs is considered a moderate elevation, and >200 WBCs is a marked elevation.
- The presence of large lymphoid cells (stimulated lymphocytes) may occur following any nonspecific immune stimulus, such as infection, subarachnoid hemorrhage, infarction, and neoplasia.
- Mononuclear phagocytes may be present in normal animals. Activated monocytes (histiocytes), which contain vacuoles in the cytoplasm and are larger than the parent cells, are found only in disease states. Macrophages are simply histiocytes with phagocytized material in them. Neutrophils are seen rarely in normal CSF, unless the CSF tap resulted in trauma.
  - A mild increase in neutrophils may be the result of recent myelography, hemorrhage, infarction, neoplasia (e.g., meningioma), and acute viral infections.
  - A marked increase in the number of neutrophils usually indicates bacterial or immune disease of the nervous system.
- Eosinophils are rarely seen in CSF. If present, consider parasitic and fungal diseases as the cause, although occasionally they are seen following myelography or hemorrhage; they may be associated with tumors and idiopathic conditions.
- Tumor cells are not shed in the CSF unless the tumor is contiguous with the subarachnoid space. This is most likely to happen with lymphoma and meningioma.

Protein
- Perform protein evaluations on all CSF samples. This is the most useful chemical change in CSF.
- About 75% of the protein in CSF is albumin; the remaining 25% is mostly globulin.
  - An albumin level >75% indicates increased endothelial permeability resulting from a nonspecific disruption of the blood-brain barrier or from defective resorption of protein.
  - An abnormally high percentage of globulin indicates intrathecal antibody production. Any inflammatory disorder may produce this increase. If there is no associated elevation in the cell count, the inflammatory disorder is not affecting the meninges.
- A mixed protein elevation suggests both intrathecal antibody production and damage to the blood-brain barrier.

Interpretation

- Degenerations, anomalies, and metabolic, toxic, and nutritional diseases usually have no effect on CSF; cell type, numbers of cells, and protein level and composition are not changed in the presence of these disorders.
- In neoplasia there usually is an increase in protein levels, and there may be increased pressure. An increase in the cell count is rare, except in meningiomas, in which there may be increased neutrophils, possibly due to tumor necrosis.
- Inflammation of the CNS usually results in an increased cell count and increased protein values. The predominant type of WBC reflects the type of inflammation present. CSF pressure may be mildly elevated.
- In infarctions of the CNS, usually there is an early elevation in protein values that resolves rapidly.
- With significant hemorrhage, the RBC count may be increased; with necrosis, the WBC count may be elevated.
- In cases of trauma, RBCs and protein levels are increased. If the trauma was to the brain, CSF pressure may be elevated.

Toxicologic Screening

- *Principle:* Because the cerebrum is more susceptible than any other part of the nervous system to toxic effects, carefully screen for intoxications as part of the diagnostic evaluation of any patient with acute, monophasic cerebral dysfunction.
- *Use:* Select tests for the types of intoxications most likely to occur in the species being evaluated.

PRINCIPLES OF TREATMENT

Specific Therapy

Based on the diagnosis, consider one or more of the following specific treatments.

Antimicrobial Agents

These drugs can be useful in the treatment of bacterial, protozoal, and some fungal infections. See Tables 2 and 3 for specific agents effective in CNS disorders.

Immunosuppressive/Anti-inflammatory Drugs

The pathogenesis of many inflammatory diseases of the CNS is unknown; an immune basis is suspected in some of these disorders.

- In the absence of infection, anti-inflammatory drug therapy may reverse the inflammation and also may alleviate secondary processes (e.g., edema, vasculitis).
- Prednisone may be more effective than dexamethasone in the treatment of CNS disorders.
  - For anti-inflammatory effects, give prednisone, 0.25–0.5 mg/kg q12h; for immunosuppression, give 1–2 mg/kg q12h.

Antineoplastic Drugs

- Chemotherapy for CNS tumors is becoming an accepted treatment in small animals.
  - Results of treatment are mixed, but patients with certain tumor types (e.g., lymphoma) have shown significant improvement for a limited time (see sec. 3, ch. 5 for discussion of chemotherapy).

Toxin Removal

- Chronic intoxications of the CNS (e.g., lead poisoning) may respond to chelating drugs that facilitate removal of the toxin from the CNS.
- The second component of therapy for intoxications is removal of the source of the toxin from the environment.

Nutritional Therapy

- Nutritional deficiencies of vitamins B_1 (thiamine), B_{12} (cobalamin), and E are known to cause neurologic disorders in humans. To date, only vitamin B_1 deficiency has been documented as a cause of neurologic disorders in dogs and cats.
- Copper intoxication may cause neurologic signs in Bedlington terriers (see sec. 7, ch. 8).

Nonspecific Therapy

The goal is to relieve clinical signs by reversing the secondary effects of the disease process.

Antiedema Therapy

Edema produces local compressive effects on the nervous tissue and also has a direct effect on myelin, disrupting its attachment to axons. In cytotoxic edema, the edema fluid produces disruption of cell function.

- A number of drugs are known or suspected to be effective in the relief of CNS edema, including diuretics, corticosteroids, and antiprostaglandins.

- Local tissue hypothermia has been shown to prevent edema from developing.
- Furosemide, (1–2 mg/kg q6–8h), decreases production of CSF, which results in a decrease in intracranial pressure and relief of edema.
  - If furosemide is given simultaneously with mannitol (1 g/kg IV, once), the effects of both drugs are prolonged and the rebound effect of the osmotic agent (mannitol) is minimized.

Anti-inflammatory Drugs

Many CNS diseases produce nonspecific inflammation. Its injurious effects add to the damage from the primary pathologic process.

- In the absence of an infection, nonspecific anti-inflammatory therapy may reverse the inflammation and alleviate secondary processes (e.g., edema, vasculitis)
- Agents effective in the treatment of CNS inflammation include corticosteroids, antiprostaglandins, and other nonsteroidal anti-inflammatory drugs (NSAIDs). The most widely used are corticosteroids, of which prednisone appears to be the most beneficial in the CNS.

Restoration of Blood Flow

Many CNS diseases cause secondary effects resulting in ischemia or hypoxia. Decreased oxygenation of CNS tissue can result in further loss of neural function.

- Drugs that may act to restore circulation include: vasodilators, calcium channel blockers, and opiate antagonists. Data on effectiveness of these drugs remain inconclusive, and they are not routinely used in veterinary practice.

Analgesia

Although pain is not a major feature of brain diseases in veterinary medicine, it does occur in some patients, especially those with brain stem lesions involving CN V. Pain alleviation will facilitate recovery of the patient.

- Drugs used for analgesia include corticosteroids, sedatives, and analgesics such as morphine, Demerol, pentazocine, and aspirin.

Surgical Therapy

Difficulty in approaching the brain stem surgically makes this an uncommon mode of therapy for brain diseases in veterinary practice; however, brain biopsy is becoming more common.

Decompression

- This is the primary reason that surgery is performed in brain diseases.
- Attempts may be made to decompress or remove tumors, abscesses, and hematomas. The results are generally quite poor with brain stem lesions, more mixed with cerebral and cerebellar lesions.

Biopsy

- Because of the compactness of the brain stem, and the vital structures it contains, brain stem biopsy is not recommended without an operating microscope.
- Cerebral and cerebellar biopsies are more commonly performed, with minimal morbidity or mortality.

Factors Affecting Prognosis

Anatomic Location of the Disease

- In general, brain stem disorders carry a poor prognosis, primarily because of the vital structures contained in the brain stem.
- Diseases confined to the cerebellum usually are less severe symptomatically than are diffuse diseases, and there is a better ability to compensate for the injury.
- Cerebral diseases are intermediate in prognosis; they are more likely to produce permanent sequelae than are cerebellar diseases, but they are less likely to be fatal than brain stem diseases.

Severity of Injury

- More severe injuries are less likely to heal completely than are mild injuries.
- White matter injuries are more capable of recovery than are gray matter injuries. As a rule, mild white matter injuries produce ataxia, moderate white matter injuries produce paresis, and severe white matter injuries produce paralysis; thus the neurologic examination can provide clues to the severity of injury.
- The vital structures contained in the brain stem are mainly composed of gray matter. Thus a brain stem injury resulting in respiratory or cardiovascular impairment is less likely to improve than would a similar injury affecting white matter. Regardless of severity of injury, brain stem diseases carry guarded prognoses.
- Injuries to the cerebellum carry a guarded prognosis if the severity of the injury results in secondary brain stem compromise.

Progressiveness of Disease

The final determining factor in establishing a prognosis is the ability to stop the progression of the disease.

- Some disorders are self-limiting (e.g., those due to trauma); in these conditions, location and severity are most important.
- In progressive diseases, a disorder with a reversible etiology carries a much better prognosis than a disorder without a reversible etiology.
- If a cerebral disease is extracranial and reversible, there is a high probability of complete recovery. If the etiology can be reversed, even a structural disorder may have minimal sequelae.
- In patients with functional disease (e.g., epilepsy), the goal of therapy is to limit clinical signs and provide an acceptable quality of life for pet and owner.
- Patients with nonprogressive, postnatally acquired cerebellar and vestibular injuries appear to have a remarkable capacity to compensate for their clinical disabilities. Patients with congenital lesions rarely improve clinically.

FOCAL BRAIN DISEASES

Disorders affecting the brain can be divided into two major groups: focal and disseminated. Focal diseases usually cause asymmetric clinical signs and are generally the result of a mass lesion. Most disseminated brain diseases (discussed later) also affect other parts of the neuraxis, but brain signs are often the predominant clinical feature.

Neoplasia

Etiology

Replacement or compression of neural tissue, vascular compromise, ventricular obstruction, and secondary inflammation contribute to the development of CNS signs in patients with brain neoplasms.

Tumor Types

- *Cats:* Meningiomas, lymphosarcoma, and bony neoplasms are the most common.
- *Dogs:* Choroid plexus tumors, meningiomas, reticulosis (CNS lymphoma), astrocytoma, oligodendroglioma, and metastatic neoplasms are the most common.

Clinical Signs

Tumors are most commonly seen in middle-aged and older animals.

- Clinical signs reflect the location of the tumor.
  - Except for lesions of the cerebellopontine angle, most neoplasms affect only a single brain area in the early stages of the disease process.
  - Patients with cerebral neoplasms often have signs that are acute in onset; the first clinical sign may be a seizure.
  - In patients with brain stem or cerebellar neoplasms that produce vestibular signs there is an acute onset of clinical disease.
- Other neurologic signs associated with neoplasia are more variable in onset.
  - Metastatic diseases tend to have a more rapid onset than primary tumors because there is a high incidence of secondary vascular injury associated with metastases.
- Neoplasms tend to cause a relentless progression of clinical signs, usually with an orderly progression of neurologic deficits.
- In the early stage of the disease, the principal signs of extramedullary brain stem neoplasms are cranial nerve deficits. Intramedullary brain stem neoplasms produce early involvement of the limbs.
- If the lesion is at the cerebellopontine angle, paradoxical vestibular syndrome can occur. Sudden death from respiratory paralysis may occur, especially in the later stages of the disease, usually as a result of brain herniation.

- Superficial cerebral tumors such as meningiomas may produce only seizures.
- If the neoplasm is slow-growing and located in a clinically silent region of the cerebrum, signs of other neurologic deficits may not develop for months.
- In the late stages, signs include stupor and coma, which may be rapid in onset if there is brain herniation.

Diagnosis

Differentiate brain tumors from traumatic and vascular injuries, abscesses, granulomas, and aberrant parasite migrations.

CSF Analysis
- Pressure: Elevated intracranial pressure is seen in many intramedullary tumors. Extramedullary tumors may produce little change in pressure until the very late stages of the disease. In general, posterior fossa tumors affect intracranial pressure less than tumors of the middle and anterior cranial fossae, possibly because they cause less impedance of the flow of CSF.
- Protein: Protein levels generally are elevated in patients with tumors, especially choroid plexus tumors and lymphoma. On electrophoresis, elevations are predominantly of albumin.
- Cytology: An elevated WBC count occurs in CNS lymphoma (lymphocytes and macrophages) and meningiomas (neutrophils). Cytologically, necrotic meningiomas resemble brain abscess, except that, in the latter, neutrophils are normal and microorganisms are absent.

Radiography
- Skull radiographs usually are normal in patients with brain tumors. The exceptions are meningiomas and bony tumors; these tumors will result in changes in bone density.

Ophthalmoscopic Examination
- Optic nerve edema may be seen in CNS lymphoma or astrocytoma.
- Rarely, tumor infiltration of the optic nerve occurs with some CNS tumors (e.g., oligodendrogliomas).

CT/MRI
These image-enhancing techniques are the diagnostic tests of choice for accurately localizing a neoplasm and confirming the diagnosis. However, their use is limited by cost and lack of availability.

Therapy

Currently, therapy is directed at relief of clinical signs rather than tumor destruction; only a few tumors (e.g., superficial meningiomas in cats and dogs and chondroid osteomas in dogs) are accessible for surgical removal.

- Corticosteroid therapy can decrease edema and, when given in conjunction with anticonvulsants, can reduce intracranial pressure in patients having seizures. Frequently there is initial clinical improvement, but in later stages the disease becomes refractory to treatment.

KEY POINT ▶ A sudden decrease in corticosteroid dosage can precipitate edema and death.

- Results have been mixed using radiation therapy to treat brain tumors in dogs. Mean survival time was increased but quality of life was not always improved.
- Chemotherapy is being used in some animals, but lack of agents that cross the blood-brain barrier is a major limiting factor.

Prognosis

- The prognosis for all brain neoplasms is grave.
- Typically, patients with extramedullary tumors (e.g., meningiomas) survive longer than those with intramedullary or metastatic tumors.

Vascular Disease

Vascular disease of the brain is seen primarily in dogs. It is rare in cats, although feline ischemic encephalopathy has been reported as an idiopathic disorder of the middle cerebral artery.

Etiology

Vascular injury to the brain may result from hemorrhage or infarction.

Hemorrhage
- Extravasation of blood into the parenchyma of the CNS produces a mass effect and results in necrosis and inflammation.
- CNS hemorrhage may be seen in arteriovenous malformations, bleeding disorders, and vascular neoplasms and also may be idiopathic.

Infarction
- Infarction results in loss of function of a discrete area of the CNS, with some associated edema and necrosis. In general, infarctions are not as destructive as CNS hemorrhage.
- Infarction may occur with sepsis, vasculitis (Rocky Mountain spotted fever, disseminated intravascular coagulation [DIC]), atherosclerosis (secondary to hypothyroidism), hypercoagulable states (secondary to hypoproteinemia), and for no discernible cause.

Clinical Presentation

- The history usually includes acute onset of severe focal signs. The patient stabilizes rapidly and, if it survives the first 48 hours, slowly improves.
- Limb signs often are severe (usually more so than in other brain disorders), with profound extensor rigidity.
- Animals with brain stem or cerebellar "strokes" have significant torticollis. Most signs are asymmetric.
- Often there is an associated systemic disorder, and the animals will have other clinical signs.
- There appears to be a high incidence of brain-heart syndrome in patients with CNS vascular injuries, and cardiac arrhythmias and/or myocardial infarction may be seen.

Diagnostic Tests

Hematology
- Initially, search for a systemic disorder that may have resulted in hemorrhage or vasculitis.
- Obtain a hemostasis screen, bleeding time, and activated clotting time.
- Evaluate the CBC for evidence of sepsis or vasculitis.

Serum Biochemistries
- Renal failure and hypothyroidism are associated with vascular diseases of the CNS. Evaluate a biochemical profile, if evidence supports a diagnosis of hypothyroidism, evaluate a baseline T_4 and possibly a thyroid-stimulating hormone (TSH) response test (see sec. 4, ch. 1).

CSF Analysis
- The CSF may be normal, but usually there is an albuminocytologic dissociation. Occasionally there will be an increase in the number of cells.
- With hemorrhage near the subarachnoid space, xanthochromia, free blood, and erythrophagocytosis by neutrophils and macrophages are seen.
- With severe necrosis and malacia there are increased numbers of WBCs.
- The primary cell type is mononuclear (lymphocytes and macrophages), resulting in a diagnosis of non-suppurative inflammation.

CT/MRI
These image-enhancing techniques are the best tools currently available for accurately localizing a mass and determining cause. However, their use is limited by cost and availability.

Treatment

Supportive Therapy
- Give corticosteroids for edema and inflammation.
- Unless the patient is in shock, moderate fluid restriction is indicated to prevent further edema.
- Monitor for cardiac arrhythmias.
- Give nutritional support if needed. Treat any systemic electrolyte disturbances that may develop.

Specific Therapy
- If possible, treat the underlying metabolic disorder. (See Specific Therapy in the previous discussion of Principles of Treatment and refer to appropriate chapters in this book.)

Prognosis

- If the animal has no underlying disease and survives the first 48 hours, the prognosis is fair to good.
- Long-term recovery depends on the success of treatment for the underlying disorder.
- As a rule, patients with cerebellar infarcts make the best recovery and patients with brain stem hemorrhage the poorest.

Brain Abscess

Etiology

Brain abscesses are focal accumulations of pus in the CNS with clinical signs of a rapidly progressive mass lesion, often with necrosis and edema of adjacent neural tissue. They are relatively uncommon in dogs and cats.

Clinical Signs

- The onset of signs generally is acute to subacute, and the clinical course is rapidly progressive.
- Signs are usually focal and referrable to the area of the nervous system involved.
  - The most common locations are the cerebellopontine angle (direct extension from otitis interna) and the frontal lobe of the cerebrum (direct extension from chronic sinusitis).
- Often there is a prior history of inner ear, respiratory, or oral infection.
- Abscesses of hematogenous origin frequently are multiple and can occur in any part of the brain, especially in the cerebrum and hypothalamus.
- The brain abscess may be extradural, especially as a sequela to inner ear infection.

Diagnosis

The differential diagnosis for brain abscesses includes trauma, vascular injury, tumors, granulomas, and aberrant parasite migrations.

CSF Analysis
This is the test of choice for the diagnosis of brain abscesses.

- The most common finding is an increase in the number of cells, usually neutrophils, which may contain phagocytized organisms.
- Cultures may be positive and Gram stains may reveal the organism.
- Protein values are elevated, usually due to local globulin production.
- If the abscess is extradural, CSF may be normal.

CT/MRI
- The appearance of the abscess on CT and MRI may resemble that seen with hemorrhage or certain tumors; therefore, these procedures may not be able to establish the diagnosis definitively.

Treatment

Specific Therapy
- Antimicrobial drugs are the basis of specific therapy. Higher drug dosages are often required for CNS infections.
- Choose a drug based on its ability to penetrate the blood-brain barrier and its availability in parenteral and oral forms (see Tables 2 and 3).
- Use Gram staining and culture of CSF to select the most appropriate drug.
- If no organism is found, use a broad-spectrum antimicrobial agent, preferably a bactericidal rather than a bacteriostatic drug.

Supportive Therapy
- Although inflammation is associated with brain abscesses, the use of steroids is contraindicated.
  - These drugs impair the immune system and normalize the blood-brain barrier, diminishing the ability of drugs to penetrate the CNS.

TABLE 2. Antimicrobial Drug Dosages for CNS Infections

Drug	Dose (mg/kg)	Route	Frequency (hours)
Amphotericin B	0.15–0.5	IV	48
Ampicillin	5–22	IV	6
Carbenicillin	10–30	IV or IM	4–6
Cefotaxime	6–40	IM or IV	4–6
Cephalexin	20–30	PO	8
Cephapirin	20–30	IV or IM	8
Chloramphenicol	10–15	PO	4–6
Cloxacillin	8.8–20	IV or PO	4–8
Flucytosine	50	PO	8
Gentamicin	2	IV or IM	8
Metronidazole	10–15	PO	8
Penicillin (aqueous)	10,000–22,000 units/kg	IV	4–6
Rifampin	10–20	PO	8–12

IV = intravenous; IM = intramuscular; PO = per os.

- Patients with brain abscesses treated with steroids have a higher incidence of sequelae than patients not receiving steroids, although they may show a more rapid initial improvement. NSAIDs (e.g., aspirin), may be beneficial in these cases. In addition, proper fluid therapy and nutritional support are essential.

Prognosis

- In most cases, the prognosis is grave, possibly because of delay in diagnosis or inability to surgically drain the abscess.
- Cerebellar herniation may occur as a terminal event.

Otitis Media/Otitis Interna

See sec. 5, ch. 23 for discussion of this disorder.

Hydrocephalus

Etiology

Hydrocephalus is a pathologic accumulation of fluid within the ventricular system of the brain.

- It may occur as a primary condition (e.g., congenital hydrocephalus) or may be secondary to another disorder.
- Secondary hydrocephalus can result from obstruction of the ventricular system (internal hydrocephalus) or inhibition of CSF resorption at the arachnoid villi (external hydrocephalus). Meningitis, neoplasia, and head trauma are common underlying causes.

Clinical Signs

- Hydrocephalus can be occult (thus it can be an incidental finding on MRI or at necropsy), or it may result in clinical signs of cerebral dysfunction.
- Primary (congenital) hydrocephalus:
  - Common signs include seizures, visual deficits, and dementia.
  - Some affected animals have an open fontanelle, but this finding is not diagnostic, because it can occur as a normal variant in healthy toy breeds of dogs. The calvarium may be dome-shaped and prominent.
  - Bilateral divergent strabismus, referred to as the

TABLE 3. Antimicrobial Drug Penetration of the Blood-Brain Barrier

| Drug Class | Penetration | | |
	Good	Intermediate	Poor
Microbicidal	Metronidazole Trimethoprim	Ampicillin Carbenicillin Methicillin Oxacillin Penicillin Ticarcillin Some cephalosporins Cefuroxime Cefotaxime Ceftazidime Ceftriaxone Moxalactam Vancomycin	Aminoglycosides First-generation cephalosporins Clindamycin
Microbistatic	Chloramphenicol Sulfonamides	Flucytosine Tetracyclines	Amphotericin B Erythromycin Some tetracyclines

"setting sun" sign, may be present; ocular motility is normal in these cases.

- Secondary hydrocephalus causes rapidly progressive signs of diffuse cerebral dysfunction owing to precipitous elevations of intracranial pressure.

Diagnosis

Differential diagnoses include metabolic, nutritional, degenerative, and inflammatory disorders.

Skull Radiography

- Thinning of the calvarium, often with loss of the bony gyral pattern, is seen. Contrast ventriculography provides a definitive diagnosis.

Enhanced Imaging

- In patients with open fontanelles, ultrasonography with positioning of the ultrasound probe over the opening can diagnose hydrocephalus.
- In other patients, MRI or CT can establish the diagnosis.

CSF Analysis

- Increased intracranial pressure is an inconsistent finding. Generally, CSF is normal unless the hydrocephalus is secondary.

Serum Biochemistries

- Many hydrocephalic dogs are marginally hypoglycemic; therefore, if neurologic abnormalities persist in a dog that is treated for hypoglycemia, consider hydrocephalus and/or hepatoencephalopathy as underlying causes.

Treatment

- Long-term therapy with low-dose, maintenance prednisone or furosemide has had some success. The mechanism appears to be decreased production of CSF.
- Surgical drainage has been beneficial in some cases. This requires implantation of a permanent drain system (placement of a ventriculovenous shunt).
- The prognosis is fair if hydrocephalus is diagnosed and treated early.

Prognosis

- Affected animals may always be mentally dull and have limited ability to learn.

Lissencephaly

Etiology

There is retention of the early fetal pattern of the telencephalon due to restricted growth of the primor-

dial cells. Thus the gyri and sulci fail to form, and the surface of the brain is nearly smooth. Paradoxically, the gray matter of the cortex is thicker than normal, but the periventricular gray matter may appear attenuated owing to the much smaller total number of axons in the cerebrum.

Clinical Signs

- Signs include dementia, seizures, blindness, and severe behavior changes.
- Most affected animals are symptomatic at birth or shortly after.

Diagnosis

- The diagnosis is established at necropsy.

Treatment

No treatment is available.

Cerebellar Hypoplasia

Etiology

- Cerebellar hypoplasia may be genetic, related to in-utero viral (Table 4) or toxic injury, or idiopathic. The condition is present at birth and is nonprogressive.
- The genetic form has been reported in Airedales, Irish setters, and chows. It also has been reported in bull terriers, Weimaraners, dachshunds, and Labrador retrievers, but no inheritance pattern has been shown in these breeds.
- Other CNS malformations (e.g., hydranencephaly) may occur concurrently.
- It is known to affect cats also and probably can occur in other species.
- Even when the condition is related to in-utero infection, not all members of a litter will be affected.

Clinical Signs

- See Clinical Signs and Neurologic Examination at the beginning of this chapter.

Diagnosis

- The diagnosis is based on clinical signs of cerebellar dysfunction, exclusion of acquired causes, and static course. Most diagnostic tests are normal.
- The majority of patients have signs limited to the cerebellum.
- MRI/CT allow visualization of an abnormally small cerebellum. However, the cerebellum may be normal

TABLE 4. Infectious Cerebellar Hypoplasia in Domesticated Animals

Species	Infection		
	Virus	Type	Origin
Feline	Parvovirus (see sec. 2, ch. 7) (panleukopenia)	Granuloprival	In utero; early postnatal
Canine	Herpesvirus (see sec. 2, ch. 9)	Segmental dysplasia	Early postnatal

in size grossly in some patients; therefore, this test is not definitive.

Treatment

No treatment is currently available.

Prognosis

■ Many of these animals make functional pets even though they do not show any clinical improvement.

Cerebellar Abiotrophy

Etiology

Cerebellar abiotrophy is a group of inherited, slowly progressive, degenerative diseases of the cerebellum reported in many canine breeds, including Kerry blue terriers, Gordon setters, Labrador retrievers, golden retrievers, cocker spaniels, Cairn terriers, Great Danes, Airedales, Finnish harriers, Samoyeds, and Bern running dogs (Table 5). It also has been reported in cats. In contrast to cerebellar hypoplasia, cerebellar abiotrophies reflect cell dysfunction and death in previously normal tissue; thus they are frequently progressive in course.

Clinical Signs

■ Most animals are normal at birth, with signs starting at 2 months of age or older.
■ Because the disease usually is confined to the cerebellum, affected animals show only cerebellar signs, which are slowly progressive, eventually incapacitating the animal.

Diagnosis

■ Diagnosis is based on the history and clinical signs and exclusion of similar disorders in the differential diagnosis.
■ Diagnostic tests are normal, as the cerebellum is normal in size grossly.

Craniocerebral Trauma

General Principles of CNS Trauma. When a traumatic injury occurs to the spinal cord or brain certain events result. Some of these events are immediate and do not progress; the degree of recovery in these cases is based on the severity and location of the tissue damage. Other events, however, are reversible or preventable. These injuries are secondary, occurring minutes, hours, or days after the initial trauma. Because these secondary injuries often are responsive to therapy and may be fatal if not treated, it is essential to recognize and reverse these events.

Craniocerebral Trauma. Head trauma affecting the CNS is referred to as craniocerebral trauma (CCT), regardless of the precise site of injury. In the majority of animals with head trauma there is no CNS damage; however, when CCT does occur, it can result in severe disability or death. The goal of clinical management is to treat reversible injuries while preventing further, secondary damage.

Etiology

The most common cause of CCT in small animals is a motor vehicle accident. Other causes include blunt trauma (e.g., being hit by a bat or swing, child falling on the animal), animal fights, falls, and gunshot wounds.

Pathogenesis

Trauma to the CNS results in immediate and direct tissue injuries (*primary events*) that initiate a cascade of *secondary* (metabolic) *events* that worsen the neurologic disease and produce systemic effects such as increased intracranial pressure, systemic hypertension, myocardial necrosis, cardiac arrhythmias, pulmonary edema, and the need for increased nutritional support.

Primary Events
■ Necrosis/lacerations: The events that occur at the time of trauma usually involve direct mechanical injury (e.g., contusion) to fiber tracts and cell membranes. These mechanical disruptions may not be capable of repair.
■ Transient neuronal disruption (concussion): At the time of injury, some cells undergo physiologic disruption of function from hypoxia, acidosis, or unknown causes. This loss of CNS function, without structural injury, is transient and completely reversible.
■ Seizures: Seizures may occur at the time of injury or any time thereafter, resulting in elevated intracranial pressure, hypoxia, acidosis, and edema.

Secondary Events
■ Increased intracranial pressure: This usually is due to edema and hemorrhage and results in decreased cerebral blood flow by compression of vessels, which decreases outflow of CSF, further elevating pressure.
  • If not corrected, this condition can result in herniation of brain contents and death.
■ Edema: Edema can be intracellular and extracellular.
  • Intracellular edema results from hypoxia, which produces CNS acidosis. Treat by maintaining blood flow and using buffers (bicarbonate) to minimize the effects of the acidosis.
  • Extracellular edema results from leakage of fluid across the blood-brain barrier.
■ Hypoxia: Hypoxia results from decreased tissue perfusion, mainly caused by tissue swelling.
■ Hypercarbia (increased CO_2) and vascular changes: Systemic hypercarbia results in venodilation, which

---

TABLE 5. Canine Cerebellar Abiotrophy

Breed	Age of Onset	Disease Progression
Beagle, Samoyed, Irish setter	Birth	Minimal
Kerry blue terrier	9–16 weeks	Rapid
Gordon setter	6–36 months	Slow
Rough-coated collie	2–12 weeks	Rapid
Airedale, Finnish harrier, Bernese mountain dog, Labrador and golden retriever, cocker spaniel, Cairn terrier, Great Dane	4–12 weeks	Variable

decreases cerebral perfusion pressure and oxygenation, exacerbating cerebral edema.
- Some patients develop arterial spasms.

Clinical Signs

■ Assess clinical signs of CNS trauma according to the scale given in Table 6.

Treatment

In head trauma patients without evident neurologic abnormalities, observation is indicated, but treatment may not be necessary.

Surgical Therapy

■ Surgery is usually not needed except for depressed skull fractures that are compressing neural tissue and for open wounds that may serve as a source of infection:
- Elevate fractures to allow decompression and debride open wounds to prevent infection.

Emergency Measures

■ Elevate the head to facilitate passive emptying of

TABLE 6. Clinical Rating Scale for Evaluation of Patients with Craniocerebral Trauma (CCT)

Criteria	Score
Motor Activity	
Normal gait and reflexes	6
Hemiparesis, tetraparesis, or decorticate activity	5
Recumbent, intermittent extensor rigidity	4
Recumbent, constant extensor rigidity	3
Recumbent, intermittent extensor rigidity/ opisthotonus	2
Recumbent, hypotonic, depressed or absent spinal reflexes	1
Brain Stem Reflexes	
Normal PLR and OVR	6
Slow PLR and normal to reduced OVR	5
Bilateral/unresponsive miosis and normal to reduced OVR	4
Pinpoint pupils and reduced to absent OVR	3
Unilateral/unresponsive mydriasis and reduced to absent OVR	2
Bilateral/unresponsive mydriasis and reduced to absent OVR	1
Level of Consciousness	
Occasionally alert and responsive	6
Depressed/delirious, but capable of response to stimulus	5
Obtunded/stuporous, but responds to visual stimuli	4
Obtunded/stuporous, but responds to auditory stimuli	3
Obtunded/stuporous, but responds to noxious stimuli	2
Coma—i.e., unresponsive to noxious stimuli	1

Total Score	Prognosis
3–8	Grave
9–14	Poor to guarded
15–18	Good

Adapted from scale of Dr. A. Shores, Michigan State University.
PLR = pupillary light reflexes; OVR = oculovestibular reflexes.

the venous sinuses, decrease intracranial pressure enhance resorption of CSF, and maintain cerebral blood flow.
■ Give oxygen to help reverse cerebral edema and prevent hypercarbia.
■ Because of their deleterious effects, control seizures with anticonvulsive agents, preferably the short-acting drug diazepam.
■ In animals with stupor or coma, intubation/hyperventilation is the quickest way to reverse both hypercarbia and hypoxia.

Drug Therapy

■ **Corticosteroids:** Corticosteroids stabilize the blood-brain barrier, preventing the development of further edema, and lessen the inflammatory response that results from tissue necrosis, decreasing secondary demyelination.
■ Administer methylprednisolone, 1–2 mg/kg daily, for 5–7 days following injury. Give the initial dose IV.
■ **Diuretics:** Osmotic diuretics such as mannitol, carbonic anhydrase inhibitors, and furosemide help to reverse CNS edema.
■ Give furosemide, 2–4 mg/kg q6–8h.
- If the patient's condition is deteriorating rapidly, add mannitol to the treatment regimen, 1.25 g/kg IV, given as a single dose.
■ **Anticonvulsants:** Administer intravenous benzodiazepines (e.g., diazepam, lorazepam) for active seizures, followed by oral anticonvulsants (see sec. 10, ch. 3).
- If the patient remains seizure-free, taper the drug dosage and discontinue in 6 months.

Supportive Therapy

■ Give fluids and monitor for electrolyte imbalance and hypernatremia.
■ Turn the animal frequently to prevent bedsores.
■ If the patient is unable to eat, initiate hyperalimentation as soon as possible.

Prognosis

■ If injuries are limited to the peripheral nervous system (PNS), the prognosis is fair.
■ Animals with CNS injury that are in a coma for >48 hours usually do not recover.
■ In general, the prognosis for CTT is best determined by stabilization (or deterioration) of signs and by location in the CNS of the injury.

Idiopathic Vestibular Disease

■ In cats, idiopathic vestibular disease (IVD) occurs most frequently in the summer and early fall (75% of reported cases occur between June and September) but may be seen any time of year in both dogs and cats. It can occur at any age in cats.
■ Because IVD usually affects middle-aged and older dogs, it is also called geriatric or senile vestibular syndrome in dogs. It is the second most common cause of peripheral vestibular disease in dogs, accounting for 39% of all cases.
■ There is no sex predilection.

Clinical Signs

- Signs usually are acute or peracute in onset, often peaking in less than 24 hours.
- Reflecting the vestibular involvement, common signs include loss of balance, severe (often incapacitating) disorientation, ataxia, head tilt, and nystagmus. Constant, rotary nystagmus is the most common form seen.
- The nystagmus disappears after several days; the ataxia gradually resolves but may persist for 3–6 weeks.
- The disease may cause nausea initially; many patients (about 25%) vomit during the first 24 hours. The nausea may persist, making some patients anorectic for several days.

Diagnosis

Diagnostic tests are normal.

Treatment

- There is no treatment that can alter the course of the disease.
- Supportive therapy is important to prevent self-injury and to maintain adequate nutrition.

Prognosis

The prognosis generally is excellent. There rarely are any sequelae (except occasionally a mild head tilt), and recovery occurs in all cases.

Idiopathic Trigeminal Neuropathy

Also called canine dropped jaw syndrome, this is a condition of unknown pathogenesis that produces motor dysfunction of CN V. No age, breed, or sex predilection has been described. The disease appears to occur more often in the fall.

Clinical Signs

- Signs are acute or peracute in onset. Sensory abnormalities are rare.
- The patient appears unable to close its mouth, and the owner may complain that the animal is dysphagic.
- Atrophy of the masticatory muscles is an uncommon sign.
- Motor cranial nerves other than CN V, especially sympathetic innervation to the eyes, are affected rarely.
- Because the disease is confined to the PNS, limb strength and spinal reflexes are normal.

Diagnosis

Differential Diagnosis

- Any disease that affects the brain stem may produce similar signs. However, patients with brain stem involvement have other neurologic signs (e.g., weakness), which facilitates the diagnosis.
- It is important to exclude rabies (the principal differential) from the diagnosis.

- Trauma and tumors may affect CN V. However, these conditions usually involve sensory as well as motor fibers, are generally unilateral, and are associated with significant muscle atrophy.

Diagnostic Tests

- Motor nerve conduction velocity of CN V is slowed. If there is axonal involvement, electromyography (EMG) may be abnormal.
- Generally, other tests are normal.

Treatment

- The primary therapy is supportive care.
- Instruct the owner to feed the dog with its head elevated.
- Avoid using corticosteroids because they do not change the course of the disease.

Prognosis

The prognosis is excellent. Recovery has occurred in 4–8 weeks in all reported cases.

Sensory Trigeminal Neuropathy

This is a disorder of unknown pathogenesis with an acute onset and characterized by inability to prehend food and by facial analgesia. Pathologically there is a loss of CN V fibers without inflammation. The condition is unresponsive to steroids and may be a variant of idiopathic trigeminal neuropathy.

Idiopathic Facial Paralysis

This disorder is associated with unilateral or bilateral paralysis of CN VII. Although clinical signs are primarily referable to CN VII, careful testing may reveal other (often subclinical) cranial nerve involvement.

Clinical Signs

- There is an acute onset of unilateral or bilateral facial paralysis, including loss of eye blink, drooping lip, and sagging of the ear(s).
- Often, owners report excessive salivation, because of the loss of lip tone.
- If innervation to the lacrimal gland is affected, the eye and the nostril on the affected side will be dry.

Diagnosis

Differential Diagnosis

- Facial paralysis has been associated with endocrine dysfunction (e.g., hypothyroidism and hyperadrenocorticism), drug toxicity (especially from Lysodren), other toxins (e.g., lead poisoning), tumors, and middle ear infections. In the last two conditions, there usually are other signs.
- Pure isolated facial paralysis usually is idiopathic.

Diagnostic Tests

- Evaluate for endocrine disease, especially thyroid function (TSH test) (see sec. 4, ch. 1).
- EMG can confirm localization and rule out involvement of other nerves.

- Obtain skull radiographs if neoplasia or infection of the middle ear is a potential cause. Otherwise, radiography rarely is helpful.

Treatment

- If an etiology can be detected, initiate specific therapy. Otherwise, treat secondary effects such as dry eye (keraconjunctivitis sicca; see sec. 11, ch. 9).
- In humans, corticosteroids are routinely used, but they are not recommended for veterinary patients.
- Prognosis: Most patients recover in 1–2 months.

DISSEMINATED BRAIN DISEASES

Infectious Encephalitis

Inflammatory disease is the most common type of disseminated brain disorder. There are many causes of infectious encephalitis in small animals; the most important are listed below:

- In cats:
  - Feline infectious peritonitis (see sec. 2, ch. 3)
  - Toxoplasmosis (see sec. 2, ch. 13)
  - Systemic fungal diseases (primarily cryptococcosis) (see sec. 2, ch. 12)
  - Rabies and pseudorabies (see sec. 2, ch. 8)
- In dogs:
  - Canine distemper (see sec. 2, ch. 6)
  - Granulomatous meningoencephalitis
  - Systemic fungal diseases (see sec. 2, ch. 12)
  - Toxoplasmosis (see sec. 2, ch. 13)
  - *Neosporum caninum* encephalitis (sec. 2, ch. 13)
  - Rabies and pseudorabies (see sec. 2, ch. 8)

Diagnostic Tests

CSF Analysis
This is the diagnostic test of choice for inflammatory diseases of the CNS. Encephalitis causes an increase in the number of WBCs; the highest counts are seen in granulomatous and bacterial diseases.

- In systemic fungal, protozoal, and parasitic infections eosinophils may be present.
- Protein levels may be increased, mostly composed of globulins. In some viral diseases, the protein elevation may be minimal (e.g., in canine distemper and rabies).
- Organisms can be identified in bacterial and fungal diseases.

Ophthalmoscopic Examination
- Many of the inflammatory diseases of the CNS also affect the eye, causing concurrent chorioretinitis, uveitis, corneal changes, and other evidence of ophthalmic disease.
- The eye is most commonly affected in viral and granulomatous disease (see sec. 11, chs. 6 and 8).

Serology
- Testing for antibodies can sometimes help to identify the specific causative agent.

- The principal limitation is the time needed to obtain results. Also, CSF analysis is a more reliable indicator of CNS involvement.

CT/MRI
CT/MRI are more helpful for identifying mass lesions than disseminated inflammations.

Treatment

Treatment is directed at eliminating the causative infectious agent whenever possible. Administer antimicrobial agents for a period no shorter than for that recommended for a similar infection located outside the CNS.

- When choosing a drug, be sure that the agent can cross the blood-brain barrier.
- Give general supportive therapy along with specific therapy.

Granulomatous Meningoencephalitis (GME)

GME is an idiopathic inflammatory disease of the CNS that is seen primarily in dogs and that also occurs in cats. The designation *reticulosis* was coined because it was theorized that the cellular infiltrates were derived from the mononuclear-phagocytic cell line (reticuloendothelial system). It appears that reticulosis is in fact two (at least) separate diseases: an inflammatory condition called GME and a primary CNS lymphoma (see under Neoplasia).

Etiology/Pathology

- The lesions in GME may be focal or disseminated and are characterized by proliferation of vascular adventitial cells in the brain.
  - In the disseminated form (inflammatory reticulosis), there is accumulation of lymphoid, mononuclear, polymorphonuclear, plasma, and giant cells.
  - In the local form (neoplastic reticulosis), the proliferation is associated with accumulations of mitotic reticulohistiocytic and lymphoid cells.
- GME occurs most commonly in the subcortical white matter. Although lesions may occur in any portion of the CNS, there is a predilection for the cerebrum and the cerebellopontine angle. The lesions tend to coalesce, appearing as focal or multifocal masses.
- A large group of cases have the histopathologic characteristics of both processes.
- Although lesions may occur in the eye (ocular form), systemic involvement is rare.

Incidence and Prevalence

- GME is the most common inflammatory disease of the canine nervous system after canine distemper virus encephalitis.
- There is a predilection for GME in female toy-breed dogs; in one study 50% of dogs with GME were poodles or poodle crosses.
- GME occurs mainly in young and middle-aged dogs (1–8 years) but may occur at any age.

Clinical Signs and Clinical Course

- Onset usually is rapid, but indolent cases have been reported. In most cases, death occurs within 2 months; however, survivals up to 2 years are documented.
- Clinical signs vary but can be grouped according to the categories of focal, disseminated, and ocular.

Focal Form

- This form mimics an expanding mass.
- Clinical signs reflect the site of the granuloma; the most common site is the cerebellopontine angle.
- This form is intermediate in progression and there is partial response to therapy. Duration of illness may be up to 6 months but usually is less.
- Although signs are referable to the largest mass, at necropsy the disease usually is seen to be more widespread.

Disseminated Form

- This is the most rapidly progressive and diffuse form, often characterized by meningitis, neck pain, and fever.
- Because this is a multifocal disease, various neurologic signs may be seen.

Ocular Form

- There is acute visual loss in the affected eye(s), with loss of the pupillary light reflex when the eye is illuminated (optic neuritis).
- This form is rare and is the slowest to progress, often remaining static for months. With the passage of time, the disease becomes more disseminated in the CNS, and at necropsy multiple lesions are found.

Diagnosis

- The diagnosis can be confirmed only by histopathology.
- Base a tentative diagnosis on clinical signs, CSF analysis, and exclusion of other disorders.
- The principal differential for the ocular form of GME is the syndrome of acute retinal degeneration, which is seen in toy breeds of dogs.

Diagnostic Tests

- CSF Analysis: The WBC count is elevated, consisting predominantly of mononuclear cells (800 ± 300/μl in cisternal fluid and 533 ± 256/μl in lumbar fluid). There is a mixture of cell types (10–20% neutrophils, 10–20% monocytes and macrophages, and 60–80% lymphocytes and plasma cells). Eosinophils are not seen; if they are present, consider another diagnosis. In some cases, large anaplastic-type mononuclear cells may be seen.
  - Protein values generally are elevated (40–1000 mg/dl).
  - Pressure usually is normal.
  - The CSF is rapidly normalized by steroid therapy; avoid treating with steroids before collection.
- Serology: Consider blood testing for fungal and protozoal infections that can cause similar CSF analysis findings.

- Electroencephalography (EEG): Look for evidence of diffuse multifocal cerebral involvement, which is seen in most cases.

Treatment

- Administer prednisolone (1–2 mg/kg/day); other immunosuppressive drugs such as cyclophosphamide and azathioprine are being evaluated.
- Preliminary reports suggest promising results with radiation therapy.
- The success of therapy is limited to temporary remission.

Prognosis

GME almost invariably is a progressive fatal disease.

Pug Encephalitis

This is a chronic form of GME that affects all brain regions in adult pugs. It bears many similarities to GME histologically (diffuse perivascular infiltration of mononuclear cells); however, there is a higher incidence of associated malacia.

Etiology

- There is a familial tendency, and immunosuppression with secondary CNS infection is suspected.

Clinical Signs

- Onset of CNS signs occurs in young adult pugs (9 months to 4 years of age).
- Often the earliest signs are cerebral, including seizures and dementia.
- Circling, head tilt, nystagmus, and other brain stem signs are common. Cerebellar signs (e.g., head tremor) may be seen.

Diagnosis

- On CSF analysis there are increased protein values and a mixture of inflammatory cells. Eosinophils may be present, but this is atypical of classic GME.

Treatment

- Corticosteroids may alleviate the clinical signs for short periods, but antimicrobial agents have no effect.

Prognosis

- The disease is invariably fatal.

Meningitis

Etiology

- Bacterial infection of the meninges can occur as a result of septicemia, local invasion, and bite wounds. Viral and protozoal infections are rare causes.
- An immune-mediated meningitis is suspected but not proven.

■ Sterile vasculitis/meningitis has been reported in young dogs.

History/Clinical Signs

■ There may be a history of a systemic illness or a bite wound near the spine.
■ The primary signs are hyperesthesia, neck pain, depression, and fever (103–106°F).
■ Extension of nasal sinus and inner ear infections may be a source of meningitis.

Neurologic Examination

■ Ataxia and mild paresis may be seen in all four limbs.
■ Spinal reflexes usually are normal.

Diagnosis

■ In the CBC, neutrophilic leukocytes may be seen in bacterial and immune-mediated meningitis; leukopenia is present in viral infections.
■ Radiographs are normal unless the meningitis is secondary to bony infection of the spine.
■ On CSF analysis, there is normal to increased pressure, normal to increased numbers of WBCs (cell type depending on the etiology), and increased protein levels.
■ Bacterial or fungal organisms may be identified cytologically or cultured.

Treatment

■ For bacterial meningitis, administer antibiotic therapy (see Tables 2 and 3) as determined by culture and sensitivity testing of CSF or other foci of infection.
■ For immune-mediated meningitis, give prednisone long-term for immunosuppression.

Prognosis

■ The prognosis is fair to good for patients with bacterial infections and immune vasculitis that are identified early and treated properly.
■ The prognosis is poor to grave for patients with other types of meningitis.

Cerebellitis/Nonsuppurative Encephalitis

This is a condition of unknown etiology that affects mainly young and middle-aged dogs. It is also called the white dog shaker syndrome because it is seen primarily in breeds of dogs with white hair coats (e.g., bichon frisé, white poodle, Maltese terrier, West Highland white terrier).

It may be a diffuse demyelinating disorder or, because of the unusual lack of lesions, a generalized neurotransmitter deficiency disease.

Clinical Signs

■ The principal sign is acute onset of diffuse tremors of the entire body, often so severe that the animal is disabled.

■ Hyperthermia may occur as a result of the tremors.
■ A characteristic finding is chaotic and random eye movement (opsoclonus) that resembles severe, uncoordinated pathologic nystagmus.

Diagnosis

■ Base the diagnosis on clinical signs, physical and neurologic examinations, and exclusion of similar CNS disorders.
■ All diagnostic tests are normal.

Treatment

■ Corticosteroids generally are effective in reversing the clinical signs.
  • Administer prednisone, 2–3 mg/kg, PO, for several weeks, gradually tapering the dosage.
■ Do not discontinue therapy too early, or signs may recur.

Prognosis

■ The prognosis is good.
■ Generally, recovery is complete if treatment is early and vigorous; however, some dogs (about 25%) will have residual tremors that persist for life or that require protracted therapy.

CNS Intoxications

Usually there is an acute onset of abnormal consciousness in combination with seizures. Signs usually are static; any progression is attributed to the metabolic consequences of seizures (e.g., brain edema, hypoxia, acidosis).

General principles of therapy for intoxications are:

■ Identify and remove the source.
■ Whenever possible, inactivate or remove the toxin.
■ Reactivate or replace injured enzyme systems.
■ Provide supportive therapy.

Intoxications commonly seen in small animal medicine are discussed here.

Encephalopathy Due to Sepsis

■ Septicemia may result in a diffuse encephalopathy (CNS micro-abscesses, infarction, and hemorrhage) without serum biochemical changes or any other recognizable cause for the encephalopathy.
■ The encephalopathy is probably the result of CNS intoxication from the by-products of bacteria and WBCs.

Clinical Signs
■ Signs include an acute decrease in the level of consciousness and multifocal seizures, accompanied by other evidence of sepsis (e.g., fever, shock).

Diagnosis
■ Cytologically, there usually is neutropenia with a degenerative left shift.
■ CSF analysis usually is normal, although there may be evidence of meningitis.
■ EEG may show diffuse or multifocal abnormalities.

Treatment

■ Correct the underlying septicemia and provide adequate supportive therapy.

Lead Intoxication

Etiology

■ Sources of lead include lead-painted walls in old buildings, dry wall (plasterboard or sheetrock), caulking material, batteries, crank case oil, and grease.
■ Lead levels in the soil can be high as a result of the long-term use of leaded gas.
■ Animals that are chewers or diggers may develop lead poisoning.

Clinical Signs

■ Lead intoxication usually occurs in young animals.
■ Generally there is an acute onset of gastrointestinal (GI) signs (diarrhea, occasionally constipation), colic, and CNS signs such as dementia, blindness, hysteria, and seizures.
■ Pharyngeal and laryngeal paralysis may also be seen.
■ Lead intoxication alters cerebral metabolism and leads to edema, hypoxic changes, and eventually (if untreated) cerebral necrosis.
■ The primary differential is canine distemper.

Diagnosis

■ On the CBC there may be many nucleated RBCs, mild anemia, and marked basophilic stippling.
■ Metal-dense material may be visible radiographically in the GI tracts of animals that have recently ingested lead.
■ Definitive diagnosis is based on measurement of blood lead:

KEY POINT ▶ When testing for lead poisoning, be sure to use unclotted, whole blood, because lead attaches to the red cell membrane. Do not use EDTA as the anticoagulant because it chelates lead and gives a falsely low reading

• Blood levels > 40 μg/dl in the presence of clinical signs are highly suggestive of intoxication.
• Blood levels > 60 μg/dl are diagnostic of lead poisoning, even without signs.

Treatment

■ Whenever possible, determine the source of the lead and prevent further exposure.
■ Prior to therapy, take radiographs of the abdomen to determine if there is lead in the GI tract. If lead is present remove with cathartics or enemas prior to EDTA therapy.
■ Remove lead from tissues using chelation therapy.
  • Give calcium disodium EDTA (Calcium Disodium Versenate; Riker), 100 mg/kg/day, divided into four daily doses (maximum daily dose = 2 g). Dilute to 1.0% solution in 5% dextrose in water and administer SC for 5 days (20 total treatments).
  • Alternatively, give D-penicillamine (Cuprimine; Merck Sharp & Dohme), 110 mg/kg/day, PO, once or divided q6–8h for 14 days. Penicillamine is less

effective than calcium disodium EDTA and frequently causes vomiting.
■ If seizures persist, institute appropriate anticonvulsant therapy (see sec. 10, ch. 3).
■ If the animal shows progressive decreases in the level of consciousness after therapy is started, administer dexamethasone, 0.1 mg/kg/q24h, to decrease cerebral edema.

Prognosis

■ The prognosis is good with early diagnosis and treatment.

Organophosphate (OP), Carbamate, and Chlorinated Hydrocarbon (ClHC) Intoxication

Etiology and Pathophysiology

■ These chemicals are commonly used insecticides. OPs and carbamates are found in flea collars, wormers, and insecticide spray and dips; ClHCs are found in dips and sprays.
■ OPs and carbamates are anticholinesterase drugs that produce signs by allowing uninhibited excitation of synapses. Although most of the effects of these drugs occur at the neuromuscular junction, the signs usually are classified as seizures.
■ ClHCs cause a true cerebral encephalopathy.

Clinical Signs and History

■ Usually there is a history of contact with the insecticide.
■ Insecticide intoxication is characterized by excessive salivation, miotic pupils, seizures, and/or whole body trauma.
■ OPs may produce vomiting and diarrhea.
■ Farm dogs and cats can be poisoned by eating stool from horses and cattle that have licked OP-impregnated salt blocks.

Diagnosis

■ OP and carbamate intoxication: RBC and serum cholinesterase levels are reduced.
■ ClHC intoxication: Analyze a fat biopsy for presence of the drug.

Treatment

■ Stop seizures with intravenous diazepam or phenobarbital to effect (see sec. 10, ch. 3).
■ For OP intoxication, administer atropine (0.2 mg/kg, IM or SC) or pralidoxime (2-PAM) (20 mg/kg IV over a 2-minute period; subsequent doses q8–12h, IM or SC). *Do not* use 2-PAM in carbamate intoxications.
■ Supportive therapy: Administer fluids to aid in diuresis and elimination of toxins. Bathe animal to remove any external residual toxins.

Prognosis

■ The prognosis is good with early diagnosis and treatment; however, recovery may take several weeks.

Strychnine Intoxication

Because the sale of strychnine is now illegal in the United States, this intoxication is most likely to occur in free-roaming animals in rural areas where farmers or ranchers have saved supplies of strychnine products for eradication of feral animals.

Pathophysiology

■ Strychnine is antagonistic to glycine, a putative inhibitory neurotransmitter.

Clinical Signs and History

■ Look for a history of other dogs or cats in the area with similar signs.
■ There is acute onset of hypertonic contractures of muscles (tremors and spasms) that may resemble seizures.
■ Hyperthermia due to the muscle contractions may be seen. Stress or noise causes flailing of limbs and exacerbation of other signs.

Neurologic Examination

■ There are severe extensor spasms and opisthotonus.
■ All limbs are in an extreme rigid, hypertonic state.

Diagnosis

■ Base the diagnosis on clinical signs and potential for exposure.

Treatment

■ Control muscle spasms with diazepam (Valium).
■ If diazepam is ineffective, administer intravenous sodium pentobarbital or phenobarbital to effect, while monitoring for respiratory depression.
■ Use fluid therapy to help eliminate the toxin from the animal's system.
■ If the strychnine was ingested within the last 12 hours, perform gastric lavage, followed by administration of activated charcoal to adsorb the toxin.

Prognosis

■ The prognosis is fair if treatment is started early.
■ If treatment is delayed and protracted seizures have occurred, the prognosis is poor.

Ethylene Glycol Poisoning

Ingestion of ethylene glycol, the active component of antifreeze products, initially causes progressive CNS depression characterized by disorientation, stupor, and coma, followed by renal failure (see sec. 8, ch. 1 for discussion of diagnosis and treatment).

Thiamine Deficiency

Etiology/Pathophysiology

■ Thiamine is a water-soluble vitamin (B_1) that is a cofactor in the decarboxylation of pyruvate and alpha-ketoglutarate, which is essential for aerobic metabolism.
■ Deficiency of thiamine blocks the aerobic metabolic pathways of the CNS. As a result, there is conversion to glycolysis, local production of lactic acid, and neuronal dysfunction. In carnivores, the end result is hemorrhagic necrosis of the CNS, centered in the midbrain.
■ Because vitamin B_1 cannot be manufactured by mammals, it must be available in the diet. Also, it must be added to commercial foods to replace that lost in processing.

■ Thiamine supplementation is especially necessary for cats, which do not store the vitamin in large quantities. Furthermore, if cats are fed uncooked fish with reddish flesh (e.g., tuna, salmon), which contain a thiamine-inactivating enzyme (thiaminase), vitamin B_1 deficiency can result.

Clinical Signs

■ Signs are acute in onset and can include progressive seizures and dementia, blindness with normal pupils, stupor and coma, and episodes of opisthotonus.
■ In cats signs can include fixed dilated pupils, paralysis of the extraocular muscles, and vestibular crises consisting of rigid extension of all four limbs with the head and neck ventroflexed between the front limbs. These crises are sometimes considered vestibular seizures.
■ In the early stages, the signs wax and wane, but then progress.

Diagnosis

■ In the differential diagnosis, rule out inflammations, toxic injuries, and vascular disorders.
■ Base the diagnosis on clinical signs and history.
■ Routine laboratory tests are normal, but serum assayed for thiamine metabolites can confirm the deficiency.

Treatment

The manifestations of thiamine deficiency are completely reversible with early treatment.

■ Inject thiamine (cats, 5–30 mg/day; dogs, 10–100 mg/day), followed by dietary correction.
■ Continue vitamin supplementation (oral) for 1–2 weeks after release from the hospital if the animal is anorectic.
■ Avoid giving intravenous dextrose prior to thiamine therapy; this may cause exacerbation of signs.

Prognosis

■ The prognosis is excellent with proper treatment; if untreated, the condition is fatal.

Metabolic Encephalopathies

Various metabolic disorders may secondarily impair CNS function, especially affecting the cerebrum because of its high energy requirement. Metabolic encephalopathies are characterized by altered consciousness (confusion, delirium, stupor, and coma) and, occasionally, by altered motor and ventilatory responses. For additional information concerning the metabolic causes of encephalopathy in the list that follows, refer to sections/chapters shown in parentheses.

■ Fuel deprivation:
  • Hypoxia: respiratory dysfunction, ischemia (sec. 6)
  • Hypoglycemia: excess insulin, decreased gluconeogenesis, excess utilization (sec. 4, chs. 4 and 5)

■ Endogenous neurotoxins
  • Uremia: renal failure (sec 8, ch. 1)
  • Hepatic encephalopathy (hyperammonemia): portosystemic shunts, liver failure (sec. 7, ch. 8)
■ Endocrine dysfunction: Cushing's syndrome, Addison's disease, thyrotoxicosis, hypothyroid myxedema (sec. 4, chs. 1 and 3)
■ Acid-base, water, and ionic imbalances (sec 1, ch. 5)
  • Acid-base: acidosis, alkalosis, CO_2 excess from pulmonary insufficiency
  • Water: Hypo-osmolar (diuretic therapy, hyponatremia) or hyperosmolar (hypernatremia, hyperglycemia) states
  • Ions: hypercalcemia, hypocalcemia (sec. 4, ch. 2)
■ Exogenous neurotoxins or deficiency states
  • Toxins: anticholinergics, mold intoxication, lead, sedative-depressants (barbiturates, benzodiazepines), salicylates
  • Deficiency states: thiamine deficiency

Lysosomal Storage Disease (LSD)

See Table 7 for a list of types of LSD seen in dogs and cats.

Etiology

■ Lysosomes are membrane-bound cytoplasmic particles found in all cells that contain hydrolytic enzymes. They are responsible for degradation of protein, polysaccharides, and nucleic acids. Rare genetic defects cause lysosomal deficiency and produce secondary lysosomal engorgement with undegraded material. As a result, cell function is compromised.
■ LSD is most likely to occur in purebred animals with historical inbreeding in the affected line.

Clinical Signs

■ Affected animals are normal at birth, with signs developing during the first year of life
■ Usually only a single member of a litter is affected, and its development lags behind that of the others.
■ Signs are those of a disseminated process and include ataxia tremors, paresis, visual loss, seizures, and behavior changes. Although age of onset and progression of disease vary, they often are related. As a rule, the younger the animal at the onset of clinical signs, the more rapid the progression of disease.
■ More than one body system (liver, skin, hemopoietic) may be affected.

TABLE 7. Lysosomal Storage Disease in Dogs and Cats

Disease	Breed	Age at Onset	Other Involvement
Ganglioside GM₁ Beta-galactosidase deficiency	Siamese, Korat, DSH cats	4–6 months	Cornea Retina Liver Pancreatic acinar cells
	Beagles, mixed-breed dogs	2–4 months	Liver Kidney Spleen Lymph nodes
Ganglioside GM₂ Hexosaminidase deficiency	German short-haired pointers	6 months	None
	DSH cats	4–10 weeks	Skeleton Cornea Liver Bone marrow Spleen Kidney
Sphingomyelin lipidosis (sphingomyelinase deficiency)	Siamese, DSH cats	3–6 months	Stunted growth Liver Lung Spleen Lymph nodes Kidney Bone marrow Adrenal glands
Glucocerebrosidosis (glucocerebrosidase deficiency)	Sidney silky terriers	7 months	Liver
Neuronal ceroid lipofuscinosis	English setters DSH cats	14–18 months	Lymph nodes Salivary glands Prostate Kidney
Globoid cell leukodystrophy	Cairn terriers, West Highland white terriers, beagles, blue tick hounds, poodles	11–30 weeks	None

DSH = domestic short-haired.

Diagnosis

- Diagnosis is based on history, clinical signs, and laboratory demonstration of abnormal storage products in cells and tissues such as blood, bone marrow, CSF, lymph nodes, rectal smooth muscle, and brain.
- Necropsy can confirm the diagnosis.

Treatment

LSD is always progressive and fatal.

- The only treatment is prevention through control of breeding and genetic counseling.

Supplemental Readings

Bailey CS, Higgins RJ: Comparison of total white blood cell count and total protein content of lumbar and cisternal cerebrospinal fluid of healthy dogs. Am J Vet Res 46:1162, 1985.

Bruyette DS, Tomlinson JL: Canine cerebral abscess: A case report and discussion. Vet Med Small Anim Clin:1706, 1983.

Carrillo JM, Sarfaty D, Greenlee P: Intracranial neoplasm and associated inflammatory response from the central nervous system. J Am Anim Hosp Assoc 22:367, 1986.

Cordy DR: Canine granulomatous meningoencephalitis. Vet Pathol 16:325, 1979.

Cuddon PA, Smith-Maxie L. Reticulosis of the central nervous system in the dog. Compend Contin Educ Pract Vet 6:23, 1984.

deLahunta A: *Veterinary Neuroanatomy and Clinical Neurology,* 2nd Ed. Philadelphia: W. B. Saunders, 1983.

Eichenwald HF: Bacterial meningitis: Is there a best antimicrobial therapy? Eur J Pediatr 146:216, 1987.

Fankhauser R, Fatzer R, Luginbuhl H, McGrath JT: Reticulosis of the central nervous system (CNS) in dogs. Adv Vet Sci Comp Med 16:35, 1972.

Gelb LD: Infections: Bacteria, fungi, and parasites. *In* Pearlman AL, Collins RC, eds. *Neurobiology of Disease.* New York: Oxford University Press, 1990, pp 417–434.

Greene CE: Infections of the Central Nervous System. *In* Greene CE, ed.: *Clinical Microbiology and Infectious Disease of the Dog and Cat.* Philadelphia: W. B. Saunders, 1984, p 284.

Hudson MD: Bacterial meningitis: A case study and review. J Am Anim Hosp Assoc 12:88, 1976.

Kornegay JN: Cerebellar vermian hypoplasia of dogs. Proc Am Coll Vet Intern Med 4(II):23, 1986.

Kornegay JN: Cerebrospinal fluid collection, examination, and interpretation in dogs and cats. Compend Contin Educ Pract Vet. 3:85, 1981.

Meric JM. Canine meningitis: A changing emphasis. J Vet Intern Med 2:26, 1988.

Sarfaty D, Carrillo, Greenlee PG. Differential diagnosis of granulomatous meningoencephalomyelitis, distemper, and suppurative meningoencephalitis in the dog. J Am Vet Med Assoc 188:387, 1986.

Shores A. Cranio-cerebral trauma: Emergency management and prognosis. Proc Am Coll Vet Intern Med 6:3, 1988.

Schunk KL, Averill DR: Peripheral vestibular syndrome in the dog: A review of 83 cases. J Am Vet Med Assoc 182:1354, 1893.

Vandevelde M: Morphologic and histochemical characteristics of GME and reticulosis: One disease or two? The Bern perspective. Proc Am Coll Vet Intern Med 4(II):81, 1986.

Whitby M, Finch R: Bacterial meningitis. Rational selection and use of antibacterial drugs. Drugs 31:266, 1986.

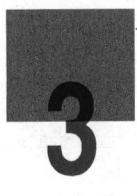

3 Seizures, Narcolepsy, and Cataplexy

William R. Fenner

Paroxysmal disorders are characterized by sudden changes in consciousness or behavior. In veterinary medicine they include two groups of disorders: seizures (epilepsy) and sleep disorders (narcolepsy).

SEIZURE DISORDERS

Definitions

Seizure—An abnormal, excessive, paroxysmal synchronous discharge in a population of neurons that results in a period of clinical abnormality. A seizure is a symptom of dysfunction in the gray matter of the brain, not a disease itself.

Epilepsy—A condition of recurring seizures, regardless of the cause. Epilepsy is *symptomatic* if a cause can be found, and *idiopathic* if the cause remains unknown. Between 2% and 3% of dogs and 0.5% of cats are epileptic.

Status epilepticus—Generalized seizures continuing for 30 minutes or more without interruption, with no return to consciousness between seizures.

Cluster seizures—Two or more seizures occurring in the same 24-hour period.

Acute symptomatic seizures—Seizures occurring in close temporal association with a known cause of seizures (e.g., within 1 week of an acute central nervous system [CNS] insult such as head trauma or encephalitis or at the time of an acute systemic metabolic or toxic insult, such as hypoglycemia, uremia, and lead poisoning).

Remote symptomatic seizures—Seizures in individuals with a CNS insult known to substantially increase the probability of subsequent epilepsy, such as head trauma, vascular insult, encephalitis, and congenital malformations occurring weeks to months prior to the first seizure.

Idiopathic Seizures—Seizures in the absence of seizure provoking insult.

Facilitating Conditions. A variety of drugs and physiologic states are known to lower the seizure threshold (increase the possibility of a seizure). These drugs and metabolic states do not usually produce epilepsy by themselves, but unmask it in an animal that has a tendency toward epilepsy.

KEY POINT ▶ Phenothiazine tranquilizers (e.g., acepromazine) lower the seizure threshold and are contraindicated in patients with epilepsy.

- Cyclical estrogen fluctuations *increase* the frequency of seizures in epileptic patients.

Inhibiting Conditions. Certain drugs and physiologic states are known to raise the seizure threshold (decrease the possibility of a seizure). This is known as an *antiepileptic* effect. In an animal that has a tendency toward epilepsy, these drugs and metabolic states may be sufficient to mask the disorder.

- Cyclical progesterone fluctuations *decrease* the frequency of seizures in epileptic patients.
- Drugs that inhibit the actions of seizures are covered later in the discussion of antiepileptic drugs under Treatment.

Etiology

Symptomatic Seizures

Changes in the metabolic state of the brain can change the available precursors for neurotransmitters.

- Some metabolic diseases decrease the available precursor for (CNS) *inhibition;* these metabolic diseases may cause epilepsy.
- Diseases that decrease the available precursor for CNS *excitation* can cause depression.
- A physical injury in a localized brain region (e.g., a tumor) that affects mostly inhibitory neurons may produce epilepsy.
- The relative frequency of symptomatic epilepsy varies with the species (dog ≅ 20% of cases; cat ≅ 50%).

Structural Symptomatic Seizures. These seizures are the result of brain injury. A disturbance of cerebral anatomy results in recurring seizures. This may result from the disruption of inhibitory interneurons or increased excitability of neurons (Table 1).

Metabolic Symptomatic Epilepsy. These disorders cause epileptiform phenomena. These are reversible insults to a normal brain that result in clinical seizures. The seizures occur only during periods of abnormal metabolic function. When the underlying disorder is corrected, the seizures do not recur (see Table 1).

Idiopathic Epilepsy. This condition appears to be related to an inherent imbalance in neurotransmitter levels. The underlying cause is not understood. In the

TABLE 1. Structural and Metabolic Causes of Symptomatic Epilepsy

Species	Structural Causes	Metabolic Causes
Canine	Canine distemper	Hypoglycemia
	Encephalitis	Hepatoencephalopathy
	Toxoplasmosis	Hypoxia
	Systemic fungal infections	Thiamine deficiency
	Lysosomal storage	Hypernatremia
	disorders	Moldy foodstuff
	Hydrocephalus	Renal failure
	Granulomatous	Hypocalcemia
	meningoencephalitis	Poisoning
	Aujesky's disease	Ethylene glycol
	Rabies	Lead
	Systemic vasculitis	Organophosphate
	Neoplasia	Carbamate
	Trauma	
	Abscess	
	Infarction	
Feline	Infectious peritonitis	Hypoglycemia
	Polioencephalomyelitis	Hepatoencephalopathy
	Toxoplasmosis	Hypoxia
	Systemic fungal infections	Thiamine deficiency
	Lysosomal storage	Hypernatremia
	disorders	Moldy foodstuff
	Hydrocephalus	Renal failure
	Granulomatous	Hypocalcemia
	meningoencephalitis	Poisoning
	Aujesky's disease	Ethylene glycol
	Rabies	Lead
	Neoplasia	Organophosphate
	Trauma	Carbamate
	Abscess	
	Infarction	

dog, about 80% of all cases of epilepsy are idiopathic; in the cat, only 50% of cases are idiopathic.

Clinical Features
Stages

Aura—The period immediately preceding the seizure. The aura is usually short and characterized by behavioral changes such as restlessness, crying, and hiding.

Ictus—The actual clinical seizure. This stage generally is brief, lasting less than 2 minutes: however, there may be clusters of several seizures. The clinical seizure may consist of abnormal consciousness, muscle tone, and autonomic function; involuntary muscle movement; and altered sensation and behavior.

Postictus—The period of neuronal recovery following a seizure. The postictal period is of variable duration but usually lasts less than 30 minutes. Clinical signs are usually behavioral. Weakness and blindness may occur.

Classification

Seizures may be classified according to clinical appearance or etiology. Each method has its advantages and disadvantages. A combination of the two methods is probably preferable. For an etiologic classification, see Etiology. Classification according to clinical appearance is as follows.

Partial Seizures (focal or local). These begin in a discrete cortical area, the seizure focus, and have restricted or asymmetric clinical manifestations. They may progress to a generalized seizure.

Simple Partial. These often are asymmetric and are rarely associated with loss of consciousness. The patient may have partial (focal) motor seizures characterized by local muscle involvement.

Complex Partial. These involve alterations of consciousness plus abnormal complex behavior, they are also called psychomotor, temporal lobe, and limbic seizures.

Generalized Seizures. These are bilaterally symmetric in the brain from the onset. There does not appear to be any localization of the seizures.

Generalized Convulsive. These are associated with involuntary, uncontrolled motor activity. The most common are tonic/clonic (grand mal) seizures, which involve the entire body, usually have autonomic release, are always characterized by loss of consciousness, and have no localizing signs.

Generalized Nonconvulsive. These are also called absence and petit mal seizures. The primary clinical sign is loss of consciousness. There is no spontaneous motor activity during these seizures; rather, there is a transient collapse. This type of seizure is easily confused with narcolepsy.

Diagnostic Approach

The goal in the work-up of a patient with seizures is to distinguish seizures with a discernible cause from those without a known cause. If a cause can be found, treatment may result in relief of the secondary problem of epilepsy.

KEY POINT ▶ Because many patients having a single seizure will never have a second, it is imperative that the diagnostic work-up include a follow-up period without therapy to determine if the patient is epileptic.

History

Always begin with a careful history.

- As a rule of thumb, the longer the patient has been epileptic, the less likely that a cause for the seizures will be found.
- Carefully determine seizure; type focal seizures are a common feature of structural diseases.
- Ask about interictal (between seizures) behavior, because change in seizure type and interictal dementia are common features of extracranial diseases.

Neurologic Examination

The neurologic examination is the best clue to the presence of structural disease.

- In some cases of idiopathic epilepsy, the postictal neural examination may be abnormal; therefore, reexamination is necessary to determine whether the abnormal results persist.
- In patients with metabolic disease, the seizure may

unmask a prior CNS injury that was clinically silent. In these patients, the neural examination may be abnormal.

- If examination results are normal, metabolic symptomatic epilepsy and functional epilepsy are probable diagnoses (15% of structural causes of epilepsy in humans are associated with a normal neurologic examination).
- If examination results are abnormal, a vigorous diagnostic evaluation is mandatory.

Laboratory Tests

- A complete blood count (CBC), serum biochemical profile, bile acid measurement, urinalysis, and fecal examination are recommended for all epileptic patients.
- Electroencephalography is indicated, although it is sometimes difficult to obtain and interpret. If there are interictal EEG abnormalities, eliminate the diagnosis of idiopathic epilepsy and vigorously pursue an etiology.
- Skull radiographs may be helpful if you suspect congenital hydrocephalus, head trauma, or a tumor of the calvarium.
- Collect cerebrospinal fluid (CSF) if the client allows it (see sec. 10, ch. 1). Because this procedure requires anesthesia in small animals, some clients are reluctant to have it performed.
- Perform ophthalmoscopy on all epileptic patients and look for evidence of systemic illness or inflammatory diseases.
- Reserve computerized tomography (CT) and magnetic resonance imaging (MRI) for patients with an abnormal neural examination or refractory seizures. If there is an open fontanel, cranial ultrasonography may be helpful.

Principles of Antiepileptic Therapy

The first principle in the treatment of epilepsy is to treat the cause if one can be found. If this is not possible, then treat the patient's symptoms (the seizures) with antiepileptic drugs.

Long-term oral antiepileptic therapy is designed to prevent, or control, seizures. This is accomplished by establishing and maintaining blood levels of a drug that inhibits the development or propagation of seizure discharges in the CNS.

KEY POINT ▶ It is important from the beginning of treatment that you and the client have the same definition of seizure control.

Seizure Control. The author defines each step in control as a 100% increase in the interictal time (the time between seizures). Achieve the first step. If inadequate, a second step of control should be attained. This method gives clients specific goals and allows them to see progress. If you cannot define control, clients will be unhappy because they cannot judge progress. Also, be realistic from the beginning. Current estimates of the success of antiepileptic therapy in veterinary patients range from 50% to 80% of cases.

Treatment Objectives

- Decrease number of seizures.
- Decrease severity of individual seizures.
- Increase time between seizure episodes.
- Decrease postictal effects.
- Avoid drug toxicity.
- Use a single drug.

These objectives still leave the client without any concrete specific goals. This is why you achieve control in steps.

KEY POINT ▶ Essential to treating epilepsy is client education and accurate information. Provide all owners of epileptic animals with a calendar for recording seizure activity. This will enable accurate assessment of the effects of therapy.

Starting Therapy

The decision when to begin therapy is arbitrary. You should, however, be certain that the patient is epileptic, (i.e., more than one seizure). I normally wait for the third seizure. This allows two interictal periods to be used as a baseline for judging the effectiveness of therapy. Use the interictal period to decide when to start drugs. My guidelines are:

- *Isolated seizures*—Start therapy if there is more than one seizure every 4–6 weeks. Because seizures may occur irregularly, another guideline is no more than 10–12 seizures in 1 year.
- *Cluster seizures*—Start therapy if there is more than one cluster every 2–3 months. Because clusters may occur irregularly, another guideline is to start therapy if there are more than 4–6 cluster seizures in 1 year.

Loading Dose. When initiating therapy, begin at a maintenance dose and wait for serum levels to equilibrate or use a loading dose to establish blood levels rapidly. The loading dose is calculated as follows:

Loading dose = volume of distribution (liters/kg) × desired level (mg/liter or μg/ml)

Pharmacokinetic Principles

- The time interval between drug doses should not exceed the half-life of the drug if the drug is to accumulate in the body at steady-state levels.
- However, to avoid wide fluctuations in serum levels and adverse consequences of a missed dose, an interval equal to ½ the drug's half-life is the minimum recommended. For example, administer a drug with a 24-hour half-life q12h. This is especially important in dogs because this species appears to be a rapid metabolizer of many antiepileptic drugs.
- A long half-life increases the risk of drug toxicity. This can be a problem with cats, which are slow metabolizers of antiepileptic agents, and in dogs when using potassium bromide (half-life about 24 days).

Serum Monitoring

KEY POINT ▶ Regular monitoring of antiepileptic drug serum levels is essential for control of epilepsy.

Serum monitoring allows evaluation of compliance and validation of the drug's effectiveness.

- Begin serum monitoring after a steady-state level has been attained. This usually takes five half-lives (e.g., 5 days for a drug with a 24-hour half-life).
- Measure serum levels at the same relative time in each patient. Begin measuring serum concentrations after peak induction has occurred.
- To monitor serum levels of phenobarbital, obtain a sample 14 days after initiating therapy. To adjust the dose to the target range, use the formula:

$$X = \frac{current\ dose \times desired\ blood\ level}{current\ blood\ level}$$

The value X is an approximation of the dose required to reach the desired blood level.

- The therapeutic range is a guideline whose upper and lower limits are based on patient response. Determine a target value within the guidelines and maintain serum concentrations within 20% of the target value.
- Take samples every 6–9 months, as well as whenever a seizure occurs. If there are signs of toxicity, modify the dosage based on your findings.

Interpreting Results. The therapeutic range is a statistical concept derived from a large population of patients. It is designed to be used only as a guideline. The bottom of the therapeutic range is the serum concentration above which most patients will have a decrease in seizure activity (i.e., seizure control is established). The top of the therapeutic range is the serum concentration at which most patients will be expected to have dose-related side effects.

- Serum levels may be measured at their peak (time of highest blood level). This is the best time to look for toxicity, but it provides no information about lowest daily (minimum therapeutic) level.
- Serum levels may be measured on the slope or halfway between trough and peak. Theoretically, this is the best overall time, as it allows evaluation of absorption and clearance. However, it gives no information about minimum therapeutic levels and requires multiple samples.
- Finally, *trough* level may be measured. This is the lowest serum level of the day. Trough levels are best for evaluation of minimal effective dose; they do not evaluate a toxic dose. When establishing control, the trough is the best sample to take; therefore, it is currently the most commonly used method.

Enzyme induction

Many antiepileptic drugs induce the enzymes responsible for their own metabolism, which then shortens their half-life. For this reason, steady-state blood levels often fall during the first week(s) of therapy. Do not assume that an increase in seizure activity means drug failure; it may mean dose failure. If you do not know the serum levels, you do not know if a drug has truly failed.

Toxicity

In general, the more drugs used, the greater the chance of drug toxicity. Many studies have shown that the use of multiple antiepileptic drugs usually potentiates toxicity and rarely improves control. Toxicity is usually dose-related: as the dose increases, so does the chance for toxicity. However, some patients may have true idiosyncratic reactions to a drug, displaying toxicity at very low doses.

Choosing a Drug

Various drugs are used in the treatment of epilepsy. Your first decision is which one to use and why. Choose a drug known to be effective in controlling seizures.

KEY POINT ▶ At proper serum levels, more than 60% of dogs can be controlled with phenobarbital. Other drugs appear to be less effective and have greater side effects.

- The ability to maintain blood levels and ease of administration are essential factors in drug choice. These factors diminish the value of phenytoin, carbamazepine, and possibly valproate.
- Veterinary studies have documented the relatively high toxicity of primidone compared with other commonly used antiepileptics.
- Many antiepileptic drugs produce side effects that do not endanger the animal's health but make it less acceptable as a companion.
  - Potassium bromide causes profound sedation.
  - Phenobarbital and primidone cause hyperactivity in about 40% of patients.
- Phenobarbital and potassium bromide are the least expensive drugs.
- Based on all factors, the author's choice in most cases is phenobarbital.

Changing Therapy

KEY POINT ▶ Always try to stay with one drug.

- Increase drug dosage to the point of control or toxicity; that is, consider changing drugs only after failure to control seizures or if there are signs of toxicity (i.e., serum levels in the toxic range).
- Begin administration of the new drug while maintaining the original drug at therapeutic levels. When therapeutic levels of the new drug are reached, gradually reduce administration of the first drug (taper over 1 month).
- If a patient is receiving antiepileptic therapy and is presented because of seizure relapse, draw a blood sample to measure drug serum levels before prescribing any drugs.
- The majority of antiepileptic drug failures are due to inadequate serum levels and in many cases can be corrected by dosage adjustment and client education.

■ There is always some correlation between serum drug levels and seizure frequency. If no consistent relationship occurs, reassess the diagnosis.

Ending Therapy

■ Factors that influence the potential for seizure recurrence when antiepileptic therapy is ended include
  • Type of seizure
  • The number of drugs tried before control is established
  • The number of seizures that occur before control is established
  • The final drug used to effect control
■ Patients with complex partial seizures with secondary generalization have the worst prognosis. If this group is considered as having the highest chance of relapse, then:
  • Patients with complex partial seizures without secondary generalization have the lowest chance of relapse.
  • Patients with generalized seizures have an intermediate chance of relapse.
■ Do not discontinue therapy until the patient is seizure-free for about 18 months.
■ If the final drug is phenobarbital, the patient may have withdrawal seizures unrelated to recurrence of epilepsy.

Antiepileptic Drugs—Indications and Clinical Use

Table 2 lists dosages and therapeutic half-lives of commonly used antiepileptic drugs.

KEY POINT ▶ Remember that the recommended initial dosages are guidelines; they will be accurate in only about 50% of cases.

Barbiturates

All barbiturates appear to induce *pharmacodynamic tolerance* (i.e., neurons adapt to the sedative effects of phenobarbital over time). This tolerance can develop rapidly. This is important for several reasons:

■ Initial sedation will resolve over a period of 1–2 weeks and lowering the drug dose is not necessary.
■ The patient may begin to require progressively higher drug doses to control the epilepsy.
■ Pharmacodynamic tolerance to barbiturates may result in the necessity for higher doses of anesthetics.

Barbiturates also induce *drug disposition tolerance*. This is the result of enzyme activation in the liver, which speeds up the detoxification of barbiturates. As a result, serum levels decline and a higher dose is required to maintain a given serum concentration. This generally develops in the first 2 weeks of therapy.

KEY POINT ▶ Phenobarbital is the antiepileptic of choice in veterinary medicine.

Phenobarbital. Phenobarbital is indicated in all seizure types.

■ The advantages of phenobarbital are that it is safe, effective, and inexpensive.
■ Disadvantages are its side effects, variable absorption, and the fact that it is a controlled drug.

Metabolism and Dosage

■ Phenobarbital is eliminated primarily by hepatic biotransformation. Elimination half-life in the dog is about 40 hours.
■ The initial dosage in dogs and cats is 5 mg/kg/day in divided doses.
■ The maintenance dosage is based on serum levels and clinical effects. Although the therapeutic range is 15–45 mg/liter, serum levels >30 mg/liter are recommended by some for adequate control.
  • For most dogs, a trough phenobarbital level of around 25 mg/liter is ideal for the initial step of control.

Adverse Effects

■ The principal adverse effect of phenobarbital is sedation. Most animals develop a tolerance to this side effect. (i.e., sedation abates while serum levels remain the same or increase). Tolerance generally requires 7–10 days to occur.

TABLE 2. Drugs Used in the Treatment of Epilepsy

Drug (Product Name)	Initial Dosage	Half-Life	Therapeutic Range
Phenobarbital	2.5 mg/kg q12h	40 hours	15–45 μg/ml (canine); 10–30 μg/ml (feline)
Primidone (Mylepsin; Fort Dodge—and Klonopin; Roche)	5–10 mg/kg q8h	40 hours (phenobarbital)	15–45 μg/ml (phenobarbital)
Potassium bromide	8–10 mg/kg q12h	24 days	1–1.5 mg/ml
Diazepam (Valium; Roche)	1–2 mg/kg q8h (canine); 0.16–0.33 mg/kg q8h (feline)	2–4 hours (canine); 15–20 hours (feline)	0.5–0.7 μg/ml
Valporic Acid (Depakote, Depakene; Abbott)	60 mg/kg q8h	1.5–2 hours (canine); 8.5 hours (feline)	50–100 μg/ml
Clorazepate (Tranxene; Abbott)	1–2 mg/kg q12h		
Phenytoin (Dilantin; Parke-Davis)	25 mg/kg q8h	1–2 hours (canine); 2–9 days (feline)	10–20 μg/ml
Clonazepam	0.5 mg/kg q12h	6–19 hours (after enzyme saturation)	0.015–0.07 μg/ml

- Another adverse effect, which is idiosyncratic, is hyperexcitability. About 40% of dogs on phenobarbital develop hyperexcitability or restlessness.
- A final adverse effect is dependence. Sudden withdrawal of the drug may precipitate seizures, even in normal animals. Because of this, use caution when ending therapy.
- Enzyme induction may occur in dogs on barbiturate therapy. Although this is not actually an adverse effect, it may affect the ability to control seizures.

Primidone (Mylepsin; Ft. Dodge)

Metabolism. A congener of phenobarbital, primidone is metabolized to phenobarbital and phenylethylmalonic acid (PEMA). All three drugs—primidone, phenobarbital, and PEMA—have antiepileptic properties. Based on efficacy, primidone appears more effective by a factor of 10 than phenobarbital, which is a factor of 10 more effective than PEMA. This is misleading, however, because the extremely short half-life of primidone in the dog makes it almost impossible to maintain therapeutic blood levels of either primidone or PEMA. Because of this, about 90% of the efficacy of primidone in the dog is from its major metabolite (phenobarbital). A longer half-life (7 hours) may make primidone useful in cats.

KEY POINT ▶ Primidone is a hepatotoxic drug, producing hepatic necrosis, hepatic lipidosis, and obstruction of bile canaliculi in clinical patients and experimental animals.

Dosage

- In dogs, a dosage of 10–15 mg/kg q8h results in peak primidone levels of 4–7 μg/ml and peak phenobarbital levels of 10–20 μg/ml.
- In cats, administer 20 mg/kg q12h. Cats have less ability than dogs to convert the parent drug, resulting in higher serum primidone concentrations and lower phenobarbital levels when primidone is given at the same dosages as dogs.
- Serum PEMA levels are similar in cats and dogs.
- The dose equivalency of primidone to phenobarbital is 250 mg primidone = 65 mg (or 1 grain) phenobarbital.

Adverse Effects. Disadvantages of primidone include the following:

- It is a potent hepatotoxic drug.
- The liver must produce the drug's clinically important metabolites.

Phenytoin (Dilantin; Parke-Davis)

Metabolism. The bioavailability of phenytoin generally is poor, owing to its poor absorption and low solubility. Following oral administration, peak serum levels are reached in 4–7 hours. Phenytoin is highly protein-bound (75%), with a wide half-life range (dogs, 3 hours; cats, 72 hours; humans, 22 hours). The elimination of phenytoin is by metabolism. Therapeutic serum levels in humans are 10–30 μg/ml. In dogs, therapeutic antiarrhythmic levels are 10–20 μg/ml;

according to one report, therapeutic antiepileptic levels are ≥3 μg/ml.

Dosage

- In dogs, give 25 mg/kg q8h to reach serum levels >3 μg/ml. For levels >10 μg/ml, give 35 mg/ml q8h.
- Phenytoin is toxic in cats and is not recommended, although dosages of 2 mg/kg q8h have been used with claimed success.

Diazepam (Valium, Roche)

This drug is a minor tranquilizer (benzodiazepine type) that also has antiepileptic properties.

Metabolism. The metabolism of diazepam involves conversion to two active metabolites. Diazepam is highly lipid-soluble and rapidly acts on the CNS. The elimination half-life for diazepam averages 3.2 hours. The amount of unmetabolized diazepam in serum samples ranges from 1 to 21%, depending on the route of administration. It appears that diazepam and its metabolites do not induce microsomal enzymes. The parent drug diazepam and its metabolites have antiepileptic effects of the same order of magnitude.

KEY POINT ▶ Diazepam is effective long term in cats only.

Dosage

- Continuous oral administration of 1–2 mg/kg q8h in the dog results in maximum plasma concentrations of 100–800 ng/ml of diazepam and steady-state plasma concentrations of 600–1100 ng/ml of desmethyldiazepam. These ranges are in the therapeutic levels. Oxazepam levels do not exceed 100–200 ng/ml.
- The dosage for cats is 0.25–0.5 mg/kg q2h. Some clinicians consider diazepam the preferred antiepileptic in cats, with a control rate of 75%.
- Diazepam appears to induce pharmacodynamic tolerance in dogs, but not in cats. There may be tolerance to the antiepileptic effects, which can develop as rapidly as 2 weeks. As a result, initial sedation will resolve over 1–2 weeks; therefore, lowering the drug dose is not required.
- Progressively higher doses of drug may not control the epilepsy if tolerance develops.
- Tolerance also has been demonstrated for the metabolites in dogs, but not in cats. Benzodiazepines do not induce drug disposition tolerance.

Potassium Bromides

Potassium bromide is now being used as an adjunct antiepileptic. It is not recommended as a "stand-alone" drug. Any patient that has serum phenobarbital levels >35 mg/liter and inadequate seizure control is a candidate for potassium bromide therapy.

Metabolism and Dosage

- Potassium bromide has a prolonged half-life (up to 24 days); thus it takes about 4 months to reach steady-state levels.
- Begin dosage of 20 mg/kg (10 mg/lb) daily, usually divided q12h.

- Therapeutic serum levels are 1–1.5 mg/ml. Monitor serum levels 6 weeks after starting therapy. Reassess levels every 6 months.

Adverse Effects
- Drowsiness may occur, but no serious side effects have been reported.
- Fictitious hyperchloremia—because bromide is a halogen, serum chemical profile tests may detect bromide on routine testing and report it as chloride. Use of ion-specific electrodes allows verification of chloride levels.

Emergency Therapy

Cluster Seizures. In general, outbreaks of cluster seizures are easier to manage than status epilepticus. They usually respond to intravenous fluids and diazepam. The principles of therapy are the same as for status epilepticus, but the results usually are more rewarding.

Status Epilepticus. This is a condition in which generalized seizures occur rapidly, one after the other, with no return of consciousness between the seizures. The specific cause of most episodes of status epilepticus is unknown. It is known that systemic metabolic derangements and inflammatory brain injuries may predispose to status epilepticus, as does a sudden drop in antiepileptic serum levels.

Diagnostic Approach

- Establish that epileptic seizures are present; rule out vestibular disease, narcolepsy, tetanus, hypocalcemia, hypoglycemia, organophosphate intoxication.
- If this is the first seizure episode, perform the same diagnostic tests that you would on any first-time seizure patient.
- If the patient is a confirmed epileptic, treat like any confirmed epileptic patient that presents with exacerbation of seizures.
- Indicated diagnostic tests include:
  - Neurologic examination
  - Measurement of antiepileptic serum levels
  - Monitoring of glucose, calcium, and acid/base status
  - CSF tap and EEG (following recovery)

General Therapy

Catheterization. Place an intravenous catheter for rapid delivery of drugs and to provide metabolic support.

Check Serum Drug Levels. Collect laboratory samples prior to initiation of therapy and check serum phenobarbital levels in all animals currently on therapy with drugs containing phenobarbital.

- If serum phenobarbital levels are inadequate (<15–45 mg/liter), adjust drug dosage appropriately.

Initiate Therapy. If the patient is a *naive* epileptic (i.e., first-time seizure patient), administer thiamine and dextrose. If the patient is a confirmed *idiopathic* epileptic, administer IV fluids immediately.

- Administer thiamine (B-complex vitamins)—*dogs,* 24–100 mg IV; *cats,* 25 mg IV. Give before administering any dextrose-containing solution, because thiamine is an essential coenzyme in CNS glucose utilization; if dextrose-containing fluids are given to a thiamine-deficient animal, this may promote CNS acidosis and increase the potential for cavitating necrosis from seizures.
- Administer 1 gm/kg of 10% dextrose IV over 35 minutes.
- Administer IV fluids, using a fluid administration pump (if available). Place the patient on maintenance fluid therapy, using lactated Ringer's solution or normal saline unless the animal is dehydrated (see sec. 1, ch. 5). If the patient is hypoglycemic, add dextrose to make a 5% dextrose solution.
- Because antiepileptic drugs usually are administered in the IV fluids, monitor the fluid administration rate closely to avoid over- or underdosing. (If a fluid pump is not available, use a Buretrol device (Baxter) to prevent overdose.)

Specific Seizure Therapy

Begin antiepileptic drug therapy if the patient's seizures are not controlled by the preceding measures. In actively seizuring patients, most antiepileptic drugs are administered intravenously to facilitate a rapid onset of action.

Phase One. At the time of the seizure, short-acting antiepileptics with minimal side effects are administered to immediately control seizures, while rapidly establishing serum levels of a maintenance drug to preserve control. This therapy is effective in the majority of patients.

- Administer a bolus dose (0.7–3.0 mg/kg) of diazepam IV.
- At the same time, administer phenobarbital (12–36 mg/kg, slowly IV).
  - The onset of action of phenobarbital is about 15–30 minutes; therefore, phenobarbital is given simultaneously with the diazepam to provide a sustained antiepileptic effect as the serum levels of diazepam decline.
  - The lower dosage achieves serum concentrations close to 15 mg/liter; the higher dosage will achieve serum concentrations close to 45 mg/liter.
- To calculate a precise loading dose (appropriate only if the patient was not previously receiving phenobarbital) based on the desired serum level of phenobarbital, multiply the serum level times the dog's effective volume of distribution ($BW_{kg} \times 0.8$) to determine the dosage. For example, to achieve a serum level of 25 mg/liter in a 15-kg animal:

$$25 \times (15 \times 0.8) = 300 \text{ mg or 6 gr of phenobarbital}$$

Steroids. For some patients who have suffered a prolonged course of seizure activity prior to being placed on this treatment protocol, administer 1.0 mg/kg of a corticosteroids such as dexamethasone (Azium; Schering) q12h for 1–2 days. This may minimize edema, necrosis, and inflammation within the brain.

Phase Two

- If the seizures stop following the above therapy, continue to administer maintenance phenobarbital at the calculated dose.
- If the seizures continue, but at a lower frequency than before, initiate regular administration of diazepam at a dose of 0.1–0.5 mg/kg IV, q6h for 48 hours. Continue to administer maintenance phenobarbital at the calculated dose.
- If any seizure lasts longer than 60 seconds, administer an additional dose of diazepam (0.1–0.5 mg/kg).

Phase Three. This phase of therapy is designed for *refractory patients* (i.e., patients that failed to respond to the initial IV boluses of diazepam and phenobarbital).

Step One—Diazepam Drip. Administer diazepam at the rate of 0.1 mg/kg/h in a 5% dextrose/0.9% NaCl drip.

- Cardiovascular and respiratory depression may occur with IV administration of diazepam. Other adverse effects include sedation, ataxia, dizziness, limb hypotonia, increased appetite, weight gain, and increased salivary and bronchial secretions.

Step Two. If the patient has three or more seizures while receiving the diazepam drip, administer pentobarbital IV.

- Give an initial bolus adequate to induce general anesthesia. The recommended dosage is 2–3 mg/kg slowly IV, but if the patient has been on phenobarbital prior to admission, much higher levels of pentobarbital may be required to reach a satisfactory plane of anesthesia because of barbiturate tolerance.
- Maintain the anesthesia for 24 hours, using additional boluses if required. Intubate the animal and place it on a respirator.

Supportive Care. Supportive measures during seizure therapy include:

- Oxygen therapy
- Soft bedding and repositioning every 2 hours
- Temperature monitoring
- Pulse/ECG monitoring

Sequelae of Seizures

Systemic Sequelae

Systemic sequelae include hypoxemia, hyperthermia, hypotension, carbon dioxide retention, systemic acidosis, cardiac arrhythmias, pulmonary edema, myocardial necrosis, hyperglycemia (early), and hypoglycemia (late in the course of the seizure).

Neurologic Sequelae

Neurologic sequelae include clinical, EEG, and pathologic changes and alterations in seizure patterns (e.g., increase in the number of focal seizures).

SLEEP DISORDERS

Two sleep disorders occur in dogs and cats: the first and most commonly recognized is cataplexy; the second is narcolepsy (see Definitions). Purebred breeds of dogs in which narcolepsy has been reported include the beagle, cocker spaniel, dachshund, Doberman pinscher, Irish setter, Labrador retriever, and poodle. Genetic studies of Labradors and Dobermans support a recessive inheritance with complete penetrance. In the hereditary form of the disease, signs generally appear at 1–6 months of age. In acquired forms of sleep disorders, signs may not appear until the animals are mature.

Definitions

Cataplexy—A disorder characterized by brief episodes of muscle paralysis with loss of tendon reflexes. The animal may not be asleep during these episodes and will appear alert and able to follow objects with its eyes. Clinical signs are due to motor inhibition, are short in duration, and are completely reversible. The episodes are initiated during periods of excitement by activities such as eating, playing, and sexual arousal.

Narcolepsy—A disorder characterized by excessive daytime sleepiness. Unless associated with cataplectic attacks, this disorder may be difficult to diagnose.

Etiology

Both of these disorders are believed to represent abnormalities of neurotransmitter balance. Abnormalities in the ability to release or turn over serotonin could produce the signs seen in both conditions.

Clinical Signs

The physical examination, including the neurologic examination, is usually normal except during an actual attack.

- Onset of signs is rapid in both conditions; they may last from a few seconds to 30 minutes. During attacks, the muscles are hypotonic.
- Partial attacks of cataplexy may involve only the pelvic or thoracic limbs.
- Animals can usually be aroused from the episode by loud noises, petting, or other external stimuli.
- Frequently associated rapid eye movement (REM) sleep-like events will be observed during episodes, (e.g., ocular motility, twitching of facial muscles, whining).
- Affected animals may have many episodes in one day.

Diagnosis

Differential Diagnosis

Consider a variety of neurologic and non-neurologic conditions in the differential diagnosis of sleep disorders:

Cataplexy—myasthenia gravis, hypoglycemia, hypocalcemia, hypokalemia, adrenal insufficiency, polymyositis, non-motor epilepsy (lapse attacks/drop attacks), syncope
Narcolepsy—hypothyroidism, chronic hypoxia, obesity, other metabolic illness.

Diagnostic Tests

Food-Elicited Cataplexy Test
Method
1. Place 10 pieces of food (each 1 cubic centimeter), 30.5 cm apart, in a row.
2. Record the time required to eat all the pieces and the number, type, and duration of any cataplectic attacks that occur.
   a. In a complete attack the patient drops completely to the ground with head resting on the floor.
   b. In a partial attack the patient drops the hindquarters, forequarters, or both to the ground, but does not drop its head.

Interpretation
- Normal dog—A normal dog will eat all food in less than 45 seconds and will have no attacks.
- Cataplectic dog: A cataplectic dog will take >2 minutes to eat the food and will have 2–20 attacks.

Pharmacologic Tests
- Yohimbine challenge:
  - Give 25–50 μg/kg of yohimbine as an IV bolus. A positive test is a 90% reduction in the number or severity of cataplectic attacks.
  - A response should be present 20–30 minutes after administration. The total effect will last 4 hours.
- Imipramine (Tofranil) challenge:
  - Give 0.5 mg/kg of imipramine as an IV bolus. There will be a general improvement in arousal.
  - This test is *not* specific for narcolepsy.
- Physostigmine challenge:
  - Give 0.025 mg/kg of physostigmine salicylate (Antilirium) IV; 5–15 minutes after the injection, repeat the food-elicited cataplexy test.
  - You may repeat the test using increasing doses of physostigmine (0.05 mg/kg, 0.075 mg/kg, and 0.10 mg/kg).
  - This test consistently produces signs in affected patients, causing up to a 300% increase in the number and duration of episodes. The signs increase in severity and frequency in a dose-dependent manner. The effects of each dose last 15–45 minutes.
- Arecoline challenge:
  - Give 0.15 mg/kg of arecoline hydrochloride subcutaneously, then repeat the food-elicited cataplexy test as in the physostigmine challenge.
  - The results are similar to those with the physostigmine challenge; the effects last about 1 hour.
- Atropine response:
  - Give 0.1 mg/kg atropine sulfate IV and repeat the food-elicited cataplexy test as in the physostigmine challenge.

- A marked decrease in the number of cataplectic attacks should be observed.

Treatment

The primary goal of therapy in dogs is to decrease the severity and frequency of the cataplectic attacks. The excessive drowsiness seen with pure narcolepsy usually is of less concern to the client, and therefore treatment of non-cataplectic narcoleptics is not a major therapeutic goal.

Client Education
- Explain that cataplexy is not a fatal disease.
- Inform clients that choking on food and airway obstruction have not been reported.
- Advise client to avoid situations where the attacks could endanger the patient: for example, no hunting, walks only on leash or in fenced-in yard, no swimming.
Another concern of clients is the expense of therapy.

Drug Therapy
- As a general rule, use drugs that block serotonin uptake, decrease concentrations of dopamine, decrease turnover of norepinephrine, or have anticholinergic properties. In addition, the drug must be able to cross the blood-brain barrier.
- Many patients develop drug tolerance, and therapy will need to be changed as it becomes ineffective.
- Monoamine oxidase inhibitors are contraindicated in dogs because of possible toxic cardiovascular side effects.

Several effective drugs are available:

- Yohimbine—currently the drug of choice:
  - Give 50–100 μg/kg SC q12h or q8h.
- Imipramine—an anticataplectic drug:
  - Give 0.5–1.0 mg/kg three times daily PO and titrate dose based on clinical effect.
- Methylphenidate (Ritalin):
  - Give 5–10 mg PO on a daily basis and titrate the dose from there.
  - This drug primarily is used as a supplement to imipramine.
- Dextroamphetamine:
  - Give 5–10 mg of this drug PO on a daily basis. Titrate the dose based on clinical efficacy.
  - This drug may be used as a supplement to imipramine.

Prognosis

The disease is not fatal and the prognosis is good.

- Many animals (e.g., Doberman pinschers and Labrador retrievers) that are afflicted with the inherited form improve with increasing age.
  - The prognosis is variable for client satisfaction, because the disease is not curable and even with rigorous therapy many patients remain symptomatic.

Supplemental Readings

Brown SA: Anticonvulsant therapy in small animals. Vet Clin North Am: [Small Anim Pract] 18:1197, 1988.

Frey HH: Anticonvulsant drugs used in the treatment of epilepsy. *In* Indrieri RJ, ed: Epilepsy: Problems in Veterinary Medicine 1:558, 1989.

Hauser WA, Rich SS, Annegers JF, Anderson VE: Seizure recurrence after a first unprovoked seizure: An extended follow-up Neurology 40:1170, 1990.

Lane SB, Bunch SE: Medical management of recurrent seizures in dogs and cats. J Vet Intern Med 4:26, 1990.

Oliver JE: Protocol for diagnosis of seizure disorders in companion animals. J Am Vet Med Assoc 172:822, 1978.

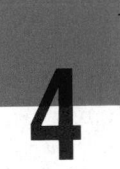

Spinal Cord Disorders

Patricia J. Luttgen

The term *spinal cord disorders* (see Table 1 for classification and examples) broadly refers to all diseases affecting the spinal cord. Clinically, spinal cord disorders cause dysfunction in one or more limbs and/or the tail.

KEY POINT ▶ Disorders of the spinal cord do not cause signs referable to diseases above the foramen magnum such as mentation change, cranial nerve deficits, and vestibular and cerebellar ataxia.

Differentiate spinal cord disorders from peripheral nerve disorders, which present with many of the same clinical signs (see sec. 10, ch. 5). Disorders of the spinal cord can seriously impair the quality of life of afflicted animals.

ETIOLOGY

Spinal cord disorders can arise from numerous insults and may be associated with particular signalments (breed, age, sex) and neuroanatomic localizations.

TABLE 1. Classification and Examples of Spinal Cord Disorders

Category	Examples
Degenerative	Myelopathy of German shepherds
	Hereditary spinal muscular atrophy of Brittany spaniels
	Hereditary ataxia of smooth-haired and Jack Russell terriers
Anomalous	Spinal dysraphism
	Spina bifida
	Myelodysplasia
Metabolic	Globoid cell leukodystrophy
	Hypervitaminosis A in cats
Neoplastic	Intramedullary ependymoma
	Extramedullary intradural meningioma
	Extradural vertebral osteosarcoma
Inflammatory	Feline infectious peritonitis
	Canine distemper myelitis
	Toxoplasmosis
Granulomatous	Granulomatous meningoencephalitis
Immune-mediated	Steroid-responsive meningitis/vasculitis
Toxic	Tetanus
	Strychnine
Traumatic	Intervertebral disc herniation
	Fracture/luxation of spinal column
	Caudal cervical spondylomyelopathy
Vascular	Fibrocartilaginous embolization
	Progressive hemorrhagic myelomalacia
	Caudal aortic embolization

Many of these disorders result in relatively predictable patterns of onset (acute versus chronic) and clinical signs (progressive versus nonprogressive).

Degenerative Disorders

Degenerative conditions usually present in an insidious manner and invariably are progressive in nature. Many of these conditions are inherited and are seen in young animals (e.g., spinal muscular atrophy of Brittany spaniels and hereditary ataxia of Jack Russell and smooth-haired fox terriers). Other disorders seem to be related to aging and may be familial in nature such as the degenerative myelopathy seen in older, large-breed dogs, particularly the German shepherd.

Anomalies

Anomalies of the spinal cord usually are first recognized when ambulation begins. However, traumatically induced "decompensation" may be required for minor lesions to be recognized clinically. Spinal cord anomalies can be inherited, such as spinal dysraphism in Weimaraners, or they can be congenital, such as myelomeningocele. The majority of these conditions are nonprogressive, but they may become progressive if additional disease conditions are superimposed.

Vertebral anomalies that compromise the stability of the vertebral column or the canal size may cause spinal cord dysfunction secondary to compression. For example, hemivertebra may lead to spinal luxation, and malarticulation/malformation of articular facets may lead to spinal canal stenosis.

Metabolic Conditions

Metabolic disorders that affect the nervous system generally present in a chronic progressive manner, with signs referable to more than the spinal cord. However, dogs afflicted with globoid cell leukodystrophy may display signs of spinal cord disease prior to development of other neurologic signs. Also, hypervitaminosis A in cats may result in extensive cervical and thoracic vertebral new bone formation with secondary compression of the spinal cord.

Neoplasia

Neoplastic conditions of the spinal cord can affect animals of all ages and breeds. Initial presentation of clinical signs varies, depending on the type and location of the tumor. Signs usually become progressive, given time. Two major types of tumors affect the spinal cord:

intramedullary and extramedullary. Intramedullary tumors such as astrocytoma and ependymoma arise from the spinal cord itself, causing damage by derangement of the normal anatomy. Extramedullary tumors arise from tissues surrounding the spinal cord and cause damage by compression. Extramedullary tumors can be located intradurally, (e.g., meningiomas and nerve root tumors) or extradurally (e.g., vertebral osteosarcomas and multiple myeloma). See sec. 9, ch. 6 for discussion of neoplasia of the axial skeleton.

Infection

Numerous infectious agents can affect the spinal cord and surrounding structures of animals of all breeds and ages. Presentation of clinical signs varies, depending on the inciting agent, the location of the lesion, and the degree of spinal cord involvement. Often inflammatory disease of the central nervous system (CNS) is not confined to the spinal cord, and clinical signs of brain involvement also will be present.

Bacterial

Primary bacterial meningitis or meningomyelitis is infrequently diagnosed in dogs and cats. When present, bacterial infection is most commonly introduced secondary to infection of surrounding tissues or to trauma. For example, bacterial discospondylitis causes discomfort from disc and vertebral body infection and, if extensive, secondary compression of the spinal cord. Infection of the lumbar epaxial muscles seen with grass awn migration can extend through the intervertebral foramen to cause secondary meningitis.

Viral

Viral myelitis is a relatively common problem in dogs and cats. Clinical presentation and neuroanatomic localization vary. Typically, encephalitic signs are associated with rabies infection, but this virus may cause signs of myelitis as well. All ages of dogs are susceptible to canine distemper virus (CDV). Previous vaccination does not preclude "breaks" in immunocompetency due to other illnesses or disease states. Signs of spinal cord disorder without associated encephalitic signs may occur. In cats, coronavirus (feline infectious peritonitis) and retrovirus (feline leukemia virus and feline immunodeficiency virus) infections frequently cause signs of spinal cord disorder with or without signs of brain involvement. For a discussion of these viral diseases of dogs and cats, see appropriate chapters.

Fungal

Fungal myelitis has been reported in patients with cryptococcosis, blastomycosis, histoplasmosis, and coccidioidomycosis. Multiple levels of the nervous system usually are involved simultaneously (e.g., eyes, brain, spinal cord); however signs are limited to the spinal cord in some patients. Systemic mycoses are discussed in sec. 2, ch. 12.

Rickettsial

In addition to other clinical signs, the tick-borne rickettsial diseases ehrlichiosis and Rocky Mountain spotted fever (see sec. 2, ch. 10) have been reported to cause nervous system dysfunction. Signs referable to spinal cord dysfunction include ataxia, upper motor neuron limb dysfunction, and hyperesthesia resulting from meningitis and myelitis.

Protozoal

The main protozoal disease causing spinal cord disorders in dogs and cats is toxoplasmosis (see sec. 2, ch. 13). Encephalitis, ocular involvement, and myositis may be present. Fortunately this rarely occurs in pet animals, owing to decreased predation of the intermediate hosts.

Granulomatous Meningoencephalitis

This disorder is suspected to be caused by an infectious agent that has not been definitively identified. Both acute and chronic onset of signs have been reported. The disease is invariably progressive in nature, and disseminated CNS involvement is the general rule (see sec. 10, ch. 2); however, signs limited to the spinal cord have been reported. The cervical area seems to be the preferred site of infection in the spinal cord.

Immune-Mediated Disorders

Immune-mediated steroid-responsive meningitis/vasculitis has been reported in numerous dogs. Clinical signs are typical of spinal meningitis, including neck stiffness, hyperesthesia, and fever. Signs are usually acute in onset and are progressive if the dog is untreated.

Toxins

Strychnine and tetanus directly affect the spinal cord in dogs and cats. These toxins act in a similar manner: tetanus toxin decreases the release of the inhibitory neurotransmitters, gamma-aminobutyric acid and glycine in the spinal cord, whereas strychnine competitively blocks the inhibitory effect of glycine. Clinical onset is usually acute, and the disease progresses to a state of severe tetany.

Trauma

Trauma is probably the main cause of spinal cord disorders in dogs and cats. Trauma can arise from external sources (e.g., being hit by a car or a bullet) or from internal sources (e.g., disc herniation or a pathologically collapsed vertebra). Whatever the source, the onset of clinical signs usually is acute and nonprogressive. However, progressive signs may be seen if disc nucleus herniates slowly or instability of the spinal column allows further luxation to occur.

Vascular Disorders

Vascular conditions resulting in ischemia of the spinal cord most often cause acute nonprogressive spinal cord dysfunction. In dogs, fibrocartilaginous embolization seems to be the main etiologic agent. In cats, caudal aortic embolization secondary to cardiomyopathy is the most common cause.

CLINICAL SIGNS

KEY POINT ▶ Ascending proprioceptive fibers in the spinal cord are the most sensitive to compressive lesions; therefore, incoordination (sensory ataxia) of one or more limbs is commonly the initial sign of spinal cord disease.

As compression increases, the descending upper motor neurons (UMNs) in the spinal cord are affected, resulting in a loss of muscle strength in one or more limbs.

- If the lesion is located in the cervical or thoracolumbar area, UMN signs of exaggerated myotatic reflexes (e.g., patellar reflex) will be apparent in the limbs caudal to the lesion.
- If the lesion is located in the cervicothoracic or lumbosacral area and it causes compression so severe that it damages the ventral horn cells in the ventrolateral gray matter of the spinal cord, lower motor neuron (LMN) signs of decreased or absent myotatic reflexes may be present in the corresponding limbs (cervothoracic lesion = forelimbs; lumbosacral lesion = hindlimbs).

KEY POINT ▶ The ascending spinal cord pain fibers are the most resistant to compressive lesions; therefore, a lack of deep pain perception as demonstrated by a lack of visible response to a noxious stimulus applied to a limb or tail caudal to a suspected compressive lesion indicates severe damage to the spinal cord.

Deep Pain. Test for deep pain by presenting a noxious stimulus to the affected limb or tail. Presence of deep pain is indicated by the animal's demonstration of conscious perception of the pain (e.g., crying, turning the head toward the leg.)

DIAGNOSIS

History

The history establishes the signalment and the nature of onset and progression of clinical signs. Because many spinal cord disorders are relatively predictable in these areas, the history can identify general differential possibilities that should be considered before performing the physical examination. For example, chronic progressive disease in an old German shepherd suggests degenerative myelopathy, neoplasia, or chronic disc herniation. Acute nonprogressive disease in a young dog suggests trauma such as disc herniation or vascular insult such as fibrocartilaginous embolization.

Lesion Localization (Neurologic Examination)

The neurologic examination establishes the presence or absence of neurologic dysfunction. When dysfunction is established, localize the affected areas of the spinal cord. For this purpose, the spinal cord is divided into four major areas: cervical (C): C1–C5 cord segments; cervicothoracic (CT): C6–T2 cord segments; thoracolumbar (TL): T3–L3 cord segments; and lumbosacral (LS) coccygeal: L4–S3 cord segments and caudal.

- C lesions classically present with UMN tetraplegia, or with UMN hemiplegia if the lesion is asymmetric.
- CT lesions cause tetraplegia with LMN signs in the forelimbs and UMN signs in the hindlimbs. However, there are many exceptions because of the large amount of extradural space in the area. CT lesions may cause only UMN forelimb signs if not of sufficient severity to interrupt LMN cell body function. If the lesion affects the CT area of the spinal cord asymmetrically, one forelimb may show more dysfunction than the other or hemiplegia may be present.
- TL lesions typically cause UMN paraplegia (normal forelimb responses; UMN hindlimb responses).
- LS lesions cause LMN paraplegia (normal forelimb responses; LMN hindlimb and perineal responses). If coccygeal segments also are involved, the tail will show LMN motor dysfunction as well. It is possible for LS lesions to affect only the sacral and/or coccygeal segments without affecting the lumbar cord segments that contribute to the femoral and sciatic nerves. In these cases, the animal will have LMN perineal and/or tail responses while maintaining motor function of the hindlimbs.

Minimum Data Base

Establishing an animal's minimum data base (MDB) is essential for assessment of the animal's overall health prior to general anesthesia for neurologic testing.

KEY POINT ▶ The MDB for neurologic patients consists of a complete physical examination (including neurologic, otic, and ophthalmic evaluation), complete blood count (CBC), serum biochemical analysis, urinalysis, fecal analysis, and electrocardiogram. Routinely test for heartworms in endemic areas.

Specialized Laboratory Examinations

Specialized tests may be indicated, based on physical examination findings and/or MDB results. Examples include fine-needle aspiration cytology of enlarged lymph nodes, tests for infectious diseases (e.g., feline leukemia, feline immunodeficiency, feline infectious peritonitis, canine distemper, toxoplasmosis, erlichiosis, and fungal infections; see sec. 2, chs. 1, 2, 3, 6, 13, 10, and 12, respectively), and resting and challenge endocrine function tests (see sec. 4).

Electrodiagnostic Tests

Electrodiagnostic tests useful in the diagnosis of spinal cord disease include electromyography (EMG), motor and sensory nerve conduction velocity (MNCV and SNCV, respectively) studies, spinal cord evoked potentials (SCEPs), and somatosensory evoked potentials (SSEPs). These evaluations generally require specialized equipment and referral to a veterinary neurologist.

- Epaxial and limb EMG is useful in verifying the presence of denervation potentials and more specifically in localizing lesions.
- MNCV and SNCV studies of peripheral nerves help to rule out peripheral nerve and muscle diseases that present with many of the same clinical signs as spinal cord disease (see sec. 10, chs. 5 and 6 for discussion of peripheral nerve and muscle disorders, respectively).
- SCEPs and SSEPs evaluate the integrity of the ascending spinal cord tracts to determine the extent of functional damage.

Imaging Techniques

KEY POINT ▶ Neuroradiography is the single most important technique used for diagnosis of spinal cord disorders.

Spinal radiography is especially important if surgical treatment of the condition is being considered.

Plain Films

Plain spinal films often are sufficient to diagnose problems such as vertebral fracture/luxation, disc herniation, vertebral neoplasia, vertebral anomalies, and discospondylitis. Avoid causing further injury to the animal during these procedures. When plain radiographs are inconclusive, specialized procedures can be used.

Myelography

Myelography is the most commonly performed special neuroradiographic procedure and is particularly helpful in differentiating intramedullary and extramedullary spinal cord lesions. With the introduction of new contrast agents, post myelographic complications, such as seizures and contrast-induced meningitis, have been markedly reduced. However, myelography is contraindicated in the presence of CNS inflammation (encephalitis, myelitis, meningitis) or if increased intracranial pressure is suspected. See sec. 1, ch. 4 for myelography technique and interpretation.

Discography

Discography, in which contrast media is injected into an intervertebral disc nuclear area, is useful in cases of LS stenosis. Combined with EMG, this technique can add valuable information to confirm the presence of a chronic (type II) disc herniation at the LS junction. Fluoroscopic guidance is useful, but not absolutely necessary, to confirm needle placement prior to injection of contrast media.

Epidurography and Sinus Venography

These modalities have had limited diagnostic usefulness; now, with ready accessibility to newer imaging techniques at referral centers, these techniques are seldom performed.

Specialized Imaging Techniques

Computerized fluoroscopy, computed tomography (CT), and/or magnetic resonance imaging (MRI) are now available in many referral centers. In human medicine, these modalities provide detailed information about the precise nature, location, and extent of conditions affecting the spinal cord. With greater accessibility, these tests are now being applied in veterinary medicine.

Cerebrospinal Fluid (CSF) Analysis

CSF analysis is the test of choice for establishing an inflammatory cause of spinal cord disease; furthermore, it provides nonspecific information that is helpful in the diagnosis of degenerative, metabolic, neoplastic, and vascular conditions, including the following:

- Degenerative, neoplastic, and occasionally vascular problems may cause albumino-cytologic dissociation of CSF (increased protein levels in the presence of normal cell counts).
- Neoplastic cells rarely are seen in the CSF of patients with CNS neoplasia. However, globoid cells may be identified in cases of globoid cell leukodystrophy.
- Inflammatory conditions of the spinal cord cause increases in CSF protein and variable increases in cell numbers and type, depending on the specific etiologic agent causing the insult.

For further details concerning CSF collection technique and abnormalities in specific infectious and inflammatory conditions of the CNS, see sec. 10, ch. 1.

TREATMENT

The management of spinal cord disorders depends on the causative agent and the degree of irreversible damage caused. Often only palliative treatment can be provided.

Medical Therapy

Spinal Cord Trauma

Medical therapy to combat the effects of acute spinal cord trauma (e.g., edema, ischemia) currently is based on the use of anti-inflammatory and hyperosmotic agents. However, the benefits of hyperoxygenation to

duce CNS edema should not be forgotten in the rush
o the pharmacy shelf.

Anti-inflammatory Agents

Glucocorticosteroids are the most useful anti-inflammatory agents. Unfortunately, their vigorous use to
save" a spinal cord may result in significant hemorrhagic or ulcerative gastroenteritis and pancreatitis.
Consequently, the simultaneous administration of H_2-
receptor antagonists (e.g., cimetidine or ranitidine)
and intestinal protectants such as sucralfate are recommended (see sec. 7, ch. 4 for dosages).

The two most commonly used glucocorticosteroids
re dexamethasone and the newer and apparently
uperior agent methylprednisolone sodium succinate
Solu-Medrol; Upjohn). The general principles of administration are similar for both drugs. Best results in
pinal cord trauma cases are obtained when large doses
re administered immediately after injury, followed by
rapid dosage tapering. The maximum amount of time
hat glucocorticosteroids are beneficial following spinal
ord injury appears to be 2–3 days; longer administration is of little benefit and enhances the likelihood of
erious gastroenteritis and pancreatitis.

Dexamethasone. The relative value of dexametha-
one versus dexamethasone sodium phosphate is still
being debated.

- For both types, administer 2–4 mg/kg IV immediately after severe trauma.
- Base the total dosage and tapering of dosage on the
patient's response to therapy.

Solù-Medrol. This highly soluble, fast-acting glucocorticosteroid is especially effective when administered
immediately following spinal cord trauma.

- In experimental models, a dosage of 30 mg/kg administered q6–8h during the first 12–24 hours following injury has shown remarkable sparing action on
the spinal cord compared with dexamethasone, mannitol, dimethyl sulfoxide (DMSO), naloxone, and
thyrotropin-releasing hormone.
- The dosage is usually tapered rapidly over the course
of 2 days.
- If additional glucocorticosteroid therapy is necessary,
methylprednisolone sodium succinate may be continued in reduced dosages, or less expensive dexamethasone or prednisone may be substituted.

Hyperosmotic Solutions

Hyperosmotic solutions have been widely used to
combat post-traumatic brain edema, but their use in
cases of spinal cord trauma does not appear to be as
successful. *Mannitol* is the most commonly used hyperosmotic agent for CNS trauma.

- Give one or two doses of 1–2 gm/kg IV. Be cautious
when considering further administration, because of
possible rebound paradoxical CNS edema.

Other Drugs

Many drugs have been investigated as adjunctive
therapy in cases of spinal cord trauma. The most
notable is DMSO, currently more commonly used in
large animal species than in small.

- DMSO appears to have many beneficial effects on
damaged CNS tissues, including anti-edema properties, stabilization of cell membranes, and reduction
of metabolic demands of affected tissues.
- Recommended dosage is 0.5–2.5 gm/kg, IV, q8h.

Other investigated drugs, such as antioxidants, calcium channel blockers, and vasodilators, are not recommended at this time.

Infection

Antimicrobial Agents

Antimicrobial drugs may be indicated if specific
infectious agents are identified or suspected. Treatment
of systemic mycoses, toxoplasmosis, and rickettsial
infections are discussed in detail in section 2, chapters
12, 13, and 10, respectively.

In cases of *meningitis* or *myelitis,* select antimicrobials that are known to cross the blood-brain barrier
readily (i.e., highly lipid soluble in the un-ionized
state).

- Examples of antimicrobials with good penetrating
abilities include trimethoprim-sulfonamide combinations, rifampin, metronidazole, chloramphenicol,
and certain imidazoles such as itraconazole.
- Drugs with intermediate penetrating abilities in the
normal CNS may have improved penetrating abilities
when the CNS is inflamed. These include the penicillin family (e.g., amoxicillin, carbenicillin), the
newer-generation tetracyclines (e.g., doxycycline,
minocycline), and certain cephalosporins.
- Avoid drugs that penetrate poorly, such as the
aminoglycosides, amphotericin B, and ketoconazole.

Treatment of *discospondylitis* presents a unique challenge because of the difficulty of presenting sufficient
antimicrobial concentrations to the affected disc
space and vertebral bodies. *Staphylococcus* is the organism most frequently reported. *Brucella canis, Nocardia, Streptococcus canis, Corynebacterium diphthe-
roides,* and various fungi also have been isolated. Most
infections arise via hematogenous spread from infected
tissues.

- If possible, base selection of antimicrobial drugs on
positive culture results (blood, urine, or the affected
disc space) or a positive *Brucella* agglutination test.
Otherwise, assume that the causative organism is
coagulase-positive *Staphylococcus* and administer
beta-lactamase–resistant antibiotics (e.g., cephra-
dine, cloxacillin), which reach sufficient therapeutic
levels in bone and pus.
- Clinical symptoms usually improve after only a few
days of therapy, but several weeks of drug administration are required to effect a "cure." In some
cases, antimicrobials alone are not effective, and
surgical intervention is required.

Degenerative Disorders/Neoplasia

- Glucocorticosteroids have been recommended in degenerative conditions for slowing the degenerative

process and as chemotherapeutic agents in certain types of neoplasia such as lymphosarcoma.

■ Other chemotherapeutic agents usually are not effective in CNS neoplasia.

■ Radiation therapy has been beneficial in the treatment of neoplasia, and protocols such as whole body hyperthermia combined with radiation therapy are under investigation.

Intoxication

Tetanus. In tetanus cases, several medications are utilized. Penicillin, tetracycline, and metronidazole have been shown to be effective against *Clostridium* organisms.

■ Administer penicillin G (20,000–100,000 IU/kg q6h, IV or IM) as the first line of attack.

■ Tetracycline (22 mg/kg q8h, PO or IV) is recommended as an alternative because of the variable effect of penicillins on vegetative forms.

■ Metronidazole (dog, 10 mg/kg q8h, PO; cat, 250 mg total, q12–24h, PO) has shown excellent efficacy. It is bactericidal against most anaerobes and reaches effective levels in necrotic tissues.

■ Equine tetanus antitoxin (100–500 IU/kg, IV, usually administered only once) may combat the neurotoxin if given early enough; however, anaphylactic reactions are common, necessitating an initial test dose (0.1–0.2 ml) given SC or ID.

■ Chlorpromazine (0.5–2.0 mg/kg q8–12h, given IM, IV, or PO) is effective against the hyperexcitability sometimes observed.

Diazepam (dog, 5–10 mg total, q2–4h, given PO, IV, or IM; cat, 2.5–5 mg total, q2–3h, PO) blocks the effect of the toxin on the spinal cord but has a very short duration of action. Barbiturates also may be used to combat the tetany.

Strychnine Intoxication. When strychnine intoxication is suspected, further gastrointestinal absorption should be blocked by aspiration of stomach contents and oral administration of binding agents, such as activated charcoal, that prevent absorption of the toxin.

■ Diazepam therapy also can be used to block the action of the toxin at the spinal cord level (see sec. 10, ch. 3 for dosage).

■ Barbiturates may be necessary to combat seizures (see sec. 10, ch. 3 for dosage).

Principles of Surgical Treatment

Surgical intervention is helpful most frequently in cases of compressive extramedullary spinal cord disease rather than in cases of intramedullary disease such as spinal cord laceration and neoplasia. The primary goals of neurosurgical intervention are:

■ Decompression of the spinal cord and nerve roots
■ Stabilization of the vertebral column.

The decision for neurosurgical intervention is based on:

■ A thorough understanding of the historical presentation of dysfunction (i.e., acute versus chronic onset, progressive versus nonprogressive course)
■ The localization and extent of neurologic deficits
■ Radiographic studies done under anesthesia.

When indicated, surgical intervention is most valuable in the early stages of a problem, especially in acute compressive conditions such as disc herniation, in which the functional outcome often parallels the speed with which surgical decompression is performed. In chronic progressive conditions, such as caudal cervical myelopathy, surgery performed in the early stages of disease is far more rewarding than surgery performed after significant dysfunction has been allowed to develop. Chronic compression causes irreversible damage to the spinal cord which surgery cannot correct and may even worsen by decompensating a chronically compensated condition.

KEY POINT ▶ When recommending spinal cord surgery for a paralyzed animal, warn the owner that extensive postoperative physiotherapy and nursing care may be necessary.

How a particular extramedullary problem affects the spinal cord depends a great deal on the level of the spinal column involved. The spinal cord fills only approximately half of the available canal space in the cervical area, in contrast to the thoracolumbar area, where it fills almost the entire available canal space. There is also a great deal of extradural space in the last two lumbar canal spaces because of the tapering of the spinal cord into the cauda equina. Consequently, a spinal subluxation of one-fourth the canal space in the cervical area may cause very little if any clinical dysfunction, but significant hindlimb paralysis if the same degree of luxation occurs in the thoracolumbar area. (See sec. 9, ch. 5 for details on treatment of spinal fractures and luxation).

In general, extramedullary compressive lesions have a better prognosis than intramedullary destructive lesions. It is possible to debulk some intramedullary tumors, but surgery has no application in the majority of intramedullary diseases (i.e., degenerative, anomalous, and infectious disorders; traumatic lacerations; vascular accidents). In comparison, there are many surgical alternatives for the treatment of compressive extramedullary disease such as disc herniation.

The long axonal tracts in the spinal cord vary in their sensitivity to pressure depending on their size. Clinical signs parallel the degree of compression and can be used as a prognostic guide.

■ Sensory ataxia in animals with non-neoplastic extramedullary compression is a good prognostic sign because it indicates compression affecting only the proprioceptive fibers. Most of these animals will not require surgery unless there is a fracture or other injury that may potentially destabilize the spinal column in the future, or unless chronic pain from nerve root entrapment or irritation of the meninges is a problem.

▪ Paresis or more severe paralysis indicates the presence of a greater degree of spinal cord compression and a guarded prognosis is justified initially. Many of these patients improve if deep pain perception is still present and surgery is performed immediately.

▪ The prognosis usually is grave when superficial and deep pain perception are lost. However, transient loss of deep pain, which cannot be differentiated clinically from irreversible loss, can frequently be seen in the hours immediately following an acute insult to the spinal cord. In an animal with spinal fractures, if vertebral displacement, seen radiographically, is severe, it is likely that the loss is irreversible; advise the owner that surgical intervention probably will not be beneficial. However, in cases in which radiography indicates that the spinal cord may be intact, a significant percentage will improve if surgery, combined with aggressive medical therapy, is performed within a few hours of injury. If deep pain has been absent for several hours to days, surgical decompression is of little value.

KEY POINT ▶ Accurately assess for the presence or absence of deep pain sensation prior to recommending surgery on paralyzed animals. The animal must exhibit conscious perception of pain, not just a withdrawal reflex.

Surgical decompression of the spinal cord usually is performed via hemilaminectomy or dorsal laminectomy in the thoracolumbar spine, depending on the site of the lesion. Cervical cord decompression for disc herniation usually is performed via ventral slot decompression (through the vertebral body). Dorsal decompression of the cervical cord is used less frequently.

Disc fenestration is performed by some surgeons as a prophylactic procedure to prevent recurrence of disc herniation. The efficacy of fenestration is controversial. Disc fenestration does not decompress the spinal cord.

Spinal cord surgery requires advanced skills and equipment, and can cause significant harm to the animal if improperly performed.

Physiotherapy and Nursing Care

KEY POINT ▶ Regardless of the nature of the spinal cord disorder, physiotherapy and good nursing care are extremely important to avoid the development of secondary problems and to hasten return to a functional state.

Physiotherapy can include:

▪ Daily periods of swimming
▪ "Towel walking"
▪ Limb manipulations
▪ Muscle massage

Nursing care should include:

▪ Frequent evacuation of the bladder (q4–6hs) to prevent urinary tract infections and secondary bladder dyssynergia

▪ Padded clean bedding or pet waterbed to prevent decubital ulceration
▪ Daily baths to prevent secondary dermatitis

PROGNOSIS

The prognosis depends to a great extent on the etiologic agent involved.

▪ Degenerative conditions vary in the rate of progression but invariably lead to severe disability.
▪ Anomalous conditions usually have a nonprogressive course and thus their prognosis depends on the extent of spinal cord injury.
▪ Some metabolic conditions, such as globoid cell leukodystrophy, cannot be treated and lead to a chronic degenerative state; others, such as nutritional disorders, can be reversible if proper therapy is initiated promptly.

Neoplasia

The prognosis for neoplastic conditions varies greatly.

Intramedullary Tumors

Intramedullary tumors usually have a poor prognosis.

▪ Surgical removal is not possible or feasible in most cases.
▪ Chemotherapeutic agents, including glucocorticosteroids, may slow progression but do not affect a cure.
▪ Radiation therapy can provide some relief but seldom a cure.

Nerve Root Tumors

Nerve root tumors have a variable prognosis depending on their location (intramedullary, extramedullary, or both) and extent of involvement.

▪ The prognosis is poor when multiple nerve root tumors are present but can be good if only one nerve root is involved and surgical removal can be performed.

Extramedullary Tumors

Some extramedullary tumors, including lymphosarcoma and meningioma, are very sensitive to chemotherapy and/or radiation therapy. In combination with surgical debulking, good results can be obtained.

Vertebral Tumors

Vertebral tumors such as osteosarcoma and multiple myeloma have a poor prognosis.

▪ These tumors compromise the structural integrity of the spinal column, leading to secondary spinal cord compression from proliferative bone and/or pathologic collapse.

■ Surgical and chemotherapeutic protocols may be used, but pathologic collapse of the spinal column is usually the end result. (See sec. 9, ch. 6 for more information about tumors of the axial skeleton.)

Infection

In general, infectious problems have a guarded prognosis unless a specific causative agent can be identified and/or response to antimicrobial therapy occurs. Under the best of circumstances, it is difficult to obtain significant levels of appropriate antimicrobials in the CNS, disc space, and vertebrae, and prolonged administration usually is required. If the spinal cord parenchyma is directly involved, the prognosis is poorer.

■ *Granulomatous meningoencephalitis* is initially very steroid-responsive. Unfortunately, relapses are common and the disease usually proves fatal (see sec. 10, ch. 2).
■ Glucocorticosteroids are the therapy of choice for immune-mediated *meningitis/vasculitis,* but the results are highly variable.

Toxicity

■ *Strychnine* toxicity can be fatal if aggressive therapy is not begun immediately.

Trauma/Vascular Accidents

The prognosis in cases of spinal cord trauma is highly variable, as discussed previously. The same is true for vascular accidents. The prognosis depends on the location and extent of spinal cord involvement.

■ The prognosis is good if the cervical or thoracolumbar area is involved (i.e., UMN paralysis).

■ In patients with fibrocartilaginous embolization, the cervicothoracic and lumbosacral areas are predisposed sites (i.e., LMN paralysis of one or more limbs). As in caudal aortic embolization, which mainly affects the lumbosacral spinal cord, the prognosis is guarded to poor until response to therapy and time prove otherwise.

PREVENTION

In general, degenerative, anomalous, metabolic, neoplastic, and vascular disorders of the spinal cord cannot be prevented.

■ Certain infectious conditions (e.g., canine distemper, feline leukemia) can be reasonably prevented by a regular vaccination program.
■ Most cases of external trauma (hit by car) and toxicity can be prevented if pets are restricted to fenced backyards and leash walks.
■ Keeping susceptible dogs from jumping excessively or becoming obese will help prevent disc herniations.

Supplemental Readings

Greene CE: *Infectious Diseases of the Dog and Cat.* Philadelphia: W. B. Saunders, 1990.
LeCouteur RA, Child G: Diseases of the spinal cord. *In* Ettinger SJ, ed.: *Textbook of Veterinary Internal Medicine,* 3rd Ed. Philadelphia: W. B. Saunders, 1989, p 624.
Luttgen PJ: Paraplegia. *In* Ford RB, ed.: *Clinical Signs and Diagnosis in Small Animal Practice.* New York: Churchill Livingstone, 1988, p 295.
Oliver JE Jr, Hoerlein BF, Mayhew IG: *Veterinary Neurology.* Philadelphia: W. B. Saunders, 1987.

5 Peripheral Nerve Disorders

Linda G. Shell
Karen R. Dyer

ANATOMY AND PHYSIOLOGY

The peripheral nervous system (PNS) is composed of 12 pairs of cranial nerves (see sec. 10, chs. 1, 2), and 36 pairs of spinal nerves that arise from the spinal cord. Spinal nerve fibers give rise to the peripheral nerves, which usually are composed of both sensory and motor fibers. Sensory nerve fibers are activated by peripheral receptors (Fig. 1). Impulses are transmitted up the peripheral nerve to the spinal cord. Some disorders affect only the sensory nerve fibers or ganglia, causing clinical signs such as hyperesthesia and analgesia, proprioceptive deficits, and self-mutilation (Table 1). In many cases sensory losses may be difficult to detect.

Motor or efferent nerve fibers arise from nerve cell bodies in the gray matter of the spinal cord. They carry information from the central nervous system (CNS) to the striated muscles (see Fig. 1). Motor deficits, characterized by limb weakness, muscle atrophy, and reduced spinal reflexes, occur with injury to any of the following: lower motor neuron in the gray matter of the spinal cord, ventral nerve root, spinal nerve, peripheral motor nerves, neuromuscular junction, and muscle (see Fig. 1). Disorders of the neuromuscular junction and muscle are discussed in sec. 10, ch. 6.

Neuropathy is a general term denoting pathologic changes and/or functional disturbances in the PNS. *Polyneuropathy* refers to involvement of several nerves, usually resulting in bilaterally symmetric signs.

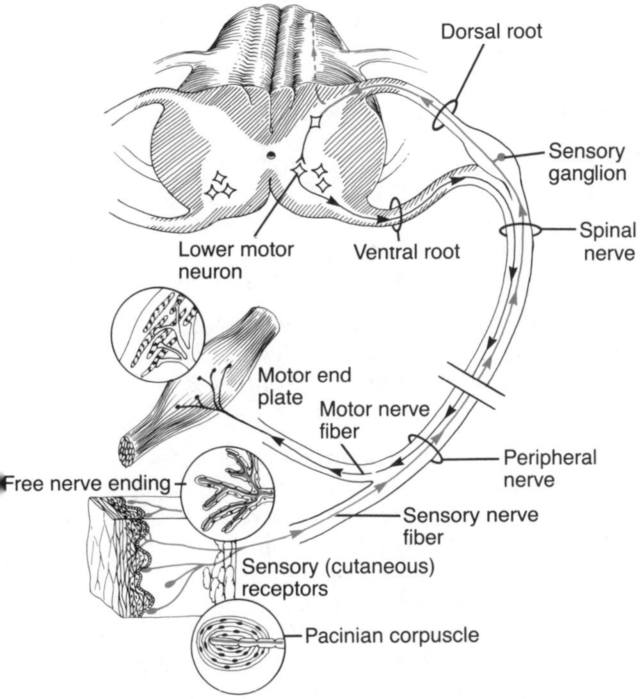

CLINICAL SIGNS

Motor nerve disorders generally cause weakness and muscle atrophy; sensory nerve disorders cause hyperesthesia or anesthesia, self-mutilation, and other abnormalities (see Table 1). The clinical signs of motor nerve disorders are similar to those of muscle disorders and can be distinguished using muscle enzyme determinations and muscle and nerve biopsies (see sec. 10, ch. 6).

KEY POINT ▶ Many common peripheral nerve disorders are manifested as one of the following clinical problems: acute flaccid quadriplegia, chronic progressive quadriparesis, monoparesis or monoplegia, and sensory disturbances (Table 2).

PRINCIPLES OF DIAGNOSIS

- The *history* allows classification of the disease process as acute or chronic and progressive or nonprogressive.

Figure 1. Impulse pathways in peripheral and spinal nerves.

TABLE 1. Clinical Signs of Motor and Sensory Nerve Deficits

Motor Nerve Deficits
Weakness/paralysis
Muscle atrophy
Reduced reflexes
Reduced muscle tone

Sensory Nerve Deficits
Hyperesthesia/anesthesia
Self-mutilation
Loss of proprioception
Dysmetria
Reduced reflexes

TABLE 2. Differential Diagnosis Based on Clinical Signs of Neuropathy

Problem	Differential Diagnosis
Monoparesis or Monoplegia	
Acute onset	Trauma to nerve root or peripheral nerve
	Fibrocartilaginous infarct
	Intervertebral disc herniation to lateral side
Chronic onset	Tumor of nerve root or peripheral nerve
	Intervertebral disc herniation to lateral side
	Joint disease
Acute Flaccid Quadriplegia	Acute polyradiculoneuritis (Coonhound paralysis)
	Tick paralysis
	Botulism
	Post-vaccinal polyneuropathy
	Acute idiopathic polyneuropathy
	Protozoal infection
Chronic Progressive Quadriparesis	
Immature	Globoid cell leukodystrophy
	Giant axonal neuropathy (German shepherds)
	Progressive axonopathy (Boxers)
	Hypertrophic neuropathy (Tibetan mastiffs)
	Motor neuron diseases (Brittany spaniels, rottweilers)
Mature	Chronic relapsing polyradiculoneuritis
	Distal denervating disease
	Distal polyneuropathy (Doberman pinschers)
	Distal symmetric polyneuropathy
	Hypertrophic neuropathy
	Metabolic neuropathy
	Neoplastic neuropathy
	Toxic neuropathy
	Nutritional neuropathy
	Various myopathies
Sensory Disturbances	
Immature	Acral mutilation in pointers
	Sensory neuropathy (long-haired dachshunds)
Mature	Sensory neuropathy (ganglioradiculoneuritis)

- Perform a careful *physical examination* to detect signs of involvement of other systems (e.g., endocrine disorders) that may influence the peripheral nerves.
- Perform a *neurologic examination* (see sec. 10, ch. 1) to localize the process to the PNS if reduced muscle mass and tone and reduced spinal reflexes are seen in the physical examination.
- *Laboratory data:*
  - Basic studies usually consist of a hemogram, blood chemistry profile, and urinalysis to evaluate for metabolic, endocrine, and neoplastic disorders.
  - Elevated muscle enzymes, creatine kinase, aldolase, lactate dehydrogenase (LDH), and serum glutamate oxaloacetate transaminase (SGOT), may help the physical examination distinguish muscle disorders from peripheral neuropathies.
  - Low cholinesterase levels may suggest exposure to organophosphates.
  - Blood and tissue samples can be analyzed for heavy metal levels.
- *Needle electromyography (EMG) studies* record electrical activity in skeletal muscle (see sec. 10, ch. 1). They are used to confirm the presence and to determine the distribution of peripheral nerve and muscle disorders and can be performed on the awake or anesthetized patient.
  - Spontaneous activity, or denervation potentials, such as fibrillations and positive sharp waves, are found in many neuropathies.
- *Nerve stimulation studies* can determine the location and nature of peripheral nerve abnormalities (see sec. 10, ch. 1).
  - Reduction of the conduction velocity or a change in amplitude, duration, or waveform of the evoked action potential suggests pathologic conditions.
  - Nerve conduction studies are recorded using specialized electrodiagnostic equipment (usually by a specialist at a referral center) under general anesthesia. Both motor and sensory nerves can be evaluated.
- *Muscle biopsy* specimens not only distinguish different muscle disorders but can also differentiate nerve from muscle disorders if histochemical staining is used (see sec. 10, ch. 6).
- *Sensory and motor nerve biopsies* involve removing a fascicle of the nerve several centimeters in length, leaving the rest of the nerve intact. Because special handling and processing are required, these biopsies are probably best performed by a specialist at a referral center.
- *Spinal fluid analysis* occasionally is beneficial in diagnosis of disorders of the nerve roots such as acute polyradiculoneuritis and protozoal diseases.

PRINCIPLES OF TREATMENT

KEY POINT ▶ The key to treatment is to find the cause. Unfortunately, a specific cause of many of the acquired peripheral neuropathies may not be obvious even after extensive diagnostic procedures.

Treatment often must rely on supportive care. In all peripheral nerve disorders that cause decreased mobility and muscle wasting, the following measures are important:

- Use waterbeds or heavily padded surfaces for bedding, to prevent decubital ulcer formation.
- Flex and extend the joints several times a day to prevent tendon and muscle contraction.
- Maintain proper nutritional intake.
- Ensure frequent and complete bladder evacuation.
- Corticosteroids are indicated only for those neuropathies associated with immune-mediated diseases such as systemic lupus erythematosus.

CLASSIFICATION

A wide range of disease processes, varying from simple trauma to more complex inherited disorders, can affect the peripheral nerves. For the purpose of this discussion, peripheral nerve disorders are categorized according to their etiology, that is, anomalous/inherited/congenital, metabolic, neoplastic, nutritional, inflammatory/immunologic, idiopathic, traumatic, and toxic.

SPECIFIC PERIPHERAL NERVE DISORDERS*

Anomalous/Inherited/Congenital Disorders

Anomalous causes of peripheral nerve disease usually are noticed before one year of age. For each of the following anomalies, signalment and clinical signs are keys to a presumptive diagnosis, and thus only additional procedures are described under Diagnosis.

KEY POINT ▶ Many anomalous causes of neuropathies are breed-specific and are not treatable.

Globoid Cell Leukodystrophy

This is caused by an inherited (autosomal recessive) deficiency of the enzyme beta-galactocerebrosidase that results in cell damage to oligodendrocytes and Schwann cells in the CNS and PNS, respectively.

- *Signalment:* West Highland white and Cairn terriers, beagles, poodles, Pomeranians, cats <1 year of age.
- *Clinical Signs:* Progressive pelvic limb ataxia, hypermetria, and head tremors. Nystagmus, blindness, and anorexia may develop prior to death.
- *Diagnosis:* Nerve biopsy demonstrating segmental demyelination, axonal degeneration, and endoneural globoid cell accumulation; biochemical evaluation of beta-galactocerebrosidase enzyme activity in leukocytes, brain, and spinal cord.

Giant Axonal Neuropathy in German Shepherds

This is an inherited (probably autosomal recessive) neuropathy characterized primarily by distal axonal swellings filled with neurofilaments in the PNS and CNS.

- *Signalment:* German shepherds 1–2 years of age.
- *Clinical Signs:* Progressive symmetric paraparesis followed by loss of patellar reflexes, distal muscle atrophy, hypalgesia in the pelvic limbs, weak bark, vomiting, regurgitation from megaesophagus, and aspiration pneumonia. Some dogs have a curly coat.
- *Diagnosis:* Spontaneous needle EMG activity in distal muscle groups; decreased amplitude of evoked action potential on nerve stimulation; giant axonal swellings on nerve biopsy.

*Grouped according to etiology.

Hypertrophic Neuropathy in Tibetan Mastiffs

This inherited (autosomal recessive trait) chronic demyelinating disease of the PNS is most likely due to an inability of the Schwann cells to form and maintain a myelin sheath.

- *Signalment:* Tibetan mastiffs 7–12 weeks old.
- *Clinical Signs:* Pelvic limb weakness that rapidly progresses to generalized weakness, hyporeflexia, hypotonia, and recumbency. Some dogs may regain some strength.
- *Diagnosis:* Occasional spontaneous needle EMG activity; slowed motor nerve conduction velocities; Schwann cell proliferation and relatively little axonal degeneration on nerve biopsy specimen.

Progressive Axonopathy of Boxers

Progressive axonopathy is an inherited (probably autosomal recessive trait) neuropathy characterized by axonal degeneration and demyelination and remyelination in the PNS. The CNS also is affected, having large axonal spheroids.

- *Signalment:* Boxer dogs <1 year of age.
- *Clinical Signs:* Slowly progressive pelvic limb ataxia with a swaying hypermetric gait; hypotonia; loss of patellar reflex and conscious proprioception; mild muscle atrophy. Thoracic limb involvement and mild cerebellar signs may occur late in the course.
- *Diagnosis:* Normal or slightly reduced motor nerve conduction velocities; small or absent evoked muscle action potential; histopathologic changes on nerve biopsy; necropsy.

Acral Mutilation and Nociceptive Loss in Pointers

This is a suspected inherited (probably autosomal recessive) nociceptive defect.

- *Signalment:* Pointers 3–4 months old.
- *Clinical Signs:* Biting and licking at paws progressing to mutilation of paws; normal gait, posture, and spinal reflexes, with loss of pain sensation in digits of pelvic limbs.
- *Diagnosis:* Normal EMG activity and sensory and motor nerve conduction velocities; pathologic changes of the primary sensory neurons include degeneration of nerve fibers in the dorsal roots and peripheral nerves and reduced number of cell bodies in spinal ganglia, with the remaining cell bodies appearing smaller than normal.

Sensory Neuropathy in Long-Haired Dachshunds

This is a familial disorder (possibly autosomal recessive trait) characterized by degeneration of large and small, myelinated and unmyelinated, sensory and autonomic nerve fibers.

- *Signalment:* Young long-haired dachshunds. (Signs begin at 3 months.)
- *Clinical Signs:* Slowly progressive pelvic limb ataxia, urinary incontinence, loss of conscious propriocep-

tion, and decreased pain perception over the entire body; normal patellar reflexes but absent flexor reflexes.

- *Diagnosis:* Reduced sensory and normal motor nerve conduction velocities; loss of myelinated fibers in sensory nerves and widespread unmyelinated fiber pathology on nerve biopsy.

Motor Neuron Diseases in Brittany Spaniels and Rottweilers

These disorders are characterized by progressive degeneration and eventual loss of the motor neurons in the gray matter of the spinal cord and the motor nuclei of the brain stem.

- *Signalment:* Young Brittany spaniels and rottweilers.
- *Clinical Signs:* Progressive weakness, muscle atrophy, and hyporeflexia. Megaesophagus and head tremors have been observed in some affected Rottweilers.
- *Diagnosis:* Histopathology of the spinal cord and brain.

Metabolic Disorders

Metabolic disorders do not always produce a clinically evident peripheral neuropathy; however, do not overlook the presence of hypothyroidism, hyperadrenocorticism, diabetes mellitus, hyperinsulinism, uremia, and hepatopathy. Additionally, there is increased incidence of neuropathies in patients with neoplasms.

KEY POINT ▶ Evaluate all animals with signs of a chronic neuropathy for an underlying endocrine or metabolic abnormality.

Diabetes Mellitus

Diabetes mellitus can cause nerve fiber degeneration, although the exact pathophysiology is not fully understood. Clinical signs consist of weakness (especially of the pelvic limbs) and mild muscle atrophy. A plantigrade stance is common in cats. The diagnosis is based on clinical signs and laboratory evidence of diabetes mellitus (see sec. 4, ch. 4), needle EMG, denervation potentials, decreased motor and sensory nerve conduction velocities, and thinning of the myelin sheath on nerve biopsy. Neurologic signs usually improve over weeks to months with proper control of the diabetes mellitus (as described in sec. 4, ch. 4).

Hypothyroidism

Hypothyroidism (see sec. 4, ch. 1 for detailed description) occasionally is associated with polyneuropathies, but the pathophysiology is not understood. Most likely there is a relationship between thyroid hormone activities and neuronal metabolism.

- *Clinical Signs:* Slowly progressive weakness, muscle wasting, and normal or reduced spinal reflexes. Cranial nerve disturbances, such as facial paresis and vestibular dysfunction, may also be found. Other clinical signs of hypothyroidism, such as obesity,

mental depression, and dermatological lesions, are not always present.

- *Diagnosis:* Needle EMG changes and decreased motor nerve conduction velocities; thyroid-stimulating hormone test.
- *Treatment:* Replacement hormone therapy may improve the neurologic signs.

Hyperinsulinism

Hyperinsulinism results in hypoglycemia and most commonly is caused by pancreatic islet cell tumors. Profound hypoglycemia most frequently causes CNS disturbances such as seizures (see sec. 4, ch. 5); however, a few cases of muscle atrophy and weakness due to a neuropathy have been documented. Because insulinomas generally are malignant, do not overlook the possibility that the neuropathy is the result of a paraneoplastic effect. (Diagnosis and treatment of hyperinsulinism are described in sec. 4, ch. 5.)

Paraneoplastic Neuropathies

These neuropathies may occur more often than realized. The pathogenesis is poorly understood, but there is an unusually high incidence of peripheral neuropathy in human patients with carcinomas. More evidence exists for immune reaction to shared antigen than for elaboration of neurotoxin by neoplastic cells.

- *Clinical Signs:* Weakness (especially in the pelvic limbs), decreased muscle tone, and reduced spinal reflexes. Decreased sensory and motor nerve conduction velocities also may be seen. Demyelination, ganglioneuritis, and axonal atrophy may be observed on nerve histopathology.
- *Diagnosis:* Identification of a primary neoplasm and the elimination of other causes.
- *Treatment:* Removal of the underlying neoplasm if possible.

Nutritional Causes

Nutritionally caused neuropathies are uncommon in veterinary medicine; however, look for vitamin B deficiency, because of diet or impaired absorption, especially in idiopathic cases.

Neoplastic Causes

Progressive lameness or monoparesis resulting from neoplasia usually occurs in middle-aged and older patients. The nerves to the forelimb are most frequently affected.

Nerve Sheath Tumors

These are the most common primary tumor affecting the PNS. Schwannomas (malignant transformation of Schwann cells) are the most common type; tumors arising from endoneural and epineural fibroblasts (neurofibromas, neurofibrosarcomas) also occur.

- *Signalment:* Mature dogs; rarely cats.
- *Clinical Signs:* Signs vary with tumor location. Spinal

nerve roots of the brachial plexus are most susceptible. Neoplastic cells invade adjacent spinal nerve roots, causing dysfunction of multiple peripheral nerves. Proliferation of neoplastic cells within the spinal canal can result in a compressive myelopathy.

KEY POINT ▶ Vague lameness progressing to weakness and muscle atrophy of the affected limb is the most common sign of a nerve sheath tumor.

■ *Diagnosis:* Needle EMG denervation potentials; histopathology
■ *Treatment:* Surgical excision of tumor and/or amputation of the affected limb. Recurrence is common.

Lymphosarcoma

KEY POINT ▶ Lymphosarcoma is the most common tumor of non-neural origin affecting the PNS.

Lymphosarcoma is more common in cats than in dogs. Clinical signs and diagnosis are similar to those of nerve sheath tumors except that other signs of multicentric lymphosarcoma may be present. Treatment consists of chemotherapy (see sec. 3, ch. 6) and/ or surgical removal of the tumor. Peripheral nerve damage may be permanent.

Inflammatory and Immune-Mediated Disorders

These disorders can affect the neuromuscular junction, peripheral nerves, spinal nerves and roots, and ventral horn cells in the gray matter of the spinal cord.

Protozoal Infection

Organisms such as *Toxoplasma gondii* and *Neospora caninum* can cause inflammatory and degenerative changes in peripheral nerves and dorsal and ventral nerve roots, as well as muscle. Dogs <4 months of age are frequently presented for hind limb hyperextension, but others may be presented for acute or chronic flaccid weakness. (See sec. 2, ch. 13 for diagnosis and treatment of infections.)

Acute Polyradiculoneuritis (Coonhound Paralysis)

This is one of the most common peripheral nerve disorders in dogs. It is characterized by a mild lymphocytic radiculitis with demyelination of the ventral (and occasionally the dorsal) spinal roots. Immune-mediated destruction of the myelin is suspected.

■ *Signalment:* Adult dogs of any age, breed, or sex; frequently observed in hunting dogs 7–14 days after contact with a raccoon.
■ *Clinical Signs:* Pelvic limb weakness progressing to hyporeflexic or areflexic quadriparesis or quadriplegia within 1–2 days; rapid muscle atrophy. Thoracic limb weakness occasionally develops first. Responses to mild pain stimuli often are exaggerated. Some dogs develop facial paralysis, change in bark, and dysphagia. Respiratory muscle paralysis occurs occasionally, requiring the use of a respirator.

■ *Diagnosis:* Needle EMG denervation potentials; normal or slowed motor nerve conduction velocities.

KEY POINT ▶ Differential diagnoses for coonhound paralysis include botulism, tick paralysis, and protozoal infection of nerve and muscle (see sec. 2, ch. 13).

■ *Treatment:* Supportive care (e.g., physical therapy, bladder evacuation). Recovery usually is complete but may take weeks or months. Complications include cystitis, aspiration pneumonia, tendon contracture, and decubital ulcers.

Brachial Plexus Neuritis

This is a rare weakness of the thoracic limbs that has been compared to serum neuritis in humans. In one case, a newly instituted horse meat diet was incriminated as the cause of the allergic neuritis. Flexor reflexes in the thoracic limbs are reduced or absent and muscle atrophy is present.

Postvaccinal Polyneuropathy

This disorder is rare and occurs 7–10 days after rabies vaccination. Clinical signs are similar in appearance to those of acute polyradiculoneuritis. Spontaneous recovery usually occurs over a period of weeks to months.

Idiopathic Disorders

The causes of many acquired peripheral nerve disorders often are unknown. There are many single case reports but very few series of cases of the majority of these disorders. To consolidate these disorders, they are grouped here according to the predominant site of pathology. Many of the cases described under a single heading actually may have multiple, but as yet unknown, causes.

Idiopathic Neuropathies Affecting the Neuronal Cell Body

Lower Motor Neuron Disease. This disorder, characterized by an acute loss of ventral horn cells within the spinal cord, was reported in nine dogs in New Zealand.

■ *Clinical Signs:* Acute onset of paraparesis or quadriparesis that progressed over 2–4 weeks until euthanasia was performed. Sensory and autonomic function were preserved.
■ *Diagnosis:* Spinal cord histopathology

Sensory Neuropathy Ganglioradiculitis. This has been reported in several dogs with progressive ataxia and decreased patellar reflexes.

■ Variable degrees of facial hypalgesia, dysphagia, and prehension difficulty may occur.
■ Few to no needle EMG changes, normal to slightly reduced motor nerve evoked action potentials, and reduced sensory nerve evoked action potentials and conduction velocity were found.

■ Histopathology showed degeneration of sensory neurons within dorsal root and cranial nerve ganglia.

Dysautonomia. Dysautonomia is characterized histopathologically by a loss of neurons in all autonomic ganglia, some cranial nerve ganglia, and occasionally ventral horn cells. It is more common in cats in the United Kingdom, but isolated cases have been observed in other countries. A disorder with similar features has been reported in six dogs.

■ *Clinical Signs:* Mydriasis, megaesophagus, constipation, dry mucous membranes, bradycardia, and protrusion of the nictitating membrane. Pupillary pharmacologic testing showed increased sensitivity to direct-acting parasympathomimetics or sympathomimetics.
■ *Treatment:* Recovery is possible after months to years of supportive care.

Idiopathic Neuropathies Affecting the Proximal Axon

Acute Idiopathic Polyneuropathy. This was reported in 14 dogs.

■ *Clinical Signs:* Acute onset of generalized flaccid paralysis, similar to that described for acute polyradiculoneuritis (coonhound paralysis) except that there was no known exposure to raccoons or other neurotoxins.
■ *Treatment:* Most dogs recovered spontaneously. Those that died had mononuclear inflammation of the nerve roots and extensive peripheral nerve demyelination.

Chronic Relapsing Polyradiculoneuritis. This chronic form of acute polyradiculoneuritis has been reported in both dogs and cats.

■ *Clinical Signs:* Insidious onset with periods of remissions and subsequent relapses.
■ *Diagnosis:* Needle EMG changes; reduced motor and sensory nerve conduction velocities.

Idiopathic Neuropathies Affecting the Distal Axon

Distal Denervating Disease. This disorder was reported in 10 dogs with diffuse muscle atrophy and areflexia. Eight of the 10 dogs recovered spontaneously in 1–5 months. Needle EMG changes and abnormal motor nerve evoked action potentials were present. Histologically, distal degeneration of motor axons was found.

Distal Polyneuropathy in Doberman Pinschers. This chronic, progressive distal axonopathy begins with persistent rear limb flexion ("bicycling" motions) when the dog is standing. One or both rear limbs may be affected, with changes of the gastrocnemius muscles predominating. Progression over months to years may produce generalized weakness, muscle atrophy, and proprioceptive deficits. Diagnosis is based on breed, clinical signs, EMG changes, and muscle biopsy.

Distal Symmetric Polyneuropathy. This disorder was reported in a 12-month-old male Great Dane with progressive weakness and atrophy of limb muscles distal to the stifle and elbow. EMG abnormalities were confined to the distal limb muscles. Evoked muscle action potentials were absent.

Hypertrophic Neuropathy. This disorder was reported in a 12-year-old male mixed-breed dog that had remitting and relapsing bouts of quadriparesis. No ancillary studies were reported. A demyelinating peripheral neuropathy with Schwann cell proliferation and "onion bulb" formation (indicating demyelination and remyelination of the nerve) was diagnosed.

Traumatic Injury

Traumatic injuries to peripheral nerves are common causes of monoparesis or monoplegia.

Nerve Injuries

Nerve injury can occur from automobile trauma, intramuscular injections, fractures and repair of fractures, lacerations, and bite wounds. Tables 3 and 4 list the nerves that can be injured, their site of origin, and

TABLE 3. Signs of Nerve Injury in the Thoracic Limb

Nerve	Origin	Clinical Signs	Reflexes Affected
Suprascapular	C6-7	No gait changes; pronounced atrophy of supraspinatus and infraspinatus muscles	None
Radial	C6–T1	1. Injury proximal to branches that supply triceps muscle: Unable to support weight; limb collapses; may carry the limb if musculocutaneous nerve is functional; atrophy of muscle	Reduced to absent triceps and extensor carpi radialis reflexes
		2. Injury distal to branches that supply triceps muscle: Can support some weight but knuckles on dorsum of paw	
Musculocutaneous	C6-8	No gait changes; slight straightening of angle-to-elbow joint	Reduced withdrawal and biceps reflexes
Median and ulnar	C8–T2	Slight carpal extension ("dropped carpus")	Reduced carpal flexion on withdrawal reflex
Axillary	C6-8	None	Reduced shoulder flexion on withdrawal reflex

TABLE 4. Signs of Nerve Injury in the Pelvic Limb

Nerve	Origin	Clinical Signs	Reflexes Affected
Femoral	L4–6	Unable to support weight; limb collapses or may be carried; short stride; lack of pain perception on medial surface of thigh, stifle, leg, and paw; atrophy of quadriceps muscle	Reduced to absent patellar reflex
Sciatic	L6–S1-2	Supports weight on limb but knuckles on dorsum of paw; unable to flex or extend hock; atrophy of biceps femoris, semimembranosus, semitendinosus, cranial tibial, gastrocnemius and other muscles; lack of pain perception on caudal and lateral sides of leg	Reduced to absent withdrawal reflex
Peroneal	L6–S1	Straightening of hock; knuckles on dorsum of paw and fetlock	Reduced to absent hock flexion on withdrawal reflex
Tibial	L6–S2	Increased flexion to hock ("dropped" hock)	None
Obturator	L4–6	Abduction of limb on slippery surface	None

the clinical signs associated with each injury. Injuries are commonly classified as neurapraxia, axonotmesis, and neurotmesis.

Neurapraxia. Neurapraxia is a temporary loss of physiologic function without physical disruption of the nerve fibers. It results in weakness with intact pain perception. Motor function usually returns to normal within days to weeks.

Axonotmesis. Axonotmesis is severance of nerve fibers (axons) within a nerve, usually producing motor and sensory deficits. Following disruption of the axons, the distal axonal fragments degenerate. The proximal axonal segment must regrow along the intact connective tissue sheath at the rate of 1–3 mm/day or about one inch per month. Because the connective tissue sheath is intact, axonal regeneration may result in functional recovery, but this may take weeks to months, depending on the extent and the location of the injury. If the proximal axon segment is more than 12 inches from the muscle it innervates, it is unlikely that it will be able to make anatomic contact with the muscles because the connective tissue sheath shrinks and muscle fibers become fibrotic with time.

Neurotmesis. Neurotmesis is severance of axons and the connective tissue sheath. Axonal regeneration is hampered because there is no scaffold of connective tissue to guide the direction of growth of the axons. Without surgical intervention to appose the two severed ends of the nerve, it is unlikely that any function will return.

KEY POINT ▶ The closer the injured nerve is to the muscle it innervates, the better the prognosis.

Nerve Root or Brachial Plexus Avulsions

These avulsions are common sequelae of road traffic accidents or jumping from moving vehicles. It is more common for the nerve roots to be torn or avulsed from the spinal cord than for the brachial plexus to be severed (injured). Occasionally motor nerve roots (ventral nerve roots) are affected and sensory nerve roots (dorsal nerve roots) are spared.

■ *Clinical Signs:* Sudden onset of a combination of the nerve injuries to the forelimb is described in Table 3. Signs of radial nerve injury are almost always present.
• Damage to the T1–T3 ventral nerve roots may cause an ipsilateral Horner's syndrome.
• Damage to C8 and T1 nerve roots may result in loss of ipsilateral panniculus reflex.
• Damage to C5, C6, and C7 nerve roots may cause ipsilateral paralysis of the diaphragm.

TABLE 5. Possible Causes of Toxic Neuropathy in Humans and Animals

Chemical Agents
Organophosphorus compounds
    Parathion
    Malathion
    Tri-ortho-cresyl phosphate
    Di-isopropyl fluorophosphate
Acrylamide
Lindane
Polychlorinated biphenyls
Carbon tetrachloride
Methylbutyl ketone
Zinc pyridinethione
Carbon disulfide
N-hexane
Chlorophenothane

Heavy Metals
Arsenic
Lead
Gold
Thallium
Mercury

Drugs
Vincristine
Vinblastine
Doxorubicin
Chloramphenicol
Ampicillin
Erythromycin
Tetracycline
Nitrofurantoin
Diphenylhydantoin

- *Diagnosis:* History of trauma and clinical signs of monoparesis, needle EMG denervation potentials 5 days postinjury; changes in motor nerve conduction velocities within 3 days of injury.
- *Treatment:*
  - Daily physical therapy helps to prevent tendon and muscle contraction.
  - A sock, boot, or bandage may be used to prevent abrasions.
  - Regrowth of injured nerves (axonotmesis or neurotmesis) is slow and may take months. Serial monthly examinations are recommended.
  - Consider amputation if there is self-mutilation or unacceptable improvement in motor abilities after 6–8 months.

Toxic Neuropathies

Toxic neuropathies are diagnosed infrequently; however, the list of agents with the potential to cause neuropathies is quite extensive (Table 5). Suspect toxic causes when there is history of exposure.

Chemical Agents

Certain organophosphorus compounds can cause a delayed neuropathy in sensitive species.

- *Clinical Signs:*
  - Signs of generalized motor unit disease develop within 2–3 weeks after exposure.

- Long, large-diameter axons in the peripheral nerves and the spinal cord undergo distal degeneration ("dying-back"), causing a mixture of lower motor neuron clinical signs (muscle atrophy, weakness, reduced spinal reflexes) and upper motor neuron signs (weakness, exaggerated spinal reflexes).
- *Treatment:* There is no treatment for the delayed neuropathy. Partial recovery may occur if the nerves regenerate.

Drugs

Nitrofurantoin, vincristine, vinblastine, and doxorubicin can have adverse effects on peripheral nerves; however, reports in veterinary literature are scant.

Heavy Metals

Arsenic, lead, and mercury appear to be uncommon causes of neuropathies in animals.

Supplemental Readings

Chrisman CL: Peripheral nerve disorders. *In* Ettinger ST, ed.: *Textbook of Veterinary Internal Medicine,* Vol. 1, 3rd ed. Philadelphia: W. B. Saunders, 1989, p 719.
Duncan ID: Peripheral nerve disease in the dog and cat. Vet Clin North Am [Small Anim Pract] 10(1):177, 1980.

6 Neuromuscular Disorders

G. Diane Shelton

Neuromuscular disorders of dogs and cats are disorders of the motor unit. The motor unit is the morphologic and functional unit of skeletal muscle and includes:

- Motoneuron, consisting of the cell body and axon extending along a peripheral nerve
- Neuromuscular junction
- Myofibers innervated by the motoneuron

KEY POINT ▶ Weakness is the clinical sign common to all neuromuscular disorders, with the clinical expression varying considerably in severity and distribution.

This chapter focuses on disorders of the neuromuscular junction and muscle. Disorders of peripheral nerves are discussed in sec. 10, ch. 5.

TABLE 1. Causes of Neuromuscular Diseases

Hereditary Disorders
Canine X-linked muscular dystrophy
  Golden retriever
  Irish terrier
Congenital myasthenia gravis (MG)
  Jack Russell terrier
  Springer spaniel
  Smooth fox terrier
Familial canine dermatomyositis
  Collie
  Shetland Sheepdog
Hereditary myopathy of Labrador retrievers
Hereditary myotonia of Chows

Acquired Disorders
Autoimmune
  Generalized MG
  Focal MG
  Masticatory muscle myositis
  Polymyositis
Metabolic
  Glycogen metabolism and glycolytic pathway
  Lipid metabolism and oxidative phosphorylation
  Electrolyte alterations
  Hyperthermia—malignant and exercise-related
Endocrine
  Hypothyroidism
  Hypoadrenocorticism and hyperadrenocorticism
Neoplastic/paraneoplastic
Infectious
  Toxoplasma gondii
  Neospora caninum
  Hepatozoon canis
Toxic or drug-induced
  Tick paralysis
  Botulism
  Organophosphate toxicity
  Drugs affecting neuromuscular transmission
Ischemia

ETIOLOGY

Underlying causes of disorders of muscle and neuromuscular transmission are listed in Table 1 and include hereditary or suspected hereditary disorders and acquired disorders with autoimmune, metabolic, endocrine, neoplastic/paraneoplastic, infectious, toxic or drug-induced, and ischemic etiologies.

Hereditary Disorders

Several neuromuscular diseases have a known or suspected genetic basis.

Canine X-Linked Muscular Dystrophy

Canine X-linked muscular dystrophy in golden retrievers has strikingly similar phenotypic and genotypic similarities to Duchenne muscular dystrophy (DMD) in humans. Onset of clinical signs in affected males is about 10 weeks of age. Affected animals show stunting, weakness, gait abnormalities, and muscle atrophy with hypertrophy of proximal limb muscles. Serum creatine phosphokinase (CK) levels are dramatically elevated (>10,000 units/liter, compared with normal levels of <100 units/liter). As in humans with DMD, affected dogs lack the Duchenne gene transcript and its protein product, dystrophin. A similar X-linked myopathy is reported in Irish terriers, although the molecular defect is not described. Dystrophin deficiency has also been reported in cats.

Congenital Myasthenia Gravis

A congenital familial form of myasthenia gravis (MG), inherited as an autosomal recessive trait, is described in Jack Russell terriers, springer spaniels, and smooth fox terriers. Failure of neuromuscular transmission results from a deficiency in muscle acetylcholine receptor (AChR) content, but unlike the acquired form of MG, it is not related to the presence of autoantibodies to AChR.

Familial Canine Dermatomyositis

Familial canine dermatomyositis is well documented in young collies and less well characterized in Shetland sheepdogs. In collies the inheritance pattern appears to be autosomal dominant with variable expression. Initially there is a variably severe dermatitis on the skin of the face, ears, distal extremities over bony prominences, and tail tip that may be followed by an inflammatory myopathy of the masticatory muscles and muscles distal to the elbow and stifle. There is evidence of an immunologic pathogenesis in DM, but exact mechanisms are uncertain.

Hereditary Myopathy of Labrador Retrievers

Although this disorder of Labrador retrievers is commonly referred to as type II myofiber deficiency or "muscular dystrophy," at present the underlying pathologic mechanism is unknown. The disorder typically presents as progressive muscle weakness with exercise intolerance and abnormalities of gait and posture. There is, however, a wide variation in clinical presentations and pathologic findings. This may be more than one disorder affecting young Labradors. The mode of inheritance has been determined to be autosomal recessive. Within muscle biopsy specimens, variable morphologic features have been reported; some biopsies show changes typical of neuropathic disease, whereas others show myopathic changes. The fiber type proportions are also variable. To date, pathologic changes in the spinal cord and peripheral nerves have not been found, even in cases where histologic changes within the muscle biopsy suggest an underlying neuropathic disorder.

Hereditary Myotonia of Chows

Clinical signs, noted when pups first ambulate, are due mainly to a myotonia and include stiffness on rising and walking, especially after rest. The mode of inheritance has been determined to be autosomal recessive.

Acquired Neuromuscular Disorders

Autoimmune

Some of the most commonly occurring neuromuscular disorders of dogs are in this group. Included are MG, masticatory muscle myositis, and polymyositis. Although considered in the hereditary group, dermatomyositis in collies and shelties is also postulated to have an autoimmune basis.

Acquired Myasthenia Gravis. Acquired MG is not uncommon in dogs but is rare in cats. Acquired MG probably is the best defined of all the neuromuscular disorders with respect to mechanisms of injury and pathogenesis. It is now well documented that acquired MG is associated with autoantibodies directed against the nicotinic acetylcholine receptor (AChR) on the postsynaptic membrane of the neuromuscular junction. As a consequence of autoantibody binding, there is loss of AChRs resulting in impaired neuromuscular transmission and marked muscle weakness. AChR loss is a result of:

- Increased endocytosis due to cross-linking of AChRs by antibody
- Complement activation leading to focal lysis of the postsynaptic membrane
- Direct inhibition of AChR function by bound antibodies

Masticatory Muscle Myositis. Masticatory muscle myositis is a focal inflammatory myopathy that selec-tively affects the muscles of mastication. This selective distribution may be attributed to histochemical and biochemical differences between canine masticatory and limb muscles that provide the basis for a selective immune-mediated response. Although the role of auto-antibodies is not yet determined, autoantibodies against cytoplasmic and sarcolemmal proteins of masticatory muscle type 2M proteins have been demonstrated by immunocytochemical methods both within muscle biopsy sections and indirectly in the serum in cases of MMM.

Extraocular Muscle Myositis. Another focal inflammatory myopathy is described in which the cellular infiltration is localized to canine extraocular muscles with lack of involvement of the masticatory muscles. An immune-mediated condition is suggested by a marked lymphocytic cellular infiltrate, bilateral muscle necrosis, and a rapid response to corticosteroid therapy alone. Although the specific immune mechanism is not known for this disorder, myofiber-specific antigens may play a role in the selective involvement of the extraocular muscles.

Polymyositis. Not as common as masticatory muscle myositis, PM is a generalized inflammatory myopathy in which muscle damage is probably the result of cell-mediated immunity. An association has been reported with systemic lupus erythematosus and with an immune-mediated arthritis/polymyositis complex (see sec. 3). PM also may be associated with malignancies; it has been reported as a paraneoplastic disorder associated with thymoma.

Metabolic

These myopathies are associated with primary abnormalities of muscle metabolism, including defects in glycogen metabolism (glycolytic pathway) and lipid metabolism (fatty acid oxidation, oxidative phosphorylation, or mitochondrial enzyme defects).

Enzyme Deficiencies. In contrast to human studies, relatively few metabolic defects have been documented in dogs. These defects include pyruvate dehydrogenase deficiency in Clumber and Sussex spaniels; alpha-1,4-glucosidase (acid maltase) deficiency in Lapland dogs; generalized glycogen storage disease due to amylo-1,6-glucosidase (debranching enzyme) deficiency in German shepherds; and deficiency of phosphofructokinase, a key regulatory enzyme in the glycolytic pathway, in English springer spaniels.

Malignant Hyperthermia. This hypermetabolic disorder of skeletal muscles has been described in dogs and in one cat. Hyperpyrexia usually occurs following administration of certain anesthetic agents, particularly halothane and quaternary amide muscle relaxant drugs. An exercise-related hyperthermia is described in an English springer spaniel. Studies currently are in progress to define a previously unreported exercise-related hyperthermia in young Labrador retrievers (Dr. D. Brass, personal communication).

Electrolyte Imbalances. Alterations in the levels of serum K^+ and Ca^{++} due to underlying metabolic disorders can affect the excitability of neurons and muscle fibers, resulting in an increase or decrease in membrane excitability and resultant episodes of muscle weakness. A condition analogous to hyperkalemic periodic paralysis in humans has been described in a young American pit bull. Studies in cats have shown that certain diet types (e.g., acidifying diets containing insufficient potassium) and diseases (especially renal disease) are associated with an increased occurrence of hypokalemia and clinically evident weakness that resolves following potassium administration. Alterations in the levels of serum phosphate and magnesium may also result in neuromuscular dysfunction although they are poorly described. Electrolyte disorders and their therapy are discussed in sec. 1, ch. 5.

Endocrine

Myopathies can be associated with endocrine disorders, especially hypothyroidism and glucocorticoid excess. In hypothyroidism (see sec. 4, ch. 1), peripheral neuropathies and myopathies are reported to occur, whereas myopathy and myotonia are associated with hyperadrenocorticism (see sec. 4, ch. 3). Muscle weakness, probably as a consequence of hyperkalemia, is frequently associated with hypoadrenocorticism (see sec. 4, ch. 3).

Neoplastic/Paraneoplastic

An association between neoplasia and neuromuscular disorders is suspected but not proven. Thymoma is sometimes associated with MG and polymyositis in dogs. Thymoma may also be diagnosed after the diagnosis of MG is established and should be considered if AChR antibody titers remain elevated for long periods. Consider evaluating AChR antibody titers prior to surgery in all dogs with a suspected thymoma. Positive AChR antibody titers and clinical signs of MG have been reported in two cases of canine osteosarcoma and in single cases of cholangiocellular carcinoma and anal sac adenocarcinoma. Postulated mechanisms of paraneoplastic-associated muscle damage include:

- Autoantibodies produced against tumor antigens that cross-react with muscle components
- The liberation of myotoxic substances by the neoplasm
- The possibility that the neoplasm and the underlying muscle disorder have a common pathogenesis

Parasitic

Although not common clinically, parasitic myositis can be caused by protozoa such as *Toxoplasma gondii*, *Neospora caninum*, and *Hepatozoon canis*. Infection may be diagnosed on a muscle biopsy (further discussion of protozoa is found in sec. 2, ch. 13). Other parasites, such as *Trichinella spiralis*, *Sarcocystis*, and *Hammondia*, elicit minimal inflammation and may be found incidentally in muscle biopsies.

Toxic or Drug-Induced

Neuromuscular blockade may be the result of various neurotoxins.

- Neurotoxins that inhibit the evoked release of acetylcholine (ACh) at the neuromuscular junction are secreted by ticks such as *Dermacentor* and *Ixodes* species, resulting in tick paralysis.
- Ingestion of the exotoxin of *Clostridium botulinum* results in clinical signs of botulism by a similar mechanism.
- Organophosphate insecticides containing long-acting anticholinesterases reversibly or irreversibly bind acetylcholinesterase (AChE), permitting continuous cholinergic stimulation with accumulation of ACh at central, muscarinic, and nicotinic cholinergic synapses. "Myasthenia-like" syndromes are reported with organophosphate intoxication.
- Several drugs have been shown to reduce the safety margin of neuromuscular transmission, including aminoglycoside antibiotics, antiarrhythmic agents, phenothiazines, methoxyflurane, and magnesium given parenterally or in cathartics. These agents can potentiate neuromuscular blocking agents used during surgical procedures and may worsen or unmask preexisting disorders of neuromuscular transmission.
- PM may occur rarely in association with certain drug therapies. In human medicine, the drug most often implicated has been D-penicillamine. PM can occur as part of a generalized allergic drug reaction in Doberman pinschers following trimethoprim-sulfadiazine administration; however, this has not been confirmed by muscle biopsies or electromyographic studies.

Ischemic

Ischemia as a result of thromboembolic disease and vascular occlusion is the most common cause of ischemic myopathy and neuromyopathy in dogs and cats. Circulation may be partly or completely compromised; the severity of clinical signs varies with the degree of occlusion.

CLINICAL SIGNS

KEY POINT ▶ Muscular weakness is the clinical sign common to all neuromuscular disorders. Expression of muscular weakness may be limited to certain muscle groups or may be generalized and varies considerably in severity.

Generalized signs of motor system involvement include:

- Gait abnormalities
- Paresis or paralysis
- Exercise-related weakness

Other clinical signs that may occur concurrently with generalized weakness or in the absence of detectable weakness include:

- Masticatory dysfunction
- Dysphagia (pharyngeal dysfunction)
- Regurgitation (esophageal dysfunction)

■ Dysphonia and dyspnea (laryngeal dysfunction) indicating involvement of selected motor units serving visceral functions

DIAGNOSIS

A thorough history and careful general physical and neurologic examinations are critical to the evaluation of neuromuscular disorders. Perform routine and special diagnostic testing procedures based on the differential diagnosis. Following the examination, it should be possible to localize the disorder tentatively to the motor unit.

History

Look for:

■ Exposure to chemical agents
■ Recent illnesses and particularly recent medications
■ Exposure to different geographic locations

Physical and Neurologic Examinations

Following a careful general physical examination including a thorough evaluation of the cardiovascular system, perform a complete neurologic evaluation:

■ Weakness (motor sign) is common to all motor unit abnormalities.
■ Evaluate muscle strength by observing the animal's gait as it walks and, if necessary, after more strenuous exercise.
■ Examine for stiffness of movement, seen in inflammatory myopathies, myotonias, and MG.
■ The presence of ataxia (sensory sign) suggests an underlying neuropathic disorder with involvement of large myelinated proprioceptive fibers or their cell bodies in sensory ganglia.
■ Assess muscle tone and spinal reflexes.
■ Note the presence of muscle atrophy or swelling.

Because the clinical expression of weakness varies considerably in severity and distribution, other tests such as wheelbarrowing, hopping, or hemiwalking may be necessary to define a paresis.

Clinical signs such as dysphagia, regurgitation, dysphonia, and dyspnea may indicate selective involvement of motor units. These clinical signs may occur in the absence of generalized weakness and may indicate disorders of motor units originating in cranial nerves.

KEY POINT ▶ Differentiate vomiting from regurgitation because a wrong assessment may lead to an inappropriate diagnosis.

Routine and Special Laboratory Examinations

Perform a complete blood count (CBC), serum chemistry profile (including electrolytes), and urinalysis in all cases to evaluate possible underlying metabolic abnormalities. Although not indicated in all instances, other laboratory assays may assist in obtaining a diagnosis.

Serum Creatine Kinase (CK) Assay

Serum CK levels are elevated in muscle disorders associated with damage to myofibers and membranes. Although CK is a sensitive indicator of the presence and severity of myonecrosis, modest elevations in CK can occur in neuropathies.

KEY POINT ▶ An elevation of serum CK is not diagnostic of myositis. Perform a muscle biopsy to confirm the diagnosis.

Thyroid and Adrenal Function Tests

Myopathies can occur secondary to disorders of both the thyroid and adrenal gland. Hypothyroidism can occur concurrently with autoimmune neuromuscular disorders such as acquired MG and an optimal clinical response may rely on the treatment of both disorders.

Antinuclear Antibody (ANA) Assay

A positive ANA titer in association with an inflammatory myopathy suggests an underlying systemic autoimmune disorder. A subset of canine patients with myasthenia gravis also have positive ANA titers.

Serum Toxoplasma gondii and Neospora caninum Titers

Serology, as described in sec. 2, ch. 13, may be useful in the evaluation of inflammatory myopathies and peripheral neuropathies caused by protozoa. However, demonstration of the organism in a muscle biopsy specimen is diagnostic.

Plasma Cholinesterase Levels

Myasthenia-like syndromes and delayed neuropathies are associated with organophosphate toxicity.

Serum Antibodies Against Masticatory Muscle Type 2M Fibers

The demonstration of autoantibodies against masticatory muscle type 2M fibers in fresh-frozen muscle sections by immunocytochemical methods using the immunoreagent staphylococcal protein A–horseradish peroxidase is useful in the diagnosis of masticatory muscle myositis. Direct methods demonstrating the presence of antibodies bound to myofibers within a muscle biopsy and indirect methods for demonstrating antibodies circulating within the patient's serum are available.*

Serum Antibodies Against Nicotinic AChRs

Demonstration of autoantibodies against muscle AChRs by immunoprecipitation radioimmunoassay is the diagnostic test of choice* for acquired MG. This assay is sensitive and specific and demonstrates an

---

*Assays are available from the Comparative Neuromuscular Laboratory, Basic Science Building, Room B200, University of California–San Diego, La Jolla, CA 92093-0614 (phone: 619-534-1537).

immune response specifically against muscle AChRs. It is particularly valuable in cases of focal myasthenia in which muscle weakness is localized to pharyngeal or esophageal musculature in the absence of detectable generalized weakness. Serial serum antibody titers also are important in following clinical response to treatment because there is good correlation between serum titers and response to treatment.

KEY POINT ▶ Previous corticosteroid administration can lower serum antibody levels in assays for masticatory muscle myositis and MG. Collect serum prior to corticosteroid therapy.

Edrophonium Chloride Challenge Test

A presumptive diagnosis of generalized MG in dogs and cats may be based on an increase in muscle strength following IV administration of edrophonium chloride (Tensilon; Roche) at a recommended dosage of 0.1–0.2 mg/kg. The most dramatic response to edrophonium chloride is in MG; however, responses are variable: some patients with MG fail to respond, whereas some patients with neuropathic disorders show an increase in muscle strength.

KEY POINT ▶ Do not eliminate a diagnosis of MG based on a negative response to edrophonium. Serum AChR antibody titers can confirm the diagnosis.

- In cases of focal MG, if the palpebral reflex is absent or decreased, administration of the edrophonium chloride may result in an improved blink.
- During treatment of generalized MG with anticholinesterase drugs, edrophonium chloride may be useful in differentiating a myasthenic crisis (underdosing) from a cholinergic crisis (overdosing).
  - In a myasthenic crisis, rapid improvement usually follows IV administration of edrophonium chloride.

Electrodiagnostic Evaluation

Electrodiagnostic testing is a valuable adjunct to the neurologic examination. It provides:

- Information on the location of a lesion within the motor unit (e.g., axon, neuromuscular junction, or muscle)
- Information on the distribution and severity of the disease process
- Guidance to appropriate muscle groups and peripheral nerves for subsequent biopsy

Electrodiagnostic testing includes:

- Evaluation of muscles by electromyography
- Evaluation of peripheral nerves by measurement of motor and sensory nerve conduction velocities and compound muscle and nerve action potentials (see sec. 10, ch. 5).
- Measurement of evoked potentials following repetitive nerve stimulation, which is useful in the diagnosis of disorders of neuromuscular transmission if performed appropriately

In normal dogs stimulus rates >5/second resulted in large decrements and variations between dogs. Use of stimulus rates >5/second is not recommended for clinical use because it can result in an inaccurate diagnosis of MG.

Muscle Biopsy

Muscle biopsy allows direct examination of portions of most motor unit components (e.g., intramuscular nerve branches, neuromuscular junction, and myofibers) and of supportive, connective, and vascular tissues. Using fresh-frozen sections, histologic and cytologic detail is preserved, and many biochemical and immunochemical reactions within cells and tissues can be localized. Frozen sections also may be used in specific biochemical assays for enzymes and substrates.

KEY POINT ▶ For maximum information from a muscle biopsy, specimens should be flash-frozen in isopentane or Freon precooled in liquid nitrogen. Do not place muscle biopsy specimens in formalin.

Appropriate sampling and transport methods are essential to the diagnostic value of the muscle specimen. Selection of the muscle(s) for biopsy is also important.

- Sample an involved muscle; however, avoid end-stage muscle because essential diagnostic features may no longer be present.
- The site of a localized disorder determines which muscle(s) should be sampled; however, in generalized disorders (e.g., polyneuropathy and polymyositis), it is desirable to sample standard muscles (e.g., vastus lateralis in dogs and cats).
- Following collection, wrap the muscle specimen in a saline-dampened gauze sponge, place in a watertight container, and transport on cold packs to the laboratory.
- Delivery to the laboratory for processing within 24 hours is critical for optimal results.

KEY POINT ▶ To ensure correct methods of sampling and transportation, it is important to consult with the person who will be examining biopsy specimens prior to the biopsy procedure. Once a muscle biopsy sample has been placed in formalin it is too late.

Special Radiographic Studies

Because dysphagia as a result of oropharyngeal dysfunction and megaesophagus is a major problem in certain neuromuscular disorders, contrast studies that evaluate the dynamic swallowing process and motility throughout the esophagus are indicated. These studies should be attempted only if appropriate fluoroscopy and video recording equipment is available. (See sec. 7, ch. 2 for discussion of diagnosis and management of esophageal disease.)

KEY POINT ▶ If a large air-filled pharynx or a megaesophagus is visualized on plain radiographs, do not perform a barium swallow. If a contrast agent is absolutely necessary, use a small amount of dilute barium solution to minimize chance of barium aspiration.

TREATMENT

Selective breeding and prevention is the treatment of choice for the *hereditary* neuromuscular disorders. New techniques in molecular genetics, available at selected research centers, allow the identification of underlying genetic defects and carrier animals. Gene replacement therapies are currently in experimental testing stages and may be available in the future for treatment of some of these disorders. *Acquired* neuromuscular disorders in many instances are secondary to diverse underlying medical problems such as hypothyroidism (see sec. 4, ch. 1), adrenal gland dysfunction (see sec. 4, ch. 3), electrolyte disorders (see sec. 1, ch. 5), and protozoal infection (see sec. 2, ch. 13); direct treatment, if possible, to resolution of the primary problem. Specific treatment is available for some neuromuscular disorders. These are described below.

Generalized MG

Anticholinesterase Drugs

These drugs are the cornerstone of treatment for MG. They inhibit enzymatic hydrolysis of ACh at the neuromuscular junction, thereby increasing the effective concentration of ACh and the duration of its effect in the synaptic cleft and prolonging the interaction of released ACh with remaining AChRs.

- If the animal can tolerate oral medication, administer pyridostigmine bromide syrup (Mestinon; Roche) at a dose of 0.5–3.0 mg/kg q8–12h, beginning at the low end of the dosage scale and gradually increasing.
- If delivery of drugs is a problem owing to megaesophagus or pharyngeal dysfunction, give injectable neostigmine (Prostigmin; Roche) at a dosage of 0.04 mg/kg IM q6h until the animal is able to handle oral medication.
- Initiate concurrent treatment for aspiration pneumonia (sec. 6, ch. 21) if this disorder is present.

KEY POINT ▶ In the treatment of MG, it is important to titrate dosages to fit each animal's needs; requirements may vary from day to day in response to activity levels and stress.

Corticosteroids

Corticosteroids are not recommended as initial therapy in MG. Although it is true that MG is an autoimmune disease, clinical signs of weakness can be controlled in most cases with anticholinesterase drugs.

Contraindications

- Some dogs become weaker with corticosteroid therapy, possibly precipitating a myasthenic crisis.

- In many dogs with MG, there is spontaneous remission within variable periods of time; therefore, generalized immunosuppression may not be warranted, particularly in light of the side effects of these drugs in dogs.

Indications

- If muscle strength is not greatly improved following anticholinesterase treatment and aspiration pneumonia is not present, administer prednisone (1.0 mg/kg q12h), gradually tapering to alternate-day dosage.
- Other autoimmune disorders, for which a specific treatment for the underlying clinical signs is not available, may occur concurrently with MG. In these cases, immunosuppression with corticosteroids is warranted.

Other Immunosuppressive Treatments

Reserve agents such as azathioprine and cyclophosphamide (see sec. 3, ch. 5) and therapies such as plasmapheresis for the rare refractory cases that do not respond to conventional therapy.

Management of Pharyngeal and Esophageal Problems

KEY POINT ▶ Early recognition of regurgitation due to megaesophagus is important in the successful management of MG; management includes alteration in methods of delivery of food and water.

Megaesophagus. When regurgitation due to megaesophagus is present:

- Administer anticholinesterase drugs 1 hour prior to feeding.
- Deliver food and water with the animal in an upright position (see sec. 7, ch. 2).
- Ensure that the animal remains upright for at least 10 minutes following feeding.

Placement of a Percutaneous Gastrostomy Tube. Placement of a gastric feeding tube (see sec. 1, ch. 3) is recommended for bypassing the dysfunctional pharynx and esophagus in patients that do not respond to elevated feeding.

KEY POINT ▶ In the absence of severe aspiration pneumonia and with appropriate management, the prognosis for complete remission of MG is good. In many animals, the megaesophagus resolves and regurgitation is eliminated. Continue treatment until serum AChR antibody titers are normal.

Focal MG

Megaesophagus and pharyngeal dysfunction in the absence of detectable generalized weakness may occur in MG. The diagnosis in these cases is made by demonstration of positive serum AChR antibody titers.

- The single most important part of treatment is elevation of food and water (see previous discussion).
- The value of anticholinesterase drugs in focal MG is not known; however, lower doses may be of some benefit in controlling regurgitation.
  - In the absence of generalized weakness, monitoring drug response is difficult and overdosages may occur.
- Because the majority of dogs with the focal form of MG go into spontaneous remission, it is not known whether the benefits of corticosteroids outweigh the risks; however, as in generalized MG, in focal MG the presence of concurrent autoimmune disorders without a specific therapy warrants the use of corticosteroids.

Immune-Mediated Inflammatory Myopathies

Masticatory Muscle Myositis

- During the acute stages of MMM, masticatory muscle swelling and trismus (spasm) usually resolve rapidly subsequent to immunosuppressive doses of glucocorticoids (prednisone, 1.0–1.5 mg/kg PO q12h).
- Determine response to therapy by ability to open the jaw and by serial determinations of serum CK levels.
- If the response is favorable, decrease dosage after 1–2 weeks to 0.5 mg/kg PO q12h; then gradually decrease to the lowest effective alternate-day dosage.
- Relapses are common.

KEY POINT ▶ In acute MMM, glucocorticoids usually produce rapid resolution. In chronic MMM, glucocorticoid therapy may improve jaw mobility even though a significant proportion of muscle is replaced by fibrous connective tissue.

Polymyositis

- Treat dogs with polymyositis with immunosuppressive doses of corticosteroids in the absence of aspiration pneumonia or underlying infectious agent. Initiate a treatment regime similar to that for MMM.
- In refractory cases other immunosuppressive agents such as azathioprine or cyclophosphamide (see sec. 3, ch. 5 for dosages) may be used concurrently.

Supplemental Readings

Cardinet GH III: Muscle biopsy techniques for the evaluation of neuromuscular (motor unit) disorders. San Diego: Proceedings of the 7th Annual ACVIM Forum, 1989, p 373.

Carpenter JL, Schmidt GM, Moore FM, et al.: Canine bilateral extraocular polymyositis. Vet Pathol 26:510, 1989.

Le Couteur RA, Dow SW, Sisson AF: Metabolic and endocrine myopathies of dogs and cats. Semin Vet Med Surg [Small Anim] 4:146, 1989.

Miller LM, Lennon VA, Lambert EH, et al.: Congenital myasthenia gravis in 13 smooth fox terriers. J Am Vet Med Assoc 182:694, 1983.

Sharp NJH, Kornegay JN, Lane SB: The muscular dystrophies. Semin Vet Med Surg [Small Anim] 4:133, 1989.

Shelton GD: Disorders of neuromuscular transmission. Semin Vet Med Surg [Small Anim] 4:126, 1989.

Shelton GD, Cardinet GH III: Pathophysiologic basis of canine muscle disorders. J Vet Intern Med 1:36, 1987.

Shelton GD, Cardinet GH III: Canine masticatory muscle disorders. In Kirk RW, ed.: Current Veterinary Therapy X. Philadelphia: W. B. Saunders, 1989, p 816.

Shelton GD, Willard MD, Cardinet GH III, Lindstrom J: Acquired myasthenia gravis: Selective involvement of esophageal, pharyngeal, and facial muscles. J Vet Intern Med 4:281, 1990.

Simms MH, McLean RA: Use of repetitive nerve stimulation to assess neuromuscular function in dogs. Prog Vet Neurol 1:311, 1990.

Ophthalmology

David A. Wilkie

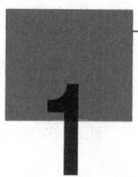

Introduction

David A. Wilkie

To properly evaluate and treat the patient with ocular disease, the clinician must have an accurate understanding of ophthalmic anatomy (Fig. 1).

OPHTHALMIC EQUIPMENT

The instruments and other equipment necessary for ophthalmic examination and surgery can be generally categorized as basic and advanced.

Diagnostic Equipment

Basic

- Penlight
- Direct ophthalmoscope with Finoff transilluminator
- Indirect lens (20 diopter)

- Tonometer (Schiøtz)
- Miscellaneous—
  - Schirmer tear test strips
  - Fluorescein stain
  - Nasolacrimal cannula (23 gauge)
  - Dilating agent (e.g., tropicamide)
  - Topical anesthetic (e.g., proparacaine)
  - Graefe forceps for third eyelid manipulation
  - Kimura spatula for cytology

Advanced

- Biomicroscope (slit lamp)
- Indirect ophthalmoscope
- Indirect lenses (15, 20, and 30 diopter)
- Applanation tonometer
- Gonioscopy lens

Surgical Equipment

Basic

- Magnifying loupes (4–6 ×)
- Colibri corneal forceps (0.3 mm teeth with tying platform)
- Bishop Harmon forceps (0.3 or 0.8 mm teeth)
- Barraquer needle holder (curved, without lock device; 9 mm × 0.85 mm jaws)
- Westcott tenotomy scissors
- Stevens tenotomy curved scissors
- Barraquer eyelid speculum
- Beaver blade handle
- Bard-Parker blade handle
- Desmarres chalazion clamp
- Strabismus hooks (two)
- Jamieson calipers

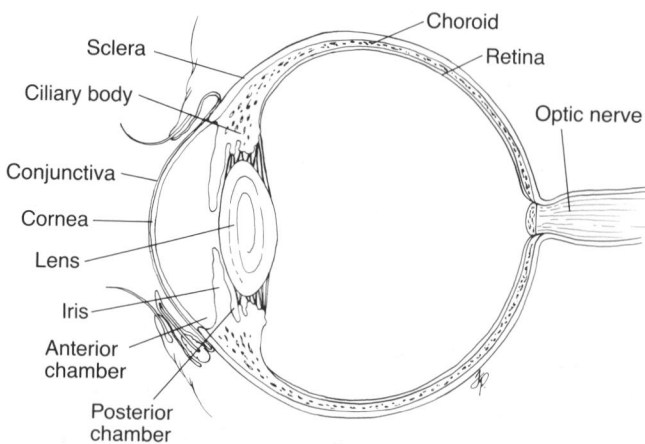

Figure 1. Normal ophthalmic anatomy.

- Jaeger eyelid plate
- Irrigating cannula (23 gauge)

Advanced

- Operating microscope
- Right and left corneal section scissors
- Lens loop
- Angled tying forceps
- Carter sphere introducer
- Castroviejo cyclodialysis spatula
- Various intraocular forceps

Other

- Suture material
  - 7-0 Vicryl or Dexon—ophthalmic spatula needle
  - 9-0 Nylon
  - 6-0 Monofilament—ophthalmic cutting needle (nylon, Surgilene, prolene)
- Blades
  - #64, 63, and 65 Beaver blades
  - #11 and 15 Bard-Parker blades
- Irrigating solutions
  - Ophthalmic balanced salt solution (BSS)
  - Lactated Ringer's
- Weck-cel surgical spears
- Prosthesis implants (19 mm)

OPHTHALMOLOGY TECHNIQUES

The general veterinarian in private practice should be able to perform the following routine ophthalmic procedures:

- Culture of the eye
- Schirmer tear test
- Examination of the nictitating membrane (third eyelid)
- Direct ophthalmoscopy
- Indirect ophthalmoscopy
- Fluorescein stain of the cornea
- Nasolacrimal irrigation
- Schiøtz tonometry
- Conjunctival/corneal cytology

In addition, based on the information obtained by these diagnostic tests, the clinician should be able to arrive at a diagnosis and formulate a plan for further diagnostic tests or treatment.

Culture

Indications

- Chronic, nonresponsive corneal ulcer
- Acute, severe melting corneal ulcer
- Purulent ocular discharge
- Infectious blepharitis

Equipment

- A sterile, moist, synthetic culture swab is preferable but a sterile cotton swab can be used.

Technique

The general principles and techniques for obtaining a culture from the eye are the same as for other organs.

1. Using a sterile swab moistened in transport media, obtain the sample in an aseptic manner from the area of concern; for example:
   a. If the lesion is a corneal ulcer, touch the swab to the ulcer (do not place in the conjunctival fornix).
2. Do not use a topical anesthetic for this procedure because it will interfere with the growth of organisms.
3. Label the sample and submit for aerobic and possibly fungal culture and sensitivity testing. It should be streaked onto nutrient agar as soon as possible.

Schirmer Tear Test

Indications

- Assessment of normal tear production
- Chronic pigmentary keratitis
- Epiphora, including chronic mucoid epiphora

Equipment

- Commercially available Schirmer tear test strips

Technique

1. Place the notched end of the test strip in the lower conjunctival fornix. Do not touch this end.
2. Hold the eye closed and allow the strip to remain in place for exactly 1 minute. If convenient, both eyes may be tested at the same time.
3. Remove the strip and, using the standard measurement on the package, measure and record tear production. Normal dogs secrete 15 mm or more in 1 minute.
4. Do not use topical anesthetic for this test because the objective is to measure the response of the eye to an irritant. This requires the response of the ophthalmic branch of cranial nerve (CN) V as the afferent arm and the parasympathetic fibers in CN VII as the efferent arm.

Examination of the Nictitating Membrane

Indications

- Chronic conjunctivitis
- Suspicion of a foreign body
- Mass lesion of the nictitating membrane (third eyelid)

Equipment

- Topical anesthetic
- Atraumatic forceps

Technique

1. Examine the palpebral surface of the third eyelid by gently retropulsing the globe and allowing the nictitating membrane to prolapse passively while

the lower eyelid is retracted. This is useful for assessing the mobility of the third eyelid and for protecting the eye when obtaining a conjunctival scraping.
2. Examine the bulbar surface of the third eyelid. This requires topical anesthesia.
   a. The topical anesthetic of choice is proparacaine (Alcaine), which provides 10–15 minutes of anesthesia. Apply 2 drops of anesthetic and wait 2–3 minutes for the full effect.
   b. After anesthetizing the surface, gently grasp the leading edge of the third eyelid with small non-toothed forceps. Take care to avoid damaging the cornea.
   c. Gently pull the third eyelid up and out to allow examination of the posterior surface.
3. Examine all surfaces and the inner and outer fornices of the third eyelid for a foreign body and for lymphoid follicles, which indicate a chronic inflammatory process.

Direct Ophthalmoscopy

This technique provides an upright image of the fundus and associated structures and magnifies the image 15–18 times. In small animals, the field of view is narrow and therefore difficult to use for general screening of the eye.

Indications

- Examination of the ocular fundus
- Detailed examination with higher magnification of specific areas such as the optic nerve and blood vessels.

Equipment

- Dilating agent, (e.g., tropicamide)
- Charged, direct ophthalmoscope

Technique

1. Turn on the ophthalmoscope and use the rheostat to adjust the light intensity.
2. Turn the diopter wheel to the zero (0) setting. This usually is the proper setting to view the fundus.
3. Darken the examination room.
4. Place the ophthalmoscope to your eye, and from a distance of 12–24 inches obtain the tapetal reflection. While looking through the ophthalmoscope move toward the animal's eye, observing for any interference with the tapetal reflection, which may indicate opacity of the transmitting media, cornea, aqueous humor, lens, or vitreous. When you are 1–2 inches from the patient's cornea, the retina, optic nerve, retinal vessels, and tapetum will be clearly in focus.
5. Locate a blood vessel and follow it to the optic nerve. Evaluate the optic nerve and blood vessels and scan the fundus for abnormalities of color, clarity, size, and shape. Use the diopter wheel to adjust the focus, and to evaluate raised and depressed lesions (numbers in red indicate negative

or deeper; those in black are positive or more superficial).

Indirect Ophthalmoscopy

Although practice is required to become proficient in this technique, once it is mastered it is more useful than direct ophthalmoscopy for screening the fundus in small animals. Also, the equipment needed is less expensive. Indirect ophthalmoscopy provides an inverted, reversed image magnified 3–5 times. This image, although of a lower magnification than with direct ophthalmoscopy, has a much larger field of view and is better for routine screening of the eye.

Indications

- Examination of the ocular fundus

Equipment

- Dilating agent (e.g., tropicamide)
- Light source (e.g., penlight)
- Indirect, hand-held 20-diopter lens

Technique

1. Dilate the patient's pupil with 1–2 drops of tropicamide (Mydriacyl). Allow 10–15 minutes for complete dilation (the effect will last 8–12 hours in dogs).
2. Begin the examination at arm's length from the patient, having an assistant restrain the patient and hold the eyelids open.
3. Darken the examination room.
4. With a focal light source (e.g., a penlight or direct ophthalmoscope) held at arm's length from the patient, obtain the tapetal reflection.
5. Holding the lens in the other hand, place the lens 1–2 inches in front of the patient's eye, in the path of the light. The fundus should appear as a virtual image in front of the lens.
   a. It is important to look at the image that is in front of the lens and not at the lens or the eye.
6. To view other areas of the fundus, you must move yourself, the light source, and the lens while keeping all of these in alignment. Remember that because the image is inverted you must move in the opposite direction to the image.
7. If the image is lost, move the lens out of the light beam and start again.

Fluorescein Stain of the Cornea

Fluorescein is a hydrophilic drug that binds to the corneal stroma, but not to the epithelium or to Descemet's membrane.

Indications

- Red or painful eye
- An obvious corneal irregularity
- Ocular trauma or a foreign body
- Assessment of nasolacrimal duct function

Equipment

- Prepackaged fluorescein strips (commercially available)
- Sterile ocular collyria (eyewash solution)
- Cotton balls

Technique

1. Remove the fluorescein strip from the package, holding it by the green end. Fold the strip lengthwise to create a trough.
2. Place 2–3 drops of sterile eyewash solution on the strip and tilt it to allow the stain to drip onto the eye. Do not touch the eye with the strip because this may result in an iatrogenic area of stain retention.
3. With the eyewash solution, gently irrigate excess stain from the eye onto a cotton ball; examine the eye for stain uptake, using a penlight. Visualization of the fluorescein uptake is improved by using a blue or Wood light, which excites the fluorescein molecules, making them fluoresce green.

Assessment of Nasolacrimal Duct Function

1. To evaluate the patency of the nasolacrimal duct, perform the previously described steps, but do not rinse the fluorescein from the eye. The stain should appear at the nares within 5 minutes.
2. A positive test is definitive for a patent nasolacrimal duct but does not prove that both puncta are patent. A negative test suggests a problem, and irrigation of the duct is indicated.

Nasolacrimal Duct Irrigation

- This procedure can be performed on a minimally restrained dog, using only topical anesthesia.
- Sedation or general anesthesia usually is required for cats.

Indications

- Epiphora without an obvious etiology
- Failure of passage of fluorescein stain
- Mucopurulent ocular discharge

Equipment

- Topical anesthetic
- Syringe (3–6 ml)
- Nasolacrimal duct cannula (23 or 25 gauge)

Technique

1. Apply a topical anesthetic and connect a nasolacrimal duct cannula to a syringe filled with eyewash solution.
2. While an assistant restrains the animal's head, elevate and roll the upper eyelid in the medial canthus to expose the superior punctum.
3. Place the thumb or index finger on the plunger of the syringe, in preparation for injection. Hold the syringe loosely so that no injury will result if the patient should jerk its head.
4. Gently insert the cannula in the punctum and, without forcing, allow it to seat itself in the duct.

Apply gentle pressure to the plunger and observe fluid emerging from the inferior punctum.
5. Occlude the lower punctum, tip the nose down and continue flushing. Fluid should now appear at the nostril.

KEY POINT ▶ Do not use excessive force when placing the catheter or when irrigating.

6. If a patent duct cannot be established and the epiphora is severe, consider medical therapy such as topical antibiotics or anti-inflammatories and repeated irrigation or general anesthesia to further pursue the problem.

Schiøtz Tonometry

Schiøtz tonometry is a fast and inexpensive method for determining intraocular pressure. It is recommended that every veterinary practice have a functioning tonometer and that every clinician is familiar with its use.

Indications

- Red or painful eye
- Breeds predisposed to glaucoma
- Predisposed breeds with a history of glaucoma in the opposite eye
- Follow-up in animals with medically controlled glaucoma

Equipment

- Topical anesthetic
- Calibrated Schiøtz tonometer
- Conversion chart

Technique

1. Anesthetize the eye with topical proparacaine.
2. To assemble the tonometer, place the shaft in the housing and attach the 5.5 gm weight. Hold the instrument vertically and check that the plunger slides freely within the hollow sleeve.
3. Use the metal calibration standard to test the accuracy of the tonometer. When the instrument is placed on the standard it should read zero (0) on the scale (i.e., the 5.5 gm weight does not indent the metal standard).
4. While an assistant gently elevates the patient's nose, elevate the upper eyelid and place the tonometer foot plate on the cornea. Keep the tonometer vertical and on the center of the cornea. The tonometer should rest on the eye and does not need to be pushed down.
5. Take three readings and average them. Using the conversion chart, convert the averaged value to an approximation of the intraocular pressure, matching the weight used with the reading obtained.
6. Normal values for dogs are 15–27 mm Hg; the variation in both eyes should be no greater than 5 mm Hg.

Cytology

Cytology is a simple, fast, and inexpensive method for characterizing the type of inflammatory process and in many cases to obtain a diagnosis.

Indications

- Obtain a sample for Gram stain
- Characterize the type of inflammation, i.e., neutrophilic, lymphocytic, eosinophilic
- Aid in the diagnosis of feline conjunctivitis (e.g., for *Chlamydia, Mycoplasma*)
- Obtain samples for fluorescent antibody testing

Equipment

- Topical anesthetic
- Platinum spatula or other instrument suitable for sample collection
- Microscope
- Microscope slides
- Stain

Technique

1. Place a topical anesthetic in the animal's conjunctival sac.
2. Gently retropulse the globe and retract the lower eyelid, thus exposing the third eyelid.
3. Using a spatula or other suitable instrument, scrape the palpebral surface of the third eyelid and the adjacent palpebral conjunctiva. Avoid damaging the surface, but use sufficient force to exfoliate cells.
4. Place the cells on a glass slide and streak them to form a monolayer.
5. Submit the slide for Gram staining (to characterize the type of bacteria); for Giemsa, Wright's, or Diff-Quik staining (to examine for cell type, inclusion bodies, etc.); for fluorescent antibody testing (*Chlamydia,* herpesvirus).

OCULAR MANIFESTATIONS OF SYSTEMIC DISEASE

Ophthalmic clinical signs frequently are manifestations of systemic disease (Table 1). For many of these ophthalmic signs, specific ocular causes must be differentiated from the systemic ones provided in Table 1. For a more complete discussion of these diseases and their treatment, refer to appropriate chapters in this book.

TABLE 1. Presenting Ophthalmic Clinical Signs and Associated Systemic Diseases

Ophthalmic Clinical Sign	Associated Systemic Disease
Keratitis sicca	Hypothyroidism Autoimmune disease Drug-induced (sulfonamides) Facial nerve paralysis Otitis media/interna Canine distemper virus
Anterior uveitis/ chorioretinitis	Infectious (bacteria, rickettsia, mycoses, viruses) Trauma Neoplasia Autoimmune disease
Glaucoma	Anterior uveitis Neoplasia Trauma Hyphema
Cataract	Trauma Diabetes mellitus Nutritional disorder Radiation Inflammatory diseases (see anterior uveitis/ chorioretinitis)
Retinal detachment	Trauma Infectious (bacteria, rickettsia, mycoses, viruses) Neoplasia Autoimmune diseases Systemic hypertension (renal disease, pheochromocytoma, hyperthyroidism, idiopathic) Hyperviscosity
Blindness	Trauma Neoplasia Reticulosis Infectious (bacteria, rickettsia, mycoses, viruses) Autoimmune diseases Other central nervous system diseases
Horner's syndrome	Thoracic mass Spinal cord trauma (C1–T2) Neck trauma Otitis media/interna Orbital mass lesion
Hyphema	Coagulopathy Trauma Hypertension (renal disease, pheochromocytoma, hyperthyroidism, idiopathic) Infectious diseases Neoplasia

2 Diseases of the Eyelid

Susan E. Kirschner

Diseases of the eyelid result in a variety of clinical signs. Initially, the eyelids alone may be affected, but because of their close proximity to the cornea and conjunctiva, disease of these structures frequently results. Because corneal and conjunctival involvement is often more severe and more obvious, eyelid disease may be overlooked. Manage concurrent conjunctival and corneal disease as described in sec. 1, chs. 2 and 3, respectively, in this section (sec. 11).

Diseases of the eyelid can be broadly categorized by their appropriate treatment (i.e., surgery or medical therapy), as listed in Table 1.

Anatomy

- The eyelid functions to protect and moisten the cornea and to remove debris. The eyelid is covered by skin and lined internally by palpebral conjunctiva.
- The eyelid is closed by the orbicularis oculi muscle, which is innervated by the palpebral branch of the facial nerve. Paralysis of this nerve results in inability to close the eyelids. Spasm of the orbicularis oculi muscle results in spastic entropion.
- The eyelids are opened by the levator palpebrae and Mueller's muscle, which are innervated by the oculomotor nerve and by postganglionic sympathetic fibers, respectively. Paralysis of either of these nerves results in ptosis, or drooping of the eyelid.
- The meibomian glands line the conjunctival surface of the eyelid margin. They open onto the eyelid margin, where they secrete an oily fluid that helps prevent evaporation of the precorneal tear film. Distichia and ectopic cilia originate from the meibomium glands.

TABLE 1. Classification of Eyelid Diseases According to Type of Therapy

Surgery
Ankyloblepharon
Coloboma
Entropion
Ectropion
Distichiasis/ectopic cilia
Lagophthalmos
Neoplasia

Medical Treatment
Bacterial blepharitis
Chalazion/hordeolum
Allergic blepharitis
Parasitic and fungal blepharitis

Principles of Eyelid Surgery

- The skin covering the eyelids is thin and easily traumatized. Perform clipping and aseptic preparation gently. A povidone-iodine solution diluted with saline solution to a 1:10 concentration is appropriate for preparing the eyelids for surgery.
- The eyelids have an extensive blood supply, and injured tissue heals well; therefore, remove only clearly necrotic tissue. Removal of excess tissue can result in abnormal lid function.
- Close eyelid skin incisions with 4-0–6-0 monofilament nonabsorbable suture in a simple interrupted pattern. Close conjunctival wounds with 6-0–8-0 absorbable suture material. Remove nonabsorbable sutures 2 weeks following surgery.
- An Elizabethan-type collar may be necessary to prevent self-trauma.

KEY POINT ▶ Accurate closure of the eyelid margin is the most important component of eyelid defect repair.

ANKYLOBLEPHARON

Ankyloblepharon is a condition seen in neonatal puppies in which the eyelids do not open properly.

- This condition may result in a subpalpebral infection called ophthalmia neonatorum.
  - If infection occurs, gently massage the eyelids to open a portion of the palpebral fissure. Occasionally, scissors or a scalpel blade is required to partially open the eyelids.
  - Lavage the subpalpebral area with a 1% povidone-iodine solution and apply a topical antibiotic solution or ointment (e.g., triple antibiotic, erythromycin, gentamicin) 3–4 times daily.
- If the infection is left unattended, the cornea may ulcerate or perforate.
- If the entire palpebral fissure is opened prematurely, corneal damage may result from exposure and desiccation.
  - To protect against corneal desiccation, use an artificial tear ointment 4–6 times daily.

COLOBOMA

In this disorder, which affects kittens and occasionally puppies, a portion of the lid margin does not form.

- The major clinical signs are epiphora and blepharospasm.

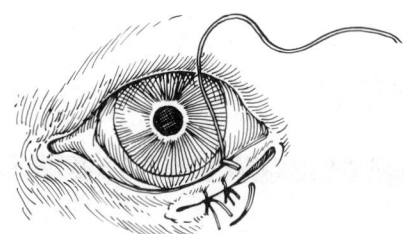

Figure 1. Correction of ventral entropion.

- Coloboma may be confused with entropion because eyelid hairs often contact the cornea.
- Many cases can be corrected by slightly everting the lid with entropion correction surgery, thus preventing corneal trauma by facial hairs.
- Extensive colobomas require a pedicle flap or other reconstructive surgical procedure performed by a veterinary ophthalmologist.

ENTROPION

Entropion usually is observed in young dogs and is common in the chow, Shar pei, and hunting breeds. It can also occur in cats.

- Clinical signs vary from conjunctivitis with mild serous discharge to severe blepharospasm with corneal ulceration and purulent discharge.
- Diagnosis is made by examination of the eyelids. When the eyelid is rolled inward, facial hairs often directly contact the cornea.
- Correct neonatal entropion in the Shar pei with temporary everting sutures at 3–5 weeks of age. Failure of this technique indicates the need for permanent surgical correction.

Classification

KEY POINT ▶ Entropion may be anatomic, anatomic with a secondary eyelid spasm, or primarily spastic.

Classification of entropion is made when the eyelids are relaxed. This may require topical anesthesia, palpebral nerve blocks, or general anesthesia.

- *Anatomic entropion*—The eyelid rolls inward even when the eyelids are relaxed.
  - Surgical correction is indicated.
- *Anatomic entropion with secondary spasm*—Blepharospasm exaggerates entropion such that a portion of the rolling is from an anatomic abnormality, with the remainder due to squinting.
  - Surgically correct the anatomic portion of the entropion; additional temporary everting sutures may be required until the spasm cycle is broken.
- *Spastic entropion*—Blepharospasm results in rolling inward of the eyelid margin. Under anesthesia or when the eyelids are relaxed, the entropion resolves.
  - Correct with temporary everting sutures and treatment of the underlying cause of the spasm.

Surgical Procedures

Techniques

Correction of Anatomic Entropion
Ventral or Dorsal Eyelid Entropion

1. Remove an ellipse of skin parallel to and 2–3 mm from the lid margin (Fig. 1). The amount of skin removed depends on the severity of the entropion.
2. Remove the tissue with a scalpel or by crushing the selected tissue with a hemostat and then removing the crimped tissue with scissors.
3. Close the skin routinely with monofilament nylon sutures (e.g., 4-0) in a simple interrupted pattern.

Lateral Entropion

1. Remove a V-shaped area of skin (Fig. 2*A*) at the lateral canthus.
2. If the lateral canthus is extremely lax, dissect the underlying orbicularis oculi muscle free (Fig. 2*B*) and suture it to the lateral orbital rim with 4-0–5-0 nonabsorbable monofilament suture material.
3. Close the skin with 4-0–5-0 nonabsorbable sutures in a simple interrupted pattern.

Medial Entropion

1. Evert the skin with an elliptical incision, as for ventral entropion.
2. Alternatively perform a medial canthoplasty. Make a V-shaped incision along the eyelid margin that encompasses the caruncle (Fig. 3*A*). Take care not to injure the underlying lacrimal canaliculi.

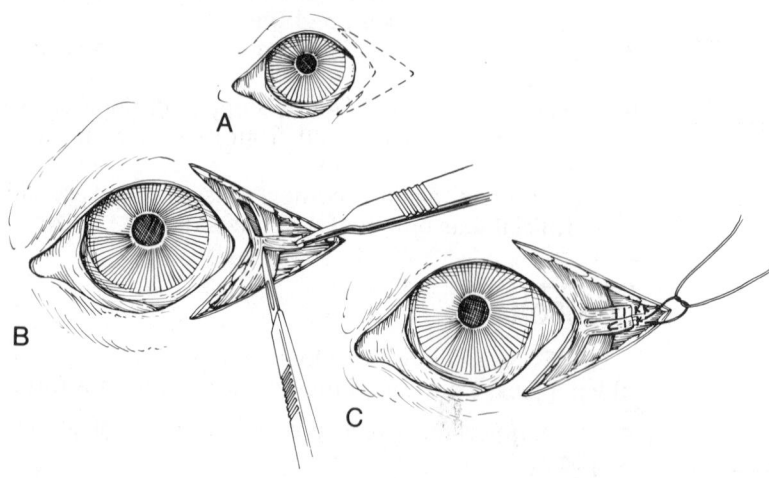

Figure 2. Correction of lateral entropion. *A*, Area of skin to be removed; *B*, orbicularis oculi dissected free; and *C*, sutured to the lateral orbital rim.

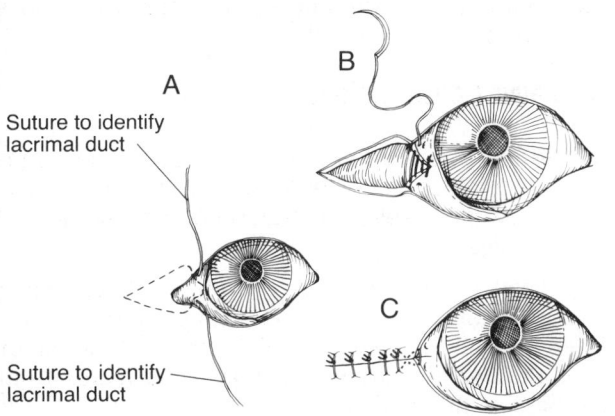

Figure 3. Correction of medial entropion by medial canthoplasty. *A,* Mark the lacrimal canaliculus with a suture—then make a V-shaped incision along the eyelid margin, encompassing the caruncle. *B and C,* Close the incision in two layers, creating horizontal closure.

3. Close the incision by suturing the upper lid to the lower lid to create a horizontal closure (Fig. 3*B* and *C*). This has the effect of correcting the entropion and slightly shortening the palpebral fissure.

Temporary Everting Sutures for Spastic Entropion and for Neonatal Entropion in Shar peis

1. Use minimal anesthesia for very young puppies (occasionally, light inhalation anesthesia via a mask is required).
2. In older dogs, inject a short-acting anesthetic such as sodium thiamylal or ketamine and diazepam.
3. Place 1–2 4-0–5-0 nylon sutures in a mattress pattern in each eyelid. Sutures should be partial thickness only. Make the first bite 1–2 mm from the eyelid margin. Place the second bite at a sufficient distance to cause eversion of the eyelid margin when the suture is tied (Fig. 4).
4. Leave the sutures in place for 3–4 weeks. Premature suture removal may result in recurrence of the entropion.

ECTROPION

■ Ectropion may be caused by excessive eyelid length or by decreased tone of the eyelid muscles. This results in sagging of the lower eyelid, with exposure of conjunctiva. In addition, ectropion can result iatrogenically from over-correction of entropion.
■ Increased conjunctival exposure often results in chronic conjunctivitis or exposure keratitis. Poor lid-to-cornea fit may exacerbate keratoconjunctivitis sicca (KCS) because of abnormal tear distribution.
■ Most cases of ectropion can be corrected by a full-thickness wedge resection of the affected portion of the eyelid (see under Neoplasia for procedure).
■ Shortening of the palpebral fissure via a permanent lateral tarsorrhaphy is beneficial in many dogs.

DISTICHIASIS

Distichiasis is a condition in which hairs that originate from the meibomian glands and emerge from their ducts contact the cornea and cause irritation. It is common in cocker spaniel, golden retriever, and Shih Tzu breeds and occasionally is seen in St. Bernards and other breeds.

KEY POINT ▶ Reserve surgical removal for animals in which epiphora, blepharospasm, or corneal disease are significant clinical signs and when other ocular disease has been ruled out.

■ The most common complication of distichiasis surgery is recurrence 3–5 months postoperatively.

Surgical Procedures

Technique

Cryoepilation

1. Evert and stabilize the lid with a chalazion clamp and freeze a 3-mm band along the base of the meibomian glands, on the palpebral surface of the eyelid, below each abnormal cilia. Freeze time varies, depending on whether nitrous oxide or liquid nitrogen is used. In general, the ice ball should extend to the lid margin, taking care not to freeze the full thickness of the lid.
2. A double freeze-thaw cycle is most effective.
3. To minimize swelling, administer a systemic anti-inflammatory agent (e.g., a single dose of flunixin meglumine, 0.25–0.5 mg/kg, IV) prior to surgery.

Technique

Electroepilation

Reserve this time-consuming technique for cases in which only a few hairs are to be removed.

1. Insert an electrolysis stylet along the hair shaft into the base of the follicle.
2. Apply low amperage (2–4 mA) coagulating current until a small amount of meibomian gland material bubbles out of the duct opening.

ECTOPIC CILIA

■ Ectopic cilia are hairs originating from the meibomium gland that emerge through the conjunctival surface of the eyelid.

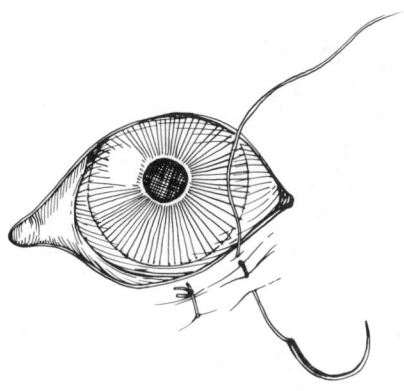

Figure 4. Temporary lid-everting sutures.

- The most common clinical signs are blepharospasm and corneal ulceration.
- The most common location is the central upper eyelid, 2–4 mm from the eyelid margin.

Technique

Removal

1. Excise the hair and its root en bloc with a #15 scalpel blade.
2. Stabilize the eyelid during the procedure with a chalazion clamp.
3. The conjunctival wound may be left open.

LAGOPHTHALMOS

- Lagophthalmos is a condition in which the eyelids cannot completely close. The most common cause is anatomic exophthalmos, seen in brachycephalic breeds. In these breeds, blink frequency often is decreased, exacerbating the problem.
- It also is associated with buphthalmos (progressive enlargement of the eye), palpebral nerve palsy, and ectropion.
- Corneal disease, including ulceration, pigmentation, neovascularization, and keratinization, may result.
- Treat surgically by permanent closure of a portion of the palpebral fissure. Attempt to shorten the palpebral fissure to expose any corneal surface.

Technique

1. Excise the eyelid margin of the ventral and dorsal lids at the lateral or medial canthus.
2. Close the eyelids in two layers, as described for wedge resection under Neoplasia.

NEOPLASIA

Diagnosis

- The most common tumor in the dog is meibomian gland adenoma. Other tumors seen in the eyelids include papilloma, meibomian gland adenocarcinoma, melanoma, histiocytoma, and squamous cell carcinoma and basal cell tumors.
  - Meibomian gland tumors originate in the base of the gland but often emerge from the meibomian gland duct on the eyelid margin.
- Tumors occurring in the eyelids of cats include melanoma, fibrosarcoma, neurofibroma, and squamous and basal cell carcinoma.
  - Squamous cell carcinomas usually are seen in white cats and appear as nonhealing ulcerative lesions. They are locally aggressive and have a high recurrence rate.
  - Melanomas of the eyelids have been known to metastasize in cats.
- In dogs, most eyelid tumors are benign and are removed to prevent irritation or injury to the cornea or conjunctiva.
- In cats, most eyelid tumors are malignant and carry a guarded prognosis.

- For additional information on skin tumors in dogs and cats, see sec. 3, ch. 9.

Preoperative Considerations

KEY POINT ▶ One-fourth of the upper eyelid and one-third of the lower lid can be removed without severe distortion of the palpebral fissure.

- The most common cause of recurrence of meibomian gland adenoma is incomplete removal of the tumor. Keep in mind that even though the bulk of the tumor is at the eyelid margin, the tumor originates from the base of the meibomian gland.

Surgical Procedures

- A full-thickness wedge resection of the eyelid is sufficient to remove most tumors.
- Cryosurgery also can be used to treat many eyelid tumors.
  - Although there is a slightly higher recurrence rate with this technique than with excision, it is a relatively safe, simple procedure that may be performed with local anesthesia combined with tranquilization.
- Submit all excised tissues for histopathology.

Technique

Wedge Resection

1. Using a scalpel blade, incise the skin in a pie-shaped wedge with the base at the eyelid margin. Alternatively, crush along the incision line with hemostats and cut along the crimped line with scissors. Use a tenotomy or Metzenbaum scissors to complete the incision.
2. Close the incision in two layers:
   a. Close the subconjunctival tissue with 6-0 or 7-0 absorbable sutures, with the knots buried within the eyelid.
   b. Close the skin with 6-0 sutures (Fig. 5) beginning at the lid margin.
3. Close the eyelid margin with a figure-of-eight 6-0 suture, and the remainder of the skin with sutures

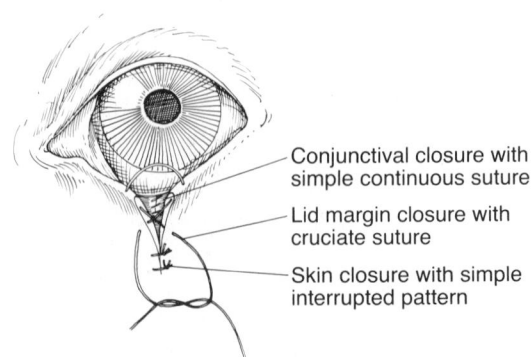

Conjunctival closure with simple continuous suture

Lid margin closure with cruciate suture

Skin closure with simple interrupted pattern

Figure 5. Closure for wedge resection of the eyelid. Close the subconjunctiva with 6-0 or 7-0 absorbable suture in a simple continuous pattern; the lid margin with a cruciate suture; and the remainder of the skin with 6-0 suture, in a simple interrupted pattern.

in a simple interrupted pattern. Alternatively, a horizontal mattress or simple continuous pattern can be used to close eyelid margins.

Technique

Cryosurgery

1. Perform a double freeze-thaw cycle. Treat an area extending 3–5 mm beyond the tumor.
2. For meibomian gland tumors, place the probe on the conjunctival surface of the eyelid.

BACTERIAL BLEPHARITIS

- In blepharitis, the eyelids and lashes are crusted with mucopurulent discharge and are erythematous and swollen. The conjunctiva usually is inflamed, and there may be an associated nonulcerative keratitis.
- Blepharitis can also be a manifestation of various generalized inflammatory skin diseases (see sec. 5), including pyoderma, atopy, dermatomycosis, demodicosis, and autoimmune diseases.

Treatment

- Apply a topical bactericidal ophthalmic solution or ointment (e.g., neomycin, bacitracin, polymyxin B) 3–4 times daily.
- Instruct the owner to give eyelid scrubs, using dilute baby shampoo once a day.
- In severe or chronic cases, give systemic antibiotics as described for pyoderma.
- If there is associated nonulcerative keratitis, consider giving topical corticosteroids once or twice a day.
- If associated with pruritus or other signs of atopy, give systemic antihistamines (e.g., diphenhydramine hydrochloride) twice a day.
- If a good response is not seen within 2 weeks, swab the meibomian gland secretions or upper conjunctival cul-de-sac for culture and sensitivity testing, and perform thyroid function testing.

KEY POINT ▶ Bacterial blepharitis can be difficult to cure. Inform the owner that some dogs require periodic eyelid scrubs and antibiotic therapy on a long-term basis.

CHALAZION/HORDEOLUM

- Chalazion is a granuloma of the meibomian gland.
  - Treat with surgical curettage of the granuloma via the conjunctival surface of the eyelid.
- Hordeolum is an infection or abscess of a meibomium gland or of an eyelash that results in a focal swelling of the lid.
  - Treat with hot packs and systemic antibiotics.
  - To hasten resolution, apply a topical antibiotic/corticosteroid solution or ointment, such as dexamethasone 0.1%, neomycin, polymyxin B, AK-TROL (Akorn, Inc.), q6h–8h.

ALLERGIC BLEPHARITIS

- The annual usually present with acute swelling of the eyelids that may be pruritic but that is rarely painful. There may be a serous discharge.
- Chronic or recurrent allergic blepharitis may be a manifestation of atopy.
- Treat with systemic antihistamines such as diphenhydramine (Benadryl, 0.5 mg/kg q12h, PO) or corticosteroids (Prednisone, 0.5–1.0 mg/kg q12h, PO) and with topical corticosteroids.
  - Cold compresses help to decrease pruritus.
- For further information on allergy testing and treatment for atopy, see sec. 5, ch. 7.

PARASITIC OR FUNGAL BLEPHARITIS

- The eyelids may be infected by cutaneous parasites such as *Demodex* and *Sarcoptes* or by dermatophytes (ringworm).
- In dogs in which periocular alopecia and skin lesions are present but in which the conjunctiva is relatively spared, perform skin scrapings, dermatophyte cultures, and skin biopsies (see sec. 5, ch. 3, 4, and 5).

Supplemental Readings

Bistner S, Aguirre G, Batik G: *Atlas of Veterinary Ophthalmic Surgery.* Philadelphia: W.B. Saunders, 1977, chs. 3–5.

Lavach JD, Gelatt KN: Diseases of the eyelids. Part II. Compend Contin Educ Pract Vet 1:485, 1979.

Roberts SM, Severin GA, Lavach JD: Prevalence and treatment of palpebral neoplasms in the dog: 200 cases (1975–1983). J Am Vet Med Assoc 189:1355, 1986.

Wheeler CA, Severin GA: Cryosurgical epilation for the treatment of distichiasis in the dog and cat. J Am Anim Hosp Assoc 20:877, 1984.

3

Conjunctiva

Cecil P. Moore

ANATOMY AND PHYSIOLOGY

- Conjunctival mucosa covers the inner aspect of the eyelids, the third eyelid, and the anterior sclera. Conjunctiva extends from the lacrimal caruncle medially to the lateral canthus temporally.
- Normal conjunctiva is semitransparent and appears moist and glistening. Numerous small, branching blood vessels are visible within the conjunctiva.
- Sensory innervation to the conjunctiva is via ophthalmic and maxillary branches of the trigeminal nerve.
- The conjunctiva serves as a protective external physical and immunologic barrier for the eye.
- Epithelial goblet cells within the conjunctiva produce mucus, which contributes to the preocular tear film, harbors immunoglobulin, and traps foreign material and debris.

The term *conjunctivitis* describes nonspecific inflammation of the ocular mucous membrane that covers the sclera (bulbar conjunctiva) and lines the inner surface of the eyelids (palpebral conjunctiva). Conjunctivitis is the most common cause of "red eye" in animals. To accurately assess the small animal patient presented with conjunctivitis it is important to recognize inherent species differences in susceptibility and to establish whether the disorder is primary or secondary. For example, feline conjunctivitis is generally caused by a primary ocular infection. Canine conjunctivitis, however, usually is secondary to ocular surface irritants, tear film deficiencies, or foreign bodies.

Additional pertinent information is found in other chapters in this text. Conjunctival disease is often associated with viral infections (see sec. 11, ch. 6), diseases of the cornea (see sec. 11, ch. 4), diseases of the lacrimal apparatus (see sec. 11, ch. 9), and diseases of the eyelids (see sec. 11, ch. 2).

ETIOLOGY OF CONJUNCTIVITIS

Causes of conjunctivitis are numerous. Frequently, more than one etiologic factor plays a role in the clinical course of the disease.

KEY POINT ▶ Regardless of the primary cause, bacterial infection is a common complicating factor in conjunctivitis cases.

Infectious Agents

Infectious agents cause severe conjunctivitis in cats by infecting epithelial cells. Feline herpesvirus and *Chlamydia psittaci* cause the most serious and common ocular infections in cats (see sec. 2, ch. 4). *Mycoplasma felis*, *Staphylococci* spp., *Streptococci* spp., and coliform organisms are bacterial causes of usually less severe forms of feline conjunctivitis.

Gram-positive aerobic bacteria are most commonly isolated from cases of canine conjunctivitis. Opportunistic bacterial infections are common in dogs following conjunctival irritation from other causes. Canine distemper virus (see sec. 2, ch. 6) causes conjunctivitis and dacryoadenitis.

Tear Film Deficiency

Tear film deficiency results in dehydration with accompanying inflammation of the conjunctiva and cornea. Aqueous tear deficiency, or keratoconjunctivitis sicca, occurs more frequently in dogs than in cats (see sec. 11, ch. 9). Although less common than aqueous deficiency, inadequacy of the lipid or mucus components may, when present, complicate the surface disease. Poor eyelid conformation, as with exophthalmos and lagophthalmos, potentiates exposure and drying and is a further complicating factor.

Foreign Bodies

Foreign bodies of the conjunctiva can include plant material, synthetic material, and metallic substances. Plant awns and weed seeds may become embedded in the fornices of the conjunctiva or migrate behind the third eyelid. Embedded plant material is quite reactive and stimulates an intense pyogranulomatous inflammation. By contrast, synthetic material, such as glass and plastic, or certain metals, such as lead and stainless steel, are minimally reactive. Depending upon the location and rigidity of the material, conjunctival foreign bodies may cause direct frictional irritation and resulting surface tissue ulceration.

Trauma

Trauma to the conjunctiva may be blunt, resulting in bruising of an intact membrane, or penetrating with puncture or laceration. In cases of conjunctival trauma, examine the eye thoroughly for the presence of foreign bodies and intraocular lesions.

Chemical Irritants

Chemical irritants that damage the conjunctiva include noxious gases, alkalis, and acids. Alkaline substances, e.g., lye, fresh lime, or ammonia, cause the most serious injuries. When chemical injury has occurred, evaluate the eye for associated corneal and/or anterior uveal involvement.

Environmental Irritants

Environmental irritants, such as dust, particles of sand or plant material, wind, and solar irradiation, are causes of conjunctivitis in small animals. These are particularly common causes in hunting dogs and outdoor working dogs.

Immune-mediated Conjunctivitis

Immune-mediated conjunctivitis results from acute allergic chemosis, atopy (see sec. 5, ch. 7), follicular conjunctivitis, and conjunctivitis resulting from eosinophilic or plasmacytic infiltrates.

Proliferative Diseases

Proliferative diseases are categorized as non-neoplastic or neoplastic. Episcleritis and idiopathic granulomatous disease are the main non-neoplastic proliferative disorders (see sec. 11, ch. 4). Conjunctival epithelial hyperplasia, granulation tissue, and pigmentary infiltrates are examples of additional proliferative conditions. Conjunctival neoplasms may be primary or secondary. Papillomas, squamous cell carcinomas, and hemangiomas are the most common primary tumors. Less common primary neoplasms are hemangiosarcomas, mastocytomas, and melanomas. Adenomas, adenocarcinomas, fibromas, fibrosarcomas, lymphosarcomas, and melanomas are tumors that may secondarily involve the conjunctiva.

Other Eye Diseases

Other eye diseases, either ocular surface disorders or intraocular diseases, are frequently associated with conjunctival inflammation. Surface diseases with associated conjunctivitis include episcleritis, keratitis, and eyelid disease (e.g., chalazia, entropion, ectropion, cilia disorders). Conjunctival inflammation is characteristic of uveitis and glaucoma, although deeper episcleral injection is a hallmark of these intraocular diseases.

Iatrogenically Induced Conjunctivitis

Iatrogenically induced conjunctivitis is caused when topically administered therapeutic agents or surgical manipulations cause conjunctival inflammation. A number of drugs may cause conjunctivitis because of irritation from their active ingredients, vehicles, or preservatives. Surgical procedures result in conjunctivitis from direct trauma (e.g., manipulation, dissection, thermal injury, exposure during or following surgery).

CLINICAL SIGNS OF CONJUNCTIVITIS

- *Hyperemia* occurs with vasodilation of conjunctival vessels resulting in the appearance of a red eye. The redness is intensified when conjunctival hemorrhage or episcleral vascular injection is also present.

- *Ocular discharge* is characteristic of conjunctivitis and is serous, mucoid (catarrhal), or mucopurulent. The type of discharge may change as conjunctivitis progresses—from serous (mild) to mucopurulent (severe).
- *Chemosis* is swelling or "puffiness" of the conjunctiva caused by edema of the mucous membrane.
- *Pain* with conjunctivitis varies with the severity of the ocular disease. Squinting and tearing are characteristic of most cases of conjunctivitis. Photophobia and blepharospasm generally occur only when other eye disease is present, such as ulcerative keratitis or uveitis.
- *Tissue proliferation* is a variable finding of subacute or chronic conjunctival disease. Conjunctival lymphoid follicular hyperplasia may develop in dogs as a nonspecific immune response to persistent antigenic stimulation. In cats, conjunctival follicles are associated with chlamydial conjunctivitis (see sec. 2, ch. 4). Diffuse thickening of the conjunctiva may occur from epithelial hyperplasia or from chronic inflammatory cell infiltrates. Focal, acquired, proliferative lesions may be either granulomas or neoplastic lesions.

DIAGNOSIS OF CONJUNCTIVITIS

History

History includes possible systemic illnesses; environment and habits; possible exposure to infectious or chemical agents; possible trauma; and previous ocular diseases, including the medications administered.

Physical Examination

Physical examination is performed to rule out multisystemic diseases.

Cultures

Cultures are indicated for the definitive diagnosis of ocular infection. Subsequent susceptibility testing is important in selecting the optimal antimicrobial agent. When culturing for fungi, *Mycoplasma, Chlamydia,* or viral agents, it is important to consult with the laboratory in advance regarding any special requirements for submitting culture samples.

KEY POINT ▶ When the need for cultures is anticipated, samples are collected prior to applying topical agents or manipulating ocular surface tissues.

Ophthalmic Examination

Ophthalmic examination is thorough and aimed at identifying other forms of eye disease and confirming the presence of conjunctival disease. If confirmed, establishing the cause completes the process. Components of the complete ophthalmic examination are as follows:
- Inspect the external ocular surfaces and the anterior portion of the globe directly using a focal light

source with magnification. The focused light is also used to check for pupil symmetry and light response.

- Perform the intraocular examination with a focused light and an ophthalmoscope. Opacities of the normally clear ocular media (cornea, intraocular chambers, lens) are noted. Funduscopy is done to determine if abnormalities of the retina, choroid, or optic nerve are present.
- Measure aqueous tear production with Schirmer tear test strips as described in sec. 11, ch. 9. The diagnosis of aqueous tear deficiency must be ruled out because this is a common occurrence in small animals, particularly in dogs, and results in chronic conjunctivitis with a tenacious mucopurulent ocular discharge.

KEY POINT ▶ The Schirmer tear test strips measure reflex tear production that is evaluated prior to application of any local solutions including topical anesthetic agents.

- Apply fluorescein stain to determine if surface ulceration is present. Nasolacrimal duct patency can also be established by allowing fluorescein stain to gravitate into the external nares.
- Following application of a topical anesthetic, examine for foreign bodies. Use blunt-tipped forceps to probe the conjunctival fornices. Lift the third eyelid to allow inspection behind this eyelid.
- Employ tonometry to rule out the possibility of other intraocular causes of red eye, e.g., glaucoma (elevated pressure) and uveitis (low pressure). Indentation (Schiøtz) or applanation tonometry produces accurate intraocular pressure readings in small animal patients (see sec. 11, ch. 7).

Cytology

Cytology of conjunctival scrapings may provide a definitive diagnosis of inflammatory or neoplastic disease. Immunofluorescence testing of cytologic specimens can confirm viral or chlamydial infection. Fine needle aspirates of masses can also provide the cytologic material for a definitive diagnosis.

Biopsy

Biopsy of the conjunctiva is indicated when cytology has not allowed the differentiation of inflammatory from neoplastic processes. Conjunctival biopsy is also needed to determine goblet cell density in suspected cases of preocular mucin deficiency.

TREATMENT

The goals for therapy of conjunctival disease are as follows:

- Correct or remove the underlying cause
- Control secondary infection
- Remove exudates and clean the eye and periocular area
- Ensure a moist and well-hydrated ocular surface
- Reduce inflammation and discomfort

Treat Primary Cause

Because the primary causes of conjunctivitis in small animals are numerous, specific treatments vary considerably. Depending upon the circumstances, the following treatments may apply:

- Treat infection with a specific antimicrobial agent
- Remove foreign materials
- Surgically remove or correct for irritants (hairs or masses) that rub the eye
- Remove offending allergens when possible
- Treat for atopy (see sec. 5, ch. 7)
- Treat tear deficiencies medically (see sec. 11, ch. 9).

See Table 1 for more specific treatment recommendations.

KEY POINT ▶ The following procedures are beneficial as symptomatic treatment and may be used as adjuncts when treating the primary disease, when awaiting results of diagnostic tests or, when treating empirically in nonspecific or undiagnosed cases of conjunctivitis.

Antimicrobial Therapy

To control or prevent secondary pathogenic or opportunistic bacterial infections, broad-spectrum antibiotic ophthalmic drops or ointments are applied topically. Avoid prolonged, indiscriminate application of topical antibacterial agents because this may encourage development of antibiotic-resistant bacterial strains or secondary fungal infections. This practice can predispose the animal to medication hypersensitivity.

Cleanse Discharges

Use an eyewash solution (e.g., Dacriose, CooperVision) to irrigate the ocular surface, remove exudates, and clean the eye and periocular area. Clip the periocular hairs. Use cotton swabs moistened with saline to soak and remove exudates.

Moisten/Hydrate Eye

Ensure that the conjunctival and corneal surfaces are kept moist. If applied three to four times daily, antibacterial ointments have sufficient lubricating property to ensure continuous moistening of swollen or injured conjunctival tissues. When severe chemosis results in exposure of swollen conjunctiva, temporary tarsorrhaphy sutures are placed until the acute swelling subsides (see sec. 11, ch. 2). In cases in which the Schirmer tear test values are subnormal, artificial tear solutions are applied topically four to six times daily. Lacrimostimulants may be indicated (see sec. 11, ch. 9).

Anti-Inflammatory Therapy

Systemic anti-inflammatory drugs may be used in selected cases to minimize acute swelling, discomfort, and self-trauma. In cases of ocular trauma in dogs, systemic nonsteroidal anti-inflammatory drugs may be beneficial to reduce chemosis, hyperemia, and associ-

TABLE 1. Treatment of Specific Causes of Conjunctivitis

Causes	Treatments
Infectious Agents	
Bacterial	
Chlamydia felis	Tetracycline ointment (q6–8h × 14–28 days) (Terramycin, Pfizer; Achromycin, Lederle; Aureomycin, Lederle)
Mycoplasma felis	Tetracycline ointment (q6–8h × 10–14 days)
	or
	Erythromycin ointment (q6–8h × 10–14 days) (Erythromycin, Pharmafair)
	or
	Chloramphenicol ointment (q6–8h × 7 days) (Chlorbiotic, Schering-Plough)
Streptococcus spp.	Triple antibiotic (TA) ointment (q6–8h × 10–14 days) (Neobacimyx, Schering-Plough; TriOptic-P, SmithKline; Vetropolycin, Pitman-Moore; or equivalent)
Staphylococcus spp.	TA or gentamicin (Gentocin, Schering-Plough) (as per TA above)
Coliforms	TA or gentamicin (as per TA above)
Viral	
Feline herpesvirus	Idoxuridine or trifluridine (see sec. 2, ch. 4 and sec. 11, ch. 4)
	Symptomatic therapy (see text)
Canine distemper virus	Symptomatic therapy (see text)
Keratoconjunctivitis Sicca	Treat cause if determined (see sec. 11, ch. 9)
Many causes	Topical cyclosporine (see sec. 11, ch. 9)
	Topical or oral pilocarpine (see sec. 11, ch. 9)
	Topical antibiotics as needed
	Artificial tears (see sec. 11, ch. 9)
	Lubricant ointments (see sec. 11, ch. 9)
Foreign Bodies	Remove using magnification
	Irrigate eye
	Symptomatic therapy (see text)
	Complete eye examination
Trauma	
Bruise/focal puncture	Symptomatic therapy (see text)
Laceration	Symptomatic therapy (see text)
	± Surgical repair
Chemical Irritants	Copious irrigation
	Symptomatic therapy (see text)
Environmental Irritants	Flush eyes
	Topical corticosteroid (CS) solution (q6–8h reduced to q12h as response noted, then discontinue) only if fluorescein stain results are negative
	Lubricant ointment (q8h reduced to q24h as response noted, then discontinue)
	± Antibiotics (see TA above)
	Avoid re-exposure
Immune-Mediated Disorders	
Acute chemosis	Topical and systemic CS
Atopy	Topical ± systemic CS, antihistamines, desensitization (see sec. 5, ch. 7)
Follicular conjunctivitis	Topical ± intralesional CS, ± abrade follicles
Eosinophilic infiltrate	Topical ± intralesional CS (see sec. 11, ch. 4)
Plasmacytic infiltrate	Topical ± intralesional CS (see sec. 11, ch. 4)
Proliferative Diseases	
Inflammatory	Topical ± intralesional or systemic CS
Neoplastic	Surgery ± radiation or cryosurgery
Other Ocular Diseases	
Surface diseases	
Eyelid disorders	Medical ± corrective surgery (see sec. 11, ch. 2)
Keratitis	Medical ± surgery (see sec. 11, ch. 4)
Episcleritis	Topical ± intralesional or systemic CS (see sec. 11, ch. 4)
Intraocular diseases	
Uveitis	Treat cause if determined (see sec. 11, ch. 6)
	Topical CS and atropine
	Systemic anti-inflammatory agents
Glaucoma	Determine if primary or secondary (see sec. 11, ch. 7)
	Topical hypotensive agents (see sec. 11, ch. 7)
	Systemic hypotensive agents (see sec. 11, ch. 7)
Iatrogenic	
Topical agents	Discontinue use of irritating medications
Surgical procedures	Symptomatic treatment until surgical site heals

ated ocular pain. In dogs with normal renal function, flunixin meglumine (Banamine, Schering) may be given as a single dose IV of 0.5–1.0 mg/kg. This procedure may be followed by oral aspirin at a dosage of 10 mg/kg twice daily until signs of inflammation subside. Monitor the animal closely for the side effects of gastric erosion and ulceration from these drugs or simultaneously protect the stomach with an H_2-blocker, such as cimetidine (see sec. 7, ch. 4). Flunixin and aspirin are not given in cases in which hemorrhage is the primary manifestation of the conjunctival disease.

Topical corticosteroids may reduce the swelling and hyperemia of an inflamed conjunctiva.

KEY POINT ▶ Topical corticosteroids are contraindicated in cases of primary infectious conjunctivitis or corneal ulceration.

Topical 5% sodium chloride may be applied to reduce chemosis; however, it is not applied in eyes producing marginal amounts of aqueous tear because it will further dehydrate the ocular surface.

CONJUNCTIVAL SURGERY

Surgery of the conjunctiva may be performed for one of the following reasons:

- Trauma repair
- Diagnostic procedure
- Focal lesion resection
- Repair of fibrotic adhesions
- Grafting procedure.

Because the last category applies primarily to the treatment of ulcerative keratitis, refer to section 11, chapter 4 for a discussion of conjunctival flaps and grafts.

Laceration Repair

Preoperative Considerations

- Examine the eye carefully for other damage (e.g., corneal, scleral, intraocular lesions) and evaluate for the presence of retained ocular foreign bodies. Radiographs of the head and orbit allow the clinician to determine the presence of radiopaque foreign bodies.

KEY POINT ▶ If the traumatized eye is opaque, ultrasound imaging may be indicated to determine the integrity of the globe and the extent of any intraocular damage.

- Because of the conjunctiva's rapid reparative characteristic, many punctures and small lacerations heal spontaneously without the need for suturing. Conjunctival lacerations 7–8 mm or greater or those associated with eyelid lacerations are sutured.

Surgical Procedure

Objectives
- Cleanse and disinfect wound.

- Remove surface foreign material and tissue debris.
- Explore wound to determine if a foreign body was retained and to determine if deeper structures were damaged.
- Suture conjunctival wound, if necessary, to restore mucous membrane integrity and function.
- Prevent secondary infection.

Equipment
- Eyelid retractors (e.g., Barraquer wire speculum)
- Small rat-tooth forceps (e.g., Bishop-Harmon forceps)
- Ophthalmic needle holders (Castroviejo)
- Conjunctival or Stevens tenotomy scissors
- Braided 6-0 or 7-0 absorbable suture material (e.g., Dexon, Vicryl) with microcutting needle

Technique

1. Following general anesthesia, insert eyelid retractors and flush the conjunctiva with 1:50 betadine:saline solution; explore the wound for foreign bodies and for damage to deeper structures.
2. After assessing the extent of conjunctival defect and confirming that surgical repair is needed, minimally debride the margins of the wound and gently undermine adjacent conjunctiva.
3. Close the conjunctival wound in a continuous pattern; space suture bites 2 mm apart.

Postoperative Care and Complications

- Apply topical antibiotics (e.g., neomycin, bacitracin, polymyxin B) three to four times daily for 10 days.
- Administer systemic antibiotics for 1 week.
- If the eye is painful, apply fluorescein stain to determine the presence of corneal erosion or ulceration.

Biopsy

Preoperative Considerations

- Conjunctival biopsy is a diagnostic procedure that allows histopathology studies to distinguish inflammatory from neoplastic diseases and to determine goblet cell densities in suspected cases of preocular mucin deficiency.
- In tractable animals, conjunctival biopsy procedures can usually be performed following serial applications of topical anesthetic (e.g., 0.5% proparacaine).
- Subconjunctival or intralesional local anesthetic may be injected for deeper biopsies or for lesions of the palpebral, perilimbal, or third eyelid conjunctiva. Sedation and systemic analgesia may be needed in some cases.

Surgical Procedure

Objectives
- Remove a representative sample of conjunctiva for histopathology study.
- Minimize the resulting defect and avoid distorting the conjunctiva.

Equipment
- Small rat-tooth forceps
- Curved conjunctival or tenotomy scissors (e.g., Stevens, Westcott)
- Vial of 10% buffered formalin

Technique

1. Following local anesthesia, grasp the desired area of conjunctiva with rat-tooth forceps and tent slightly.
2. Using small curved scissors excise a 3 mm × 4 mm specimen.
3. Gently spread the specimen onto a flat surface, such as a small Styrofoam pad or a section of wooden tongue depressor.
4. Immediately fix the specimen in 10% buffered formalin.

Postoperative Care and Complications

- A small amount of hemorrhage is anticipated but is usually minimal, as fibrin quickly seals the wound.
- Defects resulting from biopsy that are less than 4 mm × 4 mm usually heal uneventfully with topical antibiotic treatment. Larger defects should be sutured as described in Laceration Repair.
- Remove discharges and cleanse the eye as needed. This may be necessary three to four times the first day but is reduced over the following 5 days to once daily.
- Apply topical antibiotic ointment (e.g., neomycin, bacitracin, polymyxin B) to the affected eye three times daily for 7 days.

Mass Removal

Preoperative Considerations

- Surgical excision alone may be curative for cysts, dermoids, ectopic hairs, focal granulomas, and certain neoplasms of the conjunctiva (e.g., papillomas and adenomas).
- Surgical excision is an important adjunct in the treatment of inflammatory pseudotumors and more aggressive neoplasms, such as squamous cell carcinomas or adenocarcinomas.
  - Chemotherapy, immunotherapy, cryosurgery, hyperthermia, or beta-irradiation may be needed in addition to local excision.
  - Definitive therapy depends upon the specific diagnosis.
- General anesthesia is usually required for effective removal of conjunctival masses.

Surgical Procedure

Objectives
- Surgically remove conjunctival masses that interfere with ocular function, threaten preservation of the globe, or pose a threat to survival of the animal.
- Debulk a mass to increase efficacy of adjunctive treatments (e.g., cryosurgery, radiation, immunotherapy, hyperthermia, chemotherapy).

Equipment
- Same as that listed for Laceration Repair.
- Vial of 10% buffered formalin

Technique

1. Grasp the mass with forceps and elevate; undermine and excise with small curved tissue scissors.

2. Small conjunctival wounds, i.e., less than 5 mm in diameter, generally do not require suturing and heal in 2–4 days.
3. Conjunctival wounds 5 mm in diameter or larger are sutured with 7-0 braided absorbable material (Vicryl) in a continuous pattern.
4. To allow primary closure for wounds greater than 5 mm in diameter, it may be necessary to undermine and slide adjacent conjunctiva.
5. Large defects are repaired by a pedicle graft of adjacent healthy conjunctiva similar to that of a swinging cutaneous pedicle graft.
6. For conjunctival mass lesions involving the cornea, see Figure 1, in section 11, chapter 4.

Postoperative Care and Complications

- Remove discharges and cleanse the eye as needed.
- Apply topical antibiotic ointment (e.g., neomycin, bacitracin, polymyxin B) to affected eye three times daily for 7 days.
- Prevent self-trauma with restraint collar.
- Large defects of the conjunctiva that heal by second intention may result in extensive granulation and scarring, with possible symblepharon formation.

Symblepharon Repair

Preoperative Considerations

- Symblepharon results from the fibrosis of two apposing ulcerated epithelial surfaces.
- Neonatal conjunctivitis of kittens, caused by feline herpesvirus, is a common cause in cats (see sec. 2, ch. 4).
- Postinflammatory adhesions may reduce or obliterate the conjunctival fornices resulting in immobility of the globe.
- Abnormal tear dynamics account for chronic epiphora.
- Corneal involvement results in scarring and opacification, which reduces vision.

Surgical Procedure

Objectives
- Remove scar tissue and free adhesions, thereby restoring normal anatomic relationships and functions of the ocular surface structures.
- Prevent readhesion and minimize postoperative scarring.

Equipment
- Colibri forceps
- Beaver blade (#64) with handle
- Instruments as listed for Laceration Repair

Technique

1. When extensive corneal opacification is present, perform a lamellar keratectomy (see Fig. 1, sec. 11, ch. 4).
2. Incise the perilimbal bulbar conjunctiva with a #64 Beaver blade, undermine and free adhesions with small curved scissors, and elevate the conjunctiva as a mobile circumlimbal flap.

3. Perform sufficient dissection and removal of sub-conjunctival scar tissue to allow re-establishment of the conjunctival fornices.
4. Free the third eyelid by dissecting between the third eyelid, the globe, and the eyelids, if necessary.
5. Place a bandage soft contact lens over the corneal surface behind the third eyelid.
6. Apply a broad-spectrum antibiotic ophthalmic ointment into the conjunctival cul de sac.
7. Place a corneal-scleral conformer over the globe and the front side of the third eyelid.
   a. A conformer may be constructed using a commercially available corneal-scleral protector (Crouch corneal protector, Storz Instrument, St. Louis).
   b. The corneal protector may be reduced to an appropriate size by trimming the perimeter with utility scissors, smoothing the cut margins with a file or fine sandpaper, rinsing the plastic of sanded particles, and sterilizing with gas.
8. Secure the corneal protector with three temporary tarsorrhaphy mattress sutures.

Postoperative Care and Complications

- Place a restraint collar on the animal to prevent self-trauma.
- Immediately administer postoperatively a mild sedative/analgesic.
- Remove discharges and cleanse the eye as needed.
- Tarsorrhaphy sutures prevent topical treatment of the eye, and broad-spectrum systemic antibiotics are administered for 1 week. Oral amoxicillin works well for this purpose.
- Remove tarsorrhaphy sutures and remove conformer and contact lens in 14 days.
- Following removal irrigate the eye and initiate topical treatment with an antibiotic ointment three times daily for 1 week or until the ocular surface has a negative reaction to fluorescein stain.
- Initiate topical antibiotic/corticosteroid (e.g., neomycin, bacitracin, dexamethasone) treatment three times daily *after* the surface has completely healed (i.e., negative results with fluorescein stain).
- Gradually reduce the frequency of topical treatments, and discontinue after 3 weeks.
- Additional corneal scarring and readhesion of conjunctival surfaces are the main complications with symblepharon surgery; however, the contact lens and corneal conformer minimize these problems and result in marked improvement in ocular function.

Conjunctival Grafts

See section 11, chapter 4.

Supplemental Readings

Brooks DE: *Veterinary Ophthalmology.* Philadelphia: Lea & Febiger, 1991, p 290.

Gerding PA, McLaughlin SA, Troop M: Pathogenic bacteria and fungi associated with external ocular diseases in dogs: 131 cases (1981–1986). J Am Vet Med Assoc 193:242, 1988.

Moore CP: *Current Veterinary Therapy X. Small Animal Practice.* Philadelphia: W. B. Saunders, 1989, p 673.

Nasisse MP: *Veterinary Ophthalmology.* Philadelphia: Lea & Febiger, 1991, p 529.

4 Diseases of the Cornea and Sclera

Thomas J. Kern

Disorders of the cornea comprise a large proportion of ocular complaints presented to veterinarians. Acquired corneal disorders such as ulcerative keratitis, melanosis, and pannus are leading causes of preventable blindness in dogs and cats. The high frequency of corneal disorders should not lull practitioners into forgetting the importance of rigorous diagnosis and attentive management.

Disorders of the sclera are less common. Their diagnosis may be more difficult than corneal disorders and they may be presented at a more advanced stage.

CONGENITAL DISORDERS

Dermoids

Dermoids are islands of skin embryologically misplaced on the cornea (especially the temporal cornea) and conjunctiva and occasionally malpositioned on the eyelids. They contain epidermis, dermis, fat, sebaceous glands, and hair follicles.

Etiology
- In Burmese cats, dermoids are an inherited condition that frequently involves the eyelids.
- Generally this is considered a spontaneous nonheritable condition in dogs, although some breeds (e.g., German shepherd) appear to be afflicted at a higher frequency than others; thus a genetic basis cannot be completely ruled out.

Clinical Signs
- Dermoids' surface irregularity promotes chronic blepharospasm and epiphora; the hairs cause corneal and conjunctival irritation.

Diagnosis
- On ocular examination, the typical appearance of skin on the cornea or conjunctiva is diagnostic.

Treatment
- Remove by keratectomy. If removal is complete, corneal scarring is present but minimal.
- If the conjunctiva also must be resected, suture the edges of the conjunctiva to the limbus, using 7-0 Vicryl, to discourage postoperative adhesion of the conjunctiva to the cornea.

Microcornea

Etiology
Microcornea usually is associated with complicated *microphthalmos,* a condition with both genetic and environmental causes.

- Inherited microphthalmos syndromes have been characterized in the Australian shepherd, collie, Shetland sheepdog, Old English sheepdog, Akita, American cocker spaniel, miniature schnauzer, Doberman pinscher, Samoyed, Cavalier King Charles spaniel, and Lancashire heeler.
- Multiple heritable ocular defects associated with partial albinism and deafness occur in the Great Dane and collie. Teratogenic influences on the dam during early pregnancy (e.g., viral or other illnesses, live virus vaccines, drugs) may be responsible.
- Microphthalmos occurs less frequently in cats than in dogs; its causes are poorly characterized.

Clinical Signs
- The cornea appears abnormally small and often is misshapen.

Diagnosis
- Measure the horizontal and vertical diameters of the cornea and compare with those of the normal contralateral eye, if present, or with the eye of a normal animal of similar breed.

Treatment
- Treatment is neither available nor warranted. If the condition is associated with microphthalmos, vision may be impaired.

Corneal Opacities

Persistent Pupillary Membrane-Associated Opacities

Etiology
- An embryologic cleavage defect results in the attachment of strands of iris to the endothelial surface of the cornea. Where attachment occurs, endothelium is absent and Descemet's membrane is abnormal, resulting in permanent nonprogressive opacity.
- The condition is inherited in basenjis and probably in other breeds; the mode of inheritance is uncertain. (see sec. 11, ch. 6).

Axial Geographic Subepithelial Opacities in Puppies

Etiology
- The cause(s) of these variably prominent, well-circumscribed corneal opacities is unknown.
- They are commonly noted during examination of certain breeds (collie, Shetland sheepdog, English springer spaniel) for inherited ocular disorders and thus have an uncertain genetic basis.

Clinical Signs

- Most obvious in the "exposure strip" of axial cornea, these superficial opacities are usually bilateral, relatively symmetric, painless, and irregular.
- Typical appearance is that of a nonulcerated geographic axial corneal opacity of variable density.

Diagnosis

- The presence of a typical corneal opacity in a dog < 1 year of age suggests the diagnosis.
- The absence of fluorescein dye retention rules out ulcerative keratitis and the lack of corneal vascularization rules out an old corneal scar.

Treatment

- Do not treat. Most opacities substantially disappear by maturity.
- A residual faint opacity may remain near the nasal and temporal limbus.

Colobomatous Defects of the Sclera

Etiology

- Scleral defects occur as part of the spectrum of inherited ocular anomalies in collies, Shetland sheepdogs, and Australian shepherds.
  - The collie/Shetland sheepdog anomaly is said to be due to a simple recessive gene with variable expression; a different mode of inheritance has been postulated for the colobomas.
  - The Australian shepherd defect is inherited as an incompletely penetrant recessive trait.
- Optic disc and peripapillary colobomas occur in basenjis; inheritance may be autosomal dominant.
- Great Danes that are the progeny of two harlequin parents are afflicted with colobomatous microphthalmos similar to that in Australian shepherds.
- Posterior pole colobomas of the optic disc and surrounding sclera of unknown cause are seen occasionally in domestic short- and longhaired cats.

Clinical Signs

- In collies and Shetland sheepdogs, the only commonly visible external sign of the defect is relative to absolute microphthalmos. Choroidal hypoplasia, scleral ectasia, optic nerve coloboma, and retinal detachment may be present in the fundus. Blindness is present with retinal detachment and/or optic nerve coloboma.
- Affected Australian shepherds (and Great Danes) usually have mostly white coat color and unilateral or bilateral microphthalmos. In many microphthalmic eyes there are large equatorial staphylomas (i.e., areas of pitted and thinned sclera posterior to the ciliary body). Iris anomalies (heterochromia, corectopia, persistent pupillary membranes, pseudopolycoria) often are present, as are cataracts, retinal dysplasia, and retinal detachment.
- Basenjis with optic disc colobomas have abnormal vision and may have persistent pupillary membranes, although the two defects may not be related.
- Cats afflicted with posterior segment optic nerve coloboma and scleral ectasia are blind in the affected eye, the external appearance of which is normal except for tonic mydriasis.

Diagnosis

- Indirect ophthalmoscopy provides panoramic views of the ocular fundus and is the most sensitive and practical means of diagnosis.

Treatment

- Therapy for these defects is neither indicated nor available.
- Discourage breeding of affected animals.

ACQUIRED DISORDERS

Corneal Degenerations and Dystrophies

KEY POINT ▶ Corneal dystrophy is a hereditary congenital or acquired, usually bilateral, corneal opacity typically unassociated with neovascularization. Degenerations are often but not invariably unilateral abnormalities, frequently (but not necessarily) associated with neovascularization, which are secondary to other ocular or systemic disorders.

Corneal degenerations and dystrophies may affect epithelium, stroma, or endothelium (epithelial dystrophies are discussed under Corneal Ulceration). In some animals, differentiation between the two disorders is difficult.

Stromal Dystrophy

Etiology

- Stromal corneal dystrophy is a genetic disorder afflicting many breeds of dogs, including the collie, Siberian husky, Cavalier King Charles spaniel, beagle, Airedale terrier, cocker spaniel, Alaskan malamute, bearded collie, bichon frise, German shepherd, Lhasa apso, mastiff, miniature pinscher, Weimaraner, pointer, and Samoyed.
- One line of Manx cats was reported with an inherited bilateral stromal dystrophy.

Clinical Signs

- At least two forms of stromal dystrophy occur in dogs:
  - One form is a bilaterally symmetric oval axial or paraxial subepithelial/anterior stromal crystalline opacity.
  - The second form, in which a deeper stromal opacity involves more peripheral portions of the cornea, occurs in Siberian huskies and occasionally in other breeds.
  - Corneal neovascularization is absent in both forms. Age of onset varies according to breed and individual animals, from 6 months to old age.
- Affected Manx cats developed progressive stromal edema leading to bullous keratopathy and recurrent epithelial erosion.

Diagnosis

- *Dogs:* The typical crystalline, usually bilateral, corneal opacity (fluorescein dye–negative) unassociated with corneal neovascularization or other corneal pathologic changes suggests of stromal dystrophy.

- Rule out causes of corneal degeneration, which may appear similar, including keratoconjunctivitis sicca (KCS), lagophthalmos, eyelid defects, and endocrinopathy (e.g., hypothyroidism).
▪ *Cats:* Progressive corneal edema in Manx cats suggests the diagnosis.

Treatment
▪ Treatment in dogs is rarely indicated or necessary. Keratectomy may remove superficial opacities, but recurrence is likely.
▪ Do not breed affected animals.

Stromal Degenerations

Etiology
Ocular causes of stromal degenerations include:

▪ Ulcerative and nonulcerative keratitis
▪ Corneal exposure
▪ Dryness secondary to keratoconjunctivitis sicca or lagophthalmos

KEY POINT ▶ Systemic diseases suspected to cause degenerations include primary hyperlipidemia, secondary hyperlipidemia (especially associated with hypothyroidism), and hyperadrenocorticism (implicated in calcific degeneration or "band keratopathy").

Clinical Signs
▪ The central (axial) to paracentral opacities are often bilaterally symmetric and range from crystalline to dense yellow-white; they may be indistinguishable from primary corneal dystrophy.
▪ In calcific degeneration, the cornea feels "gritty" when touched with a cotton-tipped applicator.
▪ Neovascularization is often although not invariably present.

Diagnosis
▪ The presence of a typical lesion (with or without neovascularization) in the presence of (or with a history of) a previous condition (e.g., ulcer, other keratitis, lagophthalmos) suggests degeneration rather than dystrophy.

KEY POINT ▶ Do not assume that concurrent primary or secondary hyperlipidemia or hyperadrenocorticism is the cause unless ocular causes of degeneration have been ruled out. Even then, a causal relationship may be uncertain.

▪ Clinical differentiation of these two conditions frequently is difficult.

Treatment
▪ Treatment is rarely indicated or necessary.
▪ Consider keratectomy for large, dense axial lesions that interfere with vision.
  - Prognosis is guarded, as recurrence is possible; in addition, postoperative corneal opacity may be significant.
▪ For calcific degeneration, consider keratectomy for

superficial lesions. Topical application of 1–4% EDTA q4-6h may be helpful.

Endothelial Dystrophy

Etiology
▪ Endothelial dystrophy is a breed-related, acquired disease resulting in premature loss of corneal endothelial cells to a level below that required to maintain normal corneal stromal deturgescence.

Clinical Signs
▪ *Dogs:* Progressive bilateral corneal edema may affect Boston terriers, Chihuahuas, and occasionally other breeds. It can begin focally or in a diffuse pattern and progress from the peripheral to the central cornea or vice versa.
  - Initially painless, the condition frequently results in recurrent corneal erosion when stromal and epithelial edema become extensive. Corneal neovascularization usually is absent.
▪ *Cats:* Endothelial dystrophy causing progressive bilateral corneal edema has been reported rarely in domestic shorthaired cats.

Diagnosis
▪ Endothelial dystrophy is presumptively diagnosed when bilateral corneal stromal edema is present unassociated with signs of uveitis or glaucoma.

KEY POINT ▶ Determine intraocular pressure (IOP) to rule out uveitis (decreased IOP) or glaucoma (elevated IOP) (see sec. 11, chs. 6 and 7).

▪ Corneal ulceration, if present, usually is superficial and insufficient to cause the degree of stromal edema observed.

Treatment
▪ For severe stromal and epithelial edema, consider treatment with topical 5% sodium chloride (Muro-128) q4–6h to discourage corneal erosion development.
▪ When erosions occur, debride nonadherent epithelium and administer topical broad-spectrum antibiotics and 1% atropine.

Endothelial Degeneration

Etiology
▪ Intraocular inflammation or hemorrhage, primary and secondary glaucoma, anterior lens luxation, and corneal injury may cause endothelial degeneration.
▪ Natural infection with canine adenovirus-1 (infectious canine hepatitis) or vaccination with modified live vaccines containing adenovirus-1 or adenovirus-2 may result in immune-mediated anterior uveitis and endothelial destruction 7–10 days following exposure.
  - The proportion of dogs affected can be high (in natural infection, about 20%), low (adenovirus-1 vaccination), or very low (adenovirus-2 vaccination).

Clinical Signs
▪ Chronic focal or diffuse corneal edema (giving the cornea a ground-glass appearance) with or without

superficial or deep corneal neovascularization characterizes endothelial degeneration. If the edema resolves, only transient endothelial dysfunction occurs.

KEY POINT ▶ Corneal endothelial cells in many adult domestic animals have little to no regenerative capacity. Repair occurs by hypertrophy and migration of remaining endothelial cells.

- Most dogs with adenovirus-mediated uveitis present with generalized corneal edema after resolution of transient uveitis.
  - A small proportion of affected dogs, especially sight hounds and Arctic breeds, quickly develop intractable secondary glaucoma.

Diagnosis

- Diffuse, moderate to severe generalized corneal edema strongly suggests endothelial dysfunction.
- Perform a careful ocular examination to rule out antecedent causes (e.g., inflammation, glaucoma, hyphema, lens luxation).

Treatment

- Direct treatment toward prevention by effectively controlling the causative or attendant conditions (e.g., glaucoma, uveitis, hyphema) before irreversible endothelial degeneration occurs.

Prognosis

- Most dogs with adenovirus-related endotheliopathy recover endothelial function, and the corneal edema resolves within a few weeks.
- Corneal edema secondary to other causes has a variable prognosis for resolution.

Corneal Ulceration

Loss of one or more corneal epithelial layers commonly is termed *corneal erosion or abrasion*. Full-thickness loss of epithelium with at least some stromal loss is termed *ulceration*.

- Simple corneal ulceration is that which heals uneventfully in a normal time period (3–5 days).
- Complicated corneal ulceration involves delayed healing associated with infection or other pathologic processes.
- Progressive corneal ulceration involves a deepening or enlarging area.

Etiology

Traumatic Injury. This is probably the most common cause of ulcerative keratitis in dogs and cats.

- Blunt trauma may cause focal or diffuse damage to any or all corneal layers. Corneal laceration may be partial or full-thickness. Aqueous loss, anterior chamber collapse, and iris prolapse may ensue.
- Most traumatic corneal erosions and ulcers heal rapidly; however, some become persistent if epithelial basement membrane damage is severe or if a foreign body persists in the conjunctival fornix.
- Traumatic injury may begin a cascade of pathologic complications resulting in complicated ulceration.

Bacterial Infection. At least minor epithelial injury is required for colonization to occur; bacteria do not adhere to normal epithelial cell membranes.

- Pathogenic and normally nonpathogenic commensal organisms may infect the cornea. *Staphylococci* and *streptococci* are the ocular bacterial organisms most frequently isolated from normal eyes of dogs and cats.
- Topical antibiotic or corticosteroid therapy may result in overgrowth of pathogenic fungi, yeasts, and bacteria. However, infection of corneal ulcers by fungal agents is rare in dogs and cats.

Pseudomonas

- *Pseudomonas* infection commonly results in corneal melting, perforation, and loss of the eye.
  - Proteolytic enzymes produced by the bacteria, inflammatory cells, and response to infection by the cornea itself cause stromal proteoglycan and collagen destruction, giving the affected cornea a mucoid appearance as melting occurs.

Feline Herpesvirus (FHV)

- FHV infection is an important cause of corneal ulceration in cats (see sec. 2, ch. 4). Superficial ulcers may be small, punctate, or linear branching fernlike figures classically described as dendrites. Larger, geographic superficial to deep ulcers form from coalescence of smaller focal ulcers. Stromal ulcers, descemetoceles (i.e., a circular loss of stroma down to Decemet's membrane), and perforations may develop.

Epithelial Dystrophy (Erosion, Indolent Ulcer, Boxer Ulcer)

- An apparently inherited corneal epithelial basement membrane dystrophy has been recognized in boxers and probably occurs in other breeds. A different inherited epithelial dystrophy afflicts Shetland sheepdogs. Affected dogs are usually middle-aged or older.
- Trauma and chronic corneal inflammation may result in acquired epithelial basement membrane abnormalities.
- Endocrinopathies such as diabetes mellitus, hyperadrenocorticism, and hypothyroidism may be associated with fragile corneal epithelium that may be susceptible to injury and prone to delayed healing.

Neurotrophic Keratitis. This condition develops following denervation of the cornea's sensory nerve supply from the ophthalmic branch of the trigeminal nerve. The presence of sensory nerves and the neurotransmitters and other substances involved have a beneficial influence on the maintenance of epithelial integrity.

Corneal Dryness. This condition occurs secondary to:

- Aqueous tear deficiency (KCS)
- Qualitative tear film abnormalities (mucin deficiency).
- Exposure from lagophthalmos due to conformational abnormalities of eyelid closure or facial nerve palsy (see sec. 11, ch. 9).

Endocrinopathies. Endocrinopathies such as diabetes mellitus, hypoadrenocorticism, and hypothyroidism have been associated with corneal ulceration in dogs; a causative role in the development of ulcers has not been established.

Idiopathic Corneal Ulceration. An idiopathic form is unique to the cat and is associated with corneal sequestrum formation ("mummification").

- Following chronic, usually superficial, unilateral or bilateral corneal ulceration a brown or black discoloration of the stroma develops; the discolored plaques of degenerate cornea remain in place or slough away after weeks or months.
- The presence of a corneal sequestrum is associated with pain and corneal neovascularization.
- Concurrent herpesvirus infection has been demonstrated in some cats.

Clinical Signs

- Blepharospasm, photophobia, and epiphora are stimulated by painful sensations from damaged epithelium as well as from secondary ciliary muscle spasm.
- Corneal opacity results from stromal and epithelial edema and infiltration by inflammatory cells into the affected area.
- Corneal surface depression is present if stromal loss, including descemetoceles, has occurred.
- Neovascularization denotes complicated ulceration in which healing has been delayed by ocular (e.g., KCS, eyelid defects, infection) or nonocular factors (e.g., self-trauma, inappropriate medical therapy).
  - Superficial neovascularization usually suggests a corneal or external complicating factor and appears as tree-like individual vessels infiltrating focal sectors of cornea.
  - Deep (ciliary) neovascularization denotes intraocular inflammation and appears as an advancing ring of fine vessels evenly infiltrating the peripheral cornea for its entire circumference.
- In epithelial dystrophy, the fluorescein dye–positive stained area is surrounded by a halo of poorly adherent or nonadherent epithelium that stains less brilliantly than the center, where epithelium is absent.
  - Corneal neovascularization is absent unless previous traumatic manipulation (e.g., chemical cauterization) has been performed. This is in contrast to chronic corneal ulceration due to traumatic, infectious, and other causes, which routinely incite neovascularization.
  - Blepharospasm and photophobia, if present, frequently are minimal.
- Miosis occurs as an axon reflex from stimulation of corneal, conjunctival, and periocular branches of the ophthalmic nerve (see sec. 11, ch. 6).
- Aqueous flare (i.e., the presence of large amounts of serum proteins in the anterior chamber) indicates iridocyclitis (anterior uveitis) with breakdown of the blood-aqueous barrier (see sec. 11, ch. 6).
- Hypotony (reduced intraocular pressure) usually accompanies moderate to severe anterior uveitis and

results from reduced aqueous production and, possibly, increased aqueous outflow.

Diagnosis

History
Important aspects include:

- Time and circumstances of onset
- Presence and duration of discharge and blepharospasm
- Change in the eye's appearance between onset and presentation
- Current and previously treated ocular disorders

Ocular Examination and Accessory Diagnostic Tests

- Collect samples for corneal culture before instilling any diagnostic solutions.
- The hallmark of corneal ulceration is retention of fluorescein dye, which stains corneal stroma, tear, and aqueous humor.
  - To rule out KCS, perform Schirmer's tear test (Iolab Pharmaceuticals) before fluorescein dye application.

KEY POINT ▶ Descemetoceles demonstrate an annular pattern of dye retention along their walls, but exposed Descemet's membrane in the center does not stain.

- Before applying topical anesthesia, test corneal sensitivity with a cotton-tipped swab.
- Following topical anesthesia, obtain scrapings for cytology and Gram staining from ulcers showing rapid progression, soft edematous margins, or a yellow inflammatory cell infiltrate.
- Because sequestra have been noted in cats experimentally infected with FHV, submit diagnostic tests (viral isolation or immunofluorescence testing of conjunctival scrapings; see sec. 2 ch. 4) to rule out herpesvirus infection.
- The diagnosis of epithelial dystrophy is suggested by the presence of a chronic nonadherent epithelial margin with only mild discomfort.

Treatment

KEY POINT ▶ Ocular corticosteroid administration is contraindicated in the presence of corneal ulceration.

KEY POINT ▶ Use of topical anesthetics for *diagnostic* purposes is safe; however, because they are toxic to corneal epithelium, their use in *treatment* is contraindicated.

Simple Erosions and Superficial Ulcers
- Instill topical broad-spectrum antibiotics (e.g., bacitracin, neomycin, polymyxin). Treat with ointments q6h or with aqueous solutions at least q4h.
- Instill topical 1% atropine ointment or solution, to effect, to maintain mydriasis and, presumably, ciliary muscle paralysis (e.g., q6–8h initially, followed by q12–24h, and then every other day).

TABLE 1. Antibiotic Selection Based on Gram Stain of Corneal Scapings

Gram Stain Finding	Antibiotics*		
	Topical	Subconjunctival	Systemic
Gram-positive cocci	Bacitracin (Neosporin; Burroughs Wellcome) or cefazolin (Kefzol; Eli Lilly)	Methicillin (Staphcillin; Squibb), 100 mg, or gentamicin (Gentocin; Schering), 10–40 mg, or tobramycin (Tobrex; Alcon Labs.), 10–30 mg	Ampicillin (Omnipen; Wyeth-Ayerst) or gentamicin or cefazolin or tobramycin
Gram-negative rods	Gentamicin or tobramycin	Gentamicin, 10–40 mg, and/or carbenicillin, 250 mg, or tobramycin, 10–30 mg	Chloramphenicol (Chloromycetin Palmitate; Parke-Davis) or gentamicin or tobramycin
Mixed infections	Bacitracin and gentamicin	Methicillin, 100 mg, and gentamicin, 20 mg	Gentamicin or tobramycin

*Product name and manufacturer are given in parentheses following the first mention of the generic drug.
Modified from Kern TJ: Ulcerative keratitis. Vet Clin North Am [Small Anim Pract] 20(3):653, 1990.

■ Schedule follow-up examinations every few days until epithelialization is complete.

Deep and/or Progressive Ulceration
Medical Management

Base the choice of topical and subconjunctival antibiotics on corneal cytologic findings (Table 1).

■ Supplement topical 1% atropine therapy with:
  • Topical fortified gentamicin or tobramycin drops (Tables 2 and 3) applied q1–2h
  • Subconjunctival antibiotic injection (see Table 1).
■ Consider treatment of acetylcysteine or sodium EDTA (0.15 M) q1–2h if corneal melting is apparent or suspected. Efficacy of these drugs is uncertain.

Surgical Management

■ Objectives:
  • Prevent ulcer progression.
  • Repair perforation.
  • Protect the corneal surface.
  • Retard melting.
■ Protective Procedures:

KEY POINT ▶ Protective procedures do not provide blood supply or cells to aid in the healing of corneal ulceration. They do interfere with treatment and further evaluation of corneal ulceration.

  • Nictitans Flap—Indications include postproptosis corneal coverage and, possibly, conservative treatment of recurrent superficial erosion following debridement; contraindications include deep or infected ulcers, descemetoceles, and uncorrected perforations.
  • Temporary Tarsorrhaphy—Indications and contraindications are the same as for nictitans flap.
■ Conjunctival Flap (supportive procedure):
  • *Indications*—Deep ulcers, infected ulcers following short-term intensive antibiotic therapy, descemetoceles, sutured corneal wounds that leak, and, rarely, recurrent epithelial erosions.
  • *Type*—Depending on the extent and location of the lesion, the flap may be a pedicle graft (Fig. 1), Fornix-based hood (180°) flap (Fig. 2), or circumferential (360°) flap.

Technique

Conjunctival Flap

1. Carefully debride any necrotic or melting corneal stroma from the ulcer and its margin, using a #64 Beaver blade.
2. Form flaps by making a conjunctival incision at the limbus. Bluntly dissect the conjunctiva from the underlying connective tissue (episclera) using tenotomy scissors.
3. Free the conjunctival graft by cutting it from its limbal attachment.
4. Suture pedicle and hood grafts to the cornea, using 7-0 Vicryl or smaller suture material. Attempt to achieve epithelial to epithelial apposition of the

TABLE 2. Formulas for Fortified Antibiotics in Artificial Tears

Drug	Form	Quantity of Antibiotic	Quantity of Artificial Tears (ml)	Final Volume (ml)	Final Concentration (mg/ml)
Gentamicin (Gentocin injectable; Schering)	100 mg/ml	2.5 ml (250 mg)	15	17.5	14
Gentamicin (Gentocin injectable; Schering)	50 mg/ml	5 ml (250 mg)	12.5	17.5	14
Tobramycin (Nebcin; Eli Lilly)	40 mg/ml	5.5 ml (220 mg)	15	20.5	11
Bacitracin (Bacitracin sterile USP; Quad Pharmaceuticals)	50,000 IU/vial	150,000 U (3 vials)	15	15.6	9600 IU/ml
Cefazolin (Kefzol; Eli Lilly)	1 g/vial	3 ml (1 vial)	15	18	50

Reprinted with permission from Kern TJ: Ulcerative keratitis. Vet Clin North Am [Small Anim Pract] 20(3):655, 1990.

TABLE 3. Formulas for Fortified Forms of Proprietary Topical Ophthalmic Antibiotics

Drug	Bottle Concentration (mg/ml)	Bottle Volume (ml)	Parenteral Antibiotic Added	Final Concentration (mg/ml)
Gentamicin (Gentocin ophthalmic solution; Schering)	3	5	50 mg (1 ml of 50 mg/ml solution)	11
Tobramycin (Tobrex; Alcon)	3	5	10 mg or 40 mg/ml	4 or 9

Reprinted with permission from Kern TJ: Ulcerative keratitis. Vet Clin North Am 3(20):565, 1990.

conjunctiva and cornea. To relieve tension, the graft can be sutured to the limbus with two sutures.

5. Suture complete 360° flaps in a horizontal mattress pattern, top half to the bottom half, along the center of the cornea but not directly to the cornea.
6. Remove sutures in 10–14 days.
7. Separate the graft from its blood supply and trim points of adhesion of the flap to the previous corneal defect with tenotomy or iris scissors under topical anesthesia 1 week after suture removal.

▪ Cyanoacrylate tissue adhesive application (supportive procedure):
  • *Indications*—Small partial- or full-thickness perforations, small descemetoceles, and deep stromal ulcers.

Technique

Tissue Adhesion

1. Sedate or anesthetize the animal as necessary.
2. Debride the lesion as necessary to remove necrotic tissue, nonadherent epithelium, and adherent mucus.
3. Instill a topical anesthetic (Alcaine; Alcon, Inc.; Ophthaine; Solvay Animal Health, Inc.; Ophthetic; Allergan Pharmaceuticals).

4. Insert an eyelid speculum.
5. Dry the corneal site of application with a cotton-tipped swab or cellulose sponge.
6. Apply a very thin layer of adhesive (Ophthalmic Nexaband) through a 30-gauge needle. Application of excessive amounts of adhesive can result in failure of the plug to adhere to the cornea.
7. Wait several minutes for adhesive to polymerize before removing the speculum. Instill lubricant ointment until blinking returns.
8. Epithelialization occurs underneath the adhesive, which is extruded spontaneously by most animals within a few weeks. Excessive neovascularization may overgrow the plaque, necessitating manual removal under topical anesthesia.

▪ Reconstructive procedures are indicated for descemetoceles and perforating corneal wounds. Commonly used types (described later) include sutures, pedicle flaps, and free conjunctival grafts.

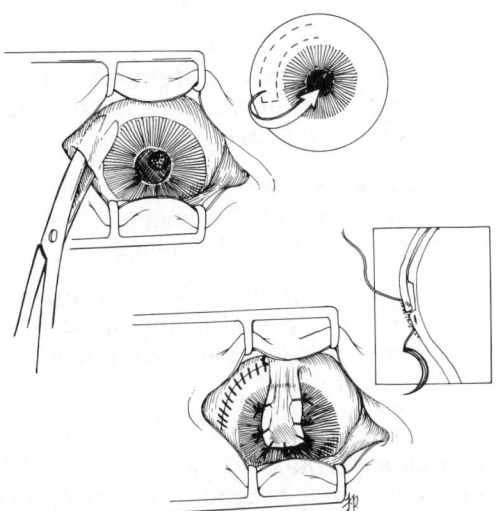

Figure 1. Pedicle graft. *A,* Using Stevens tenotomy scissors, the bulbar conjunctiva is elevated, incised, and dissected free of the globe. A pedicle of conjunctiva is created and rotated, epithelial surface up, to cover the corneal defect.

B, The conjunctival pedicle is sutured to the cornea, covering the defect, using simple-interrupted sutures. An attempt is made to ensure that the epithelial margins of the conjunctival graft and the cornea are in apposition (see inset Fig. 2 B).

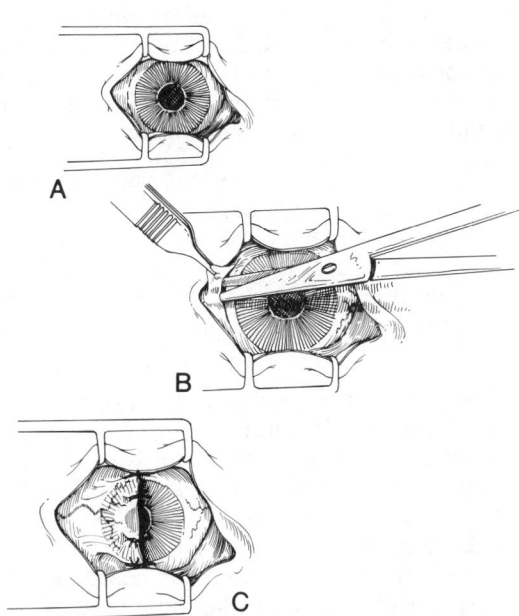

Figure 2. Fornix-based hood (180°) flap. *A,* A corneal ulcer is present and is to be repaired with a hood-graft from the adjacent bulbar conjunctiva.

B, The bulbar conjunctiva adjacent to the corneal defect is elevated and Stevens tenotomy scissors are used to incise and dissect free this portion of conjunctiva. *C,* The conjunctiva is then advanced over the defect and sutured in place using simple interrupted sutures. Sutures are placed in the cornea to stabilize the graft over the corneal defect and in the limbus to relieve tension.

Sutures—Technique

1. Suture perforating wounds and small descemetoceles directly with 7-0–9-0 absorbable (e.g., polyglactin 910—Vicryl, Ethicon) or nonabsorbable (monofilament nylon) sutures, using a horizontal mattress or simple interrupted pattern (Fig. 3).
2. Remove nonabsorbable sutures in 10–14 days.

Technique

Pedicle Flap

1. Raise a pedicle of bulbar conjunctiva, rotate, and then suture it to the edges of the deep corneal wound with absorbable suture material (e.g., polyglactin or polyglycolic acid-Dexon) (see Fig. 1).
2. After 2–4 weeks, trim adhered flap connection to the limbus, leaving an island of conjunctiva to be incorporated into the scar.

Free Conjunctival Graft—Technique

1. Dissect an island of conjunctiva slightly larger than the corneal defect from the bulbar or palpebral conjunctiva, and suture it to the cornea directly over the defect.
2. The grafted conjunctiva will become incorporated as a translucent portion of the cornea.

■ Referral reconstructive procedures:
  • Corneoconjunctival transposition and autogenous corneal grafting are forms of lamellar corneal graft requiring special instrumentation and expertise.
  • Penetrating keratoplasty (corneal transplant) has few indications in veterinary medicine.

Chronic Superficial Erosion

■ After instilling a topical anesthetic, debride the nonadherent epithelium with a wet or dry cotton-tipped applicator back to the junction with normally adherent epithelium. Frequently, most of the corneal epithelium is removed in the process.

KEY POINT ▶ The use of cauterants such as phenol, aqueous and tincture of iodine, trichloroacetic acid, and others is unnecessary and harmful. These agents incite excessive neovascularization that retards rather than accelerates epithelial healing.

■ Instill topical broad-spectrum antibiotic drops (q3–4h) or ointments q6h, until healing is complete.
■ To maintain mydriasis, administer topical 1% atropine drops or ointment to effect; apply q8h until dilatation occurs, followed by once daily to every other day.
■ If the erosion has not healed, or nearly so, within 10 days, consider the following options:
  • Contact lenses and collagen shields
  • Keratatomy
  • Drugs

Contact Lenses and Collagen Shields. Insertion of a soft contact lens (Duragel; Veterinary Hydrophilics) or collagen shield (Opti-Cor; Pitman Moore) following simple debridement frequently is effective.

■ *Indication:* Chronic corneal ("indolent") erosion
■ *Contraindications:* KCS; bacterial keratitis

Technique

1. Following topical anesthesia, debride nonadherent epithelium with a cotton-tipped swab.
2. Insert soft contact lens or collagen shield (diameter, 15 mm; Base curve, 8.4–8.8 mm). Optional partial temporary tarsorrhaphy.
3. Administer a topical broad-spectrum antibiotic and 1% atropine solutions as described for simple erosions. Apply an Elizabethan collar.
4. Remove contact lens weekly and stain with fluorescein to monitor ulcer healing. Reinsert the contact lens or insert a new one after cleaning and disinfection; repeat process until healed. Collagen shields degrade and disappear within a few days of insertion. Insert a new shield if erosion has not healed.

Superficial Punctate or Linear Keratotomy (Anterior Stromal Puncture). The resultant small, visually insignificant scars are believed to secure the epithelium to the stroma.

Technique

1. Sedate the animal.
2. Instill a topical anesthetic to effect.
3. Debride nonadherent epithelium with a cotton-tipped swab.
4. Under magnification (Optivisor or similar device), make a series of shallow punctures or linear cuts with a sterile 25-gauge needle, spaced approximately 0.5 mm apart throughout the debrided area and extending 1 mm onto the surrounding epithelium.
5. Instill a topical broad-spectrum antibiotic and 1% atropine as described for simple erosions.

Superficial Keratectomy to Remove the Affected Area of Stroma, Epithelium, and Basement Membrane. Disadvantages include:

■ The need for general anesthesia
■ Proficiency in the surgical technique
■ Possible permanent corneal thinning

Drugs. Drugs not yet commercially available but showing promise for medical management of chronic corneal erosions include epidermal growth factors, fibronectin, and aprotinin.

Corneal Sequestra
Surgical Management

■ Perform keratectomy to remove sequestra that lie in the *superficial* half of the cornea; deeper keratectomy encourages iatrogenic corneal perforation.
■ Sequestra may recur at the operated site or at other sites.
■ For large or deep sequestra, consider performing a conjunctival pedicle graft to support and reconstruct the wound.

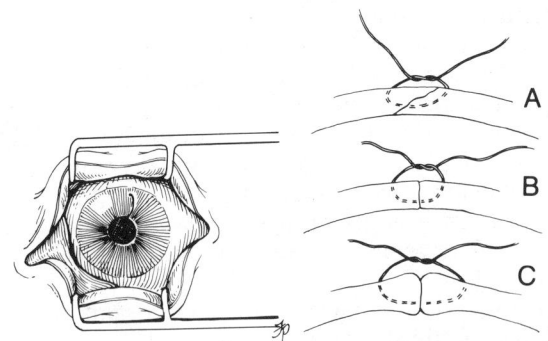

Figure 3. Repair of corneal laceration. Note that all sutures are placed to a depth of approximately 2/3 of the corneal thickness. *A,* Closure of oblique edges of the laceration.

B, Closure of vertical wound edges.

C, Closure of edematous wound margins. Note that the sutures extend beyond the edematous edge and into healthy cornea.

Nonulcerative Corneal Disorders

Chronic Superficial Keratitis (CSK)

Etiology
- The specific cause of CSK is unknown.
- Its predominance in a small spectrum of dog breeds (German shepherd, greyhound, occasionally others) and in mixed-breed dogs originating from these strongly implicates a genetic predisposition for immune-mediated disease.

Clinical Signs
- Superficial, bilaterally symmetric neovascularization, usually beginning inferotemporally, with or without melanosis is a hallmark. Pain is not a common sign.
- Rarely, corneal ulceration develops.
- Corneal degeneration, manifested by oval crystalline opacities, may develop with chronicity.

Diagnosis
- Diagnosis is based on the presence of typical corneal signs in a German shepherd, greyhound, or mixed-breed dog of their extraction, in the absence of other causes of chronic superficial keratitis (e.g., tear deficiency, eyelid abnormalities).

Treatment
- Administer corticosteroids topically (and, intermittently, subconjunctivally) to control this incurable condition.
  - For initial management administer a subconjunctival injection of 5 mg of betamethasone acetate and sodium phosphate (Betavet Soluspan; Schering Veterinary), triamcinolone acetonide (Kenalog-40; Squibb), or methylprednisolone acetate (DepoMedrol; Upjohn).
  - Supplement with a topical corticosteroid ointment or solution on a regimen of reducing frequency (e.g., q3–4h tapering to q8h over 4 weeks).
  - Long-term topical therapy is essential to maintain control; even short periods of owner noncompliance will result in relapse.
  - Only neovascularization responds to this therapy; melanosis and corneal degeneration do not.
- Consider instillation of 1 drop of 2% cyclosporine in oil (see sec. 11, ch. 9) q12h. Over many months,

this may reduce corneal melanosis in many conditions, including CSK, by a poorly understood mechanism. CSK is believed to be a T-lymphocyte–mediated disease and has been reported to respond in some instances to cyclosporine therapy.
- Plesiotherapy with strontium-90–generated beta-radiation is an effective adjunctive treatment for neovascularization. However, this is only available through specialty practices and teaching institutions.

KEY POINT ▶ Do not perform keratectomy for removal of corneal pigmentation. Complications include delayed epithelialization, recurrence of CSK, and corneal perforation.

Feline Eosinophilic Keratitis

Etiology
- The etiology is unknown.

Clinical Signs
- Corneal neovascularization, which is frequently bilateral and symmetric, leads to formation of a pink-white plaque covered by a granular, crumbled cheese–like material. The superior temporal, inferior temporal, and inferior nasal quadrants are most frequently involved.
- This lesion is unique to the cat.
- Corneal ulceration is present rarely.

Diagnosis
- Corneal scrapings contain combinations of eosinophils, mast cells, and mixed inflammatory cells.

KEY POINT ▶ The presence of eosinophils or mast cells is pathognomonic for feline eosinophilic keratitis.

Treatment
- Intensive topical corticosteroid therapy frequently is successful.
  - Give dexamethasone 0.1% (Decadron; Merck, Sharp and Dohme) or prednisolone 1% (Econopred Plus; Alcon) as an ointment or solution, q3–4h. Monitor progress closely if epithelial erosion was present.
  - If needed, combine topical corticosteroids with administration of subconjunctival betamethasone, triamicinolone, or methylprednisolone (3–6 mg per eye). This combination controls the condition in most cats.
  - Once the disease is in remission, reduce frequency of topical therapy to minimal levels; discontinue if remission is maintained.
  - Some affected cats will have relapses, requiring chronic topical corticosteroid administration at a minimal effective frequency.
- Administer megestrol acetate (Ovaban; Schering) (0.5 mg/kg q24h until effect, and then 1.25 mg 1–3 times weekly) *only* to cats that have not responded to topical and subconjunctival corticosteroids.
  - Side effects of oral megestrol acetate include weight gain, behavior changes, diabetes mellitus, and mammary gland hypertrophy and neoplasia.

Corneal Melanosis

Etiology

- Among domestic animals, only dogs commonly develop corneal pigmentation, which apparently develops through migration of limbal melanocytes into the basal epithelial layers and anterior stroma.

KEY POINT ▶ Melanosis develops in response to chronic irritation from many causes, including KCS, eyelid deformities, lagophthalmos, and CSK.

Clinical Signs

- Superficial corneal pigmentation develops focally or over large areas; corneal neovascularization usually precedes or accompanies melanosis.

Diagnosis

- The typical appearance of a variably melanotic cornea is diagnostic.
- Rarely, melanosis must be distinguished from iris prolapse (anterior synechiae are also apparent) or, at the limbus, epibulbar melanoma.

Treatment

- Identify and treat the underlying causes of melanosis if possible (e.g., KCS) or definitively correct them (e.g., entropion, nasal fold trichiasis).
- Rarely, perform superficial keratectomy to improve corneal clarity when vision is reduced, but only after correcting the inciting cause.
- Consider long-term topical therapy for KCS with 2% cyclosporine, (see sec. 11, ch. 9) which may retard or reduce corneal melanosis (evidence of benefit is anecdotal).

Scleral Inflammation

Fibrous Histiocytoma; Proliferative Keratoconjunctivitis of Collies; Nodular Granulomatous Episclerokeratitis

Etiology

- This condition probably is a genetic disorder of collies, but has been noted in other breeds. Clinical and pathologic features of both inflammation and neoplasia are present.

Clinical Signs

- Bilaterally symmetric scleral/episcleral nodules, especially at the temporal limbus, are hallmarks.
- The eyelids, planum nasale, and other mucocutaneous junctions (lips, anogenital areas) may be involved.
- If the cornea is invaded, corneal opacity develops, often with a leading edge of crystalline corneal degeneration.

Diagnosis

- The presence of typical lesions in a collie is presumptive evidence.
- Obtain a biopsy of atypical lesions.
- The histologic appearance is that of fibroplasia with extensive histiocytic proliferation.
- Differential diagnosis includes lymphosarcoma and other neoplasms.

Treatment

- Corticosteroids are the initial treatment of choice. For dogs with ocular lesions only, combine intensive topical corticosteroid therapy (dexamethasone 0.1% or prednisolone 1%) with subconjunctival injection of 3–6 mg per eye of triamcinolone, betamethasone, or methylprednisolone acetate.
  - Recurrence is discouraged with long-term topical steroid treatment at the minimally effective frequency.
- For dogs with ocular and oral, nasal, and/or genital lesions, administer oral prednisone (1.1 mg/kg q12h); taper to the effective minimal dose and frequency. Indefinite treatment may be required.
- For dogs with corticosteroid-unresponsive lesions, administer azathioprine (Imuran; Burroughs Wellcome) 2.2 mg/kg q24h, PO, for 14 days followed by 1 mg/kg every other day for 14 days; then give 1 mg/kg once weekly for 4 weeks and discontinue.
  - Indefinite treatment at a low frequency may be required.
  - Monitor leukocyte and platelet counts in animals on azathioprine therapy. Discontinue treatment if a significant reduction in either is observed.
- Discourage breeding of affected dogs.

Scleritis; Episcleritis; Ocular Nodular Fascitis

Etiology

- The cause is unknown; an immune-mediated etiology is suspected.

Clinical Signs

- Nodular, diffuse infiltrative, and necrotizing forms have been recognized.
  - Nodular lesions resemble fibrous histiocytomas, but often are unilateral and affect dogs other than collies.
  - Diffuse thickening and inflammation of the sclera may be associated with scleral necrosis and moderate to severe uveitis.

Diagnosis

- The diagnosis is based on clinical signs, histopathology, and response to therapy.
- Differential diagnosis includes lymphosarcoma and other neoplasia.

Treatment

- Treatment plan is similar to that for fibrous histiocytoma.

Scleral Wounds

Etiology

Blunt or perforating trauma may cause rupture of the globe through the sclera although the cornea is spared.

Clinical Signs

- Chemosis, conjunctival or external ocular hemorrhage, hyphema, and eyelid swelling in a traumatized small animal suggest scleral perforation.

Treatment

- Surgical repair of small wounds may result in preservation of the globe, and even of vision if the repair is performed promptly.

■ Enucleation or evisceration with intraocular prosthesis implantation is indicated if the scleral laceration is large or if other ocular injuries prevent comfortable retention of the globe.

Corneoscleral Neoplasia

Primary—Epibulbar Melanoma

Etiology

■ These benign neoplasms probably arise from conjunctival or episcleral melanocytes.
■ The German shepherd is a predisposed breed, but the disorder has been reported in numerous other breeds.

Clinical Signs

■ A nonpainful, pigmented mass near the limbus, involving sclera (and, later, adjacent cornea), slowly enlarges, expanding horizontally and vertically into surrounding sclera.

Diagnosis

■ The typical appearance suggests the diagnosis.
■ Epibulbar melanomas should be distinguished (not always easily) from uveal melanomas, which may expand through the sclera.

Treatment

■ Small, superficial lesions may be resectable. Because scleral grafting may be necessary, consider referral to a specialist.
■ Observe for a long period to assess the growth rate and characteristics of individual tumors.
  • In dogs, these normally benign neoplasms may be safely observed until/unless deeper extension causes uveitis or glaucoma, prompting enucleation.
  • Recommendations in cats are similar, although based on fewer reported cases.

Secondary

Etiology

■ Primary or secondary intraocular neoplasms may extend through the sclera and into the orbit.

■ Rarely, episcleral metastasis of a distant primary or multicentric neoplasm may occur.

Clinical Signs

■ Masses may be obvious extensions of intraocular tumors. Episcleral masses may mimic episcleritis or fibrous histiocytoma.

Diagnosis

■ Relationship to an intraocular tumor is presumptive evidence. Association of a scleral mass with a visible intraocular tumor suggests that the scleral mass is an extension of it.
■ For histopathological evaluation, completely excise solitary masses.

Treatment

■ Consider palliative and diagnostic enucleation of a painful globe.

Supplemental Readings

Cooley PL, Dice PF: Corneal dystrophy in the dog and cat. Vet Clin North Am [Small Anim Pract] 20(3):681, 1990.

Dice PF, Cooley PL: Use of contact lenses to treat corneal diseases in small animals. Semin Vet Med Surg (Small Anim) 3:46, 1988.

Kern TJ: Ulcerative keratitis. Vet Clin North Am [Small Anim Pract] 20(3):643, 1990.

Kirschner SE: Persistent corneal ulcers: What to do when they won't heal. Vet Clin North Am [Small Anim Pract] 20(3):627, 1990.

Moore CP: Surgery of the conjunctiva. In Bojrab MJ, ed.: Current Techniques in Small Animal Surgery, 3rd Ed. Philadelphia: Lea & Febiger, 1990, p 76.

Munger RJ: The conjunctiva. In Slatter DH, ed.: Textbook of Small Animal Surgery. Philadelphia: W. B. Saunders, 1985, p 1469.

Slatter DH: Cornea and sclera. In Fundamentals of Veterinary Ophthalmology, 2nd Ed. Philadelphia: W. B. Saunders, 1990, p 257.

Slatter DH: Cornea and sclera. In Slatter DH, ed.: Textbook of Small Animal Surgery. Philadelphia: W. B. Saunders, 1985, p 1509.

Vestre WA: Surgery of the cornea. In Bojrab MJ, ed.: Current Techniques in Small Animal Surgery, 3rd Ed. Philadelphia: Lea & Febiger, 1990, p 947.

5 Diseases of the Lens

Margi Gilmour
David A. Wilkie

ANATOMY

The normal canine and feline lens is composed of an outer elastic capsule, epithelial cells beneath the anterior capsule, and fibers formed by the migration of epithelial cells to the lens equator, where the cells elongate and create a regular arrangement of fibers. The regular arrangement of these fibers accounts for the transparency of the lens. The lens is posterior to the iris; anterior to the vitreous to which it is attached; and suspended by zonules, which arise from the ciliary body and attach to the lens capsule at the equator.

CONGENITAL ANOMALIES

Etiology

Lens development takes place early in embryogenesis and is complete in the dog by day 30 of gestation. Any genetic abnormality affecting lens development or any insult to the bitch or queen early in gestation, including infectious, nutritional, chemical, or drug-related, can result in congenital lens anomalies. These abnormalities are often associated with other congenital ocular anomalies, including microphthalmia (small globe), persistent pupillary membranes, retinal dysplasia, retinal detachment, and optic nerve hypoplasia.

Clinical Signs

Examples and features of congenital lens anomalies include the following.

- *Microphakia* (small lens). With the pupil dilated, the equator of the lens and fine zonules, attaching at the equator and originating from elongated ciliary processes, are visible.
- *Coloboma* (notch defect). With the pupil dilated, a notch defect may be visible in any quadrant of the equatorial zone, with or without zonular attachments.
- *Cataract.* See the cataract discussion in this chapter.
- *Lens luxation.* Often associated with microphakia (see discussion this chapter).

Diagnosis

- Clinical signs
- Present at birth. Microphakia and coloboma are always congenital. Cataract and lens luxation, unless associated with microphakia, may not be congenital.

An accurate history and early examination are helpful in differentiating congenital from acquired abnormalities.

Treatment

- Determine concomitant ocular anomalies and their significance to vision.
- Microphakia and coloboma alone require no treatment.
- Cataract, if impairing vision, may be amenable to surgical removal once the integrity of the retina and optic nerve has been ascertained by fundic examination, electroretinogram, ocular ultrasound, and visual-evoked potential.
- Removal of a luxated lens is indicated if it is inciting uveitis and/or glaucoma, impairing vision, or interfering with corneal endothelial cell function.

Prevention

Congenital anomalies are not necessarily inherited anomalies. Careful inquiry into affected littermates and prevalence of problems in previous matings may raise the suspicion for an inherited defect. If the cause of the abnormality cannot be determined, discourage the use of this and related animals for breeding.

CATARACT

Etiology

Cataract is an opacity of the lens resulting from pathologic changes in lens protein composition or disruption of lens fiber arrangement.

KEY POINT ▶ Cataract must be distinguished from nuclear sclerosis. Nuclear sclerosis is a normal aging change seen in all dogs and cats 6 years of age or older, produced by compression of central lens fibers.

Etiologies of cataract development include the following:

- *Hereditary.* This is the most common cause of cataract in the dog (Table 1). Location, progression, and mode of inheritance of cataracts varies among breeds. The majority of inherited cataracts are bilateral but often asymmetric in onset and progression.
- *Inflammatory.* This is a common cause of cataract in the cat. Because the lens needs the aqueous and

TABLE 1. Breed List of Inherited or Familial Cataracts in the Dog*

Afghan hound	French bulldog	Papillon
Alaskan malamute	German shepherd	Pembroke Welsh corgi
Beagle	German shorthaired pointer	Pointer
Bedlington terrier	Giant Schnauzer	Pomeranian
Belgian Tervuren	Golden retriever	Poodle (toy, miniature, standard)
Bernese mountain dog	Grean Dane	Puli
Bichon frise	Ibizan hound	Rhodesian Ridgeback
Border collie	Irish setter	Rottweiler
Border terrier	Irish water spaniel	St. Bernard
Borzoi	Irish wolfhound	Samoyed
Boston terrier	Italian greyhound	Schipperke
Bouvier des Flandres	Keeshond	Scottish terrier
Cairn terrier	Kerry blue terrier	Siberian husky
Cavalier King Charles spaniel	Labrador retriever	Silky terrier
Chesapeake Bay retriever	Lakeland terrier	Staffordshire bull terrier
Cocker spaniel	Lhasa apso	Standard schnauzer
Collie	Manchester terrier	Tibetan terrier
Curly-coated retriever	Miniature pinscher	Welsh Springer spaniel
Dachshund	Miniature schnauzer	Welsh terrier
English Cocker spaniel	Norfolk terrier	West Highland White terrier
English Springer spaniel	Norwegian elkhound	Whippet
English toy spaniel	Norwich terrier	Wire Fox terrier
Field spaniel	Old English sheepdog	Yorkshire terrier

*From Rubin LF: *Inherited Eye Diseases in Purebred Dogs.* Baltimore: Williams & Wilkins, 1989.

vitreous humors for nutrition and removal of metabolic wastes, intraocular inflammation can result in capsular and cortical opacities. Posterior synechia from anterior uveitis can result in anterior capsular cataracts.

■ *Metabolic.* Diabetes mellitus in dogs frequently results in rapid (days to weeks) onset of bilateral cataracts, because of a shift in metabolic pathways, an accumulation of sorbitol causing an osmotic gradient, and a subsequent disruption of lens fibers. The cataracts are irreversible.

■ *Traumatic.* Severe blunt trauma to the eye can result in cataract formation from concussive effects or can be secondary to inflammation and/or lens luxation. Penetrating injuries that puncture the anterior lens capsule (e.g., cat claw injuries) result in a focal or diffuse cataract, depending upon the severity of the capsular tear. Uveitis may occur secondary to rupture of the lens capsule and exposure of antigenic lens material.

■ *Nutritional.* Puppies and kittens hand fed exclusively milk-replacement formula that is deficient in required amino acids, the most frequently cited being arginine, can develop bilateral cataracts.

■ *Toxic.* Electric shock, radiation therapy involving the ocular region, and certain drugs have been reported to cause cataracts.

Clinical Signs and Diagnosis

KEY POINT ▶ For a thorough examination of the lens, mydriasis is mandatory because some of the most significant changes occur in the extreme periphery (equatorial zone) of the lens. Topical tropicamide 1% (Mydriacyl, Alcon) results in mydriasis in 15–20 minutes and lasts 6–8 hours.

■ Any *opacity,* anywhere in the lens or its capsule observed after dilation of the pupil, is a cataract.

■ The degree of *visual impairment* is dependent upon the extent of cataract development in one or both eyes.

■ Cataracts must be distinguished from nuclear sclerosis. Nuclear sclerosis is a bilaterally symmetric, well-defined, homogeneous haze to the center of the lens observed in animals older than 6 years. Sclerosis is not a true opacity, and it does not obstruct a dilated examination of the fundus or cause clinically significant visual impairment.

■ A focal cataract can be localized with respect to anterior or posterior by comparing the nasal/temporal direction of movement of the cataract with that of the eye. Anterior cataracts will move in the same direction as the globe; posterior cataracts will appear to move in the opposite direction of the globe. Thus—if the animal looks temporally—an anterior opacity will move temporally and a posterior opacity will move nasally. By localizing cataracts, one can help determine if they are inherited and predict progression. For example, nuclear cataracts are generally static, whereas equatorial cataracts, where new lens fibers are forming, are generally progressive.

Stage of Development

Incipient

Focal or multifocal opacities of the lens causing no clinical loss of vision and not impairing tapetal reflection or view of the fundus.

Immature

Significant lenticular opacity. Tapetal reflection remains, but an incomplete view of the fundus is present. Vision is affected depending upon the extent of lens involvement.

Mature

Dense lenticular opacity with no tapetal reflection or fundus visible, resulting in total vision loss in the affected eye.

Hypermature

As lens protein degenerates and liquefies the lens can become smaller in the anterior-posterior axis, resulting in a wrinkled anterior capsule and deep anterior chamber.

Resorbing

As lens protein degenerates and liquefies it can leak through the capsule. This is usually associated with hypermature cataracts but can occur in immature and mature cataracts as well. The process is faster in young dogs. A resorbing lens has varying amounts of clear, liquefied cortex with the remaining lens material often taking on a sparkling appearance. Although in some animals vision is regained by significant lens resorption, the process generally results in mild-to-severe lens-induced uveitis because of the antigenicity of the leaking lens protein. Dogs with lens-induced uveitis may show a range of clinical signs typical of uveitis (see sec. 11, ch. 6).

Treatment

KEY POINT ▶ There is no medical treatment to eliminate cataracts. Surgical removal of cataracts is a referral procedure.

- Cataracts secondary to inflammation are generally not amenable to surgery.
- Because of the surgical risks, the cost to the owner, and most animals' ability to function well in their environment without vision, cataract surgery is considered elective. The exception is a traumatic cataract that has released cortical material into the anterior chamber, which will incite severe uveitis if not removed.
- Success rates for cataract surgery vary depending upon pre-existing uveitis and glaucoma predisposition, and the surgical procedure and expertise. Success rates cited in the literature are with phacofragmentation (see Surgical Procedures), 95% at 1 month following surgery; 86% at 2 years; and 71% at 4 years; with extracapsular extraction, 80% at 1 month following surgery, with one study showing 69% at 6 months and 38% at 2 years.

Pre-operative Considerations

- For owners expressing an interest in cataract surgery, refer them to a veterinary ophthalmologist early, while the fundus is still visible and before lens-induced uveitis develops.
- The animal should be healthy. If diabetic, the condition should be well-regulated.
- The eyes are examined for concurrent uveitis, glaucoma, abnormal iridocorneal angle, keratitis, and retinal disease.
- If the fundus is not visible through the cataract, an electroretinogram is performed to evaluate for progressive retinal atrophy. An ocular ultrasound is carried out to evaluate for retinal detachment.

Surgical Procedures

- The most common technique for cataract removal in veterinary ophthalmology is *extracapsular extraction*. This removes the lens and a portion of the anterior lens capsule, leaving the posterior lens capsule.
- Lens removal can be performed through a 120–160° corneal or corneoscleral incision, removing the anterior lens capsule and delivering the remaining lens cortex and nucleus. This technique generally results in greater postoperative inflammation because of the collapse of the globe and failure to adequately remove the cortical material.
- *Phacofragmentation* (phacoemulsification) uses an ultrasound-driven needle to emulsify and aspirate lens material. Phacofragmentation requires a smaller corneal incision and less surgical time. It prevents collapse of the globe and results in less postoperative inflammation.
- Implantation of an *intraocular lens (IOL)* following cataract removal is becoming more common in veterinary ophthalmology. The benefit of an IOL is still a matter of debate. IOLs may increase the risk of postoperative complications. Animals without IOLs often function well in their environments with little complaint from owners. A successful IOL provides the animal with a return of more normal vision, however.
- Laser surgery, where available, can be used postoperatively to create, by capsulotomy, a clear visual axis when posterior capsular opacities interfere with vision.

Postoperative Considerations

Complications of cataract surgery can occur 1 week to several years postoperatively. Patients are evaluated frequently for several months following surgery. A long-term, 6-month re-evaluation schedule is maintained for life.

- *Immediate postoperative complications* include anterior uveitis, glaucoma, and retinal detachment.
- *Long-term complications* include chronic low-grade uveitis, glaucoma, corneal endothelial damage with associated corneal edema, fibrous metaplasia across the posterior capsule with opacification of the capsule, posterior synechia, production of new cortical material from remaining epithelial cells, and retinal detachment.
- Re-evaluation includes tonometry to determine intraocular pressure (IOP) and a dilated examination of the posterior capsule and fundus.

Prevention

- Incidence of inherited cataracts can be reduced by discouraging breeding of affected animals and carriers and by encouraging breeders to have yearly Certified Eye Registration Foundation (CERF) examinations.

- Nutritional-based cataracts can be prevented by supplementing commercial milk replacers with blenderized, complete dog food.
- Inflammatory cataracts can often be prevented by prompt, appropriate treatment of uveitis (see sec. 11, ch. 6).

LENS LUXATION

Etiology

- *Primary zonular degeneration.* This is an inherited trait in many terrier breeds and has familial tendencies in other breeds (Table 2). Lens luxation usually occurs at middle age with no predisposing ocular disease.
- *Glaucoma.* Chronic glaucoma results in a buphthalmic (enlarged) globe that can stretch and break the lenticular zonules, causing the lens to luxate.

KEY POINT ▶ A primary lens luxation can also cause glaucoma, making it difficult to distinguish which occurred first in some cases.

- *Uveitis.* Chronic uveitis may weaken zonules owing to inflammatory cell infiltration.
- *Cataracts.* Advanced cataracts may cause degenerative changes in the zonules or zonular attachments.
- *Trauma.* Severe ocular trauma may cause lens luxation; however, it is not a common cause unless there is underlying zonule pathology.

Clinical Signs

- The clinical signs of lens luxation vary depending upon whether the lens luxates anteriorly or posteriorly. Many times it is the secondary ocular changes that result in the clinical presentation, rather than the lens luxation itself.
- In many eyes with luxated lenses, the vitreous will liquefy and can be found in the anterior chamber. Vitreous appears as filmy, white material suspended in the aqueous humor. Its presence, in the absence of lens luxation, may indicate early zonular breakdown and an animal's predisposition to lens luxation.

Anterior Lens Luxation

- A penlight beam directed parallel to the iris will reveal the lens positioned in the anterior chamber, anterior to the iris and often blocking the pupil.

- Blue light (Wood's lamp) will cause a clear lens to fluoresce, simplifying the examination.
- A focal area of corneal edema may result from the lens' touching the posterior cornea and damaging the corneal endothelium. This may be a permanent change.
- Secondary glaucoma can occur from pupillary occlusion by the lens or attached vitreous or from occlusion of the aqueous outflow through the iridocorneal angle.

Posterior Lens Luxation

- The edge of the lens may be seen through the pupil resulting in an "aphakic crescent" between the pupil margin and the edge of the lens.
- The lens may fall into the vitreal chamber where it can be seen on the floor of the chamber, trapped in the vitreous or adhered to the retina.
- Without support of the lens, the iris may tremble with eye movement (iridodonesis). The anterior chamber will be deep.

Diagnosis

- Based on ophthalmic examination
- Tonometry to identify primary or secondary glaucoma
- Ocular ultrasound (if intraocular structures cannot be observed because of corneal or aqueous opacity).

Treatment

- Acute anterior lens luxation is a surgical emergency requiring immediate referral. The pupil is *not* to be dilated. Surgical complications include uveitis, corneal edema, dyscoria, synechia, glaucoma, vitreous entrapment in the incision, and retinal detachment.
- If surgery is not an option and pupillary block has resulted in secondary glaucoma, a short-acting mydriatic such as 1% tropicamide (Mydriacyl, Alcon) can restore aqueous flow through the pupil.
- Posterior lens luxation rarely results in a clinical problem unless the lens subsequently moves anteriorly. Removing a lens from the vitreal chamber is difficult and results in disruption of the vitreous and possible retinal damage. Over time the lens often adheres to the inferior retina. A miotic agent, such as topical 2% pilocarpine, can initially prevent the lens from luxating anteriorly.

TABLE 2. Breed List of Inherited or Familial Lens Luxation in the Dog*

Australian cattle dog	Lakeland terrier	Sealyham terrier
Border collie	Manchester terrier	Siberian husky
Cairn terrier	Miniature schnauzer	Skye terrier
Cardigan Welsh corgi	Norfolk terrier	Smooth Fox terrier
Chihuahua	Norwegian elkhound	Tibetan terrier
German shepherd	Norwich terrier	Welsh terrier
Greyhound	Pembroke Welsh corgi	West Highland White terrier
Irish setter	Poodle (toy)	Whippet
Jack Russell terrier	Scottish terrier	Wire Fox terrier

*From Rubin LF: *Inherited Eye Diseases in Purebred Dogs.* Baltimore: Williams & Wilkins, 1989.

■ No specific treatment for lens luxation in the buphthalmic globe is indicated (see sec. 11, ch. 7).

Prevention

■ Examine the contralateral eye carefully for evidence of lens subluxation, such as a deep or shallow anterior chamber, iris tremor, aphakic crescent, or vitreous in the anterior chamber.

■ Advise owners to watch the animal's eye at risk for signs of lens luxation and to call immediately if noted.

Supplemental Readings

Curtis R: Lens luxation in the dog and cat. Vet Clin North Am [Sm Anim Pract—Sm Anim Ophthalmol] 20:755–773, 1990.

Dziezyc J: Cataract surgery—current approaches. Vet Clin North Am [Sm Anim Pract—Sm Anim Ophthalmol] 20:737–754, 1990.

Gwin RM, Gelatt KN: The canine lens. *In* Gelatt KN, ed.: *Veterinary Ophthalmology*. Philadelphia: Lea & Febiger, 1981, p 435–473.

Rubin LF: *Inherited Eye Diseases in Purebred Dogs*. Baltimore: Williams & Wilkins, 1989.

6 Uvea

David A. Wilkie

ETIOLOGY OF ANTERIOR UVEITIS

Anterior uveitis is inflammation of the anterior uvea, which consists of the iris and ciliary body. Anterior uveitis is associated with pain and has potentially severe systemic and ophthalmic sequelae. Anterior uveitis has numerous etiologies, many of which are systemic diseases (Table 1).

KEY POINT ▶ If no primary ocular etiology of anterior uveitis can be ascertained, systemic disease must be considered. This approach applies whether the uveitis is unilateral or bilateral.

- *Corneal ulceration* often results in reflex anterior uveitis. Uveitis occurs as the result of stimulation of the ophthalmic branch of cranial nerve V and does not indicate infectious keratitis.
- *Trauma* can result in anterior uveitis as the result of a direct penetration of the globe or a concussive effect. Uveitis may be associated with other ophthalmic abnormalities, such as corneal ulceration, hyphema, lens luxation, retinal detachment, proptosis, and globe rupture. See appropriate chapters for further discussion of these abnormalities.
- *Infectious causes* of anterior uveitis are numerous and include bacteria, fungi, rickettsia, and protozoal organisms (see Table 1). These organisms result in

anterior uveitis by direct infections of the eye, immune-mediated responses, or circulating endotoxins. Many of these infectious agents also cause posterior segment (retina, choroid) involvement (see sec. 11, ch. 8). Direct infection of the eye can occur from penetrating trauma or blood-borne infection. Although anterior uveitis is commonly associated with infectious causes, the organism itself is generally not present within the eye.

- *Lens-induced anterior uveitis* results from traumatic rupture of the lens capsule or from leakage of the lens material through an intact capsule as noted with a hypermature cataract. Lens protein is antigenic and, if released, will result in mild-to-severe anterior uveitis. Cataracts are discussed in section 11, chapter 5.
- *Autoimmune anterior uveitis*, unassociated with lens protein leakage, is observed in the uveodermatologic syndrome (formerly Vogt-Koyanagi-Harada syndrome or VKH). This syndrome is observed in dogs and results in anterior and posterior uveitis, poliosis (depigmentation of the hair), and vitiligo (depigmentation of the skin). See section 5, chapter 9 for discussion of the dermatologic manifestations.

CLINICAL SIGNS (Table 2)

- *Miosis* is a smaller than normal pupil that is the result of contraction of the iris sphincter muscle. Spasm of the iris sphincter muscle, along with the ciliary body musculature, results in pain, noted clinically as photophobia (intolerance of light).
- *Flare* results from a breakdown in the blood-aqueous humor barrier and a subsequent leakage of plasma protein (with or without cells) into the eye. It is observed clinically as a haze in the anterior chamber (Fig. 1).
- *Hypotony* is a decrease in the intraocular pressure below the normal range of 15–25 mmHg—the result of a decrease in the production of aqueous humor.
- *Cells* are released into the anterior chamber in severe

TABLE 1. Systemic Infectious Etiologies of Anterior Uveitis—Dog and Cat*

Mycotic
　Blastomycosis, cryptococcosis, histoplasmosis, coccidioidomycosis, aspergillosis, others
Rickettsial
　Ehrlichiosis, Rocky Mountain spotted fever
Toxoplasmosis
Feline infectious peritonitis (FIP), feline immunodeficiency virus (FIV), feline leukemia virus (FeLV)
Lyme disease
Bacteremia/septicemia
Brucellosis
Aberrant parasitic migration
　Heartworm, roundworm, hookworm, others
Canine distemper
Infectious canine hepatitis
Prototer canine hepatitis
Prototothecosis
Mycobacteriosis
Leptospirosis
Leishmaniasis

*For a description of each disease see the appropriate chapters.

TABLE 2. Clinical Signs of Anterior Uveitis

Discharge (serous, mucoid)	Redness
Blepharospasm	Photophobia
Miosis	Hypotony
Corneal edema	Aqueous flare
Keratitic precipitates	Hyphema
Hypopyon	Blindness

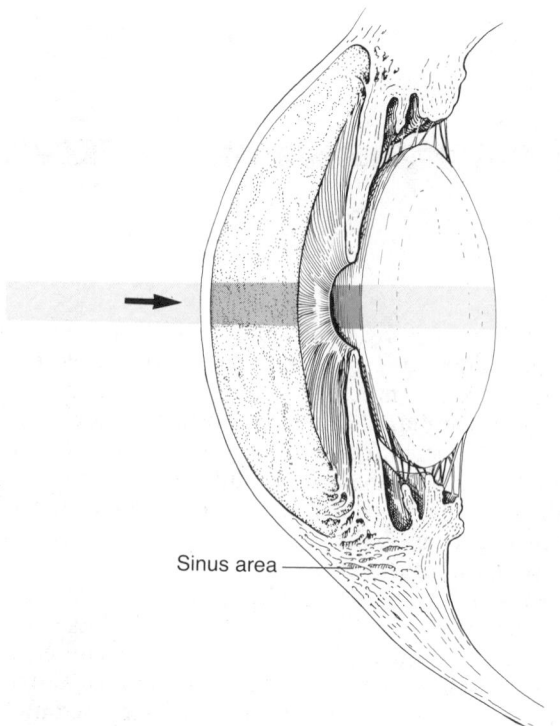

Sinus area

Figure 1. Using a bright, focused light source, aqueous flare is seen as a continuation of the light beam through the normally dark-appearing anterior chamber.

uveitis. The inflammatory cellular response can be polymorphonuclear or granulomatous. In addition, red blood cells (i.e., hyphema) or neoplastic cells can enter the anterior chamber.

■ *Hyperemia* or redness may be seen on examination of the conjunctival, episcleral, and iris blood vessels in eyes with anterior uveitis.

DIAGNOSIS

■ A complete *history* is essential to detect previous or concurrent problems that may be associated with anterior uveitis. The history includes both ophthalmic and systemic problems.

■ *Ophthalmic examination*
  • A *penlight examination* is performed to evaluate pupil size, symmetry, and response to light. The severity along with the character of the uveitis is assessed by the degree of aqueous flare and the cellular response. The clarity of the clear media of the eye, cornea, aqueous humor, lens, and vitreous is also assessed. All abnormalities are described and diagramed in the medical record.
  • *Tonometry* is the determination of the intraocular pressure (IOP). Eyes with anterior uveitis have a decreased IOP (hypotony). A normal or elevated IOP indicates the potential for, or the presence of, glaucoma. The tonometer of choice for the general practitioner is the Schiøtz tonometer (see sec. 11, ch. 7).

KEY POINT ▶ The clinical signs of anterior uveitis and glaucoma can be similar. Both diseases can be present together in the same eye. Determination of IOP is therefore essential.

  • *Fundic examination*, either by direct or indirect ophthalmoscopy, is performed to determine the presence or absence of posterior segment involvement. Anterior uveitis in combination with posterior uveitis is termed panuveitis and is strongly suggestive of systemic disease, especially those infectious in nature (see Table 1). Posterior segment changes indicating active inflammation include retinal hemorrhage, retinal detachment, vasculitis, and infiltration by granulomatous or neoplastic cells. If the posterior lesions are chronic in nature, they will appear as tapetal hyper-reflectivity, pigment clumping and depigmentation of the nontapetal region, and atrophy of the retinal vasculature (see sec. 11, ch. 8).
  • *Fluorescein stain* is performed to examine for a corneal ulcer. Corneal ulcers can result in a secondary anterior uveitis. If detected, the ulcer must be characterized with regards to depth, severity, and infection (see sec. 11, ch. 4). In addition, the etiology must be determined and eventually eliminated. Anterior uveitis, resulting from a corneal ulcer, resolves once the ulcer is healed.

■ *Complete physical examination* is an essential part of the diagnostic evaluation of a patient with anterior uveitis. The examination includes palpation of all the external lymph nodes, auscultation of the cardio-pulmonary system, palpation of the abdomen, and determination of the body temperature.

■ *Biochemical profile, urinalysis,* and *complete blood count* are parts of the routine screening that is performed on all patients with anterior uveitis of unknown cause and patients with concomitant systemic abnormalities.

■ *Serology,* for the specific infectious diseases listed in Table 1, is performed as indicated by the findings of the history, physical examination, ophthalmic examination, biochemical profile, urinalysis, and complete blood count.

■ *Radiography* of the thorax and abdomen is performed to evaluate for the presence of systemic mycosis, disseminated neoplasia, or other organ system involvement.

■ *Cytology* of intraocular or extraocular samples may be indicated in selected instances. Intraocular samples include both the aqueous and vitreous humors. Of these, the vitreous humor sample is the most diagnostic but also the most traumatic to obtain. Anterior chamber samples are frequently not diagnostic. The indication for vitreocentesis is panuveitis in a blind eye for which the diagnosis cannot be obtained by alternate methods.
  • Using general anesthesia, a 20-gauge needle is inserted 4–5 mm posterior to the corneal-scleral junction superior-temporally.
  • The needle is directed towards the center of the eye and 0.5–1.0 ml of fluid is aspirated for culture and cytology.

▪ Extraocular cytology includes aspirates of regional lymph nodes or mass lesions.

TREATMENT

The treatment of anterior uveitis includes nonspecific approaches directed towards decreasing the inflammation and sequelae and specific ones directed towards eliminating the underlying etiology when one has been identified.

Nonspecific (Table 3)

▪ *Mydriatic-cycloplegics* are used to paralyze the iris sphincter and ciliary body musculature. This effect will decrease the pain associated with anterior uveitis and the tendency towards formation of posterior synechia. The mydriatic-cycloplegic of choice is topical 1% atropine (parasympatholytic). Atropine is administered to effect (pupil dilation) but not to exceed a treatment frequency of four times/day. This results in maximum drug effects with minimal side effects.

KEY POINT ▶ Atropine is contraindicated in anterior uveitis when accompanied by secondary glaucoma.

▪ *Topical anti-inflammatory drugs* include both corticosteroids and nonsteroidal agents. Topical medication does not penetrate beyond the iris and ciliary body. Its use is therefore limited to problems of the anterior segment of the eye.

- *Corticosteroids.* The topical corticosteroid of choice for the treatment of anterior uveitis is 1% prednisolone acetate ophthalmic suspension (Econopred). This agent achieves the highest intraocular level of the ophthalmic corticosteroids. If unavailable, 0.1% dexamethasone solution or 0.05% dexamethasone ointment can be applied. The frequency of treatment varies according to the severity of the uveitis, ranging from one to 6 times/day.

KEY POINT ▶ Topical corticosteroids delay healing and potentiate infection and collagenase ulceration. Topical corticosteroids are contraindicated for anterior uveitis associated with corneal ulceration.

Topical corticosteroids are also absorbed systemically and alter adrenal and hepatic function.

- *Nonsteroidal.* Topical nonsteroidal ophthalmic drugs are now available. The indications for their use are similar to those for topical corticosteroids. They are used as supplements to topical corticosteroids or as substitutes when topical corticosteroids are contraindicated (e.g., in diabetes mellitus). As with topical corticosteroids, nonsteroidal agents may delay the healing of a corneal ulcer. Frequency of administration is four times/day.

TABLE 3. Dosages of Commonly Used Ocular Anti-Inflammatory Agents

Drugs	Trade Names	Dosages
Topical		
Corticosteroids		
1.0% Prednisolone acetate suspension	Econopred Plus	1–6×/day
0.1% Dexamethasone solution	Decadron	1–6×/day
0.05% Dexamethasone ointment	Decadron	1–6×/day
NSAIDs		
0.03% Flurbiprofen	Ocufen	4×/day
1.0% Suprofen	Profenal	4×/day
Atropine		
1.0% Atropine		1–4×/day
Systemic		
Corticosteroids		
Prednisolone/prednisone		*Dog*
Immunosuppressive		1.0 mg/kg PO q12h × 7–14 days, then taper
Anti-inflammatory		0.5 mg/kg PO q12h × 3–5 days, then taper
NSAIDs		
Acetylsalicylic acid	Aspirin	*Dog*
		10–25 mg/kg PO q12h
		Cat
		80 mg PO q48–72h
Flunixin meglumine	Banamine	*Dog*
		0.25–0.5 mg/kg IV single dose
		Cat
		Do not use
Phenylbutazone	Butazolidin	*Dog*
		13 mg/kg PO q8h × 48 h, then taper
		Cat
		10–14 mg/kg q12h PO
Immunosuppressive		
Azathioprine	Imuran	*Dog*
		2.2 mg/kg to q48h, then taper
Cyclophosphamide	Cytoxan	*Dog*
		50 mg/m² PO q24h × 4 days/week

■ *Systemic anti-inflammatory drugs* include corticosteroids, nonsteroidal agents, and immunosuppressive drugs.

• *Corticosteroids.* Systemic corticosteroids are indicated in the management of noninfectious posterior uveitis and in severe anterior uveitis as a supplement to topical corticosteroids. The dosage is dependent upon the underlying disease. An immunosuppressive dose is indicated for animals with uveodermatologic syndrome and an anti-inflammatory dose is indicated for most other cases (see Table 3). The side effects of systemic corticosteroids include polyphagia/polyuria/polydyspia, infection potentiation, altered carbohydrate metabolism, and adrenal suppression. Therapy with systemic corticosteroids begins at a high dose to achieve a response followed by a tapered dose to maintain effect and to decrease adverse side effects.

• *Nonsteroidal.* Systemic nonsteroidal anti-inflammatory drugs (NSAIDs) include aspirin, flunixin meglumine, and phenylbutazone. They are indicated to decrease inflammation and facilitate pupil dilation. In small animal ophthalmology, flunixin meglumine is administered as a single dose (0.25–0.5 mg/kg IV) prior to ocular surgery to decrease postsurgical ocular inflammation. If prolonged therapy with NSAIDs is required, aspirin is the drug of choice. Side effects of NSAIDs include gastrointestinal ulceration and hemorrhage and acute renal papillary necrosis. Systemic NSAIDs are not used in combination with systemic corticosteroids and must be used with caution in patients with questionable renal fuction.

• *Immunosuppressive Drugs.* Systemic immunosuppressive therapy may be required when animals fail to respond to corticosteroids or NSAIDs or when the required levels of these drugs result in systemic toxicity.

Specific

Specific therapy is dependent upon the etiology of the uveitis. See appropriate chapters for treatment of the systemic diseases that cause anterior uveitis.

SEQUELAE

■ *Secondary glaucoma* results from the obstruction of the outflow pathway of the aqueous humor. This can occur at the pupil from posterior synechia, at the drainage angle from anterior synechia, or in the trabecular meshwork from deposits of inflammatory debris and fibrosis. Control of this type of secondary glaucoma through medical therapy is often extremely difficult to achieve (see sec. 11, ch. 7).
■ *Synechiae* are adhesions from the iris to adjacent structures, such as the cornea or lens. Synechiae can result in abnormal pupillary light response, misshapen pupil, glaucoma, pigmentation of the cornea or lens, and blindness.
■ *Cataracts* can occur subsequent to anterior uveitis. The lens is dependent upon the aqueous humor for nutrients and waste product removal. Anterior uveitis results in altered lens metabolism and a buildup of inflammatory by-products that may cause opacification of the lens and capsule (cataract). The cataract that occurs secondary to intraocular inflammation is usually not amenable to surgical removal (see sec. 11, ch. 5).
■ *Corneal edema* occurs from the failure of the corneal endothelial cell pump/barrier. Corneal endothelial cells are responsible for the maintenance of corneal deturgesence, which is essential to corneal transparency. Endothelial cells need the aqueous humor for nutrients and waste product removal. Anterior uveitis may alter the function of these cells, resulting in diffuse corneal edema. Corneal endothelial cells in the adult dog and cat have little regenerative capabilities, thus damage may be permanent.
■ *Blindness* secondary to severe anterior uveitis is common and results from secondary glaucoma, cataract formation, synechia, pigment migration, or posterior segment (retina, choroid) changes.
■ *Phthisis bulbi* occurs as a result of atrophy of the ciliary body and a sustained decrease in aqueous humor production. Chronic hypotony (i.e., low IOP) results, and the eye decreases in size.

PREVENTION

Although prevention of anterior uveitis is usually not possible, the sequelae of anterior uveitis can be prevented by accurate diagnosis and appropriate and rapid treatment. Therapy directed towards the etiology will not only aid the management of the ocular disease but may also prevent the serious and life-threatening complications of the systemic disease.

Supplemental Readings

Blouin P: Uveitis in the dog and cat: Causes, diagnosis, and treatment. Can Vet J 25:315–323, 1984.
Crispin SM: Uveitis in the dog and cat. J Small Anim Pract 29:429–447, 1988.
Martin CL: Ocular signs of systemic disease. Mod Vet Pract 689–694, 799–804, 1982.
Morgan RV: Vogt-Koyanagi-Harada syndrome in humans and dogs. Compend Cont Ed Pract Vet 11:1211–1218, 1989.
Patnaik AK, Mooney S: Feline melanoma: A comparative study of ocular, oral, and dermal neoplasms. Vet Pathol 25:105–112, 1988.
Peiffer RL: Inherited ocular diseases of the dog and cat. Compend Cont Ed Pract Vet 4:152–165, 1982.
Swanson JF: Uveitis. *In* Kirk RW, ed: *Current Veterinary Therapy X.* Philadelphia: W.B. Saunders, 1989, pp 652–655.
Wilcock BP, Peiffer RL: The pathology of lens-induced uveitis. Vet Pathol 24:549–553, 1987.
Wilcock BP, Peiffer RL: Morphology and behavior of primary ocular melanomas in 91 dogs. Vet Pathol 23:418–424, 1986.

7 Glucoma

David A. Wilkie

Glaucoma is an increase in the intraocular pressure (IOP) beyond that compatible with maintenance of normal ocular physiology and function.

ANATOMY

See section 11, chapter 1.

ETIOLOGY

- *Primary glaucoma* is not associated with any other event or problem within the eye. It is usually breed related and often hereditary in nature. A list of predisposed breeds is given in Table 1.

KEY POINT ▶ When glaucoma is primary, it signifies that the opposite, unaffected eye is also at risk for developing glaucoma. Studies indicate an incidence of 50% involvement of the contralateral eye within 2 years following the diagnosis of glaucoma in the first eye.

- *Secondary glaucoma* is the result of an antecedent event within the eye. The etiologies of secondary glaucoma include anterior uveitis, anterior lens luxation, neoplasia, hyphema, and trauma.
  - *Anterior uveitis* can cause glaucoma through obstruction of the flow of aqueous humor. This results from peripheral anterior or posterior synechiae or from deposition of inflammatory debris in the iridocorneal angle. Anterior uveitis is discussed in detail in section 11, chapter 6.
  - *Anterior lens luxation* can obstruct the flow of aqueous humor from the posterior to the anterior chamber or to the iridocorneal angle. The etiologies of anterior lens luxation include hereditary (in terriers), neoplasia, anterior uveitis, and trauma (see sec. 11, ch. 5). Anterior lens luxation can also be the result of chronic glaucoma with enlargement of the globe (buphthalmos) and tearing of the lens zonules and secondary luxation.
  - *Intraocular neoplasia,* whether primary or secondary, can block the flow of the aqueous humor through the shedding of neoplastic cells into the iridocorneal angle or the displacing of normal intraocular structures (see sec. 11, ch. 6).
  - *Hyphema* can result from trauma, systemic hypertension, congenital ocular anomalies, vascular disorders, or bleeding disorders (see sec. 11, ch. 6). Red blood cells can obstruct the trabecular mesh-work of the iridocorneal angle resulting in glaucoma.
  - *Trauma* can result in anterior uveitis, anterior lens luxation, hyphema, or damage to the iridocorneal angle, all of which may lead to secondary glaucoma.

CLINICAL SIGNS

- *Acute glaucoma* is a true medical and possibly a surgical emergency. A diagnosis of acute glaucoma is made based on the history and clinical signs (Table 2). If in doubt, it is better to err on the side of a diagnosis of acute rather than chronic glaucoma.
- *Chronic glaucoma* implies the presence of ophthalmic changes that have resulted in the irreversible loss of vision (Table 3). The clinical changes most indicative of chronic glaucoma are retinal and optic nerve degeneration and buphthalmos.

DIAGNOSIS

KEY POINT ▶ Although the history, breed, and clinical signs are all important in the determination of glaucoma, the definitive diagnosis can be made only through measurement of the IOP.

Measurement of IOP requires a tonometer. The Schiøtz tonometer is the most useful for general practice. Digital tonometry had been advocated but is extremely inaccurate and unreliable. Normal IOP in the dog and cat is 15–25 mm Hg.

Once the diagnosis of glaucoma is made based on IOP, the etiology must be established (i.e., primary vs. secondary) and the degree of ocular damage assessed. Depending on the history and associated ocular changes, the glaucoma can be classified as either acute or chronic.

TREATMENT

KEY POINT ▶ In order to treat glaucoma appropriately, the clinician must answer two specific questions (Fig. 1). Is the glaucoma primary or secondary? Is the glaucoma acute or chronic?

Treatment can be grouped into medical and surgical approaches. If the glaucoma is acute, a return of a

TABLE 1. Breeds Predisposed to Primary Glaucoma

American and English Cocker spaniel
English Springer spaniel
Miniature poodle
Beagle
Basset hound
Siberian husky
Norwegian elkhound
Samoyed
Malamute
Chow Chow
Shar Pei
Afghan
Other

portion of, or all of, the animal's vision is then possible. In acute glaucoma, immediate aggressive medical therapy is required to reduce the IOP to within normal range. Failure of medical therapy to lower and maintain IOP at a normal level indicates the need for surgical intervention and the possible referral to a veterinary ophthalmologist.

The only treatment that is appropriate for chronic glaucoma is surgery, the goal of which is aimed primarily at reducing the IOP in order to relieve discomfort. The most cost-effective means of reducing IOP is surgery. The surgery of choice is either the placement of an intraocular silicone prosthesis or an enucleation.

Medical

Medical therapy of acute glaucoma includes some, or possibly all, of the following agents (Table 4). The decision as to which medications to choose varies according to the severity of the glaucoma, the etiology, and the response to the initial therapy.

■ *Osmotic agents* act to dehydrate the vitreous and aqueous humors and thereby decrease the IOP. In order to be effective, they require an intact blood-eye barrier and therefore do not work well in eyes with uveitis or hyphema.

KEY POINT ▶ The initial drug of choice for rapidly decreasing IOP in the treatment of acute glaucoma is an osmotic agent. The osmotic agent of choice is 20% mannitol, administered intravenously (Table 4).

Water is withheld from the animal for 3–4 hours following osmotic administration. The IOP begins decreasing within 20 minutes, with the maximum effect at 2 hours—the duration of effect is approximately 6

TABLE 2. Clinical Signs of Acute Glaucoma

Episcleral hyperemia
Diffuse corneal edema
Dilated pupil
Slow-to-absent pupillary light response
Weak-to-absent menace response
Epiphora
Blepharospasm

TABLE 3. Clinical Signs of Chronic Glaucoma

Episcleral hyperemia
Diffuse corneal edema
Corneal striae
Dilated pupil
Absent pupillary light response
Absent menace response
Epiphora
Blepharospasm
Retinal degeneration
Optic nerve cupping
Buphthalmia

hours. An alternative osmotic agent is oral glycerin, but emesis is a frequent side effect.

■ *Carbonic anhydrase inhibitors* (CAIs) work to decrease the IOP by blocking the enzyme responsible for the active production of aqueous humor. The CAIs of choice, based on their efficacy and low frequency of side effects, are dichlorphenamide and methazolamide. These are administered orally q8–12h (see Table 4). In addition to the eye, carbonic anhydrase can be found in the kidney, red blood cells, and lungs. Potential side effects of oral carbonic anhydrase inhibitors include metabolic acidosis and hypokalemia, manifested as panting, depression, vomiting, diarrhea, and collapse. If any of these side effects are noted, CAI therapy is discontinued. Symptoms should resolve within 24 hours, and therapy can be reinstituted at a decreased dosage.

■ *Autonomic agents* include parasympathomimetics, sympathomimetics, and sympatholytics. All of these drugs are administered topically q8–12h (see Table 4). These drugs are synergistic and can, if needed, be applied to the same eye, provided their administration is 5–10 minutes apart.

• *Parasympathomimetics* result in contraction of the iris sphincter and ciliary body musculature. Contraction of the longitudinal ciliary musculature increases the outflow of aqueous humor. The parasympathomimetic of choice is 2% pilocarpine (see Table 4). Transient topical irritation is often exhibited following administration but resolves 24–48 hours following initiation of therapy. Parasympathomimetics are contraindicated in animals with active anterior uveitis that results in secondary glaucoma. Parasympathomimetics exacerbate the pain and symptoms of anterior uveitis.

• *Sympathomimetics* increase the outflow of aqueous humor. Their mechanism of action differs from that of the parasympathomimetics and the two are synergistic. The sympathomimetic agent of choice is 0.1% dipivefrin HCl (Propine), a prodrug of epinephrine (see Table 4). Alternately, 1.0% epinephrine HCl can be administered either alone or in combination with 2% pilocarpine (E-Pilo-2). Side effects are minimal and include mild topical irritation, which is avoided with the use of 0.1% dipivefrin HCl.

• *Sympatholytics* decrease the active production of aqueous humor. The sympatholytic agent of choice

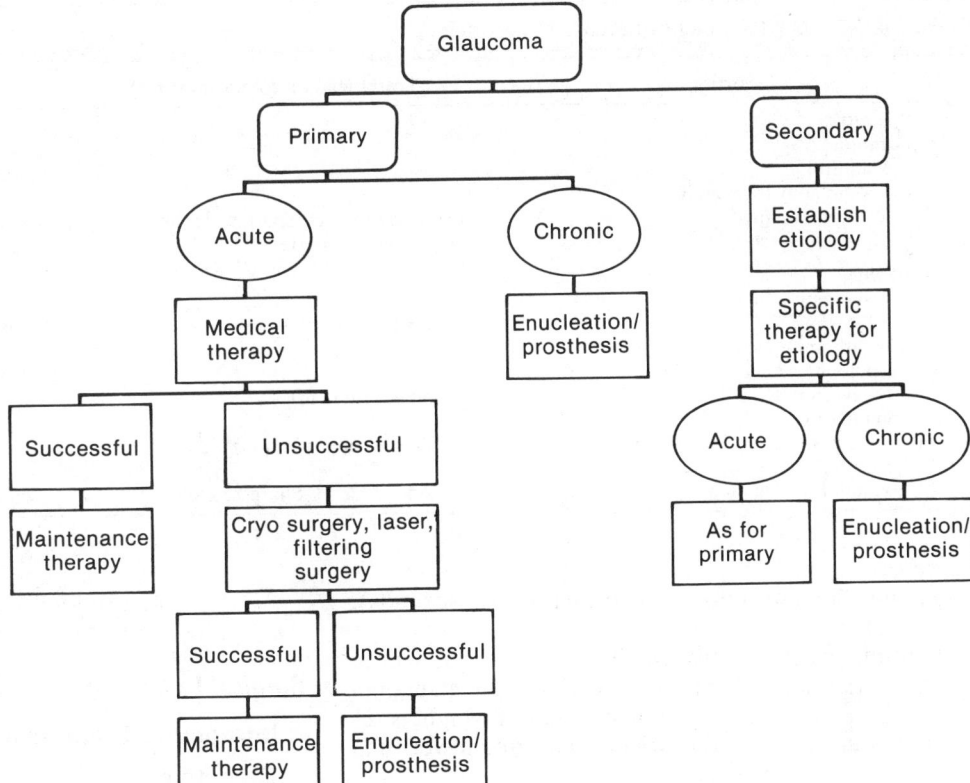

Figure 1. Treatment algorithm for glaucoma.

is a nonselective beta-blocking agent, 0.5% timolol maleate (Timoptic). Although disagreement exists over the efficacy of topical timolol maleate in small animal patients, information indicates that it has some IOP lowering ability. Side effects have not been observed in small animals, but potentially systemic absorption could cause bronchoconstriction and bradycardia, both of which are side effects in humans.

Plan of Action for Medical Treatment

When presented with a patient with acute glaucoma, mannitol is administered first, followed by maintenance therapy with an oral CAI and topical pilocarpine, provided no contraindications for these medications are present. The IOP is monitored every 2–4 hours for the next 24 hours. If, following the initial reduction in IOP with mannitol, the IOP increases and exceeds 30 mm Hg, mannitol therapy can be repeated. Medical therapy can be increased to include all of the aforementioned topical medications. When administering multiple topical medications, space each treatment 5 minutes apart. The failure of this aggressive, maximal therapy to lower and maintain IOP within the normal range indicates the need for surgical intervention.

Surgical

- *Cyclocryosurgery* involves the transscleral freezing of a portion of the ciliary body. This procedure is designed to selectively destroy an area of the ciliary processes, thereby decreasing the production of aqueous humor. It works best in conjunction with medical therapy and is indicated primarily in the

case of an acute glaucomatous eye in which IOP is not effectively controlled with medical therapy alone.

Surgical Procedure

Cyclocryosurgery

Objectives
- Reduce the intraocular pressure to a level compatible with maintaining vision.
- Relieve the discomfort associated with glaucoma.

Equipment
- Liquid nitrogen *or* nitrous oxide cryogen unit with an ocular probe, 2.5 mm in diameter.

Technique

1. The animal is anesthetized and placed in lateral recumbency. A single dose of systemic flunixin meglumine (Banamine) is administered 0.25 mg/kg IV. Systemic flunixin meglumine is not used in combination with methoxyflurane anesthesia, because this step may exacerbate its renal toxicity.
2. An eyelid speculum is used to obtain adequate exposure of the globe (Fig. 2).
3. The cryoprobe is placed on the conjunctiva, 4–5 mm posterior to the limbus, in the superior or inferior temporal quadrant of the eye (Fig. 2). Care is taken to avoid the long posterior ciliary arteries found at the 3- and 9-o'clock positions.
4. The cryoprobe is activated, and the site is frozen. The actual freezing time varies according to the cryounit. Approximate freeze times and probe tip temperatures are for nitrous oxide, 2 minutes, −60 to −80°C, and for liquid nitrogen, until the ice ball

TABLE 4. Medical Treatment of Acute Glaucoma

Drug	Trade Names (Manufacturer)	Dosages
Systemic		
Osmotic Drugs		
Mannitol		0.5–1.0 gm/kg, IV
Carbonic anhydrase inhibitors		
Dichlorphenamide	Daranide (Merck Sharp & Dohme)	2–4 mg/kg, q8–12h, PO
Methazolamide	Neptazane (Lederle)	2–4 mg/kg, q8–12h, PO
Topical		
Parasympathomimetics		
Pilocarpine 2%	Isopto Carpine (Alcon)	q8–12h
Sympathomimetics		
Epinephrine 1%		q8–12h
Dipivefrin HCl 0.1%	Propine (Allergan)	q8–12h
Combination		
Pilocarpine 2%: Epinephrine 1%	E-Pilo-2 (Cooper/Vision)	q8–12h
Sympatholytics		
Timolol maleate 0.5%	Timoptic (Merck Sharp & Dohme)	q8–12h

extends 1 mm into the cornea (<30 seconds), −185°C.

5. Multiple sites are frozen. The number of freeze sites varies according to the severity of the glaucoma and the cryoprobe. In general, four to eight sites are frozen with liquid nitrogen, requiring fewer than does nitrous oxide.

Following surgery, the IOP is monitored. Medical therapy for glaucoma is prescribed, based on the response of the IOP to cryosurgery. Any postoperative discomfort is controlled using oral nonsteroidal anti-inflammatory drugs, such as aspirin (10 mg/kg PO bid).

- *Laser surgery* (cyclocoagulation) has been advocated for the control of canine glaucoma. The laser used is a neodymium:yttrium-aluminum-garnet laser (Nd:YAG). The energy is delivered transsclerally, resulting in ciliary body atrophy and fibrosis. The production of aqueous humor is consequently reduced. The indications for cyclocoagulation are similar to those for cyclocryosurgery, but it is thought that cyclocoagulation has fewer intraocular side effects than cyclocryosurgery. The cost of the Nd:YAG laser and the skill required to use it result in this surgery being a referral procedure exclusively.
- *Filtering procedures* are designed to provide an alternate outflow pathway for the aqueous humor. The aqueous is usually redirected to the subconjunctival tissue space through either a filtering hole or an implantation of a filtering device. Although the initial success with this procedure may be high, most filtering procedures ultimately fail owing to fibrosis of the new outflow pathway. Filtering procedures work best in conjunction with medical and surgical therapies and for a short time only. Animals requiring a filtering procedure are referred to an appropriate specialist.

KEY POINT ▶ This procedure is indicated only for chronic glaucomatous eyes that are irreversibly blind. Intraocular prosthetic implants are contraindicated in cases of intraocular neoplasia, infectious panophthalmitis, and midstromal or deeper corneal ulceration.

Surgical Procedure

Intraocular Prosthesis

Objectives
- Relieve pain associated with chronic glaucoma
- Maintain cosmetic appearance of the eye

Equipment
- Routine ocular surgical pack with a cyclodialysis spatula
- Sterile intraocular silicone implant (Jardon Corp. Southfield, MI 48076). The implant is 2 mm larger than the horizontal dimension of the cornea of the normal eye. In the dog, a 19-mm prosthesis generally is satisfactory.
- Sphere introducer

Technique

1. The animal is anesthetized and placed in lateral recumbency. Systemic flunixin meglumine is administered as discussed in the cryosurgery section.
2. An eyelid speculum is used to obtain adequate exposure of the globe.
3. An incision is made in the superior conjunctiva, 4–5 mm posterior to the limbus (Fig. 3A). The incision is continued 120° around the globe.
4. The conjunctival and episcleral tissues are dissected to the level of the sclera.
5. An incision is made in the superior sclera, 4–5 mm posterior to the limbus.
6. A cyclodialysis spatula is introduced into the globe between the fibrous and vascular tunics and is used to gently separate these tunics. Care is taken to avoid injury to the cornea (Fig. 3B).
7. The scleral incision is enlarged (Fig. 3C).
8. The intraocular contents are removed (Fig. 3D), leaving only the fibrous tunic (cornea and sclera).
9. The silicone implant is placed within the globe.
10. The sclera and conjunctival tissues are closed with 6-0 absorbable suture (e.g., Vicryl, Ethicon) in

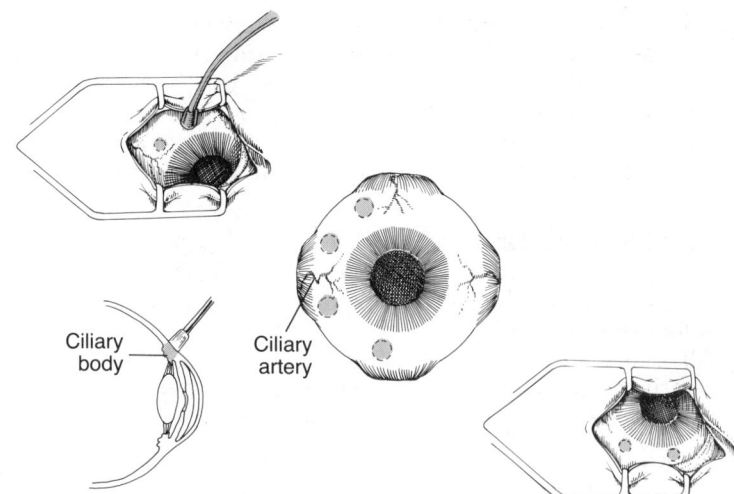

Figure 2. Cryosurgery selectively destroys portions of the ciliary body (at areas indicated) and effects a decrease in the production of aqueous humor. Take care to avoid freezing the long posterior ciliary arteries.

Ciliary body

Ciliary artery

simple interrupted and simple continuous patterns, respectively.

Postoperative Care

■ Topical, broad-spectrum antibiotic ointment 4 times per day
■ Warm, moist compresses twice daily for 5–7 days
■ Systemic nonsteroidal anti-inflammatory agents as required
■ As the surgical procedure removes the aqueous humor (the primary source of corneal nutrition) the cornea will vascularize over the 2–4 weeks following surgery.
■ Evaluate the eye 2 weeks after surgery. Note the progression of corneal vascularization and the absence of corneal ulceration. Determine the IOP in the contralateral eye of patients with primary glaucoma at this time.

KEY POINT ▶ An enucleation is indicated in the animal with eyes with chronic glaucoma that is irreversibly blind and in which an intraocular prosthetic implant is contraindicated.

Surgical Procedure

Enucleation

Objectives
■ Relieve the pain associated with glaucoma

Equipment
■ Routine ocular surgical pack

Technique

1. The eyelids are aseptically prepared and sutured closed.
2. The skin is incised 5–6 mm away from the eyelid margin 360° around the eyelids. Using sharp dissection, the incision is continued to the level of the extraocular muscles.
3. The extraocular muscles are severed at their attachment to the sclera.

4. The optic nerve and blood vessels are clamped and severed and the pedicle is ligated with 3-0 to 4-0 absorbable suture.
5. If desired, insertion of an intraorbital silicone prosthesis to minimize the postsurgical "sunken" appearance of the orbit can be performed at this time. A 24- to 34-mm prosthesis is used, nearly filling the orbital space.

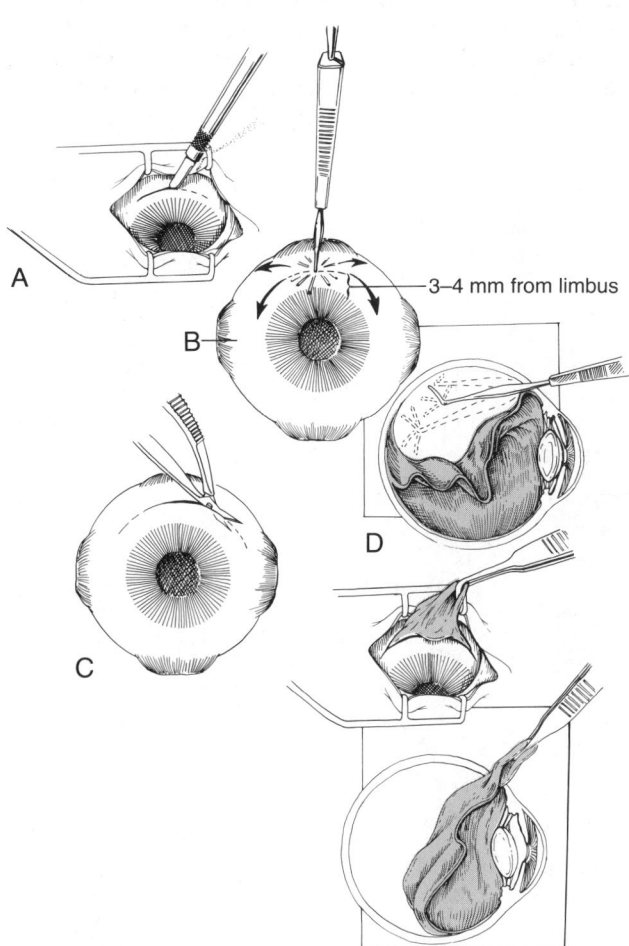

A

B — 3–4 mm from limbus

D

C

Figure 3. Preparation of globe for intraocular prosthesis. See text for details.

6. The extraocular muscles, periorbita, subcutaneous tissues, and skin are closed in a routine manner. The orbital space and subcutaneous tissues are closed utilizing continuous 4-0 absorbable sutures and the skin is closed utilizing 5-0 or 6-0 nonabsorbable sutures in an interrupted or continuous pattern.

Postoperative Care

■ Postoperative systemic antibiotics are indicated for eyes enucleated for infectious panophthalmitis or penetrating keratitis.

■ All enucleated eyes are submitted to a qualified veterinary pathologist for examination.

■ Sutures are removed 10–14 days following surgery.

Pharmacologic ablation, in my opinion, is an unacceptable method for the management of glaucoma. It involves the intravitreal injection of a substance toxic to the eye in the hope that this approach will result in the destruction of the ciliary body, thereby lowering the intraocular pressure. This is an irreversible, inaccurate, and sometimes painful procedure. In addition, the end result is usually a noncosmetic phthisic globe, often requiring enucleation.

PREVENTION

■ Evaluate IOP in all breeds predisposed to the development of primary glaucoma, as part of the routine yearly physical examination. A sustained, gradual increase in IOP, even if still within normal limits, is sufficient cause to initiate preventive topical therapy.

■ An animal with primary glaucoma in one eye is examined for the IOP in the opposite eye, two to three times per year.

■ An animal with primary glaucoma in one eye receives preventive treatment in the opposite eye. This can consist of a systemic CAI administered to control the affected eye, which will also lower the IOP in the opposite eye. Alternatively, the unaffected eye may be treated topically, if systemic CAI's are not required for the affected eye.

■ All eyes with lens luxation or subluxation, anterior uveitis, or hyphema must have the IOP determined. If possible, the primary problem is eliminated in an effort to avoid secondary glaucoma.

Supplemental Readings

Brooks DE, Dziezyc J: The canine glaucomas: Pathogenesis, diagnosis, and treatment. Compend Cont Ed Pract Vet 5:292, 1983.

Nasisse MP, Davidson MG, MacLachlan NJ, et al.: Neodymium:yttrium, aluminum, and garnet laser energy delivered transsclerally to the ciliary body of dogs. Am J Vet Res 49:1972, 1988.

Ridgway MD, Brightman AH: Feline glaucoma: A retrospective study of 29 clinical cases. J Am Anim Hosp Assoc 25:485, 1989.

Roberts SM, Severin GA, Lavach JD: Cyclocryotherapy—Part I. Evaluation of a liquid nitrogen system. J Am Anim Hosp Assoc 20:823, 1984.

Roberts SM, Severin GA, Lavach JD: Cyclocryotherapy—Part II. Clinical comparison of liquid nitrogen and nitrous oxide cryotherapy on glaucomatous eyes. J Am Anim Hosp Assoc 20:828, 1984.

Whitley RD, Shaffer KW, Albert RA: Implantation of intraocular silicone prosthesis in dogs. Compend Cont Ed Pract Vet 7:802, 1985.

8 Diseases of the Retina, Choroid, and Optic Nerve

Nicholas J. Millichamp
Joan Dziezyc

EVALUATION OF THE POSTERIOR SEGMENT

The posterior segment of the eye includes the vitreous humor; the retina and its vasculature; and the choroid, sclera, and optic nerve. The fundus is the portion of the posterior segment that can be seen with an ophthalmoscope. Considerable variation exists in the appearance of the normal fundus in the dog and cat. To fully appreciate subtle differences in normal fundi, consult available atlases detailing their appearance.

Generally, the fundus is divided into the brightly colored and reflective tapetal region, occupying the upper and more temporal area, and the darkly pigmented nontapetal region, occupying the lower area and completely surrounding the tapetal area. Apart from these fundic regions, examine the retinal blood vessels and the optic nerve head (optic disc).

Ophthalmoscopy is the technique used to examine the fundus. The technique is ideally performed after dilating the pupil (except in an animal with ocular hypertension, glaucoma, or lens luxation), with a short-acting parasympatholytic drug such as tropicamide hydrochloride (Mydriacyl 0.5%, Alcon).

- *Direct ophthalmoscopy* with a hand-held ophthalmoscope is commonly used in practice. Unfortunately, this technique yields limited information about the fundic appearance even in the hands of experienced ophthalmologists. Small lesions and variations in contrast between normal and abnormal areas of the fundus are often overlooked when utilizing the direct technique.
- *Indirect ophthalmoscopy,* utilizing a 20D planoconvex lens held 2–3 inches from the animal's eye and illuminated with a penlight held at arm's length from the animal, is more useful as a diagnostic technique.

KEY POINT ▶ Indirect ophthalmoscopy enables the examiner to quickly scan a large area of the fundus and to recognize obvious lesions.

- *Ocular ultrasonography* is utilized to evaluate the structures of the posterior segment when opacities of the ocular media prevent an ophthalmoscopic examination.
- *Electroretinography* employs a light stimulus of varying intensity and frequency to elicit a retinal response from rod and/or cone photoreceptors. This test evaluates the functional integrity of the retina and is a procedure that requires referral to the appropriate specialist.

DISEASE OF THE VITREOUS HUMOR

The vitreous is a gel comprised mostly of water with lesser quantities of mucopolysaccharides and proteins. The normal adult vitreous is transparent and lacks blood vessels. The vitreous cannot itself become inflamed. However, products of inflammation or other abnormalities of adjacent tissues can result in exudate or hemorrhage that enter the vitreous and are seen by ophthalmoscopy.

Etiology

- *Retention of the fetal hyaloid artery* or its remnants may be seen in an adult dog as a fine gray strand arising from the optic disc or inserting onto the posterior pole of the lens.
- *Persistent hyperplastic primary vitreous/persistent tunica vasculosa lentis* is inherited in some breeds, notably the Doberman pinscher. The hyaloid artery is retained and is hyperplastic and associated with vessels that ramify over the posterior lens surface. Blood vessels and associated posterior lens capsular pigmentation and opacities (cataracts) or intralenticular hemorrhage is observed clinically. Surgical therapy yields poor results. Discourage the use of these animals for breeding.
- *Asteroid hyalosis* is a unilateral or bilateral degenerative change associated with aging in dogs. Calcium-lipid complexes are deposited on the vitreous protein matrix. These appear as multiple white sparkles that oscillate slightly with eye movements. Asteroid hyalosis does not significantly impair vision, and no treatment is indicated.
- *Cholesterosis bulbi* or synchysis scintillans is a less common entity in which white cholesterol crystals are deposited in the vitreous secondary to intraocular inflammation. The vitreous often will become liquefied *(syneresis)* as a result of posterior segment inflammation. The cholesterol deposits sink to the bottom of the vitreous cavity. When the eye moves, the deposits swirl in the liquid vitreous, before settling again under gravity. The initial cause of

ocular inflammation and vitreous liquefaction may often have subsided by the time cholesterosis bulbi is detected. Vision is not affected by the cholesterosis bulbi per se, although it may be compromised by the underlying inflammatory disease.

- *Vitreous hemorrhage* most commonly occurs in the dog and cat as a sequel to ocular trauma, intraocular surgery, retinal detachment, or systemic coagulopathy. If the hemorrhage is severe, blindness may result.
- *Exudate and cellular infiltrate* appear as hazy, white, or gray material in the vitreous or on the posterior capsule of the lens. Pigment may also be deposited in the vitreous. Cellular infiltrate may become dense enough to obscure a view of the retina. Anterior uveitis or chorioretinitis is investigated.
- Other possible vitreous opacities include posterior lens luxation; retinal detachment; foreign bodies; parasites *(Dirofilaria)*; and neoplasms arising from the ciliary body, retina, choroid, or optic nerve.

Clinical Signs

KEY POINT ▶ Opacities of this otherwise clear medium are the most commonly observed clinical findings that indicate disease of the vitreous.

The effect on the animal's vision depends upon the severity and density of the opacities.

Diagnosis

- *Ophthalmoscopic examination* with a focal light source (penlight) or an ophthalmoscope will reveal the nature of the opacities (asteroid hyalosis, hemorrhage, pigment).
- *A blood clotting profile* is indicated when vitreous hemorrhage occurs unassociated with ocular trauma or intraocular surgery.
- *Physical examination, complete blood count,* and *serum biochemistry* and *serology evaluations* for infectious inflammatory disease (see Chorioretinitis) are performed in cases in which vitreous exudate or cellular infiltrate is seen.
- *Ultrasonography* is indicated in ruling out a diagnosis of coexisting retinal detachment, posterior segment neoplasia, or foreign bodies.

Treatment

- *Vitreous hemorrhage* resorbs slowly over the course of several weeks. Coagulopathy is treated systemically when possible.
- *Exudate and infiltrate* decrease by treating the underlying inflammatory disease with systemic antibacterial, antifungal, and anti-inflammatory drugs (NSAIDs), as indicated. Corticosteroids can be used in dogs and cats once infectious etiologies are ruled out (prednisone or prednisolone, 1–2 mg/kg, q12–24h, PO). Nonsteroidal anti-inflammatory drugs (aspirin, 25 mg/kg, q12h, PO in dogs only) often improves ocular inflammatory disease.

CONGENITAL CHORIORETINAL AND OPTIC NERVE DISEASES

Etiology

Many of these diseases occur most frequently in dogs and are inherited. Other possible congenital causes include inflammation and necrosis in the developing retina *in utero* due to infectious diseases, radiation, and teratogens.

- *Collie eye anomaly (CEA)* is a disorder that occurs commonly in collies and less often in Shetland sheepdogs and some other breeds. CEA affects the retinal pigment epithelium; the choroid; and, in severe cases, the retina and optic nerve. The disease is usually asymmetric in the two eyes. The most characteristic lesion is choroidal hypoplasia, which appears as a pale area of fundus temporal to the optic nerve. The lesion is one of depigmentation of the retinal pigment epithelium and choroid, exposing hypoplastic choroidal blood vessels overlying the sclera. Occasionally, hazy white corneal opacities accompany the chorioretinal lesions. In severe cases, colobomata (a gap or hole due to incomplete development) may occur in the optic nerve or choroid. Retinal detachment or intraocular hemorrhage is found in the most severe cases.

KEY POINT ▶ The developmental abnormalities do not worsen after birth. Retinal detachment associated with optic nerve colobomata, however, may occur at any age.

- *Retinal or vitreoretinal dysplasia* occurs in cats and dogs. The disease may be inherited (often recessively) in the dog or may be a sequel to intrauterine infection (canine herpesvirus, feline panleukopenia). In the dog, inherited retinal dysplasia may be manifested as bilaterally asymmetric, small focal folds in the outer layers of the retina that do not result in retinal elevation. These folds are observed in the cocker spaniel and the Labrador retriever. The folds may appear as small dark dots, streaks, or circles in the tapetal fundus and gray or dark spots or streaks in the nontapetal fundus. In some breeds (Sealyham and Bedlington terriers, Labrador retrievers, springer spaniel), the lesion is severe, and the dog is blinded by the retina lying unattached in abnormally formed vitreous.
- *Multiple ocular anomalies* are seen most commonly in Australian sheepdogs. Affected animals may have microphthalmia, iris colobomas, cataracts, retinal dysplasia or detachment, and uvea-lined defects (staphylomas) in the sclera.
- *Optic nerve hypoplasia* if bilateral may be noted by breeders or owners in animals a few weeks old. Affected eyes lack pupillary light reflexes and are blind. Ophthalmoscopy reveals a small optic nerve head with normal retinal vasculature.

Clinical Signs

Vision may be affected in dogs with severe congenital lesions. The pupillary light reflexes may also be varialy affected, depending upon the severity of the lesions.

Diagnosis

Congenital abnormalities of the fundus are most readily diagnosed by the ophthalmoscopic appearance at 4 to 8 weeks of age.

Treatment and Prevention

The mode of transmission in the inherited diseases is often as an autosomal recessive trait (e.g., CEA and retinal dysplasia in most breeds). Intrauterine infections are prevented by vaccination of breeding animals and by avoidance of infection and exposure of pregnant animals to ionizing radiation and teratogenic toxins.

KEY POINT ▶ There is no treatment for congenital chorioretinal disease, although breeding affected dogs must be discouraged.

ACQUIRED CHORIORETINAL AND OPTIC NERVE DISEASE

Chorioretinal Degeneration

Etiology and Clinical Features

- *Progressive retinal atrophy (PRA)* includes several genetic retinal diseases in which the ultimate outcome is degeneration and loss of retinal structure with varying degrees of blindness. The different forms of PRA are all progressive and bilaterally symmetric. The disease occurs commonly in many pure breed and mix breed dogs. The inheritance in most instances in the dog is autosomal recessive. PRA also occurs in various breeds of cat, although it has been best characterized in the Abyssinian.
- PRA may primarily affect the photoreceptors (rods/cones) or the adjacent layer of retinal pigment epithelium. Pigment epithelial dystrophy or central PRA, which occurs in Europe is extremely rare in the United States. PRA affecting the rods or cones can be distinguished by the age of onset. In early onset PRA (rod, rod-cone dysplasias), affected dogs show signs of night blindness during the first year of life. Affected breeds include the collie, Irish setter, miniature schnauzer, elkhound, miniature dachshund. In late onset PRA (progressive rod-cone degeneration), night blindness may be noticed at any age from 1 year until several years. Breeds affected include the miniature poodle, Cocker spaniel, and Labrador retriever. The typical ophthalmoscopic appearance of diffuse retinal degeneration is an increased reflectance of light from the tapetal fundus (tapetal hyper-reflectivity). Retinal blood vessels are narrowed or lost, and depigmentation and patchy hyperpigmentation in the nontapetal fundus may be seen. In advanced cases, atrophy of the optic nerve occurs.
- *Sudden acquired retinal degeneration (SARD)* is a degeneration of the retina that occurs in dogs. The basic defect that causes the degeneration is unknown.

Dogs of any age that are otherwise normal may be affected. Obese, middle-aged dogs are most prone to the disorder. The most characteristic feature of SARD is the rapid and complete loss of vision, often within a few days or at most weeks. The disease usually affects both eyes equally.

KEY POINT ▶ The photoreceptors are ultrastructurally abnormal at the time when blindness is first noted, although the fundus appears ophthalmoscopically normal.

Ophthalmoscopic signs of retinal degeneration (tapetal hyper-reflectivity, vascular attenuation) appear over several months. The electroretinogram is extinguished at the time of presentation, which distinguishes the disease from optic neuritis, pituitary neoplasia, and CNS blindness.

- *Nutritional deficiency* or taurine deficiency in the cat, especially in the cat fed dog food that is deficient in taurine (an essential amino acid in the cat), results in feline central retinal degeneration. The typical early lesion is a focal area of tapetal hyper-reflectivity in the temporal fundus. With progression of the lesion, a similar area appears nasally and the two patches join to form a horizontal band above the optic disc. Continued deficiency results in diffuse atrophy throughout the retina. Restoration of a taurine-rich diet halts the degeneration in the early stages, although the fundic lesion remains visible throughout the cat's life. Cats with taurine deficiency rarely show any evidence of blindness until the disease is advanced. For discussion of the cardiac effects of taurine deficiency in cats, see section 6, chapter 8.
- *Chronic glaucoma* results in diffuse retinal atrophy because of ischemia and pressure necrosis of initially the inner and later the outer retina (see sec. 11, Ch. 7).
- *Inflammation* that subsides or is successfully treated often results in focal lesions of chorioretinal degeneration in the affected areas. These appear as focal hyper-reflective areas in the tapetal fundus or depigmented areas in the nontapetum. Vision is affected to an extent commensurate with the area and region of the fundus involved (central vs. peripheral retina).

Clinical Signs

- *Blindness* is a characteristic feature of retinal degeneration. Night blindness may be noted first in PRA that progresses to complete visual loss. Blindness may be sudden when caused by SARD and slowly progressive when caused by glaucoma.
- *Mydriasis* may be observed. Pupillary light reflexes may be incomplete and sluggish in advanced cases of PRA and can be absent in SARD.

Diagnosis

- *Ophthalmoscopy* allows the diagnosis of retinal degeneration when typical lesions are present.
- *Electroretinography (ERG)* may help one to make a diagnosis of PRA before typical ophthalmoscopic signs are seen and to confirm a diagnosis of SARD.

The ERG is a test of retinal function for which referral to an ophthalmology center is necessary.

Treatment

No treatment is available for PRA or SARD. Chorioretinal degeneration due to glaucoma (see sec. 11, ch. 7) or inflammation (see Chorioretinitis) can be limited by controlling the primary disease process. A deficiency of taurine in the diet can be corrected to halt progression of the disease (see sec. 6, ch. 8).

Prevention

Progressive retinal atrophy in either dogs or cats can be prevented by selective breeding of unaffected dogs and of those dogs believed not to be carriers of the PRA gene. All purebred dogs used for breeding are evaluated yearly by a board-certified veterinary ophthalmologist and registered through the Canine Eye Registry Foundation (CERF) as phenotypically normal.

Chorioretinitis

Chorioretinitis is inflammation of the retina and choroid. Although inflammation may begin in either of the two layers, their proximity often results in spread and involvement of both. Clinically, the differentiation is of little importance.

Etiology

Numerous causes of, or diseases associated with, chorioretinitis are recognized in the dog and cat. Chorioretinitis may develop as an extension of anterior uveitis (see sec. 11, ch. 6) or as an isolated entity. Systemic diseases that can cause unilateral or bilateral chorioretinitis are listed in Tables 1 and 2. Refer also to the appropriate chapters elsewhere in this book for specifics on these diseases.

Clinical Signs

- *Vision* may be affected in severe cases of chorioretinitis, especially with concurrent optic nerve inflammation. In mild cases of chorioretinitis, visual deficits may not be noticed.
- *The tapetal fundus* areas of chorioretinal exudate or edema appear as hazy gray areas that may have discrete borders and appear elevated. If cellular infiltrate is also present, the areas may appear darker and obscure the underlying tapetum.
- *The nontapetal fundus* areas of exudate or cellular infiltrate appear gray or white. Perivascular cuffing appears as a hazy white border to retinal vessels.
- *Hemorrhages* may be seen at various depths in the retina.
- *Exudative retinal detachments* may occur.
- *Associated ocular disease* may include anterior uveitis (see sec. 11, ch. 6) and exudate or hemorrhage in the vitreous.

Diagnosis

KEY POINT ▶ The presence of either unilateral or bilateral chorioretinitis indicates a systemic disease until proved otherwise.

TABLE 1. Diseases Associated with Chorioretinitis in Dogs

Viral	Distemper
Fungal	Blastomycosis
	Coccidioidomycosis
	Cryptococcosis
	Histoplasmosis
	Aspergillosis
	Geotrichosis
Bacterial	*Brucella canis*
	Borrelia burgdorferi
Algal	Protothecosis
Rickettsial	Ehrlichiosis
	Rocky Mountain spotted fever
Parasitic	Toxoplasmosis
	Neosporum caninum
	Leishmaniasis
	Migrating fly larvae
	Toxocara canis larva migrans
Immune-mediated	Autoimmune chorioretinitis
	Uveodermatologic syndrome
Neoplastic	Lymphosarcoma
	Multiple myeloma
	Metastatic neoplasia
Toxic	Miscellaneous toxins (often undiagnosed)

- *Physical examination* is concentrated on finding any evidence of inflammatory or neoplastic disease elsewhere in the body.
- *Evaluate complete blood count, serum biochemistry profile, and urinalysis* for evidence of underlying systemic disease.
- *Evaluate thoracic and abdominal radiography* for evidence of systemic mycosis or neoplasia.
- *Evaluate serology* to rule in or out the various infectious causes of chorioretinitis as described in the chapters on viral diseases, systemic mycoses, and toxoplasmosis.
- *Evaluate lymph node aspirate and skin biopsy samples* in animals with lymphadenopathies or cutaneous lesions.
- *Evaluate vitreous by paracentesis* for cytology and culture, but *only as a last resort* in cases in which al

TABLE 2. Diseases Associated with Chorioretinitis in Cats

Viral	Feline infectious peritonitis
	Feline leukemia virus
	Feline immunodeficiency virus
Bacterial	Tuberculosis
Fungal	Blastomycosis
	Cryptococcosis
	Histoplasmosis
Parasitic	Toxoplasmosis
	Migrating fly larvae
Immune-mediated	Autoimmune chorioretinitis
Neoplastic	Lymphosarcoma
	Metastatic neoplasia
Toxic	Miscellaneous toxins (often undiagnosed)

other less invasive systemic diagnostic techniques have been performed and the eye is irreversibly blind.

Treatment

The retina and choroid are inaccessible to most topical medications.

KEY POINT ▶ To effectively treat chorioretinitis, drugs must be given systemically.

Underlying systemic disease is treated appropriately (as described in the appropriate chapters in this book). If all evidence of infectious disease is ruled out, systemic corticosteroids or NSAIDs are given to control the inflammation. Additional therapy with immunosuppressive drugs, such as azothiaprine (Imuran) may be indicated in immune-mediated chorioretinitis (see sec. 11, ch. 6).

Retinovascular Disease

The retinal or choroidal vasculature may be affected in the aforementioned congenital chorioretinal diseases, retinal degenerations, and chorioretinitis. Vascular disease also may occur unrelated to these other entities.

Etiology

- *Coagulopathies,* including canine ehrlichiosis, warfarin and aspirin toxicity, von Willebrand's disease, autoimmune hemolytic anemia, and immune-mediated thrombocytopenia in dogs, may cause retinal hemorrhage (see sec. 3, ch. 2).
- *Systemic hypertension* in dogs and cats may result in retinal hemorrhage and transudative retinal detachment (see sec. 6, ch. 11).
- *Congenital cardiac anomalies* may cause engorgement of retinal venules (see sec. 6, ch. 12).
- *Hyperviscosity syndrome* due to macroglobulinemia in dogs with myelomas and polycythemia causes engorgement of the retinal blood vessels (see sec. 6, ch. 1).
- *Anemia* in cats has been associated with retinal hemorrhage.
- *Hyperlipidemia* in cats and dogs results in pink-colored retinal blood vessels.

Clinical Signs

Retinal and vitreous hemorrhage and retinal detachment may result in acute blindness and loss of the pupillary light reflex.

Diagnosis

- *Ophthalmoscopy* reveals retinal hemorrhage, vessel engorgement, increased tortuosity, and color change.
- *Clotting profile and complete blood count* assess clotting time, clotting factor deficiencies, thrombocytopenia, and anemia. Coagulopathies are described in section 3, chapter 2.
- *Blood pressure measurement* (see sec. 6, ch. 11) is indicated in any older dog or cat with retinal hemor-

rhage or detachment. Renal disease, cardiac disease, and hyperthyroidism are investigated in animals with hypertension (see appropriate chapters for each).

Treatment

Therapy in all acquired forms of retinovascular disease is directed at the underlying cause. In most cases, retinal hemorrhage resorbs spontaneously, during a few days to weeks, once the disease is under control.

Retinal Detachment

Retinal detachment is separation of the neural retina from the retinal pigment epithelium. Unilateral detachments may exist undetected.

KEY POINT ▶ Retinal detachments are often caused by systemic disease in dogs and cats.

Detachments may be partial or complete (infundibular) and arise near the periphery of the retina or adjacent to the optic nerve.

Etiology

- *Congenital developmental disease* includes both CEA and retinal dysplasia.
- *Inflammation* results in accumulations of serous fluid or cellular infiltrate or granulomas between the retina and retinal pigment epithelium, causing detachment. The same causes of chorioretinitis apply to retinal detachment (see Tables 1 and 2).
- *Hypertension* (see sec. 6, ch. 11) causes the accumulation of transudate within and beneath the retina.
- *Tears* in the retina associated with cataract formation, intraocular surgery, or liquefaction of the vitreous may allow vitreous to penetrate between the retina and RPE.
- *Traction* on the retina may result from fibrous tissue that forms in the retina or vitreous secondary to intraocular hemorrhage or chorioretinitis.
- *Neoplasia or granuloma* of the choroid or orbit may indent the sclera and detach the retina.
- *Ethylene glycol* toxicity in cats (see sec. 8, ch. 1) may result in serous retinal folding and detachment.

Clinical Signs

- *Sudden blindness* occurs if bilateral; visual deficits occur if unilateral, depending upon the extent of the detachment.
- *The pupil is often dilated,* and the pupillary light reflexes are weak to absent.
- *A translucent, folded, gray or white sheet of tissue* with retinal blood vessels may be observed behind the lens.

Diagnosis

- *Ophthalmoscopy* reveals focal retinal detachment. Complete retinal detachment can usually be seen clearly with a focal light source.
- *Blood pressure measurement* is performed to diagnose hypertension (see sec. 6, ch. 11).
- *Ultrasonography* may support the diagnosis of retinal

detachment in cases of intraocular neoplasia or hemorrhage. It is also indicated to detect retinal detachment in eyes with opacities of otherwise clear ocular media (cornea, lens, vitreous).

- *Serology* is indicated if infectious disease is suspected.

Treatment

- *Appropriate therapy for a systemic disease* (hypertension) once diagnosed sometimes results in retinal reattachment, especially if the detachment is not chronic. This response may result in a return of vision and is more likely in dogs than in cats.
- *Systemic corticosteroids* are used after infectious disease and hypertension have been diagnostically ruled out (see sec. 11, ch. 6).
- *Systemic NSAIDs* are indicated in retinal detachment, although avoided in cases associated with intraocular hemorrhage (see sec. 11, ch. 6).
- *Retinal reattachment surgery* is indicated in recent detachments associated with small retinal tears. This procedure is performed at some referral centers. In retinal detachments with 360° tears, surgery is not indicated.

ACQUIRED OPTIC NERVE DISEASE

The optic nerve may be involved in several chorioretinal diseases, including chorioretinitis and retinal degeneration.

Optic Neuritis

Optic neuritis is inflammation of the optic nerve. The condition may be recurrent in nature and often results in atrophy of the optic nerve and permanent blindness, regardless of therapy.

Etiology

- *Inflammatory and infectious etiologies* are similar to those causing CNS disease (see sec. 10, ch. 2) and chorioretinitis (see Tables 1 and 2).
- *Neoplasia* (canine GME, feline lymphosarcoma) affecting the CNS may cause optic neuritis (see sec. 10, ch. 2).
- *Ocular trauma* (ocular proptosis) causes optic neuritis.
- *Orbital inflammatory disease* may, in severe cases, result in optic neuritis.
- *Immune-mediated optic neuritis* may be presumed in cases in which no underlying systemic cause can be identified.
- *Miscellaneous toxins* may potentially cause optic neuritis, although diagnosis is rarely possible.

Clinical Signs

- *Acute blindness* is present with bilateral optic nerve involvement, although no visual deficit may be noted if the neuritis is unilateral.
- *Mydriasis* and absence of the pupillary light reflex are evident.

Diagnosis

- *Ophthalmoscopy* allows the diagnosis of intraocular optic neuritis and helps differentiate optic neuritis from retinal detachment as a cause of sudden blindness.
- *The optic disc appears hazy, elevated, and edematous.* The edema often radiates into the peripapillary retina when the inflammation involves the intraocular portion of the nerve. Hemorrhages may be present at the disc or in the adjacent retina or vitreous. Vitreous exudate may obscure the optic disc.
- *Ophthalmoscopic signs may not be present* if the neuritis does not involve the optic disc.
- *Chorioretinitis* can be a concurrent finding.
- *Electroretinography* is indicated to rule out SARD in cases in which the optic nerve appears normal.
- *Ultrasonography* can detect nerve swelling when the retrobulbar nerve is involved.
- *Neurologic examination* and cerebrospinal fluid (CSF) analysis are employed to diagnose concomitant neurologic disease (see sec. 10, ch. 1).
- *Evaluate the complete blood count and serology findings* for evidence of infectious etiologies.

Treatment

- Wherever possible, infectious etiologies are diagnosed and treated appropriately (see appropriate chapters).
- In cases in which infectious etiologies are ruled out, administer systemic corticosteroids (prednisone, 2 mg/kg q24h, PO). Failure to limit the inflammation results in optic atrophy and vision loss.

Papilledema

Papilledema is the bilateral swelling of the optic nerve, due to reduced blood and axoplasmic flow from the optic disc. The term is loosely applied in dogs and cats to any form of optic disc edema.

Etiology

- *Pressure applied to the optic nerve* by tumors or granulomas of the nerve or within the orbit can cause stasis of axoplasmic and optic nerve blood flow and can result in papilledema.
- *Neoplasia and inflammation of the CNS* can cause papilledema in dogs and cats by increasing CSF pressure and increasing pressure within and around the optic nerve.

Clinical Signs

- *Vision is usually unaffected.* However, blindness may occur in the absence of optic neuritis when inflammatory or neoplastic lesions significantly damage the central optic pathways, including the visual cortex (see sec. 11, ch. 11).

Diagnosis

- Attempt to differentiate papilledema from optic neuritis.
- *Ophthalmoscopic appearance of a swollen optic disc,*

usually with normal vision, is likely to indicate papilledema. This is unlike optic neuritis in which vision is affected.

- *The optic disc* protrudes into the vitreous. The retinal blood vessels leaving the optic disc appear to cascade over the edge of the disc. The margins of the optic disc appear hazy and indistinct. Hemorrhages may occasionally be observed in the adjacent retina.
- *Perform globe retropulsion* to determine whether a space-occupying lesion is present in the orbit.
- *Neurologic examination* can help localize CNS lesions.
- *Ultrasonography, radiology, and computed tomography (if available)* can be used to locate orbital space-occupying lesions.
- *Exploratory orbitotomy* is a difficult technique that can be employed to localize and diagnose any masses detected with the previous methods.

Treatment

- Because papilledema is often associated with CNS tumors, the prognosis is guarded to poor.
- Orbital tumors may occasionally be surgically removed during exploratory orbitotomy.
- *Exenteration of the eye and orbital contents* is indicated when a mass is localized near the globe.

Optic Nerve Atrophy

Atrophy of the optic nerve may occur as a sequel to other ocular diseases.

Etiology

- Advanced inherited retinal degenerations can occur.
- Glaucoma causing ischemia of the optic nerve at the scleral lamina cribrosa, resulting in atrophy and "cupping."
- Optic neuritis can be either severe or recurrent.
- Optic nerve trauma (traumatic ocular proptosis) can occur.
- Orbital inflammation or neoplasia may be noted.

Clinical Signs and Diagnosis

- Blindness is evident in the affected eye.
- The pupil is mydriatic, and the pupillary light reflexes are absent.
- Ophthalmoscopy confirms the diagnosis. The optic disc appears small and gray, with a loss of retinal blood vessels. The outline of the scleral lamina cribrosa may become visible, particularly in cats. In dogs, the margins of the disc may appear to spread from the disc owing to peripapillary gliosis (hypertrophy of neuronal supporting cells).

Treatment

No treatment is effective once the optic nerve undergoes atrophy.

NEOPLASIA OF THE POSTERIOR SEGMENT

Most tumors of the posterior segment in dogs and cats result from metastasis from other sites. The most common secondary tumor is malignant lymphoma. Primary tumors are rare but include malignant teratoid medulloepitheliomas, melanomas, and optic nerve meningiomas. Therapy entails enucleation or exenteration of the orbit, depending upon the localization of the tumor to the globe.

Supplemental Readings

Barnett KC: *Color Atlas of Veterinary Ophthalmology*. Baltimore: Williams & Wilkins, 1990.

Curtis R, Barnett KC: Canine posterior segment. *In* Gelatt KN, ed.: *Veterinary Ophthalmology*, 2nd ed. Philadelphia: Lea & Febiger, 1991.

Millichamp NJ: Retinal degeneration in the dog and cat. Vet Clin North Am [Sm Anim Pract] 20:799, 1990.

Rubin LF: *Atlas of Veterinary Ophthalmology*. Philadelphia: Lea & Febiger, 1974.

Rubin LF: Inherited eye diseases. *In Purebred Dogs*. Baltimore: Williams & Wilkins, 1989.

Slatter D: *Fundamentals of Veterinary Ophthalmology*, 2nd ed. Philadelphia: W.B. Saunders Company, 1990.

Walde I, Schäffer EH, Köstlin RG: *Atlas of Ophthalmology in Dogs and Cats*. Philadelphia: B.C. Decker Inc., 1990.

9 Diseases of the Lacrimal Apparatus

Renee L. Kaswan

Common disorders of the lacrimal apparatus include insufficient tearing (i.e., keratoconjunctivitis sicca), prolapse of the gland of the nictitating membrane (third eyelid), and overflow tearing (i.e., epiphora). Keratoconjunctivitis sicca (KCS) occurs when tear secretion is deficient, and the cornea and conjunctiva become desiccated. Aqueous tear deficiency leads to excessive mucus buildup; secondary bacterial conjunctivitis; recurrent corneal ulcers; corneal pigmentation, vascularization, and keratinization; and dense corneal scars. Traditionally a difficult disorder to manage, KCS has been one of the most frequent causes of canine visual loss. Introduction of topical cyclosporine (Optimmune; Scherig-Plough) promises to greatly reduce the morbidity of KCS and to increase the convenience of treatment.

Prolapse of the nictitating membrane gland is a cosmetic problem. The major significance of prolapse management is that the gland is replaced, not removed, to avoid KCS.

Epiphora, or overflow tearing, can be a cosmetic problem or an indication of ocular pain that requires the clinician to investigate its etiology. Irritation of the eye, distichiasis (eyelashes touching the eye), trichiasis (misdirected facial hairs touching the eye), entropion (inward rolling of the lid margin), and dacryocystitis (inflammatory blockage of the nasolacrimal drainage duct) cause epiphora.

ANATOMY AND PHYSIOLOGY

Lacrimal Glands

- There are two lacrimal glands in cats and dogs: the nictitans gland and the orbital lacrimal gland. They each produce approximately one half of the tear volume.
- The *nictitans gland* is the lacrimal gland of the nictitating membrane. The nictitans gland is wrapped around the vertical cartilage of the third eyelid (Fig. 1).
- The *orbital lacrimal gland* lies internal to the lateral orbital ligament, directly below the zygomatic process of the frontal bone.
- Parasympathetic innervation of the lacrimal gland originates with the trigeminal nerve, courses through the inner ear with the facial nerve, and distributes superficially as divisions of the facial nerve (see sec. 11, ch. 11).

Tear Film

- Tears provide the cornea with physical lubrication as well as essential proteins, vitamins, epithelial growth factors, and hormones. Because the cornea is avascular, the lacrimal glands have evolved to produce the nutrients and regulatory proteins necessary to sustain a healthy, transparent cornea.
- The tear film is composed of three transparent layers of fluid—inner mucus, middle aqueous, and outer lipid—which coat and protect the cornea.
- Tears flow from the excretory ducts of the lacrimal glands and coat all the exposed surfaces of the conjunctiva and cornea. The overflow exits through the nasolacrimal drainage system.

KERATOCONJUNCTIVITIS SICCA

Etiology

KEY POINT ▶ Despite a list of known etiologies of canine KCS (Table 1), in most animals KCS is considered to be either idiopathic or immune-mediated.

Serology has identified numerous KCS–affected dogs with positive rheumatoid factor, antinuclear antibodies, and hypergammaglobulinemia. Lacrimal gland biopsy specimens typically reveal multifocal to diffuse mononuclear cell infiltration, with varying degrees of fibrosis and atrophy. Paradoxically, many glands have few focal inflammatory lesions and large areas of apparently normal acinar tissue, except that the acinar cells have reduced numbers of secretory granules. These dysfunctional acini are the proposed target of cyclosporine intervention.

Clinical Signs

KEY POINT ▶ KCS is the most common cause of canine conjunctivitis. Misdiagnosed cases treated with virtually any topical medication will show transient improvement, however. Suspect KCS in any dog with chronic or recurrent conjunctivitis, keratitis, or corneal ulceration.

- Chronic mucoid-to-mucopurulent discharge is the hallmark of KCS. Secondary bacterial overgrowth

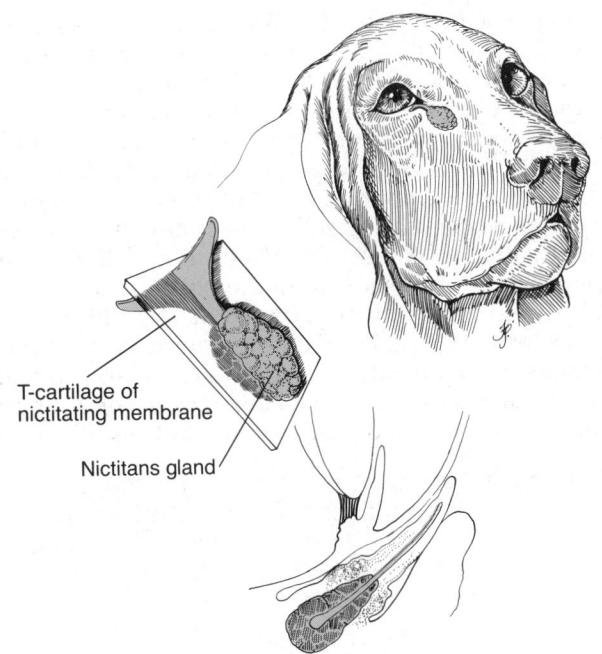

Figure 1. *In-situ* representation of the nictitans gland. Note how it wraps around the vertical cartilage of the nictitating membrane or third eyelid *(below)*.

T-cartilage of nictitating membrane

Nictitans gland

may be misleading and cause the primary diagnosis of KCS to be overlooked. If this problem occurs, the dog may be treated endlessly for conjunctivitis without resolving the underlying cause.

- In KCS, blepharitis and conjunctivitis occur with hyperemia, chemosis, thickened conjunctiva, periocular crust, and pruritus.
- The cornea appears dull and opaque. Corneal scarring varies in severity. Signs of scarring include vascularization, pigmentation, surface granulation, keratinization, and fibrosis. Exophthalmic breeds and highly pigmented dogs exhibit corneal scarring most severely.
- *Blindness commonly occurs due to corneal opacification.*
- Superficial or deep-melting ulcers may occur. Ulcers are more common in acute cases of KCS, in which the cornea has not become thick and keratinized.
- Pain is highly variable and warrants examination for corneal ulcers. Common signs of pain include blepharospasm, photophobia, and eye rubbing.
- KCS, less frequent in cats, occurs with similar but less dramatic signs. In cats, fright may cause transient sympathomimetic inhibition of tearing. This temporary condition must be distinguished from KCS by clinical signs.

Diagnosis

The Schirmer tear test (STT) is indicated in all animals suspected of keratoconjunctivitis, even when the cornea does not appear dry. Before administering any ocular drops, place the 5 × 30 mm commercial STT filter paper strip (Alcon Pharmaceuticals) in the medioventral cul-de-sac for 1 minute. Normal wetting for dogs and cats is 20 ± 5 mm/min. Typically, KCS cases wet less than 10 mm/min, with the majority of

symptomatic cases less than 5 mm/min on repeated trials. Diagnosis of KCS can be made when decreased STT values occur together with mucopurulent conjunctivitis, corneal inflammation, ulceration, or pigment deposition.

Treatment

Traditionally, KCS management has focused on tear replacement, tear conservation, and neurologic tear stimulation. Surgical transposition of the parotid salivary duct to the eye is a last resort for medically unmanageable cases. A radically new management approach uses a topically applied immunosuppressive agent, cyclosporine, intended to reverse immune-mediated destruction of the lacrimal gland and restore normal tear production.

Topical Cyclosporine

KEY POINT ▶ The initial treatment of choice for KCS is topical cyclosporine.

Unexpectedly, cyclosporine also increases tearing in the KCS associated with facial nerve paralysis, sulfonamide toxicity, and nictitans gland removal.

- *Ophthalmic cyclosporine* is an investigational product introduced for KCS treatment. It is a noncytotoxic (reversible) T-cell inhibitor utilized primarily in human organ transplantation.

Advantages of Ophthalmic Cyclosporine
- *Production of natural tears.* Cyclosporine appears to interrupt the pathologic process in the lacrimal glands, allowing them to resume tear production. Because tears contain antibodies, vitamins, amino acids, mucin, growth regulatory hormones, and many other constituents essential to corneal health, production of natural tears is a major advantage over artificial tears. Comparison of tear composition in cyclosporine-treated dogs with that produced by normal dogs shows the seven major tear proteins are conserved by cyclosporine.
- *Anti-inflammatory effects.* Cyclosporine is an im-

TABLE 1. Characteristics of Keratoconjunctivitis Sicca of Various Etiologies

Cause	Common Characteristics
Idiopathic or immune-mediated	Frequently associated with atopy, otitis externa, hypothyroidism, rheumatic diseases, deficient salivation (xerostomia)
Congenital alacrima	Usually unilateral, extreme xerosis, small breeds
Neurologic	Associated with other neurologic signs (e.g., facial nerve loss, deficient blink, head tilt, lip droop); commonly associated with otitis media (see sec. 5, ch. 23)
Drug-induced	Sulfadiazine, sulfasalazine, phenazopyridine, atropine (usually transient)
Distemper virus	In puppies with inadequate vaccinations; recent clinical infection (see sec. 2, ch. 6)

munosuppressive drug that reduces corneal vascularization, granulation, pigmentation, and conjunctival inflammation—similar to the activity of corticosteroids. However, unlike corticosteroids, cyclosporine does not activate collagenase in the presence of corneal ulcers.

- *Dosage frequency.* Cyclosporine is usually given twice daily in both eyes. Tear supplementation requires much more frequent dosing.

Method of Use

Currently, cyclosporine is recommended for twice-daily use. The dose frequency, vehicle, and concentration are expected to change with further investigation prior to approval by the Food and Drug Administration (FDA) and commercial introduction. A topical broad-spectrum antibiotic (neomycin:bacitracin:polymyxin B) may be used 4 times daily in conjunction with cyclosporine for 2 weeks to decrease secondary bacterial conjunctivitis while cyclosporine takes effect.

Monitoring

The patient is re-evaluated using STT results and clinical signs, 2–4 weeks after beginning treatment, and monthly, until clinical control is achieved. Following 6 weeks of treatment, if signs have not improved, increase dosing to q8h. If the STT is greater than 20 mm/min, on reevaluation, decrease to once daily or, occasionally, alternate-day dosing.

KEY POINT ▶ Measure the STT approximately 3 hours after dosing cyclosporine because the effect on the STT is lost in most cases in 12–24 hours.

When treatment is interrupted for 24 hours, signs recur in 90% of dogs that have been treated for over a year. Recapture of cyclosporine efficacy occurs rapidly, with the STT increasing after approximately 3 hours and the keratitis decreasing, usually, within 1 week after resuming treatment.

Precautions

KEY POINT ▶ Ophthalmic cyclosporine is currently approved for investigational use in dogs and humans only and not for commercial use.

With instruction, a licensed pharmacist can compound a sterile preparation of cyclosporine suitable for ophthalmic use in dogs. Although extra-label drug use is routine in veterinary medicine, an awareness of the increased liability of such use must be balanced with the anticipated benefit for the patient.

Because cyclosporine does not inhibit neutrophil activity, it will not likely interfere with immune response to bacteria. Under certain conditions, however, cyclosporine exacerbates viral (e.g., feline herpes keratitis) and fungal infections which is similar to the findings associated with corticosteroids. Fortunately, dogs are not affected by viral keratitis and are seldom affected by mycotic keratitis.

Response Rate

End-stage lacrimal gland pathology cannot be reversed with cyclosporine. The etiology of KCS does not accurately predict the response to therapy—positive responses have been seen in every known etiology.

Treatment failure has, likewise, occurred in all types of KCS. Although investigated, no sex or breed predilection for response has been discerned.

About 70% of all dogs with KCS respond positively to cyclosporine treatment within 2–4 weeks. An additional 10–15% of dogs respond to long-term treatment, with the slowest reported onset of response being one dog who began tearing following 8 months of twice-daily treatment. About 10–15% of dogs will not tear; however, they may show resolution of corneal scarring and mucoid conjunctivitis. Approximately 10% of dogs do not benefit clinically, requiring return to traditional methods of treatment, such as artificial tears, corticosteroids, pilocarpine, acetylcysteine as needed, or parotid duct transposition surgery as a last resort.

KEY POINT ▶ Increased lacrimation in response to cyclosporine therapy is related to the initial STT. Those dogs with STT of > 2 mm/min wetting had a much greater response (87–100%) than those with STT of < 2 mm/min (29–59%).

Artificial Tears

- *Artificial tears supplementation* or methylcellulose and polyvinylalcohol increase artificial tear viscosity and surface tension, which increase ocular surface wetting time. Table 2 lists commonly used artificial tear preparations. In dogs, ointments are usually preferred to solutions because of their lower cost and decreased dosing frequency. Preservative-free products are also preferred. Artificial tears are applied as often as reasonably possible, from 4–12 times daily, depending upon the severity of disease and the client's compliance.

Tear Stimulants

- *Tear stimulants* or pilocarpine 2% dosed at 1 drop/5 kg body weight twice daily on feed can be used in an attempt to stimulate the parasympathetic supply to the lacrimal gland and maximize its output. If the initial dosage is ineffective, it may be increased by 1 drop per day, to effect or until toxicity develops.

KEY POINT ▶ The first sign of pilocarpine toxicity is hypersalivation, followed by vomiting and diarrhea. Severe bradycardia and death can occur with overdosage.

Gastrointestinal discomfort is a side effect in humans that cannot be evaluated in dogs. Pilocarpine's effect diminishes over time. Treatment is long-term. Approximately 20% of dogs respond positively.

Mucolytics

- *Mucolytics* or acetylcysteine 5% Mucomyst (diluted 1:1 with artificial tears) solution may be applied topically once or twice daily to reduce the heavy mucus accumulation on the eye. Package directions indicate a shelf life of 5 days; however, it can be refrigerated and used provided it is not discolored.

TABLE 2. Artificial Tear Solutions and Ointments

Product Names	Principal Ingredients	Preservatives
	Solutions	
Adsorbotear	HEC, Adsorbobase	Thimerosal, EDTA
Akwa Tears	PVA	Benzalkonium Cl, EDTA
Comfort	HEC	Benzalkonium Cl, EDTA
Isopto	HPMC 0.5%	Benzalkonium Cl, EDTA
Lacril	HPMC 0.5%, GEL, PSB	Chlorobutanol
Cellufresh	CMC 0.5%	No preservative
Celluvisc	CMC 1.0%	No preservative
Murocel	MC 1.0%, PG	Parabens
Murocel	HPMC 1.5%, DEX	Parabens
Muro Tears	HEC, PVA	Benzalkonium Cl, EDTA
Neo-Tears	HEC, Lipids	Thimerosal, EDTA
Teargard	HPMC 0.5%	Thimerosal, EDTA
Tearisol	HPMC 1.0%	Benzalkonium Cl, EDTA
Tears Naturale	HMC, DEX	Benzalkonium Cl, EDTA
Tears Naturale II	HMC, DEX	Polyquaternium-1
Tears Renewed	MC, DEX	Benzalkonium Cl, EDTA
Tears Naturale Free	HPMC 0.3%, DEX	No preservative
Vit-A-Drops	Vitamin A, PSB	EDTA
Celluvisc	CMC 1.0%	No preservative
Hypotears	PVA 1%, HEC, DEX	Benzalkonium Cl, EDTA
Liquifilm Forte	PVA 3%	Thimerosal, EDTA
Liquifilm Tears	PVA 1.4%	Chlorobutanol
Neo-Tears	PVA, HEC	Thimerosal, EDTA
Refresh	PVA 1.4%	No preservative
Tears Plus	PVA 1.4%	Chlorobutanol
	Ointments	
Akwa Tears	Petrolatum, Lanolin	No preservative
Dry Eyes	Petrolatum	No preservative
Duratears	Petrolatum, Lanolin	No preservative
Hypotears	Petrolatum	No preservative
Lacri-Lube	Petrolatum, Lanolin	Chlorobutanol

CMC = carboxymethyl cellulose, DEX = dextran, GEL = gelatine, HEC = hydroxyethyl cellulose, EDTA = ethylenediaminetetra acetic acid, HPMC = hydroxypropyl methyl cellulose, MC = methyl cellulose, PSB = polysorbate 80, PVA = polyvinyl alcohol, PG = propylene glycol.

Topical Antibiotics

■ Topical broad-spectrum *antibiotics* are advised whenever corneal ulcer or secondary bacterial conjunctivitis, notably a purulent discharge, develops (see sec. 11, ch. 3). Because a bacterial overgrowth, not a specific pathogen, is involved, ocular culture is rarely needed.

Topical Corticosteroids

■ Topical *corticosteroids* can be provided judiciously to decrease inflammatory signs. Prior to application, a corneal fluorescein stain is evaluated to ensure the absence of corneal ulceration. Because corneal ulcers can occur intermittently in KCS, and because corticosteroids activate collagenase that can melt an ulcer and cause ocular perforation, the high risk of steroids must be conveyed to the owner, balanced with the need for anti-inflammatory drugs. In general, topical cyclosporine is better as an anti-inflammatory agent, because it avoids the risk of a melting corneal ulcer that is associated with corticosteroids. Some ophthalmologists prefer concurrent cyclosporine and corticosteroids in patients with dense pigmentary keratitis.

Surgical Treatment

■ When medical management fails, the *parotid salivary duct can be surgically transposed* to the lateral conjunctival surface. Referral to an ophthalmologist is recommended.

PROLAPSE OF THE GLAND OF THE THIRD EYELID

Hypertrophy and prolapse of the nictitating membrane gland, i.e., gland of the third eyelid, also called "cherry eye," presents an unattractive appearance often accompanied by recurrent conjunctivitis.

KEY POINT ▶ Removal of the third eyelid gland precipitates KCS in a predisposed individual. Because this gland provides half the lacrimation, its removal is contraindicated.

The gland can be repositioned surgically (Fig. 2). Alternatively, topical corticosteroids and antibiotics can be administered to combat the conjunctivitis, and the appearance can be ignored.

Surgical Procedure

Objectives

- Replace the gland of the nictitans in its normal position.
- Restore normal nictitans function.
- Preserve function of the gland of the nictitans.

Equipment

- Eyelid speculum
- Standard ophthalmic surgical pack

Technique

1. Expose globe for repositioning of nictitating membrane and nictitans gland (Fig. 2A).
2. Extend nictitating membrane and incise palpebral conjunctiva of the fornix (Fig. 2B).

3. With 3-0 nonabsorbable monofilament suture, take a long bite of the periosteum along the orbital rim. The needle should traverse medially to laterally through the rim and not perpendicularly (toward eyeball).
4. Pass the suture back through the incision then dorsally through the prolapsed gland, exiting on the dorsal bulbar face (Fig. 2C).
5. Reflect the nictitating membrane downward.
6. Pass the suture back through the exit hole in the apex of the gland taking a horizontal bite through the dorsal prominence of the gland.
7. The final pass of suture begins again at the previous exit hole and passes ventrally through the gland, exiting through the conjunctival incision, within which both suture ends are securely tied (Fig. 2D).

Postoperative Care and Complications

- Topical broad-spectrum antibiotics 4 times daily for 7 days
- Complications are uncommon, but include reprolapse of the gland and infection of the surgical site. Reprolapse is treated surgically, repositioning the gland. Infection is managed with systemic antibodies.

EPIPHORA

Epiphora is the overflow of tears down the face. It can be an important sign of ocular pain, or it can be a cosmetic problem (staining of facial hair) associated with nasolacrimal duct dysfunction.

When corneal ulceration or uveitis are present, the underlying etiology is investigated further, as described in sec. 11, chs. 4, 6.

- *Aberrant hair* can also cause epiphora. When facial hairs lie in the tear film (trichiasis), they act like a wick and draw tears onto the face. Distichia (abnormal eyelashes) and entropion (rolling inward of the

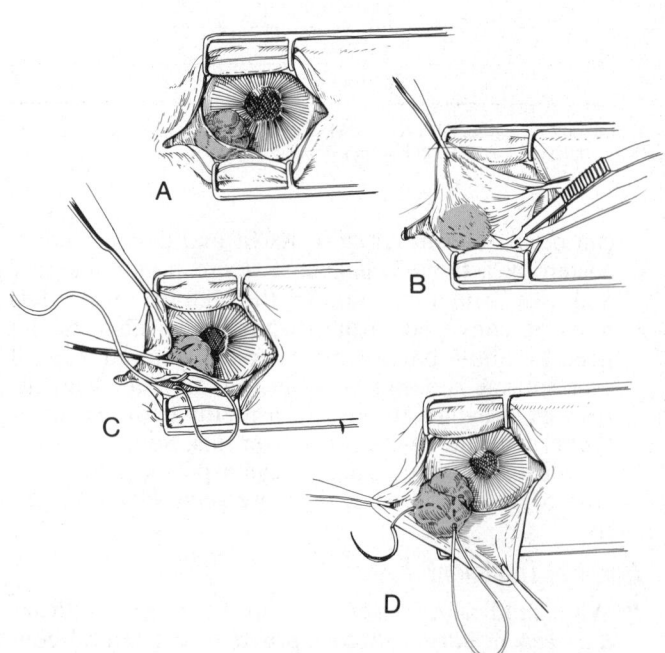

Figure 2. Procedure for repositioning of nictitating membrane and gland. See text for explanation. (From Kaswan RL, Martin CL: Surgical correction of the third eyelid prolapse in dogs. J Am Vet Med Assoc 186:83, 1983.)

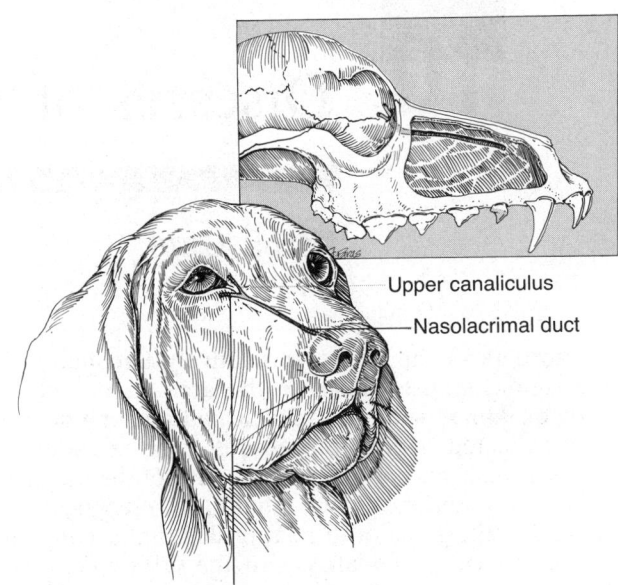

Figure 3. Anatomic representation of the canaliculi and nasolacrimal duct.

Upper canaliculus

Nasolacrimal duct

Lower canaliculus

lid margin) also cause epiphora, and surgical correction is advised (see sec. 11, ch. 2).

■ *Dacryocystitis*, inflammation and obstruction of the nasolacrimal outflow duct (Fig. 3), may cause epiphora. Careful irrigation of the duct with a lacrimal cannula is advised. Topical antibiotic-corticosteroid preparations are indicated. In the case of recurrent nasolacrimal duct obstruction, anesthetize the animal and place an indwelling monofilament nylon suture (2-0 to 4-0, depending on size) for 2 weeks to maintain patency while using topical antibiotic-corticosteroid preparations.

■ *Imperforate inferior punctum* is seen in some dogs, especially Cocker spaniels. The nasolacrimal system is normal except for a conjunctival membrane covering the inferior nasolacrimal canaliculus. Grasp the conjunctiva over this area and excise. Then irrigate the nasolacrimal system. This procedure can often be performed using topical anesthesia. Give topical antibiotic-corticosteroids for 5–7 days following the correction.

■ *Nasolacrimal punctal malposition* may occur in exophthalmic dogs with tight lid/globe conformation. With medial entropion, the ventral punctum may roll inward, such that the tears are not drained efficiently. Medial entropion correction can be used (see sec. 11, ch. 2).

Supplemental Readings

Lavach JD: The lacrimal system. *In* Slatter DH, ed.: *Textbook of Small Animal Surgery*, vol. II. 1496–99. Philadelphia: W.B. Saunders, 1985, pp 1496–1499.

Jensen HE: Keratitis sicca and parotic duct transposition. Compend Cont Ed Pract Vet 9:721–726, 1979.

Kaswan RL, Salisbury MA: A new perspective on canine keratoconjunctivitis sicca. Vet Clin North Am [Sm Anim Pract] 20:583–613, 1990.

Kern TJ: Disorders of the lacrimal system. *In* Kirk RW, ed.: *Current Veterinary Therapy IX*. Philadelphia: W.B. Saunders, 1986, pp 634–641.

10 Diseases of the Orbit

Mary B. Glaze

Disorders of the orbit are relatively uncommon in companion animals. Because the area cannot be directly examined without sophisticated imaging devices or complicated surgical procedures, even the simplest of lesions can pose a diagnostic and therapeutic challenge. In addition to the ability to recognize the changes in the globe-orbit relationship that accompany orbital diseases, familiarity with the orbital contents, boundaries, and neighboring structures is essential to the initial clinical evaluation and diagnostic planning.

ORBITAL ANATOMY
Orbital Cavity

- The orbit is a cone-shaped cavity that surrounds the eye and its supporting structures.
- Only the medial wall and part of the orbital roof are bony in the dog and cat. The floor of the orbit is muscular, with the exception of a small shelf of maxillary bone in the cat. The lateral aspect is completed by a ligament that bridges the space between the frontal and zygomatic bones.
- Three prominent openings at the apex of the orbit permit the passage of its major vessels and nerves.
- When the mouth is opened, the dorsal aspect of the ramus of the mandible moves rostrally, compressing the orbital contents.
- Neighboring structures include the oral cavity, teeth, tongue, zygomatic salivary gland, mastication muscles, paranasal sinuses, and nasal turbinates. Diseases of these structures may extend into the orbit and must always be considered when evaluating orbital disease.

Orbital Contents

- The contents of the orbit are enclosed by a fibrous membrane, the periorbita, which attaches to the orbital wall at the optic foramen and extends to the orbital rim. The periorbita contains sympathetically innervated smooth muscle fibers.
- The anterior limit of the orbit is formed by a sheet of connective tissue, the orbital septum, which extends from the periorbita at the orbital margin to blend with the tarsus of the lid.
- Of the seven extraocular muscles, six originate at the orbital apex. The inferior oblique arises from the anteromedial orbital wall.
- The orbital fat pad cushions the orbital contents and is found between the periorbita and the surrounding structures. Fat is also located within the periorbita between the extraocular muscles.

- In addition to numerous arteries, veins, and autonomic nerves, the second, third, fourth, and sixth cranial nerves and the ophthalmic branch of the trigeminal nerve traverse the orbit.
- The nictitans occupies the ventronasal portion of the orbit and moves primarily in relation to globe movements.
- The lacrimal gland is contained within the periorbita near the superotemporal aspect of the globe.
- The zygomatic salivary gland occupies the lateral orbital floor, just behind the orbital margin and outside the periorbita.

ALTERATIONS IN THE GLOBE-ORBIT RELATIONSHIP

The position of the eye within the orbit depends upon the orbital dimensions, the relative globe size, and the volume of the other orbital contents. The normal brachycephalic dog or cat has a shallow orbit and prominent eye. Larger orbits and less prominent eyes are found in mesaticephalic and dolichocephalic breeds. As a general rule, the feline globe nearly fills the orbit and predisposes the animal to alterations in the globe-orbit relationship early in the course of orbital disease.

KEY POINT ▶ The first clinical sign of orbital disease is often a change in the position or the direction of the globe relative to the orbital rim and to the other eye.

EXOPHTHALMOS

Exophthalmos refers to the abnormal protrusion of a normal-sized eye. The condition is distinguished from buphthalmos (enlarged eye) by comparing the corneal diameter of the animal's affected eye with the normal eye. Exophthalmos must also be differentiated from contralateral enophthalmos, the exaggerated palpebral fissures of euryblepharon and facial paralysis, and the characteristically prominent globe of the brachycephalic dog and cat.

Causes of exophthalmos in dogs and cats encompass a spectrum of developmental disorders, inflammatory processes, neoplasias, traumatic lesions, cystic disorders, and skeletal diseases.

Developmental Disorders
Congenital Cysts

- Orbital cysts develop in association with other ocular anomalies, appearing as appendages of microphthalmic eyes or entirely supplanting a recognizable globe.

- These cysts are rare, nonheritable consequences of defective ocular organogenesis.
- If asymptomatic and cosmetically acceptable, no treatment is warranted. Excise large, exposed cysts to prevent secondary drying and irritation.

Craniofacial Deformities

- *Cyclopia* is a rare lethal anomaly in which the orbits and their contents are fused into a single structure. The anomaly is characterized by a single midline orbit and a dysplastic eye, which may appear as a single or bilobed sphere. The nose and maxilla are rudimentary. Obviously there is no treatment for this lethal anomaly.
- *Orbital malformation* and a subsequent divergence of the ocular axes accompany hydrocephalus (see sec. 10, ch. 2 for further discussion of hydrocephalus).

Etiology
Both genetic and teratogenic influences are incriminated in congenital hydrocephalus. The enlarging lateral ventricles alter orbital development and cause ventrolateral displacement of the eyes.

Clinical Signs
The affected animal demonstrates behavioral abnormalities, often in association with an enlarged skull, an open fontanelle, and a bilateral ventrolateral strabismus.

Diagnosis
Rule out strabismus secondary to oculomotor disease from the differential diagnoses and confirm the diagnosis of hydrocephalus.

Treatment
Orbital malformation and strabismus are not treatable.

Arteriovenous Malformations

Etiology
Rarely, fistulas may develop between orbital or periorbital vessels. The cause is unknown.

Clinical Signs
Exophthalmos is associated with a pulsatile murmur auscultated over the orbit. The bruit diminishes when the carotid artery is compressed. The exophthalmos may be exacerbated in response to postural changes.

Diagnosis
Perform an orbital contrast venography in the anesthetized patient. Immediately before and during radiography, inject 5 to 10 ml of contrast medium into the angularis oculi vein, using a 21-gauge needle or catheter. Perform a contrast study on the normal side for comparison.

Treatment
Surgical attempts at ligation and resection are frequently unsatisfactory. One report described severe intraoperative hemorrhage and postoperative recurrence of the lesion in a dog.

Acquired Disorders

Acquired disorders are more common than congenital orbital diseases as causes of exophthalmos in dogs and cats. Acute lesions associated with discomfort and swelling of conjunctiva and eyelids are usually inflammatory, whereas slowly progressive, nonpainful disorders are secondary to space-occupying lesions.

KEY POINT ▶ In instances of acquired exophthalmos, document the rapidity of onset and the presence or absence of pain, especially that noted upon opening the mouth.

Inflammatory/Infectious Disorders

Orbital Cellulitis/Orbital Abscess
Orbital inflammatory disease is a common cause of *acute, painful,* unilateral exophthalmos.

Etiology
Orbital inflammation is usually the result of trauma or infection or the extension of a disease process from neighboring structures.

- Trauma—Trauma produces both septic and nonseptic inflammation. Infections follow breaching of the oral mucosae or eyelids by bite wounds or foreign objects, such as bones. Blunt trauma may damage the osseous and soft tissues of the orbit. Occasionally, a foreign body will be retained within the orbit, causing recurrent inflammation.
- Infection—Bacteria, fungi, and parasites infect the orbit primarily or extend from the paranasal sinuses and nasal cavity. Orbital fungal pyogranulomas are observed with blastomycosis, cryptococcosis, and coccidioidomycosis. In cats, *Aspergillus* and *Penicillium* have been implicated in orbital cellulitis secondary to sinusitis. Larvae of *Dirofilaria immitis* and *Ancylostoma* species produce primary orbital cellulitis by invading canine orbital tissues. The nasal mite *Pneumonyssus caninum* is a documented cause of orbital cellulitis and sinusitis in a dog. Even *Cuterebra* larvae occasionally invade the orbit.
- Extension of Disease—Disorders of the teeth, frontal or paranasal sinuses, nasolacrimal system, temporal and pterygoid muscles, or zygomatic salivary and lacrimal glands may cause secondary orbital inflammation or infection. Inflammation of the posterior sclera may also affect adjacent orbital tissues.
- Rare proliferative inflammatory disorders referred to as pseudotumors may mimic orbital neoplasms and include fibrous histiocytoma, undifferentiated inflammatory pseudotumor, and eosinophilic granuloma.

Clinical Signs
Orbital inflammation is characterized by a relatively *acute* unilateral exophthalmos, with chemosis, third eyelid protrusion, and *pain on opening the mouth*. The animal may be febrile and exhibit an inflammatory leukogram. Abscesses may produce swelling or discoloration behind the last upper molar.

Diagnosis
Diagnosis is based upon history and physical examination, including a thorough evaluation of the oral cavity. Consider sedation in animals in obvious pain. Hematology, radiography, cytology, and culture of orbital aspirates may be of benefit in some cases.

Radiographically localize orbital foreign bodies

with four views: lateral, ventrodorsal, oblique, and frontal. Place a ring of wire around the limbus as a helpful point of reference.

Treatment
- Administer a broad-spectrum systemic antibiotic for at least 10 days. Response to antibiotic therapy is generally rapid, with resolution within 1 week.
- Protect the corneal surface with an antibiotic ophthalmic ointment in cases of extreme exophthalmos.
- Alleviate the acute swelling and discomfort with compresses and a systemic nonsteroidal anti-inflammatory agent (aspirin, 10–25 mg/kg, q12h, PO in dogs). Corticosteroid therapy is controversial owing to the potential for sepsis in some patients.
- If no response is seen within 24 to 48 hours, establish ventral drainage through the mouth.
- Incise the mucous membrane behind the last upper molar with a #15 Bard-Parker scalpel blade.
- Carefully insert a hemostat through the pterygoid muscle and open gently in the retrobulbar space.

KEY POINT ▶ This procedure can damage the optic nerve, globe, or major orbital vasculature and must be performed carefully.

Eosinophilic Myositis
Inflammation and swelling of the muscles of mastication may compromise the orbital space and push the globe forward.

Etiology
The finding of myofibril-specific antibodies in affected dogs suggests an autoimmune disorder.

Clinical Signs
Temporal and masseter muscle swelling causes fever, pain on opening the mouth, difficulty eating, and trismus. The German shepherd appears most susceptible. The condition is more often bilateral than unilateral. Acute episodes may last 10 to 20 days. Recurrences lead to muscle atrophy and decreased prominence of the globe. Blindness is a rare complication.

Diagnosis
Confirm the clinical diagnosis with temporal muscle biopsy samples, which demonstrate mononuclear and eosinophilic infiltrates (see sec. 10, ch. 6). The finding of peripheral eosinophilia is inconsistent.

Treatment
Administer oral prednisone, beginning with a daily dose of 1 mg/kg for 1 to 2 weeks. Continue treatment for a total of 4 to 6 weeks, reducing the dose by half each week. Treatment must precede the onset of muscle atrophy to prevent recession of the globe into the orbit.

Extraocular Polymyositis
An unusual myositis involving only the extraocular muscles occurs in the dog.

Etiology
The etiology has not been determined. Localization to the extraocular muscles suggests an immune mechanism directed against specific muscle fiber antigens.

Clinical Signs
Dogs 6 to 18 months of age demonstrate bilaterally symmetric, nonpainful exophthalmos. The globes appear otherwise normal. Optic nerve compression by the swollen extraocular muscles may cause visual impairment.

Diagnosis
Complete blood counts and serum chemistry values are normal. Confirm the clinical diagnosis with extraocular muscle biopsy to demonstrate muscle necrosis, severe lymphocytic and histiocytic inflammation, and mild neutrophilic infiltration that are seen histopathologically.

Treatment
Administer oral prednisone (same dosage as that for eosinophilic myositis) in decreasing doses over a 2-week period. Response to therapy is rapid, but rare relapses can occur.

Neoplasia

KEY POINT ▶ Most orbital neoplasms are aggressive and malignant tumors that are diagnosed in the advanced stages of development.

Affected animals usually do not survive longer than 3 years from the time of diagnosis.

Etiology
Both primary and secondary orbital tumors occur in dogs and cats. Primary neoplasms arise from an assortment of tissues within the orbit, including epithelium; bone; nerves; vessels; and connective, hemolymphatic, and glandular tissues. Secondary tumors extend from adjacent structures or metastasize from distant sites.

In dogs, 90% of orbital tumors are malignant and 75% are primary.

Clinical Signs
Gradual, painless exophthalmos is accompanied by periocular swelling, third eyelid protrusion, and globe deviation. Secondary lagophthalmos may cause corneal drying. Compression of the globe can cause retinal detachment with subsequent abnormalities of the pupillary light response and blindness. Primary orbital neoplasia is typically unilateral. Metastatic disease may affect both orbits, however.

The mean age of dogs with orbital neoplasia is 8 years, ranging from 18 months to 15 years. Older cats experience a similar risk as do dogs, yet orbital lymphosarcoma and multicentric fibrosarcoma occur in cats less than 2 years of age.

Diagnosis
- Perform a complete physical examination to evaluate for other neoplastic changes.
- Substantiate the clinical diagnosis with radiography and orbital ultrasonography.
- Evaluate adjacent structures, such as the nasal cavity and sinuses, radiographically.
- Perform thoracic radiography for metastatic disease.
- With the animal heavily sedated or anesthetized, obtain orbital aspirates for cytologic evaluation using a 1-inch, 22-gauge needle attached to a 12-ml syringe. The direction of deviation of the exophthalmic globe suggests the tumor's location and the site for needle entry. For example, lateral strabismus suggests a

medial space-occupying mass. To reach the mass, insert the needle medial to the third eyelid, penetrate the conjunctiva, and aspirate gently along the medial orbital wall. Other orbital quadrants may be sampled in a similar manner. For masses directly behind the eye, surgically prepare the lateral aspect of the orbit and insert the needle just posterior to the angle formed by the lateral orbital ligament and the zygomatic arch. If available, ultrasound-guided orbital aspiration helps to minimize complications and ensure accurate needle placement.

Treatment

Surgical resection of the neoplasm is the treatment of choice. Orbitotomy and excision may be attempted in cases of circumscribed primary tumors. If the extent of involvement precludes total excision of the tumor, orbital exenteration is performed. Many tumors respond to adjunct chemotherapy or radiation therapy (see sec. 3).

Surgical approaches to the orbit are described elsewhere. Refer patients requiring exploratory orbitotomy to a veterinary ophthalmologist or surgeon.

Orbital Trauma

Traumatic Proptosis

Complete displacement of the globe from the orbit is a true emergency. Treatment begins as soon as the animal's systemic condition allows.

Etiology

The depth of the orbit dictates the force necessary to displace the globe. Proptosis most commonly occurs in the brachycephalic dog because of its shallow orbit and exaggerated palpebral fissure. Excessive restraint may be sufficient to dislodge the globe. In contrast, the feline eye is rarely displaced from its well-proportioned orbit except in severe head trauma.

Clinical Signs

The globe rests in front of the eyelids, its proximity to the orbit determined by the extent of the extraocular muscle damage, the integrity of the optic nerve, and the degree of retrobulbar hemorrhage. Chemosis and subconjunctival hemorrhage are often present. Prolonged exposure of the cornea leads to ulceration.

Diagnosis

Perform a thorough physical examination to assess the other effects of head trauma. Examine the eye closely for intraocular damage. Palpate the orbital rim for fractures, and radiograph if indicated. Apply fluorescein dye to the cornea to document ulceration.

Treatment

Once the animal's general condition is stabilized from the effects of the trauma, the eye is repositioned as soon as possible. Reserve enucleation for ruptured globes or for those with severed optic nerves.

Surgical Procedure
Objectives

- Manipulate the eyelids to place them anterior to the globe.
- Protect the cornea from exposure.

Equipment

- Two strabismus hooks
- Ophthalmic forceps and needle holder
- Tubing or other material suitable for use as stents

Technique

1. Anesthetize the patient.
2. Irrigate the globe and surrounding tissues with sterile physiologic saline.
3. Elevate the eyelid margins with either a blunt probe, such as a strabismus hook, or simple interrupted 4-0 nonabsorbable suture material placed over stents. Sutures enter the eyelid 5 mm from the margin and exit through the meibomian gland openings to prevent corneal damage. As the eyelids elevate, apply gentle counterpressure against the cornea with a moistened cotton ball or the flat surface of a scalpel handle to replace the globe within the orbit.
4. Suture the eyelid margins together, leaving a slight separation at the medial canthus to facilitate topical therapy with broad-spectrum antibiotics and 1% atropine ointments 2 or 3 times daily.
5. Administer an oral broad-spectrum antibiotic, such as ampicillin, for 7 days. Avoid systemic sulfonamides, which may reduce tear production.
6. Administer an initial IV or IM injection of dexamethasone (0.2 mg/kg). Continue oral prednisone therapy (1.0 mg/kg) for 5 days to reduce orbital swelling.

KEY POINT ▶ Do not inject medication into the retrobulbar area. Do not aspirate orbital contents or the globe itself.

7. Remove the eyelid sutures when the orbital swelling resolves, usually in 2 to 3 weeks. Orbital swelling is evaluated by retropulsing the globe. Use the unaffected eye for comparison.

Prognosis

An animal with an eye tightly positioned against the eyelids, a miotic pupil, a minimal amount of extraocular muscle damage, and an absence of hyphema has the best prognosis.

Potential sequelae include lateral strabismus, chronic keratitis due to lagophthalmos or low tear production, phthisis bulbi, and blindness. A deviated globe may spontaneously realign as the extraocular muscles fibrose after several weeks to months.

Orbital Hemorrhage/Emphysema
Etiology

Less severe orbital trauma may result in lagophthalmos due to retrobulbar and subconjunctival hemorrhage. Fractures of the sinus wall may cause air to collect beneath the conjunctiva. Entry of air through the nasolacrimal duct may lead to orbital emphysema after routine enucleation.

Clinical Signs and Diagnosis

Mild-to-moderate exophthalmos is associated with lagophthalmos, chemosis, subconjunctival hemorrhage or emphysema, and lid swelling.

Treatment

Confine the patient to limit further hemorrhage. Use cold compresses to reduce acute swelling. Apply topical methylcellulose artificial tear ointments frequently (4–6 times daily) to protect the corneal surface from drying (see Table 2). Administer oral or parenteral corticosteroids as described for the proptosed globe. Avoid nonsteroidal anti-inflammatory drugs, such as aspirin, which inhibit platelet function.

Arteriovenous Fistula

Orbital vascular fistulas may develop secondary to trauma. Clinical signs and diagnostic procedures are similar to those described for developmental vascular anomalies.

Cystic Diseases

Acquired orbital cysts are uncommon consequences of trauma to orbital glands and incomplete excision of secretory tissues during enucleation.

Zygomatic Mucocele

Leakage of saliva from the zygomatic salivary gland or its duct is an uncommon cause of exophthalmos in the dog.

Etiology

The condition may occur spontaneously or after orbital trauma.

Clinical Signs

A painless swelling beneath the inferior temporal or nasal conjunctival fornix is commonly associated with prominence of the third eyelid. The mucosa behind the last upper molar may protrude.

Diagnosis

Aspirate fluid from the lesion. The mucocele contains a clear, straw-colored, or blood-tinged tenacious material. Perform a zygomatic sialogram to confirm the clinical and cytologic diagnosis.

Treatment

The treatment is surgical and the location of the swelling dictates the approach for removal of the mucocele. Approach mucoceles beneath the inferior conjunctival cul-de-sac transconjunctivally, making an incision between the nictitans and the lower eyelid or through the eyelid surface. Lateral mucoceles require a limited orbitotomy, the details of which are described in other texts.

Mucocele Following Enucleation

Cystic swelling of the orbit may follow enucleation if mucus or tear-producing tissues are not completely excised.

Etiology

Retained conjunctival goblet cells or glandular tissue from the third eyelid may cause cystic swelling of the orbit.

Clinical Signs

As fluid accumulates within the orbit, the overlying skin distends. A fistula may develop, draining seromucoid fluid.

Diagnosis

Clinical signs are suggestive. Perform aspiration cytology to rule out the finding of postsurgical infection.

Treatment

Explore the orbit to remove retained secretory tissue, approaching anteriorly through the eyelids.

Other Causes of Exophthalmos

Anecdotal reports attribute the causes of exophthalmos to the hormonal influences of estrus and to the edema caused by hypoproteinemia or systemic hypertension.

ENOPHTHALMOS

Enophthalmos refers to the recession of the eye within the orbit. The condition must be differentiated diagnostically from the relative enophthalmos that accompanies periorbital swelling or edema of the eyelids and conjunctiva.

Enophthalmos may be accompanied by mucoid-to-mucopurulent discharge, because of the exaggerated conjunctival cul-de-sac, and by ptosis and entropion, because of the eyelids losing the support of the underlying globe. With rare exception, restoration of the globe's normal position within the orbit is seldom successful.

Causes of enophthalmos include developmental abnormalities, retraction of the globe due to pain, atrophy of orbital tissues following debilitating disease or trauma, and loss of smooth muscle tone in the periorbita.

Developmental Disorders

Microphthalmos/Anophthalmos

The microphthalmic globe fails to develop to normal size in dogs and occasionally in cats. Anophthalmos refers to a rare condition in which all ocular tissues are absent.

Etiology

Microphthalmos is inherited in several breeds of dog, including the Australian shepherd, miniature schnauzer, Old English sheepdog, Akita, Cavalier King Charles spaniel, Samoyed, American Cocker spaniel, Bedlington and Sealyham terriers, beagle, Labrador retriever, and Doberman pinscher. Multiple ocular defects, including microphthalmos, occur associated with partial albinism and deafness in the Great Dane and collie. Teratogenic influences during early pregnancy may affect ocular development. Causes of microphthalmos in cats are poorly characterized.

Clinical Signs

The anomaly is characterized by varying degrees of enophthalmos. Because orbital development is influenced by globe size during skeletal maturation, the orbit may also appear small and the palpebral fissure narrowed. Accompanying ocular defects include persistent pupillary membranes, cataracts, colobomas, retinal dysplasias, and orbital cysts. Multiple ocular anomalies may render the globe sightless, but on occasion small globes may be structurally and functionally normal.

Diagnosis

Diagnosis is based upon clinical signs. Differentiate microphthalmos from phthisis bulbi, an acquired atrophy of the globe. Evidence of scarring, inflammation, and normal-sized orbit accompany atrophy. Anophthalmos is diagnosed only after serial histologic examination of orbital tissue has excluded the possibility of microphthalmos.

Treatment

There is no treatment for microphthalmos. Enucleate if chronic irritation and discharge accompany the condition. Eliminate affected animals from breeding programs.

Breed-Related Enophthalmos

Etiology

The large orbits and deeply set eyes inherited as conformational traits of dolichocephalic breeds, such as the Doberman pinscher, Irish setter, and Golden retriever, may create a relative enophthalmos.

Clinical Signs and Diagnosis

The globe appears normal but deeply set within the orbit. The nictitans may be prominent. Mucoid-to-mucopurulent discharge, ptosis, and entropion are common sequelae.

Treatment

The condition is incurable. Manage secondary conjunctivitis with intermittent applications of topical antibiotic-corticosteroid ointment. Correct accompanying entropion.

Acquired Disorders

Acquired enophthalmos is common, particularly in response to ocular pain and as a consequence of severe or recurrent inflammation of the globe itself.

Ocular Pain

The retractor bulbi muscle pulls the eye into the orbit when pain is present. The phenomenon is more apparent in the dog than the cat.

Etiology

Any painful ocular disorder may cause enophthalmos, especially ulcerative keratitis, anterior uveitis, and acute glaucoma.

Clinical Signs

In addition to enophthalmos, the animal demonstrates other nonspecific signs of ocular pain: excessive tearing, eye rubbing, blepharospasm, photophobia, and nictitans protrusion.

Diagnosis

Examine closely for ectopic cilia, foreign body, corneal ulcer, or intraocular disease. Pain associated with ocular surface disorders, such as ulcers, may decrease following topical application of 0.5% proparacaine.

Treatment

Treat the underlying ocular disease.

Changes in Orbital Volume

Reduction in retrobulbar tissue mass or damage to the bony or soft-tissue structures forming the walls of the orbit causes the globe to recede.

Dehydration/Cachexia

Loss of retrobulbar fat causes a mechanical sinking of the globe into the orbit. Pronounced weight loss and dehydration secondary to vomiting, diarrhea, or other debilitating conditions decrease the retrobulbar fat pad. Reduced orbital tissue mass may also be a feature of aging. Dehydration is treated, but enophthalmos secondary to cachexia and loss of retrobulbar fat may not be reversible.

Atrophy Following Inflammation or Trauma

Reduction of the orbital tissue mass effectively enlarges the orbit, resulting in enophthalmos.

Etiology

Atrophy of the temporal, masseter, and pterygoid muscles is relatively common in dogs following myositis or as an idiopathic phenomenon (see sec. 10, ch. 6). Brain stem infections or injuries may produce alterations in the trigeminal motor nucleus and result in atrophy of the muscles of mastication. Similar lesions may develop as a consequence of trauma to the trigeminal nerve at the base of the ear or fractures in the temporomandibular joint or skull at the oval foramen. Chronic or recurrent orbital inflammation may lead to atrophy of orbital contents; trauma or inflammation of the globe may lead to phthisis bulbi.

Clinical Signs and Diagnosis

Atrophy of the masticatory muscles alters the facial appearance, exaggerating the skull's bony protuberances. The animal is unable to open the mouth widely and often has difficulty prehending food. Enophthalmos and passive nictitans prolapse may cause visual impairment.

The phthisical globe is small and blind, with a thickened sclera, opaque cornea, and profound disorganization and scarring of the intraocular structures.

Treatment

Consult a veterinary ophthalmologist regarding autogenous fat transplants or implantable beads (strictly a cosmetic procedure) to modify the degree of postinflammatory or post-traumatic enophthalmos.

There is no effective treatment for phthisis bulbi. Control secondary conjunctivitis with regular irrigation and intermittent topical antibiotic-corticosteroid ophthalmic preparations. Phthisical globes in cats are enucleated because of the potential for post-traumatic ocular sarcoma.

Sympathetic Denervation

Horner's syndrome and feline dysautonomia cause loss of sympathetic tone in the periorbita, with varying degrees of enophthalmos (see sec. 11, ch. 11).

Supplemental Readings

Barr F: *Diagnostic Ultrasound in the Dog and Cat.* Oxford: Blackwell Scientific Publications, 1990, p 167.

Bistner SI, Aguirre G, Batik G: *Atlas of Veterinary Ophthalmic Surgery.* Philadelphia: W.B. Saunders, 1977, p 245.

Kern TJ: Orbital neoplasia in 23 dogs. J Am Vet Med Assoc 186:489, 1985.

Martin CL, Kaswan RL, Doran CC: Cystic lesions of the periorbital region. Compend Contin Educ Pract Vet 9:1021, 1987.

McCalla TL, Moore CP: Exophthalmos in dogs and cats. Compend Contin Educ Pract Vet 11:911, 1989.

Szymanski C: The eye. *In* Holzworth J, ed.: *Diseases of the Cat.* Philadelphia: W.B. Saunders, 1987, p 677.

Wolf ED, Wilkie DA: Exploratory surgery of the orbit. *In* Bojrab MJ, ed.: *Current Techniques in Small Animal Surgery.* Philadelphia: Lea & Febiger, 1990, p 126.

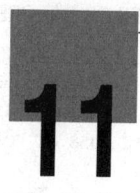

11 Neuro-Ophthalmology

Randall H. Scagliotti

Abnormal ocular clinical signs may appear as the result of disorders in the neuroanatomic pathways that subserve the sense of vision. The visual sense performs optimally when sufficiently protected eyes receive the proper amount of light while holding images steady on the retina. The neuroanatomic components that mediate vision in this fashion include the visual sensory system, those responsible for pupillary behavior, and those subserving the proper positioning and movement of the eyeballs and eyelids.

Diagnosis of abnormal neuro-ophthalmic clinical signs is dependent upon an understanding of the normal neuro-ophthalmic responses and the neuroanatomic pathways that mediate them. This chapter emphasizes the interpretation and neuroanatomic localization of neuro-ophthalmic signs. Specific diseases of the nervous system and eyes are discussed in other chapters of this book.

NEURO-OPHTHALMIC ANATOMY

- The pertinent neuroanatomy is summarized in Table 1.
- The pathways that modulate the pupillary light responses are depicted in Figure 1. Note the unequal crossing of afferent pupillary fibers both at the chiasm and the posterior commissure. This finding accounts for the anisocoria (unequal pupil size) apparent with lesions in the afferent arm of the light reflex.

CLINICAL SIGNS OF NEURO-OPHTHALMIC IMPORTANCE

- *Absence of reflex blinking* is present with an eyelid closure abnormality.

TABLE 1. Summary of Neuro-Ophthalmic Anatomy

Nerve	Nerve Type	Nerve Cell Body Location Gross	Microscopic	Ganglia	Distribution	Function
Optic (CN II)	SSA	Retina to ventral diencephalon	Ganglion cell layer of retina	—	Lateral geniculate body Pretectal nucleus	Vision Innervates parasympathetic nucleus of CN III (miosis)
Oculomotor (CN III)	SE	Ventral mesencephalon	Motor nucleus of oculomotor nerve	—	Median, dorsal, ventral recti, ventral oblique levator palpebrae muscles	Ocular motility Lid elevation
	GVE	Ventral mesencephalon	Parasympathetic nucleus of CN III	Ciliary ganglion	Iris sphincter muscle Ciliary muscle	Miosis Regulates lens curvature
Trochlear (CN IV)	SE	Dorsal mesencephalon	Motor nucleus of trochlear nerve	—	Dorsal oblique muscle	Ocular motility
Trigeminal (CN V)	SA	Cavum trigeminale of dura/petrous temporal bone to v. metencephalon	Trigeminal ganglion, ganglion (gasserian or semilunar)	—	Ophthalmic division, orbit Maxillary division, eyelids	Sensory to orbit, eyeball, and eyelid Sensory to eyelids
Abducent (CN VI)	SE	Ventral metencephalon	Motor nucleus of abducent nerve	—	Lateral rectus muscle Retractor bulbi muscle	Ocular motility Globe retraction, third eyelid up
Facial (CN VII)	SVE	Ventral myelencephalon	Motor nucleus of facial nerve	—	Orbicularis oculi Muscles of face	Eyelid closure Facial expression
	GVE	Ventral myelencephalon	Parasympathetic nucleus of CN VII	Pterygopalatine ganglion	Lacrimal gland	Tear secretion
Vestibulocochlear (CN VIII)	SP	Myelencephalon	Vestibular ganglion	—	Semicircular canals, utricle, sacculus	Coordinates eye with head movement, equilibrium
Glossopharyngeal (CN IX)	GVE	Myelencephalon	Parasympathetic nucleus of CN IX	Otic ganglion	Parotid salivary gland	Salivary secretion used for PDT

CN = cranial nerve; SE = somatic efferent; GVE = general visceral efferent; SVE = special visceral efferent; SA = somatic afferents; SSA = special somatic afferents; SP (SSA proprioception) = special proprioception; PDT = parotid duct transposition.

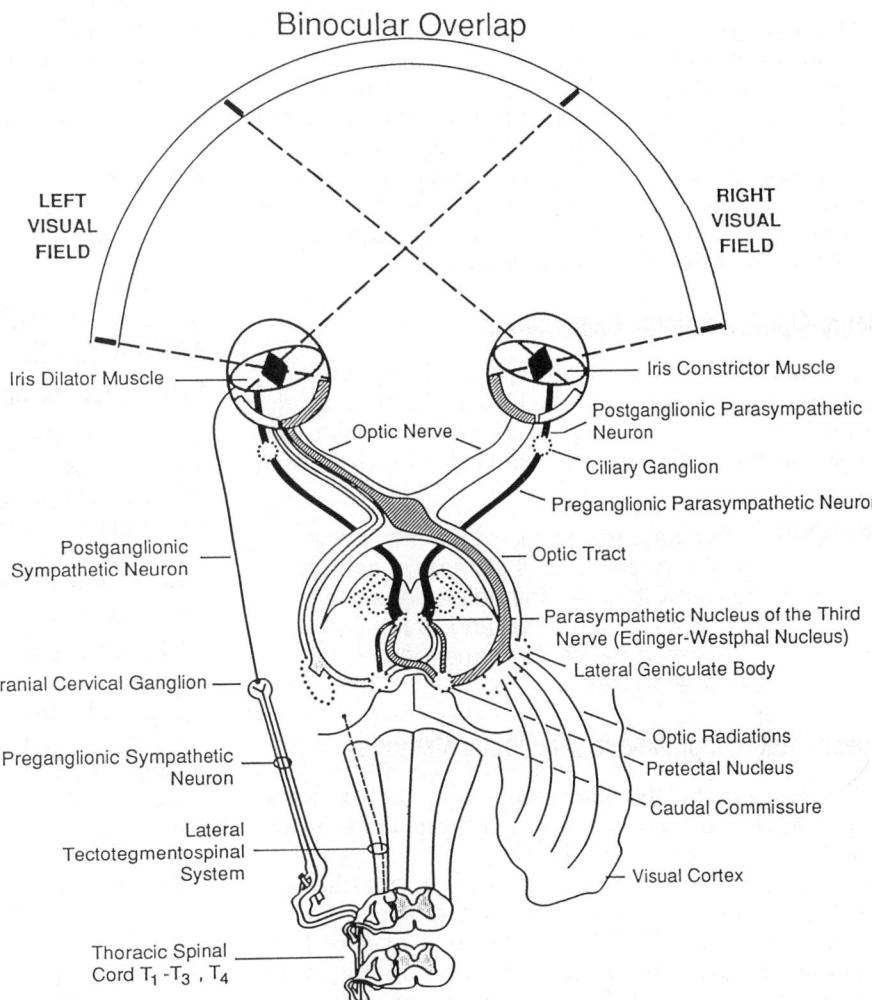

Binocular Overlap

LEFT VISUAL FIELD

RIGHT VISUAL FIELD

Iris Dilator Muscle

Optic Nerve

Iris Constrictor Muscle

Postganglionic Parasympathetic Neuron

Ciliary Ganglion

Preganglionic Parasympathetic Neuron

Postganglionic Sympathetic Neuron

Optic Tract

Parasympathetic Nucleus of the Third Nerve (Edinger-Westphal Nucleus)

Lateral Geniculate Body

Cranial Cervical Ganglion

Optic Radiations

Preganglionic Sympathetic Neuron

Pretectal Nucleus

Caudal Commissure

Lateral Tectotegmentospinal System

Visual Cortex

Thoracic Spinal Cord T$_1$-T$_3$, T$_4$

Figure 1. Pathways modulating the pupillary light response.

- *Ptosis or blepharoptosis* is a sign indicating insufficient opening of the eyelids. This sign must be differentiated from *pseudoptosis,* which occurs when the upper eyelid droops over an eye that is abnormal in size, shape, or position (see sec. 11, ch. 2).
- *Decreased tear production* (as determined by a Schirmer tear test of less than 10 mm wetting/min) may indicate a disorder of either the afferent arm (trigeminal nerve) or efferent arm (general visceral efferents of the facial nerve) of the corneolacrimal reflex. This disorder must be differentiated diagnostically from injury to the lacrimal gland proper (see sec. 11, ch. 9).
- *Decreased parotid salivary gland production* may result from glossopharyngeal nerve injury. Parotid secretion must be adequate in the event that the parotid salivary duct is to be transpositioned to an eye for treatment of keratoconjunctivitis sicca as discussed in sec. 11, ch. 9.
- *Loss of corneal/adnexal pain or tactile sensation* occurs with trigeminal sensory neuropathies.
- *Anisocoria,* not present as a result of anatomic or mechanical problems of the iris, is usually the result of neuropathology in the pupillary light reflex pathway or efferent sympathetic pathway, both of which control pupillary behavior.

- *Strabismus* (eyes that deviate while focusing on the same object) indicates a problem with ocular alignment.
- *Nystagmus* is the involuntary, repetitive, to-and-fro movement of one or both eyes that includes smooth sinusoidal oscillations (pendular nystagmus) and alternation of slow drift and corrective quick phase oscillations (jerk nystagmus). Nystagmus occurs in any plane and may be either acquired or congenital.
- *Blindness* is the congenital or acquired inability to see due to any disorders of the organs of sight or to lesions in the areas of the brain responsible for the sense of vision.

DIAGNOSIS

History

General History. Elicit information on prior neurologic disturbances, systemic illnesses, head or neck diseases, and drug use. Although a symptom rather than a sign, a history of pain can be surmised if there has been rubbing of the face and eye along standing surfaces or furniture or with paws. Often, head and eye pain leads to altered behavior. Infrequently, aggression is noted, but most often patients with pain become secretive and reclusive.

Ocular History. Establish the specific nature of any ocular secretion; the presence of inflammation about the eye, eyelids, and orbit; and the abnormalities in globe position and motility. The nature of a vision disturbance is often characterized by owners as a loss of night or day vision or a difficulty with near or far objects or with still or moving objects.

Neuro-Ophthalmologic Examination

In addition to a complete physical examination, perform a thorough neurologic examination as described in section 10, chapter 1, with particular emphasis on the evaluation of cranial nerves II through IX.

KEY POINT ▶ Evaluate the status of the ear, nose, mouth, pharynx, and paranasal sinuses, because they are intimately linked in disease to each other and to the eye. They often cause abnormal neuro-ophthalmic signs.

Special Neuro-Ophthalmic Diagnostic Methods

- *Duction tests* involve alternating eye patches, while the unpatched viewing eye is led through secondary and tertiary positions of gaze.
- In the passive forced duction test, an anesthetized eye is grasped at the limbus with forceps and the eye is forcibly moved in the direction of gaze limitation. In the active forced duction test, a tug on the grasped eye is felt if the nerve supply to the muscle is intact.
- *Swinging flashlight test* takes place in a dark room. Light is directed at one eye and then quickly moved to the other eye. If the second pupil dilates, an afferent lesion is present.
- *Schirmer tear tests* (see sec. 11, ch. 9) are used to measure reflex tearing (Schirmer 1 in the unanesthetized eye) and basal secretion (Schirmer 2 in the anesthetized eye).
- *Corneal sensitivity* is quantitatively measured with the Cochet and Bonnet anesthesiometer.
- *Pharmacologic drug testing* is employed to determine if anisocoria caused by lesions of the efferent sympathetic system or the efferent arm of the pupillary light reflex is of central or peripheral origin.
- *Cerebrospinal fluid pressure and analysis* assess the status of the CNS when lesions are thought to be central in origin (see sec. 10, ch. 1).
- *Electroretinography (ERG)* differentiates retinal pathology from disorders of postretinal anatomy (see sec. 11, ch. 8).
- *Ocular and orbital ultrasonography* aids the diagnosis in problems involving anisocoria and globe position and/or in motility problems involving orbital vascular disorders.
- *Radiographs* include bilateral lateral oblique, ventrodorsal, and frontal open mouth and frontal ("skyline") views in order to assess the integrity of the skull and sinuses.

- *Optic nerve thecograms/basal cisternograms and myelograms* uncover and detail filling defects in the CNS spaces.
- *Computerized axial tomography (CAT)* provides images of orbital and intracranial CNS disorders.
- *Magnetic resonance imaging (MRI)* is the most exquisite image available for soft tissue diseases of the orbit and brain.

SPECIFIC NEURO-OPHTHALMIC ABNORMALITIES
Eyelid Closure Abnormalities

Failure of the reflex closure of the eyelids may result from central or peripheral disorders that affect the afferent arm of the blink reflex (the optic nerve and/or trigeminal nerve) or the efferent arm (the facial nerve), which innervates the orbicularis oculi muscle. Diagnosis requires separate testing of the various nerve components of the reflex.

- The *corneal blink reflex* is a closure of the eyelids in response to a tactile or painful stimulus on the unanesthetized cornea that is afferently mediated by the trigeminal nerve and efferently mediated by the facial nerve. Cortical perception of a noxious stimulus results in head withdrawal as well as reflex blepharospasm. Presenting the stimulus outside the visual field avoids the optic nerve. Diseases affecting the afferent and/or efferent arm centrally or peripherally cause the loss of this reflex.
- The *dazzle reflex* is a *subcortical* reflex afferently mediated by the optic nerve and produces a *bilateral partial eyelid closure* (blink or squint) in response to a bright light shined on one eye at a time. The bright light must be from a powerful source (halogen power with a Finoff transilluminator or fiberoptic light). Care is taken to avoid stimulating the trigeminal nerve endings. This reflex is lost in complete lesions of the optic nerves and in certain mesencephalic lesions that may not demonstrate other neurologic deficits.
- The *menace response* is a rapid eyelid closure, with or without head withdrawal, in response to a threatening or unexpected image suddenly appearing in the near visual field. This response is *cortical*, afferently mediated by the optic nerve and requires intact peripheral and central visual pathways, including the cerebellum and facial nerves.

KEY POINT ▶ The menace response, (cortical) may be lost when the corneal blink and dazzle reflexes (subcortical) persist.

- Diffuse cerebellar cortical degenerative lesions cause a failure of the menace response bilaterally without visual deficits.
- Large unilateral cerebellar lesions cause ipsilateral unilateral menace-response deficits without a loss of vision.

Eyelid Opening Abnormalities

Neuroanatomic diagnosis of ptosis is dependent upon clinical signs and evidence of neuropathic, neuromus-

ular, or myopathic disease. Consider the following
our types:

Oculomotor ptosis results from injury to the oculomotor nerve at any level from the cerebral cortex to
the levator palpebrae superioris muscle. Oculomotor
ptosis is exaggerated in the lateral two thirds of the
eyelid during eyebrow elevation in the dog, if the
facial nerve, which innervates the levator anguli oculi
medialis muscle, remains intact. This muscle assists
in lifting the nasal portion of the eyelid and erects
the long tactile hairs (pili supraorbitales) of the
eyebrow. Lesion localization is enhanced if the other
functions produced by the general visceral efferent
fibers and the remaining somatic efferent fibers of
the third cranial nerve are also disturbed.

▪ *Oculosympathetic ptosis* is a component of *Horner's
syndrome* and results from damage along the efferent
sympathetic pathway. The lower lid often has an
"upside-down ptosis," which creates a narrowed
palpebral fissure. It must be diagnostically differentiated from oculomotor ptosis. All or some of the
other signs of Horner's syndrome (ipsilateral miosis,
enophthalmos, protrusion of the third eyelid) may
be present.

▪ *Myopathic ptosis* is usually an acquired condition
caused by damage to the levator muscle by inflammation, infiltration, or orbital trauma.

▪ *Neuromuscular ptosis* is a myasthenia gravis (MG)–
induced abnormality not yet reported in veterinary
medicine. Decreased palpebral relexes in dogs with
MG have been recorded, however.

Abnormalities of the Trigeminal Somatic Sensory System

Neuroanatomic diagnosis of trigeminal neuropathy
involves the analysis of the abnormal objective signs
and any associated neurologic signs.

▪ *Loss of the trigeminoabducent reflex* results from
damage to the trigeminal nerve or nucleus or to the
abducent nerve or its nucleus. The trigeminoabducent reflex retracts the eye into the orbit, after a
noxious stimulus, by direct action of the retractor
bulbi muscles. This indirectly causes the third eyelid
to protrude by direct contraction of the lateral rectus
muscle, which has a slip of ligament attached to the
third eyelid.

▪ *Loss of the corneolacrimal reflex* occurs in corneal
anesthesia (see Tear Insufficiency).

▪ The *corneal blink reflex* to noxious stimulation of the
cornea and adnexa can be lost in trigeminal injury
while the voluntary blink is retained, provided the
seventh cranial (facial) nerve remains intact.

Tear Insufficiency

Loss of reflex tearing (low Schirmer 1 tear test values
in the unanesthetized eye) occurs with disorders (inflammation, infection, neoplasia) of the trigeminal
nerve (afferent arm of the corneolacrimal reflex) or of
the facial nerve (efferent arm), along its convoluted
course to the lacrimal gland (see sec. 11, ch. 9).

▪ *Middle ear* disease (chronic otitis media) can injure
the *major petrosal nerve* containing the general visceral efferents of the facial nerve, which innervates
the lacrimal gland.

▪ *Lateral orbit* disease can injure the *zygomaticotemporal nerve,* an eyelid sensory nerve (a branch of the
maxillary nerve of the fifth cranial [trigeminal]
nerve), containing lacrimal gland general visceral
efferents of the facial nerve.

▪ *Cerebellopontine angle* disease (tumors) can affect
the facial and vestibulocochlear nerves, as they cross
this site together. The disease can result in hearing
loss, vestibular disease, facial paralysis, "dry eye,"
or any combination thereof.

▪ *Ophthalmic nerve* (fifth cranial nerve branch) disease
results in corneal anesthesia, loss of the *corneolacrimal reflex,* and diminished Schirmer 1 tear test
findings.

Parotid Salivary Gland Insufficiency

Determine parotid duct secretion prior to parotid
duct transpositioning for treatment of keratoconjunctivitis sicca. The bitter taste of atropine sulfate
ophthalmic solution applied directly to the buccal mucosa immediately stimulates reflex parotid secretion.
A pulse-like squirting of parotid secretion from the
parotid duct papilla indicates adequate secretion. If
the secretion slowly flows from the duct orifice without
the pulse-like squirting, successful transposition is more
problematic.

▪ *Disease of the middle ear* can injure the general
visceral efferents of the *minor petrosal nerve* and the
otic ganglion, located in the auditory tube of the
middle ear.

▪ *Disease of the external ear,* especially that which
ossifies the external canal and leads to periauricular
tissue damage, can injure the *auriculotemporal nerve*
of the mandibular division of the fifth cranial nerve.
This sensory nerve carries glossopharyngeal postganglionic general visceral efferents from the otic ganglion that innervate the superficial parotid gland,
situated between the ear and angle of the mandible.

Anisocoria

Lesions of the pupillary pathways result in all or
some of the following clinically detectable disturbances, depending upon the lesion site and extent:
abnormalities in pupillary diameters and, in the cat,
sometimes shape; abnormalities in response to dark
adaptation; abnormalities in the pupillary light reflex;
and abnormalities in vision (Table 2).

Anisocoria in Ambient Light

▪ Unilateral pupillary pathway lesions result in anisocoria of variable degrees. Some disorders (feline
spastic pupil syndrome and the feline hemidilated
pupil) result in dyscoria.

▪ Unilateral lesions of the afferent arm of the pupillary
light reflex create small *(subtle)* anisocorias. Horner's
pupils, which are similar in appearance to those in
anisocoria, are distinguished on the basis of associ-

TABLE 2. Neuropathic and Other Causes of Anisocoria—Differential Signs and Tests

Disease	Pupil Affected Side	PLR D / i	SFT	Dazzle Reflex	Menace Response	DAD Test	Tonometry	PT	Diagnostic SLB	Funduscopy	Vision	Special tests
1. Anterior uveitis	Miotic	± ±	−	+	±	Unequal	Hypo	No	+	−	Poor	−
2. Glaucoma (advanced)	Dilated (fixed)	− −	−	−	−	Unequal	Hyper	No	±	+	Blind	−
3. Afferent arm lesions												
a. Retina/optic nerve	Dilated	− −	+	−	−	Equal	Normo	No	−	±	Blind	−
b. Chiasm	± Dilated	± ±	−	± +	± +	Equal	Normo	No	−	−	Variable	−
c. Optic tract	Miotic	+ +	−	+	+	Equal	Normo	No	−	−	Homonymous hemianopia	−
4. Efferent arm lesions												
a. Atrophic iris disease	Dilated	− +	−	+	+	Variable	Normo	Yes	+	−	Normal	PT
b. Traumatic iridoplegia	Dilated	− +	−	+	+	Unequal	Hypo/normo	Yes	±	−	May be poor	PT
c. Pharmacologic blockade (atropine-induced mydriasis)	Dilated	− +	−	+	+	Equal	Normo	Yes	−	−	Normal	PT
d. Postganglionic denervation	Dilated	− +	−	+	+	Dog—unequal Cat—equal	Normo	Yes	−	−	Normal	PT
e. Preganglionic/central denervation	Dilated	− +	−	+	+	Unequal	Normo	Yes	−	−	Normal	PT
5. Efferent sympathetic nerve lesions												
a. Preganglionic denervation	Miotic	+ +	−	+	+	Unequal	Normo	Yes	−	−	Normal	PT
b. Postganglionic denervation	Miotic	+ +	−	+	+	Unequal	Normo	Yes	−	−	Normal	PT
6. Polyneuropathy												
a. Spastic pupil syndrome	Variable	± ±	−	+	+	No	Normo	No	−	−	Normal	+FeLV

PLR = pupillary light reflexes; D = direct (in affected, stimulated eye) light reflex; I = indirect (in nonaffected, unstimulated fellow eye) light reflex; X = swinging flashlight test; DAD test = dark adaptation test; PT = pharmacologic test; SLB = slit lamp biomicroscopy; SFT = swinging flashlight test; SLB = slit lamp biomicroscopy; FeLV = feline leukemia virus; Hypo = < 15 mm Hg; Hyper = > 25 mm Hg; and Normo = 15-25 mm Hg.

ated clinical signs and response to dark adaptation. Horner's anisocoria partially or completely disappears in bright light.

■ *Large differences* in pupil size occur with unilateral lesions of the efferent arm of the pupillary light reflex.

Anisocoria in Darkness

■ Unilateral and bilateral lesions of the afferent arm of the pupillary light reflex dilate maximally and equally in darkness.

KEY POINT ▶ This response distinguishes lesions of the afferent arm and efferent arm of the pupillary light reflex in cats from all other pupillary abnormalities, including those leading to a mechanical restriction of the iris (synechia).

■ In cats, unilateral and bilateral lesions of the efferent arm of the pupillary light reflex dilate maximally and equally in darkness.
■ In dogs, anisocoria persists in darkness. The smaller pupil is ipsilateral to the lesions in the ciliary ganglion or short ciliary nerves.
■ Anisocoria of Horner's syndrome becomes more pronounced in darkness.
■ Cats with the feline spastic pupil syndrome (i.e., FeLV-associated anisocoria), if the eyes dilate at all in darkness, will dilate only slightly while retaining a relative anisocoria.

Anisocoria in Optic Nerve Dysfunction

■ A complete unilateral prechiasmal lesion, which involves the retinal portion and/or prechiasmal optic nerve, creates anisocoria with the smaller pupil contralateral to the side of the lesion (see Table 2).
■ Lesions of the chiasm lead to anisocoria when the fiber destruction is asymmetric. The pupillary light reflex may be paradoxical (i.e., the pupil of the eye opposite to that which is stimulated will constrict to a greater extent than the eye under stimulation). This response reverses when the opposite eye is stimulated (see Table 2).
■ A unilateral lesion of the optic (postchiasmal) tract always appears with a subtle anisocoria with the smaller pupil ipsilateral to the side with the lesion (see Table 2).

Anisocoria in Oculomotor Dysfunction

Injury to the oculomotor nerve general visceral efferent fibers (efferent arm of the pupillary light reflex) leads to anisocoria without blindness (see Table 2).

Anisocoria in Oculosympathetic Dysfunction

Lesions in the efferent sympathetic pathway lead to the signs of Horner's syndrome with anisocoria its most diagnostic sign (see Table 2). Any or all of the other signs of Horner's syndrome, including oculosympathetic ptosis resulting in a narrowed palpebral fissure, third eyelid protrusion, and enophthalmos, may be present.

Ocular Alignment and Motility Abnormalities

Ocular Alignment

Strabismus may be congenital or acquired and results either from central dysfunction, as is commonly observed in Siamese cats, or from peripheral abnormalities to the motor nerves of the eye (III, IV, and VI). It can also occur with disorders of the extraocular muscles and the neuromuscular junction.

■ *Comitant strabismus* is a deviation that does not vary either with different positions of gaze or with either eye fixating.
■ *Incomitant strabismus* is an ocular deviation that varies when the direction of gaze changes and/or when either eye fixates.

Ocular Motility

■ The ability of one eye to rotate while it is viewing is referred to as *duction*.
■ The extent of rotation with both eyes viewing is referred to as *version*.
■ If the *range of movement* is restricted during version and/or duction, *muscle paresis must be distinguished from mechanical restriction to ocular motility*. This differentiation is accomplished by performing passive and active forced duction tests (see special neuro-ophthalmic diagnostic methods).
■ In *oculomotor nerve dysfunction*, somatic efferent lesions (see Table 1) lead to ptosis and an inability to rotate the eye upwards, downwards, or inwards. When the unaffected eye is fixating straight ahead (primary position of gaze), the eye is held in a position of divergent strabismus. The eye can be returned to midline by having the gaze directed to the side opposite the paralysis. The strabmismus, therefore, is incomitant.
■ In *trochlear nerve dysfunction*, paralysis of the trochlear nerve results in extorsion (outward rotation) of the eye, which is increasingly apparent as the gaze is directed outward. Because the dorsal oblique muscle acts as an intorter during outward gaze, the unopposed ventral oblique extorts the eye. This extorsion results in a deviation of the dorsal retinal vessels temporally. In the cat, temporal deviation of the dorsal aspect of the slit-like pupil is observed.
■ In *abducent nucleus and nerve dysfunction*, lesions of the abducent *nucleus* cause ipsilateral palsy of the horizontal gaze (dysfunction of lateral rectus muscle). The eyes do not cross the midline. The trigeminoabducent reflex can be lost if the motoneurons to the retractor oculi muscles are disturbed. The vestibulo-ocular reflex (see sec. 10, ch. 1) is abnormal.
  • Lesions of the abducent *nerve* usually cause paralysis of both the lateral rectus and retractor oculi muscles. This effect results in an ipsilateral convergent (incomitant) strabismus when the normal eye is fixating in its primary position, along with ipsilateral palsy on horizontal gaze—only now the contralateral eye crosses the midline.

Nystagmus

Nystagmus (see sec. 10, ch. 1) is a normal response to vestibular and optokinetic stimuli. Pathologic nystagmus occurs in disorders of systems (vestibular and optokinetic), which stabilize images of objects on the retina during head rotations or stabilize images of moving objects on the retina (pursuit system).

- *Congenital nystagmus* is caused by metabolic dysfunction or structural abnormalities of the brain or eye.
  - *Sensory congenital nystagmus* is either jerk or pendular and associated with disease in the visual sensory system (cataracts, persistent hyperplastic primary vitreous, retinal detachment).
  - *Motor congenital nystagmus* is either jerk or pendular type and lacks any primary disease of the visual sensory system. Any decrease in vision is secondary to the nystagmus.
- *Acquired nystagmus* is often associated with other neurologic signs. *Vestibular nystagmus* is an acquired jerk nystagmus caused by imbalance within the vestibular apparatus, with the corrective quick phases directed away from the side of the lesion.
  - In *peripheral vestibular disease,* the nystagmus is mixed because the axis around which the eye rotates relates to the geometric relationships of the semicircular canals. Vertical-torsional nystagmus indicates posterior or anterior semicircular canal irritation, depending upon the direction of the corrective quick phase's vertical movement. Horizontal-torsional nystagmus occurs from complete unilateral labyrinthitis. Positional nystagmus can also be seen.
  - In *central vestibular disease* the nystagmus is more purely torsional, horizontal, or vertical. Positional nystagmus can be present.

Blindness

Blindness may be complete or partial and represents a loss of visual acuity and/or visual fields. Blindness can be categorized according to the lesion site as ocular, brain stem, or cerebral blindness. The resulting blindness can be unilateral or bilateral.

- *Ocular blindness* is caused by any eye disorder that interrupts the path of light through the eye or the retinal processing of light as determined by focal illumination for the anterior segment and by ophthalmoscopy for the posterior segment. Lack of funduscopic abnormalities does not diagnostically rule out the retina as the site of the lesion.
  - Retinal causes of vision loss are most frequently bilateral and include nyctalopia (night blindness), hemeralopia (day blindness), and generalized retinal atrophy or degeneration. Electroretinography differentiates the retinal diseases (see sec. 11, ch. 8).
  - The essential features of ocular blindness of *retinal* origin include a loss of the reflex eyelid closure to bright illumination (dazzle reflex) and to threatening gestures (menace response), abnormal pupillary reflexes (positive swinging flashlight test with unilateral retinal disease), anisocoria (only with unilateral or asymmetric retinal disease) and large pupils (with bilateral retinal disease), and normal extraocular movements of the eyes.

- *Brain stem blindness* may be caused by inflammation, infection, neoplasia, or vascular accidents in those areas of the brain stem and the intracranial and intraorbital portion of the optic nerve that are important vision relay centers to the cortex and those areas responsible for visually guided behavior (see sec. 10, ch. 2).
  - The essential features include a loss of the dazzle reflex and menace response; abnormal pupillary reflexes; anisocoria (only with unilateral disease); and extraocular eye movements or positions, which may be abnormal.
  - Other neurologic signs of brain stem disease may be present (see sec. 10, ch. 2).
- *Cerebral blindness* is a generalized term describing the blindness that is caused by a disorder to any area of the cerebral cortex responsible for vision.
- *Cortical blindness* indicates selective loss of the visual occipital cortex. In some instances, cerebral blindness includes cortical blindness.
  - The essential features of both include the loss of reflex eyelid closure to threatening gestures (menace response); retention of the reflex constriction of the pupils to illumination (pupillary light reflexes); retention of the integrity of the ocular structures, especially the retinas as verified by ophthalmoscopy; and retention of the full extraocular movements of the eye.
  - Visual occipital cortex loss must be distinguished from the loss of function in the motor cortex. In motor cortex lesions, images are seen, but the response may be inappropriate to the visual challenge (walks off a visual cliff, while visually aware of the cliff).

TREATMENT

Treatment depends upon the nature of the lesion, the location, the extent, and the duration. Treatment often involves a combination of modalities, including both surgical and medical. Refer to other chapters in this text for specific treatment for other various ocular and neurologic diseases.

PROGNOSIS

In general, patients with diseases of neuro-ophthalmic importance have their best prognoses when the diseases are purely of an inflammatory nature. Patients with disorders of an infectious or vascular nature carry more guarded prognoses. A patient with a neoplastic disease, although often successfully treated, has a poor prognosis.

Supplemental Readings

De Lahunta A: *Veterinary Neuroanatomy and Clinical Neurology.* Philadelphia: W.B. Saunders, 1983, p 279.
Scagliotti RH: Current concepts in veterinary neuro-ophthalmology. Vet Clin North Am [Sm Anim Pract] 10:417, 1980.
Scagliotti RH: Neuro-ophthalmology. *In* Gelatt KN, ed.: *Textbook of Veterinary Ophthalmology,* 2nd ed. Philadelphia: Lea & Febiger, 1991, pp 706–743.

Disorders of Avian and Exotic Pets

Barbara L. Oglesbee

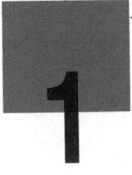

Avian Techniques

Barbara L. Oglesbee

RESTRAINT

For General Physical Examination (Fig. 1)

- Hold the bird's head firmly with one hand, placing the thumb and second finger under the mandibles and the first finger on the crown.
- With the other hand, grasp the bird with a towel wrapped securely around the body.

For Radiography

- Anesthesia with isoflurane may be necessary and reduces stress from the procedure.
- Use an acrylic positioning board (Silverdust, El Granada, CA).

Dorsoventral View (Fig. 2A)

- Lock the head in an acrylic shield.
- Extend the wings fully and place masking tape proximal to the carpus and on the primary feathers.
- Tape the legs in full extension.
- Align the keel bone over the spinal column.

Lateral View (Fig. 2B)

- Position the bird with the right side down.
- Lock the head in an acrylic shield.
- Pull the wings dorsally and tape with masking tape proximal to the carpi.
- Tape the legs caudally, with the right leg slightly anterior to the left leg.
- Restrain the tail with masking tape.

OPENING THE MOUTH

- A mouth speculum (Lafeber Co., Odell, IL) can be used to keep the mouth open (Fig. 3A).
  - This procedure can cause cracking of the beak in some birds.
- Alternatively, loops of gauze can be used (Fig. 3B):
  - Restrain the bird in a towel with one hand (see Fig. 1); with the other hand, pull down on a gauze loop placed over the upper beak.

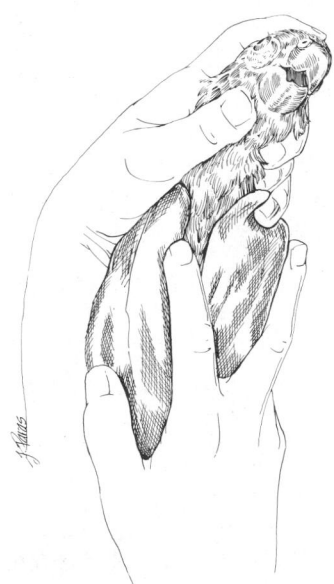

Figure 1. Restraint of parrot using towel.

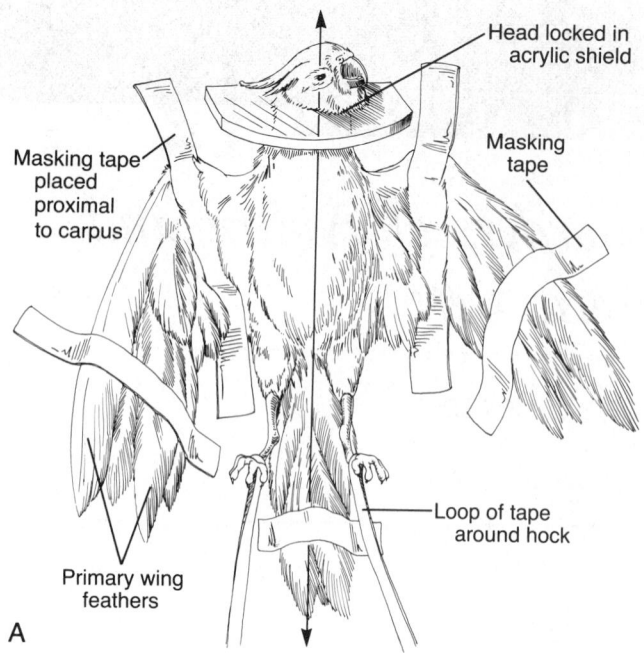

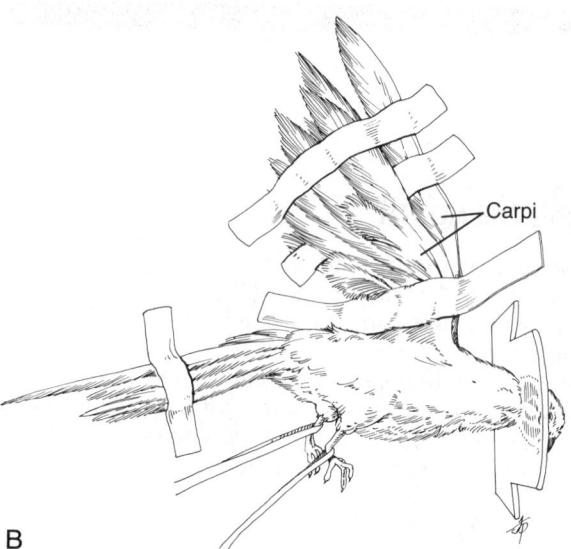

Figure 2. Restraint and positioning for radiography: *A,* dorsoventral view; *B,* lateral view.

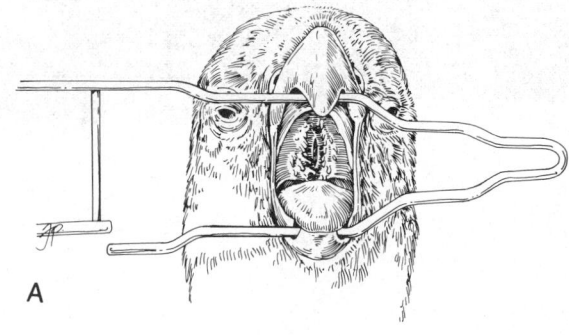

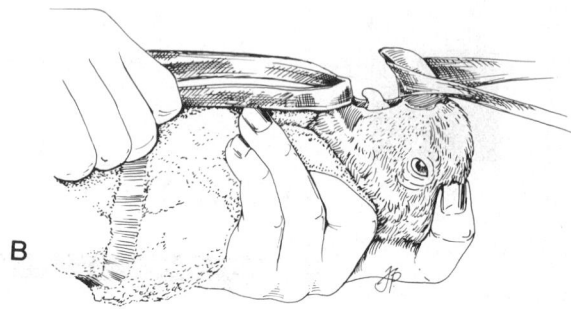

Figure 3. Opening the mouth using *(A)* a mouth speculum and *(B)* loops of gauze.

- Palpate the tube within the crop to check position.
- Expel the contents of the syringe while monitoring the pharynx for reflux of food.
- Withdraw the tube and immediately release the bird.

- Instruct an assistant to pull a second gauze loop over the upper beak.

FORCED ALIMENTATION

- Hold the bird in an upright position, using towel restraint if necessary (see Fig. 1).
- Hold the mouth open with a speculum or gauze loops (see Fig. 3).
- Gently pass a rigid feeding tube (Lafeber Co., Odell, IL) or soft rubber catheter with attached, gruel-filled syringe from the right side of the mouth into the crop (Fig. 4).

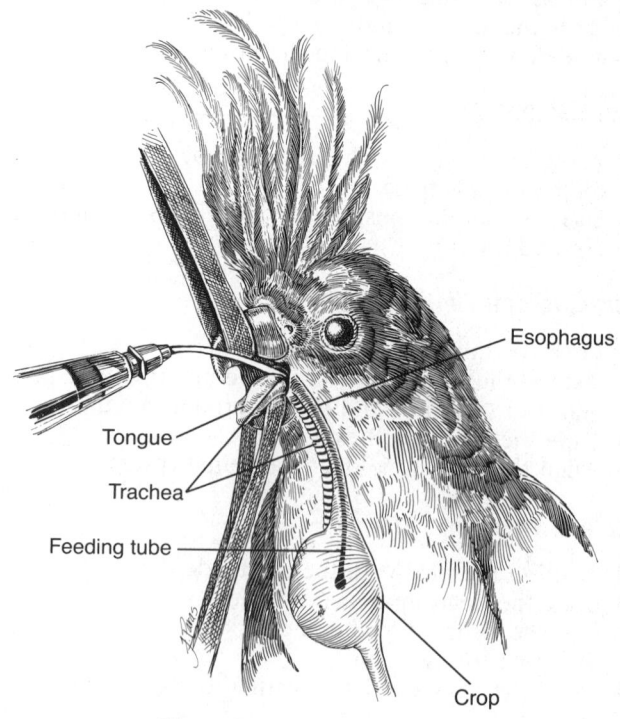

Figure 4. Forced alimentation.

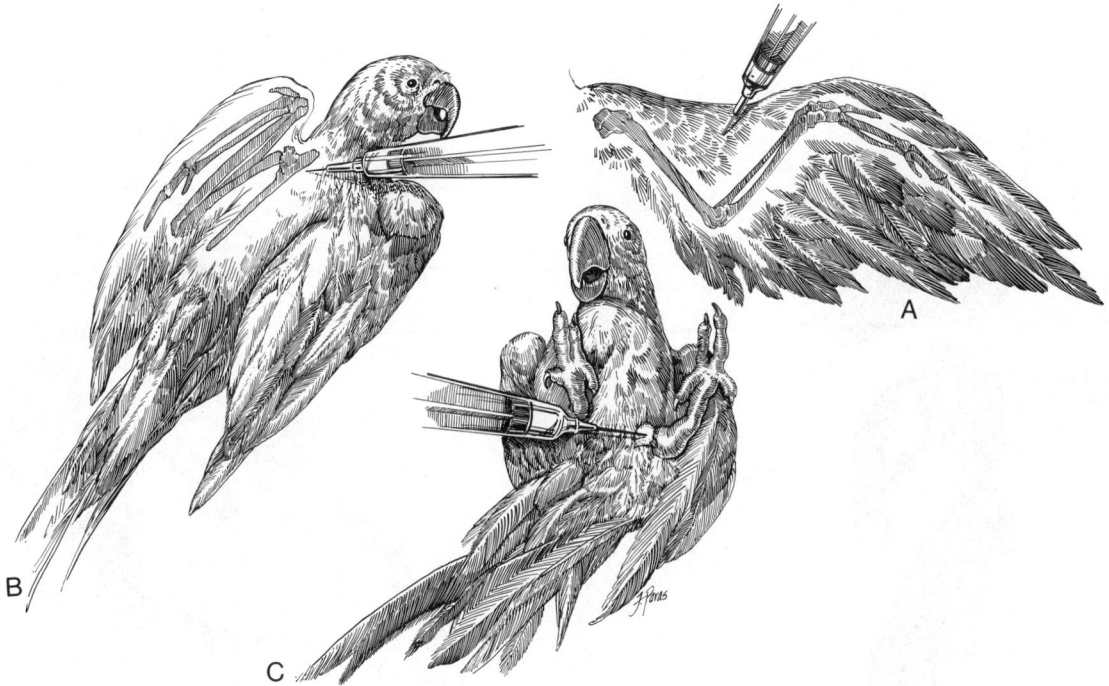

Figure 5. Subcutaneous fluid injection sites: *A*, wing web; *B*, interscapular region; *C*, groin.

SUBCUTANEOUS FLUID INJECTION

- Always use warmed fluids (98°F).
- Divide volume of fluid into multiple sites, including

the wing webs (Fig. 5*A*), interscapular region (Fig. 5*B*), and groin (Fig. 5*C*).

COLLECTION OF SAMPLES FOR CULTURE

Via the Choana (Fig. 6*A*)

- Hold the bird upright and open its mouth with a speculum or gauze loops (see Fig. 3).
- Insert a cotton-tipped swab into the most rostral portion of the choana.

Via the Cloaca (Fig. 6*B*)

- Restrain the bird in a towel.
- To avoid trauma to the mucosa, moisten the cotton-tipped swab with transport media or sterile saline solution prior to insertion into the cloaca.

VENIPUNCTURE SITES

KEY POINT ▶ To prevent hematoma formation, always apply firm pressure following venipuncture.

The following sites are recommended for blood collection and infusion of bolus fluids.

Jugular Vein

Birds Under 100 g (Fig. 7*A*)

- Use a hypodermic needle (25 or 27 gauge) and syringe (1 ml) for blood collection.
- The jugular vein is highly movable; make sure that the neck is in full extension.

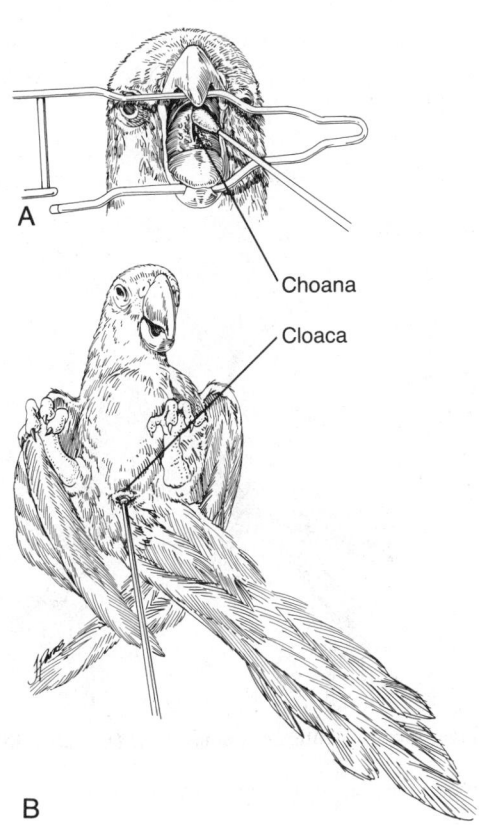

Choana

Cloaca

Figure 6. Collection of culture samples from *(A)* the choana and *(B)* the cloaca.

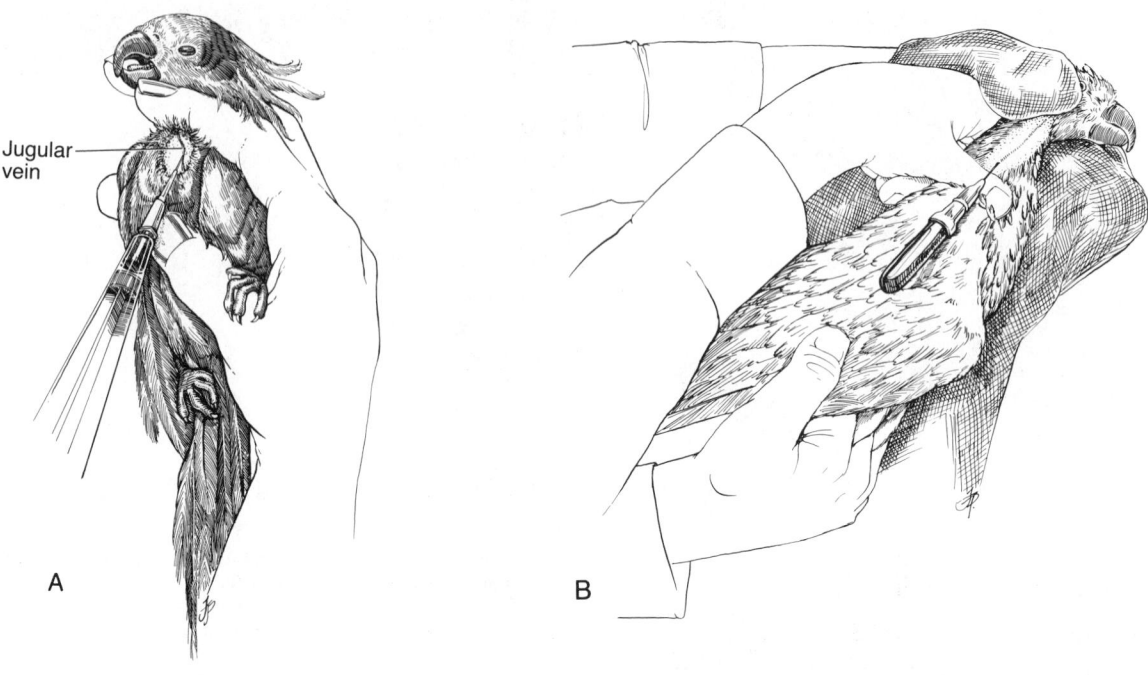

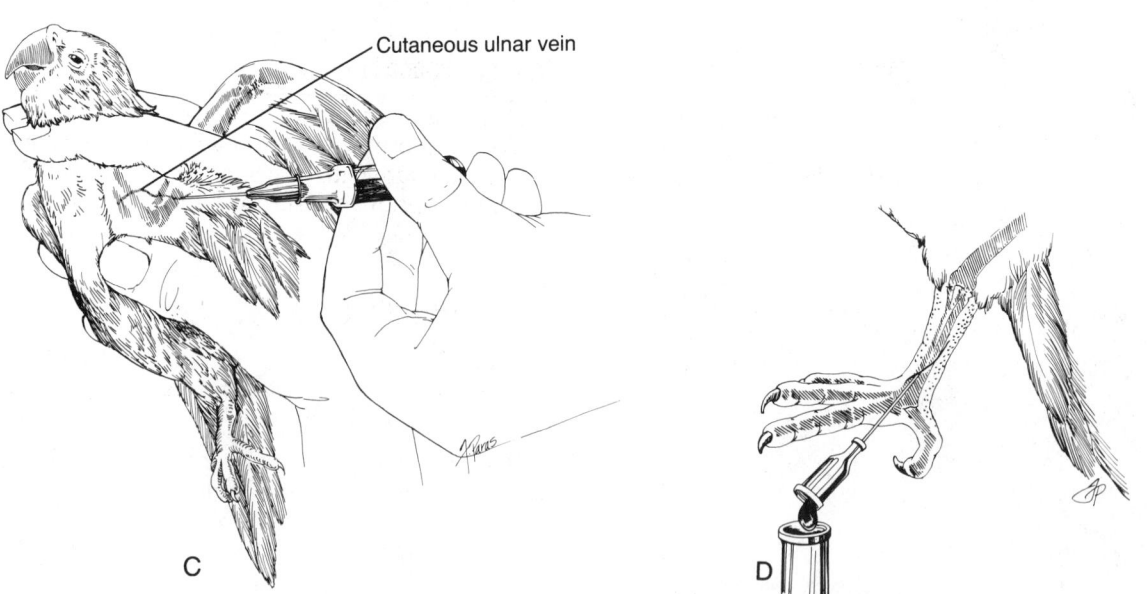

Figure 7. Venipuncture sites: *A,* jugular vein, birds under 100 g; *B,* jugular vein, larger birds; *C,* cutaneous ulnar vein; *D,* caudal tibial vein.

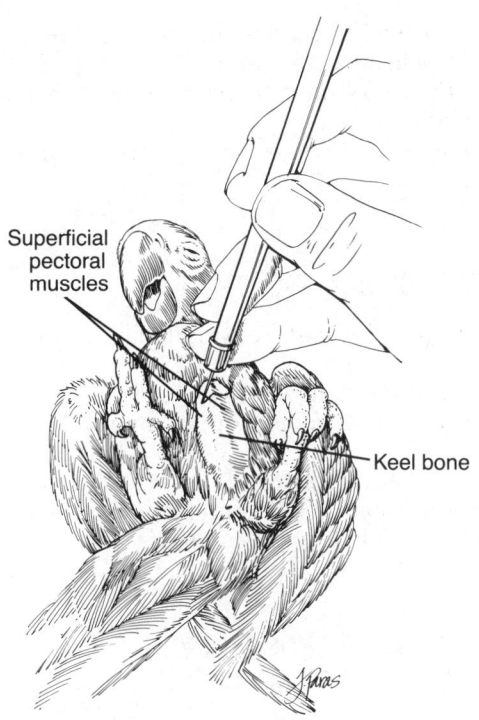

Superficial pectoral muscles

Keel bone

Figure 8. Intramuscular injection.

Larger Birds (Fig. 7B)

- If an assistant is not available, larger birds (e.g., parrots) may require anesthetization with isoflurane.
- With the right hand, the assistant holds the feet and the right wing pulled caudally; with the left hand. He/she restrains the bird's head.
- Using a larger needle (22–27 gauge) and syringe (3 ml) for blood collection, apply firm pressure to the right jugular vein at the thoracic inlet.

Cutaneous Ulnar Vein (Fig. 7C)

- The cutaneous ulnar vein crosses the ventral surface of the humeroradioulnar joint.

- To collect blood, cannulate the vessel with a 25-gauge needle and allow the blood to flow freely into a microcollection tube (Microtainer; Becton-Dickinson, Rutherford, NJ) or aspirate with a 1-ml syringe.

Caudal Tibial Vein (Fig. 7D)

- The caudal tibial vein passes on the medial side of the tibiotarsus just above the tarsal joint.
- To collect blood, cannulate vessel with a 25-gauge needle and allow blood to flow into a microcollection tube.

INTRAMUSCULAR INJECTION (Fig. 8)

- If necessary, use towel restraint (see Fig. 1).
- Inject into the superficial pectoral muscles on either side of the keel bone. Alternate sides with subsequent injections.

SINUS INJECTION/FLUSH

Sinus Injection (Fig. 9A)

- Restrain the head firmly in a normal upright position.
- Insert the needle percutaneously into the sinus slightly above the commissure of the beak, midway between the upper beak and the medial canthus of the eye.

Sinus Flush (Fig. 9B)

- Position the head so that it is slightly lower than the body, and restrain firmly.
- Press the syringe (without needle) against the nares opening.
- Inject 0.25–1.0 ml (depending on the size of the bird) of saline solution/antibiotic mixture into the nares.
- If the flushing procedure is successful, the mixture

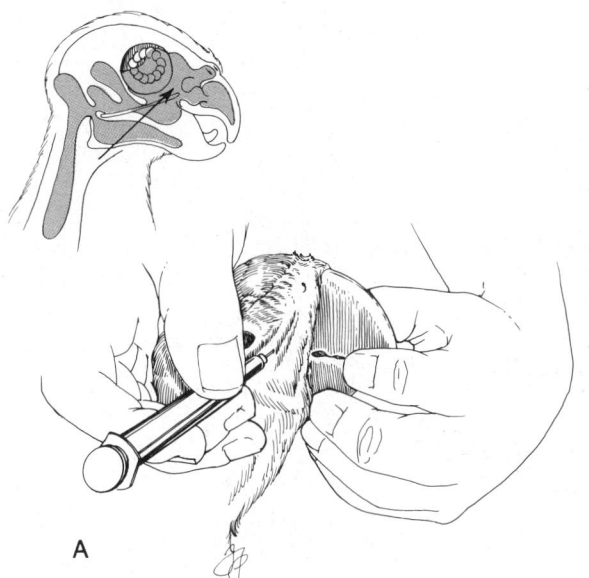

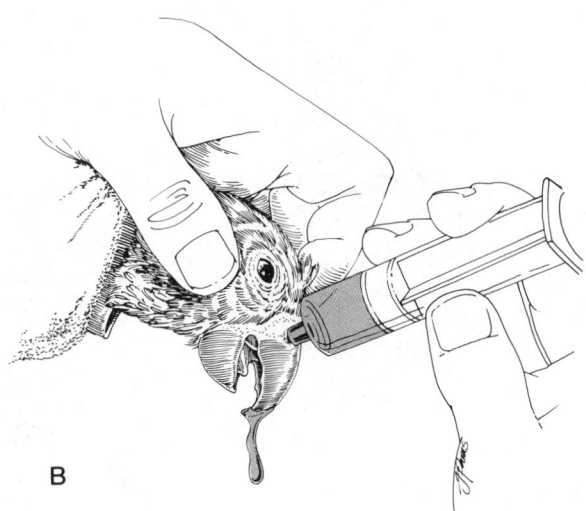

A

B

Figure 9. *A,* Sinus injection; *inset,* diagram of sinuses showing injection site *(arrow). B,* Sinus flush.

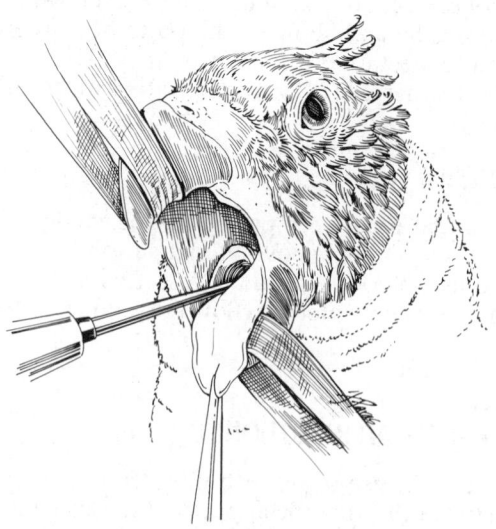

Figure 10. Tracheal injection/wash.

will flow freely from the choana, opposite nares, and ipsilateral eye.

■ Perform alternate flushes into each nares until all of the mixture is used and/or no further exudate is produced.

TRACHEAL INJECTION/WASH (Fig. 10)

■ Restrain the bird firmly.
  • For tracheal injection the bird may be held with the face upward, if desired.
  • For tracheal wash, hold the bird in an upright position.
■ Open the bird's mouth, using gauze loops or a speculum (see Fig. 1).
■ Insert an open-ended tomcat catheter with attached syringe into the tracheal opening:
  • For tracheal injection—inject medication.

  • For tracheal injection—inject medication.
  • For tracheal wash—inject 1.0 to 2.0 ml of 0.9% NaCl/kg B.W. into the trachea, and then aspirate immediately.
■ This method also may be used for tracheal endoscopy.

CROP SUPPORTER (Fig. 11)

■ Cut cast padding and Vetwrap longitudinally on each end.
■ Apply cast padding across the crop.
■ Position the longitudinal cuts above and below each wing.
■ Secure in back with tape.
■ When applying the Vetwrap, maintain slight pressure inward to aid in crop emptying.

PREPARATION FOR ENDOSCOPY OF THE ABDOMINAL AIR SAC (Fig. 12)

■ Anesthetize the bird with isoflurane.
■ Place the bird in lateral recumbency, right side down.
■ Extend the wings out over the back; have an assistant hold them in this position.
■ Pull the left leg as far caudally as possible.
■ Push the right leg under the body to aid in maintaining true lateral recumbency.
■ Pluck the area anterior to the proximal one-third of the femur free of feathers and perform a sterile scrub.
■ Apply clear drapes (3M, St. Paul, MN) over the area.
■ Make a stab incision with a #15 scalpel blade through the skin anterior to the proximal one-third of the femur and caudal to the last rib.

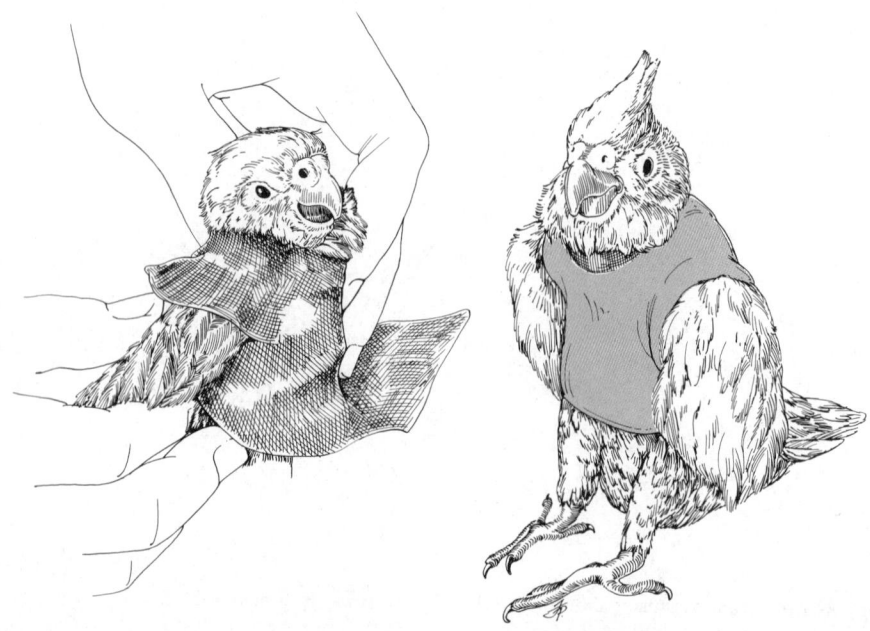

Figure 11. Crop supporter.

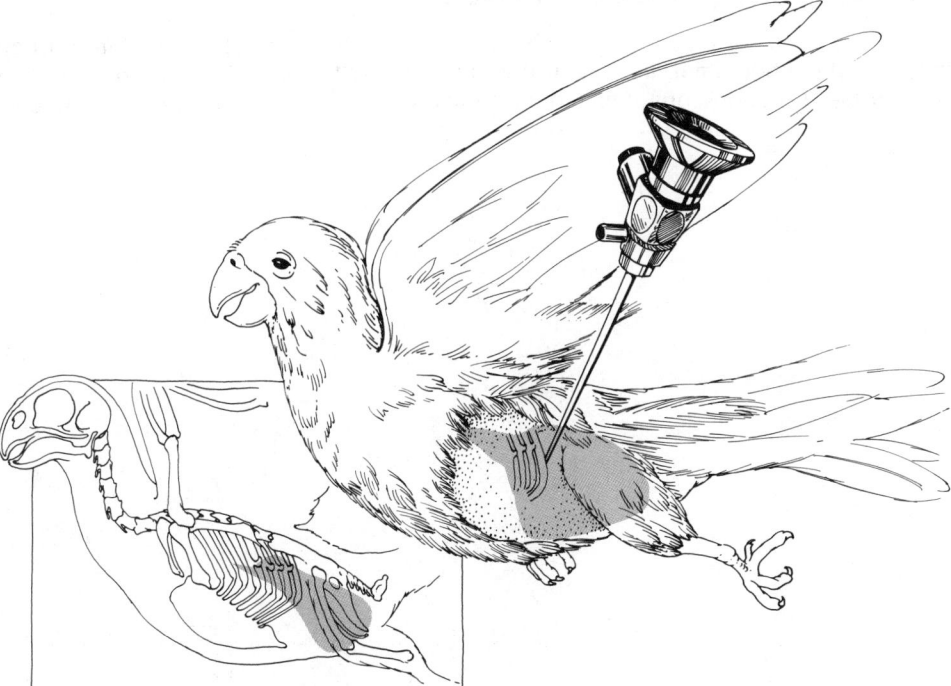

Figure 12. Preparation for endoscopy of the abdominal air sac; *inset,* trocar/cannula site *(arrow).*

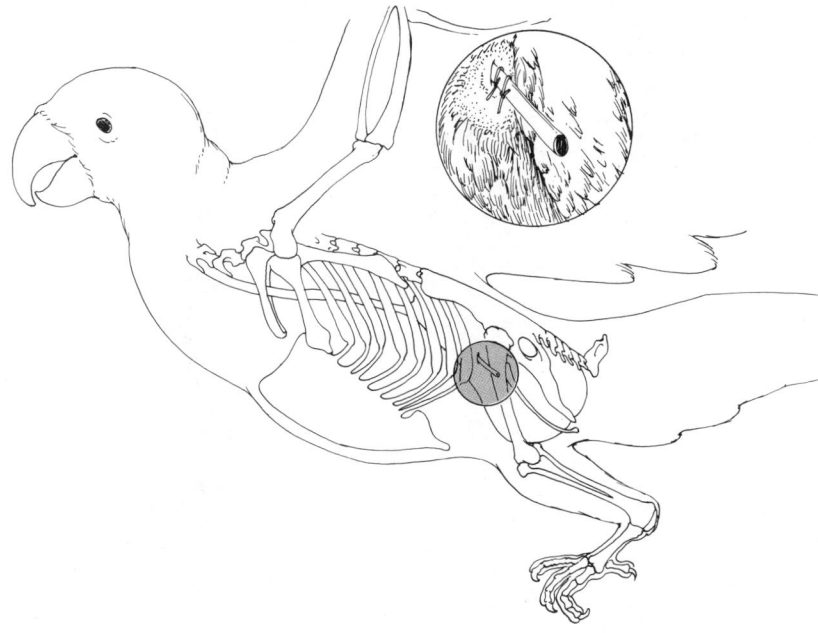

Figure 13. Abdominal breathing tube placement. Enlargement of placement site is shown in *inset.*

- Bluntly separate the underlying musculature and peritoneum, using straight mosquito forceps.
- Introduce the trocar/cannula through the opened musculature to visualize the air sacs.

PLACEMENT OF ABDOMINAL BREATHING TUBE
(Fig. 13)

- Enter the abdominal air sac using the technique described for endoscopy. Once the air sac is entered, the bird will begin breathing normally through the opening.
- Hold open the abdominal musculature/peritoneum with the inserted mosquito forceps.
- Place a sterilized rubber catheter (1–2½″ in diameter, depending on the size of the bird) in the opening and suture it in place with nonabsorbable suture material.
- The catheter can be left in place for up to 2 weeks. If obstruction with mucus or exudate occurs, flush with a 0.9% saline solution.

2 Avian Infectious Diseases

Barbara L. Oglesbee
Cynthia L. Bishop

ASPERGILLOSIS

Aspergillosis is an infectious but not contagious disease of pet and wild birds that is caused by the ubiquitous soil saprophyte *Aspergillus.* Infection generally occurs via inhalation of spores, resulting in primary lesions in the thoracic and abdominal air sacs and in the large airways (syrinx). Dissemination to other organ systems often occurs. Two forms of the disease, acute and chronic, commonly are seen.

- The *acute form,* which is seen most often in wild birds or psittacines under poor sanitary conditions, occurs following inhalation of an overwhelming number of spores. Severe dyspnea may result, with rapid progression to death.
- The *chronic form,* seen most often in psittacines, follows a stressful event or immunosuppressed state. Signs are often nonspecific and depend on the location of the infection and the immune status of the bird.
- The most common species isolated is *Aspergillus fumigatus. A. flavus, A. niger* and other species play a lesser role.

KEY POINT ▶ Aspergillosis is an opportunistic disease, requiring predisposing immunosuppressive factors such as stress, malnutrition, and environmental factors.

Etiology

Predisposing factors include the following:

- *Stress* may occur in shipping, quarantine, or capture of wild birds. Stress also may result from a prolonged illness, such as chlamydiosis, or following a traumatic event such as an injury or smoke inhalation.
- *Malnutrition* or vitamin deficiencies, especially hypovitaminosis A, often occurs in birds on diets consisting of seed only.
- *Prolonged antibiotic or corticosteroid use* may cause underlying immunosuppression. For example, aspergillosis may occur following treatment for chlamydiosis owing to the immunosuppressive effects of tetracycline in conjunction with the debilitated state of a diseased bird.

KEY POINT ▶ Suspect aspergillosis in cases in which respiratory signs do not respond to or worsen with antibiotic treatment.

- *Environmental factors:*
  - Poor ventilation in conjunction with damp litter (especially corn cob litter) soiled with feces promotes spore formation.
  - Poor sanitation, such as occurs when nest boxes and incubators are inadequately cleaned, can predispose birds to aspergillosis.

Clinical Signs
Acute Form

- Signs include anorexia, dyspnea, and cyanosis.
- Sudden death may occur without signs.

Chronic Form

The onset is insidious and signs vary, depending on the location of the infection.

- *Respiratory system*—Signs are common and depend on the area affected.
  - Signs include a change in voice, reluctance to talk, and a respiratory click that can be heard when lesions involve the main airways, especially the syrinx.
  - Severe dyspnea often occurs if the lesions are large enough to occlude the trachea or main stem bronchi. In some cases, these may be the only lesions present.
  - Mucoid to mucopurulent discharge seen with aspergillus infections.
  - The thoracic and abdominal air sacs may be involved, resulting in dyspnea or exercise intolerance.
  - In some cases, respiratory signs may be absent, even though lesions are seen on endoscopy or necropsy.
- *Liver and kidneys*—Diarrhea, anorexia, and polyuria may be seen. Green discoloration of the urates (biliverdinuria) and hepatomegaly are occasionally seen.
- *Nervous system*—Ataxia, torticollis, and paralysis may indicate central nervous system (CNS) involvement. Compression of the sciatic nerve by a granulomatous *Aspergillus* lesion has resulted in unilateral paralysis.
- *Nonspecific signs*—Weight loss, muscle wasting, depression, and lethargy often are the only clinical signs.

Diagnosis

History

- The history may identify an underlying environmental or immunosuppressive factor.

Physical Examination

- Examine the mouth and nares for mucus and exudates. Take samples from the trachea or choana for fungal culture.
- Palpate the breast muscles and weigh the bird for evidence of weight loss and muscle wasting.
- Palpate the abdomen for evidence of organomegaly.
- Auscultate the trachea or chest for congestion and for the presence of a respiratory click.

Complete Blood Count (CBC)/Serum Biochemical Profile

- A severe leukocytosis of 25,000–100,000 white blood cells (WBC) per μl often is present.
- The differential count usually reveals heterophilia with a left shift, monocytosis, lymphopenia, and anemia of chronic disease.
- Increased serum total protein with an increased globulin portion may be present in chronic disease.
- Serum glutamate oxaloacetic transaminase (SGOT), lactate dehydrogenase (LDH), and creatine phosphokinase (CPK) levels usually are increased, especially with hepatic involvement.

Endoscopy

Endoscopy is invaluable for the diagnosis of aspergillosis.

- When there are episodes of severe dyspnea, tracheal endoscopy may reveal a single lesion occluding the trachea or syrinx.
- If a thick, white discharge or plaque is visualized in the trachea, obtain a sample for culture on Sabouraud's dextrose agar.
- Endoscopy of the abdominal air sacs may reveal diffuse cloudiness or the presence of white or yellow plaques. These plaques may become covered with a green/gray pigmented mold; obtain samples via air sac lavage for culture and cytology.

Radiography

- Radiographic changes often are not visible in early cases.
- In advanced disease, radiographic abnormalities can include loss of definition of the air sacs, asymmetry of the air sacs due to air sac collapse or hyperinflation, and focal densities in the lungs or air sacs.
- Hepatomegaly or renomegaly may be visible radiographically, when there is involvement of these organ systems.

Treatment

Treatment is most successful when lesions are confined to the trachea, syrinx, and main stem bronchi, and when aggressive treatment is instituted early.

Antifungal Agents

- Administer amphotericin B (Fungizone; Squibb), 1.5 mg/kg q8h, IV, for 3–7 days. Mask the bird with isoflurane anesthesia and maintain an IV catheter for each injection.
  - If the main airways are involved, amphotericin B may be given by intratracheal injection, using a tomcat urinary catheter (Sherwood Medical) at a dosage of 1 mg/kg, q12h, for up to 1 month.
  - For mycotic air sacculitis, make a solution of 1 mg of amphotericin B per ml of 0.9% saline and nebulize q12h for 15 minutes.
  - Amphotericin B is potentially nephrotoxic and may cause bone marrow suppression.
- Give 5-fluorocytosine (Ancobon; Roche Labs), 100–250 mg/kg q12h, PO, in conjunction with or following amphotericin B treatment. Give the higher dosage for active infections; the lower dosage often is used prophylactically for 10–14 days in high-risk patients.
- Administer ketoconazole (Nizoral; Janssen), 25mg/kg q12h, PO, for 2–6 weeks in conjunction with or following amphotericin B treatment.
- Give fluconazole (Diflucan; Roerig), 5–10 mg/kg q24h, PO, for up to 6 weeks, with or after amphotericin B.

Antibiotic Therapy

- Antibiotic treatment based on culture and susceptibility testing may be necessary if a secondary bacterial infection is present.

Supportive Care

- Fluid therapy, forced alimentation (see sec. 12, ch. 1), nebulization, and heat are imperative for successful treatment.

Prognosis

- The prognosis is poor to grave, depending on the severity of the disease.

Prevention

- Because *Aspergillus* is an opportunistic pathogen, attempt to reduce predisposing immunoppressive factors such as stress and malnutrition.
- Place birds on prolonged antibiotic therapy or other birds at risk on 5-fluorocytosine prophylactically (as previously described).

KEY POINT ▶ To avoid inhalation of an overwhelming number of Aspergillus spores, house birds in a well-ventilated area. Do not use organic materials as bedding in nest boxes.

CHLAMYDIOSIS

Avian chlamydiosis is known as psittacosis when occurring in psittacine species and ornithosis when occurring in passerine species. The incidence in pet birds is high and is reported at 15–30% of those tested.

Etiology

Avian chlamydiosis is caused by the obligate intracellular parasite *Chlamydia psittaci*. The organism infects many species of wild, domestic, and exotic birds, domestic mammals, and humans. Manifestation of this disease varies from subclinical to fatal, depending on the strain of *C. psittaci* involved and the species of bird affected.

Life Cycle and Transmission

Chlamydiae have a biphasic life cycle.

- Infectious, extracellular *elementary bodies* are shed in oral/nasal secretions and feces and may survive outside the host for a month or longer. Dissemination may occur via shared food dishes or aerosolized fecal dust.
- Elementary bodies are inhaled or ingested and enter host cells where they undergo cellular rearrangement to form *reticulate bodies*, the replicating form of the organism.
- Following replication, initial bodies reorganize to form *infectious* elementary bodies, which are released upon rupture of the host cell. Elementary bodies may then be disseminated to cells of the liver, spleen, lungs, intestines, kidneys, gonads, and CNS.

Clinical Signs

KEY POINT ▶ Clinical signs vary greatly, depending on the organ system affected, virulence of the organism, and immune status of the host.

- *Inapparent carriers* are common. These may be birds that have recovered from clinical illness or that may have never shown signs. High numbers of organisms may be intermittently shed from the feces or nasal/oral secretions, putting other pet birds and humans at risk.
  - These carriers may develop clinical signs when stressed or otherwise immunocompromised.

Acute Form

- The acute form of the disease is seen more often in young psittacines. Signs may include:
  - Liver/gastrointestinal (GI) signs such as inappetence, green/gray diarrhea, biliverdinuria (lime-green urates), and occasionally vomiting or regurgitation
  - Respiratory signs, including serous to purulent nasal/ocular discharge, labored breathing, blepharitis, and conjunctivitis
  - Nonspecific signs, including ruffled feathers, weight loss, and depression
- Without treatment, signs may progress over a period of a few weeks, leading to prostration and death.

Chronic Form

- Nonspecific signs such as muscle wasting and poor feathering may be the only signs observed.
- Occasionally, mild respiratory, gastrointestinal, or

CNS signs (e.g., torticollis, seizures, rear limb paresis/paralysis) may be seen alone.

Diagnosis

History

- Recently imported birds may be at higher risk, owing to the increased exposure and stress associated with quarantine.

KEY POINT ▶ Recently acquired birds are not the only ones at risk; birds may harbor the disease for months and even years prior to manifestation of clinical signs.

Physical Examination

- Findings may be normal in inapparent carriers.
- Suspect chlamydiosis in birds with poor feathering, weight loss, or signs of GI or respiratory disease.

CBC/Serum Chemistry Profile

- Leukocytosis, often >40,000 WBC/μl demonstrating heterophilia with a left shift and toxic heterophils usually is seen in acute disease. Relative monocytosis and reactive lymphocytes are often present.
- The WBC count may be normal in subclinical cases.
- A low packed cell volume (PCV) is common in both acute and chronic disease.
- Serum protein usually is elevated as a result of chronic inflammatory stimulation.
- SGOT, LDH, bile acids and/or uric acid levels may be elevated, depending on the organ system affected.

Radiography

- Hepatosplenomegaly is the most common radiographic feature.
- Diffuse clouding of the air sacs may be present with airsacculitis.
- Often, no radiographic abnormalities are seen with chronic disease.

Antigen Capture

Enzyme-Linked Immunosorbent Assay (ELISA)
- The ELISA (IDEIA antigen system, California Avian Laboratories, Citrus Heights, CA) or the Kodak Surecell test (Eastman Kodak, Clin. Prod. Div., Rochester, NY), may be used to detect chlamydial antigen in naso-ocular discharges, pharyngeal swabs, and feces. The chlamydial organisms do not have to be viable for antigen to be detected.
- Shedding of organisms is often intermittent, producing false-negative results.
- There is some evidence that choanal sampling is preferable, because intermittent shedding may be more common in the feces than in naso-oral secretions.
- Shedding is temporarily inhibited in birds tested within 2–3 weeks of treatment with erythromycin (e.g., Ornacyn, available in pet stores), doxycycline, tetracyclines, penicillins, chloramphenicol, tylosin and quinolones.

■ False-positive results also are common owing to cross-reactivity with some gram-negative bacteria. Confirm positive ELISA results using another method of testing.

Blocking Antibody ELISA (BELISA)

■ The BELISA (California Avian Lab, Citrus Heights, CA) is performed on 50 μl of serum. This sensitive assay detects serum IgG and IgM from 1–2 weeks to 12 months following infection.
■ A positive assay indicates that the patient has mounted an immunological response to *C. psittaci* within the past year (or possibly longer). Therefore, a positive BELISA indicates active disease or past exposure, with no current disease.
■ In one study, 50% of the pet bird population as a whole tested positive.

Serology

Direct Complement Fixation (DCF)

■ In the DCF test (Texas Veterinary Medical Diagnostic Lab., College Station, TX), single serum samples are of value if the titer is sufficiently high or low.
■ Titers up to 1:8 are considered negative, 1:16–1:32 is suspicious, and >1:64 is positive. A fourfold rise in titer over a 4-week period is considered most significant. Titers may remain high following successful treatment.
■ Young birds, budgerigars, cockatiels, canaries, and finches with chlamydiosis may not produce antibody titers high enough to be detectable by DCF, making negative results unreliable in these birds.

Latex Agglutination

■ This test detects serum IgM, which indicates a current infection.
■ False-negative results are common in cockatiels, lovebirds, budgerigars, and some young birds, as well as in later stages of the disease.

Isolation on Culture

■ Isolation requires live *Chlamydia* organisms.
■ Success is highly dependent on proper transport medium, transport conditions, and previous antibiotic treatment.
■ The chlamydial agent may be propagated in tissue culture, mice, or embryonated chicken eggs. Obtain postmortem samples from the spleen, liver, or air sacs.
■ Isolation may be possible from antemortem exudate or fecal samples; however shedding often is intermittent. This is the most reliable postmortem confirmation.

Fluorescent Antibody (FAB) Staining

■ Perform staining on conjunctival scrapings, choana or cloacal swabs, or impression smears of the heart, lungs, liver, spleen, air sacs, or intestinal contents.
■ High numbers of organisms must be present in order for this test to be positive, and nonspecific reactions are common.

■ The FAB test is most reliable as a postmortem confirmation of chlamydiosis.

KEY POINT ▶ False-negative results are common in ELISA, DCF, latex agglutination, and FAB testing for *Chlamydia* organisms owing to intermittent shedding, administration of inhibitory antimicrobials, and production of low antibody titers in the face of active disease. Positive results with the BELISA may only indicate exposure. Base the diagnosis of chlamydiosis on a combination of these diagnostic tests, clinical signs, hematology, serum biochemical profile and radiography.

Treatment

Tetracyclines are the most effective antibiotics against *Chlamydia*.

KEY POINT ▶ Tetracyclines are effective only when the organism is actively dividing, necessitating a 45-day treatment regimen.

■ Chlortetracycline (CTC)–medicated feed, achieving a therapeutic blood concentration of 1 μg/ml for 45 days, is the most common federally approved treatment.
  • CTC-impregnated seeds (Keet Life; Hartz Mountain) and pelleted foods (Lafeber Products, Zeigler Brothers, Inc.) are commercially available, or a 1% CTC cooked mash may be prepared.
  • Reduce dietary calcium to 0.7% of the diet, because calcium interferes with CTC absorption.
  • This treatment regimen may not be effective, however, due to poor acceptance of these food mixtures.
  • Secondary enteric mycotic or bacterial infections owing to alterations of the normal enteric flora are a common problem.
■ Doxycycline (Vibramycin syrup/suspension; Pfizer) appears to be more effective clinically than CTC. It is available only in an oral or intravenous (IV) form in the United States. The IV form should *not* be injected IM or subcutaneously.
  • Administer the oral form of doxycycline at a dose of 25 mg/kg q12h, or 50 mg/kg q24h for 45 days if this dosage is tolerated without vomiting.

Supportive Care

■ Many birds with acute chlamydiosis are seriously ill and require supportive care such as fluid therapy, forced alimentation (see sec. 12, ch. 1), and heat, as well as antibiotic therapy if secondary bacterial infection is present.

Prevention

■ Imported psittacine birds receive CTC-treated food for a 30-day period while in quarantine. Continue this treatment for at least 15 additional days following quarantine.
■ Because inapparent carriers are common and an accurate screening test is not available, it is difficult

to prevent the introduction of *Chlamydia* organisms into a flock when purchasing new birds. A combination of serology and antigen capture to screen for chlamydiosis is recommended, with repeated yearly testing.

PSITTACINE VIRAL DISEASES

Psittacine Beak and Feather Disease (PBFD)

PBFD is an infectious, usually fatal disease characterized by feather loss, feather dystrophy, occasional beak deformity, and destruction of the thymus and bursa. Originally believed to affect only white and pink cockatoos and a few other South Pacific psittacine birds, the disease has now been reported in over 30 species of psittacines and is believed to be capable of causing disease in many others. Death is attributed to secondary bacterial, viral, or mycotic infections, or general debilitation warranting euthanasia, and typically occurs within several months following the onset of signs in the acute form; however, it may occur after several years with the chronic form of the disease.

Etiology

- PBFD is caused by a nonenveloped, single-stranded DNA virus (PBFDV) that is structurally similar to the porcine circovirus (PCV) and chicken anemia agent (CAA).
  - It has been proposed that these viruses be placed in a new family of animal viruses called Circodnaviridae.

Transmission

- Virus may be recovered in the feces, crop secretions, and feather dust of infected birds. Being nonenveloped, PBFDV is thought to be extremely stable in the environment and may be resistant to many disinfectants.
- Infection may occur by inhalation or ingestion of the virus.
- PBFDV is believed to spread throughout the body of an infected bird via circulating WBCs. There is evidence that inapparent carriers may exist.

KEY POINT ▶ Feather dust is a major method of transmission and environmental persistence of PBFDV. Feather dust may be dispersed through natural air flow and may contaminate food dishes, cages, bird carriers, insects, and human clothing.

Clinical Signs

PBFDV may cause peracute, acute, or chronic disease.

Peracute Form
- This form is seen in neonates, most often cockatoos and African gray parrots, and may be associated with crop stasis, pneumonia, diarrhea, weight loss, and rapid death. There are few feather lesions.

Acute Form
This form is seen in birds as young as 30 days of age, when feathers begin to replace neonatal down.

- Feather lesions include fractures, necrosis, hemorrhage, curvature, and premature shedding of affected feathers.
- GI signs include diarrhea, crop stasis, and anorexia. There may be few feather lesions, especially in young cockatoos, lovebirds, and African gray parrots.
- Death may follow the onset of clinical signs within days to several weeks.

Chronic Form
- This form usually is recognized in psittacines <3 years of age, but has been reported in birds as old as 20 years. Birds may live for months to years before succumbing to secondary infections or chronic debilitation.
- Progressive feather abnormalities may be accompanied by beak lesions.
  - Feather lesions include retained feather sheaths, bleeding within the pulp cavity, fractured feathers, clubbed feathers, circumferential constrictions within the feather shaft, curled or deformed feathers, and stress lines within feather vanes.
  - Feather loss typically begins with powder down feathers. Contour, crest, wing, and tail feather loss is roughly symmetric and progresses with each molt. Some birds become completely bald and remain so until death (months to years).
  - Beak lesions often occur in galahs and Mollucan and sulfur-crested cockatoos but are not routinely seen in other species. Lesions may include oral ulceration, and elongation and fractures of the beak, often accompanied by secondary mycotic or bacterial infections. Beak lesions usually occur following chronic feather loss but can also occur in birds with mild feather lesions. In cockatoos, the beak may appear shiny and black owing to absence of powder that settles on the beak during preening.

Diagnosis

Histopathology
- In affected feathers typically there are ballooning degeneration and necrosis of epithelial cells in the epidermal collar and in the epidermal basal and intermediate zones of the developing rachis.
- Nonsuppurative inflammation, characterized by perivascular accumulations of heterophils, plasma cells, lymphocytes, and macrophages are the primary lesions seen in the feather pulp.
- Beak lesions histopathologically are similar to those seen in the feather shafts.
- The thymus and bursa typically are atrophied, with focal areas of necrosis and degeneration. These lesions are thought to cause immunosuppression.

Hematoxylin and Eosin (H&E) Stain
- Basophilic intranuclear and intracytoplasmic inclusion bodies may be seen with H&E staining in the feathers, pulp, and follicular epithelium. These were once considered diagnostic for PBFDV; however,

other viruses (e.g., avian polyomavirus) may induce similar intranuclear inclusion bodies.

DNA Probe

- A highly sensitive and specific viral DNA probe for the detection of PBFDV infection is commercially available. Birds latently infected can be detected by submitting 0.2 to 0.5 ml of whole unclotted blood. This test allows veterinarians to screen for birds subclinically infected with PBFDV.*

Treatment

- There is currently no effective treatment for PBFDV.
- Provide supportive care (e.g., good nutrition, debridement of lesions, beak trimming, heat) and antimicrobial therapy for secondary bacterial and fungal infections for chronically infected patients.
- Limited success in reducing clinical signs has been reported with the use of various immune stimulants such as human gammaglobulin preparations (Gamimune N; Cutter Biologicals, Berkeley, CA).

Prevention

KEY POINT ▶ Using the DNA probe, test all birds for PBFDV prior to admission to the aviary.

- Isolate all birds testing positive for PBFDV to prevent contact with noninfected birds.
- Exercise care to prevent feather or fecal dust from infected birds contaminating noninfected birds, particularly psittacine neonates.
- An experimental vaccine for PBFDV has been developed and tested, and a commercial product currently is being developed.

Budgerigar Fledgling Disease (Polyomavirus)

Budgerigar fledgling disease (BFD) is responsible for major economic losses in commercial budgerigar aviaries. Polyomavirus also has been reported to cause acute death in large psittacine birds, including Moluccan cockatoos, Eclectus parrots, and painted conures, and in passerine birds.

Budgerigars that survive BFD infection may develop feather abnormalities commonly referred to as "French molt." The lesions of French molt, however, also may be caused by PBFDV.

Transmission

- Polyomavirus may be present in feces, feather dust, and oronasal and oral secretions. These contaminated materials may be inhaled or ingested by susceptible birds.
- Infected hens may pass the virus to offspring through the egg.
- Inapparent carriers are common and are believed to be responsible for spread of this virus. Clinically normal parents may transmit polyomavirus to their offspring, some of which also become inapparent carriers.

Clinical Signs

Hatchling Budgerigars <15 Days Old

- Signs include abdominal enlargement, delayed crop emptying, subcutaneous hemorrhage, retarded growth, and abnormal feathers.
- Sudden death is common. Reported mortality rates vary from 30–100% of affected hatchlings.

Budgerigars >15 Days Old

- Signs are similar to those described for hatchlings; however, the mortality rate is much lower.

Neonatal Parrots

- Clinical signs usually develop at the time of weaning but may be seen anywhere from 14–120 days of age.
- Sudden death with and without clinical signs is common; birds that develop clinical signs usually die within 12–48 hours.
- Signs include diarrhea, delayed crop emptying, depression, anorexia, hemorrhage at the base of feathers and at injection sites, polyuria, and posterior paresis and paralysis.

Diagnosis

- Gross pathologic changes include hydropericardium, cardiomegaly, pale kidneys, ascites, hepatomegaly, splenomegaly, and diffuse petechial and ecchymotic hemorrhages in the subcutis, intestines, myocardium, epicardium and serosal surfaces.
- Histopathologic demonstration of karyomegaly with basophilic intranuclear inclusion bodies in the kidneys, liver, spleen, heart or feather follicles suggests BFDV.
- Confirmatory diagnosis requires the identification of viral antigen using virus-specific antibodies or the detection of viral nucleic acid using virus-specific DNA probes.
  - Highly specific and sensitive viral DNA probes (Avian Research Associates, Inc. Laboratory, Milford, OH) can detect polyomavirus in infected tissue, cloacal swabs, and fresh feces of birds shedding virus. Birds that are shedding the polyomavirus can be identified by submitting a cloacal swab for testing.

KEY POINT ▶ Perform polyomavirus-specific DNA probe testing for definitive diagnosis of BFD and to distinguish this disease from PBFD.

Treatment

- Provide supportive care, as described for PBFD.

Prevention

KEY POINT ▶ Perform DNA probe testing on all birds prior to entrance into an aviary. Isolate birds testing positive.

- Follow the general principles described for PBFDV.
- Disinfection with chlorine solution (50 ml/liter of water) or prolonged contact with iodophors inactivates the BFD virus.

Pacheco's Disease

Also known as *herpes hepatosplenitis,* Pacheco's disease (PD) causes an acute, necrotizing hepatosplenitis

---

*Positive results in birds with lesions suggest active infection. Birds without lesions are retested in 90 days. If positive, bird is considered a carrier; negative, virus is eliminated and bird is considered immune.

that usually is rapidly fatal. The hallmark of PD is sudden death in birds that appear clinically normal until just prior to death. All species of psittacines of all ages, both imported and domestically raised, are susceptible.

Etiology

- Several strains of antigenically unrelated herpesvirus (HV) may cause PD; HV persists by inducing latent disease, with periodic reactivation and shedding.

Transmission

- Although the exact route of PD virus transmission is unknown, this virus can be recovered in high numbers in the feces and pharyngeal secretions of symptomatic and asymptomatic carrier birds. Thus, direct contact with contaminated aerosols and fecaloral routes is the most likely route of virus transmission.
- HV is an enveloped virus and is relatively unstable in the environment. Anecdotal reports suggest that humans can serve as vectors, even with relatively long time intervals between bird exposure. An incubation period of 3–7 days is common.

KEY POINT ▶ Asymptomatic carriers of viruses that cause Pacheco's disease are common and often are incriminated in disease outbreaks. Imported and domestically raised Nanday and Patagonian conures, macaws, and Amazon parrots have been suggested as carriers.

Clinical Signs

- Sudden death without premonitory signs is most commonly encountered and has been reported most frequently in Amazon parrots, cockatoos, lovebirds, pionus parrots and parakeets.
- Nonspecific signs, especially seen in macaws and conures, include lethargy, anorexia, vomiting, diarrhea (sometimes hemorrhagic), biliverdinuria, nasoocular discharge, and occasionally CNS signs.
- Signs often progress to death within several days; however, recovery has been reported in some birds with clinical signs consistent with PDV.

Diagnosis

Antemortem Diagnosis

- Virus isolation from feces may reveal infection; however, viral shedding may be intermittent, making it ineffective for the detection of carrier birds.
- Serologic testing is not commercially available.

KEY POINT ▶ No reliable test is currently available for the identification of carrier birds with PD virus.

Postmortem Examination

- Gross lesions may include hepatomegaly, splenomegaly, hemorrhagic enteritis, sinusitis, pneumonia, airsacculitis, and congestion and hemorrhage in the spleen, liver, and kidneys. Gross lesions may not be apparent in birds with peracute death.

- Histopathologic lesions often include hepatic and splenic necrosis.
- Virus may be isolated from liver, spleen, small intestine, and pancreas.

KEY POINT ▶ Basophilic and eosinophilic Cowdry type A inclusion bodies, often present in the liver, spleen, kidneys, and pancreas suggest herpesvirus infection.

Treatment

- Oral administration of acylovir (Zovirax; Burroughs-Wellcome) (80 mg/kg q8h) or the intravenous form given IM (40 mg/kg q8h) has been reported to decrease morbidity and mortality during PD outbreaks.
  - The intravenous form can cause muscle necrosis at the injection site; do not use for >72 hours.
- Supportive care including fluids, heat, assisted alimentation, and antibiotic therapy for secondary infections may be of some benefit.

Prevention

- Do not mix susceptible species with suspect carriers.
- Sanitation is critical in disease prevention because viral spread within an aviary occurs primarily by contact with contaminated feces and pharyngeal secretions.
  - Thoroughly clean water and feed dishes followed by treatment with a disinfectant. HV typically is inactivated by desiccation and through contact with most disinfectants.
  - Instruct all aviary personnel to practice sound hygiene by washing and disinfecting hands prior to entering the aviary and after handling individual birds or cages.
- Reduce stress to help prevent shedding and spread of the virus.

Vaccination

Provisionally licensed PD virus vaccines are currently available from Maine Biological Labs. (Waterville, ME) and Biomune, Inc. (Lenexa, KS). Two vaccinations subcutaneously in the inguinal area 4–8 weeks apart followed by yearly boosters are recommended. However, adverse reactions have been reported.

KEY POINT ▶ The potential for serious adverse reactions to PD virus vaccines limits their use to high-risk birds only.

- Sudden death has been reported at a rate of 1 per 10,000 birds vaccinated (this estimate may be conservative).
  - Most deaths have been reported in small species receiving *simultaneous PDV and poxvirus vaccine IM*. There are anecdotal reports of death within 48 hours of PDV vaccination alone in larger psittacines.
  - Granuloma formation at the injection site, sometimes large enough to require surgical debridement, can occur. This appears to be most common in cockatoos.
  - Other anecdotal reports include decreased fertility

and increased dead-in-the-shell chicks from vaccinated hens. The relation of these incidents to vaccination has not been substantiated.

Other Herpesviruses

Thirteen different herpesviruses are known to affect birds. The pathogenicity, host spectrum, and relation of these viruses largely are unknown.

- The only HV of known clinical significance in psittacine birds (besides those that cause PD) is Amazon tracheitis virus.
  - This virus causes a pseudomembranous tracheitis, pharyngitis and sinusitis.
  - Signs include dyspnea, change or loss of voice, abnormal respiratory signs, and occasionally hemoptysis.
  - Diagnosis is based on virus isolation or the presence of typical Cowdry type A inclusion bodies in the tracheal mucosa at necropsy.
  - Treatment is similar to that discussed for PDV.
- Based on histologic findings, another herpesvirus has been reported as the suspected etiology of wartlike lesions occurring on the feet of cockatoos.
  - Limited success has been reported in these cases with treatment with topical application of acyclovir cream.

Poxviruses

Two forms of clinical disease caused by avian poxviruses are commonly encountered:

- Dry, or cutaneous, pox is characterized by discrete nodules on unfeathered skin.
- The more common wet, or diphtheritic, pox is characterized by fibronecrotic lesions in the respiratory system, conjunctiva, and pharynx.

The type of disease that develops may depend on the strain of infecting virus, route of infection and species, and age or condition of the host.

Recently imported Amazon parrots, especially bluefronted Amazons and Pionus parrots, are among the most susceptible species and typically develop the diphtheritic form of the disease. Passeriformes (canaries, finches) may develop either form.

Etiology

- Avipoxviruses replicate in the cytoplasm of epithelial cells, inducing characteristic intracytoplasmic, lipophilic inclusion bodies called *Bollinger bodies.*
- Host susceptibility and virulence of the virus varies with the strain of avipoxvirus. Most poxvirus strains are relatively host-specific.

Transmission

- Poxvirus is incapable of penetrating intact epithelium. Entrance into the host is gained through preexisting traumatic lesions or is often introduced into a flock via mosquito vectors.
- Virus is shed in epithelial crusts and exudates during active infection, and in feces, skin, and feather quills during recovery and in latent infections.

- Virus transmission may occur through direct contact with affected birds or through contact with contaminated soil, food or cages.
- Aerosol transmission may be responsible for the diphtheritic (wet) form, whereas contamination of skin wounds or mosquito bites is most likely to result in the cutaneous (dry) form.
- Poxviruses are very resistant to desiccation, humidity, and light and may survive for up to 1.5 years in the environment.
- Recurrence of poxvirus lesions has been reported in some species.
- It is postulated that asymptomatic carriers of poxvirus may exist.

Clinical Signs

Diphtheritic (Wet) Pox

- Yellow to gray/brown fibronecrotic plaques may occur on the mucosa of the mouth, choana, beak, esophagus, and trachea.
  - Multiple plaques may coalesce, forming tightly adherent diphtheritic membranes, which, if forcibly removed, leave a raw, hemorrhagic surface.
- Respiratory epithelium may be affected, with resulting dyspnea, rales, serous to purulent naso-ocular discharge, lethargy, and anorexia.
- Death due to secondary bacterial bronchopneumonia is extremely common. Sudden death from septicemia occasionally is seen in recently imported Amazon parrots.

Cutaneous (Dry) Pox

- Signs include papules, pustules, and scabs on the unfeathered portions of the skin.
  - Secondary bacterial and fungal infections are common and may result in swelling or abscessation.
  - If no secondary bacterial infection occurs, the lesions may resolve without scarring in 10–14 days.
- In canaries and finches, wartlike lesions are common on unfeathered skin.

Diagnosis

- Clinical lesions suggest the diagnosis.
- Differential diagnoses for diphtheritic lesions include hypovitaminosis A, aspergillosis, and trichomoniasis (see sec. 12, ch. 5).
- Epithelial hyperplasia with ballooning degeneration and intraepithelial vesicles seen on histopathologic examination suggest avian pox.
- Intracytoplasmic lipophilic Bollinger bodies are pathognomonic.

Treatment

Cutaneous Pox

- Base treatment of secondary fungal or bacterial infections on culture and susceptibility testing.

Diphtheritic Pox

- Birds often have systemic illness, and mortality rates are high.
- Provide supportive care (see sec. 12, ch. 1), such as supplemental heat, fluid therapy, and assisted alimentation, if mouth lesions are present.

- Prophylactic administration of systemic broad-spectrum antibiotics may prevent secondary bacterial infections.
- If bronchopneumonia is present, nebulization is recommended (see sec. 12, ch. 4).

Prevention

Vaccination. Vaccination of all susceptible species is the best prevention currently available. Vaccines are available for psittacine birds, canaries, pigeons, and domestic fowl.

- The psittacine poxvirus vaccine is a killed, oil emulsion, adjuvanted vaccine conditionally licensed for production by Maine Biological Labs. (Waterville, ME).
  - Administer two inoculations, SC, 4–8 weeks apart (large birds 0.50 ml; small birds [<100 g], 0.25 ml).

KEY POINT ▶ Simultaneous vaccination with psittacine poxvirus vaccine and PD virus vaccine has resulted in death in some small birds.

- A vaccine for use in canaries is available from Biomune, Inc. (Lenexa, KS). Vaccination protocol is the same as for psittacine pox.
  - Vaccination of canaries during an outbreak may increase spread of the virus owing to the stress of handling and to direct bird-to-bird spread, with the veterinarian as a mechanical vector.

Disinfection. Effective disinfectants include 1% potassium hydroxide (KOH), 2% sodium hydroxide (NaOH), and 5% phenol.

- To control an outbreak, replace all wood items in the aviary and clean and disinfect all equipment, nets, cages, and breeding containers.

Reoviruses

There are 11 avian serotypes of reoviruses that are antigenically distinct from each other and from reoviruses isolated from mammals. Of the common pet birds, African gray parrots are most commonly affected, giving rise to the term *Ghana gray syndrome* to describe this often fatal viral disease. Cockatoos also are commonly affected, and less severe reovirus infections may be seen in several New World psittacine parrots.

Etiology

- Avian reoviruses have been isolated or identified by electron microscopy from asymptomatic psittacine and passerine birds in quarantine stations.
- Infections in Old World species tend to be fatal, whereas New World species appear to be less susceptible to infections and often recover.

Transmission

- Both horizontal and egg transmission of reovirus occurs in chickens. However, little is known about transmission in psittacine birds; horizontal transmission through oral and respiratory routes is believed to occur.
- The incubation period in experimental studies is 2–15 days. Following natural exposure, replication of the virus occurs in the gastrointestinal mucosa, followed by viremia (24–48 hours) and spread to other organ systems.

Clinical Signs

- Severity of the disease, and thus clinical signs, varies, depending on the age of the host, the virulence of the virus, the route of infection, and the presence or absence of secondary infections.
- Signs include anorexia, depression, yellow-orange urates, diarrhea, dyspnea, and occasionally paresis, hindlimb paralysis, and bloody nasal discharge.

Diagnosis

- Gross pathologic changes include hepatosplenomegaly with pale yellow mottling and multifocal gray-white foci.
- The typical histologic lesion is disseminated or focal coagulative necrotizing hepatopathy.
- A tentative histologic diagnosis may be confirmed by isolating the virus in cell culture from feces, liver, or spleen.

Treatment

- Supportive care is the only treatment currently available.

KEY POINT ▶ The prognosis for Old World avian species with clinical signs is poor. Death often occurs within 3–4 days after development of clinical signs. Infected New World species often survive with appropriate supportive care.

Control

- There is currently no serologic test or commercial vaccine available for reoviruses affecting pet birds.
- Strict quarantine of newly arrived birds, especially birds of African descent, may help to prevent flock exposure. However, epidemiologic evidence suggests the existence of an asymptomatic carrier state.
- Viral infectivity can be reduced by prolonged contact with phenols, aldehydes, ethanol, halides, 0.5% iodine solution, and a temperature of 158°F.

Adenoviridae

Adenovirus infections have been associated with depression, diarrhea, anorexia, and acute death in budgerigars, Amazon parrots, macaws, cockatoos, lovebirds, and red-rumped parakeets. Adenovirus infections typically produce eosinophilic and basophilic intranuclear inclusion bodies.

Adenovirus infections in psittacines commonly are referred to as *inclusion body hepatitis* or *inclusion body pancreatitis,* depending on the predominant organ system involved.

Clinical Signs

- Signs generally are nonspecific and vary with the organ system affected. Signs include lethargy, depression, fluffed feathers, yellow urates, diarrhea, anorexia, and sudden death.

Diagnosis

- An enlarged, friable liver is the most consistent feature recognized on gross necropsy examination.
- Base definitive diagnosis on histologic examination of affected tissues from necropsy specimens. Histologically, there is diffuse necrosis of parenchymatous organs with the presence of eosinophilic and basophilic intranuclear inclusion bodies.

Treatment

- There is no specific treatment.
- General supportive care may be beneficial (warmth, fluids, forced alimentation, and antibiotic therapy for secondary infection).

Control

- Disinfect cages and supplies with an aldehyde disinfectant (requires 1 hour of contact) to prevent spread of the disease.
- Quarantine all new birds and strictly isolate affected birds.

Newcastle Disease Virus (Paramyxovirus-1)

Newcastle disease virus (NDV) is of extreme economic importance to the poultry industry. Current United States Department of Agriculture (USDA) quarantine stations were created to prevent the introduction of virulent form of this virus into the United States. Hundreds of psittacine birds were destroyed because of an outbreak of Newcastle disease in the 1970s. If a suspect bird is brought into an aviary, the USDA can legally destroy every bird in the aviary as a precaution.

KEY POINT ▶ Smuggling of birds into the United States is the main source of NDV-infected birds. Newcastle disease should not be a problem for the serious aviculturist who does not expose an aviary collection to birds of questionable origin.

Etiology

- There are nine serotypes of avian paramyxovirus (PMV). The most significant pathogens are virulent serotypes of PMV-1, which has been isolated from most species of domestic, aviary, and wild birds.

Transmission

- The respiratory and oral routes of transmission are equally important.
- Fecal contamination of eggshells may lead to viral spread. The virus infects the red blood cells and then is spread throughout the body.

- The incubation period typically is 4–7 days.

Clinical Signs

- Clinical signs depend on the virulence of the strain of virus involved.
- Predominant clinical signs in psittacine birds include fluffed feathers, conjunctivitis, and CNS signs (e.g., ataxia, wing and head tremors, paralysis of extremities).
- The mortality rate is 22–55% of affected birds.
- Survivors may develop chronic NDV infection. Virus has been isolated from oral and cloacal swabs 84 days postexposure in conures, and 1 year postexposure in Amazon parrots.

Diagnosis

- Serologic testing using hemagglutination inhibition (HI) can indirectly diagnose avian paramyxovirus infection. Antibodies typically appear 8 days following infection.
  - HI is not specific for PMV-1 (cross-reaction may occur with other paramyxoviruses); however, suspect NDV in birds demonstrating high titers.
- Base definitive diagnosis on virus isolation from feces or oral secretions of live birds, or from infected organs at necropsy.

Treatment

- No treatment is available. Inform the USDA of any birds positively diagnosed with NDV.

Prevention

All birds legally presented for importation into the United States are placed in a USDA-approved quarantine station for 30 days, at which time samples are taken to detect hemagglutination (HA) viruses including PMV and influenza. Birds with isolates of hemagglutination (HA) viruses that are pathogenic to chickens are refused entry.

KEY POINT ▶ The best prevention against NDV in psittacine birds is avoidance of contact with birds that may have been smuggled into the country.

- No vaccine is available for psittacine birds.

SUSPECTED VIRAL DISEASES

Proventricular Dilatation Syndrome (PDS)

Other names for this disease include *myenteric ganglioneuritis, infiltrative splanchnic neuropathy,* and *macaw wasting disease.* The disease originally was seen only in macaws but has now been reported in many psittacine species. Both ultrastructural findings and epidemiologic evidence suggest that PDS has a viral etiology. Avian serositis virus, believed to be in the Togaviridae family, has been associated with neurologic lesions that resemble those seen with PDS. The disease does appear to have a protracted course, with low virulence and extended incubation periods. The potential mode of transmission is unknown at this time.

Clinical Signs

- Signs include intermittent regurgitation, diarrhea, depression, passage of undigested seeds, progressive weight loss, abdominal distension, and occasionally systemic neurologic signs.
- Birds with a severely dilated proventriculus may develop secondary aspiration pneumonia following repeated bouts of regurgitation.
- Once signs develop, the disease is invariably fatal.

Diagnosis

Antemortem Diagnosis
- Diagnosis may be based on clinical signs and radiographic identification of an enlarged proventriculus.
  - Contrast radiography is usually necessary to positively identify a dilated proventriculus.
- Rule out other causes of regurgitation, proventricular dilatation, or passage of undigested food, such as GI foreign bodies, proventricular outflow obstruction (e.g., tumors, granuloma), proventriculitis, enteritis, crop disorders, impaction, pancreatitis, and liver and kidney disease.

Postmortem Diagnosis
The diagnosis usually is made by identification of characteristic lesions on necropsy.

- Gross pathologic changes include proventricular dilatation, ventricular ulcers, and undigested food in the lower GI tract.
- Histologic lesions are common in the GI tract and neurologic tissues.
  - GI lesions include endoventriculitis, muscle atrophy, lymphocytic leiomyositis, and smooth muscle degeneration.
  - Lesions may be found in the brain and peripheral nerves. Peripheral nervous tissue is affected most often, and lesions include mononuclear cell infiltrates in the mesenteric plexus ganglia and in the intrinsic and extrinsic nerves of the proventriculus and ventriculus, and intranuclear and intracytoplasmic eosinophilic inclusion bodies in nerve cells of intestinal ganglia.
  - Other, less frequently encountered nervous tissue lesions include multifocal lymphocytic encephalitis with gliosis; neuronophagia and perivascular cuffing in the cerebellum, medulla oblongata, brain stem, cerebrum, spinal cord and meninges; visceral ganglioneuritis; and lymphocytic poliomyelitis.

Treatment

- There are some reports of prolonged survival with supportive care and a soft gruel diet. In the majority of cases, however, PDS is invariably fatal.

Prevention

- There is little information concerning PDS, including preventive measures.
- If it is determined that the syndrome is caused by an infectious agent, diagnostic tests and vaccines may be available in the future.

Papillomatosis

Papillomas are proliferative, wartlike lesions that may occur on mucosal surfaces of the intestinal tract, including the oral cavity, esophagus, crop, proventriculus, and cloaca. Lesions are most commonly identified on the cloacal mucosa. Macaws, Amazon parrots, and conures are the species most frequently affected.

Etiology

- A viral etiology is suspected because papillomas often appear to spread through groups of birds and it is known that papillomaviruses cause wartlike growths in other species.

Clinical Signs

Clinical signs vary with the location of the lesions.

- Signs of cloacal papillomas include straining to defecate, flatulence, malodorous and bloody stools, persistent enteric bacterial infections, and reduced fertility.
  - Cloacal papillomas may resemble granulation tissue and can be difficult to distinguish from cloacal prolapse.
- Oral papillomas may cause wheezing, dyspnea, excessive salivation, dysphagia, and persistent oral bacterial infections.
- Signs of esophageal, crop, and proventricular papillomas include vomiting, regurgitation, and weight loss.

Diagnosis

- Base the diagnosis on the appearance of the lesions, biopsy, and histopathology.

Treatment

In some cases, the size and appearance of lesions wax and wane without treatment. Treatment is indicated when clinical signs are evident, or, in the case of cloacal papillomas, if self-mutilation occurs.

- Remove surgically by ligation and resection, electrocautery, or cryosurgery. The technique used depends on the extent of the lesion.
  - Circumferential lesions of the cloaca may require more than one procedure.
  - Take care to avoid the development of postoperative strictures.
- Treat secondary bacterial infections prior to surgical removal.
- The effectiveness of autogenous vaccines is somewhat controversial; however, their use often is recommended to reduce recurrences.

Prevention

- Because papillomas may be caused by an infectious agent, carefully examine the cloaca and mouth of all

birds being added to a collection for the presence of papillomas. Those with lesions should be denied entry.
- It may be difficult to detect birds that have had papillomas surgically removed. It is unknown if a carrier state exists.

BACTERIAL DISEASES

Gram-Negative Infections

Bacterial infections requiring treatment are commonly encountered in avian medicine, especially in birds that have been stressed, are on a poor nutritional plane, or are housed in unsanitary conditions. Normal flora in most pet bird species consist primarily of gram-positive bacteria; gram-negative bacteria generally are primary or potentially opportunistic pathogens. Normal psittacine flora include *Lactobacillus, Bacillus*, nonhemolytic *Streptococcus, Micrococcus, Staphylococcus, Corynebacterium*, and *Streptomyces* spp.

Etiology

Commonly encountered gram-negative pathogens include *Escherichia coli* and *Enterobacter, Klebsiella, Pseudomonas, Salmonella, Proteus, Pasteurella*, and *Campylobacter* spp.

Clinical Signs

Clinical signs depend on the organ system affected.

- Respiratory, gastrointestinal, or nonspecific signs such as inappetence, lethargy, and ruffled feathers may be seen alone or concurrently.
- Septicemia, especially from invasion of enteric pathogens, is extremely common in pet birds.
  - Suspect septicemia in any severely depressed bird.

Diagnosis

- A CBC, in conjunction with choanal or cloacal Gram staining, is a useful screening tool to detect underlying problems in healthy birds.
- Perform a Gram stain and culture on samples collected from suspected sites of infection.

Respiratory System
- The rostral portion of the choana is a readily accessible site for collecting specimens from the upper respiratory system.
- Other techniques for isolation of respiratory microbial agents include aspiration of the sinuses and transtracheal washing (see sec. 12, ch. 1).
- Direct culture of the air sacs or air sac flushing may be performed via laparoscopy.

Gastrointestinal System
- Readily accessible sites for isolation of microbial agents include the crop, cloaca, and fresh feces.
- In large birds, the proventriculus and ventriculus may be cultured directly using a pediatric bronchoscope.

Other Organ Systems
- Organ systems such as the urogenital tract and liver, both common sites of bacterial infection, are accessible only by more invasive techniques, such as laparoscopy or exploratory laparotomy.

KEY POINT ▶ Septicemic birds usually are severely depressed and are unable to withstand invasive procedures. Aggressive empirical treatment with antibiotics is indicated for these birds.

Treatment

Treatment is indicated when gram-negative bacteria are isolated from a bird with system-specific signs or signs of septicemia.

KEY POINT ▶ Identification of gram-negative organisms on samples taken from clinically healthy birds does not necessarily warrant treatment. Monitor these birds for the development of clinical signs and shifts in bacterial flora.

Selection of Antibiotics
Whenever possible, select antibiotics based on culture and susceptibility testing.

Kirby Bauer Susceptibility Test
- Bacterial isolates are classified as susceptible based on serum concentrations of antimicrobial agents that are achievable in humans.
  - Because it may not be possible to achieve these high levels in pet birds, this test may not accurately predict the efficacy of the antibiotic chosen in vivo.
- Determining the minimum inhibitory concentration (MIC) of antibiotics allows a more accurate assessment of antimicrobial efficacy in pet birds; however, this test is not readily available. For this reason, the Kirby Bauer test is still commonly used.
- When choosing an antibiotic based on standard Kirby Bauer testing:
  - The bacterial isolate should be susceptible to the antibiotic.
  - The antibiotic preferably should be bactericidal, known to penetrate into the site of infection, and effective at very low serum concentrations.
- An identified bacterial isolate may not be the primary pathogen responsible for the septicemic state; nevertheless, treat with the appropriate antibiotic to prevent secondary infection.
- Antibiotics and dosages commonly used in pet birds are listed in Table 1.

Route of Administration
Oral Administration
- Direct oral administration of medications often is used in pet birds, especially for palatable solutions or suspension. However this method is difficult for some owners. Instruct owners on the proper restraint techniques. But even then, birds sometimes spit out the medication, and aspiration also is a possibility.
- Addition of medications to a favorite food is a stress-free method; however, the addition of food may decrease the drug's bioavailability.

TABLE 1. Antibiotics for Use in Avian Patients

Generic Name	Product Name (Mfr)	Dose	Comments
Amikacin (250 mg/ml)	Amiglyde (Bristol)	20 mg/kg q12h IM	Potentially nephrotoxic Synergistic w/penicillins Effective against most gram-negative bacteria
Carbenicillin (injectable)	Geopen (Roerig)	• 100 mg/kg q12h IM • 100 mg/kg q12h IT • 1 ml/10 ml saline for neb	Synergistic w/aminoglycosides Freeze following reconstitution until use Good activity against gram-negative bacteria
Carbenicillin (tablets)	Geocillin (Roerig)	• 100–200 mg/kg q12h PO	Very unpalatable; must be crushed and gavaged or hidden in food Not water-soluble
Cefotaxime	Claforan (Hoechst-Roussel)	100 mg/kg q6–8h IM	Broad-spectrum, low toxicity Good against gentamicin-resistant gram-negative isolates Synergistic w/aminoglycosides Reconstituted drug lasts 12 weeks in freezer, 10 days in refrigerator
Cephalexin (suspension)	Keflex (Eli Lilly)	30–50 mg/kg q6h PO	Variable efficacy against gram-negative isolates Dosing schedule may be impractical
Chloramphenicol palmitate (suspension)	Chloromycetin Palmitate (Parke Davis)	75 mg/kg q8h PO	Palatable; well tolerated; effective in neonatal enteric infections Erratic absorption
Ciprofloxacin (tablets)	Cipro (Miles)	20–40 mg/kg q12h PO	Broad-spectrum activity against gram-negative isolates including *Pseudomonas* spp Well absorbed orally Water-soluble—crush tablets and make into solution for direct oral dosing
Enrofloxacin	Baytril (Haver)	15 mg/kg q12h IM	Similar activity to Cipro Irritating when injected IM—do not use for >3–5 days
Gentamicin	Gentocin (Schering)	10 mg/kg q12h IM 10 mg/kg q12h IT 1 ml/10 ml saline for neb	More nephrotoxic than amikacin when given IM Use IT or by neb as adjunctive therapy in respiratory infections (not absorbed)
Sulfachlorpyridazine (soluble powder)	Vetisulid (Solvay)	¾ tsp per 2 qts drinking water	Fairly effective against gram-negative enteric infections, especially *E. coli*
Trimethoprim sulfamethoxazole (suspension)	Bactrim (Roche)	2 ml/kg q12h PO	Good against many gram-negative and gram-positive isolates Excellent for hand-feeding neonates May cause emesis in some birds, especially macaws

IM = intramuscularly; IT = intratracheally; neb = nebulization; PO = orally (per os).

■ Administration of antibiotics via the drinking water is the least preferred method because many antibiotics are unpalatable and are not water-soluble, and ingestion of the medication often is sporadic.
■ Although there are several disadvantages to oral administration, in many flock situations, or when owners cannot hospitalize the bird or otherwise administer parenteral antibiotics, consider using one of the above methods.
■ When a bird is hospitalized and the intestinal tract is functioning properly, oral medications may be administered via gavage tube.

Parenteral Administration
■ Many antibiotics commonly used in avian medicine are poorly absorbed when given orally, necessitating parenteral administration.
■ Use injectable antibiotics:
  • When a bird is unwilling to take oral medications
  • When gastrointestinal motility is altered

  • In critically ill or septicemic birds.
■ The advantages of this method include precise dosing, rapid development of therapeutic serum concentrations, and relatively stress-free administration.
■ Many practitioners teach their clients to administer IM injections to their pets (the technique for IM injection is described in sec. 12, ch. 1).

Monitoring
Assess antibiotic effectiveness by monitoring the resolution of clinical signs, serial hemograms and Gram staining. Serial Gram stains during and following antibiotic administration are important, as development of secondary infections, especially yeasts, are common.

Gram-Positive Infections

Gram-positive infections occur infrequently in pet birds. Pathogens include beta-hemolytic *Streptococcus*, *Staphylococcus aureus*, and *Listeria* spp. Diagnosis and treatment follow the same principles as outlined above for gram-negative infections.

Avian Tuberculosis

Etiology

Tuberculosis in psittacines, unlike that in mammals, usually is a primarily alimentary disease.

- Although a few cases of *Mycobacterium tuberculosis* and *M. bovis* have been reported in pet birds, the causative agent usually is *M. avium.*
- Seven serotypes have been reported; the most common isolate in the United States is serotype 1.
- These gram-positive, acid-fast granulated rods are capable of causing disease in birds, pigs, guinea pigs, rabbits, and humans.
- Brotorgeris parakeets (especially gray-cheeked parakeets) are particularly susceptible, followed by Amazon parrots, budgerigars and Pionus parrots.

Transmission

- Transmission occurs primarily by ingestion of fecal-contaminated food, water, or soil; an aerosol route or wound contamination also is possible. The organism is capable of surviving in soil for up to 2 years.
- Following ingestion, the organisms penetrate the GI mucosa and colonize under the serosa.
- A primary bacteremia occurs (usually without clinical signs) and the organisms are phagocytized (but not killed) by mononuclear phagocyte cells of the liver, spleen, and bone marrow. Multiplication within these cells causes a local reaction by the cell-mediated immune system, characterized by focal or diffuse infiltration of epithelioid cells and multinucleated giant cells. These nodules frequently contain necrotic centers, which may calcify with time.
- Release of the organisms from the liver results in a secondary bacteremia, with localization in lungs, kidneys, gonads, and intestines. Tubercles in the intestinal wall may open into the intestinal lumen, resulting in shedding of large numbers of organisms in the feces.

Clinical Signs

- Clinical signs include chronic weight loss (despite a good appetite), depression, chronic diarrhea, and poor feathering.
- Abdominal distension due to hepatomegaly and dilated, fluid-filled, thickened intestines is common.

- Subcutaneous and periorbital masses may be seen.
- Lameness due to endosteal bone proliferation occasionally is reported.
- Signs often are nonspecific and slowly progressive.

Diagnosis

Hematology and Serum Biochemistry

- Severe leukocytosis (20–44,000) with marked heterophilia and monocytosis is common.
- A left shift may persist for months (unlike bacterial infections in which a left shift is a grave sign and rarely persists for more than a few days).
- Anemia and polychromasia usually are present.
- Aspartate aminotranferase (AST) levels usually are elevated.

Histopathologic Lesions

- On postmortem examination, in addition to the grossly visible nodules previously described, diffuse infiltration of epithelioid or giant cells may result in a grossly thickened firm intestine, hepatomegaly, or splenomegaly.
- Histologically, the intestinal villi may be club-shaped and swollen and filled with epithelioid cells containing acid-fast rods.
- Definitive diagnosis is based on the presence of acid-fast rods and epithelioid cells on biopsy or postmortem slide preparations. The liver is generally the most reliable source.
  - Acid-fast staining or culture of feces may also demonstrate the organism, although false-negative results are common.
  - Culture require 3–6 weeks for results.
- Indirect diagnosis with intradermal tuberculin and slide agglutination tests also frequently produce false-negative results.

Treatment

- Euthanasia often is recommended because of the potential human health hazard, especially to immunocompromised owners.
- Successful treatment of pet birds with *M. avium,* mimicking human treatment protocols, has been reported.

Supplemental Reading

WJ Rosskopf, RW Woerpel: Successful treatment of avian tuberculosis in pet psittacines. Proceedings, Association of Avian Veterinarians, 1991.

3 Avian Dermatology

Elizabeth V. Hillyer

BASIC ANATOMY AND PHYSIOLOGY

An understanding of the structure and function of avian skin and feathers is necessary when working with avian dermatologic problems.

Skin

Avian skin, consisting of epidermis and dermis, is histologically similar to that of mammals but is relatively thin. It is devoid of true glandular structures.

Cutaneous Glands

There are four types of true cutaneous glands in birds:

- Meibomian glands of the eyelids
- Uropygial gland
- Glands of the external ear
- Mucus-producing glands around the vent

Uropygial Gland. The uropygial gland is a bilobed, holocrine gland located at the base of the tail.

- As birds preen, they spread uropygial gland secretions on the feathers; these secretions aid in waterproofing and in suppressing the growth of microorganisms.
- Amazon parrots and some other psittacines lack a uropygial gland.

Incubation Patch

- During the breeding season, most avian species develop an incubation or "brood" patch over the ventral abdomen. In this area the feathers are sparse and the dermis becomes thickened and vascular in order to increase local body heat production for egg incubation.
- The brood patch may occur in one or both sexes, depending on the species of bird.

Feathers

Feather follicles are found in the dermis and may extend into the subcutis. The structure resembles that of hair follicles.

- Feathers of birds are specialized epithelial derivatives that provide flight, waterproofing, flotation, insulation, and display for breeding purposes. Feathers grow in tracts on the body called *pterylae;* the featherless tracts between pterylae are called *apteria.*
- There are seven types of feathers: contour, semiplume, down, powder down, hypopenna, filoplume, and bristle.
  - Contour feathers are the largest feathers and include the flight feathers and the external layer of feathering on the trunk.
  - Semiplume and down feathers provide thermal insulation.
  - Powder down feathers, which are found in many species of birds including psittacines, shed 1-mm granules of keratin, a white powdery substance that aids in waterproofing. Psittacines that produce a large amount of "powder" include many cockatoo species, cockatiels, and African gray parrots.

The Molt

- During the molt, the "old" feathers are pushed out by the growth of new feathers. Following emergence of the new "pin" or "blood" feathers, the vascular pulp retracts back to the base of the follicle. Only the powder down feathers are continuously growing. Most species of birds molt once a year after the breeding season.
- Some species molt two or three times a year; other species molt continuously throughout the year.
- The molt is influenced by light exposure and controlled by hormones. Birds kept indoors may not show a regular molting pattern.
- The growth of new feathers results in an increase in protein mobilization and basal metabolic rate.

KEY POINT ▶ The molting period is physically demanding for birds, and may be a particularly stressful time for those on a poor nutritional plane. Malnourished birds may not undergo normal molting.

- Dietary protein restriction during the molt in house sparrows has been shown to decrease intensity and duration of the molt.

Feather Color

- Feather color in birds is produced both by pigments and by what is termed *structural color*. Structural color is produced by interference, resulting in iridescence, or by scattering of light, resulting in noniridescent color such as the blue of budgerigars.
- Pigmentary colors include melanins, carotenoids, and porphyrins.
  - Carotene pigments, which originate from plant

Adapted from Hillyer EV, Quesenberry KE, and Baer K: *Basic Avian Dermatology.* Proceedings of the Association of Avian Veterinarians, 1989.

material, are found in fat globules in the feathers. They are responsible for yellow, orange, and red colors; these bright colors will be muted in the plumage of birds lacking a dietary source of carotenoids.

- Dietary deficiencies that result in abnormal pigmentation of feathers include deficiencies in lysine, folic acid, iron, choline, and riboflavin.

Basic Recommendations for Healthy Skin and Feathers

1. Instruct clients on the proper diet for birds. The diet should contain good sources of carotenoids such as mangoes, nectarines, and orange and dark green vegetables (e.g., carrots, sweet potatoes, squash, broccoli, watercress).
2. Do not keep birds in the kitchen, because cooking fumes can coat the feathers.
3. Daily misting with warm water will encourage normal preening and keep the feathers healthy.

KEY POINT ▶ Use only water on the feathers on a routine basis. Avoid the use of commercial mite and lice sprays and other products that coat the feathers.

HISTORY

A complete history is important in the diagnosis of feather and skin disorders.

Diet

- Question the client about types, amounts, and frequency of food offered.
  - Is there a source of protein? of carotenoids?
  - Does the bird eat offered foods?

Environment

- Obtain a description of cage set-up and surroundings.
- Determine the daily routine and the amount of interaction with people and with other birds.
- Is the bird getting adequate sleep (8–12 hours)?
- Has there been a change in routine?

Medical History

- Ascertain whether the bird has had previous medical problems or ongoing problems in addition to skin or feather abnormalities.
  - Does the bird show breeding behavior?
  - Important facts regarding the current dermatologic problem include duration of signs, initial appearance of lesions, progression of lesions, previous treatment and response to same.
- Determine whether there is self-trauma. It is important to ascertain whether skin and feather lesions are self-induced because this will help to guide the differential diagnosis.
- Table 1 classifies common dermatologic problems and their causes; Table 2 groups common problems

TABLE 1. Classification and Causes of Dermatologic Problems

Problem	Possible Etiologies
Feather loss without picking	*Knemidocoptes* mites, psittacine beak and feather disease, polyomavirus Genetic (e.g., baldness in Lutino cockatiels) Altered molt (e.g., with malnutrition) Endocrine abnormality
Feather picking	Behavioral/environmental problem Frustrated courtship/breeding behavior Primary skin disease Malnutrition causing pica Internal disease such as hepatopathy
Skin mass	Feather cyst/folliculoma Lipoma Xanthoma Other neoplasms
Uropygial mass	Abscess or impaction Squamous cell papilloma Squamous cell carcinoma Adenoma/adenocarcinoma
Facial lesions	*Knemidocoptes* mite infection Poxvirus Trauma, insect bite Papillomavirus
Foot and leg lesions	*Knemidocoptes* mite infection Scaly leg syndrome of canaries Amazon foot skin necrosis syndrome Pox-, polyoma, and herpesvirus

by species; Table 3 lists common and scientific names of selected species.

FEATHER PROBLEMS

Pseudoproblems

The following normal avian behaviors and anatomic features often are perceived as abnormal by new bird owners.

- Normal molting mistaken for excessive feather picking:
  - During the molt, birds spend long periods preening to open up new feather shafts. Clues to the fact that a molt is underway are: the presence of pin feathers on the head (where the solitary cage bird cannot reach to preen) and the presence of many feathers on the cage bottom.
  - If the bird appears normal, with healthy skin and feathers, "excessive" feather picking probably is secondary to a normal molt.
- Dandruff:
  - Pieces of normal feather shaft, which fall to the cage bottom during preening of new feathers, may be misinterpreted as dandruff.

TABLE 2. Common Dermatologic Conditions in Different Avian Species

Species	Dermatologic Condition
Canary (*Serinus canarius*)	*Knemidocoptes* mite infection Feather cysts Scaly leg syndrome
Budgerigar (*Melopsittacus undulatus*)	*Knemidocoptes* mite infection Lipomas Fibrosarcoma Feather cysts Uropygial gland conditions
Cockatiel (*Nymphicus hollandicus*)	*Giardia* infection/featherpicking Genetic baldness in lutino cockatiels Feather cysts
Conures (*Aratinga* spp and *Nandayus nenday*)	Feather picking Self-mutilation
Amazon parrot (*Amazona* spp)	Foot skin necrosis syndrome Lipomas Feather picking
Cockatoo (*Cacatua* spp)	Feather picking Psittacine beak and feather disease Papillomas
Rose-breasted cockatoo (*Eolophus roseicapillus*)	Lipomas
Macaw *Ara* spp	Feather picking

- Bare areas:
  - Sometimes the owner is concerned about the apteria (i.e., normal featherless areas) between the feather tracts.
- Dark or "bruised" skin:
  - Because avian skin is thin, the color of dark

TABLE 3. Names of Selected Avian Species

Common Name	Scientific Name
Canary	*Serinus canarius*
Lady Gouldian finch	*Peophila g. gouldiae*
Hill mynah	*Gracula religiosa*
Budgerigar	*Melopsittacus undulatus*
Cockatiel	*Nymphicus hollandicus*
Galah or rose-breasted cockatoo	*Eolophus roseicapillus*
Sulfur-crested cockatoo	*Cacatua galerita*
Lesser sulfur-crested cockatoo	*Cacatua sulfurea*
Major Mitchell's cockatoo	*Cacatua leadbeateri*
Little corella	*Cacatua sanguinea*
Moluccan cockatoo	*Cacatua moluccensis*
Ringneck parakeet	*Psittacula eupatria*
Plum-headed parakeet	*Psittacula cyanocephala*
Peach-faced lovebird	*Agapornis roseicollis*
Fischer's lovebird	*Agapornis fischeri*
African gray parrot	*Psittacus erithacus*
Timneh gray parrot	*Psittacus erithacus timneh*
Gray-cheeked parakeet	*Brotogeris pyrrhopterus*
Quaker parakeet	*Myiopsitta monachus*
Blue-fronted Amazon	*Amazona aestiva*
Yellow-headed Amazon	*Amazona ochrocephala* spp
Yellow-naped Amazon	*Amazona ochrocephala auropalliata*
Hooded crane	*Orus monacha*

underlying muscle is visible through the skin; some owners become alarmed at this color.

Broken Blood Feather

KEY POINT ▶ When a growing feather, or *blood feather*, breaks along the vascular shaft, it may continue to bleed until the feather is pulled from the base. Birds can die from blood loss due to a bleeding blood feather.

Instruct owners on how to pull a bleeding feather if there is not enough time to reach the clinic.

- Firmly stabilize the limb in one hand; then, using a hemostat or needle-nose pliers, firmly grasp the feather at the base and pull it out.
  - The feather should separate at the epidermis; however, if the vascular dermis should tear, resulting in bleeding, apply pressure to the area until bleeding stops.

Feather Loss Without Plucking

This is less common than feather picking.

Etiology

Possible causes of spontaneous feather loss include:

- *Knemidocoptes* mite infection
- Previous damage to feather follicles
- Genetic causes (e.g., baldness in lutino cockatiels)
- Altered molt (e.g., with malnutrition)
- Abnormal growth of feathers, such as occurs with psittacine beak and feather disease (PBFD) and polyomavirus infection (see sec. 12, ch. 1).
- Endocrine disturbances such as hypothyroidism (uncommon in pet birds)

Clinical Signs

- Feather loss can occur anywhere on the body.
- The skin may be normal or may be thickened.
- The owner usually relates that the bird is not picking, scratching, or rubbing.

Diagnosis

- Obtain a thorough history including:
  - Rate and pattern of feather loss
  - Previous feather picking or self-trauma
  - Other medical problems
  - Specific details of diet and management
- Perform a thorough physical examination, paying particular attention to skin and feathers.
  - Examine pin feathers carefully for signs of abnormal growth, such as would occur with PBFD.
- Consider a serum biochemical analysis, complete blood count (CBC), and whole body radiography to screen for systemic disease. Poor feathering may be a sign of chronic systemic disease.
- Perform skin biopsy (including several abnormal follicles) for diagnosis of PBFD, hypothyroidism, malnutrition, and prior damage to follicles.
- Consider a thyroid-stimulating hormone (TSH) re-

sponse test (see discussion of hypothyroidism under Endocrine Diseases).

Feather Picking and Self-Mutilation

Feather picking refers to the plucking or mutilation of feathers by the bird. Psittacine birds are most commonly affected. Self-mutilation of skin and underlying muscle can also occur.

KEY POINT ▶ Feather picking and self-mutilation are two of the most common, frustrating, and time-consuming conditions encountered by the avian practitioner.

Etiology

■ Feather picking by psittacine birds, which are very social creatures, may be the result of jealousy, boredom, fear, frustration, and other emotions.
■ Feather picking may begin as the result of a behavioral or medical problem and develop into a "vice."
■ Feather picking that begins during the breeding season and involves the breast, abdominal, and leg regions may be a manifestation of exaggerated or frustrated courtship and brooding behavior. The role of sex hormones in eliciting true pruritus in birds has not been elucidated.
■ True bacterial or mycotic folliculitis is rare in cage birds.
■ Many bird owners worry about external parasites when they see their birds preening (normal) or feather picking (abnormal). Caution owners that commercial feather lice and mite spray is greatly overused and is mostly ineffective.

KEY POINT ▶ External parasites such as *Knemidocoptes* and feather lice are rarely a cause of feather picking.

■ Malnutrition may result in pica, manifested as feather mutilation.
■ Internal diseases such as intestinal parasitism, liver disease, and airsacculitis may result in feather picking.
   • Intestinal giardiasis is associated with feather picking in cockatiels. The mechanism is uncertain, but possible causes include a hypersensitivity reaction and malabsorption of essential nutrients.
   • Intestinal candidiasis as detected by fecal Gram stain commonly is seen in association with feather picking. The cause and effect of this association is uncertain.
■ Food allergy, especially to sunflower seeds, is suspected in some birds.
   • In one case, feather picking stopped when the owner eliminated the large quantity of oranges the bird was eating daily.

Diagnosis

KEY POINT ▶ Investigate the possibility of underlying medical problems before attributing feather picking to behavioral causes. The basic data base ideally includes fecal parasite examination, fecal Gram stain, CBC, serum biochemical analysis, whole body radiography, and skin biopsy.

■ Obtain a thorough history, including:
   • Diet and management practices
   • Any environmental changes
   • Pattern and timing of feather picking
   • Other medical problems
■ In the physical examination, look for the hallmark sign of feather picking: normal feathering on the head (inaccessible to the beak) with areas of feather loss or feather mutilation elsewhere on the body.
■ Perform a fecal examination for intestinal parasites, including a direct fecal smear and fecal flotation. For cockatiels, a trichrome stain of the feces is useful to detect *Giardia* organism.
■ Obtain samples for fecal or cloacal Gram stain. Submit a fecal culture if abnormal numbers of gram-negative bacteria are seen.
■ Serum biochemical analysis and CBC are indicated to screen for systemic disease, especially if feather picking is chronic or there is evidence of self-mutilation.
■ Whole body radiography is useful to evaluate internal organs.
■ To perform a skin biopsy in birds:

1. Make an elliptical incision with a #11 blade or obtain a sample with a biopsy punch (Acu-Punch; Acuderm, Inc., Ft. Lauderdale, FL).
2. Close the incision with 5–0 absorbable suture in a simple continuous pattern.

■ Elevated gamma globulins on serum protein electrophoresis (EPH) suggest an underlying infectious or inflammatory condition.
■ If necessary, perform abdominal laparoscopy to investigate abnormalities seen on radiographs.
■ A liver biopsy, via laparoscopy or keyhole skin incision, is useful if results of blood tests and radiography suggest liver disease.

Treatment

KEY POINT ▶ There is no single effective treatment for feather picking. Tailor treatment to the individual bird and owner, and prepare the owner for the possibility of long-term therapy involving a series of therapeutic trials.

   • If possible, identify and treat underlying medical problems.
   • Consider treatment for giardiasis in all feather-picking cockatiels, even if no *Giardia* organisms are found, because they are shed intermittently.
   • Give metronidazole (20 mg/kg q12h, PO) for 7–10 days.
   • Some birds respond to injectable metronidazole (Flagyl IV RTU; Schiapparelli Searle) (20 mg/kg q24h, IM, for 2 days).
■ Correct management practices when appropriate; for example:

- Improve caging
- Move the cage to the center of family activity
- Turn on the radio or television when leaving the bird alone
- Provide toys and "activity foods" such as chicken bones, corn on the cob, and pine cones.
- Be sure that birds get 8–12 hours of sleep at night.
- Some birds, particularly cockatiels and conures, may benefit from the presence of a cagemate. However, warn the owner that the birds may not be socially compatible and the original bird may be less interactive with humans if it bonds with the new cagemate.
  - Any new bird should be quarantined for a minimum of 30 days prior to introduction.
- Make any necessary diet corrections, including vitamin supplementation.
  - Birds on a marginal diet should receive at least one injection of vitamins A, E, and D₃ (Injacom 100; Hoffman-La Roche Inc.) because intestinal absorption of nutrients is reduced with hypovitaminosis A.
  - Subsequent supplementation with vitamin A is indicated if dietary modifications are difficult to institute.
- Antihistamines may relieve pruritus and have the additional benefit of causing mild drowsiness.
  - Give hydroxyzine hydrochloride (Atarax; Roerig) at a dose of 2 mg/kg q8h, PO, or 1.5–2.0 mg per 4 oz of drinking water daily; adjust the dosage as necessary to minimize drowsiness and maximize the antipruritic effect.
- Tranquilizers such as diazepam (Valium; Roche) (0.5–1 mg/kg q8h, PO) and phenobarbital (2 mg/kg q8–12h, PO) may be temporarily beneficial.
- Drugs used for neurodermatitis in humans and other mammals show some promise in birds. Examples include fluoxetine hydrochloride (Prozac; Dista), and narcotic antagonists such as naltrexone (Trexan; Du Pont). Dosage regimens have not been established for avian patients.
- Levamisole phosphate has been used in birds as an immunostimulant, coupled with injections of polyvalent avian bacterin.
- The administration of thyroxine may stimulate a molt and produce new feather growth. Use only if the bird has ceased feather picking and is on an adequate nutritional plane.
- Use anti-inflammatory and hormonal therapy with caution; avoid in birds with suspected liver disease.
  - Testosterone, megesterol acetate, or medroxyprogesterone may reduce feather picking in some birds.
  - Side effects include hepatomegaly and anorexia. Corticosteroid administration can be fatal in some birds; the reason for this is not known.
- Use Elizabethan and tube collars with discretion because they can prevent normal preening and eating behaviors.
  - Hospitalize birds for 8–24 hours for observation; placement of a collar may elicit extreme listlessness and anorexia or, conversely, hyperexcitability.
  - Some birds will not tolerate a collar; others may

benefit early in the course of treatment to prevent the development of feather picking into a "vice."
- Radical beak grinding or notching the upper beak interferes with a bird's ability to pull and mutilate feathers. Usually the beneficial effect is temporary.

Prevention

- Owner education regarding nutrition, management, and the social needs of birds may help to reduce the incidence of feather picking. However, this disorder also is seen in apparently well–cared for and socially well-adjusted birds.

INFECTIOUS DISEASES

Viral Diseases

Most viral diseases are discussed elsewhere in this section.

Herpesvirus

Herpesvirus (HV) is known to cause papilloma-like growths on the legs and feet of Moluccan and lesser sulfur-crested cockatoos. The lesions are self-limiting.

Bacterial Diseases

- Bacterial infection of the skin and feathers is uncommon in birds.
- Superficial infection may occur secondary to self-trauma.
- Base the diagnosis on skin biopsy and culture.

Bacterial Folliculitis

- Bacterial folliculitis is rare in birds.
- One report describes *Aeromonas* folliculitis in a lovebird with acute pruritus on the ventral surface of the wings. Pulp samples from a blood feather showed numerous gram-negative rods and grew *Aeromonas* on culture.
  - Clinical signs resolved following a course of amikacin therapy.

Septic Exudative Dermatitis

- This syndrome is characterized by epidermal erosion and ulceration with dermal hyperemia and edema focused primarily in the patagial area (the fold of skin that stretches from the carpus to the humeral region in birds).
- Staphylococci are the most common isolates on bacterial culture.
- Perform a skin biopsy and culture for diagnosis.
- Treat aggressively with systemic and local antibiotics; treatment may be unsuccessful owing to the self-mutilation that occurs as a result of scar formation and contraction.

Avian Tuberculosis

- A granulomatous dermatitis is seen in some cases of avian tuberculosis infection.

- On histopathology, large foamy macrophages containing *Mycobacterium avium* bacilli are seen in the dermis and subcutis.
- Systemic therapy for tuberculosis is necessary (see sec. 12, ch. 2).

Parasitic Infection

Scaly Face and Leg Mite

KEY POINT ▶ Scaly face and leg mite is the only external parasite seen commonly in cage birds.

Etiology

Knemidocoptes pilae is a mite that lives in the skin. It is seen most commonly in budgerigars and canaries but also has been reported in Lady Gouldian finches, cockatiels, Amazon parrots, and ringneck parakeets.

Canaries often are presented with thickened, erythematous scales on the legs and feet. This condition appears to be multifactorial; *Knemidocoptes* infection, low environmental humidity, and hypovitaminosis A and other nutritional deficiencies may all be contributory.

Clinical Signs

- Keratinaceous, proliferative, honeycomb-like lesions occur around the beak, cere, and vent and on the legs and feet. Lesions in canaries are predominantly on the legs and feet.
- In chronic infections, deformed growth of beak and nails may occur.

Diagnosis

- Infection can be latent for 2 years and longer.
- The history often does not include exposure to new birds.
- The gross appearance of the lesions usually is diagnostic.
- If necessary for confirmation, perform a gentle skin scraping of affected areas and examine them microscopically for the mite.

Treatment

- Ivermectin (Ivomec; Merck) is the treatment of choice.
  - For budgerigars and canaries, place 1 drop of the bovine preparation (Ivomec) on the skin over the jugular vein; the drug is absorbed percutaneously.
  - For larger birds, give a single dose of ivermectin, 200 μg/kg, SC or PO; repeat 2 weeks later.
- If lesions are proliferative, gently debride loose scales with mineral oil on a cotton swab.
- Clip nails and beak as necessary. Several corrective beak trims may be necessary.
- For scaly leg mite infection in canaries (see Etiology), consider vitamin A supplementation as well as ivermectin therapy.

Prevention

- Treat cagemates of affected birds.

Red Mite

Red mite infection is seen occasionally in cage birds. Canaries are most commonly affected. The mite may be found on budgerigars and other psittacines.

Etiology

Dermanyssus gallinae is a nocturnal feeder that leaves the host during the day.

Clinical Signs

- Signs include restlessness at night and manifestations of anemia such as weakness, lethargy, and decreased appetite.

Diagnosis

- Cover the cage with a white cloth at night. In the morning the mites, which appear red owing to the ingestion of blood, can be seen on the inner surface of the cover.

Treatment

- Remove the bird from the cage during the day and clean the cage and cage parts thoroughly.
- In cases of chronic infection, give general supportive care and, if indicated, treat for anemia with iron and vitamin supplementation.

Feather Lice

- Rarely, feather lice are found on cage birds. The lice are grossly visible on the feathers.
- Treat by dusting lightly with carbaryl powder (Sevin; Southern Agricultural Insecticides, Inc.).

ENDOCRINE DISEASES

Hypothyroidism

Several hypothyroid birds have been identified in a large volume of avian samples (Lothrop, 1989). All are older Amazon parrots with obesity, molting problems, and mild anemia. Dramatic feather loss or feather picking is not part of the presentation (Lothrop, 1989).

Etiology/Clinical Signs

- Because thyroid hormone plays an important role in the molt and in overall body metabolism, hypothyroidism in cage birds may contribute to an abnormal molt, dry skin, high serum cholesterol levels, enlarged fatty deposits, and lethargy.
- Budgerigars with iodine-deficiency goiter may become hypothyroid. Clinical signs are usually the result of thyroid enlargement and include voice change, squeaking, and regurgitation.

Diagnosis

- Base the diagnosis of goiter in budgerigars on clinical signs and a positive response to iodine supplementation.
- Perform thyroid function testing by administering TSH IM (small birds, ¼ IU; large birds such as macaws, 1 IU); measure T_4 at the baseline and 6 hours post-TSH administration. Submit samples to a laboratory that routinely handles avian specimens and has established normal values for birds.
  - Measurement of basal T_4 alone is not conclusive because low basal T_4 can result from a variety of illnesses, drugs, and stress.

- Perform a routine serum biochemical profile and CBC in birds suspected of being hypothyroid.
- Whole body radiography is helpful to rule out other, underlying disease.

Treatment

- Supplement iodine in budgerigars with goiter.
- Recommended dosages for thyroid supplementation in birds range from ¼ to 1 tablet of 0.1 mg sodium levothyroxine per 4 oz of drinking water; use the lower dosage for birds that drink large quantities of water.

Prevention

- Routinely supplement iodine in all budgerigars.

Hyperadrenocorticism

Pituitary tumors have been reported in birds, but there are no clinical reports of spontaneous hyperadrenocorticism (Cushing's syndrome). However, iatrogenic Cushing's syndrome does occur.

KEY POINT ▶ In psittacines and other avian species that have been studied, corticosterone (not cortisol) is the principal corticosteroid in adults.

Etiology

- In mammals, hyperadrenocorticism is the result of excessive production of cortisol by the adrenal cortex, either caused by a tumor or secondary to excessive production of adrenocorticotropic hormone (ACTH) by a pituitary gland tumor (see sec. 4, ch. 3).
- Iatrogenic Cushing's syndrome occurs secondary to the administration of systemic or topical corticosteroids. Clinical signs are the same as in spontaneous Cushing's syndrome; however, the adrenal glands are hypofunctional as the result of negative feedback from exogenous corticosteroids.
- The use of a cream or ointment containing triamcinolone acetate (Panolog; Solvay Animal Health, Inc.) for feather picking has been incriminated as a cause of iatrogenic Cushing's syndrome.

Clinical Signs

- Signs in birds with iatrogenic Cushing's syndrome include sparse feathering and increased subcutaneous fat deposition. Polyuria-polydipsia (PU/PD) is common.

Diagnosis

- Determine if the bird has PU/PD or shows other signs of Cushing's syndrome.
- Obtain a history of all treatments, including drug dosages and frequency of use.
- Perform a physical examination; give particular attention to the skin and feathers.
- The ACTH response test may be useful. In iatrogenic

Cushing's syndrome, baseline and post-ACTH cortisol values are low.

- Based on one study the avian ACTH response test protocol is administration of 15 IU of ACTH IM; measure corticosterone at the baseline and 90 minutes post-ACTH. Use a laboratory that routinely handles avian samples; check for preferred protocol.
- In birds with PU/PD, perform a serum biochemical profile and CBC to check blood glucose levels, renal function, and hepatic values.

Treatment

- Discontinue exogenous corticosteroid therapy in birds with iatrogenic Cushing's syndrome.
  - Administer prednisone, starting at slightly less than the physiologic replacement dose (0.25 mg/kg q24h) and gradually taper the dose for 1–3 months.
  - Mineralocorticoid administration usually is not necessary.
- Treatment of spontaneous hyperadrenocorticism in birds has not been reported (see sec. 4, ch. 3 for treatments used in dogs and cats).

Prevention

- Use systemic and topical corticosteroids with caution in avian patients.

Baldness in Canaries

A syndrome of testosterone-responsive baldness in male canaries has been reported. The incidence is as high as 60% in some flocks.

- Treatment consists of testosterone, 2.5 mg/kg, IM or PO, once weekly for 6 weeks.
  - Testosterone is contraindicated in birds with liver disease.

NUTRITIONAL DISEASES

A nutritionally complete diet is important in the normal molting process and for the health and coloration of the feathers and skin.

Etiology

Pet birds often are fed an all-seed diet without vitamin or mineral supplementation; as a result, adequate dietary protein, essential fatty acids, copper, zinc, and vitamins A, E, and B, may be lacking.

KEY POINT ▶ Hypovitaminosis A is one of the most important nutritional deficiencies in pet birds.

Clinical Signs

- Dermatologic changes in malnourished birds include dull, ragged feathers and thickened, scaly skin, especially on the face, feet, and around the vent.
- Delay or interruption of the molt related to malnutrition results in feathers that are worn and frayed because they are not replaced.

■ Malnourished birds are prone to reproductive disorders and upper respiratory and gastrointestinal infections.

Diagnosis

■ Base the diagnosis on a complete dietary history.
■ The physical examination demonstrates the aforementioned dermatologic changes.
■ Evaluate a serum biochemical profile, CBC, and whole body radiographs to rule out underlying systemic diseases.

Treatment

■ Educate the owner about proper management and feeding of pet birds.
  • Converting from an all-seed to a well-rounded diet often is a difficult and lengthy undertaking. Dispense high-quality avian vitamin and mineral supplements and instruct the owner on their proper use.
■ Initially, give a supplemental vitamin A, E, and D_3 preparation (Injacom-100; La Roche) by injection, because oral vitamins are poorly absorbed from the gastrointestinal (GI) tract in birds with hypovitaminosis A. The recommended protocol is 0.1 ml/200 g body weight, IM, once weekly for two to four doses depending on severity of clinical signs.
  • Scale up for small birds such as budgerigars (0.03 ml, IM) increase to a maximum of 0.2 ml for larger birds such as macaws.
■ To avoid overdosing, give oral vitamin A as beta-carotene (pro-vitamin A) via a proper diet.
  • For an average size Amazon parrot that refuses to eat vegetables, give 1 drop from a capsule of 5000 IU vitamin A once weekly for 4–8 weeks. Caution the owner against exceeding this dosage because of possible vitamin A toxicity.

NEOPLASTIC DISEASES

Cutaneous Papillomatosis

Cutaneous papillomas have been reported in African gray parrots, yellow-headed Amazons, cockatiels, budgerigars, and Quaker parakeets.

■ Affected sites include head, neck, oral commissures, feet, and uropygial gland.
■ Diagnosis and treatment is with excisional biopsy, if possible.

Squamous Cell Carcinoma

Squamous cell carcinoma (SCC) is a malignancy of squamous epithelial cells and can occur in the skin, oral cavity, crop, and esophagus.

■ In birds, SCC is most common in the skin of the wing, beak, and uropygial gland.
■ SCC is most common in older birds and has been reported in many species of psittacines.
■ Cutaneous SCC usually appears as a poorly defined,

raised, proliferative, and sometimes ulcerated cutaneous mass.
■ Use exfoliative cytology or histopathology for diagnosis.
■ Attempt complete excision of the tumor if possible.

Uropygial Gland Adenoma and Adenocarcinoma

SCC is the most common neoplasm of the uropygial gland; however, adenomas and adenocarcinomas also occur.

■ Adenomas are reported in budgerigars and canaries; adenocarcinomas have been seen in budgerigars, a yellow-fronted parrot, a peach-faced lovebird, and a plum-headed parakeet.
■ Diagnosis of uropygial gland neoplasia is by exfoliative cytology or biopsy of the lesion.
■ Surgically resect adenomas.
■ The prognosis for birds with adenocarcinoma is poor, especially if there is radiographic evidence of metastasis or local bony invasion.
  • Consider surgical excision of uropygial gland adenocarcinoma if the lesion is amenable to total excision.

Lipoma

Lipomas occur most commonly in budgerigars and rose-breasted cockatoos and occasionally in Amazon parrots.

Etiology

■ Lipomas are benign tumors arising from lipocytes; they may represent altered fat storage or lipocytic hyperplasia in the obese bird. High dietary fat levels or hypothyroidism may predispose to their development.

Clinical Signs

■ Lipomas appear as smooth, raised masses growing in the subcutis; the yellow color is often visible through the skin. They occur primarily over the sternum and abdominal regions.
■ Subcutaneous lipomas can become very large and may occur in multiple locations.

Diagnosis

■ Establish the duration and rate of growth of the mass(es).
■ Physical appearance of the tumor is usually diagnostic (see above).
■ If the diagnosis is questionable, perform fine-needle aspiration and cytology. However, there is no way to distinguish hyperplastic fat cells from lipoma cells on cytology (or histopathology).
■ Perform a TSH response test if hypothyroidism is suspected (see previous discussion under Hypothyroidism).

Treatment

■ Dietary management may help to reduce the size of lipomas.

- Gradually reduce the amount of oats offered to small seed eaters such as budgerigars, and the amount of sunflower seeds offered to larger seed eaters such as cockatoos.

Provide supplemental iodine to budgerigars.

Administration of thyroxine may help to shrink lipomas.

- Dosage for budgerigars is half of a 0.1 mg tablet per 4 oz of drinking water.
- Administer thyroxine to larger parrots only if the TSH response test is abnormal (see under Hypothyroidism for dosage).

Surgical removal of lipomas may be beneficial if the overlying skin is necrotic, the bird picks at the area, or a lipogranuloma is suspected. Weigh the risk of anesthesia and surgery against the benefits of surgical removal.

Prevention

Recommend varied diets for pet birds; instruct owners to avoid offering a preponderance of oats or sunflower seeds.

Provide supplemental iodine for budgerigars.

Liposarcoma

Liposarcoma, a malignant neoplasm of lipocytes, has been reported in budgerigars and cockatiels.

- Liposarcomas are less common than lipomas. They occur in similar areas but tend to be poorly encapsulated, firmer, and more highly vascularized than lipomas.
- A definitive diagnosis of liposarcoma is made by tissue biopsy; aspiration cytology may not be diagnostic.
- The treatment of choice is surgical excision; however, complete excision may be difficult because these tumors are locally invasive and there is a potential for metastasis.

Fibrosarcoma

- Fibrosarcoma is a malignant tumor of mesenchymal origin. This tumor is one of the most common malignancies of budgerigars and also occurs in cockatiels, parrots, and macaws.
- Fibrosarcomas are locally invasive and may metastasize to the liver, lungs, and bones. They can occur anywhere on the body but often are found on extremities.
- Use aspiration cytology as an aid to diagnosis.
- The treatment of choice is total excision or amputation of the affected extremity.

Lymphohistiocytic Tumors

- Lymphoid neoplasms are relatively uncommon in cage birds. Cutaneous manifestations have been reported; the periorbital area is the most common site.
- Perform aspiration cytology for diagnosis. A full systemic medical evaluation is important.
- Possible treatments include excision and chemotherapy.

Xanthoma

Xanthoma ("yellow mass") is not a true neoplasm. Xanthomas have been seen in poultry, budgerigars, cockatiels, a rose-breasted cockatoo, a gray-cheeked parakeet, and a green-wing macaw.

Xanthomas are characterized microscopically by dermal infiltration with large numbers of macrophages containing lipid particles. There may be cholesterol clefts and multinucleated giant cells.

Etiology

- In dogs and cats, xanthomas usually are associated with abnormal concentrations or composition of plasma lipids, as with diabetes mellitus or hereditary hyperlipoproteinemia of cats.
- Toxic amounts or toxic substances in dietary fat may contribute to the development of xanthomatosis in birds.

Clinical Signs

- Xanthomas become a clinical problem if they are large or if the bird self-traumatizes the area.
- Xanthomas appear as yellow, thickened, featherless areas of skin that may be vascular and friable. The lesion may be discrete or diffuse (xanthomatosis).
- Xanthomas generally occur on the dorsum or wings, but they can be found anywhere on the body and may overlie a tumor or lipoma.

Diagnosis

- Review the dietary history for evidence of overfeeding of foods high in fat. Determine if there is self-trauma.
- The gross appearance of the tumor often is diagnostic.
- A definitive diagnosis is made by tissue biopsy.

Treatment

- No treatment is necessary for small xanthomas.
- If the xanthomas are large or bleeding, attempt surgical excision.
  - If surgical excision is not possible, consider the use of low-energy radiation therapy (20–30 Gy) and hyperthermia.
- Although pre-existing xanthomas will probably be unaffected, correction of the diet is important in long-term management.

Cutaneous Cysts

Cutaneous cysts are benign lesions defined as having an epithelial wall surrounding secretory or keratinaceous contents.

- *Follicular cysts*, also known as feather cysts, are much more common than epidermal cysts and occur in many passerine and psittacine species.
- *Epidermal cysts* are reported in budgerigars. These lesions are lined with stratified squamous epithelium filled with keratin and are found in the dermis or subcutis.

Etiology

- Follicular cysts are the result of congenital or acquired obstruction of follicular orifices, resulting in accumulation of keratinaceous debris in follicles. In some cases the cyst may actually contain a feather shaft, representing an ingrown feather.
- Follicular cysts in canaries may have a hereditary basis because they occur most commonly in strains bred for dense and curled feathering, such as Norwich canaries.
- Microscopically, canary follicular cysts resemble benign neoplasms of follicular cells and some authors have proposed calling them "folliculomas."

Clinical Signs

- Follicular cysts usually occur on the wings of psittacines and on the wings or dorsum of canaries.
- They appear as firm, raised, yellow skin masses that generally are movable over the underlying muscle.
- Self-trauma occurs in some instances.

Diagnosis

- Establish the duration and progression of the lesions and any history of self-trauma.
- The physical appearance of cutaneous cysts generally is diagnostic.
- Keratin debris is seen with aspiration cytology.
- Tissue biopsy is necessary for definitive diagnosis of follicular cysts and epidermal cysts.

Treatment

- If the cutaneous cysts are large or if the bird is picking at the area, surgical treatment is required.
  - Lancing or excision of the cyst can be performed.
  - General anesthesia and careful hemostasis are important.
  - Recurrence is possible with either technique.

  Lancing
- Lance the cyst and express its contents.
- Carefully curet and flush the cyst cavity.
- Leave open to heal.

  Excision
- Excise the cyst and close the skin routinely.
  - In canaries, excision of an entire feather tract may be necessary.

GENETIC CONDITIONS

Two dermatologic conditions are thought to be hereditary: feather follicle cysts in canaries (see previous discussion) and a syndrome of baldness in Lutino cockatiels.

OTHER DISEASES

Allergies

The presence of allergies in birds is difficult to prove. However, histopathologic lesions suggestive of hyper-sensitivity or allergic reaction have been seen. In many instances feather picking has been attributed to food allergy to seeds, particularly sunflower seeds.

Amazon Foot Skin Necrosis Syndrome

The yellow-naped Amazon parrot is most commonly affected.

Etiology

- The cause of this disorder is unknown.
- Possible causes include bacterial or viral infection, allergy, sensitivity to cigarette smoke, and an immune-mediated disorder.

Clinical Signs

- This syndrome occurs in birds of all ages.
- Affected birds usually present for self-trauma to the feet.
- Irregular patches of erythema or brown or black discoloration occur on the unfeathered skin of the legs and feet.
- Bleeding and crusting of the feet occur secondary to self-trauma.

Diagnosis

- Obtain a history, giving particular attention to changes in diet, management, or environment that may have precipitated the problem. Often, no cause is identifiable.
- Physical examination is usually normal except for skin changes on the legs and feet.
- The diagnosis is based on the gross appearance of the lesions.
- Perform a serum biochemical profile and CBC to assess overall organ function.
- Consider whole body radiography to evaluate for underlying disease.
- Biopsy of the affected skin usually is not possible because lesions are located on the extremities where there is minimal excess skin for closure of the surgical site.

Treatment

- Various treatment regimens have been used.
- Long-term management usually is necessary; recurrence has been noted after apparent recovery.
- There is no known prevention.

Drug Therapy
- Anti-pruritic drugs
  - Therapy with an antihistamine, hydroxyzine hydrochloride (Atarax; Roerig) has had some success; give 2 mg/kg q8h or 1.5–2.0 mg per 4 oz of drinking water, and adjust the dosage to minimize drowsiness but relieve pruritus.
  - Other antihistamines such as benadryl have minimal unwanted side effects and may be useful (extrapolate from canine and feline dosages).
  - Use corticosteroids with caution in birds.
- Broad-spectrum antibiotics—Consider giving a combination of trimethoprim-sulfa (30 mg of the com-

bined dosage/kg q12h, IM, SQ, or PO), especially if cutaneous lesions are extensive.
▪ One affected bird is reported to have responded to oral therapy with ketoconazole (Nizoral; Janssen Pharmaceutica).

Topical Treatment

▪ Topical disinfection with dilute chlorhexidine or dilute betadine can be used to clean the skin.
▪ Antibiotic and antifungal creams are preferred to ointments, which tend to coat the feathers.
▪ Use topical corticosteroids with caution.
▪ Leg and foot bandages may be necessary to minimize self-trauma.
▪ An Elizabethan collar helps to prevent self-trauma; however, this usually does not prevent self-trauma of the feet unless the collar is very wide.
▪ Instruct the owner on routine sanitation of the cage and environment.

French Molt

French molt is a term used generically to describe various conditions causing an abnormal molt. In North America, it is generally used to identify a syndrome in smaller psittacines (budgerigars, cockatiels, lovebirds) in which the primary feathers and tail feathers do not develop beyond pin-feather stage following a molt. Affected birds are labeled "runners" or "creepers" because they cannot fly.

▪ French molt is caused by a variety of etiologic agents, including viruses (PBFD virus, polyomavirus), parasites, and genetic and environmental influences.
▪ There is no treatment.

Oiled Birds

Occasionally the avian clinician is presented with a pet bird with oiled feathers. Generally this occurs because the bird accidentally landed in a household oil or because a well-meaning owner doused the bird with an oily substance because it was "picking at itself" (often normal preening behavior).

▪ A coating of oil disrupts the thermoregulatory and waterproofing functions of the feathers; ingestion of oil during preening may be harmful to the bird.
▪ Treatment consists of initial stabilization of the patient with heat, fluids, and nutritional support.

▪ Once the patient is stable, remove the oil using warm water and a dilute solution of a dishwashing detergent such as Dawn (Procter & Gamble) or Lux Liquid Amber (Lever).
  • After washing, blow-dry or towel-dry the bird carefully and place it in a warm environment until fully dry.

Glue Traps

Careless placement of pest control "glue traps" has resulted in unintended entrapment of pet birds.

▪ Instruct owners to bring trapped birds immediately into the veterinary hospital and to leave the bird attached to the trap unless it can be easily removed.
▪ On arrival, release the bird from the trap by gently pulling the feathers out of the glue, taking care not to rip the bird's skin.
▪ Remove the glue from the feathers; an automobile cleaner, Armor All Protectant (Armor All Products), is effective when sprayed onto the feathers and is relatively nontoxic.
  • Protect the eyes when spraying.
▪ Gently massage the feathers until the glue is removed; if necessary, rinse the feathers with warm water.

Supplemental Readings

Clubb SL: Therapeutics: Individual and flock treatment regimens. *In* Harrison GJ, Harrison LR, eds.: *Clinical Avian Medicine and Surgery.* Philadelphia: W. B. Saunders, 1986, p 327.

Feldman EC, Nelson RW: *Canine and Feline Endocrinology and Reproduction.* Philadelphia: W. B. Saunders, 1987.

Galvin C: The feather picking bird. *In* Kirk RW, ed.: *Current Veterinary Therapy VIII.* Philadelphia: W. B. Saunders, 1983, p 646.

Graham DL: Feather and beak disease: Its biology, management, and an experiment in its eradication from a breeding aviary. Proc Assoc Avian Vet, 1990, p 8.

Harrison GJ: Disorders of the integument. *In* Harrison GJ, Harrison LR, eds.: *Clinical Avian Medicine and Surgery.* Philadelphia: W. B. Saunders, 1986, p 509.

Lothrop C: Personal communication, 1989.

Ritchie BW, Niagro FD, Latimer KS, et al.: Advances in understanding the PBFD virus. Proc Assoc Avian Vet, 1990, p 12.

Turrell JM, McMillan MC, Paul-Murphy J: Diagnosis and treatment of tumors of companion birds. I. AAV Today 1:109, 1987.

Turrell JM, McMillan MC, Paul-Murphy J: Diagnosis and treatment of tumors of companion birds II. AAV Today 1:159, 1987.

Zenoble RD, Kemppainen RJ: Endocrinology of birds. *In* Kirk RW, ed.: *Current Veterinary Therapy IX.* Philadelphia: W. B. Saunders, 1986, p 702.

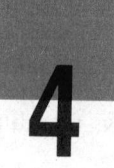

4 Avian Respiratory System

Richard R. Nye

GENERAL ANATOMIC CONSIDERATIONS

The avian respiratory system is a unique gas exchange system compared to that of other domestic animals.

- The lungs are tightly adhered to the body wall and have an essentially uniform volume throughout the respiratory cycle.
- Air moves unidirectionally through the lung, allowing a high efficiency of gas exchange.
  - The first passage of air through the trachea into the primary bronchus and lung is not through the gas-exchange region, but enters the posterior air sacs.
  - The same air then re-enters the lungs, where gas exchange takes place.
  - The "used" air moves to the anterior air sacs on the next inhalation and moves out the trachea on the subsequent exhalation.
- The high efficiency is derived from the action of the air sacs, unidirectional air flow through the lung, small air capillary diameter, a cross-current relationship between parabronchial gas and blood, counter-current relationship between blood and air capillaries, and a high diffusion capacity of the lung for oxygen.
- Air sacs are hollow spaces divided by a thin layer of simple squamous epithelium supported by a small amount of connective tissue. They appear as clear, shiny membranes when healthy. Air exchange does not occur in the air sacs.
- Most birds have four paired and one unpaired pulmonary air sacs with diverticula. They may also have cervicocephalic, pharyngeal, and tracheal air sacs.
  - The cervicocephalic air sacs are located in the neck and head region and arise from the sinuses ventral to the tympanic area (Fig. 1).
  - The body air sacs are interconnected with the lungs and the pneumatic bones (ribs, vertebrae, humerus, coracoid, clavicle, sternum, ilium, ischium, and pubis).
- A diaphragm, which divides the thoracic and abdominal contents as in mammals, is not present in birds. Birds breathe by expanding and contracting the rib cage, which acts in conjunction with the air sacs, like a bellows.
- The complexity of the avian respiratory system must be considered when treating infections and administering inhalant anesthetics. Accessibility of drugs to all areas of the respiratory system can be limited, predisposing it to chronic disease and often necessitating concurrent systemic and topical (i.e., nebulization) treatment.
- Because of the high efficiency of the avian gas exchange system, inhalant anesthetic induction, changes in depth of anesthesia, and recovery all occur more rapidly in birds than in mammals.

DISEASES OF THE UPPER RESPIRATORY SYSTEM

The upper respiratory system includes the nares, nasal passages, paranasal sinuses (infra- and supraorbital), choana, pharynx, laryngeal prominence that contains the glottis, and the cervicocephalic air sacs.

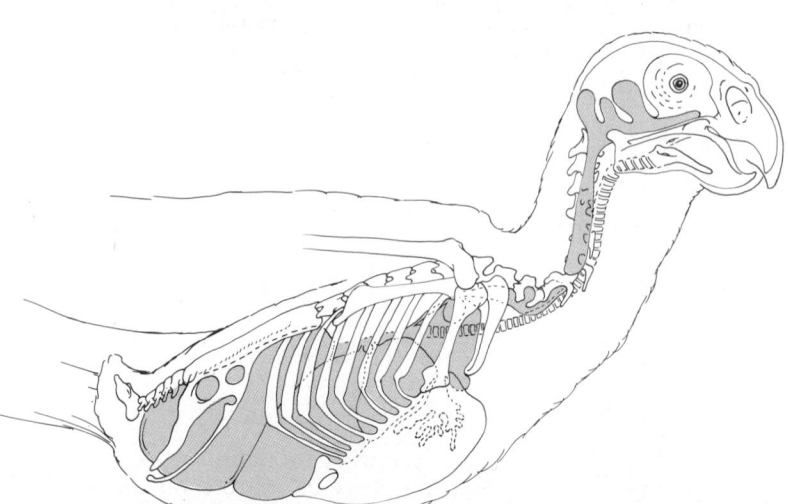

Figure 1. Air sac anatomy.

Disorders of the Nares and Nasal Passages

Etiology

Underlying causes or predisposing factors leading to diseases of the nasal passages include nutritional, mechanical, parasitic, environmental, infectious, traumatic, and neoplastic.

■ *Hypovitaminosis A* is the principal nutritional cause of nasal disease in birds. It is commonly seen in birds fed inadequate diets, such as all-seed diets.
  • Hypovitaminosis A can cause squamous metaplasia of the respiratory epithelium, manifested clinically by secondary invaders such as gram-negative bacteria and fungi.
■ *Mechanical obstruction* of the nares can be caused by dried exudates, foreign material, or thickening of the cere.
  • Introduction of foreign material (e.g., seeds, seed hulls, dust, feathers, air gun (BB) pellets) into the nares causes sneezing and nasal discharges.
  • Cere thickening (brown hypertrophy) can block the nares and obstruct nasal air movement. This benign thickening is believed to be due to hormonal influences in older, laying budgerigar hens.
■ *Parasites* such as *Cnemidocoptes pilae* mites can cause deposits of honeycomb crusts around the outside of the nares, sometimes obstructing air flow.
■ *Environmental factors* such as airborne particles from smoking, cooking, and heating and air-conditioning units, decreased humidity, perfumes, and aerosols can cause irritation of the nasal membranes.
■ *Infectious agents* such as bacteria, fungi, *Chlamydia, Mycoplasma,* and viruses can attack the nasal membranes, causing sneezing, serous or mucous discharge, nasal obstruction (plugs), and distortion of the nares.
■ *Trauma* to the nares or nasal passages can cause tissue damage and can lead to secondary infection or obstruction.
■ *Neoplasia* of nasal membranes or nasal structures can cause signs of nasal disease. Tumor types reported include fibromas, fibrosarcomas, squamous cell carcinoma, adenosarcomas, and osteogenic sarcomas.
  • Nasal tumors in birds are frequently inoperable.

Clinical Signs

■ Sneezing is usually the first sign of nasal irritation.
■ Nasal discharge is the most common sign and can be present with or without sneezing and matting of the feathers around the nares.
■ Chronic sinusitis can lead to changes in the size of the nares. Damage to the germinal layer of cells at the beak-cere border creates ridges or depressions in the surface of the beak.
■ Anatomic distortion of one or both nares can occur, causing mild to severe dyspnea.
  • Plugging of the nares with inspissated exudate, without any distortion, also may occur.
■ Honeycomb crusting around the nares (which can extend to all nonfeathered areas around the head,

feet, vent, and uropygial gland usually is present with *C. pilae* infestation.

KEY POINT ▶ Signs of nasal disease usually are not indicative of systemic disease, but rather of inflammation of the upper respiratory system only. However, be sure to assess the health status of the entire bird.

Diagnosis

History
■ Identify factors relating to dietary, environmental, traumatic, or mechanical causes.
■ Determine potential exposure to infectious disease agents.

Physical Examination
■ Examine the nares for the presence of nasal exudate.
  • An active discharge will often stain or mat the feathers around the nares.
  • Pressure near the nasal opening may express exudate that was not previously visible.
  • Transillumination of the nasal passages with a bright focal light source may reveal the presence of fluid or solid tissue.
■ Examine the choana for mucus and evidence of postnasal discharge. Also examine the connection between the nasal passages and the choana (i.e., the sphenopalatine cleft), which is visible at the most rostral portion of the choanal slit.
■ Use a small, blunt thumb forceps or dental cure to remove caseous material or debris from the nasal opening. (Sometimes the material is solid tissue and cannot be removed in this way.)

Laboratory Studies
■ Following removal of nasal material, perform culture and sensitivity tests, accompanied by a Gram stain; the sphenopalatine cleft appears to be a better location for culture specimens than the nasal passage. However, both locations may yield a potpourri of bacterial contaminants that are of no clinical significance.
■ Cytology or microscopic evaluation of the nasal exudate can be helpful in ruling out the presence of fungi, *Chlamydia,* mycobacteria, yeasts, and foreign material. Scrapings of crusts from around the nares (or other featherless areas) will reveal *C. pilae* mites.
■ Histopathology of biopsied nasal tissue can help to identify neoplastic processes, or deep infections such as chronic fungal sinus infections.

Radiography
Radiography can identify metallic foreign bodies and space-occupying lesions in the nares or nasal passages.

Treatment

KEY POINT ▶ In all birds with diseases of the nares or nasal passage, make necessary corrections in the diet when deficiencies are suspected, especially of vitamin A.

■ Initially, an injection of a vitamin A supplement is helpful (Injacom 100) (0.1 to 0.2 ml/100 gm body weight), followed by daily addition to the food of a powdered multivitamin product.

- When there are mild signs of nasal disease, flush the sinuses via the nares with 3–5 ml of a dilute solution of Nolvasan (30 ml per gal water) or sterile saline (with or without antibiotics) (see sec. 12, ch. 1 for techniques). If foreign material is present, remove as much as possible before flushing.
- Ophthalmic antibiotic ointments or drops (Gentocin Ophthalmic Ointment or Gentocin Durafilm; Schering) work well when infused into the nares once or twice daily.
  - For chronic or resistant infections, add systemic antibiotics to the treatment based on culture and sensitivity that results.
- When the results of cultures are negative, nasal flushing as described above, followed by a nasal decongestant, is effective (1–2 drops of 2.5% Neo-Synephrine q12h).
- Remove any inciting environmental agents from the surroundings.
- Provide increased humidity with a humidifier or by placing the bird in a "steamed-up" bathroom. This is especially helpful in cases of acute sneezing or respiratory distress.
- If a fungal infection (e.g., aspergillosis) is determined, use a topical antifungal amphotericin B ointment (Fungizone; Squibb) infused into the nares q12h.
- For *C. pilae* mites, use 1% ivermectin (Ivomec; Merck) at a dose of 200 μg/kg, PO or topically over the jugular vein; repeat in 2–3 weeks.
- Flush traumatic wounds with antibiotics diluted in sterile saline and treat topically with ophthalmic antibiotic ointment. Leave the wounds open to allow healing by second intention.
- Because tumors of the nasal area are very vascular, surgical removal is difficult if not impossible. Control of hemorrhage is the main problem.
- For chronic problems that do not respond to topical or systemic antimicrobial therapy, sinus trephination is recommended. (See appropriate text sources for surgical technique.)

Prevention

Education of the owner is the best prevention. Instruct the owner to:

- Provide food items high in vitamin A or add avian multiple vitamin supplements to the existing diet (see sec. 12, ch. 5).
- Avoid exposure of the bird to airborne irritants.
  - Do not smoke in the same room as the bird.
  - Do not keep the cage in or near the kitchen. Use an air purifier or a fan with a filter. Sudden deaths have been attributed to using Teflon-coated pons, cooking gas, and electronic oven cleaning.
  - Do not house a susceptible bird with powder-producing birds such as cockatoos, cockatiels, and African gray parrots.
- Provide adequate humidity, preferably with a humidifying unit placed in the vicinity of the bird.
- Avoid traumatic injuries (e.g., choose the proper cage mate; do not allow the bird out of the cage unsupervised).

Disorders of the Paranasal Sinuses

Etiology

Underlying causes of predisposing factors leading to disease of the paranasal sinuses (infraorbital and supraorbital) include infections and neoplasms.

- *Infectious causes* include gram-negative bacteria, fungi, mycoplasma, and *Mycobacterium avium*.
- Neoplasms of the infra- or supraorbital sinus tissues are usually highly malignant and include undifferentiated sarcomas, fibrosarcomas, and osteogenic sarcomas.

Clinical Signs

- Swelling above or below the eye is the most common clinical feature.
- Occasionally an ocular discharge accompanies the swelling.
- Exophthalmos may be present, with the eye displaced upward, downward, or outward. If the disorder is long-standing, the cornea may be dry and cloudy.

Diagnosis

KEY POINT ▶ Paranasal sinus disease usually is determined from physical examination and confirmed by surgical exploration or aspiration of the affected sinus.

- Examine the periocular area for swelling; palpate to determine whether the swelling is solid, fluid, or air (most abscesses in birds are caseous and firm).
- Aspirate the swollen area for cytology and culture.
  - If air is obtained, this indicates a problem related to the cervicocephalic air sac system.
  - If a clear liquid is aspirated, as is the case with many canaries and budgies, a viral or mycoplasma etiology is suggested, and cytology and culture usually are not rewarding.
- Surgical exploration (lancing and/or curettage) may provide a definitive diagnosis or differentiate an abscess from neoplasia.
- Culture and sensitivity testing of the sinus cavity is recommended for abscessation. Special stains may be required to rule out mycobacteria (acid-fast stain) and fungi (new methylene blue stain).
- Biopsy of solid tissue masses is indicated for a definitive diagnosis and prognosis.

Treatment

- Most paranasal sinus swellings require surgical intervention to remove caseated material, fluid, or isolated solid tissue masses.
  - Incision over the swelling with an electrosurgical wire helps to minimize hemorrhage.
  - After removal of the material, which may require curettage or dissection, flush the sinus once or twice daily with sterile saline (with or without antibiotics) or with a dilute solution of Nolvasan, then infuse the sinus with an appropriate ophthalmic antibiotic ointment. Aggressive flush

ing is necessary to keep the affected area open for treatment.

If the causative agent is a fungus, an ointment containing an antifungal such as amphotericin B (Fungizone; Squibb) is indicated.

- Prognosis for a cure is poor, and aggressive curettage or excision may be necessary.

If mycobacteria are found to be the cause, excision of the affected tissue may not be possible because of the invasiveness of the disease (see sec. 12, ch. 2 for treatment protocol).

- The treatment of tuberculosis cases is controversial because of the possible health significance in humans; however, *Mycobacterium avium* has rarely been reported to cause disease in humans.

Suspect mycoplasma infection when sterile fluid is present in the paranasal sinuses, especially in canaries and budgies.

- Remove the fluid, infuse with dilute Nolvasan, and administer tylosin (Tylan plus vitamins; Elanco) (½ g. powder in 1 qt of water for 10 days). This has had good clinical results in many cases.

For sinus infections without caseated exudate accumulations, inject an antibiotic such as Gentocin (50 mg/ml) directly into the affected sinus. The amount depends on the drug chosen and the size of the bird.

Disorders of the Oral Cavity

Etiology

Diseases of the oral cavity (choana, pharynx, laryngeal prominence with glottis) may obstruct the glottis or upper airway, causing respiratory distress or dyspnea. Underlying factors leading to diseases of the oral cavity and adjacent structures include nutritional, infectious, parasitic, and neoplastic.

- The primary *nutritional factor* is hypovitaminosis A (as discussed previously for nasal disease).
- *Infectious agents* including bacteria, fungi yeasts, and viruses (e.g., avian pox) can cause conditions such as mechanical blockage in the oral cavity and adjacent structures that result in respiratory distress.
- *Parasites* (e.g., trichomonads) in the oral cavity can lead to inflammation and accumulation of caseated deposits around the glottis, causing dyspnea.
- *Neoplasms,* including oral papilloma (see sec. 12, ch. 2), involving tissues in the oral cavity can cause signs of respiratory difficulty.

Clinical Signs

Common signs include:

- Inspiratory or expiratory dyspnea manifested as open-mouth breathing, labored respiratory effort, horizontal posture, and tail bobbing
- Wasting or weight loss due to decreased appetite or inability to swallow food
- Crusty exudates at the commissures of the mouth
- Coughing and wheezing
- Abnormal respiratory sounds, such as squeaking, clicking, or moist sounds
- Distortion of the palate, tongue, or beak with abscesses, pustules, or keratin cysts

Diagnosis

History
- Identify predisposing or causative factors.
- Determine the duration of the problem and any previous treatment.
- Determine whether the bird is newly imported, caged alone, previously owned, and so forth.

Physical Examination
- Examine the oral cavity for exudates, abscesses, and keratin cysts.
- Palpate the breast musculature for evidence of muscle wasting (prominent keel bone), indicating chronic disease.
- Auscultate the chest for evidence of lower respiratory disease. Auscultation generally is unremarkable in birds with upper respiratory problems.

Laboratory Studies
- Culture and sensitivity testing with a Gram stain is helpful in determining whether bacteria, fungi, or yeast are involved in the disease process.
  - Take samples from the choana, glottis, and any associated abscesses. Frequently, these apparent abscesses are sterile keratin cysts associated with hypovitaminosis A.
- Cytologic examination of oral deposits or plaques may reveal the presence of trichomonads in a wet mount preparation.
- Histopathological examination is indicated for solid tissue masses.

Surgery
Surgical exploration of nodules in the oral cavity can differentiate abscesses from solid tumors.

Treatment

- Papillomas in the oral cavity usually involve the choana and glottis. Surgically excise these growths and submit for histopathology.
- Apply silver nitrate to surface of tissue (3 to 4 treatments are adequate). Debulking with electrocautery is also recommended.
  - Other neoplasms involving the oral cavity usually are not amenable to surgical excision. Tumors usually involve the palatine tissue and are highly malignant. Osteogenic sarcoma and fibrosarcomas frequently are seen.
- For palatine, lingual, or sublingual abscesses or keratin cysts, lancing and curettage are necessary (culture is optional).
  - Following the removal of exudates, infuse the area with antibiotic ophthalmic ointment and inject an appropriate dose of vitamin A. Systemic antibiotics may be indicated by the overall condition of the bird.
- In trichomoniasis, the plaques of necrotic tissue containing the parasite usually extend deeply into the surrounding tissue and cannot be easily excised. Surgically debulk these lesions and then treat with metronidazole (Flagyl; Rhone-Poulenc), 25 mg/kg q12h, PO, for 10 days.
- Virus-induced lesions rarely cause respiratory diffi-

culty unless they involve the glottis (as with avian pox). Symptomatic therapy (e.g., debridement) to provide an open airway and antibiotics to reduce secondary infection are necessary (see sec. 12, ch. 2).

Disorders of the Cervicocephalic Air Sacs

Etiology

The principal manifestations of cervicocephalic air sac dysfunction are overinflation and rupture. Factors contributing to overinflation of the cervicocephalic air sacs include infectious, traumatic, parasitic, and congenital.

- Infectious agents such as bacteria, viruses, fungi, mycoplasma, and yeasts can cause infections in the upper respiratory system that extend to the cervicocephalic air sacs.
- Trauma can lead to rupture of the air sacs and subcutaneous emphysema.
- Parasites (i.e., threadworms) have been reported in the cervical air sacs but were not incriminated as a cause of clinical problems.
- Congenital anomalies are suspected in neonates with rupture or overinflation of the cervicocephalic air sacs, although bacteria and yeasts have occasionally been cultured from affected birds.

Clinical Signs

- The skin over the head and/or neck is distended with air.
- Depending on the degree of distension, there may or may not be dyspnea.

Diagnosis

- Diagnosis is made by visual observation of the distended skin.
- Confirm the presence of air by needle aspiration.
- Culture the affected air sac to rule out infectious causes.

Treatment

- Surgical correction:
  - Needle aspiration provides immediate relief and when repeated as needed may resolve the condition in some birds.
  - Excision of a circular piece of skin over the inflated area (2 cm or larger) and leaving it open gives longer-lasting results than aspiration.
  - Placement of a permanent valve (a small piece of Silastic tubing sutured to the skin) also has been successful.
  - Microsurgical repair of the infraorbital sinus/cervicocephalic junction has been suggested (Harrison and Harrison, 1986); however, this is a difficult procedure, requiring the skill of an experienced microsurgeon.
  - The prognosis for these surgical procedures providing a permanent cure is guarded.
- If cultures are positive, institute appropriate antimicrobial therapy.

DISEASES OF THE TRACHEA AND SYRINX

The trachea is composed of complete cartilaginous rings (unlike the mammalian trachea) and resists compression or crushing.

Etiology

The underlying causes or factors leading to disease of the trachea and syrinx include mechanical, nutritional, infectious, parasitic, traumatic, and neoplastic.

- *Mechanical factors* include inhalation of foreign material, usually food-related (such as gavage, seeds or seed hulls) but occasionally pieces of hyperkeratotic plaque that have been dislodged from the oral or tracheal mucosa. Dried mucus plugs, at the level of the syrinx, have been reported. The presenting sign is a sudden and severe dyspnea.
  - Extrarespiratory causes such as thyroid hyperplasia or enlargement due to infection or neoplasia are common causes of progressive dyspnea.
- *Nutritional factors* center around hypovitaminosis A and subsequent squamous metaplasia. This can lead to hyperkeratotic plaques on the tracheal mucosa or thickened deposits at the level of the syrinx.
- *Infectious agents* include bacteria, viruses, fungi, and yeasts, which can cause inflammation and exudate formation resulting in narrowing of the main airway and respiratory difficulty.
  - Specific agents include *Chlamydia* spp, diphtheritic avian pox, Amazon tracheitis virus, Newcastle disease virus and other avian paramyxoviruses and *Aspergillus* and *Candida* spp (see sec. 12 ch. 2).
- *Parasitic organisms* of clinical significance that invade the trachea include tracheal and air sac mites (*Sternostoma tracheacolum*) and gapeworms (*Syngamus trachea*).
- *Trauma* to the trachea can cause damage to the tracheal rings and narrowing of the airway, leading to dyspnea.
- *Neoplasia* of the trachea and syrinx is rare.

Clinical Signs

Common signs include:

- Acute, sudden onset of severe inspiratory dyspnea, sometimes open-mouth breathing (gasping)
- Gradual onset of inspiratory or expiratory dyspnea, characteristic expiratory squeak in thyroid hyperplasia
- Coughing and wheezing
- High-pitched, or sucking, or clicking respiratory sounds
- Change in or loss of voice

Diagnosis

History
- If possible, identify predisposing or causative factors.
- Determine the duration of the problem and exposure to possible sources of infection.
- Always question the quality of the diet.

Physical Examination
- Evaluate the severity of the dyspnea and assess the urgency of therapy.
- In small, light-skinned birds, the trachea can be transilluminated.
- In cases of tracheitis, auscultate for moist rales from excess mucus in the trachea and oral cavity.

Laboratory Studies
- Obtain specimens for culture and sensitivity testing of the trachea, using a small, sterile cotton-tipped swab (Calgi-Swab; Spectrum Labs.). Introduce the swab through the glottis and into the trachea.
  - When the procedure is accompanied by a Gram stain, the presence of bacteria (gram-negative), yeasts, and fungal hyphae can be determined.
- Airway cytology of tracheal washings or exudate (see sec. 12, ch. 1 for techniques) may reveal inflammatory cells, degenerate epithelial cells, and possibly the causative agent.

Radiography
- If indicated, obtain radiographs to determine the presence of material at the level of the syrinx, ascertain the architecture of the trachea, and assess involvement of lower respiratory structures.

Endoscopy
- In birds with acute respiratory distress, endoscopy of the trachea and syrinx may reveal obstruction of the airway by accumulation of exudates, which can occur with hypovitaminosis A, aspergillosis, certain viral infections, inhalation of foreign material, and damage to the tracheal rings.
- Endoscopy can be performed quickly under isoflurane anesthesia, or an abdominal breathing tube can be placed (see sec. 12, ch. 1).

Treatment

KEY POINT ▶ In cases of acute inspiratory dyspnea, which is a life-threatening condition in birds, institute immediate therapeutic measures.

- For acute dyspnea, immediate action is required.

Inhalation of Foreign Material
- Foreign material in the trachea of birds smaller than cockatiels frequently causes death.
- In cockatiels, in which surgical removal is not possible, attempt to push the foreign body into the thoracic cavity with a small cotton-tipped swab such as a Calgi-swab (Spectrum Labs.); follow with long-term systemic antibiotic therapy.
- In larger birds, visualize foreign bodies by endoscopy and remove with long alligator forceps or biopsy forceps. If this is not possible, surgical removal is indicated.
  - Use an abdominal breathing tube to maintain anesthesia.

Surgical Technique

1. The surgical approach for removal of tracheal foreign bodies is cranial or caudal to the foreign body.
   a. For foreign material in the syrinx, make the approach through the distal trachea.
2. Make a transectional incision, separating the tracheal rings. Avoid cutting the rings longitudinally, which can lead to tearing and, on closure, stricture.
3. Close the incision with fine 5-0 or 6-0 suture material such as Vicryl, Maxon, or PDS, using a single interrupted pattern.

Infection
- Treat infections of the trachea (tracheitis) by placing the bird in a nebulizer (therapy unit plus nebulizing chamber; Corners Ltd.) with the appropriate solution for 30 min twice daily.
  - For bacterial infections as determined from culture, nebulization with 10 ml sterile saline, 1 ml Gentocin (50 mg/ml) and 0.5 ml acetylcysteine (Mucomyst) is effective.
  - For severe inflammation, add 0.25 ml dexamethasone.
  - For fungal infections, add amphotericin B instead of Gentocin (see sec. 12, ch. 2 for treatment of aspergillosis).
  - For viral tracheitis, it is important to reduce inflammation and keep the trachea open. Death due to asphyxiation by excess mucus accumulation is common in birds with acute viral infections.
- Nebulization can be accompanied by intratracheal injections of appropriate antimicrobial agents diluted in saline. For noninfectious tracheal or syringeal deposits, injections of sterile saline alone may be effective (see sec. 12, ch. 2 for intratracheal injection technique).
- Treat chronic infections with aggressive application of nebulization and systemic antibiotics.
  - If fibrinous exudates are present in the trachea or syrinx, attempt to remove them surgically, as previously described.
- For parasitic infections, give ivermectin (Ivomec; MSD Agvet), 200 to 400 µg/kg, PO or SC.

Neoplasms
- For neoplasia of the trachea or syrinx, euthanasia is recommended, because surgical incision is not possible.

Nutritional Deficiency
- If an underlying nutritional deficiency is suspected, treat hypovitaminosis A with Injacom 100 (Roche), 0.1 ml/300 g body weight.

DISEASES OF THE LOWER RESPIRATORY SYSTEM

The lower respiratory system includes the major bronchi, lungs, air sacs (excluding the cervicocephalic sacs), and pneumatic bones. Because the air sacs are poorly supplied with blood and lack cilia and glandular secretions to aid in removal of infectious agents and foreign material, they are relatively susceptible to disease. Note that air sacs do not communicate directly with one another.

Etiology

Underlying causes or predisposing factors leading to diseases of the bronchi, lungs, and air sacs include mechanical, environmental, infectious, parasitic, and neoplastic.

- *Mechanical factors* include inhalation of foreign material (e.g., blood, gavage solution, hand-rearing formula), resulting in acute dyspnea.
  - With aspiration of large volumes of material death usually is instantaneous. Smaller volumes can cause aspiration pneumonia or airsacculitis.
- *Environmental factors* include airborne irritants and toxins. The resultant inflammation can cause excess mucus production, chronic lung changes (e.g., thickening of bronchi and parabronchi), and airsacculitis.
  - Inhalation of toxins (e.g., carbon monoxide, polymer fumes from Teflon) can cause acute pulmonary hemorrhage and death.
  - Allergies can cause inflammation of lung tissue, with peribronchial thickening and edema.
- *Infectious agents* such as gram-negative bacteria, viruses, fungi, and mycobacteria can lead to pneumonia and pulmonary or air sac granulomas.
- *Parasites* in the bronchi, lungs, and air sacs may cause coughing, wheezing, and abnormally slow, deep respirations.
- *Neoplasia* of the bronchi and lungs is uncommon but should be considered. Rhabdomyoma/sarcoma, leiomyoma/sarcoma, and mesotheliomas of lung tissue have been reported.

Clinical Signs

Common signs include:

- Acute or severe dyspnea with horizontal posture, tail bobbing, and accentuated breathing movements
- Coughing and wheezing
- Audible moist rales or dull breathing sounds
- Concurrent upper respiratory problems

Diagnosis

History

- Identify factors related to possible mechanical, environmental, infectious, or parasitic causes.
- Check whether the bird has recently been hand- or gavage-fed or has recently undergone laparoscopy.
- It is important to know if the bird has been recently imported or has been exposed to imported birds.

Physical Examination

- The bird usually will be fluffed and in a slumped or horizontal posture.
- There may be audible respiratory sounds.
- Breathing movements may be obvious and can be very exaggerated, depending on the severity of the problem.
- Extrarespiratory factors may contribute to the dyspnea.
- Auscultation may help to identify fluid movement in the airways, although referred upper respiratory sounds frequently complicate the interpretation of auscultated sounds. Inflamed air sacs frequently make a crackling sound like crumpled cellophane.

KEY POINT ▶ Many diseases that create respiratory symptoms are extrarespiratory; because birds lack a complete diaphragm, organomegaly, ascites, tumors or egg binding may cause mild to severe respiratory distress.

Laboratory Studies

- Clinical pathology aids assessment of severity: A high white blood cell (WBC) count, degenerative cell changes, and anemia can indicate the severity and duration of the illness.
- Perform serology (e.g., for *Aspergillus, Chlamydia*) or other tests to rule out psittacosis and aspergillosis.
- Cytology of air sac smears is useful for identification of bacteria (e.g., *Chlamydia, Mycobacterium* spp) and fungi.
- Histopathology of birds necropsied from multiple-bird facilities with a history of respiratory disease can be useful. For example, moist or wet avian pox can be diagnosed (see sec. 12, ch. 2).

Radiography

- Radiography is the most important diagnostic tool to assess the integrity of the lower respiratory system.
- Evaluate the lungs and bronchi for anatomic changes such as pulmonary densities, bronchial and peribronchial thickening.
- Radiographic changes indicating air sac disease may be subtle (e.g., diffuse densities, feathery-appearing densities, rounding of the caudal air sac borders); or the changes may be obvious, including discrete densities (granulomas), thickening of air sacs seen as definite lines, and hyperinflation of one side indicating disease on the other.
- Assess changes in extrarespiratory structures (heart, liver, spleen, kidneys, proventriculus and gizzard, reproductive organs, and intestines) to rule out other causes of respiratory signs; for example, heart disease can cause pulmonary edema.

Endoscopy

- Endoscopy can be used to visualize the caudal borders of the lungs and directly examine the abdominal air sacs. During this procedure, samples for culture, cytology, and biopsy can be procured.
  - The point of entry for the endoscope is the abdominal air sac (see sec. 12, ch. 1 for technique).

Treatment

- Tailor treatment for lower respiratory diseases to the suspected cause as determined by diagnostic evaluation. While waiting for laboratory results, treat the symptoms.
  - Initially, administer a broad-spectrum antibiotic such as cefotaxime (Claforan; Hoechst-Roussel) (50–100 mg/kg q6–8h) or enrofloxacin (Baytril; Haver/Diamond) (15–30 mg/kg, q12h, IM or SQ).
  - If a fungal infection is suspected, give an antifungal agent such as fluconazole tablets at 5 to 10 mg/kg SID or itraconazole at 5 to 15 mg/kg SID or BID with food.

- If dyspnea is severe, nebulization with saline or antibiotic/antifungal combinations (as described earlier) is indicated for 20–30 min twice a day.
- Confirm suspected mycoplasmal infections by response to treatment with tylosan powder (Tylan; Elanco); culture and isolation frequently are unrewarding.
▪ If radiology and endoscopy identifies an isolated granulomatous mass, success of treatment depends on the specific location of the mass.
  - If the mass is in the lung tissue proper, surgical removal is difficult, if not impossible.
  - Granulomas in the air sacs offer a better prognosis if surgical removal is possible.
▪ The cause of the granulomas is an important factor in deciding treatment and predicting outcome (for suggested therapy for aspergillosis and chlamydiosis see sec. 12, ch. 2).
▪ If acute dyspnea is caused by inhalation of gavage material, attempt to clear the airways with air via an endotracheal tube or by flushing saline into the trachea (5–10 ml have been used without any problems in Amazon parrots). Follow with oxygen therapy using a face mask.
  - Inhalation of large volumes of gavage material, usually is fatal; if only a small amount of material is aspirated, administer long-term antibiotic therapy in the hope that the body will wall off the inhaled material.
▪ Treat respiratory parasites with ivermectin (Ivomec; MSD Agvet) at a dosage of 200 to 400 μg/kg, PO or SC. This will eliminate air sac mites and lung worms.
▪ Control exposure to environmental factors such as smoking; dust from heating or air conditioning ducts; dust from birds such as cockatoos, cockatiels, and African gray parrots; cooking odors; and aerosols.
▪ Primary neoplasia of the lung is uncommon. Surgical removal of pulmonary tumors is risky because of inaccessibility and risk of blood loss.

Disorders of the Pneumatic Bones

▪ The pneumatic bones (ribs, vertebrae, humerus, coracoid, clavicle, sternum, ilium, ischium, and pubis) connect with the major air sacs; although extension of infection from these sacs may occur, it is uncommon and is not clinically significant.
▪ Infections within the pneumatic bones appear to have a hematogenous origin.

EXTRARESPIRATORY DISEASES

Various conditions in extrarespiratory organs may mimic respiratory disease; for example, thyroid and ultimobranchial body disorders, heart-base tumors, cardiomegaly, hepatomegaly, splenomegaly, gonadal conditions (disease and nondisease), and pancreatic and kidney diseases (see sec. 12, ch. 5).

Supplemental Readings

Arnall L, Petrak ML: *In* Petrak ML, ed.: *Diseases of Cage and Aviary Birds,* Philadelphia: Lea & Febiger 1982, p 395.
Graham DL: The avian respiratory system: AAV Proceedings, 1987, p 143.
Harrison GJ, Harrison LR: *Clinical Avian Medicine and Surgery.* Philadelphia: W. B. Saunders, 1986.
McDonald SE: Anatomical and physiological characteristics of birds and how they differ from mammals. AAV Proceedings, 1990, p 372.
Walsh M: Upper respiratory diseases in avian species: The rhinal cavities, sinuses, and cervicocephalic air sac system. AAV Proceedings, 1984, p 151.
Walsh MT, Martinez D: Lower respiratory system of psittacines. AAV Proceedings, 1985, p 155.

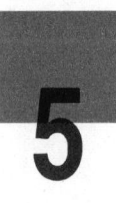

5 Avian Digestive System Disorders

Barbara L. Oglesbee
Scott McDonald
Ken Warthen

DISORDERS OF THE BEAK

General Principles

Normal Structure and Function

- The beak includes the bones of the upper and lower jaws and their keratinized sheaths or rhamphotheca. This horny covering functionally replaces the lips and teeth of mammals.
- The shape of the beak varies, depending on how the species feed and live.
  - In psittacines, the upper beak is massive and curved, and the lower beak is small and horseshoe-shaped (this is why psittacines are called hook-bills).
- The beak is adapted to cracking large nuts and seeds as well as tearing and shredding wood from trees to provide nest sites.
- Histologically, the horny beak resembles skin, and consists of dermis and modified epidermis. The stratum corneum of the epidermis is very thick; its cells contain free calcium phosphate and hydroxyapatite crystals in addition to abundant keratin.
  - The horny tissue of the beak is continuously being replaced during normal wear and tear.

Normal Beak Growth

- Many bird owners erroneously believe that the upper beak grows only from the cere and continues to the tip (or edges), where it is then worn off (and that the process is similar in the lower beak). On the contrary, beak tissue grows continuously outward (toward the surface) over much of the beak.
  - As the keratinized epithelium reaches the surface, it is worn off or may move distally a short distance before it is shed.
  - Beak tissue truly moves rostrally only toward the edges and tip.

Beak Overgrowth

Many pathologic conditions can change the normal outward appearance of the beak, adversely affecting its primary functions of food gathering, prehension, preening, and protection. Regardless of the etiology,

overgrowth may take various forms, the most common of which are listed here.

- The tip of the upper beak is overgrown.
- The tip of the lower beak is overgrown.
- The tips of the upper and lower beaks are overgrown, as well as the edges along one or both sides.
- The edge of one side of the beak is overgrown.
- Malocclusion of the beak causes the upper beak to angle off to one side, whereas the lower beak is directed in the opposite direction. The condition is referred to as *scissors beak*. The tips and outer edges usually are overgrown owing to a lack of occlusal wear.
- The upper beak is shortened and does not extend out over the tip of the lower beak (prognathism).
- An area of the beak may appear bulged or swollen.

Beak Trimming

When the underlying condition has been identified and treated, corrective beak trimming usually is necessary.

- Depending upon the size of the bird, use human fingernail trimmers, cuticle nippers, Roscoe nail trimmers, or an electric hobby tool (Dremel) with a coarse sanding bit.
- Anesthesia usually is not required; however, be aware that some birds stress easily during this procedure, especially when using a hobby tool, and deaths have been reported.

Nutritional Disorders

An *all-seed diet* is deficient in vitamin A, which is important in maintaining the health and integrity of epithelial tissues. Hypovitaminosis A may cause hyperkeratosis of epithelial surfaces.

Clinical Signs

- Signs include beak thickening and overgrowth. The surface of the beak is hard and thickened, and appears flaky and chipped instead of smooth.

Diagnosis

- Base the diagnosis on clinical signs and a history of a seed-based diet.

Treatment

KEY POINT ▶ Place all pet birds on a commercial pelleted diet whenever possible.

- Supplement this diet with fruits, vegetables, whole-grain baked goods or cereals, and small amounts of lean cooked meats or eggs.
- If the bird will not convert to a commercial diet, then use a commercial avian vitamin supplement.
- Perform beak trims as necessary.

Bacterial and Mycotic Infection

Superficial or deep bacterial and mycotic infections occasionally are seen. These usually are secondary to trauma, beak and feather disease (BFD), chronic rhinitis, or other systemic diseases. Gram-negative enteric organisms (e.g., *Pseudomonas, Escherichia coli, Klebsiella* spp) are the most common bacteria cultured. *Aspergillus fumigatus* is the mycotic agent most commonly identified. Psittacine (BFD) virus and *Knemidokoptes* are among the most common causes of beak deformity.

Clinical Signs

- The surface of the beak appears brittle and crumbly instead of smooth and hard. This may involve the entire beak or be localized.
- The bird is reluctant to eat, crack seeds, and play with toys. The beak may seem painful.
- Areas of localized necrosis may be found on the beak surface or on the underside of the upper beak.

Diagnosis

- Perform Gram and new methylene blue stains of lesions.
- Obtain bacterial and fungal cultures of lesions.

Treatment

KEY POINT ▶ Bacterial and mycotic infections of the beak usually are secondary to systemic disease or nutritional deficiencies. Whenever possible, identify and treat the primary disease.

- Debride localized necrotic areas with the bird under anesthesia.
- Base antibiotic therapy on culture and sensitivity testing. Pending culture results, begin antibiotic therapy with a broad-spectrum antibiotic such as cefotaxime (Claforan; Hoechst-Roussel) or enrofloxacin (Baytril; Haver/Diamond) (see sec. 12, ch. 2 for dosages). Long-term systemic therapy usually is required in addition to local debridement.
  - The poor success rate may be due in part to the sparse vascular supply to the horny layers of the beak.
- For localized *Aspergillus* infection, give 5-flucytosine (Ancobon; Roche), 100 mg/kg q12h, PO. Treatment for months may be required.
  - The prognosis is guarded if the fungal disease is systemic (see sec. 12, ch. 2).

Trauma

Beak damage from trauma can occur in all species and is the result of aggressive behavior between individual birds housed together, flying into walls or windows, or struggling following beak entrapment. A split lower beak may result from a fall, injury from another bird, biting with excessive force, or beak trimming.

Clinical Signs

- An inability to eat and manipulate food or toys may be the only presenting signs. Thorough inspection of the beak may be required to identify trauma, because some injuries are not obvious.
- The beak may seem painful.
- Hemorrhage, cracks, punctures, avulsions, or complete amputation may be present.

Treatment

Treatment varies with the type of injury. If the bird is reluctant to eat, forced alimentation may be necessary until the beak is sufficiently healed.

Cracked Upper Beak Tip
- Remove the tip with nail clippers or grind it with a hobby tool.
- Apply ammonium sulfate or ferric subsulfate powder to control hemorrhage.

Split Lower Beak
- If the crack extends throughout the entire length of the beak, dividing it into two movable segments, nothing can be done to permanently fuse the pieces back together.
  - Wire and dental acrylics can only temporarily repair the crack.
- Birds can eat a normal diet with this condition; cracking seed or pellets is not a problem.
- Occasional trimming of the lower beak segments may be necessary because of inadequate occlusion with the upper beak.

Puncture Injury Penetrating the Horny Layer
- Initially treat as an open wound and debride damaged and necrotic areas with the bird under general anesthesia.
- Administer topical and systemic antifungal or antibiotic agents, based on culture and sensitivity testing.
- Defects in the horny layer may later be filled or patched with acrylic compounds.

Beak Avulsions
- Avulsion of the distal one-third:
  - Treat initially as an open wound (as described above).
  - Cover the open end with acrylics as a temporary patch if necessary.
  - Regeneration of the beak is possible, but the beak may never appear totally normal.
- Damage to the proximal one-third of the beak usually is not reversible.
- If the injured birds can be kept alive with forced alimentation, the damaged beak may scar over and the bird may adapt to a soft-food diet.

- Avulsion of the entire upper or lower beak is not reversible. Affected birds usually die of starvation, secondary infection, or require euthanasia.
  - Successful utilization of beak prosthetic devices has been reported but is rare.

Prevention

- Do not leave birds uncaged unless they are closely supervised.
- Keep apart birds that exhibit obvious aggressive tendencies toward each other. This is a common problem in breeding pairs of cockatoos. Sexually active males may attack females that are not sexually receptive, and beaks are commonly bitten. Preventive measures include:
  - Large flight cages.
  - Clipping wings of male but not female bird.
  - Nest boxes with two separate entrances.

Neoplasia

Neoplasia of the beak is encountered infrequently, usually in older birds. Fibrosarcoma, fibroma, and squamous cell carcinoma are the most common types.

Clinical Signs

- *Fibrosarcoma* usually appears as a well-demarcated, fleshy protrusion from the horny layer.
- *Squamous cell carcinoma* appears as a focal area of hemorrhage or ulceration.
- Common signs include weight loss and inability to eat.

Diagnosis

Base the diagnosis on histopathologic examination of excised tissues.

Treatment

- Surgical excision or debulking of beak tumors is rarely successful.
- Cryosurgery or radiation therapy may be beneficial, but the prognosis is guarded.

Environmental Factors

- To maintain a normal appearance of the beak, chewing on hard objects and rasping of the outer horny layer of the beak is necessary.
- Lack of access to materials necessary for normal beak wear can result in beak overgrowth or a flaky, chipped surface.
- Ample amounts of wood should be available for the bird to chew on. This may be in the form of perches, nest boxes, or wood toys.
- Other items suitable for chewing include rawhide, lava stones, mineral blocks, and leather.

Growth and Developmental Abnormalities

These conditions are usually seen in pre-weaned or recently weaned birds. The exact causes are unknown.

- The most common presentations are:

  - *Scissors beak,* a lateral deviation of the upper beak seen most often in macaws
  - *Prognathism,* which affects the architecture of the upper beak and is seen most often in cockatoos
- Treatment by construction and application of a simple, durable prosthesis allows the redirection of beak growth (see AAV, 1989).

DISORDERS OF THE ORAL CAVITY

Normal Structure and Function

- Because birds lack a soft palate, which separates the nasal and oral parts of the pharynx in mammals, the oral cavity and pharynx of birds form a single cavity called the *oropharynx.*
- The roof of the mouth, or hard palate, is located immediately behind the upper beak.
  - Rostrally, the palate resembles a hard, fleshy cushion against which the tongue can manipulate objects.
  - Caudally, the palate is divided into two folds containing numerous caudally directed papillae, which is referred to as the *choana.* The choana communicates directly with the nasal passageway.
- The floor of the oropharynx is occupied by the tongue and the glottis.
  - The psittacine tongue is thick, blunt, and dextrous.
  - The glottis lies on the midline directly behind the tongue.
  - Papillae are distributed over the laryngeal prominence and posterior floor of the pharynx. Birds do not have an epiglottis.
- The surface of the oropharynx is lined by stratified squamous epithelium that is keratinized in regions subject to abrasion, such as the papillae.
  - *Salivary glands* are not visible grossly and are distributed over the palatine folds, base of the tongue, laryngeal prominence, and pharynx. These glands produce primarily mucus and thus are often referred to as mucous glands.
  - The large amount of watery saliva produced in mammals is not present in psittacines. Therefore, the oral mucosa is normally only slightly moist, and the tongue is dry.

KEY POINT ▶ Because diseases of the oral cavity are common in psittacine birds, routinely inspect the mouth during examination.

Hypovitaminosis A

Hypovitaminosis A, which is generally the result of an unsupplemented all-seed diet, can cause squamous metaplasia of the oral epithelium and subsequent hyperkeratosis of the mucous glands. Keratin-filled cystic structures may be found on the palatine folds, base of the tongue, laryngeal prominence, and pharynx. These lesions often coalesce and become secondarily infected to form large abscesses.

Lesions are more likely to be seen in large psittacines

(e.g., Amazon and African gray parrots, macaws, cockatoos) than in small species (e.g., budgerigars, cockatiels).

Clinical Signs

- Signs include white or yellow cysts and abscesses in the oral mucosa.
- If the lesions become secondarily infected, anorexia, general malaise, and weight loss may be present.
- Accompanying respiratory signs include blepharitis, conjunctivitis, uveitis, rhinitis, sinusitis, and dyspnea.

Diagnosis

- The diagnosis is usually based on the history and physical examination.
- Biopsy can confirm the presence of keratin-filled cysts and squamous metaplasia of the mucous glands

Treatment

- Change the diet as previously described under Nutritional Disorders.
- Administer a single injection at a dose of 0.05 ml/100 g, IM, of vitamins A and D_3 (Injacom 100; Roche).
- Lance and drain any oral abscesses and perform a Gram stain and bacterial and fungal culture on the abscess contents; perform curettage of lesions.
- Administer systemic antibiotic or antifungal agents, as indicated by culture.
- Provide supportive therapy, such as forced alimentation and fluid therapy, as needed.

Prevention

- Provide a diet adequate in vitamin A or add vitamin supplementation, as described under Nutritional Disorders.
  - Cod liver oil and dark green and yellow vegetables are good sources of vitamin A.

Psittacine Pox

- See section 12, chapter 2 in this section for discussion of this disorder.

Oral Candidiasis

Candida albicans is a secondary invader that affects the mouth, esophagus, and crop. Factors predisposing to oral candidiasis include poor sanitation, malnutrition, coexisting disease, and prolonged antibiotic therapy. Cockatiels and macaws are most commonly affected.

Clinical Signs

Clinical signs vary with the severity of the disease and include:

- Anorexia, general malaise, and weight loss
- Vomiting, expelled food, and mucus evident on the feathers of the head

- Wet feathers surrounding the mouth, halitosis, and oral hemorrhage
- Poor feeding response in hand-fed baby birds

Diagnosis

- Examine the oral mucosa for the presence of lesions that typically appear as a thickening of the oral mucosa associated with a mucoid exudate.
  - Lesions may progress to focal or widespread mucosal necrosis, forming diphtheritic membranes or white caseated plugs.
- Perform a Gram or new methylene blue stain on exudate from oral lesions; look for budding yeasts.
- Perform a fungal culture of oral lesions.

Treatment

KEY POINT ▶ Candidiasis is usually a secondary invader. Correct predisposing factors in conjunction with specific antifungal treatment.

- Most cases respond to nystatin (Mycostatin; Squibb), 1 ml/300g q8h, PO.
- Occasionally, nystatin-resistant strains of *Candida* are seen. In these cases, give 5-flucytosine (Ancoban; Roche), 100 mg/kg q12h, PO, or ketoconazole (Nizoral; Janssen), 25 mg/kg q12h, PO.
- Continue treatment until all lesions are healed (usually 1 month or longer).

Prevention

- Provide a clean environment, including food and water. Do not leave soft foods in the cage for longer than 12 hours.
- Thoroughly disinfect utensils when feeding baby birds. Soak utensils in chlorhexidine solution (Nolvasan; Fort Dodge), 2 oz/gallon of water.
- Do not save powdered baby foods once they are reconstituted beyond one feeding because the number of yeast and bacterial colonies is greatly increased.
- If long-term antibiotic therapy is indicated (e.g., to treat chlamydiosis), give antifungal agents such as nystatin and ketoconazole prophylactically.
  - Chlorhexidine added to the drinking water at 20 ml/gallon is effective and has no adverse effects.

Bacterial Infections

Bacterial infections of the mouth usually are secondary to predisposing conditions that encourage the growth of *C. albicans*. Common pathogens include *E. coli* and *Salmonella*, *Proteus*, *Pseudomonas*, *Enterobacter*, and *Citrobacter* spp.

Clinical Signs

- Lesions are variable but can appear similar to those of candidiasis (e.g., mucoid exudate, abscess formation).

Diagnosis and Treatment

Bacterial culture of the mouth is performed routinely in avian practice. The choana is the most common site cultured.

- Large numbers of enteric bacteria present in clinically ill psittacines with accompanying oral lesions is significant.
- Administer systemic antibiotic therapy, based on susceptibility testing.

Prevention

- Treat any underlying systemic disease.
- Provide a clean environment and offer fresh food, as described previously under Oral Candidiasis.

Oral Papillomas

See discussion of oral papillomas in section 12, chapter 2 in this section.

Trichomoniasis

T. gallinae is a flagellated protozoan parasite. Trichomoniasis usually occurs in aviaries with many birds and is rarely seen in individual pet birds. Infection may extend into the esophagus, crop, lungs, and oral cavity. The budgerigar is the most common psittacine affected. Outbreaks are reported in neonatal Amazon parrots, conures, and cockatiels.

Clinical Signs

- White, sticky plaques may coalesce to form yellow, caseous masses on the choana, tongue, or pharyngeal mucosa.
- Common signs include anorexia and weight loss.
- Moisture around the beak and halitosis may occur.

Diagnosis

- Perform a saline wet mount of oral exudate for microscopic examination.
  - Organisms are flagellated and pear-shaped and move in a spiral motion. Thousands may be seen on one slide.
  - In psittacine birds, organisms often are not present on wet mounts of oral exudates, especially in the early stages.
- Highest numbers of organisms are found on wet mount smears from lungs of recently deceased birds.

Treatment

Give metronidazole (Flagyl-Searle), 30 mg/kg, PO, for 10 days. Crush the tablets and mix with a palatable liquid.

KEY POINT ▶ Treat birds with oral lesions that suggest trichomoniasis with metronidazole, even when this organism is not positively identified.

Prevention

- In an aviary, quarantine and examine all new budgerigars for the presence of organisms in the pharynx and crop prior to introduction to the flock.

Trauma

Trauma to the mouth is rare, but when it occurs, lacerations or bite wounds to the tongue are most common. The next most common injury is laceration or crushing injury to the intermandibular space as a result of the bird's being hooked or caught on items such as chains or toys.

KEY POINT ▶ Hemorrhage in tongue lacerations can be profuse and life-threatening. Immediate treatment is required.

Treatment

- Anesthesia may be required to immobilize the patient for treatment; isoflurane is recommended.
- Control hemorrhage via direct pressure or cauterization. Intubate the bird if aspiration of blood is a potential threat.
- Clean, debride, and suture injuries, as required.
- Administer systemic broad-spectrum antibiotics prophylactically.

DISORDERS OF THE ESOPHAGUS AND CROP

Normal Structure and Function

The Esophagus

- The avian esophagus is thin-walled and distensible. It courses down the right side of the neck, the opposite to that of mammals.
- The esophagus is lined by incompletely keratinized, stratified squamous epithelium, with numerous subepithelial mucous glands.

The Crop

- The crop is a dilatation of the esophagus found in many (but not all) species of birds. It is prominent in psittacines.
- The crop is located just cranial to the thoracic inlet. It is firmly attached to the underlying skin and thus can easily be seen and palpated externally.
  - The crop in parrots is oriented transversely across the neck. Food enters from the right side and exits caudally on the midline.
- When the proventriculus and ventriculus are full, food may be stored in the crop. Stored food undergoes softening and swelling, but no chemical digestion takes place.
  - Food eventually is moved caudally from the crop by powerful smooth muscle contractions of the crop and the esophageal wall.
- The crop (and proventriculus) is much larger in preweaned psittacines than in adults, in order to accommodate a fluid diet compared to solid foods later on.
  - As a bird is weaned, it is not uncommon for it to lose 10–15% of its body weight owing to shrinkage of these organs and the change in diet.

Crop Stasis

Many environmental, dietary, and systemic conditions can lead to crop stasis.

- Management factors include dehydration, low ambient temperature, change in formula or in the consistency or amounts being fed, and unsanitary feeding methods.

■ Medical conditions that cause crop stasis include bacterial or fungal ingluvitis (inflammation of the crop), foreign bodies, tumors (including papillomas), obstruction within the alimentary tract distal to the crop, and generalized systemic disease (e.g., polyomavirus infection).

■ *Sour crop* refers to crop stasis in baby birds caused by bacterial or yeast infection.

Clinical Signs

Hand-Fed Chicks

■ The crop may be enlarged and pendulous and may fail to empty or do so extremely slowly.
■ Feeding response varies from normal to absent.
■ Vomiting or regurgitation may occur.
■ Initially, birds are alert and active, but depression and listlessness occur as the disease progresses.
■ There is failure to gain weight or loss of body weight.
■ The number of droppings decreases.
■ There may be discoloration or necrosis of the skin overlying the crop.
■ Complete crop fistulas result in leakage of formula.

Adult Birds

■ The enlarged crop fails to empty or does so slowly.
■ Varying degrees of weight loss, weakness, depression, and anorexia are seen.
■ Vomiting may occur; expelled food may collect on feathers of the head and neck.

Diagnosis

History

■ Question the owner regarding housing, ambient temperature, humidity, and diet.

Physical Examination

■ Palpate the crop to determine the amount and consistency of its contents, degree of thickness, muscle tone, fibrous or necrotic areas, and abscesses.
■ Examine the skin over the crop for discoloration and necrosis.
  • Transillumination of the crop may reveal its contents.
  • The lower esophagus extends through the thoracic inlet and cannot be examined externally.
■ Examine the mouth for oral lesions, which, if present, often extend into the esophagus and crop. This is often the case with bacterial and yeast infections, trichomoniasis, and occasionally papillomas.
■ Endoscopy can visualize the interior of the crop and esophagus, but general anesthesia is required. This is not a routine procedure because the degree of visualization is limited by the presence of mucus and fluids and rarely provides information not evident on external examination.
■ In birds over 800 g, examination of the proventriculus (i.e., with a pediatric bronchoscope) can identify proventriculitis, tumors, and foreign bodies that can cause crop stasis.
■ Perform a Gram stain and culture of exudate or food material from the esophageal or crop wall.
  • Large numbers of gram-negative bacteria and budding yeasts are abnormal.
■ Perform a complete blood count (CBC) and serum chemistry profile to rule out systemic disease.

■ Radiographs (plain films or contrast studies) may reveal obstruction caused by foreign bodies or tumors.
■ Histopathologic examination of tissues from chicks at necropsy can be important in the management and treatment of outbreaks of disease in aviaries. Biopsy of individual birds is of limited value.

Treatment

The primary goal of therapy is to alleviate crop stasis which, if not corrected, leads to dehydration, starvation, secondary infections, and eventually, death. Treatment and management in neonates can be extremely labor-intensive and time-consuming. If at all possible, evaluate and stabilize these birds in the hospital, and then instruct the client in home treatment. Most clinics simply do not have the personnel, housing, or time to provide 24-hour nursing care.

KEY POINT ▶ Regardless of the cause of crop stasis, do not feed solid food (adult birds) or formula (chicks) until crop motility returns.

Measures to Restore Crop Motility

■ Add warm water or lactated Ringer's solution to the crop to break down impacted food. This may stimulate emptying of the crop.
■ If crop motility does not return, manually empty the crop contents.
  • Insert a large catheter (metal or rubber) into the crop via the mouth and aspirate the contents.
  • If the above method fails, hold the bird upside down and milk the contents; however, there is a high risk of death from aspiration or stress with this method.
■ Rinse the crop with several flushes of normal saline or warm water, after emptying contents.
■ To treat dehydration, administer 25–50 ml/kg of subcutaneous fluids daily until crop motility returns.
■ Administer oral fluids such as lactated Ringer's solution and Pedialyte (Ross Labs) in place of solid food or formula until motility begins to return. Frequent dosing of small amounts is recommended so as not to stretch the crop.
  • If the crop fails to empty adequately during this time, remove the solution contents once daily to prevent putrefaction.
■ As motility begins to return, add formula to the oral fluids. Begin with a very dilute solution and gradually increase the concentration until a normal consistency is achieved.
■ Digestive enzymes such as Pancrezyme powder (Daniels) may be effective to prevent clumping. Sprinkle a small amount (~⅛ tsp) on the formula just prior to feeding.
■ Administer broad-spectrum antibiotic and antifungal agents as indicated by Gram staining or to prevent secondary infections.

Environmental Factors

■ House birds in an incubator or brooder (95–98°F for hatchlings; 94–97° for neonates up to 7 days old; 90–94°, up to 14 days old; 85–90°F for chicks more than 14 days old).

- Maintain relative humidity above 50%.
- Feed birds a consistent formula type or brand. Formula temperature should be approximately 98–100°F.

Prolonged Crop Stasis

- Overfeeding or prolonged stasis in neonates can result in a pendulous, atonic crop.
- A "crop bra" can provide support for the crop and facilitate emptying:
  - Place a piece of Vetwrap under the crop. Bring the ends upward, and cut longitudinally; join the cranial strips over the neck and connect the caudal strips behind the shoulders. This device can be worn for more than 1 month (see Fig. 11, sec. 12, ch. 1).

Prevention

- To prevent crop stasis in hand-fed neonates, provide a clean, warm brooder, feed a good hand-feeding formula, and practice sanitary handling techniques:
  - Clean the brooder daily; follow ambient temperature guides as previously described.
  - Use a commercial hand-feeding formula or a proven home recipe. Do not switch arbitrarily from one formula to another.
  - Feed birds on a regular schedule.
  - Feed amounts appropriate for the size of the bird; do not overfill the crop.
  - Maintain consistent formula viscosity and temperature.
  - Make fresh formula for each feeding.
  - Disinfect utensils and bowls used for food preparation and delivery after each feeding.
  - Use separate feeding syringes for each bird.
  - Instruct caretakers to wash hands prior to handling each bird.
- If there is a history of candidiasis in the aviary or for an individual bird, administer nystatin, 5 ml/8 oz of formula prophylactically until weaning.
- Correct other predisposing factors for bacterial and fungal infections, as previously described.

Foreign Bodies

The powerful beaks and persistent chewing habits of psittacines can lead to ingestion of foreign bodies, which may lodge in the crop.

Clinical Signs

- Crop stasis or delayed crop emptying may be seen.
- Regurgitation or repeated attempts at regurgitation may occur.

Diagnosis

- Palpate the crop. Many rigid objects large enough to lodge in the crop are palpable externally.
- Transillumination of the crop may reveal its contents.
- Radiograph the cervical area. In some cases, contrast (barium or air) radiography may be necessary to visualize the object.

Treatment

- Retrieve smaller foreign bodies by passing a forceps into the crop through the mouth or by percutaneously manipulating the object into the esophagus for removal through the mouth.
  - General anesthesia is usually required in all birds except neonates.
- Surgical removal via *ingluviotomy* (incision into the crop) may be required to remove the object.
  - Close the crop wall with 4–0 to 6–0 silk sutures in an inverting, interrupted Lembert pattern.
  - Close the skin using a simple interrupted suture pattern.
- Wood chips and seed hulls are sometimes ingested by formula-fed neonates or parent-fed birds. Large amounts may require surgical removal, but small pieces have been successfully digested using cellulase-containing enzyme tablets (available at health-food stores).
  - Crush the tablets and add to formula (1 tablet/4 oz formula); give until the chips/hulls are broken down (usually 2–3 days).

Goiter

Etiology

- Budgerigars fed a seed diet without vitamin/mineral supplementation may develop iodine-deficient thyroid dysplasia.

Clinical Signs

All clinical signs are attributed to the space-occupying effects of the enlarged glands; excessive thyroid hormone is not produced. Signs include:

- Regurgitation
- Crop stasis or delayed crop emptying
- Respiratory click

Diagnosis

Base the diagnosis on the clinical signs and history.

- The thyroid glands cannot be palpated externally because they are contained within the thoracic cavity.

Treatment

- Inject sodium iodide (Butler), 0.02 ml/30 g, IM.
- Maintain budgerigars on oral Lugol's iodine (Strong Iodine solution; Humco) in the drinking water, 1 drop/oz of water daily for 1 week, and then once weekly thereafter.

Prevention

- For budgerigars, switch to a commercial pelleted diet, or supplement the existing diet with a commercial avian vitamin/mineral preparation.

Thermal Burns

Crop burns in neonates are caused by feeding hand-rearing formula at a temperature >105°F. The formula usually was heated in a microwave oven and not sufficiently stirred or tested for temperature.

Clinical Signs

- Birds usually remain bright and alert and maintain a normal feeding response despite the presence of full-thickness necrosis of the crop and overlying skin. Therefore, these birds are usually not presented for evaluation until the caretaker notices formula leaking from the crop fistula onto the chest feathers.
- Necrosis and fistula formation may not be seen until several days after the burn occurs.

Diagnosis

- Base the diagnosis on the clinical signs and history.

Treatment

- After anesthetizing the bird with isoflurane, debride all necrotic edges of the skin and crop.
- Close the crop wall and skin as described for ingluviotomy under Foreign Bodies.

DISORDERS OF THE PROVENTRICULUS AND VENTRICULUS

Normal Structure and Function

Proventriculus

- The proventriculus, or glandular stomach, is continuous with the esophagus at the level of the base of the heart and contains digestive (pepsinogen-secreting) and mucous glands.
- A strong muscular sphincter separates the proventriculus from the ventriculus.

Ventriculus

- The ventriculus, or muscular stomach (also known as the "gizzard"), consists primarily of smooth muscle.
- The epithelium secretes keratinous fluid that hardens to provide a surface against which food may be ground. Grit within the proventriculus aids in this grinding action; however, in most psittacines, grit may not be essential for digestion of food.

Foreign Body Impaction

Ingested objects small enough to bypass the thoracic inlet may lodge in the proventriculus or ventriculus. The pyloric valve, a valve-like structure separating the ventriculus from the duodenum, helps to restrict larger solid objects from leaving the ventriculus. Small objects tend to collect in the ventriculus, owing to its blind pouch–like relationship to the remainder of the digestive tract.

Etiology

- Unweaned chicks typically are presented for ingestion of nesting substrates such as wood chips and shavings (especially young macaws), or for accidental swallowing of feeding instruments (e.g., tubes, spoons, gavage needles).
- In weaning-age chicks, there may be impaction of seed hulls and other food objects that have been swallowed whole.
- Adults commonly present with a history of ingesting toys, cage parts, perch materials, or carpet fibers.
- Over-consumption of grit can cause impaction. If grit is provided, a small amount (10–20 pieces) given every few months is adequate.

KEY POINT ▶ Do not offer gravel or grit free-choice to pet birds. Ill or otherwise stressed birds may overconsume grit, a common cause of impaction of the ventriculus.

Clinical Signs

- Early signs include crop stasis, decreased fecal output, and regurgitation.
- If the impaction is partial, chronic regurgitation, weight loss in adults, and decreased weight gain in neonates may be seen.
- Endotoxemia and hypoglycemia may lead to anorexia, lethargy, depression, seizures, and death.

Diagnosis

- Rule out crop impaction and foreign bodies (described previously).
- Obtain radiographs of the abdominal area. Some objects may be visible on scout films, but contrast radiography often is necessary, using barium sulfate administered at 25 ml/kg into the crop via a gavage tube. The entire gastrointestinal (GI) tract should be delineated by the barium within 2½ hours.
- It may be possible to visualize and retrieve the object via rigid endoscopy. Insert the endoscope through the crop via an ingluviotomy at the level of the thoracic inlet and direct it through the esophagus into the proventriculus.
- In larger birds, a flexible endoscope can be inserted through the oral cavity.

Treatment

- If the foreign body consists primarily of cellulose-containing materials (e.g., wood) the impaction may respond to cellulase-containing digestive enzymes.
- Small nontoxic objects lodged in but not obstructing the ventriculus may be ground down and enzymatically digested by natural processes. Limited amounts of fine gravel grit will expedite the process.
- If the object is visible via endoscopy, it usually can be removed using blunt-jawed grasping forceps.
- Gastric lavage may be used to flush out many objects lodged in the proventriculus.

Technique

1. Anesthetize the bird using isoflurane, intubate for maintenance, and place the bird in lateral recumbency.
2. Fully extend the head and neck and insert a well-

lubricated, soft rubber catheter through the mouth and down into the proventriculus.
3. Position the head so that it is lower than the body and attempt to flush the foreign material out through the mouth, using warm water or saline solution.

■ Proventriculotomy may be necessary to remove larger foreign bodies (Harrison, 1986).

Prevention

■ In neonates, use only large, noningestible or, alternatively, easily digestible nesting substrates. Also, use only long, flexible feeding tubes to allow easy retrieval if syringe disconnection should occur.
■ Monitor parent-reared chicks for signs of nestbox substrate ingestion.
■ When chicks begin feeding on their own, monitor for ingestion of unhulled seeds. Offer only small particles of fresh foods.
■ Restrict adult birds from access to toys, cage parts, and other miscellaneous small objects. Remove coarse, shaggy bark from perches.
■ Avoid feeding chitinous insects to pet birds.

Proventricular Dilatation Syndrome (PDS)

See ch. 2 in this section for a discussion of PDS.

Papillomatosis

See ch. 2 in this section for a description of this disorder.

Candidiasis
Etiology

Candida albicans is a secondary invader, primarily of the mouth, esophagus, and crop, and has been discussed earlier as a cause of oral lesions and crop stasis. This mycotic overgrowth may also occur in the lower digestive tract, particularly in the proventriculus. Lesions usually are not found in the lower digestive tract alone but are an extension of esophageal or crop candidiasis.

Clinical Signs

Common signs include delayed crop emptying, vomiting, diarrhea, and weight loss.

Diagnosis

■ Endoscopic examination of the proventriculus (described above) may reveal rough, thickened, white mucosa characteristic of candidiasis. Similar gross lesions usually are visible in the crop.
■ Perform a Gram stain and fungal culture on samples obtained from the crop and fresh feces or from the proventriculus during endoscopic examination.
  • Although *C. albicans* may be part of the normal intestinal flora, large numbers of budding yeasts on Gram stains of these samples is abnormal and warrants treatment.

Treatment

■ See Treatment under Oral Candidiasis.

Bacterial Proventriculitis

Common pathogens of bacterial proventriculitis include *E. coli*, *Klebsiella*, *Enterobacter*, and *Salmonella* spp.

Clinical Signs

■ Signs include vomiting, regurgitation, delayed crop emptying, and weight loss.

Diagnosis

■ Perform the diagnostic procedures outlined under Oral Candidiasis.
■ The CBC may demonstrate leukocytosis with heterophilia.

For further discussion of gram-negative bacterial infections, see ch. 1 in this section.

DISORDERS OF THE INTESTINES
Infectious Diseases

Bacterial enteritis, *Mycobacterium avium*, and viral enteritis are common causes of diarrhea, vomiting, and weight loss in pet birds (see sec. 12, ch. 2).

Giardiasis
Etiology

The trophozoite and cyst forms of the flagellated protozoan parasite *Giardia* is found in the crop and duodenum.

■ The incidence is estimated to be 70% in cockatiels, 55% in budgerigars, and 25% in lovebirds.
■ Giardiasis occurs less frequently in conures, Amazon parrots, cockatoos, and macaws.

Clinical Signs

■ Diarrhea (often voluminous), mucus-covered feces, or the passing of undigested food may be seen, due to malabsorption caused by giardiasis.
■ Weight loss may be gradual or sudden, with losses of 20–30% of body weight.
■ Pruritus, especially along the wing webs, axillary region, and back, is a common finding in cockatiels with intestinal giardiasis. This is often manifested by feather picking and occasionally self-mutilation.
  • Although the exact relationship is unknown, a hypersensitivity reaction is believed to be responsible.
  • Relief from pruritus is often noted within hours of treatment for giardiasis.
■ Paresis/lameness has been reported in birds with heavy *Giardia* infections. Malabsorption of vitamin E and selenium is the suspected cause.

Diagnosis

- Perform a direct saline smear assay on fresh feces to identify *Giardia* trophozoites and cysts.

KEY POINT ▶ Because *Giardia* organisms are shed intermittently, false-negative test results are common.

- To increase the probability of detecting *Giardia* organisms, collect feces for several days in polyvinyl alcohol and then stain them with trichrome stain. (California Avian Laboratories, Citrus Hill, CA.)
- The CBC may demonstrate a peripheral eosinophilia.
- Hypoproteinemia may be noted on the serum biochemical profile as a result of intestinal malabsorption.

Treatment

- Give metronidazole (Flagyl; Searle), 25–30 mg/kg q12h, PO, for 7–14 days. Crush the tablets and mix with a palatable liquid.
- If lameness or paresis is present, give vitamin E/selenium (Seletoc; Schering), 0.1 ml/kg, IM, every 3–14 days.

Helminthiasis

Intestinal helminths are most frequently a problem in newly imported birds or birds in captive breeding colonies.

Etiology

- Ascarids are commonly found in cockatiels, cockatoos, budgerigars, and other Australian parakeets. Ascaridiasis can be a persistent problem in captive breeding colonies, particularly if the birds have access to a wood or concrete floor. The life cycle is direct, as in mammals.
- *Capillaria* spp. (intestinal threadworm) can be found in all species of pet birds but is most common in macaws, conures and Australian birds. The worms may be found in the mouth, esophagus, and small intestines. The life cycle is direct.
- Cestodes are found primarily in Old World psittacines (e.g., cockatoos, African gray parrots). They may be responsible for hemorrhagic enteritis and chronic wasting in African gray parrots. They have an indirect life cycle, with arthropod or annelid worms as intermediate hosts.

Clinical Signs

- Clinical signs are generally nonspecific, with weight loss, diarrhea, and general unthriftiness predominating.

Diagnosis

- Avian helminth eggs are detected by routine salt/sugar fecal flotation, as for dogs and cats.

Treatment

- Ivermectin (Ivomec 1% solution; Merck) is effective against intestinal nematodes when given at a dose of 200 μg/kg, IM as a single dose, or diluted 1:9 with propylene glycol and given at 0.22 ml/kg, PO, every 2 weeks.
- Levamisole (Tramisol; American Cyanamid) is effective against most intestinal nematodes when given at 20 mg/kg, IM, every 2 weeks or as a solution of 10 ml/gallon drinking water if treating entire flock (use as only source of drinking water for 1–3 days).
- For cestodes, give praziquantel (Droncit Injectable, 56.8 mg/ml; Haver/Diamond) at a dose of 0.16 ml/kg, IM.
- Administer fenbendazole (Panacur Paste; Hoechst-Roussel) at a dose of 20–50 mg/kg, PO for ascarids (one dose and then repeat in 2 weeks) and for capillaria (once daily for 5 days).

DISORDERS OF THE LIVER

Infectious Diseases

Etiology

Infectious disorders such as chlamydiosis, viral disease, bacterial hepatitis, and occasionally *Mycobacterium avium* are the most common causes of liver diseases in pet birds. This is especially true in larger psittacines such as parrots, macaws, and cockatoos, although cockatiels and budgerigars also may be affected.

Diagnosis

- Indicators of liver disease include green-yellow urates (biliverdinuria), hepatomegaly (palpable or radiographically evident), and serum biochemical profile indicators such as increased levels of serum glutamate oxaloacetic transaminase (SGOT), bile acids, lactic dehydrogenase (LDH), and cholesterol and decreased serum albumin levels.
- Liver biopsy often is necessary for definitive diagnosis with identification of a specific etiologic agent.
- See ch. 2 of this section for specific diagnostic tests, treatment, and prevention of infectious disease.

Fatty Liver Syndrome (FLS)

FLS, or hepatic lipidosis, is commonly seen in budgerigars, cockatiels, and some Amazon parrots. Gradual excessive triglyceride accumulation in the liver may cause the destruction of normal liver cells and lead to cirrhosis.

Etiology

- The etiology of FLS is unknown; however, it appears to be primarily a nutritional problem.
  - Most birds with FLS are obese and on a high-fat diet consisting primarily of seeds.
- Unlike FLS in cats, anorexia does not appear to play a role in the development of this disorder.

Clinical Signs

- Signs often include diarrhea, biliverdinuria, obesity, poor feathering, and abdominal enlargement.
- Budgerigars frequently have overgrown, soft, friable beaks, with focal areas of hemorrhage.

- Sudden death has been reported in budgerigars, cockatiels, and Amazon parrots, with hepatic lipidosis as the only identifiable lesion on necropsy.

Diagnosis

- Palpate and, if indicated, obtain radiographs of the abdomen to detect hepatomegaly.
- Increased SGOT, bile acids, LDH, and cholesterol levels may be present on the serum biochemistry profile.
- Liver biopsy is necessary to confirm the diagnosis.

Treatment

- Place the bird on a strict low-fat diet. Eliminate seeds from the diet or reduce the amount to a maximum of 25%.
  - For large birds, add more cereal grains.
  - Ideally, a commercial avian pellet formula should make up at least 40% of the diet, the remainder consisting of vegetables, fruits, and grains/legumes.
- Lactulose (Cephulac; Marion Merrell Dow), given at a dose of 0.3 ml/kg q8–12h, PO, may help to stimulate the appetite and decrease the colonic absorption of toxins that cause hepatic encephalopathy.

Hepatic Fibrosis

Etiology

- Hepatic fibrosis is a common sequela to chronic liver disease.
- The primary insult can be infectious (e.g., bacterial, viral, chlamydial) or noninfectious (e.g., FLS). Fibrosis can persist after elimination of the primary insult.

Diagnosis

- Liver biopsy is required for definitive diagnosis of hepatic fibrosis.

Treatment

- Colchicine has been reported to decrease clinical signs of chronic liver disease (Hoefer, 1991) by interfering with collagen precursor synthesis.

Aflatoxicosis

Etiology

- Avian aflatoxicosis is caused by the ingestion of toxic metabolites from molds such as *Aspergillus flavus* and *A. parasiticus*. Foods in which these molds may be found include peanuts and peanut products, cereals, breads, cheeses, beans, and meat.
- Aflatoxins frequently are hepatoxic and may be carcinogenic.

Clinical Signs

- Signs generally are nonspecific and include anorexia, weight loss, and depression.

Diagnosis

- Base the diagnosis on history, clinical signs, and fungus isolation from feed or the GI tract.
- Gross and histopathologic lesions from postmortem or liver biopsy confirm the diagnosis.
  - Chronic lesions include biliary hyperplasia, cirrhosis, generalized fatty degeneration, and portal fibrosis.
  - Acute lesions include massive hepatocyte necrosis and hepatic hemorrhage.

Treatment

- No specific therapy is available.
- Activated charcoal may help to eliminate the toxin from the intestinal tract.
- Oral selenium may act as a competitive inhibitor of aflatoxins in the liver.
- Vitamin A is believed to provide some protection prophylactically against aflatoxins.

Hemochromatosis

Etiology

Hemochromatosis, defined as excessive deposition of iron in hepatic parenchymal cells with resultant cellular damage, is common in mynahs and toucans. Iron is normally absorbed from the intestines at a rate dependent on the body's needs, and then recycled with minimal excretion from the body.

- In hemochromatosis, there is excessive uncontrolled absorption and storage of iron.
- The mechanism of this defect in iron metabolism is not understood, but affected birds will absorb and store even small amounts of iron in the diet.

Clinical Signs

- Signs include weight loss, dyspnea, and abdominal swelling from severe hepatomegaly and ascites.

Diagnosis

- Diagnosis is based on clinical signs, elevated SGOT and LDH levels, and serum iron levels in excess of 150 μg/100 ml (the ideal maximum normal value).

Treatment

- For symptomatic control of ascites, periodically remove abdominal fluid and administer diuretics.
- Successful long-term treatment has been reported with weekly phlebotomies (Worell, 1991).

Prevention

Many commercial mynah pellets contain excessively high levels of iron.

- Place mynahs and toucans on a diet consisting of a low-iron kibbled dog food such as Science Diet Senior or Maintenance dog food (Hill's Pet) or Scenic Low Iron Pelleted Ration (Marion Zoological) with freshly diced fruits such as grapes, apples, and melons.

Neoplasia

Primary and metastatic neoplasms have been reported in all psittacines; they are particularly prevalent in budgerigars.

- Primary tumors seen include bile duct carcinoma, hepatocellular carcinoma, hepatoma, fibrosarcoma, and hemangiosarcoma.
- Hepatomegaly usually is palpable or visible on radiographs.
- Diagnosis is confirmed by biopsy.
- Treatment is ineffective.

DISORDERS OF THE PANCREAS

Etiology

- As in liver disease, many infectious agents (e.g., bacteria, *Chlamydia*, viruses) may target the pancreas alone (e.g., many viral infections) or concurrently with other organ systems (see sec. 12, ch. 1).
- Noninfectious causes of pancreatitis include nutritional factors; pancreatitis may be seen secondary to egg yolk peritonitis (see sec. 12, ch. 6).
- In some cases, pancreatitis diagnosed at necropsy showed an intense inflammatory process without infectious etiology in birds on high-fat (seed) diets.
- There is a possible correlation between hypercalcemia occurring in hens in breeding condition (serum calcium levels usually are 20 times normal prior to ovulation) and the onset of pancreatitis (hypercalcemia is known to be a cause of pancreatitis in humans).

Clinical Signs

- Signs include anorexia, polyuria-polydipsia, diarrhea, and listlessness.

Diagnosis

- Serum amylase levels may be consistently elevated, and lipemia, hypercalcemia, and hyperglycemia may be present.
- Radiography may reveal decreased abdominal detail.
- In one confirmed case an abdominal tap revealed the presence of blood and serum in the abdomen.

Treatment

- Treatment is similar to that for dogs and cats, and includes fluid therapy (nothing per os), antibiotic therapy, and maintenance on a low-fat diet (see sec. 7, ch. 10).

Supplemental Readings

Campbell TW: Mycotic diseases. *In* Harrison GH, Harrison LR, eds.: *Clinical Avian Medicine and Surgery*. Philadelphia: W. B. Saunders, 1986, p 466.

Clipsham R: Surgical beak restoration and correction. AAV Proceedings, 1989, p 164.

Gould J: Liver disease in psittacines. AAV Proceedings, 1989, p 125.

Harrison GJ: Selected surgical procedures. *In* Harrison GH, Harrison LR, eds.: *Clinical Avian Medicine and Surgery*. Philadelphia: W. B. Saunders, 1986, p 577.

Hillyer EV: Bile duct carcinoma in two of ten Amazon parrots with cloacal papillomas. J Assoc Avian Vet 5(2):193, 1991.

Hoefer HL: Hepatic fibrosis and colchicine therapy. J Assoc Avian Vet 5(4):193, 1991.

Hoefer HL, Moroff S: The use of bile acids in the diagnosis of hepatobiliary disease in the parrot. AAV Proceedings, 1991, p 118.

Worell A: Phlebotomy for treatment of hemochromatosis in two sulfur-breasted toucans. AAV Proceedings, 1991, p 9.

6 Avian Obstetrical Medicine

Walter J. Rosskopf
Richard W. Woerpel

This chapter describes the problems encountered in female pet avian species while forming, developing, and delivering eggs. Obstetric problems are common in birds (Table 1).

ANATOMY OF THE FEMALE REPRODUCTIVE TRACT

The gross anatomy of the female reproductive tract is relatively simple (Fig. 1).

Ovary

- In most pet bird species, only the left ovary is functional.
  - The inactive ovary is a miniature white botryoid organ; the cortex consists of a wall of small, white developing follicles and a medulla of highly vascular connective tissue.
  - The active ovary contains numerous follicles, containing varying amounts of yolk material.
- The ovary is intimately associated with the ventral surface of the cranial pole of the left kidney.
- The size and appearance of the ovary varies, depending on the physiologic state of the bird.

Oviduct

- Usually, the left oviduct is functional and the right side is vestigial.
- Anatomically the oviduct is divided into five parts: the infundibulum, magnum (pars albuginea), isthmus, shell gland (pars calcigerous), and vagina (pars terminalis). The term *uterus* has been used synonymously for the term *oviduct* in birds; others consider the *shell gland* the uterus.
- The size of the oviduct varies, depending on the physiologic state and age of the bird.
  - The virgin oviduct may be microscopic in size; the mature oviduct is considerably larger.
  - A gravid oviduct may occupy much of the abdominal cavity.
- The oviduct is suspended by a cranial and a caudal ligament, through which it receives its well-developed blood supply.

NORMAL EGG FORMATION

- The *development of ova* is influenced by several factors. When sexual maturity has been achieved, most avian species respond to increasing periods of daylight with follicular maturation.
- *Follicular growth* is controlled by follicle-stimulating hormone (FSH). After an ovum begins growing within a follicle, maturation takes several days. Yolk is deposited as concentric rings, representing daily maturation.
- *Ovulation* is controlled by luteinizing hormone (LH). No structure analogous to a mammalian corpus luteum develops.
- The funnel-shaped *infundibulum* is closely associated with the ovary. It engulfs extruded ova, and here fertilization occurs. The infundibulum propels the ovum down the oviduct.
  - If the engulfing procedure does not occur (injury, disease, drug therapy, obstruction, or other cause of nervous dysfunction), the ovum will fall into the body cavity or be resorbed.
- The longest portion of the oviduct is the highly glandular *magnum*. Pressure on the secretory glands causes the magnum to secrete mucin and albumin around the ovum.
- The ovum is next propelled into the short, nonglandular *isthmus,* where the two shell membranes are secreted loosely around the ovum and albumin.
- The *shell gland* is a comparatively short, dilated

TABLE 1. Common Obstetric Problems by Species

Condition	Species*											
	1	2	3	4	5	6	7	8	9	10	11	12
Metritis				C		C		C				
Egg peritonitis			C	O	C		C	C	R	C	C	R
Egg binding			C	C	C	R	C	C	R	O		R
Cloacal prolapse		R					C					
Cloacal papilloma		C									C	O
Lipomatosis			C		C	C						
Abdominal hernia			C	R	C		O	O				
Other tumors	R		C									
Prolonged egg laying			C	O	C		C	C		C		
Ectopic eggs	R		R									
Oviduct prolapse				O	R	O		R				

R = rare; O = occasionally seen; C = commonly encountered.
*1 = African gray parrots; 2 = Amazon parrots; 3 = budgerigars; 4 = canaries; 5 = cockatiels; 6 = cockatoos; 7 = ducks; 8 = finches; 9 = gray-cheeked parakeets; 10 = lovebirds; 11 = macaws; 12 = conures.

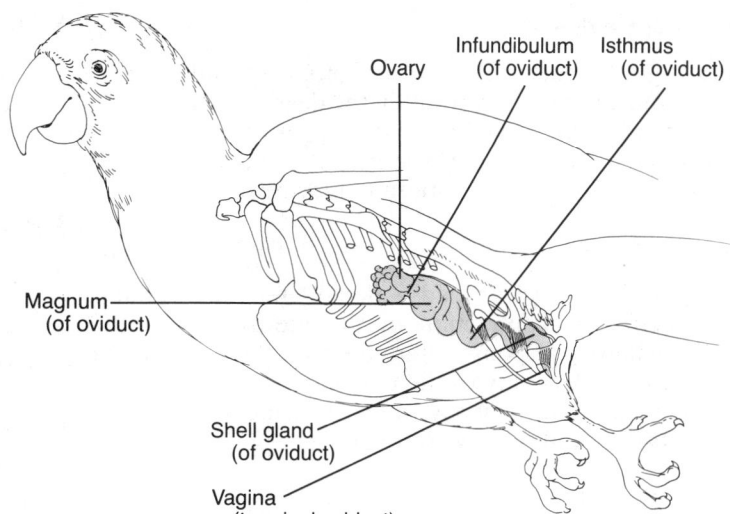

Figure 1. Reproductive anatomy of the female bird.

portion of the oviduct, with glandular mucosa. Albumin is secreted here also, along with the shell and shell pigments (if present).

- While the egg is in the shell gland and before calcification proceeds further, water and vitamins and mineral salts pass through the semipermeable egg membranes into the egg and migrate toward the yolk, the site of lowest water concentration.

■ The terminal portion of the oviduct, the *vagina,* is a muscular portion that communicates with the cloaca. This area is responsible for forcefully expelling the ova and is calcium- and oxytocin-responsive.

■ Oviduct disease can be transferred to the egg contents (bacteria, fungi, viruses). Hypermotility of the oviduct and uterus, or calcium deficiencies, can result in a soft-shelled egg.

■ *Egg transit time*—In most bird species, the ovum spends about 15 minutes in the infundibulum, 3 hours in the magnum, 1½ hours in the isthmus, and 20–21 hours in the shell gland and passes through the vagina almost instantly. Thus, egg formation usually takes 24–26 hours.

PHARMACOLOGIC INFLUENCES ON EGG PRODUCTION

There are no anatomic structures to prevent the egg from undergoing reverse peristalsis. Physical disturbance of a laying hen and certain drugs can result in egg peritonitis or eggs that are soft-shelled, shell-less, or misshapen.

■ Adrenergic drugs cause relaxation of the oviduct, and cholinergic drugs cause constriction.

■ Acetylcholine, oxytocin, and vasotocin produce expulsion of uterine eggs.

■ In order for a shell to be produced, metabolic CO_2 must be converted to HCO_3^- within the shell gland catalyzed by carbonic anhydrase.

- Drugs such as sulfonamides and acetazolamide

inhibit carbonic anhydrase and result in eggshell thinning.

NUTRITIONAL INFLUENCES ON EGG PRODUCTION

Nutritional status has profound effects on egg-producing and laying.

■ *Protein deficiency* may result in reduced numbers of eggs and in high chick mortality.

■ The formation of specialized medullary bone in the tibia and femur of females is stimulated by the action of estrogens and androgens; as a result, more calcium is made available for eggshell formation. However, breeding birds fed a *calcium-deficient* diet may pass thin-shelled eggs and have an increased incidence of egg binding.

- Calcium also has profound effects on *uterine contractibility.* Calcium used for eggshell formation may result in borderline blood calcium status with insufficient calcium available for uterine contraction.

■ *Vitamin D₃ deficiency* may exacerbate signs of calcium deficiency and may be associated with poor bone development and splay legs.

DISEASES THAT INFLUENCE EGG PRODUCTION
Chronic Disease

■ Overt disease may be precipitated by the production of ova or egg laying in female birds with borderline health status.

■ A chronically ill bird is less likely to form ova, but surprisingly, many seriously ill birds, especially small birds such as budgerigars, cockatiels, and lovebirds, continue to lay eggs. In contrast to mammals, female birds tend to sacrifice themselves in egg laying. It is theorized that this phenomenon occurs because male birds can successfully raise young alone.

Bacterial Metritis

- Low-grade bacterial metritis, often secondary to systemic disease, may result in the death of neonates.
- Such infections can have adverse effects on shell formation and uterine contractility. Egg binding, uterine rupture, and septicemia may result.

Egg Peritonitis

- Egg peritonitis (described in detail later) may result in ineffective contraction of the uterus (i.e., the inflammatory response interferes with the peristaltic and expulsive ability of the oviduct).
- Recovered birds may have adhesions and abdominal distension, influencing subsequent egg laying efforts.

Cloacal Abnormalities

Cloacal abnormalities that may impair the ability to normally pass ova include weak cloacal musculature, papillomatosis, and cloacal strictures and scar formation.

- *Weak cloacal musculature or internal attachments*— A weakened cloaca may develop into a full-blown prolapse after the expulsive efforts of egg laying. The degree of cloacal prolapse varies.
  - Treatment of prolapse is described in detail later in this chapter.
- *Papillomatosis* (see sec. 3, ch. 9) can be a serious problem in obstetrics. It is considered viral in origin and may have a venereal route of transmission. Serious anatomic disruption may occur, destroying the bird's reproductive abilities.
- *Cloacal strictures and scar formation* can occur following egg laying, infection, injury, papilloma surgery, episiotomy, and cloacoliths.
  - When practical, a pre-breeding examination should include a vent and cloacal examination.

Abdominal Hernias

- Birds that have had previous heavy egg-laying episodes may develop large abdominal hernias, interfering with subsequent egg laying; the abdominal musculature may completely separate. This is particularly common in cockatiels.
- Imbrication of abdominal musculature may be necessary. An elliptical area of skin is removed from sternum to vent and the peritoneum and skin are sutured together, effectively tightening the area.
- Achieving muscle-to-muscle repair may be impossible if the condition is chronic and contraction of muscle tissue is severe.

Abdominal Tumors

- Lipomas and xanthomas that involve the abdomen are common in budgerigars and cockatiels.
- Massive lipomas are common in rose-breasted cockatoos. These growths may damage abdominal muscle tone and can influence egg laying, resulting in egg binding.

- Tumors of the kidneys and gonads may push the gizzard ventrally, mimicking the appearance of an egg.
  - In some birds, both abdominal masses and eggs may be present; radiographs of the abdomen can differentiate abdominal masses from retained eggs, unless the eggs have no shells.

Recurrence of Historical Problems

- Carefully observe birds with a history of previous egg-laying problems.
- Recurrences of uterine or cloacal prolapses, egg peritonitis, or ectopic eggs are common.

Miscellaneous Problems

- Conditions that may influence obstetric procedures include congenital deformities, injuries (e.g., leg injury), previous egg-laying status (heavy egg layers tend to repeat), age (e.g., very old, very young), uterine structural status (e.g., strictures), nutritional status, and general health.

PROLONGED EGG LAYING

Prolonged egg laying is a common problem in cockatiels, lovebirds, and budgerigars. This process can be detrimental. According to its owner, one cockatiel laid 30 eggs in 1½ months. Certain individual birds tend to be multiple egg layers; others of the same species rarely or never lay eggs.

Etiology

- Extremely close attachment of the bird to an owner, with a resultant display of masturbatory activity, may stimulate the process, especially if the owner encourages it.
- *Double clutching effect*—Usually, when the number of eggs laid constitute a clutch, hormonal levels change and the female shifts into "broodiness" until the eggs are ready to be hatched, completing the cycle. Continuous removal of eggs as they are laid disrupts this cycle, causing repeated laying.

Behavioral Modification

- Discourage mating behavior with the owner.
- Do not remove eggs until brooding is complete (usually 21 days).
- Change the bird's environment (e.g., move to another room); the mild stress may stop the egg-laying cycle.

Medical Therapy

- If behavioral methods are ineffective, administration of medroxyprogesterone (Depo-Provera; Upjohn) may break the egg-laying cycle.
- The effect is only temporary (3 weeks to several months) and may be associated with undesirable side effects such as depression, polyuria, weight gain, liver compromise with elevated serum glutamate oxaloacetic transaminase (SGOT) levels, lowered

resistance to disease (with latent problems becoming overt) and, in rare cases, diabetes mellitus.
■ In most cases, the drug works well in routine clinical use. The author has used Depo-Provera repeatedly in some birds, with minimal side effects at the dose range suggested in Table 2.
■ Injections may be repeated with return of laying so long as side effects are acceptable.

Surgical Treatment: Hysterectomy

Hysterectomy is the method of choice for permanent alleviation of chronic egg laying. However, initially attempt conservative methods because clients may be concerned about surgical risk, loss of "intactness" of the bird, and loss of breeding potential.

In most birds, ovarian development is under uterine control, and removal of the uterus will inhibit future follicle release; however, continued production of ova and subsequent yolk peritonitis occasionally occur following simple hysterectomy. In psittacines, partial hysterectomy (i.e., removal of 2/3 of uterus) is usually effective.

Indications

Consider hysterectomy if:
■ Side-effects of Depo-Provera are unacceptable.
■ The owner objects to use of long-acting steroids.
■ There are concurrent problems such as severe uterine disease, repeated egg binding or a life-threatening egg binding episode, and recurring or chronic peritonitis.

KEY POINT ▶ Most small birds normally experience "menopause" and stop laying eggs after a few years; but this varies.

Technique

1. Perform a left lateral lapartomy approach. To avoid hemorrhage, the ovary is left intact.
2. Bluntly dissect the infundibulum away from the ovary.
3. Ligate the artery leading from the ovary. Place a ligature around the uterus at the junction of the uterus with the cloaca.
4. Transect the uterus after tying off or cauterizing any other vessels contained in the suspensory ligaments.
   a. Electrocautery is a necessity in most small birds. In larger birds, blunt dissection and simple ligation may suffice.
5. Close the abdominal wall with absorbable sutures in a simple interrupted pattern.
6. Close the skin with absorbable or nonabsorbable sutures in a simple continuous pattern.

TABLE 2. Suggested Dose Ranges for Depo-Provera

Weight of Bird	Dose (mg/g)
<150 g	0.05
150–300 g	0.04
300–700 g	0.03
700 g	0.025

7. Depo-Provera is given to stop egg formation until hormonal control ceases.

EGG PERITONITIS (YOLK PERITONITIS)

Peritonitis due to the escape of yolk material into the peritoneal cavity is a common condition in many avian species, including cockatiels, budgerigars, lovebirds, ducks, and macaws. Generalized peritonitis may result, with adhesions between the various organs, especially between loops of intestine. Subsequent inflammation may occur in vital areas such as the adrenal glands, liver, and pancreas.

Etiology

■ It has been postulated that yolk excites only a mild histiocytic response and is gradually resorbed by the peritoneum, and that yolk peritonitis occurs when the yolk (a good bacterial growth medium) becomes contaminated by bacteria.
■ Alternatively, it is theorized that the yolk causes a foreign body reaction or is itself caustic.
■ Peritonitis can occur when ova extruded from the ovary fail to enter the infundibulum of the oviduct.
■ Rupture of the oviduct may result from infection of surrounding tissues and weakening of the ovarian wall, stasis of normal or abnormal eggs, obstruction of the oviduct (egg binding, mechanical blockage as from cystic hyperplasia of the oviduct or neoplasia of the oviduct), or, in rare cases, injury.
■ Reverse peristalsis of the oviduct may occur. Many apparently normal cockatiels develop egg peritonitis immediately following egg laying. An ovum just starting to enter the infundibulum is driven into the body cavity when the expulsive egg laying process is occurring simultaneously.

Clinical Signs

■ Common signs include abdominal distension, depression, lethargy, and anorexia.

Diagnosis

Base the diagnosis of egg peritonitis on clinical signs, a complete blood count (CBC), radiography, abdominocentesis, and laparotomy.

■ A history of egg laying may be helpful; however, egg peritonitis can occur just prior to the onset of laying.
■ Abdominal radiographs often reveal a typical "ground glass" appearance. Calcified egg material is rarely present within the peritoneal cavity.
■ A CBC is useful for diagnosing egg peritonitis. A severe inflammatory response (marked leukocytosis, heterophilia with a left shift, toxic heterophils) often mimics chlamydiosis, septicemia, tuberculosis, or generalized aspergillosis. Table 3 lists typical hemograms seen in confirmed cases.
■ Abdominocentesis is helpful when ascites is present. Aspirated fluid may contain yolk material, heterophils, macrophages, and bacteria.
■ Laparotomy, which often is necessary for treatment (discussed later), can confirm the diagnosis.

TABLE 3. Typical Hemograms of Birds with Confirmed Egg Peritonitis

	Budgerigar	Cockatiel	Scarlet Macaw	Scarlet Macaw
WBC (per μ)	29,000	24,000	120,000	2000
Bands (%)	3		6	6
Heterophils (%)	87	90*	75*	92*
Lymphocytes (%)	8	8	14	2
Monocytes (%)	2		5	
Eosinophils (%)		2		
Basophils (%)				
PCV (%)	55	60	48	31
SGOT (μ/liter)	850	1750	1200	2300
Outcome	Resolved	Resolved	Died postoperatively	Degenerative picture; resolved after surgery

*Toxic heterophils.
WBC = white blood cells; PCV = packed cell volume; SGOT = serum glutamate oxaloacetic transaminase.

Complications

- *Diabetes mellitus* may be an aftermath of yolk peritonitis, especially in cockatiels. Transient diabetes may occur, in which resolution appears to correlate with cessation of pancreatic inflammation.
- The presence of apparent yolk in serum, or *yolk emboli,* appears to have been responsible for stroke-like symptoms seen in several cockatiels with yolk peritonitis.
  - Lipemia and liver damage may be associated with this phenomenon.
  - Most cases resolve after a week or so with supportive care alone.

Treatment

- If yolk peritonitis is mild, most birds recover with initial corticosteroid therapy and broad-spectrum antibiotics, and supportive care (e.g., vitamins, forced alimentation, heat, and fluids as indicated).
- Aspirin is an effective anticoagulant in birds. Dissolve one 5-grain tablet in 30 ml of water or juice.
  - A typical dose is 0.05 ml of the mixture given q8h to a 100 g bird.
- If massive amounts of yolk collect, laparotomy may be required after medically stabilizing the patient. Surgery may be postponed for long periods while the patient's condition stabilizes.
  - A scarlet macaw (see Table 3) was presented with a degenerative left shift and was near death from yolk peritonitis. After stabilization (e.g., WBC = 12,000 μl, PCV = 47%, no toxic heterophils), several inspissated yolks were removed and a large opening in the oviduct was closed.
- Birds with chronic peritonitis may require long periods of treatment; monitor with hematology and microbiology.
  - Warn owners that future problems may occur because of uterine and abdominal damage.
- Treat diabetes with long-term insulin therapy, if indicated.

EGG BINDING

KEY POINT ▶ Eggbinding is one of the most common emergency conditions encountered in pet birds.

Birds may be presented in various stages of this condition, ranging from slight distress to moribund.

Etiology

- The obstruction may be caused by developing or fully formed eggs, concretions of egg material, calculi, or excessive secretions from the mucosa of the oviduct itself.
- Obstruction by a developing egg is the condition most frequently seen in clinical practice.
  - Inability to expel the egg may be due to low blood calcium levels, resulting from a calcium-deficient diet or from over-production of eggs that drain calcium reserves.
  - Other causes include uterine damage from peritonitis, infection, or injury.
  - Occasionally, a larger than normal egg or an egg presented laterally is the cause.
- The most commonly affected species are budgerigars, canaries, finches, cockatiels, and lovebirds; however, any species can be susceptible.

Clinical Signs

Signs depend on the species of bird and the position of the egg.

- Most egg-binding occurs at the distal part of the oviduct (the uterus).
- Eggs trapped below the pelvis may crush the kidneys or cause intestinal blockage. The lack of "give" between the surface of the egg and the pelvic outlet makes this condition potentially life-threatening in a short period of time (Fig. 2).
- In small birds such as canaries or finches, sudden death without prior clinical signs is common.
- Larger birds may perch unsteadily with ruffled feathers and half-closed eyes. Birds may make frequent tail-wagging and abdominal straining movements and may move back and forth to the nest.
- Eventually, because of complications from intestinal blockage, kidney compromise, or ureter blockage, there are signs of pain, and the bird moves to the cage bottom.
- Hashold described egg-bound canaries as "having hanging wings and tail, making them look as if they had a swelling over the root of the tail, whereas

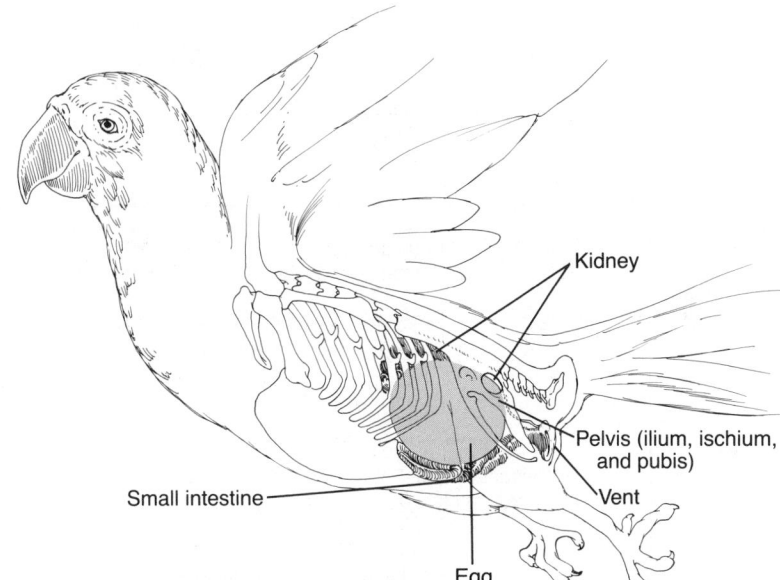

Figure 2. Anatomic landmarks associated with egg binding.

budgerigars often sit on the tail with legs far apart and with the wings and body erect, like penguins."

Diagnosis

Diagnosis is usually made by clinical signs, palpation, and radiography.

- If an egg is palpable in a heavily producing cockatiel found on the bottom of the cage, it is usually easy to diagnose egg binding.
- In large birds such as parrots, macaws, and cockatiels, eggs can be easily distinguished by digital palpation against the pelvic girdle.
- In small birds such as canaries and finches, normal soft tissue structures such as the gizzard may be pushed downward, making palpation difficult.
- Distinguishing the presence of an egg from an intra-abdominal mass, ascites, hernias, or lipomas may be difficult; in these cases, abdominal radiography is indicated.
- If an egg is not easily palpable, consider yolk peritonitis, septicemia from stress of over-production, leg injuries, and other causes in a "downer" egg-producing female.
- The presence of an egg is not conclusive evidence of egg binding.
  - Observe the bird for clinical signs of egg binding before undertaking corrective measures.

Treatment

Treatment and manipulative procedures in egg binding vary with the severity of the condition and the location of the egg.

- Choose a procedure based on its ability to relieve the patient's distress with the least amount of stress and shock potential.
- Because the condition may have been unattended for an extended period of time, there may be difficult manipulative and surgical problems.

- For purposes of discussion of treatment, egg binding is divided into the following categories:
  - Precloacal binding
  - Cloacal binding
  - Postcloacal binding
  - Egg binding with prolapsed oviduct (Fig. 3)

KEY POINT ▶ Avoid the use of anesthesia, which is unnecessary in the early stages of egg binding and can be dangerous in birds in late, critical stages. If an anesthetic is necessary, isoflurane is the agent of choice.

Many birds that are not egg-bound show discomfort in the laying process, similar to labor in mammals. Treat with calcium and oxytocin, as described for early oviduct binding.

Early Stages of Cloacal Binding

Birds in the early or incipient stages of cloacal binding are not immediately at risk.

- Briefly attempt to deliver the egg by working the thumb and forefinger between the egg and rib cage and then pushing outward and downward. Outward pressure prevents pain and shock from pressure on the kidneys.
- Relax the vent by gentle steam heat or use K-Y jelly to lubricate the cloaca.
- To stimulate uterine contraction and prevent hemorrhage, administer an intramuscular injection of calcium (Calphosan; Glenwood), 0.15–0.25 ml/100 g, and oxytocin, 0.025 ml/100 g 20 USP units/ml).
- If indicated, give antibiotics and corticosteroids prophylactically.

Early Stages of Oviduct Binding

In the early stages of oviduct binding, only mild signs of distress are present, and the bird is alert and

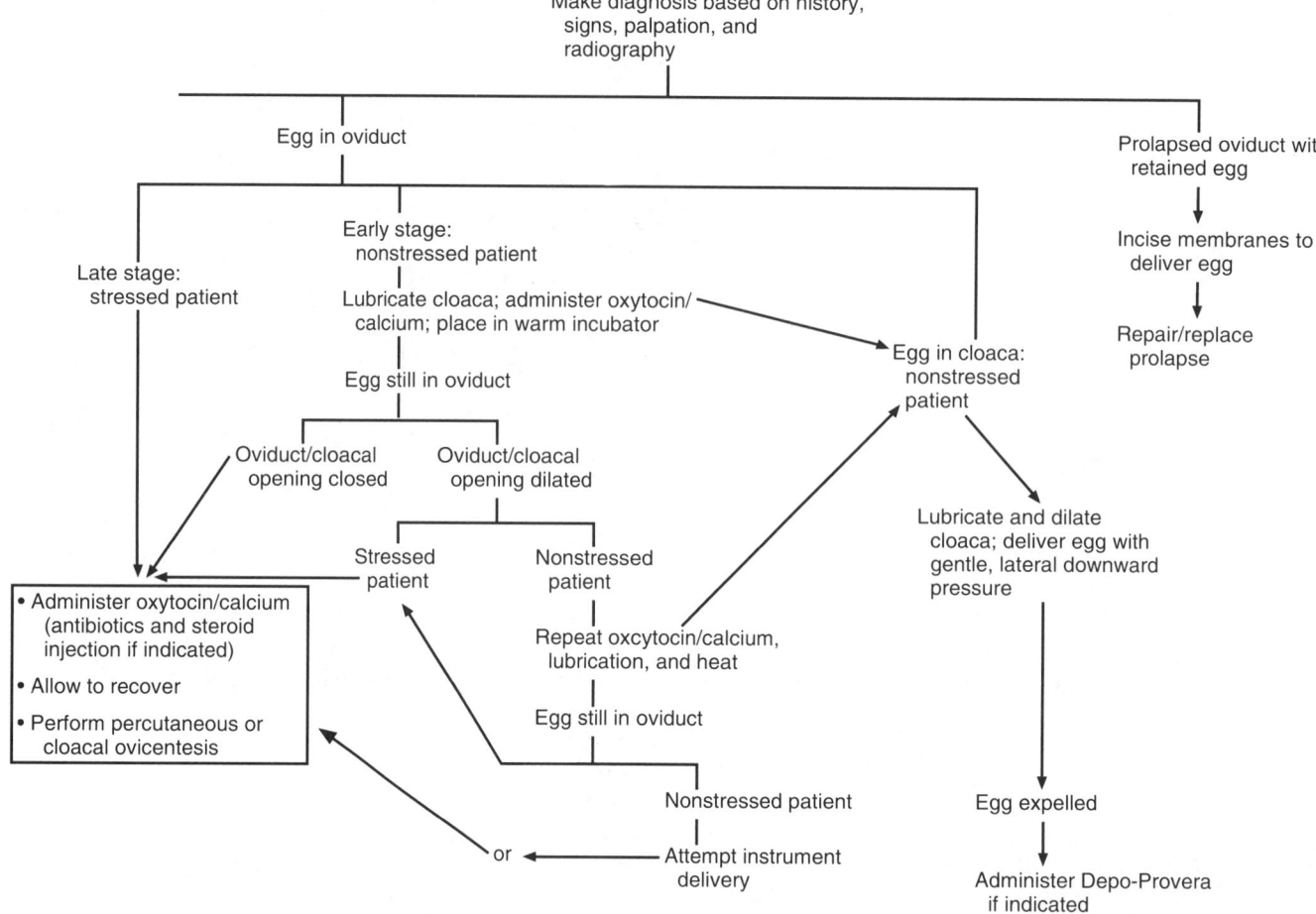

Figure 3. Flow chart for the treatment of egg binding.

active. However, because symptoms may be masked and rapid deterioration can occur, immediate medical therapy is recommended.

- Place the bird in a warm environment (e.g., incubator).
- Administer calcium and oxytocin at the dosages given previously for early stages of cloacal binding.
  - In mild cases of uterine inertia, an egg will be produced within 20–30 minutes.
- If an egg is not produced in an hour, the egg has not moved appreciably, and the bird does not demonstrate signs of further distress, repeat treatment.
- After careful observation, perform the manipulative procedures described previously for cloacal binding, if indicated.
- If gentle manual pressure does not produce results, attempt an instrumental delivery.

Technique

1. Clean the cloaca and dilate it with a hemostatic forceps or small vaginal speculum.
2. When the oviduct is visualized, insert a sterile probe between the oviduct and eggshell.
3. With a rotating motion, dilate the oviduct while applying gentle pressure just cranial to the egg to promote its passage. If necessary, insert a small amount of K-Y jelly in the oviduct to facilitate delivery.

- If other methods fail, perform *ovocentesis*. When the bird shows signs of life-threatening stress during manipulative procedures, it is better to perform ovocentesis or simply break the egg purposefully to relieve pressure.
  - Insert an 18-gauge needle in the eggshell and aspirate its contents with a syringe.
  - Collapse the egg within the oviduct by the application of gentle lateral to medial pressure.
  - Once collapsed, the egg can be removed with forceps. This may have to be done piece by piece; however, it is safer to rely on the action of calcium and oxytocin to expel the eggshell, especially if the bird is in poor condition. The egg often is passed in 1–2 days.

KEY POINT ▶ Do not apply dorsal-to-ventral pressure when pushing the egg toward the pelvis in an attempt to collapse it, because crushing of the ureters or kidneys may occur.

Late Stages of Oviduct Binding

The most common egg-binding presentation encountered clinically occurs with the egg inside the distal oviduct and with the oviduct-cloacal opening undilated, similar to uterine inertia occurring in mammals. Because birds with this condition often are presented in a semicomatose state and near death, expert and expeditious management is imperative.

Attempts to dislodge the egg can result in near-collapse and severe stress with panting. Surgical correction (e.g., laparotomy), requiring anesthesia and extensive manipulation, is dangerous. As an alternative to these methods, the following approach is recommended. This sequence relieves pressure on vital organs with a minimum of shock potential in an already compromised animal and is preferable to invasive techniques such as laparotomy and episiotomy.

- Handling the bird as little as possible, administer the following drugs:
  - An antibiotic such as piperacillin (Pipracil; Lederle), 100 mg/kg q12h, IM
  - Dexamethazone (Azium; Schering), 2–4 mg/kg
  - Calcium (Calphosan; Glenwood), 0.15–0.25 ml/100 g
  - Oxytocin (20 USP units/liter), 0.025 ml/100 g (to control hemorrhage)
- To treat dehydration, administer parenteral or intravenous fluids (see sec. 12, ch. 1).
- Place the bird in an incubator for a few minutes to allow recovery from stress.
- Perform *percutaneous ovocentesis* or manual collapse of the egg if it doesn't implode.

Technique

1. Wipe the abdomen with alcohol.
2. Push the egg ventrally toward the abdominal wall, so that the skin is stretched taut over the egg.
3. Insert an 18-gauge needle percutaneously into the egg to quickly tap off the contents. This may collapse the egg if it is thin-shelled; otherwise, apply firm lateral-to-medial (not ventral-to-dorsal) pressure to collapse the egg.
4. Place the bird into an incubator to allow recovery. The collapsed egg usually is passed within 1–2 days.
5. Another oxytocin and calcium injection may be necessary after uterine inflammation subsides.

Egg Binding with Uterine Prolapse

If the egg is presented beyond the cloacal opening and wrapped in the oviduct, the length of time that the tissues of the oviduct have been exposed determines the ease of removal and the anticipated postsurgical sequelae.

Technique

1. Make a small incision at the least vascular point over the egg. Using a pair of mosquito forceps, gently separate the incision.
2. In many cases, gentle manipulation is all that is necessary to remove the egg after incising the oviduct membrane. If the egg is excessively large, perform ovocentesis.
3. If possible, suture the oviduct with 6–0 catgut or Dexon in a simple continuous pattern.
4. If the prolapsed oviduct has dried out, debride the necrotic tissue before suturing. In small birds this can be extremely difficult and the prognosis may be grave, especially if another egg is quickly formed and travels through the injured oviduct.
   a. Ectopic eggs (described later) and egg peritonitis with soft or nonshelled yolks released into the abdomen are common sequelae.
5. Using a saline-soaked cotton swab, manipulate the oviduct back into position through the oviduct-cloacal opening.
6. Administer oxytocin at the dosage previously given for early stages of cloacal binding to promote uterine shrinkage, control bleeding, and expel accumulated blood from the oviduct.

Episiotomy

This procedure usually is performed if the egg is valuable and egg aspiration and collapse or purposeful breaking of the egg must be avoided.

Technique

1. Extend the vent opening laterally on one side only.
2. Remove the egg and suture the incision with 4–0 Dexon on a tapered needle.
3. Use careful technique to prevent stricture formation postoperatively.

ECTOPIC EGGS

Ectopic eggs (eggs free within the peritoneal cavity) occur occasionally, especially in small birds such as budgerigars and cockatiels. Diagnosis is usually made by laparotomy after all the usual methods to cause expulsion of the egg have failed.

A thirteen-year-old African gray parrot that had never laid an egg was presented with a distended abdomen. The bird never appeared to strain or showed discomfort. Radiographs revealed a single large, thick-shelled egg. After 2 weeks, the egg was tapped, the contents were removed, and the egg was collapsed. Oxytocin and calcium were given. After a waiting period in which no contractions were noted, the egg was not expelled. Laparotomy revealed an ectopic egg that was removed through a midline incision. Interestingly, no hole was observed in the oviduct, which had apparently already healed. Several similar cases have been seen in budgerigars.

OVIDUCT PROLAPSE

Oviduct prolapse (uterine prolapse) after egg laying is a common problem in budgerigars, cockatoos, and, occasionally, other birds. The oviduct may prolapse alone, or concurrent with cloacal prolapse.

Oviduct Prolapse with Intact Cloaca

- If the mucosa appears healthy, thoroughly clean exposed tissues with normal saline solution. Push the oviduct back through the cloaca into the body cavity with a lubricated cotton swab.
  - Administer oxytocin (see under Early Stages of

Cloacal Binding for dosage) to hasten oviduct shrinkage.
■ If the oviduct has become desiccated or necrotic, a full or partial hysterectomy (see below) may be necessary.

Oviduct Prolapse with Cloacal Prolapse

Usually, simple replacement of the cloaca and oviduct is insufficient because the oviduct has become desiccated or necrotic or because the cloacal-oviduct opening is damaged, resulting in continual prolapse of the oviduct back into the cloaca following cloacal replacement or repair.

■ The prolapse may not be visible externally, and the oviduct will undergo necrosis if the condition is not recognized. For this reason, a *partial hysterectomy* is recommended. This technique has worked well as a salvage operation in inexpensive pet birds.

Technique

1. Apply overlapping mattress sutures through the viable part of the exposed uterus.
2. Using a lubricated cotton swab, debride necrotic tissue and reposition the partial uterus.

■ In some cases, a laparotomy may be performed to replace the oviduct so that a complete hysterectomy can be performed.
■ If the bird is too ill to be considered a surgical candidate, the uterus may be replaced inside the cloaca and held in place by transverse sutures in the cloaca until it is considered safe to perform laparotomy.
  • Carefully observe the bird to make sure that its droppings are passed regularly during this stabilization period.

KEY POINT ▶ If it is safe to administer the drug, give medroxyprogesterone (Depo-Provera) (see Table 2) after any serious obstetric problem to prevent ovulation.

CLOACAL PROLAPSE

Minor Prolapses

■ Minor prolapses of the cloaca often are held in place with pursestring or two transverse stay sutures placed perpendicular to the vent (Fig. 4). Be careful to leave an opening large enough to allow feces to pass normally.
  • Sutures may be wire, silk, Vetafil, or other non-absorbable material.

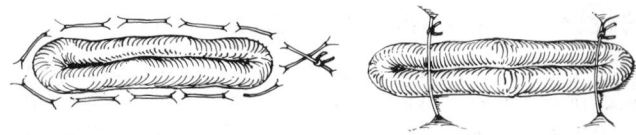

Figure 4. Cloacal suturing techniques. *Left,* Pursestring suture; *right,* transverse suture.

■ Remove sutures after 3 days.
■ Once the swollen tissue is reduced, the oviduct and/or cloaca may heal.

Cloacopexy

If serious damage has occurred to the cloacal attachments, prolapse of the cloaca and oviduct may continue following suture removal. In these cases cloacopexy is recommended. This technique effectively prevents recurrence of the prolapse. Birds can return to immediate reproductive activity. However, if the uterus is very thin-walled, permanent repair is much more difficult to achieve.

Technique

1. Make a midline abdominal incision.
2. Outline the cloaca by having an assistant, wearing a finger cot, push the cloaca into the incision site.
3. Dissect the fat pad (analogous to the falciform ligament in the dog) away from the cloacal wall.
4. Suture the anterolateral walls of the ventral cloaca with 3–0 Vicryl to the posterior ribs and, if necessary, to the cartilage of the ventral sternum. Apply sufficient tension to slightly invert the vent opening.
5. Suture the lateral and ventral cloaca to the abdominal musculature, with 3–0 Vicryl in a simple interrupted pattern.

Complications

Failure may occur if:

■ The adipose pad is not dissected away
■ The lumen of the cloaca is not penetrated
■ Rapidly absorbed suture material is used
■ The ribs or ribs plus sternum are not used to anchor at least two sutures
■ The sutures tear through a thin-walled cloaca

CLOACAL MUCOSAL RESECTION

Cloacal mucosal prolapse with necrotic or desiccated tissue is common in cockatoos and is seen in other avian species. Treatment consists of mucosal resection as performed in mammals.

Supplemental Readings

Altman RB: Surgery of the urogenital system. Proceedings of the 14th Annual Veterinary Surgical Forum, American College of Veterinary Surgeons, 1986, p 94.
Blackmore DK (Rev. by Cooper JE): Diseases of the reproductive system. *In* Petrak ML, ed.: *Disease of Cage and Aviary Birds,* 2nd Ed. Philadelphia: Lea & Febiger, 1982, p 458.
Flammer K: Avicultural medicine of psittacine birds. Vet Clin North Am [Small Anim Pract] 14(2):381, 1984.
Harrison GJ: Selected surgical procedures. *In* Harrison GJ, Harrison LR, eds.: *Clinical Avian Medicine and Surgery.* Philadelphia: W. B. Saunders, 1986, p 577.
Harrison GJ: Reproductive medicine. *In* Harrison GJ, Harrison LR, eds.: *Clinical Avian Medicine and Surgery.* Philadelphia: W. B. Saunders, 1986, p 620.
Harrison GJ, Davis CS: Captive behavior and its modification. *In* Harrison GJ, Harrison LR, eds.: *Clinical Avian Medicine and Surgery.* Philadelphia: W. B. Saunders, 1986, p 20.

Reece RL: Reproductive diseases. *In* Burr EW, ed.: *Companion Bird Medicine*. Ames: Iowa State Press, 1987, p 89.

Rosskopf WJ Jr: Surgery of the avian digestive tract. Proceedings of the 14th Annual Veterinary Surgical Forum, American College of Veterinary Surgeons, 1986, p 100.

Rosskopf WJ Jr, Woerpel RW: Pet avian obstetrics. AAV Proceedings, 1987, p 213.

Rosskopf WJ Jr, Woerpel RW: Cloacal conditions in pet birds with a cloaca-pexy update. AAV Proceedings, 1989.

Rosskopf WJ Jr, Woerpel RW, Pitts BJ: Surgical repair of a chronic cloacal prolapse in a greater sulfur-crested cockatoo (*Cacatua galerita*). VM/SAC, 1983, p 719.

Rosskopf WJ Jr, Woerpel RW, Howard EB, Gendron AP: Egg-yolk peritonitis in a cockatiel. Mod Vet Pract 63(5):420, 1982.

7 Avian Neurologic Disorders

Katherine Quesenberry

Neurologic disease is common in cage and aviary birds. Methods of diagnosis and treatment are limited by anatomic variations, size of the patient, and lack of normal baseline data. Although there are many possible etiologies of neurologic disease, certain neurologic syndromes and diseases occur relatively frequently. Diagnosis of these more common syndromes is based on history, clinical signs, selected diagnostic tests, and response to therapy.

GENERAL HISTORY AND CLINICAL SIGNS

History

There are several important points to include in the general history of a bird with neurologic disease.

- Dietary history is important because nutritional deficiencies are factors in many diseases.
  - Ask for specific details, such as:
  - What is the regular diet?
  - What vitamin and mineral supplements are being given?
  - Is adequate calcium provided for heavy egg layers?
- What is the home environment of the bird, especially as related to exposure to trauma and toxins?
  - Is the bird always caged or is it allowed free flight in the house?
  - Does the bird chew on any painted surfaces, metal objects, or plants?
  - What type of toys are kept in the cage?
- Is the bird a recent purchase or a long-term pet? Is there exposure to other birds?
- When was the onset of the disorder and what has been the duration and progression of clinical signs?

Clinical Signs

Clinical signs associated with neurologic disease in birds are similar to those seen in mammals.

- The most common clinical signs are seizures, ataxia, paresis, paralysis, head tilt, circling, abnormal mentation, nystagmus, intention tremors, and visual deficits. Weakness and ataxia can be manifested as falling off the perch.
- It may be difficult to distinguish weakness secondary to severe systemic disease from that associated with neurologic disease.
- The presence or absence of other neurologic deficits may be helpful in determining which body system is involved.
- Unilateral or bilateral lameness or wing droop may indicate a peripheral nerve deficit. Rule out fractures and other musculoskeletal abnormalities as a cause.

Neurologic Evaluation

Assessment of cranial nerve function is basic to a thorough neurologic examination.

- Assess vision in each eye by slowly moving a hand or an object toward the bird from behind on each side. A bird with visual deficits will not react until the object is very close or its face is touched.
- The pupillary light reflex is difficult to evaluate because of the presence of striated muscle in the iris. A widely dilated pupil that reacts minimally to changes in light intensity may indicate a visual deficit.
- Check facial sensation by touching various parts of the face with hemostats. Assess the palpebral reflex as in mammals.

PRINCIPLES OF TREATMENT

KEY POINT ▶ Special nursing care is necessary for birds with neurologic disease.

- Birds with neurologic disease usually require special *nursing care* in the hospital and at home.
  - Keep ataxic or seizuring birds in cages without perches. Provide soft bedding.
  - Use small, shallow, or covered water bowls to prevent accidental drowning.
  - Remove sharp objects, chains, and potentially dangerous toys from the cage.
  - Make food easily accessible by spreading it on the floor or by providing several large containers in the cage.
- *Supplemental fluids* and *gavage feeding* are necessary for anorectic birds (see sec. 12, ch. 1).
- Give *antibiotics* if bacterial disease is suspected or if there is a risk of secondary bacterial infection. If possible, use antimicrobials that cross the blood-brain barrier (e.g., trimethoprim-sulfate, quinolones, chloramphenicol).
- *Anti-inflammatory drugs* (corticosteroids) usually are beneficial in the treatment of acute head trauma. Be conservative in administration because of the potential for adrenal suppression and immune compromise.
- Give *supplemental calcium* if there is a dietary calcium deficiency or if blood calcium concentrations are below normal.
- Administer *chelating agents* such as calcium ethylenediaminetetraacetate (EDTA) in birds with sus-

pected heavy metal toxicity. Many birds improve with therapy even when lead toxicity cannot be confirmed. Side effects are rare.

■ *Anticonvulsants* such as diazepam (Valium) (0.05–2.0 mg/kg, IM or IV) are sometimes helpful in controlling seizures of suspected central nervous system (CNS) origin.

■ Give parenteral *vitamins* to birds with suspected dietary vitamin deficiencies. Vitamin D_3 (Injacom 100; La Roche) is especially important in African gray parrots and birds with hypocalcemia. Multivitamin B-complex and thiamine also may be beneficial.

METABOLIC/NUTRITIONAL DISORDERS

Hypocalcemia

KEY POINT ▶ African gray parrots are predisposed to a hypocalcemic syndrome.

Hypocalcemia frequently is associated with neurologic abnormalities.

Etiology

■ Deficiency of dietary calcium usually is present.

■ Deficiency of vitamin D_3 or parathyroid dysfunction also may be factor, especially in African gray parrots.

Clinical Signs

■ Common neurologic signs include seizures, weakness, paresis, ataxia, head tilt, circling, visual deficits, abnormal mentation, and anorexia.

■ Seizures are the most common clinical sign and may be triggered by sudden noise and excitement. The seizure lasts several seconds and occurs as an acute onset of tetanic spasms with extensor rigidity, wing flapping, vocalizations, and, occasionally, nystagmus.

■ Skeletal abnormalities, including pathologic fractures and nutritional bone disease, are associated with calcium deficiency; these may or may not accompany the neurologic signs.

Diagnosis

Base the diagnosis on the history, clinical signs, blood chemistry analysis, and response to therapy.

■ To determine proper treatment, a full chemistry analysis, or blood calcium concentration is necessary.
  • Total serum calcium concentrations usually are very low (1.5–6.0 mg/dl.)

■ Obtain radiographs to assess bone quality and soft tissue abnormalities and identify any metal densities in the gastrointestinal (GI) tract and soft tissues that may indicate lead toxicity.
  • The proventriculus and intestinal loops may appear slightly dilated on radiographs. Calcium deficiency may be a factor in decreased smooth muscle contraction and motility of the GI tract.

• Radiographs usually are unremarkable in African gray parrots with hypocalcemia.

■ Consider and investigate other potential etiologies (e.g., lead toxicity).

Treatment

■ Provide supplemental calcium orally or parenterally.
  • In severely debilitated birds, initiate treatment with parenteral calcium gluconate, 100 mg/kg one to four times daily.
  • If seizures are infrequent and the danger of aspiration during seizures is minimal, give oral calcium supplements such as Neocalglucon (Sandoz), 1 ml/30 ml of drinking water.

■ During initial therapy, give supplemental vitamin D_3 (Injacom 100; LaRoche), 0.1–0.2 ml/100 g, IM; repeat in 3–4 days.

■ Provide general supportive care and control continuous or severe seizures with diazepam (Valium) as needed, at a dose of 0.5–2.0 mg/kg, IM or IV.

■ Correct the diet to provide adequate calcium and vitamins.

Prognosis

■ The prognosis is good in most birds; however, African gray parrots with calcium levels less than 2.0 mg/dl usually respond poorly to treatment. Improvement usually is slow and gradual.

Miscellaneous Disorders

Gout

Gout can cause peripheral gait abnormalities that may appear neurologic in origin. Gout is most common in older parakeets but also occurs in other species.

■ Ataxia, weakness, and a stiff gait are common signs. Clinical signs may occur before subcutaneous uric acid deposits (tophi) are visible in the joints and legs.

■ Uric acid levels may be mildly to significantly elevated on serum chemistry analysis.

Liver Disease

■ Weakness, ataxia, and abnormal mentation occasionally are seen with severe *liver disease* (see sec. 12, ch. 5).

Yolk Emboli

■ Neurologic abnormalities occasionally occur in hens with egg yolk peritonitis. Clinical signs may result from *yolk emboli* to the CNS (see sec. 12, ch. 6).

Hypoglycemia

■ Hypoglycemia can cause severe depression and neurologic deficits.

KEY POINT ▶ Measure whole blood glucose concentration by rapid Chemstrip analysis in any bird presenting with acute seizures or weakness.

Lipemia

- Signs of central neurologic abnormalities can occur in birds with severe *lipemia*.

Other Nutritional Factors

- Deficiency in vitamins E, B-complex, C, and A and selenium are related to neurologic disorders.
- Because specific vitamin deficiencies are difficult to confirm, give supplemental multivitamins if a deficiency is suspected.

IDIOPATHIC EPILEPSY

Idiopathic epilepsy has been described as a clinical syndrome in lovebirds and red-lored Amazon parrots.

- Phenobarbital, available as an elixir (4 mg/ml), is variably effective in controlling clinical signs.
  - Give in the drinking water, 1.5–2.5 ml/4 oz of water, or give orally, 0.5–0.8 ml/kg q12h.

NEOPLASIA

CNS Neoplasia

Primary tumors of neural tissue origin occur infrequently in birds. Occurrences are most common in budgerigars. Meningiomas and glioblastoma have been reported.

Clinical Signs

- Common signs include ataxia, weakness, wide-based stance, and postural abnormalities.
- Depression, nystagmus, abnormal mentation, and visual deficits often are present.

Diagnosis

- Clinical diagnosis of CNS neoplasia is extremely difficult. Static or progressive clinical signs indicating CNS system involvement with failure to respond to therapy suggest neoplasia.
- In larger birds, computed tomography (CT) of the brain can be diagnostic.
- Diagnosis usually is determined at postmortem examination.

Treatment and Prognosis

- No treatment is available.
- The prognosis is poor.

Paresis Secondary to Renal or Gonadal Neoplasia

KEY POINT ▶ Tumors of renal tissue origin are common in budgerigars 4 years of age and older and are associated with progressive unilateral limb paresis.

Gonadal tumors are less common than renal tumors; Clinical signs may resemble those of renal neoplasia.

Etiology

- Viral etiology in renal adenocarcinomas has been suggested.

Clinical Signs

- Progressive paresis or paralysis of the leg occurs on the involved side from pressure of the tumor on the sciatic nerve.
- Muscle atrophy may be severe in the affected leg.
- Polyuria may be an early or late clinical sign.

Diagnosis

Base the diagnosis on history, clinical signs, and physical examination.

- Palpate the abdomen carefully on the affected side to detect the presence of a smooth soft tissue mass.
- Obtain radiographs of the abdomen to identify a soft tissue mass in the area of the kidney.
  - Barium contrast radiography may show ventral or lateral displacement of bowel loops in the area of the kidney or gonad.

Treatment and Prognosis

- No treatment is available.
- Parakeets usually die within several months of the onset of clinical signs.

INFECTIOUS DISEASES

Viruses

Several viruses affect the avian nervous system (see sec. 12, ch. 2).

- *Paramyxovirus* is a common cause of neurologic disease in many species of wild and domestic birds.
- Macaw-wasting syndrome (proventricular dilatation syndrome) occurs primarily in macaws but affects other psittacine species.
- Neurologic deficits are sometimes seen in birds with *polyomavirus*.
- Other suspected viral causes of neurologic disease have been reported.
  - Budgerigar *encephalitis* has been reported in Germany. An adenovirus is the suspected etiology.
  - *Reovirus* affects several avian species. Ataxia, paresis, and paralysis can occur, along with the typical signs of depression, swollen abdomen, diarrhea, biliverdinuria, edema, and weight loss.

Bacteria/Fungi

Neurologic signs resulting from bacterial and fungal infections are sometimes seen.

- Bacterial encephalitis secondary to systemic infection can produce multifocal neurologic disease.
  - Neurologic signs secondary to salmonellosis are especially common in pigeons.

- Neurologic disease associated with fungal infections is rare. Weakness associated with severe aspergillosis (see sec. 12, ch. 2) or candidiasis may mimic neurologic disease.
- *Chlamydia psittaci* (psittacosis) infections can cause CNS lesions and neurologic signs. Typical signs of psittacosis (see sec. 12, ch. 2) may or may not be present.

Parasites

Parasitic causes of neurologic diseases are rare in birds.

- Possible etiologies include microfilaria, protozoa (e.g., *Plasmodium, Atoxoplasma* spp), sporozoa *(Sarcocystis)* and nematode migration.
- Diagnosis is made on postmortem examination.

TOXICITIES

Lead Toxicity

Lead toxicity is a common cause of neurologic disease in caged birds. Other aspects of lead toxicity, as pertaining to dogs and cats, are discussed elsewhere.

KEY POINT ▶ Sources of lead that can cause lead toxicity in birds include surfaces or objects painted with lead-based paint, stained glass, mirror backing, champagne bottle foil, lead-weighted objects (including some bird toys), lead wires, and leaded gas fumes.

Clinical Signs

- Signs of acute lead ingestion include depression, anorexia, gastroenteritis (usually hemorrhagic), crop stasis, regurgitation, dehydration, and hemoglobinuria.
- Neurologic signs may be acute or latent in onset. Signs include seizures, ataxia, weakness, paresis, paralysis, circling, head tilt, nystagmus, blindness, and severe depression.

Diagnosis

Establish the diagnosis based on the history, clinical signs, supportive diagnostic tests, and response to therapy.

- Measure blood lead concentration. Lead concentrations of ≥15 μg/dl suggest lead toxicity.
- Although this test is not widely available, measurement of δ-aminolevulinic acid dehydratase enzyme activity is a highly specific test for lead toxicity. Because lead inhibits this enzyme, levels < 86 units indicate lead exposure.
- Obtain radiographs to screen for the presence of metal densities in the GI tract and soft tissues. The presence of a metal density in a bird with typical clinical signs suggests lead toxicity.
  - The absence of lead in the GI tract does not exclude a diagnosis of lead toxicity, because small amounts of lead may be absorbed prior to the onset of clinical signs.
- Many birds with lead toxicity have mild to severe anemia. Measure packed cell volume (PCV) before collecting blood for CBC or serum chemistry analysis. Basophilic stippling is uncommonly seen in avian RBCs.

Treatment

- Chelation therapy is indicated in any bird with suspected lead toxicity. Calcium EDTA is effective and is the most commonly used chelating agent.
  - Give EDTA, IM or SC, after diluting with saline, at a dose of 30–50 mg/kg q12h for 5 days.
  - Persistence of an elevated blood lead level or clinical signs can necessitate a second course of therapy in some birds.
- Other chelating agents are potentially useful in birds.
  - Dimercaptosuccinic acid (DMSA), which can be given orally, chelates lead in soft tissues more quickly than EDTA.
  - D-Penicillamine, another oral chelating drug, is used for chelation therapy in mammals.
- Oral magnesium sulfate (Epsom salt) may help to bind lead particles in the GI tract and inhibit further absorption. Dosage is empirical (e.g., a pinch dissolved in dextrose or added to food given q12h).
- Supportive therapy includes supplemental fluids, antibiotics, iron supplementation, vitamins, and tube feeding.
- Anticonvulsants are rarely necessary to control seizures.

Prognosis

- Birds with lead toxicity usually respond quickly to chelation therapy. Clinical signs may diminish significantly after 1–2 days of therapy.
- Consider other etiologies of neurologic disease if a bird with suspected lead toxicity is refractory to treatment.

Other Toxicities

Other heavy metals occasionally cause neurologic disease in cage birds. Diagnosis usually is made by tissue analysis at necropsy.

- Exposure to organophosphates and other pesticides may cause incoordination, severe depression, and diarrhea.
- Toxicity from exposure to marijuana, alcohol, and other drugs has been reported.
- Neurologic signs may be seen immediately before death with Teflon toxicity (see sec. 12, ch. 4).

TRAUMATIC INJURY

Head Trauma

- Head trauma can cause mild to severe neurologic signs.
- Treatment depends on the severity of clinical signs.

- Administer anti-inflammatory doses of corticosteroids in acute cases.
■ Provide general supportive therapy as needed.
■ The prognosis depends on the severity of the injury and the response to therapy.

Peripheral Nerve Trauma

■ Musculoskeletal injury can result in peripheral nerve damage.
■ Treatment and prognosis depend on the extent of tissue damage.

Supplemental Readings

Gaskin JM: Psittacine viral diseases: A perspective. J Zoo Wildlife Med 20(3):249, 1989.

Gerlach H: Viral diseases. *In* Harrison GJ, Harrison LR, eds.: *Clinical Avian Medicine and Surgery.* Philadelphia: W. B. Saunders, 1986, p 408.

Labonde J: Pet avian toxicology. AAV Proceedings, 1988, p 159.

Lyman R: Neurologic disorders. *In* Harrison GJ, Harrison LR, eds.: *Clinical Avian Medicine and Surgery.* Philadelphia: W. B. Saunders, 1986, p 486.

Mautino M: Avian lead intoxication. AAV Proceedings, 1990, p 245.

McDonald S: Lead poisoning in psittacine birds. *In* Kirk RW, ed.: *Current Veterinary Therapy IX.* Philadelphia: W. B. Saunders, 1986, p 713.

Rosskopf W, Woerpel R: Epilepsy in peach-faced and pied peach-faced lovebirds. AAV Proceedings, 1988, p 225.

Rosskopf WJ, Woerpel R: Epilepsy in red-lored Amazons *(Amazona autumnalis).* AAV Proceedings, 1985, p 141.

Quesenberry KE, Hillyer EV: Neurologic disorders in caged birds: A retrospective review of cases. AAV Proceedings, 1988, p 170.

Walsh MT: Seizuring in pet birds. AAV Proceedings, 1985, p 121.

8 Ferrets

Elizabeth V. Hillyer
Susan A. Brown

Clinical Techniques

Elizabeth V. Hillyer

RESTRAINT

- Because most pet ferrets are gentle and tractable, it is possible to use *minimal restraint* when performing a physical examination; this is preferable because ferrets (like cats) are calmer on the examination table when light restraint is used.
- Use *firm restraint* to administer vaccinations and perform procedures such as ear cleaning.
  - Control the head by a circumferential grip around the caudal aspect of the mandibles or by holding the scruff of the neck. Restrain the rump tightly on the table with the ferret's hind legs underneath; do not allow legs to stretch out (Fig. 1).
  - An alternative is to suspend the ferret in the air by the scruff (Fig. 2). Stroke the abdomen with a downward motion to relax the ferret. This hold has a calming effect on most ferrets, although very young ferrets and some females may resist.
- *Aggressive* ferrets, such as nursing females or ferrets raised with little human contact, are uncommon.
  - Restrain these ferrets by the scruff of the neck, using the techniques previously described.
  - Avoid the use of leather gloves, which are awkward; use sedation, if necessary.

DIAGNOSTICS

Blood Collection

There are several suitable sites for blood collection in ferrets:

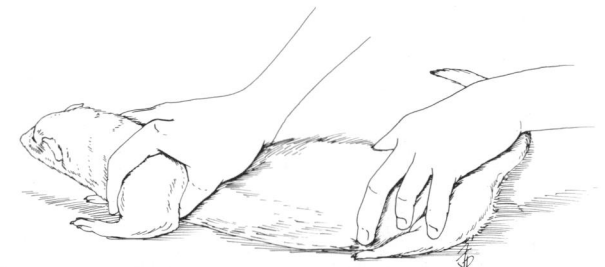

Figure 1. Proper method for restraining a ferret on an examination table.

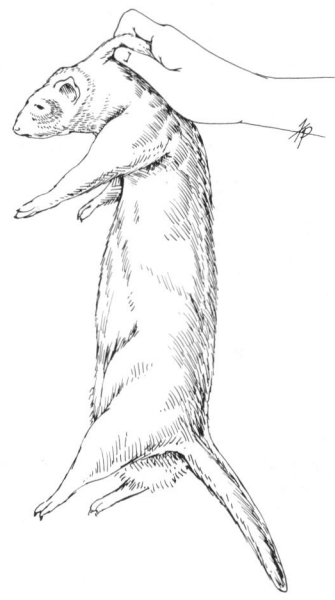

Figure 2. "Scruffing" a ferret.

- Toenail
- Cephalic vein
- Lateral saphenous vein
- Jugular vein
- Cranial vena cava
- Ventral tail artery

Cardiac puncture and retro-orbital bleeding are not recommended.

Indications

- Perform cephalic or lateral saphenous venipuncture to obtain small amounts of blood for rapid determination of packed cell volume (PCV) or blood glucose by reagent strip (Chemstrip bG; Boehringer Mannheim, Indianapolis, IN).
- Use the jugular vein or cranial vena cava for blood collection for a complete blood count (CBC) and biochemical analysis.
- Use the jugular vein to collect blood for transfusion.

Other Considerations

- Sedation:
  - Sedation is rarely required for a toenail clip or for cephalic or lateral saphenous venipuncture.
  - Collection of blood from other sites may require

sedation or the assistance of two persons for restraint in addition to the person drawing blood.
■ If necessary, clip the hair over the venipuncture site to see the vein.
■ Because the normal hematocrit of ferrets is high, draw three times as much blood as the volume of plasma or serum required. See Tables 1 and 2 for blood values reported in normal ferrets.

Techniques

Toenail Clip
Clipping a toenail is a rapid means of obtaining a few drops of blood. However, it is painful and should be reserved for use in emergencies.

Cephalic Vein
■ Collect blood from the cephalic vein in ferrets using the same restraint technique as for dogs and cats.
■ Use Lo-Dose U-100 insulin syringe (Becton Dickinson, Rutherford, NJ) with 28-gauge needle to obtain 0.3–0.4 ml of blood.
■ An alternative technique is to place a 25-gauge needle in the vein and collect blood directly from the hub into small blood collection tubes.

Lateral Saphenous Vein
■ The lateral saphenous vein in ferrets has the same orientation as in dogs and cats; however, it lies more distally, just proximal to the hock.
■ Use a Lo-Dose insulin syringe as described above, to obtain a small blood sample.

Jugular Vein
■ Position the ferret in dorsal or sternal recumbency at the edge of the table. Extend the ferret's head with the front legs held out of the path of the venipuncturist.
■ It may be helpful to wrap the ferret in a towel, place the animal in dorsal recumbency, and feed it Nutri-Cal (Evsco Pharmaceuticals) (a nutritional supplement very palatable to ferrets) during the procedure.
■ Use a 3-ml or larger syringe with a 25-gauge needle for small ferrets and a 22-gauge needle for larger ferrets.

Collection of Blood for Transfusion
The jugular vein is the preferred site for collection of large volumes of blood for transfusion.

■ Although the normal blood volume of ferrets has not been reported, a conservative estimate is 60 ml/kg.

TABLE 1. Hematologic Values Reported in Normal Ferrets

Parameter		Albino Ferrets* Male	Albino Ferrets* Female	Fitch Ferrets† Male	Fitch Ferrets† Female	Fitch Ferrets, Male‡ Orbital	Fitch Ferrets, Male‡ Cardiac
PVC (%)	Mean	55.4	49.2	43.4	48.4	52.1	53.1
	Range	44–61	42–55	36–50	47–51	47–57.5	48–59
Hemoglobin (g/dl)	Mean	17.8	16.2	14.3	15.9	16.8	16.9
	Range	16.3–18.2	14.8–17.4	12–16.3	15.2–17.4	14.5–18.5	15.4–18.5
RBC ($\times 10^6$/mm³)	Mean	10.23	8.11			11.3	11.3
	Range	7.3–12.18	6.77–9.76			9.7–12.4	10.1–13.2
Platelets (10^3/mm³)	Mean	453	545				
	Range	297–730	310–910				
Reticulocytes (%)	Mean	4.0	5.3				
	Range	1–12	2–14				
WBC ($\times 10^3$mm³)§	Mean	9.7	10.5	11.3	5.9	6.3	6.2
	Range	4.4–19.1	4.0–18.2	7.7–15.4	2.5–8.6	2.8–13.4	1.7–11.9
Differential (%)	Mean			0.9	1.7		
Bands	Range			0–2.2	0–4.2	0–2	0–1
Neutrophils	Mean	57.0	59.5	40.1	31.1		
	Range	11–82	43–84	24–78	12–41	22–75	24–72
Lymphocytes	Mean	35.6	33.4	49.7	58.0		
	Range	12–54	12–50	28–69	25–95	20–72	26–73
Monocytes	Mean	4.4	4.4	6.6	4.5		
	Range	0–9	2–8	3.4–8.2	1.7–6.3	0–4	1–4
Eosinophils	Mean	2.4	2.6	2.3	3.6		
	Range	0–7	0–5	0–7	1–9	0–3	0–3
Basophils	Mean	0.1	0.2	0.7	0.8		
	Range	0–2	0–1	0–2.7	0–2.9		
MCV	Mean					46.3	47.1
	Range					42–55.9	42.6–51
MCH	Mean					14.9	15.0
	Range					14–16.4	13.7–16
MCHC	Mean					32.3	32.0
	Range					26.9–35	30.3–34.9

*Data from Thornton et al., 1979.
†Data from Lee et al., 1982.
‡Data from Fox et al., 1986.
§At the authors' practice, WBC counts are lower than reported here, ranging from 2800 to 6000 per mm³.
PCV = packed cell volume; RBC = red blood cells; WBC = white blood cells; MCV = mean corpuscular volume; MCH = mean corpuscular hemoglobin; MCHC = mean corpuscular hemoglobin concentration.
Reprinted with permission from Fox JG: *Biology and Diseases of the Ferret.* Philadelphia: Lea & Febiger, 1988, p 163.

TABLE 2. Serum Chemistry Values Reported for Normal Ferrets

Parameter		Albino Ferrets*	Fitch Ferrets†	Fitch Ferrets, Male‡	
				Orbital	Cardiac
Sodium (mmol/L)	Mean	148	152	152	154
	Range	137–162	146–160	153–164	152–156
Potassium (mmol/L)	Mean	5.9	4.9	4.5	4.4
	Range	4.5–7.7	4.3–5.3	4.1–5.2	4.1–4.9
Chloride (mmol/L)	Mean	116	115	121	121
	Range	106–125	102–121	118–125	118–126
Calcium (mg/dl)	Mean	9.2	9.3	9.2	8.5
	Range	8.0–11.8	8.6–10.5	7.5–9.9	8.7–9.4
Inorganic phosphorus (mg/dl)	Mean	5.9	6.5	5.8	5.6
	Range	4.0–9.1	5.6–8.7	4.8–7.2	52–7.6
Glucose (mg/dl)	Mean	136	101	115	115
	Range	94–207	62.5–134	99–125	107–138
BUN (mg/dl)	Mean	22	28	16	15
	Range	10–45	12–43	11–25	11–25
Creatinine (mg/dl)	Mean	0.6	0.4	0.6	0.5
	Range	0.4–0.9	0.2–0.6	0.4–0.8	0.4–0.7
Total protein (g/dl)	Mean	6.0	5.9	6.9	6.6
	Range	5.1–7.4	5.3–7.2	6.3–7.7	6.2–7.1
Albumin (g/dl)	Mean	3.2	3.7	4.0	3.9
	Range	2.6–3.8	3.3–4.1	3.3–4.4	3.5–4.2
Total bilirubin (mg/dl)	Mean	<1.0		<1.0	<1.0
	Range			0–0.1	0–0.1
Cholesterol (mg/dl)	Mean	165		165	148
	Range	64–296		129–209	119–201
SAP (IU/L)	Mean	23	53		
	Range	9–84	30–120		
ALT (IU/L)	Mean		170	108	109
	Range		82–289	86–145	78–149
SGOT (IU/L)	Mean	65		85	117
	Range	28–120		57–165	74–248
CO₂	Mean			23.9	24.9
	Range			16–28	20–28
Globulin (g/dl)	Mean			2.3	2.2
	Range			1.8–3.1	2–2.9
AG (g/dl)	Mean			1.7	1.8
	Range			1.2–2.1	1.3–2.1
LDH	Mean			408	460
	Range			221–618	241–752
Alkaline phosphatase	Mean			44	42
	Range			34–66	31–64
Triglycerides	Mean			19	18
	Range			11–30	10–32

*Combined values for male and female ferrets from Thornton et al., 1979.
†Combined values for male, female, and castrated ferrets from Lee et al., 1982.
‡Data from Fox et al., 1986.
BUN = blood urea nitrogen; SAP = serum alkaline phospatase; ALT = alanine aminotransferase; SGOT = serum glutamate oxaloacetic transferase; AG = albumin to globulin ratio; LDH = lactate dehydrogenase.

Therefore, it is safe to draw 12 ml/kg from healthy ferrets.
■ Sedate and place the donor ferret in dorsal recumbency.
■ Using a butterfly catheter, collect the blood into a syringe with acid-citrate-dextrose (ACD) solution added as an anticoagulant (1.0 ml of ACD per 6 ml of blood).
■ Transfer the blood immediately to the recipient.

Cranial Vena Cava

KEY POINT ▶ Blood collection from the cranial vena cava requires complete immobility of the ferret; otherwise, do not attempt the procedure.

■ A contraindication for use of this site is suspected intrathoracic disease (e.g., mediastinal mass, megaesophagus).

Technique

1. Place the ferret in dorsal recumbency; instruct two assistants to restrain the ferret. Precise positioning facilitates the procedure.
2. Palpate the manubrium and locate the notch on both sides between the manubrium and the first rib.
3. Using a 3-ml syringe with a 25-gauge needle, enter the skin at either notch and direct the needle at a shallow angle toward the opposite hip.
4. Locate the vein by gently aspirating as the needle enters the thorax.

Ventral Tail Artery

Technique

1. Place the ferret in dorsal recumbency and prepare the site aseptically.
2. Using a 22- to 25-gauge needle, collect 1–3 ml of blood from the artery that runs along the ventral midline of the tail.
3. Insert the needle about 2–3 cm from the anus and direct the needle toward the body at a 30° angle to the skin.
4. Gently insert the needle to the bone; withdraw it slowly while applying a slight vacuum to the syringe.

Radiography

- Use standard radiographic techniques. Sedation may be necessary for correct positioning.
- When interpreting films, it helps to consider the ferret an "elongated cat." Ferrets have several radiographic peculiarities:
  - The cardiac silhouette is globoid, with a prominent right ventricle.
  - The kidneys are relatively short (about two lumbar vertebrae in length).
  - Splenomegaly is a common radiographic finding.
- For barium-contrast radiography of the gastrointestinal (GI) tract, give 15 ml/kg of a 20% barium solution (usually by syringe). Normal GI transit time is about 3 hours.

Bone Marrow Aspiration

- The indications, guidelines, and techniques for bone marrow sampling are the same as for dogs and cats, but the procedure may be more difficult owing to the ferret's small size.
- Potential sites include the iliac crest, proximal femur, and humerus; the first two sites are preferable.
- After sedating the animal, use a 20- or 22-gauge spinal needle with stylet to aspirate the bone marrow.

Splenic Aspiration

Fine-needle aspiration of the spleen is a rapid means of evaluating splenic cytology. In dogs, the only contraindication is suspected hemangiosarcoma of the spleen. The procedure has been performed successfully in ferrets. Sedation rarely is necessary.

Techniques

1. Place the ferret in dorsal recumbency.
2. Palpate the spleen and position it against the ventral or left lateral body wall.
3. Clip and prepare the site aseptically.
4. Using a 25-gauge needle attached to a 3-ml syringe, enter perpendicular to the skin and aspirate from the spleen.
5. When a small amount of bloody fluid is seen in the needle hub, withdraw the needle and prepare slides routinely for cytology.

Cystocentesis

- Use the same technique as for dogs and cats; a 25-gauge needle is preferable.

THERAPEUTICS

Intravenous Therapy

- For *small-volume* (0.3–0.4 ml) intravenous therapy, use a Lo-Dose insulin syringe injected into the cephalic or lateral saphenous vein. Sedation is rarely needed for a single injection.
- An *indwelling catheter* can be placed in the cephalic, lateral saphenous, or jugular vein. Sedation may be necessary.
  - Because of the ferret's small size, flush with small volumes of heparinized saline solution to keep the catheter patent.
- *Peripheral catheters* can be placed more rapidly than jugular catheters (see below) and are useful in emergency situations and for surgery.

Technique

1. Clip and prepare the site aseptically.
2. Tent the skin over the vein and make a small hole in the skin with an 18-gauge needle, taking care to avoid the vein.
3. Insert a short indwelling catheter (20–24 gauge) through the hole and into the vein and tape it in place routinely.
   a. A skin hole is unnecessary if using a 24 gauge, ¾-inch catheter (Sureflo; Terumo Corp., Tokyo).

- Placement of a *jugular catheter* generally requires sedation.
- Place the ferret in dorsal recumbency and clip and prepare the site aseptically. Make a small skin hole over the jugular vein as described previously.
- Either a short or long catheter can be used; 20-gauge or smaller is suitable.

Subcutaneous and Intramuscular Injections

- Administer subcutaneous and intramuscular injections in the same sites and using the same techniques as for dogs and cats.

Fluid Therapy

- The daily fluid requirement for ferrets has not been reported but can be estimated at roughly 70 ml/kg/day. Adjust for dehydration and fluid loss.
- Administer fluids SC over the dorsal cervical and thoracic region.
- Reserve intravenous fluid therapy for ferrets in critical condition and for intraoperative and postoperative therapy, because catheter placement usually requires sedation.

Blood Transfusions

- Indications for blood transfusions in ferrets are the same as for dogs and cats. Calculate the required blood transfusion volume using the same formula.
- Draw blood for transfusion purposes from the jugular vein of the donor (described earlier) and transfer immediately to the recipient.
  - As many as three transfusions from the same donor are considered safe; blood groups have not been identified in ferrets.
- Administer fresh blood transfusions through an indwelling catheter or via a butterfly catheter into the jugular vein. If the vein is inaccessible, administer into the peritoneal cavity or via the intraosseous route into the proximal femur.
  - Prior to transfusion, give a rapidly-acting corticosteroid such as dexamethasone sodium phosphate, 6–8 mg/kg once, IV, or prednisolone sodium succinate (Solu-Delta-Cortef; Upjohn), 22 mg/kg once, IV as a slow bolus infusion.

Oral Therapy

- Oral medications are most easily given to ferrets in liquid form.
- Crush medications formulated only in tablet or capsule form and mix with Nutri-Cal and administer by syringe.
- Alternatively, medications can be hidden in Linatone (Lambert Kay LP), a liquid nutritional supplement.

Nutritional Support

- Most ferrets must be force-fed dietary supplements by syringe. Once they acquire a taste for a given supplement, it may be possible to offer it in a bowl.
- When indicated, give nutritional support as an adjunct to specific medical therapy.
  - To supplement the diet of a ferret with a poor appetite, give Nutri-Cal, 1–3 ml q6–8h.
- For an anorexic animal, try Isocal or Isocal HCN (Mead Johnson Nutritionals), or mix either product with strained meat baby food (50:50) and give 5–15 ml q6–8h.

Drug-Dosing Guidelines

- Use feline dosages (scaled down for size) to calculate most drug dosages in ferrets, with the following exceptions.
  - Give chloramphenicol at a dose of 50 mg/kg q12h, IV, SQ, IM, or PO.
  - Give aspirin at a dose of 0.5–22 mg/kg q8–24h (canine dosage).
  - Most ferrets can become lethargic on captopril (Capoten, Squibb). Start with a very low dose, such as 1/8th of a 12.5 mg tablet q48h. Some ferrets will not tolerate more than every-other-day therapy with captopril.
  - Give ivermectin (Ivomec; Merck Sharp & Dohme) at a dose of 0.4 mg/kg, SQ or PO, once; repeat this dose in 2–4 weeks if necessary.

Urinary Catheterization

Both male and female ferrets are very difficult to catheterize. Even with anesthesia, attempts to pass a urinary catheter are usually unsuccessful.

- Catheterization of females is done blindly using a tomcat catheter.
- To catheterize a male ferret, use an open-ended tomcat catheter, a small-gauge canine urinary catheter, or a red rubber feeding catheter (# 3.5 Fr). Prolapse the penis and find the urethral opening, which lies ventral to the tip of the penis.
  - Usually the catheter will pass only 1–2 cm into the urethra. This may be sufficient to allow retrograde flushing of urethral calculi into the bladder.

Sedation and Anesthesia

Dosages for injectable agents used in ferrets are listed in Table 3.

- Acepromazine is useful for sedation. A combination of ketamine and acepromazine is effective and safe for minor surgery. Ketamine used alone does not produce effective muscle relaxation.
- A tiletamine-zolazepam preparation (Telazol; Fort Dodge) gives variable muscle relaxation but is useful for immobilization for procedures such as venipuncture, radiography, and electrocardiography.
- The administration of isoflurane (AErrane; Anaquest) by face mask is the most convenient method to immobilize a ferret to perform procedures such as venipuncture and radiography. Induction and recovery are rapid.
- Preanesthetic agents rarely are necessary in ferrets. If needed, give atropine, 0.04 mg/kg, IV, SC, or IM.
- Halothane and isoflurane are useful gas anesthetics for surgery.
- Halothane can be used for routine surgery. Isoflurane is the anesthetic of choice for ferrets with cardiac or liver disease and for debilitated animals.
  - For induction of anesthesia, place the ferret in an induction chamber or hold a face mask over the nose and gradually increase the concentration of gas (use the same concentrations as for dogs and cats).

TABLE 3. Drugs Recommended for Chemical Restraint of Ferrets

Drug	Dosage (mg/kg)	Route
Acepromazine	0.1–0.5	IM, SC
Ketamine†	25–35	IM, SC
plus acepromazine†	0.2–0.3	
Ketamine	10–20	IM
plus diazepam	1–2	
Ketamine	10–25	IM
plus xylazine‡	1–2	

*Use lower doses for sedation.
†Use this combination for minor surgery.
‡Avoid xylazine in sick ferrets.
IM = intramuscular; SC = subcutaneous.

- Endotracheal intubation is facilitated by the use of a small laryngoscope blade (Miller blade #0, North American Drager, Telford, PA) to expose the glottis. A 2.5–3.0 mm endotracheal tube usually is suitable.
  - Follow basic principles of anesthesia for small animals, and provide supplemental heat during surgery; an intravenous drip with isotonic electrolyte solution supplemented with 2.5% dextrose is recommended during long procedures.

Infectious Diseases of the Ferret

Susan A. Brown

VIRAL DISEASES

Canine distemper and influenza are the two most common viral diseases in the ferret. Influenza is transmissible between humans and ferrets. Canine distemper causes 100% fatality in the ferret; distemper vaccination of ferrets is imperative.

Canine Distemper

Etiology

Canine distemper virus (CDV), a large RNA paramyxovirus, can be transmitted to ferrets directly from affected animals of any species and through contact with fomites such as shoes or clothing. The normal incubation period for CDV in the ferret is 7–10 days; however, incubation for some strains of CDV may take up to 21 days. For discussion of CDV in dogs, see sec. 2, ch. 6.

Clinical Signs

- Early in the disease the only sign is a mild conjunctivitis, either unilateral or bilateral.
- As the disease progresses, signs include a high fever (>40°C), anorexia, and profuse mucopurulent naso-ocular discharge.

KEY POINT ▶ Ferrets develop a distinct pattern of thickening and crusting of the integument of the chin and lips and a pronounced hyperkeratosis of the footpads. Crusting may also include the rectal and inguinal area.

- Other signs include central nervous system (CNS) disturbances, diarrhea, and severe depression.

Diagnosis

KEY POINT ▶ Diagnosis of CDV is based primarily on the signs, which are unlike those of any other disease in the ferret.

- Differential diagnoses early in the disease include influenza and bacterial conjunctivitis. Once the disease has progressed, concurrent integumentary lesions around the chin and lips are pathognomonic.
- The history usually reveals that the animal is unvaccinated or is overdue for booster vaccination. There may be no evidence of direct exposure to another affected animal because fomite transmission can occur.
- Physical examination findings include the clinical signs previously described.
- A fluorescent antibody test can detect distemper antigen in blood smears and conjunctival scrapings, but it is a moderately insensitive test.

Treatment

KEY POINT ▶ There is no treatment for canine distemper; euthanasia is recommended in all cases.

- In a multiple animal household, remove all clinically affected animals and euthanize them. Vaccinate the remaining animals immediately.
- Disinfect the household thoroughly using 0.2% Roccal, 0.75% phenol, or 2–5% sodium hydroxide.

Prevention

KEY POINT ▶ Vaccination is the most effective prevention for canine distemper in ferrets.

- Vaccinate all ferrets in the household or facility using an attenuated canine distemper vaccine of chick embryo tissue culture origin. Fromm D (Solvay) or FerVac-D (United Vaccine) is a safe and effective vaccine that has been tested on ferrets. Give 1 ml, SC, using the following schedule:
  - If the dam is vaccinated, vaccinate the kit initially at 8 weeks of age and repeat vaccination every 2–3 weeks until the kit is 14 weeks of age.
  - If the dam is unvaccinated, vaccinate the kit initially at 6 weeks of age and repeat as above.
- Revaccinate annually. Although some sources claim immunity for 3 years, outbreaks have been known to occur 18 months after vaccination.
- It is not recommended to use canine vaccines that contain parvovirus, adenovirus, or other viruses, because the ferret is not susceptible to these diseases. Also, it is not necessary to vaccinate for leptospirosis unless there is frequent exposure to wild rodents.
- Vaccinate any new animals brought into a facility or household containing ferrets immediately and quarantine for 4 weeks prior to exposure to the other animals.

Influenza

Etiology

The domestic ferret is susceptible to the same influenza viral strains that affect humans. Influenza virus from affected humans and other ferrets can infect ferrets by contact with naso-ocular discharges and inhalation of aerosolized droplets. Ferrets can transmit influenza to humans.

Clinical Signs

KEY POINT ▶ Influenza generally causes only mild illness and discomfort in ferrets and is self-limiting in an otherwise healthy animal.

- Clinical signs are essentially the same as in humans with influenza and include any combination of the following:
  - Sneezing with the presence of a clear, serous nasal discharge.
  - Mild conjunctivitis with serous ocular discharge and, rarely, crusting around the eyes.
  - Nonproductive coughing, that occurs more frequently at night and may be loud and paroxysmal.
  - Diarrhea and, rarely, vomiting.
  - Listlessness, fever, and poor appetite (rarely, anorexia).
- The clinical course of the disease is 7–14 days.
- Severe illness or death may occur in neonates and in ferrets with concurrent immunosuppressive disease such as lymphosarcoma.

Diagnosis

Diagnosis is based primarily on the history and physical examination.

- Differential diagnoses include the very early stages of canine distemper, GI rotavirus infection, and lymphosarcoma.
- The history usually indicates recent exposure to a human or another ferret with influenza (the incubation period is 2–10 days).
- Physical examination reveals the clinical signs previously described.
- The overall physical condition remains good, although slight or moderate dehydration may be present if the animal is not eating or drinking normal amounts.
- If mucopurulent ocular or nasal discharge is noted, consider early canine distemper or a secondary bacterial infection.

Treatment

- *Supportive care* generally is sufficient.
  - Encourage the ferret to eat and drink. Offer strained meat baby food if the animal refuses the regular diet.
  - If indicated, give an oral electrolyte solution (e.g., Gatorade, Pedialyte), which is palatable to ferrets.
- If sneezing or coughing is excessive and interferes with eating or sleeping, give an *antihistamine* such as chlorpheniramine (Chlor-Trimeton), 1.0–2.0 mg/kg q8–12h, or diphenhydramine (Benadryl; Parke-Davis), 0.5–2.0 mg/kg q8–12h.
- Antibiotics are *not* necessary unless secondary bacterial infection is present.

Prevention

Good hygiene is the key to prevention.

- If influenza is present in ferrets or humans, advise clients to wash their hands frequently and to avoid holding the ferret near the face. Remember the disease can be transmitted from animals to humans, and vice versa.

- In the veterinary hospital, do not allow influenza-infected personnel to handle ferrets especially if the animal is debilitated by serious disease.

Rabies

Etiology

Rabies is caused by a rhabdovirus that results in a fatal disease in ferrets. It is transmitted through contact with an infected animal's saliva (see sec. 2, ch. 8).

Clinical Signs

KEY POINT ▶ Very little is known about rabies in naturally infected ferrets.

There is no recorded case of rabies transmitted by a ferret to a human. It is known that ferrets may become naturally infected; however, there is some question about how easily they can contract the disease and the length of the incubation period. Information about clinical signs is derived primarily from experiments with laboratory-infected ferrets. Signs are variable and include:

- Behavioral abnormalities that range from hyperactivity and anxiety to lethargy
- Posterior paresis.

Diagnosis

Diagnosis is based on a history of known or potential exposure to rabies and clinical signs.

- Sacrifice of the suspect animal may be necessary in order to protect humans and other animals in its environment.
- Differential diagnoses include brain hypoxia from severe seizures, insulinoma, Aleutian disease, intervertebral disc disease, and botulism.
- History may include possible exposure to a rabid animal.
- The ferret usually is unvaccinated; however, vaccination breaks have been known to occur in other animals.
- The physical examination reveals the clinical signs previously described.
- Postmortem laboratory testing confirms the diagnosis by examination of the brain tissue with fluorescent antibody staining (FAS) or virus isolation, as in dogs and cats (see sec. 2, ch. 8).

Treatment

- There is no treatment for rabies.
- Euthanize a clinically ill animal suspected to have rabies and have the brain examined as previously described.

KEY POINT ▶ The incubation period for naturally occurring rabies in the ferret is unknown; therefore, the 10-day quarantine period used in dogs is no guarantee that a ferret with potential exposure to rabies is healthy.

Prevention

- Vaccination is the only prevention. Immunity is excellent.
- Administer Imrab (Pitman-Moore), an inactivated rabies vaccine approved for use in ferrets, at a dose of 1 ml, SC.
- Vaccinate initially at 3 months of age and revaccinate annually.

Aleutian Disease
Etiology

Several strains of a parvovirus known as the Aleutian disease virus (ADV) affect both minks and ferrets. Transmission is by direct contact or through fomites contaminated with any infected body fluid including blood.

ADV produces a progressive immune complex–mediated disease with antigen-antibody complex deposition in various organs of the body. The lesions caused by these deposits include inflammation and lymphocytic and plasma cell infiltration of tissues.

The disease is prevalent in the ferret population, but the percentage of ferrets that develop clinically evident illness is low. In a survey of 700 ferrets, 10% were positive, but only two animals developed clinically active disease. Some ferrets may have natural immunity to the disease.

Clinical Signs

KEY POINT ▶ The clinical signs of Aleutian disease are extremely variable, and the incubation period can be as long as 200 days. Some ferrets become asymptomatic carriers.

- Posterior paresis may be the initial presenting sign. Initially, the ferret appears bright and alert. As the disease progresses, the paresis affects the forelimbs, and wasting occurs that may continue for weeks or even months.
- Dark, tarry stools, lethargy, and urinary incontinence is seen in later stages of the disease.
- Appetite is not lost unless the ferret is severely debilitated.
- A slow wasting disease exists without neurologic signs in ferrets.

Diagnosis

- Diagnosis is based primarily on clinical signs and a positive ADV test.
- Differential diagnoses include lymphosarcoma, gastric foreign body, tuberculosis, intervertebral disc disease, systemic mycoses, and rabies (in cases with behavioral changes and sudden paralysis).
- The history is of little value because the presence of asymptomatic carriers makes it difficult to detect specific exposure to the disease.
- The physical examination reveals the signs previously described.
- FAS serum is the test of choice for antemortem diagnosis. The FAS technique developed for ADV in minks appears to be accurate for diagnosis in ferrets.
  - This test may be used in clinically normal animals

for detection of inapparent carriers, but false-positive and -negative results are possible occasionally. Retesting in 2 to 4 weeks is necessary in suspected cases.
- Serum protein electrophoresis may demonstrate hypergammaglobulinemia >20% of the total serum protein.
- Histopathology, particularly of the kidney, liver, lymph nodes and spleen, shows lymphocytic plasmacytic infiltration and perivascular cuffing.

Treatment

KEY POINT ▶ There is no effective treatment for Aleutian disease. Euthanasia is recommended for all clinically affected animals. However it is not necessary to euthanize healthy animals that test FAS-positive, because they may never become clinically ill.

- Corticosteroid therapy and supportive care have prolonged the life of some ADV infected ferrets, but clinically active disease is invariably fatal.

Prevention

- Breeding colonies
  - Test all ferrets and remove serologically positive animals from the population.
  - Quarantine and test any new additions.
  - Because of potentially long incubation period, retest ADV-negative animals in 6 months before adding them to the colony.
- Pets
  - It is not necessary to test a ferret used as a pet unless it has been exposed to a clinically ill animal.
  - Retest ADV-positive animals in 6 months, because occasionally a positive result may revert to a negative titer.
  - It is unnecessary to euthanize an ADV-positive nonbreeding ferret or remove it from contact with other ferrets if it is clinically normal. Advise the client, however, that there is a slight possibility that the pet may become clinically ill.
- Do not house ferrets in close proximity to minks.

Rotavirus

Rotavirus infects the GI tract and causes a bright green or yellowish-green diarrhea. Rotavirus is described under *Gastrointestinal System* in this chapter.

Lymphosarcoma

A viral agent is being sought for this disease, and it is discussed elsewhere.

BACTERIAL DISEASES
Common Pyogenic Infections
Etiology

Staphylococcus, Streptococcus, Escherichia coli, and other common bacteria from the environment can be introduced through penetrating wounds, punctures, abrasions, and contact with mucous membranes by inhalation or ingestion.

- Abscessation is a common form of bacterial infection in ferrets. The abscesses may occur in any part of

the body including the subcutis, mouth, vagina, anal glands, and mucous membranes.
■ Deeper infections may occur in the uterus, mammary tissue, and lungs, primarily from *E. coli.*

Clinical Signs

■ Body temperature may be >40°C in bacterial sepsis.
■ Bacterial vaginitis causes a thick mucopurulent yellow to green vaginal discharge with little odor. Fever is absent, and the animal does not appear systemically ill.
■ Bacterial metritis may or may not cause a vaginal discharge; depression, fever, and partial or total anorexia are present.
■ Bacterial mastitis causes depression, fever, and anorexia. One or more mammary glands are swollen, discolored, and warm to the touch. Mastitis occurs primarily in the lactating female.
■ Bacterial pneumonia causes lethargy, fever, anorexia, and eventually dyspnea, sometimes accompanied by mucopurulent nasal discharge and coughing.
■ Bacterial conjunctivitis causes a thick mucopurulent ocular discharge and swelling of the conjunctiva; corneal ulcerations may be present.
■ Bacterial dermatitis causes thickened, irritated areas of skin. The ferret frequently licks and chews at these areas until they become denuded and ulcerated.

Diagnosis

■ Diagnosis is based primarily on clinical signs and demonstration of bacteria on routine bacterial cultures.

Treatment

■ Treatment consists of appropriate antibiotic therapy and, if necessary, surgical drainage or excision of the affected tissue.
■ Initially, before culture and sensitivity testing results are available, or when obtaining a culture is not feasible, use one of the broad-spectrum antibiotics in Drug-Dosing Guidelines under Clinical Techniques.
■ Provide supportive treatment as needed, such as fluid therapy and nutritional support.

Specific Treatment
■ Lance and thoroughly flush *cutaneous abscesses* with an antiseptic solution. Keep the area open and flush twice daily until healing by second intention occurs.
  • Administer oral antibiotics for 7–10 days.
■ Infected mammary glands frequently require surgical removal.
  • Remove kits from the mother and hand-raise or place them with a foster mother.
  • Give oral antibiotics to the affected female and apply hot packs to the abdominal area two or three times daily for 2 days.
  • If there is no clinical response to medical therapy, consider surgical removal of the affected mammary tissue. Because of potential for severe toxicity and

life-threatening disease, do not delay surgery if there is no improvement with medical therapy.
  • Do not breed females with a history of mastitis.
■ For *metritis* and *pyometra,* perform ovariohysterectomy.
■ For *pneumonia,* start oral antibiotic therapy immediately.
  • If possible, first perform a tracheal culture.
  • If pleural effusion is evident on radiography, perform thoracic aspiration for culture and sensitivity testing and cytology.
■ For *conjunctivitis,* use a broad-spectrum ophthalmic ointment.
  • Perform fluorescent corneal stain tests to detect corneal ulcers.
■ For *anal gland infection,* initially give oral antibiotics for 3–7 days until the swelling regresses and some healing occurs. Then excise both anal glands.
■ To prevent abrasions to mammary tissue and nipples that can cause *mastitis,* provide an opening with smooth edges into the nest box that is large enough for the ferret to pass through easily.

Campylobacteriosis Infection

■ *Campylobacter* organisms primarily cause GI disease (see under *Gastrointestinal System* in this chapter).

Salmonellosis

Salmonella organisms are gram-negative bacteria that can cause gastroenteritis in ferrets (see *Salmonella* under *Gastrointestinal System* in this chapter).

Botulism

■ Botulism is a rarely encountered disease in the domestic ferret caused by the ingestion of food contaminated with the *Clostridium botulinum* toxin. *C. botulinum* is commonly found in the soil.
■ Food contaminated with soil or uncooked food can be the source of the infection.

Tuberculosis

■ Clinical cases of tuberculosis in the ferret are infrequently reported; however, ferrets are extremely susceptible to bovine, avian, and human *Mycobacterium tuberculosis* infections.
■ The disease generally is transmitted by ingestion of contaminated meat (poultry or beef) or milk, or by contamination of food from the droppings of infected wild or pet birds (see sec. 2, ch. 11 for information about tuberculosis in dogs and cats).

FUNGAL INFECTIONS
Dermatomycoses
Etiology

Microsporum canis and *Trichophyton mentagrophytes* are the most common causes of superficial mycotic infections in ferrets. Dermatophytes are transmitted by direct contact with infected animals or contaminated bedding, caging, and other materials.

Clinical Signs

Like other species, young ferrets are more commonly infected than mature ferrets.

- The lesions are consistent with those seen in other species (see sec. 5, ch. 3). Circular areas of alopecia are thickened, scaly, and inflamed and may be pruritic.

Diagnosis

- Diagnosis is based on the identification of the fungal agent on skin scrapings, fungal culture, or a positive Wood's light examination (see sec. 5, ch. 3).

Treatment

- Dermatomycosis usually is self-limiting and resolves without therapy.
- In refractory cases, treat with lime-sulfur dips weekly and give griseofulvin (Fulvicin; Schering), 25 mg/kg q24h, PO (see sec. 5, ch. 3 for details of management of dermatophyte infections).

Other Fungal Infections

Blastomycosis, histoplasmosis, cryptococcosis, coccidioidomycosis, and aspergillosis have been reported rarely in domestic ferrets.

- Consider these infections in the differential diagnosis of any systemic disease that involves wasting, granulomatous lesions, persistent or recurring draining wound tracts, and chronic respiratory disease refractory to treatment.
- Diagnosis is based on the demonstration of the fungal organism by histopathology or cytology from biopsies or aspirates (see sec. 2, ch. 12).
- Complement fixation and precipitation tests have been used with varying success.
- Treatment is the same as described for the dog and cat (see sec. 2, ch. 12).

Hematopoietic System

Elizabeth V. Hillyer

SPLENOMEGALY

The spleen is readily palpable in most ferrets, and splenomegaly (enlarged spleen) is a frequent finding. Splenomegaly can be an incidental finding in an otherwise healthy animal, or it may occur in association with a wide variety of disease conditions.

Etiology

- About 10% of ferrets with enlarged spleens have lymphoma.
- Splenic histopathology in most cases shows extramedullary hematopoiesis (also seen in normal spleens) and congestion.
- In ferrets that do not have lymphoma, splenomegaly can occur in conjunction with infectious, endocrine, and systemic conditions including (but not restricted to) influenza, enteritis, GI obstruction, cardiomyopathy, insulinoma, and adrenal tumors.
- Idiopathic hypersplenism has been reported but is rare.

Clinical Signs

- Clinical signs usually are due to the primary disease condition; for example, ferrets with insulinoma and splenomegaly have signs referable to the insulinoma.
- Abdominal discomfort due to splenomegaly, which occurs in dogs, is rare in ferrets.
- Abdominal distenstion may occur.

Diagnosis

- Diagnosis is based on evaluation of the spleen in addition to a search for other diseases.
- Monitor asymptomatic ferrets with splenomegaly with periodic CBC evaluation and splenic aspiration.

Differential Diagnosis

- Perform a CBC and platelet count to evaluate for cytopenia(s), which may indicate *hypersplenism*.
  - Hypersplenism is characterized by one or more cytopenias that resolve only with splenectomy. The bone marrow is hypercellular, and in many cases there is splenomegaly.
  - There is one reported case of idiopathic hypersplenism in ferrets.
- Perform a fine-needle aspiration of the spleen using a 25-gauge needle and submit it for cytologic evaluation (see under Clinical Techniques in this chapter).
  - Splenic aspiration is contraindicated if splenic *hemangiosarcoma* is suspected; however, this is rare in ferrets.
- Splenitis was diagnosed by histopathology in a young ferret with fever, depression, splenomegaly, and neutrophilic leukocytosis.

Further Diagnostic Testing

- The choice of other tests depends on the clinical signs and includes serum biochemical profile, fasting blood glucose assay, urinalysis, serum insulin assay, thoracic and abdominal radiography, echocardiography, abdominal ultrasonography, and bone marrow aspiration.

Treatment

Treatment depends on the primary disease condition. Usually splenectomy is *not* necessary.

- Indications for splenectomy are the same as for other species and include hypersplenism, splenitis, splenic abscess, torsion, rupture, and neoplasia.
- To perform splenectomy, follow the surgical guidelines for splenectomy in dogs and cats (see sec. 3, ch. 4).
- Administer antibiotics and fluid therapy pre- and postoperatively.

ANEMIA

The clinical approach to anemia in ferrets is the same as for other species. Anemias are classified as regenerative or nonregenerative; treatment is aimed at the specific cause.

Etiology

There are many causes of anemia in ferrets, as in other companion animal species.

- *Regenerative anemias* usually are the result of blood loss or hemolysis.
  - The most common causes of blood loss in ferrets are trauma, external parasites such as fleas, and GI bleeding due to ulcers, foreign bodies, or enteritis/colitis.
  - Hemolysis is rare. Theoretically, lead or zinc toxicity can cause hemolysis in ferrets. Autoimmune diseases are not documented and would be difficult to diagnose due to lack of ferret-specific reagents.
- *Nonregenerative anemia* occurs when bone marrow hematopoiesis is disrupted.
  - The most common cause in ferrets is estrogen toxicity due to persistent estrus. Ferrets are very sensitive to estrogen myelotoxicity which can occur from 4 weeks following the onset of estrus. An estrogen-secreting ovarian remnant or adrenal tumor also may cause estrogen toxicity. All cell lines are affected, resulting in anemia, leukopenia, and thrombocytopenia. Anemia is worsened due to bleeding from thrombocytopenia.
  - Bone marrow infiltration by neoplastic cells (e.g., in lymphoma) can result in nonregenerative anemia.
  - Anemia of chronic disease is seen in ferrets. Potential causes are similar to those in other species.

Clinical Signs

Clinical signs include weakness, lethargy, and inappetence.

- A swollen vulva is present in ferrets with persistent estrus and some cases of adrenal neoplasia (see under Neoplasia in this chapter).
- An observant owner may report melena if GI bleeding is present.

Diagnosis

KEY POINT ▶ Anemia in an intact female ferret with a swollen vulva for more than 4 weeks most likely is due to estrogen toxicity.

History

- Obtain a careful history regarding possible blood loss, toxicity, and foreign body ingestion. Determine the duration of vulvar swelling (if present).

Physical Examination

- Mucous membranes are pale; jaundice may be seen with hemolysis.
- A soft systolic murmur is common in anemic ferrets.
- Examine females for a swollen vulva, an external indication of estrus, or elevated serum estrogens.
- Ferrets suffering from estrogen toxicity will also have signs of thrombocytopenia such as petechiae, ecchymoses, and melena. When anemia is severe, usually it is due to blood loss from thrombocytopenia.
- Hair loss is common, especially on the rump in hyperestrogenism.
- Palpate the spleen, because splenomegaly may indicate hypersplenism and subsequent anemia.
- Check carefully for fleas.

Laboratory Studies

- Evaluate the packed cell volume (PCV) and red blood cells (RBCs) on a peripheral blood smear as a minimum data base. If possible, obtain a CBC, platelet count, and reticulocyte count.
- Bone marrow aspiration is indicated (see under Clinical Techniques in this chapter), particularly if the anemia is nonregenerative, to identify infiltrative processes and assess the morphology of RBC precursors.
- Draw a blood level if lead poisoning is suspected.
- If the anemia is not severe and the cause is not apparent, draw blood for serum biochemical analysis to evaluate for chronic renal or metabolic disease.

Radiography

Consider

- Thoracic radiography to identify the presence of intrathoracic neoplasia.
- Abdominal radiography if intra-abdominal neoplasia or if GI bleeding or obstruction is suspected.
- Abdominal ultrasonography to diagnose an adrenal tumor.

Treatment

The objectives of treatment are:

- Treat the anemia.
- Treat the cause of the anemia.

Anemia Therapy

- Give supportive care such as oxygen therapy, subcutaneous fluids, and nutritional supplementation.
- Provide iron with a product such as Pet-Tinic (SmithKline), 0.2 ml/kg q24h.

■ Use standard criteria to determine if a blood transfusion is necessary (i.e., status of the patient, acuteness of blood loss, PCV). Consider a transfusion if the PCV <15% (see under Clinical Techniques in this chapter for blood transfusion techniques).

Treatment of the Cause of Anemia

■ Arrest external bleeding.
■ Treat fleas with any product that is safe for use in cats (see sec. 5, ch. 6).
■ Correct the underlying cause of GI bleeding, including medical therapy for GI ulceration (see under Gastrointestinal System in this chapter), surgery to remove GI foreign body, and antibiotics and supportive care for enteritis/colitis.
■ Treat lead poisoning following the same protocols recommended for cats (see sec. 5, ch. 6).
■ For diagnosis and treatment of adrenal tumors see discussion of neoplasia in ferrets.
■ Anemia secondary to neoplasia is associated with a poor prognosis. Some cases of lymphoma may respond to treatment (see Neoplasia in this chapter).
■ For anemia of chronic disease, treat the underlying primary disease process.
■ To correct estrogen toxicity, terminate estrus and provide supportive care until the bone marrow is functional. Broad-spectrum antibiotic therapy is important for control of sepsis in leukopenic patients.

KEY POINT ▶ In ferrets with estrogen myelotoxicity, ovariohysterectomy can be performed to terminate estrus if the PCV and platelet count are adequate; however, the safest method is hormonal stimulation of ovulation.

Termination of Estrus

■ Administer human chorionic gonadotropin (hCG) (Pregnyl; Organon) in a single injection of 1000 USP (or 100 IU), IM. Repeat this dose in 1–2 weeks if vulvar swelling has not diminished.
■ Alternatively, give gonadotropin-releasing hormone (GnRH) (Cystorelin; Sanofi) at a dose of 20 μg, IM or SC; repeat in 2 weeks if necessary.
■ GnRH and hCG are effective only after the tenth day of estrus. Bone marrow toxicity is not immediately reversible with termination of estrus; the PCV continues to fall for a few days to weeks.
■ Monitor the PCV as a useful guide to therapy and prognosis:
  • PVC >25%—the prognosis is good and termination of estrus is the only therapy required.
  • PVC 15–25%—the prognosis is guarded because the PVC level can decrease further after termination of estrus.
  • PVC <15%—the prognosis is poor, and aggressive supportive care is indicated, including multiple blood transfusions until bone marrow function is restored.

Prevention

■ Some causes of anemia in ferrets can be prevented. Instruct owners about proper husbandry techniques to avoid trauma, foreign body ingestion, and flea infestation.

KEY POINT ▶ To prevent estrogen myelotoxicity, spay all female ferrets not used for breeding.

Neoplasia

Elizabeth V. Hillyer
Susan A. Brown

INSULINOMA

Insulinomas, or pancreatic beta-cell tumors, are the most common tumors in ferrets. More than 30% of ferrets over 3 years of age are affected; the disease is most commonly diagnosed in ferrets 3–7 years of age. Adrenal neoplasia (discussed later) is found concurrently in up to 50% of these animals.

Etiology

The cause(s) of the high incidence of insulinomas in ferrets is unknown.

■ Possible etiologies include genetics (ferrets in the United States come from a small gene pool) and diet.

Histology

■ Histologic examination may reveal multiple tissue changes including hyperplasia, adenoma, and adenocarcinoma of beta cells, even within a single tissue specimen.

Clinical Signs

■ Episodic lethargy, depression, "stargazing," and posterior paresis may be seen during periods of hypoglycemia. Because various counterregulatory mechanisms compensate for hypoglycemia, early signs may be subtle and transient.
  • As the disease progresses, and in periods of inadequate feeding, signs become more pronounced and may progress to stupor or coma. Seizures can also occur.
■ The most alarming clinical signs during episodes of hypoglycemia are profuse hypersalivation and pawing at the mouth, which are indicative of nausea.
■ Splenomegaly is common; the mechanism for this is not known (see Splenomegaly under Hematopoietic System in this chapter).

Diagnosis

The differential diagnosis for hypoglycemia in ferrets includes hepatic insufficiency, starvation, and laboratory error.

Fasting Serum Glucose

- A carefully monitored fast of 4–6 hours is sufficient.
- Normal fasting serum glucose is 90–110 mg/dl. Ferrets with insulinoma may have a fasting serum glucose of 20–85 mg/dl.
- If necessary, obtain several samples over a period of several days.

KEY POINT ▶ *Do not fast the animal for >6 hours,* because prolonged fasting may cause collapse, coma, or even seizures in an affected animal. Feed the ferret as soon as possible following collection of blood.

Blood Insulin Values

- Values >275 pmol/liter (or 38 μU/ml) are considered elevated in ferrets. However, because insulin and glucose are in a constant dynamic state, a random insulin value may be normal (relative rather than absolute hyperinsulinemia), especially if the ferret is severely hypoglycemic at the time.

KEY POINT ▶ Base a presumptive diagnosis of insulinoma on clinical signs and demonstration of hypoglycemia in the absence of other causes of hypoglycemia and in the presence of elevated or normal insulin levels. Definitive diagnosis is made with surgical removal and histopathologic examination of a pancreatic tumor.

Serum Biochemical Profile and CBC

- These values usually are normal except for low blood glucose levels.
- A slight elevation in alanine aminotransferase (ALT) levels (180–250 IU/liter) may be seen; the cause is unknown.

Treatment

KEY POINT ▶ Insulinoma is a progressive disease in ferrets, requiring constant monitoring and adjustment of medication. Instruct owners on how to recognize the signs of hypoglycemia and to manage at home (see later, under Medical Therapy).

Surgical Removal

Surgical removal or debulking of pancreatic tumors is palliative and may provide at best only temporary remission of signs.

- Follow canine protocols (see sec. 4, ch. 5), taking care to avoid hypoglycemia.
- Administer intravenous dextrose (2.5–5.0%) during anesthesia and surgery.
- Gently palpate to locate tumor nodules, which are firmer than the surrounding tissue; nodules may be solitary or multiple.

- If no visible or palpable nodules are found, perform a pancreatic biopsy to look for random neoplastic cells.
- Perform a complete abdominal exploratory examination; insulinomas can metastasize to the spleen (uncommon), regional lymph nodes, and liver, and concurrent adrenal tumors (discussed later) are common.
  - If the spleen is enlarged and appears irregular or mottled, consider performing splenectomy with biopsy.

Complications
- *Iatrogenic pancreatitis* is rarely a problem in ferrets; however, as a precaution, withhold food and water for 24 hours postoperatively; give 2.5–5.0% dextrose as an intravenous drip during fasting.
  - Monitor blood glucose 1–4 times daily, depending on physical examination findings.
- *Transient diabetes mellitus* may occur postoperatively. Hyperglycemia and glucosuria may be present for several days to 3 weeks after surgery; generally no treatment is required.
  - However, two ferrets that remained diabetic, requiring daily insulin treatment, have been reported.

Medical Therapy

Medical treatment is necessary as the disease progresses. Frequent feeding is the first step in treatment. Add prednisone and diazoxide as clinical signs necessitate. Corticosteroids promote hepatic gluconeogenesis and antagonize the effects of insulin at the cellular level. Ferrets appear to tolerate corticosteroids well; side effects are minimal at lower dosages.

- Feed frequent, high-quality protein meals, especially after exercise or a long sleep. Avoid foods high in sugar (except as stated below) as these foods will cause short energy bursts followed by a period of hypoglycemia 1–2 hours later.
- Chromium has been reported to stabilize blood glucose and insulin levels in humans. Brewer's yeast which is a rich source of chromium, has been beneficial in some ferrets with insulinoma.
  - Give ⅛–¼ tsp of brewer's yeast q12h in soft food such as strained meat baby food or Isocal, a liquid human nutritional supplement (Mead Johnson Nutritionals).
- When frequent feedings no longer control clinical signs, give prednisone or prednisolone (Pediapred; Fisons) at a starting dosage of 0.25–1.0 mg/kg/day divided q12h, PO. As clinical signs worsen, increase the dosage up to 4 mg/kg/day divided q12h, PO.
- When frequent feedings and glucocorticoids no longer control clinical signs, add diazoxide (Proglycem; Medical Market Specialties), 10 mg/kg/day, PO, divided q8–12h. Decrease the prednisone dosage to 2 mg/kg/day, divided q12h. Gradually increase diazoxide dosage to 60 mg/kg/day, as needed.
  - *Warning:* Diazoxide can cause hypertension; lethargy, depression, and nausea can occur.

Treatment of Hypoglycemia

Hypoglycemic episodes require specific therapy.

- Mild to moderately severe hypoglycemic episodes often can be treated successfully at home. Instruct the client to give the ferret honey, corn syrup, or Nutri-Cal (Evsco).
  - If the ferret has collapsed, rub honey or corn syrup on the gingiva (taking care not to be bitten!).
  - Once the animal is stabilized, feed a high-protein meal.
- Severe hypoglycemic episodes that do not respond to home therapy or that result in seizures require treatment in a hospital (see sec. 4, ch. 5 for treatment of hypoglycemia in dogs and cats). Intravenous fluids with dextrose and parenteral corticosteroids may be necessary.
  - If seizures continue, give 1 or 2 intravenous 1-mg boluses diazepam.
  - A continuous intravenous drip of diazepam, at 1–1.5 mg/hour, may be necessary to control status epilepticus.
  - Perform emergency surgery to remove the insulinoma nodules when the seizures have been controlled.

Prognosis

- The prognosis is guarded, but with surgery and medical treatment ferrets have had a good quality of life for >2 years after diagnosis of insulinoma.

ADRENAL NEOPLASIA

Adrenal tumors are common in ferrets, occurring with approximately the same frequency as insulinomas and often concurrently. Adrenal tumors have been found in ferrets as young as 1 year of age, although typically they occur between 2 and 5 years of age. These tumors occur twice as commonly in females as males.

Etiology

- Adrenal tumors in ferrets appear histologically to arise from adrenocortical tissue; hyperplasia, adenomas, and adenocarcinomas are seen. The left adrenal gland is most commonly affected.
- Possible causes of the high incidence of adrenal neoplasia in this species include early neutering, inbreeding, and lack of exposure to normal seasonal photoperiods.
- Hyperadrenocorticism in ferrets causes a variety of clinical signs (see below) and is probably due to excessive secretion of more than one adrenocortical hormone or hormones other than cortisol. Pituitary-dependent hyperadrenocorticism has not been documented in ferrets.

Clinical Signs

- Signs include bilaterally symmetric alopecia, usually starting at the tail base and progressing cranially. There may be a history of alopecia and spontaneous hair regrowth.
- Pruritus often is reported, along with excessive dryness of the skin and small excoriations. Thinning and softening of the skin are common.
- An enlarged vulva, mimicking estrus, may be the only sign in spayed females. Mucoid to mucopurulent vulvar discharge may be present. Castrated males may resume sexual activity and have the strong body odor and oily hair coats of intact males. Mammary hyperplasia can occur in either sex.
- Atrophy of abdominal musculature and mobilization of fat to the ventral abdomen, leading to a pendulous appearance, may be seen.
- Atrophy of hindlimb musculature and rear limb paresis can occur.
- Polyuria/polydipsia is uncommon.
- Collapse, anemia, and petechiation, mimicking estrogen toxicity, are seen in some ferrets with advanced adrenal disease (see discussion of Anemia under Hematopoietic System in this chapter).

Diagnosis

- A history of symmetric truncal hair loss, with or without pruritus, suggests the diagnosis.
- On physical examination, an enlarged left adrenal may be palpable cranial and medial to the left kidney; right adrenal tumors are more difficult to palpate.

KEY POINT ▶ Ultrasonography is the most practical and reliable technique to detect an adrenal tumor.

- Ultrasonography can identify a mass in the region of the adrenal gland; in addition, the liver often is hyperechoic.
- The CBC usually is normal except for a mild thrombocytopenia in some ferrets. Rarely the CBC will show leukopenia, anemia, and thrombocytopenia, probably resulting from estrogen myelotoxicity.
- The serum biochemical profile usually is normal except for low blood glucose levels in animals with concurrent insulinoma (discussed previously).
- Protocols for the adrenocorticotropic hormone (ACTH) stimulation test and the low-dose dexamethasone suppression test have been reported in ferrets; however, these generally are not useful in diagnosing adrenal tumors, probably because cortisol is not the primary hormone secreted by most of these tumors.
- Adrenal mineralization has not been seen on abdominal radiography, as occurs in dogs.
- Exploratory surgery is a valuable diagnostic tool.

Treatment

Adrenal tumors can be treated successfully medically or surgically. To date, there is insufficient experience with medical therapy to accurately compare success rates of the two techniques.

Adrenalectomy

Follow the protocol described for dogs (see sec. 4, ch. 3).

- Use a ventral midline approach in order to perform complete exploratory surgery.
- Palpate both adrenal glands carefully for firm, nodular changes.
  - Visual changes, such as dark circular lesions and small raised cysts, may be present in the absence of gross enlargement.
  - Adrenal changes may be subtle, especially in younger ferrets and because the adrenal glands are surrounded by fat.
- Usually only the left adrenal gland is affected, and removal is relatively straightforward. If the tumor is right-sided, removal can be difficult owing to the proximity of the vena cava and the aorta.
  - Check for accessory adrenal tissue, usually located near the vena cava, which is present in up to 15% of ferrets.

KEY POINT ▶ Always perform complete abdominal exploratory surgery. Observe and palpate the pancreas at surgery for the presence of insulinomas, which often are found concurrently with adrenal neoplasia. Hypoglycemia due to insulinoma may be masked by excessive adrenocorticosteroid production.

- Administer dexamethasone immediately postoperatively at a dose of 1 mg/kg, IM. Follow with prednisone, 0.25 mg/kg q12h, PO, for 5 days, and then 0.1 mg/kg q12h for 10 days. Long-term corticosteroid therapy usually is not necessary.

Medical Therapy

Medical treatment is an alternative when surgery is unsuccessful or is not possible, if the ferret is young, or if there is bilateral adrenal involvement.

- Give mitotane (also known as o,p′-DDD) (Lysodren; Bristol-Myers Oncology) at a dose of 50 mg, q24h, PO, for 7 days, and then q72h until clinical signs resolve.
  - Have the dosage prepared by a pharmacist who mixes the crushed tablets with cornstarch and divides them into 50-mg aliquots in #1 capsules.
  - To administer, coat the capsules with vegetable oil or Linatone (Lambert Kay LP), push into the back of the throat, and follow with Nutrical diluted with water to promote swallowing.
- Watch for side effects from Lysodren, which are similar to those in dogs (see sec. 4, ch. 3).
  - If side effects occur, discontinue Lysodren and administer predisone, 1.0–1.25 mg, PO.

Long-Term/Postoperative Care and Complications

- Monitor fasting serum glucose levels every 1–3 months during Lysodren therapy and after adrenalectomy, even if no pancreatic nodules were evident during surgery.

KEY POINT ▶ If an insulinoma is present and if the adrenal gland tumor was secreting cortisol, as cortisol levels drop with treatment serum glucose levels may also fall, causing a hypoglycemic crisis.

Prognosis

Adrenal tumors appear to have a very low rate of metastasis in ferrets.

- With proper treatment, a full resolution of clinical signs can be expected.
- Even without treatment, ferrets may survive up to 2 years or longer following diagnosis, although the hair loss is generally progressive.
- Hair loss may resolve spontaneously, only to recur the following year.
- The second adrenal gland may eventually also become involved.

LYMPHOSARCOMA

Lymphosarcoma (lymphoma) is common in ferrets of all ages. Similar to the disease in cats and dogs (see sec. 3, ch. 6), lymphoma in ferrets may be solid, disseminated, or leukemic. The most commonly affected organs are the spleen, liver, cranial mediastinum, and lymph nodes.

Etiology

- A viral etiology is suspected, and research is currently under way to isolate the causative agent.

Clinical Signs

Clinical signs are variable, depending on the organ system involved.

- Lymphoma tends to be a more acute, fulminant disease in younger animals.
- Some ferrets are totally asymptomatic; lymphoma may be an incidental finding during evaluation for another medical problem.
- Common signs include:
  - Weight loss despite a normal appetite.
  - Splenomegaly.
  - Lethargy and inappetence.
  - Dyspnea, tachypnea, and exercise intolerance with mediastinal and sternal lymph node involvement.
  - Peripheral lymphadenopathy.
  - Acute collapse, often with pyrexia.
  - Cutaneous masses.

Diagnosis

The method of diagnosis depends on the organ system involved.

- Perform a thorough history and physical examination.
- Evaluate a serum chemistry profile, CBC, and platelet count. If the ferret is anemic, perform a reticulocyte count.
  - The serum chemistry profile may disclose elevated liver enzymes if the liver is involved; paraneoplastic syndromes are uncommon in ferret lymphoma.

- The CBC may be normal or may reveal an absolute or relative lymphocytosis, occasionally with abnormal lymphocytes. Anemia, leukopenia, and thrombocytopenia are also seen. Persistent absolute lymphocyte counts >3500 are considered suspicious; follow with a bone marrow biopsy or lymph node biopsy if lymphadenopathy is present.
- Perform thoracic and abdominal radiography and ultrasonography to evaluate for the presence of intrathoracic and intra-abdominal masses.
- Perform a biopsy, if possible, or fine-needle aspiration, of affected tissues for histologic and cytologic examination.
  - Fine-needle aspiration of the spleen frequently is inconclusive.
  - The popliteal lymph node is the most accessible peripheral node for excisional biopsy, which is the most helpful diagnostic tool if peripheral lymphadenopathy is present.
- Perform bone marrow aspiration to identify infiltration by neoplastic cells (see Clinical Techniques in this chapter). This procedure is most helpful in cases in which persistent lymphocytosis occurs without lymphadenopathy.

Treatment

Splenectomy

- If the spleen is involved, perform a splenectomy (see sec. 3, ch. 4) to reduce the overall tumor load.

Chemotherapy

Chemotherapy for lymphoma may be successful. In general, protocols have been adapted from feline medicine (see sec. 3, ch. 5, and ch. 6).

- Limitations in developing protocols for ferrets include difficulty in administering intravenous medications and in dosing accurately because of the ferret's small size.
- Intravenous chemotherapeutic agents are given via butterfly catheter or small-gauge needle with the ferret under sedation; face-mask administration of isoflurane is the most convenient and rapid method.

Protocols

- One of the authors (SAB) has successfully treated (up to 4 years in remission) ferrets with lymphoma using the following protocol:
  - Administer cyclophosphamide (Cytoxan; Bristol-Myers Oncology), at a dose of ¼ of a 25-mg tablet, PO, once every 3 weeks for 3 doses.
  - Administer vincristine (Oncovin; Eli Lilly) once weekly for 4 weeks, IV, at a dose of 0.05 mg for ferrets up to 1 kg and 0.10 mg for ferrets 1 kg and over. Administer via a butterfly catheter and flush before and after treatment with 3 ml of isotonic saline.
  - Administer prednisone at a dose of 2 mg/kg q24h, PO. Continue daily treatment with prednisone for 4–5 weeks, and then discontinue with a gradually tapering dose.

KEY POINT ▶ Monitor the CBC weekly. If the white blood cell (WBC) count falls below 2000 WBC/μl, or the RBC count falls below 4 million/liter, discontinue vincristine for 1 or more weeks until the WBC count increases to at least 3000 WBC/μl.

- Another protocol that was successful in one ferret included oral prednisone, L-asparaginase, given IP, and oral cyclophosphamide.
- At one author's (EVH) institution, ferret lymphoma treatment has been most successful using modifications of feline lymphoma protocols. Drugs used include prednisone, methotrexate, cyclophosphamide, vincristine, and L-asparaginase.

OTHER TYPES OF NEOPLASIA

- Tumors of the *reproductive tract* in ferrets include granulosa cell tumors, luteomas, and leiomyomas in intact females and in remnant tissue in spayed females. Sertoli cell tumors have been seen in intact males.
- *Hepatic hemangiosarcomas* and *hemangiomas* occur in ferrets.
- Tumors of the *GI tract* are rare.
- Tumors of the *skin* and *subcutis* are discussed in Dermatologic Diseases in this chapter.
- Other tumors reported in ferrets include chordoma (a malignant tumor arising from the embryonic remains of the notochord), chondroma, osteoma, osteosarcoma, mesothelioma, thymoma, schwannoma, renal and pancreatic carcinoma, and fibrosarcoma.

Dermatologic Diseases

Susan A. Brown
Elizabeth V. Hillyer

SEASONAL CHANGES IN THE SKIN AND HAIR COAT

Ferrets may have dramatic seasonal changes in the hair coat length, thickness, and color triggered by photoperiod changes. This is particularly true in intact animals. If one is unfamiliar with these changes, normal coat alterations may be interpreted incorrectly as a medical problem.

KEY POINT ▶ Although individual animals may exhibit different patterns of coat change each successive year, ferret coats generally get shorter and darker in the summer months and longer, thicker, and lighter in the winter months.

Hair Coat

- Hair thinning (along with up to 40% weight loss) occurs in the spring when the photoperiod is increasing. There may be a 1-day dramatic loss of the undercoat or, more commonly, gradual hair loss and regrowth.

- The coat may also change color and facial masks may appear or disappear.
■ Normal thinning of the hair coat in spring and summer is diffuse, without any areas of focal alopecia. This condition is retained through the summer, with regrowth of the undercoat in the fall.
■ Females in estrus and males "in season" may show an even more marked hair loss and a dry, lackluster coat.
  - Males typically lose hair in the inguinal area due to constant rubbing to mark territory; the abdomen often is wet with urine.
■ Neutered animals can experience the same coat cycles, although usually less dramatically. There may be no coat changes in neutered animals or in animals kept under unchanging lighting conditions.
■ Neutering or spaying a ferret can cause dramatic, but temporary, hair thinning postoperatively, particularly if the animal was in season at the time of surgery. The preoperative color pattern may not return.
■ At any time of the year, regrowth of hair that has been shaved for medical procedures is slow in ferrets, but it is particularly so in the winter and summer when no active hair growth is occurring.

Skin

■ Ferrets in estrus may exhibit a bluish discoloration of the skin, most noticeable on the abdomen and the face. This discoloration is caused by new hairs growing through the dermis.
  - If ovariohysterectomy is performed while a ferret is in estrus, the discoloration may occur within 10 days following surgery.
■ In ferrets with alopecia of any cause, hair regrowth is often preceded by a blue to purple discoloration of the skin that can alarm the owner.
■ Hyperkeratosis of the foot pads severe enough to result in growth of pseudonails may occur in ferrets over 2 years of age. It is seen most often in animals that are housed on carpeting or linoleum surfaces.
■ A small amount of petroleum jelly or Vitamin E oil placed on the pads daily is helpful.

INFECTIOUS DISEASES

Bacterial Infections

Cutaneous bacterial infections in ferrets usually are manifested as abscesses or a diffuse, ulcerative pyoderma.

Abscesses

■ Abscesses usually occur as the result of a puncture wound or a serious bite but may also develop in the inguinal fat following a traumatic injury, (e.g., being stepped on).

■ Diagnosis and treatment of abscesses are discussed in Infectious Diseases in this chapter.

Ulcerative Pyoderma

Ulcerative pyoderma is the second most commonly encountered form of bacterial dermatitis in the ferret.

Etiology

■ Various bacteria can cause ulcerative pyoderma; however, the most common agents are *Staphylococcus* and *Streptococcus* spp.

Clinical Signs

■ Focal alopecia with diffusely hyperemic, thickened ulcerated skin may occur over any area of the body.

Diagnosis

■ Perform a cutaneous punch biopsy (see sec. 5, ch. 15) to rule out cutaneous mast cell tumor, which may have a similar gross appearance.
■ Perform a bacterial culture for susceptibility testing.

Treatment

■ Administer systemic antibiotics based on culture and susceptibility testing. Antibiotics effective in the treatment of pyoderma in ferrets include amoxicillin-clavulanate (Clavamox; SmithKline), 13–25 mg/kg q8–12h, PO, and cephalexin (Keflex; Dista), at 15–30 mg/kg q8h, PO.
■ Topical treatment may include twice-weekly cleansing with an antibacterial shampoo containing chlorhexidine or benzoyl peroxide. Daily application of an antibacterial cream may be beneficial if the lesion is small and localized.

Canine Distemper Virus (CDV) Infection

Dermatologic lesions are quite prominent with CDV infection in ferrets.

■ Dermatologic signs begin with a rash on the skin around the lips, chin, eyes, and sometimes the inguinal area. With time, crusts and skin thickening may appear.
■ Hyperkeratosis of the foot pads occurs as the disease progresses.
■ See Infectious Diseases in this chapter for a detailed discussion of CDV in ferrets.

Dermatomycoses

■ *Microsporum canis* and *Trichophyton mentagrophytes* are the most common causes of superficial mycotic infections in the ferret.
■ See Infectious Diseases in this chapter for diagnosis and treatment.

EXTERNAL PARASITES

Fleas

- Flea infestation is the most common external parasite problem encountered in pet ferrets. Clinical signs are similar to those seen in cats (see sec. 5, ch. 6).
- All flea products approved for use in cats are safe to use in ferrets, with the exception of flea collars, because they come off easily and can be ingested.

Ear Mites

Ear mite infection in ferrets is caused by *Otodectes cyanotis,* the same parasite that infects cats and dogs.

Clinical Signs

- Ferrets, unlike dogs and cats, rarely exhibit pruritus, even with heavy mite infestation.
- Ferrets normally have a large volume of dark reddish brown ear wax, mimicking the character of wax present with *O. cyanotis* infestation in cats. However, with heavy infestations wax production may be excessive and cause plugging of the external ear canal.
- Occasionally, *O. cyanotis* infestation may be exacerbated by a secondary bacterial infection. Otitis media may result, accompanied by head tilt, circling, and pain (see sec. 5, ch. 23 for management of otitis media as in cats).
- With chronic ear mite infestation, a bluish pigment may appear on the inner surface of the pinnae. There may be thickening of the tissue in the areas of pigmentation. This pigmentation is not harmful, is a response to chronic irritation, and usually fades with treatment of the mites.

Diagnosis

- Examine all ferrets for the presence of ear mites, as the incidence of infestation is high.
  - Mites in the ear canal frequently can be observed with the naked eye, using a bright light source.
  - Otoscopic examination is often difficult owing to the uncooperative nature of the patient and small ear canal.
- Confirm the diagnosis by microscopic examination of ear wax.

Treatment

- Thoroughly clean the ears. Divide 1 mg/kg of ivermectin (Ivomec; Merck-Sharp & Dohme Agvet) into two doses and instill into each ear. Repeat in 2 weeks.
  - Bathe the animal within 24–48 hours following treatment. Wash all bedding and treat any other affected mammals in the household (see sec. 5, ch. 21).
- Other ear mite remedies approved for use in cats also may be used in ferrets (see sec. 5, ch. 21). These treatments usually involve daily topical application, a task often difficult for clients to perform.

Sarcoptic Mange

Etiology

Sarcoptes scabei mites are transmissible between dogs and ferrets. Transmission is by direct contact with infected hosts or their bedding. See sec. 5, ch. 5 for discussion about sarcoptic mange in dogs and cats.

Clinical Signs

- Lesions commonly are confined to the feet, which become hyperemic, swollen, and intensely pruritic, with crusting around the nails and toes.
- Generalized alopecia, scaling, and pruritus occur rarely.

Diagnosis

- As in other mammals, diagnosis is based on a positive skin scraping. Several areas should be scraped.
- A common differential diagnosis is contact allergy. Similar lesions have been observed on the feet of ferrets housed in plastic-floor cages. These resolve when the cage bottom is changed to one of wire or wood.

Treatment

- Give ivermectin (Ivomec; Merck Sharp & Dohme Agvet), 0.2–0.5 mg/kg, SC, once every 2 weeks for three treatments.
- Wash all bedding and treat all potential contact hosts in the household.

ENDOCRINE ALOPECIA

Tail Alopecia

Etiology

The etiology of tail alopecia in the ferret is unknown but is suspected to be caused by hormonal fluctuations, because the disease responds to changes in the photoperiod. Hair loss occurs most commonly in the fall when the photoperiod is becoming shorter, but may be seen any time of year under artificial lighting conditions. Hair regrowth usually occurs in 2–8 weeks. The same pattern of alopecia is not always repeated annually.

Clinical Signs

- Hair loss, ranging from diffuse hair thinning to complete alopecia, occurs from the base to the tip of the tail.

KEY POINT ▶ Alopecia occurs only on the tail. If it extends to the body, suspect another form of endocrine alopecia.

- Comedones and a brown, waxy scale may accompany the alopecia.

Diagnosis

- Diagnosis is based on clinical signs.
- Differential diagnoses include the early stages of

other endocrine alopecias; however, these conditions include hair loss on the body as well as the tail.

Treatment

- No treatment is necessary because hair regrowth will occur when the photoperiod changes. Artificially lengthening the photoperiod may speed hair regrowth in some cases.
- If the tail exhibits excessive amounts of waxy scaling or comedones, clean the tail weekly with a mild shampoo.

Estrus Alopecia

Alopecia may be seen in intact females that have been in estrus for 1 month or longer.

Clinical Signs

- Hair loss is bilaterally symmetric, beginning over the shoulders and flanks, and may eventually progress to involve the entire body. Hairs epilate easily, and the underlying skin appears normal.
- A grossly enlarged vulva indicates a state of estrus. Be aware that the ferret may also be anemic and thrombocytopenic.

Diagnosis

- Diagnosis is based in clinical signs in an intact female.

Treatment

- Administer hCG or perform an ovariohysterectomy.
- Hair regrowth is rapid following ovulation or surgery; however, changes in hair length, color, or thickness are common.

Adrenal Neoplasia

- Bilaterally symmetric alopecia that may extend over 80% of the body is a common sign of adrenal neoplasia in ferrets (see Adrenal Neoplasia in this chapter).

Hypothyroidism

- Hypothyroidism has not been documented in ferrets.

NEOPLASIA

Neoplasia of the skin and subcutaneous tissues commonly occurs in ferrets 3 years of age and older. Since metastasis is a possibility, complete removal or biopsy is recommended. Skin masses are removed and examined immediately.

Mast Cell Tumors

Mast cell tumors are the most common skin tumors and are frequently benign in ferrets.

- Individual tumors appear as slightly raised, flat, button-like cutaneous masses typically ranging in size from 2 to 10 mm. The tumors are tan in color or may become hyperemic with a dark flaky crust due to scratching if pruritus is present.

- Mast cell tumors have occasionally been associated with patchy or generalized alopecia which resolves with surgical removal of the tumor.
- See sec. 3, ch. 7 for information about mast cell tumors in dogs and cats. Remove these tumors because of metastases to lung and spleen.

Other Neoplasms

- Other less common neoplasms of the skin and subcutaneous tissues include squamous cell carcinoma, basi-squamo-sebaceous carcinoma, sebaceous gland adenoma and adenocarcinoma, basal cell carcinoma, myxosarcoma, perianal gland adenocarcinoma, neurofibrosarcoma, leiomyosarcoma, lymphoma, and histiocytoma.
- Adenocarcinomas often metastasize to liver and lungs. Remove promptly and completely.
- Diagnosis, treatment, and prognosis for these tumors in ferrets is the same as for dogs and cats (see sec. 3, ch. 9).

Cardiovascular Diseases

Elizabeth V. Hillyer

Characteristics of the Normal Ferret Heart

- The heart extends from the sixth rib to the caudal border of the seventh or eighth rib (compared to cats where it extends from the second to the sixth rib).
- Cardiac auscultation is therefore centered more caudally in the thorax than in cats.
- The heart rate averages 180–250 beats per minute.
- A pronounced sinus arrhythmia is common; temporary bradycardia is common during auscultation, almost to the point of transient sinus arrest.

Cardiomyopathy

Cardiomyopathy most frequently affects ferrets 2 years of age or older. Dilatative and hypertrophic forms can occur. In the New York State area, the dilatative form is common; in the Midwest, hypertrophic cardiomyopathy is common.

Etiology

The cause(s) of cardiomyopathy in ferrets is not known. Nutritional problems may be a factor.

Clinical Signs

- Ferrets appear to compensate well for early cardiac insufficiency, perhaps because a slight decrease in activity is not readily apparent to owners.
- A cardiac murmur or radiographic evidence of cardiomegaly may be detected as an incidental finding prior to the development of clinical signs.
- Ferrets in heart failure generally present with tachypnea and dyspnea.
- Weight loss is common, and anorexia and lethargy occur late in the disease.
- Coughing generally is not noted.

■ Abdominal distention due to ascites may be present.

Diagnosis

■ Obtain a dietary history as part of the clinical history.
■ Perform a complete physical examination:
  • Evaluate for sluggish capillary refill time.
  • Auscult the heart for murmurs or arrhythmias.
  • Observe for tachypnea or dyspnea and auscult the lungs for crackles or wheezes.
  • Palpate the abdomen and check for the presence of fluid.

KEY POINT ▶ Proceed with further testing only if the ferret is stable. Otherwise, administer furosemide and oxygen therapy. If there is pleural effusion, thoracocentesis may be necessary.

■ Obtain thoracic radiographs to evaluate the heart and lungs. The heart is normally globoid in shape with rounded right and left ventricles.
  • Pulmonary edema and pleural effusion may be present.
■ Obtain abdominal radiographs to evaluate the size of the liver and spleen and to detect abdominal effusion.
■ Evaluate a serum biochemical profile, CBC, and urinalysis to detect other systemic diseases and electrolyte abnormalities.
■ Perform standard six-lead electrocardiography (ECG) if possible (Table 4 lists normal ferret ECG parameters). Usually sedation is necessary.
  • Sedation with ketamine or a ketamine-diazepam combination (see Table 3) will raise the heart rate. The heart rate tends to decrease with ketamine-xylazine sedation; therefore, avoid using xylazine in ferrets with suspected cardiac disease.
■ If thoracic or abdominal effusion is present, submit fluid for cytologic examination. Perform centesis as in cats; however, take into consideration the relatively caudal position of the heart in ferrets.

TABLE 4. Electrocardiography Data Reported for 27 Clinically Normal Ferrets*

Parameter	Value
Average age	5.2 months
Male:female ratio	1.25
Heart rate	233 ± 22 beats per min
Rhythm	
Normal sinus	67%
Sinus arrhythmia	33%
Mean electrical axis (frontal plane)	+77.22 ± 12
Lead II	
P amplitude	0.122 ± 0.007 mV
P duration	0.024 ± 0.004 sec
P-R interval	0.047 ± 0.003 sec
QRS duration	0.043 ± 0.003 sec
R amplitude	1.46 ± 0.84 mV
Q-T duration	0.12 ± 0.04 sec

*All ferrets were sedated with ketamine-xylazine. Adapted from Fox JG: *Biology and Diseases of the Ferret.* Philadelphia: Lea & Febiger, 1989, p 170; and Edwards J: Unpublished data, 1987.

■ The most useful diagnostic tool in ferrets with myocardial disease is echocardiography.
  • Contractility, wall thickness, and chamber size can be examined.
  • Valve function and blood flow can be evaluated using various Doppler techniques.

Treatment

Treatment depends on diagnostic (especially echocardiographic) findings. Base the treatment protocol on the same parameters for cats (see sec. 6, ch. 8).

■ Consider oxygen therapy for ferrets that are dyspneic.
■ If necessary, perform thoracocentesis and abdominocentesis to relieve dyspnea. Administer supportive care such as subcutaneous fluids (e.g., 0.45% saline and 2.5% dextrose) and nutritional support for ferrets that are inappetent.

Drug Therapy

■ Ferrets tolerate diuretics well. Administer furosemide (Lasix; Hoechst-Roussel) 2 mg/kg q8–12h; increase or decrease the dosage as necessary. In severe cases, hydrochlorothiazide diuretics may be used at feline dosages.
■ If cardiac contractility is poor, administer digoxin (Lanoxin; Burroughs Wellcome). The recommended dose is 0.01 mg/kg q12h; start at 75% of lean body weight (as for dogs) and watch for potential side effects (see sec. 6, ch. 15).
■ Vasodilator therapy with captopril (Capoten; Squibb) may be useful, although ferrets are sensitive to the drug's hypotensive effects. Start at a low dose (i.e., ⅛ of a 12.5-mg tablet) given q48h. If possible, gradually increase the dosage—that is, give the same dosage q24h or q12h.
  • The vasodilator enalapril (Vasotec; Merck Sharp & Dohme) has fewer side-effects in dogs and cats and may be useful in ferrets. Preliminary trials are promising using a dosage of ⅛ of a 2.5-mg tablet q24h.
■ A bronchodilator may help to relieve dyspnea; give aminophylline, 4.4–6.6 mg/kg q12h, PO or IM.
■ For hypertrophic cardiomyopathy and tachycardia, give a beta blocker such as propranolol, 0.2–1.0 mg/kg q8–12h, PO.
■ If the diet is deficient in taurine, although supplementation is not harmful, its benefit is doubtful.
■ Salt-free diets may be beneficial; however, they are unpalatable to ferrets. Instead, instruct the owner to avoid feeding snacks, treats, or food items with a high-salt content.

Prevention

There are no means of preventing cardiomyopathy other than ensuring that ferrets are fed a good diet.

Prognosis

- The prognosis depends on the severity of disease and the initial response to treatment.
- Many ferrets do well for months on the appropriate medications.
- Ferrets with dilatative cardiomyopathy respond better to treatment than canine patients with similar echocardiographic findings.

Other Cardiac Diseases

As experience with pet ferrets increases, it is likely that different types of cardiac disease will be recognized. Third-degree heart block (of unknown etiology) and various forms of valvular disease, including mitral and tricuspid insufficiency and endocarditis, have been reported in ferrets.

- The approach to these conditions in ferrets is the same as for other companion animals; use the drug dosages given previously for cardiac myopathies.

Heartworm Disease

Natural and experimental heartworm infections have been reported in ferrets. The disease in ferrets resembles the canine form. However, because of the ferret's small size, the presence of even 1 adult worm in the heart can be lethal. Reported adult worm burdens range from 1 to 10.

Etiology

- Heartworm disease in ferrets is caused by *Dirofilaria immitis*, the canine heartworm. *D. immitis* is a filarial nematode that is transmitted via mosquitoes.
- Ferrets that are housed outdoors in endemic areas are at greatest risk of infection; however, ferrets kept indoors also can become infected.

Clinical Signs

Heartworm infection in ferrets is usually not detected until cardiac failure occurs.

- Presenting signs include terminal congestive heart failure, ascites, lethargy, inappetence, grade I–II systolic murmur, and coughing.

Diagnosis

Antemortem diagnosis is difficult.

- If the history is compatible with cardiac failure, inquire about possible mosquito exposure.
- Physical examination findings are referable to heart failure and include depression, dehydration, pale mucous membranes, dyspnea, moist lung sounds, ascites, and hypothermia. Black tarry feces may be seen.

KEY POINT ▶ Minimize stress in ferrets suspected of heartworm disease. Delay further diagnostic tests until heart failure is stabilized (see previous discussion about cardiomyopathy).

- Thoracic radiographs show right ventricular enlargement, enlarged main pulmonary artery, tortuous pulmonary arteries, pulmonary infiltrate (edema), and pleural effusion.
- Abdominal radiographs may show hepatomegaly, splenomegaly, and ascites.
- If possible, draw blood for the modified Knott's test for microfilaria and for an enzyme-linked immunosorbent assay (ELISA) for *Dirofilaria* antigen.
  - Reported incidence of microfilaremia in infected ferrets ranges from 2% in a group of naturally infected ferrets to 50% in a group of experimentally infected ferrets.
  - The ELISA may be helpful in some cases; however, most test kits are unreliable if the adult worm burden is < 5. A commercial assay (Cite; IDEXX, Inc., Portland, ME) purportedly can detect very low adult worm burdens. Check with company for test protocol for ferrets.
- If possible, evaluate a serum biochemical profile, CBC, and urinalysis to detect other systemic disease.
- If pleural or abdominal effusion is present, submit fluid for cytology. A modified transudate is found with cardiac failure.
- Echocardiography may enable visualization of the worm(s); nonselective venous angiography is a more invasive means of visualizing *Dirofilaria* but may be helpful if the ferret is stable enough to tolerate the procedure.

Treatment

- The initial goal of treatment is stabilization of the patient's heart failure (see previous discussion of cardiomyopathy).
  - Oxygen therapy, furosemide, aminophylline, and thoracocentesis may be helpful.
  - Also, consider subcutaneous fluid therapy and supportive care.
- Adulticide therapy may be attempted. Follow canine protocols and hospitalize the ferret for treatment because of possible adverse reactions (common in dogs). To date, the author does not know of any symptomatic ferrets that survived more than 2 months after treatment. This may be because of the mechanical problems associated with the large size of the adult *Dirofilaria* relative to the ferret host.
  - To decrease the incidence of thromboembolism, give heparin 200 units/kg q12h, IM or SC, for 5 days starting the day before thiacetarsamide therapy.
  - Administer thiacetarsamide (Caparsolate; Sanofi), 2.2 mg/kg q12h, IV, for 2 days.
  - Three or four weeks after adulticide therapy, give the microfilaricide ivermectin (Ivomec; Merck Sharp & Dohme) as a single dose of 0.05 mg/kg, PO or SC. (the bovine form of ivermectin can be diluted 1:10 in propylene glycol and given orally at this dose).
  - If there is evidence of thromboembolism, give prednisone, 1 mg/kg, PO, daily for 7–14 days.

Prevention

KEY POINT ▶ Because of the high mortality associated with heartworm disease in ferrets, prevention is imperative in endemic areas.

- House all ferrets in endemic areas in structures with mosquito-proof screening.
- Follow the same guidelines for heartworm prevention in ferrets as for dogs.
  - Ivermectin at the dose given previously suppresses the maturation of *D. immitis* in ferrets. Administer once monthly for a period beginning 1 month before and continuing to 2 months after possible mosquito exposure.
  - A daily dose of diethylcarbamazine (Dec Tabs; Wendt) of 5–11 mg/kg also is effective. Do not give DEC to microfilaremic ferrets.

Gastrointestinal System

Elizabeth V. Hillyer

Characteristics of the Normal Ferret Digestive Tract

Teeth

- The permanent teeth erupt between 50 and 74 days of age. The dental formula for the permanent teeth is 2(I3/3, C1/1, Pm3/3, M1/2).
- All premolars and molars have two roots, except for the third upper premolar, or carnassial tooth, which has three roots, and the second lower molar, which has one root.

Gastrointestinal (GI) Tract

- The GI tract is that of a carnivorous animal with a simple stomach and a relatively short small intestine.
  - The duodenum ends at the jejunoileum; there is no distinction between the jejunum and the ileum.
  - Ferrets do not have a cecum.
  - The junction of the jejunoileum and the colon is gauged by the pattern of anastomosis of the jejunal artery with the ileocolic artery.
- GI transit time for food is approximately 3–4 hours.

Anal Sacs

- The anal sacs lie between the external and internal anal sphincter muscles; the ducts open at 4 and 8 o'clock near the mucocutaneous junction.

Nausea and Vomiting

- Ferrets, like other carnivores, are able to vomit. Ferrets are prone to experiencing nausea as the result of GI diseases such as gastric ulcers and GI foreign bodies. Hypoglycemia also can cause nausea (see discussion of insulinoma).
- Signs of nausea include hypersalivation and pawing at the mouth.
- Tooth grinding may indicate abdominal discomfort.

DENTAL DISEASE

- Dental tartar and periodontal disease are common, especially in older ferrets on a soft diet.
- Dental abscesses are seen, even in young ferrets.
- Follow basic medical and surgical treatment principles for dental diseases in dogs and cats (see sec. 7, ch. 1).

SALIVARY MUCOCELE

Ferrets have six paired salivary glands: parotid, submandibular, sublingual, molar, zygomatic, and lingual.

- Salivary mucocele has been reported in young ferrets but is an uncommon finding in clinical practice.

MEGAESOPHAGUS

Megaesophagus is rare in ferrets.

- The etiology of megaesophagus in ferrets is unknown (see list of possible causes in dogs in sec. 7, ch. 2).
- Presenting signs are the same as for dogs with megaesophagus.
- The diagnosis is generally evident on thoracic radiography.
- Follow canine treatment protocols. The prognosis is poor.

GASTROINTESTINAL PARASITES

- Although gastrointestinal parasites are uncommon in ferrets, routine fecal testing is recommended especially in young animals and those with diarrhea or rectal prolapse.

Etiology

- Coccidiosis is seen most frequently in immature animals and may cause severe diarrhea and dehydration.
- Other internal parasites are rare and include *Giardia* and ascarids.

Treatment

- Treat with anthelmintics, following protocols and dosages for cats (see sec. 7, ch. 6).

GASTRIC AND DUODENAL ULCERS

Gastric and duodenal ulcers have been reported in laboratory ferrets and are seen occasionally in pet ferrets. Clinical signs are often vague and the diagnosis is difficult.

Etiology

- The etiology is not known; however, environmental stress may be a predisposing factor.
- Bacteria *(Helicobacter mustelae)* have been associated with the disease. A similar organism *(H. pylori)* is associated with gastric ulcer disease in humans.

Clinical Signs

- Clinical signs include anorexia, lethargy, hypersalivation, tooth grinding, vomiting, and melena.

Diagnosis

- A barium series or endoscopic examination of the stomach with biopsy may be necessary for a definitive diagnosis.
- It is important to consider other causes of nausea and upper GI bleeding such as a GI foreign body, which is much more common than gastric ulcers in ferrets.

Treatment

- Affected ferrets may require hospitalization for supportive care in addition to ulcer therapy.
- Antibiotic therapy is important because of the possible role of an infectious agent. Amoxicillin is used in humans with gastric ulcers due to *H. pylori*. In ferrets, give amoxicillin 20 mg/kg q12h, SC or PO. Metronidazole may be efficacious at a dose of 20 mg/kg q12h, PO.
- Bismuth subsalicylate (Pepto-Bismol; Procter & Gamble) interferes with *H. pylori* colonization in humans. In ferrets, give 0.25 ml/kg q4–6h, PO.
- Cimetidine may be difficult to administer because the elixir is unpalatable to ferrets and it is difficult to dose the tablets accurately. The parenteral preparation (10 mg/kg q8h) can be used in a hospital setting.
- Sucralfate (Carafate; Marion Merrell Dow) is useful in ulcer therapy. Give ⅛ of a 1-g tablet q6h, PO.
- Feed bland foods such as strained meat baby food and meat baby food mixed with Isocal (Mead Johnson Nutritionals). Most ferrets will accept these foods after an initial period of force-feeding by syringe.

GI FOREIGN BODIES

GI obstruction caused by foreign body ingestion is one of the most common problems in pet ferrets because of their inquisitive nature.

Etiology

- Foreign bodies generally are found in younger ferrets; trichobezoars may cause obstruction in older animals.

KEY POINT ▶ Until proved otherwise, suspect the presence of a GI foreign body in any young ferret presented for anorexia—even if no vomiting is reported. Rubber objects are the most common foreign bodies.

- Because ferrets enjoy chewing on rubber, most GI foreign bodies in ferrets are rubber objects.
- Obstruction with cloth, plant material, and hairballs may also occur.

Clinical Signs

- One or several episodes of vomiting may be reported; however, vomiting often is not observéd. Other signs of nausea include hypersalivation and pawing at the mouth.
- Intermittent or total anorexia occurs in ferrets with GI obstruction. Sometimes chronic wasting is the only clinical sign.
- Signs include lethargy, hindlimb weakness, dehydration, infrequent defecation, small stools, and melena may occur.

Diagnosis

History

- Identify any possibility of foreign body ingestion.

Physical Examination

- Palpate the abdomen thoroughly to detect intestinal gas, a firm mass, or the presence of a painful area.

Laboratory Studies

- The serum biochemical profile, urinalysis, and CBC usually are normal except for evidence of dehydration. Anemia is seen in some ferrets with melena.

Abdominal Radiography

- Look for radiodense foreign material in the GI tract. To improve visualization of a suspected foreign body, be sure to fast the ferret prior to radiography.
- Excessive gas and intestinal distension may indicate GI obstruction.
- Diagnosis is generally evident from physical examination and plain radiographs; thus, barium contrast radiography is rarely necessary.

Treatment

Surgical removal is the treatment of choice. However, in early, mild cases of suspected partial GI obstruction, administration of a feline hairball product q8h for 3 days may promote passage of a small foreign body. If the ferret is ill, do not delay surgery!

Surgical Therapy

- Follow routine preoperative, operative, and postoperative procedure principles to perform gastrotomy or enterotomy (see sec. 7, chs. 5 and 7). Ferret tissues are thinner than those of a pup or kitten of equivalent weight. Use 4-0 or 5-0 suture material to close the GI tract.

Prevention and Prognosis

KEY POINT ▶ Instruct owners to "ferret proof" the house if ferrets are allowed to roam. In particular, restrict access to rubber toys and rubber objects.

- To prevent trichobezoar formation, administer a feline hairball laxative product (2–4 cm) three or four times a week, PO.

Prognosis

- The prognosis is good with prompt therapy.

ROTAVIRUS

- Rotavirus causes diarrheal illness in the young of several species, including humans, cattle, swine, sheep, and rats.
- Rotavirus has caused several outbreaks of diarrhea with high mortality among ferret kits 2–6 weeks of age, and has been named "ferret kit disease."
- In adult ferrets, rotavirus infection is rarely fatal but causes the passage of bright green diarrhea with mucus for several days.
- There is no readily available antemortem test for the disease, although rotavirus particles can be identified in feces by electron microscopy.
- Treatment includes supportive care, especially fluid therapy, and antibiotics to prevent secondary bacterial infection.

SALMONELLA

Salmonella typhimurium infection generally is acquired through exposure to contaminated raw meat and meat by-products. It is uncommon in pet ferrets.

- Clinical signs include lethargy, anorexia, fever, and diarrhea that usually is bloody. Conjunctivitis and anemia also are seen.
- Diagnosis of salmonellosis is based on clinical signs and a positive fecal culture.
- Treatment includes supportive care and antibiotic therapy guided by results of culture and sensitivity testing.
  - Intravenous fluids and therapy with rapidly acting intravenous corticosteroids may be necessary for ferrets that are presented in shock.
- Other details of salmonellosis, including its public health significance, are discussed elsewhere in this text.

EOSINOPHILIC GASTROENTERITIS

This is a newly recognized syndrome of unknown etiology in ferrets. Histopathologic findings are compatible with parasitic infection; however, extensive microscopic studies have failed to identify an etiologic agent.

- Clinical signs include intermittent vomiting, inappetence, diarrhea, and weight loss.

- On physical examination, mesenteric lymph nodes may be enlarged and the intestines may feel thickened.
- A marked peripheral eosinophilia is present. If eosinophilic gastroenteritis is suspected, perform abdominal exploratory surgery, because definitive diagnosis depends on intestinal biopsy.
- Treat with two doses (400 µg/kg SC) of ivermectin (Ivomec; Merck Sharp & Dohme Agvet) given 2 weeks apart.
- If ivermectin is ineffective, consider prednisone, which is the treatment of choice for dogs and cats with eosinophilic enteritis.

PROLIFERATIVE BOWEL DISEASE (PBD)

Proliferative colitis in ferrets was first reported in 1982; a similar disease is now recognized to affect the jejunoileum. A disseminated form of PBD with lesions in extraintestinal sites has also been reported. This is a disease primarily of young ferrets 4–14 months of age.

Etiology

Intracellular *Campylobacter*-like organisms (CLOs) are seen with Warthin-Starry staining in the apical portion of colonic crypt epithelial cells. Although *C. jejuni* can be cultured from some ferrets with the disease, current research indicates that CLOs probably are not *Campylobacter* spp.

Clinical Signs

- Acute and chronic forms of the disease can occur.
- Diarrhea, often with mucus and blood, is a constant finding. Defecations are frequent and small; ferrets often cry out when they defecate. The rectum may be partially prolapsed.
- Other signs include lethargy, depression, inappetence, weight loss, dehydration, and pyrexia.
- Neurologic signs such as ataxia and muscle tremors also may be present.

Diagnosis

- The colon or jejunoileum may be palpably thickened on physical examination.
- Perform direct fecal and fecal flotation tests to rule out GI parasitism.
- A tentative diagnosis of proliferative bowel disease is based on clinical signs and physical examination. Definitive diagnosis requires intestinal or colonic biopsy, but this is rarely warranted because response to therapy usually is good if initiated early. Biopsies can be obtained during laparotomy or endoscopically (i.e., colon).

Treatment

Treat mild cases on an out-patient basis. Hospitalization for supportive care may be necessary with severe disease.

- Chloramphenicol is the drug of choice (50 mg/kg

q12h, PO, IV, IM, or SC). Treat for at least 2 weeks; longer therapy often is necessary to prevent relapse.
- Metronidazole (20 mg/kg q12h, PO) may be efficacious.

KEY POINT ▶ Proliferative bowel disease is the prime differential diagnosis for young ferrets with diarrhea. Therefore, chloramphenicol therapy is routine when GI parasitism has been ruled out.

- Supportive care, including subcutaneous fluids and nutritional support, is necessary for dehydrated and debilitated ferrets.

Prevention and Prognosis

- There is no prevention.
- The prognosis is good with timely therapy.
- Some ferrets will improve temporarily and then relapse at the end of the treatment period. Use a long-term course of antibiotic therapy in these animals.

RECTAL PROLAPSE

Rectal prolapse is common in younger ferrets.

- Diarrhea often is seen in conjunction with rectal prolapse.
- Causes include GI parasitism (e.g., coccidiosis), proliferative colitis, and other diseases that may cause straining or diarrhea.
- Perform direct fecal and fecal flotation tests to screen for parasites.
- Medical treatment is similar to that for other species, namely anthelmintics and antibiotics; chloramphenicol is the drug of choice if proliferative bowel disease is suspected. Surgical correction is usually unnecessary.

Surgical Correction—Techniques

1. Flush the prolapsed tissues and replace them into the rectum.
2. Place a pursestring suture in the anus with a small opening to allow passage of feces. Keep the pursestring suture in place for 2–5 days.
   a. Small prolapses of less than 5 mm often resolve on medical therapy without the need for a pursestring suture.
3. For ferrets with chronic prolapsed rectum, surgery may be necessary to reduce the size of the anal opening. Excise a small triangular wedge of anal mucosa and routinely close the defect by suturing.

ANAL SAC ABSCESS

- Clinical signs and physical findings in ferrets with an abscessed anal sac are the same as in dogs and cats.
- The recommended treatment is lancing and drainage of the abscess or surgical removal of both anal sacs (see sec. 7, ch. 12).

Anal Sacculectomy

KEY POINT ▶ Perform anal sac removal to decrease the musky odor or as treatment for anal sac abscesses. For odor reduction, neutering is done simultaneously because the scent glands in the skin and the perianal sebaceous and apocrine glands are under hormonal control.

Technique

1. Grasp the anal sac opening and hold it closed with mosquito forceps. Make a circumferential skin incision around the duct opening.
2. Applying gentle caudal traction to the anal sac, use a scalpel blade or gauze to tease away the surrounding fascia.
3. Do not suture the incisions.

Alternative Techniques

1. Make small, arc-like incisions just lateral to the duct openings.
2. Dissect the subcutaneous tissues bluntly to reveal the neck of the anal sac; grasp the opening and hold it closed with mosquito forceps.
3. Dissect the sac free of surrounding tissues, using gentle traction.
4. Do not suture the incision.

Urogenital System

Elizabeth V. Hillyer

REPRODUCTIVE SYSTEM

Characteristics of the Normal Ferret Reproductive System

Ferrets reach sexual maturity during the first breeding season after birth. The breeding season runs from March to August.

Males

- Males (hobs) have a large, J-shaped os penis.
- There is disagreement regarding the presence of a prostate gland; according to recent studies, a prostate gland is located at the base of the urinary bladder surrounding the urethra and may be difficult to visualize in young males.
- During the breeding season, testicle size is twice that in the fall and winter months.

Females

- A swollen vulva is an external sign of estrus.
- Female ferrets (jills) are seasonally polyestrous and are induced ovulators.
- If mating is unsuccessful, pseudopregnancy will result, lasting 41–43 days.

■ Approximately 50% of females remain in heat if they are not bred. Because the resulting prolonged elevation of serum estrogens can cause bone marrow toxicity and pancytopenia (see discussion of Anemia under Hematopoietic System in this chapter), termination of estrus is recommended.

Estrus Termination

■ Terminate estrus after day 10 by administration of a single intramuscular injection of 1000 USP units (or 100 IU) of hCG; repeat this dose, if necessary, 1–2 weeks later.
■ Alternatively, give GnRH at a dose of 20 μg, IM or SC, following the same schedule.

Castration and Ovariohysterectomy

■ Follow the same protocols and procedures as for cats (see sec. 8, chs. 11 and 15).
■ Castration can be open or closed; use scrotal incisions.
■ Note that the ovarian pedicles contain large amounts of fat.

Pyometra

■ Pyometra is uncommon in pet ferrets because generally they are neutered prior to being sold as pets.
■ Persistent estrus may predispose ferrets to the development of pyometra; therefore, screen affected females for evidence of estrogen toxicity, especially to detect thrombocytopenia preoperatively, prior to treatment (see discussion of Anemia under Hematopoietic System in this chapter).
■ Clinical signs, diagnosis, and treatment are the same as for dogs and cats (see sec. 8, ch. 14).

Vulvar Swelling in "Spayed" Females

As previously mentioned, vulvar swelling is an external sign of estrus in female ferrets.

■ In a female that purportedly is spayed, a swollen vulva indicates the presence of remnant ovarian tissue or another source of estrogens such as an abnormal adrenal gland (see Endocrine Diseases in this chapter).

Diagnosis

A simple test for the presence of functional ovarian tissues is the hCG challenge test.

■ To stimulate ovulation, administer 1000 USP units (or 100 IU) of hCG, IM, after the vulva has been swollen for at least 10 days; vulvar swelling should diminish.
■ Measure serum progesterone 5–7 days after hCG administration. (In dogs and cats, postovulatory progesterone levels increase >1 ng/ml if functional ovarian tissue is present.)

Pregnancy Toxemia (Eclampsia)

Pregnancy toxemia, or eclampsia, is a condition that occurs in late pregnancy and most commonly affects primiparous females.

■ The cause of eclampsia in ferrets is not known.
■ Affected ferrets usually are presented in an acute state of shock.
■ Aggressive supportive care and an emergency cesarean section are indicated.
■ The disease results in high mortality of jills and kits.

Mastitis

■ See Dermatologic Diseases in this chapter.

URINARY SYSTEM

Characteristics of the Normal Ferret Urinary System

■ The normal urine pH is 6.5–7.5.
■ Normal values for urine specific gravity have not been reported.
■ There is evidence that proteinuria may be normal in ferrets (7–33 mg/dl in males; 0–32 mg/dl in females) and that bilirubinuria can occur in the absence of liver disease.
■ Both male and female ferrets are difficult to catheterize, owing to the small size of the urethra (see Clinical Techniques in this chapter).

Polycystic Kidneys

Unilateral or bilateral polycystic kidneys are relatively common in ferrets (see sec. 8, ch. 1 for a description of this disease in dogs and cats). The condition usually is discovered as an incidental finding in middle-aged and older ferrets.

Etiology

■ The cause of polycystic kidneys in ferrets is unknown but is probably congenital, as in other species.

Clinical Signs

■ Usually no clinical signs are apparent.
■ In ferrets with severe renal involvement, clinical signs are due to renal insufficiency and include lethargy, inappetence, polyuria/polydipsia, vomiting, and melena.

Diagnosis

■ Palpate the kidneys for irregular shape.
■ Perform a serum biochemical profile, CBC, and urinalysis if renal disease is suspected.
■ Abdominal radiography usually is not helpful unless the kidneys are very irregular.
■ Intravenous pyelography may be helpful.
■ Abdominal ultrasonography is the most useful tool for detection of polycystic kidneys.
■ Renal cysts may be an incidental finding during abdominal surgery.

Treatment

■ No treatment is necessary in asymptomatic cases.
■ If the affected kidney becomes very enlarged, con-

sider unilateral nephrectomy (if the opposite kidney is functional).
■ Supportive care such as subcutaneous fluid admtration may temporarily improve the status of azotemic animals. Other therapy for chronic renal failure in dogs and cats may be helpful.

HYDRONEPHROSIS

■ Hydronephrosis is uncommon in ferrets. Iatrogenic hydronephrosis may occur as the result of inadvertent ligation of a ureter during ovariohysterectomy (see sec. 8, ch. 1 for information about hydronephrosis in dogs and cats).

CYSTITIS

■ Bacterial cystitis without urinary calculi is rare in pet ferrets. Follow treatment protocols for cystitis in dogs (see sec. 8, ch. 3).

UROLITHIASIS

Urinary tract calculi composed of struvite (magnesium ammonium phosphate hexahydrate) can occur in pet ferrets. Evidence suggests that the incidence of urolithiasis is increased in ferrets fed commercial dog food (see below).

Etiology

■ The cause of urinary calculi in ferrets, including the role of nutritional factors, is not known. However, most affected ferrets were being fed commercial dog food, low-quality cat food, or ferret chow. Calculi are rare in ferrets fed a high-quality feline diet such as Iams (Iams Co.) or Science Diet Kitten Chow (Hill's Pet).
■ Usually no growth occurs on bacterial culture.

Clinical Signs

Clinical signs depend on the location of the urolith(s):

■ Cystic calculi result in dysuria and hematuria.
■ Urethral calculi may cause obstruction in both male and female ferrets.
■ Renal calculi may be asymptomatic or may result in renal failure.

Diagnosis

■ On physical examination, cystic calculi are often palpable. The urinary bladder wall may be thickened; in cases of obstruction, the bladder is distended and firm.
■ Abdominal radiography can confirm the presence of urinary tract calculi (struvite calculi are radiodense).

Treatment

KEY POINT ▶ The bladder is very fragile in ferrets. Handle ferrets with obstruction gently to avoid bladder rupture.

■ Treatment of urinary obstruction may be difficult because urinary catheters are difficult to pass in ferrets.
  • If attempts at catheterization are unsuccessful, perform transabdominal cystocentesis to empty the bladder.
  • Consider a cystotomy for anterograde urethral catheterization and flushing. A perineal urethrotomy may be necessary.
■ Remove cystic calculi surgically using the same technique as for dogs and cats (see sec. 8, ch. 4).
  • Close the bladder with 4–0 or 5–0 absorbable suture material.
  • Submit the calculi for analysis and culture; results will guide subsequent therapy.
■ The efficacy of a diet to dissolve stones (Feline S/D; Hill's Pet) in ferrets is not known. Do not feed this diet for prolonged periods, because of its low protein level.

Prevention

■ Postoperative care and prevention of urolithiasis in ferrets may include antibiotic therapy. The choice of initial antibiotics includes trimethoprim sulfate (15–30 mg/kg q12h SC or PO), chloramphenicol (50 mg/kg q12h IV, SC, IM, or PO), and amoxicillin-clavulinic acid (Clavamox; SmithKline).
  • Adjust antibiotic selection and dosage according to culture and sensitivity test results and diet change.
■ Although there is no concrete evidence linking the disease in ferrets to feline urinary syndrome (FUS), the same high-quality feline diets that are used in the prevention of FUS are recommended.

PARAURETHRAL CYSTS AND URINARY TRACT OBSTRUCTION

Urethral obstruction in male ferrets may occur secondary to extraluminal pressure from a paraurethral cyst.

Etiology

■ Although prostatic disease is not reported in ferrets, and it has been hypothesized that ferrets do not have a prostate gland, it is possible that paraurethral cysts represent prostatic tissue.
■ All affected ferrets had concurrent adrenal neoplasia; hormones secreted by adrenal may cause this condition.

History and Clinical Signs

■ The history and clinical signs are compatible with urinary tract obstruction.

Physical Examination

■ On physical examination, a large, firm, caudal abdominal mass is palpable. With careful palpation this

mass is found to be bilobed, representing the urinary bladder and a cystic structure.
■ Hair loss and other signs of adrenal neoplasia may occur.

Diagnosis

■ Evaluate abdominal radiographs to rule out obstruction from cystic calculi.
■ If available, ultrasonography is useful to evaluate adrenals and any masses. Cystocentesis may be necessary to empty the urinary bladder.
■ Abdominal exploratory surgery with biopsies is necessary for a definitive diagnosis.

Treatment

■ The abnormal structures are usually nonresectable owing to their size and their position near the urethra and ureters.
■ After obtaining a wedge biopsy, attempt to resect as much of the structure as possible.
  • Typically, the structures are cavitary with multiple small pockets of cystic or purulent material.

  • If an abscess is suspected it may be necessary to marsupialize the abscess cavity.
  • On biopsy, these structures are composed of cystic or abscessed glandular tissue representing either the urethra or prostate gland.
■ Biopsy or remove abnormal adrenal tissue.

Prognosis

■ The long-term prognosis is guarded. The paraurethral cysts may regress after the adrenal gland disease is controlled.

Supplemental Readings

Besch-Williford CL: Biology and medicine of the ferret. Vet Clin North Am [Small Anim Pract] 17:1155, 1987.

Fox JG: Biology and Diseases of the Ferret. Philadelphia: Lea & Febiger, 1988.

Fox JG, Hotaling L, Ackerman BP, Hewes K: Serum chemistry and hematology reference values in the ferret (Mustela putorius furo). Lab Anim Sci 36:583, 1986.

O'Rourke LG: Practical blood transfusions. In Kirk RW, ed.: Current Veterinary Therapy VIII. Philadelphia: W. B. Saunders, 1983, p 408.

Randolph RW: Medical and surgical care of the pet ferret. In Kirk RW, ed.: Current Veterinary Therapy X. Philadelphia: W. B. Saunders, 1989, p 765.

9 Rabbits

Katherine E. Quesenberry

Rabbits are popular pets for both children and adults. They are easily litter trained and require a minimum of maintenance. Management of diseases in pet rabbits differs from that of laboratory rabbits in the emphasis on the individual animal and the approach to therapy. This chapter stresses diagnosis and management of problems commonly encountered in pet rabbits. Refer to the Supplemental Readings for more comprehensive information.

BIOLOGIC CHARACTERISTICS

Rabbits, hares, and pikas are members of the order Lagomorpha. Lagomorphs have six incisors in contrast to the closely related rodents, which have four incisors. The additional incisors are small, rounded teeth located directly behind the upper incisors.

- All domestic rabbits are descendants of the European wild rabbit, *Oryctolagus cuniculus.*
- The two main genera of rabbits are *Oryctolagus,* the European wild rabbits, and *Sylvilagus,* the cottontail rabbits. These genera differ in chromosome number and cannot interbreed.
- Domestic rabbit breeds were developed as early as the 18th century. Today there are over 60 recognized breeds.
  - Giant breeds, which average more than 5 kg in body weight, include the American Checkered Giant, the Flemish Giant, and the Giant Chinchilla rabbits.
  - Medium breeds, which average from 3.5 to 5 kg in body weight, include the Californian, the Silver Marten, and the Rex rabbits.
  - Small breeds, which average less than 3.5 kg in body weight, include the Netherland Dwarf, the Jersey Wooly, and the Polish rabbits.
  - Specific information concerning breeds can be obtained from the American Rabbit Breeders Association, 1925 S. Main, P.O. Box 426, Bloomington, IL 61702.

Anatomic and Physiologic Characteristics

- Females of several breeds of rabbits have a pendulous dewlap. This area is a frequent site of moist dermatitis, especially in obese rabbits kept in humid, warm environments.
- Teeth are open rooted and grow continuously. There are 2/1 incisors, 0/0 canines, 3/2 premolars, and 2-3/3 molars. Malocclusion and overgrowth of the incisors, premolars, and molars are common.

- The gastrointestinal tract has a simple glandular stomach, a long intestinal tract, and a large cecum.
  - The cecum is the site of bacterial synthesis of B-vitamins.
  - About one third of the normal stool output is composed of soft stools called cecotrophs. Cecotrophs are consumed primarily at night by domestic rabbits as an important source of B-vitamins, electrolytes, and nitrogen.
- Veins are thin-walled and fragile. Hematoma formation after venipuncture is common.
- The skeletal system is light and delicate in comparison with most mammals. The skeleton comprises 8% of the total body weight in rabbits, as opposed to 13% of the total body weight in cats.
- Inguinal canals remain open throughout life.
- Female rabbits (i.e., does) have four to five pairs of mammary glands and nipples. Nipples are not present in male rabbits (i.e., bucks).

KEY POINT ▶ Red, pink, or orange discoloration of the urine occurs periodically in healthy rabbits. The color may be caused by the presence of a porphyrin pigment or a food-related metabolite excreted in the urine.

- Calcium and phosphorus are excreted primarily through urine in rabbits. Calcium is excreted in the bile in most other mammals.
- In rabbits, high total leukocyte counts may not be characteristic of acute inflammation from infectious causes. Instead, the distribution of the white blood cells shifts from a normally high lymphocyte/low neutrophil ratio to neutrophilia and lymphopenia.

Reproductive Characteristics

- Females mature sexually at 4 to 8 months of age, depending on breed. Males mature at 6 to 10 months of age.
- Females have a silent estrus and are induced ovulators.
- Gestation lasts for an average of 30 to 33 days.
- Pseudocyesis may last 17 days.
- Litters are usually born (i.e., kindled) at night. Litter size averages four to ten young (i.e., kits).
- Does normally nurse their young once or twice daily. Weaning occurs at 4 to 6 weeks of age.
- Rabbit milk is approximately 13% protein, 9% fat, and 1% lactose.

TABLE 1. Normal Physiologic Parameters

Temperature	38–40° C
Heart rate	130–325 beats/minute
Respiratory rate	32–60/min
Life span	5–9 years
Blood volume	55–65 ml/kg
Food consumption	50 g/kg/day
Water consumption	
General population	50–100 ml/kg/day
Breeding does	<900 ml/kg/day

Normal Parameters

Normal physiologic parameters are listed in Table 1. Normal hematology, serum chemistry, and urinalysis values are listed in Tables 2, 3, and 4.

PATIENT MANAGEMENT

Caging

- Cages or hutches can be purchased or constructed. Cages should be large enough to allow free movement. Small breeds, which weigh 2 kg, require a minimum of 1.5 ft² of floor space per animal. Large breeds, which weigh 5 kg or more, require at least 5 ft² of floor space per animal. Cages should be easy to clean.
- Both wire and hard flooring may predispose the rabbit to the development of sore hocks. If mesh flooring is used, either 1 × ½ in² or ⅝-in² mesh is recommended. There should be no rough edges in the cage. Provide clean, soft bedding such as straw in one area of the cage.
- Rabbits can be housed indoors or outdoors at temperatures ranging from 40° to 80°F. Rabbits are very susceptible to heat stroke in ambient temperatures above 85° F. If outdoor housing is used, provide ventilation or protection from direct sunlight. In temperatures below 40° F, provide heat or protection from cold.

Restraint

KEY POINT ▶ Rabbits must be restrained firmly for most procedures. Inadequate restraint

TABLE 3. Normal Serum Chemistry Values

Serum protein	5.4–8.3 g/dl
Albumin	2.4–4.6 g/dl
Globulin	1.5–2.8 g/dl
Glucose	75–155 g/dl
Blood urea nitrogen	13–29 mg/dl
Creatinine	0.5–2.5 mg/dl
Total bilirubin	0.0–0.7 mg/dl
Cholesterol	10–80 mg/dl
Total lipids	243–390 mg/dl
Calcium	5.6–12.5 mg/dl
Phosphorus	4.0–6.9 mg/dl
Sodium	131–155 mEq/liter
Potassium	3.6–6.9 mEq/liter
Chloride	92–112 mEq/liter
Bicarbonate	16–38 mEq/liter
Amylase	166.5–314.5 U/liter
Alkaline phosphatase	4–16 IU/liter
Glutamic pyruvate transaminase	48–80 IU/liter
Glutamic oxalocacetic transaminase	14–113 IU/liter
Lactic dehydrogenase	34–129 IU/liter

can result in a spinal fracture in the rabbit if it is allowed to kick with its hind legs.

- Grasp the rabbit with the hindquarters supported in one arm and the rear legs held firmly between the fingers. The other hand holds the rabbit firmly by the scruff at the base of the neck.
- For examination or treatment, hold the rabbit to the table with firm, gentle downward pressure at the pelvic and thoracic girdles (see Fig. 1).
- The ventrum and anal area can be examined by cradling the rabbit on its back in one arm. Hold the rear legs firmly between the fingers of one hand and the forelegs between the fingers of the other hand (Fig. 2).
- For jugular venipuncture, restraint is similar to that for a cat. Extend the neck up and the forelegs down over a table edge. Press the pelvic girdle firmly to the table to control the rear legs.

Diagnostic Techniques

A thorough history and complete physical examination are necessary to rule out certain diagnoses.

- Measure physical parameters, including heart rate, temperature, and respiratory rate. Auscultate the lungs and palpate the abdomen thoroughly.

TABLE 2. Normal Hematologic Values

Erythrocytes	5.1–7.9 × 10⁶m³
Hematocrit	33–50%
Hemoglobin	10.0–17.4 g/dl
Mean corpuscular volume	57.8–66.5 μm³
Mean corpuscular hemoglobin	17.1–23.5 pg
Mean corpuscular hemoglobin concentration	29–37%
Platelets	250–650 × 10³/mm³
Leukocytes	5.2–12.5 × 10³/mm³
Neutrophils	20–75%
Lymphocytes	30–85%
Monocytes	1–4%
Eosinophils	1–4%
Basophils	1–7%

TABLE 4. Normal Urinalysis Values

Urine volume	
Large	20–350 ml/kg/day
Average	130 ml/kg/day
Specific gravity	1.003–1.036
Average pH	8.2
Crystals present	Ammonium magnesium phosphate, calcium carbonate monohydrate, anhydrous calcium carbonate
Casts, epithelial cells, or bacteria present	Absent to rare
Leukocytes or erythrocytes present	Occasional
Albumin present	Occasional in young rabbits

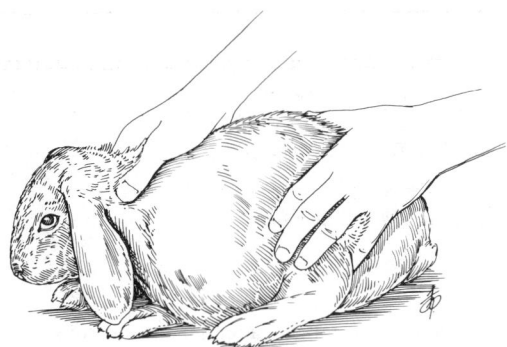

Figure 1. Proper method for restraining a rabbit.

- Check feet and hocks for evidence of erythema and ulceration.
- Check both the incisors and the molars with an otoscope for evidence of malocclusion.

Blood Collection

- Use a small-gauge needle (i.e., 22-gauge or smaller) for venipuncture to prevent hematoma formation.
- The ear vein can be used for blood collection in large rabbits. Some clinicians use a vacutainer system for rapid withdrawal. In most medium- and small-breed rabbits, the ear vein is very small and will thrombose easily. Thrombosis may lead to local sloughing of the pinna.
  - Plucking the hair over the vein is easier than shaving fine fur.
- Blood is easily collected from the lateral saphenous vein. This vein lies in the middle portion of the lateral aspect of the tibia.
- The jugular vein can be used for venipuncture in many rabbits. Jugular venipuncture is sometimes difficult in females with heavy dewlaps. The vein usually is not visible; it lies superficially in the jugular furrow. Pluck the hair from the midneck region, and extend the head up for venipuncture as described under restraint.

Treatment Techniques

- Subcutaneous fluid administration is acceptable in noncritical cases. Estimate daily maintenance fluids at 100 ml/kg/24 hours.
- An indwelling catheter is preferred in critical cases.
  - Small-gauge catheters (i.e., 22- to 24-gauge) can sometimes be placed in the cephalic or lateral saphenous vein in medium-to-large rabbits.
  - Jugular catheters can be difficult to insert and may require a cutdown procedure.
  - Vascular access ports are used by some clinicians for long-term venous access.
- Administer oral medications into the lateral cheek pouch. Use liquid or paste preparations when possible, because rabbits have a long, narrow oropharynx that makes pill administration difficult.
- Force-feed anorectic animals with a paste nutritional supplement (e.g., Nutri-Cal; Evsco Pharmaceuticals,

Buena, NJ), a commercial nutritional formula, or a gruel made of moistened rabbit pellets.
- Place nasogastric tubes in medium-to-large rabbits. The technique that follows is similar to that for placing a tube in a cat.
  - Using manual restraint, place two to three Ophthaine topical anesthetic drops (Solvay Veterinary, Inc., Princeton, NJ) in the mucosa of one nare. Wait 5 minutes, then repeat application.
  - Lubricate the tip of a small infant feeding tube (e.g., 5 Fr., Bard-Parker, Becton, Dickenson and Company, Rutherford, NJ) with topical lidocaine (Xylocaine) jelly. Pass the tube medially along the nasal passage to the level of the last rib. The tip of the tube is located in the distal esophagus.
  - Secure the free end of the tube to the skin above the nose and eye with a butterfly tape and suture. An Elizabethan collar may be necessary to prevent the rabbit from dislodging the tube.
- *Lactobacillus* spp. may aid in the treatment of enteritis by
  - Repopulating the gastrointestinal tract with healthy bacterial flora
  - Decreasing intestinal or cecal pH
  - Competing with bacterial pathogens for mucosal attachment sites
  - Commercial products in paste form are available for administration (e.g., Bene-Bac, Pet-Ag, Inc, Elgin, IL). Powdered products can be added to food, but many rabbits object to the taste.
- Commonly used antibiotics are listed in Table 5.

Tranquilization and Anesthesia

- Injectable tranquilizers are suitable for short diagnostic or surgical procedures. Drugs and dosages are

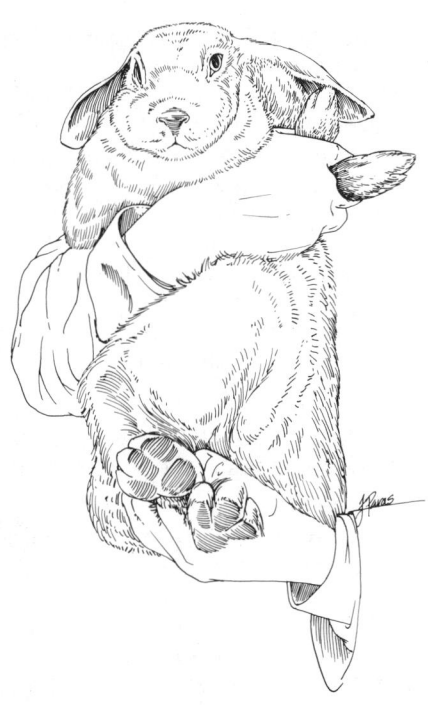

Figure 2. To examine the ventrum and anal area, cradle the rabbit as shown. Be sure to provide support to the hind limbs.

TABLE 5. Commonly Used Drugs

	Dose	Comments
Antimicrobials		
Benzathine, penicillin G (Benza-Pen, SmithKline Beecham, Exton, PA)	84,000 IU/kg q7d × 3 days SC	For treatment of *Treponema cuniculi*
Cephalexin (Keflex Pediatric Drops, Dista Products, EI Lilly, Indianapolis, IN)	11–22 mg/kg q8h	May induce enteritis and diarrhea
Chloramphenicol	25 mg/kg q12–8h PO 30 mg/kg q12–q8h IV, IM	
Ciprofloxacin (Cipro, Miles Pharmaceuticals, West Haven, CT)	5–20 mg/kg q12h PO	Make a suspension in water for easier administration; suspension is stable for 14 days
Enrofloxacin (Baytril, Haver/Diamond Scientific, Shawnee, KS)	5–20 mg/kg q12h PO, IM	Manufacturers recommend one time only use of injectable formulation
Gentamicin (Gentocin, Shering-Plough, Kenilworth, NJ)	1.5–2.5 mg/kg q8h IV, IM, SC	
Griseofulvin (Fulvicin, Schering-Plough, Kenilworth, NJ)	25 mg/kg divided q12h PO × 4–6 weeks	If using Gris-PEG, decrease dose by 50%
Procaine Penicillin	40,000 IU/kg q24 hr SC	
Sulfadimethoxine (Albon, Hoffman-LaRoche, Nutley, NJ)	50 mg/kg PO first dose, then 25 mg/kg q24h PO × 5–20 days	For treatment of coccidiosis
Tetracycline	50–100 mg/kg q8h PO	
Trimethoprim/sulfa	30 mg/kg q12h PO, IM, SC	
Anthelmintics/Insecticides		
Lime sulfur solution	2% dip 1–2 times/week × 4 weeks	Used in young animals for treatment of mites, fleas, fungal dermatitis
Ivermectin	400 μg/kg q7d × 2–3 weeks	Effective against ear and fur mites
Piperazine	200 mg/kg; repeat in 2–3 weeks	
Pyrantel pamoate	5–10 mg/kg; repeat in 2–3 weeks	
Tranquilizers		
Diazepam	1–4 mg/kg IV, IM	Used in combination with ketamine
Ketamine HCl (Fort Dodge, Fort Dodge, IA)	25–40 mg/kg IM 5–20 mg/kg IV	Should be used in combination with diazepam, xylazine, or acepromazine; ketamine/diazepam provides good relaxation and sedation
Xylazine (Rompun, Haver/Diamond Scientific, Shawnee, KS)	5–10 mg/kg	Used in combination with ketamine; not recommended for routine use

listed in Table 5. I prefer to use ketamine and Valium in combination given IM or IV.

■ Inhalant anesthesia is necessary for long or painful surgical procedures. Clinically, isoflurane is very safe and is the preferred inhalant anesthetic. Halothane is potentially hepatotoxic and is associated with anesthetic-related deaths.

■ Anesthesia in rabbits can be induced by face mask or in an induction chamber. The concentration of isoflurane is gradually increased over several minutes until a surgical plane of anesthesia is reached. Anesthesia is usually maintained at 1.5 to 2% isoflurane in oxygen.

KEY POINT ▶ Intubation is attempted in surgical procedures lasting longer than 20 to 30 minutes.

■ The long, narrow oropharynx and the propensity for laryngospasm make intubation extremely difficult. The following technique is successful in larger rabbits.

• Induce anesthesia with isoflurane. Give a low, IV dose of ketamine and valium in combination after the rabbit has begun to relax (2–10 mg and 0.5–1.0 mg, respectively).

• Place the rabbit in sternal recumbancy. Extend the neck straight up and forward.

• Using a short, flat-blade laryngoscope (i.e., Miller blade), place the tip of the blade at the base of the tongue. Hook the base of the blade against the top front incisors, and use the blade as a lever to allow visualization of the glottis.

• Pass a small endotracheal tube along the blade into the opening of the glottis. Depending on their size, most rabbits require a 2.5- to 5.0-mm endotracheal tube. The glottis cannot be seen while trying to pass the tube.

■ A face mask is used for maintenance of anesthesia during short procedures or if intubation attempts are unsuccessful.

■ All rabbits should be closely monitored during any anesthetic episode.

NUTRITION

Nutritional Requirements

Most rabbits are fed a balanced commercial ration. Consequently, specific nutrient deficiencies are rare. The nutritional requirements of rabbits are published by the National Research Council (NRC) in the series Nutrient Requirements for Domestic Animals. Further research indicates that higher levels of dietary fiber (20 to 25%) are beneficial to maintenance. Recommendations for the percentages of dietary protein, fiber, fat, and energy vary during growth, lactation, reproduction, and maintenance (Table 6).

KEY POINT ▶ Insufficient indigestible dietary fiber is an underlying factor in many disease problems.

- Inadequate fiber causes decreased colonic-cecal motility, slowing overall gastrointestinal transit time. Decreased motility and prolonged retention of food material in the cecum may lead to enteritis and diarrhea.
- High-starch, low-fiber diets provide high levels of fermentation products for cecal bacteria. The number of bacterial pathogens may increase, resulting in increased toxin production.
- Hairballs (i.e., trichobezoars) are common in rabbits that are fed inadequate amounts of roughage. Fiber stimulates gastrointestinal motility and mechanically helps to move fur through the upper gastrointestinal tract. Fur-chewing or barbering is common in rabbits on low-fiber diets.

Some commercial rations have as little as 12% crude fiber. Fiber can be supplemented by feeding free-choice grass hay (e.g., timothy, orchard grass) or legume hay (e.g., alfalfa, clover). High-fiber pelleted feeds, which are 22.5% fiber, are available (Lab Rabbit Chow HF 5326, Ralston Purina Co., St. Louis, MO).

DERMATOLOGIC PROBLEMS

Dermatitis/Alopecia

Etiology

- Mange, fur, and ear mites will cause localized or diffuse dermatitis and/or alopecia. The area involved depends on the type of mite (see Ear Mites; Fur and Mange Mites).
- Dermatophytosis is associated with alopecia and a scaly dermatitis, particularly around the head and ears (see Superficial Mycosis).
- Fur-barbering is common in rabbits on diets deficient in roughage. There is a high incidence of barbering in does during breeding season; this is probably related to hormonal influences.

- Ptyalism, alopecia, and dermatitis around the mouth are associated with malocclusion.
- Moist dermatitis of the dewlap is common in females during breeding season, especially when they are kept in warm or humid environments.
- Moist dermatitis with erythema and ulceration of the ventral abdomen and perineal area results from urine scald. Urine scald is associated with urinary incontinence, cystitis, excessive calcium in the urine, or poor management and unclean caging.
- Treponematosis causes a scaly dermatitis in the genital area. The nose, lips, and periorbital area are less commonly involved.

Clinical Signs

- Mite infestations produce clinical signs characteristic of the mite involved. (See Ear Mites, Fur and Mange Mites.) Pruritis is common with sarcoptic mite infestations.
- Dermatophytes cause a partial alopecia with slight scaliness and erythema. Rabbits are usually pruritic.
- Fur-barbering is characterized by alopecia of the dewlap, back of the neck, and paws. The underlying skin is normal.
- Moist dermatitis of the dewlap or ventral abdomen is typically erythematous with scaling and ulceration. The fur around the alopecic areas is moist.

Diagnosis

Diagnosis is based on determination of the primary etiologic agent.

- Examine skin scrapings of scaly areas for evidence of adult mites or eggs.
- Culture fur and keratin debris for fungal organisms.
- Submit a skin biopsy specimen for histologic examination if the etiologic agent cannot be determined by other diagnostic tests.
- Examine the teeth in rabbits with excessive ptyalism and alopecia around the mouth (see Malocclusion).
- Radiograph rabbits with urine scald for evidence of cystic calculi.
- Submit a urine sample for urinalysis and bacterial culture and sensitivity testing.
- Submit a serum chemistry analysis to check for elevations in serum calcium, blood urea nitrogen, and creatinine concentrations.

Treatment

Treatment is based on etiology (see Ear Mites; Fur and Mange Mites; Hairballs; Malocclusion; Treponematosis; Cystitis; Superficial Mycosis).

- Correct the diet to include adequate roughage if fur-barbering is suspected. Ovariohysterectomy is effective in females with a suspected hormonal basis for fur-barbering.
- Treat adult rabbits with suspected mite infestations with ivermectin (see Table 5).
- Steroids are rarely used for pruritic dermatitis in rabbits.
- Treponematosis is treated with penicillin (see Treponematosis).

TABLE 6. Nutritional Recommendations

Stage	Crude Protein (%)	Fat (%)	Crude Fiber (%)
Maintenance	13	3	15–25
Lactation	18	5	12
Pregnancy	18	3	14
Growth	15	3	14

- Dermatophytosis is treated with topical or oral antifungal agents, depending on the extent of lesions.

Ear Mites (Psoroptes cuniculi)

Etiology

- Ear mites are common ectoparasites in both pet and laboratory rabbits.
- *P. cuniculi* is a large, nonburrowing mite that spends its 3-week life cycle on the host rabbit.
- Mites have biting mouthparts and cause inflammation by biting and chewing the epithelial surface of the skin.

Clinical Signs

- Infestation with psoroptic mites is usually confined to the inner epithelial surface of the ear. Lesions begin in the concha and eventually extend to the inner surface of the pinna. Other areas, such as the dewlap and feet, are sometimes involved.
- Lesions consist of thick, dry, flaky, gray-to-tan crusts on the inner surface of the ear pinna. The underlying epithelial surface is raw, inflamed, and hemorrhagic.
- Psoroptic mites cause intense pruritus. Affected rabbits will shake their heads or scratch their ears with the rear feet.

Diagnosis

- Psoroptic mites are large and sometimes visible with the unaided eye.
  - Use an otoscope to detect movement of the mites within the ear canal.
  - Microscopic examination of crusts and exudate usually reveals mites and eggs.
- Check rabbits with mild cases of otitis for the presence of mites.

Treatment

- Clean the ears of all crusts and exudate. Nolvamite, a mild otic cleansing agent (SmithKlein Beecham, Exton, PA; Fort Dodge, Fort Dodge, IA) is used to soften the crusts prior to removal.
  - Lesions are usually very painful.
  - Tranquilization is sometimes necessary for cleaning.
- If ivermectin is used, ears can be cleaned in 1 to 2 weeks after pain subsides and lesions heal.
- Psoroptic mites are susceptible to topical acaricides (e.g., Mitox Liquid; SmithKline Beecham, Exton, PA). Continue treatment for at least 3 weeks.
- Apply topical antibiotics if a secondary bacterial infection is present. Topical anti-inflammatory agents may be beneficial once bacterial infection is under control.
- Ivermectin is effective against ear mites (see Table 5). Treatment is repeated in 3 weeks. A combination therapy of ivermectin and topical acaricides can be used for severe infestations.

Prevention

- Psoroptic mites are easily transmitted between rabbits. Isolate affected rabbits from healthy rabbits.

- Keep cages and bedding clean to minimize spread through contaminated fomites.

Fur and Mange Mites

Etiology

- *Cheyletiella parasitivorax* is the common fur mite of rabbits. Infestations with other species of *Cheyletiella* occasionally occur. *Listrophorus gibbus* is a less common fur mite and is considered nonpathogenic.
  - Cheyletid mites are nonburrowing, obligate parasites with an approximate 35-day life cycle.
  - Infestation can be inapparent.
  - Cheyletid mites may cause a self-limiting, transitory dermatitis in humans.
  - The cheyletid mite is a known vector of rabbit myxomatosis in Australia.
- Mange mites (e.g., *Sarcoptes scabiei, Notedres cati*) occur infrequently in rabbits.

Clinical Signs

- Lesions produced by cheyletid mites consist of a scaly dermatitis with a flaky grayish white exudate. Mites primarily inhabit the dorsal trunk and scapular region. The underlying skin may appear erythematous and inflamed. Pruritus is not a major clinical sign.
- Other areas of the body can be involved in severe infestations. Rabbits may act as if they are depressed and in pain.
- Mange mites produce a crusty dermatitis with alopecia.
- Intense pruritus results from mites burrowing in the epidermis.

Diagnosis

- Identify cheyletid mites through microscopic examination of skin scrapings. Alternatively, a strip of cellophane tape can be pressed to the skin and fur in scaly areas and examined under a microscope.
- Deep skin scrapings are necessary to find mange mites. Results are sometimes falsely negative. Differential diagnosis is then based on the typical clinical signs of each type of mite.

Treatment

- Topical acaricides, including pyrethrins, carbamates, and lime sulfur solution dips (see Table 5), are effective against fur and mange mites. Products and treatment regimens that are safe for use in cats are usually safe for use in rabbits.
- Ivermectin is effective against mange and fur mites (see Table 5).
- The treatment period should extend through the life cycle of the mite.
- Cheyletid mites can exist off the host for short periods. Treat the home environment with parasiticides and eliminate potential fomites. Any cats kept in contact with infested rabbits should be examined or treated for mites.

Myiasis (Cuterebriasis)
Etiology

Myiasis (fly larval infestation) is common in rabbits kept outdoors. Incidence is highest in the summer and fall.

- Several species of *Cuterebra* affect rabbits. Cuterebrid larvae burrow into subcutaneous tissue and migrate to preferred body sites. Areas commonly involved include the ventral cervical region *(Cuterebra horripilum),* and the inguinal, hindquarter, and axillary regions *(Cuterebra buccata).*
- Blowflies or screwworms invade preexisting wounds. These include *Cochliomyia, Callitroga,* and *Wohlfahrtia* spp.

Clinical Signs

- Rabbits may appear to be in pain, reluctant to move, or lame.
- One or more firm, fistulated, subcutaneous swellings are present on physical examination. Frequently, the larvae are seen in the fistula surrounded by necrotic tissue.
- Secondary bacterial infections of the lesions are common.
- The eye can also be involved; this is known as ophthalmomyiasis.
- Severe infestation with multiple cuterebrid larvae can cause extreme debilitation and death.

Diagnosis

Diagnosis is based on a history of outdoor housing, clinical signs, and presence of larvae in wounds.

Treatment

- Remove larvae intact with hemostats if possible. Avoid rupture of the larvae. Ether can be applied topically to anesthetize the larvae before removal.
- Thoroughly debride wounds of necrotic tissue. Daily cleaning and debridement is usually necessary until healing occurs. With large wounds, complete excision of the necrotic area is preferred.
- Observe affected rabbits carefully for several weeks for the development of additional lesions.
- Antibiotic therapy is recommended for secondary bacterial infections.

Prevention

- Keep outdoor rabbits in screened hutches, especially during summer and fall.

Superficial Mycosis
Etiology

- *Trichophyton mentagrophytes* is the most common dermatophyte affecting rabbits. Infections with *Microsporum* spp. and other dermatophytes are much less frequent.
- Infection occurs through direct contact with infected animals, contaminated fomites, or asymptomatic carriers.

Clinical Signs

- Lesions usually appear on the head and ears and can extend to the feet, neck, and other areas.
- Lesions consist of areas of alopecia with erythema and scaly dermatitis. Rabbits are usually pruritic. Alopecic areas may be circular with slightly raised edges.

Diagnosis

Dermatitis resulting from dermatophytosis must be differentiated from other possible etiologies, including mites, fur-barbering, and bacterial dermatitis.

- Submit samples of fur from the edge of the lesion for fungal culture.
  - *T. mentagrophytes* does not fluoresce with ultraviolet light.
- The organisms can be demonstrated with either PAS or silver stains in histologic sections of skin biopsy specimens of affected rabbits.

Treatment

Treatment of dermatophytosis is directed toward elimination of the organism while preventing spread of disease. Other animals and humans, especially children, are susceptible to infection.

- Topical antifungal agents, such as Conofite (Pitman-Moore, Mundelein, IL), can be applied daily for 3 to 4 weeks.
- Lime sulfur solution dips (2–3%) given every 5 to 7 days are often effective for treating fungal dermatosis. Continue treatment for 4 weeks.
- Griseofulvin is effective if given daily for 4 weeks or until the infection clears (see Table 5). Give griseofulvin with fats to enhance absorption. Gris-PEG, an ultramicronized formulation for improved absorption, is given at one half the normal dose.
- Instruct owners to wear gloves when handling or treating affected animals because of the zoonotic disease potential.
- Check other animals in the household for evidence of dermatophytosis.

Prevention

- Prevent contact with infected animals.
- Strict sanitation is necessary to eliminate spread through fomites.

Sore Hocks/Ulcerative Pododermatitis
Etiology

- Sore hocks usually occur as a result of management-related problems. Soiled or wet bedding, abrasions from flooring, sedentary behavior caused by excessive weight, small cages that restrict movement, and abrasions from thumping are predisposing factors.
- Lesions involve the plantar surface of the hocks and may be unilateral or bilateral. Forepaws are less commonly affected.
- Secondary bacterial infections are common with severely ulcerated lesions.

Clinical Signs

- Early lesions are areas of erythema and thinning fur on the plantar surface of the hock.
- Lesions progress to raw, ulcerative sores with scabs. Mucoid or purulent exudate is present with secondary bacterial infections.
- Severe lesions cause lameness and reluctance to move. Rabbits may be anorectic and depressed.

Diagnosis

Diagnosis is based on clinical signs. If wounds appear to be infected, submit samples for bacterial culture and sensitivity testing.

Treatment

- Correct the predisposing management and environmental factors.
- Thoroughly clean and debride wounds. A nonocclusive antibiotic cream can be applied topically.
- Topical astringents such as Domeboro solution (Miles, Inc., West Haven, CT) are beneficial in treating moist wounds. Apply the solution daily until the wound appears dry.
- Protect wounds with sterile, soft, padded bandages.
- Healing is often prolonged. Clean the wound with an antibacterial soak, topical antibiotics, and bandaging, daily or every other day.

Prevention

- Wire flooring should be smooth, nonabrasive, and of sufficient width to prevent abrasions. An area of soft, dry bedding such as hay or several thicknesses of newspaper is placed in one area of the cage.
- Cages are clean and of sufficient size to allow free movement.
- Check the feet and hocks periodically for signs of inflammation.

RESPIRATORY DISEASE

Respiratory disease is common in pet rabbits and usually is associated with pasteurellosis. However, respiratory disease can result from many interrelated factors and is precipitated by stress.

Rhinitis/Paranasal Sinusitis

Etiology

- The primary infectious agent of paranasal sinusitis and rhinitis in rabbits is *Pasteurella multocida* (see Pasteurellosis). Other less common bacterial etiologies include *Bordetella bronchiseptica* and *Staphylococcus aureus*.
- Infections can be transmitted from the doe to offspring or by direct contact with infected rabbits. Infections may also be spread through airborne transmission.
- Intermittent episodes of rhinitis with mucopurulent nasal discharge are common with pasteurellosis.

Chronic disease may be subclinical and precipitated by stress.

Clinical Signs

- Nasal discharge may be serous or mucopurulent.
- Accompanying acute or chronic conjunctivitis with a serous-to-mucopurulent ocular discharge is common. One or both eyes may be affected.
- Many rabbits have no other clinical signs. Rabbits with severe disease may be anorectic and lethargic.

Diagnosis

Diagnosis of rhinitis is based on clinical signs and isolation of the etiologic agent through bacterial culture and sensitivity testing.

- Submit a swab of nasal or conjunctival exudate for bacterial culture and sensitivity testing. Small-tipped culturette swabs are convenient for sample collection (e.g., Mini-tip Culturettes; Becton Dickinson, Cockeysville, MD). Culture of nasal exudate in *Pasteurella*-infected rabbits is frequently negative.
- An antibody ELISA test for *Pasteurella* is available (see Pasteurellosis).

Treatment

KEY POINT ▶ Treatment of upper respiratory disease secondary to pasteurellosis can be frustrating, especially with chronic infections (see Pasteurellosis).

- Give antibiotics, which are the most efficacious against *Pasteurella* (see Pasteurellosis), at the first signs of respiratory disease. The antibiotic choice may change based on results of bacterial culture and sensitivity testing.
- If conjunctivitis is present, apply an ophthalmic antibiotic, such as chloramphenicol ophthalmic (Aveco, Fort Dodge, IA) or Gentocin Ophthalmic (Schering-Plough, Kenilworth, NJ) topically three to four times daily for 10 to 14 days. If possible, flush the nasolacrimal duct of the affected eye or eyes. A topical ophthalmic anesthetic is necessary for this procedure.
- Long-term therapy may be necessary with chronic disease. The incidence of recurrence is high.

Prevention

General preventive measures are described in the section on *Pasteurellosis*.

Pasteurellosis

Etiology

- Pasteurellosis is an endemic bacterial disease of rabbits. It is caused by *Pasteurella multocida*, a small, gram-negative, bipolar-staining rod.
- Infection is spread by direct contact with infected rabbits, contaminated fomites, aerosolization, or from does to offspring during birth and nursing.
- Bacteria colonize the soft palate and nasal turbinates

and may produce a lifelong infection. Infection may be subclinical with intermittent episodes of mucopurulent nasal discharge, usually precipitated by stress.

- Spread from the nasal cavity can occur through several routes:
  - The eustachian tube to the middle or inner ear, meninges, and brain
  - The nasolacrimal duct to the conjunctival sac
  - The trachea to the lungs
  - The lymphatics or blood stream to the peripheral lymph nodes, reproductive tract, or other organs.

Clinical Signs

Clinical signs of disease depend on the site and chronicity of infection.

- Respiratory signs associated with pasteurellosis include rhinitis, conjunctivitis, and pneumonia.
- Abscesses of the joints and mandible and subsequent osteomyelitis are common.
- Neurologic signs, including head tilt, torticollis, nystagmus, and facial nerve deficits, can be seen with infections of the middle or inner ear, meninges, or brain.
- Abscesses can occur in various organs and in subcutaneous tissue. Exudate is typically white, thick, and caseous.
- Peracute death may occur from septicemia or pneumonia in young and weanling rabbits.

Diagnosis

- Submit bacterial cultures from exudate, blood, or tissue samples. Isolation of *P. multocida* is sometimes difficult. Many carrier animals will have negative cultures of nasal swab samples.
- Several laboratory animal research centers have developed an ELISA test to detect antibodies to *P. multocida*. The test requires whole blood or serum and is reported as positive, negative, or suspect. One laboratory offering the test is the Rabbit Research Center, Oregon State University, Lab Animal Resource Center 101, Corvallis, OR 97331-4701.

Treatment

KEY POINT ▶ Successful treatment of pasteurellosis is difficult. Antibiotics often only suppress clinical signs.

- Fluorinated quinolones are the most clinically effective in the treatment of pasteurellosis. Enrofloxacin is given (5–15 mg/kg, SID to BID). Pills are crushed and mixed with water or jam PO. Injectable form is given with cherry syrup PO. Ciprofloxacin tablets also can be given in cherry syrup (crushed and same dose as enrofloxacin).
  - Continue treatment for 14 to 30 days. Long-term therapy may effectively rid the animal of *Pasteurella* organisms.
- Other antibiotics have been used with varying degrees of success. Chloramphenicol, trimethoprim sulfate, penicillin, and aminoglycosides may be effec-

tive. The choice of antibiotic should be based on culture and sensitivity testing.

- Rabbit colonies have been treated with tetracycline added to drinking water at 300 mg/l. Feed additives also have been used (e.g., sulfaquinozaline at 225 gm/ton, furazolidone at 50 gm/ton). Success has been variable.
- Debride abscesses and drain them surgically. If possible, complete excision of subcutaneous abscesses is preferred.
- Mandibular or joint abcesses require extensive debridement and wound care (see Mandibular and Joint Abscesses).
- Daily management includes thorough cleaning and flushing until healing is well advanced.
- Debilitated rabbits require supplemental fluids, force-feeding, and general nursing care.

Prevention

- Pasteurellosis is an endemic disease in rabbits, and control is difficult. Colonies are kept *Pasteurella*-free through serologic testing and strict isolation and sanitation procedures.
- Prevention involves isolation of healthy animals from rabbits with clinical signs of disease. Eliminate rabbits with evidence of disease from breeding colonies.
- Closely examine pet rabbits for signs of respiratory disease before purchase.

Pneumonia

Pneumonia can be acute or chronic and may occur alone or accompany upper respiratory disease.

Etiology

- Pasteurellosis is the most common cause of pneumonia in rabbits. The infection spreads to the lungs from the upper respiratory tract through the trachea or, less frequently, through the bloodstream.
- Other less common causes of bacterial pneumonia include *B. bronchiseptica* and *S. aureus*.
- Stress is an important factor in disease. Sudden temperature changes, poor sanitation, or poor ventilation in high-ammonia areas contribute to the development of disease.

Clinical Signs

- Chronic pneumonia is characterized by labored breathing, weight loss, cachexia, and anorexia.
- Clinical signs are often inapparent until disease is advanced.
- Acute death is common in young rabbits.

Diagnosis

Diagnosis of pneumonia is based on clinical signs and supportive diagnostic tests.

- Auscultate the chest for the presence of crackles, expiratory wheezes, or decreased lung sounds over areas of consolidation or abscess.
- Thoracic radiographs may reveal lung lobe consolidation, air bronchograms, or well-delineated soft-tissue densities if pulmonary abscesses are present.
- A complete blood count may show a relative increase

in heterophil numbers or a reversal of the lymphocyte/heterophil ratio, indicating an inflammatory response.
■ Tracheal washes are very difficult in rabbits because of the anatomy of the oropharynx.
■ Postmortem lesions may include acute fibrinopurulent pneumonia, pleuritis, and septicemia.

Treatment

The prognosis of pneumonia is extremely guarded to poor in most rabbits.

■ Parenteral antibiotic therapy is preferred in rabbits with severe pneumonia.
■ Supportive therapy includes supplemental fluids, vitamins, and force-feeding of anorectic animals.
  • If an indwelling catheter can be placed, give fluids intravenously. Subcutaneous fluid administration is used if catheter placement is too stressful.
■ Force-feed anorectic animals. Hold recumbent animals sternal while feeding.
■ Additional supportive measures include providing oxygen therapy in severely dyspneic rabbits, periodic turning of recumbent animals to prevent hypostatic congestion, and application of ophthalmic ointments.
■ Euthanasia is often elected in severely debilitated rabbits with advanced disease.

GASTROINTESTINAL DISEASES

Diarrhea/Enteritis

Etiology

■ Dietary factors

KEY POINT ▶ Lack of roughage in the diet is a major predisposing factor in diarrhea.

  • Diets high in digestible carbohydrates contribute to overgrowth of pathogenic bacteria by supplying a ready source of fermentable products. Toxins produced by these bacteria are primary factors in enterotoxemia.
■ Bacterial pathogens
  • *Clostridium spiroforme* is the primary pathogen implicated in bacterial enteritis in rabbits. *C. spiroforme* is a gram-positive, anaerobic, spore-forming rod. It can be present as normal gastrointestinal flora. However, with a ready supply of fermentation products, *C. spiroforme* produces iota toxin, which causes severe enterotoxemia.
  • *Escherichia coli* is the second important pathogen associated with enteritis in rabbits. *E. coli* is not part of the normal gut flora but is often found in large numbers in the cecum of rabbits with diarrhea. The bacteria attach to the mucosal epithelium, causing necrosis and disruption of normal intestinal and cecal function.
  • *Bacillus piliformis,* which causes Tyzzer disease, is associated with acute diarrhea and death, primarily in young weanling rabbits. *B. piliformis* may be a subclinical inhabitant of the gut. With stress, the bacteria proliferate and cause severe epithelial necrosis of the cecum, colon, and distal ileum.
  • A *Campylobacter*-like bacteria has been associated with proliferative enterocecocolitis in rabbits.
■ Viruses
  • Rotavirus may be present as normal flora. Occasionally, the virus may act as a mild pathogen by destroying cells that produce disaccharidases and by contributing to carbohydrate overload.
■ Parasites
  • Intestinal coccidiosis is primarily a disease of young rabbits. Several species of intestinal *Eimeria* infect rabbits. Diarrhea produced secondary to intestinal coccidiosis is usually mild. However coccidia may predispose the rabbit to bacterial enteritis (see Coccidiosis). The highly pathogenic *Eimeria stieda* infects the liver.
  • Helminth parasites are rarely a problem in domestic rabbits. The only parasite that occurs commonly is the pinworm, *Passalurus ambigus.*
■ Management-related factors
  • Antibiotic therapy can cause suppression of normal gut flora and overgrowth of pathogenic bacteria. Diarrhea is associated with antibiotics that are active against gram-positive aerobes and selective gram-negative anaerobes. Antibiotic-induced diarrhea has been associated with lincomycin, clindamycin, erythromycin, ampicillin, amoxicillin, cephalexin, and penicillin.
  • Stress is a major factor in diarrhea. Stress-related hormonal release may have a direct effect on intestinal motility and digestion, allowing overgrowth of pathogenic organisms.
  • Hairballs are associated with diarrhea. Hairballs slow gastrointestinal motility, prolonging retention of fermentable food.

Clinical Signs

■ The severity of diarrhea varies from chronic, soft stool to profuse, liquid malodorous feces.
■ Rabbits with mild diarrhea may be otherwise normal. Severe diarrhea may be accompanied by lethargy, weight loss, anorexia, and dehydration.
■ Intestinal gas is often palpable on physical examination.
■ Sudden death may be the only clinical sign in peracute disease.

Diagnosis

Diagnosis of the primary etiology is based on clinical signs, history, and specific tests.

■ Dietary history is very important. Determine the fiber content of the normal feed and the amount of supplemental roughage.
■ Identify bacterial pathogens performing aerobic and anaerobic bacterial culture and sensitivity testing of the feces.
■ Check for coccidiosis by performing a direct fecal smear or fecal flotation, especially in young rabbits.
■ Serum chemistry analysis often reveals electrolyte and metabolic abnormalities in animals with moderate-to-severe diarrhea.

Treatment

- Correct the diet in animals on marginal or deficient dietary fiber levels.
- Give oral *Lactobacillus* supplements daily (see Treatment Techniques).
- Broad-spectrum antibiotics, such as the fluorinated quinolones, trimethoprim/sulfa or chloramphenicol, are indicated if bacterial enteritis is suspected. Oral antibiotics are effective in mild-to-moderate diarrhea. Give antibiotics parenterally in rabbits with severe clinical signs. Avoid antibiotics that may induce enteritis.
- Supportive fluid therapy with lactated Ringer's solution is indicated in moderate-to-severe diarrhea. Oral electrolyte-replacement formulas are used by some clinicians.
- Force-feed anorectic animals.
- If young rabbits test positive for coccidiosis, administer appropriate therapy (see Coccidiosis).

Prevention

- Instruct owners to feed their rabbits proper diets with adequate indigestible fiber content.
- Minimize stress in young or weaning rabbits. Sudden temperature changes, changes in food, overcrowding, or poor sanitation contribute to disease.
- Isolate diseased animals from healthy rabbits.
- Screen young rabbits for coccidiosis or give prophylactic therapy.

Anorexia/Refusal to Eat

Etiology

KEY POINT ▶ Malocclusion and gastric hairballs are the two most common causes of anorexia in rabbits.

- Anorexia may accompany any systemic infectious disease, especially enterotoxemia or pasteurellosis.
- Metabolic abnormalities such as kidney disease are often accompanied by anorexia.
- Anorexia and lethargy can be seen with lead poisoning and other toxicities.

Clinical Signs

Clinical signs vary according to specific etiology (see Malocclusion; Hairballs).

- Rabbits with malocclusion, hairballs, and occasionally lead poisoning often have no other clinical signs. Most remain alert and active.
- Excessive salivation is common in rabbits with malocclusion.
- Some rabbits with hairballs become depressed, lethargic, dehydrated, and develop diarrhea.

Diagnosis

- Perform a thorough oral examination in all anorectic rabbits. Examine the back molars with an otoscope. Sedation is not usually necessary.
- A hairball is often palpable as either a soft and compressible or firm mass in the cranial abdomen.
- Contrast radiography of the abdomen can be used to confirm the presence of a hairball (see Hairballs).
- A complete blood count and serum chemistry analysis are indicated in rabbits with suspected infectious or systemic diseases.

Treatment

- Molar malocclusion requires sedation for dentistry. Overgrown incisors can be clipped using manual restraint.
- Hairballs can be managed medically in most rabbits (see Hairballs).
- Manage specific infectious and metabolic diseases according to the etiology.
- Force-feed a nutritional supplement or a gruel made from rabbit pellets three to four times daily until the appetite returns.
- Most anorectic rabbits will begin to eat leafy greens, vegetables, fruit, or hay before pellets. Always provide access to these foods.

Malocclusion

Etiology

- Malocclusion of the teeth as a result of prognathism is a common problem in pet rabbits. It is a genetically-linked autosomal recessive trait, but it can occur sporadically in breeding stock.
- Other factors, such as diet, infection of the tooth root, or trauma, may play a lesser role in the development of malocclusion.
- Overgrowth of incisors, molars, or both can occur.

Clinical Signs

- Incisor malocclusion is usually noticed by the owner. Rabbits may stop eating or have difficulty prehending food.
- Rabbits with molar malocclusion are reluctant to eat or completely anoretic. Often, a rabbit will reject pellets but continue to eat soft foods.
- Many rabbits with malocclusion salivate excessively. The owner may note hair loss around the mouth or moist dermatitis on the chin or dewlap.
- Incisor malocclusion is occasionally seen in weanling rabbits but usually has a later onset. Molar malocclusion is usually first noted at 2 to 3 years of age.

Diagnosis

Diagnosis is based on oral examination. Skull or dental radiographs are sometimes needed.

- Use an otoscope to examine the cheek teeth.
- Usually the lateral edges of the upper cheek teeth overgrow and abrade the buccal mucosa. The medial edges of the lower cheek teeth overgrow and cut or entrap the tongue.
- Skull or dental radiographs are helpful in evaluating the roots of the teeth for evidence of infection. Anesthesia is usually necessary to obtain good positioning.

Treatment

- Incisors can be cut with a diagonal cutter, rongeur, or dental drill. Both pairs of upper incisors should be clipped. *Do not use Resco-type nail clippers to cut incisors, because excessive trauma and loosening of the roots can result.*
- Molar malocclusion requires dentistry with sedation. The procedure is usually short and can be done using an injectable tranquilizer. Gas anesthesia requires a face mask or endotracheal tube, making it difficult to work in the very limited space in the oral cavity.
  - Place the rabbit in sternal recumbency with an assistant extending the neck and head forward.
  - Loop strips of gauze around both upper and lower incisors to hold the mouth open. The assistant holds the gauze around the lower molars in one hand. The second hand is placed on top of the rabbit's head, holding the gauze looped around the top incisors and forcing the head and neck into extension. Make sure the nostrils are not occluded and the neck is extended or the rabbit will have difficulty breathing.
- Use a short vaginal speculum to spread open the oral cavity. Check both lateral and medial edges of upper and lower molars.
- A small bone rongeur can be used to clip the sharp edges of the cheek teeth. Use a tongue depressor to push the tongue to one side while clipping the medial edges of the lower cheek teeth. This method is quick and easy, but leaves rough edges and may cause fractures of the teeth.
- A dental drill will round and smooth sharp edges. Use a tongue depressor or the vaginal speculum to isolate the arcade and prevent damage to the tongue or buccal mucosa.

Prevention

- Most rabbits with incisor malocclusion need their incisors clipped every 3 to 4 weeks. Many owners are willing to do this procedure at home.
- Check rabbits with molar malocclusion every 2 to 3 months. Dentistry may be needed as often as every month or only once yearly.
- Rabbits with malocclusion should not be bred.

Hairballs (Trichobezoars)

Etiology

KEY POINT ▶ Inadequate dietary roughage is associated with an increased incidence of hairballs in rabbits. Rabbits on low-roughage diets also have an increased incidence of fur-chewing.

- Other factors may contribute to formation of hairballs. Long-haired breeds may consume large amounts of hair while grooming during shedding season. Hormonal influences in breeding season may contribute to aggression and fur-barbering. Mineral deficiencies may cause pica of hair. Boredom may also be a factor.
- Rabbits are unable to vomit, contributing to accumulation of hair.

Clinical Signs

- Anorexia is the primary clinical sign associated with trichobezoars. Often rabbits remain alert and active, with no other signs.
- With chronic problems, weight loss, depression, palpable intestinal gas, and a decreased amount of feces may be noted.
- Diarrhea may be present in some animals (see Diarrhea/Enteritis).
- Acute pyloric obstruction causes severe depression, lethargy, bloating, dehydration, hypothermia, and shock.

Diagnosis

KEY POINT ▶ Suspect a hairball in an anorectic but otherwise alert rabbit with a history of inadequate dietary fiber and excessive shedding.

- Palpation of a soft mass in the stomach area in an anorectic rabbit is evidence of a hairball. The stomach of a healthy rabbit is normally full. However, a rabbit that has been anorectic for several days should have an empty stomach.
- Radiographs are not necessary but may be used to confirm a diagnosis. An enlarged stomach may be visible on plain radiographs. Contrast radiography of the upper gastrointestinal tract may outline the hairball. Barium is given at a standard small-animal dose of 10 to 14 ml/kg orally into the cheek pouch.
- Ultrasound examination can be used to detect a mass in the stomach area.
- A complete blood count and serum chemistry analysis may be indicated in severely ill or debilitated animals.

Treatment

- Medical management is successful in most rabbits in my experience. Although some clinicians advocate routine surgical removal of hairballs, the risk of surgical or anesthetic complications is increased considering the debilitated condition of most of these rabbits.
  - The proteolytic enzymes bromelin and papain will dissolve rabbit fur. These enzymes are present in fresh (not heat-processed) pineapple juice. Pineapple juice is given orally at 10 ml/day for 3 to 5 days in a medium-sized rabbit. The treatment is repeated in 3 to 5 days if anorexia has not resolved. As an alternative, bromelin or papain enzyme tablets can be purchased from a health-food store and administered orally. Dosage is empirical at 1 to 2 tablets daily for 3 to 5 days.
  - Give the rabbit oral cat laxatives (e.g., Laxatone; Evsco Pharmaceuticals, Buena, NJ) at 1 to 2 ml/day for 3 to five days to aid in fur passage.
  - Force-feed nutritional supplements or slurried rabbit pellets until the rabbit's appetite returns.
  - Offer free-choice hay and fresh vegetables at all times.
- Surgical intervention is necessary in rabbits with clinical signs of acute pyloric obstruction. In my

experience, the mortality rate is very high even with surgical intervention.

Prevention

- Give pineapple juice or enzyme tablets to heavy shedders for 2 to 3 consecutive days every few months.

KEY POINT ▶ Correct the diet to include adequate dietary fiber (see Nutrition).

- Routinely brush long-haired rabbits or heavy shedders.

Coccidiosis
Etiology

- Coccidia are host-specific protozoan parasites.
- There are at least ten different species of intestinal *Eimeria*. Pathogenicity varies according to species. *Eimeria magna* is the most pathogenic species affecting the small intestine.
- Hepatic coccidiosis results from infection with the highly pathogenic *Eimeria stieda*.
- Coccidiosis is primarily a disease of young and weanling rabbits. Natural immunity develops against each *Eimeria* species after exposure. There is no cross-protection in immunity between different *Eimeria* species. Adult animals can become ill if exposed to a species against which they have no immunity.
- The severity of disease is determined by the age at time of exposure, the species of *Eimeria* involved, the number of oocysts ingested, and the environmental stress factors.

Clinical Signs

- Intestinal coccidiosis is often subclinical or causes only mild-to-moderate diarrhea. However, coccidia may predispose the rabbit to the development of bacterial enteritis (see Diarrhea/Enteritis).
- Severe diarrhea and death may occur with heavy infections.
- Hepatic coccidiosis is associated with anorexia, weight loss, abdominal enlargement, diarrhea, icterus, and acute death.

Diagnosis

Diagnosis is based on identification of *Eimeria* oocysts in a fecal sample.

Treatment and Prevention

The age of the host and the severity of clinical signs are factors to consider in treatment. Animals with light parasite burdens may develop immunity and recover without therapy.

- Therapy with coccidiostats is more prophylactic than therapeutic. Coccidia are susceptible to treatment only during a specific period in the protozoan life cycle. Clinical signs are usually inapparent during this period.
- Coccidiostats may slow multiplication until host immunity develops.

- Sulfonamides are effective in prophylaxis. Sulfaquinoxaline is the only drug approved for use in commercially raised rabbits in the United States; however, other sulfa drugs are more effective.
  - Administer sulfaquinoxaline in the feed at 0.025 to 0.03% continuously for 4 to 5 weeks during weaning or add it to the drinking water at 0.025 to 0.1% in alternating 2-week periods for 4 to 8 weeks during weaning.
  - Give sulfadimethoxine orally at 50 mg/kg once, then at 25 mg/kg, daily for 21 days.
  - Add amprolium (9.6% solution) to the drinking water at 5 ml/gallon for 21 days.
  - Add sulfamethazine to the feed at 0.05 to 1.0%.
- Sanitation is of utmost importance for effective therapy and prevention. Routinely disinfect cages, food bowls, and water bottles.
- Screen rabbits for shedding of coccidial oocysts. Separate or cull carriers from colonies.
- Check all young rabbits for coccidia.

UROGENITAL/REPRODUCTIVE DISEASES
Uterine Adenocarcinoma/Hyperplasia
Etiology

- Uterine adenocarcinoma is the most frequent type of tumor occurring in domestic rabbits.
- Adenocarcinoma rarely occurs in does younger than 3 years of age. The incidence in rabbits older than 3 years of age ranges from 50 to 80% in certain breeds. Uterine adenocarcinoma is rare in Rex, Belgian, and Polish breeds, suggesting a genetic component to the disease.
- Endometrial changes resulting from senile atrophy of the glandular epithelial cells and stroma may precede neoplasia, although a direct association has not been proven. Estrogen may play a role in enhancement of tumor growth.
- Endometrial changes that may precede neoplastic changes include endometriosis; endometritis; and papillary, cystic, or adenomatous hyperplasia.

Clinical Signs

- Uterine adenocarcinoma is a slow-growing tumor with a 5- to 24-month clinical course. Metastasis occurs late in the clinical course, after 10 to 12 months. Metastasis occurs locally to the peritoneum, lymph nodes, and liver before hematogenous spread.
- Clinical signs are usually inapparent during the early hyperplastic stages. Owners may notice increased aggressiveness in some does.
- Decreased reproductive performance is an early sign in breeding rabbits. Small litter size, stillbirths, dystocia, litter desertion, and infertility are seen.
- Pet owners may notice blood in the urine or a bloody discharge from the vaginal area.
- Cystic mastitis occurs in association with uterine changes in some does.

Diagnosis

- Recall that affected does are usually 3 years of age or older.

- An enlarged, thickened uterus or multiple rounded caudal abdominal masses may be palpable on physical examination. It is sometimes difficult to differentiate a mass from abdominal fat in small does.
- An enlarged uterus is usually observed on abdominal radiographs.
- Abdominal ultrasonography can also be used for identification of the uterine mass and for detection of metastases.

Treatment

- Ovariohysterectomy is successful if done before metastasis has occurred.
- Prognosis is poor after metastasis has occurred. Euthanasia is recommended.

Prevention

- Consider ovariohysterectomy in does older than 3 years of age with evidence of cystic mastitis or increased aggressive behavior.
- Some clinicians recommend routine ovariohysterectomy of does before 3 years of age, excluding breeds of very low incidence (Belgian, Rex, and Polish breeds).

Mastitis

Etiology

Mastitis in rabbits can be either septic or nonseptic.

- Septic mastitis is most common in lactating does. Trauma to the mammary gland and poor sanitation predispose to infection.
- *Staphylococcus* and *Streptococcus* spp are the most commonly isolated bacteria. *E. coli* and *Pseudomonas, Pasteurella,* and *Klebsiella* spp may also cause mastitis.
- Nonseptic, cystic mastitis is seen in nonbreeding females. It may be associated with increased estrogen, uterine hyperplasia, and uterine adenocarcinoma.

Clinical Signs

- In septic mastitis, the affected gland is swollen, erythematous, and warm to the touch. The tissues later become cyanotic. Infection spreads until all glands are affected.
- Systemic signs of septic mastitis include pyrexia, depression, anorexia, death of neonates, and death of the doe.
- In cystic mastitis, glands became swollen, firm, and bluish in color with a clear-to-dark serosanguineous discharge from the teat. Rabbits are not systemically ill.

Diagnosis

- Diagnosis of septic mastitis is based on clinical signs, history of lactation or pseudocyesis, and isolation of bacteria on culture of gland tissue or exudate.
- Diagnosis of cystic mastitis is based on history of a nonbreeding doe, usually older than 3 years of age,

with no known trauma to the glandular tissue. Culture and sensitivity testing of the discharge is negative for bacterial growth.

Treatment

- Antibiotic therapy is indicated in septic mastitis. Therapy is based on culture and sensitivity testing. Warm compresses 2 to 3 times daily may also be helpful. Surgical drainage or excision may be necessary with mammary abscesses.
- Cystic mastitis will resolve with ovariohysterectomy. Severely affected glands may be surgically excised.

Prevention

- Keep lactating does in a clean environment. Make sure there are no sharp surfaces or wire edges that may traumatize the teats.
- Routinely examine lactating does for evidence of inflammation or teat injuries.
- Cystic mastitis can be prevented by routine ovariohysterectomy.

Dysuria/Hematuria

Etiology

- Red, pink, or orange discoloration of the urine occurs periodically in healthy rabbits. The color may be the result of a porphyrin pigment or a food-related metabolite excreted in the urine.
- Thick, white urine indicates the presence of large quantities of mineral precipitates. Unlike other mammals, calcium absorption and blood calcium concentration are directly related to dietary calcium intake in rabbits. Excessive calcium intake will result in excretion of large amounts of calcium in the urine. Calcium is excreted in the bile in other mammals.
- Hematuria occurs commonly with cystitis. Frank blood independent of or at the end of urination may indicate the presence of uterine adenocarcinoma.
- Cystic calculi occur in both male and female rabbits. Calculi are usually composed of calcium carbonate and may be associated with high dietary calcium intake.

Clinical Signs

- Rabbits with urinary pigment changes or excessive calcium in the urine usually have no other clinical signs.
- Dysuria and stranguria may accompany cystitis and cystic calculi.
- Lethargy, anorexia, and depression may be seen in rabbits with cystitis or cystic calculi.

Diagnosis

- Differentiate hematuria from pigment changes in the urine by simple dipstick analysis. If urine discoloration is intermittent, dispense dipsticks for owners to check the urine at home.
- Measure blood calcium concentrations in rabbits excreting large amounts of urinary calcium. Blood

calcium concentrations often reach as high as 19 mg/dl.

■ Urinalysis, serum chemistry analysis, complete blood count, and urine culture are indicated in rabbits with clinical signs of cystitis, cystic calculi, or hematuria.

■ Distinguish between hematuria and hemorrhagic vaginal discharge occurring secondary to uterine adenocarcinoma by physical examination, history, and urinalysis. Uterine adenocarcinoma is likely in an older doe with a thickened uterus or multiple abdominal masses.

■ Perform radiography if cystic calculi are suspected. Calculi are usually radiopaque and therefore visible in the bladder or urethra. Large amounts of calcium sediment may be visible in the bladder in rabbits excreting large amounts of calcium.

Treatment

Treatment is not necessary in rabbits with pigment-based changes in urine color.

■ Attempt to lower dietary calcium levels in rabbits with consistently high blood calcium concentrations. Grass hay (e.g., timothy) has a lower calcium content than legume hay (e.g., alfalfa). Decrease the amount of pelleted feed, which is alfalfa-based, and substitute grains and grass hay.

■ Treat rabbits with simple bacterial cystitis with antibiotics. A 3-week course of chloramphenicol or trimethoprim sulfate is usually effective. The urine should be recultured after 4 to 6 weeks.

■ Cystic calculi must be removed surgically (see sec. 8, chap. 7). Submit calculi for stone analysis.

■ Lower dietary calcium intake postoperatively to help prevent recurrence.

Prevention

For prevention, lower dietary calcium intake, especially in older rabbits. Most pelleted diets exceed dietary calcium requirements. Substitute grass hay for alfalfa hay in the diet.

Treponematosis

Etiology

■ *Treponema cuniculi* is the etiologic agent of rabbit syphilis.

■ *T. cuniculi* is a spiral-shaped bacterium transmitted by direct contact between breeding rabbits or from doe to offspring.

■ Cold environmental conditions may predispose to development of the disease.

Clinical Signs

■ Most lesions occur on the external genitalia. The nose, eyelids, lips, and perineal area are less commonly involved. Initial lesions consist of erythematous vesicles that progress to papules, ulcerations, scaliness, and dry crusty lesions.

■ Nasal lesions in pet rabbits are commonly mistaken as dermatophyte lesions.

■ Rabbits remain alert, responsive, and active.

■ The incidence of abortions, metritis, and infertility may increase in breeding females.

Diagnosis

Diagnosis is based on history, clinical signs, and response to therapy. Supportive diagnostic tests are done as needed.

■ Perform fungal cultures and skin scrapings to rule out dermatophytes and ectoparasites.

■ *Treponema* organisms can be identified by darkfield microscopic examination of skin scrapings. The organisms can also be demonstrated histologically with silver stains of skin biopsy sections.

■ Serologic tests are available to determine the presence of antibodies against *T. cuniculi*. These include the rapid plasma reagin test (RPR), the Venereal Disease Research Laboratory (VDRL) slide test, and the Wasserman complement fixation test.
  • A fluorescent antibody test against treponemal antigen is also used. An ELISA test is available from some laboratories to screen for antibodies against *Treponema*. These tests are used for screening in rabbit breeding colonies.

Treatment

■ *T. cuniculi* is susceptible to penicillin. Give long-acting three injections of benzathine penicillin G at 42,000 to 84,000 IU/kg IM at weekly intervals. Response is rapid; lesions dramatically regress, usually after one injection.

Prevention

■ Screen rabbits in breeding colonies for treponematosis.

■ The incidence of disease in pet rabbits is low. Preventive serologic screening is not necessary.

NEUROMUSCULAR/SKELETAL DISEASES

Mandibular and Joint Abscesses

Etiology

■ Abscesses of the mandible and joints occur frequently in pet rabbits, and usually are caused by *Pasteurella multocida*. Bacteria spread hematogenously from the initial infection site (see Pasteurellosis).

■ Overgrowth of the cheek teeth may sometimes accompany mandibular abscesses. Infection may spread from the oral cavity along the tooth root.

■ Soft-tissue abscesses occasionally occur in the oral cavity secondary to a penetrating wound from a foreign body.

Clinical Signs

■ Joint abscesses are most frequent in the distal limb joints. The swellings are large, firm, and warm to the touch. Rabbits may be lame, depending on which joints are involved.

- Mandibular abscesses occur as firm swellings in the ventral facial area. Abscesses are sometimes quite large before they are apparent to the owner. Excessive ptyalism may be an early symptom.
- Affected rabbits may refuse to eat if mandibular abscesses are accompanied by dental disease.
- Many rabbits remain active and alert with no other clinical signs.

Diagnosis

- Thick, white purulent exudate is present on fine needle aspirate. Cytologic examination of the exudate shows bacteria, neutrophils, and proteinaceous debris.
- Radiographs are necessary to determine whether bone involvement is present.
- Bacterial culture and sensitivity testing are indicated if treatment is elected. Submit tissue samples at the time of surgical debridement.

Treatment

The prognosis for successful therapy is guarded. With bony involvement, the prognosis is poor.

- Simple lancing of mandibular abscesses is ineffective because of the thick, viscous nature of the exudate. Surgically debride the area vigorously using general anesthesia. Place drains at the surgical site, allow them to remain for 2 to 3 days, and flush the area thoroughly twice daily with sterile saline or dilute chlorhexidine solution. Use sterile cotton swabs to remove necrotic tissue and exudate. Continue flushing the area after the drains are removed.
- Recurrence is common, and serial surgical debridements are usually necessary.
- Joint abscesses are difficult to debride surgically and drain because of the caseous nature of the exudate.
- Amputation of the affected limb may be the most effective therapy for abscesses involving the joint and surrounding bone. Rabbits adapt well to amputation of either a fore or rear limb.
- Disease may recur in other joints, even if amputation of the affected limb has been performed. Hematogenous spread of the bacterial infection to other joints may occur at any time during the clinical course.
- Long-term antibiotic therapy is necessary. Some rabbits respond to fluoroquinolone therapy in combination with surgical debridement or amputation.
- The owners must be committed to the time required for wound management and nursing care. Daily wound debridement, cleaning, flushing, and bandage changes are necessary.

Torticollis/Head Tilt/Ataxia

Etiology

- Bacterial infection of the inner ear, middle ear, or meninges is the most common cause of torticollis in pet rabbits. The primary etiologic agent is *Pasteurella multocida*.
- *Encephalitozoon cuniculi* is another common cause of torticollis and incoordination in rabbits.
- Vascular lesions and toxicities (e.g., lead poisoning) are less common causes of head tilt and incoordination.

Clinical Signs

- Onset may be acute or slowly progressive. The head tilt may be mild or accompanied by torticollis, incoordination, and the inability to stand.
- Some rabbits have no other clinical signs. Other rabbits become depressed, anorectic, and lethargic.
- Rabbits with severe depression, positional nystagmus, and facial nerve deficits may have brain or meningeal lesions.

Diagnosis

Diagnosis is based on clinical signs. Establishment of the exact etiology may be difficult.

- Carefully examine both ear canals for evidence of infection.
- A complete blood count may show an inflammatory response, which may indicate an infectious etiology.
- Skull radiographs may aid in diagnosis. Anesthesia is usually necessary for proper positioning. Bony changes in the bulla may indicate osteomyelitis.
- Serology can be used to detect antibodies against *E. cuniculi* or *P. multocida*. A positive serologic test is not diagnostic of the etiology but is helpful in ruling out some possible causes.
- Often, the etiologic agent cannot be established, and a tentative diagnosis is based on response to therapy. Rabbits with pasteurellosis often improve with long-term antibiotic therapy and supportive care. Rabbits with parasitic migrations may remain unchanged or improve gradually. Rabbits with clinical signs secondary to encephalitozoonosis are usually unresponsive to treatment or they deteriorate clinically.
- Final etiology may be determined only on postmortem examination.

Treatment

- Give antibiotics for 4 to 6 weeks. Choose an antibiotic that penetrates the blood-brain barrier and is effective against pasteurellosis (e.g., chloramphenicol, enrofloxacin, ciprofloxacin).
- If exudate is visible in the ear canal, clean and flush the ear thoroughly. Tranquilization or anesthesia may be necessary. Administer a topical antibiotic in the ear canal 3 to 4 times daily. Systemic antibiotics are given concurrently.
- An oral *Lactobacillus* supplement is recommended during long-term antibiotic therapy.
- Supportive care is necessary in rabbits that are laterally recumbent or have severe torticollis. Recumbent rabbits should be turned every 6 to 8 hours or propped up sternally to prevent hypostatic congestion of the lung. Apply eye lubrication several times daily if the blink reflex is diminished. Hand-feeding may be required. Keep rabbits on clean, dry bedding to prevent urine scalding and contact dermatitis.
- Inform owners about the amount of supportive care needed in recumbent rabbits. Many owners elect

euthanasia when faced with the difficulties and the time required for long-term nursing care.

■ Steroids are sometimes used if other treatments fail or if diagnostic test results are negative for pasteurellosis. Give prednisolone orally 0.25 to 0.5 mg/kg q12h for 3 days, q24h for 3 days, then on alternate days. Give antibiotics concurrently.

■ Euthanasia is often selected in debilitated rabbits if there is no clinical improvement after several days of therapy.

Encephalitozoonosis

Etiology

■ *E. cuniculi* is an obligate intracellular microsporidian parasite prevalent in domestic and wild rabbits. The organism infects mice, rats, hamsters, and guinea pigs less commonly.

■ The major route of transmission is ingestion of spore-contaminated urine. Vertical transmission through the placenta is suspected.

■ The organism becomes established in the kidney 30 to 40 days after ingestion. Signs of kidney disease are not evident. Infection progresses to the brain after several weeks at which time neurologic signs may be evident.

Clinical Signs

■ Infections are usually chronic and latent. Diagnosis is usually confirmed on necropsy.

■ In some rabbits, clinical signs of torticollis, ataxia, seizures, paresis, and death may occur.

Diagnosis

Etiology is based on clinical signs and antemortem testing of rabbits exhibiting neurologic signs or on postmortem examination.

■ Several serologic tests are available to detect the presence of *E. cuniculi*. These include a complement fixation test, an indirect fluorescent antibody test, and an India ink immunoreaction test. An ELISA test has also been developed for detection of antibodies against the organism. These tests are usually available through laboratory animal research centers.

■ If serologic testing is not available, presumptive diagnosis is made based on clinical signs and response to therapy. Clinical signs of encephalitozoonosis are similar to those of the neurologic form of pasteurellosis. However, rabbits with encephalitozoonosis usually decline rapidly despite aggressive antibiotic therapy and supportive care. Death often occurs within several days of onset of clinical signs. If more than one rabbit is exposed, there may be multiple deaths.

Treatment

■ There is no effective therapy for encephalitozoonosis.

Prevention

■ Identify carriers in rabbit colonies and breeding facilities through serologic testing and culling of animals that test positive.

■ Eliminate urine contamination between cages through proper sanitation procedures.

■ Prevent possible contact between pet rabbits housed outdoors and wild rabbits or rodents by elevating cages off the ground or housing pets in a rodent proof enclosure.

Vertebral Fractures

Etiology

■ The rear leg muscles of rabbits are well developed for strong kicking and thumping.

■ If rabbits are poorly restrained with inadequate control of the rear legs, animals may kick suddenly, resulting in fracture of their spinal vertebrae.

Clinical Signs

■ Clinical signs of a fractured back include partial or complete paralysis of the rear legs and loss of normal bladder and bowel function.

■ Signs are acute in onset and directly related to a traumatic incident.

■ Other etiologies may cause clinical signs similar to a vertebral fracture. Multifocal infection of the spinal cord secondary to pasteurellosis, parasite migration, or vascular thrombosis within the cord can cause neurologic deficits; however, the clinical onset is usually more chronic and slowly progressive than that in a fracture.

Diagnosis

■ Diagnosis is based on history and clinical signs.

■ Radiographs of the vertebral column are necessary to confirm the presence of a fracture.

Treatment

■ Prognosis for recovery is guarded to poor. Euthanasia is usually recommended.

■ If steroids are given, use anti-inflammatory dosages on a decreasing dosing schedule as outlined in the section on Torticollis.

■ Surgical stabilization is impractical because of the poor prognosis and degree of nursing care necessary.

■ Some owners will try long-term supportive care to see if neurologic function will return. They must be instructed on manual expression of the bladder and general nursing care.

Long Bone Fractures/Joint Luxations

Etiology

■ The skeleton of the rabbit is light and fragile. The tibia, radius, and ulna fracture easily with trauma.

■ Traumatic joint luxations of the elbow or stifle joint occasionally occur.

Clinical Signs

- Rabbits with long bone fractures or luxations are acutely lame.
- Fractures are usually palpable on physical examination. Joint luxations are palpable as firm swellings.

Diagnosis

- Diagnosis is based on history, clinical signs, and physical examination.
- Radiographs are necessary to evaluate fractures for surgical repair or to confirm the presence of joint luxations.

Treatment

- Splints used in combination with padded bandages are usually adequate for stabilization of metatarsal, metacarpal, and phalangeal fractures. Bandage the foot in a functional position. Contour a moldable splint or casting material (e.g., Hexcelite NS; Hexcel Medical, Dublin, CA) along the plantar surface.
- With joint luxations, anesthesia is needed to manipulate the joint into normal position. A lateral or caudal splint is then applied. Many luxations are unstable and will not remain in normal position. Surgery may be elected to stabilize the joint. How-

ever, many rabbits compensate well with a permanently luxated joint.

- Long bone fractures are more difficult to manage. Surgical reduction and stabilization are sometimes successful, but complications can occur because of the fragility of the bones. Bones may splinter or shatter during attempted reduction. Surgical procedures may need to be modified and used in combination with restricted cage rest until healing occurs. Severely comminuted or open fractures are sometimes best managed with limb amputation.

Supplemental Readings

Cheeke PR: *Rabbit Feeding and Nutrition.* Orlando: Academic Press, 1987.

Cheeke PR, Patton NM, Lukefahr SD, et al: *Rabbit Production.* Danville: The Interstate Printers and Publishers, 1987.

Harkness JE, Wagner JE: *The Biology and Medicine of Rabbits and Rodents.* Philadelphia: Lea & Febiger, 1989.

Kraus AL, Weisbroth SH, Flatt RE, et al: Biology and diseases of rabbits. *In* Fox JG, Cohen BJ, Loew FM, eds.: *Laboratory Animal Medicine.* Orlando: Academic Press, 1984, p 207.

National Research Council (NRC): *Nutrient Requirements of Rabbits.* Washington, D.C.: National Academy of Sciences, 1977.

Schoeb TR, Fox JG: Enterocecocolitis associated with intraepithelial *Campylobacter*-like bacteria in rabbits *(Oryctolagus cuniculus).* Vet Pathol 27:73, 1990.

Toth LA, Krueger JM: Hematologic effects of exposure to three infective agents in rabbits. J Am Vet Med Assoc 195:981, 1989.

Weisbroth SH, Flatt RE, Kraus AL, eds.: *The Biology of the Laboratory Rabbit.* New York: Academic Press, 1974.

Basic Husbandry and Medicine of Pocket Pets

Nancy L. Anderson

All small rodents commonly kept in people's homes for companionship and enjoyment are considered pocket pets. This chapter provides the information needed to treat the most frequently encountered pocket pets, including mice, rats, gerbils, hamsters, guinea pigs, and chinchillas.

HUSBANDRY

Caging and Sanitation

- The best cages for pocket pets are made of stainless steel, hard plastic, or glass. These materials are easily cleaned and sanitized and are resistant to gnawing and corrosion by urine and fecal matter. Minimum floor space and height requirements and environmental requirements are listed for each species in Table 1. With the exception of guinea pigs, all species need cages with secure lids.
- Guinea pigs can be housed in open-topped enclosures with walls higher than 10 inches. Take care to ensure that dogs, cats, wild animals, and small children do not have unsupervised access to these cages.
- Clean cages as needed, usually 1 to 3 times per week for most rodents. A scrub brush, dish soap, and water work well. If cages are not kept clean, ammonia, other irritants, moisture, and bacteria rise to harmful levels, predisposing the animals to disease.
- Disinfect the cage twice a month with 1 part sodium hypochlorite mixed in 30 parts water. Let the bleach solution stand for at least 15 minutes. Rinse the cage well after disinfection.

- All solid-floored cages need bedding. Shredded paper, nonresinous wood shavings, wood wool, and corn cobs are all acceptable. Provide at least 2 inches of bedding. Most rodents enjoy burrowing in deeper bedding when it is provided in one corner of a cage. Filling a cage with bedding usually leads to poor sanitation as a result of owners' failure to recognize buildup of hidden wastes such as moisture from leaking water bottles, cached foods, urine, and feces.
- Successful use of wire-mesh floors is dependent on the dimensions of the mesh. Size the openings to be just large enough for an adult to retract a tarsal joint back through the mesh. Larger holes make it difficult for the animals to walk and cause pressure sores. Smaller openings cause injuries such as tibial fractures and self mutilation because animals struggle to free caught appendages. Bedding over the wire floor prevents waste from dropping out of the cage and therefore is not recommended. Wire-bottom cages do not work well for breeding because neonatal rodents require nesting material to maintain moisture levels and prevent dehydration. Young rodents often cannot walk correctly on mesh sized for adult feet.
- All pocket pets require visual security. Tubes, jars, and cans, made of nontoxic, nonabrasive substances work well as cage furniture. Provide objects for gnawing. Rodents possess open-rooted teeth. Constant wear is necessary to maintain normal dentition. Mice, rats, gerbils, and hamsters enjoy and benefit from exercise wheels.
- A good room temperature range for most pocket pets is 70 to 75°F. Keep rodents that are suffering

TABLE 1. Caging and Environmental Requirements for Pocket Pets

	Rat	Mouse	Guinea Pig	Chinchilla	Hamster	Gerbil
Air changes/hour	10–15	10–15	10–15	>6	>6	>6
Minimum cage floor space/animal (square inches)	35	15	101	288	20	36
Minimum cage height (inches)	>6	>5	>10	>12	>6	>6
Recommended room temperature (°C)	21.1–26.6	21.1–29.4	18.3–23.8	15.5–21.1	18.3–23.8	21.1
Maximum–minimum room temperature (°C)	18.3–29.4	18.3–31	12.7–32.2	10–23.8	12.7–23.8	18.3–29.4
Room humidity (%)	50–70	30–70	40–70	40–60	30–70	30–50
Cage-cleaning frequency (in days)	2–7	2–7	3–4	7	3–7	14
Light cycle–hours light:hours dark	12–14 : 10–12	12 : 12	12 : 12	>12.5 : 11.5	12 : 12	12 : 12

from disease at 85° to 90°F unless hyperthermia is of concern (e.g., in some chinchillas).

- Hamsters, guinea pigs, and chinchillas that are exposed to cool temperatures may hibernate for a few days or until the ambient temperature rises.
- Heart rates may be less than 5 beats per minute.
- Hibernation does not occur if room temperatures are kept above 65°F.

Nutrition

KEY POINT ▶ Feed pocket pets appropriately labeled laboratory animal chow (Table 2). Seed diets are deficient in protein and contain excessive fat.

- Seeds, as well as vegetables and other foods, may be fed as treats, but should not provide more than 15% of calories. Intermittent exposure to vegetables and seeds causes mild, transient diarrhea.
  - Store food in tightly sealed containers at less than 60°F; keep food refrigerated if possible.
- Feed diets within 90 days of milling to ensure the highest nutritional value. Encourage owners to check dates on packages and ask pet store managers about receiving dates on bulk items.
- If possible, feed all pocket pets except guinea pigs from overhead racks. These devices reduce waste and eliminate fecal contamination of food. Many owners are resistant to using these devices. Covered hoppers, heavy crocks, or stainless-steel bowls that are attached to the side of the cage to eliminate spillage are acceptable and recommended for guinea pigs.
- Feed breeding females and their litters from the floor of their cages until the young are large enough to reach overhead feeders or crawl in and out of crocks.
  - Usually, the cage is cleaned and a 10- to 13-day food supply is left in the cage 1 to 2 days before parturition to minimize cannibalism of neonates as a result of stress associated with cage cleaning.

KEY POINT ▶ Change water daily

- Open crocks are not acceptable because of contamination that leads to disease and spillage that leads to dehydration and poor sanitation. Sipper tubes and water bottles work well. Clean tubes and bottles daily with dish soap and water, and disinfect them weekly. Guinea pigs blow food into their sipper tubes. This practice necessitates more frequent cleaning. Some water bottles have special valves to minimize backflow. Supplement guinea pigs' water daily with 200 mg vitamin C per liter. If the water is not dechlorinated, it will inactivate the vitamin C.

Quarantine

- Quarantine all newly acquired animals in a different room from current pets for a minimum of 30 days. Feed and handle quarantined animals last. Recommend that caretakers wash their hands and change clothes before handling current pets. Avoid introductions of adult animals because this frequently results in fighting. Place animals together while they are young and allow them to mature together. More than one male pocket pet per cage leads to aggression, except in rats.

HISTORY AND PHYSICAL EXAMINATION

A systematic history and physical examination is mandatory in managing problems in pocket pets. Many

TABLE 2. Dietary Information for Pocket Pets

	Rat	Mouse	Guinea Pig	Chinchilla	Hamster	Gerbil
Recommended diet	Laboratory rodent chow	Laboratory rodent chow	Guinea pig chow	Chinchilla chow	Hamster chow	Laboratory rodent chow
Supplements and treats	<15% of calories, avoid seeds	<15% of calories, avoid seeds	Vitamin C 200 mg/L, drinking water, cabbage/kale	Ad lib grass, hay	<15% of calories, avoid fats and seeds	<15% of calories, avoid fats and seeds
Food consumption (gm food/100 gm body weight/day)	5–10	15	3–6	3–6	10–12	5–8
Water consumption (ml water/100 gm body weight/day)	10–12	15	10–40		8–30	4–7
Recommended protein (%)	12–27	16–20	18–30		15–25	16–22
Recommended fat (%)	5–25	5–25			3–5	2–4
Recommended carbohydrate (%)		45–55	16		8	
Recommended minimum fiber (%)			16–18			

TABLE 3. Normal Physiologic Data for Pocket Pets

	Rat	Mouse	Guinea Pig	Chinchilla	Hamster	Gerbil
Life span (years)	2–4	1–3.5	3–6	8–10	1.5–2.5	3–5
Heart rate (bpm)	250–600	325–780	150–400	40–100	250–600	360
Respiratory rate (breaths/minute)	33–127	60–230	42–130	40–80	33–155	70–120
Body weight (gm) Male	300–520	38–42	900–1200	450–600	85–110	60–110
Female	250–300	30–35	700–900	550–800	95–120	50–80
Birth weight (gm)	5–6	0.5–1.5	60–115	30–50	2–3	2.5–3
Body temperature (°C)	35.9–38.2	35.5–38	37.2–40	36.1–37.8	36.2–37.5	38.1–38.4
Gender determination in neonates	At 7 days, the anogenital distance of males is 5 mm, of females 2.5 mm Females show nipples at 8–15 days	Visualize testicles through skin in neonates	Anogenital distance in males is 10 mm, in females, 5 mm			

syndromes are the result of poor husbandry and ignorance of the owner. Pets that have been isolated from other rodents or acquired from a private breeder are less likely to suffer from infectious disease than animals recently obtained from a pet store, laboratory, or wholesaler. (See Table 3 for normal physiologic data.)

Obtain the following information about the pet:

- Species, age, and gender (species and gender may be obvious or the owner may not know this information)
- Origin (e.g., private individual, breeder, pet shop, research laboratory, supply house)
- Length of ownership, owner's previous experience
- Environment, caging (ask owner not to clean cage before coming to hospital), cleaning, temperature, humidity, photoperiod, person responsible for care
- Diet: brand, dating on packages, storage, supplements, type of feeder and waterer and method of cleaning, feeding schedule, person responsible for feeding
- Cagemates, other pets, quarantine history, presence of aggressive behavior

- Dates of unusual activity: breeding, parturition (Table 4), cannibalism, abnormal urination or defecation
- Medical history, previous weights
- Purpose for ownership
  - Pet, breeder, display, education
- Purpose for visit
  - Purchase examination, check-up, problem
- Become familiar with normal behavior, locomotion, haircoat, and stools, of each of the pocket-pet species.
- Observe the pet in its cage for mentation, activity, locomotion, dyspnea, head tilt, haircoat, and any grossly observable abnormalities.
- Note respiratory and heart rates prior to handling when possible.
- Observe the absence or presence of cagemates and their condition.

KEY POINT ▶ If dyspnea or severe depression is detected, warn the owner that the animal has a grave prognosis and could die from the stress of an examination.

- Handle such animals as little as possible. Initially,

TABLE 4. Reproductive Data for Pocket Pets

	Rat	Mouse	Guinea Pig	Chinchilla	Hamster	Gerbil
Age at puberty Males (days)	42–110	35–50	60–120	240–540*	45–98	70–85
Females (days)	42–110	50–60	60–90	240–540*	30–84	65–85
Length of estrous cycle (days)	4–5	4–5	15–17	41	4	4–6
Gestation (days)	21–23	19–21	63–68	105–115	15–18	24–26
Average litter size	6–14	10–12	3–4	2–3	6–8	4–6
Age at weaning (days)	21	18–28	14–28	36–48	20–25	20–30
Litter development	Eyes open 12–17 days	Eyes open 10–14 days	Precocious; eats solid food by 5 days	Precocious	Ears open 4–5 days; eyes open 14–16 days	Eyes open 16–20 days

*Fall babies breed 1 year later. Normal breeding season is November through May.

treat severely ill animals symptomatically, then perform a complete physical examination after the pet's condition has stabilized.

■ Evaluate the cage.
  • Note the type of diet and bedding, as well as the level of sanitation, and compare these to what was described in the history.
  • Observe the quantity and quality of feces and urine.
  • Diarrhea, soft stools, absence of stools, copious urine, and discolored urine can all be signs of illness.
  • Coprophagia is a normal behavior in rodents.
  • Check the diet and water supply for freshness, quantity, source, and accessibility.
  • Evaluate the presence and suitability of cage furniture or its absence.

■ Examine the animal itself.
  • An accurate weight in grams is extremely important for evaluating an animal's body condition, calculating drug dosages, and monitoring treatment. The easiest method of weighing a pocket pet is to place it in a box and then subtract the weight of the container from the total.

■ Restraint of pocket pets is easy with experience. Pets that have been frequently and gently handled by the owners require only minimal restraint. Gentle pressure directs the animal as needed. Grasp less cooperative patients (except chinchillas and guinea pigs) by the scruff over the back of the neck with the thumb and forefinger (Fig. 1). Take care to pinch enough skin to prevent the animal from turning around, yet leave enough slack for respiration. Hold the base of the tail, if present, between the fourth and fifth fingers to provide additional restraint with small specimens.

■ Hold docile guinea pigs with the palm of one hand supporting the chest while the other hand supports the hindquarters (Fig. 2). Place the thumb and forefinger of the first hand in the axillas for additional control. Take care to minimize damage to the fur when handling chinchillas since they epilate easily. Grasp the animal by the tail and scoop it up into the palm of the same hand (Fig. 3). If necessary, grasp the thorax just behind the axillas.

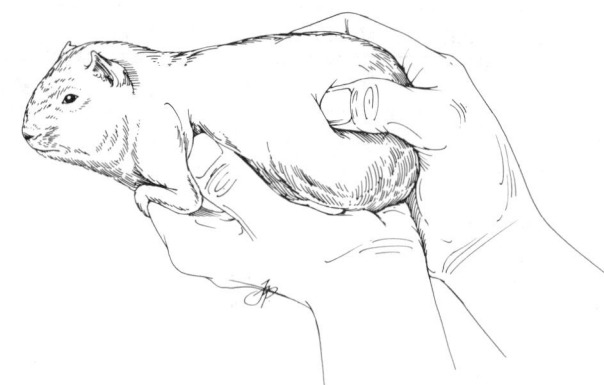
Figure 2. Proper method for restraint of guinea pig.

■ Appropriately sized towels placed over the head are especially effective in calming uncooperative rodents. Many physical examinations are completed by wrapping a patient in a towel and exposing only needed areas. Even oral, ophthalmic, and aural examinations can be accomplished with minimal effort if the animal is given the chance to relax in its new "burrow."

■ Remove particularly aggressive patients from their cages by scooping them up in a can or bucket; then slide them out onto a slick surface, and pick them up or transfer them to a holding area or scale.

KEY POINT ▶ Lift the hindquarters of mice and rats by the base of their tails to facilitate scruffing. Never use the tip of the tail for restraint.

■ Once the animal is properly restrained, examine the head. Assess the cranial nerves. Check the nose for the presence and character of discharge. Examine the mouth for ptyalism, swellings, overgrown incisors, or discharges. Place an avian speculum across the mouth just caudal to the incisors to inspect the oral cavity. Use a light source and a pair of hemostats as retractors to improve access. Alternatively, use an otoscope with a pediatric head to examine the molars of rodents heavier than 100 gm. Introduce the otoscope head through the diastema. Then direct

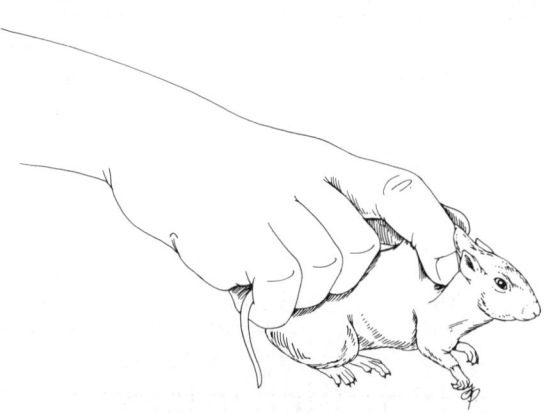
Figure 1. "Scruffing" a mouse.

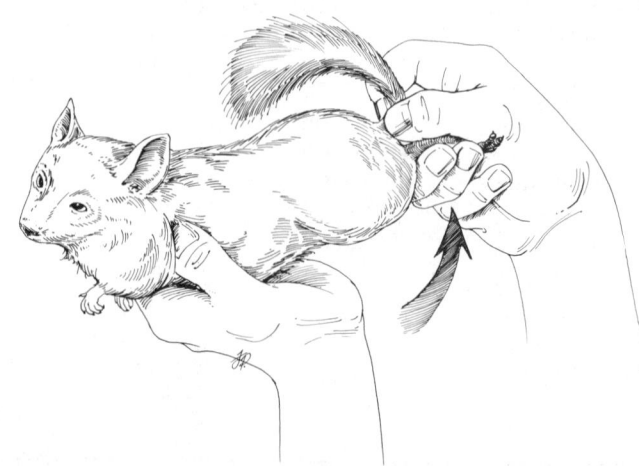
Figure 3. Proper method for restraint of chinchilla.

the tongue ventrally to allow a clear view, unless food material is present. This procedure is particularly useful in guinea pigs and chinchillas, which commonly suffer from overgrown molars and premolars. Examine the cheek pouches of hamsters for swelling, impaction, or discharge.

■ An ophthalmic exam, including a fundic examination, is important.
  • Use a slit lamp to identify superficial pathology, especially corneal ulcers or foreign bodies.
  • If indicated, perform fluorescein stain and conjunctival scrapings or cultures.
  • Note the presence of conditions such as discharge, asymmetry, and exophthalmos.

KEY POINT ▶ Gerbils, rats, and mice produce red tears (i.e., chromodacryorrhea) with stress or disease. Do not confuse them with hemorrhage.

■ Guinea pigs suffering from hypovitaminosis C often produce dry, white tears.
■ Check ears for discharge, foreign bodies, and mites. Bluish discoloration of the ears is a sign of cyanosis. Bright red injected coloration is associated with septicemia. Sores behind the ears and on the neck are often a sequela of aural disease.
■ Evaluate submandibular, axillary, inguinal, and popliteal lymph nodes for size and consistency. Enlargements usually indicate infectious or neoplastic disease.
■ Reevaluate respirations and heart rate after the stress of handling and compare with the resting rate noted when the animal was in the cage. Note dyspnea or respiratory sounds. Auscultate animals heavier than 200 gm. Count every third or fourth beat and multiply by the appropriate factor to record heart rates of up to 500 beats per minute.
■ Palpate the abdomen. Pay special attention to differentiating pregnancy from the bladder, kidneys, abdominal masses, enlarged cecum, and fecal balls in the colon. While palpating the abdomen, examine the mammary chain of all female rodents for signs of mastitis, lactation, or neoplasia. Also check male mice and rats for mammary neoplasia. Mammary tissue extends from the base of the neck to the base of the tail. Gerbils normally have an elliptic sebaceous gland on their ventral midline. Do not confuse this gland with neoplasia or infection. Check the rectum and perineal area for signs of diarrhea, prolapse, irritation, parasites, and bite wounds.
■ Evaluate the urogenital tract for signs of inflammation, foreign bodies, urine scalding, and vaginal discharge. Locate and palpate the testicles in males. The easiest method of determining the gender of pocket pets is to compare the anogenital distance, which is twice as long in males as in females. Other characteristics that allow the determination of sex are as follows:
  • Visualization or palpation of testicles indicates a male
  • Two external openings (i.e., anus and urethra) indicates a male
  • Three openings (i.e., anus, vagina, and urethra) indicates a female

  • Penis extruded from prepuce with manipulation indicates a male
■ Examine the skin and fur for conditions such as crusts, alopecia, masses, herniations, and wounds. Check the tail and feet for swellings, coloration, sores, length of toenails, and condition of footpads.
■ Evaluate the extremities for trauma or other abnormalities.

DIAGNOSIS

Skin and Ear

■ Apply cellophane tape to crusted areas of the skin and view under a microscope as an aid in diagnosing ectoparasites such as lice, mites, and fleas. Skin scrapings are beneficial in detecting mites and dermatophytes. Dermatophytes are best diagnosed through culture of broken hairs or crust on dermatophyte test medium. Culture pustules and biopsy skin lesions when indicated.
■ Use tracheal swabs to obtain ear samples from animals heavier than 25 gm. Mix the debris with mineral oil and view under low magnification to test for ear mites, or roll onto a glass slide and Gram stain to look for bacterial or yeast infections.

Urine and Fecal Collection

■ Collect urine by placing the rodent in a clean, mesh-bottomed cage with a plastic liner. When enough urine has been produced, collect it from the bottom of the cage with hematocrit tubes or a syringe and 25-gauge needle. Perform cystocentesis on nonpregnant animals heavier than 100 gm with a 27- to 25-gauge needle.
■ Collect feces over several hours to provide a volume sufficient for fecal flotation. Flotation allows the detection of nematodes and some trematodes and cestodes. Cellophane tape applied to the perineal area and viewed under a microscope often detects oxyurid eggs. Use a fresh saline smear or fecal sedimentation to diagnose protozoal parasites. Fecal cultures are useful in diagnosing bacterial diarrheas.

Radiology

■ Radiology is an extremely useful tool. Machines capable of exposures as low as 40 KVP and 3 to 10 MAS can be used to x-ray mice. Most radiograph machines are capable of generating diagnostic radiographs of guinea pigs, chinchillas, and mature rats at settings usually used for kittens. Positioning is accomplished with masking tape or Velcro straps. Sedate unruly individuals. Techniques used in cats for contrast studies of both urinary and gastrointestinal systems are easily modified for use in pocket pets.

Blood Samples

■ Obtain small blood samples by trimming a clean toenail close to the quick and collecting blood into hematocrit tubes.

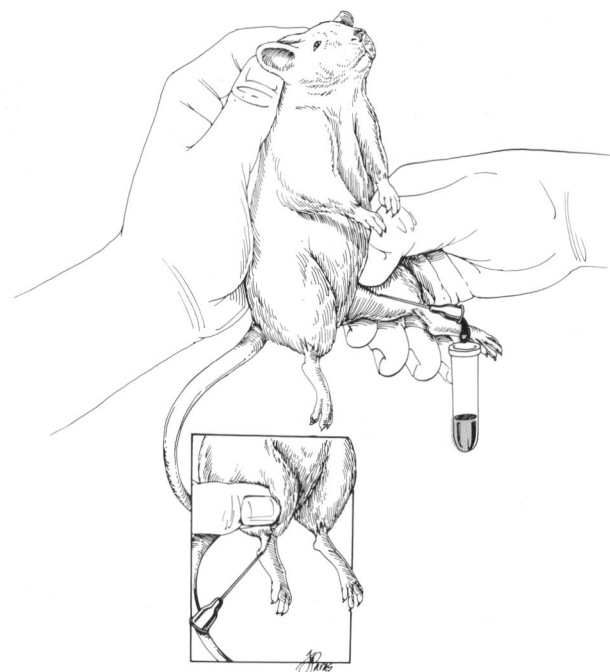

Figure 4. Medial saphenous venipuncture; *inset*, lateral tarsal venipuncture.

■ Use lateral or medial saphenous veins to obtain larger samples in animals heavier than 100 gm. Liberally clip the area to allow exposure of the vessel before attempting venipuncture. Place a 25- to 27-gauge needle in the vein and collect blood into microtainers or hematocrit tubes as it drips from the hub of the needle (Fig. 4). Take extreme care not to collapse and lacerate the vein with overzealous aspiration if a syringe is attached to the needle.
■ It is also possible to use the cephalic vein in guinea pigs.
■ Jugular veins are good alternatives in thin animals that are under sedation.
■ An alternative technique that is useful in smaller

animals is to coat the skin over the vein with a thin layer of petroleum jelly, and then to puncture the vessel. Blood is collected with a hematocrit tube as it exits the wound. Samples up to 1% of the animal's weight are considered safe even in stressed animals.

KEY POINT ▶ Attempt tail or orbital sinus bleeding only as a last resort in mice, rats, gerbils, and hamsters; do not use the tail in hamsters. These techniques are often not acceptable to owners.

■ To bleed the tail, warm the tail with water or compresses in order to dilate the tail vessels. In large rats, the vessels are cannulized with a needle, and blood is drawn in the usual fashion. In smaller animals, the tip of the tail is amputated or lacerated. Blood from the wound is collected as described previously. Orbital bleeding works best in mice. A microhematocrit tube is used to puncture the conjunctiva at the medial canthus. Aim the tip caudomedially and advance it 1 to 3 mm. If blood does not begin to fill the tube immediately, abort the attempt. Reserve cardiac sampling for extreme emergencies and perform it only using sedation. See Tables 5 and 6 for hematologic and serum chemistry values for pocket pets.

ROUTINE PROCEDURES

Oral Medications: Nutritional Support

■ Incorporate oral medications into a treat, or administer them in liquid form. If the medication is palatable, administer it by placing the tip of a dosing syringe into the diastema.

KEY POINT ▶ Take care not to place the tip into the contralateral cheek pouch or the animal will store the medication and expel it later.

■ Administer medication in small amounts. Ensure that the animal swallows the medication in its mouth before more is administered. This technique is useful

TABLE 5. Normal Hematologic Values for Pocket Pets

Indices	Rat	Mouse	Guinea Pig	Chinchilla	Hamster	Gerbil
Erythrocytes ($\times 10^6$/mm³)	7–10	7–12.5	4.5–7	5.2–10.7	4.0–10	7.0–10
Packed cell volume (%)	35–49.3	35–49	37–55	27–54	31–57	41–52
Hemoglobin (mg/dl)	11–18	10–20	11–16.5	8–15.4	10–19	12.1–16.9
Leukocytes ($\times 10^3$/mm³)	5–17.2	4–12	7–19	4–11.5	3–11	4.3–12
Neutrophils (%)	9–50	5–40	15–60	9–45	10–42	3–41
Lymphocytes (%)	50–85	30–90	30–72	19–98	50–95	32–97
Monocytes (%)	0–5.0	0–10	3–12	0–6	0–3	0–9
Eosinophils (%)	0–6.0	0–8.0	1–5.0	0–9.0	0–4.5	0–4.0
Basophils (%)	0–1.5	0–1.5	0–3.0	0–1.0	0–1.1	0–2.0
Total protein (g/dl)	5.6–7.6	3.5–7.2	4.4–6.2	5.0–6.0	4.5–7.5	4.3–12.5
Platelets ($\times 10^3$/mm³)	500–1300	100–1000	250–850	254–740	200–670	400–638

TABLE 6. Normal Serum Chemistries for Pocket Pets

Indices	Rat	Mouse	Guinea Pig	Chinchilla	Hamster	Gerbil
Sodium (mEq/L)	135–155	112–193	132–156	130–155	128–144	144–158
Potassium (mEq/L)	4–8	5.1–10.4	4.5–8.9	5–6.5	3.9–5.5	3.8–5.2
Chloride (mEq/L)		82–114	98–115	105–115		
Calcium (mg/dl)	5.3–13	3.2–8.5	3–12	5.6–12.1	5–13.2	3.7–6.2
Phosphorus (mg/dl)	5.3–8.3	2.3–10.4	3–12	4–8	3–9.9	3.7–7.0
Albumin (g/dl)	3.4–4.8	2.5–4.8	2.1–3.9	2.5–4.2	2.6–4.9	1.8–5.5
Globulin (g/dl)	1.3–3.0	0.6	1.7–2.6		2.7–4.2	1.2–60
Glucose (mg/dl)	50–217	60–250	60–125	60–120	40–200	50–135
Blood urea nitrogen (mg/dl)	6–23.9	17–28	9–31.5	10–25	12–25	17–27
Creatine (mg/dl)	0.2–0.8	0.3–1.0	0.5–2.2		0.1–1.0	0.6–1.4
Alanine aminotransferase (IU/l)	16–89	26–77	10–25	10–35	22–128	
Aspartate aminotransferase (IU/l)		54–269		96	28–122	
Alkaline phosphatase (IU/l)	16–125	45–222	18–28	3–47	45–187	
Total bilirubin (mg/dl)	0.2–0.6	0.1–0.9	0.3–0.9	0.4	0.1–0.9	0.2–0.6
Cholesterol (mg/dl)	40–130	25–82	20–66	40–100	25–180	90–150

for force-feeding pellet gruels to anorexic pets if the caregiver is patient. Medication or food that is administered too quickly will be either spit out or aspirated.

- For rodents that are intractable or for unpalatable substances, use a stomach tube.
  - Metal feeding needles, red Brunswick urinary catheters, or infant feeding tubes work well. Selection of method is based on the size of the animal and individual preference. Metal feeding needles with ball tips are frequently used in patients that weigh less than 100 gm (Fig. 5). The metal provides the necessary stiffness to pass a tube of small diameter. The ball at the end of the needle makes it difficult to pass the tube into the trachea. These tubes have the potential to create esophageal tears with improper use or restraint.
  - Measure the length from the tip of the nose to the last rib. Ventroflex the head slightly, and place the tip of the needle through the diastema and over the tongue. If the tube does not pass easily down the esophagus to the premeasured distance, check the tube size or reposition the tube before attempting further advancement. The needle is easily palpable percutaneously if it is placed correctly. It is usually safe to administer up to 3 ml/100 gm body weight.

- Larger animals are easily and safely provided with stomach tubes with flexible catheters (Fig. 6). Use a speculum to prevent the rodent from damaging the tube; an otoscope head, avian speculum, or piece of wood or plastic with a hole drilled in the center works well. Measure and mark the tube for the distance from the tip of the nose to the last rib. Place the otoscope head in the mouth and over the tongue. Pass the tube while holding the speculum in place and slightly ventroflexing the head. Resistance is the result of malpositioning or inappropriate tube size. If other speculums are used, they are placed in the diastema. The tube must pass over the tongue before it can be advanced down the esophagus. This is difficult in some animals. Palpate the throat to confirm the presence of the feeding tube in the esophagus.

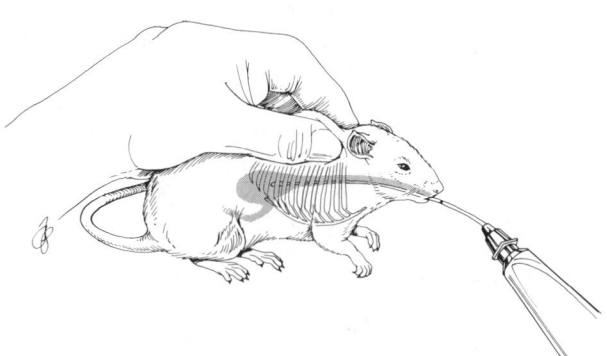

Figure 5. Proper placement of a metal feeding tube.

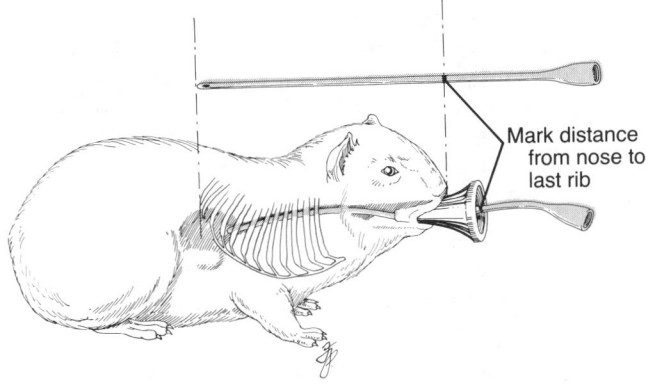

Figure 6. Measurement and use of a flexible catheter as a feeding tube.

Mark distance from nose to last rib

KEY POINT ▶ Because placing a stomach tube is a blind procedure, check the placement of all stomach tubes with a small volume of sterile saline before administering the medication. Misplaced medications are fatal.

■ This route is also useful for administering nutrition to anorectic patients. Place a pharyngostomy tube if repeated stomach tubings are necessary, using the technique for cats. Flush pharyngostomy tubes with water at least every 4 to 6 hours. Nasogastric tubes are difficult to place and keep patent because of their small size. Securely suture all tubes to the skin. Place a tube collar made of x-ray film and use rear leg hobbles to prevent removal of tubes.

■ Nutritional support is critical in rodents because of their high metabolic rate. Provide supplements in animals that are anorexic for longer than 12 hours. If the gastrointestinal tract is capable of digestion, use a slurry of pellets mixed with a high-calorie supplement. If the tube is too small for this mixture, use avian hand-feeding formula or a mixture of vegetable, cereal, and meat baby foods in place of the pellets. If the ability of the gastrointestinal tract to tolerate enteral feeding is in question, first try isotonic electrolyte or dextrose solutions. Parenteral nutrition is used successfully in research animals and may be feasible in select pets.

Subcutaneous Injections

■ Subcutaneous injections and fluids are safer and easier to administer than is stomach intubation. Give both injections and fluids over the shoulder blades, or in folds of skin on the flank of some species.
  • Avoid administering irritating substances to rats and mice, because their mammary tissue extends into these areas, and the resulting inflammatory response is thought to increase the occurrence of mammary cancer.

KEY POINT ▶ In general, avoid streptomycin and the carrier procaine in all pocket pets because of a high incidence of toxicity and hypersensitivity reactions.

Intramuscular Injections

■ Give intramuscular injections in the semimembranosus and semitendinous muscles. Inject only small volumes of nonirritating substances, or tissue damage with resulting self-mutilation often occurs. Use the epaxial or triceps muscles if repeated injections are necessary.

Intraperitoneal Injections

KEY POINT ▶ Use intraperitoneal injections only as a last resort for large volumes of fluids or irritating injections that cannot be given intravenously.

■ Express the bladder, and prepare the abdomen.
■ Restrain the rodent with its head down to move its abdominal organs cranially. Give the injection 0.5 to 2 cm lateral to the midline in the caudal abdomen. Aspirate before injecting to insure that the injection is not being given into the bladder or bowel. Never use this technique in pregnant animals.

Intravenous Injections

■ Give injections into any of the veins previously described, as well as into penile veins in hamsters and guinea pigs. Placement of intravenous catheters is possible in animals heavier than 100 gm. Spinal needles placed in the femur or tibia work well as intraosseous catheters.
■ Give boluses of fluids every 2 to 4 hours, followed by a dilute heparin flush. A pediatric intravenous pump is used for continuous infusion. Maintenance of catheters in active individuals is extremely difficult.

ANESTHESIA

Premedication and Patient Preparation

■ In chinchillas and guinea pigs, withold food for 6 hours before anesthesia. Withold food from smaller, mature rodents for 2 hours and from immature animals for 0 to 0.5 hours depending on age and condition.
■ Use heat lamps and heating pads to prevent hypothermia. Have a prewarmed incubator available for recovery. Preoperative or intraoperative warmed subcutaneous or intravenous fluids are strongly recommended. Place intravenous or intraosseous catheters whenever possible.
■ Administer atropine preoperatively to reduce airway secretions. Acepromazine or diazepam work well as premedications for other anesthetics. Avoid acepromazine in gerbils because it potentiates seizures. See Table 7 for anesthetic drugs and dosages.

Monitoring

■ Surgical anesthesia is reached when toe, tail, and ear pinches do not generate a withdrawal reaction.
■ Depth of anesthesia is best monitored by pulse and respiratory rate and character. Pulses drop to within normal ranges after induction. Further reduction, especially to less than 80% of the original stabilized value, is an indication to lighten anesthesia.
■ Attach electrocardiograph leads to even the smallest patients by clamping alligator clips onto the hubs of all-metal 27-gauge needles or steel sutures placed through the skin at the usual sites. Tape cables to the table to maintain placement. Doppler units taped over the chest provide accurate heart rates. Pulse oximeters are easier to use, more sensitive, and more expensive than the instruments mentioned previously. These instruments are easily taped to the patient's ear, foot, or tail and provide heart rates as well as information regarding oxygenation.
■ Respirations are often shallow and rapid during induction. They become deep and regular as surgical anesthesia is reached.

TABLE 7. Injectable Anesthetic Drug Dosages for Pocket Pets

Agent and Effect	Rat	Mouse	Guinea Pig	Chinchilla	Hamster	Gerbil
Atropine sulfate (parasympatholytic)	0.04 mg/kg, IM, SC	0.04–0.1 mg/kg, IM	0.1–0.2 mg/kg, IM, SC	0.2 mg/kg, IM, SC	0.04 mg/kg, IM, SC	0.04 mg/kg, IM, SC
Acepromazine (sedation)	1–2 mg/kg, IM					DO NOT USE
Diazepam (sedation)	3–5 mg/kg, IM	3–5 mg/kg, IM	0.5–3 mg/kg, IM		3–5 mg/kg, IM	3–5 mg/kg, IM
Ketamine hydrochloride (light sedation)	22 mg/kg, IM	22 mg/kg, IM	22–64 mg/kg, IM	40 mg/kg, IM	40 mg/kg, IM	40–60 mg/kg, IM
Ketamine hydrochloride (heavy sedation)	25–40 mg/kg, IM	44 mg/kg, IM	44–256 mg/kg, IM*		40–150 mg/kg, IM*	70–200 mg/kg, IM*
Ketamine hydrochloride/ xylazine (anesthesia)	60–80 mg/kg/7–12 mg/kg, IP, IM	80 mg/kg/16 mg/kg, IP, IM	35–40 mg/kg/4–8 mg/kg, IP, IM	35–40 mg/kg/ 4–8 mg/kg, IM	50–100 mg/kg/10 mg/kg, IP	50 mg/kg/2 mg/kg, IP
Ketamine hydrochloride/ acepromazine/ xylazine (anesthesia)	22 mg/kg/0.75 mg/kg/2–5 mg/kg, IM	44 mg/kg/0.75 mg/kg/2–5 mg/kg, IM	22–64 mg/kg/ 0.75 mg/kg/2–5 mg/kg, IM	40 mg/kg/0.5 mg/kg/0 mg/ kg, IM		DO NOT USE
Ketamine hydrochloride/ diazepam (anesthesia)			35–40 mg/kg/5–10 mg/ kg, IM			
Innovar-vet (0.4 mg/ml fentanyl and 20 mg/ml droperidol) (sedation)†	0.13–0.16 ml/kg, IM	0.2–0.3 ml/kg, IM	0.22–0.88 ml/kg, IM‡		DO NOT USE	
Innovar-vet (0.4 mg/ml fentanyl and 20 mg/ml droperidol) (anesthesia)†	0.3–0.5 ml/kg, IM	0.3–0.5 ml/kg, IM				
Nalorphine (reverses fentanyl)	2–5 mg/kg, IV					
Pentobarbital sodium (anesthesia)§	25–40 mg/kg, IP, IV	40–80 mg/kg, IP, IV	30–40 mg/kg, IP, IV	30 mg/kg, IV 35–40 mg/kg, IP	50–90 mg/kg, IP	30 mg/kg, IV 40–60 mg/kg, IP
Thiopental sodium (anesthesia)§	25–50 mg/kg, IP	25 mg/kg, IV 50 mg/kg, IP	20 mg/kg, IP		20–40 mg/kg, IV	

*Wide dosage ranges are due to marked individual variation. Use lower dosages first.
†Dosages listed are for agent directly from bottle. Dilute at least 1 : 10 with sterile saline to reduce chance of inflammation at injection site.
‡Up to 33% of guinea pigs receiving dosages at the higher end of the range will have inflammation at injection site.
§Dilute concentration to less than 10 mg/ml before injection.

KEY POINT ▶ Some chinchillas and guinea pigs hold their breath while being induced with gas anesthetics and then take deep rapid breaths. If the concentration of anesthetic gases is high enough, this behavior results in death.

- The risk of this behavior is reduced by premedication with tranquilizers, initial induction with nitrous oxide with later addition of primary anesthetic gas after relaxation, and low induction settings. Changes in respirations, especially erratic or apneustic patterns and decreased respiratory rates, indicate deepening anesthesia.
- The corneal reflex varies markedly among individuals and anesthetic agents. If the animal has a corneal reflex after induction and then loses it, lighten anesthesia.

Inhalation Anesthesia

- Most pocket pets are not intubated for anesthesia because their small size requires special equipment and expertise. When necessary, as in prolonged oral or thoracic procedures, intubation is accomplished with the animal in dorsal or ventral recumbency, depending on the clinician's preference. Small non-cuffed or Cole endotracheal tubes work well. A stylet is usually required to provide enough stiffness for the tube to pass the larynx. Extend the animal's head and neck. Grasp the tongue with forceps and use gentle traction. The tip of the tube is then advanced above the tongue and just past its base. The hard palate is used to deflect the tip of the tube ventrally into the glottis.
- This is a blind procedure that is difficult to master. Use of a laryngoscope is helpful in larger rodents.

- Another technique is to place an over-the-needle catheter in the trachea and move it up retrograde through the larynx to act as a guide.
- The catheter is removed after the endotracheal tube is in place.

KEY POINT ▶ If intubation is utilized, it is extremely important that the tube be checked for patency. Rodents produce copious respiratory secretions, which frequently clog endotracheal tubes.

- The small diameter allows these tubes to collapse or kink, resulting in asphyxia of the patient. Check patency at least every 2 minutes by applying positive-pressure ventilation at 10 to 15 cm H_2O and watching for excursion of the chest wall. If extending the head and neck does not result in air flow, suction the tube. If this is either not successful or impossible, remove the tube and continue anesthesia with a mask, or reintubate the animal with a new tube. The small diameter of the trachea makes tube-induced tracheitis a life-threatening situation.
- Purchase small face masks from laboratory supply houses or make them from syringe cases and latex gloves (Fig. 7). Induction in anesthetic chambers is also possible.
- All pocket pets maintained on gas anesthesia require some form of nonrebreathing system. Usual induction is achieved between 2 and 3% for isoflurane and 2 and 4% for halothane. Maintenance for isoflurane and halothane varies from 0.25 to 2%. There is marked individual variation in the amount of anesthetic required for induction and maintenance. Use of 50% nitrous oxide in oxygen reduces anesthetic concentration requirements for other gases.

Injectable Anesthesia

- Doses and routes for injectable anesthetics are listed in Table 7. Needed doses for injectable anesthetics

are tremendously variable among species and individuals. Most injectable anesthetics provide safe sedation for minor procedures, but very few induce safe surgical anesthesia on a consistent basis.

- Ketamine in combination with diazepam is easily obtainable, is given intramuscularly, and has a wide margin of safety, but it does not provide good analgesia.
- Droperidol–fentanyl combinations are reversible and give better muscle relaxation and analgesia than ketamine but may cause muscle necrosis with resulting self-mutilation.
- Intraperitoneal (IP) injections of barbiturates provide surgical anesthesia but have a low margin of safety and a significant mortality rate.

Euthanasia

- Euthanasia is easily performed by an overdose of inhalant anesthetic in an induction chamber. Induction by inhalant anesthetic through a mask or chamber followed by an overdose of barbiturates given IP or IV is another option. Euthanasia by IP injection of barbiturates alone causes pain in some animals.

SURGERY

Principles

- Surgical techniques for pocket pets are similar to those for cats and birds.
- Hemostasis is critical because of small blood volumes.
- Electrosurgery for incisions and cautery is highly recommended.
- If necessary, give fresh blood transfusions drawn from a donor of the same species and mixed with sodium heparin (1000 IU/ml) at a rate of 0.005 ml per 1 ml of blood and administer directly into an intravenous line.
- The lack of a filter creates a potential for thrombosis.
- Transfusion reactions are possible.

Common Procedures

- The most common surgeries are laceration repair and removal of dermal or subcutaneous masses.
  - Most rodents will not gnaw on skin sutures.
  - If this occurs, use steel sutures, subcuticular sutures, or tissue glue.
  - If an animal still chews at its suture line, physical restraint such as a tube or Elizabethan collar is required.

Castration

- Castration is a common procedure in guinea pigs. This is usually done when owners want to house more than one male together or do not wish to breed their female any longer.

Technique

1. Make a skin incision over each testicle or make one incision on the midline just cranial to the prepuce.

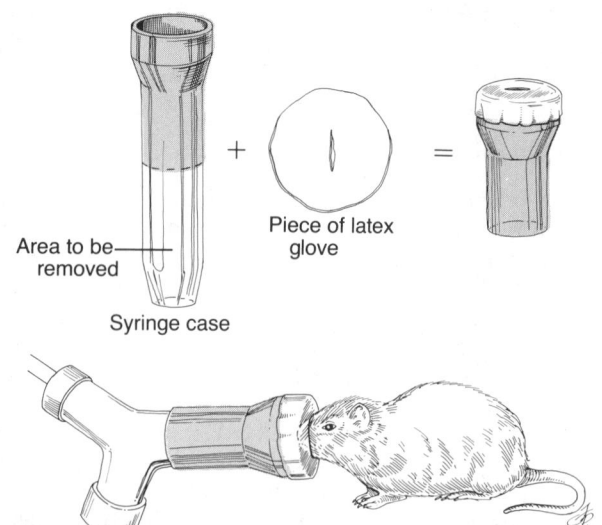

Area to be removed

Piece of latex glove

Syringe case

Figure 7. A nose cone for anesthesia delivery can be made from a cut-down plastic syringe case and material from a latex glove. Syringe cases from 12 to 60 cc can be used, depending on the size of the patient.

2. Remove the testicles via a closed technique. All rodents possess open inguinal rings and can eviscerate if a closed technique is not used.

- Some surgeons suture the rings partially closed for extra security. This technique is also applicable to other rodent species.
- Common abdominal surgeries include cystotomy for urolith removal in guinea pigs and rats, and cesarean section in guinea pigs and chinchillas because of dystocia.
- Use similar techniques to those described in dogs and cats (see sec. 8, chs 4 and 15). Preplaced stay sutures are recommended to define incision edges for closure. Use 4/0 polyglactin 910 or chromic gut swaged on a taper needle and suture in a simple, interrupted pattern to close the body wall. Close the skin with a subcuticular (absorbable) suture or interrupted skin monofilament, nonabsorable suture.
- Fracture fixation is best accomplished with intramedullary pinning or Kirschner apparatuses. Rodents gnaw on bandages until they remove them. If they are unable to remove a splint, self-mutilation often results in self-amputation. If a cast or splint is necessary, physical restraint is required. Healing usually takes 3 to 6 weeks.

Dental Procedures

- Incisors can be trimmed with nail trimmers, but this technique often fractures the tooth, creating abscesses of the root. Instead, use a high-speed dental burr or a flat cutting disk on a Dremel handtool. Trim molars with high-speed drills or pediatric rongeurs. A mouth speculum that deflects the tongue and other soft tissues is essential to prevent lacerations and provide working space (Fig. 8). Use tracheal intubation to prevent aspiration pneumonia when working on molars.
- If a tooth is abscessed, extract both it and the occlusal tooth.
  - Approach cheek teeth through an incision in the cheek.
  - Use a fine dental elevator to loosen the teeth.
  - Patience and firm but gentle pressure is needed, or the root or surrounding bone will fracture.
  - The roots of the maxillary incisors curve dramati-

cally back into the head. Take care to follow the curve of the tooth.
- In chinchillas, the roots of the molars can impact, causing swelling of the mandible or exophthalmos and epiphora. These teeth are extremely difficult to extract without causing extensive bony and soft-tissue damage. Discourage the breeding of animals suffering from malocclusion, unless acquired as a result of trauma or infection, because this trait is hereditary.

MOUSE

Most pet and laboratory mice are derived from *Mus musculus,* which is the common house mouse. Mice sold in the pet trade are randomly bred and less likely to suffer from the genetic problems associated with inbred laboratory animals. Mice possess brown fat tissues between their scapulae known as hibernating glands; these are thought to provide an energy store. The spleen in male mice is 50% larger than that of females. There are normally five pairs of mammary glands; three are thoracic and two are inguinal.

Dermatology

Ectoparasites

- *Alopecia and pruritus,* especially on the back of the head and dorsal midline, are usually associated with lice (i.e., *Polyplax serratus*), mites, or fleas.
- Mites (e.g., *Mycoptes musculinus, Myobia musculini, Radfordia affinis*) often also are associated with greasy fur and folliculitis. Transmission is by direct contact. Ectoparasites are usually seen in new acquisitions. Fleas are transmitted by other household pets such as cats and dogs.
- Diagnosis is based on clinical signs, history, visualization of the parasite, skin scrape, and cellophane-tape test.
- Pyrethrin powder or dichlorvos strips are used to treat for fleas and lice. Ivermectin is recommended for the treatment of mites (Table 8).
- Change the bedding and thoroughly clean the cage between treatments to prevent reinfestation.

Dermatophytosis

- Alopecia also may be the result of dermatophytes (see sec. 5, ch. 3). Lesions are often hyperkeratotic.
- Diagnosis is made by skin scrape or culture.
- Treatment is with lime sulfur dip or griseofulvin (Table 9).

Viral Diseases

- Ectromelia (i.e., mousepox) is a pox virus that causes acute mortality in weanling mice. Older mice suffer the chronic form and develop rashes and ulcerative lesions of the neck and tail, conjunctivitis, and alopecia. As the disease progresses, edema of the face and limbs occurs. Often, there is dry gangrene of the appendages. Asymptomatic carriers exist. Transmission is by direct contact through an abrasion

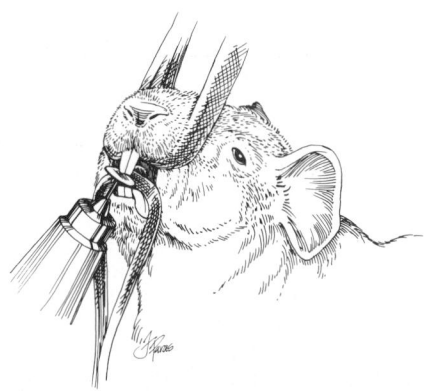

Figure 8. Proper technique for dental trimming.

TABLE 8. Parasiticide Drug Dosages for Pocket Pets

Agent	Rat	Mouse	Guinea Pig	Chinchilla	Hamster	Gerbil
Dichlorvos strip (5 cm long)	Suspend 6 inches above cage for 24 hours, 2 times per week for 3 weeks	See rat	See rat	See rat	See rat	See rat
Flea powders	3–5% malathion or 0.5% pyrethrin powder 3 times per week for 3 weeks	See rat	5% carbaryl powder or 0.1% pyrethrin powder 1 time per week for 3 weeks	See guinea pig	See rat	See rat
Ivermectin	200 µg/kg every 7 days for 3 weeks, SQ, PO	See rat	See rat	See rat	200–500 µg/kg every 14 days for 3 treatments, SQ, PO	See rat
Lime sulfur dip	Dilute 1 : 40; dip every 7 days for 6 weeks	See rat	See rat	See rat	See rat	See rat
Malathion	0.5% spray or 2% dip every 7 days for 3 weeks	See rat	See rat	See rat	See rat	See rat
Mebendazole	40 mg/kg every 7 days PO for 3 weeks	See rat				
Methyridine	100 mg/kg, SQ					
Niclosamide	100 mg/kg repeat in 2 weeks, PO	See rat	See rat	200 mg/kg, repeat in 2 weeks, PO	See rat	See rat
Piperazine adipate	200 mg/kg, q24h for 7 days, wait 7 days and repeat, PO or 0.5 gm/L in drinking water for 3 weeks					200–600 mg/kg, q24h for 7 days, wait 7 days and repeat, PO
Piperazine citrate	2–5 mg/ml drinking water for 7 days, wait 7 days and repeat	See rat	See rat	See rat	See rat	See rat
Quinacrine hydrochloride	75 mg/kg, q8h					
Thiabendazole	200 mg/kg, q24h for 5 days, PO	100 mg/kg every 7 days for 4 treatments, PO				

or inhalation. It is most likely to occur in laboratory rodents or in new shipments from large supply houses.

■ Diagnosis is by serology or finding intracytoplasmic inclusion bodies associated with clinical signs and focal necrosis of the liver, spleen, and pancreas.
■ An intradermal vaccine is available.
■ There is no treatment. Quarantine survivors permanently or euthanize them.
■ Reovirus is primarily a diarrheal disease of suckling mice that also results in an oily haircoat caused by excessive fecal fat which is not absorbed in the gut.

Bacterial Disease

■ Ulcerative dermatitis is a common syndrome caused by *Staphylococcus aureus* and resulting in pododermatitis, mastitis, and abscesses in other areas.
■ Treatment consists of antibiotics that are chosen based on culture and sensitivity tests.

TABLE 9. Antibiotic, Antifungal, and Antiprotozoal Drug Dosages for Pocket Pets

Agent	Rat	Mouse	Guinea Pig	Chinchilla	Hamster	Gerbil
Ampicillin	20–100 mg/kg, q12h IM, SC, PO	20–100 mg/kg, q12h IM, SC, PO	DO NOT USE	DO NOT USE	DO NOT USE	6–30 mg/kg, q8h, PO
Carbenicillin	100 mg/kg, q12h, PO	100 mg/kg, q12h, PO				
Cephaloridine	10–25 mg/kg, q24h, IM, SC	10–25 mg/kg, q24h, IM, SC	10–25 mg/kg, q8–24h, IM		10–25 mg/kg, q24h, IM	
Chloramphenicol palmitate	50 mg/kg, q8h, PO	50 mg/kg, q8h, PO	50 mg/kg, q8h, PO	50 mg/kg, q8h, PO	50 mg/kg, q8h, PO	50 mg/kg, q8h, PO
Chloramphenicol succinate	30 mg/kg, q8h, IV, IM	30 mg/kg, q8h, IV, IM	30 mg/kg, q8h, IV, IM	30 mg/kg, q8h, IV, IM	30 mg/kg, q8h, IV, IM	30 mg/kg, q8h, IV, IM
Dimetridazole	0.1% in drinking water					
Gentamicin	5 mg/kg, q24h, IM, SC	5 mg/kg, q24h, IM, SC	5 mg/kg, q24h, IM, SC	5 mg/kg, q24h, IM, SC	5 mg/kg, q24h, IM, SC	5 mg/kg, q24h, IM, SC
Griseofulvin	25 mg/kg, q24h, PO	25 mg/kg, q24h, PO	15 mg/kg, q24h, PO			
Metronidazole					70 mg/kg, q8h	
Neomycin	2.6 mg/ml drinking water = 10 gm/gallon = 2650 mg/l	2.6 mg/ml drinking water = 10 gm/gallon = 2650 mg/l	12–16 mg/kg, q12h, PO		100 mg/kg, q24h, PO, or 0.5 mg/ml drinking water = 500 mg/l = 1.9 gm/gallon	2.6 mg/ml drinking water = 10 gm/gallon = 2650 mg/l
Oxytetracycline	3–5 mg/ml drinking water	3–5 mg/ml drinking water	5 mg/kg, q12h, IM		3–5 mg/ml drinking water	
Sulfadiazine and trimethoprim	30 mg/kg, q12–24h, PO, SC	30 mg/kg, q12–24h, PO, SC	30 mg/kg, q24h, PO, SC	30 mg/kg, q24h, PO, SC	30 mg/kg, q24h, PO, SC	30 mg/kg, q24h, PO, SC
Sulfamethazine or sulfamerazine	1 mg/ml drinking water	1 mg/ml drinking water	1 mg/ml drinking water	1 mg/ml drinking water	1 mg/ml drinking water	0.8 mg/ml drinking water
Sulfamethizole and trimethoprim			15 mg/kg, q12h, PO	15 mg/kg, q12h, PO	15 mg/kg, q12h, PO	15 mg/kg, q12h, PO
Tetracycline	20 mg/kg, q12h, PO	20 mg/kg, q12h, PO	20 mg/kg, q12h, PO 0.2–0.35 mg/ml drinking water	20 mg/kg, q12h, PO	55–65 mg/kg, q8h, PO 0.4 mg/ml drinking water	15–20 mg/kg, q8h, PO 20 mg/kg, q4h, IM
Tylosin	10–20 mg/kg, q24h, IM 100 mg/kg, q4h–12h, PO	10–20 mg/kg, q24h, IM 100 mg/kg, q12h–24h, PO			2–8 mg/kg, q12h, IM 66 mg/l drinking water	

- Use of chloramphenicol is recommended pending results of tests (see Table 9). Hot packing, local drainage, and topical medications are also beneficial in selected cases.
- Mastitis may also be caused by *Escherichia coli,* or *Pasteurella, Klebsiella, Pseudomonas,* or *Streptococcus* species. Mastitis is usually secondary to poor sanitation, abrasive bedding, or overly aggressive young.
- Preputial gland abscesses are fairly common in males and are usually due to *E. coli* or *S. aureus.*
- Local flushing and topical treatment are usually adequate.
- Subcutaneous abscesses can be the result of the aforementioned bacteria, *Actinobacillus* species or *Corynebacterium kutscheri. Corynebacteria* species are associated with widespread abscesses, septic arthritis, gangrene, and ulcerated, draining tracts.

- Diagnosis is based on finding gram-positive pleomorphic rods on Gram stain and culture.
- The bacteria are usually sensitive to ampicillin, chloramphenicol, and tetracycline (see Table 9).

Neoplasia

- Lymphoma and mammary neoplasia are common causes of subcutaneous masses. Both tumors frequently are of viral origin. Some of these viruses are transmitted vertically. Mammary neoplasia is usually malignant in mice, and metastasis to the lungs is common.
- Consider thoracic radiographs before surgery.
- Give a guarded prognosis for long-term survival.
- Other possibilities for subcutaneous masses are fungal granulomas, nodules from the *Psorergates simplex* mite, hematoma, hernia, non-neoplastic lymphadenopathy, or emphysema.

■ Use culture, cytology, radiology, and biopsy to determine the etiology.

Otitis

■ Otitis externa is usually due to mites, although bacterial and fungal infections are also common.
■ Clinical signs include erythema, pruritus, waxy debris, and excoriations behind the ears.
■ Diagnosis of mites is by visualization of the parasites through otoscopic examination or ear swab.
■ Treatment requires cleaning debris from ears with a commercial cleanser followed by administration of ivermectin given twice at a 2-week interval or by topical acaricides used daily for 3 to 4 weeks (see Table 9).
■ Bacterial and fungal otitis is diagnosed with Gram stain and cultures.
■ Treatment is similar to that used in cats.
■ Otitis media and otitis interna are usually caused by hematogenous spread or local invasion of bacteria from a primary abscess.
■ Clinical signs include head tilt, circling, facial nerve paralysis, and otitis externa, as well as signs associated with the original infection.
■ Rule out mouse hepatitis virus as the cause of head tilt (see Gastroenterology).
■ If treatment of the primary disease is successful, the otitis media usually resolves, although a residual head tilt may persist.
■ If a cluster of *Pseudomonas*-related otitis occurs in a population, evaluate the water source and produce for contamination.
■ Use sodium hypochlorite in the drinking water at 10 ppm to control an outbreak while water quality is being restored.
■ Damage to the pinnae can be associated with trauma, dermatitis, pox virus, allergy, and vasculitis.
■ Dry gangrene is a common response and is usually self-limiting.

Miscellaneous

■ Bilateral alopecia around the muzzle with no other abnormalities is usually caused by friction from overhead feeders.
■ Alopecia occurring in smaller, weaker individuals is often the result of fur barbering. Removal of the mice in best condition from the cage results in normal appearance of fur-barbered mice in 2 to 3 weeks.
■ Tail-head alopecia and scabbing are usually the result of aggression. Separate affected individuals, or additional trauma will occur.
■ Other rare causes of alopecia are endocrinopathies, leprosy, and hereditary alopecia in nude mice.

Ophthalmology

Epiphora

■ Epiphora is a common condition of pet mice. The primary causes in pets owned for longer than 2 months are ammonia fumes and overgrown incisors.
■ Ammonia causing contact irritation is diagnosed by examining an uncleaned cage and checking for odor.

■ Treatment is improved sanitation.
■ Overgrown incisors are easily diagnosed by oral examination. Treatment is trimming affected teeth and providing opportunities for gnawing.
■ Foreign bodies and the resulting ulcers can cause epiphora. An eye examination, including fluorescein stain, allows diagnosis of the problem. Treat by removing the foreign body and administering an ophthalmic antibiotic (gentamicin, tetracycline or chloramphenicol in affected eye, TID to QID).
■ In newly acquired pets, epiphora is often the result of an upper respiratory infection. *Pasteurella pneumotropica* is the most common pathogen.
■ The clinical signs for *Salmonella* species, other bacterial respiratory infections, *Mycoplasma*, Sendai virus, lymphocytic choriomeningitis, and mousepox often begin with conjunctivitis and epiphora, leading to mucopurulent oculonasal discharge.

Retinal Degeneration

■ Retinal degeneration can be either hereditary or a result of exposure to high-intensity lighting in albino mice. The resulting blindness is often undetected because patients adapt well and behave normally in their cages.

Miscellaneous

■ Cataracts are usually hereditary or postinflammatory.
■ Other hereditary ophthalmic conditions are posterior lens capsule rupture, eyelid malformation, optic nerve hypoplasia, microphthalmos, and retinal dysplasia.

Respiratory

Pneumonia

■ *Murine respiratory mycoplasmosis (MRM)* is one of the most common respiratory diseases of pet mice. It is caused by *Mycoplasma pulmonis*. The infection remains dormant for long periods of time and is activated by stress. There are many asymptomatic carriers, and transmission is by aerosol and direct contact. The infection can spread hematogenously, especially to the middle ear, uterus, or joints.
■ Clinical signs are dyspnea described as chattering, mucopurulent oculonasal discharge, hunched posture, and anorexia. Animals with a chronic history of this disease are often cachexic.
■ Radiology aids in determination of the extent and severity of pneumonia and the absence or presence of distant foci of infection.
■ Treatment with tylosin is successful in controlling the disease if it is not too advanced. Tetracycline and chloramphenicol have also been used (see Table 8).
■ Many patients need nutritional support.
■ Mice with pyometra or other abscesses require surgery.
■ Recovered animals are carriers, and stress will elicit clinical signs. Strictly quarantine these animals.

- A common cause of pneumonia in newly acquired mice is *Sendai virus.* Fatalities are seen in suckling or weanling mice.
- Transmission is by aerosol or direct contact.
- Clinical signs in adults are caused by secondary bacterial infections that occur as a result of viral depression of immunity, and are similar to those in MRM.
- Diagnosis is based on clinical signs, self-limiting disease, and serology.
- Treat with antibiotics to control the secondary bacterial infection, and provide supportive care as needed.
- Control is achieved in breeding situations by stopping operations for 4 to 6 weeks.
- There is a killed vaccine available.
- Recovered animals are resistant to reinfection.
- Common primary or secondary pathogens causing respiratory signs in mice are *Streptococcus pneumoniae, Corynebacterium kutscheri, Pasteurella pneumotropica, Pseudomonas aeruginosa,* and *Klebsiella pneumoniae.* Treatment is empirical or based on culture and sensitivity results from a tracheal swab sample.

Neoplasia

- Dyspnea is often the result of metastasis of mammary adenocarcinomas to the lungs. Primary lung tumors, usually pulmonary adenomas, occur frequently.

Other

- Although not frequently diagnosed, cardiac problems can result in signs of respiratory disease. Radiology is a useful diagnostic tool.

Gastroenterology

Parasites

- Tapeworms usually do not cause clinical signs in mice. Occasionally, heavy burdens result in diarrhea or weight loss. The chief concern is the zoonotic potential of one species *(Hymenolepis nana)* that is directly transmissible to humans.
- Diagnosis is made by visualization of eggs in the feces. Treat by niclosamide (see Table 8), improved sanitation, and removal of indirect hosts (e.g., fleas, beetles, roaches).
- Pinworms *(Syphacia obvelata, Aspiculuris tetraptera)* cause anal pruritus and, in severe cases, rectal prolapse.
- Diagnosis is based on clinical signs and the cellophane-tape test.
- Treat with piperazine or mebendazole every 7 to 10 days for 3 treatments (see Table 8), and provide improved sanitation.
- The protozoal parasite *Spironucleus muris* causes diarrhea and slow growth associated with a pot-bellied appearance in young mice.
- Diagnosis is by fecal wet mount, and false-negative findings are common. The intestinal contents are frothy.
- Treat with dimetridazole or oxytetracycline (see Table 9). Supportive care to combat dehydration and hypothermia is extremely important.
- Control is achieved with immaculate sanitation.
- *Giardia* species, and rarely *Eimeria falciformis,* show signs similar to those with *Spironucleus. Giardia* is zoonotic. Treat with dimetridazole. Treat *Eimeria* species with sulfadiazine and trimethoprim (see Table 9). Most other protozoas are considered nonpathogenic.
- *Cystocerus fasciolarus* causes nonpathologic cysts of the liver. These cysts are the infective form of *Taenia taeniaeformis* in carnivores.

Diarrhea

- Diarrhea in young mice is usually caused by mastitis or viral infection. Lethal intestinal virus of infant mice (LIVM) is seen in mice 10 to 20 days of age.
- This virus may be a variant of mouse hepatitis virus. Mortality can reach 80%.
- Clinical signs are yellow diarrhea that mats on the perineal region causing obstipation and perineal necrosis, anorexia, and stunted growth.
- Transmission is aerosol or feco-oral from the mother.
- Treat supportively, and quarantine survivors.
- Epizootic diarrhea of infant mice (EDIM) is clinically similar to LIVM. This disease usually affects mice younger than 2 weeks of age but can occur up to 21 days of age.
- There is a low mortality rate, and nursing continues through the infection.
- Transmission is feco-oral.
- Diagnosis is based on clinical presentation.
- Treat supportively. Survivors are usually growth-stunted. Quarantine them from other mice.
- Mouse hepatitis virus is a corona virus. Most infections are latent. Outbreaks of yellow diarrhea and encephalitis secondary to viral hepatitis occur in mice 7 to 13 days of age. Older animals show clinical signs of infertility, jaundice, and hemoglobinuria as a result of a slowly progressive hepatitis.
- Diagnosis is based on clinical presentation, serology, and the presence of syncytial giant cells in the epithelium of the small intestine.
- Treat supportively, and quarantine affected individuals. The prognosis is grave.
- Although less commonly seen in pet mice, reovirus occurs in older suckling mice. It is characterized by an oily diarrhea that results in a greasy haircoat. Other signs are conjunctivitis, stunted growth, and tremors. Transmission is by ingestion.
- Diagnosis is based on clinical signs, histology, and serology.
- Treat supportively. The long-term prognosis is grave. Initial survivors are weak, jaundiced, suffer from alopecia, and eventually die.
- Transmissible murine colonic hyperplasia (MCH) caused by *Citrobacter freundii* is characterized by diarrhea followed by rectal prolapse and stunted growth. Transmission is feco-oral.
- Diagnosis is made by clinical signs and fecal culture.
- Treat with neomycin, tetracycline, or sulfamethazine until sensitivity results are available (see Table 9).

Severe thickening of the distal one half of the colon is observed at necropsy.

- Salmonellosis, also known as mouse typhoid, is transmitted by latent carriers or contaminated feed or bedding. Incubation lasts for 3 to 6 days.
- Clinical signs are lethargy, anorexia, purulent conjunctivitis, arthritis, and diarrhea.
- Diagnosis is based on clinical signs and fecal culture. Treat supportively. Use of antibiotics is controversial.
- Quarantine survivors.
- Sanitation is extremely important because *Salmonella* species are zoonotic. Necropsy reveals erythema of the distal ileum and congestion of the spleen and liver. The more chronic infections show necrotic foci in the liver, spleen, and lymph nodes. Use a reputable fresh laboratory chow from a known source to minimize the chance for introducing the disease in a closed population. Thoroughly wash all produce and then dip it in a dilute bleach solution. Rinse completely before feeding.
- Tyzzer disease is caused by *Bacillus piliformis*. Transmission is feco-oral.
- Clinical signs are precipitated by stress and consist of anorexia, diarrhea, and a high mortality rate in weanlings.
- Diagnosis is made by clinical signs or pathology.
- Tetracycline used for 4 to 5 days (see Table 9) in addition to reducing stress is helpful in controlling the disease. Necropsy reveals enteritis and multiple gray-yellow necrotic foci in the liver.

Theriogenology

- Breeding systems vary; from 1 to 6 females may be placed with one male. All animals are housed together, and youngsters are removed after weaning. Females in proestrus have swollen vulvas. Vaginal plugs are present postcopulation.
- Female mice that have been bred within 4 days will abort if a new male mouse is placed in the cage. This is known as the Bruce effect. Inappropriate light cycle, inappropriate age, crowding (i.e., Whitten effect), and poor nutrition are the most common causes of infertility in pet mice. Pyometra caused by *Pasteurella pneumotropica, Mycoplasma* species, or other bacteria is also common.
- Desertion of litters is usually a result of stress, lack of nesting materials, agalactia, or mastitis.

Urology

- Aged male mice may develop urethral obstruction from proteinaceous plugs of inspissated ejaculum. *E. coli* or *Proteus* or *Pseudomonas* species are the most frequently cultured pathogens. Prior to complete obstruction, chronic hematuria may be noticed by the owner.
- Antibiotics, which are chosen based on the results of urine culture, are often curative with early presentation. Complete obstruction requires surgery.
- Glomerulonephritis is very common in geriatric mice. It is frequently secondary to chronic viral infection. Clinical signs are anorexia, lethargy, dehydration, and cachexia. Urinalysis shows proteinuria. As the disease progresses, the urine becomes isosthenuric, the blood urea nitrogen and creatinine levels rise, and other electrolyte abnormalities typical of chronic renal failure occur.
- Treat supportively. Prognosis for long-term survival is grave.
- A coccidia (e.g., *Klossiella muris*) is occasionally found in the urine. The clinical significance of its presence is unknown.
- Mice can be asymptomatic carriers of leptospirosis. This condition is rarely seen in pet mice.
- Diagnosis is based on dark-field microscopy of urine, serology, or histopathology. Euthanasia of carriers is recommended.

Musculoskeletal System

- Infectious polyarthritis or mouse rheumatism is caused by *Streptobacillus moniliformis*. In humans, it is known as rat-bite or Havernill fever. Transmission is by direct contact. Clinical signs are cachexia, keratitis, edema and ulceration of the appendages, and ankylosing arthritis.
- Diagnosis is based on the bacterial culture findings and the presence of caseous pericarditis and arthritis on necropsy.
- Treat with an antibiotic chosen through the results of culture and sensitivity tests. Use penicillin while awaiting results. Supportive care is important. Animals that recover remain arthritic. Control is achieved through quarantine and sanitation.

Neurology

- The most frequently diagnosed neurologic disease in pet mice is head tilt resulting from bacterial otitis media (see Otitis). The second most common cause of neurologic signs is trauma.
- Diagnosis is based on history and clinical signs. Consider neoplasia in aged mice with slowly progressive signs.
- Lymphocytic choriomeningitis is a zoonotic arenavirus. Transmission is aerosol, transplacental, or by direct contact, fomites, or insect vectors. Acute signs usually occur in mice that are 3 to 6 weeks old. Approximately 20% of infected individuals show acute clinical signs which include lethargy and photophobia followed by convulsions and paralysis. Animals that are latently infected later develop glomerulonephritis. Mice infected after weaning and prior to 1 year of age lose weight, appear arthritic, and show signs of conjunctivitis and photophobia. The virus runs its course in several weeks. Animals that recover show no residual signs.
- Diagnosis is based on clinical signs and the presence of immunofluorescent antibody (IFA) as well as pleural effusion, enlarged spleen, and fatty liver found on necropsy. Treat supportively. House survivors separately.
- Prevent the disease by improving sanitation, providing pest control, and cleaning produce. Consider euthanasia because of the zoonotic potential of the virus.

- Mouse poliomyelitis/encephalomyelitis, also known as Theiler disease, causes clinical signs in 1 : 10,000 infected mice. Two thirds of normal mice are carriers. Transmission is by oral or respiratory routes. Mice younger than 4 weeks of age show signs of encephalitis. Mice that are 6 to 10 weeks of age are weak in the rear legs and progress to paralysis. The tail may remain mobile. Affected mice continue to eat and be alert. Albino mice are predisposed to show clinical signs.
- Diagnosis is based on clinical signs, serology, or histopathology that shows necrosis of the ganglionic cells of the anterior horn of the spinal cord.
- Treat supportively. Consider euthanasia because of poor prognosis.
- Seizures in mice commonly result from otitis media, trauma, liver or kidney failure, toxins, bacterial meningitis, neoplasia, or viral encephalitis.

Hematology

- Leukemia in mice is usually viral in origin. Transmission is transmammary or transplacental.
- Clinical signs are anemia, dyspnea with thymic involvement, and those signs that are compatible with chronic disease.
- Diagnosis is based on a complete blood count, bone marrow aspirate, or histopathology. Prognosis is grave.
- *Eperythrozoon coccoides* is a rickettsial red blood cell parasite of mice. Affected mice are usually asymptomatic. Occasionally, infected individuals develop fever, anemia, and splenomegaly. Transmission is through the louse, *P. serratus*. Control is achieved by extermination of the louse.
- Treat with tetracyclines.

RAT

Pet rats are derived from the Norwegian or Brown Rat breed *(Rattus norvegicus)* which did not originate from Norway but from Asia. Breeds of rats are called strains when they are extensively inbred and called stocks when the strains are hybridized. Rats have brown fat as discussed in the section on mice. They do not possess a gallbladder. Their mandibular symphysis is normally articulated. Rats are neophobic, therefore make gradual changes in food or environment when possible.

Dermatology

- Fleas, mites (e.g., *Radfordia ensifera, Ornithonyssus bacoti*), lice (i.e., *Polyplax spinulosa*), ear mites (i.e., *Notoedres muris*), and dermatophytes cause similar signs in both mice and rats. Treatment also is similar (see Mouse).
- Subcutaneous masses in rats are similar to those in mice. *Pasteurella pneumotropica* is a very common pathogen in mastitis and subcutaneous abscesses.
- Treat with chloramphenicol until culture results are available (see Table 9). Fifty to ninety percent of adult female rats and approximately 15% of male rats develop mammary cancer. Always perform histopathology. Most, but not all of these tumors are fibroadenomas, which are benign.
- Prognosis for long-term survival after surgical removal is good. Interstitial cell tumors of the testes cause subcutaneous swellings in the inguinal region. Rats with squamous cell carcinomas of the Zymbals gland of the external ear canal have a poor prognosis for long-term survival.
- Ulcerative dermatitis occurs in rats as well as mice. *S. aureus* is the causative agent. *Corynebacterium kutscheri* follows a similar course in rats and mice (see Mouse).
- Ringtail is the formation of constrictive bands of fibrous tissue around the tail in nestling rats. These bands result in gangrene of the distal tail. This disease occurs when humidity is less than 40%.
- Treat by making a longitudinal incision of the ring to release the stricture, and apply topical DMSO, steroid, and antibiotic solution (10 ml DMSO, 6 ml of 50 mg/ml amikacin, 4 ml of 2 mg/ml dexamethasone) four times daily.
- To prevent the condition, keep humidity above 50%, use solid-bottom cages, and provide ample nesting material. Prognosis for retention of the distal tail is guarded.

Ophthalmology

- Epiphora and blepharospasm are most commonly caused by ammonia fumes, overgrown incisors, or foreign bodies (see Mouse).
- Sialodacryoadenitis virus is a coronavirus that is endemic in many rat populations.
- Clinical signs vary from mild keratoconjunctivitis to blepharospasm, chromodacryorrhea, severe uveitis, hyphema, buphophthalmus, periorbital swelling, and pneumonia. The clinical course of the disease lasts for 10 to 14 days. Rats maintain normal activity levels and appetite.
- Treatment is not necessary for mild infections. Place rats showing marked ocular disease or discomfort on the appropriate ophthalmic ointments (e.g., atropine, antibiotic, steroid) based on presentation. Administer antibiotics to animals suffering from respiratory signs. Recovery is usually complete unless the eye ruptures or self-mutilation occurs.
- Control is achieved by not introducing new animals for 4 weeks.
- In contrast to mice, Sendai virus rarely causes clinical signs in rats.
- Mucopurulent ocular discharge is associated with mycoplasmosis, *Streptococcus pneumoniae, Pseudomonas* sp., and other less common bacterial or viral pneumonias.
- Cataracts are either primary hereditary defects or occur secondary to severe uveitis or diabetes mellitus. Retinal dystrophy and colobomas are also inheritable traits in rats. Retinal degeneration occurs in rats housed under intense lighting.

Respiratory

- Murine respiratory mycoplasmosis (MRM) is extremely common in pet rats. Its presentation is similar to the disease in mice (see Mouse).

- *S. pneumoniae* is normal flora for rats. However, during stressful situations, bacteremia may occur, resulting in pneumonia. Clinical signs are similar to MRM. Differentiation is based on culture and the presence of extensive fibrinopurulent pleural effusion on necropsy.
- Ampicillin controls clinical signs if the disease is not too advanced (see Table 9). Prevent the condition by minimizing stress.
- *C. kutscheri* and *Pasteurella pneumotropica* show similar signs to MRM (see Mouse). There is a serologic test for *C. kutscheri*. See the Mouse section for a discussion of *P. aeruginosa*.
- *Pneumocystosis carinii* is an uncommon protozoa that infects the lung. Cysts and trophozoites live in the alveoli. Clinical signs occur only in immunocompromised or geriatric individuals. Signs are cachexia, cyanosis, and dyspnea.
- Diagnosis is based on clinical signs, tracheal wash, response to therapy, or histopathology.
- Treat with sulfadiazine/pyrinrethamine (see Table 9).

Cardiovascular System

- Myocardial degeneration is fairly common in geriatric rats. Diagnosis is based on radiographs of the chest and clinical signs.
- Treat supportively. Use furosemide and digitalis at cat doses to alleviate pulmonary edema.
- Polyarteritis nodosa is an idiopathic condition of geriatric rats that results in thickening and tortuosity of arteries, especially in the mesentery, pancreas, and testicles. Affected areas are predisposed to clot formation and aneurysms.

Gastroenterology

Parasites

- Nematodes *(Syphacia muris),* cestodes, and intestinal protozoal parasites infestations are similar to those in mice.
- *Capillaria hepatica* has no clinical significance other than causing yellow streaks on the liver which are found at necropsy. Transmission is by cannibalism.

Dental

- The causes and treatment of malocclusion are similar to those for mice.

Diarrhea

- Epizootic diarrhea of suckling rats is a viral disorder found in rats 7 to 14 days old. The infection causes a mild diarrhea. Most animals recover. Occasionally, stunting occurs. Treat supportively.
- Salmonellosis in rats is similar to that in mice.

Theriogenology

- Breeding is accomplished by taking a female showing signs of estrus (e.g., lordosis, hyperactivity, quivering ears, and swollen vulva) to a male rat's cage for 24 hours or by keeping 1 male with up to 6 females and removing the females just prior to parturition. Check females for a postcopulatory plug to confirm breeding. House females individually while raising young. A vaginal discharge is seen 1.5 to 4 hours prior to labor. Parturition is accompanied by stretching and extension of the rear legs. All neonates are usually delivered within 1 to 2 hours.
- Infertility is usually the result of age, malnutrition (e.g., protein, vitamin E), uterine infection, or improper light cycle, temperature, or humidity.
- Litter desertion is usually the result of stress. Inadequate nesting material or agalactia are other significant causes of abandonment and death. To prevent cannibalism, remove male rats from the cage prior to parturition and do not return them until after weaning is complete.
- Rat virus infection is a parvovirus that is usually inapparent unless individuals are infected *in utero*. Small litters or jaundiced stunted neonates are often the only clinical signs. Transmission is both vertical and horizontal.
- Diagnosis is made by serology and histopathology. Permanently quarantine all in-contact animals.

Urology

- Urolithiasis is fairly common in older rats. Stones are usually composed of ammonium magnesium phosphate or calcium carbonate.
- Clinical signs are anorexia, stranguria, hematuria, and abdominal distension. Urinary obstruction can occur.
- Diagnosis is based on clinical signs, urinalysis, and radiographs.
- Treat by surgically removing uroliths, provide antibiotics chosen based on culture and sensitivity, and provide acidification of the urine. Recurrences are common.
- Two extremely common conditions recognized in geriatric rats are nephrocalcinosis and chronic progressive nephropathy. Clinical signs are compatible with those of chronic renal failure. Enlarged or small, irregular kidneys may be found on physical or radiographic examination. Urinalysis shows isosthenuria and marked proteinuria.
- Definitive diagnosis is based on renal biopsy.
- Treat supportively. Prognosis for long-term survival is grave.
- *Trichasomoides crassicauda* is an uncommon parasite of the urogenital tract. The adult worms usually reside in the kidney, but they may occasionally wander into the genital tract. The ova are passed in the urine.
- Clinical signs are hematuria and stranguria. Infrequently, the resulting proliferative mucosa of the bladder may be palpated as an abdominal mass.
- Treatment is somewhat successful with methyridine (see Table 8). Sanitation is critical in control of this disease.
- *Klossiella muris* is an incidental coccidia of the urinary tract.

Neurology

- Many geriatric pet rats suffer from chronic progressive radiculoneuropathy.

- Clinical signs are compatible with cauda equina syndrome, including posterior paresis progressing to paralysis, urine retention, and incontinence. Prognosis is grave.
- Treat supportively or euthanize.
- *Streptobacillus moniliformis,* a normal bacteria found in the oral, nasal, and pharyngeal cavities of rodents, is found in 43% of middle ear infections and 35% of chronic pneumonias in rats. The bacteria is nonpathogenic for gerbils and guinea pigs.
- Clinical signs vary with the site of infection. Head tilt and circling, septic arthritis, and respiratory disease are commonly seen.
- Diagnosis is based on culture because the clinical signs mimic many other diseases, especially MRM and *Pseudomonas* infection (see Mouse).
- Head tilt in rats may also be due to trauma or neoplasms, especially pituitary adenomas.

Hematology

- *Hemobartonella muris* is a red blood cell parasite of rats that is nonpathogenic unless the rat is immunocompromised or splenectomized. Transmission is through the louse, *P. spinulosa.*
- Clinical signs result from hemolytic anemia and hemoglobinuria.
- Treat with tetracyclines (see Table 9).

HAMSTER

Mesocricetus auratus, better known as the Golden or Syrian hamster, is a primarily nocturnal rodent that originated in the Middle East. Almost all hamsters in the United States are the offspring of three siblings that were imported in the 1930's. Many color variations are available. Long-haired hamsters are affectionately called teddy-bear hamsters. The stomach has two compartments: a nonglandular forestomach that functions like a rumen and a glandular stomach. Hamsters are very territorial. They possess flank glands, which are larger in males, that they rub against objects to mark their area. Females are larger than males. They use this size advantage to attack males, except during estrus. Do not allow groups to estivate together, or recently awakened individuals may cannibalize sleeping hamsters.

KEY POINT ▶ Hamsters are extremely sensitive to antibiotics.

- Penicillins, clindamycin, lincomycin, streptomycin, tylosin, erythromycin, and cephalosporins kill the hamster's normal intestinal flora. Overgrowth of pathogenic bacteria, particularly *Clostridium difficile,* causes a diarrhea that is almost always fatal within 3 to 7 days. Even antibiotics supposed to be safe can have this effect. Treat by discontinuing antibiotics (gram-negative antibiotics are continued if a specific gram-negative pathogen is cultured), providing a *Lactobacillus* supplement, and giving supportive therapy.

Dermatology

- Hamsters are susceptible to *Demodex creceti* and *D. aurati* mites. *D. creceti* is limited to skin folds. *D. aurati* causes hyperpigmentation, alopecia, and seborrhea sicca at the dorsal midline. *Demodex* is carried by many normal-appearing hamsters.
- Clinical signs are secondary to immunosuppression as a result of stress, chronic infection, or malnutrition.
- Diagnosis is based on clinical signs and deep skin scrapings.
- Treat with amitraz every 2 weeks for two treatments past two consecutive negative skin scrapings. Use the manufacture's recommended dilution for dogs.
- *Sarcoptes* mites infrequently cause facial alopecia. Diagnosis is based on skin scrapings. Treat with ivermectin (see Table 8). Do not confuse this condition with alopecia caused by contact with feeders or fur-barbering.
- *Notoedres* mites affect only the external ear canal in female hamsters. They affect the ears, feet, genitalia, and tail in males. Diagnosis is made by ear swabs, skin scrapings, or both. Treat with ivermectin (see Table 8).
- Other less common causes of alopecia in hamsters are dermatophytosis, endocrinopathies, and genetic defects.
- Dermal subcutaneous masses are usually abscesses caused by *Pasteurella pneumotropica, S. aureus,* or *Streptococcus* spp. Treatment is based on culture and sensitivity tests. Use chloramphenicol until culture results are available. Other frequent causes of subcutaneous swellings are distended cheek pouches, testicles, mastitis, hernias, neoplasia, and lymphadenopathy.

Ophthalmology

- Epiphora and conjunctivitis are most frequently the result of ammonia, incisor overgrowth, a foreign body, *Pasteurella* sp., *Streptococcus* sp., or lymphocytic choriomeningitis (see Rat; Mouse). Mucopurulent discharge is usually secondary to bacterial infection resulting from one of these conditions.
- Hamsters are predisposed to rupture of the eye secondary to trauma or infection. Surgical enucleation is advised. Electrosurgery is extremely helpful in controlling bleeding, but do not use it on the stump of the optic nerve and vessels because of the risk of thermal injury to the brain. Place Gelfoam in the socket to enhances clot formation.

Respiratory

- Hamsters are susceptible to the common cold.
- Clinical signs include nasal discharge, sneezing, otitis media, fever, and pneumonia. Uncomplicated cases last 5 to 7 days. Complications are usually the result of secondary bacterial infections.
- Treat supportively. Use of antibiotics is indicated if copious nasal discharge, dyspnea, anorexia, or lethargy is observed. Overuse of antibiotics may cause diarrhea-related deaths in hamsters that might have recovered uneventfully if left untreated.

- Most dyspnea in hamsters is secondary to trauma. Hamsters often bite when startled. Reflex actions on the part of humans, especially children, cause hamsters to be flung against hard objects.
- Diagnosis is made by history and the presence of fresh epistaxis.
- Treat supportively. Emergency shock therapy, consisting of supplemental heat, oxygen, parenteral fluids, and glucocorticoids is frequently required. Prognosis varies from good to grave based on the presence or absence of internal injury.
- Sendai virus can cause death in suckling hamsters housed with mice. Adults show no clinical signs (see Mouse).
- Primary bacterial pneumonias are most frequently caused by *Yersinia pseudotuberculosis, P. pneumotropica,* or *Streptococcus.* Clinical signs are compatible with those of pneumonia as seen in other species, as well as weight loss and conjunctivitis. All three agents have a tendency to form distant abscesses, especially in the uterus.
- Diagnosis is based on clinical signs and culture of a tracheal swab or abscess.
- Treat with chloramphenicol until sensitivity results are available. Animals with internal abscesses require surgery; however, anesthesia in these individuals is very risky. Recovered individuals are carriers and must be quarantined from other rodents. Prognosis is guarded.

Cardiology

Of geriatric hamsters, 73% suffer from cardiac thromboses. Most thromboses occur in the left atrium and are secondary to degenerative cardiomyopathy, cardiac amyloidosis, sepsis, or vascular disease as a result of calcification of the great vessels. Congenital myocardial necrosis also occurs.

- Clinical signs are cyanosis, dyspnea, and acute death. Enlargement of the cardiac silhouette and pulmonary edema can sometimes be seen on radiographs.
- Furosemide and digitalis (cat dose) temporarily alleviate clinical signs in some individuals.

Gastroenterology

Parasites

- Hamsters can carry the zoonotic tapeworm *Hymenolepis nana* (see Mouse).
- Treat with niclosamide (see Table 8) and provide improved sanitation.
- Pinworms (*Aspic tetraptera, Syphacia muris, S. obvelata*) occur in hamsters as well as in mice.
- Treat with piperazine (see Table 8).

Dental

- Hamsters are predisposed to dental caries. A large percentage of affected teeth abscess, causing facial swelling, ptyalism, and anorexia.
- Diagnosis is based on clinical signs, oral examination, skull radiographs, and culture results.
- Treat by tooth extraction and antibiotic therapy based on sensitivity. Prognosis is variable, depending

on the condition of the animal, the tooth affected, and the extent and nature of the abscess (see Mouse).
- Overgrown incisors occur as in mice.

Oral

- Hamsters' cheek pouches are very distensible. Impaction of the pouches occurs on occasion.
- Clinical signs vary from ptyalism to abscess. In simple cases, removal of the material from the pouch with fine forceps is sufficient. Sedation is not usually required.
- In cases involving fungal or bacterial infection of the pouch, remove the material, have it Gram stained and cultured, and flush the pouch with dilute iodine solution. If cellulitis is present, use systemic antibiotics. Fistulas often heal spontaneously.

Diarrhea

- Proliferative ileitis (i.e., wet-tail disease) is thought to be caused by *Campylobacter fetus jejuni,* with or without concurrent bacterial or viral infections. Over 90% of animals showing clinical signs die. The highest morbidity and mortality rates occur in hamsters 3 to 8 weeks of age. Teddy-bear hamsters may be more susceptible to infection than short-haired varieties. Transmission is feco-oral.
- Clinical signs include diarrhea that mats on the ventrum and perineum, anorexia, dehydration, and hunched posture. The abdomen frequently seems uncomfortable for the animal on palpation, and bowel loops are often distended secondary to ileal obstruction or intussusception. Rectal prolapse occurs.
- Treat with neomycin, gentamicin, metronidazole, or tetracycline (see Table 9). Supportive care is critical. Prognosis is grave. Gross findings on necropsy include gas and yellow diarrhea in the distal intestinal tract, thickened ileum and distal jejunum, peritonitis, and liver abscesses.
- Other bacterial diarrheas are commonly caused by *E. coli,* Tyzzer disease, or *Salmonella* sp. (see Mouse).

Liver

- Hamsters older than 1 year of age often develop liver cysts that are derived from the biliary duct. Less frequently, similar cysts arise from the pancreas, epididymis, and seminal vessicles; therefore, it is sometimes called polycystic disease. No clinical signs are associated with cysts in these structures. Abdominal palpation reveals cystic structures in the cranial abdomen, which are felt as crepitus.
- No treatment is recommended.

Theriogenology

- Timing is critical in preventing injury to the male when breeding hamsters. Transfer the female to the male's cage in the early evening 3 days after a creamy, viscous vaginal discharge is noticed. Monitor the pair carefully. Remove the male immediately if the female is aggressive. Remove the male after mating or after 1 to 2 hours even if mating has not occurred. Two days after successful copulation, a gray, malodorous discharge is observed. Pregnancy is highly likely if there is no translucent estrus discharge 5 to 9 days postbreeding. Pseudopregnancies last 8 to 12 days. Normal gestation is 15 to 16 days. There is normally a hemorrhagic discharge, and the female may pant prior to parturition. Rarely, hamsters suffer from pregnancy toxemia (see Guinea Pig).

- Infertility may be secondary to pyometra (see *P. pneumotropica* and lymphocytic choriomeningitis).
- Cannibalism is most frequently the result of stress or mastitis.

Urology

Almost 90% of geriatric hamsters develop renal amyloidosis. The disease tends to develop more rapidly in females.

- Clinical signs are edema and ascites caused by protein loss in the urine, as well as the typical signs of chronic renal failure.
- Treat supportively. Prognosis for long-term survival is grave.

Neurology

- Head tilt is usually secondary to otitis media. Also consider lymphocytic choriomeningitis or neoplasia as differential diagnosis (see Rat).
- Hamsters fed all-seed diets and deprived of exercise often develop cage paralysis syndrome. Usually, pets are presented for acute posterior paresis, which in reality was slowly progressive. The distinction is important in ruling out trauma. In mild cases, the hamster is able to move its hind legs but is unable to support its weight.
- Vitamin D and E supplementation as well as nutritional improvement and opportunity to exercise is curative in 1 to 2 weeks. In severe cases, recovery is negligible or incomplete.

Hematology

Lymphoma and lymphosarcomas are often viral in origin and are diagnosed through biopsy or fine needle aspiration of affected lymph nodes. Lymphadenopathy may also be secondary to lymphadenitis caused by *S. moniliformis*. Prognosis for long-term survival is grave (see Rat).

GERBIL

The Mongolian gerbil *(Meriones unguiculatus)* originated in the deserts of Mongolia and northern China. Gerbils alternate between periods of activity and rest throughout the day. Peak periods of activity are in the late evening. Seed storage and burrowing are important, naturally occurring behaviors. Most gerbils are brown with cream-colored abdomens (i.e., agouti). Several color variations are available (black, black and white). Gerbils drum their hind legs when alarmed. In general, gerbils are nonaggressive. However, introduction of unfamiliar adults results in fighting.

Dermatology

- Rarely, *Demodex* mites cause alopecia in gerbils.
- Diagnosis is based on skin scrapings.
- Treat with rotenone ointment or amitraz dips every 2 weeks for 3 to 6 treatments. Use the manufacturer's recommended dilution for dogs.
- Acute moist dermatitis is the result of a secondary *S. aureus* infection. The primary cause is bite wounds if the infection is at the base of the tail. If the infection is on the face, look for inflammation of the Harderian glands. The gland secretion is viscous and causes matting. The staphylococcal infection originates from under the mats. Attempts at grooming spread the infection to the feet and abdomen.
- Diagnosis is based on clinical signs and culture.
- Tetracycline or chloramphenicol are effective treatments when combined with warm, moist compresses to remove dried debris. Remove possible irritants from cage (e.g., pine or cedar shavings, ammonia). Occasionally, surgical removal of a chronically infected or irritated gland is needed.
- Alopecia of the facial area, especially when it is symmetric, is usually the result of self-trauma from feeders, cage bars, or overzealous burrowing.
- Treat by changing cage construction or provide better visual security.
- Gerbils that catch their tails in crevices or are inappropriately restrained by their tails often present with avulsion of the skin from their tail.
- Treat by controlling hemorrhage and treating shock.
- Amputate the tail after stabilization to prevent ascending infection. In some animals, the infection is localized to the distal tail, which is sloughed in approximately 3 to 4 weeks.
- Generalized alopecia is normal in some weanling gerbils. The hair grows in as the animals mature.
- Melanomas are most frequently found on the ears, feet, or base of the tail.
- Diagnosis is based on biopsy results.
- Treat by surgical removal.
- Sebaceous gland disease is usually the result of bacterial infections or neoplasia.
- Diagnosis is based on cytology, culture and biopsy results, and response to antibiotic therapy.
- Treat infections with parenteral or topical antibiotics, depending on the severity of signs.
- Sebaceous gland adenomas, basal cell tumors, and squamous cell carcinomas are the most frequently encountered neoplasm.
- Treat by surgical excision.
- Radiograph the thorax to diagnose metastases. Prognosis for long-term survival is based on tumor type, stage, and character.

Ophthalmology

- Chromodacryorrhea and epiphora occur as in mice.

Gastroenterology

Parasites

- Tapeworms (i.e., *H. nana* and *H. diminuta*) and pinworms (i.e., *S. obvelata, Dentostomella translucida, A. tetraptera*) occur as in mice.

Dental

- Incisor overgrowth occurs as in mice.

Diarrhea

- *Salmonella* spp. cause transient diarrheas in gerbils. Most recover. There is no carrier state. Animals that die have a fibrinosuppurative peritonitis. The source of infection is usually unwashed greens, contaminated feed, or carrier rodents of another species.
- Treat supportively. Use antibiotics in severe cases based on culture and sensitivity findings.
- Tyzzer disease, caused by *B. piliformis*, is mostly seen in 3- to 7-week-old weanlings and recently postpartum females.
- Clinical signs are anorexia, lethargy, rough haircoat, and sometimes diarrhea. Necropsy shows yellow-gray nodules in the liver and hemorrhage at the ileocecal junction.
- Diagnosis is based on necropsy or response to therapy.
- Treat with oxytetracycline (see Table 9) and supportive care.

Liver

- Hepatic lipidosis and gallstones are frequent sequelae to lipemia found in gerbils fed diets that are more than 2% fat.

Theriogenology

- Breeding is most successful if animals are paired at weaning and kept in these pairs. Male gerbils aid in raising the young. Pairing of older animals causes fighting. An average of 20% of neonates fail to survive to weaning. This is usually the result of agalactia and crushing.
- Chronic hemorrhagic discharge from the vulva is usually the result of cystic ovaries or ovarian tumors.
- Diagnosis is made through normal urinalysis by cystocentesis and abnormal vaginal cytology followed by exploratory laparotomy. Most tumors occur in individuals older than 2 years of age and consist of granulosa cell tumors or theca cell tumors. Leiomyomas of the uterus also cause similar clinical signs.
- Ovariohysterectomy is curative for cystic ovaries and tumors if they have not metastasized.

Urology

- Most gerbils older than 2.5 years of age develop chronic renal failure.
- Clinical signs are polyuria, polydypsia, weight loss, and anorexia. Urinalysis shows proteinuria, hematuria, casts, and an increase in white and red blood cells.

- Treat supportively. Prognosis for long-term survival is grave.

Neurology

- Up to 50% of gerbils in certain family lines suffer spontaneous epileptiform seizures. The seizures are induced by stress and are self-limiting. Seizures usually start as the gerbil reaches 2 months of age.
- Treatment is unnecessary.

Hematology

- Basophilic stippling of red blood cells is a normal finding in gerbils.

CHINCHILLA

Chinchilla laniger and *Chinchilla brevicaudata* are nocturnal rodents from the Andes mountains in South America. They are prone to overheating. Most chinchillas kept in the United States are the descendants of 11 animals. Chinchillas are commercially raised for their pelts as well as for pets. The most common pelt color is gray; the most valuable coat color is black. Chinchillas are sensitive to antibiotics (see Hamster); therefore, avoid the use of penicillins, lincomycin, erythromycin, and cephalosporins. Female chinchillas have a separate vaginal opening that is different from the rodents mentioned previously.

Dermatology

- Chinchillas require dust baths to keep their skin in condition. Use commercially available chinchilla dust only. Sand substitutions do not condition the coat and occasionally cause conjunctivitis. Offer dust at least once a week.
- Dermatophytosis occurs as in guinea pigs.
- Fur-chewing is a serious problem in chinchillas that are farmed for pelts and is often seen in pet chinchillas that are recent culls from a ranch. The etiology of fur-chewing is unknown. Some cases seem to be related to chronic disease, malnutrition, poor caging, or stress. Theories for undiagnosed cases include genetic abnormality, undiagnosed dermatophytosis, and adrenal, pituitary, or thyroid gland abnormalities.
- Diagnostics such as skin scrape, fungal culture, fecal examination, complete blood count profile, and biopsy are recommended. In general, if changes in diet and husbandry do not elicit a response, or an underlying, treatable disease condition is not discovered, prognosis for cure is grave.
- One source advocates plucking all remaining underfur in chewed areas in an attempt to stimulate new hair growth. Place collars after this procedure and leave in place until the fur has grown in completely.
- Mastitis is fairly common.
- Diagnosis is made by the presence of hot, swollen mammary glands and positive cultures of the milk. Suspect mastitis if previously healthy neonates become restless, then lethargic.
- Treat with antibiotics based on culture and sensitiv-

ity. Administer sulfa drugs until sensitivity results are available. Local hotpacking is beneficial. Occasionally, surgical drainage is required. Foster neonates to another female if possible. Use puppy or kitten milk replacers to hand-raise babies.

- Cystic subcutaneous masses may be caused by the intermediate stage of *Multiceps serialis*. Transmission is by ingestion of feed contaminated with canine feces.
- Diagnosis is made by histopathology or cytology. Treat by surgical removal of the masses.
- Otitis caused by *Pseudomonas* spp. occurs as in rats.

Ophthalmology

- Conjunctivitis occurs as in mice.
- Cataracts are congenital or developmental.
- Asteroid hyalosis occurs as a degenerative change.

Respiratory

- Pneumonia occurs as in guinea pigs.

Gastroenterology

Parasites

- Tapeworms (i.e., *H. nana*) occur as in mice.

Dental

- Malocclusion of incisors and cheek teeth occurs.

Diarrhea

- Diarrhea is most often caused by *Coccidia* spp., *Giardia* spp., or a bacterium.
- Clinical signs range from soft stools and weight loss to fluid diarrhea, dehydration, bloating, septicemia, and sudden death.
- The protozoal parasites are best diagnosed on fresh saline smear or necropsy. Bacterial diarrheas are most often the result of contaminated feed and are diagnosed through fecal culture. *Pseudomonas aeruginosa*, *E. coli*, *Salmonella enteritidis*, and *Pasteurella* spp. are the most common isolates.
- Treat supportively and use appropriate antiprotozoal or antibiotic drugs.
- *Pasteurella pseudotuberculosis* causes either acute death from septicemia or a chronic weight loss with intermittent diarrhea. Enlarged mesenteric lymph nodes are a hallmark of this disease.
- Diagnosis is based on clinical signs, histopathology, and culture.
- Treat with sulfa drugs until sensitivity results are available. Prognosis for recovery is poor. Necropsy shows yellow-to-white necrotic foci in the liver.

Theriogenology

- Check male chinchillas four times per year for penile hair rings. Roll back the prepuce and expose the penis. Roll hair rings off the penis after application of a water-soluble lubricant.
- Treat ulcerations topically or systemically as needed.
- Dystocia is fairly common in chinchillas (see Guinea Pig).

- Suspect metritis when postpartum vaginal discharge, failure to return to a normal estrus cycle, anorexia, weight loss, polydypsia, polyuria, and chewing at flank and abdomen are present.
- Diagnosis is based on history, physical examination, abdominal radiographs, culture, ultrasound, and complete blood count. It is usually caused by bacteria introduced by the male or spread from an internal abscess. Retained placentas, macerated fetuses, and dystocia are predisposing factors towards metritis.
- Treat with ovariohysterectomy after stabilization. Females used only for breeding may be treated with antibiotics alone, but the prognosis is poor.
- Female chinchillas are aggressive towards male chinchillas when not in estrus. Breeding systems usually have separate cages for females and an interconnecting run for the male. Females are kept out of the male's run either by their larger size or by collars. The young are precocious and do not need a nest. Chinchillas only produce two litters per year.

Neurology

- Chinchillas seem to be particularly sensitive to *Listeria monocytogenes*. Clinical signs can mimic *P. pseudotuberculosis* and include anorexia, lethargy, abortion, generalized central nervous system signs, hepatitis, mild enteritis, and mild emphysematous pneumonia. Necropsy shows yellow foci in the liver.
- Diagnosis is based on culture.
- Treat with sulfa drugs (see Table 9) until sensitivity results are available. The prognosis is poor.

GUINEA PIG

Guinea pigs *(Caviae porcellus)* are nocturnal rodents that originated in the Andes mountains. They are known for their dietary need for vitamin C. They are used as a food source in their native lands. There are three basic types: English, which have short hair; Abyssinian, which have short, cowlicked hair; and Peruvian, which have long hair. Male guinea pigs are known as boars, and the females are called sows.

Guinea pigs become neophobic as they mature. Offer a variety of foods early in life, and make changes in diet or environment gradually. Guinea pigs stampede when excited. Square cages and strategically placed barriers on external walls prevent the trampling of small or weak guinea pigs.

The smooth muscle of the bronchial tree is quite developed in guinea pigs. This places them at high risk for asthmatic-type anaphylactic reactions.

Both male and female guinea pigs have one pair of inguinal mammary glands; however, only the female's are well developed.

KEY POINT ▶ Antibiotic toxicity (see Hamster). Guinea pigs may also be sensitive to tetracyclines.

Dermatology

- Fleas occur as in mice.
- Lice (i.e., *Gliricola porcelli*, *Gynopus ovalis*) usually

cause no clinical signs except occasional alopecia, seborrhea, and trauma secondary to pruritus.

- Treat with ivermectin, 5% malathion dust, or pyrethrin shampoo (see Table 8).
- The mite *Trixacarus caviae* causes severe pruritus and is zoonotic. It mainly affects the dorsal midline and is difficult to find on skin scrapings. Treat with excellent sanitation and ivermectin (see Table 8). *Chirodiscoides caviae* lives on the hair shaft of the perineal regions. It is often asymptomatic.
- Treat with 5% carbaryl or lime sulfur dip (1 : 40) (see Table 8). Sanitation is critical in preventing reinfestation.
- About 6 to 13% of guinea pigs are carriers of *Trichophyton mentagrophytes*.
- Clinical signs are alopecia and seborrhea sicca, usually starting on the face and spreading along the dorsum.
- Treat with griseofulvin (see Table 9) combined with topical povidone-iodine or chlorhexadine shampoos.
- Other causes for alopecia are fur-barbering, alopecia of the flanks in late-gestation females, and generalized alopecia of some young at weaning. Subclinical hypovitaminosis C causes a poor haircoat and seborrhea sicca, as well as anorexia and large, malodorous stools.
- "Lumps" is the common name for cervical lymphadenitis, which is characterized by lymphadenopathy in the ventral neck region. *Streptococcus zooepidemicus* and *S. moniliformis* are the two most frequently cultured pathogens. Transmission is through abrasions of the oral mucosa. The enlarged lymph nodes are filled with purulent exudate.
- Treat with chloramphenicol until culture results are available. If surgery is required, attempt to remove encapsulated abscesses intact. If this is not possible, excellent drainage is required. The infection may spread, causing otitis, arthritis, or upper respiratory tract infection. Recovered individuals are carriers. Quarantine both sick and recovered animals.
- Mammary tumors occur in the inguinal areas. About 30% are adenocarcinomas; the rest are usually benign fibroadenomas. Other possible diagnoses for masses under the skin are hernias, neoplasias, granulomas, hematomas, or other abscesses.
- Diagnosis is based on cytology or histopathology. Use thoracic radiography to determine the presence of metastases.
- Pododermatitis and sore hocks are very common in guinea pigs. Predisposing factors are untrimmed toe nails, poor sanitation, and wire flooring. *S. aureus* is the most commonly cultured pathogen.
- Clinical signs range from small ulcers on the soles of the feet to abscesses and gangrene. Radiography is essential in determining bony involvement. Untreated cases develop into osteomyelitis, which is very difficult to cure.
- Treat mild cases by improving sanitation and grooming. Place affected individuals in solid-floored cages with paper bedding. Use sulfa drugs (see Table 9) until culture results are available. Surgically remove or curette abscesses, and use topical therapy and hotpacking. Amputation may be necessary.
- Dermal neoplasms are not common, except for benign trichofolliculomas, which occur in the lumbosacral area.
- Diagnosis is based on histopathology.
- Treat by surgical excision.

Ophthalmology

- Conjunctivitis and epiphora occur as in mice.
- Inclusion-body conjunctivitis is caused by *Chlamydia psittaci* and is self-limiting in 3 to 4 weeks.
- White, dry ocular discharge is an early sign of hypovitaminosis C.
- Pea-eyes are the result of subscleral fatty deposits or protrusion of the lacrimal gland through the lower conjunctiva.
- Treatment is not required.
- Cataracts are either congenital or developmental.
- Corneal or scleral calcification is an incidental finding. A thorough workup, including profile and radiographs, is recommended to ensure that the calcification is not generalized.
- A contagious form of diabetes mellitus exists in guinea pigs.
- Clinical signs are rare, but include cataracts. Urine glucose is greater than 100 mg/dl, but blood glucose remains within normal limits.
- No treatment is necessary, but strictly quarantine all contact animals.

Respiratory

- Pneumonia in guinea pigs is usually due to *S. pneumoniae*, *S. zooepidemicus*, or *Bordetella bronchiseptica*. *S. aureus*, *P. aeruginosa*, *Klebsiella pneumoniae*, and *Pasteurella multocida* are also frequently cultured.
- Clinical signs and diagnosis are similar to those in other pocket pets (see Mouse), with the addition of *Bordetella* tracheitis. Many respiratory infections in guinea pigs are secondary to hypovitaminosis C and stress. Weanlings are particularly susceptible. Transmission is aerosol or by direct contact or fomites.
- Necropsy reveals a ventrally dependent pneumonia with suppurative bronchitis. Either radiography or ultrasound is recommended to rule out abscesses, pleural effusion, or pericardial effusion in refractory cases.
- Treat with chloramphenicol (see Table 9) and vitamin C (see Table 10) until cultures are available. Cats, dogs, rabbits, and rats are reservoirs for *Bordetella* sp. Vaccines for *Bordetella* sp. are available. As in other rodents, respiratory infections may lead to otitis interna/media. *Bordetella* sp. also cause pyometra and abortions.
- Rhinitis is most frequently a sign of upper respiratory tract disease, but it may also be associated with allergies or volatile irritants.
- Diagnosis of allergies is made by exclusion and through response to antihistamines or environmental changes.
- About 30% of guinea pigs older than 3 years of age develop bronchogenic papillary adenoma.
- Diagnosis often is made when thoracic radiography is done for another problem.

- Occasionally, clinical signs are seen as a result of pressure on the heart or great vessels.
- Dyspnea is most frequently the result of heat stress or trauma. Other causes are pregnancy toxemia, gastric bloat, volatile irritants, pleural effusion, pneumonia, or pulmonary edema.

Cardiology

- Rhabdomyomatosis is seen on necropsy as pale foci located on the endomyocardium and valves. Histopathology identifies these areas as myocardial cells that have stored excessive glycogen. Do not confuse these areas with thrombi, abscesses, or neoplasia. Their clinical significance is unknown.

Gastroenterology

Parasites

- *Paraspidodera uncinata* is the cecal pinworm of guinea pigs. Infested animals are generally asymptomatic, but heavy infestations can cause diarrhea and weight loss.
- Diagnosis is based on fecal or cellophane-tape test.
- Treat with piperazine (see Table 8).
- Coccidiosis caused by *Eimeria caviae* is a fairly common cause of diarrhea in guinea pigs recently purchased from pet stores.
- Clinical signs are colitis, diarrhea, dehydration, and death.
- Diagnosis is based on fecal examination. White plaques may be present. Necropsy shows petechiation and thickening of the colon.
- Treat supportively and administer sulfa drugs (see Table 9).
- *Cryptosporidium wrairi* and *Giardia* spp. are found rarely. They cause a chronic enteritis. *Balantidium* species are thought to be nonpathogenic.

Dental

- Malocclusion in guinea pigs is diagnosed on oral examination. Clinical signs are ptyalism and anorexia. The premolars are the most commonly affected teeth.
- Gingivitis secondary to hypovitaminosis C causes similar clinical signs, but the teeth appear normal.
- Long-standing scurvy predisposes to malocclusion.
- Treat the same as for other rodents (see Dental Procedures).

Diarrhea

- Hypovitaminosis C (i.e., scurvy) is associated with soft, malodorous feces. Degeneration of the epithelium of the intestinal tract adversely affects digestion and absorption and allows secondary bacterial infections.
- Diagnosis of scurvy is based on other clinical signs, the exclusion of other causes of diarrhea, and response to vitamin C therapy (see Table 10).
- Salmonellosis is usually contracted through contaminated feed.
- Clinical signs range from sudden death to diarrhea

TABLE 10. Miscellaneous Injectable Medications for Pocket Pets

Agent	Dose	Route
Dexamethasone	0.6 mg/kg	IM
Prednisone	0.5–2.2 mg/kg	IM, SC
Oxytocin	0.2–3.0 IU/kg	IV, IM, SC
Vitamin A	500–5000 IU/kg	IM, SC
Vitamin B complex	0.02–0.2 ml/kg	IM, SC
Vitamin C	20–200 mg/kg	IM, SC
Vitamin D	200–400 IU/kg	IM, SC
Vitamin E/selenium*	0.1 ml/100–250 gm of body weight	SC
Vitamin K	1–10 mg/kg	SC

*Bo-Se: 2.18 mg sodium selenite and 50 mg vitamin E per ml, (Schering-Plough Animal Health, Kenilworth, NJ).

and anorexia. The diarrhea is frequently light-colored. Sepsis is common and is associated with conjunctivitis, shock, pneumonia, abortion, and neurologic signs.
- Diagnosis is based on culture of feces or other appropriate tissue sample.
- Treatment is controversial, because recovered individuals remain carriers. Use sulfa antibiotics (see Table 9) until sensitivity results are available. Supportive care is essential.
- *E. coli, Arizona,* and *Clostridium* are other commonly cultured diarrhea-causing organisms.
- *Yersinia pseudotuberculosis* either causes an acutely fatal diarrhea or localizes into regional lymph nodes.
- Diagnosis is based on culture.
- Treat by surgical removal or drainage of abscessed lymph nodes. Mesenteric lymph node involvement necessitates abdominal surgery. Treat with sulfa drugs until culture results are available (see Table 9).

Theriogenology

- One male is usually housed with 4 to 6 female guinea pigs for breeding purposes. Signs of estrus are vulvar swelling, lordosis, and opening of the vaginal closure membrane. Fetuses are palpable at 4 to 5 weeks of gestation. Parturition occurs within 48 hours after the symphysis has reached 15 mm. Neonates weighing less than 60 gm have a grave prognosis for survival, even with intensive care. Neonates normally do not nurse for 12 to 24 hours after birth. Litters with five or more fetuses usually result in abortion.
- Dystocia commonly occurs in females bred after the age of 6 to 9 months. After this age, the symphysis fuses and is unable to open the 2 to 3 cm required to allow passage of a fetus. Dystocia is commonly the result of obesity, large fetal size, fetal malpresentation, subclinical ketosis, or uterine inertia. On presentation, check the pelvic symphysis. If active contractions are present and the symphyseal gap is less than 2 cm, perform a cesarean section. Normal parturition is very rapid, with only 3 to 7 minutes between fetuses.
- Perform a cesarean section if active straining does not produce a fetus within 15 to 20 minutes. Radio-

graph sows with histories of weak or only a few strong contractions to ascertain the stage of pregnancy and evaluate the sizes of the fetuses. If well-developed skeletons of appropriate size are seen, give oxytocin (see Table 10) and calcium. Poorly developed fetuses indicate that abortion, ketosis, or a nonreproductive disorder is causing clinical signs.

- Pregnancy toxemia is usually seen in obese sows with large litters in late pregnancy. Other risk factors are disease or diet change causing anorexia, genetics, stress, and first litter.
- Clinical signs are tachypnea, depression, malodorous breath, seizures, and icterus. A urine pH of less than 6 with marked proteinuria is compatible with pregnancy toxemia. A marked hyperkalemia and elevation of liver enzymes often occurs. Thrombocytopenia may be present.
- Treat with intravenous saline, dextrose, glucocorticoids, and calcium. Surgical abortion of the fetuses may be attempted, but the anesthesia risk is quite high. Prognosis for survival is grave. Do not rebreed affected females. Do not breed sows heavier than 500 to 900 gm.
- Large litters can cause a hemorrhagic syndrome. Compression of the portal vein and liver causes hepatic dysfunction, which results in vitamin K and clotting factor deficiency.
- Treat with vitamin K supplementation (see Table 10). Response is poor in severely compromised patients. Affected individuals are at risk of developing ketosis. Prognosis is guarded.
- Vaginitis in guinea pigs is frequently caused by foreign bodies, usually bedding.
- Diagnosis is made on vaginal examination.
- Treatment is local flushing.
- Vaginal discharge can also be the result of pyometra, uterine torsion, urinary tract infection, or urogenital neoplasia.
- Diagnosis is based on abdominal palpation, vaginal cytology and culture, urinalysis, abdominal radiography, ultrasonography, and exploratory.
- Treatment varies with the condition and is similar to that used in cats.
- Ovarian teratomas and uterine tumors are occasionally diagnosed and usually respond well to ovariohysterectomy.
- Male guinea pigs are prone to preputial foreign bodies.
- Diagnosis is based on preputial discharge and physical examination.
- Treat by removing foreign bodies and performing local flushing. Chronic problems require a change in bedding.
- Male guinea pigs produce sebaceous secretions in the folds around the perineal area. Clean these areas with soap and water semi-annually to prevent severe localized pyodermas.
- Treat pyodermas with topical therapy and oral antibiotics.

Urology

- Bacterial cystitis and urolithiasis are relatively common problems in guinea pigs.

- Diagnosis is based on a history of stranguria, hematuria, painful abdomen, and anorexia, in addition to abdominal palpation, urinalysis, urine culture, and abdominal radiography, and ultrasonography.
- Treatment consists of antibiotics based on culture results and the surgical removal of stones if present. Prevention of recurrence is difficult if the stones are not secondary to bacterial infection. Addition of vitamin C to drinking water as well as change of brand of diet are somewhat successful in preventing recurrence of metabolic stones.
- *Klossiella cobayae* is a coccidia that lives in the renal tubules. It has no clinical significance.

Musculoskeletal

- The most common orthopedic problem in guinea pigs is overgrown toenails. This leads to pododermatitis and sore hocks, as well as to degenerative joint disease and a predisposition to tibial fractures. Tibial fractures are the most common fracture seen in guinea pigs. They most frequently result when a guinea pig catches its foot and struggles to free it. Surgically repair the fracture by producing internal fixation with an IM pin.
- Signs of hypovitaminosis C or scurvy start to develop in guinea pigs as early as 10 to 15 days after being placed on 100% deficient diets. Early signs are soft malodorous stools, weight loss, poor haircoat, and anorexia. Later, petechiae, gingivitis, cutaneous and oral sores, swollen costochondral junctions, joint pain and hemorrhage resulting in lameness, and conjunctivitis become apparent. Treat supportively and administer parenteral vitamin C (25 mg/day).

Neurology

- Lymphocytic choriomeningitis occurs as in mice.
- Guinea pig paralysis syndrome starts with mild pyrexia and urinary incontinence, followed by weight loss and posterior paresis that progresses to paralysis. The etiology is unknown, but the condition appears nontransmissible.
- Treat supportively. Prognosis for long-term survival is grave.
- Head tilt is usually the result of otitis or trauma (see Mouse).

Hematology

- Cavian leukemia is viral in origin. The liver, spleen, and lymph nodes are the primary organs involved. There is no treatment. Quarantine exposed individuals. Death usually occurs within 5 days of discovery of lymphoblasts in the peripheral blood.
- Neutrophils normally have red granules. Kurloff bodies are normally occurring eosinophilic intracytoplasmic inclusion bodies that are found in mononuclear cells. They are seen most frequently in females and appear to positively correspond with estrogen levels.
- Metastatic calcification occurs in most guinea pigs older than 1 year of age. It is more severe in females than in males. The stomach is one of the first organs affected. Dysfunction in motility causes obstruction.

The tendency appears to be exacerbated by high-calcium and low-phosphorus diets.

Supplemental Readings

Battles AH: The biology, care, and diseases of the syrian hamster. Compend Contin Educ Prac Vet 7(10):815, 1985.

Bauck L: Ophthalmic conditions in pet rabbits and rodents. Compend Contin Educ Prac Vet 11(3):258, 1989.

Collins BR: Common diseases and medical management of rodents and lagomorphs. *In* Jacobson ER, Kollias GV, eds.: *Contemporary Issues in Small Animal Practice: Exotic Animals.* New York: Churchill-Livingstone, 1988, p 261.

Fox JG, Cohen BJ, Loew FM, eds.: *Laboratory Animal Medicine.* New York: Academic Press, 1984.

Grossblatt N, ed.: *Guide for the Care and Use of Laboratory Animals.* Washington, DC: U.S. Government Printing Office, 1978.

Harkness JE, Wagner JE: *The Biology and Medicine of Rabbits and Rodents.* 2nd ed. Philadelphia: Lea & Febiger, 1983.

Holmes DD: *Clinical Laboratory Animal Medicine: An Introduction.* Ames, IA: The Iowa State University Press, 1984.

Jacobson ER, Kollias GV, Peters LJ: Dosages for antibiotics and parasiticides used in exotic animals. Compend Contin Educ Prac Vet 5(4):319, 1983.

Merry C: An introduction to chinchillas. Vet Tech 11:315, 1990.

Peters LJ: The guinea pig: An overview, part 1. Compend Contin Educ Prac Vet 3(4):334, 1981.

Peters LJ: The guinea pig: An overview, part 2. Compend Contin Educ Prac Vet 3(5):403, 1981.

Schuchman SM: The individual care and treatment of rabbits, mice, rats, guinea pigs, hamsters, and gerbils. *In* Kirk RW, ed.: *Current Veterinary Therapy. Small Animal Practice.* 10th ed. Philadelphia: W. B. Saunders, 1989, p 738.

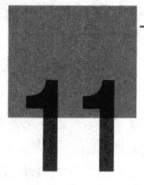

11 Reptiles

Donald Gillespie

ANATOMY AND PHYSIOLOGY

Snakes and Lizards

- Snakes have six rows of teeth, four in the upper jaw attached to the maxillary and palatine bones and two in the lower jaw (one in each mandible). All teeth, including poisonous fangs, can be shed and replaced throughout the snake's life.
- Snakes have no eyelids, differentiating them from the legless lizards. The eyes are covered by a fixed, transparent convex scale, the *spectacle,* which is shed with the skin when the snake sloughs.
- Snakes have no external auditory meatus, whereas lizards do. There is an inner ear.
- All reptiles have a righting reflex. The loss of this reflex helps to determine the stage of anesthesia.
- Two families of snakes possess heat receptors: Boiids and pit vipers.
- Snakes have poor visual acuity, but they are quick to detect movement.
- The snake uses its tongue to explore its environment. The tips of the tongue pick up scent particles and place these in contact with "taste buds" in Jacobson's organ, which lies on the roof of the mouth.
- The glottis can be carried forward to the elastic ligament of the mandibular synthesis to enable the snake to breathe during the somewhat protracted period while swallowing whole prey.
- In snakes, the trachea leads to the only functional lung, the right lung. The left lung forms an abdominal air sac in some species. There is no diaphragm.
- The heart has three chambers (two atria and one ventricle), from which emerge three main trunks: the pulmonary aorta and the right and left aorta. The heart can be palpated one-quarter of the way down the length of the snake. Heart rate varies with species and body temperature, but 40–70 beats per minute is a good rule of thumb.
- Male snakes and lizards possess paired copulatory organs called *hemipenes.* Boas and pythons usually can be sexed by observing the development of the spurs on either side of the cloacal vent. These appendages are remnants of pelvic limbs. The pelvic spurs and hemipenes can be seen radiographically.
- The snake's stomach is fusiform. All other reptiles have an S-shaped simple stomach.
- The liver is fusiform in snakes and bilobed in other reptiles. A gallbladder is present in all reptiles.
- The spleen often is attached to the pancreas, which is located next to the duodenum.

Chelonians

- Turtles may be divided into three categories (all of the below are commonly called turtles):
  - *Fresh-water turtles,* or *terrapins,* and their relatives (including *box turtles*). They can be identified by their feet, which possess flexible wrists and ankles and usually have distinct toes that are normally webbed and tipped with sharp claws.
  - *True tortoises.* Most tortoises are native to areas that have hot, dry summers. Their feet normally have no identifiable wrist or ankle motion; these joints are stiffened. The front feet possess large claws which are blunted because the animals walk "tip-toe" on these claws. The hind feet are stump-like with flattened soles, resembling an elephant's foot.
  - *Sea turtles.* All are salt-water species that possess distinctive oar-like or flipper-like feet on which the toes are scarcely distinguishable.
- The body is enclosed by a pair of bony shells. The top shell is called the *carapace* and through evolution has incorporated the rib cage. The bottom plate is called the *plastron.*
- The entire shoulder girdle and pelvic girdle are incorporated within the bony shell, an anatomic feat accomplished only in this animal.
- It is difficult to sex baby turtles until they reach a 4-inch shell length.

Sexual Dimorphism
Males
- The cloacal opening is located external to the rim of the carapace.
- The tail is usually longer and thicker than in females.
- In tortoises and box turtles, the plastron is usually concave.
- In the eastern box turtle, the eyes are red.
- In many species of fresh-water turtles, the nails are extraordinarily long on the front feet.
- Many varieties have sexual tubercles on the lower part of the mandible.

Females
- The cloacal opening is located within the rim of the carapace.
- The tail often is short and thin.
- In tortoises and box turtles, the plastron is flat.
- In the eastern box turtle, the eyes are brown.

VENOMOUS REPTILES
- Because of *liability* and other factors, dealing with privately owned venomous animals is *not* recommended.

- The practitioner is liable for problems in the clinic.
  - Have owners handle venomous reptiles, at least initially. Instruct clients regarding their responsibility for injuries that may occur during examination and treatment of the reptile.
- Proper procedures dictate established safety protocols and availability of appropriate antivenin, which usually is not kept by the client or clinician, especially for foreign species.
  - The clinician may be asked to perform procedures such as devenomation by venom duct ligation (which may later regrow and restore the reptile to its original danger potential). The question of inherent liability for performing the operation may arise years later; performance of this procedure is probably unethical.

HUSBANDRY

Temperature

- Table 1 lists ideal ambient temperatures for reptiles and amphibians.

KEY POINT ▶ Prolonged exposure to the high end of optimal temperatures can cause heat stress, secondary infections, anorexia, and, finally, maladaptation.

- Digestive enzymes are temperature-dependent and become inactive at lower temperatures; food literally will putrify in the digestive tract without being absorbed, resulting in emesis.
  - In general, metabolism is temperature-dependent, as is immunity. Optimal or slightly higher than optimal temperatures aid in resistance to infectious processes.

KEY POINT ▶ Most tropical reptiles become sluggish and reluctant to eat if the ambient temperature falls below 72°F.

- To maintain temperature, place a heating tape or pad under the cage.
  - Use heat lamps only if they can be carefully monitored, because they generate considerable heat that can burn an animal.
- Secure a thermometer to the cage to check the ambient temperature.

Housing

Snakes and Lizards

- Aquariums with a screened top are suitable for housing.

TABLE 1. Ideal Ambient Temperatures (Degrees Fahrenheit) for Various Reptiles

Alligators	80–90°
Iguanas	80–90°
Chameleons	55–75°
Turtles	75–85°
Tortoises	80–90°
Snakes	75–90°

- Do not use any screening on the sides because snakes can abrade the nose on it. Occasionally this occurs on screened tops, requiring the substitution of Plexiglas modules.
- The snake should be able to stretch two-thirds of its length.
- Do not use wood cages because it is difficult to disinfect them, and wood can harbor mites.
- Take care when selecting *substrates*.
  - Do not use soil which can readily become infested with bacteria and helminth eggs.
  - If using peat moss, bark, leaf litter, wood chips, sawdust, or ground corn cob, do not allow it to become damp, making it an ideal medium for microorganisms.
  - Gravel is suitable but must be washed and disinfected once a month; common household bleach is effective and inexpensive.
  - Substrates such as sand, small gravel, kitty litter, and ground corncobs can cause obstruction of the pharynx and cloaca.

KEY POINT ▶ The safest substrate and the easiest to use is newspaper or paper toweling; both are disposed of readily and are nonabrasive.

- Provide arboreal (tree-dwelling) species with limbs and twigs for climbing. Change these periodically because they can harbor mites.
- Provide a "hiding place" for reptiles, such as a small plastic box or piece of bark.
- Disinfect cages once a month. The halogens, quaternary ammonium compounds, hexachlorophene, chloroxylenol, and chlorhexidene are safe.
  - Do not use phenols and coal tar disinfectants.

Chelonians

- A turtle bowl, glass baking dish, or aquarium is suitable for small turtles. One square foot of space is required for every 4 linear inches of turtle.
- Fill the enclosure with water to a depth of 1 inch for small turtles. More is needed for larger turtles. Provide a large rock so that the turtle can dry off.
- Too much moisture can cause bacterial and fungal growth on the shell. For this reason, never cover the enclosure.
- Never place the aquarium or other enclosure in direct sunlight or in drafts, because of possible overheating and rapid cooling, respectively.
- Placing a lamp with a 60-watt bulb 8–12 inches above the dry area can provide warmth and a drying effect.
- Place tortoises in terrariums.

Water and Humidity

Snakes and Lizards

- When practical, provide a water bowl large enough to accommodate the entire reptile without causing the water to overflow; soaking in water aids ecdysis (shedding).
  - Larger specimens have to be soaked, as needed, in containers such as garbage cans.
- Snakes will drink from a bowl. Lizards such as geckos

and anoles lap water from vegetation; spray their enclosures lightly twice a day.

▪ Keep the humidity at 35–60%, depending on the species; desert species prefer the lower range, and forest dwellers and tropical species require higher humidity. Excessive humidity can cause blister disease.

Chelonians

▪ Because aquatic turtles must have water to eat, keep the water level deep enough to allow the animal to submerge its head.

▪ Allow 1–2 hours for eating; then clean the enclosure so that organic debris does not accumulate.
  • It is best to feed turtles in an area separate from housing and clean the enclosure weekly.

▪ To prevent human exposure to *Salmonella* organisms, do not clean turtle enclosures in a kitchen or other human food preparation area. Pour all water into the toilet.

▪ Tortoises require a shallow, nontippable water pan, preferably large enough to permit soaking.

Photoperiod

▪ The photoperiod varies with the species; in general, a 14-hour light cycle and a 10-hour dark cycle is suitable, lengthened or shortened to correspond to the time of year.

FEEDING RECOMMENDATIONS

Snakes

▪ Most snakes kept as pets will eat rodents. The size of the rodent, of course, depends on the size of the snake.
  • Pinkies (baby mice) are used to feed small snakes, whereas adult rats or rabbits are suitable for large boas and pythons.
  • When feeding growing boas and pythons, offer rodents slightly larger than the snake's head to stimulate the head to grow in proportion to the body.

KEY POINT ▶ Contrary to popular belief, snakes will accept stunned or freshly killed food. Live rodents can inflict serious bite wounds and kill snakes by severing the spinal cord, particularly in boa constrictors.

  • Occasionally it is necessary to offer the food on the end of a pair of long forceps to stimulate the snake to strike.
▪ Offer food to growing snakes once a week. Feed adult snakes every two weeks. Larger boas and pythons may be fed once every 3–4 weeks.
▪ Occasionally newly acquired snakes or those debilitated by illness will not eat.
  • Force-feeding may be accomplished with the natural diet rolled in raw egg or with chicken hearts stuffed with bone meal rolled in raw egg.
  • Some "picky" eaters may be stimulated to eat by offering chicks or other small birds.

▪ It is recommended to feed birds to pythons at regular intervals, because they may become anorexic on a rodent diet alone.
▪ Offer snakes such as garter snakes and racers guppies or goldfish (in a water bowl), earthworms, or small insects weekly.
▪ Reluctant water snakes, indigo snakes, and hognose snakes often can be induced to eat by offering poikilothermic prey such as frogs, toads, fish, and anoles. In fact, the main diet of hognose snakes is toads.
▪ Other snakes such as vine snakes feed primarily on anoles and other lizards.

Lizards

▪ Feed all lizards at least two or three times weekly; feed immature animals and those that do not attain a foot or more in length as adults daily. Most lizards are carnivorous except for iguanids, which are the most frequent type of pet lizard.

Iguanids

▪ Iguanids are herbivores as adults (2½–3 feet or longer); however, young growing iguanids need approximately 25% of their diet as animal matter such as young mice, dog food, and occasionally crickets, mealworms, and various cooked meats without bones. Offer this several times weekly; to avoid spoilage, do not leave in the cage more than 4–6 hours. The remaining 75% is the same as that for adults.
▪ Base the bulk of adult iguanids' diet on legumes. Convenient sources include bean sprouts, alfalfa pellets, and alfalfa hay.
▪ Also offer frozen mixed vegetables, broken down into daily serving portions and thawed as needed; these mixtures contain both legumes and brightly colored vegetables such as carrots and corn that attract attention to the food. (The basis of this attraction is that brightly colored flowering plants are the best quality forage available to reptiles in arid regions.)
▪ Legumes should be about 75% of the diet; the balance should be dark green leafy vegetables such as spinach, kale, and broccoli; fresh green cuttings such as dandelions, rose petals, and good-quality lawn grass; and other fruits and vegetables.
▪ Feed a good-quality vitamin–trace mineral product (e.g., Vionate; Pitman-Moore) and a primary calcium supplement.

KEY POINT ▶ Note that most vitamin supplements have minimal amounts of calcium and should not serve as the primary calcium supplement.

▪ Feeding dog or cat food to adult iguanids generally is not recommended because of the following:
  • Dog and cat foods may be too rich in protein and minerals and can lead to gout or urinary tract stones.
  • Often lettuce is used in combination with dog or cat food; inevitably the iguanid consumes lettuce as the staple dietary item, resulting in a diet

deficient in protein, calcium, vitamin D_3, and other essential nutrients that can lead to secondary hypoparathyroidism and fibrous osteodystrophy.

- Excessive loss of calcium mobilized from bones to compensate for dietary insufficiency can result in cystic calcium urate stones.

Insectivorous Lizards

- Offer geckoes and other insectivorous lizards fruit flies, fly larvae, small crickets, and mealworms.
  - Larger insectivores including chameleons may be offered giant mealworms, cockroaches, and pinkies.
  - Individuals will show certain preferences, and insect sources other than those mentioned can be offered.
- Improve the nutritional content of the insects by maintaining them for at least 1 week on a medium such as laying mash, alfalfa pellets, and commercial insect chows made specifically for this purpose.
  - Place sliced apple, carrot, or potato in the medium as a moisture source.
  - The content of calcium, protein, and other nutrients in insects has been measured and shown to increase substantially with this system.

KEY POINT ▶ A calcium source must be included in the diet of insectivores and iguanids, especially during laying season.

- Some hobbyists use fine gravel composed of calcium carbonate both as a substrate and as a calcium source for geckoes. However, animals may ingest too much of this material, resulting in colonic impaction, cloacal prolapse, and possibly death.
- Suitable calcium sources include:
  - A mineral block placed in the drinking water
  - or the addition of ¼–1 teaspoon of liquid calcium gluconate per ounce of drinking water.
  - "Dust" food sources with calcium carbonate powder (and a vitamin–trace mineral supplement) prior to feeding.

Carnivorous Lizards

- Offer carnivorous lizards such as the tegu and monitor whole prey including stunned rodents, quail, and chicken, on a rotating basis, as 75–80% of the diet.
- Other dietary items include various meats or insects when these animals are young.
- Feed a vitamin–trace mineral supplement regularly.

Agamids

- For agamids (skinks), animal matter as described for iguanids can comprise 50% of the diet; the remaining portion should be dark green leafy vegetables, carrots, tomatoes, and fruit.
- Provide a calcium source such as bone meal, calcium gluconate, or a mineral block in the water dish, along with a vitamin–trace mineral supplement.

KEY POINT ▶ Regular, voracious feeding usually is a good indicator of general health in all reptiles.

Chelonians

KEY POINT ▶ Turtles and tortoises may be fed daily or every other day. Large specimens may only need weekly feedings. Exposure for 10–15 minutes to unfiltered sunlight or a black lamp often is needed as a physiologic stimulation of appetite in tortoises and diurnal lizards.

Hatchlings and Young Animals

- In hatchlings, a delicate touch may be required to induce feeding, which may be delayed 1–2 weeks until the yolk sac is totally resorbed internally.
- Small aquatic species often will start feeding on earthworms broken into pieces, tubifex worms, and stunned or killed guppies.
- Once feeding occurs on a regular basis, decrease insects and worms and add whole prey or turtle pellets.
- For baby tortoises and omnivorous turtles, grinding the diet is essential, as is adding bright colors, such as red via strawberries and rose petals, and yellow and orange, via vegetables such as corn and carrots.

For discussion of adult feeding recommendations, turtles divide into general categories of aquatic turtles (carnivores), omnivores such as box turtles, and tortoises (herbivores).

Aquatic Turtles

Aquatic turtles are primarily carnivorous but will eat some plant matter.

- Offer sliders and painted turtles good-quality commercial turtle pellets and whole fish (live or freshly killed). Feed insects, earthworms, and plant matter as 25% of the diet.
- Offer more carnivorous species such as musk, mud, big-headed, and snapping turtles a variety of whole live fish as well as insects, earthworms, and meat.
- Some species such as mata-mata turtles eat fish exclusively, which they literally vacuum up by means of a large hyoid apparatus.
- It is essential to rotate fish types. Exclusive feeding of goldfish has been associated with mortality in several turtle species including mata-mata turtles.
- Obtain fresh-water fish from a clean source to avoid carriers of bacterial or parasitic diseases.
- Fish may be fed high-quality food sources to improve their nutritional content similar to the method described for insects.
- Do not give frozen fish on a regular basis as it lacks viscera and must be supplemented with vitamin E and thiamine owing to loss of these vitamins during the freezing process.

Box Turtles and Other Omnivorous Turtles

- Turtles such as box, wood, Blanding, and Muhlenberg species can be fed canned or dry dog food as 50% of the diet, and offer vegetables, fruits, earthworms, and insects as the balance of the diet.
  - Vegetables include carrots, tomatoes, kale, water-

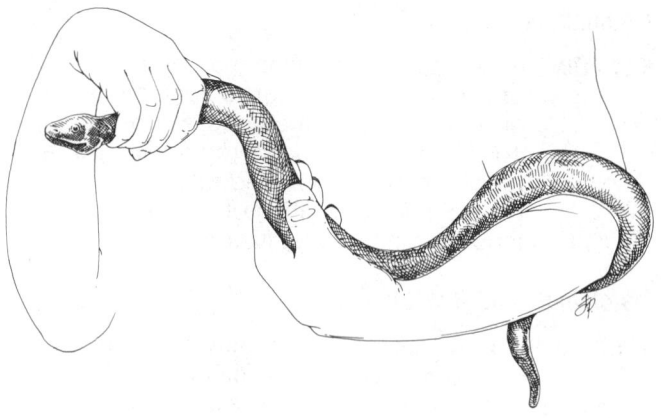

Figure 1. Proper restraint of a nonaggressive, nonvenomous snake.

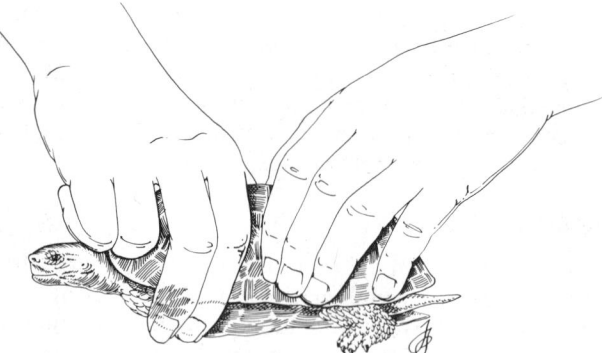

Figure 3. Proper restraint of a turtle.

cress, string beans, corn, endive, spinach, and thawed frozen mixed vegetables.
- Fruits include bananas, apples, oranges, peaches, strawberries, cantaloupes, watermelons; offer petals from garden flowers to difficult eaters.
- Supply vitamin–trace mineral supplements.

Tortoises

- Feed tortoises a regimen similar to that for iguanids and other herbivorous reptiles.
- Certain tortoises, such as those from the Galapagos Islands, are prone to goiter, which requires the addition of Lugol's iodine, one to several drops once or twice weekly, empirically as a preventative.

Crocodilians

- Similar to carnivorous turtles or lizards, offer crocodilians balanced whole prey items such as fish, frogs, rodents, and birds, on a rotating basis for variety.
- Feed specimens less than 2 feet in length daily or every other day; and feed large specimens weekly or every 2 weeks.
- Supplement frozen fish with vitamin E (50–100 IU/kg of fish fed) and thiamine (50–100 mg/kg of fish fed) to avoid deficiencies from loss of these vitamins during frozen storage.

CLINICAL TECHNIQUES

Blood Collection

Snakes

Most snakes a foot or more in length can be sampled using this technique.

- Restrain as shown in Figure 1.
- Approach the ventral tail vein on the midline about one third of the distance caudal between the cloaca and tail end. This avoids damage to the hemipene area.
  - Direct the needle at a 45° angle until reaching the vertebra, and then withdraw slowly while using gentle aspiration on the syringe. Use 25- or 27-gauge needles in small specimens, and 22- or 20-gauge needles in snakes 3 feet and longer.
- Alternatively, open the mouths of boas and pythons with a soft spatula or tongue depressor to collect from the buccal veins on the inside of the mouth (Fig. 2).

KEY POINT ▶ Cardiocentesis is not recommended because of the risk of hemopericardium even with atraumatic collection.

Chelonians

- Restrain as shown in Figure 3.
- Jugular veins are variable but blood collection is possible after proper positioning in many tortoises (Fig. 4). Administer ketamine (10–20 mg/kg, SC) if necessary.
- Toenail clip and microhematocrit tube collection is possible in most chelonians as a last resort after attempting other sites.
- The occipital sinus of most turtles, even smaller specimens, yields appreciable amounts of blood for analysis. By fixing the turtle's head in an extended

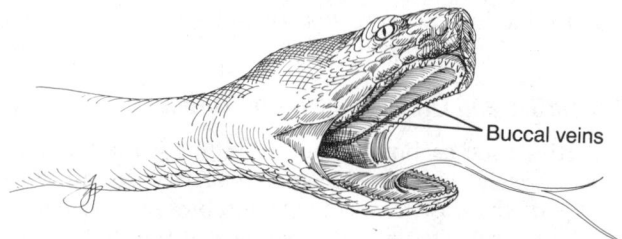

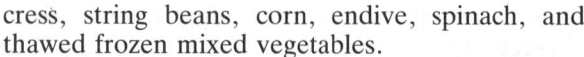

Figure 2. Venipuncture sites for the dorsal buccal veins of a snake.

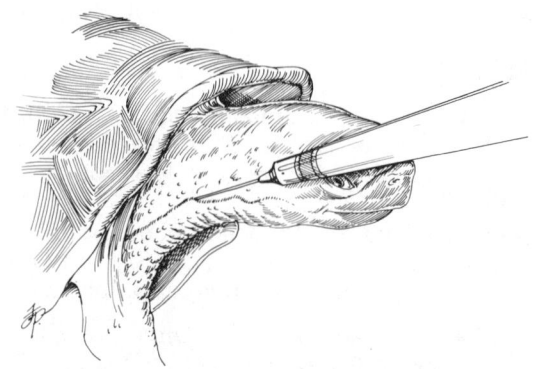

Figure 4. Jugular venipuncture site in a turtle.

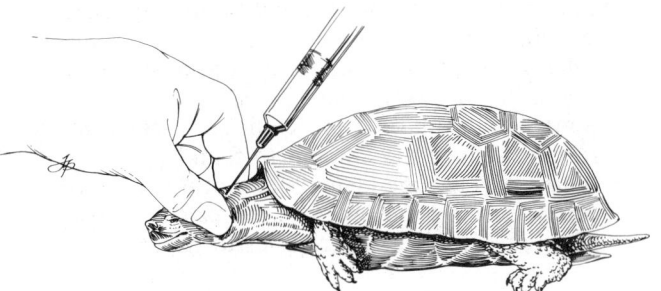

Figure 5. Occipital sinus aspiration in a turtle.

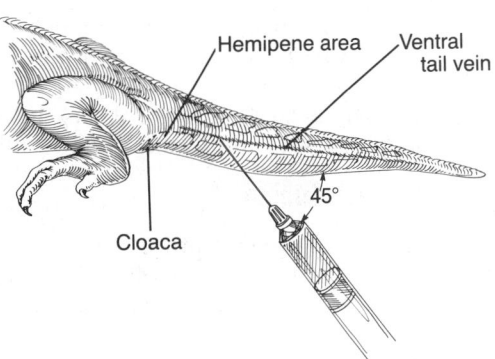

Figure 7. Venipuncture of ventral tail vein of a lizard.

position against the plastron, a stable platform is created to enter the occipital sinus, which should be palpable (Fig. 5). Ketamine and/or gas anesthesia may be necessary in active turtles to ensure atraumatic collection.

- Using gentle technique, slowly advance a syringe with a small-gauge needle into the sinus with slight aspiration of the syringe. Once blood enters the syringe, maintain its position and then withdraw the needle slowly without aspiration.
- Complications include hemorrhage from improper restraint or technique and pithing of the spinal cord; however, with patience and experience, this is a safe and reliable technique.
- This site may be used for collection of cerebrospinal fluid (CSF) and for euthanasia injection in all reptiles.
■ Cardiocentesis is not recommended for turtles because of the risk of hemopericardium.

Lizards and Crocodilians

■ Restrain lizards as shown in Figure 6.
■ Crocodilians and lizards may be bled from the ventral tail vein, as described for snakes (Fig. 7).
■ Blood also may be collected from the lateral tail veins and jugular veins in larger crocodilian specimens.
■ Cardiocentesis is not recommended because of the risk of hemopericardium.
■ Toenail clip and hematocrit tube blood collection can be used in smaller specimens and in larger specimens when blood cannot be obtained by venipuncture.

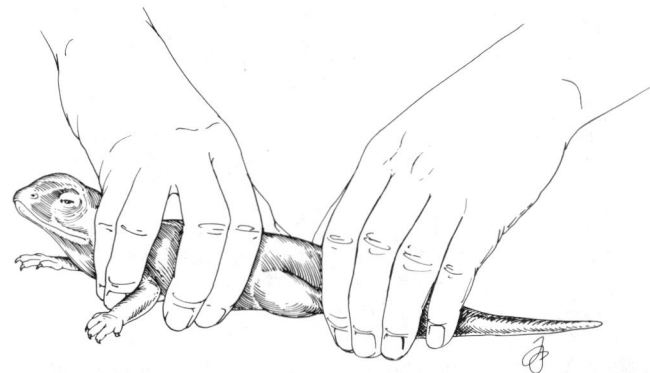

Figure 6. Proper restraint of a lizard.

Oral Examination

Snakes

Snakes often can be examined orally by use of a soft spatula, credit card, or padded tongue depressor.

■ Insert the speculum into the lateral aspect of the mouth and with a steady, gentle twisting motion position it transversely.
■ Alternatively, grasp the skin on the ventral midline mandible and exert steady downward pressure to compel a snake to open its mouth.
■ While opening the mouth, grasp the head gently behind the mandible and loosely around the neck to avoid excessive twisting or thrashing.

Lizards and Crocodilians

■ Perform oral examination of lizards by using the same techniques described for snakes.
■ Techniques for oral examination of crocodilians is the same as for lizards and snakes, except that *total restraint* (chemical if needed), is recommended, because many specimens struggle and attempt to bite.

Chelonians

Turtles can present a special challenge, depending on their strength and physical condition.

■ Extend the turtle's head carefully by placing fingers in back of the head and exerting gentle pressure cranially. Tip the turtle ventrally or press the back hinge plate of mud or box turtles to assist in inducing the turtle's head to come out of the shell enough to be grasped by the fingers.
  • Ketamine (10–20 mg/kg, SC) may be needed for aggressive species, (e.g., most aquatic turtles) and if manual restraint alone is traumatic. For simple oral examination, many aquatic turtles will attempt to bite when approached and, hence, present the mouth open.
■ Once the chelonian's head is in a fixed extended position, use paper clips (the size depends on the size of the specimen) to gently open the mouth.
  • Insert the paper clip between the mandible and maxilla and then, with a gentle prying action, open the mouth and insert the clip transversely to hold the mouth open.

- Next, insert a hemostat, wooden block, tongue depressor, or other device to open the mouth farther if needed.
- If the paper clip is large enough, it may be left in place to allow passage of a small stomach tube.

Insertion of Stomach Tubing

In debilitated or anorexic reptiles, stomach tubing often is a desired route for delivery of medications and nutritional supplements (see Feeding Recommendations).

Snakes

■ Restrain as shown in Figure 1.

KEY POINT ▶ Intubate snakes to the level of the stomach (about one-fourth of the length of the body), or they usually will regurgitate.

■ After opening the mouth, place the tube in the back of the mouth and direct it caudally, taking care to avoid catching the tube on the dorsal and ventral rows of the recurved teeth.
  - Normally, at this point the snake will attempt to retract the head and coil. This usually necessitates the presence of a second person to straighten the neck to allow easy passage of the tube.
■ Use gentle pressure or gravity to deliver the medications or supplements, and then apply a small amount of air to clear the contents of the stomach tube.
■ Kink the tube and withdraw it; again, avoid catching the tube on the recurved teeth.
■ Restrict handling of the snake for several hours (preferably 24–48 hours), to prevent regurgitation.

Other Reptiles

■ For chelonians, lizards, and crocodilians, follow the general principles of stomach tubing outlined for snakes.
  - Exceptions include measurement and then placement of the tube to a point just past the mid-coelomic area.
  - Turtles have a keratinized beak and no teeth (for the tube to catch on).
  - Crocodilians have a waterproof flap arrangement in the caudal pharynx that must be opened manually prior to passage of the stomach tube.
■ Stomach tubing may be used for force-feeding of whole food items such as fish, mice, and chicks in carnivorous reptiles, and of small sections of leafy dark green vegetables in anorexic reptiles.
  - Whole food items have the advantage of being considerably more difficult to regurgitate than liquid feedings.
  - Liquid or tablet/capsule medications may be injected or placed into these food items concurrently.
  - Avoid overfeeding; several pieces once to several times weekly usually is sufficient.
  - After several weeks of force-feeding, make every effort to get the patient to eat voluntarily to avoid stress and psychological damage and the dependence associated with this technique.

- When giving liquid nutritional supplements, avoid overfilling of the stomach, or regurgitation may result. Total stomach capacity for most animals is 25–50 ml/kg of body weight.
- Start at 10 ml/kg per feeding; if regurgitation results, reduce the amount to 5 ml/kg.
- Alternatively, feed small amounts of Nutri-Cal orally several times weekly; this calorie-dense supplement is difficult for reptiles to expel.

Injections

KEY POINT ▶ Because of the renal portal venous system in reptiles and (probably) amphibians, administer injectable medications in the front half of the body. This ensures body-wide drug distribution prior to excretion and avoids concentration of nephrotoxic drugs too rapidly in the kidneys.

Snakes

Intramuscular (IM) and Subcutaneous (SC) Injections

The preferred area for IM and SC injections is the paralumbar area (Fig. 8, *top*).

■ Advance the needle (the smallest gauge possible) to the hub and then make the injection.
■ Enter between rather than through the scales, and slowly withdraw the needle, pinching the scales with

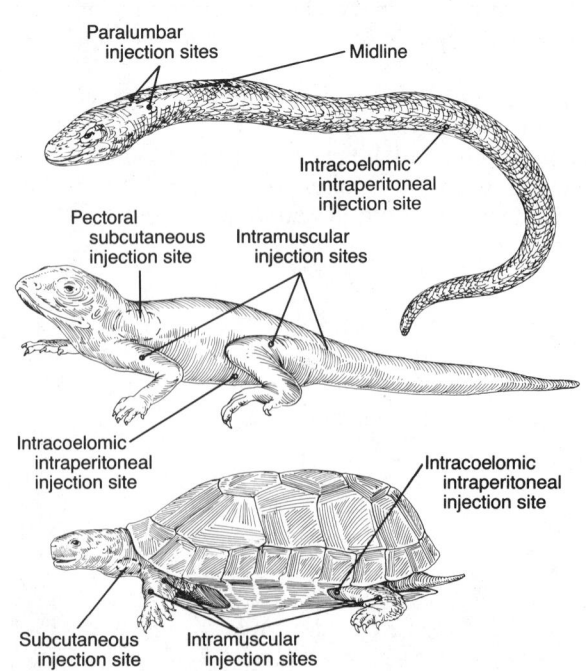

Figure 8. Common injection sites in a snake *(top)*, lizard *(center)*, and turtle *(below)*.

the fingers to avoid leakage (which can occur because of the tight nature of reptile skin).

■ SC fluids advance cranially in the paralumbar area from the point of injection. This allows a considerable volume to be injected at a single point and then repeated on the other side of the paralumbar area.

Intraperitoneal (IP) Injections

The injection site is between the ventral scutes in the mid-coelomic region.

■ IP injections are not recommended for routine use because of the potential for organ damage and peritonitis. Some clinicians advocate IP fluid injections because of apparent lack of absorption by the SC route, but this is not correct.

■ IP injection has been used for administration of euthanasia drugs when intravenous and intracardiac delivery is not possible. However, owing to slow absorption, euthanasia may take several to 24 hours by this route.

Intracardiac (IC) Injections

■ IC injections are not recommended because of the potential for trauma (see Blood Collection).

■ The IC route, however, is useful for administration of euthanasia drugs.
  • Position the snake in dorsal recumbency; the heart is located one-fourth to one-third of the body length caudal to the head. The location varies among species.
  • The heart can be visualized beating slowly beneath a ventral scute, often on the lateral aspect. This may take several minutes to envision properly.

Chelonians

SC and IM Injections

■ Injections can be made in the skin between the neck and medial aspect of the front limbs (SC injections) or on the medial aspect of the front limbs (IM injection) (Fig. 8, *center*).
  • Avoid giving SC and IM injections on the lateral aspect of the front limbs or axillary region, because this often results in hemorrhage.

■ By grasping the front foot and fixing it to the lateral carapace or plastron with the thumb, most aquatic turtles can be given SC and IM injections by one person, with the hand out of range of the biting jaws and with the turtle securely restrained.

■ An exception is the soft-shelled turtle, whose neck length is sufficient to reach the fingers in this position. For these animals, approach the leathery skin of the neck on the dorsal and ventral midline and pinch to trap the head inside the shell.
  • With the head secured, quickly make the injection and withdraw the fingers caudally.

IP Injections

■ Grasp a rear leg and fix it against the plastron caudally.

■ Make the injection in the space proximal to the leg underneath the skin and muscle, which is the coelomic or peritoneal cavity.

■ Stones, impactions, and eggs can be palpated in this space.

IC Injections

■ Make the injection after drilling a hole with an IM pin on the midline at the first one-third of the plastron, between growth plates.

■ IP injection or injection into the vein in the occipital sinus region (see Blood Collection) is recommended for chelonians, especially for administration of euthanasia drugs.

Intravenous (IV) Injections

■ A dorsal tail vein has been described for blood collection and intravenous drug administration in large sea turtles and may be a potential site in large fresh-water species.

Lizards and Crocodilians

■ SC injection in lizards is difficult because of their tight skin but usually can be made in the cervical and shoulder areas (Fig. 8, *center*).
  • As in snakes, use a small needle and place it to the hub prior to injection.
  • For some lizards and crocodilians, SC injection is impractical; thus, oral or IP administration of fluids and IM injection of other medications are preferred.

■ IM injections are usually given in the lateral aspect of the arm or forearm of the front limbs.

■ IP injections are given in the same location and for the same reasons as in snakes.

■ Occipital sinus injection has been attempted in lizards and crocodilians with variable results.

Euthanasia

■ Euthanasia drugs for reptiles may be administered at the same rate as for birds and mammals, using the occipital sinus, IC or less preferably IP or coelomic route.
  • It may take several hours for the reptile to die.

■ An alternative method for humane euthanasia is sudden decapitation after induction of anesthesia.

KEY POINT ▶ Do not use hypothermia (placement of small reptiles in freezer) for euthanasia. Clients may be inclined to do this to save costs. This method is not only inhumane but is also unreliable; in several cases, a reptile was still alive after > 48 hours when removed for disposal.

RADIOLOGY

Snakes

■ Obtain lateral radiographs (usually the most useful view for diagnosis) by taping the snake in a stable position on the film cassette; take sequential exposures running cranial to caudal.
  • Small tape markers placed on the skin during this process help ensure that the whole body is radiographed.
  • Give ketamine (10–20/kg, IM or SC) if necessary to maintain the position of active patients.

■ Ventrodorsal (VD) exposures often can be made by

allowing the snake to coil on a large cassette with minimal or no restraint.
  • Hold, tape, or sedate larger patients and radiograph sequentially from cranial to caudal, as described for the lateral view.

Chelonians

■ Obtain AP views by holding the turtle in a vertical plane so that the x-ray beam travels parallel to the longitudinal axis from head to tail, or the same is achieved by horizontal projection of the x-ray beam.
  • Patients must usually be strapped or taped to boards of different sizes or to large wooden spoons to achieve good position without exposure of operator's hand to the primary beam.
  • Water turtles often are very active and move the feet constantly while being held. Use tape wrapped around the shell to contain the leg movement, or sedate prior to positioning.
■ Normal lung fields on the lateral view are of black density throughout the cranial two-thirds to three-fourths of the turtle's length in the dorsal aspect of the coelomic cavity.
  • Pneumonia is seen as an alveolar pattern of soft tissue density, usually concentrated in the cranial one-third to one-half of the lung area.
■ On the AP view there is normally some soft tissue density on the midline of the dorsal aspect of the coelomic cavity owing to normal hilar region anatomic structures.
  • Pneumonia is seen as an extension of this soft tissue density toward the lateral shell edges. This alveolar pattern often extends at least halfway toward the lateral shell edges, and in severe cases extends to the lateral shell margins, with miliary densities in the central region.
■ In desert tortoises, tracheal culture and radiography are essential for differentiating lower respiratory disease from simple upper respiratory infections and/or allergies commonly seen when animals are kept in a climate different from that of their natural environment.
■ VD views are useful for visualization of stones, eggs, and foreign bodies. This view often can be accomplished with minimal or no restraint.

Lizards and Crocodilians

■ Because of their body shape, these animals can be radiographed with conventional holding techniques used in mammals and birds.
  • Use of tape and precise collimation can result in accurate lateral radiographs.
  • Crocodilians of any size are usually easier to handle when sedated with ketamine (10–20 mg/kg, SC or IM).
  • As in chelonians, VD views are useful for visualizing bladder stones, eggs, and foreign bodies, with minimal restraint.
  • Place the crate or cage of aggressive reptiles directly over the film cassette(s), eliminating the need for handling.

ENVIRONMENTAL DISEASES

Temperature-Related Diseases

Chronic Hypothermia

Reptiles may live a considerable length of time and even eat at less than optimal temperatures; however, adverse effects include:

■ Impaired digestive enzyme function
  • A proven cause of emesis in reptiles
  • Implicated as a cause of necrotizing gastroenteritis secondary to putrefaction
■ Visceral and articular gout, resulting from impaired protein metabolism and excretion and possible temperature effect on solubility of excreted waste products such as urates
■ Increased susceptibility to infections (impaired humoral and cellular immunity)

Hyperthermia

Higher than optimal temperatures are poorly tolerated. Adverse effects include:

■ Functional thyroid hypertrophy
■ Decreased spermatogenesis
■ Skeletal muscle atrophy
■ Sudden death

Humidity-Related Diseases

■ Long-term high humidity may cause:
  • Blister disease, characterized by fluid-filled skin vesicles that rapidly become purulent (most commonly seen in lizards)
  • Shell plate sloughing in turtles
■ Long-term low humidity may result in dehydration, causing:
  • Dysecdysis (difficulty in shedding)

KEY POINT ▶ Treat dysecdysis with soaks and misting with water and wetting agents at shedding time. Avoid manual manipulation, especially of eye caps in snakes.

  • Visceral and articular gout

Light-Related Diseases

■ Suboptimal light may induce complete anorexia.
■ Nocturnal species will not feed in the absence of darkness.
■ The proper photoperiod is required for breeding success.
■ Induce reluctant feeders to feed by placing under wide-spectrum lights, such as Grolux (Sylvania Corp.) and Vita-Lite (Dyna-Lite Lamps).
■ Because wide-spectrum lights may retain visible light when the ultraviolet portion burns out, periodic replacement is necessary.
■ Some diurnal geckoes, chameleons, and other lizards may require a black light in addition to wide-spectrum ultraviolet light in order to induce feeding.

Population Dynamics

- Generalized edema is a sign of high population pressure in iguanid lizards, which are highly territorial. The edema is believed to be induced by adrenocortical insufficiency.
- Population pressure in crocodilians can cause depletion of liver glycogen, resulting in hypoglycemia. Hypoglycemia may cause mydriasis, tremors, and cataleptic-like seizures.
  - Treat with oral or parenteral glucose (3 g/kg).

Nutritional Disorders

Because of a generally poor understanding of reptilian nutrition, nutritional disorders are common.

Hypovitaminosis A

- Commonly seen in young terrapins on dried insect and lettuce diets.
- Clinical signs include swollen, shut eyes. The harderian glands (accessory lacrimal glands) of turtles are highly developed solute excretory organs with a high vitamin A requirement. Squamous metaplasia with keratin plugging is a prominent feature of this disease.
- Squamous metaplasia may occur in respiratory epithelium and bile ducts.
- Secondary bacterial infections are common.

Hypovitaminosis D

- Clinical signs include rickets and osteomalacia and (in chelonians) soft shells.

Hypervitaminosis D

- Hypervitaminosis D, caused by overzealous dietary supplements or prolonged exposure to sunlamps, may lead to:
  - Metastatic calcification of soft tissues including aortic arches, joints, and viscera.
  - Mobilization of calcium from bone, resulting in osteopenia.

Hypovitaminosis E

- Vitamin E deficiency usually is seen in fish-fed reptiles. Oily fish such as mackerel contain long-chain unsaturated fatty acids that compete for vitamin E.
- The disease has also been reported in rodent-fed snakes and may relate to obesity in laboratory rodents.
  - Adverse effects include:
  - Steatitis (i.e., induration and inflammation of fat with acid-fast ceroid accumulation)
  - Skeletal muscle degeneration and necrosis

Hypovitaminosis K

- Vitamin K deficiency is manifested as bleeding gingiva responsive to vitamin K therapy.

Hypovitaminosis C

- Vitamin C deficiency may be the underlying cause of ulcerative stomatitis.

- Vitamin C is often included in therapy for stomatitis and respiratory infections in reptiles (see Infectious Diseases).

Thiamine or Vitamin B Deficiency

- This deficiency is seen primarily in iguanas.
- Thiaminase present in frozen fish can cause deficiency in reptiles fed an all-fish diet.
- Clinical signs include posterior limb and tail paresis and trembling.
- Distinguish from calcium deficiency by radiology.

Nutritional Secondary Hyperparathyroidism

- This disorder is most commonly seen in herbivorous lizards and is commonly encountered in carnivorous reptiles on boneless meat diets.
- Monostotic or polyostotic fibrous osteodystrophy may result. Lizards with this condition often appear well nourished because the resultant fibrous thickening of bones gives them a well-muscled appearance.
- Cystic calculi are the most common manifestation of secondary hyperparathyroidism in tortoises and are commonly seen in herbivorous lizards.

  Treatment
- The following can be instituted:
  - Supplement the diet with 900 mg calcium carbonate ($CaCO_3$) per 100 g of meat; 150 mg $CaCO_3$ per 100 g of live food, or 100 mg $CaCO_3$ per kg of body weight given once IM.
  - Alternatively, give direct oral supplementation 50–100 mg $CaCO_3$ per kg of body weight two–three times weekly.

Iodine Deficiency

- Iodine deficiency is most commonly seen in giant tortoises that originate from volcanic islands where they have adapted to a diet of vegetation with sequestered volcanic iodine.
- Iodine deficiency may be induced by a goitrogen such as potassium nitrate in overfertilized grass and anionic goitrogens in hay, lettuce, kale, and spinach.
- Iodine deficiency may result in:
  - Colloid goiter
  - Myxedema (commonly seen in captive aquatic turtles fed a diet of meat and lettuce, which are deficient in trace minerals)

  Treatment
- Add 0.5% iodized salt to the diet (0.15 mg available iodine per kg of food), or kelp tablets as a natural source.

Constipation

- Constipation can result from feeding heavily furred rodents or thickly feathered birds to reptiles that get inadequate exercise.

  Treatment
- Provide the following:
  - Give dioctyl sodium sulfosuccinate (1–5 mg/kg of 1:20 dilution) or mineral oil (1–5 mg/kg), PO.

- Alternatively, infuse mineral oil into the cloaca and gently "milk out" the fecal masses.

Vomiting

- The two most common causes of vomiting in reptiles are postprandial handling and low ambient temperatures (see Temperature-Related Diseases).
- Other causes include neoplasms, parasitism, and bacterial infections.

Maladaptation Syndrome

- Maladaptation syndrome is used to describe all the problems that can result from failure to properly simulate the natural environment, ranging from uncomplicated inanition-dehydration to infections secondary to loss of tissue integrity, including ulcerative stomatitis, ulcerative dermatitis, and necrotizing gastroenteritis.
- Proper husbandry and nutrition (described previously) are the key factors in treatment and prevention.

INFECTIOUS DISEASES

Viral Infections

- Reptiles are known to develop antibody titers against a number of *arboviruses,* including western equine encephalomyelitis and eastern equine encephalomyelitis. They are believed to be important overwintering hosts for the equine encephalomyelitides.
- C-type viruses have been isolated from splenic tissue cultures from a viper with myxofibroma of the mediastinum. The role in reptilian tumor induction is not known.
- Inclusion body disease of boa constrictors is characterized by pantropic eosinophilic cytoplasmic inclusions and appears associated with pneumonia, neurologic disorders, and systemic infection. Virus is associated with the syndrome but is not a verified etiologic agent.

Bacterial Disease

Atypical Mycoplasmosis

- Atypical, or nontuberculous, mycobacterial infections are ubiquitous in aquatic poikilotherms.
- The causative mycobacteria are gram-positive, acid-fast organisms classified as Runyan groups III (slow-growing nonphotochromogens including *Mycobacterium xenopei*) and IV (rapidly growing organisms including *M. chelonei, fortuitum, marinum, piscium,* and *thamnopheos*). They grow best at room temperature and can be cultured on Lowenstein-Jensen and other *Mycobacterium* media.
- Like tuberculosis in humans, some form of host debilitation is required to induce disease.
- Mycobacteriosis tends to occur sporadically in collections; stagnant water is the usual reservoir, and diseased fish and amphibians can infect reptiles.
- *Mycobacterium* organisms can cause

- Pneumonia
- Alimentary disorders
- Dermatitis

Pneumonia

- Clinical signs include dyspnea, mouth breathing, loss of swimming equilibrium, and chronic wasting.
- Histologic lesions include miliary or large granulomas in the lung.
- The diagnosis is based on histopathology, acid-fast stains, and culture of tracheal washes.

Alimentary Disorders

- Clinical signs include anorexia, emesis, diarrhea, and chronic wasting.
- Histologic lesions include miliary or large granulomas in the GI tract; small, 1-mm miliary liver granulomas are most common.
- The diagnosis is made by laparotomy or by histopathology at necropsy.

Dermatitis

- Clinical signs include cutaneous granulomas and chronic ulcers, as well as chronic debilitation.
- The diagnosis is based on acid-fast stains or culture of impression smears and on biopsy of the granulomas or ulcers.

Treatment of Mycobacteriosis

- Kanamycin has been reported to be effective with piscine (fish), but no other successful therapy has been reported.
- In general, treatment is not recommended because of the zoonotic potential of mycobacterial infection.

Nocardiosis

- Septicemic lesions reported in snakes in which organisms with the morphologic appearance and staining characteristics of *Nocardia* have been identified.

Dermatophilus Infection

- Depigmented multiple small nodules in the skin of Australian bearded lizards have been reported, in which large numbers of *Dermatophilus*-like organisms were identified.

Ulcerative Stomatitis

- The pathogenesis of this disease is controversial. Several bacteria have been implicated, including *Aeromonas hydrophila, Pseudomonas* spp, and *Klebsiella.*
  - It is hypothesized that malnutrition, and specifically vitamin C deficiency, makes the oral epithelium vulnerable to invasion by a variety of organisms.
  - Stomatitis may be a manifestation of a more serious problem such as pneumonia and septicemia.
- In general, ulcerative stomatitis is considered a secondary complication rather than a primary disease.

Treatment

- Therapy can include the following:
  - Improvement in the plane of nutrition, including administration of ascorbic acid (100–250 mg/kg q 24h, PO, or 10–20 mg/kg, SC).
  - Topical debridement and medication using C povidone-iodine or hydrogen peroxide

- Broad-spectrum antibiotics

Septicemia

In the presence of maladaptation syndrome, many gram-negative organisms can invade the host, including *Aeromonas*, *Pseudomonas*, *Proteus*, *Klebsiella*, and various fungi.

Hemorrhagic Septicemia
- This is the septicemia of *Aeromonas hydrophila* as transmitted by the snake mite, *Ophionyssus natricis*.

Subcutaneous Ulcerative Disease (SCUD)
- This disease of turtles has been attributed to *Citrobacter freundii*, although *Serratia* spp. may play a role in the initial invasion of skin.
- Installation of ultraviolet lights and the addition of chloramphenicol (Chloromycetin; Parke-Davis) (250 mg/20 gallons of water) to the water two or three times weekly has been successful in controlling outbreaks.
- Parenteral chloramphenicol therapy (see dosage in Medications) also may be effective.

Pneumonia

- This is a common disease in captive reptiles and probably represents, in part, invasion of the lungs of a maladapted host by the same organisms capable of causing septicemia.
- Although the majority of these are gram-negative organisms, *Peptostreptococcus* and other gram-positive bacteria are occasionally encountered.

Diagnosis
- The following are considered:
  - Because of the variability of etiologic agents, perform laryngeal swabs or washes in an attempt to isolate the organism. The ease of access of the reptilian glottis in its anterior position makes this a practical technique.
  - Give ketamine (Ketalar; Parke-Davis) 10 mg/kg, SC, to facilitate cooperation of the patient.

Treatment
- Antibiotics based on sensitivity results
- Improved husbandry

Enteritis

- The intestinal tract often is invaded in maladaption states by *Pseudomonas*, *Aeromonas*, *Salmonella*, and other bacteria. These organisms can be isolated from healthy reptiles, and their role in enteritic and septicemic conditions is not well understood.
- Primary pathogenic bacteria probably exist but have not been well described.

Abscess

- Abscesses are common in captive reptiles and include primarily gram-negative organisms. These must be distinguished from mycotic granulomas and parasite migration.

Treatment
- Treatment includes drainage and debridement owing to the caseous nature of the reptilian inflammatory exudate.

Fungal Diseases
Mycotic Stomatitis
- *Cladosporidium* has been isolated from lesions identical to those of Ulcerative Stomatitis (discussed previously).

Mycotic Pneumonia
- This disorder is common in tortoises and less so in snakes.
- Possible causes include *Aspergillus*, *Beauveria*, *Geotrichum*, *Mucor*, and *Paecilomyces* spp.

Carrier States

Reptiles can be asymptomatic carriers of a variety of organisms of potential public health significance.

Salmonellosis
- When red sliders and painted turtles were part of the pet industry, 15–30% of all cases of salmonellosis in the United States were attributed to pet turtles.
  - Causes of infection in these turtles included the sewage-contaminated settling ponds where many were raised and the slaughter-house offal that they were fed.
- All reptiles harbor strains of *Salmonella* that are potentially pathogenic in humans. There is no known effective treatment to eliminate the carrier state.

Spirochetes
- *Leptospira*, *Treponema*, and *Spirochaeta* spp. are found in reptiles, with no apparent harmful effects.
- The importance of reptiles as a reservoir of these bacteria is unknown.

Subcutaneous Phycomycosis
- *Basidiobolus haptosporus* organism causes subcutaneous phycomycosis in humans and is an inhabitant of the lizard gastrointestinal tract.

PARASITIC DISEASES
Ectoparasites

Mites
- 250 species of mites are known to infect reptiles.
- Blood-feeding habits of mites can kill a reptile in several weeks, or in a few days if infection is heavy.
- Many of these mites are intermediate or transport hosts for a variety of Blood Parasites (see below).
- *Aeromonas hydrophila*, which is transmitted by the snake mite, *Ophionyssus natricis*, can cause hemorrhagic septicemia.

Treatment
- Pyrethrum flea products generally are safe and effective.
- Other treatment regimens include ivermectin (0.2 mg/kg, PO or SC, every 14 days; Ivomec; Merck

Sharp and Dohme, Agvet) or cat flea collars placed in the cage (see Anthelmintics and Parasiticides under Medications).

Ticks

- Numerous species are found in reptiles, and they present the same potential threats as mites.
- *Ornithodoros* is the most commonly encountered tick.
- Painting the tick with 70% isopropyl alcohol followed by mechanical removal and antiseptic swabs is an effective treatment.

Endoparasites

Parasites can be found in almost every body organ in reptiles. For the purposes of this discussion, they are listed according to the anatomic area in which they are seen.

Blood Parasites

- Reptiles are host to a large number of blood parasites, which are generally well-tolerated but can, on occasion, induce anemias, thrombosis, and other diseases (see Table 2)

Muscle

- Microsporidia
  - *Pleistophora* has been associated with tuatara deaths resulting from extensive myositis.
  - *Glugea,* a muscle parasite of snakes and turtles, is transmitted by trematodes and is not known to be pathogenic.
  - *Sarcocystis* (Sarcosporidia) is reported in reptiles but is not believed to be pathogenic.
  - Plerocercoids (spargana of pseudophyllidean cestodes) may be found on or in muscle and are usually well tolerated.
  - Migrating ascarid larvae may be found in muscle.

Kidneys

- *Myxidium* (Microsporidia) occasionally is found in the renal tubules of snakes and turtles; its pathogenicity is unknown.
- Digenetic trematodes are common in aquatic reptiles and may be extensive enough to induce uremia.

Gallbladder

- *Eimeria* may cause cholecystitis in snakes.
- In aquatic reptiles, digenetic trematodes are seen and may cause cholecystitis.

TABLE 2. Blood Parasites

Organ Affected	Parasite Type/Name	Host(s)	Vector	Clinical Significance	Comments
Red blood cells (RBC)	Hemococcidia (*Schellackia* spp)	Lizards	Mites	Unknown—gains access to blood after gastrointestinal proliferation	Gametocytes, are independent
RBC, endothelial cells	Hemogregarines (*Karyolysus* spp)	Lizards	Mites	Unknown	Gametocytes of all hemogregarines develop attached to each other
RBC, intestinal submucosa, liver, lungs	Hepatozoan spp	All reptiles	Arthropods	Unknown	
RBC, lungs	*Haemogregarina* spp	Turtles, snakes	Leeches, ticks	Induces anemia if >4% of RBC affected	
RBC	Hemosporidia (*Haemoproteus* spp)	Lizards, snakes, turtles	Unknown	Unknown	All hemosporidia have motile zygotes
RBC	*Simondia* spp	Turtles	Arthropods	Unknown	
RBC, leukocytes, endothelium	*Plasmodium* spp	Lizards	Arthropods	Can be pathogenic in young animals	Over 30 species infective
RBC	Piroplasmida (*Nuttallia* spp)	Turtles	Arthropods	Unknown	
Blood	Trematodes (*Spirorchis* spp)	Turtles	Snails (intermediate host)	Unknown	
Blood	Filarial nematodes (*Macdonaldius* spp)	Snakes (especially Mexican species)	Arthropods	Postcaval thrombosis	Exposure to ambient temp >96.8° F (36.0° C) for >24 h may be effective treatment
	Other filarial spp	All reptiles	Arthropods	Generalized edema, dermal lesions, subcutaneous swelling	More than 50 species occur in reptiles

Oral Cavity

- Monogenetic trematodes are seen in turtle parasites; there is no known pathogenicity.
- Digenetic trematodes are present in the oral cavities of many aquatic reptiles and may induce dyspnea.

Urinary Bladder

- Monogenetic trematodes frequently are present in the turtle bladder and are not known to be pathogenic.

Liver

Plerocercoids

- Snakes serve as intermediate hosts after acquiring *Spirometra* infection from ingestion of prey.
- Damage usually is mechanical, and heavy infestations may result in liver failure, with clinical signs such as anorexia, depression, and emesis.
- Multifocal nodules may be found in the liver at necropsy.
- Niclosamide (Yomesan; Mobay Corp.) is not effective; however, praziquantel (Droncit; Mobay), 5–8 mg/kg, IM or PO, repeated in 2 weeks, may be effective.

Tetrathyridia

- Reptiles are secondary intermediate hosts; mammals the definitive hosts. Transmission is via ingestion of infected arthropods.
- Cysts of cestodes of the family Mesocestoididae found in the liver of affected lizards may be numerous enough to cause hepatic failure.
- Similar clinical signs and necropsy lesions are observed as for plerocercoids.
- Treatment usually is not effective; praziquantel may be tried at the dosage listed above.

Capillariasis

- Snakes and lizards may acquire *Capillaria* infection by direct transmission or by prey ingestion.
- Mechanical damage to hepatic bile ducts occurs with heavy infestations, resulting in clinical signs of liver failure such as depression and anorexia.
- The double operculated eggs may not always be visible on fecal examination.
- Treatment includes thiabendazole, fenbendazole, and ivermectin.

Acanthocephaliasis

- Larval acanthocephalan parasites may be found in the livers of snakes and turtles.
- Transmission occurs by ingestion of intermediate hosts such as arthropods or snails.
- Most infections are subclinical or self-limiting in captive collections.
- No current chemotherapeutic agent exists for treatment.

Lungs

Pentastomes (Tongue Worms)

- Reptiles are the main host, and mammals, birds, and insects may serve as intermediate hosts.

- Because humans can be infected as intermediate hosts, these parasites present a public health threat.
- Adult worms live in the lungs and may cause severe tissue damage.
- Eggs are coughed up and passed in the feces.
- Genera include
  - *Armillifer,* found in pythons and vipers.
  - *Porocephalus,* found in boas and rattlesnakes.
  - *Kiricephalus,* found in colubrid snakes.
- In a variety of reptile species, migrating larvae can cause plaques and aneurysms. With heavy pulmonary infestation, clinical signs such as anorexia, lethargy, and dyspnea may be seen.
- Diagnosis is based on the presence of finding aortic lesions at necropsy or thin-walled eggs containing larvae with hooklets in lung washings.
- No safe effective treatment currently exists.
- Prevention by avoiding feeding affected intermediate hosts such as wild-caught rodents is the best measure.

Lung Mites

- *Entonyssus* parasitism is not known to induce disease.

Nematodes

- *Rhabdias* infection is common in wild snakes recently captured from the southeastern United States. Spirurid larvae are occasionally encountered.
- When *Rhabdias* organisms are seen in mucoid oral secretions of recently imported snakes, aspirate and examine microscopically for embryonated eggs.
  - To treat, give levamisole (Ripercol-L; American Cyanamid) (5–8 mg/kg) or fenbendazole (Panacur, Hoechst-Roussel) (50 mg/kg) and repeat in 2 weeks. Ivermectin has been associated with treatment failures.
  - Perform a tracheal wash and treat secondary bacterial infections if indicated.
- Digenetic trematodes occasionally may be seen in aquatic reptiles.

Skin and Connective Tissue

- *Dracunculus* occasionally induces ulcers and swelling in snakes. Mechanical removal is the only effective therapy.
- Plerocercoids.
- Filarial nematodes are seen but have no known clinical significance.

Intestines

Parasites of reptiles are comparable to those in mammals with respect to family representations, with the addition of several new groups.

Coccidia

- A large number of coccidia are found in reptiles including *Eimeria, Isospora, Globidium, Cyclospora, Caryospora, Wenyonella, Tyzzeria* and the micrococcidia *Cryptosporidium.*
- These can at times be pathogens, especially with massive infections due to poor husbandry and fecal contamination.
- These organisms tend to be highly species-specific.
- Treatment has been effective with sulfadimethoxine

(Bactrovet; Pitman-Moore), 90 mg/kg, PO, the first day, and then 45 mg/kg q24h, PO, for the next 6 days.

Monogenetic Trematodes

- During their life cycle, these trematodes affect a single host. They can be found in the GI tract, respiratory system, and urinary bladder of many species. If present in massive numbers they can cause intestinal obstruction.
- After detection of ova on fecal examination, treat with praziquantel, at 5–8 mg/kg, IM or PO, and repeat in 2 weeks; or give fenbendazole (Panacur; Hoechst-Roussel), 50 mg/kg q24h PO, for 3–5 days.

Digenetic Trematodes
Renifers

- Renifers are commonly found in wild and captive snakes, with amphibians serving as the intermediate host. They often are seen in the oral cavity during the physical examination.
- Although usually not a source of clinical problems, renifers can migrate into the lungs and air sac, causing focal lesions that may result in secondary bacterial pneumonia.
- Diagnosis is based on the presence of flukes in the oral cavity or operculated eggs on tracheal/lung washings and fecal sedimentation.
- Treat as for monogenetic trematodes.

Styphylodora

- This digenetic trematode is found in the urinary system of various snakes. Most infections are subclinical, although massive infection can result in renal failure and death.
- The diagnosis is based on the presence of operculated eggs in urine or urine sediment, or multifocal pale nodules in the kidneys at necropsy. The life cycle is unknown but probably involves an intermediate host.
- Efficacy of treatment is unknown but may be attempted as for monogenetic trematodes.

Ova Spirorchis

- Eggs of this vascular trematode of turtles pass into the gut where heavy infestations may contribute to malabsorption.
- Eggs may be trapped in terminal blood vessels of the spleen, liver, heart, kidney, and shell.
  - Shell lesions may result over the carapace and plastron in the form of pitted ulcerations.
- The diagnosis is based on the presence of operculated eggs on fecal sedimentation or in tissues.
- No treatment currently exists, but most infections are self limiting. Prevention requires limiting exposure to the intermediate host (snails) in the environment or diet.

Acanthocephaliasis

- Acanthocephala (thorny-headed worm) is found in aquatic reptiles from the ingestion of snail and crustacean intermediates.
- Infections can be massive and cause intestinal obstruction.
- There is no effective treatment.

Sarcodines

- Amebiasis is a threat in all reptile collections. *Entamoeba invadens* is the only proven pathogenic

sarcodine of reptiles; however, the Hartmanella group ameba of the genera *Acanthamoeba* and *Hartmanella* occasionally may be pathogenic, perhaps as secondary invaders.
  - *Entamoeba invadens* must be distinguished from other nonpathogenic *Entamoeba* species that inhabit reptiles.
- The disease usually is introduced by carriers (e.g., turtles, aquatic snakes).
- Clinical signs include hemorrhagic diarrhea, rapid dehydration, and terminal convulsions.
- Lesions include hemorrhagic colitis, with later extension to the small bowel and up the portal vein, causing focal hepatic necrosis.
- Amebic pneumonia and occasionally nephritis may occur.
- To treat, give metronidazole (Flagyl; Searle), 50 mg/kg, and repeat in 1–2 weeks; or give the same dose q24h for 3 days (do not exceed a total dose of 400 mg).

Trichomonads

- Numerous commensals are reported in this group; however, *Monocercomonas* has been reported to be pathogenic for snakes and lizards.

Cestodes

- Genuses represented are *Acanthotaenia*, *Ophiotaenia*, *Oochoristica*, *Cyclophyllidea* and *Proteocephalus*.
- Like mammalian cestodes, reptilian cestodes are well adapted to their hosts and rarely cause problems.
- Various crustaceans and insects serve as intermediates.
- Intestinal obstruction occasionally results. Treatment with niclosamide (Yomesan; Farbenfabriken Bayer A.G., Germany) and praziquantel (Droncit; Mobay) have been reported to be effective.

Nematodes
Over 500 species are represented in reptilian intestines.

- Eight genera of spirurids are encountered in the stomach and (less frequently) esophagus, including *Physaloptera* and *Gnathostoma*. Infection may be massive in horned lizards (*Phyrynosoma*) owing to ingestion of ants.
- Ascarids are represented by seven genera, including *Ophidascaris*, *Ascaris*, and *Hexametra*. Unlike mammalian ascarids, visceral migrations are not a prominent feature, perhaps because carrier hosts in the form of amphibians serve as intermediates. These parasites are large and may rarely cause obstruction.
  - Treatment with levamisole, fenbendazole, or ivermectin is usually effective (always repeat treatment in 2 weeks).
- Genera of reptilian strongyles, which are not as pathogenic as mammalian species, include *Oswaldocruzia* (hookworm of lizards), *Kalicephalus* (hookworm of snakes) and *Strongyloides*. All have direct life cycles and are found in the esophagus and small intestine.
- About 150 species of oxyurids are found in the reptile colon. Most are seen in lizards and tortoises and cause few problems.

- Cammalanoidea are stomach worms in turtles.
- Heterakoidea are parasites of snakes, lizards, and occasionally turtles.
- Capillarids are abundant in lizards and snakes.
- Anisakids are parasites of crocodilians, turtles, and occasionally lizards and snakes.

MISCELLANEOUS DISEASES

Congenital Disorders

- Multiple cartilaginous exostosis has been reported in lizards.
- Achondroplastic dwarfism can occur in turtles.

Cardiovascular Disease

Congestive Heart Failure

This is probably a common cause of mortality among aged reptiles, owing to the highly efficient nature of the reptilian heart combined with high susceptibility of the myocardium to injurious agents such as parasite larvae, bacteria, and endocarditis.

Arterial Lesions

Fatty Streaks

- Up to 12% of reptile aortas have fatty streaks, which often occur as a normal result of aging or excessive fat in the diet.
- Normally no clinical signs occur with this condition, which is a necropsy finding.

Medial Calcification

- As a result of aging or hypervitaminosis D, hyaline and fatty degeneration of the subendothelial muscular arterial tissue occurs followed by calcification. Lesions are usually found in the aorta and its larger branches, resulting in severely restricted or blocked blood flow.
- This condition is most often seen in lizards. Active, egg-laying females are less severely affected, perhaps because of the mobilization of calcium during eggshell formation.
- Clinical signs vary according to the degree of ischemia in the affected organ (e.g., dyspnea with pulmonary involvement; lethargy and anorexia with aortic involvement).
- Diagnosis is based on observation of affected radiopaque vessels on radiography.
- Once lesions are radiographically apparent, there is no effective clinical treatment.
- Prevention consists of feeding diets balanced with respect to the calcium:phosphorus ratio and avoiding oversupplementation of vitamin D.

Kidney Disease

Basement Membrane Disease

- Generalized thickening of glomerular tubular basement membranes is often associated with necrotizing processes such as bacterial, fungal, protozoan, and parasitic infections. The most common etiology is bacterial sepsis secondary to abscesses, infectious stomatitis, or pneumonia.

- Clinical signs include lethargy and anorexia.
- Metastatic calcification in hepatic, pericardial, and other periarticular areas may be seen radiographically if renal failure occurs.
- Serum uric acid levels are often elevated.
- Treatment consists of maintaining hydration with subcutaneous or intraperitoneal fluids and identification and treatment of the underlying infection.

Glomerulosclerosis

- Glomerulosclerosis is seen in up to 15% of reptile necropsies.
- Unlike mammalian glomerulosclerosis, tubular degeneration is not a feature because of the presence of a renal portal blood supply.
- Chronic bacterial infections appear to be a major cause because of hematogenous dissemination from abscesses, infectious stomatitis, or pneumonia.
- Clinical signs, radiographic lesions, and blood values are similar to those of basement membrane disease if renal failure occurs. Treatment also follows the same guidelines.
- This condition has also been reported in iguanas with signs of lameness or a stilted gait, similar to systemic lupus erythematosus in mammals.

Pancreatitis

- Regenerative pancreatitis may occur in reptiles as a result of migrating parasites, abscesses, calculi, and hematogenous or pancreatic duct bacterial infections.
- Clinical signs can include lethargy, anorexia, and emesis, although subclinical episodes are more common.
- No reliable values exist for reptiles with regard to use of amylase and lipase in antemortem diagnosis of pancreatitis. Biopsy at laparotomy and necropsy lesions are current standard diagnostic tools.
- This disorder previously was reported as pancreatic adenocarcinoma because of the bizarre appearance of regenerating acinar tissue.
- If severe pancreatic damage occurs, diabetes mellitus may follow, with clinical signs of weight loss, polyuria, glycosuria, and hyperglycemia.
- Conceivably, insulin could be used for control, but no guidelines exist at present.
- Spontaneous diabetes is not a common clinical finding in reptiles.

Liver Disease

Giant Cell Hepatitis

- This typical regenerative activity may occur secondary to hepatopathies such as lipidosis, hydropic degeneration, and hepatic necrosis. The long list of etiologies for these conditions includes:
  - Obesity due to overfeeding resulting in fatty change
  - Plant and bacterial toxins involved in hydropic degeneration
  - Parasitic, bacterial, viral, and fungal infections resulting in hepatic necrosis

- Clinical signs include lethargy, anorexia, weight loss, and, with severe involvement, emesis and icterus.
- Serum biochemical abnormalities accompanying liver disease may include increased values of total bilirubin, alkaline phosphatase, and aspartate aminotransferase. Other diagnostic measures include laparotomy and hepatic biopsy.
- Administer specific as well as symptomatic therapy such as diet control, elimination of toxins from the environment, and treatment of specific infections.
- Force-feeding and parenteral fluid therapy including fat and water-soluble vitamin supplementation may be needed during periods of anorexia and emesis.

Cirrhosis

- Chronic severe episodes of hepatic necrosis may lead to a continuous cycle of fibrosis and additional necrosis, resulting in cirrhosis. Chronic fibrotic changes may not be accompanied by corresponding increases in liver enzymes.
- Clinical signs include progressive anorexia and death.
- Diagnosis is confirmed by biopsy via laparotomy or by necropsy.

Amyloidosis

Amyloidosis is most commonly reported to accompany necrotizing processes. A variety of tissues may be involved, including myocardium, glomeruli, and liver.

- Signs of this progressive disease become apparent when target organs contain enough amyloid to affect normal function. Older animals are most often affected.
- The diagnosis is based on the presence of amyloid on periodic acid–Schiff stain at biopsy or necropsy.
- No effective treatment currently exists.

Spinal Osteoperiostitis

- Osteoperiostitis usually is encountered in boas, but may occur in all snakes.
- Affected specimens are reluctant or unable to move normally, and palpation reveals hard swellings along the ribs or spine.
- Radiography may show involvement of one or many vertebral bodies, with proliferative and osteolytic lesions that can result in spondylosis or pathologic fractures.
- There is no effective treatment. The progressive nature of the disease usually ultimately results in death of the affected reptile; or euthanasia may be required.

Dystocia

Clinical Signs

- In snakes and lizards, dystocia usually manifests as persistent swelling or lumps in mid- or caudal abdomen. Anorexia and reduced activity may be present.
- In turtles and tortoises, dystocia usually manifests as anorexia and straining.

- Live bearers such as vipers, boas, and elephant trunk snakes may exhibit swelling over the posterior third of the body and may have anorexia while being active during the last quarter of gestation.

Diagnosis

- Differentiate normal eggs, which often can be removed by medical management, from tumors, abscesses, calculi, impactions, and inspissated eggs.
  - Radiology may reveal ovoid masses with a clearly defined, slightly calcified line (like the edge of a normal egg). Other masses may appear round or ovoid but will not have the clearly delineated appearance of a normal egg.
  - Ultrasonography performed with good resolution scanning heads and experience often can distinguish abdominal masses from normal eggs or fetuses in live bearers.
  - Malformations have been reported in hatching snakes radiographed in the last trimester of pregnancy; therefore, ultrasonography, rather than radiography, is recommended to verify pregnancy in these species.

Medical Management

The following protocol is recommended for dystocia with normal retained eggs.

- Apply warm water soaks for 30 minutes to 1 hour daily.
- Provide appropriate nesting material with proper ambient temperatures.
- Administer 10% calcium gluconate solution at 50 mg/kg IM q24h. Increase in increments of 50 mg/kg over several days to 1 week not to exceed 200 mg/kg total daily dose.
- To remove all eggs, give oxytocin (Sussex) (1–2 IU for small reptiles; 5–20 IU for large reptiles), q24h, IM or SC, for several days up to 1 week, as needed.
- Used in combination with calcium, proper environment management, and patience, > 80% of normal eggs can be passed from reptiles.
- Vasotocin at a dose of 0.01–1.0 mg/kg, IM or SC, appears to be much more specific for reptile oviduct stimulation than oxytocin; however, this drug is not currently available through veterinary commercial suppliers.

Surgical Management

- Celiotomy is recommended (see Common Surgical Procedures).

MEDICATIONS
Antibiotics
Chloramphenicol (Elase-Chloromycetin; Parke-Davis)

- *Dosage:* 40 mg/kg, SC, daily for 5–10 days.
- *Disadvantages*
  - Owing to widespread use, many bacterial pathogens have developed resistance.
- *Indications:* Antibacterial (anaerobes and *Campylobacter*). Distributes through body, especially CNS.

- The bacteriostatic nature of this drug often does not allow decisive control of severe infections.

Gentamicin (Gentocin; Schering)

- *Dosage:*
  - 2.5 mg/kg q72h, SC, for 3–5 treatments for snakes, tortoises, and crocodilians.
  - 10 mg/kg q48h, SC, for 3–5 treatments for aquatic turtles.
- *Indications:* Because of the likelihood of mixed infections, especially with anaerobes in ulcerative stomatitis, combine with another bactericidal drug with a complementary spectrum, such as a beta-lactam, cephalosporin, and trimethoprim-sulfa.
- *Disadvantages:* Gentamycin is extremely nephrotoxic and can cause proximal tubular nephrosis. Hydration with SC fluids is mandatory; administer approximately 20 ml/kg (up to 100 ml total) at each treatment.

Amikacin (Amikin; Bristol)

- *Dosage:* 2.5 mg/kg q72 h, SC, for 3–5 treatments.
- *Indications*
  - Combination therapy in mixed infections (as outlined under gentamicin) is beneficial.
  - Overuse (especially in the wholesale and retail trade) has resulted in the development of resistant bacterial strains; therefore, reserve for gentamicin-resistant infections, as determined by culture and sensitivity testing.
- *Disadvantages:* This drug is not as nephrotoxic as gentamicin, but it is a potentially toxic drug; follow fluid recommendations for gentamicin.

Ampicillin (Polyflex; Bristol)

- *Dosage:* 25 to 100 mg/kg q24h, SC, for 7–10 days, and up to several weeks if needed.
- *Indications*
  - Use in combination with other antibiotics in mixed infections.
  - If the reptile has not been previously treated, use as an initial antibiotic.

Oxytetracycline (LA-200; Pfizer)

- *Recommended Dosage:* 6–10 mg/kg q24h, IM, as an empirical dose.
- *Disadvantages:* Not recommended because of possible irritation and necrosis at the injection site as well as widespread resistance of reptilian bacterial pathogens.
- *Indications:* Inexpensive antibiotic used orally and as an injection.

Trimethoprin-Sulfadiazine (Di-Trim; Burroughs Wellcome)

- *Dosage:* Total dose of 30 mg/kg q48h, SC.
- *Indications/Advantages*
  - This bactericidal agent is active against a wide variety of bacterial pathogens.
  - Unless the patient is already dehydrated, hydration usually is not necessary.

- May be used in combination with penicillins and aminoglycosides.

Carbenicillin (Pyopen; SmithKline) and Piperacillin (Piperacil; Lederle)

- *Dosage:* 100 mg/kg q24h, SC, for 5–7 days.
- *Indications*
  - A broad gram-negative spectrum of activity includes *Proteus, Pseudomonas, Klebsiella,* and *Enterobacter* spp.
  - Often used in combination with aminoglycosides.

Penicillin G Procaine/Benzathine (Flo-Cillin; Fort Dodge)

- *Dosage:* 10,000 IU/kg q24h or 20,000 IU/kg q48h, SC, for 5–10 days.
- *Indications:* Use in mixed infections in combination with trimethoprim-sulfa and aminoglycosides.

Anthelmintics and Parasiticides

Thiabendazole (Omnizole; Merck)

- *Dosage:* 50 mg/kg, PO; repeat in 2 weeks.
- *Disadvantages:* Can cause gastrointestinal impactions and fluid and electrolyte shifts; has been reported to be fatal in king snakes.
- *Indication:* Broad-spectrum anthelmintic for nematodes.

Fenbendazole (Panacur; Hoechst-Roussel)

- *Dosage:* 50 mg/kg, PO; repeat in 2 weeks. Give orally via stomach tube or place inside preferred food items.
- *Indications:* Safe, broad-spectrum anthelmintic; do not use against cestodes.

Niclosamide (Yomesan; Haver-Lockhart)

- *Dosage:* 150 mg/kg; do not use more than once a month.
- *Indication:* Tapeworm infestations.

Levamisole (Ripercol-L; American Cyanamid)

- *Dosage:* 5 mg/kg, SC, repeat in 2 weeks. For accurate use in small specimens, dilute the 13.1% solution 1:10 to 1:100.
- *Disadvantages:* Use caution when using in sick or debilitated animals (no adverse reactions have been seen by author).
- *Indication:* Broad-spectrum anthelmintic especially against lungworms.

Ivermectin (Ivomec; Merck Sharp and Dohme, Agvet)

- *Dosage:* 0.2 mg/kg, SC, or preferably PO in snakes and lizards.
- *Indications:* Broad-spectrum anthelmintic and against mites up to 2 weeks.

KEY POINT ▶ Do not use ivermectin in turtles or tortoises because of reported toxicities.

■ *Disadvantages:* Not effective against cestodes, acanthocephalans, or protozoans.

Metronidazole (Flagyl; Searle)

■ *Dosage:* 50 mg/kg as a single dose or q24h for 3 days; repeat in 1–2 weeks. Do not exceed a total dose of 400 mg.
■ *Advantages:* For unknown reasons, appears to function as an appetite stimulant, especially in snakes.
■ *Indications:* Treatment of protozoan and anaerobic infections.

Cat Flea Collars

■ *Dosage:* For ectoparasites, place one-third of a collar in the cage for 3–4 days.
■ *Advantages:* Safer than Vapona strips.
■ As an alternative, warm water baths are safe and fairly effective to drown mites.

Vitamins and Minerals

Ascorbic Acid Injection USP (Sussex Drugs)

■ *Dosage:* 10–20 mg/kg, SC.
■ *Indications:* Use as adjunctive treatment in ulcerative stomatitis.

Calcium Gluconate Injectable 10% (Sussex Drugs)

■ *Dosage:* 100–200 mg/kg, SC or IM, in divided doses. Repeat daily if needed, until oral supplementation with calcium gluconate or calcium carbonate is initiated.
■ *Indication:* Corrects calcium deficiency.

Cyanocobalamin (Vitamin B₁₂) (Sussex Drugs)

■ *Dosage:* Dosage has not been established. Suggested doses are 0.02–2.0 ml, depending on body size.
■ *Indication:* B_{12} supplement; possible appetite stimulant.

Vitamin A (Sussex Drugs)

■ *Dosage:* 1000–50,000 units, IM, once, depending on body size.
■ *Disadvantages:* Overdosage can cause signs of hypervitaminosis A, such as exostosis, hepatomegaly, and skin exfoliation.
■ Alternatively, consider correcting deficiencies with oral supplementation and balanced diet.
■ *Indication:* Correct vitamin A deficiency.

Vitamin B Complex (Sussex Drugs)

■ *Dosage:* 0.1–0.2 ml/kg, SC, daily or as needed.

Vitamin K (Sussex Drugs)

■ *Dosage:* 0.5 mg/kg, IM, as needed.

Vitamin E (Sussex Drugs)

■ *Dosage:* 50–100 IU/kg, IM, as needed.

Thiamine (Vitamin B) (Sussex Drugs)

■ *Dosage:* 50–100 mg/kg, SC or IM, as needed.

ANESTHESIA

General Anesthesia

Ketamine Hydrochloride (Ketalar; Parke-Davis)

Doses of 10–50 mg/kg are given, SC or IM, with variable induction, duration, and recovery.

■ A dose of 10–20 mg/kg works well for restraint and diagnostic procedures such as blood collection, stomach tubing, tracheal wash, and radiology, appropriate for outpatient procedures.
  • Animals can usually move, eat, and drink after this dose but will be tranquilized for about 24 hours.
■ A dose of 50 mg/kg is adequate for restraint and minor surgical procedures but is best combined with regional or gas anesthesia for internal surgery or extended procedures.
  • Patients usually will be immobilized for 24 hours and tranquilized for 48–72 hours.
  • If repeat dosage is needed, use increments of 25 mg/kg at 30-minute intervals twice only, or use alternative anesthetic drugs.

Tiletamine–Zolazepam Hydrochloride (Telazol; A. H. Robins)

■ Effects are similar to those of ketamine-diazepam combination, with rapid onset of action (5–10 minutes) but often a more prolonged recovery time.
■ Dose range is 1–3 mg/kg, SC or IM.
■ Although results are satisfactory, there is no advantage over ketamine alone and/or supplemental agents.

Diazepam (Valium; Roche)

■ A total dose alone of 25 mg is reported to be satisfactory for reproductive examination of American alligators.
■ Use as a supplemental drug for ketamine at ¼–½ of the mammal dose (0.1 mg/kg).

Succinylcholine (Anectine; Burroughs Wellcome)

■ Use for immobilization only; supplement with anesthetic drugs for painful procedures.
■ Doses of 0.25–1.0 mg/kg, SC or IM, have been reported for use in tortoises and crocodilians, but has been used less frequently in recent years because of apnea and some fatalities in reptile patients.

Gallamine (Flexadil; American Cyanamid)

■ This drug is reported to have been used safely in field translocations of large crocodilians.
■ The main use appears to be for immobilization of large monitors, chelonians, or crocodilians in zoologic collections.

- Recommended dosages are 2.0 mg/kg, IM, for animals <10 kg; 1.0 mg/kg, IM, for animals 10–200 kg; and 0.5 mg/kg, IM, for animals >200 kg.
- Administer with atropine; drug effects can be reversed with neostigmine.
- Gallamine is fairly inexpensive, and it is not a controlled drug.

Inhalation Procedures

- Give 5% isoflurane (AErrane; Anaquest) or halothane (Fluothane; Fort Dodge) and oxygen in a clear plastic bag or tube or induction chamber. Fill chamber with gas and seal. Induction time is 30–60 minutes.
- Induction time is greatly shortened (15–30 minutes) and depth of anesthesia is increased with an initial injection of 10–20 mg/kg of ketamine, SC or IM.
- Keep the patient warm on a water blanket.
- Surgical anesthesia is determined by loss of the righting reflex.
- Pull the reptile's body out of the chamber, leaving the head in, or use face mask or endotracheal tube.
- Maintenance levels are 2–3% halothane or isoflurane; 3–5% may be needed if gas induction is used alone.
- Recovery of the righting reflex usually occurs within 1 hour, even with ketamine supplementation. Tranquilization may still be evident, however, for 24 hours.
- To control apnea during or following gas anesthetic use, discontinue the gas anesthetic and apply gentle manual ventilation two–four times per minute along with small doses of doxapram IV. Normal respiration usually begins within 3–5 minutes.

Hypothermia

- This procedure is inhumane in the light of modern anesthetics and stressful on the reptile's overall metabolism. Hypothermia also may predispose to pneumonia.

Regional Anesthesia

Lidocaine (1%) Without Epinephrine

- Manual restraint is required.
- Indications include use for removing small growths, suturing lacerations, and amputating digits or tails.

COMMON SURGICAL PROCEDURES

Soft Tissue Surgery

Celiotomy

Indications

- Tumor removal—frequently required in long term captive snakes
- Obstruction—usually concretions or decaying food in GI tract
- Cystic calculi removal—cystotomy, especially in tortoises and iguanas
- Dystocia—removal of inspissated eggs; hysterectomy

- Exploratory celiotomy—biopsies

Approach
Snakes

- Make an incision in the convergence of the abdominal scutes and lateral scales through the skin, abdominal muscle, and coelomic membrane.

Turtles

- An orthopedic or hobby rotary saw instrument usually is required for an osteotomy of the plastron.
- Radiographs are essential for accurate location and sizing of the square or rectangle cut and to avoid the pelvic bones.
- During cutting, avoid overheating of the shell by periodic use of saline or other isotonic solution on the site and avoid cutting too slowly with the instrument, which may cause it to skip and injure the operator.
- Once the plastron is incised and removed with a chisel, make an incision through the abdominal muscles and the coelomic membrane. Avoid the dual paramedian ventral abdominal veins; however, they can be ligated without causing harm.

Lizards and Crocodilians

- In most lizards the skin and muscle are tightly adherent; approach as one continuous layer when making an incision.
- A large midline ventral abdominal vein can be ligated, but a paramedian approach is preferred. Make a "T" at the end of the paramedian incision by a transverse lateral incision or incisions (cranial or caudal), as needed, for greater abdominal exposure.

Closure
Snakes

- Close with a simple continuous layer of Vicryl or Dexon in the muscle layer.
- Suture the skin with the same material in a simple interrupted or slightly everting pattern. Avoid apposing the skin too tightly or excessive scarring will result.
- Remove sutures after the next shed is complete.

Turtles

- After suturing of abdominal muscle wall, replace the osteotomized plastron using epoxy resin and boat or autobody fiberglass cloth built in layers.
- Avoid getting the resin along the osteotomy edges.
- The fiberglass-epoxy patch is a semipermanent patch that may have to be sanded away to allow shell growth in turtles. This dust is harmful, and goggles and face mask are essential during removal.
- Other restorative materials such as dental acrylics may be used if the clinician has access to and skill with these materials.

Lizards and Crocodilians

- Close the abdomen with a single layer of simple interrupted sutures in the skin because of the tight adherence of the skin and muscle.
- Use Dexon or Vicryl with protective bandaging; in large reptiles, use monofilament stainless steel sutures.

Cloacal/Hemipene Prolapse

Cloacal Prolapse

Most cloacal prolapses can be reduced under manual restraint. Use of 50% dextrose to reduce edema does not usually produce visible results.

Technique

1. Lubricate the prolapse with an antibiotic or antibiotic-cortisone ointment and gently replace in stages.
2. Place a pursestring suture (monofilament nylon or polypropylene) in the cloaca and insert a blunt smaller-diameter instrument.
3. After completing the suture, remove the instrument, resulting in a restricted opening. This allows feces and urates to pass while helping to prevent recurrence of the prolapse.
4. Investigate and correct bacterial, parasitic, and mechanical causes of irritation, and give broad-spectrum antibiotics for 7–10 days.
5. Remove the pursestring suture after 10–14 days.

Results

All cloacal prolapses treated by the author have been reducible manually and have not necessitated colopexy or resections, except for occasional massive devitalized prolapses in moribund animals that died shortly after presentation.

Hemipene Prolapse

Hemipenes prolapse normally during breeding as a conduit or guide for seminal fluid; occasionally the reptile can not retract the organ, after which the hemipene quickly becomes dried and edematous.

- Usually the organ can be gently replaced by a cotton swab after lubrication with an antibiotic ointment.
- If this fails, amputation is required after one or several interrupted transfixing sutures are placed at the base of the organ.
- In turtles, impaired breeding activity may result because they usually only have one hemipene.
- In snakes and lizards, there should be no impairment because the reproductive structures, including internal organs, are paired.

Orthopedic Surgery

Bone Fracture Repair

- Aseptic technique is essential during orthopedic surgical procedures.
- Internal fixation in most reptiles is limited to the use of intramedulary (IM) pins or Kirschner-Ehmer apparatus using small IM pins or hypodermic needles. To provide additional stability, coaptation with splinting of the legs to the body for lizards (Fig. 9), and limbs inside the shell for tortoises, often is used with IM pins.
- Fractures due to secondary hyperparathyroidism can be reduced with internal fixation; often, however,

coaptation may be used while the deficiency is being corrected.

- Diet analysis and adequate calcium intake can ensure proper healing.
- Bones heal over a period of months, as opposed to weeks in mammals. It is essential to monitor the progress of healing via radiography.

Shell Fracture Repair

- Chelonian shells often are damaged by automobiles or carnivore trauma.
  - Advise clients to provide complete protective screening for turtles and tortoises that are allowed outdoor access to prevent trauma from curious, free-ranging dogs.
- Often shell injuries are accompanied by massive contamination and secondary infection. Completely resolve these complications before attempting final repair.
  - Clean daily with large volumes of isotonic solutions, followed by use of Silvadene (Merrell Dow) or Kymar (Schering-Plow) ointment for 5–10 days.
  - Cover large defects temporarily with bandage ma-

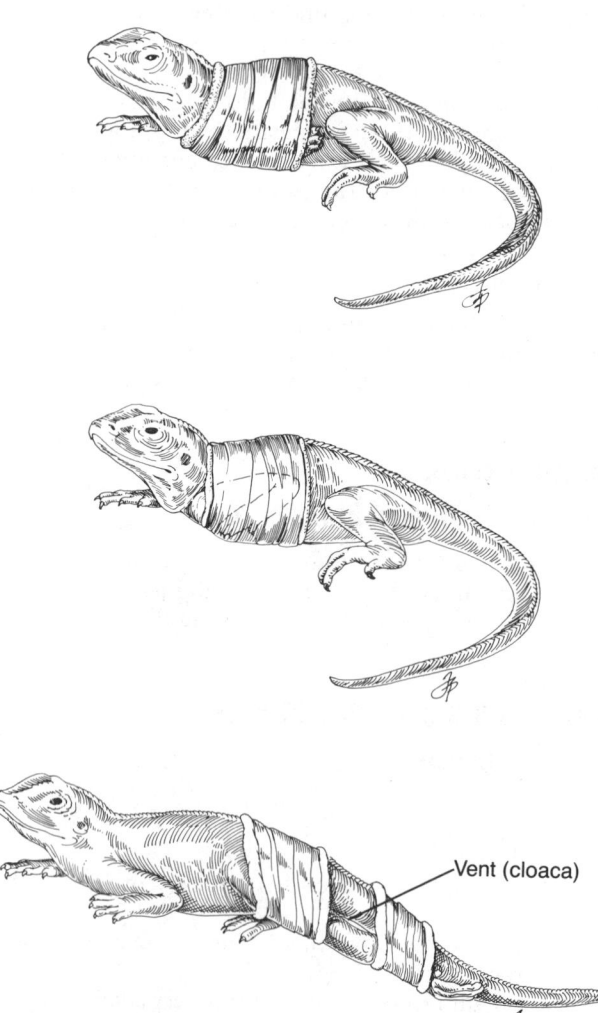

Figure 9. Three methods for applying external splints on a lizard.

Vent (cloaca)

terial between cleanings to prevent further contamination.

- Give broad-spectrum antibiotics for 10–14 days.

■ Similar to plastron osteotomy, cover large defects with fiberglass and epoxy resin or dental acrylics. Small defects can be completely filled using hoof or dental acrylics.

■ As in osteotomy, removal of the patch around growth rings may be necessary in growing chelonians.

■ This patch is semipermanent; it may be >1 year before there is radiographic evidence of bone healing.

Supplemental Readings

Barnard SM: 1986. Color atlas of reptilian parasites. Part I. Protozoans. Compend Cont Educ Pract Vet 8(3):145, 1986.

Barnard SM: Color atlas of reptilian parasites. Part II. Flatworms and roundworms. Compend Cont Educ Pract Vet 8(4):259, 1986.

Barnard SM: Color atlas of reptilian parasites. Part III. Miscellaneous endoparasites and ectoparasites. Compend Contin Educ Pract Vet 8(5):287, 1986.

Barnard SM: Color atlas of reptilian parasites. Part IV. Pseudoparasites. Compend Cont Educ Prac Vet 8(6):265, 1986.

Fowler ME: *Zoo and Wild Animal Medicine,* 2nd Ed. Philadelphia: W. B. Saunders, 1986, p 99.

Frye FL: *Biomedical and Surgical Aspects of Captive Reptile Husbandry.* Bonner Springs, Kansas: Veterinary Medicine Publishing, 1981.

Jacobson ER, Kollias GV (eds.): *Contemporary Issues in Small Animal Practice,* Vol. 9. *Exotic Animals.* New York: Churchill Livingstone, 1988, p 1.

Wallach JD, Boever WJ: *Diseases of Exotic Animals. Medical and Surgical Management.* Philadelphia: W. B. Saunders, 1983, p 978.

Index

Note: Page numbers in *italics* refer to illustrations; numbers followed by t indicate tables.

1413